CONTENTS

Maternity & Women's Health Care

Maternity & Women's Health Care

EIGHTH EDITION

DEITRA LEONARD LOWDERMILK, RNC, PHD, FAAN

Clinical Professor, School of Nursing
University of North Carolina at Chapel Hill
Chapel Hill, North Carolina

SHANNON E. PERRY, RN, CNS, PHD, FAAN

Professor, School of Nursing
San Francisco State University
San Francisco, California

Mosby
An Affiliate of Elsevier

Mosby
An Affiliate of Elsevier
11830 Westline Industrial Drive
St. Louis, Missouri 63146

MATERNITY & WOMEN'S HEALTH CARE
ISBN 0-323-02008-9

NOTICE

Pharmacology is an ever-changing field. Standard safety precautions must be followed, but as new research and clinical experience broaden our knowledge, changes in treatment and drug therapy may become necessary or appropriate. Readers are advised to check the most current product information provided by the manufacturer of each drug to be administered to verify the recommended dose, the method and duration of administration, and contraindications. It is the responsibility of the appropriately licensed health care provider, relying on experience and knowledge of the patient, to determine dosages and the best treatment for each individual patient. Neither the publisher nor the author assumes any liability for any injury and/or damage to persons or property arising from this publication.

Previous editions copyrighted 1977, 1981, 1985, 1989, 1993, 1997, 2000

International Standard Book Number 0-323-02008-9

Senior Editor: Michael S. Ledbetter
Senior Developmental Editor: Laurie K. Muench
Publishing Services Manager: Catherine Jackson
Project Manager: Jeff Patterson
Designer: Teresa McBryan Breckwoldt

Printed in the United States of America

Last digit is the print number: 9 8 7 6 5 4 3

CONTRIBUTORS

KATHRYN RHODES ALDEN, RN, MSN, IBCLC
Clinical Assistant Professor School of Nursing
University of North Carolina at Chapel Hill
Chapel Hill, North Carolina;
Lactation Consultant, Rex Healthcare
Raleigh, North Carolina

DEBBIE FRASER ASKIN, MN, RNC
Assistant Professor, Faculty of Nursing
University of Manitoba
Winnipeg, Manitoba, Canada

ANGELINE BUSHY, PHD, RN, CS, FAAN
Professor & Bert Fish Chair, School of Nursing
University of Central Florida
Orlando, Florida

CATHERINE CASHION, RN, C, MSN
Clinical Nurse Specialist
University of Tennessee Health Science Center
Department of Obstetrics & Gynecology
Division of Maternal-Fetal Medicine
Memphis, Tennessee

GAYLE TART DAVIS, BSN, MSN, EDD, CPNP
Associate Professor, School of Nursing
University of North Carolina at Chapel Hill
Chapel Hill, North Carolina

KAREN F. DORMAN, RNC, MS
Research Instructor, School of Medicine
University of North Carolina at Chapel Hill
Chapel Hill, North Carolina

LIENNE D. EDWARDS, PHD, RN
Associate Professor of Nursing
University of North Carolina at Charlotte
Charlotte, North Carolina

ANNE H. FISHEL, PHD, RN, CS
Professor, School of Nursing
University of North Carolina at Chapel Hill
Chapel Hill, North Carolina

CATHERINE INGRAM FOGEL, PHD, RNC (WHCNP), FAAN
Professor, School of Nursing
University of North Carolina at Chapel Hill
Chapel Hill, North Carolina

KATHLEEN K. FURNISS, RNC, MSN, NP
Women's Health Nurse Practitioner
Women's Health Initiative
Newark, New Jersey;
Associates in Women's Health Care
Wayne, New Jersey

CYNTHIA GARRETT, RNC, MSN
Clinical Systems Analyst
University of North Carolina Healthcare System
Chapel Hill, North Carolina

S. KIM GENOVESE, RNC, BSN, MSN, MSA
Acting Director of Nursing
Associate Professor, School of Nurisng
Purdue University, North Central
Westville, Indiana

PAT MAHAFFEE GINGRICH, RN-C, MSN, WHNP
Instructor, School of Nursing
North Carolina Central University
Durham, North Carolina

SHARRON S. HUMENICK, PHD, MPH, BSN, RN, LCCE, FAAN
Professor and Chair, Department of Maternal Child Nursing
Virginia Commonwealth University
Midlothian, Virginia

CAROLE KENNER, DNS, MSN, BSN, RNC
Associate Dean, Academic Advancement
Professor of Clinical Nursing, College of Nursing
University of Illinois at Chicago;
Consultants with Confidence, Inc.
Chicago, Illinois

SHARON E. LOCK, PHD, ARNP
Associate Professor, College of Nursing
University of Kentucky
Lexington, Kentucky

JANE McATEER, BSN, MN
Professor of Nursing
College of San Mateo
San Mateo, California

MARGARET S. MILES, RN, PHD
Professor, School of Nursing
University of North Carolina at Chapel Hill
Chapel Hill, North Carolina

MARY COURTNEY MOORE, RN, RD, PHD
Research Assistant Professor, School of Medicine
Vanderbilt University
Nashville, Tennessee

MAUREEN A. NALLE, PHD, RN
Assistant Professor, College of Nursing
University of Tennessee
Knoxville, Tennessee

KELLY PELOSI, RNC
Registered Nurse, Labor & Delivery
Western Wake Medical Center
Cary, North Carolina;
Duke University Health System
Durham, North Carolina

KAREN A. PIOTROWSKI, RNC, MSN
Assistant Professor of Nursing
D'Youville College
Buffalo, New York

JUDITH H. POOLE, PHD, BSN, BA, MN
Perinatal Clinical Nurse Specialist
Presbyterian Healthcare System
Charlotte, North Carolina

CHRISTENA RAINES, RN, WHNP
Nurse Practitioner
Center for Women's Health
Oxford, North Carolina

ANGELA SAMMARCO, PHD, RN
Assistant Professor of Nursing
College of Staten Island
City University of New York
Staten Island, New York

REBECCA BURDETTE SAUNDERS, PHD, RNC
Associate Dean, The Graduate School
University of North Carolina at Greensboro
Greensboro, North Carolina

SUSAN SPERAW, RN, MN, PHD
Associate Professor, College of Nursing
University of Tennessee
Knoxville, Tennessee

SUSAN MARTIN TUCKER, MSN, RN, PHN, CNAA
Nursing and Health Care Consultant
Quality Management and Perinatal Systems
Windsor, California

MARCIA VAN RIPER, RN, PHD
Associate Professor, School of Nursing
University of North Carolina at Chapel Hill;
Carolina Center for Genome Sciences
Chapel Hill, North Carolina

WENDY WETZEL, RN, MSN, FNP, HNC
Nurse Practitioner
A Woman's Place
Flagstaff, Arizona

JAN LAMARCHE ZDANUK, RNC, MSN, CNS, FNP-BC
Certified Family Nurse Practitioner
Private Practice
Fort Worth, Texas

CONSULTANTS

MARY ANNE ANDERSON, RN, C, LCCE, MA
Instructor
Contra Costa College
San Pablo, California

ANGELINE BUSHY, PHD, RN, CS, FAAN
Professor & Bert Fish Chair, School of Nursing
University of Central Florida
Orlando, Florida

VICKIE E. CARTER, RN, MSN, CPNP, CS
Adjunct Faculty, School of Nursing
University of Indianapolis;
Certified Pediatric Nurse Practitioner
Old Schoolhouse Pediatrics, Inc.
Indianapolis, Indiana

SHIRLEY S. CHANG, RN, MS, PHD
Professor of Nursing
Evergreen Valley College
San Jose, California

DUSTY DIX, RN, MSN
Clinical Instructor, School of Nursing
University of North Carolina at Chapel Hill
Chapel Hill, North Carolina

MARIAN L. FARRELL, PHD, CRNP, CNS, CS
Associate Professor of Nursing
University of Scranton
Scranton, Pennsylvania

MILDRED G. HARVEY, BSN, MSN, RNC
Obstetric Clinical Nurse Specialist
Obstetric Nursing Consultant
Lakeland, Tennessee

EDWARD L. LOWDERMILK, BS, RPH
Pharmacist Consultant
Lowdermilk Associates
Chapel Hill, North Carolina

RHONDA R. MARTIN, MS, RN
Clinical Instructor
University of Tulsa
Tulsa, Oklahoma

LISA MURPHY, RNC, BSN, MS
Nursing Instructor
Trinity Valley Community College
Kaufman, Texas

KRISTEN D. PRIDDY, RNC, MSN, CNS
Clinical Instructor, School of Nursing
University of Texas at Arlington
Arlington, Texas

DEBORAH A. REDD-TERRELL, BSN, MS, CFNP, CS
Assistant Professor, School of Nursing
Harry S. Truman College
Chicago, Illinois

DONNA B. ROWE, BSN, RN, NCI
Nurse Clinician
James A. Taylor Student Health Service
University of North Carolina at Chapel Hill
Chapel Hill, North Carolina

BARBARA C. RYNERSON, MS, APRN, BC
Associate Professor Emerita
School of Nursing
University of North Carolina at Chapel Hill
Chapel Hill, North Carolina

MARTHA SLEUTEL, PHD, RN, CNS
Assistant Professor of Nursing
Angelo State University
San Angelo, Texas

SUE A. TEDFORD, MNSC, CNS, APN
Level III Coordinator
Jefferson School of Nursing
Pine Bluff, Arkansas

PREFACE

Women's health care encompasses reproductive health care and the unique physical, psychologic, and social needs of women throughout their life span. The specialty of women's health and maternity nursing offers both challenges and opportunities. Nurses are challenged to assimilate knowledge and develop technical and critical thinking skills needed to apply that knowledge to practice. Each woman, with her individual needs that must be identified and met, presents a challenge. However, the opportunities are sufficiently extraordinary to make this one of the most fulfilling specialties of nursing practice.

The goal of nursing education is to prepare today's students to meet the challenges of tomorrow. This preparation must extend beyond mastery of facts and skills. Nurses must be able to combine clinical competence with caring and critical thinking. They must address both the physiologic and psychosocial needs of their clients. They must look beyond the condition and see the woman as an individual with distinctive needs. Above all, they must strive to improve nursing practice on the basis of sound evidence-based information. In a time of a nursing shortage and shrinking financial resources for health care, nurses can use evidence-based practice to produce measurable outcomes that can validate their unique and necessary role in the health care delivery system.

Maternity & Women's Health Care was developed to provide students with the knowledge and skills they need to become clinically competent, think critically, and attain the necessary sensitivity to become caring nurses. ***Maternity & Women's Health Care*** has been a leading maternity nursing text since it was first published in 1977, and we are proud of the continued support this text has received. With this eighth edition, we have a responsibility to continue this leading tradition.

This eighth edition has been revised and refined in response to comments and suggestions from educators, clinicians, and students. It includes the most accurate, current, and clinically relevant information available. We have had the assistance of expert faculty, nurse clinicians, and specialists from other health disciplines who authored, reviewed, and revised the text. Many exciting updates and new additions will be noted throughout the book; they demonstrate the various dimensions of women's health care and areas of rapid and complex changes such as genetics, fetal assessment, and alternative therapies. However, we have retained the underlying philosophy that has been the strength of previous editions: our belief that pregnancy and childbirth and developmental changes in a woman's life are natural processes. We have also retained a strong integrated focus on the family and evidence-based practice.

The text is also used as a reference for the practicing nurse. The most recent recommendations based on evidence from research and clinical experts have been included from professional organizations such as the Association for Women's Health, Obstetric, and Neonatal Nurses; the National Association of Neonatal Nurses; the American College of Obstetricians and Gynecologists; the American Academy of Pediatrics; the American Diabetes Association; and the Centers for Disease Control and Prevention.

APPROACH

Professional nursing practice continues to evolve and adapt to society's changing health priorities. The ever-changing health care delivery system offers new opportunities for nurses to alter the practice of maternity and women's health nursing and to improve the way care is given. Consumers of maternity and women's health care vary in age, ethnicity, culture, language, social status, marital status, and sexual preference. They seek care with obstetricians, gynecologists, family practice physicians, nurse-midwives, nurse-practitioners, and other health care providers in a variety of health care settings, including the home. Increasingly, many are self-treating, using a variety of alternative and complementary therapies.

Nursing education must reflect these changes. Clinical education must be planned to offer students a variety of maternity and women's health care experiences in settings that include hospitals and birth centers, the home health setting, clinics and private physician offices, shelters for the homeless or women in need of protection, prisons, and other community-based settings. The changing needs of nursing students also must be addressed. Today's nursing students are challenged to learn more than ever before and often in less time than their predecessors. Students are diverse. They may be new high school graduates, college students, or older adults with families. They may be male or female. They may have college degrees in other fields and be interested in changing careers. They may represent various cultures; English may not be their primary language.

This eighth edition of ***Maternity & Women's Health Care*** is designed to meet the needs of women during their reproductive years and beyond, as well as the needs of students in all types of nursing programs, including accelerated ones. This edition presents tighter, more focused content in a clearly written and easily read manner while retaining the comprehensiveness of previous editions.

To ensure a logical and consistent presentation of material, ***Care Management*** has been used as an organizing framework for discussion in the nursing care chapters. This approach incorporates the nursing process and collaborative care strategies to demonstrate how nursing care is combined with care from other health care providers to give the most comprehensive care to women and newborns. Assessments, nursing diagnoses, expected outcomes, nursing and collaborative interventions, and evaluations of care are highlighted throughout the chapters for emphasis. Nursing plans of care reinforce the problem-solving approach to client care. In chapters that focus on complications of childbearing and reproductive conditions, medical care is often the priority for client care. Therefore, in these discussions, the specific condition and medical therapy are discussed first, followed by the nursing care management.

Health care today emphasizes ***wellness.*** This focus is an integral part of our philosophy. Likewise, the developmental changes a woman experiences throughout her life are considered natural and normal. In women's health care, the goal is promotion of wellness for the woman through knowledge of her body and its normal functioning throughout her life span, while developing an awareness of conditions that require professional intervention. The unit on women's health care emphasizes the wellness aspect of care but also includes information about common gynecologic problems as well as gynecologic cancers. This unit has been placed before the units on pregnancy because many of the aspects of assessment and care can be applied to later chapters. Pregnancy and childbirth are also part of a natural developmental process. We believe that students need to thoroughly understand and recognize the normal processes before they can identify complications and comprehend their implications for care. We present the entire normal childbearing cycle before discussing potential complications. Although childbearing is a normal process, complications may occur. When making assessments, the nurse must be alert for ***Signs of Potential Complications;*** therefore we have included these signs as special boxes in chapters that cover uncomplicated pregnancy and childbirth.

Teaching for Self-Care is an essential component of nursing care of women and newborns. In recognition of integrative health care models that provide both traditional and nontraditional health care and in seeking to provide options for women that encourage them to take more responsibility for their health, we have thoroughly updated Chapter 4, **Alternative and Complementary Therapies.** The chapter on women's health promotion and screening emphasizes teaching for self-care to promote wellness and encourage preventive care. A **NEW** Chapter 3, **Genetics,** addresses issues of concern in both obstetrics and women's health, for example breast and colon cancer, both common in women. It also provides new information on genetic transmission, the Human Genome Project, and the role of the nurse in genetics. A **NEW** Chapter 28, **Care of the Newborn at Home,** focuses on anticipatory guidance and care for infants at home. Special boxed features highlight teaching for self-care throughout the text. To implement ***preventive care,*** perinatal and women's health nurses must be able to recognize signs and symptoms of emergent problems. Throughout the discussion of assessment and care, we alert the nurse to signs of potential problems and provide boxed information highlighting warning signs and emergency situations.

Today's perinatal and women's health nurses will encounter women from diverse backgrounds. Chapter 2, **Community Care: The Family and Culture,** has been revised to integrate discussions of home-, community-, and family-focused nursing in relation to culture and perinatal outcomes. This chapter also stresses the importance of assessing both the nurse's and the client's cultural beliefs. Cultural implications are integrated throughout in the text and in ***Cultural Considerations*** boxes to emphasize the wide range of ethnic diversity and its effects on maternity and women's health. English-Spanish ***Guidelines/Guías*** boxes provide students with common terms to make assessments and provide teaching. Community aspects of care are also integrated throughout nursing care chapters to emphasize that care can take place wherever the woman and her family may be.

To truly meet the specific needs of each woman, the nurse must include family members and significant others in the plan of care. ***Family dynamics*** are rarely more prominent than in pregnancy and childbirth. The nurse is often the family's primary advocate. Integrated family considerations throughout the chapters on pregnancy, labor and birth, postpartum, and newborn care demonstrate the importance of the entire family. Issues concerning grandparents, siblings, and different family constellations are also addressed.

Nursing research is an integral part of nursing education and practice. ***Research*** boxes are incorporated throughout the text to demonstrate the effect of research utilization on the practice of maternity and women's health nursing. Conclusions from research studies on care practices are described and highlighted. Students and practicing nurses will be challenged to think critically and improve nursing practice by questioning traditional nursing practices that have no scientific basis. **NEW *Evidence-Based Practice*** boxes are included for each unit and integrate findings from several studies on selected clinical practices and discuss implications for changing practice.

Maternity and women's health nurses confront ethical and legal challenges daily. Nurses need to develop a reflective stance that assesses new reproductive and women's health technologies and policies in light of their potential to influence human well-being. Although we have chosen not to include separate chapters on legal or ethical issues, highlighted information on ethical considerations and legal tips throughout the text emphasize these issues as they relate to maternity and women's health nursing.

FEATURES

The eighth edition features a contemporary design and spacious presentation. Students will find that the logical, easy-to-follow headings and attractive full-color design highlight important content and increase visual appeal. More than 750 color photographs and drawings throughout the text illustrate important concepts and techniques to further enhance comprehension. Each chapter begins with a list of ***Learning Objectives*** designed to focus students' attention on the important content to be mastered, and ***Key Terms*** that alert students to new vocabulary are boldfaced and defined within the chapter. Each chapter consistently ends with ***Key Points*** that summarize important content. ***Critical Thinking Exercises*** guide the students in applying their knowledge and in increasing their ability to think critically about maternity and women's health care issues. **NEW** to each chapter is a list of resources including websites and or contact information for organizations and educational resources available for the topics discussed. References have been updated significantly, with most citations being less than 5 years old and all chapters having citations within 1 year of publication. In addition the following are more of the outstanding features:

- ***Care Management*** is used as the consistent framework throughout to discuss collaborative care and specifically nursing care incorporating the five steps of the ***Nursing Process.***
- ***Plans of Care*** help students apply the nursing process in the clinical setting and use only NANDA-approved nursing diagnoses, describe expected outcomes for client care, provide rationales for interventions, and include evaluation of care.
- ***Care Paths, Protocols, and Procedures*** provide students with examples of various approaches to implementation of care.
- English-Spanish ***Guidelines/Guías*** boxes provide common English-to-Spanish phrases for client assessments and teaching.
- ***Teaching for Self-Care*** boxes emphasize guidelines for the client to practice self-care and provide information to help students transfer learning from the hospital to the home setting.
- ***Emergency*** boxes alert students to the signs and symptoms of various emergency situations and provide interventions for immediate implementation.
- ***Signs of Potential Complications*** boxes alert students to signs and symptoms of potential problems and are included in chapters that cover uncomplicated pregnancy and childbirth.
- ***Nurse Alerts*** highlight critical information for the student.
- ***Research*** boxes include a brief summary of the study and a discussion of application to practice.
- ***Evidence-Based Practice*** is incorporated throughout in **NEW** boxes that integrate findings from several studies on selected clinical practices and changing practice. In addition, research findings summarized in the ***Cochrane Pregnancy and Childbirth Database*** that confirm effective practices or identify practices that have unknown, ineffective, or harmful effects are integrated throughout the text and identified by this icon ❊ in the margin.
- ***Alternative and Complementary Therapies*** are discussed for many women's health and pregnancy-related problems and are identified in the text by a **NEW** icon in the margin.
- ***Cultural Considerations*** boxes describe beliefs and practices about pregnancy, childbirth, parenting, and women's health concerns and the importance of understanding cultural variations when providing care.
- ***Legal Tips*** and ***Ethical Considerations*** are integrated throughout to provide students with relevant information to deal with these important areas in the context of maternity and women's health nursing.
- ***Medication Guide*** boxes include key information about medications used in maternity and women's health care, including their indications, adverse effects, and nursing considerations.

ORGANIZATION

The eighth edition of ***Maternity & Women's Heath Care*** comprises eight units organized to enhance understanding and learning and to facilitate easy retrieval of information.

Unit One, Introduction to Maternity and Women's Health Nursing, begins with an overview of contemporary issues in maternity and women's health nursing practice. It then addresses the community as a unit of care, incorporating family theory, cultural aspects of care, and home care in relation to maternity and women's health nursing. The unit continues with one **NEW** chapter on genetics that provides essential discussion about genetics in relation to maternity and women's health care. The last chapter in the unit describes alternative and complementary therapies, providing an overview of the important therapies that can be used instead of or in addition to traditional techniques used in maternity and women's health care.

Unit Two, Women's Health, is a revised and expanded unit on women's health. Eight chapters discuss health promotion, screening, and physical assessment, and then present common reproductive concerns. The chapter on assessment and health promotion incorporates normal anatomy and physiology of the female reproductive system and integrates health promotion for common women's health problems. There are separate chapters on reproductive problems and concerns, sexually transmitted infections and other infections, contraception and abortion, infertility, violence, problems of the breast, and structural disorders and neoplasms of the female reproductive system.

Unit Three, Pregnancy, describes nursing care of the woman and her family from conception through preparation for childbirth. Nursing care during pregnancy includes both physiologic and psychologic aspects of care. A separate chapter on maternal and fetal nutrition emphasizes the important aspects of care, highlights cultural variations on diet, and stresses the importance of early recognition and management of nutritional problems. The preparation for childbirth chapter has been updated and revised significantly to include information on incorporating doula care during pregnancy and labor and birth.

Unit Four, Childbirth, focuses on collaborative care among physicians, nurse-midwives, nurses, and women and their families during the processes of labor and birth. Separate chapters deal with the nurse's role in management of discomfort during labor and childbirth and fetal monitoring. These chapters familiarize students with current childbirth practices and focus on evidence-based interventions to support and educate the woman and her family.

Unit Five, Postpartum, deals with a time of significant change for the entire family. The mother requires both physical and emotional support as she adjusts to her new role. The chapter on transition to parenthood discusses family dynamics in response to the birth of a child and describes ways nurses can facilitate parent-infant adjustment.

Unit Six, The Newborn, has been extensively revised and addresses physiologic adaptations of the newborn and assessment and care of the newborn. Information on the nutritional needs of the newborn and nursing care associated with breastfeeding and formula feeding are highlighted in a separate chapter. A **NEW** chapter on care of the newborn at home includes anticipatory guidance for the first few weeks at home and home follow-up care.

Unit Seven, Complications of Childbearing, discusses the conditions that place the woman, fetus, infant, and family at risk. This unit has been extensively revised and updated and includes a chapter on high risk assessment of pregnancy complications and eight other chapters on hypertensive disorders, antepartal hemorrhagic disorders, endocrine and metabolic problems, medical-surgical problems, obstetric critical care, mental health problems and substance abuse, labor and birth complications, and postpartum complications. Care management focuses on achieving the best possible outcomes, as well as supporting the woman and family when expectations are not met.

Unit Eight, Newborn Complications, addresses the most common acquired conditions of the neonate and hematologic disorders and congenital anomalies. It then describes the nursing care for high risk newborns, emphasizing the care of the preterm infant. All chapters have been greatly revised and updated. This unit addresses the continuing trend of providing care to moderately compromised newborns in the newborn nursery. A separate chapter on loss and grief discusses care management of the family experiencing a fetal or neonatal maternal loss.

TEACHING AND LEARNING PACKAGE

Several ancillaries to this text have been developed to assist instructors and students in the teaching and learning process.

For the instructor an ***Instructor's Resource*** is available either **online** or on **CD-ROM** and includes the following:

- The ***Instructor's Manual*** is keyed chapter by chapter to the text to help coordinate course objectives to chapter content and includes an outline of content with course guidelines, suggested learning activities, and a summary of key concepts. Sample syllabi are provided that include proposed class schedules and reading assignments for 5- to 7-week courses as well as 14- to 16-week courses so that educators can use the text in the most essential manner or in a more comprehensive way. The manual also provides over 10 case study presentations, many with community-based applications that can be used to foster critical thinking skills.
- The ***Test Bank*** is provided in Word format both with and without answers and includes over 900 questions that parallel the NCLEX format.
- The ***Image Collection*** provides easy access to electronic images from the main textbook. Each image can be imported to a slide presentation (e.g., PowerPoint) to enhance lecture materials.

For the student, the following are available to enhance the understanding of content from the main text:

- The ***Study Guide*** includes Chapter Review Activities and Critical Thinking Exercises to reinforce learning and evaluate comprehension. The *Study Guide* can be used for homework assignments or for remedial practice. The exercises in the guide were developed to assist students in synthesizing knowledge of maternity and women's health care and to foster critical thinking.

- The ***Maternity & Women's Health Care CD-ROM*** included in the text is an exciting, interactive program that provides students with a resource to solve critical thinking case studies, review questions, and review vocabulary. The vocabulary review includes a sound card so that students can easily hear and practice the correct pronunciations.

An exciting **NEW** resource for instructors and students is ***EVOLVE*** provided through Elsevier's website at http://evolve.elsevier.com/Lowdermilk/MatWmnHlth/. Evolve provides online access to **free** learning resources and activities designed specifically for the textbook you are using in your class. The resources will provide you with information that enhances the material in the book and much more. The ***Evolve*** website has two components available:

Evolve Learning Resources

- ***Weblinks*** for both students and instructors allows access to information and resources based on topics covered in this edition of *Maternity & Women's Health Care.*
- The ***Instructor's Online Resource*** includes the *Instructor's Manual, Test Bank,* and *Image Collection* for the instructor and is passcode protected.

Evolve Course Management System (CMS)

The CMS is available to instructors upon adoption of the eighth edition of *Maternity & Women's Health Care.*

- Instructors and students will have **full** access to a comprehensive suite of communication and organization tools, including discussion boards, e-mail, chat rooms, calendars, address books, task organizers, and more.
- Instructors will have **exclusive** access to the course management tools that allow them to customize their course content, build online tests, create assignments, enter grades, post announcements, manage student groups, and much more.

ACKNOWLEDGMENTS

The eighth edition of ***Maternity & Women's Health Care*** would not have been possible without the contributions of many people. First, we want to thank the many nurse educators, clinicians, and nursing students in the United States, Canada, Australia, and Taiwan whose comments and suggestions about the manuscript led to this collaborative effort by an outstanding group of contributors. A special thanks goes to these contributors, many of whom are new to this edition, whose names are listed in the Contributor list. Their expertise and knowledge of current clinical practice and research have added to the relevancy and accuracy of the materials presented. Karen Piotrowski, Kitty Cashion, and Kathy Alden deserve special recognition for their continuing extra efforts. We acknowledge the contributions to the chapter on Alternative and Complementary Therapies from The American Holistic Nurses' Association, and Phillip Fenske, LAc. We also thank Pat Gringrich for contributing to the Research boxes, Jane McAteer for developing Plans of Care, Martha Lebron and Laurie Muench for assisting with Spanish translations, and Ed Lowdermilk for his assistance with Medication Guides and verification of other medication information.

We are also appreciative of the critiques given by the reviewers, especially their attention to validating the accuracy of content and their challenge to present content differently and to include new ideas. These combined efforts have resulted in a revision that incorporates the most recent research and current information about the practice of maternity and women's health care.

We offer thanks for shared expertise and photographs to the staffs of University of North Carolina Women's Hospital; University of North Carolina School of Nursing; the staff of Spa Health Club of Chapel Hill, NC; Nurses Certificate program in Interactive Imagery; Jane Stansbury, SRS Medical Systems, Inc.; Phil Wilson, Momentum, Inc.; Leonard Nihan, Sea-Band International; Gayle Kipnis, RNC, CHTP, HNC; Tina Whitehorn; Polly Perez, Cutting Edge Press; and Barbara Harper, Global Maternal/Child Health Association.

We would also like to thank the following photographers: Marjorie Pyle, RNC, Lifecircle, Costa Mesa, CA; Kim Molloy, Knoxville, IA; Jonas N. McCoy, Raleigh, NC; Michael S. Clement, MD, Mesa, AZ; Leslie Canerday, San Jose, CA; Ed Lowdermilk, Chapel Hill, NC; and Amy and Ken Turner, Cary, NC.

Special words of gratitude are extended to Michael Ledbetter, our editor; Laurie Muench, our developmental editor; Jeff Patterson, our project manager; and Teresa Breckwoldt, our designer, for their encouragement, inspiration, and assistance in preparation and production of this text. These talented and hardworking people helped change our manuscript into a beautiful book by editing the manuscript, designing an attractive format for our special features, and overseeing the production of the book from start to finish. We are especially thankful to Laurie Muench who always had time to answer our questions, kept track of innumerable details, found just the right photo or resource, obtained that elusive permission, and always reassured us that we were doing a great job.

Deitra Leonard Lowdermilk
Shannon E. Perry

CONTENTS

UNIT EIGHT
NEWBORN COMPLICATIONS

CHAPTER 38
Acquired Problems of the Newborn, 1051

CHAPTER 39
Hemolytic Disorders and Congenital Anomalies, 1082

CHAPTER 40
Nursing Care of the High Risk Newborn, 1112

CHAPTER 41
Grieving the Loss of a Newborn, 1150

CHAPTER 1

Shannon E. Perry

Contemporary Maternity Nursing and Women's Health Care

http://evolve.elsevier.com/Lowdermilk/MatWmnHlth/

LEARNING OBJECTIVES

- Describe the scope of maternity and women's health nursing.
- Evaluate contemporary issues and trends in maternity and women's health nursing.
- Describe sociopolitical issues affecting the care of women and infants.
- Compare selected biostatistical data among races and countries.
- Examine social concerns in maternity and women's health care.
- Explain quality management and standards of practice in the delivery of nursing care.
- Debate ethical issues in perinatal nursing.
- Examine the *Healthy People 2010* goals related to maternal and infant care (U.S. Department of Health and Human Services, 2000).

Maternity nursing focuses on the care of childbearing women and their families through all stages of pregnancy and childbirth, as well as the first 4 weeks after birth. A perinatal nurse today may function as a nurturer, educator, physical care provider, critical thinker, support person, counselor, case manager, or researcher (MacMullen & Dulski, 1999). Throughout the prenatal period, nurses, nurse practitioners, and nurse-midwives provide care for women in clinics and physicians' offices and teach classes to help families prepare for childbirth. Nurses care for childbearing families during labor and birth in hospitals, in birthing centers, and in the home. Nurses with special training may provide intensive care for high risk neonates in special care units and for high risk mothers in antepartum units, in critical care obstetric units, or in the home. Maternity nurses teach about pregnancy; the process of labor, birth, and recovery; and parenting skills and provide continuity of care throughout the childbearing cycle.

Women's health nursing focuses on the physical, psychologic, and social needs of women throughout their lives. The concept *women's health* emphasizes the overall experience of women: general physical and psychologic well-being, childbearing functions, and diseases. Women's health nurses specialize in and investigate conditions unique to women (such as reproductive malignancies and menopause) and sociocultural and occupational factors that may be related to women's health problems (such as poverty, lower wages, rape, incest, sexual harassment, and family violence). They may also provide care for women and their families during the childbearing cycle. The Vision for Women and Their Health of the International Confederation of Midwives is an excellent model for nurses who care for women and children (Box 1-1).

Nurses caring for women have helped make the health care system more responsive to women's needs. The changing health care delivery system offers opportunities for nurses to alter nursing practice and improve the way care is delivered through **managed care,** integrated delivery systems (IDSs), and redefined roles. Nurses have been critically important in developing strategies to improve the well-being of women and their infants and have led the efforts to implement clinical practice guidelines and to practice using an evidence-based approach. Through professional associations, nurses can have a voice in setting standards and in influencing health policy by actively participating in the education of the public and of state and federal legislators.

Tremendous advances have taken place in the care of mothers and their infants during the past 150 years (Box 1-2). However, in the United States, serious problems exist related to the health and health care of mothers and infants. Lack of access to prepregnancy and pregnancy-related care for all women and the lack of reproductive health services for adolescents are major concerns. One sixth of all Americans, 44.3 million people, have no health insurance (Sheridan-Gonzalez, 2000).

Racial and ethnic diversity are increasing within North America. Within 40 years, an estimated 50% of the population will be European-American, 22% will be African-American, 18% will be Hispanic, and 10% will be Asian-American (Gary et al., 1998). This presents a

BOX 1-1 The Vision for Women and Their Health

International Confederation of Midwives envisions a world where:

- Women are respected and treated as persons in their own right in all societies
- Women stand as equal partners with men in the world order
- Women are recognized as crucial to the health of any nation
- Women and their families are part of a health care system with high quality care and easy access when needed
- Women have the right to choose from among safe options for care throughout their lives including high quality state-of-the-art care from competent providers who truly care about the woman and her health
- Women are educated and empowered to delight in a strong sense of self, to trust their bodies, to plan their pregnancies, and to make wise choices in their health care
- Women experience a reasonable standard of living including a clean and safe environment, healthy food, and a reasonable place to live
- Women need have no fear for their lives or the lives of their babies when they are pregnant
- Women believe that birth is normal and prefer to avoid unnecessary intervention

From International Confederation of Midwives. Accessed from http://www.internationalmidwives.org/vision.htm on June 15, 2002.

BOX 1-2 Historic Overview of Milestones in the Care of Mothers and Infants

1847—James Young Simpson in Edinburgh, Scotland, used ether for an internal podalic version and birth; the first reported use of obstetric anesthesia

1861—Ignaz Semmelwies wrote *The Cause, Concept and Prophylaxis of Childbed Fever*

1906—First program for prenatal nursing care established

1908—Childbirth classes started by the American Red Cross

1909—First White House Conference on Children convened

1911—First milk bank in the United States established in Boston

1912—U.S. Children's Bureau established

1916—Margaret Sanger established first American birth control clinic in Brooklyn, NY

1923—First U.S. hospital center for premature infant care established at Sarah Morris Hospital in Chicago

1933—*Natural Childbirth* published by Grantly Dick-Read

1941—Penicillin used as a treatment for infection

1953—Virginia Apgar, an anesthesiologist, published Apgar scoring system of neonatal assessment

1958—Edward Hon reported on the recording of the fetal ECG from the maternal abdomen (first commercial electronic fetal monitor produced in the late 1960s)

1958—Ian Donald, a Glasgow physician, was the first to report clinical use of ultrasound to examine the fetus

1959—*Thank You, Dr. Lamaze* published by Marjorie Karmel

1960—American Society for Psychoprophylaxis in Obstetrics (ASPO/Lamaze) formed

1960—International Childbirth Education Association founded

1960—Birth control pill introduced in the United States

1962—Thalidomide found to cause birth defects

1963—Title V of the Social Security Act amended to include comprehensive maternity and infant care for women who were low income and high risk

1965—Supreme Court ruled married people have the right to use birth control

1967—Rh_o(D) immune globulin produced

1967—Reva Rubin published article on Maternal Role Attainment

1968—Rubella vaccine available

1969—NAACOG (Nurses Association of the American College of Obstetricians and Gynecologists) founded; renamed AWHONN (Association of Women's Health, Obstetric and Neonatal Nurses) and incorporated as a $501(c)_3$ organization in 1993

1972—WIC (Special Supplemental Food Program for Women, Infants, and Children) started

1973—Abortion legalized

1974—First standards for obstetric, gynecologic, and neonatal nursing published by NAACOG (Nurses Association of the American College of Obstetricians and Gynecologists)

1975—The Pregnant Patient's Bill of Rights published by the International Childbirth Education Association

1978—Louise Brown, first test-tube baby, born

1991—Society for Advancement of Women's Health Research founded

1992—Office of Research on Women's Health authorized by U.S. Congress

1993—Human embryos cloned at George Washington University

1993—Family and Medical Leave Act enacted

1998—Newborns' and Mothers' Health Act went into effect

2000—Working draft of sequence and analysis of human genome completed challenge for health care providers to provide culturally sensitive health care.

Although the United States has made great strides in public health, significant disparity exists in health outcomes among people of various racial and ethnic groups. In addition, people may have lifestyles, health needs, and health care preferences related to their ethnic or cultural backgrounds. They may have dietary preferences and health practices that are not understood by caregivers. To meet the health care needs of a culturally diverse society, the nursing workforce must reflect the diversity of its clients.

This chapter presents a general overview of issues and trends related to the health and health care of women and infants.

CONTEMPORARY ISSUES AND TRENDS

Structure of Health Care Delivery

Changes in the health care market are influencing the way health care providers can care for their clients. Health spending in the United States increased 6.9% in 2000 and accounts for 13.2% of the total output of the nation (Pear, 2002). A national nursing shortage exists; the number of professional nurses in hospitals has declined, and unlicensed assistive personnel and multiskilled workers have been substituted. The role of the nurse is evolving from primary caregiver to leader of the interdisciplinary care team. Documentation of client outcomes has become essential (see later discussion). Advanced practice roles will increase as nurses assume more responsibility for client care.

Integrative Health Care

Integrative health care encompasses complementary and alternative therapies in combination with conventional Western modalities of treatment. Many popular alternative healing modalities offer human-centered care based on philosophies that recognize the value of the client's input and honor the individual's beliefs, values, and desires. The focus of these modalities is on the whole person, not just on a disease complex. Clients often find that alternative modalities are more consistent with their own belief systems and also allow for more client autonomy in health care decisions. Complementary and alternative therapy will be identified throughout the text with a icon.

Increasing numbers of American adults are seeking alternative and complementary health care, which exceeds visits paid to U.S. primary health care physicians. Approximately 45% of the general population use complementary therapies (King et al., 1999), and most of these users do not tell their physicians. Annual expenditures related to alternative therapies are estimated at $27 billion, approximately half of which is out-of-pocket expense not covered by medical insurance (Eisenberg et al., 1998).

Childbirth Practices

Prenatal care may promote better pregnancy outcomes by allowing early risk assessment and promoting healthy behaviors such as improved nutrition and smoking cessation. In 2000, 83.2% of all women received early prenatal care, whereas 3.9% had late or no prenatal care (Hoyert et al., 2001). Women can choose physicians or nurse-midwives as primary care providers. In 1997, physicians attended 92% of all births, and nurse-midwives attended 7% of all births (Curtin & Park, 1999). Women can give birth in a hospital labor room (rather than a delivery room), in a birthing room, in a freestanding birthing center, or at home. In 1997, approximately 99% of births in the United States occurred in the hospital (Curtin & Park, 1999); home births made up 0.64% of all births, and births in freestanding birthing centers were 0.28% of all births (Curtin & Park, 1999). In contrast, in British Columbia, Canada, 6.6% of births occurred at home, and in Ontario, 4.5% were home births. Cesarean births increased to 22.9% of live births in the United States in 2000, whereas the rate of vaginal births after cesarean (VBACs) declined (Hoyert et al., 2001). Women who choose nurse-midwives as their primary providers participate actively in childbirth decisions and receive fewer interventions such as epidural analgesia for labor and episiotomy.

Changes are occurring in the conduct of the second stage of labor (from 10-cm dilation to birth of the baby); positions are varied, with more emphasis on upright posture. The arbitrary limit of 2 hours for the second stage is less rigid as delayed pushing (waiting until the forces of labor propel the fetus down in the birth canal instead of encouraging pushing as soon as the cervix is 10 cm dilated) is instituted. Delayed pushing conserves the energy of the mother, results in fewer instrumental deliveries, and is less costly. The rates of episiotomy are declining, resulting in fewer severe perineal lacerations; midwives perform fewer episiotomies than do physicians.

The method of analgesia varies, depending on the condition and choice of the mother and preferences of the providers. Mothers typically are awake and aware during labor and birth. Contrasting philosophies exist regarding analgesia during labor. Some women prefer to experience the sensations of birth with little or no analgesia; others opt for epidural analgesia to provide comfort and control over their behavior during the experience.

With family-centered care, fathers, partners, grandparents, siblings, and friends may be present for labor and birth. Fathers or partners may be present for cesarean births. Doulas–trained and experienced female labor attendants–provide a continuous, one-on-one, caring presence throughout the labor and birth. Newborn infants remain with the mother and may breastfeed immediately after birth. Parents participate in the care of their infants in nurseries and neonatal intensive care units.

Childbirth education and parenting classes encourage the participation of a support person, teach breathing and relaxation techniques, and give general information about birth, infant development, and parenting. Other classes or parent support groups may be organized for the weeks and months after birth.

In some cases, a woman labors, gives birth, and recovers in the same room (labor-delivery-recovery); she may stay in the same room for the entire birth experience (labor-delivery-recovery-postpartum). Instead of having one nurse care for the baby and another nurse care for the mother, some hospitals have one nurse care for both the mother and baby (couplet or mother-baby care). In some hospitals, central nurseries have been eliminated, and babies "room-in" with their mothers. Many hospitals use lactation consultants to assist mothers with breastfeeding.

Discharge of a mother and baby within 24 hours of birth has resulted in a growing need for follow-up or home care. In some settings, discharge may occur as early as 6 hours after birth. Legislation has been passed to ensure that mothers and babies are permitted to stay in the hospital for at least 48 hours after vaginal birth and 96 hours after cesarean birth. Focused and efficient teaching are necessary to enable the parents and infant to make the transition safely from the hospital to the home. Nurses may use follow-up telephone calls or home visits to assist families needing information and reassurance.

Neonatal security in the hospital setting is receiving increasing attention. A number of cases of "baby-napping" and sending home the wrong baby have been reported. Parents have expressed concerns for their infant's safety. Security systems are being placed in nurseries, and nurses are required to wear photo identification or some other security badge.

Certified Nurse-Midwives

Certified nurse-midwives (CNMs) are registered nurses with education in the two disciplines of nursing and midwifery. **Certified midwives** (direct-entry midwives) are educated only in the discipline of midwifery. In the United States, certification of midwives is through the American College of Nurse-Midwives, the professional association for midwives in the United States. The Royal College of Midwives is the professional association for midwives in the United Kingdom. In Canada, the Association of Ontario Midwives is the professional association, and the College of Midwives of Ontario is the regulatory body for midwives in Ontario; the other provinces of Canada have similar regulatory bodies. Many national associations belong to the International Confederation of Midwives, which comprises 83 member associations from 70 countries in the Americas and Europe, Africa, and the Asia-Pacific region.

Views of Women

Women must be viewed holistically and in the context in which they live. Their physical, mental, and social factors must be considered because these interdependent components influence women's health and illness. Even the language used to describe women and their problems must be examined (Freda, 1995). For example, practitioners describe women who have an "incompetent cervix," who "fail to progress," and who have an "arrest" of labor or describe a fetus with intrauterine growth "retardation." They also "allow" women a "trial" of labor. Freda suggests that practitioners use the phrases "women who have recurrent premature dilation of the cervix" or "fetuses whose intrauterine growth has been restricted." A movement has arisen to refer to spontaneous pregnancy loss as a miscarriage instead of the more politically charged "abortion," especially when talking to clients (Freda, 1999).

Breastfeeding in the Workplace

Women are a significant proportion of the workforce. Companies are recognizing that it is good business to retain good employees and are making provisions for women returning to work after childbirth. Lactation rooms that provide space and privacy for pumping are available at many work sites and on college campuses (see Fig. 27-12). In some instances, breastfeeding women bring their babies to work. Since 1999, by law, women may breastfeed in federal buildings and on federal property. Some states have enacted legislation to ensure that mothers can breastfeed their babies in public places. These efforts may help mothers breastfeed longer and meet the recommendation of the American Academy of Pediatrics that breastfeeding continue for at least 1 year.

Family Leave

The Family and Medical Leave Act of 1993 provides for up to 12 weeks' unpaid leave to eligible employees for birth, adoption, or foster placement; for care of a child, spouse, or parent who is seriously ill; or for the employee's own illness. This is of great benefit to women because they are usually the primary caretakers of family members.

International Concerns

Female genital mutilation, infibulation, and circumcision are terms used to describe procedures in which part or all of the female external genitalia are removed for cultural reasons (Parkin, 2001). Worldwide, many women undergo such procedures. With the growing number of immigrants from African and other countries where female genital mutilation is practiced, nurses will increasingly encounter women who have undergone the procedure. The International Council of Nurses and other health professionals have spoken out against the procedures as harmful to women's health.

Health of Women

Various factors and conditions affect the health of women. Race is a major factor: Caucasian women have a life expectancy at birth of 80.0 years in contrast with 75.0 years for African-American women (Hoyert et al., 2001). In 2003, there will be an estimated 211,300 new cases of invasive breast cancer in women in the United States, and 39,800 women are expected to die of the disease (American Cancer Society, 2003). Early detection of breast cancer through breast self-examination and mammography can reduce the mortality rate resulting from this type of cancer. However, through lack of information or lack of insurance and access, many women never have mammograms. Wide disparity exists between Caucasian women and women of other races and between older and younger women in their rates of mammography, detection and treatment of breast cancer, and survival rates.

The population has grown older; approximately 50 million women are older than 50 years of age; 51 is the median age for menopause. Hormone replacement therapy for menopausal women has been used for many years and has benefits and risks (see Chapter 7).

Violence is a major factor affecting women. Violence includes battery, rape or other sexual assaults, and attacks with various weapons. The incidence of violence has increased, possibly because of better assessment and reporting mechanisms. Approximately 8% of pregnant women are battered; the incidence of battering increases during pregnancy. Violence is associated with complications of pregnancy such as bleeding. Alcoholism in and substance abuse by the woman and her abuser are associated with violence and homelessness, which affect a growing number of women and children, placing them at risk for a variety of health problems.

The rates of pregnancy and abortion among adolescents have declined (Hoyert et al., 2001) but are still higher in the United States than in any other industrialized country. Single mothers, the majority of whom are adolescents, gave birth to almost one third of the babies born in the United States in 2000 (Hoyert et al., 2001).

Cases of perinatally transmitted acquired immunodeficiency syndrome (AIDS) peaked in 1992; the rate of AIDS among infants declined from 8.9 per 100,000 births in 1992 to 2.8 per 100,000 births in 1996. Of mothers who tested positive for the human immunodeficiency virus (HIV) before giving birth, 91% received zidovudine. This contributed to the decrease in infants infected with the virus (Lindegren et al., 1999) and is the rationale for the call for universal screening of pregnant women.

Healthy People 2010 Goals

Healthy People 2010 is the agenda of the United States for improving health. It has two overarching goals: to increase the quality and years of healthy life and to eliminate health disparities. In *Healthy People 2010*, the 467 objectives to improve health are organized into 28 specific focus areas, including one related to maternal, infant, and child health (Box 1-3).

BOX 1-3 ***Healthy People 2010*, Focus Area 16, Maternal, Infant, and Child Health**

Goal: Improve the health and well-being of women, infants, children, and families.

Fetal, infant, and child deaths
Maternal death and illness
Prenatal care
Obstetric care
Risk factors
Developmental disabilities and neural tube defects
Prenatal substance exposure
Breastfeeding, newborn screening, and service systems

From US Department of Health and Human Services. (2000). *Healthy People 2010* (conference edition, in two volumes). Washington, DC: USDHHS.

Trends in Fertility and Birth Rate

Fertility trends and birth rates reflect women's needs for health care. In 2000 the **fertility rate,** births per 1000 women from 15 to 44 years of age, was 67.6, an increase of 3% (Hoyert et al., 2001). The highest birth rates occurred among women between 20 and 29 years of age (Table 1-1). The **birth rate,** number of live births in 1 year per 1000 population, was 14.8 in 2000 (Hoyert et al., 2001). In 2000 the proportion of births by unmarried women varied widely among racial groups in the United States: African-American, 68.5%; Hispanic, 42.5%; and Caucasian, 22.1% (Hoyert et al., 2001). Births to unmarried women are frequently related to less favorable outcomes, such as low birth weight or preterm birth, because a large number of these women are teenagers (79% of teenagers who gave birth in 2000 were unmarried). In 1997, the latest year for which data on abortion are available, among teenagers, only an estimated 55% of pregnancies resulted in live birth, whereas 29% were induced abortions, and 15% resulted in fetal loss (Hoyert et al., 2001).

Number of Low-Birth-Weight Infants

The risks of morbidity and mortality increase for newborns weighing less than 2500 g (5 lb, 8 oz)–**low-birth-weight (LBW) infants.** Multiple births contribute to the incidence of LBW. In 1999, 3.1% of births were multiple births. In 2000 the incidence of LBW infants increased to 7.6%, the highest rate since 1973 (Hoyert et al., 2001). For African-American births, the incidence of LBW infants was 12.9%, whereas the rate was 6.6% for Caucasian births and 6.4% for

TABLE 1-1 **Birth Rate According to Age—2000**

AGE (YR)	RATE PER 1000 WOMEN
10-14	0.9
15-17	27.2
18-19	79.5
20-24	112.5
25-29	121.7
30-34	94.2
35-39	40.3
40-44	7.9

Data from Hoyert, D. et al. (2001). Annual summary of vital statistics: 2000. *Pediatrics, 108*(6), 1241-1255.

Hispanic births (Hoyert et al., 2001). African-American infants are more than twice as likely as Caucasian infants to be of LBW and to die in the first year of life.

Infant Mortality in the United States

A common indicator of the adequacy of prenatal care and the health of a nation as a whole is the **infant mortality rate,** the number of deaths of infants younger than 1 year of age per 1000 live births. The **neonatal mortality rate** is the number of deaths of infants younger than 28 days of age per 1000 live births. The **perinatal mortality rate** is the number of stillbirths plus the number of neonatal deaths per 1000 live births. The U.S. infant mortality rate for 2000 was 6.9, the lowest ever recorded (Hoyert et al., 2001). The disparity in infant mortality rate between African-American infants and Caucasian infants has increased over time (Chima, 2001). The infant mortality rate continues to be higher for African-American infants (14.1 per 1000) than for Caucasian infants (6.0 per 1000) (Guyer et al., 1999). Limited maternal education, young maternal age, unmarried status, poverty, lack of prenatal care, and smoking appear to be associated with higher infant mortality rates. Poor nutrition, smoking and alcohol use, and maternal conditions such as poor health or hypertension also are important contributors to infant mortality. A shift from the current emphasis on high-technology medical interventions to a focus on improving access to preventive care for low-income families is necessary.

International Infant Mortality Trends

The infant mortality rate of Canada ranks fifteenth and that of the United States ranks twenty-third when compared with those of other industrialized nations (Hoyert et al., 2001). Even though the infant mortality rate decreased in the United States, it did not keep pace with the rates of other industrialized countries. One reason for this is the high rate of LBW infants in the United States in contrast with the rates in other countries.

Maternal Mortality Trends

Worldwide, approximately 1600 women die each day of problems related to pregnancy or childbirth; many of these deaths are preventable. In the United States in 2000, the annual **maternal mortality rate** (number of maternal deaths per 100,000 live births) was 9.8 (Minino et al., 2002). The rates have significant racial differences: "African-American women are four times more likely and Hispanic women are 1.7 times more likely than Caucasian women to die of pregnancy-related complications" (Jones, 2000). The predominant causes of these deaths are hemorrhage, infection, pregnancy-induced hypertension, and ectopic pregnancy. Ectopic pregnancy is the leading cause of first trimester maternal mortality. *Healthy People 2010* proposed a goal of 3.3 maternal deaths per 100,000. To achieve this goal, early diagnosis and appropriate intervention must occur. Worldwide strategies to reduce maternal mortality rates include improving access to skilled attendants at birth, providing postabortion care, improving family planning services, and providing adolescents with better reproductive health services (Liljestrand, 2000).

Involving Consumers and Promoting Self-Care

Self-care is appealing to both clients and the health care system because of its potential to reduce health care costs. Maternity care is especially suited to self-care because childbearing is essentially health focused, women are usually well when they enter the system, and visits to health care providers can present the opportunity for health and illness interventions. Measures to improve health and reduce risks associated with poor pregnancy outcomes and illness can be addressed. Topics such as nutrition education, stress management, smoking cessation, alcohol and drug treatment, improvement of social supports, and parenting education are appropriate for such encounters.

Efforts to Reduce Health Disparities

Significant disparities in morbidity and mortality rates are experienced by African-Americans, Native Americans, Hispanics, Alaska natives, and Asians/Pacific Islanders. Shorter life expectancy, higher infant and maternal mortality rates, more birth defects, and more sexually transmitted infections are found among these groups. For pregnancy-induced hypertension, the rate for African-American women of 3.6 deaths per 100,000 live births was more than five times the rate of 0.7 for Caucasian women (Murphy, 2000). The disparities are thought to result from a complex interaction among biologic factors, environment, and health behaviors. Disparities in education and income are associated with differences in occurrence of morbidity and mortality. The National Institutes of Health has a commitment to improve the health of minorities and provides funding for research as well as training of minority researchers. The National Institute of Nursing Research has included the goal of reducing disparities in its strategic plan and supports research for that purpose. The nation must make a concerted effort to eliminate health disparities.

Emphasis on High-Technology Care

Advances in scientific knowledge and the large number of high risk pregnancies have contributed to a health care system that emphasizes high-technology care. Maternity care has branched out to preconception counseling, more and better scientific techniques to monitor the mother and fetus, more definitive tests for hypoxia and acidosis, and neonatal intensive care units. Point-of-care testing is available. Robotic aids may become common (Eckberg, 1998). Virtually all women are monitored electronically during labor despite the lack of evidence of efficacy of such monitoring.

Telemedicine is an umbrella term for the use of communication technologies and electronic information to provide or support health care when the participants are separated by distance. Telemedicine permits specialists, including nurses, to provide health care and consultation when distance separates them from those needing care. For example, Baby CareLink (Gray et al., 2000) is an Internet-based program that incorporates teleconferencing and the World Wide Web to enhance interactions among health care providers, families, and community providers. It includes distance learning, virtual home visits, and remote monitoring of the infant after discharge. This technology will save billions of dollars annually for health care.

Strides are being made in identifying genetic codes, and genetic engineering is taking place. Women's health has expanded to emphasize care of older women, new cancer-screening techniques, advances in the diagnosis and treatment of breast cancer, and work on an AIDS vaccine. In general, high-technology care has flourished, whereas "health" care has become relatively neglected. These technologic advances also have contributed to higher health care costs. Nurses must use caution and prospective planning and assess the effect of the emerging technology.

Community-Based Care

A shift in settings, from acute care institutions to the home, has been occurring. Even childbearing women at high risk are cared for in the home. Technology previously available only in the hospital is now found in the home. This has affected the organizational structure of care, the skills required in providing such care, and the costs to consumers. Home health care also has a community focus. Nurses are involved in providing care for women and infants in homeless shelters, in caring for adolescents in school-based clinics, and in promoting health at community sites, churches, and shopping malls. Nursing education curricula are increasingly community based.

Increase in High Risk Pregnancies

The number of high risk pregnancies has increased, which means that a greater number of pregnant women are at risk for poor pregnancy outcomes. Escalating drug use (ranging from 11% to 27% of pregnant women, depending on the geographic location) has contributed to higher incidences of prematurity, LBW, congenital defects, learning disabilities, and withdrawal symptoms in infants. Alcohol use in pregnancy has been associated with miscarriages, mental retardation, LBW, and fetal alcohol syndrome.

The two most frequently reported maternal medical risk factors are hypertension associated with pregnancy and diabetes. The multiple birth rate is increasing; in 1999, multiple births accounted for 3.1% of all births (Hoyert et al., 2001). The cesarean birth rate increased to 22.9% for 2000, making it unlikely that the *Healthy People 2010* goal of 15% can be accomplished (Hoyert et al., 2001).

High Cost of Health Care

Health care is one of the fastest-growing sectors of the U.S. economy. Even though the United States spends proportionately more on health care than any of the other 190 countries that make up the World Health Organization, it ranks 37th in quality (Rubin, 2000). A shift in demographics, an increased emphasis on high-cost technology, and the liability costs of a litigious society contribute to the high cost of care. Most researchers agree that the cost of caring for the increased number of LBW infants in neonatal intensive care units contributes significantly to the overall health care costs.

Midwifery care has helped contain some health care costs, but not all insurance carriers reimburse nurse practitioners and clinical nurse specialists as direct care providers or reimburse for all services provided by nurse-midwives, a situation that continues to be a problem. Nurses must become involved in the politics of cost containment because they, as knowledgeable experts, can provide solutions to many of the health care problems at a relatively low cost.

Early postpartum discharge programs also are used to reduce costs. The American Academy of Pediatrics has published minimal criteria for early discharge of a newborn (American Academy of Pediatrics Committee on Fetus and Newborn, 1995) (see Chapter 23).

Limited Access to Care

Barriers to access must be removed so pregnancy outcomes can be improved. The most significant barrier to access is the inability to pay. Lack of transportation and dependent child care are other barriers. In addition to a lack of insurance and high costs, a lack of providers for low-income women exists because many physicians either refuse to take Medicaid clients or take only a few such clients. This presents a serious problem because a significant proportion of births are to mothers who receive Medicaid.

TRENDS IN NURSING PRACTICE

The increasing complexity of care for maternity and women's health clients has contributed to specialization of nurses working with these clients. This specialized knowledge is gained through experience, advanced degrees, and certification programs. Nurses in advanced practice (e.g., nurse practitioners and nurse-midwives) may provide primary care throughout a woman's life, including during the pregnancy cycle. In some settings, the clinical nurse specialist and nurse practitioner roles are blended, and nurses deliver high-quality, comprehensive, and cost-effective care in a variety of settings. Lactation consultants provide services in the postpartum unit or on an outpatient basis, including home visits.

Nursing Interventions Classification

When the National Institute of Medicine proposed that all client records be computerized by the year 2000, a need for a common language to describe the contributions of nurses to client care became evident. Nurses from the University of Iowa developed a comprehensive standardized language that describes interventions that are performed by generalist or specialist nurses. This language is included in the Nursing Interventions Classification (NIC) (McCloskey & Bulechek, 2000). Interventions commonly used by maternal-child nurses include those in Box 1-4.

Evidence-Based Practice

Evidence-based practice–providing care based on evidence gained through research and clinical trials–is being increasingly emphasized. Although not all practice can be evidence based, practitioners must use the best available information on which to base their interventions. The first

BOX 1-4 Childbearing Care Interventions

WOMEN'S HEALTH
- Abuse Protection Support
- Active Listening
- Anticipatory Guidance
- Behavior Modification
- Body Image Enhancement
- Coping Enhancement
- Counseling
- Decision-Making Support
- Emotional Support
- Family Planning: Contraception
- Health Education
- Health Screening
- Health System Guidance
- Medication Management
- Nutritional Counseling
- Pelvic Floor Exercise
- Risk Identification
- Teaching: Disease Process
- Teaching: Individual
- Teaching: Safe Sex
- Telephone Consultation
- Urinary Bladder Training
- Weight Management
- Weight Reduction Assistance

OBSTETRIC
- Birthing
- Bleeding Reduction: Antepartum Uterus
- Bleeding Reduction: Postpartum Uterus
- Bottle Feeding
- Breastfeeding Assistance
- Cesarean Section Care
- Childbirth Preparation
- Electronic Fetal Monitoring: Antepartum
- Electronic Fetal Monitoring: Intrapartum
- Environmental Management: Attachment Process
- Family Integrity Promotion: Childbearing Family
- Family Planning: Contraception
- Grief Work Facilitation: Perinatal Death
- High Risk Pregnancy Care
- Intrapartal Care
- Intrapartal Care: High Risk Delivery
- Invasive Hemodynamic Monitoring
- Labor Induction
- Labor Suppression
- Newborn Care
- Newborn Monitoring
- Parent Education: Childbearing Family
- Parent Education: Childrearing Family
- Postpartal Care
- Pregnancy Termination Care
- Prenatal Care
- Resuscitation: Fetus
- Resuscitation: Neonate
- Risk Identification: Childbearing Family
- Surveillance: Late Pregnancy

NEONATAL
- Acid-Base Management: Metabolic Acidosis
- Acid-Base Management: Metabolic Alkalosis
- Acid-Base Management: Respiratory Acidosis
- Acid-Base Management: Respiratory Alkalosis
- Airway Management
- Artificial Airway Management
- Attachment Promotion
- Bottle Feeding
- Breastfeeding Assistance
- Caregiver Support
- Code Management
- Critical Path Development
- Developmental Enhancement
- Discharge Planning
- Electrolyte Management
- Emotional Support
- Family Involvement
- Feeding
- Fluid Management
- Fluid Monitoring
- Fluid/Electrolyte Management
- Hyperglycemia Management
- Hypoglycemia Management
- Hypothermia Treatment
- Immunization/Vaccination Administration
- Infant Care
- Kangaroo Care
- Mechanical Ventilation
- Medication Administration: Oral
- Medication Administration: Parenteral
- Multidisciplinary Care Conference
- Newborn Care
- Nonnutritive Sucking
- Pain Management
- Parent Education: Childbearing Family
- Resuscitation: Neonate
- Teaching: Infant Care
- Tube Care: Umbilical Line

From Iowa Intervention Project. McCloskey, J., & Bulechek, G. (Eds.). (2000). *Nursing interventions classification (NIC)* (3rd ed.). St. Louis: Mosby.

consensus initiative of the Coalition for Improving Maternity Services, the *Mother-Friendly Childbirth Initiative,* is an evidence-based model that focuses on prevention and wellness as alternatives to costly programs of screening, diagnosis, and treatment (*The Mother-Friendly Childbirth Initiative,* 1997). The Association of Women's Health, Obstetric, and Neonatal Nurses (AWHONN) *Standards and Guidelines for Professional Nursing Practice in the Care of Women and Newborns* (1998) includes an evidence-based approach to practice. Discussion of nursing care and research boxes throughout this text provide examples of evidence-based practice in perinatal and women's health nursing.

The incorporation of research findings into practice is essential in developing a science-based practice. AWHONN has conducted six research-based practice projects (Box 1-5). These projects were conducted in several states, and staff nurses were involved in their implementation and in data collection. The AWHONN practice guidelines incorporate evidence-based practices for second-stage labor management, continence for women, breastfeeding support, midlife well-being, perianesthesia care, neonatal skin care, and cardiac health. By using such guidelines and published reports, nurses can develop protocols and procedures based on published research and incorporate an evidence base into their practice. AWHONN research priorities include the aforementioned topics as well as family violence, fetal surveillance, genetics, infertility, and early parenting (Box 1-6).

BOX 1-5 AWHONN Research-Based Practice Programs

Transition of the Preterm Infant to an Open Crib
Management of Women in Second-Stage Labor
Continence for Women
Neonatal Skin Care
Cyclic Pelvic Pain and Discomfort Management
Setting Universal Cessation Counseling, Education, and Screening Standards: Nursing Care for Pregnant Women Who Smoke (SUCCESS)

Cochrane Pregnancy and Childbirth Database

The Cochrane Pregnancy and Childbirth Database was first planned in 1976 with a small grant from the World Health Organization to Dr. Iain Chalmers and colleagues at Oxford. In 1993, the Cochrane Collaboration was formed, and the Oxford Database of Perinatal Trials became known as the **Cochrane Pregnancy and Childbirth Database.** The Cochrane Collaboration oversees up-to-date, systematic reviews of randomized controlled trials of health care and disseminates these reviews. The premise of the project is that these types of studies provide the most reliable evidence about the effects of care.

The evidence from these studies should encourage practitioners to implement useful measures and to abandon those that are useless or harmless. Studies are ranked in six categories:

1. Beneficial forms of care
2. Forms of care that are likely to be beneficial

BOX 1-6 AWHONN Research Priorities for Women's and Neonatal Health

STRATEGIES TO PROMOTE HEALTHY BEHAVIORS IN WOMEN ACROSS THE LIFESPAN

- Prevention of unintended pregnancy
- Cardiovascular health, including smoking cessation
- Weight management and nutrition
- Menstrual and menopausal adjustment and symptom management
- Cancer screening and risk reduction
- Chronic illness self-care (e.g., diabetes)
- Social risks (poverty, addiction, sexual risks, violence)
- Promotion of women's mental health and stress management

REDUCING HEALTH DISPARITIES

- Delivery of culturally competent care
- Enhancing access to and utilization of health care
- Reducing disparities in rates of low birth weight
- Improving breastfeeding rates among low-income and minority women
- Reducing genetically determined risk through appropriate screening

MODELS OF NURSING CARE DELIVERY

- Strategies to increase diversity of the nursing work force
- Effect of work force diversity on patient outcomes
- Comparative studies of quality, patient outcomes, and cost across:
  - Providers (physicians, nurses, advanced practice nurses)
  - Delivery settings (medical centers, birth centers, primary care, home care)
  - Practice decisions and decision-making (levels and types of clinical decision-making and interventions)
- Staff development and support models
- Models of care delivery in prenatal and antepartum care

Approved by AWHONN Research Committee, July 2001.

3. Forms of care with a trade-off between beneficial and adverse effects
4. Forms of care with unknown effectiveness
5. Forms of care that are unlikely to be beneficial
6. Forms of care that are likely to be ineffective or harmful

Practices that have been reviewed by the Collaboration will be identified with a ❊ throughout this text.

Outcomes-Oriented Practice

Outcomes of care (that is, the effectiveness of interventions and quality of care) are receiving increased emphasis. **Outcomes-oriented care** measures effectiveness of care against benchmarks or standards based on results achieved by others. It is a measure of the value of nursing using quality indicators such as cost, length of stay, and client satisfaction (Oermann & Huber, 1999). The Outcome Assessment Information Set (OASIS) is an example of an outcome system important for nursing. Its use is required by the Centers for Medicare and Medicaid Services, formerly the Health Care Financing Administration (HCFA), in all home health organizations that are Medicare accredited. The Nursing Outcomes Classification (NOC) is an effort to identify outcomes and related measures that can be used for evaluation of care of individuals, families, and communities across the care continuum (Johnson, Maas, & Moorhead, 2000). An example of outcomes classification is provided in Box 1-7.

BOX *1-7* **Nursing Outcomes Classification**

BREASTFEEDING ESTABLISHMENT: INFANT (1000)
Domain—Physiologic Health (II)
Class—Nutrition (K)
Scale—Not adequate to Totally adequate (f)
Definition: Proper attachment of an infant to and sucking from the mother's breast for nourishment during the first 2 to 3 weeks

BREASTFEEDING ESTABLISHMENT: INFANT	**NOT ADEQUATE 1**	**SLIGHTLY ADEQUATE 2**	**MODERATELY ADEQUATE 3**	**SUBSTANTIALLY ADEQUATE 4**	**TOTALLY ADEQUATE 5**
Indicators					
100001 Proper alignment and latch on	1	2	3	4	5
100002 Proper areolar grasp	1	2	3	4	5
100003 Proper areolar compression	1	2	3	4	5
100004 Correct suck and tongue placement	1	2	3	4	5
100005 Audible swallow	1	2	3	4	5
100006 Swallowing a minimum of 5 to 10 minutes per breast	1	2	3	4	5
100007 Minimum eight feedings per day (on demand)	1	2	3	4	5
100008 Six or more urinations per day (after infant 2 to 3 days of age)	1	2	3	4	5
100009 Two or more loose, yellow, seedy stools per day	1	2	3	4	5
100010 Age-appropriate weight gain	1	2	3	4	5
100011 Infant contentment after feeding	1	2	3	4	5
100012 Other ____________ *(Specify)*	1	2	3	4	5

Outcome Content References:

Lawrence, R. (1994). *Breastfeeding: A guide for the medical professional* (4th ed.). St. Louis: Mosby.
Minchin, M. (1989). Positioning for breastfeeding. *Birth: Issues in Perinatal Care and Education, 16*(2), 67-80.
Neifert, M., & Seacat, J. (1986). A guide to successful breastfeeding. *Contemporary Pediatrics, 3,* 1-14.
Page-Goertz, S. (1989). Discharge planning for the breastfeeding dyad. *Pediatric Nursing, 15,* 543-544.
Righard, L., & Alade, M. (1992). Sucking technique and its effect on success of breastfeeding. *Birth: Issues in Perinatal Care and Education, 19,* 185-189.
Riordan, J., & Auerbach, K. (1993). *Breastfeeding and human lactation.* Boston: Jones and Bartlett.
Shrago, L., & Bocar, D. (1990). The infant's contribution to breastfeeding. *Journal of Obstetric, Gynecologic, and Neonatal Nursing, 19,* 209-213.
Walker, M. (1989). Functional assessment of infant breastfeeding patterns. *Birth: Issues in Perinatal Care and Education, 16,* 140-147.

From Johnson, M., Maas, M., & Moorhead, S. (Eds.). (2000). *Nursing outcomes classification (NOC)* (2nd ed.). St. Louis: Mosby.

Best Practices as Goal of Care

A program or service that has been recognized for excellence is considered to be a **best practice.** A best practice must provide a better or a new way to achieve goals and be sound from operational, clinical, and financial perspectives. To determine best practices, information is collected from similar institutions. Staff members then identify solutions that have been successful in addressing specific needs and select one that incorporates the best resolutions of the problem that fit the agency's unique population and mission characteristics. The agency continually compares its performance against the best in the industry and the best of a specific function.

Clinical Benchmarking

Clinical benchmarking is a process used to compare one's own performance against the performance of the best in an area of service. Benchmarking supports and promotes continual quality improvement and helps the organization remain competitive in the health care market.

The Best Practices Network uses collaborative benchmarking, which involves sharing strategies and outcomes and leads to the development of new best practices (Reclaiming benchmarking, 1999/2000). Areas of practice routinely monitored in perinatal nursing include hospital length of stay, maternal mortality rate, infant mortality rate, cesarean birth rate, epidural rate, and episiotomy rate.

A Global Perspective

Advances in medicine and nursing have resulted in increased knowledge and understanding in the care of mothers and infants and reduced perinatal morbidity and mortality rates. However, these advances have affected predominantly the industrialized nations. As the world becomes smaller because of travel and communication technologies, nurses and other health care providers are gaining a global perspective and participating in activities to improve the health and health care of people worldwide. Nurses participate in medical outreach, providing obstetric, surgical, ophthalmologic, orthopedic, or other services (Fig. 1-1); attend international meetings; conduct research; and provide international consultation. International student and faculty exchanges occur (Fig. 1-2). More articles about health and health care in various countries are appearing in nursing journals. Several schools of nursing in the United States are World Health Organization Collaborating Centers.

STANDARDS OF PRACTICE AND LEGAL ISSUES IN DELIVERY OF CARE

Nursing standards of practice in perinatal and women's health nursing have been described by several organizations, including the American Nurses Association (ANA), which publishes standards for maternal-child health nursing; AWHONN, which publishes standards of practice and education for perinatal nurses (Box 1-8); ACNM, which publishes standards of practice for midwives; and the National Association of Neonatal Nurses (NANN), which publishes standards of practice for neonatal nurses. These standards reflect current knowledge, represent levels of practice agreed on by leaders in the specialty, and can be used for clinical benchmarking.

In addition to these more formalized standards, agencies have their own policy and procedure books that outline standards to be followed in that setting. In legal terms, the **standard of care** is that level of practice that a reasonably prudent nurse would provide. In determining legal negligence, the care given is compared with the standard of care. If the standard was not met and harm resulted, negligence occurred. The number of legal suits in the perinatal area has typically been high. As a consequence,

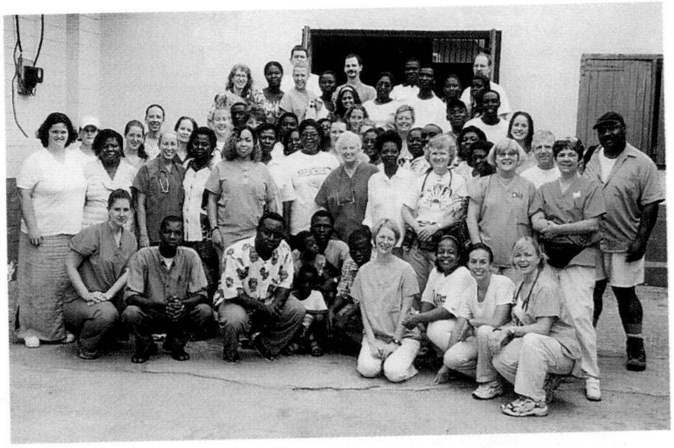

FIG. 1-1 Students and faculty from the United States and Ghanaian community workers participating in a Health Mission in Ghana, West Africa. (Courtesy Shannon Perry, San Jose, CA.)

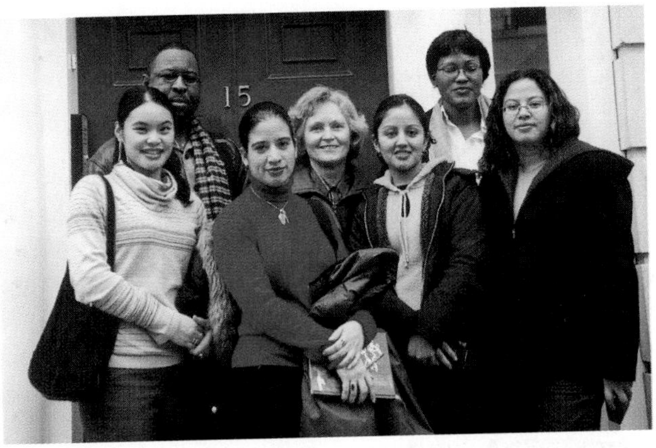
15

FIG. 1-2 Students and faculty visit the Royal College of Midwives during an international community service learning experience. (Courtesy Shannon Perry, San Jose, CA.)

BOX 1-8 **Standards of Care for Women and Newborns**

STANDARDS THAT DEFINE THE NURSE'S RESPONSIBILITY TO THE CLIENT

Assessment
Collection of health data of the woman or newborn

Diagnosis
Analysis of data to determine nursing diagnosis

Outcome Identification
Identification of expected outcomes that are individualized

Planning
Development of a plan of care

Implementation
Performance of interventions for the plan of care

Evaluation
Evaluation of the effectiveness of interventions in relation to expected outcomes.

STANDARDS OF PROFESSIONAL PERFORMANCE THAT DELINEATE ROLES AND BEHAVIORS FOR WHICH THE PROFESSIONAL NURSE IS ACCOUNTABLE

Quality of Care
Systemic evaluation of nursing practice

Performance Appraisal
Self-evaluation in relation to professional practice standards and other regulations

Education
Participation in ongoing educational activities to maintain knowledge for practice

Collegiality
Contribution to the development of peers, students, and others

Ethics
Use of Code for Nurses to guide practice

Collaboration
Involvement of client, significant others, and other health care providers in the provision of client care

Research
Use of research findings in practice

Resource Utilization
Consideration of factors related to safety, effectiveness, and costs in planning and delivering client care

Practice Environment
Contribution to the environment of care delivery

Accountability
Legal and professional responsibility for practice

Source: Association of Women's Health, Obstetric, and Neonatal Nurses (AWHONN). (1998). *Standards and guidelines for professional nursing practice in the case of women and newborns* (5th ed.). Washington, DC: AWHONN.

malpractice insurance costs are high for physicians, nurse-midwives, and nurses who work in labor and delivery.

LEGAL TIP Standard of Care

When you are uncertain about how to perform a procedure, consult the agency procedure book and follow the guidelines printed therein. These guidelines are the standard of care for that agency.

Risk Management

Risk management is an evolving process that identifies risks, establishes preventive practices, develops reporting mechanisms, and delineates procedures for managing lawsuits. Nurses should be familiar with concepts of risk management and their implications for nursing practice. These concepts can be viewed as systems of checks and balances that ensure high-quality client care from preconception until after birth. Effective risk management minimizes the risk of injury to clients and the number of lawsuits against nurses. Each facility or site develops site-specific risk management procedures based on accepted standards and guidelines. The procedures and guidelines must be reviewed periodically (Brott, 2000).

ETHICAL ISSUES IN PERINATAL NURSING AND WOMEN'S HEALTH CARE

Ethical concerns and debates have multiplied with the increased use of technology and with scientific advances. For example, with reproductive technology, pregnancy is now possible in women who thought they would never bear children, including some who are menopausal or postmenopausal. Should scarce resources be devoted to achieving pregnancies in older women? Is giving birth to a child at an older age worth the risks involved? Should older parents be encouraged to conceive a baby when they may not live to see the child reach adulthood? Should third-party payers assume the costs of reproductive technology? Potential clients, nurses, physicians, ethicists, and lawmakers must discuss and debate these questions. With induced ovulation and in vitro fertilization, multiple pregnancies occur, and multifetal pregnancy reduction (selectively terminating one or more fetuses) may be considered. Innovations such as intrauterine fetal surgery, fetoscopy, therapeutic insemination, genetic engineering, stem cell research, surrogate childbearing, surgery for infertility, "test tube" babies, fetal research, and treatment of very LBW

(VLBW) babies have resulted in questions about informed consent and allocation of resources. The introduction of long-acting contraceptives has created moral choices and policy dilemmas for health care providers and legislators; that is, should some women (substance abusers, women with low incomes, or women who are HIV positive) be required to take the contraceptives? With the potential for great good that can come from fetal tissue transplantation, what research is ethical? What are the rights of the embryo? Should cloning of humans be permitted? Discussion and debate about these issues will continue for many years. Nurses and clients, as well as scientists, physicians, attorneys, and clergy, must be involved in the discussions.

RESEARCH IN PERINATAL NURSING AND WOMEN'S HEALTH CARE

Research plays a vital role in the establishment of a maternity and women's health science. Nurses should promote research funding and conduct research on maternity and women's health, especially concerning the effectiveness of nursing strategies for these clients. Research can validate that nursing care makes a difference. For example, although prenatal care is clearly associated with healthier infants, no one knows exactly which nursing interventions produce this outcome. The research into women's health must increase. In the past, medical researchers rarely included women in their studies, so more research in this area is crucial. Many possible areas of research exist in maternity and women's health care. The clinician can identify problems in the health and health care of women and infants. Through research, nurses can make a difference for these clients.

Ethical Guidelines for Nursing Research

Nurses must protect the rights of human subjects (that is, clients) in all of their research. For example, nurses may collect data on or care for clients who are participating in clinical trials. The nurse ensures that the subjects are fully informed and aware of their rights as subjects. Research with perinatal clients may create ethical dilemmas for the nurse. For example, participating in research may cause additional stress to a woman concerned about outcomes of genetic testing or one who is waiting for an invasive procedure. Obtaining amniotic fluid samples or performing cordocentesis poses risks to the fetus. The nurse may be involved in determining whether the benefits of research outweigh the risks to the mother and the fetus. The ANA has published ethical guidelines in the conduct, dissemination, and implementation of nursing research (Silva, 1995). Following these guidelines helps nurses ensure that research is conducted ethically.

KEY POINTS

- Maternity nursing focuses on women and their infants and families during the childbearing cycle.
- Women's health nursing focuses on the special physical, psychologic, and social needs of women throughout their life spans.
- Nurses caring for women can play an active role in shaping health care systems to be responsive to the needs of contemporary women.
- Childbirth practices have changed to become more focused on the family and to allow alternatives in care.
- Home care is a cost-effective alternative locus of health care.
- *Healthy People 2010* provides goals for maternal and infant health.
- A variety of factors, including race, aging, and violence, affect women's health.
- The United States ranks twenty-third and Canada ranks fourteenth among industrialized nations in infant mortality rates.
- Evidence-based practice, outcomes orientation, best practices, and clinical benchmarking are emphasized in current practice.
- Ethical concerns have multiplied with the gradual increase in the use of technology and scientific advances.
- Research plays a vital role in establishing a scientific base for the care of women and infants.

CRITICAL THINKING EXERCISES

1. Examine health disparities in your community. Obtain statistics from your state and local health departments on racial and ethnic makeup of the state and your community; and the death rate, maternal mortality rate, and infant mortality rate according to racial and ethnic categories. What are the leading causes of death? Are these deaths preventable? What can you as a citizen and a nurse do to affect these health indicators?
2. From the list of resources provided, access at least three web sites. What information available on those sites would assist you as a nurse? Do the sites provide information appropriate for clients? Select a topic related to maternal and infant care. Do a short search of the World Wide Web by using your preferred search engine to access information on that topic that is appropriate for clients. Is information available in languages other than English? Where could you refer your non–English-reading clients for information?

RESOURCES

American Academy of Pediatrics
141 Northwest Point Blvd.
Elk Grove, IL 60007-1098
847-228-5005
www.aap.org

American College of Nurse Midwives
818 Connecticut Ave. NW, Suite 900
Washington, DC 20006
202-728-9860
www.acnm.com

American College of Obstetricians and Gynecologists
409 12th St. SW
Washington, DC 20090
www.acog.org

American Nurses Association
600 Maryland Ave. NW
Suite 100 W
Washington, DC 20024
www.ana.org; www.nursingworld.org

Association of Maternal and Child Health Programs
1220 19th St. NW, Suite 801
Washington, DC 20036
202-775-0436
www.amchp.org

Association of Ontario Midwives
www.aom.on.ca

The Association of Women's Health, Obstetric, and Neonatal Nurses (AWHONN)
2000 L St. NW, Suite 740
Washington, DC 20036
800-673-499 (United States)
800-245-0231 (Canada)
www.awhonn.org

Baby-Friendly USA
8 Jan Sebastian Way
Sandwich, MA 02563
508-888-8092
Fax: 508-888-8050
www.babyfriendlyusa.org
E-mail: info@babyfriendlyusa.org

Canadian Nurses Association
50 The Driveway
Ottawa, Ontario, Canada K2P 1E2
613-237-2133
www.can-nurses.ca

Coalition for Improving Maternity Services
CIMS National Office
P. O. Box 2346
Ponte Vedra, FL 32044
888-282-2367 or 904-285-1613
Fax: 904-285-2120
www.motherfriendly.org

College of Midwives of British Columbia
www.cmbc.bc.ca

College of Midwives of Ontario
2195 Yonge St., 4th Floor
at Eglinton Avenue
Toronto, Ontario, Canada M4S 2B2
416-327-074
Fax: 416-327-219
E-mail: adm@cmo.on.ca

Healthy Mothers, Healthy Babies Coalition
409 12th St. SW
Washington, DC 20090
202-863-2458
www.hmhb.org

Healthy People 2010
800-367-4728
www.health.gov/healthypeople

Institute for Women's Policy Research
1400 20th St. NW, Suite 104
Washington, DC 20036
202-785-5100
www.iwpr.org

International Confederation of Midwives
www.internationalmidwives.org

International Council of Nurses
3, place Jean-Marteau
CH-1201 Geneva, Switzerland
www.icn.ch

Maternity Center Association
281 Park Ave. South, 5th Floor
New York, NY 10010
212-777-5000
www.maternitycenter.com

National Association of Childbearing Centers
3123 Gottschall Rd.
Perkiomenville, PA 18074
215-234-8068
www.birthcenters.org

National Association of Neonatal Nurses (NANN)
4700 W. Lake Avenue
Glenview, IL 60025-1485
800-451-3795
Fax: 800-477-6266
www.nann.org

National Center for Health Statistics
www.cdc.gov.nchs

National Institute of Nursing Research
31 Center Dr., Room 5B-10
Bethesda, MD 20892-2178
301-496-2307
www.nih.gov/ninr

National Perinatal Association
101½ South Union St.
Alexandria, VA 22314-3323
703-549-5523
www.nationalperinatal.org

Office of Minority Health Resource Center
P. O. Box 37337
Washington, DC 20013-7337
www.omhrc.gov

Statistics Canada
www.statcan.ca/stat.html

REFERENCES

American Academy of Pediatrics Committee on Fetus and Newborn. (1995). Hospital stay for healthy term newborns. *Pediatrics, 96*(4 pt. 1), 788-790.

American Cancer Society. (2003). *Cancer facts and figures 2003.* Available at www.cancer.org. Accessed January 25, 2003.

Association of Women's Health, Obstetric, and Neonatal Nurses (AWHONN). (1998). *Standards and guidelines for professional nursing practice in the care of women and newborns* (5th ed.). Washington, DC: AWHONN.

Brott, L. (2000). Risk management and obstetrics. *Community Health Forum, 1*(1), 54-57.

Chima, F. (2001). Infant mortality, class, race, and gender: Implications for the health profession. *Journal of Health and Social Policy, 12*(4), 1-18.

Curtin, S., & Park, M. (1999). Trends in the attendant, place, and timing of births, and in the use of obstetric interventions: United States, 1989-97. *National Vital Statistics Report, 47*(27), 1-16.

Eckberg, E. (1998). Opinion: The future of robotics can be ours. *AORN Journal, 67*(5), 1018, 1020-1023.

Eisenberg, D. et al. (1998). Trends in alternative medicine use in the United States, 1970-1997. *Journal of the American Medical Association, 280,* 1569-1575.

Freda, M. (1995). Arrest, trial, and failure. *Journal of Obstetric, Gynecologic and Neonatal Nursing, 24*(5), 393-394.

Freda, M. (1999). MCN Editorial: The power of words. *MCN American Journal of Maternal Child Nursing, 24,* 63.

Gary, F., Sigsby, L., & Campbell, D. (1998). Preparing for the 21st century: Diversity in nursing education, research, and practice. *Journal of Professional Nursing, 14*(5), 272-279.

Gray, J. et al. (2000). Baby CareLinks: Using the Internet and telemedicine to improve care for high-risk infants. *Pediatrics, 106*(6), 1318-1324.

Guyer, B. et al. (1999). Annual summary of vital statistics–1998. *Pediatrics, 104*(6), 1229-1246.

Hoyert, D. et al. (2001). Annual summary of vital statistics: 2000. *Pediatrics, 108*(6), 1241-1255.

Johnson, M., Maas, M., & Moorhead, S. (Eds.). (2000). *Nursing outcomes classification (NOC)* (2nd ed.). St. Louis: Mosby.

Jones, W. (2000). Safe motherhood: Preventing pregnancy-related illness and death. Available at www.cdc.gov/nccdphp/drh/smh_aag2000.htm. Accessed August 23, 2002.

King, M., Pettigrew, A., & Reed, F. (1999). Complementary, alternative, integrative: Have nurses kept pace with their clients? *MEDSURG Nursing, 8*(4), 249-256.

Liljestrand, J. (2000). Strategies to reduce maternal mortality worldwide. *Current Opinions in Obstetrics and Gynecology, 12*(6), 513-517.

Lindegren, M. et al. (1999). Trends in perinatal transmission of HIV/AIDS in the United States. *Journal of the American Medical Association, 282*(6), 531-538.

MacMullen, N., & Dulski, L. (1999). Mother-baby nursing: Transition to the 21st century. *Mother Baby Journal, 4*(2), 7-12.

McCloskey, J., & Bulechek, G. (Eds.). (2000). *Nursing interventions classification (NIC)* (3rd ed.). St. Louis: Mosby.

Minino, A. et al. (2002). Deaths: Final data for 2000. *National Vital Statistics Report, 50*(15), 1-119.

The Mother-Friendly Childbirth Initiative. (1997). The first consensus initiative of the coalition for improving maternity services. *Journal of Nurse Midwifery, 42*(1), 59-63.

Murphy, S. (2000). Death: Final data for 1998. *National Vital Statistics Report, 48*(11), 1-105.

Oermann, M., & Huber, D. (1999). Patient outcomes: A measure of nursing's value. *American Journal of Nursing, 99*(9), 40-48.

Parkin, J. (2001). Female genital mutilation: A midwife's perspective. *British Journal of Midwifery, 9*(7), 421-424.

Pear, R. (January 8, 2002). Health spending rises 6.9%. *San Jose Mercury News,* pp. 1A, 4A.

Reclaiming benchmarking for clinicians. (1999/2000). *AWHONN Lifelines, 3*(6), 41.

Rubin, R. (2000, June 21). U.S. ranks 37th in health care. *USA Today,* p. 1.

Sheridan-Gonzalez, J. (2000). It's not my patient. *American Journal of Nursing, 100*(1), 13.

Silva, M. (1995). *Ethical guidelines in the conduct, dissemination, and implementation of nursing research.* Washington, DC: American Nurses' Association.

U.S. Department of Health and Human Services. (2000). *Healthy People 2010* (Conference edition, in two volumes). Washington, DC: Author.

CHAPTER 2

Maureen A. Nalle, Susan Speraw, and Angeline Bushy

Community Care: The Family and Culture

http://evolve.elsevier.com/Lowdermilk/MatWmnHlth/

LEARNING OBJECTIVES

- Describe the main characteristics of various contemporary family forms.
- Identify key factors influencing family health.
- Explain theoretic approaches for working with childbearing families.
- Relate the impact on and role of culture in childbearing families.
- Discuss cultural competence in relation to one's own nursing practice.
- Identify key components of the community assessment process.
- List indicators of community health status and their relevance to perinatal health.
- Describe data sources and methods for obtaining information about community health status.
- Identify predisposing factors and characteristics of vulnerable populations.
- List the potential advantages and disadvantages of home visits.
- Explore telephonic nursing care options in perinatal nursing.
- Describe how home care fits into the maternity continuum of care.
- Identify and describe common perinatal conditions amenable to home care.
- Discuss safety and infection control principles as they apply to the care of clients in their homes.
- Describe the nurse's role in perinatal home care.

INTRODUCTION TO FAMILY, CULTURE, COMMUNITY, AND HOME CARE

Health care in the United States has rapidly evolved in recent years, with notable shifts in both the nature of health priorities and the ways that health care is delivered to populations, families, and individuals. Greater emphasis is placed on the prevention of disease and disability, rather than the curative focus of past decades. Mechanisms of health care delivery also are radically different, requiring not only alterations in the way direct care delivery systems operate but also increased flexibility and adjustment in ways of relating to others.

One major shift in health care delivery is an increased emphasis on brief hospital stays that serve to reduce the financial burden for individuals, agencies, and insurance carriers. However, by minimizing inpatient length of stay, much of acute care nursing has been transferred to home-based nursing services in local communities.

In community settings, nurses must expand their knowledge base and make accommodation for a wide range of family organizational structures and unfamiliar customs. Larger societal changes have resulted in a broader definition of "family" that includes increasing numbers of single parents, same-gender couples living and raising children together, and wide acceptance of conception achieved through advanced reproductive technologies.

Through contemporary waves of immigration that began in the early 1970s, the face of America also has changed dramatically, requiring nurses to apply an extended base of cultural knowledge. The cultural diversity within the United States includes large groups of families from Central and South America in addition to Mexico, as well as populations of immigrants from Southeast Asia, Haiti, Africa, and Eastern Europe. These families bring their own rich traditions, new customs, and often histories of trauma resulting from the experiences of war and resettlement.

These shifts in the delivery of health care have been especially pronounced in childbearing. Newly immigrated families, or those living in poverty, often have limited access to care or experience cultural barriers to receiving health services (Arcia et al., 2001; Austin et al., 2002; Bushy, 2002; Kim et al., 2001). Hospital stays after childbirth may be abbreviated (Walowitz et al., 2000); follow-up care is limited.

Changing demands on the community-based nurse evolve out of these societal, economic, and health-related trends. Acuity of illness of home care clients may be far greater than that in the past, requiring the community nurse to become more adept in maternal assessment, direct care, and teaching. Assessment of the neonate requires knowledge of parameters for measuring the health of a newborn within the first days of life; skill in assisting with breastfeeding is essential. Knowledge of an ever-widening array of diverse family traditions, beliefs, and expectations related to childbearing becomes even more critical if the nurse is to facilitate effectively the transition required when a family moves through the stages of incorporating a new family member into its unique system of functioning.

This home- and community-based delivery system presents unique challenges for perinatal and maternity nurses who must incorporate community standards, cultural considerations, and family health needs into a comprehensive and holistic approach to health care, yet the integration of all of these related elements is critical to the delivery of effective nursing care. The family and each of its members, all of whom are the "client," exist within the context of the larger community; thus community and family cannot be considered apart. Furthermore, as population demographics change, nurses are assuming greater roles in assessing community health status and providing health promotion and disease prevention interventions across the perinatal health continuum. This chapter discusses the integration of home, community, and family-focused nursing in relation to culture, *Healthy People 2010,* and perinatal health outcomes.

COMMUNITY HEALTH AND WELLNESS

In the context of community-based health care, both the aggregate (group of people who have shared characteristics) and the population become the focus of intervention. Health professionals are required not only to determine health priorities but also to develop successful plans of care to be delivered in the health clinic, community health center, or the client's home.

The impetus for the shift in focus from curative modes of treatment to preventive intervention and health promotion is reflected in the publication of health goals for the nation, *Healthy People: The Surgeon General's Report on Health Promotion and Disease Prevention* (United States Department of Health, Education and Welfare [USDHEW], 1979). The most recent document, *Healthy People 2010,* established national health priorities that focused on two major goals: (1) increased quality and years of healthy life, and (2) elimination of health disparities. The 28 diverse focus areas and 467 objectives provide a systematic approach to health improvement for all people (U.S. Department of Health and Human Services [USDHHS], 2000a). The Healthy People initiative continues to shape national health policy with a focus on health promotion and disease prevention rather than on curative services (McGuire & Nalle, 2000).

The leading health indicators outlined in *Healthy People 2010* provide an important measure of the nation's health and the health of each community (USDHHS, 2000a) (see Chapter 1). Maternal-child focus areas address the most significant health issues for mothers, infants, and children, including those related to pregnant and postpartum women–maternal illness and death rates, access to prenatal care–and those affecting infant health and survival–infant mortality, birth outcomes, and prevention of birth defects (USDHHS, 2000b). Specific objectives for each maternal-child health indicator are used to track progress, highlight achievement, and identify areas for further action (Davis & Fields, 2000).

Trends in maternal and infant health in the United States reveal that progress has been made in relation to reduced infant and fetal deaths, use of prenatal care, and rates of cesarean births (see Chapter 1), but notable gaps remain in many other target areas. Some critical measures, such as low birth weight (LBW) and very low birth weight (VLBW), have increased, with significant disparities in infant mortality rates between Caucasians and other racial and ethnic groups in the United States. Despite favorable trends in early prenatal care and cesarean births, maternal mortality has not decreased significantly since 1982, with disproportionate rates among African-American and Hispanic women (USDHHS, 2000b). That many of these outcomes are preventable through access to prenatal care and use of preventive health practices clearly demonstrates the need for comprehensive, community-based care for mothers, infants, and families.

THE FAMILY IN CULTURAL AND COMMUNITY CONTEXT

The **family** and its cultural context play an important role in defining the work of maternity nurses. Family structure and function, care-seeking behavior, and relationships with providers are all influenced by culturally related health beliefs and values. Ultimately all of these factors have the power to affect maternal and child health outcomes. It therefore is important to recognize these influences, discuss current trends in families, and explore nursing implications.

Defining Family

The family has traditionally been viewed as the primary unit of socialization, the basic structural unit within a community. However, Chen and Rankin (2002) expanded on this definition, describing family as "the primary institution in society that preserves and transmits culture." Although a family is the primary cultural and socialization unit within a community, it also plays a pivotal role in health care, representing the primary target of health care delivery for maternal and newborn nurses. Most models of health behavior view family as a "system" within the larger social framework of a community. These definitions and understandings affect our approaches to health and health care of individuals within the family unit.

As one of society's most important institutions, the family represents a primary social group that influences and is influenced by other people and institutions. Most people have more continuous contact with this social group than with any other. A family is considered a fundamental social unit because it assumes most of the responsibility for socialization of its members and transmits its cultural background and core values in this context. This unique social network provides a powerful support system for each family member.

Family Organization and Structure

Census data clearly indicate significant alterations in the definition and social configuration of families over the past several decades. The Urban Institute recognizes four categories of families: the two-parent family, the single-parent family, blended families, and no-parent families (Staveteig & Wigton, 2000). A broader view of the contemporary family is offered by Brooks (2002), who defines a family as "a group of two or more persons related by blood, marriage, adoption, or emotional commitment who have a permanent relationship and who work together to meet life goals and needs." Beyond these basic characteristics, family trends are difficult to monitor, as current national data systems do not provide extensive information on family structure or caregiving patterns (Federal Interagency Forum on Children and Family Statistics, 2001).

The **nuclear family** has long represented the traditional American family in which male and female partners and their children live as an independent unit, sharing roles, responsibilities, and economic resources (Fig. 2-1). In contemporary society, this "idealized" family structure actually represents only a relatively small number of families. Two-parent families (biologic or adoptive parents) account for approximately 64% of American families, representing 72% of Caucasian, 60% of Latino, and 29% of African-American families (Staveteig & Wigton, 2000). The **binuclear family** is an alternate form of the traditional nuclear family arrangement that results from divorce. Children of remarried parents then become members of both the maternal and paternal nuclear households.

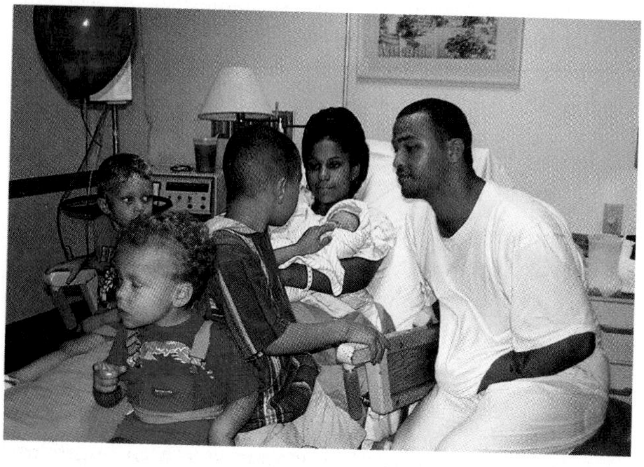

FIG. 2-1 Nuclear family. (Courtesy Marjorie Pyle, RNC, Lifecircle, Costa Mesa, CA.)

Many nuclear families have other relatives living in the same household. These **extended family** members, called *kin*, are grandparents, aunts or uncles, or other people related by blood. For some groups, such as African-American and Latin-American women, the family kin network is an important resource in terms of preventive health behavior (Clarke, L., 2001; Williams et al., 2001). The extended family is becoming more common as American society ages. The need to care for elderly parents within the same household often creates a "sandwich generation" in which parents of the nuclear family provide care for their children as well as for elderly grandparents or other relatives.

Single-parent families comprise an unmarried biologic or adoptive parent who may or may not be living with other adults. The single-parent family may result from the loss of a spouse by death, divorce, separation, or desertion; from either an unplanned or planned pregnancy; or from the adoption of a child by an unmarried woman or man. This family structure is becoming more prevalent, with current estimates at one fifth of Caucasian families, one third of Hispanics, and more than half of African-American families in the United States. Although the number of single-parent households has decreased for most groups, the number of single-parent families among African-American households has remained fairly steady at approximately 55% (Staveteig & Wigton, 2000).

Current research takes opposing perspectives on the merits and challenges of single-parent households. In many cases, the single-parent family tends to be vulnerable economically and socially, creating an unstable and deprived environment for the growth potential of children. Research demonstrates the impact of single-parenthood not only in economic instability but also in relation to health status, school achievement, and high risk behaviors for these children. Single mothers are more likely to live in poverty and have poor perinatal outcomes (USDHHS, 2000b).

In recent years, single parenting has become a frequent and acceptable choice in society. Individuals for whom the single-parent family is a chosen lifestyle often enjoy a free and open system for the development of parents and children. In these families, decision making and communication are seen as joint commitments between parent and child, and the parent-child relationship is considered a major source of life fulfillment; the most frequently identified strength was emotional closeness (Ford-Gilboe, 2000).

Reconstituted or **blended families,** those formed as the result of divorce and remarriage, consist of unrelated family members (stepparents, stepchildren, and stepsiblings) who join together to create a new household. These family groups frequently involve a biologic or adoptive parent whose spouse has not adopted the child.

Other family configurations, which are less well documented, include the 3.3 million children in families whose parents are cohabiting and an increasing number of **homosexual** (lesbian and gay) **families,** who may live together with or without children (Federal Interagency Forum on Children and Family Statistics, 2001). Children in homosexual (lesbian and gay) families may be the offspring of previous heterosexual unions, conceived by one member of a lesbian couple through therapeutic insemination, or adopted. These trends reflect the increased opportunities for alternate forms of parenthood within our society, owing both to more liberal social mores and to technologic and medical advances that offer the possibility of parenthood to single men and women. Despite increasing recognition of the biologic and psychologic needs of homosexual families, social acceptance and attitudes of health care providers often present significant barriers to quality health care (Clarke, V., 2001)

The Family in Society

The social context for the family can be viewed in relation to social and demographic trends that define the population as a whole. Current U.S. census data indicate that the racial and ethnic diversity of the population has grown dramatically in the last three decades. This increased diversity–first manifested among children, and soon to be evident in the older population–is projected to increase in the future (Federal Interagency Forum on Children and Family Statistics, 2001). Racial and ethnic minorities and immigrant families are increasingly evident in major metropolitan areas as well as in rural communities. Whereas the current statistics reflect a population that is 71% Caucasian, 12% African-American, and 13% Hispanic, it is predicted that the majority population in the United States will soon be nonwhite or Hispanic (National Alliance for Hispanic Health, 2001).

THEORETIC APPROACHES TO UNDERSTANDING FAMILIES

A family theory can be used to describe families and how the family unit responds to events both within and outside the family. Each family theory makes certain assumptions about the family and has inherent strengths and limitations. Most nurses use a combination of theories in their work with families. A brief discussion of a theory commonly used with families, systems theory, and the implications of this theory for maternal-child nursing is presented. A brief synopsis of several other theories useful in working with families is included in Table 2-1.

Family Systems Theory

Among the caring disciplines, a systems approach to understanding the family is almost universally applied. Many systems concepts are central to the delivery of holistic nursing care. These include recognition that changes occurring in one member affect the entire family, and an appreciation that nurses who work with families also enter into a systemic relationship with them. This is especially true for nurses who provide perinatal nursing care through community- or home-based agencies. Understanding how family members influence and interact with each other can help the nurse develop empathy with and respect for different ways of functioning.

When applied to families, the systems theory allows nurses to "view the family as a unit and thus focus on observing the interaction among family members rather than studying family members individually" (Wright & Leahey, 2000). Within a systems framework, the individual takes on several roles as a unique and important person in his or her own system and as part of one or more subsystems within the larger family. For example, an individual may belong to one of several subsystems, such as a child subsystem or a parental subsystem. When considering more than one generation of a family, a married woman may belong to a parental subsystem in her own home and to a subsystem of children when considered in relationship to her own older parents.

Wright and Leahey (2000) outlined the key characteristics of the family systems theory:

- A family system is part of a larger suprasystem and in turn is composed of many subsystems.
- The family as a whole is greater than the sum of its individual members.
- A change in one family member affects all family members.
- The family is able to create a balance between change and stability.
- Family members' behaviors are best understood from a view of circular rather than linear causality.

The family systems theory encourages nurses to view individual family members as part of a larger family system influenced by and influencing others. Application of these concepts can guide assessment and interventions for the family. For example, the childbearing family as a system interacts with many elements in the environmental suprasystem, including the health care community. The extent to which this suprasystem influences the family in matters such as prenatal care, childbirth education, and infant care depends on the family's boundary permeability. A relatively closed family may want instructions only from others within the family, whereas a relatively open family may be more receptive to instructions from health care providers.

Using Theories to Guide Practice

People effectively interact with each other in many ways. The nurse must understand that countless factors influence ways in which family members relate among themselves and with the health care community. Some of these factors include the natural history of the family, culture,

TABLE 2-1 **Theories and Models Relevant to Family Nursing Practice**

THEORY	SYNOPSIS OF THEORY
Family Life Cycle (Developmental) Theory (Carter & McGoldrick, 1999)	Families move through stages. The family life cycle is the context in which to examine the identity and development of the individual. Relationships among family members go through transitions. Although families have roles and functions, a family's main value is in relationships that are irreplaceable. The family involves different structures and cultures organized in various ways. Developmental stresses may disrupt the life cycle process.
Family Stress Theory (Boss, 1996)	Concerned with ways families react to stressful events. Family stress can be studied within the internal and external contexts in which the family is living. The internal context involves elements that a family can change or control, such as family structure, psychologic defenses, and philosophic values and beliefs. The external context consists of the time and place in which a particular family finds itself and over which the family has no control, such as the culture of the larger society, the time in history, the economic state of society, maturity of the individuals involved, success of the family in coping with stressors, and genetic inheritance.
McGill Model of Nursing (Allen, 1997)	Strength-based focus in clinical practice with families rather than a deficit approach. Identification of family strengths and resources; provision of feedback about strengths; assist family to develop and elicit strengths and use resources.
Health Belief Model (Becker, 1974; Janz & Becker, 1984)	The goal of the model is to reduce cultural and environmental barriers that interfere with access to health care. Key elements of the Health Belief Model include the following: Perceived susceptibility, perceived severity, perceived benefits, perceived barriers, cues to action, and confidence.
Human Developmental Ecology (Bronfenbrenner, 1979, 1989)	Behavior is a function of interaction of traits and abilities with the environment. Major concepts include ecosystem, niches (social roles), adaptive range, and ontogenetic development. Individuals are "embedded in a microsystem (role and relations), a mesosystem (interrelations between two or more settings), an exosystem (external settings that do not include the person), and a macrosystem (culture)" (Klein & White, 1996). Change over time is incorporated in the chronosystem.

roles, values, beliefs, and traditional customs. Because so many variables affect ways of relating, the nurse must be aware that most family members will interact and communicate with each other in ways that are very different from those of the nurse's own family of origin. Most families will hold at least some beliefs about health that are very different from those of the nurse; in some instances, their beliefs will conflict with principles of health care management predominant in the Western health care system. Therefore to be effective in working with families, the nurse must possess a degree of personal openness and acceptance and be willing to work with families in a way that is respectful and adapts to their ways of learning and communicating.

Because family relationships are always complex, viewing the interaction of the whole family helps nurses to understand more fully the functioning of individual family members. Family systems theory encourages nurses to view individual family members as part of a larger family system influenced by and influencing others. The extent to which this suprasystem influences the family in matters such as prenatal care, childbirth education, and infant care depends on the family's boundary permeability. A family that has recently immigrated to this country may want to receive health information only from others within the family or the immediate cultural community, whereas a family that has more experience in dealing with the American health care system may be more receptive to nurses who are culturally different. When interacting with a family, the nurse becomes part of a system with them. The behaviors and interaction style of the nurse affect not just the individual who is identified as the "client" but also contribute to family members' responses to each other. Finally, the quality of the nurse-family system strongly influences how the family will interact with the greater health care community in the future.

Knowing about the phases of the life cycle can assist nurses in providing anticipatory guidance for families. For example, helping childbearing families prepare for the birth of a newborn may minimize the development of crises. By using developmental theory, a nurse can anticipate that a family who delivers a child with a serious anomaly might experience a crisis or state of disequilibrium because the birth of an ill child is not a normative event. Because such a family may revert to a state of dependence, the nurse will realize that their need for extra support and nurturing from the nurse is a natural response to stress.

Because today's families experience a great deal of pressure, they must develop effective stress-management strategies. Maternity nurses working in community settings may care for a full range of family situations including healthy but highly stressed families and families coping with the extraordinary stress of ill infants or mothers who have recently had major surgical procedures such as cesarean births. Nurses can assist families in changing their stress levels by helping families control internal and external context factors. The nurse can intervene through educational strategies to correct misconceptions and reduce stress. Explaining normal infant growth and development (maturation) may reduce the stress of parenting.

In planning the care of a family or an individual family member, the nurse may find it useful to view the family at a developmental phase in the life cycle, facing stressful life events, and operating as a system. A family assessment tool such as the one outlined by Friedman (1998) (Fig. 2-2) can be used as a guide for assessing aspects of the family discussed in this chapter. A family **genogram** (family tree format depicting relationships of family members over at least three generations) (Fig. 2-3) provides valuable information about a family and can be placed in the nursing care plan for easy access by care providers.

By using the Health Belief Model as a guide to assessment, nurses can better address concerns specific to an individual from a different cultural group, motivating them to take action on their own behalf. Understanding a woman's concerns from her own point of view can help the nurse to provide interventions that will place women at ease in the health care setting. For example, the nurse can modify or adjust her care in assessing uterine involution as part of postpartum care for a woman who holds traditional Mexican beliefs and fears of having cold enter her uterus during a normal examination. The culturally competent nurse can close the door to the room, pull curtains to minimize air flow around the woman, position the woman so that the perineum is facing away from the door or air vents, and keep the perineum draped so that the examination takes place with a minimum of exposure.

Within the larger society, individuals and families have a variety of stressors that affect their ability to function and to engage consistently in behaviors that will promote health and wellness. These individuals and families fall into high risk or vulnerable populations. Their stresses relate to many aspects of life: ethnic and cultural minority status, immigration status, poverty, challenges with English language fluency and literacy, malnutrition, and limited access to housing. The U.S. Department of Health and Human Services (2000c) adds the following to the list of characteristics associated with vulnerability: (1) poor, isolated communities, (2) residence in areas that have health professional shortages, (3) poor utilization of preventive health care, (4) disease and illness prevalence at catastrophic rates, and (5) higher use of expensive hospital emergency care instead of lower cost routine health maintenance. Finally, Lee and Cubbin (2002) noted that high residential turnover and large numbers of households headed by females also are characteristics found among high risk or vulnerable groups.

Some families have multiple stressors, placing them at especially high risk for poor health outcomes. It should be noted, however, that not only low-income or minority groups are at high risk for morbidity and mortality. Some stressors affect families at all strata of society. Even those who are well educated and in a higher socioeconomic class can have life stressors that make them highly vulnerable to health problems. These antecedents to vulnerability include mental illness; substance use; domestic violence; and reduced access to medical care due to unemployment, loss of medical insurance, or inadequate insurance coverage. Nurses cannot make the assumption that a family is immune to vulnerability because its members live in an exclusive neighborhood, are well educated, and are fully employed. The concepts of high risk and vulnerability potentially apply to everyone.

Of particular relevance to nurses working within communities, providing home-based care, is the reality that individuals who are in high risk or vulnerable groups often lack preventive care. This is especially true for routine obstetric and pediatric care. Because people with very limited financial, social, or emotional resources must carefully assign priorities to their needs if they are to assure basic survival, "extras" such as routine health care are often neglected. Consider the single, unemployed mother who loves her family and must choose between purchasing formula for her newborn infant or paying the water bill so her children will have fresh drinking water. She is unlikely to seek medical care for herself because she is feeling fatigued or to purchase contraception that she cannot afford. This delay in seeking services often results in more severe health problems that must be managed at a future date. An unintended pregnancy for this same young mother will potentially worsen her economic, emotional, and social stress; failure to treat conditions such as anemia or depression will reduce her ability to function and to parent effectively.

The Friedman Family Assessment Model (Short Form)

Identifying Data

1. Family name
2. Address and phone
3. Family composition
4. Type of family form
5. Cultural (ethnic) background
6. Religious identification
7. Social class status
8. Family's recreational or leisure-time activities

Developmental Stage and History of Family

9. Family's present developmental stage
10. Extent of family developmental tasks fulfillment
11. Nuclear family history
12. History of family of origin of both parents

Environmental Data

13. Characteristics of home
14. Characteristics of neighborhood and larger community
15. Family's geographic mobility
16. Family's associations and transactions with community
17. Family's social support system or network (See Fig. 2-6.)

Family Structure

18. Communication patterns
    - Extent of functional and dysfunctional communication (types of recurring patterns)
    - Extent of emotional (affective) messages and how expressed
    - Characteristics of communication within family subsystems
    - Extent of congruent and incongruent messages
    - Types of dysfunctional communication processes seen in family
    - Areas of open and closed communication
    - Familial and contextual variables affecting communication
19. Power structure
    - Power outcomes
    - Decision-making process
    - Power bases
    - Variables affecting family power
    - Overall family system and subsystem power (Family power continuum placement)
20. Role structure
    - Formal role structure
    - Informal role structure
    - Analysis of role models (optional)
    - Variables affecting role structure
21. Family values
    - Compare the family to American or family's reference group values and/or identify important family values and their importance (priority) in family.
    - Congruence between the family's values and the family's reference group or wider community
    - Congruence between the family's values and family member's values
    - Variables influencing family values
    - Values consciously or unconsciously held
    - Presence of value conflicts in family
    - Effect of the above values and value conflicts on health status of family

Family Functions

22. Affective function
    - Family's need–response patterns
    - Mutual nurturance, closeness, and identification
    - Separateness and connectedness
23. Socialization function
    - Family child-rearing practices
    - Adaptability of child-rearing practices for family form and family's situation
    - Who is (are) socializing agent(s) for child(ren)?
    - Value of children in family
    - Cultural beliefs that influence family's child-rearing patterns
    - Social class influence on child-rearing patterns
    - Estimation about whether family is at risk for child-rearing problems and if so, indication of high risk factors
    - Adequacy of home environment for children's need to play
24. Health care function
    - Family's health beliefs, values, and behavior
    - Family's definitions of health–illness and their level of knowledge
    - Family's perceived health status and illness susceptibility
    - Family's dietary practices
    - Adequacy of family diet (recommended 3-day food history record)
    - Function of mealtimes and attitudes toward food and mealtimes
    - Shopping (and its planning) practices
    - Person(s) responsible for planning, shopping, and preparation of meals
    - Sleep and rest habits
    - Physical activity and recreation practices (not covered earlier)
    - Family's drug habits
    - Family's role in self-care practices
    - Medically based preventive measures (physicals, eye and hearing tests, and immunizations)
    - Dental health practices
    - Family health history (both general and specific diseases—environmentally and genetically related)
    - Health care services received
    - Feelings and perceptions regarding health services
    - Emergency health services
    - Source of payments for health and other services
    - Logistics of receiving care

Family Stress and Coping

25. Short- and long-term familial stressors and strengths
26. Extent of family's ability to respond, based on objective appraisal of stress-producing situations
27. Coping strategies utilized (present/past)
    - Differences in family members' ways of coping
    - Family's inner coping strategies
    - Family's external coping strategies
28. Dysfunctional adaptive strategies utilized (present/past; extent of usage)

Family Composition Form

Name (last, first)	Gender	Relationship	Date/place of birth	Occupation	Education
1. (Father)					
2. (Mother)					
3. (Oldest child)					
4.					
5.					
6.					
7.					
8.					

FIG. 2-2 The Friedman Family Assessment Model (short form). (From Friedman, M. [1998]. *Family nursing theory and assessment* [4th ed.]. New York: Appleton & Lange.)

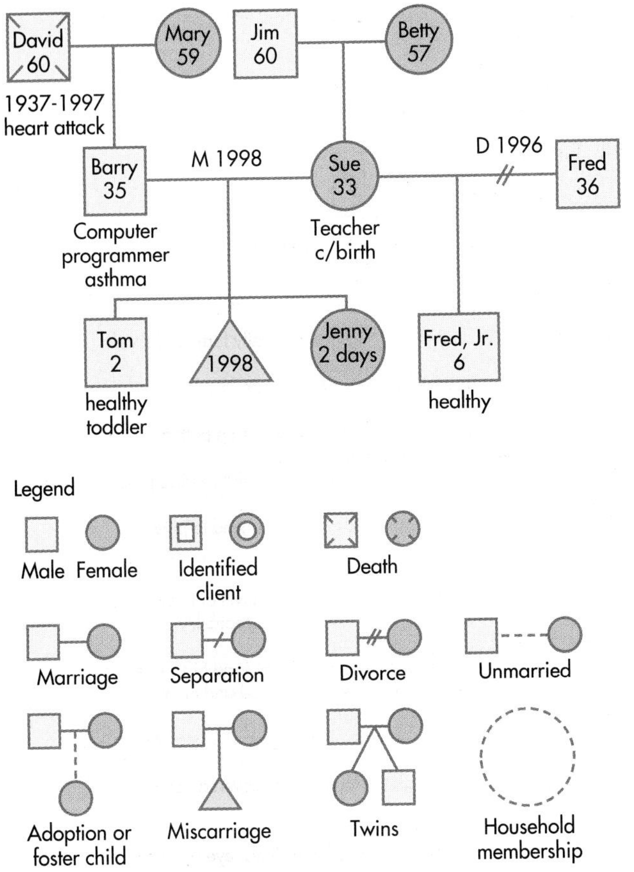
David 60
1937-1997
heart attack
Mary 59
Jim 60
Betty 57
Barry 35
M 1998
Sue 33
D 1996
Fred 36
Computer
programmer
asthma
Teacher
c/birth
Tom 2
1998
Jenny 2 days
Fred, Jr. 6
healthy
toddler
healthy
Legend
Male
Female
Identified client
Death
Marriage
Separation
Divorce
Unmarried
Adoption or foster child
Miscarriage
Twins
Household membership

FIG. 2-3 Example of a family genogram.

VULNERABLE POPULATIONS

Several broad categories of high risk or vulnerable populations are of special interest to perinatal nurses working in the community. These include the following.

Women

For women, the duration and quality of life are affected by sociocultural, economic, and physical environments (USDHHS, 2001b), and these determinants of health must be continuously monitored and evaluated (USDHHS, 2000b). The *Report Card* on women's health (National Women's Law Center [NWLC], 2001) assessed women's health across the 50 states and the District of Columbia, providing status indicators related to access to services, use of preventive health care and health promotion activities, the occurrence of certain health conditions, and an assessment of the community's impact on women's health. The report suggested that one of the primary factors compromising women's health is lack of access to acceptable-quality health care, which may take many forms: lack of health insurance, living in a medically underserved area, or an inability to obtain needed services, particularly basic services such as prenatal care. For example, some rural areas have few obstetricians, pediatricians, and nurse midwives; women may have to travel hundreds of miles for this kind of care (Bushy, 1998; 2001). Federal and state policies and programs also fail to safeguard women's interest in relation to reproductive health and health care coverage (NWLC, 2001).

Women often have lower income and less education and are therefore considered at high risk. Maternal education has been identified as a "key determinant of welfare and survival of children." It is linked to the family's ability to use health-related information and to make health care decisions, and also to infant mortality. Infant mortality is nearly two times higher for mothers without a high school education (USDHHS, 2000b).

Within the larger group of vulnerable women, a number of subgroups present challenges to the community-based perinatal nurse.

Adolescent Girls

Youth and young adults younger than 24 years are the least medically served of all age groups in the United States (USDHHS, 2001b). Lifestyle choices related to substance use, sexually transmitted infections, and human immunodeficiency virus (HIV) represent high risk behaviors with both immediate and long-term health consequences. Young women, particularly African-Americans and Hispanics, are less likely to have access to routine care and often fail to seek care because of inability to pay, lack of transportation, or confidentiality issues (USDHHS, 2000c).

Minority Women

In the United States, disparities continue to exist in terms of adult women's health and the health of their infants. Higher infant and maternal mortality are evident in African-American and Hispanic women and among some Native American and Alaskan Native communities. A significant contributing factor to these deaths is the increased rate of teen pregnancy among minority women. In 1998, Hispanics had the highest rate of teen pregnancy at 93.6/1000 births and non-Hispanic African-American teens had a pregnancy rate of 88.2/1000 (USDHHS, 2000c). Minority women, many of whom live in poverty, also have disproportionate rates of heart disease, cancer, hepatitis, and acquired immunodeficiency syndrome (AIDS), leading to mental health issues as well as to reduced life expectancy and premature death and disability (USDHHS, 2001b). Women with underlying health conditions are at especially high risk for poor obstetric outcomes for both themselves and their infants. They have high rates of preterm labor, pregnancy-induced hypertension, and often have intrauterine growth restriction resulting in the birth of infants who are small for gestational age. These are the clients for whom the community-based perinatal nurse will be providing care, and their needs are complex, demanding high levels of skill and expertise.

Older Women

Although women have a greater life expectancy than men, they are more likely to have chronic illnesses, less likely to use preventive services, and ultimately spend more on health care (USDHHS, 2001b).

Incarcerated Women

Many of these women report a history of sexual and physical abuse. The lifestyle choices of this group, including risky sexual relationships, illicit drug use, and smoking, place them at high risk for sexually transmitted infections, HIV and AIDS, other chronic and communicable diseases, and complicated pregnancies (USDHHS, 2001b). Because their relationship histories are often unstable, and because they often lack the support of family, incarcerated women, or those with a history of repeated incarceration, frequently have difficulty providing emotional stability, secure housing, and health promotion role modeling for their children. For example, of the 9500 women in prison in California, more than 7300 are mothers and have very limited access to their children (Nixon, 2002).

Migrant Women

An estimated 3 to 5 million people, 16% of whom are women, are classified as migrant farm workers in the United States (Maternal Child Health Bureau, 1997). Migrant workers establish temporary residence in various areas on a seasonal basis to obtain employment. Although many acquire temporary housing for at least 6 months, others move continuously throughout the year. They may be categorized as episodically homeless due to the seasonal nature of their employment and living arrangements.

The primary regions for migrant workers in the United States are associated with agriculture, tobacco production, fishing, and mining industries. The three primary migrant streams are East Coast states, Midwestern and Western states, and West Coast states (Bushy, 2002; Murray, Zentner, & Samiezade-Yazd, 2001). Diverse ethnic groups are represented among migrant workers: African-Americans, European-Americans, Hispanics, Haitians, and Southeast Asians.

Migrant laborers and their families face many problems, including financial instability, child labor, poor housing, lack of education, language and cultural barriers, and limited access to health and social services (Clemen-Stone, McGuire, & Eigsti, 2002). Migrant farm work is one of the most hazardous occupations in the United States because of heavy physical demands, fatigue, operation of potentially dangerous machinery, exposure to pesticides and naturally occurring irritants, and limited enforcement of Occupational Safety and Health Administration (OSHA) standards.

Poor dental health, diabetes, hypertension, malnutrition, tuberculosis, and parasitic infections are common health issues among migrant populations. Substance abuse and intimate partner violence also are significant problems. The average life expectancy of migrant workers is 49 years, compared with 79 years for the general population. This may be partially explained by the fact that most farm workers do not view illness as a problem unless the condition interferes with work.

Numerous reproductive health issues exist for migrant women, including less consistent use of contraception and increased rates of sexually transmitted infections. Migrants are less likely to receive early prenatal care and have a greater incidence of inadequate weight gain during pregnancy than do other poor women. The infant mortality rate among migrant workers is estimated to be 25 times higher than the national average (Murray et al., 2001).

Federally funded migrant health centers have been established in many regions of the United States, but they are unable to meet the demands of the 3 to 5 million migrants. Many seek care at local hospitals and clinics in the areas in which they work, but access is limited by lack of time and financial constraints. Even if services are free, the loss of wages incurred in leaving the field is a deterrent to preventive care. Lack of trust or fear of being reported to the Immigration and Naturalization Services prevents many undocumented workers from seeking care.

Rural versus Urban Community Settings

Rural refers to a town or community area that has a population of less than 2,500 or to a county with fewer than 50,000 people. A number of common characteristics define rural groups: they lack anonymity, are isolated, and tend to be content to live independently (Bushy, 2000; Murray et al., 2001). Geographic and socioeconomic factors present barriers to accessing prenatal care associated with transportation and provider inaccessibility.

Homeless Women

Although the numbers are difficult to estimate, homeless populations are becoming more evident throughout the United States. An estimated 2.5 to 3.5 million individuals are homeless nationally, with 6.5% of adults reporting homelessness each year. This includes increasing numbers of women, children, and adolescents who are disenfranchised from their homes, families, and services for various reasons, resulting in a 17% increase in the demand for family assistance (Bureau of Primary Health Care, 2001). Depending on the cause of homelessness and the availability of services, a person may be homeless for weeks or months, intermittently, or on a prolonged basis.

The multiple, interacting factors contributing to homelessness include external causes such as economic issues and unemployment and personal behavioral choices such as drug and alcohol use. The most significant causes of homelessness in the United States relate to mental illness (approximately 50%) and substance use (nearly 75% among homeless men).

Violent relationships and a history of abuse are significant contributing factors to homelessness for women.

Although the homeless population is generally higher in urban areas, a growing number of the homeless are found in rural agricultural, mining, and fishing regions, where they seek temporary employment. Often these families remain hidden within the community. Sometimes the family stays in a local hotel (paying on a daily basis while they work), lives out of their car, resides in an unoccupied building, or may camp in a national park. Couples with children form the largest group among rural homeless. Lack of visibility and community resources in rural areas frequently results in longer periods of poverty and homelessness for these families (Bushy, 2000).

Health issues among the homeless are numerous, resulting primarily from a lack of preventive care and a lack of resources in general. In most homeless groups, chronic illness, including asthma, circulatory problems, and diabetes, is rampant. Living conditions contribute to higher levels of infectious disease, such as tuberculosis and enteric infections. Anemia, obesity, and other nutritional disorders are common because of lack of cooking and food storage facilities and greater reliance on more accessible convenience foods. Dental caries is one of the most common health problems among homeless people; this affects their overall health status.

Because very few are able to access primary care, most of the homeless population are forced to use the emergency room for routine health problems. Mental health and substance abuse services for the homeless are extremely limited in many communities, in particular in medically underserved rural regions of the United States (Bureau of Primary Health Care, 2001)

For women, the emotional and psychologic trauma of the homeless experience is often exacerbated by physical or sexual assault; 36% of homeless women report being a victim of a crime while living on the streets. Approximately 24% of women become pregnant while they are homeless. Although many women are eligible for Medicaid and public health services, few receive prenatal care.

Refugees and Immigrants

Refugees are defined as those who are displaced suddenly or forced to leave their country of origin because of persecution, civil unrest, or war. Families are thus forced from their own homes to seek residence and employment elsewhere (Murray, Zentner, & Samiezade-Yazd, 2001). Often these groups are extremely impoverished and face extreme physical and emotional stress when they arrive in the United States. Some refugees have a history of arrival in a new country by precarious means, such as crossing wide oceans in fragile boats. Many survivors of such journeys have memories of relatives and friends who died at sea; many have been raped by modern pirates who prey on those who are desperate for a better life. The traumatic stress of having witnessed the murders of their families as a result of war haunts many refugees. Many have profound grief over the loss of loved ones, their homelands, and all they owned. Both refugees and immigrants are saddened by the knowledge that it will be difficult or impossible to go "home" to the people, traditions, and customs that were familiar and comforting.

Along with their profound resilience and determination, refugees and immigrants have brought rich diversity to the United States in several important dimensions, including cultural heritage and customs, economic productivity, and enhanced national vitality. At the same time, multiple challenges accompany the dramatic influx of individuals and families from other countries.

In general, refugees are more likely to live in poverty than are immigrants (Murray et al., 2001). Over time, measures of health and well-being actually decline for the immigrant population as they become part of American society (National Academy Press [NAP], 2002). Many of the conditions or illnesses that they acquire contribute to the persistence of disparities in maternal and neonatal health outcomes for both immigrants and refugees.

Implications for Nursing

Working in the community or in the home with the full spectrum of family organizational styles, vulnerable populations, and cultural groups presents challenges for the nurse. Whether it involve perinatal care focused on women and their newborns, or women's health care directed toward treatment and prevention of other health conditions such as communicable diseases and sexually transmitted infections, nursing must exhibit a high degree of professionalism. Cultural sensitivity, compassion, and a critical awareness of family dynamics and social stressors that will affect health-related decision making are critical components in developing an effective plan of care.

Although the long-term consequences of contemporary immigration for American society are unclear, the successful incorporation of immigrant families depends on the resources, benefits, and policies that ensure their healthy development and successful social adjustment. Culturally competent health care and involvement of the immigrant community in health care programs are recommended strategies for improving the access to and effectiveness of health care for this population (NAP, 2002).

The use of camp volunteers, known as "romatoras," has been effective in assisting families living in migrant worker camps to obtain prenatal, postpartum, and infant care (see Resource list at the end of the chapter). Working in partnership with health professionals such as nurses, lay camp aides have been used effectively for outreach and health education; however, more strategies are needed to link traditional practices with the formal health care system. Guidance and information about other health resources are available to health care providers through the National Migrant Resource Program and the Migrant Clinicians Network.

Nurses working with homeless women and families are challenged to treat them with dignity and respect to establish a therapeutic relationship. Case management is recommended to coordinate the services and disciplines that may be involved in meeting the complex needs of these families. Whenever possible, health services must be provided when the woman seeks treatment, as this may be the only opportunity to provide health information and intervention. Building on existing coping strategies and strengths, the health care provider helps the woman and her family to reconnect with a social support system. Nurses also have an important role in advocating for funding to support homeless health services and to improve access to preventive care for all homeless populations.

CULTURAL FACTORS RELATED TO FAMILY HEALTH

Cultural Context of the Family

Culture has many definitions. Thomas (2001) defined **culture** as "a unified set of values, ideas, beliefs, and standards of behavior shared by a group of people; it is the way a person accepts, orders, interprets, and understands experiences throughout the life course." Willis (1999) added to that explanation, stating, "Culture is an integrated dynamic system of values, beliefs and practices shaped by close ties, teachings, and common interactions from conception and throughout the lifespan." Williams et al. (2001) described culture as a "set of interlocking cognitive schemata that construct and give meaning to what people do in their everyday lives." The political, social, and economic context of people's lives also is part of the cultural experience. According to Doyle and Ward (2001), culture is influenced by religion, environment, and historic events, and plays a powerful role in the individual's behavior and patterns of human interaction. All of these definitions include the recognition that culture helps shape a person's interpretation of every life experience. Culture is not static; it is an ongoing process that influences a woman throughout her entire life, from birth to death. Culture is an essential element of what defines us as people.

Cultural knowledge includes beliefs and values about each facet of life and is passed from one generation to the next. Cultural beliefs and traditions relate to food, language, religion, art, health and healing practices, kinship relationships, and all other aspects of community, family, and individual life. Culture also has been shown to have a direct effect on health behaviors. Values, attitudes, and beliefs that are culturally acquired may influence perceptions of illness, as well as health care–seeking behavior and response to treatment (NAP, 2002). The impact of these influences must be assessed by health professionals in providing health care and developing effective intervention strategies (Williams et al., 2001).

Many subcultures may be found within each culture. *Subculture* refers to a group existing within a larger cultural system that retains its own characteristics. A subculture may be an ethnic group or a group organized in other ways. For example, in the United States, many ethnic subcultures such as African-Americans, Asian-Americans, and Latinos exist, as do subcultures within these groups. In addition, the Caucasian population in America has multiple subcultures of its own. Because every identified cultural group has subcultures, and because it is impossible to study every subculture in depth, greater differences may exist among and between groups than is generally acknowledged.

In a multicultural society, many groups can influence traditions and practices. As cultural groups come in contact with each other, acculturation and assimilation may occur.

Acculturation refers to changes that take place within one group or among several groups when people from different cultures come in contact with one another. People may retain some of their own culture while adopting some of the cultural practices of the dominant society. This familiarization among cultural groups results in some overt behavioral similarity, especially in mannerisms and dress. Language patterns, food choices, and health practices are often much slower to adapt to the influence of acculturation. Furthermore, during times of family transitions such as childbearing, or during crisis or illness, a person may rely on old cultural patterns even after she has become acculturated in many ways. This is consistent with family developmental theory that states that during times of stress, people revert to practices and behaviors that are most comfortable and familiar.

Assimilation refers to the complete loss of cultural identity. According to Friedman (1998), "assimilation denotes the more complete and one-way process of one culture being absorbed into the other." Assimilation is the process by which groups "melt" into the mainstream, thus accounting for the notion of a "melting pot," a phenomenon that has been said to occur in the United States. This is illustrated by individuals who identify themselves as being of "Irish" or "German" descent, without having any remaining cultural practices or values linked specifically to that culture, such as food preparation techniques, style of dress, or proficiency in the language associated with their reported cultural heritage.

Implications for Nursing

Nurses must be aware that some factors may prevent some health care practitioners from providing optimal care, whereas others can enhance nursing practice. Understanding the concepts of ethnocentrism and cultural relativism may help nurses care for families in a multicultural society.

Ethnocentrism refers to "the view that one's culture's way of doing things is the right and natural way" (Galanti, 1997). Essentially, ethnocentrism supports the notion that "my group is best." Although the United States is a culturally diverse nation, the prevailing practice of health care is based on the beliefs and practices held by members of the dominant culture, primarily Caucasians of European descent. This practice is based on the biomedical model that focuses on curing disease states. From this biomedical perspective, pregnancy and childbirth are viewed as processes with inherent risks that are most appropriately managed by using scientific knowledge and advanced technology. The medical perspective stands in direct contrast with the belief systems of many cultures. Among many women, birth is traditionally viewed as a completely normal process that can be managed with a minimum of involvement from health practitioners. When encountering behavior in women unfamiliar with the biomedical model, the nurse may become frustrated and impatient. The nurse may label the women's behavior inappropriate and believe that it conflicts with "good" health practices. If the Western health care system provides the nurse's only standard for judgment, the behavior of the nurse is called ethnocentric.

Cultural relativism is the opposite of ethnocentrism and refers to learning about and applying the standards of another person's culture to activities within that culture. To be culturally relativistic, the nurse recognizes that people from different cultural backgrounds comprehend the same objects and situations differently. In other words, culture determines a person's viewpoints. Cultural relativism does not require nurses to accept or personally adopt the beliefs and values of another culture; rather nurses recognize that others' behavior may be based on a system of logic different from their own. Cultural relativism affirms the uniqueness and value of every culture.

Childbearing Beliefs and Practices

Nurses working with childbearing families care for families from many different cultures and ethnic groups. To provide culturally competent care, the nurse should be aware of the spectrum of cultural beliefs and practices important to individual families. A nurse should consider all aspects of culture, including communication, space, time orientation, and family roles, when working with childbearing families.

Communication often creates the most challenging obstacle for nurses working with clients from diverse cultural groups. This is because communication is not merely the exchange of words. Instead it involves (1) understanding the individual's language, including subtle variations in meaning and distinctive dialects; (2) appreciation of individual differences in interpersonal style; and (3) accurate interpretation of the volume of speech as well as the meanings of touch and gestures. For example, members of some cultural groups tend to speak more loudly, with great emotion, and with vigorous and animated gestures when they are excited; this is true whether their excitement is related to positive or negative events or emotions. It is important, therefore, for the nurse to avoid rushing to judgment regarding a client's intent when the client is speaking, especially in a language not understood by the nurse. In these situations, it is critical that the nurse avoid instantaneous responses that may well be based on an incorrect interpretation of the client's gestures and meaning. Instead, the nurse should withhold an interpretation of what has been communicated until it is possible to clarify the client's intent. The nurse needs to enlist quickly the assistance of a person who can help and to seek to verify with the client the true intent and meaning of the communication.

Inconsistencies between the language of clients and the language of providers present a significant barrier to effective health care. Because of the diversity of cultures and languages within the U.S. and Canadian populations, health care agencies are increasingly seeking the services of interpreters (of oral communication from one language to another) or translators (of written words from one language to another) to bridge these gaps and fulfill their obligation for culturally and linguistically appropriate health care (Box 2-1). Finding the best possible interpreter in the circumstance also is critically important. A number of personal attributes and qualifications contribute to an interpreter's potential to be effective. Ideally, interpreters should have the same native language and be of the same religion or have the same country of origin as the client (Murray et al., 2001). Interpreters should have specific health-related language skills and experience and help bridge the language and cultural barriers between the client and the health care provider (Howard et al., 2001). The person interpreting also should be mature enough to be trusted with private information. However, because the nature of nursing care is not always predictable and because nursing care that is provided in a home or community setting does not always allow expert, experienced, or mature adult interpreters, ideal interpretive services sometimes are impossible to find when they are needed. In crisis or emergency situations, or when family members are having extreme stress or emotional upset, it may be necessary to use relatives, neighbors, or children as interpreters. If this situation occurs, the nurse must ensure that the client is in agreement and comfortable with using the available interpreter to assist.

When using an interpreter, the nurse respects the family by creating an atmosphere of respect and privacy. Questions should be addressed to the woman and not to the interpreter. Even though an interpreter will of necessity be exposed to sensitive and privileged information about the family, the nurse should take care to assure that confidentiality is maintained. A quiet location free from interruptions is the ideal place for interpretive services to take place. In addition, culturally and linguistically appropriate educational materials that are easy to read, with appropriate text and graphics, should be available to assist the woman and her family in understanding health care information (Simmons et al., 2002).

When using interpretive services, the nurse demonstrates respect for the woman and helps her maintain a sense of dignity by taking care to

- Respect the woman's wishes
- Involve her in the decision about who will be the most appropriate person to interpret under the circumstances
- Provide as much privacy as possible, and
- Use culturally appropriate learning aides.

Cultural traditions define the appropriate personal space for various social interactions. Although the need for personal space varies from person to person and with the

BOX 2-1 **Working with an Interpreter**

STEP 1: BEFORE THE INTERVIEW

A. Outline your statements and questions. List the key pieces of information you want/need to know.
B. Learn something about the culture so that you can converse informally with the interpreter.

STEP 2: MEETING WITH THE INTERPRETER

A. Introduce yourself to the translator and converse informally. This is the time to find out how well he or she speaks English. No matter how proficient or what age the interpreter is, be respectful. Some ways to show respect are to ask a cultural question to acknowledge that you can learn from the interpreter, or you could learn one word or phrase from the interpreter.
B. Emphasize that you do want the client to ask questions because some cultures consider this inappropriate behavior.
C. Make sure the interpreter is comfortable with the technical terms you need to use. If not, take some time to explain them.

STEP 3: DURING THE INTERVIEW

A. Ask your questions and explain your statements (see Step 1).
B. Make sure that the interpreter understands which parts of the interview are most important. You usually have limited time with the interpreter, and you want to have adequate time at the end for client questions.
C. Try to get a "feel" for how much is "getting through." No matter what the language is, if in relating information to the client, the interpreter uses far fewer or far more words than you do, "something else" is going on.
D. Stop every now and then and ask the interpreter, "How is it going?" You may not get a totally accurate answer, but you will have emphasized to the interpreter your strong desire to focus on the task at hand; if there are language problems: (1) speak slowly; (2) use gestures (e.g., fingers to count or point to body parts); and (3) use pictures.
E. Ask the interpreter to elicit questions. This may be difficult, but it is worth the effort.
F. Identify cultural issues that may conflict with your requests or instructions.
G. Use the interpreter to help problem solve or at least give insight into possibilities for solutions.

STEP 4: AFTER THE INTERVIEW

A. Speak to the interpreter and try to get an idea of what went well and what could be improved. This will help you to be more effective with this or another interpreter.
B. Make notes on what you learned for your future reference or to help a colleague.

Remember:

Your interview is a *collaboration* between you and the interpreter. *Listen* as well as speak.

Notes:

1. The interpreter may be a child, grandchild, or sibling of the client. Be sensitive to the fact that the child is playing an adult role.
2. Be sensitive to cultural and situational differences (e.g., an interview with someone from urban Germany will likely be different from an interview with someone from a transitional refugee camp).
3. Younger females telling older males what to do may be a problem for both a female nurse and a female interpreter. This is not the time to pioneer new gender relations. Be aware that in some cultures it is difficult for a woman to talk about some topics with a husband or a father present.

Courtesy Elizabeth Whalley, PhD, San Francisco State University.

situation, the actual physical dimensions of comfort zones differ from culture to culture. Actions such as touching, placing the woman in proximity to others, taking away personal possessions, and making decisions for the woman can decrease personal security and heighten anxiety. Conversely, if nurses respect the need for distance, they allow the woman to maintain control over personal space and support the woman's autonomy, thereby increasing her sense of security. For example, many Asian groups have reserved attitudes about physical contact, and this may at times create anxiety when health care is delivered.

Nurses often use touch, and frequently do so without any awareness of the emotional distress they may be causing to their clients. Johnson et al. (1999) reported in their research with South Asian women that tremendous psychologic distress is caused when a woman who has breast cancer comes into physical contact with another woman. The fear is that through physical contact, the cancer will be spread from one person to another. In the home care setting, a nurse who must provide physical care to a woman with disease may cause the woman great anxiety, as she fears that her disease will be spread to the nurse. Fears about spreading disease also may interfere with her acceptance of physical comfort and care from family members.

Time orientation also is a fundamental way in which culture affects health behaviors. People in cultural groups

CULTURAL CONSIDERATIONS

Questions to Ask to Obtain Cultural Expectations about Childbearing

1. What do you and your family think you should do to remain healthy during pregnancy?
2. What can you do or not do to improve your health and the health of your baby?
3. Who do you want with you during your labor?
4. What can he or she do to help you be most comfortable during labor?
5. What actions are important for you and your family after the baby's birth?
6. What do you and your family expect from the nurse(s) caring for you?
7. How will family members participate in your pregnancy, childbirth, and parenting?

BOX 2-2 Strategies for Care Delivery and Providing Appropriate Care

STRATEGIES FOR CARE DELIVERY

- Break down the language barriers
- Explain your rationale and reasons for suggestions
- Integrate folk and Western treatments
- Enlist the family caretaker and others
- Get consent from the right person
- Provide language-appropriate materials

PROVIDING APPROPRIATE CARE

- Ask about traditional beliefs, such as the role of hot and cold
- Be sensitive regarding translators and language barriers
- Ask about important dietary practices, particularly related to events such as childbirth
- Ask about group practices and beliefs
- Ask about a woman's fears, and those of her family, regarding an unfamiliar care setting

From Mattson, S. (2000). Providing culturally competent care: Strategies and approaches for perinatal clients. *AWHONN Lifelines, 4*(5), 37-39.

may be relatively more oriented to past, present, or future. Those who focus on the past strive to maintain tradition or the status quo and have little motivation for formulating future goals. In contrast, individuals who focus primarily on the present neither plan for the future nor consider the experiences of the past. These individuals do not necessarily adhere to strict schedules and are often described as "living for the moment," or "marching to their own drummer." Individuals oriented to the future maintain a focus on achieving long-term goals.

The time orientation of the childbearing family may affect nursing care. For example, talking to a family about bringing the infant to the clinic for follow-up examinations (events in the future) may be difficult for the family that is focused on the present concerns of day-to-day survival. Because a family with a future-oriented sense of time plans far in advance, thinking about the long-term consequences of present actions, they may be more likely to return as scheduled for follow-up visits. Despite the differences in time orientation, each family may be equally concerned for the well-being of its newborn.

Family roles involve the expectations and behaviors associated with a member's position in the larger family system (e.g., mother, father, or grandparent). Social class and cultural norms also affect these roles, with distinct expectations for men and women clearly determined by social norms. For example, culture may influence whether a man actively participates in the pregnancy and childbirth, yet maternity care practitioners working in the Western health care system expect fathers to be involved. This can create a significant conflict between the nurse and the role expectations of very traditional Mexican or Arab families, who usually view the birthing experience as a female affair (see Cultural Considerations box). The way that health care practitioners manage such a family's care molds its experience and perception of the Western health care system.

In maternity nursing and women's health care, the nurse supports and nurtures the beliefs that promote physical or emotional adaptation to childbearing. However, if certain beliefs might be harmful, the nurse should carefully explore them with the woman and use them in the reeducation and modification process. Strategies for care delivery and providing appropriate care are presented in Box 2-2.

Few families are exclusively "Asian" or "Caucasian." Instead they are often blended composites, with one partner bringing to the relationship the traditions of one culture or family of origin, whereas the other partner brings a slightly differing perspective. Even when partners are both of Asian ancestry, for example, their families of origin may come from different regions of the same country and follow completely different health practices. Table 2-2 provides examples of some cultural beliefs and childbearing practices frequently encountered by the nurse who works with women who identify themselves as European-American (Caucasian), Latin-American, Asian-American, African-American, or Native American. The cultural beliefs and customs in Table 2-2 are categorized based on distinct cultural traditions and are not practiced by all members of the cultural group in every part of the country. Women from these cultural and ethnic groups may adhere to some, all, or none of the practices listed. In using this table as a guide, the nurse should use caution to avoid making stereotypic assumptions about any person based on sociocultural-spiritual affiliations. Nurses should exercise sensitivity in working with every family, being careful to assess the ways in which they apply their own mixture of cultural traditions.

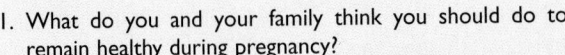

TABLE 2-2 **Traditional* Cultural Beliefs and Practices: Pregnancy, Childbirth, and Parenting**

PREGNANCY	CHILDBIRTH	PARENTING
Hispanic		
(Based primarily on knowledge of Mexican-Americans; members of the Hispanic community have their origins in Spain, Cuba, Central and South America, Mexico, Puerto Rico, and other Spanish-speaking countries.)		
Pregnancy Pregnancy desired soon after marriage Late prenatal care Expectant mother influenced strongly by mother or mother-in-law Cool air in motion considered dangerous during pregnancy Unsatisfied food cravings thought to cause a birthmark Some pica observed in the eating of ashes or dirt (not common) Milk avoided because it causes large babies and difficult births Many predictions about sex of baby May be unacceptable and frightening to have pelvic examination by male health care provider Use of herbs to treat common complaints of pregnancy Drinking chamomile tea thought to ensure effective labor	***Labor*** Use of "partera" or lay midwife preferred in some places; may prefer presence of mother rather than husband After birth of baby, mother's legs brought together to prevent air from entering uterus Loud behavior in labor ***Postpartum*** Diet may be restricted after birth; for first 2 days only boiled milk and toasted tortillas permitted (special foods to restore warmth to body) Bed rest for 3 days after birth Keep warm Delay bathing Mother's head and feet protected from cold air; bathing permitted after 14 days Mother often cared for by her own mother 40-day restriction on sexual intercourse	***Newborn*** Breastfeeding begun after third day; colostrum may be considered "filthy" or "spoiled" Olive oil or castor oil given to stimulate passage of meconium Male infant not circumcised Female infant's ears pierced Belly band used to prevent umbilical hernia Religious medal worn by mother during pregnancy; placed around infant's neck Infant protected from "evil eye" Various remedies used to treat "Mal ojo" (evil eye) and fallen fontanel (depressed fontanel)
African-American		
(Members of the African-American community, many of whom are descendants of slaves, have different origins. Today a number of Black Americans have emigrated from Africa, the West Indian Islands, the Dominican Republic, Haiti, and Jamaica.)		
Pregnancy Acceptance of pregnancy depends on economic status Pregnancy thought to be state of "wellness," which is often the reason for delay in seeking prenatal care, especially by lower-income African-Americans "Old wives' tales" include having a picture taken during pregnancy will cause stillbirth and reaching up will cause cord to strangle baby Craving for certain foods, including chicken, greens, clay, starch, and dirt Pregnancy may be viewed by African-American men as a sign of their virility Self-treatment for various discomforts of pregnancy, including constipation, nausea, vomiting, headache, and heartburn	***Labor*** Use of "Granny midwife" in certain parts of United States Varied emotional responses: some cry out, some display stoic behavior to avoid calling attention to selves Client may arrive at hospital in far-advanced labor Emotional support often provided by other women, especially own mother ***Postpartum*** Vaginal bleeding seen as sign of sickness; tub baths and shampooing of hair prohibited Sassafras tea thought to have healing power Eating liver thought to cause heavier vaginal bleeding because of its high "blood" content	***Newborn*** Feeding very important: "Good" baby thought to eat well Early introduction of solid foods May breastfeed or bottle-feed; breastfeeding may be considered embarrassing Parents fearful of spoiling baby Commonly call baby by nicknames May use excessive clothing to keep baby warm Belly band used to prevent umbilical hernia Abundant use of oil on baby's scalp and skin Strong feeling of family, community, and religion

Data from Amaro (1994), Bar-Yam (1994), Galanti (1997), D'Avanzo & Geissler (2003), Mattson (1995), Spector (2000), and Williams (1989).

Note: Most of these cultural beliefs and customs reflect the traditional culture and are not universally practiced. These lists are not intended to stereotype clients but rather to serve as guidelines while discussing meaningful cultural beliefs with a client and her family. Examples of other cultural beliefs and practices are found throughout this text.

*Variations in some beliefs and practices exist within subcultures of each group.

TABLE 2-2 Traditional* Cultural Beliefs and Practices: Pregnancy, Childbirth, and Parenting—cont'd

PREGNANCY	CHILDBIRTH	PARENTING
Asian-Americans (Typically refers to groups from China, Korea, the Philippines, Japan, Southeast Asia [particularly Thailand], Indochina, and Vietnam.)		
Pregnancy Pregnancy considered time when mother "has happiness in her body" Pregnancy seen as natural process Strong preference for female health care provider Belief in theory of hot and cold May omit soy sauce in diet to prevent dark-skinned baby Prefer soup made with ginseng root as general strength tonic Milk usually excluded from diet because it causes stomach distress Inactivity or sleeping late may cause difficult birth	***Labor*** Mother admitted by other women, especially her own mother Father does not actively participate Labor in silence Cesarean birth not welcome ***Postpartum*** Must protect self from yin (cold forces) for 30 days Ambulation limited Shower and bathing prohibited Warm room Chinese mother avoids fruits and vegetables Diet: Warm fluids Some patients are vegetarians Korean mother served seaweed soup with rice Chinese diet high in hot foods	***Newborn*** Concept of family important and valued Father is head of household; wife plays a subordinate role Birth of boy preferred May delay naming child Some groups (e.g., Vietnamese) believe colostrum is dirty; therefore they may delay breastfeeding until milk comes in
European-American (Members of the European-American [Caucasian] community have their origins in countries such as Ireland, Great Britain, Germany, Italy, and France.)		
Pregnancy Pregnancy viewed as a condition that requires medical attention to ensure health Emphasis on early prenatal care Variety of childbirth education programs available and participation encouraged Technology driven Emphasis on nutritional science Involvement of the father valued Written source of information valued	***Labor*** Birth is a public concern Technology dominated Birthing process in institutional setting valued Involvement of father expected Physician seen as head of team ***Postpartum*** Emphasis or focus on early bonding Medical interventions for dealing with discomfort Early ambulation and activity emphasized Self-care valued	***Newborn*** Increased popularity of breastfeeding Breastfeeding begins as soon as possible after childbirth ***Parenting*** Motherhood and transition to parenting seen as stressful time Nuclear family valued, although single parenting and other forms of parenting more acceptable than in the past Women often deal with multiple roles Early return to prepregnancy activities
Native American (Many different tribes exist within the Native American culture; viewpoints vary according to tribal customs and beliefs.)		
Pregnancy Pregnancy considered as a normal, natural process Late prenatal care Avoid heavy lifting Herbal teas encouraged	***Labor*** Prefers female attendant, although husband, mother, or father may assist with birth Birth may be attended by whole family Herbs may be used to promote uterine activity Birth may occur in squatting position ***Postpartum*** Herbal teas to stop bleeding	***Newborn*** Infant not fed colostrum Use of herbs to increase flow of milk Use of cradle boards for infant Babies not handled often

DEVELOPING CULTURAL COMPETENCE

In an extensive review of the literature related to cultural competence, Willis (1999) noted that **cultural competence** has many names and definitions, all of which have subtle shades of difference, but which are essentially the same: multiculturalism, cultural sensitivity, and intercultural effectiveness. Lynch and Hansen (1998) offered the following definition, one that applies especially well to the nursing profession: "Cultural competence is the ability to think, feel, and act in ways that acknowledge, respect and build upon ethnic, [socio]cultural, and linguistic diversity."

Willis (1999) noted that culturally competent professionals are able to act in ways that meet the needs of the client and are respectful of ways and traditions that may be very different from their own (see Evidence-Based Practice box). In today's society, with its ever-expanding diversity, it is of critical importance that nurses develop more than technical skill. It has always been vital that nurses develop the ability to relate to others, but the challenges of meeting the broad scope of these needs has never before been so great. Nurses at every level of preparation, and throughout their professional lives, must engage in a continual process of developing and refining attitudes and behaviors that will promote culturally competent care (Ryan, Carlton, & Ali, 2000).

In addition to issues of preserving and promoting human dignity, the development of cultural competence is of equal importance in terms of health outcomes. Nurses who relate effectively with clients are able to motivate

EVIDENCE-BASED PRACTICE

CULTURAL COMPETENCE IN CHILDBEARING

Centuries-old beliefs and traditions for assuring the well-being of the souls (*plig*) of newborns among Hmong immigrants from Laos are detailed in an ethnographic study of 27 women by Liamputtong-Rice (2000). Traditions relate to the rites of welcoming that are extended to each of the three souls believed to be part of the essential physical and spiritual health of every person. If the "soul calling" is delayed, or if any one of the souls is not successfully called out, then the child will be weak, tired, fail to thrive, or die. To assure that a child has all three of the essential souls, and that none of the souls is frightened away, the soul-calling ceremonies must be conducted by a shaman or respected elder on the third morning of life. During the ceremonies, the guardian spirits for the baby are called out, and the household spirit is informed of the new baby's arrival. Integral to the ceremony is the assignment of a name that is right for the child through the completion of complex rituals. In addition to spiritual benefits, the rites have the function of bringing the community together in support of the family.

Implications for nursing are many, because in Western societies significant conflict may exist between cultural traditions and local law. Mothers and infants are often not discharged until a birth certificate is completed, placing pressure on the family to name the child too soon. Infants who are hospitalized beyond the morning of the third day will be perceived as being at even greater risk for continued ill health or death. Ill mothers may refuse hospitalization beyond the second day, because this will prevent their participation in soul-calling ceremonies. If an infant dies during the early neonatal period, parents may not exhibit the degree of grief that nursing staff expects, yet this will fall within Hmong cultural norms because the infant will not be considered fully human until all three souls have been called forth. Understanding and respecting Hmong belief will help the perinatal nurse to make needed accommodations to reduce family stress, enhance coping, and facilitate a healthy integration of the child into Hmong family life.

A descriptive study (Rehm, 1999) of 25 parents from 19 families sought to explore the validity of assumptions commonly made by health professionals who characterize Mexican-American families as fatalistic and passive, with religious belief as central to their health-related behaviors. Families were interviewed in depth about ways in which they dealt with chronic illness in their children. Findings revealed the presence of common core religious beliefs. However, in contrast to health professionals' assumptions, Mexican-American families in the sample were neither fatalistic nor passive in their approach to seeking health care for their ill children. Through prayer, families sought to intercede with God to assure health and recovery for their children. In addition to prayer, families actively sought expert medical advice and did all that was recommended to them by health professionals. As they sought the best available care, provided medications, and administered treatments, families found that their religious faith provided them with a source of hope and consolation when their children failed to make the desired progress.

Findings indicate that nurses who misinterpret the place of religious faith in the lives of families not only risk alienating their clients, but they also fail to recognize a critical source of comfort and a potent coping resource for families under stress. In helping families to manage their worries and concerns and maintain their integrity as a functioning system, nurses must make use of each family's unique strengths and resources. Few of these are as basic or potent as the hope associated with the practice of one's own religious faith.

Raines and Morgan (2000) studied Caucasian and African-American women's expectations for the birth experience in an exploratory study. Their methods included interviews with women older than 18 years who had given birth within 3 days. Their interest was in determining differing expectations among women with regard to the degree of comfort that would be experienced during labor and birth and for personal involvement in the childbirth. Researchers found that the women from different cultural groups had expectations for their own participation and for supportive care from the nurse that varied substantially.

Nurses must take an active role in assessing the individual needs of childbearing women. To make assumptions that all women desire or need the same level of support leads to inadequate and possibly culturally insensitive care. The culturally competent nurse knows that although it is impossible to know everything about the traditional practices of every culture or cultural subgroup, it is important to ask the client about her personal preferences and needs. Gathering these data as part of the baseline assessment will allow the nurse to plan culturally appropriate interventions.

them in the direction of health-promoting behaviors. In that way, cultural competence becomes an issue of cost-effectiveness as well (USDHHS, 2001c).

A number of authors have discussed the key components of culturally competent care:

- Personal insight into the reality that there is disparity between one's own culture and that of the client
- The ability of the nurse to understand the behaviors of clients from their own unique cultural background, and educate and promote healthy behaviors in a cultural context that has meaning for the clients (Bushy, 2002; Doyle & Ward, 2001; Sebastian & Bushy, 1999)
- The ability to take abstract knowledge about other cultures and apply it in a practical way, so that the quality of service improves and policies are enacted that meet the needs of all clients (Davis, Meldrum, & Tippy, 1996)
- The ability to communicate respectfulness for a wide range of differences, including client use of nontraditional healing practices and alternative therapies
- Recognition of the importance of culturally different communication styles, problem-solving techniques, concepts of space and time, and desires to be involved with care decisions
- Ability to plan effective care that anticipates the need to address varying degrees of language ability and literacy and barriers to care and compliance with treatment (Howard, Andrade, & Byrd, 2001)

Pathways to the Development of Cultural Competence

Cultural competence proceeds along a continuum. Out of her research into nursing cultural competence, Willis (1999) devised a framework for developing competence. Her framework comprises seven steps that can move a professional from a lower level of continuum development toward higher levels of culturally competent professionalism (Box 2-3).

Programs that promote values important to the cultural identity of the community build on the values of mutual support, cohesiveness, and self-sufficiency and therefore result in better health outcomes for community members. One such program is described by Ma'at et al. (2001). Racial and Ethnic Approaches to Community Health (REACH) is a funded initiative program to reduce health disparities and/or improve health outcomes of minority Americans. Included under this umbrella is Reach Out, a faith-based breast and cervical cancer detection program conducted in African-American and Latino churches in communities in which more than half of cervical and breast cancers go undetected until disease is far advanced. In discussing the efficacy of these programs, Ma'at et al. highlighted the value of having a culturally appropriate message delivered by community leaders trained in self-help and health care advocacy. Williams et al. (2001) pointed out that the use of community advocates most effectively reaches underserved populations through a network of existing social relationships. This can be especially true in isolated communities such as those that exist in remote or rural areas. Using local health workers builds on preexisting trust relationships. Moreover, local health workers are in a position to reinforce continually health teaching and best practices in health maintenance even when nurses or other heath professionals are absent.

BOX 2-3 Willis' 7-Step Framework for Cultural Competence

Step 1	Knowledge of one's own cultural affiliation (beliefs, values, lifeways)
Step 2	Knowledge of other's cultural beliefs, values, lifeways
Step 3	Nonthreatening, non–fear-provoking interactions with others
Step 4	Tolerance
Step 5	Inclusion
Step 6	Appreciation for and acceptance of difference
Step 7	Competence

(From Willis, W. [1999]. Culturally competent care during the perinatal period. *Journal of Perinatal and Neonatal Nursing, 13*[3], 45-59.)

Integrating Cultural Competence with the Nursing Plan of Care

Shamsudin (2002), in her discussion of the effectiveness of models for delivering nursing care as applied to persons of different cultures, noted that models useful in one culture might not be readily applied to another. She observed that many nursing scholars and researchers focus almost exclusively on the interpersonal and collaborative relationship between the nurse and the client, excluding the family as central to decision making. In many cultures, family members make most of the decisions for the client, and therefore the central relationship between the nurse and client is mediated directly by the family. The nurse must recognize the cultural importance of family in supporting the client, guiding decision making, and preserving cultural integrity in the health care interaction.

Other nursing scholars also addressed the issues of cultural competence and cultural inclusion in models that guide nursing care. Engebretson and Littleton (2001) noted that all nursing care is delivered in multiple cultural contexts. These include the cultures of the client, of the nurse, of the health care system, and the larger culture of the society in which health care is delivered. If any of these cultural groups is excluded from the nurse's assessment and consideration, nursing care may fail to achieve its goals and may be culturally insensitive.

Lowe (2002) presented a unique model of care that is specific to the traditions of the Native American culture. From his perspective, nurses establish interpersonal connections and health partnerships with clients to achieve the goal of providing care that promotes harmony and balance, key elements in Native American beliefs and traditions.

Implications for Nursing

According to Huff and Kline (1999), there are four areas of focus for culturally competent care: (1) developing cultural awareness or sensitivity to differences; (2) gaining cultural knowledge of values, beliefs, and lifeways of other groups; (3) developing skills in cultural assessment as a basis for intervention; and (4) engaging in direct cultural encounters or immersion in cultural experiences. These approaches build a basis for effective care strategies, enabling the nurse to promote self-care and effective lifestyle changes (Pender, Murdaugh, & Parsons, 2002). Cross-cultural experiences also present an opportunity for the health care professional to expand cultural sensitivity, awareness, and skills.

Holistic nursing care by definition is delivered with understanding and sensitivity to the unique cultural values, beliefs, and traditions of the family. Nurses providing care within the community, especially when invited into the homes of their clients, are allowed an especially intimate view of the traditions that surround childbearing. All cultures maintain behavioral norms and expectations for each stage of the perinatal cycle. These norms and expectations evolve from a culture's view of how people stay healthy and prevent illness. A culture's economic, religious, kinship, and political structures pervade its beliefs and practices regarding childbearing. To practice with cultural competence, nurses must understand the ways in which people of different cultures perceive life events and the health care system. Clients have a right to expect that their physiologic and psychologic health care needs will be met and that their cultural and spiritual beliefs will be respected.

When nurses develop plans of care for clients who are culturally different from themselves or from the dominant culture of the community, they should be certain to include an assessment that addresses psychosocial issues related to that diversity. No nursing care plan is complete without attention to nursing diagnoses that address cultural diversity issues.

- *Compromised family coping related to*
  –immigration or refugee status
- *Impaired verbal communication related to*
  –inability to speak or understand English
- *Risk for loneliness related to*
  –separation from family and country of origin
- *Posttrauma syndrome related to*
  –impact of war, persecution, or civil and political unrest
- *Social isolation related to*
  –separation from family and friends due to immigration status
- *Chronic sorrow related to*
  –refugee status, separation from family, and death of family members

ASSESSING THE COMMUNITIES IN WHICH FAMILIES LIVE

Mothers assume much of the health-related decision making for their families (USDHHS, 2001b) with up to 83% of them having sole or shared responsibility for financial decisions affecting family health. A significant link exists between the maternal roles of health care provider and decision maker and family health behavior. Clearly it is in the context of family that health beliefs and health behaviors are formed (Rainey et al., 1999).

The health and well-being of women and children will be in jeopardy as long as the communities in which they live are ill prepared to provide the quantity and quality of services they need. Whereas the support and reinforcement available from family members can be instrumental in health behavior change (Bruhn, 2001), absence of programs and health policies is often a barrier to family health, resulting in increased health risks (Rainey et al., 1999).

Important measures of community health include access to care, level of provider services available, as well as other social and economic factors. For women and infants, access to a consistent source of care is critical. Those with a regular source of care are more likely to use preventive services and receive timely treatment for illness and injury (USDHHS, 2000c), but current statistics indicate that more than 16% of Medicaid-covered women versus 13.4% of privately insured women lack access to a usual source of care or rely primarily on emergency services. Consequently, many of these women report unmet health and/or dental needs (Almeida, Dubay, & Ko, 2001).

Methods of Community Assessment

Community, in its broadest definition, refers to a geographically defined area; its residents; their cultural, religious, and ethnic characteristics; and the activities or functions through which the needs of the residents are met. The health of individuals or groups is inextricably linked to the health status of each community.

With the community as the focus of perinatal health care, the nurse must become familiar with the neighborhoods and resources that influence clients. Community assessment is a complex although well-defined process through which the unique characteristics of the populations and their special needs are identified to plan and evaluate health services for the community as a whole. The desired outcome of this process is identification of direct service as well as advocacy needs of the targeted aggregate or group and improved health for the community as a whole (Kuehnert, 2002).

Data Collection and Sources of Community Health Data

A community assessment framework or model provides criteria for conducting a community assessment, identifies types and methods of data collection, and organizes the data of a community assessment (Ervin, 2002) (Fig. 2-4). Many models and frameworks may be used, but the actual process often depends on the extent and nature of the assessment to be performed, the time and resources available, and the way the information is to be used.

Data collection is often the most time-consuming phase of the community assessment process, but it provides an important definition and description of the community (Ervin, 2002). A broad range of health information is available for nurses in conducting a community assessment. According to the Centers for Disease Control and Prevention (CDC), the most critical indicators of perinatal health in a community are related to access to health care; maternal mortality; infant mortality; low birth weight; first trimester prenatal care; and rates for mammography, Pap smears, and other similar screening tests (USDHHS, 2000c). Nurses may use these indicators as a reflection of access, quality, and continuity of health care in a community.

Individuals and groups for whom English is a second language often lack the skills necessary to seek medical care and function adequately in the health care setting. Lack of English fluency is a barrier, and communication difficulties continue to affect access to care, particularly in such areas as making appointments, applying for services, and obtaining transportation (NAP, 2002). As a result of the increasingly multicultural U.S. population, we have a more urgent need to address health literacy as a component of culturally and linguistically competent care. Health literacy involves a spectrum of abilities, ranging from reading an appointment slip to interpreting medication instructions. These skills must be assessed routinely to recognize a problem

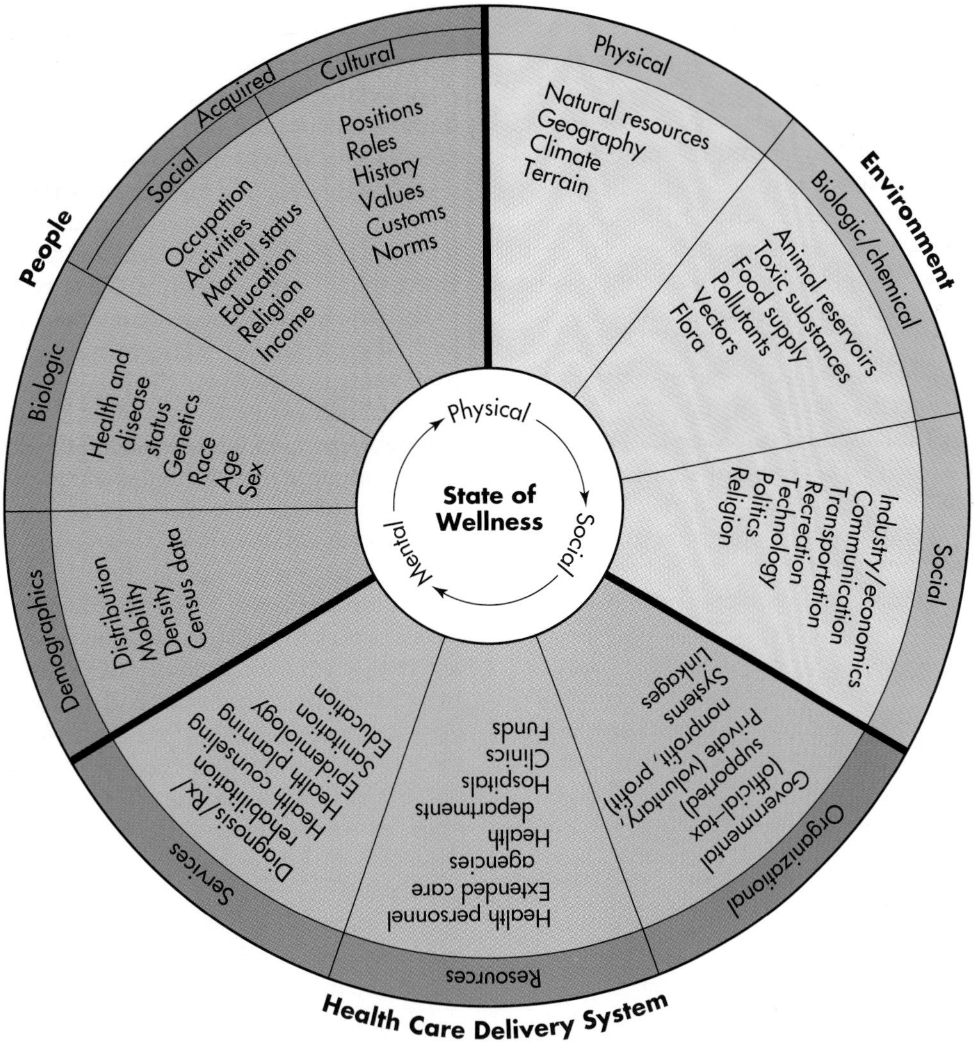
People
Environment
Health Care Delivery System
Acquired
Cultural
Social
Positions
Roles
History
Values
Customs
Norms
Occupation
Activities
Marital status
Education
Religion
Income
Biologic
Health and disease status
Genetics
Race
Age
Sex
Demographics
Distribution
Mobility
Density
Census data
Physical
Natural resources
Geography
Climate
Terrain
Biologic/chemical
Animal reservoirs
Toxic substances
Food supply
Pollutants
Vectors
Flora
Social
Industry/economics
Communication
Transportation
Recreation
Technology
Politics
Religion
Organizational
Governmental (official-tax supported)
Private (voluntary, nonprofit, profit)
Systems
Linkages
Resources
Health personnel
Extended care agencies
Health departments
Hospitals
Clinics
Funds
Services
Diagnosis/Rx/rehabilitation
Health counseling
Health planning
Epidemiology
Sanitation
Education
State of Wellness
Physical
Social
Mental

FIG. 2-4 Community health assessment wheel. (Clemen-Stone, S., McGuire, S., & Eigsti, D. [2002]. *Comprehensive community health nursing: Family, aggregate, & community practice* [6th ed]. St. Louis: Mosby.)

and accommodate clients with limited literacy skills. An excellent resource is *Teaching Patients with Low Literacy Skills*, 2nd edition (Doak, Doak, & Root, 1996).

The U.S. government census provides data on population size, age ranges, sex, racial and ethnic distribution, socioeconomic status, educational level, employment, and housing characteristics. Summary data are available for most large metropolitan areas, arranged by zip code and census tract, which usually corresponds to a neighborhood (approximately 3000 to 6000 people). Looking at individual census tracts within a community helps to identify subpopulations or aggregates whose needs may differ from those of the larger community. For example, women at high risk for inadequate prenatal care according to age, race, and ethnic or cultural group may be readily identified, and outreach activities may be appropriately targeted.

City, county, and state health departments provide annual reports of births and deaths. Maternal and infant death rates are particularly important, as they reflect health outcomes that may be preventable (McDevitt & Wilbur, 2002). Local health departments also compile extensive statistics about the birth complications, causes of death, and leading causes of morbidity and mortality for each age group. Local and state health data are compiled and reported through the Centers for Disease Control and Prevention to the National Center for Health Statistics (NCHS). From this source, the National Health Survey is published annually, describing national health trends. However, national data are only as accurate and reliable as the local data on which they are based (Doyle & Ward, 2001), so caution is needed in interpretation and application of the data to specific population groups.

Other sources of useful information are hospitals and voluntary health agencies. The March of Dimes Birth Defects Foundation, for example, has supported perinatal needs assessments in many communities across the United States. Other community health resources include health care providers or administrators, government officials, religious leaders, and representatives of voluntary health agencies. Community or county health councils exist in many areas, with oversight of specific health initiatives or programs for that region. These **key informants** often provide a unique perspective that may be inaccessible through other sources.

The perinatal health nurse also may explore community health program reports, records of preventive health screenings, and other informal data. Established programs often provide good indicators of the health promotion and disease prevention characteristics of the population.

Professional publications are a rich and readily accessible source of information for all nurses. In addition to nursing and public health journals, behavioral and social science literature offers diverse perspectives on community health status for specific populations and subgroups. The Internet has increased the availability and accessibility of national, state, and local health data as well. Use of web-based resources for health information requires some caution, however, as the reliability and the validity of the data are difficult to verify. Some guidelines for evaluation of Internet health resources can be found at the Health on the Net web site: www.hon.org. Additional health web sites are identified at the end of the chapter.

Data collection methods may be either qualitative or quantitative, including visual surveys that can be completed by walking through a community, participant observation, interviews, focus groups, and analysis of existing data. Potential clients and health care consumers may be asked to participate in focus groups or community forums to present their views on needed community services and programs. Formal surveys, either by mail, by telephone, or by face-to-face interviews, can be a valuable source of information not available from national databases or other secondary sources. Several drawbacks exist with this method: surveys are generally expensive to develop and time consuming to administer. In addition to the cost of such surveys, poor response rates often preclude a sufficiently representative response on which to base nursing interventions.

A **walking survey** is generally conducted by a walk-through observation of the community (Box 2-4), taking note of specific characteristics of the population, economic and social environment, transportation, health care services, and other resources. This method allows the nurse to collect subjective data and may facilitate other aspects of the assessment (Ervin, 2002).

Participant observation is another useful assessment method in which the nurse actively participates in the community to understand the community more fully and to validate observations.

Finally, as part of the assessment process, nurses working in multiethnic and multicultural groups need an in-depth assessment of culturally driven behaviors (Williams et al., 2001). Needs assessment for these groups should focus on epidemiologic data and population needs and interests.

Analysis and synthesis of data obtained during the assessment process helps to generate a comprehensive picture of the community's health status, needs, and problem areas, as well as its strengths and resources for addressing these concerns. The goal of this process is to assign priorities to community health needs and to develop a plan of action for correcting them. A comparison of community health data with state and national statistics may be useful in identification of appropriate target populations as well as interventions to improve health outcomes.

Successful community-based health initiatives involve understanding of community relationships and resources as well as participation of community leaders (Lauderdale, 2001). Failure to recognize and involve individuals, families, and communities in the process often results in failed or short-lived health interventions (Bruhn, 2001).

Comprehensive community assessment and the use of timely, high-quality data sources can help prevent poor birth outcomes and promote maternal health by identify-

BOX 2-4 Learning About the Community on Foot

I. Community Core

1. **History**—What can you glean by looking (e.g., old, established neighborhoods; new subdivision)? Ask people willing to talk: How long have you lived here? Has the area changed? As you talk, ask if there is an "old-timer" who knows the history of the area.
2. **Demographics**—What sorts of people do you see? Young? Old? Homeless? Alone? Families? What races do you see? Is the population homogeneous?
3. **Ethnicity**—Do you note indicators of different ethnic groups (e.g., restaurants, festivals)? What signs do you see of different cultural groups?
4. **Values and beliefs**—Are there churches, mosques, temples? Does it appear homogeneous? Are the lawns cared for? With flowers? Gardens? Signs of art? Culture? Heritage? Historical markers?

II. Subsystems

1. **Physical environment**—How does the community look? What do you note about air quality, flora, housing, zoning, space, green areas, animals, people, human-made structures, natural beauty, water, climate? Can you find or develop a map of the area? What is the size (e.g., square miles, blocks)?
2. **Health and social services**—Evidence of acute or chronic conditions? Shelters? "Traditional" healers (e.g., curanderos, herbalists)? Are there clinics, hospitals, practitioners' offices, public health services, home health agencies, emergency centers, nursing homes, social service facilities, mental health services? Are there resources outside the community but accessible to them?
3. **Economy**—Is it a "thriving" community or does it feel "seedy?" Are there industries, stores, places for employment? Where do people shop? Are there signs that food stamps are used/accepted? What is the unemployment rate?
4. **Transportation and safety**—How do people get around? What type of private and public transportation is available? Do you see buses, bicycles, taxis? Are there sidewalks, bike trails? Is getting around in the community possible for persons with disabilities? What types of protective services are there (e.g., fire, police, sanitation)? Is air quality monitored? What are the types of crimes committed? Do people feel safe?
5. **Politics and government**—Are there signs of political activity (e.g., posters, meetings)? What party affiliation predominates? What is the governmental jurisdiction of the community (e.g., elected mayor, city council with single member districts)? Are people involved in decision making in their local governmental unit?
6. **Communication**—Are there "common areas" where people gather? What newspapers do you see in the stands? Do people have TVs and radios? What do they watch/listen to? What are the formal and informal means of communication?
7. **Education**—Are there schools in the area? How do they look? Are there libraries? Is there a local board of education? How does it function? What is the reputation of the school(s)? What are major educational issues? What are the dropout rates? Are there extracurricular activities available? Are they used? Is there a school health service? A school nurse?
8. **Recreation**—Where do children play? What are the major forms of recreation? Who participates? What facilities for recreation do you see?

III. Perceptions

1. **The residents**—How do people feel about the community? What do they identify as its strengths? Problems? Ask several people from different groups (e.g., old, young, field worker, factory worker, professional, minister, housewife) and keep track of who gives what answer.
2. **Your perceptions**—General statements about the "health" of this community. What are its strengths? What problems or potential problems can you identify?

From Anderson, E., & McFarlane, J. (2000). *Community-as-partner: Theory and practice in nursing* (3rd ed.). Philadelphia: Lippincott Williams & Wilkins.
Note: Supplement your impressions with information from the census, police records, school statistics, chamber of commerce data, health department reports, etc., to confirm or refute your conclusions. Tables, graphs, and maps are helpful and will aid in your analysis.

ing aggregates at risk and giving direction to preventive interventions. Because women and children in at-risk communities require comprehensive services to improve health outcomes and quality of life (Oros, Perry, & Heller, 2000), the importance of the community assessment process cannot be overestimated. Often the outcomes of local and state assessments are used to determine policy and resource allocation, which directly or indirectly affect health for the most needy and vulnerable populations. Decisions related to funding of community health promotion initiatives also are linked to these data sources (Doyle & Ward, 2001).

Levels of Preventive Care

Population-based care involves prevention activities focused on target needs identified in the community assessment process. These levels of prevention provide a framework for nursing interventions. **Primary prevention** involves health promotion and disease prevention activities to decrease the occurrence of illness and enhance general health and quality of life. Sometimes referred to as "true prevention," primary prevention precedes disease or dysfunction and encourages individuals to achieve the optimal level of health possible. This includes the use of specific health protections such as recommended immunizations, infant car seats, and school health education to prevent tobacco use.

Early detection of health problems is the focus of **secondary prevention.** Persons who are asymptomatic or who have nonspecific disease symptoms are targeted to receive curative treatment and reduce disease prevalence (Marks & Wilcox, 1999). At this level, various methods of health screening and testing facilitate early treatment of the pathologic process. The goal is to shorten disease duration and severity, thus enabling an individual to return to normal function as quickly as possible (Murray et al., 2000).

Tertiary prevention follows the occurrence of a defect or disability that is permanent and irreversible (Murray et al., 2000). Persons who have developed disease are provided with treatment and rehabilitation to prevent complications and further deterioration and to maintain their optimal level of function.

Because most women are healthy during pregnancy, maternal-newborn nursing emphasizes primary and secondary prevention activities regardless of where care is provided. Tertiary prevention is frequently the focus for the ill client at home or in the hospital.

Primordial prevention, which refers to genetic modifications that prevent susceptibility to some conditions, is an emerging concept made possible through recent genetic research and the advances of the Human Genome Project (Marks & Wilcox, 1999).

Community Health Promotion

The emphasis on community-based health promotion has grown in recent years, with recognition that many health issues require the collaborative efforts of a diverse community network to achieve public health goals (Marks & Wilcox, 1999). Pender, Murdaugh, and Parsons (2002) also noted the benefits of community-based, coordinated health promotion programs with the potential for widespread change in community health status. These efforts are particularly relevant in relation to maternal-newborn health, which encompasses multiple public health issues: lack of health insurance, teen pregnancy, substance abuse, and the consequences of inadequate prenatal care.

Family systems and developmental theories provide a framework for the appropriate timing and content of health promotion activities. The nurse's role in this process is focused on collaboration with the family, identifying risk factors, and providing health information to facilitate positive health behaviors (McCarty & Mandle, 1998b). A similar approach is used in community health promotion, in which the nurse collaborates with an interdisciplinary team to identify health concerns and risk factors and contributes to the planning and implementation of community health promotion programs (McCarty & Mandle, 1998a). Throughout this process, the nurse must be aware of the continuous interactions and influences between individuals, the family, and the larger community that is the context for maternal and child health (Patterson, 1998).

Health promotion efforts for childbearing families are primarily focused on early intervention through prenatal care and prevention of complications during the perinatal period. Often this early exposure to health information sets the stage for a successful birth and positive outcomes for mother and baby. Involving expectant mothers and fathers in identification of their learning needs is an essential first step to securing their participation in the health promotion process.

A wide variety of strategies have been used to disseminate heath information to women in the community. Some are more successful than others. Prenatal classes are a well-established mechanism for increasing awareness of healthy behaviors during pregnancy and preparing parents for the care of themselves and their newborn during the postpartum period. Mass media efforts such as those presented by the March of Dimes "Baby Your Baby" advertisements are clear, consumer-friendly messages designed to reach a large target audience. Other venues include public health education in newspapers and magazines, and health department programs such as the Special Supplemental Program for Women, Infants, and Children (WIC), which offers a variety of health education and written information to mothers.

Many communities have organized coalitions to address specific health promotion agendas related to sharing information, educating community members, or advocating for health policies around maternal and child health issues. An example of this is Healthy Start, a community-based initiative to reduce infant mortality and improve the health and well-being of women, children, and families (Goldman & DeLaCruz, 1999). Adolescent health is another broad target area for community health promotion efforts, including both health education and policy initiatives. Issues related to adolescent sexuality, teen pregnancy, and substance abuse are particularly problematic, requiring aggressive prevention programs and community outreach (Maehr & Felice, 1999).

Community-based health promotion for childbearing families is often a challenge, because those who are most in need are less able to access such services. For example, low-income, uneducated, or homeless women, who frequently delay seeking prenatal care, also are disenfranchised in relation to other health promotion activities. Failure to address these social and environmental barriers and inability to engage the target audience often limits the benefits and sustainability of health promotion initiatives (Bruhn, 2001). Efforts should thus be focused on increasing awareness of health promotion activities as well as ensuring access for all community groups.

PERINATAL CONTINUUM OF CARE

Within the community, perinatal care is provided on a continuum. A continuum of care is defined as a range of clinical services provided for an individual or group that reflects care given during a single hospitalization or care for multiple conditions over a lifetime. Home care is one delivery component available along the perinatal continuum of care (Fig. 2-5). This continuum begins with family planning and continues with preconception care, prenatal care, intrapartum care, postpartum care, newborn care, interconception care, and infant care until the infant is 1 year old. Independent self-care, ambulatory care, home care, low risk hospitalization, or specialized intensive care may be appropriate at different points along this continuum. Home perinatal care is the focus of the following section.

Current Trends and Historical Perspectives

A priority for future decades will be the development of innovative, cost-effective methods of health care delivery. Large health care organizations are developing clinically integrated health care delivery networks. The goals of clinical integration are improved coordination of care and care outcomes; better communication among health care providers; increased client, payer, and provider satisfaction; and reduced cost. With clinical integration, the focus changes from illness to health, from the individual to the population, and from care provided in one setting to care across the continuum (Kastens, 1998). The following factors make home care an important area in perinatal services:

- Interest in family birthing alternatives
- Shortened hospital stays
- New technologies that allow sophisticated assessments and treatments to be performed in the home
- Reimbursement by third-party payers

Modern home care nursing has its foundation in public health nursing, which provided comprehensive care to sick and well clients in their own homes. Specialized maternity home care nursing services began in the 1980s when public health maternity nursing services were limited and services had not kept pace with the changing practices of high risk obstetrics and emerging technology. Lengthy antepartal hospitalizations for such conditions as preterm labor and pregnancy-induced hypertension created nursing care challenges for staff members of inpatient units. Many women expressed their concern for the negative effect of antepartal hospitalizations on the family. Although clinical indications showed that a new nursing care approach was needed, home health care did not become a viable alternative until third-party payers (i.e., public or private organizations or employer groups that pay for health care) pushed for cost containment in maternity services.

Antepartal home care that prolongs gestation and reduces neonatal intensive care hospitalization is cost-effective. Even home infusion services at a cost of $225 to $325 per day provide a substantial saving over an average ($1500 per day) hospitalization (Monical, 1998).

Communication to Bridge the Continuum

As maternity care continues to consist of frequent and brief contacts with health care providers throughout the prenatal and postpartum periods, services that link maternity clients throughout the perinatal continuum of care, including critical pathways, telephonic nursing assessments, discharge planning, specialized education programs, parent support groups, home visiting programs, nurse advice lines, and perinatal home care have assumed increasing importance. Some hospitals provide cross-training for hospital-based nurses to make postpartum home visits or to staff outpatient centers for postpartum follow-up.

Telephonic Nursing Care

Telephonic nursing care through services such as "warm lines," nurse advice lines, and telephonic nursing assessments is a valuable means of managing health care problems and bridging the gaps among acute, outpatient, and home care services. Some providers are using the Internet to communicate with clients who have an Internet service provider (ISP). Nursing care that occurs by telephone is

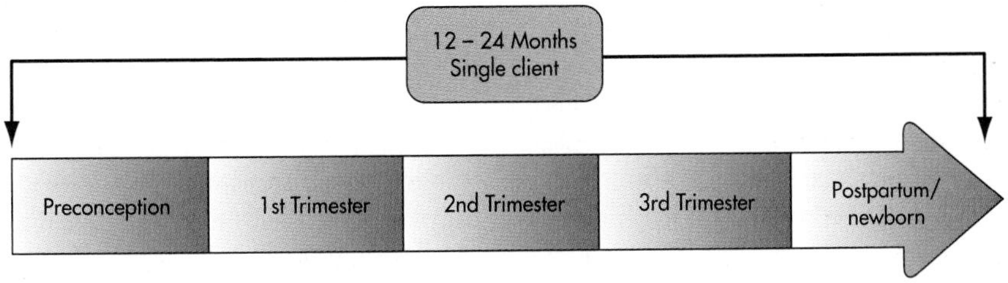
12 - 24 Months
Single client
Preconception
1st Trimester
2nd Trimester
3rd Trimester
Postpartum/
newborn

FIG. 2-5 Perinatal continuum of care.

interactive and responsive to immediate health care questions about particular health care needs. **Warm lines** are telephone lines that are offered as a community service to provide new parents with support, encouragement, and basic parenting education. Nurse advice lines, or toll-free nurse consultation services, often are supported by third-party payers or health management organization/managed care organization (HMO/MCO) nurse case managers and are designed to provide answers to medical questions. These nurses are prepared to guide callers through urgent health care situations, suggest treatment options, and provide health education (Bleich, 1998). Telephonic nursing assessments, or nurse consultation, assessment, and health education that take place during a telephone conversation, can be added to the plan of care in conjunction with skilled nursing visits or may be a separate nursing contact for the woman. Telephonic nursing assessments are commonly used after a postpartum home care visit to reassess a woman's knowledge about the signs and symptoms of adequate hydration in breastfeeding, or, after initiating home phototherapy, to assess the caregiver's knowledge regarding problems with equipment.

Guidelines for Nursing Practice

The Association of Women's Health, Obstetric, and Neonatal Nurses (AWHONN, 1998) defined home care as the provision of technical, psychologic, and other therapeutic support in the client's home rather than in an institution. The scope of nursing care delivered in the home is necessarily limited to practices deemed safe and appropriate to be carried out in an environment that is physically separated from a health care institution and its resources. Nursing practice at home is consistent with federal and state regulations that direct home care practice. The nurse demonstrates practice competence through formalized orientation and ongoing clinical education and performance evaluation in the respective home care agency. Standards for practice from key specialty organizations such as AWHONN, the American College of Obstetricians and Gynecologists (ACOG), the American Academy of Pediatrics (AAP), and the Intravenous Nursing Society (INS) provide the basis for clinical protocols and pathways and organizational programs in home care practice. The Joint Commission on Accreditation of Health Care Organizations (JCAHO) provides criteria for home care operations based on Centers for Medicare and Medicaid Services (formerly HCFA) regulations.

AWHONN (1994) developed standards of practice and identified essential knowledge and skills to provide safe perinatal home care. Health care agencies and individuals can use these to assess the nurse's skills and learning needs.

A wide range of professional health care services and products can be delivered or used in the home with technology and telecommunication. For example, telehealth and telemedicine make it possible for clients in the home to be interviewed and assessed by a specialist located hundreds of miles away. Some view home health care as an extension of in-hospital care. Essentially, the primary difference between health care in a hospital and home care is the absence of the continuous presence of professional health care providers in a client's home. Generally, but not always, home health care entails intermittent care by a professional who visits the client's home for a particular reason and/or provides care on site for fewer than 4 hours at a time. The home health care agency maintains on-call professional staff to assist home care clients who have questions about their care and for emergencies, such as equipment failure.

Perinatal Services

Home care perinatal services may be provided by hospital-based programs, independent proprietary (for-profit) agencies or nonprofit home care agencies, and official or tax-supported agencies. Innovative programs may be supported by research grants for a period of years, but ultimately they must be sponsored by an agency with long-term funding. Home visits have both advantages and disadvantages. The pregnant woman is able to maintain bed rest if indicated, and vulnerable neonates are not exposed to the weather or external sources of infection. The nurse can observe and interact with family members in their most natural and secure environment. Adequacy of resources and safety factors can be assessed. Teaching can be tailored to the actual home conditions, and other family members can be included. A home visit is less expensive than a day's hospitalization, but a 60- to 90-minute visit requires 2.5 to 3 hours of nursing time, including travel and documentation. Travel time may be even greater when a client resides in a rural area because of distance, travel, and weather-related factors (Bosch & Bushy, 1997). It is more cost effective for the health care provider to see clients in an office, where professional time is not spent in travel. Availability of nurses with expertise in maternity care may be limited, and concerns about the nurse's physical safety in some communities may limit visits.

Visits for outreach and health promotion are an integral part of community (or public) health nursing. In countries with national health systems, a nurse or midwife may see all women during pregnancy and after birth. In the United States, visits of this sort have been provided mainly to low-income families without health insurance and Medicaid recipients who use the clinics provided by local health departments (Koniak-Griffin et al., 1999; Olds et al., 1997). Until recently, private insurers did not reimburse for health promotion visits. MCOs now recognize that anticipatory guidance can be cost-effective, but home visitation programs for the most part still target specific high risk populations, such as adolescents and women at risk for preterm labor.

Home care agencies are subject to regulation by governmental and professional organizations and provide interdisciplinary services including social work, nutrition, and occupational and physical therapy. Increasingly their case loads are made up of clients who require high-technology care, such as infusions or home monitoring. Although the home health nurse develops the care plan, all care must be ordered by a physician. Additionally, interventions must meet the insurer's criteria for reimbursement, and services are limited to registered clients. Preconception care and low risk antepartum care can usually be provided more efficiently in offices and are not currently reimbursable. High risk antepartum care is often provided by home care agencies; for example, women with hyperemesis gravidarum who require parenteral nutrition may be treated at home. Conditions requiring bed rest, such as preterm labor and hypertension, are other common indications for home care. Other conditions may include cardiac disease, substance abuse, and diabetes in pregnancy.

Some insurers reimburse for at least one postpartum visit to families after early discharge or in the presence of high risk factors. Home phototherapy is used for treatment of neonatal hyperbilirubinemia and to avoid separation of mother and infant. Many other neonates who require long-term high-technology care also are managed with home care. The American Academy of Pediatrics (1998) recommends home visits as an effective early intervention strategy to improve child health in families at risk.

Client Selection and Referral

The office- or hospital-based nurse is often the key person in making effective referrals to home care. When considering a referral to home care, the following factors are evaluated:

- Health status of mother and fetus or infant: Is condition serious enough to warrant home care, and is it stable enough for intermittent observation to be sufficient?
- Availability of professionals to provide the needed services within the client's community
- Family resources, including psychosocial, social, and economic resources: Will the family be able to provide care between nursing visits? Are relationships supportive? Is third-party reimbursement available, or can it be negotiated with the insurer? Could a voluntary or tax-supported community agency provide needed care without payment?
- Cost-effectiveness: Is it more reasonable for the client to receive these services at home or to go to a local outpatient facility to receive them?

Community referrals should not be limited to women with physiologic complications of pregnancy that require medical treatment. Clients at risk (e.g., young adolescents, families with a history of abuse, members of vulnerable population groups, developmentally disabled individuals) may need follow-up care at home. In consultation with the social worker, the hospital-based nurse should become familiar with agencies in the community that accept such referrals. When the client lives in a rural area, hospital-based nurses should familiarize themselves with available formal and informal resources in that community, as these may be different from those in a more populated setting (Bushy, 2000)

Standardized referral forms simplify the referral process and ensure that all needed information will be forwarded to the home health agency. The nursing assessment should include the woman's physical and psychologic status, her level of knowledge about self-care activities, her willingness to learn, the availability of caregivers and social support in the home, and her level of comfort with home care. If the referral is for a mother and infant home care visit, the nursing assessment should include newborn data.

High-technology home care requires additional information to be collected from the chart and consultation with the referring physician and other members of the health care team before making a home care referral. These additional data include the medical diagnosis, medical prognosis, prescribed therapies, medication history, drug-dosing information, potential ancillary supplies, type of infusion access device, and the available systems of social support for the client and family. The nursing assessment and therapies data provide baseline information for the home care nurse and other types of health care providers involved in the care plan.

Whenever a referral is called in to a home health care agency, a member of the nursing or admission staff determines the agency's ability to accept the client for service. The use of telecommunication such as fax machines, cellular phones, and the internet to transmit information has eliminated delays in initiating home care services, even in more remote rural areas.

Preparing for the Home Visit

The home care nurse reviews the available clinical data, demographic information, and completed plan of care form and consults with the home care pharmacist or other health care team members who have previously contacted the woman to determine the goals of the visit. At this point, the nurse uses the medical diagnosis and place on the perinatal continuum as a starting point to organize the woman's care. The nurse reviews agency policies and procedures, professional literature about diagnosis, and community resources as part of the previsit preparation work (Box 2-5).

Before going on a home visit, the nurse contacts the woman to make necessary arrangements and obtain detailed instructions on the location of the home. Contact by telephone has several goals besides establishing a convenient time to visit and exact directions; it also sets the stage for the first home care visit.

The nurse identifies himself or herself by name, title, and agency. He or she then explains who referred the woman to the agency for home care and the purpose of the home care visits. The nurse briefly explains what will

BOX 2-5 **Protocol for Perinatal Home Visits**

PREVISIT INTERVENTIONS

1. Contact family to arrange details for home visit.
   a. Identify self, credentials, and agency role.
   b. Review purpose of home visit follow-up.
   c. Schedule convenient time for visit.
   d. Confirm address and route to family home.
2. Review and clarify appropriate data.
   a. All available assessment data for mother and fetus or infant (i.e., referral forms, hospital discharge summaries, family identified learning needs).
   b. Review records of any previous nursing contacts.
   c. Contact other professional caregivers as necessary to clarify data (i.e., obstetrician, nurse-midwife, pediatrician, referring nurse).
3. Identify community resources and teaching materials appropriate to meet needs already identified.
4. Plan the visit, and prepare bag with equipment, supplies, and materials necessary for assessments of mother and fetus or infant, actual care anticipated, and teaching.

IN-HOME INTERVENTIONS: ESTABLISHING A RELATIONSHIP

1. Reintroduce self and establish purpose of visit for mother, infant, and family; offer family opportunity to clarify their expectations of contact.
2. Spend brief time socially interacting with family to become acquainted and establish trusting relationship.

IN-HOME INTERVENTIONS: WORKING WITH FAMILY

1. Conduct systematic assessment of mother and fetus or newborn to determine physiologic adjustment and any existing complications.
2. Throughout visit, collect data to assess the emotional adjustment of individual family members to pregnancy or birth and lifestyle changes. Note evidence of family-newborn bonding and sibling rivalry; note relationships among mother, father, children, and grandparents.
3. Determine adequacy of support system.
   a. To what extent does someone help with cooking, cleaning, and other home management tasks?
   b. To what extent is help being provided in caring for the newborn and any other children?
   c. Are support persons encouraging the new mother to care for herself and get adequate rest?
   d. Who is providing helpful information? Emotional support?
4. Throughout the visit, observe home environment for adequacy of resources:
   a. Space: privacy, safe play of children, sleeping.
   b. Overall cleanliness and state of repair.
   c. Number of steps pregnant woman/new mother must climb.
   d. Adequacy of cooking arrangements.
   e. Adequacy of refrigeration and other food storage areas.
   f. Adequacy of bathing, toilet, and laundry facilities.
   g. Arrangements in home for newborn: sleeping, bathing, formula preparation (if needed), layette items, and diapers.
5. Throughout the visit, observe home environment for overall state of repair and existence of safety hazards:
   a. Storage of medications, household cleaners, and other substances hazardous to children.
   b. Presence of peeling paint on furniture, walls, or pipes.
   c. Factors that contribute to falls, such as dim lighting, broken steps, scatter rugs.
   d. Presence of vermin.
   e. Use of crib or playpen that fails to meet safety guidelines.
   f. Existence of emergency plan in case of fire; fire alarm or extinguisher.
6. Provide care to mother, newborn, or both as prescribed by their respective primary care provider or in accord with agency protocol.
7. Provide teaching on basis of previously identified needs.
8. Refer family to appropriate community agencies or resources, such as warm lines and support groups.
9. Ascertain that woman knows potential problems to watch for and who to call if they occur.
10. Ensure that used disposable items have been handled appropriately and that reusable items are cleaned and repacked appropriately in the nurse's bag.

IN-HOME INTERVENTIONS: ENDING THE VISIT

1. Summarize the activities and main points of the visit.
2. Clarify future expectations, including schedule of next visit.
3. Review teaching plan and provide major points in writing.
4. Provide information about reaching the nurse or agency if needed before the next scheduled visit.

POSTVISIT INTERVENTIONS

1. Document the visit thoroughly, using the necessary agency forms to serve as a legal record of the visit and to allow third-party reimbursement, as possible.
2. Initiate the plan of care on which the next encounter with the woman/family will be based.
3. Communicate appropriately (by telephone, letter, progress notes, or referral form) with primary care provider, other health professionals, or referral agencies on behalf of woman/family.

occur during the visit and approximately how long the visit will last. The woman should be asked to restrain any pets during the visit. Last, the nurse asks about health supplies that may be needed for the woman's care.

Before the first visit, the home care nurse collects the woman's clinical record, client education materials, medical supplies, and equipment necessary for the visit. Medications and specialized equipment should be ordered before the visit and delivered at the time of the scheduled visit.

CARE MANAGEMENT

First Home Care Visit

Making the first home care visit can be stressful for the nurse and the woman. The home care nurse is faced with an unknown environment controlled by the woman and her family. The woman and her family also experience feelings about the unknown, such as anxiety about the way the nurse will treat them or what the nurse will do during the visit. The challenge for the home care nurse is to establish a nurse-client relationship and provide the prescribed home care services within the time provided for the initial home visit. One of the most important roles of the home care nurse is modeling health-related behaviors for the client and others who are in the home during the visit.

Introductions generally begin the visit; the nurse identifies himself or herself and the home care agency. The woman introduces herself and the other family members who are present. Sometimes the woman may feel uncertain of her role or be uncomfortable in taking the lead in introductions, so other people in the home may not be introduced to the nurse. In these situations, the nurse can politely ask about other people in the home and their relationship to the woman.

In the first visit to the home, the home care nurse completes extensive documentation with the client (Fig. 2-6). Before performing any services, the nurse must obtain written agreement and consent for the home health care services. This consent-for-care serves two major purposes: agreement for care and authorization to release medical information. Many third-party payers require written documentation of the services provided; therefore the agency obtains authorization from the woman to give information to her physician and any individual or company involved in payment for the services. Agencies that bill third-party payers for the rendered services will include agreement language for assignment of benefits and financial remuneration. By agreeing to assign insurance benefits to the agency, the woman allows her insurance company to pay the home health care agency directly.

All clients have the right to participate actively in their plan of care. These client rights and responsibilities should begin the discussion about the nurse and client roles during this initial visit.

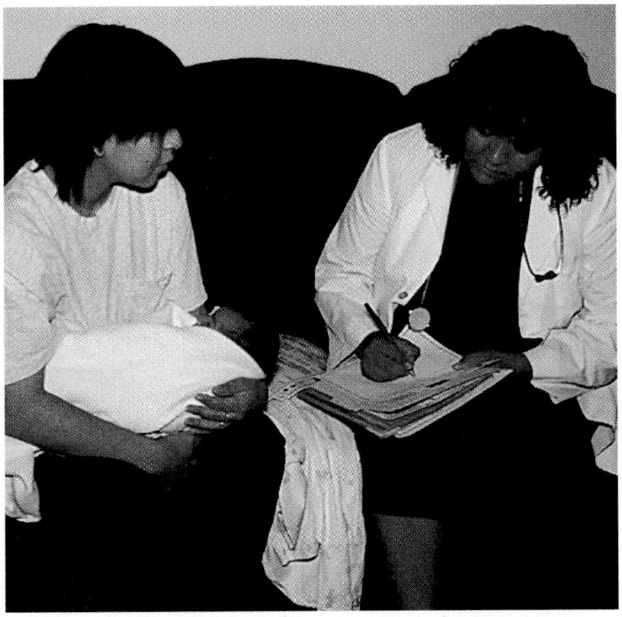

FIG. 2-6 Home care nurse visits with woman and her infant. (Courtesy Michael S. Clement, MD, Mesa, AZ.)

Assessment and Nursing Diagnoses

The primary goals of the assessment phase are to develop a trusting relationship and collect data by various methods to obtain a comprehensive client profile. It may not be feasible or appropriate to collect in-depth information about all areas of assessment during the first visit. In many instances, however, the nurse may be limited to one visit and must obtain information pertinent to the current situation in that hour.

The establishment of a trusting relationship begins with the previsit telephone call. An interview style that reflects sensitivity; a nonjudgmental, accepting attitude; and respect for the woman's rights facilitates the development of that trusting relationship. A skillful interviewer avoids barriers to communication such as false reassurance, advice giving, excessive talking, and the showing of approval or disapproval. This nurse-client relationship continues to develop over the course of home visits.

The nurse is a guest in the woman's home and should show respect for her and her belongings. Some adaptation of the home visit schedule may be made if numerous distractions interrupt a visit, such as caring for the needs of small children. The nurse may ask to have the volume of the television reduced or suggest moving to another room where it is more quiet and private.

The major areas of the assessment are demographics, medical history, general health history, medication history, sociocultural assessment, home and community environment, and physical assessment. Some of this information can be obtained from client records sent to the home care agency at the time of referral or from the previsit interview. These data will be used to develop the nursing care plan and complete the plan of care, which is required for many licensed home health care agencies. Two areas requiring further discussion are the social assessment and the home environment assessment.

Social assessment includes information regarding the number in the family and the roles of each household member, which family members or individuals have taken on the roles of caregivers, and the woman's social support network (Box 2-6). Identifying the roles of each member is helpful for developing the plan of care.

Physical assessment of the home environment is an essential element of the home care assessment. The major areas of the home environment assessment include physical features of the home, access to the home, sanitary conditions, the presence of utilities (for example, indoor plumbing, telephone, electricity), safety features, and access to transportation and emergency support. Although some of this information can be collected during an interview, physically inspecting many areas of the home essential to care is a critical part of developing an accurate nursing plan of care. Before any physical inspection, the home care nurse should ask the woman or the caregiver for permission and assistance in identifying areas in the home that will be involved in the caregiving activities. During the physical inspection, careful consideration should be taken to avoid moving personal belongings that are not affected by the care.

Each plan of care has a different emphasis in the home environment. For example, women receiving infusion therapy for hyperemesis gravidarum need a safe place to store medications and infusion supplies that are out of reach of small children living in the home. The home care nurse should incorporate the agency policies and procedures for the storage and handling of infusion supplies into her walk-through inspection. During the walk through, the home care nurse looks at the potential storage areas that are dry, that are clean, and where the temperature can be maintained. The home care nurse should include an inspection of the work areas, such as countertops, tabletops, sinks, and trash areas, that the woman or caregiver may use for mixing medications, changing infusion tubing, handling supplies, or disposing of used equipment and supplies.

The homes of clients using electronic home health care equipment, such as phototherapy equipment or infusion pumps, require physical inspection of electrical outlets, electrical cords, and extension cords that will be used. Homes with faulty electrical wiring may place the client at risk for being involved in an electrical fire; faulty wiring may require inspection and repair by a professional electrician before electronic devices are used. Findings from the assessment are incorporated into the plan of care.

Nursing diagnoses are derived from the data collected at the first home visit. Nursing diagnoses for perinatal home health care clients include the following:

- *Deficient knowledge related to*
  - –management of therapeutic regimen (e.g., nausea and vomiting, preterm labor, gestational diabetes)
  - –newborn care and feeding
- *Compromised family coping related to*
  - –lack of child care while mother is on bed rest
  - –care of newborn receiving oxygen therapy
- *Impaired parenting related to*
  - –maternal immaturity and lack of family support
- *Deficient diversional activity related to*
  - –prolonged bed rest

BOX 2-6 **Psychosocial Assessment**

LANGUAGE
Identify the primary language spoken in the home
Assess whether there are any language barriers to receiving support

COMMUNITY RESOURCES/ACCESS TO CARE
Identify primary and secondary means of transportation
Identify community agencies family currently uses for health care and support
Assess cultural and psychosocial barriers to receiving care

SOCIAL SUPPORT
Determine the people living with the pregnant woman
Identify who assists with household chores
Identify who assists with child care/parenting activities
Identify who the pregnant woman turns to for problems or during a crisis

INTERPERSONAL RELATIONSHIP
Identify the way decisions are made in the family
Identify the family's perception of the need for home care
Identify roles of adults in caring for family members

CAREGIVER
Identify the primary caregiver for home care treatments
Identify other caregivers and their roles
Assess the caregiver's knowledge of treatments and care process
Identify potential strain from the caregiver role
Identify the level of satisfaction with the caregiver role

STRESS AND COPING
Identify what the woman perceives as lifestyle changes and their impact on her and her family
Identify the changes she and her family have made to adjust to her health condition and home health care treatments

Expected Outcomes of Care

Examples of expected outcomes for perinatal clients include that the woman/family will do the following:

- Verbalize understanding of treatments.
- Report decreased anxiety about performing procedures (e.g., blood glucose monitoring).
- Use support systems to cope effectively with problems (e.g., pregnancy complications, newborn complications or treatments).
- Perform procedures accurately, as evidenced by return demonstration.
- Verbalize decreased role strain.

Plan of Care and Interventions

The nursing plan of care is developed in collaboration with the client, based on the health care needs of the individual. Home care nurses working in home health care agencies regulated by the Centers for Medicare & Medicaid Services use a plan of care that includes client demographics, the health care provider's orders, home care goals, and the level of functioning. This document is initiated at the time of referral to the home care agency and must be updated every 60 days or as specified by state regulations.

The frequency of the skilled nursing visit may vary with the individual plan of care and reimbursement criteria established by the third-party payers.

Nurse safety and infection control are two important aspects specific to home care.

Safety Issues for the Home Care Nurse

The nurse should be fully aware of the home environment and neighborhood in which the home care is being provided. Unlike hospitals, in which the environment is more predictable and controlled, the client's neighborhood and home have the potential for uncertainty. Home care nurses should take necessary safety precautions and avoid dangerous areas.

Agencies that serve clients in high crime areas may conduct a violence potential assessment by telephone before the visit and enlist the client's cooperation in minimizing risk. Others have hired full-time security personnel to accompany nurses on their visits. Personal strategies recommended for nurses visiting families with a history of violence or substance abuse include (1) self-awareness; (2) environmental assessment; (3) using listening and observation skills with clients to be aware of behavioral changes indicating aggression or lack of impulse control; (4) planning for dealing with aggressive behavior (i.e., allowing personal space and taking a nonaggressive stance); (5) making visits in pairs; and (6) having access to a cellular phone at all times.

Personal Safety

The home care nurse must be aware of personal safety behaviors before going on a home visit. Dress should be casual but professional in appearance, with a name identification tag. Limited jewelry should be worn. Valuable personal items, such as an expensive purse or coat, should not be worn on a visit. Carrying an extra set of car keys in the nursing home care bag saves time and frustration if the nurse becomes locked out of the automobile. Automobile keys spread between the fingers with sharp ends outward can be used as a weapon if necessary. The same commonsense behaviors and precautions that guide a person's behavior when alone in any setting should be followed by home care nurses.

The agency should have a copy of the nurse's home care itinerary, including contact telephone numbers if a client does not have a telephone and information on the nurse's car (make, model, color, and license plate number). Many home care nurses carry agency-provided pagers or cellular telephones that allow the agency to contact the nurse throughout the day to give information about client updates, changes in orders or services, schedule changes, and new clients who require an initial visit. The telephone also is useful to notify clients when the nurse is delayed.

The automobile used for the home care visits, whether a personal or an agency-owned vehicle, should have regular preventive maintenance checks, an adequate fuel level, and road safety items stored in the trunk. Items to carry in the vehicle include change for telephone calls and tolls, maps, emergency telephone numbers, a flashlight, a first aid kit, flares, a blanket, and equipment for inclement weather conditions. When making a visit to a client in a more remote rural setting, other travel considerations may be needed, as well as taking additional supplies or medication to the client (Bosch & Bushy, 1997).

Home care nurses should park and lock their cars in a safe place that is visible from the street and the client's home and away from hidden alleys. While driving to the client's home, the nurse should assess the neighborhood for safety, especially if the neighborhood is unfamiliar. All valuable items should be stored out of sight before leaving the office. While walking to the client's home, nurses should not walk near groups of strangers hanging out in doorways or alleys, enter into vacant buildings, or enter a yard that has an unrestrained dog. The home or building should not be entered if the nurse has any safety concerns. All home care agencies should have policies to follow for such situations.

Client's Home

Once inside the woman's home, the nurse may encounter unsafe situations such as the presence of weapons, abusive behavior, or health hazards. Each potentially hazardous situation must be dealt with according to agency policies and procedures. If abuse or neglect is reasonably suspected, the home care nurse should follow home care agency and state and federal regulations for reporting and documenting the situation. Nurses should maintain their own safety first and act accordingly throughout the visit.

Infection Control

The nurse carries the necessary supplies and equipment to provide nursing care to the woman. Home care bags should contain infection control supplies, such as personal protection equipment; disposable nonsterile, sterile, and utility gloves; disinfectants; disposable cardiopulmonary resuscitation (CPR) masks; gowns; shoe covers; caps; leak-proof and puncture-resistant specimen containers; sharps container; dry hand disinfectants; and leak-proof barriers. Proper infection control techniques should be used in stocking, storing, handling, and transporting this bag. When a procedure is to be performed, the nurse should set up a clean area for necessary supplies. A "dirty" area is designated with a trash bag for the collection of soiled equipment and supplies. Hands are washed before all supplies and equipment for the visit are removed from the bag and placed in a clean area.

The importance of infection control does not diminish because nursing care is provided in the client's home rather than in a hospital. Clients are not likely to become infected because of their home environment, but the nurse may become exposed to an infectious disease.

The CDC has recommended Standard Precaution guidelines for the protection of health care workers from blood-borne pathogens. These guidelines recommend that Standard Precautions be used whenever a treatment is performed because it is difficult to determine which clients have a communicable disease (see Box 8-4).

Handwashing remains the single most important infection-control procedure, and the caregiver is in a position to educate about the importance of this practice in preventing disease. Hands should be washed before and after each client contact. Wearing gloves does not eliminate the necessity for handwashing. If running water or clean facilities are unavailable, the hands can be cleaned with a self-drying antiseptic solution.

Using gloves reduces the incidence of exposure to blood-borne pathogens. Gloves should be selected according to the nursing activity to be performed. Nonsterile latex or vinyl gloves should be worn with each procedure that has the potential for contact with bodily substances (e.g., performing venipunctures, heel sticks on the newborn, and perineal care). Sterile gloves should be worn with clinical procedures requiring sterile technique, such as insertion of peripherally inserted central lines and certain dressing changes. General purpose utility gloves should be used for housekeeping activities, such as cleaning equipment or spills. Nonsterile and sterile gloves should be discarded after each use in a leak-resistant waste receptacle. Utility gloves may be disinfected and reused.

Disposable personal protection equipment should be removed after each use and discarded in a plastic trash container. Safety glasses or goggles can be cleaned with soap and water after each use.

Whenever specimens are collected, Standard Precautions should be used. Any specimen of bodily fluids should be placed in a leak-proof bag and secured in a puncture-proof container. The outside of the container is washed off, if it was soiled, before transporting it. Specimens should be labeled with the woman's name and additional identifying information according to the home health care agency or laboratory policies. If specimens are being transported, they should be placed in a container on a flat surface in the vehicle. An insulated container may be used to keep specimens cool in transit. The nurse should be aware of the time-sensitive laboratory procedures for certain types of specimens.

Sharps containers are puncture-proof and leak-proof containers labeled with a biohazard sign on the outside and should be used to collect needles and sharp objects. Clients are instructed to fill containers between two-thirds and three-fourths full to prevent spillage of their contents. As part of the client teaching process, information about storage and handling is covered by the home care nurse. When the container reaches its maximal capacity, it should be returned to the home health care agency and replaced. Medical waste, such as urine and secretions, can be discarded through the sewer or septic system.

Contaminated dressings and disposable supplies should be placed in a leak-proof plastic bag and securely fastened for disposal at the client's home. The client should be instructed regarding the proper disposal of medical waste in the home. Agency policies and procedures and local waste management ordinances should be consulted before the client is instructed.

Nursing Considerations

In home care, the woman or family members are responsible for administration of medications in the absence of the nurse. A careful medication history should be obtained to see if the woman is taking her medications correctly and understands the desired action and potential side effects. Sometimes when orders are changed, women continue to take both the old and new prescriptions, which can lead to dangerous overdoses or medication interactions. The culturally competent nurse ensures that there is an adequate supply and a safe place for proper storage of medications to prevent deterioration or accidental ingestion by children or pets. The nurse inquires about any other medications that the woman might be taking concurrently. Over-the-counter drugs or herbal supplements may not be considered medications by the women and not mentioned unless such information is specifically asked for. Even more important is ensuring that the client and her caregivers fully understand the information that they are exposed to by health care providers.

High-technology home care involves many diagnostic and therapeutic procedures. A focused physical assessment is always part of the visit. Nurses involved in perinatal home care must be skilled in prenatal, postpartal, and newborn assessment. Many women require additional diagnostic tests. The nurse may need to collect blood or other specimens. Portable fetal monitoring equipment or even ultrasound can be used in the home for fetal assessment. Home infusion for women with hyperemesis gravidarum often replaces hospitalization. Women with preterm labor may receive parenteral tocolytic therapy. Phototherapy or apnea monitors can be provided in the home for newborns. The power supply and wiring must be reliable. Family members may need to be taught to monitor equipment between nurse visits and to prevent accidental damage.

Medical emergencies may occur during or between the nurse's visits to the home. Prior planning and education can reduce the risk of problems. All parents of newborns should know infant CPR. There should be immediate telephone access to call for emergency medical assistance. Women and their families should be taught to recognize danger signs related to their condition. For example, women at risk for preterm labor should learn to palpate the uterus and recognize contractions in the absence of pain; women with diabetes must learn the signs of hypoglycemia and what to do if it occurs; women with preeclampsia must know the danger signs that indicate worsening of their condition and notify the health care provider immediately. In a more remote rural community that does not have an obstetrician in the region, the nurse may need to assist the client's family to arrange for "boarding" somewhere that is closer to a medical specialist.

Client and family education in home care includes information about the specific high risk condition(s) involved, implications for pregnancy outcome, and measures for self-monitoring. Verbal explanations should be supplemented with clearly written instructions. General information to promote well-being, such as about nutrition and common discomforts of pregnancy, also should be included. The need for preparation for childbirth can be addressed by using books or videos and supplemented by individual teaching at home. Coping with bed rest or other limitation of activity is a problem for many women with high risk pregnancies. The nurse may share strategies that others have used, help with time management, and provide information about support services. Teaching about infant care or the special needs of the preterm infant may be appropriate during the prenatal period.

Clear documentation of assessments, problems identified, treatments and interventions performed, and the client's responses is essential. Third-party payers base reimbursement on the nurse's written record of providing skilled nursing care and assessments that support the woman's continuing need for those services. The nurse must promptly inform the health care provider by telephone or facsimile of any significant changes. When new orders are transmitted by telephone, a written copy must be sent for the physician's signature.

The home care nurse continually reassesses the client's condition and response to the interventions during every home visit and revises the nursing diagnoses and plan of care. Nursing documentation should reflect an objective description of the nursing assessment data collected at each visit. Statements such as "no change" or "same as last visit" do not accurately reflect the monitoring of the client condition that occurred during the skilled nursing visit. Once the home care outcomes are achieved and the client is discharged from the home care agency, documentation should include information about the client's status at the time of discharge, progress toward attaining health care goals, and plans for follow-up care.

The role of the clinical record in home care has been affected by social, economic, and legal health care changes. Appropriate care should be taken to complete the necessary home health care records accurately and in a timely manner. Documentation guidelines include writing or dictating notes or using a laptop computer at the client's home or shortly after the visit.

Evaluation

Evaluation is based on the expected outcomes of care. The plan is revised as necessary.

KEY POINTS

- Contemporary American society recognizes and accepts a variety of family forms.
- The family is a social network that acts as an important support system for its members.
- Ideally, the family provides a safe, intimate environment for the biopsychosocial development of its children and adult members.
- Family theories provide nurses with useful guidelines for understanding family function.
- Family socioeconomics, response to stress, and culture are key factors influencing family health.
- The reproductive beliefs and practices of a culture are embedded in its economic, religious, kinship, and political structures.
- To provide quality care to women in their childbearing years and beyond, nurses should be aware of the cultural beliefs and practices important to individual families.
- A community is defined as a locality-based entity composed of systems of societal institutions, informal groups, and aggregates that are interdependent and whose function is to meet a wide variety of collective needs.
- Of necessity, most changes aimed at improving community health involve partnerships among community residents and health workers.
- Methods of collecting data useful to the nurse working in the community include walking surveys, analysis of existing data, informant interviews, and participant observation.

KEY POINTS—cont'd

- Vulnerable populations are groups who are at higher risk for developing physical, mental, or social health problems.
- Perinatal home care is a unique nursing practice that incorporates knowledge from community health nursing, acute care nursing, family therapy, health promotion, and client education.
- Social and economic factors affect the scope of perinatal nursing practice.
- Perinatal home care can be provided for women and infants throughout the perinatal period, beginning before conception and ending in the postpartum period.
- Perinatal home care nurses should incorporate personal safety and infection control practices in the nursing plan of care.
- Telephonic nurse advice lines, telephonic nursing assessments, and warm lines are low-cost health care services that facilitate continuous client education, support, and health care decision making, even though health care is delivered in multiple sites.
- Communication protocols among members of the home health care team are critical to diminish fragmentation and duplication of health care services.

CRITICAL THINKING EXERCISES

1. Read your local newspaper and identify articles illustrating community partnerships to meet health needs of vulnerable populations. Were these needs identified by providers or consumers? What needs are unmet?
2. Prepare education materials that could be used for teaching clients self-care for preterm labor. Describe the difference between hospital teaching and home care teaching. What follow-up is necessary?
3. The home care nurse receives a referral for home visits to a 14-year-old mother with a wound infection after cesarean birth. The new mother and her healthy preterm infant are living with the maternal grandmother in a one-bedroom apartment.
   a. What additional information is needed to develop the plan of care?
   b. How might wound care in the home differ from hospital practice?
   c. What health teaching should be provided in addition to wound care?
   d. Assuming that the wound heals promptly and the skilled nursing visits are discontinued, what other resources could be used by this family?

RESOURCES

American Medical Association
Cultural Competence Compendium (2000). *Cross-cultural health care program, guidelines for providing health care services through an interpreter, 2001.* [Online]. Retrieved from: www.xculture.org.

Center for Cross Cultural Health
www.crosshealth.com
www.umn.edu/ccch

Center for Education in Cultural Competency
www.cecp.air.org/cultural

Centers for Medicare and Medicaid Services
cms.hhs.gov

Child and Family Policy Center
www.cfpciowa.org

Community Health Status Indicators
www.communityhealth.hrsa.gov/

Community Health Status Report: Data Sources, Definitions, and Notes
www.communityhealth.hrsa.gov (July 2000)

Cultural Competency Home Page
www.cecp.air.org/cultural/default.htm

Cultural Competence: A Journey
www.bphc.hrsa.gov/cultural competence/Default.htm

Cultural Competence Works: Using Cultural Competence to Improve the Quality of Health Care for Diverse Populations
www.hrsa.gov/financeMC/cultural-competence.pdf

Culture Clues
www.depts.washington.edu/pfes/cultureclues.html

Department of Health and Human Services, Office of Minority Health (2001)
Assessing cultural competence in health care: Recommendations for national standards and an outcomes-focused research agenda. [Online]. Retrieved from: www.ohhrc.gov

Diversity Rx
www.diversityrx.org/HTML/DIVRX.htm

Federal Interagency Forum on Children and Family Statistics
www.childstats.gov

From generation to generation: The health and well-being of children in immigrant families
search.nap.edu/html/generation/summary.html

Georgetown University: National Center for Cultural Competence
gucdc.georgetown.edu/nccc/topic4.html

The Harriet and Robert Heilbrunn Department of Population and Family Health
cpmcnet.columbia.edu/dept/sph/popfam/

Health Literacy Toolbox 2000
www.prenataled.com/healthlit/hlt2k/script/index.asp

Indian Health Services
www.ihs.gov

Institute for the Support of Latino Families and Communities
www.uiowa.edu/nrcfcp/new/Latinos/1st%20latino%20page.htm

Institute for Urban Family Health
www.institute2000.org/

Kaiser Family Foundation
www.kff.org/

Maternal and Child Health Bureau
mchb.hrsa.gov/

Maternal and Neonatal Health Resources
www.jhuccp.org/mmc/mnh/index.stm

National Alliance for Hispanic Health
www.hispanichealth.org

National Association of County and City Health Officials
health-disparities.nacchoweb.naccho.org/

National Center for the Study of Adult Learning & Literacy
www.hsph.harvard.edu/healthliteracy/

The National Multicultural Institute
www.nmci.org

National Resource Center on Family Centered Practice (NRC/FCP)
www.uiowa.edu/nrcfcp/new/index.html

Online Content for Low-Income and Underserved Americans: The Digital Divide's New Frontier
www.childrenspartnership.org/pub/low_income/index.html

Population & Family Health Sciences (Johns Hopkins)
www.jhsph.edu/pfhs/

Provider's Guide to Quality and Care
erc.msh.org/quality&culture

Survey on Women's Health in the United States
www.kff.org/content/2002/20020507a/

Urban Institute: National Survey of America's Families
newfederalism.urban.org/nsaf/

U.S. Department of Health and Human Services HRSA
www.hrsa.gov/

U.S. Department of Health and Human Services, Centers for Disease Control and Prevention. CDC Fact Book 2000/2001
www.cdc.gov

REFERENCES

Allen, F. (1997). Comparative theories of the expanded role in nursing and implications for nursing practice. *Nursing Papers, 9,* 38-45.

Almeida, R., Dubay, L., & Ko, G. (2001). Access to care and use of health services by low-income women. *Health Care Financing Review, 22*(4), 27-47.

Amaro, H. (1994). Women in the Mexican-American community: Religion, culture, and reproductive attitudes and experiences. *Journal of Comparative Psychology, 16*(1), 6-19.

American Academy of Pediatrics Council on Child and Adolescent Health. (1998). The role of home-visitation programs in improving health outcomes for children and families. *Pediatrics, 101,* 486-489.

Anderson, E., & McFarlane, J. (2000). *Community-as-partner: Theory and practice in nursing* (3rd ed.). Philadelphia: Lippincott Williams & Wilkins.

Arcia, E. et al. (2001). Models of acculturation and health behaviors among Latino immigrants to the US. *Social Science & Medicine, 53*(1), 41-53.

Association of Women's Health, Obstetric, and Neonatal Nurses (AWHONN) (1994). *Didactic content and clinical skills verification for professional nurse providers of perinatal home care.* Washington, DC: AWHONN.

Association of Women's Health, Obstetric, and Neonatal Nurses (AWHONN) (1998). *Standards and guidelines for professional nursing practice in the care of women and newborns* (5th ed.). Washington, DC: AWHONN.

Austin, L. et al. (2002). Breast and cervical cancer screening in Hispanic women: A literature review using the health belief model. *Women's Health Issues, 12*(3), 122-128.

Bar-Yam, N. (1994). Learning about culture: A guide for birth practitioners. *International Journal of Childbirth Education, 9*(2), 8-10.

Becker, M. (1974). The Health Belief Model and sick role behavior. *Health Education Monographs, 2,* 409-419.

Bleich, M. (1998). Growth strategies to optimize the functions of telephonic nursing call centers. *Nursing Economics, 4*(6), 215-218.

Bosch, D., & Bushy, A. (1997). Case management: Implementing home care in rural areas. *Home Healthcare Consultant, 4*(7), 19-42.

Boss, P. (1996). *Family stress management* (2nd ed.). Newbury Park, CA: Sage.

Bronfenbrenner, U. (1979). *The ecology of human development.* Cambridge, MA: Harvard University Press.

Bronfenbrenner, U. (1989). Ecological systems theory. In R. Vasta (Ed.), *Annals of child development* (Vol. 6, pp. 187-249). Greenwich, CT: JAI.

Brooks, E. (2002). Family assessment and cultural diversity. In S. Clemen-Stone, S. McGuire, & D. Eigsti (Eds.), *Comprehensive community health nursing: Family, aggregate, and community practice* (6th ed.) (pp. 171-223). St. Louis: Mosby.

Bruhn, J. (2001). Ethical issues in intervention outcomes. *Family & Community Health, 23*(4), 24-35.

Bureau of Primary Health Care (2001). *Homeless population statistics.* Online: www.hrsa.bphc.gov

Bushy, A. (1998). Health issues of women in rural environments: An overview. *Journal of American Medical Women's Association, 53*(2), 53-56.

Bushy, A. (2000). *Orientation to nursing in the rural community.* Thousand Oaks, CA: Sage.

Bushy, A. (2001). Framing the issues: Bridging rural women's health into the new millennium rural women: Women's Health Issues: Jacob's Institute. *Women's Health, 11*(1), 26-29.

Bushy, A. (2002). *Resource manual: Rural minorities, their health issues and resources.* Kansas City, MO: National Rural Health Association.

Carter, B., & McGoldrick, M. (1999). *The expanded family life cycle: Individual, family, and social perspectives* (3rd ed.). Boston: Allyn & Bacon.

Chen, J., & Rankin, S. (2002). Using the resiliency model to deliver culturally sensitive care to Chinese families. *Journal of Pediatric Nursing, 17*(3), 157-166.

Clarke, L. (2001). La Familia: Methodological issues in the assessment of perinatal social support for Mexicans living in the United States. *Social Science & Medicine, 53,* 1303-1320.

Clarke, V. (2001). What about the children? Arguments against lesbian and gay parenting. *Women's Studies International Forum, 24*(5), 555-570.

Clemen-Stone, S. (2002). Community assessment and diagnosis. In S. Clemen-Stone, S. McGuire & D. Eigsti (Eds.), *Comprehensive community health nursing: Family, aggregate, and community practice* (6th ed.) (pp. 449-480). St. Louis: Mosby.

Clemen-Stone, S., McGuire, S., & Eigsti, D. (2002). *Comprehensive community health nursing: Family, aggregate, and community practice* (6th ed.). St. Louis: Mosby.

D'Avanzo, C., & Geissler, E. (2003). *Pocket guide to cultural assessment* (3rd ed.). St. Louis: Mosby.

Davis, M., & Fields, B. (2000). Healthy People 2010: A resource for health. *Tennessee Nurse, 63*(4), 17-18.

Davis, T., Meldrum, H., & Tippy, P. (1996). How poor literacy leads to poor health care. *Patient Care, 30*(16), 94-103.

Doak, C., Doak, L., & Root, J. (1996). *Teaching patients with low literacy skills* (2nd ed.). Philadelphia: J.B. Lippincott.

Doyle, E., & Ward, S. (2001). *The process of community health education and health promotion.* Mountain View, CA: Mayfield Publishing.

Engebretson, J., & Littleton, L. (2001). Cultural negotiation: A constructivist-based model for nursing practice. *Nursing Outlook, 49*(5), 223-230.

Ervin, N. (2002). *Advanced community health nursing practice: Population-focused care.* Upper Saddle River, NJ: Prentice Hall.

Federal Interagency Forum on Children and Family Statistics (2001). *Population and family characteristics.* Online: www.childstats.gov

Ford-Gilboe, M. (2000). Dispelling myths and creating opportunity: A comparison of the strengths of single-parent and two-parent families. *Advances in Nursing Science, 23*(1), 41-58.

Friedman, M. (1998). *Family nursing theory and assessment* (4th ed.). New York: Appleton & Lange.

Galanti, G. (1997). *Caring for patients from different cultures: Case studies from American hospitals.* Philadelphia: University of Pennsylvania.

Goldman, T., & DeLaCruz, D. (1999). The Healthy Start Initiative. In H. Wallace et al. (Eds.), *Health and welfare for families in the 21st century* (pp. 467-482). Sudbury, MA: Jones and Bartlett Publishers.

Howard, C., Andrade, S., & Byrd T. (2001). The ethical dimensions of cultural competence in border health care settings. *Family & Community Health, 23*(4), 36-49.

Huff, R., & Kline, M. (1999). *Promoting health in multicultural populations.* Thousand Oaks, CA: Sage.

Janz, N., & Becker, M. (1984). The Health Belief Model: A decade later. *Health Education Quarterly, 11*(1), 1-47.

Johnson, J. et al. (1999). South Asian women's views on the causes of breast cancer: Images and explanations. *Patient Education and Counseling, 37*(3), 243-254.

Kastens, J. (1998). Integrated care management: Aligning medical call centers and nurse triage services. *Nursing Economics, 16,* 320-322, 329.

Kim, Y. et al. (2001). Client communication behaviors with health care providers in Indonesia. *Patient Education and Counseling, 45*(1), 59-68.

Klein, D., & White, J. (1996). *Family theories: An introduction.* Newberry Park, CA: Sage.

Koniak-Griffin, D. et al. (1999). An early intervention program for adolescent mothers: A nursing demonstration project. *Journal of Obstetric, Gynecologic, and Neonatal Nursing, 28,* 51-59.

Kuehnert, P. (2002). Overview of program planning. In N. Ervin (Ed.), *Advanced community health nursing practice* (pp. 225-245). Upper Saddle River, NJ: Prentice Hall.

Lauderdale, M. (2001). Issues in securing the community's sanction before making an intervention. *Family and Community Health, 23*(4), 1-8.

Lee, R., & Cubbin, C. (2002). Neighborhood context and youth cardiovascular health behaviors. *American Journal of Public Health, 92*(3), 428-436.

Liamputtong-Rice, P. (2000). Baby, souls, name and health: Traditional customs for a newborn infant among the Hmong in Melbourne. *Early Human Development,* 57(3), 189-203.

Lowe, J. (2002). Balance and harmony through connectedness: The intentionality of Native American nurses. *Holistic Nursing Practice, 16*(4), 4-11.

Lynch, E., & Hanson, M. (1998). *Developing cross-cultural competence.* Baltimore: Paul H. Brooks Publishing.

Ma'at, I. et al. (2001). REACH 2010: A unique opportunity to create strategies to eliminate health disparities among women of color. *American Journal of Health Studies, 17*(2), 93-101.

Maehr, J., & Felice, M. (1999). Adolescent health and welfare reform. In H. Wallace et al. (Eds.), *Health and welfare for families in the 21st century* (pp. 511-524). Sudbury, MA: Jones and Bartlett Publishers.

Marks, J., & Wilcox, L. (1999). The future of prevention. In H. Wallace et al. (Eds.), *Health and welfare for families in the 21st century* (pp. 457-465). Sudbury, MA: Jones and Bartlett Publishers.

Maternal Child Health Bureau (1997). Pregnancy-related behaviors among migrant farm workers: Four states, 1989-1993. *Morbidity and Mortality Weekly Report, 46*(13), 283.

Mattson, S. (1995). Culturally sensitive prenatal care for Southeastern Asians. *Journal of Obstetric, Gynecologic, and Neonatal Nursing, 24*(4), 335-341.

Mattson, S. (2000). Providing culturally competent care: Strategies and approaches for perinatal clients. *AWHONN Lifelines, 4*(5), 37-39.

McCarty, N., & Mandle, C. (1998a). Health promotion and the community. In C. Edelman & C. Mandle (Eds.), *Health promotion throughout the lifespan.* (4th ed.) (pp. 171-192). St. Louis: Mosby.

McCarty, N., & Mandle, C. (1998b). Health promotion and the family. In C. Edelman & C. Mandle (Eds.), *Health promotion throughout the lifespan* (4th ed.) (pp. 145-170). St. Louis: Mosby.

McDevitt, J., & Wilbur, J. (2002). Locating sources of data. In N. Ervin (Ed.), *Advanced community health nursing practice: Population-focused care* (pp. 109-147). Upper Saddle River, NJ: Prentice Hall.

McGuire, S. (2002). Promoting healthy people: Public health policies and legislation. In S. Clemen-Stone, S. McGuire, & D. Eigsti (Eds.), *Comprehensive community health nursing: Family, aggregate, and community practice.* (6th ed.) (pp. 82-99). St. Louis: Mosby.

McGuire, S., & Nalle, M. (2000). Healthy people initiative: An introduction. Part 1. *Tennessee Nurse, 63*(4), 11-12.

Monical, W. (1998). Managing high risk pregnancies at home. *Home Healthcare Consultant, 5*(9) 28-31.

Murray, R., Zentner, J., & Samiezade-Yazd, C. (2001). Sociocultural influences on the person and family. In R. Murray & J. Zentner (Eds.), *Health promotion strategies through the lifespan* (7th ed.). Upper Saddle River, NJ: Prentice-Hall.

National Academy Press (2002). *From generation to generation: The health and well-being of children in immigrant families.* Online: search.nap.edu/html/generation/summary.html

National Alliance for Hispanic Health (2001). *A primer for cultural proficiency: Towards quality health services for Hispanics.* Washington, DC: Author.

National Women's Law Center (2001). *Making the grade on women's health: A national and state-by-state report card.* Online: www.nwlc.org

Nixon, K. (2002, August 30). Moms in prison: "Get on Bus" program helps keep families in touch. *Catholic San Francisco,* p. 23.

Olds, D., et al. (1997). Long term effects of home visitation on maternal life-course and child abuse and neglect. *Journal of the American Medical Association, 278*(8), 637-643.

Oros, M., Perry, L., & Heller, B. (2000). School-based health services: An essential component of neighborhood transformation. *Family and Community Health, 23*(2), 31-35.

Patterson, J. (1998). Healthy American families in a postmodern society. In H. Wallace et al. (Eds.). *Health and welfare for families in the 21st century* (pp. 31-52). Sudbury, MA: Jones and Bartlett Publishers.

Pender, N., Murdaugh, C., & Parsons, M. (2002). *Health promotion in nursing practice.* Upper Saddle River, NJ: Prentice-Hall.

Raines, D., & Morgan, Z. (2000). Culturally sensitive care during childbirth. *Applied Nursing Research, 13*(4), 167-172.

Rainey, C. et al. (1999). Views of low-income, African American mothers about child health. *Family & Community Health, 22*(1), 1-15.

Rehm, R. (1999). Religious faith in Mexican-American families dealing with chronic childhood illness. *Image: Journal of Nursing Scholarship, 31*(1), 33-38.

Ryan, M., Carlton, K., & Ali, N. (2000). Transcultural nursing concepts and experiences in nursing curricula. *Journal of Transcultural Nursing, 11*(4), 300-307.

Sebastian, J., & Bushy, A. (Eds.) (1999). *Special populations in the community: Advances in reducing health disparities.* Gaithersburg, MD: Aspen Publishers.

Shamsudin, N. (2002). Can the Neuman Systems Model be adapted to the Malaysian nursing context? *International Journal of Nursing Practice, 8*(2), 99-105.

Simmons, R. et al. (2002). Health education and cultural diversity in the health care setting: Tips for the practitioner. *Health Promotion Practice, 3*(1), 8-11.

Spector, R. (2000). *Cultural diversity in health and illness* (5th ed.). Upper Saddle River, NJ: Prentice Hall Health.

Staveteig, S., & Wigton A. (2000). *Key findings by race and ethnicity: Findings from the National Survey of America's Families.* Washington, DC: The Urban Institute. Online: www.urban.org

Thomas, N. (2001). The importance of culture throughout all of life and beyond. *Holistic Nursing Practice, 15*(2), 40-46.

U.S. Department of Health and Human Services (2000a). *Healthy people 2010: Understanding and improving health.* Washington, DC: U.S. Department of Health and Human Services, Government Printing Office.

U.S. Department of Health and Human Services (2000b). *Healthy People 2010: Chapter 16: Maternal, infant, and child health.* Online: www.health.gov/healthypeople/Document/HTML/Volume2/16MICH.htm

U.S. Department of Health and Human Services. (2000c). *CDC fact book, 2000/2001.* Atlanta, GA: Centers for Disease Control and Prevention.

U.S. Department of Health and Human Services (2000d). *Community health status report: Data sources, definitions, and notes.* Health Resources and Services Administration. Online: www.communityhealth.hrsa.gov

U.S. Department of Health and Human Services (2001a). *Changing lives, changing communities through primary health care.* Washington, DC: Health Resources and Services Administration, Bureau of Primary Health Care.

U.S. Department of Health and Human Services (2001b). *Office on Women's Health: Women's health issues: An overview.* Online: www.4woman.gov

U.S. Department of Health and Human Services (2001c). *Cultural competence works: Using cultural competence to improve the quality of health care for diverse populations.* Online: www.hrsa.gov/financeMC/cultural-competence.pdf

U.S. Department of Health, Education and Welfare. (1979). *Healthy People: The Surgeon General's report on health promotion and disease prevention.* Washington, DC: Government Printing Office.

Walowitz, P. et al. (2000). Desperately seeking synergy: The journey to systems integration of women's health services. *Women's Health Issues, 10*(4), 161-177.

Williams, M. et al. (2001). Promoting early breast cancer screening: Strategies with rural African American women. *American Journal of Health Studies, 17*(2), 65-73.

Williams, R. (1989). Issues in women's health care. In B. Johnson (Ed.), *Psychiatric mental health nursing: Adaptation and growth.* Philadelphia: Lippincott.

Willis, W. (1999). Culturally competent nursing care during the perinatal period. *Journal of Perinatal and Neonatal Nursing, 13*(3), 45-59.

Wright, L., & Leahey, M. (2000). *Nurses and families* (3rd ed.). Philadelphia: F.A. Davis.

CHAPTER 3

Marcia Van Riper

Genetics

http://evolve.elsevier.com/Lowdermilk/MatWmnHlth/

LEARNING OBJECTIVES

- Explore how recent advances in genetics have changed the field of health care.
- List the five main genetics-related activities that all nurses should be prepared to provide.
- Identify ongoing initiatives designed to improve the genetics expertise of nurses.
- Explore challenges and opportunities related to integrating genetics into nursing practice.
- Describe expanded roles for nurses in genetics and genetic counseling.
- Explore the possible benefits and risks of pharmacogenomics.
- Discuss the purpose, key findings, and potential outcomes of the Human Genome Project.
- Examine the ethical, legal, and social implications of the Human Genome Project.
- Discuss the current status of gene therapy (gene transfer).
- Explain the key concepts of basic human genetics.
- Discuss the different types of genetic testing.
- Identify genetic disorders commonly tested for in maternity and women's health nursing.
- Discuss the education and counseling needs of individuals and families who undergo genetic testing.
- Explore the availability of genetic testing to individuals and families from diverse backgrounds.
- Describe the role of genetics in cancer.
- Identify genetics resources for nurses and other health care professionals.

Recent advances in molecular biology and genetics have revolutionized the field of health care by providing the molecular tools needed to determine the hereditary component of most diseases (Collins & Mansoura, 2001; Greendale & Pyeritz, 2001). Never before has there been such a demand for genetic services, especially genetic testing. In addition, the convergence of genetics, biotechnology, and electronics has dramatically changed how these services are accessed and delivered (Lea, 2000). With growing public interest in genetics, increasing commercial pressures, and web-based opportunities for individuals, families, and communities to participate in the direction and design of their genetic health care, genetic services are rapidly becoming an integral part of routine health care (Collins & Guttmacher, 2001; Collins & McKusick, 2001).

Health care professionals in all settings and roles are caring for individuals and families who want, and deserve, high-quality genetic health care. Nowhere is this more apparent than in the area of maternity and women's health care. A growing number of health care professionals working in this area are offering and interpreting genetic tests to individuals and families. Although most of these tests are being used to determine a client's risk of having a child affected by a genetic condition such as Down syndrome or cystic fibrosis (CF), the number of tests being used to determine the presence of, or susceptibility to, adult-onset disorders (e.g., breast cancer, Huntington disease [HD], Alzheimer disease) is increasing at a rapid rate. Health care professionals working in maternity and women's health care are caring for individuals and families who are dealing with complex ethical, legal, and social issues associated with genetic testing and the experience of living with someone who has a genetic condition (Jones & Fallon, 2002; Lewis, 2002; Mahowald et al., 2001).

NURSING AND GENETICS EXPERTISE

Historically, few nurses had formal education in genetics (Hetteberg et al., 1999; Lea, Feetham, & Monsen, 2002; Williams, 1999). It was considered relatively unusual for a nurse to be caring for a client with a genetic condition. Nurses could choose whether they wanted to learn genetics and become involved in the delivery of genetic health care. Today, with genetics rapidly moving into the mainstream of health care, understanding genetics is not an option for nurses (Lea & Williams, 2001).

The pace and significance of recent genetics discoveries has made it virtually impossible for nurses not to be involved in some aspect of genetic health care. Because of their frontline position in the health care system and their long-standing history of providing holistic, family-centered care, nurses are likely to be the first health care professionals to whom individuals and families turn with questions about genetic risk and susceptibility (Lea & Williams, 2001; Tinkle & Cheek, 2002). Nurses are likely to be the first health care professionals from whom individuals and families seek guidance regarding the complexities of genetic testing and interpretation.

Increasingly, nurses from all specialty areas, as well as all practice settings, are being expected to have expertise in genetics, especially maternity, women's health, and oncology nurses. Consequently, these nurses will have significant role changes because of recent increases in genetics knowledge and technology (Jones & Fallon, 2002; Lessick & Anderson, 2000; Loud et al., 2002; Tinkle, 2002) (Box 3-1).

Expanded or New Roles

Expanded or new roles for nurses with genetics expertise are developing in many areas of maternity and women's health nursing. These areas include but are not limited to preconception counseling and preimplantation diagnosis for clients at risk for the transmission of a genetic disorder (Jones & Fallon, 2002); prenatal screening and testing (Grant, 2000; Jones, 2000; Lewis, 2002); prenatal care for women with psychiatric disorders that have a genetic component, such as bipolar disorder and schizophrenia (Carlson-Sabelli & Lessick, 2001); newborn screening and testing (Lloyd-Puryear & Forsman, 2002); the care of families who have lost a fetus or a child affected by a genetic condition (Bryar, 1997; Chandler & Smith, 1998); and the identification and care of children with genetic conditions and their families (Lessick & Anderson, 2000; Raines, 1999; Tinkle, 2002; Van Riper & Cohen, 2001; Williams, 2000). Oncology nurses are beginning to integrate genetics into all phases of care for individuals and families affected by cancer (Loud et al., 2002).

Initiatives to Improve Genetics Expertise

A number of ongoing initiatives are designed to help nurses in all stages of their nursing careers gain the knowledge, skills, and confidence they need to provide high-quality genetics health care in a wide variety of settings (Diekelmann & Diekelmann, 2000; Lea et al., 2002; Menix, 1999; Prows et al., 1999; Williams, 1999). Many of these initiatives are listed in Box 3-2. Others can be found on websites for the International Society for Nurses in Genetics (ISONG), the National Coalition for Health Professional Education in Genetics (NCHPEG), and the Genetics Programs for Nursing Faculty shown in Box 3-2.

ISONG, a nursing specialty organization dedicated to fostering the scientific and professional growth of nurses in human genetics, was founded in 1981 and incorporated

BOX 3-1 Roles of Nurses in Genetics

NURSE GENERALISTS

- Identifying individuals with genetic conditions
- Collecting and recording genetics information
- Offering genetics information
- Assessing comprehension of genetics information
- Making a genetics referral
- Obtaining informed consent or assent (in the case of a minor) for genetic testing
- Assessing the responses of family members to a genetic diagnosis
- Providing care for clients affected by or at risk for genetic conditions
- Recognizing risks for stigma and discrimination
- Identifying individual, family and community resources

(Jones & Fallon, 2002; Lea, Feetham, & Monsen, 2002; Lea & Williams, 2001; Lessick & Anderson, 2000).

ADVANCED PRACTICE NURSES

- Performing genetics health assessments
- Identifying elements of genetic family history suggestive of increased risk for genetic conditions
- Facilitating the informed consent process
- Providing genetic counseling
- Making referrals to specialists in genetics
- Providing psychosocial interventions for families who are adjusting to a recent genetic diagnosis
- Monitoring and evaluating the health of individuals with genetic conditions
- Serving as consultants to other professionals
- Collaborating with medical geneticists and other members of the genetics team
- Serving as an advocate for individuals with genetic conditions and their family members
- Developing, conducting, and evaluating genetics nursing research
- Coordinating and participating in multidisciplinary genetics studies
- Participating in the development of recommendations to address the ethical, legal, and social implications of existing and future genetics services
- Applying findings from genetics research
- Participating in public and private educational efforts in genetics

(Lea et al., 2002; Lessick & Anderson, 2000; Zawacki & Phillips, 2002).

BOX 3-2 Initiatives to Improve Genetics Expertise

GENETICS INITIATIVES FOR NURSES AND OTHER HEALTH CARE PROVIDERS

National Coalition of Health Professional Education in Genetics (NCHPEG)
www.nchpeg.org/

International Society of Nurses in Genetics (ISONG)
www.nursing.creighton.edu/isong/

SUMMER INSTITUTES

Genetics Interdisciplinary Faculty Training Program, Duke University Genetics Program for Nursing Faculty
www.gift.duke.edu/index.html

Cincinnati Children's Hospital Medical Center
www.cincinnatichildrens.org/Professional_Education/programs/Genetics_Program_for_Nursing_Faculty/GPNF/About_GPNF/default.htm

Summer Genetics Institute, Intensive Research Training, NINR
www.fmp.cit.nih.gov/ninr/

ADVANCED DEGREE PROGRAMS

Rush University, Chicago, IL
University of California, San Francisco
University of Cincinnati
University of Iowa, Ames
University of Washington, Seattle
Teacher's College at Columbia University, New York

in 1988. Through annual education conferences, newsletter communication, and credentialing efforts, ISONG strives to assure that practicing nurses around the world are adequately prepared to provide genetics health care (Jenkins, 2000). ISONG members have developed frameworks for integrating genetics into the nursing curriculum, published textbooks on genetics, developed educational resources on genetics, provided summer genetics institutes, and offered web-based genetics courses. ISONG members also have worked collaboratively with other professionals on interdisciplinary initiatives, such as NCHPEG, to promote genetics education.

NCHPEG, established in 1996 with the cooperation of the American Nurses Association (ANA), the American Medical Association (AMA), and the National Human Genome Research Institute (NHGRI) at the National Institutes of Health (NIH), is a national effort to promote health professional education and access to information about advances in human genetics (Monsen, 1999). The membership of NCHPEG is an interdisciplinary group of leaders from more than 125 diverse health professional organizations, consumer and voluntary groups, government agencies, private industry, managed care organizations, and genetics professional societies. Nursing, represented by ANA and 15 other nursing organizations, plays a key role in this initiative. Leaders from three nursing organizations (American Association of Colleges of Nursing, ISONG, and the National Institute of Nursing Research) now serve on the NCHPEG Steering Committee.

NCHPEG members have developed a list of core competencies in genetics that all health professionals should possess (Monsen, 1999). The list is constantly evaluated and revised to reflect the current status of knowledge in genetics. Members of the Core Competency and Curriculum Work Group at NCHPEG have suggested that at a minimum, each health care professional should be able to appreciate limitations of his or her genetics expertise; understand the social and psychologic implications of genetics services; and know how and when to make referrals to genetics professionals.

Genetics-Related Nursing Activities

Although many of the roles for nurses in genetics are being expanded or developed, all nurses should be prepared to collaborate in interdisciplinary clinical partnerships and provide five main genetics-related nursing activities (ISONG, 1998; Lea et al., 2002; Lea, Jenkins, & Francomano, 1998). The five main activities are as follows:

- Collecting, reporting, and recording genetics information;
- Offering genetics information and resources to clients and families;
- Participating in the informed consent process and facilitating informed decision making;
- Participating in management of clients and families affected by genetic conditions; and
- Evaluating and monitoring the impact of genetics information, testing, and treatment on clients and their families.

These activities are not limited to particular practice settings, nor are they limited to specific specialty areas.

Genetics-related activities that all nurses should be able to provide are further delineated in the *Statement on the Scope and Standards of Genetics Clinical Nursing Practice* (ISONG, 1998). This document includes standards and levels of practice for genetics nursing that were established cooperatively by ISONG and ANA. Efforts are under way to strengthen genetics knowledge and skill requirements for nursing licensure and certification examinations (Lea et al., 2002). ISONG has developed a credential to recognize advanced practice nurses in genetics for their advanced knowledge, skills, and abilities. In addition, ISONG is working cooperatively with the American Nurses Credentialing Center to develop recognition of nurses in genetics.

HUMAN GENOME PROJECT

The Human Genome Project is a publicly funded international effort coordinated by the NIH and the U.S. Department of Energy. Not only is the Human Genome Project responsible for a long list of amazing genetics discoveries, but it also has stimulated and facilitated the work of thousands of scientists worldwide. Within 24 hours after a piece of deoxyribonucleic acid (DNA) has been sequenced by Human Genome Project scientists, the results are posted on a public database (www.ncbi.nlm.nih.gov/genome/guide/human/). Anyone who has access to an Internet connection has access to this information. More important, there are no restrictions on its use or redistribution. According to Dr. Francis Collins (2001), director of the National Human Genome Research Institute, "The argument for doing this was simple: the sequence would only benefit the public fully if it could be understood, and that required making it immediately available so that all the creative minds of the planet would work on it."

When the Human Genome Project was initiated in 1990, the ultimate goal of the project was to map the **human genome** (complete set of genetic instructions in the nucleus of each human cell) by 2005. Considering that the human genome consists of approximately 3 billion base pairs of DNA, many people considered this to be an impossible task. By February 1999, less than 15% of the human genome had been sequenced. Then a turning point occurred for the Human Genome Project (Collins, 2001). A decision was made to aim for working draft coverage, rather than complete coverage, of the human genome by the spring of 2000. This decision was based on findings from an earlier study in which draft sequences of DNA were compared with finished sequences of DNA, and they were found to be very useful.

On June 26, 2000, an announcement was made at the White House that a working draft of the Human Genome Project had been completed by two groups: scientists working on the Human Genome Project and scientists from Celera Genomics, a privately funded effort. Simultaneous publications describing the initial draft sequence and analysis of the human genome appeared in *Nature* (International Human Genome Sequencing Consortium, 2001) and *Science* (Venter et al., 2001) on February 12, 2001. A substantially complete version of the human genome was announced in April, 2002. Not only was this years ahead of the original schedule, but it also was right in time for the fiftieth anniversary of the uncovering by Watson and Crick of the chemical basis of heredity with their elucidation of the double helical structure of DNA.

Current Outcomes

Two key findings from initial efforts to sequence and analyze the human genome are that (1) all human beings are 99.9% identical at the DNA level, and (2) approximately 30,000 to 40,000 **genes** (pieces or sequences of DNA that contain information needed to make proteins) make up the human genome (International Human Genome Sequencing Consortium, 2001). The finding that human beings are 99.9% identical at the DNA level should help to discourage the use of science as a justification for drawing precise racial boundaries around certain groups of people (Collins & Mansoura, 2001). The vast majority of the 0.1% genetic variations are found within and not between populations. The finding that humans have 30,000 to 40,000 genes, which is only twice as many as roundworms (18,000) and flies (13,000), was unexpected. Scientists had estimated that there were 80,000 to 150,000 genes in the human genome. It had been assumed that the main reason that humans are more evolved and more highly sophisticated than other species is that they have more genes. A new explanation for human complexity, given the relatively small number of genes, is that humans are more efficient with their genes. Humans are able to do much more with their genes than are other species. Instead of producing only one protein per gene, most human genes produce at least three proteins. In addition, the architecture of human proteins is far more complex than the architecture of worm and fly proteins.

Gene Identification and Testing

Initial efforts to sequence and analyze the human genome have proven invaluable in the identification of genes involved in disease and in the development of genetic tests. More than 100 genes involved in diseases such as HD, breast cancer, colon cancer, Alzheimer disease, achondroplasia, and CF have been identified. Genetic tests for more than 700 inherited conditions are commercially available or in research development (Burke, Pinsky, & Press, 2001).

Genetic testing involves the analysis of human DNA, ribonucleic acid **(RNA), chromosomes** (threadlike packages of genes and other DNA in the nucleus of a cell), or proteins to detect abnormalities related to an inherited condition. Genetic tests can be used to examine directly the DNA and RNA that make up a gene **(direct or molecular testing),** look at markers that are coinherited with a gene that causes a genetic condition **(linkage analysis),** examine the protein products of genes **(biochemical testing),** or examine chromosomes **(cytogenetic testing).** Cytogenetic analysis of malignant tissue has become a mainstay of oncology.

Most of the genetic tests now being offered in clinical practice are tests for single-gene disorders in clients with clinical symptoms or who have a family history of a genetic disease (Yoon et al., 2001). Some of these genetic tests are **prenatal tests** or tests used to identify the genetic status of a pregnancy at risk for a genetic condition. Current prenatal testing options include **maternal serum screening** (a blood test used to see if a pregnant woman is at increased risk for carrying a fetus with a neural tube defect or a chromosomal abnormality such as Down syndrome) and invasive procedures (amniocentesis and chorionic villus sampling). Other tests are **carrier screening tests,** which are used to identify individuals who have a gene mutation for a genetic condition but do not show symptoms of the condition, because it is a condition that is inherited in an autosomal recessive form (e.g., CF, sickle cell disease, and Tay-Sachs disease). Another type of genetic testing is **predictive testing,** which is used to clarify the genetic status of asymptomatic family members. The two types of predictive testing are presymptomatic and predispositional. Mutation analysis for HD, a neurodegenerative disorder, is an example of **presymptomatic** testing. If the gene mutation for HD is present, symptoms of HD are certain to appear if the individual lives long enough. Testing for a BRCA1 gene mutation to determine breast cancer susceptibility is an example of predispositional testing. **Predispositional** testing differs from presymptomatic testing in that a positive result (indicating that a BRCA1 mutation is present) does not indicate a 100% risk of developing the condition (breast cancer).

In addition to using genetic tests to test for single-gene disorders, genetic tests are being used for population-based screening such as state newborn screening for phenylketonuria (PKU) and other inborn errors of metabolism (IEMs) and to test for common complex diseases such as cancer and cardiovascular conditions. Genetic tests also are being used to determine paternity, identify victims of war and other tragedies, and profile criminals.

In 2001, two exciting announcements were made regarding work on genetic tests being done by scientists at the National Human Genome Research Institute (NHGRI). The first announcement reported the development of a technique, **gene-expression profiling,** that uses a special kind of DNA chip called a microarray to differentiate between breast tumors caused by inherited genetic changes and those caused by sporadic changes (Hedenfalk et al., 2001). The team of NHGRI scientists was able to differentiate quickly and accurately the BRCA1 mutation changes from BRCA2 mutation changes and from sporadic or noninherited changes. Leading cancer specialists have described these results as a breakthrough in basic science with potentially broad clinical applications.

The second announcement reported that NHGRI scientists had used gene chip technology and a form of artificial intelligence called an artificial neural network (ANN) to develop a method of genetic fingerprinting that can differentiate between several closely related types of childhood cancer (Khan et al., 2001). When the NHGRI team of scientists started the study, they were exploring more than 6000 genes. The ANN analysis eventually narrowed the number of genes needed to differentiate between the four tumor types (neuroblastoma, Ewing sarcoma, rhabdomyosarcoma, and non-Hodgkin lymphoma) to 93 genes. Of these, 41 were new genes that may provide important insights into the biology of these cancers and offer possible targets for new treatments.

Pharmacogenomics

One of the most immediate clinical applications of the Human Genome Project may be **pharmacogenomics,** or the use of genetic information to individualize drug therapy (Phillips et al., 2001). There has been speculation that pharmacogenomics may become part of standard practice for a large number of disorders and drugs by 2020 (Collins & McKusick, 2001). The expectation is that by identifying common variants in genes that are associated with the likelihood of a good or bad response to a specific drug, drug prescriptions can be individualized, based on the individual's unique genetic make-up (Roses, 2000). A primary benefit of pharmacogenomics is the potential to reduce adverse drug reactions. Considering that adverse drug reactions result in significant morbidity, mortality, and excess medical costs, pharmacogenomics could prove to be very important.

Gene Therapy (Gene Transfer)

In the early 1990s, a great deal of optimism was felt about the possibility of using genetic information to provide quick solutions to a long list of health problems (Collins & McKusick, 2001). However, the field of gene therapy, also known as gene transfer, has sustained a number of major disappointments during the past few years. Although the early optimism about gene therapy was probably never fully justified, it is likely that the development of safer and more effective methods for gene delivery will ensure a significant role for gene therapy in the treatment of some diseases (Collins & McKusick, 2001). Major challenges include targeting the right gene to the right location in the right cells, expressing the transferred gene at the right time, and minimizing adverse reactions (Brower, 2001). Some reports detail exciting possibilities regarding the application of gene therapy for hemophilia B (Kay et al., 2000) and severe combined immunodeficiency (Anderson, 2000; Cavazzana-Calvo et al., 2000). According to W. French Anderson (2000), a scientist who is very active in the field of gene therapy, "Gene therapy will succeed with time. And it is important that it does, because no other area of medicine holds as much promise for providing cures for the many devastating diseases that ravage humankind."

Potential Outcomes

Finished Sequence of the Human Genome

Although completion of a working draft sequence and analysis of the human genome represents a major milestone, a vast amount of additional work remains to be done (Collins & McKusick, 2001). First, the human genome sequence must be finished. Scientists must fill in existing gaps in the sequence and resolve any ambiguities. An understanding of the entire sequence will help to clarify which human characteristics are innate and which are acquired, as well as the interplay between heredity and environment in defining susceptibility to disease (Subramanian et al., 2001). In the long run, the greatest payoff from sequencing the entire human genome will most likely be an illumination of the molecular pathogenesis of disorders that are poorly understood, and for which treatments are largely experimental and frequently suboptimal (Collins, 2001).

Four of the 23 chromosomes in the human genome are almost completely sequenced. It is probably not surprising that these are the four smallest chromosomes: chromosome 20 (1179 genes), chromosome 21 (560 genes), chromosome 22 (978 genes), and the Y chromosome (295 genes). Chromosome 21 was the first chromosome to be sequenced. Like the Y chromosome, chromosome 21 is considered to be "gene poor" because it has a relatively small number of genes. Chromosome 20 is almost the same size as chromosome 21, but it has more than twice as many genes. Chromosomes 6, 7, 13, and 14 are in the final stages of being sequenced (Pennisi, 2002). So far, 2393 genes have been identified on chromosome 7.

Catalog of Human Variation

Another important task that must be finished is the development of a catalog of common variants. A public-private partnership has been developed to complete this catalog as quickly as possible. Most of the common variants in the genome are represented by alterations at a single nucleotide. So far, more than 3 million **single nucleotide polymorphisms,** or **SNPs** (pronounced 'snips'), have been identified and made available in public databases.

According to the National Human Genome Research Institute's talking glossary of genetic terms available at http://www.genome.gov/, SNPs are defined as common, but minute, variations that occur in human DNA at a frequency of one in every 1000 bases. A particular SNP may or may not influence a person's **phenotype** (observable traits or characteristics), depending on the SNP's nature and location. For example, a SNP in a coding region may alter an amino acid, or a SNP in a regulatory region may alter gene expression. However, most SNPs are in the **introns** or noncoding sequences of DNA. Development of a vast, dense catalog of SNPs will make it possible for researchers to look for relations or associations between particular SNPs and common diseases such as cancer, heart disease, and mental illness (Collins & Mansoura, 2001). This research will facilitate the development of individualized preventive health care based on genetic risk.

Sequences of Other Genomes

A third task that must be finished is the sequencing of other genomes such as the mouse or rat genome. The genomes of most organisms have many homologous or similar genes; therefore the identification of the sequence or function of a gene in a model organism, such as a mouse, has the potential to explain a homologous gene in human beings. Sequencing of the mouse, rat, and zebrafish genomes are already under way, and serious consideration is being given to sequencing other large-vertebrate genomes, such as the pig, dog, cow, and chimpanzee (Collins & McKusick, 2001). The mouse genome is similar in size to the human genome and has a similar gene complement. Because of this, the mouse genome will most likely be extremely helpful in efforts to unravel the causes of genetic diseases when there is a complex pattern of inheritance (Gardiner, 2002).

Ethical, Legal, and Social Implications

Before the beginning of the Human Genome Project, widespread concern about misuse of the information gained through genetics research resulted in 5% of the Human Genome Project budget being designated for the study of the *ethical, legal, and social implications (ELSIs)* of human genome research. Two large ELSI programs were created to identify, analyze, and address the ELSIs of human genome research at the same time that the basic science issues were being studied. One ELSI program was established in the NHGRI at the NIH, and another was established in the Office of Biological and Environmental Research (OBER) at the Department of Energy (DOE). The two ELSI programs are separate but complementary programs. During the past decade, issues of high priority for these programs have been privacy and fairness in the use and interpretation of genetic information; clinical integration of new genetics technologies; issues surrounding genetics research, such as possible discrimination and stigmatization; and education for professionals and the general public about genetics, genetic health care, and ELSI of human genome research. Both ELSI programs have excellent websites that include vast amounts of educational information, as well as links to other informative sites.

ELSI of Genetic Testing

According to Elizabeth Thomson (1997), a nurse who is the current program director for the ELSI Program at NHGRI, the major risk associated with genetic testing is that of gaining information that may result in increased anxiety and altered family relationships; that may be difficult to keep confidential, especially if the test results are shared with the individual; that may result in discrimination and stigmatization; and about which little, if anything, can be done. Thomson also noted that informed consent is very difficult to ensure when some of the outcomes, benefits, and risks of genetic testing remain unknown. In addition, many of the tests being used are, as yet, imperfect. That is, few have a 100% detection rate. Individuals and families who receive false-positive results (the test results indicate that a person or fetus is affected by a genetic condition when they are not) may terminate an unaffected pregnancy or undergo unwarranted extreme measures such a bilateral prophylactic mastectomy. Individuals and families who receive false-negative results (the test results indicate that a person or fetus is not affected by genetic condition when they are) may fail to follow surveillance strategies designed to improve their health outcomes because they have been falsely reassured that they are not at increased risk for a specific condition.

Factors Influencing the Decision to Undergo Genetic Testing

The decision to undergo genetic testing is seldom an autonomous decision based solely on the needs and preferences of the individual being tested. Instead, it is often a decision based on feelings of responsibility and commitment to others (Burgess & d'Agincourt-Canning, 2002; Juengst, 1998, 1999). For example, a woman who is receiving treatment for breast cancer may undergo BRCA1 mutation testing not because she wants to find out if she carries a BRCA1 mutation, but because her two sisters have asked her to be tested, and she feels a sense of responsibility and commitment to them. A female airline pilot with a family history of HD, who has no desire to find out if she has the gene mutation associated with HD, may undergo mutation analysis for HD because she feels she has an obligation to her family, her employer, and the people who fly with her.

Decisions about genetic testing are shaped, and in many instances constrained, by factors such as social norms, where care is received, and socioeconomic status. Most pregnant women in the United States now have at least one ultrasound examination, many undergo some type of multiple-marker screening, and a growing number undergo other types of prenatal testing (Grant, 2000). The range of prenatal testing options available to a pregnant woman and her family may vary significantly, based on where the pregnant woman receives prenatal care and her socioeconomic status. Certain types of prenatal testing may not be available in smaller communities and rural settings (e.g., chorionic villus sampling; FISH analysis [fluorescent in situ hybridization]). In addition, certain types of genetic testing may not be offered in conservative medical communities (e.g., preimplantation diagnosis). Some types of genetic testing are expensive and typically not covered by health insurance. Because of this, these tests may be available only to a relatively small number of individuals and families: those who can afford to pay for them.

Cultural and ethnic differences also have a significant impact on decisions about genetic testing. When prenatal diagnosis was first introduced, the principal constituency was a self-selected group of Caucasian, well-informed, middle- to upper-class women. Today the widespread use of genetic testing has introduced prenatal testing to new groups of women, women who had not previously considered genetics services. The fact that many of the women currently undergoing prenatal testing may not share mainstream U.S. views about the role of medicine and prenatal care, the meaning of disability, or how to respond to scientific risks and uncertainties further amplifies the complexity of ethical issues associated with prenatal testing.

The genetic testing experience raises fundamental questions about the mutual obligations of kin (Burgess & d'Aincourt-Canning, 2002; Juengst, 1998, 1999). Are individuals morally obligated to alert extended family members about inherited health risks? Conversely, do extended family members have a moral obligation to participate in research designed to determine genetic risk when unwanted information about themselves may be generated in the process? In a case presentation involving familial conflict over genetic testing for breast cancer, Green and Thomas (1997) raised another important question that must be considered: "Whose gene is it?" This question is likely to stimulate a great deal of debate, especially in the area of preimplantation genetic testing.

CLINICAL GENETICS

Genetic Transmission

Human development is a complicated process that depends on the systematic unraveling of instructions found in the genetic material of the egg and sperm. Development from conception to birth of a normal, healthy baby occurs without incident in most cases; occasionally, however, some anomaly in the genetic code of the embryo creates a birth defect or disorder. The science of **genetics** seeks to explain the underlying causes of **congenital disorders** (disorders present at birth) and the patterns in which inherited disorders are passed from generation to generation.

Genes and Chromosomes

The hereditary material carried in the nucleus of each of the **somatic** (body) cells determines an individual's physical characteristics. This material, called DNA, forms threadlike strands known as **chromosomes.** Each chromosome is composed of many smaller segments of DNA referred to as **genes.** Genes, or combinations of genes, contain coded information that determines an individual's unique characteristics. The "code" is found in the specific linear order of the molecules that combine to form the strands of DNA. Genes control both the types of proteins that are made and the rate at which they are produced. Genes never act in isolation; they always interact with other genes and the environment.

All normal human somatic cells contain 46 chromosomes arranged as 23 pairs of **homologous** (matched) chromosomes; one chromosome of each pair is inherited from each parent. The 22 pairs of **autosomes** control most traits in the body, and one pair of **sex chromosomes** control primarily sex determination. The large female chromosome is called the X; the tiny male chromosome is the Y. Generally the presence of a Y chromosome causes an embryo to develop as a male; in the absence of a Y chromosome, the individual develops as a female. Thus in a normal female, the homologous pair of sex chromosomes are XX, and in a normal male, the homologous pair are XY.

Homologous chromosomes (except the X and Y chromosomes in males) have the same number and arrangement of genes. In other words, if one chromosome has a gene for hair color, its partner chromosome also will have a gene for hair color, and these hair-color genes will have the same **loci** or be located in the same place on the two chromosomes. Although both genes code for hair color, they may not code for the *same* hair color. Genes at corresponding loci on homologous chromosomes that code for different forms or variations of the same trait are called **alleles.** An individual having two copies of the same allele for a given trait is said to be **homozygous** for that trait; with two different alleles, the person is **heterozygous** for the trait.

The term **genotype** typically is used to refer to the genetic makeup of an individual when discussing a specific gene pair, but at times, genotype is used to refer to an individual's entire genetic makeup or all the genes that the individual can pass on to future generations. **Phenotype** refers to the observable expression of an individual's genotype, such as physical features, a biochemical or molecular trait, and even a psychologic trait. A trait or disorder is considered **dominant** if it is expressed or phenotypically apparent when only one copy of the gene is present. It is considered **recessive** if it is expressed only when two copies of the gene are present.

As more is learned about genetics, the concepts of dominance and recessivity have become more complex, especially in X-linked disorders (Lashley, 1998). For example, traits considered to be recessive may be expressed even when only one copy of a gene located on the X chromosome is present. This occurs frequently in males because males have only one X chromosome; thus they have only one copy of the genes located on the X chromosome. Whichever gene is present on the one X chromosome determines which trait is expressed. Females, conversely, have two X chromosomes, so they have two copies of the genes located on the X chromosome. However, in any female somatic cell, only one X chromosome is functioning (otherwise, there would be inequality in gene dosage between males and females). This process, known as X-inactivation or the Lyon hypothesis, is generally a random occurrence. That is, there is a 50:50 chance as to whether the maternal X or the paternal X is inactivated. Occasionally the percentage of cells that have the X with an abnormal or mutant gene is very high. This helps explain why hemophilia, an X-linked recessive disorder, can clinically manifest itself in a female known to be a heterozygous carrier (a female who has only one copy of the gene mutation). It also helps explain why traditional methods of carrier detection are less effective for X-linked recessive disorders; the possible range for enzyme activity values can vary greatly, depending on which X chromosome is inactivated.

The pictorial analysis of the number, form, and size of an individual's chromosomes is known as a **karyotype.** Cells from any nucleated, replicating body tissue (not red blood cells, nerves, or muscles) can be used (Scheuerle, 2001). The most commonly used tissues are white blood cells and fetal cells in amniotic fluid. The cells are grown in a culture and arrested when they are in metaphase (during metaphase, the chromosomes are condensed and visible with a light microscope), and then the cells are dropped onto a slide. This breaks the cell membranes and spreads the chromosomes, making them easier to visualize. Next the cells are stained with special stains (e.g., Giemsa stain) that create striping or "banding" patterns. These patterns aid in the analysis because they are consistent from person to person. Once the chromosome spreads are photographed or scanned by a computer, they are cut out and arranged in a specific numeric order according to their length and shape. The chromosomes are numbered from largest to smallest, 1 to 22, and the sex chromosomes are designated by the letter X or Y. Each chromosome is divided into two "arms" designated by p (short arm) and q (long arm). A female karyotype is designated as 46, XX and a male karyotype is designated as 46, XY. Figure 3-1 illustrates the chromosomes in a body cell.

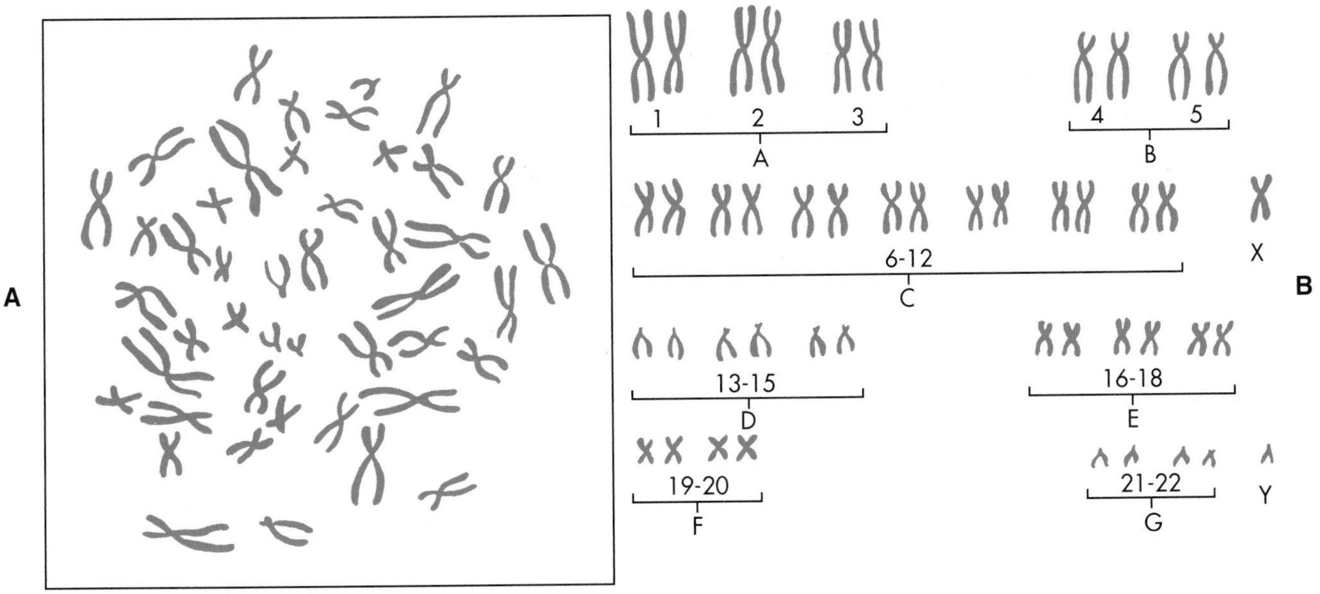
A
1
2
3
A
4
5
B
6-12
C
X
B
13-15
D
16-18
E
19-20
F
21-22
G
Y

FIG. 3-1 Chromosomes during cell division. **A,** Example of photomicrograph. **B,** Chromosomes arranged in karyotype; female and male sex-determining chromosomes.

Chromosomal Abnormalities

Chromosomal abnormalities account for approximately 4% to 7% of perinatal deaths and 0.5% to 1% of infants born with multiple anomalies (Gelehrter, Collins, & Ginsberg, 1998; Jones, 1997). Errors resulting in chromosomal abnormalities can occur during mitosis or meiosis. These errors can occur in either the autosomes or sex chromosomes. Even without the presence of obvious structural malformations, small deviations in chromosomes can cause problems in fetal development.

Autosomal Abnormalities

Autosomal abnormalities involve differences in the number or structure of chromosomes. They result from unequal distribution of genetic material during **gamete** (egg and sperm) formation.

Abnormalities of Chromosome Number. Euploidy is the term used to denote the correct number of chromosomes. Deviations from the correct number of chromosomes or the **diploid** number (2N, 46 chromosomes) can be one of two types: (1) **polyploidy,** in which the deviation is an exact multiple of the **haploid** number of chromosomes or one chromosome set (23 chromosomes); or (2) **aneuploidy,** in which the numerical deviation is not an exact multiple of the haploid set (Lashley, 1998). A **triploid** (3N) cell is an example of a polyploidy. It has 69 chromosomes. A **tetraploid** (4N) cell, also an example of a polyploidy, has 92 chromosomes.

Aneuploidy is the most commonly identified chromosome abnormality in humans. Aneuploidy occurs in at least 5% of all clinically recognized pregnancies, and it is the leading known cause of pregnancy loss (Hassold & Hunt, 2001). Aneuploidy also is the leading genetic cause of mental retardation. The two most common aneuploid conditions are monosomies and trisomies. A **monosomy** is the product of the union between a normal gamete and a gamete that is missing a chromosome. Monosomic individuals only have 45 chromosomes in each of their cells. The product of the union of a normal gamete with a gamete containing an extra chromosome is a **trisomy**. Trisomies are more common than monosomies. Trisomic individuals have 47 chromosomes in each of their cells.

During the past decade, DNA polymorphisms have been used to determine the origin of different aneuploid conditions (Hassold & Hunt, 2001). Limited data are available concerning the origin of monosomies because when an embryo is missing an autosomal chromosome, the embryo never survives. Although a great deal of variation exists among trisomies with regard to the parent and stage of origin of the extra chromosome, most trisomies are maternal meiosis I (MI) errors. This means that most trisomies are caused by **nondisjunction** during the first meiotic division. The first meiotic division involves the segregation of homologous or similar chromosomes. One pair of chromosomes fails to separate. One resulting cell contains both chromosomes, and the other contains none. The fact that most trisomies are maternal MI errors is not that surprising, because maternal MI occurs over a long time span. It is initiated prenatally, but it is not completed until the time of ovulation.

The most common trisomal abnormality is **Down syndrome,** or trisomy 21 (47, XX+21 or 47, XY +21). The incidence of Down syndrome is approximately one in every 600 to 800 live births (National Down Syndrome Society, 2002). Ninety-five percent of individuals with Down syndrome have trisomy 21 or an extra chromosome 21. Individuals with Down syndrome have various degrees of mental retardation, but most fall within the mild to moderate range. Common characteristics seen in individuals with Down syndrome are as follows:

- Oblique palpebral fissures or an upward slant to the eyes
- Epicanthal folds or small skin folds on the inner corners of the eyes
- Small, white crescent-shaped spots on the irises called Brushfield spots
- A flat facial profile that usually includes a somewhat depressed nasal bridge and a small nose
- A protruding tongue
- Small, low-set ears
- Short, broad hands with a fifth finger that has one flexion crease instead of two
- A deep crease across the center of the palm, often referred to as a simian crease
- Hyperflexibility
- Muscle hypotonia or low muscle tone

Some individuals with Down syndrome have all of these characteristics, but others have only a few. Figure 3-2 is a picture of an infant with Down syndrome who has some

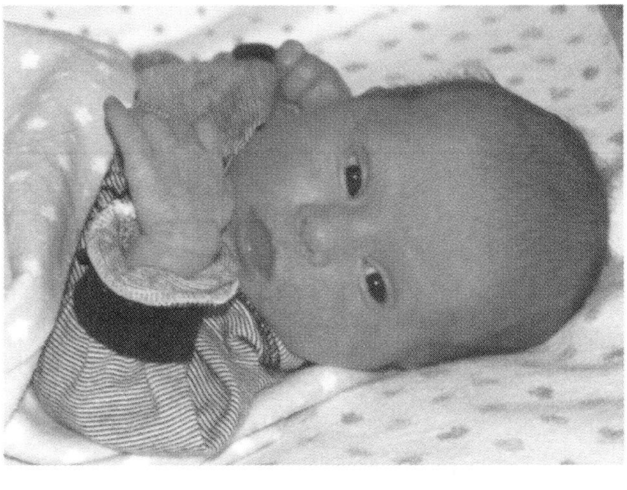

FIG. 3-2 Infant with Down syndrome. Note upward slant to eyes, flat nasal bridge, slightly protruding tongue, and mottled skin. (Courtesy Thomas and Christie Coghill, Clayton, NC.)

of the characteristics commonly associated with that syndrome (see Plan of Care).

Congenital abnormalities and diseases found in individuals with Down syndrome are the same as those that occur in the general population, but individuals with Down syndrome are affected more often and more severely by specific abnormalities and diseases than are typically developing individuals (Cohen, 1999; Van Riper & Cohen, 2001). For example, congenital heart disease occurs in 40% to 60% of individuals with Down syndrome, but only 8 of every 1000 individuals in the general population have congenital heart disease (Freeman et al., 1998). Children with Down syndrome are 10 to 30 times more likely to acquire leukemia than are typically developing children. Individuals with Down syndrome have increased susceptibility to infections and a higher mortality rate from infectious disease than do individuals who do not have Down syndrome. Detailed guidelines have been developed for the care of individuals with Down syndrome (see the Resources section at the end of this chapter).

Plan of Care — The Family with Down Syndrome

NURSING DIAGNOSIS Risk for interrupted family processes related to birth of a neonate with an inherited disorder

Expected Outcome *The couple will verbalize accurate information about Down syndrome, including implications for future pregnancies.*

Nursing Interventions/*Rationales*

Assess knowledge base of couple regarding the clinical signs and symptoms of Down syndrome and inheritance patterns *to correct any misconceptions and establish basis for teaching plan.*

Provide information throughout the genetics evaluation regarding risk status and clinical signs and symptoms of Down syndrome *to give couple a realistic picture of neonate's defects and assist with decision making for future pregnancies.*

Use therapeutic communication during discussions with the couple *to provide opportunity for expression of concern.*

Refer to support groups, social services, or counseling *to assist with family cohesive actions and decision making.*

Refer to child development specialist *to provide family with realistic expectations regarding cognitive and behavioral differences of child with Down syndrome.*

NURSING DIAGNOSIS Situational low self-esteem related to diagnosis of inherited disorder as evidenced by parents' statements of guilt and shame

Expected Outcome *The parents will express an increased number of positive statements regarding the birth of a neonate with Down syndrome.*

Nursing Interventions/*Rationales*

Assist parents to list strengths and coping strategies that have been helpful in past situations *to use appropriate strategies during this situational crisis.*

Encourage expression of feelings using therapeutic communication *to provide clarification and emotional support.*

Clarify and provide information regarding Down syndrome *to decrease feelings of guilt and gradually increase feelings of positive self-esteem.*

Refer for further counseling as needed *to provide more in-depth and ongoing support.*

NURSING DIAGNOSIS Risk for impaired parenting related to birth of neonate with Down syndrome

Nursing Interventions/*Rationales*

Assist parents to see and describe normal aspects of infant *to promote bonding.*

Encourage and assist with breastfeeding if that is parents' choice of feeding method *to facilitate closeness with infant and provide benefits of breastmilk.*

Assure parents that information regarding the neonate will remain confidential *to assist the parents to maintain some situational control and allow for time to work through their feelings.*

Discuss and role play with parents ways of informing family and friends of infant's diagnosis and prognosis *to promote positive aspects of infant and decrease potential isolation from social interactions.*

Provide anticipatory guidance about what to expect as infant develops *to assist family to be prepared for behavior problems or mental deficits.*

NURSING DIAGNOSIS Spiritual distress related to situational crisis of child born with Down syndrome

Expected Outcome *Parents seek appropriate support persons (family members, priest, minister, rabbi) for assistance.*

Nursing Interventions/*Rationales*

Listen for cues indicative of parents' feelings ("Why did God do this to us?") *to identify messages indicating spiritual distress.*

Acknowledge parents' spiritual concerns and encourage expression of feelings *to help build a therapeutic relationship.*

Facilitate visits from clergy and provide privacy during visits *to demonstrate respect for parents' relationship with clergy.*

Encourage parents to discuss concerns with clergy *to use expert spiritual care resources to help the parents.*

Facilitate interaction with family members and other support persons *to encourage expressions of concern and seek comfort.*

NURSING DIAGNOSIS Risk for social isolation related to full-time caretaking responsibilities for a neonate with Down syndrome

Expected Outcome *Parents will describe a plan to utilize resources to prevent social isolation.*

Nursing Interventions/*Rationales*

Provide opportunity for parents to express feelings about caring for a neonate with Down syndrome *to facilitate effective communication and trust.*

Discuss with parents their expectations about caring for the neonate *to identify potential areas of concern.*

Assist parents to identify potential caregiving resources *to permit parents to return to a routine at home.*

Identify appropriate referrals for home care *to provide continuity of care.*

Although the risk of having a child with Down syndrome increases with maternal age (incidence is approximately 1 in 1350 for a 25-year-old woman; 1 in 400 for a 35-year-old woman; and 1 in 30 for a 45-year-old woman), children with Down syndrome can be born to mothers of any age. Eighty percent of children with Down syndrome are born to mothers younger than 35 years (National Down Syndrome Society, 2002). The average age of mothers when they give birth to children with Down syndrome is about 27 years. The risk of a mother having a second child with Down syndrome is about 1% when the cause of the Down syndrome is trisomy 21.

During the past 30 years, fundamental changes have occurred in the care of individuals with Down syndrome (Van Riper & Cohen, 2001). These changes, which underscore the importance of the family and emphasize the need for health promotion and health protection activities, have resulted in individuals with Down syndrome living longer and enjoying an improved quality of life. The median age at the time of death has increased from 25 years in 1987 to 49 years in 1997 (Yang, Rasmussen, & Friedman, 2002). Some individuals with Down syndrome are living beyond the age of 70 years. For decades, it was assumed that the experience of living in a family that includes a child with Down syndrome was a negative experience. Findings from three large programs of research concerning families of children with Down syndrome do not provide support for this notion (Van Riper, 1999). Many families living with a child with Down syndrome have described the experience as positive and growth producing.

Other identified autosomal trisomies are trisomy 18 and trisomy 13. Trisomy 18 (Edward syndrome) is more common than trisomy 13 (Patau syndrome). Infants with trisomy 18 may exhibit more than 130 different anomalies, but some of the major phenotypic features and medical complications are small for gestational age or low birth weight; small mouth; feeding difficulties; weak cry; central nervous system manifestations including hypertonia, seizures, and apnea; craniofacial abnormalities; cardiac malformations; unusual or absent fingerprints; and extremity malformations such as clenched hands with overlapping fingers and rocker-bottom feet (Lewis, 2001; Matthews, 1999).

As with trisomy 18, infants with trisomy 13 have numerous abnormalities, the most common of which are as follows:

- Central nervous system anomalies
- Holoprosencephaly (one large eyelike structure in the center of the face due to fusion of the developing eyes)
- Craniofacial malformations such as microcephaly (small head)
- Capillary hemangiomas
- Cardiac defects
- Extremity deformities including polydactyly (extra fingers or toes)
- Renal abnormalities
- Genital abnormalities

Infants with trisomy 18 and trisomy 13 are usually severely to profoundly retarded. Although both conditions have a very poor prognosis, with the vast majority of affected infants dying within the first few days of life, a significant percentage of these infants will survive the first 6 months to 1 year of life; some children with trisomy 18 and trisomy 13 have lived to age 10 years.

Nondisjunction also can occur during mitosis. If this occurs early in development when cell lines are forming, the individual has a mixture of cells, some with a normal number of chromosomes and others either missing a chromosome or containing an extra chromosome. This condition is known as **mosaicism.**

Mosaicism in autosomes is most commonly seen as another form of Down syndrome. Approximately 1% to 2% of individuals with Down syndrome have mosaic Down syndrome.

Depending on when the nondisjunction occurs during development, different body tissues will have different numbers of chromosomes. The clinical characteristics of Down syndrome may be mild or with varying degrees of severity, depending on the number and location of the abnormal cells. An individual with mosaic Down syndrome may have normal intelligence. Mosaicism of both trisomy 18 and trisomy 13 has been reported. Both situations usually lead to a partial clinical expression of the phenotype. Infants who are mosaic for trisomy 18 or trisomy 13 usually have a longer life span than do infants with these disorders who are not mosaic.

Abnormalities of Chromosome Structure. Structural abnormalities can occur in any chromosome (Matthews, 1999). Types of structural abnormalities include translocation, duplication, deletion, microdeletion, and inversion. **Translocation** results when there is an exchange of chromosomal material between two chromosomes. Exposure to certain drugs, viruses, and radiation can cause translocations, but often they arise for no apparent reason (Lewis, 2001). The two major types of translocation are reciprocal and robertsonian. Reciprocal translocations are the most common. In a *reciprocal translocation,* either the parts of the two chromosomes are exchanged equally **(balanced translocation)** or a part of a chromosome is transferred to a different chromosome, creating an **unbalanced translocation** because there is extra chromosomal material (Nehring & Faux, 1999). In a balanced translocation, the individual is phenotypically normal because there is no extra chromosome material; it is just rearranged. In an unbalanced translocation, the individual will be both genotypically and phenotypically abnormal.

In a *robertsonian translocation,* the short arms (p arms) of two different acrocentric chromosomes (chromosomes with very short p arms) break, leaving sticky ends that then cause the two long arms (q arms) to stick together. This forms a new, large chromosome that is made of the two long arms. The individual will have 45 chromosomes. Because genes on the short arm are represented elsewhere, the individual usually does not show any symptoms. The individual may produce an unbalanced gamete (sperm or egg with too many or two few genes). This can lead to reproductive difficulties such as miscarriages or birth defects. Three percent to 4% of all cases of Down syndrome occur because one parent has a robertsonian translocation, a translocation between chromosomes 21 and 14. The child with this type of Down syndrome has an unbalanced translocation because there is an extra part of chromosome 21. The second most common robertsonian translocation occurs between chromosomes 13 and 14.

Deletions result in the loss of chromosomal material and partial monosomy for the chromosome involved (Matthews, 1999). Loss of chromosomal material at the end of a chromosome is referred to as a **terminal deletion.** In contrast, loss of chromosomal material anywhere else in the chromosome is called an **interstitial deletion.** The resulting clinical phenotype of either a terminal or an interstitial deletion will depend on how much of the chromosome has been lost and the number and function of the genes contained in the missing segment. **Microdeletions** are deletions too small to be detected by standard cytogenetic techniques. These deletions can be identified with FISH analysis. FISH technology uses a single-stranded piece of DNA with a florescent label that will adhere to its complementary piece of DNA in the chromosome being investigated.

Whenever a portion of a chromosome is deleted from one chromosome and added to another, the gamete produced may have either extra copies of genes or too few copies. The clinical effects produced may be mild or severe, depending on the amount of genetic material involved. Two of the more common conditions are the deletion of the short arm of chromosome 5 (*cri du chat* syndrome) and the deletion of the long arm of chromosome 18. *Cri du chat* syndrome, so named after the typical mewing cry of the affected infant, causes severe mental retardation with microcephaly and unusual facial appearance. Deletion of the long arm of chromosome 18 causes severe psychomotor retardation with multiple organ malformations. *Velocardiofacial syndrome,* characterized by cardiac and craniofacial abnormalities, is an example of a microdeletion. In this syndrome, a very small piece of the long arm of chromosome 22 is missing. Microdeletions in the Y chromosome have been found in men with infertility problems.

Inversions are deviations in which a portion of the chromosome has been rearranged in reverse order. Few birth defects have been attributed to the presence of inversions, but it is suspected that inversions may be responsible for problems with infertility and miscarriages. Some inversions can be detected prenatally. Inversions do not appear to occur randomly; more than 40% of all inversions involve chromosome 9 (Lashley, 1998).

Sex Chromosome Abnormalities

Several sex chromosome abnormalities are caused by nondisjunction during gametogenesis in either parent. The most common deviation in females is *Turner syndrome* or monosomy X (45,X). The affected female is missing an X chromosome. She usually exhibits juvenile external genitalia with undeveloped ovaries. She is short and often has webbing of the neck and lymphedema of her hands and feet. Intelligence may be impaired. Most affected embryos miscarry spontaneously. DNA polymorphism studies suggest that in most cases of Turner syndrome, it is the paternal X or Y that is lost (Hassold & Hunt, 2001)

The most common deviation in males is *Klinefelter syndrome,* or trisomy XXY. The affected male has an extra X chromosome and exhibits poorly developed secondary sexual characteristics and small testes. He is infertile, usually tall, effeminate, and may be slow to learn. Males who are mosaic for Klinefelter syndrome may be fertile.

Patterns of Genetic Transmission

Heritable characteristics are those that can be passed on to offspring. The patterns by which genetic material is transmitted to the next generation are affected by the number of genes involved in the expression of the trait. Many phenotypic characteristics result from two or more genes on different chromosomes acting together (referred to as **multifactorial inheritance);** others are controlled by a single gene (referred to as **unifactorial inheritance).** Defects at the gene level cannot be determined by conventional laboratory methods such as karyotyping. Instead, specialists in genetics (e.g., geneticists, genetic counselors, and nurses with advanced expertise in genetics) predict the probability of the presence of an abnormal gene from the known occurrence of the trait in the individual's family and the known patterns by which the trait is inherited.

Multifactorial Inheritance

Most common congenital malformations result from multifactorial inheritance, a combination of genetic and environmental factors. Examples are cleft lip, cleft palate, congenital heart disease, neural tube defects, and pyloric stenosis. Each malformation may range from mild to severe, depending on the number of genes for the defect present or the amount of environmental influence. A neural tube defect may range from spina bifida, a bony defect in the lumbar region of the vertebrae with little or no neurologic impairment, to anencephaly, absence of brain development, which is always fatal. Some malformations occur more often in one sex. For example, pyloric stenosis and cleft lip are more common in males, and cleft palate is more common in females.

Unifactorial Inheritance

If a single gene controls a particular trait or disorder, its pattern of inheritance is referred to as *unifactorial mendelian,* or single-gene inheritance. The number of single-gene disorders far exceeds the number of chromosomal abnormalities. This is understandable, considering that 30,000 to 40,000 genes in the haploid number (23) of chromosomes are passed on from each parent to an offspring. Single-gene disorders follow the inheritance patterns of dominance, segregation, and independent assortment described by Mendel. These include autosomal dominant, autosomal recessive, and X-linked dominant and recessive modes of inheritance.

Autosomal Dominant Inheritance. Autosomal dominant disorders are those in which only one copy of the abnormal gene is needed for phenotypic expression. The abnormal gene may appear as a result of a **mutation,** a spontaneous and permanent change in the normal gene structure, in which case the disorder occurs for the first time in the family. Usually an affected individual comes from multiple generations having the disorder. An affected parent who is heterozygous for the trait has a 50% chance of passing the abnormal gene to each offspring (Fig. 3-3, *B* and *C*). There is a vertical pattern of inheritance. Males and females are equally affected.

Autosomal dominant disorders are not always expressed with the same severity of symptoms. For example, a woman who has an autosomal dominant disorder may show few symptoms and may not become aware of her diagnosis until after she gives birth to a severely affected child. Predicting whether an offspring will have a minor or severe abnormality is not possible. Examples of autosomal dominant disorders are HD, Marfan syndrome (a connective tissue disorder with skeletal, ocular, and cardiovascular abnormalities), polycystic kidney disease, and achondroplasia (dwarfism).

Neurofibromatosis (NF) is a progressive disorder of the nervous system that causes tumors to form on nerves anywhere in the body. NF affects all races, all ethnic groups, and both sexes equally. Half of the cases of NF result from spontaneous genetic mutation, whereas the other half are inherited in an autosomal dominant manner. Two genetically distinct forms of NF include NF1, the most common type, with an incidence of 1 in 3000 (Mueller & Young, 2001), and NF2 with an incidence of 1 in 35,000. The most notable features of NF1 are the small pigmented skin lesions known as café-au-lait spots and the neurofibromata (small soft fleshy growths). Other clinical features of NF1 are axillary freckling, mild developmental delay, large head, and Lisch nodules (small harmless, raised pigmented area in the iris). Individuals with NF1 generally are able to live a normal, healthy life. Café-au-lait spots and neurofibromata can occur with NF2, but they are far less common than with NF1.

NF1 is inherited in an autosomal dominant manner with almost complete penetrance by age 5 years (Mueller & Young, 2001). **Penetrance** is defined as the proportion of heterozygotes for a dominant trait who express a trait, even mildly. Expression of NF1 is very variable. Affected members of the same family can look strikingly different as far as disease severity is concerned. The NF1 gene, located on chromosome 17, functions as a tumor suppressor. When it is missing or mutated, tumors grow. More than 100 mutations have been identified in the NF1 gene. The NF2 gene has been mapped to chromosome 22. The gene product, merlin, is thought to be a cytoskeleton protein that acts as a tumor suppressor. No treatment for NF is available, other than the surgical removal of the tumors. Once removed, the tumors may grow back.

Autosomal Recessive Inheritance. *Autosomal recessive inheritance disorders* are those in which both genes of a pair must be abnormal for the disorder to be expressed. Heterozygous individuals have only one abnormal gene and are unaffected clinically because their normal gene overshadows the abnormal gene. They are known as *carriers* of the recessive trait. Because these recessive traits are inherited by generations of the same family, an increased incidence of the disorder occurs in consanguineous matings (closely related parents). For the trait to be expressed, two carriers must each contribute the abnormal gene to the offspring (see Fig. 3-3, *C*). The chance of the trait occurring in each child is 25%. A clinically normal offspring may be a carrier of the gene. Autosomal recessive disorders have a horizontal pattern of inheritance, rather than

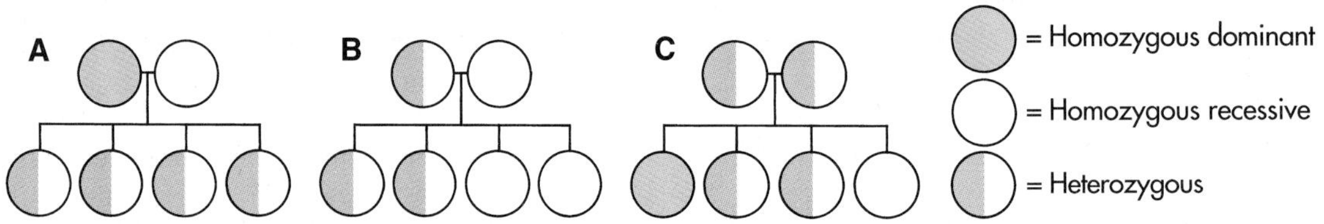
A
B
C
= Homozygous dominant
= Homozygous recessive
= Heterozygous

FIG. 3-3 Possible offspring in three types of matings. **A,** Homozygous-dominant parent and homozygous-recessive parent. Children all heterozygous, displaying dominant trait. **B,** Heterozygous parent and homozygous-recessive parent. Children 50% heterozygous, displaying dominant trait; 50% homozygous, displaying recessive trait. **C,** Both parents heterozygous. Children 25% homozygous, displaying dominant trait; 25% homozygous, displaying recessive trait; 50% heterozygous, displaying dominant trait.

the vertical pattern seen with autosomal dominant disorders. Males and females are equally affected.

Most recessive disorders tend to have severe clinical manifestations, and affected offspring do not often reproduce. If they do, all their offspring will be carriers for the disorder.

Most IEMs, such as PKU, galactosemia, maple syrup urine disease, Tay-Sachs disease, sickle cell anemia, and CF, are autosomal recessive inherited disorders.

Inborn Errors of Metabolism. More than 350 *inborn errors of metabolism* have been recognized (Jorde et al., 1999). Individually, IEMs are relatively rare, but collectively, they are common (1 in 5000 live births). Archibald Garrod first used the term, inborn errors of metabolism, in 1908 when he described variants of metabolism. Garrod recognized that IEMs illustrate our "chemical individualities." As noted previously, most IEMs are inherited in an autosomal recessive pattern. IEMs occur when a gene mutation reduces the efficiency of encoded enzymes to a level at which normal metabolism cannot occur. Defective enzyme action interrupts the normal series of chemical reactions from the affected point onward. The result may be an accumulation of a damaging product such as phenylalanine or the absence of a necessary product such as thyroxin or melanin. Many screening tests for IEMs are available.

Phenylketonuria is a relatively uncommon autosomal recessive disorder. A deficiency in the liver enzyme phenylalanine hydroxylase results in failure to metabolize the amino acid phenylalanine, allowing its metabolites to accumulate in the blood. The incidence of this disorder is 1 in every 10,000 to 20,000 births. The highest incidence is found in Caucasians (from northern Europe and the United States). It is rarely seen in Jewish, African, or Japanese populations. Screening for PKU is routinely performed on all infants through a blood test.

Tay-Sachs disease is a lipid-storage disease that occurs more commonly in Ashkenazi Jews and French-Canadians from Quebec (Lashley, 1998). It results from a deficiency in hexosaminidase. Until age 4 to 6 months, infants with Tay-Sachs disease appear normal; their facial features are considered very beautiful. Then the clinical symptoms appear: apathy and regression in motor and social development and decreased vision. Death occurs between ages 3 and 4 years. No treatment exists for Tay-Sachs disease.

X-linked Dominant Inheritance. *X-linked dominant inheritance disorders* occur in males and heterozygous females. Because the females also have a normal gene, the effects are less severe than those in affected males. Affected males transmit the abnormal gene only to their daughters on the X chromosome. Heterozygous females have a 50% chance of transmitting the abnormal gene to each offspring. Examples of X-linked dominant disorders are Fragile X syndrome (FXS) and vitamin D–resistant rickets. FXS is the most common inherited form of mental retardation. Unlike Down syndrome, FXS is not generally detectable through behavioral observation or physical examination at birth. Delays and behavioral abnormalities gradually become apparent during the first 2 years of life, but ultimately its presence can be verified only through DNA testing. FXS is caused by an inherited trinucleotide repeat expansion (CGG) at a "fragile site" (Xq27.3) on the upper end of the FMR1 gene (Lashley, 1998). Individuals who do not have FXS have approximately 6 to 50 CGG sequences (Lewis, 2001). In carriers of FXS, the CGG repeats are more than 50 but fewer than 200. These individuals are unaffected but may show subtle learning and/or emotional problems. Individuals with more than 200 CGG repeats have the full mutation FXS and typically have long, narrow faces and big ears.

X-linked Recessive Inheritance. Abnormal genes for *X-linked recessive inheritance disorders* are carried on the X chromosome. Females may be heterozygous or homozygous for traits carried on the X chromosome because they have two X chromosomes. Males are hemizygous because they have only one X chromosome carrying genes with no alleles on the Y chromosome. Therefore X-linked recessive disorders are most commonly manifested in the male, with the abnormal gene on his single X chromosome. Hemophilia, color blindness, and Duchenne muscular dystrophy are X-linked recessive disorders.

The male receives the defective gene from his carrier mother on her affected X chromosome. Female carriers (those heterozygous for the trait) have a 50% probability of transmitting the abnormal gene to each offspring. An affected male can pass the abnormal gene to his daughters, but not to his sons. The daughters will be carriers of the trait if they receive a normal gene on the X chromosome from their mother. They will be affected only if they receive an abnormal gene on the X chromosome from both their mother and father.

CANCER GENETICS

Genes that Cause Cancer When Mutated

Cancer is genetic in origin (Vogelstein & Kinzler, 1998; Zawacki & Phillips, 2002). It begins with one or more genetic mutations that make cells unstable. Three classes of genes lead to cancer if they are mutated: (1) protooncogenes, (2) tumor suppressor genes, and (3) DNA repair genes (Lashley, 1998). Mutations that go unchecked start a cascade of further genetic events that lead to uncontrolled growth and tumor formation.

Oncogenes are mutated forms of protooncogenes. The main functions of protooncogenes are to encourage and promote normal growth and development. When protooncogenes mutate to become carcinogenic oncogenes, the result is excessive cell multiplication. There are approximately 100 known oncogenes. Two examples of oncogenes are ERBB2, located on chromosome 13 and

KRAS2, located on chromosome 12. ERBB2 is involved in breast, ovarian, lung, gastric, and salivary gland cancers. KRAS2 is involved in breast, pancreatic, thyroid, colorectal, bladder, and lung cancer, as well as acute myeloid leukemia.

Tumor suppressor genes normally function to inhibit or "put the brakes on" the cell growth and division cycle. They function to prevent the development of tumors. Mutations in tumor suppressor genes cause the cell to ignore one or more of the components of the network of inhibitory signals, removing the brakes from the cell cycle. This results in a higher rate of uncontrolled growth: cancer. Examples of tumor suppressor genes include APC, located on chromosome 5 and involved with familial adenomatous polyposis of the colon (FPC); BRCA1, located on chromosome 17 and associated with hereditary breast cancer and ovarian cancer; and RB1, found on chromosome 13 and involved with familial retinoblastoma.

DNA repair genes ensure that each strand of DNA is accurately copied during cell division in the cell cycle. Mutations in DNA repair genes lead to an increase in the frequency of other mutations. Disorders associated with faulty DNA repair genes include Bloom syndrome, ataxia telangiectasia, Fanconi anemia, and hereditary nonpolyposis colon cancer (HNPCC).

People acquire mutations in genes in three main ways. The first is from the environment. Known factors in the environment that cause cancer are ultraviolet (UV) light (skin cancer) and tobacco smoke (lung cancer). The second way that people acquire mutations is by chance. Normal metabolic processes can generate chemicals that damage DNA. Third, people acquire mutations through heredity. Sometimes people are born with specific mutations in critical genes. For example, people in whom HNPCC develops were born with a mutation in a DNA repair gene.

Hereditary Breast Cancer

Breast cancer is a common disease and a central concern in women's health. Each year, approximately 200,000 women in the United States are diagnosed with breast cancer. One in nine American women will develop breast cancer in her lifetime. Hereditary breast cancer is not a common disease. It is estimated that 5% to 10% of all cases of breast cancer diagnosed before age 40 years and 1% to 4% of those diagnosed after age 40 years are associated with the BRCA1 mutation (Malone et al., 1998). Women at high risk for developing breast cancer typically have several relatives who had breast cancer diagnosed before age 45 to 50 years and one or more relatives affected with bilateral or multifocal breast cancer. Women at high risk for developing breast cancer also may have a family history of ovarian cancer or male breast cancer.

BRCA1, the first major breast cancer gene, was identified and isolated in 1994. A second breast cancer gene, designated BRCA2, was mapped to chromosome 13 in 1994 and cloned in 1995. Women and men found to carry a mutated form of BRCA1 or BRCA2 have an increased risk (somewhere between 30% and 85%) of developing breast or ovarian cancer at some point in their lives. Children of parents with a BRCA1 or BRCA2 mutation have a 50% chance of inheriting the gene mutation. Ashkenazi Jews are 10 times more likely to have BRCA1 and BRCA2 mutations than are the general population. Not all hereditary breast cancers are linked to BRCA1 and BRCA2 mutations. Scientists have suggested that more than 50% of hereditary breast cancers are not linked to BRCA1 and BRCA2 mutations; they are caused by a number of different genes.

Genetic testing for BRCA1 and BRCA2 is commercially available. The cost for testing ranges from $2100 to $2400 for full-sequence BRCA1 and BRCA2 and $357 to $395 for an analysis of relatives of an individual with an identified mutation. Based on preliminary reports, it was predicted that there would be strong interest in BRCA1 testing, both in the general population and for high risk families. To date, actual use has been less than was predicted.

Colon Cancer

In the United States, lifetime risk of colon cancer is about 6%. More than 135,000 new cases are reported each year. Colon cancer is the third leading cause of cancer-related death in women (Greenlee, Hill-Harmon, Murray, & Thun, 2001). Ten percent of cases of colon cancer are likely to involve a mutation in one of several predisposing genes. Two examples of predisposing genes are mutations in the APC tumor suppressor gene and mismatch-repair genes. Mutations in the APC tumor suppressor gene, which is located on chromosome 5, have been associated with FPC, a rare, autosomal dominant syndrome that accounts for about 1% of all colon cancer (Vogelstein & Kinzler, 1998). It is typically diagnosed clinically. Affected individuals have 100 to 1000 polyps in their colon by the time they are aged 20 to 30 years. Genetic testing is greater than 80% sensitive. Identification of high risk individuals guides surveillance strategies (sigmoidoscopy every 1 to 2 years) and the timing of a prophylactic colectomy. Low risk individuals can stop the increased surveillance.

Hereditary nonpolyposis colorectal cancer (HNPCC) results from mutations in one of many mismatch repair genes. Mutations in MSH2 and MLH1 account for 50% to 60% of HNPCC. Families at high risk for HNPCC often have three or more relatives with colorectal cancer; colorectal cancer present in at least two generations; and a diagnosis of colorectal cancer before age 50 years in at least one case. Genetic tests are available to test for MSH2 and MLH1. Testing should be done first on the affected family member. At-risk clients should be offered a prophylactic colectomy. Women may be offered a total abdominal hysterectomy with a salpingo-oophorectomy to decrease cancer risk. If colon cancer develops, a total colectomy is recommended.

GENETIC COUNSELING

Genetic counseling is a clinical genetics service that grew out of a need for professionals who could provide genetics information, education, and support to individuals and families with ongoing or potential genetic health concerns (Lea et al., 1998). Introduction of the term "genetics counseling" is usually credited to Sheldon Reed, who first used the term in 1947 when he was teaching, counseling, and doing research in genetics at the University of Minnesota. One of the first places to offer formal genetic counseling in the United States was the Dight Institute for Genetics in Minnesota (Begleiter, 2002). By 1951, genetic counseling was offered in at least 10 centers in the United States. This growth in the number of centers providing genetic counseling occurred although no formal training programs existed in clinical genetics or genetic counseling. The first class of master's degree genetics counselors graduated from Sarah Lawrence College in 1971. Now 25 master's level genetic counseling programs exist in the United States, six graduate nursing programs with advanced practice courses in genetics (see Box 3-2), and six international programs in genetic counseling (four in Canada, two in Australia, and one in the United Kingdom). The National Society of Genetic Counselors, formed in 1979, now has more than 2000 members.

Definition of Genetic Counseling

In 1975, an ad hoc committee of the American Society of Human Genetics developed a formal definition of genetic counseling. According to this definition,

> Genetic counseling is a communication process that deals with the human problems associated with the occurrence or risk of occurrence of a genetic disorder in a family. This process involves an attempt by one or more appropriately trained person to help the individual or family to (1) comprehend the medical facts including the diagnosis, probable course of the disorder, and the available management; (2) appreciate the way heredity contributes to the disorder and the risk of recurrence in specified relatives; (3) understand the alternatives for dealing with the risk of recurrence; (4) choose a course of action that seems to them appropriate in view of their risk, their family goals, and their ethical and religious standards and act in accordance with that decision; and (5) make the best possible adjustment to the disorder in an affected family member and/or to the risk of recurrence of that disorder.

Access and Referral to Genetic Counseling

Genetic counseling is typically provided by a team of genetics specialists that includes clinical geneticists (physicians with an MD or DO), medical geneticists with a PhD, genetics fellows, genetics counselors, and in a growing number of cases, advanced practice genetics nurse specialists. Cytogeneticists, biochemical geneticists, and molecular geneticists support the clinical genetics team by providing laboratory expertise that helps with the diagnosis and management of individuals and families affected by genetic conditions.

Until recently, most individuals and families interested in receiving genetic counseling went to regional genetics centers or major medical centers. Genetic counseling also was provided in outreach or satellite genetics clinics, public health clinics, and some community hospitals. Now that genetics is invading the mainstream of health care, genetic counseling is being offered in a wide variety of other settings. These include, but are not limited to, managed health care organizations, commercial facilities, and private practices. A number of specialized groups provide genetics education and counseling for individuals and families affected by specific genetic disorders, such as Down syndrome, CF, diabetes, muscular dystrophy, HD, and cancer. Genetic counseling also is offered over the Internet.

Individuals and families seek out, or are referred for, genetic counseling for a wide variety of reasons and at all stages of their lives. Some seek preconception or prenatal information; others are referred after the birth of a child with a birth defect or a suspected genetic condition; still others seek information because they have a family history of a genetic condition (Lea et al., 1998). Regardless of the setting or the individual and family's stage of life, genetic counseling should be offered and available to all individuals and families who have questions about genetics and their health. However, there is currently a shortage of appropriately trained genetics professionals who can provide genetic counseling (Begleiter, 2002; Greendale & Pyeritz, 2001). This means that many individuals and families will not be offered genetic counseling when they undergo genetic testing. Moreover, some of the genetics education and counseling that is provided will be less than adequate.

At the present time, more individuals who can provide genetic counseling are needed urgently. It has been suggested that in the near future, primary care providers will need to assume prominent roles in the provision of genetic counseling and other genetics services (Collins, 1997; Touchette, Holzman, Davis, & Feetham, 1997). This suggestion has not met with overwhelming support (Begleiter, 2002; Greendale & Pyeritz, 2001). The main criticism of this suggestion is that most primary care providers (physicians and nurses) lack an adequate understanding of genetics. This deficit reflects both rapid advances in the field of genetics and historical limitations in genetics education in medical and nursing curricula (Burke & Emery, 2002). As noted previously, a number of initiatives are under way to help nurses and other health care professionals gain the knowledge, skills, and confidence they need to provide high quality genetics health care in a wide variety of settings.

It may take years before a sufficient number of health care professionals feel comfortable and are proficient in providing genetic counseling. Until then, it is imperative that all health care professionals become familiar with existing genetics resources. Some of these resources may be in their own community, but others will be regional, national, and international resources (see Resources). As noted earlier in this chapter, at a minimum, each health care professional should be able to appreciate limitations of his or her genetics expertise; understand the social and psychologic implications of genetics services; and know how and when to make referrals to genetics professionals.

Estimation of Risk

Most families with a history of genetic disease want an answer to the following question: What is the chance that our future children will have this disease? Because the answer to this question may have profound implications for individual family members and the family as a whole, health care professionals must be able to answer this question as accurately as they can in a timely manner. In some cases, estimation of risk is rather straightforward; in other cases, it becomes rather complicated. Because of this, health care professionals should be prepared to refer families with a history of genetic disease to genetics professionals if they are at all unsure. Again, the answer to this question can have profound implications for individual family members and the family as a whole, so health care professionals must do their best to ensure that the question is answered correctly.

If a couple has not yet had children, but they are known to be at risk for having children with a genetic disease, they will be given an **occurrence risk.** Once the mating of a couple has produced one or more children with a genetic disease, the couple will be given a **recurrence risk.** Both occurrence and recurrence risks are determined by the mode of inheritance for the genetic disease in question. For genetic diseases caused by a factor that segregates during cell division (genes and chromosomes), risk can be estimated with a high degree of accuracy by application of the mendelian principles. In an autosomal dominant disorder, both the occurrence and recurrence risk is 50%, or one in two, when one parent is affected and the other is not. The recurrence risk for autosomal recessive disorders is 25%, or one in four, if both parents are carriers (they each have one recessive disease gene and one normal gene). Occasionally an individual homozygous for a recessive disease gene mates with an individual who is a carrier of the same recessive gene. In this case, the recurrence risk is 50%, or one in two. If two individuals affected by an autosomal recessive disorder mate, all of their children will be affected. For X-linked disorders, recurrence risk is related to the sex of the child. Translocation disorders have a high risk of recurrence.

A number of autosomal disorders display fairly complex patterns of inheritance, making estimation of risk somewhat difficult. For example, if a child is born with a genetic disease and there has been no history of the disease in the family, the disease may have been caused by a new mutation (this is more likely if the disease in question is an autosomal dominant disorder, such as achondroplasia). If the child's genetic disease has been caused by a new mutation, the recurrence risk for the parents' subsequent children is not higher than that for the general population. However, the offspring of the affected child may have a substantially elevated occurrence risk.

The risk of recurrence for multifactorial conditions can be estimated empirically. An empiric risk is based not on genetics theory but rather on experience and observation of the disorder in other families. Recurrence risks are determined by applying the frequency of a similar disorder in other families to the case under consideration.

An important concept to be emphasized to individuals and families during a genetic counseling session is that *each pregnancy is an independent event.* For example, in monogenic disorders in which the risk factor is one in four that the child will be affected, the risk remains the same no matter how many affected children are already in the family. Families may maintain the erroneous assumption that the presence of one affected child ensures that the next three will be free of the disorder. However, "chance has no memory." The risk is one in four for each pregnancy. Conversely, in a family with a child who has a disorder with multifactorial causes, the risk increases with each subsequent child born with the disorder.

Interpretation of Risk

The guiding principle for genetics counselors has traditionally been the principle of **nondirectiveness.** According to the principle of nondirectiveness, the individual who is providing genetic counseling respects the right of the individual or family being counseled to make autonomous decisions. Counselors using a nondirective approach avoid making recommendations, and they try to communicate genetics information in an unbiased manner. The first step in providing nondirective counseling is becoming aware of one's own values and beliefs. Another important step is recognizing how one's values and beliefs can influence or interfere with the communication of genetics information.

If the individual who is providing genetic counseling has difficulty being nonjudgmental and objective, he or she may either intentionally or unintentionally influence the decision-making process. Individuals and families also may pressure the counselor to make decisions for them with questions such as, "What would you do if you were me?" Families and individuals need education, guidance, and support throughout the counseling process. They should be given the facts and possible consequences, as well as all of the assistance they need in problem solving, but the final decision regarding a course of action must be their own.

Role of Nurses in Genetic Counseling

The role of nurses in genetic counseling continues to expand. Some nurses will play a key role in the identification of families in need of genetic counseling, and they collaborate with other health care professionals to make referrals to specialists in genetics. Other nurses take a more active role in genetic counseling. For example, these nurses might provide appropriate genetics information before, during, and after the initial genetic counseling session; construct family pedigrees of three or more generations; clarify the genetics information that family members receive during counseling sessions or from other sources such as the public library, the Internet, or support groups; help families manage the ongoing challenges associated with living with genetic disorder; make referrals to support groups and national organizations; and provide long-term follow-up of families affected by genetic conditions.

Probably the most important of all nursing functions is to provide emotional support during all aspects of the counseling process. Feelings that are generated under the real or imagined threat posed by a genetic disorder are as varied as the people being counseled. Responses may include a variety of stress reactions, such as apathy, denial, anger, hostility, fear, embarrassment, grief, and loss of self-esteem. Guilt and self-blame are universal reactions. Many look on the disorder as a stigma, especially if the disorder is visible to others. Old wives' tales, superstitions, and long-held misconceptions may influence a family's reaction to a genetic disorder.

FUTURE PROMISE OF GENETICS

Overall, the Human Genome Project and other sequencing efforts have been a huge success. Our understanding of the human genome, as well as other genomes, has grown exponentially during the past decade. The increased availability of genetic testing and other genetics services gives individuals and families unprecedented opportunities to learn whether they have heightened risks for certain diseases or the potential to transmit gene mutations to their offspring. Awareness of genetic risk also can facilitate informed health care decisions and, in some cases, can promote risk reduction behaviors that have the potential to reduce morbidity and mortality. Ultimately it is hoped that advances in molecular biology and genetics will make it possible to offer diagnostic, preventive, and treatment options not only for genetic diseases but also for common diseases such as cancer, atherosclerosis, diabetes, and Alzheimer disease.

Recent advances made possible through the Human Genome Project have been remarkable, but our ability to offer treatment options, even for single-gene disorders, remains very limited. Progress in the acquisition of genetics knowledge and the development of genetics technology continues to outpace the development of therapeutic interventions. For most genetic conditions, therapeutic interventions are nonexistent or disappointingly limited. Consequently the most useful means of reducing the incidence of genetic disorders now is preventing transmission. Only three reproductive options exist for individuals at risk for transmitting a genetic disorder: the avoidance of pregnancy; genetic diagnosis during an ongoing pregnancy; and prevention of transmission of an altered gene or genes (Jones & Fallon, 2002). For many families, none of these options is viewed as acceptable.

Dialogue among pregnant women, expectant families, health care professionals, and disability advocates concerning prenatal testing for Down syndrome and other genetic disorders is urgently needed. Clinical and technical information must be complemented by social understanding of the experience of disability in contemporary society (Asch, 1999). The picture of life with a disability should be more balanced than that currently portrayed (Marteau & Dormandy, 2001). It is critical that the voices of individuals and families living with disabilities be heard (Asch, 1999).

Nurses are in an ideal position to help individuals and families maximize the benefits of the genetics revolution, but first, nurses need (1) a working knowledge of human genetics, (2) an awareness of recent advances in the field of genetics, and (3) an understanding of the potential effects of genetics discoveries on individual and family well-being. More research is needed concerning the family experience of genetic testing. Nurses must understand why individuals and families decide to undergo genetic testing. Nurses also need to be aware of how individuals and families define and manage ethical, legal, and social issues that emerge during the genetic testing experience. The following quote by Juengst (1998) underscores why this knowledge is needed:

> The promise of accessible genetic information lies in its ability to allow individuals and families to identify, understand, and sometimes control their inherited health risks. This promise puts the individual and families that receive genetic services at the moral center of the enterprise: if genetic assessment is to be judged a success, it must be from the recipients' point of view, in terms of their ability to use the information to enrich their lives.

KEY POINTS

- Recent advances in molecular biology and genetics have revolutionized the field of health care by providing the molecular tools needed to determine the hereditary component of most diseases.
- Increasingly, nurses from all specialty areas, as well as all practice settings, are expected to have expertise in genetics.
- The major force behind the genetics revolution has been the Human Genome Project.
- All humans are 99.9% identical at the DNA level.
- Approximately 30,000 to 40,000 genes are found in the human genome.
- Most of the genetic tests being offered in clinical practice are tests for single-gene disorders.
- Pharmacogenomics will probably be the most immediate clinical application of the Human Genome Project.
- The decision to undergo genetic testing is often based on feelings of responsibility and commitment to others.
- Genes are the basic units of heredity responsible for all human characteristics. They comprise 23 pairs of chromosomes: 22 pairs of autosomes and 1 pair of sex chromosomes.
- Chromosomal abnormalities occur in both autosomes and sex chromosomes.
- Genetic disorders follow mendelian inheritance patterns of dominance, segregation, and independent assortment of normal genetic transmission.
- Multifactorial inheritance includes genetic and environmental contributions.
- Advances in genetics have complex ethical, legal, and social implications.

CRITICAL THINKING EXERCISES

1. Sylvia confides in you that several infants have been born into her family with serious anomalies. From previous conversations, you know that she is opposed to abortion and would never consider having one. Sylvia is currently 6 weeks pregnant, and her physician has urged her to have chorionic villus sampling (CVS). Sylvia asks you for information about CVS and the implications of a finding that her fetus has serious anomalies. Describe your response, keeping in mind genetics, the social and moral implications of genetic testing, and Sylvia's ethical and moral beliefs. What other information do you need? To whom could you refer her? What options does she have?
2. Select two web addresses for resources on genetics for parents from the Resources. Access the sites.
   - **a.** Compare and contrast the appearance, readability, and information contained in the sites.
   - **b.** Do you agree that these sites are appropriate for parents?
   - **c.** Is the information contained culturally relevant?
   - **d.** How could you as a nurse use this information?
3. Reisa is a 28-year-old woman whose mother, aunt, and sister have been diagnosed and treated for breast cancer. Reisa's husband would like Reisa to be tested to see if she "has the breast cancer gene" before they have children so they don't "give the gene to their daughters." What are the ethical responsibilities of Reisa to her husband and potential daughters to undergo testing? What information would the testing provide? Does Reisa need other information before making the decision to be tested? What teaching is necessary if Reisa asks about the advisability of having prophylactic mastectomies?

RESOURCES

GENETIC INFORMATION AND DATABASES

Cystic Fibrosis Foundation
www.cff.org

Down Syndrome on the Internet
www.ds-health.com/ds_sites.htm

Down Syndrome Quarterly
www.denison.edu/dsq/health99.shtml

Gene Tests
www.genetests.org/

OMIM Home Page: Online Mendelian Inheritance in Man
www3.ncbi.nlm.nih.gov/omim/

Virtual Hospital: Clinical Genetics: A self-study for health care providers
www.vh.org/Providers/Textbooks/ClinicalGenetics/Contents.html

Virtual Library on Genetics
www.ornl.gov/TechResources/Human_Genome/genetics.html

Visible Embryo
www.visembryo.ucsf.edu

Webget
www.med.upenn.edu/bioethic/webget

"Your genes, your choice"
ehrweb.aaas.org/ehr/books/index.html

GOVERNMENT PROGRAMS

CDC: Office of Genetics and Disease Prevention
www.cdc.gov/genetics/activities/ogdp.htm

Human Genome Project of the U.S. Department of Energy
www.ornl.gov/hgmis/

National Human Genome Research Institute
www.nhgri.nih.gov/

NATIONAL AND INTERNATIONAL ORGANIZATIONS

Genetic Alliance
www.geneticalliance.org

International Society of Nurses in Genetics (ISONG)
www.nursing.creighton.edu/isong/

March of Dimes Birth Defects Foundation
National Foundation/March of Dimes
1275 Mamaroneck Ave.
White Plains, NY 10605
914-428-7100
888-663-4637 (MODIMES)
www.modimes.org

Muscular Dystrophy Association of Canada
www.mdac.ca

Muscular Dystrophy Association of the United States of America
www.mdausa.org

National Cancer Institute
www.nci.nih.gov/

National Down Syndrome Congress
1800 Dempster St.
Park Ridge, IL 60068-1146
708-823-7550
800-232-6372

National Down Syndrome Society Hotline
666 Broadway
New York, NY 10012
800-221-4602

National Foundation for Jewish Genetic Diseases, Inc.
250 Park Ave., Suite 1000
New York, NY 10177
212-371-1030

National Society of Genetic Counselors
www.nsgc.org/

SITES FOR PARENTS AND FAMILIES

Alliance for Genetic Support Groups
www.geneticalliance.org

Ask NOAH About: Pregnancy
www.noah.cuny.edu/pregnancy/pregnancy.html

Family Guide to Cystic Fibrosis Genetic Testing
www.phd.msu.edu/cf/fam.html

Help4cysticfibrosis: Cystic Fibrosis Information
www.help4dysticfibrosis.com

National Down Syndrome Society
www.ndss.org

National Fragile X Foundation
www.nfx.org

National Marfan Foundation
www.marfan.org

Neurofibromatosis
www.nf.org

Osteogenesis Imperfecta Foundation
www.oif.org

World of Genetics Societies
www.faseb.org/genetics/mainmenu.htm

REFERENCES

ACMG/ASHG (1998). Laboratory guidelines for Huntington disease genetic testing. *American Journal of Human Genetics, 62,* 1243-1247.

Ad Hoc Committee on Genetic Counseling, American Society of Human Genetics (1975). Genetic counseling. *American Journal of Human Genetics, 27,* 240-242.

Anderson, W. (2000). Perspectives: Gene therapy: The best of times, the worst of times. *Science 288,* 627-628.

Asch, A. (1999). Prenatal diagnosis and selective abortion: A challenge to practice and policy. *American Journal of Public Health, 89,* 1649-1656.

Begleiter, M. (2002). Training for genetic counselors. *National Review of Genetics, 3,* 557-561.

Brower, V. (2001). Gene therapy revisited. *EMBO Reports, 21,* 1064-1065.

Bryar, S. (1997). One day you're pregnant and one day you're not: Pregnancy disruption for fetal anomalies. *Journal of Obstetric, Gynecologic, and Neonatal Nursing, 26,* 559-566.

Burgess, M., & d'Agincourt-Canning, L. (2002). Genetic testing for hereditary disease: Attending to relational responsibility. *Journal of Clinical Ethics, 12,* 361-372.

Burke, W., & Emery, J. (2002). Genetics education for primary-care providers. *National Review of Genetics, 3,* 561-566.

Burke, W., Pinsky, L., & Press, N. (2001). Categorizing genetic tests to identify their ethical, legal, and social implications. *American Journal of Medical Genetics, 106,* 233-240.

Carlson-Sabelli, L., & Lessick, M. (2001). Genetic advances in bipolar disorder. *AWHONN Lifelines, 5,* 34-41.

Cavazzana-Calvo, M. et al. (2000). Gene therapy of human severe combined immunodeficiency. *Science, 288,* 669-672.

Chandler, M., & Smith, A. (1998). Prenatal screening and women's perception of infant disability: A Sophie's Choice for every mother. *Nursing Inquiry, 5,* 71-76.

Cohen, W. (1999). Health care guidelines for individuals with Down syndrome: 1999 revision. *Down Syndrome Quarterly, 4,* 1-16.

Collins, F. (1997). Preparing health care professionals for the genetic revolution. *Journal of the American Medical Association, 278,* 1285-1286.

Collins, F. (2001). Contemplating the end of the beginning. *Genome Research, 11,* 641-643.

Collins, F., & Guttmacher, A. (2001). Genetics moves into the medical mainstream. *Journal of the American Medical Association, 286,* 2322-2324.

Collins, F., & Mansoura, M. (2001). The human genome project: Revealing the shared inheritance of all humankind. *Cancer Supplement, 91,* 221-225.

Collins, F., & McKusick, V. (2001). Implications of the Human Genome Project for medical science. *Journal of the American Medical Association, 285,* 540-544.

Demsey, S. (2000). Carrier screening for cystic fibrosis: A perinatal perspective. *Nursing Clinics of North America, 35,* 14-26.

Diekelmann, N., & Diekelmann, J. (2000). Learning ethics in nursing and genetics: Narrative pedagogy and the grounding of values. *Journal of Pediatric Nursing, 15,* 226-231.

Evers-Kiebooms, G., & Decruyenaere, M. (1998). Predictive testing of Huntington's disease: A challenge for persons at risk and for professionals. *Patient Education and Counseling, 35,* 15-26.

Freeman, S. et al. (1998). Population-based study of congenital heart defects in Down syndrome. *American Journal of Human Genetics, 80,* 213-217.

Gardiner, R. (2002). The human genome project: The next decade. *Archives of Disease in Childhood, 86,* 389-391.

Gelehrter, T., Collins, F., & Ginsberg, D. (1998). *Principles of medical genetics* (2nd ed.). Baltimore: Williams & Wilkins.

Grant, S. (2000). Prenatal genetic screening, *Online Journal of Issues in Nursing, 5,* 2. Available at www.nursingworld.org/ojin/topic13/tpc13_3.htm

Green, R., & Thomas, A. (1997). Whose gene is it? A case discussion about familial conflict over genetic testing for breast cancer. *Journal of Genetic Counseling, 6,* 245-253.

Greendale, K., & Pyeritz, R. (2001). Empowering primary care health professionals: How soon? How fast? How far? *American Journal of Human Genetics, 106,* 223-232.

Greenlee, R. et al. (2001). Cancer statistics, 2001. *CA: A Cancer Journal for Clinicians, 51,* 15-36.

Hassold, T., & Hunt, P. (2001). Too err (meiotically) is human: The genesis of human aneuploidy. *National Review of Genetics, 2,* 280-291.

Hedenfalk, I. et al. (2001). Gene-expression profiles in hereditary breast cancer. *New England Journal of Medicine, 344,* 539-548.

Hetteberg, C. et al. (1999). National survey of genetics content in basic nursing preparatory programs in the United States. *Nursing Outlook, 47,* 168-174.

Huntington's Disease Society of America (2001). *The marker.* New York: Huntington's Disease Society of America, Inc.

International Human Genome Sequencing Consortium (2001). Initial sequencing and analysis of the human genome. *Nature, 409,* 860-921.

International Society for Nurses in Genetics, ISONG (1998). *Statement on the scope and standards of genetics clinical nursing.* Washington, DC: American Nurses Association.

Jenkins, J. (2000). A historical perspective on genetic care. *Online Journal of Issues in Nursing, 5.* www.nursingworld.org/ojin/topic13/tpc13_3.htm.

Jones, K. (1997). *Smith's recognizable patterns of human malformation* (5th ed.). Philadelphia: W.B. Saunders.

Jones, S. (2000). Reproductive genetic technologies: Exploring ethical and policy implications. *AWHONN Lifelines, 4,* 33-36.

Jones, S., & Fallon, L. (2002). Reproductive options for individuals at risk for transmission of a genetic disorder. *Journal of Obstetric, Gynecologic, and Neonatal Nursing, 31,* 193-198.

Jorde, L. et al. (1999). *Medical genetics* (2nd ed.). St. Louis: Mosby.

Juengst, E. (1998). Caught in the middle again: Professional ethical considerations in genetic testing for health risks. *Genetic Testing, 1,* 189-200.

Juengst, E. (1999). Genetic testing and the moral dynamics of family life. *Public Understanding of Science, 8,* 1-13.

Kay, M. et al. (2000). Evidence for gene transfer and expression of factor IX in haemophilia B patients treated with an AAV vector. *Nature Genetics, 24,* 257-261.

Khan, J. et al. (2001). Classification and diagnostic prediction of cancers using gene expression profiling and artificial neural networks. *Nature Medicine, 6,* 673-679.

Lashley, F. (1998). *Clinical genetics in nursing practice* (2nd ed.) New York: Springer Publishing Company.

Lea, D. (2000). A new world view of genetics service models. *Online Journal of Issues in Nursing, 5.* www.nursingworld.org/ojin/topic13/tpc13_6.htm

Lea, D., Feetham, S., & Monsen, R. (2002). Genomic-based health care in nursing: A bi-directional approach to bringing genetics into nursing's body of knowledge. *Journal of Professional Nursing, 18,* 120-129.

Lea, D., Jenkins, J., & Francomano, C. (1998). *Genetics in clinical practice: New directions for nursing and health care.* Sudbury, MA: Jones and Bartlett Publishers.

Lea, D., & Williams, J. (2001). Are you ready for the genetics revolution? *American Journal of Nursing, 101,* 11.

Lessick, M., & Anderson, M. (2000). Genetic discoveries: Challenges for nurses who care for children and their families. *Journal of the Society of Pediatric Nursing, 5,* 47-51.

Lewis, J. (2002). Genetics in perinatal nursing: Clinical applications and policy considerations. *Journal of Obstetric, Gynecologic, and Neonatal Nursing, 31,* 188-192.

Lewis, R. (2001). *Human genetics: Concepts and applications.* Boston, MA: McGraw-Hill.

Lloyd-Puryear, M., & Forsman, I. (2002). Newborn screening and genetic testing. *Journal of Obstetric, Gynecologic, and Neonatal Nursing, 31,* 200, 207.

Loud, J. et al. (2002). Application of advances in molecular biology and genomics to clinical cancer care. *Cancer Nursing, 25,* 110-122.

Mahowald, M. et al. (2001). *Genetics in the clinics: Clinical, ethical, and social implications for primary care.* St. Louis: Mosby.

Malone, K. et al. (1998). BRCA1 mutations and breast cancer in the general population: Analyses in women before age 35 years and in women before age 45 years with first-degree family history. *Journal of the American Medical Association, 279,* 922-929.

Marteau, T., & Dormandy, E. (2001). Facilitating informed choice in prenatal testing: How well are we doing? *American Journal of Medical Genetics, 106,* 185-190.

Matthews, A. (1999). Chromosomal abnormalities: Trisomy 18, trisomy 13, deletions, and microdeletions. *Journal of Perinatal and Neonatal Nursing, 13,* 59-75.

Menix, K. (1999). State of the art: Continuing education in nursing and genetics. *Biological Research in Nursing, 1,* 122-127.

Monsen, R. (1999). State of the art: Interdisciplinary collaboration for health professional education in genetics. *Biological Research in Nursing, 1,* 119-121.

Mueller, R., & Young, I. (2001). *Emery's elements of medical genetics* (11th ed.) New York: Churchill Livingstone.

National Down Syndrome Society (2002). *Down syndrome myths and facts.* Available at www.ndss.org/content.cfm?fuseaction=InfoResGeneralArticle&article=29

Nehring, W., & Faux, S. (1999). Clinical genetics: An overview. *Journal of Cardiovascular Nursing, 13*(4), 19-33.

Pennisi, E. (2002). Genome centers push for polished draft. *Science, 296,* 1600-1601.

Phillips, K. et al. (2001). Potential role of pharmacogenomics in reducing adverse drug reactions. *Journal of the American Medical Association, 286,* 2270-2279.

Prows, C. et al. (1999). Preparation of undergraduate faculty to incorporate genetic content into curricula. *Biological Research in Nursing, 1,* 108-122.

Raines, D. (1999). Suspended mothering: Women's experiences mothering an infant with a genetic anomaly identified at birth. *Neonatal Network, 18,* 35-39.

Roses, A. (2000). Pharmacogenetics and the practice of medicine. *Nature, 405,* 857-865.

Scheuerle, A. (2001). Diagnosis of genetic disease. In M. Mahowald, A. Scheuerle, V. McKusick, & T. Aspinwall (Eds.), *Genetics in the clinic: Clinical, ethical, and social implications for primary care.* St. Louis: Mosby.

Subramanian, G. et al. (2001). Implications of the human genome for understanding human biology and medicine. *Journal of the American Medical Association, 286,* 2296-2307.

Thomson, E. (1997). Ethical, legal, social, and policy issues in genetics. In F. Lashley (Ed.), *The genetics revolution: Implications for nursing.* Washington, DC: American Academy of Nursing.

Tinkle, M. (2002). Cystic fibrosis carrier screening: Are nurses ready to be on the front line? *AWHONN Lifelines, 6,* 134-139.

Tinkle, M., & Cheek, D. (2002). Human genomics: Challenges and opportunities. *Journal of Obstetric, Gynecologic, and Neonatal Nursing, 31,* 30-38.

Touchette, N. et al. (Eds.) (1997). *Toward the 21st century: Incorporating genetics into primary health care.* Cold Spring Harbor, NY: Cold Spring Harbor Laboratory Press.

Van Riper, M. (1999). Living with Down syndrome: The family experience. *Down Syndrome Quarterly, 4,* 1-11.

Van Riper, M., & Cohen, W. (2001). Caring for children with Down syndrome and their families. *Journal of Pediatric Health Care, 15,* 123-131.

Venter, J. et al. (2001). The sequence of the human genome. *Science, 291,* 1304-1351.

Voglestein, B., & Kinzler, K. (1998). *The genetic basis of human cancer.* New York: McGraw-Hill.

Wertz, D. (1997). How many people seek genetic testing for cystic fibrosis, BRCA1, and Huntington's disease? *The Gene Letter, 1,* 1-3.

Williams, J. (1999). Evolution and current status of graduate programs in nursing genetics. *Biological Research in Nursing, 1,* 103-107.

Williams, J. (2000). Impact of genome research on children and their families. *Journal of Pediatric Nursing, 15,* 207-211.

Williams, J. et al. (1999). Adults seeking presymptomatic gene testing for Huntington disease. *Image: the Journal of Nursing Scholarship, 31,* 109-114.

Yang, Q., Rasmussen, S., & Friedman, J. (2002). Mortality associated with Down's syndrome in the USA from 1983 to 1997: A population-based study. *Lancet, 359,* 1019-1024.

Yoon, P. et al. (2001). Public health impact of genetic tests at the end of the 20th century. *Genetic Medicine, 3,* 405-410.

Zawacki, K., & Phillips, M. (2002). Cancer genetics and women's health. *Journal of Obstetric, Gynecologic, and Neonatal Nursing, 31,* 208-216.

CHAPTER 4

Wendy Wetzel

Alternative and Complementary Therapies

http://evolve.elsevier.com/Lowdermilk/MatWmnHlth/

LEARNING OBJECTIVES

- Describe the differences between standard (allopathic or Western) and holistic health care.
- Define the biopsychosocial and spiritual implications of holistic health care.
- Outline the advantages of a holistic philosophy.
- Compare and contrast touch, energetic, mind-body, and alternative pharmacologic healing modalities.
- Discuss the limitations of research in holistic healing.
- Identify the appropriate modalities for integrative women's health care.

It began as a quiet revolution. Consumers, feeling dismayed with the depersonalization of health care and the increasing reliance on high technology and specialization, began investigating alternatives to **standard (Western** or **allopathic) medicine.** Voicing dissatisfaction with hurried providers, decisions made by insurance companies, and increasing health care costs, some consumers turned to folk healers, spiritual healers, massage therapists, or herbalists.

It has long been argued that the current health care system is disease focused. For example, insurance companies may offer reimbursement for the treatment of various illnesses but not for health maintenance activities; new drugs for chronic illnesses appear in large numbers, but little attention is paid to the role of diet in health and in disease. Stress has been identified as a major health problem, but the treatment of choice has often been pharmaceutical agents rather than lifestyle change and stress management techniques at a fraction of the cost.

In an emerging paradigm, health is valued, and a new appreciation for the connection of body, mind, and spirit is honored and nurtured. Human values, including **spirituality** (that which brings values, meaning, and purpose to life, blending with the sense of the divine, the natural environment, other individuals, and the inner self), ethics, and partnership within health care, are blending with the finest in technology and research. In her classic work, Ferguson (1980) suggested that **holistic healing,** including **alternative and complementary therapies,** focuses on the correction of underlying disharmony in the interaction of body, mind, and spirit and demonstrates concern and compassion for the whole client, not just the client's symptoms (Box 4-1). **Holism** (a philosophy that an integrated whole has an independent reality that is greater than the sum of its parts, that patterns and processes combine to form the whole, and that evaluation, acceptance, and modulation of those patterns can lead to profound personal healing) encompasses attitude, acceptance, perception, and purpose.

Many of the popular **alternative healing modalities** offer **human-centered care,** with philosophies that recognize the value of the client's input and honor the individual's beliefs, values, and desires. The focus of these modalities is the whole person, not just a disease complex. Clients often find that alternative modalities are more consistent with their own belief systems and allow more client autonomy in health care decisions (Astin, 1998).

Although standard medical practice excels in many areas, alternative methods are often cited as being more beneficial for the treatment of chronic illness, as well as being more cost-effective because of the emphasis on preventive care and health maintenance (Peters et al., 2001; Weil, 1998a).

As consumer demand for alternatives grew, the medical community began to investigate these therapies. Current researchers suggest that increasing numbers of American adults are seeking alternative and complementary health care and estimate that more than 629 million visits were made in 1997 alone, an increase of 47% over previous use. This volume exceeds visits paid to primary health care providers. Expenditures related to alternative therapies are estimated at $27 billion, approximately half of which is out-of-pocket expense not covered by insurance (Eisenberg et al., 1998). Throughout the world, the use of traditional medicine presents unique challenges in terms of policy, efficacy, accessibility, and utilization (WHO, 2002).

BOX 4-1 **Definitions**

An understanding of the following terms used to describe alternative therapies is essential:

- **Acupressure** Massage techniques applied to specific points along certain energy pathways of the body called meridians. A form of treatment based in the theories of traditional Chinese medicine.
- **Acupuncture** A form of treatment using slender needles to stimulate points along energy pathways to correct, enhance, and rebalance the flow of body energy.
- **Alternative and complementary therapies** Nontraditional approaches to health care and healing, often philosophically different from Western medicine. Often involve interventions that are said to induce healing from within the client or improve the internal environment so that the body, mind, or spirit can heal. Often referred to as "natural healing." Can be used in place of or in conjunction with standard health care practices. Also defined as therapeutic modalities not commonly taught by U.S. medical schools or available in U.S. hospitals. Alternative healing often refers to those modalities used *in place of* conventional (or other) health care. Complementary healing refers to those modalities used *in conjunction with* conventional (or other) health care. Many therapies can be either alternative or complementary.
- **Biofeedback** Techniques that teach the client to consciously control certain body functions usually thought of as unconscious (breathing, heart rate, etc.). Often involves electronic instrumentation that provides immediate visual and auditory feedback to assist the learning process.
- **Energy healing** A variety of techniques and disciplines that are said to augment, modulate, stimulate, or remedy certain deficiencies or blocks in the human energy system.
- **Guided imagery** The use of imagination and thought processes in a purposeful way to change certain physiologic and emotional conditions.
- **Healing** The integrating and balancing of the body, mind, and spirit. May or may not effect physical healing from illness. Often perceived as improved sense of well-being, acceptance, and inner peace and harmony.
- **Healing touch** A combination of energetic healing techniques used by nurses and other health care professionals.
- **Holism** Philosophy that states that the whole is greater than the sum of its parts. In healing, refers to consideration and treatment of the whole client as a unified being. May include alternative and complementary modalities but is more a philosophic base than a modality in and of itself.
- **Holistic medicine** Health care treatment with techniques not commonly taught in U.S. medical schools or widely available in U.S. hospitals. May include a variety of disciplines involving diet, exercise, vitamin and nutritional supplements, body work, or alternative pharmacologic agents. Philosophy of medicine that encompasses holism.
- **Holistic nursing** Nursing practice that stems from the philosophy of holism, one that views the client as an integrated whole and is influenced by a variety of internal and external factors, including the biopsychosocial and spiritual dimensions of the person, an integrated whole.
- **Meditation** Any activity that focuses the attention in the present moment and, in the process, quiets and relaxes the mind and body.
- **Reflection** Looking within for solutions and answers to certain dilemmas, using intuition and inner wisdom as guides for attainment of healing.
- **Relaxation** The absence or alleviation of mental, physical, and emotional tension through purposeful activities that quiet the mind and body.
- **Spirituality** The individual's connection to one's own values, purpose, and meaning of life. May encompass organized religion or belief in higher power or authority. Recognition of wisdom, imagination, spirit, and intuition. A perception of the unity of nature and the interconnectedness of all beings; inner strength.
- **Standard (Western or allopathic) medicine** Interchangeable terms used to describe the current American health care system. With foundations in germ theory and reductionism, standard medical practice often focuses on one body system or disease complex. Treatments are often pharmaceutical or surgical and produce effects that are different from those of the disease complex.
- **Therapeutic touch** A modern interpretation of the laying on of hands for healing, as interpreted by Dolores Krieger, PhD, RN, and Dora Kunz, a noted healer. Originally taught within nursing programs.
- **Traditional Chinese medicine** Ancient methods of healing that combine herbs, energy healing, and movement as a pathway to health. Seeks to heal on deeper levels rather than just deal with symptoms.

Sources: Cassileth, B. (1998). *The alternative medicine handbook: The complete reference guide to alternative and complementary therapies.* New York: W.W. Norton; Chilton, B. (1998). Recognizing spirituality. *Image: Journal of Nursing Scholarship* 30(4), 400-401; Dossey, B. (Ed.). (1997). *Core curriculum for holistic nursing.* Gaithersburg, MD: Aspen; Dossey, B., Keegan, L., Guzzetta, C., & Kolkmeier, L. (1995). *Holistic nursing: A handbook for practice* (2nd ed.). Gaithersburg, MD: Aspen; Eisenberg, D. et al. (1998). Trends in alternative medicine use in the United States, 1990-1997. *Journal of the American Medical Association* 280, 1569-1575; Eisenberg, D., Kessler, R., & Forster, C. (1993). Unconventional medicine in the United States. *New England Journal of Medicine* 329, 246-252; Ferguson, M. (1980). *The Aquarian conspiracy.* Los Angeles: J.P. Tarcher; and Strohecker, J. (Ed.). (1994). *Alternative medicine: The definitive guide.* Puyallup, WA: Future Medicine.

Although skeptical at first, physicians, nurses, and other providers began to see the value in integrating some of these alternative methods into health care. The research and knowledge base for alternative and complementary therapies has grown and will continue to expand as the interest in and quest for healing continues.

This chapter presents an overview of alternative and complementary therapies, their place in current health care practices, current research endeavors, the role of the nurse in holistic health care, and possibilities for use in women's health care.

OVERVIEW OF ALTERNATIVE AND COMPLEMENTARY MODALITIES

Alternative health care options are many and diverse. Some modalities focus on the body structure and balance, and some, on the biochemical environment. Various treatment forms address emotional and psychologic health, and others work with the human energy field. It is beyond the scope of this chapter to address all the philosophic and procedural specifics of current alternative and complementary therapies; many texts and reference volumes provide detailed information (Cassileth, 1998; Clark, 1999; Peters et al., 2001).

Regardless of modality, several concepts are shared by many of these systems. First, there is an emphasis on the client as a whole being, capable of decision making, and an integral part of the health care team. Clients are encouraged to take responsibility for their health and healing. Equal consideration is provided for all the biopsychosocial and spiritual needs of the client. Each client is seen as a unique individual, and treatment is tailored to that specific person (Dossey, 1997; Dossey, Keegan, & Guzzetta, 2000).

Second, proper nutrition, adequate rest, relaxation, exercise, and emotional health are cornerstones of good health and are thought to promote healing. Although various philosophies advocate a variety of dietary regimens, there is agreement that nutrition is often overlooked by mainstream medicine and must be emphasized for healing to occur. Our fast-paced culture often seems to deny individuals the chance to make time for rest, relaxation, exercise, and spiritual renewal (Dossey et al., 2000; Weil, 1998b).

Third, signs and symptoms of disease states are seen as reflective of deeper processes, including those on the emotional and spiritual levels. Alternative healing modalities attempt to treat those deeper levels and the underlying causes, rather than just the symptoms. Physical symptoms are seen as signals from the mind and the spirit that change is in order (Gerber, Tiller, & Cousens, 2001; Shames & Hover-Kramer, 1997; Starn, 1998).

The road to healing therefore becomes an individual journey, encompassing the client's entire being, while addressing specific physical, mental, emotional, spiritual, and social needs.

Integrative Health Care

The health care community exists as a fluid and dynamic environment. With a variety of clinicians, from physicians and nurses, physical therapists, and mental health counselors to acupuncturists and massage therapists, energy healers and herbalists, a variety of philosophies and treatment options exist.

Western medicine excels in the treatment of acute diseases, bacterial diseases, surgical emergencies, and trauma. It has also, by necessity, become highly specialized and systematic. With the vast amount of information and research available, it is virtually impossible for one practitioner to know and absorb all of the current data. With increasing specialization in health care, providers often focus on one body system or disease, and other symptoms may be overlooked or not evaluated. Clients who seek alternative health care often do so in an attempt to find a practitioner who will address the client as a whole person and who shares the client's own philosophy, convictions, and values (Astin, 1998; Weil, 1998a).

Western medicine has been less successful in the treatment of chronic disease states, such as diabetes, heart disease, immune disorders, and environmental illnesses. Over time, the role of the mind in the health of the body has been forgotten or neglected. Chronic disease states have been treated with an increasing number of pharmaceutic agents or invasive surgery, but the root causes of such ailments have not been considered. The avenues to continued and improved health have not been fully explored (Weil, 1998b; Wetzel, Eisenberg, & Kaptchuk, 1998).

It is imperative that health care become an integrative and cooperative venture, one in which both mainstream and alternative medicine can be accessed and used. Fortunately, an environment is being created in which healing forms are used for what they do best and work side by side in harmony. Medical schools, hospitals, and health care institutions are devising integrative health care models, and these programs are expected to proliferate as the health care system responds to increased consumer demand (Wetzel et al., 1998). Barriers still exist to complete integration, including a lack of research; opposing or competing philosophies and paradigms; health care cost concerns; lack of consistency in state licensing laws; and lasting biases, attitudes, and prejudices (Peters et al., 2001; Phalen, 1998).

Research Efforts

In 1992 the National Institutes of Health (NIH) developed the Office of Alternative Medicine (OAM). Mandated by Congress, the OAM was designed to support research and evaluation of various alternative and complementary modalities and to provide information to health care consumers about such modalities. With a beginning budget of $2 million in 1992, the OAM was awarded a $20 million budget in 1998 to provide research grants; develop and maintain a research database; disseminate information to both health care providers and consumers; support, evaluate, and coordinate domestic and worldwide research; and train researchers. In 1998 Congress instituted the National Center for Complementary and Alternative Medicine (NCCAM), which incorporates the work of the OAM in its mission and function. With additional funding, NCCAM will expand its research focus (Dossey, 1998; NCCAM, 2002).

To facilitate definitions and research, the NIH established seven categories of alternative and complementary healing (Table 4-1). Although many therapies belong in more than one category, this system provides a starting point for research and data collection.

The creation of OAM and later NCCAM made a substantial statement regarding the willingness of legislators and health care officials to consider integration of these modalities into mainstream health care. Funding has been granted to researchers investigating guided imagery, biofeedback, prayer, movement (dance, yoga, qi gong, and tai chi), music, acupuncture, chiropractic, massage, homeopathy, herbs, and other therapies for a variety of disease processes and health concerns (NCCAM/OAM, 1999).

THE NURSE'S ROLE: HOLISTIC NURSING

Nursing is coming full circle. As consumers seek medical treatment that is more caring and personal, nurses are playing a key role in the rehumanization of health care. Although it was originally grounded in the holistic theories of Nightingale (Dossey, 2000), nursing has moved into highly technical areas, often losing some of the human-centered caring that was once its hallmark. Many nurses now are rediscovering the value of client-centered care that addresses the whole person, not just a diagnosis or condition. With that realization, these nurses often self-identify as holistic nurses.

Holistic nurses can be found in every area of nursing practice. Being holistic refers more to one's underlying philosophy than to the tasks assigned to a specific nurse. Holistic nurses provide care that is relationship centered rather than disease or task oriented. By seeing the client as a whole individual, nurses can then provide care that encompasses all of the needs of the individual: physical, emotional, spiritual, or social. Seeking to blend technology with healing, holistic nurses are striving to create models of health care that embrace the whole person while enhancing healing and the interconnectedness of all beings (Dossey et al., 2000). Holistic nurses recognize the need for health care to be based on the interrelated relationships between client and provider, provider and provider, and community and provider. By acknowledging the importance of these levels of relationship, nurses can develop strategies for professional and personal growth (Keegan & Dossey, 1998).

Although many holistic nurses incorporate and integrate alternative and complementary healing modalities

TABLE 4-1 National Institutes of Health Categories of Alternative Healing Modalities

CATEGORY	EXAMPLES
Alternative systems of medical practice	Acupuncture Ayurveda Environmental medicine Homeopathy Native American healing Naturopathic medicine Shamanism Traditional Chinese medicine
Bioelectromagnetic applications	Electroacupuncture Neuromagnetic stimulation devices
Diet, nutrition, lifestyle changes	Changes in lifestyle Diet Macrobiotics Megavitamins and other nutritional supplements
Herbal medicine	Herbal approaches from a variety of cultures including the Americas, Europe, and the Far East
Manual healing	Acupressure Chiropractic Massage therapy Osteopathy Reflexology Therapeutic touch/healing touch Trager method
Mind-body control	Art therapy Biofeedback Counseling Dance therapy Guided imagery and hypnosis Humor therapy Meditation Music therapy Prayer Psychotherapy Relaxation Support and self-help groups Yoga
Pharmacologic and biologic treatments	Antioxidizing agents Chelation therapy Oxidizing agents Vaccines (not currently accepted by mainstream medicine)

Sources: Dossey, B. (1998). Holistic modalities and healing moments. *American Journal of Nursing, 98*(6), 44-47; and National Center for Complementary and Alternative Medicine (NCCAM)/Office of Alternative Medicine (OAM). (2002). Internet document: http://nccam.nih.gov.

BOX 4-2 Description of Holistic Nursing

Holistic nursing embraces all nursing practice that has healing the whole person as its goal. Holistic nursing recognizes that there are two views regarding holism: that holism involves studying and understanding the interrelationships of the biopsychosocial and spiritual dimensions of the person, recognizing that the whole is greater than the sum of its parts; and that holism involves understanding the individual as an integrated whole interacting with and being acted on by both internal and external environments. Holistic nursing accepts both views, believing that the goals of nursing can be achieved within either framework.

Holistic practice draws on nursing knowledge, theories, expertise, and intuition to guide nurses in becoming therapeutic partners with clients in strengthening the client's responses to facilitate the healing process and achieve wholeness.

Practicing holistic nursing requires nurses to integrate self-care in their own lives. Self-responsibility leads the nurse to a greater awareness of the interconnectedness of all individuals and their relationships to the human and global community, and it permits nurses to use this awareness to facilitate healing.

Source: American Holistic Nurses' Association. (2000). *Mission statement.* Flagstaff, AZ: AHNA.

into their practices, these techniques are not prerequisites for holistic nursing practice. **Holistic nursing practice** rather reflects the attitudes and philosophy brought to the nursing situation, rather than the techniques or modalities used during the course of nursing care. Holistic nurses also involve themselves in self-care activities, striving to attain their own levels of wellness and integration (Box 4-2) (Dossey et al., 2000; Frisch et al., 2000; Keegan & Dossey, 1998).

LEGAL TIP

Although a vast array of alternative healing modalities are available, not all of them are within the scope of nursing practice, as defined by licensing bodies (Box 4-3). Nurses are advised to consult their own state's nurse practice act for details.

As the body of knowledge grows, more methods will be integrated into nursing practice. Many modalities require intensive training, additional certification, or both. As with basic nursing practice, certain competencies must be established before using the skill with clients. With the introduction of dozens of various modalities into health care, nurses are cautioned to examine carefully the reputation, research, and educational criteria of any program of study.

BOX 4-3 Holistic Therapies and Modalities Most Commonly Used in Nursing

- *Body therapies,* including acupressure, healing touch, massage, therapeutic touch, reflexology
- *Mind-body healing,* including art therapy, biofeedback, cognitive therapy, counseling (in cases of addiction, grief, environmental concerns, relationships, spiritual crisis, violence and sexual abuse, and wellness issues), exercise and movement, goal setting and contracts, holistic self-assessment, journaling and self-reflection, meditation, prayer, humor and laughter, imagery, music and sound therapy, play therapy, rituals of healing (combining several modalities)
- *Lifestyle modifications,* including smoking cessation, weight management

Source: Dossey, B. (1998). Holistic modalities and healing moments. *American Journal of Nursing 98*(6), 4-47; Dossey, B. (Ed.). (1997). *Core curriculum for holistic nursing.* Gaithersburg, MD: Aspen.

The North American Nursing Diagnosis Association also has acknowledged the emergence of holism with several nursing diagnoses. These include altered/risk for/potential for/enhanced spiritual well-being, spiritual distress, and energy field disturbance. The Nursing Interventions Classification Code lists several alternative modalities as nursing interventions. These include but are not limited to therapeutic touch (TT), simple massage, touch, relaxation, meditation, imagery, and hypnosis (Dossey et al., 2000; Frisch et al., 2000).

Support and Education for Holistic Nursing

In 1980 a group of nurses and supporters formed the American Holistic Nurses' Association (AHNA) to assist and support nurses in their journeys to holism. A vital force in nursing today, AHNA has established certification in holistic nursing and published a core curriculum of holistic nursing practice (Dossey, 1997). It is the mission of AHNA "to unite nurses in healing" (American Holistic Nurses Association, 2000). This is to be accomplished through the development, implementation, and evaluation of the standards, education, and research for holistic nursing. This mission is accomplished through various educational offerings, certification, and support of holistic nursing research. AHNA also supports the individual journey toward wholeness and healing by encouraging self-care and personal growth for nurses (AHNA, 2000; Frisch et al., 2000).

AHNA established criteria to guide holistic nursing practice. Although similar to standard nursing principles, the Core Values for Holistic Nursing Practice (Dossey, 1997; Frisch et al., 2000) reflect the interconnectedness and partnerships that clearly herald a new era of nursing.

Within holistic nursing, other organizations have been established to promote the use of various modalities and healing techniques. Of these, Nurse Healers–Professional Associates International, Inc. (NH-PAI), is one of the largest specialty groups. Focusing on TT with the Krieger-Kunz method, NH-PAI supports TT research and education and sets standards for the practice and scope of the method. They also have been instrumental in creating guidelines and procedures for using TT in health care settings and for practitioner and instructor competency.

Healing Touch International, Inc. (HTI), is another specialty organization that promotes education and research with various forms of **energy healing.** Healing Touch is not restricted to nurses and has grown rapidly in its use and knowledge base. National certification is available to practitioners and instructors. HTI is now recognized in the United States, Canada, and many European countries.

Although these three organizations are representative of nursing involvement in holistic care, many others exist to promote their own specialty or modality (see Resources at end of this chapter). Many welcome nurses as members and supporters. As nurses continue to integrate alternative healing into their practices, additional doors will open for education and support.

BOX 4-4 Representative Alternative Therapies Commonly Used by Nurses in Women's Health Care

TOUCH AND ENERGETIC THERAPIES

Massage
Acupressure
Therapeutic touch
Healing touch

MIND-BODY HEALING

Imagery
Meditation, prayer, reflection
Biofeedback
Other modalities that may fall outside of nurse practice guidelines unless the nurse has completed additional training or certification:
- Herbs
- Homeopathy
- Traditional Chinese medicine

ALTERNATIVE AND COMPLEMENTARY THERAPIES IN WOMEN'S HEALTH CARE

Women's health care is an emerging specialty. There is increased realization that the human female body is biochemically different from that of a male. The long-standing gender biases of Western medicine are giving way to a broader view of women's health care. In the realm of **holistic medicine,** too, an increasing number of modalities are seen as appropriate and are being integrated into care. Thousands of articles and books exist on these topics; this section addresses only an overview of a representative sample of those most often used in women's health care and specific to nursing practice (Box 4-4).

Nurses are cautioned to be informed regarding the statutes of their state nurse practice act and to seek the additional training required to integrate complementary healing into their nursing practice.

Touch and Energetic Healing

One of the most primitive yet effective healing gestures is that of touch. First recorded more than 5000 years ago by ancient Asian healers, touch has been a key element of healing through the ages. It is a natural instinct to touch that which hurts or needs comfort. The touch of a mother's hand to her child's feverish head and the touch of one friend to another in a time of crisis are clear images of this intuitive healing method.

Archaeologic data from ancient cultures, including East Indian, Asian, Native American, and other civilizations, show evidence of touch being integral to the health care systems of these eras. Healing by the laying on of hands was a key element in many spiritual traditions, including those of the ancient Egyptians, Greeks, and Celts. As medicine became a separate entity, the practice of hands-on healing declined. Early medical scientists viewed it as a superstition and characteristic of more primitive healing. Not until the twentieth century did touch became a research topic in modern medicine (Gerber et al., 2001; Oschman, 2000).

Early studies showed that touch was vital to human development and had a positive impact on immune function. Other preliminary work documented reduction in heart rate, diastolic blood pressure, and anxiety through touch. Over time, nurses have embraced touch as a therapeutic tool and have studied its effects in client care. Several forms of touch therapy have arisen from this work (Dossey, 1997; Gerber et al., 2001; Oschman, 2000; Sayre-Adams et al., 2001; Scheiber & Selby, 2000).

The use of touch for healing has many forms. Most people are familiar with massage therapy and its various methods. **Massage** involves rubbing, stroking, and manipulating the muscle groups and other connective tissue to relieve tension and pain and increase blood flow to the area, thus promoting healing. Various claims are made for the different modes of massage therapy, including increasing circulation, promoting lymphatic drainage, relieving muscle tension, aiding in recovery from certain musculoskeletal injuries, decreasing edema, and improving the functioning of certain body systems. Although simple massage is listed in the nursing intervention categories, therapeutic massage requires additional formal training, and national certification is available. Massage therapists are subject to individual state laws and regulations (Clark, 1999; Juhan, 1998).

Other forms of touch in healing combine physical touch and energetic theory. A variety of alternative and complementary therapies use an energy-based philosophy that essentially states that the human body has an energy field around and in it. That energy field not only is detectable, but also can be modulated and changed. Energy-based healing seeks to improve the health of the energy field, balance it, and restore it, so that the body then can heal. Any physical, emotional, or spiritual illness is said to be detectable in the field, as well as healed with the field (Hover-Kramer, Mentgen, & Scandrett-Hibdon, 2001; Oschman, 2000). In many respects, this is congruent with the nursing theory of Martha Rogers (1970), who spoke of the person as a four-dimensional being.

Energy healing has its roots in the writings of the ancient Hindus (who spoke of *prana*), Asians (who referred to it as *chi* or *qi*), and Greeks and early Christians. The healing ability of Christ is interpreted by some as an energetic healing form. Healing as part of a spiritual path was routinely practiced by clergy and lay persons alike within the context of their religious practices until Pope Alexander mandated a halt to the healing mission of the church in the twelfth century. Although this took healing out of the hands of the church, history records many talented healers who continued to use energetic techniques (Hover-Kramer et al., 2001; Sayre-Adams et al., 2001; Starn, 1998).

Acupressure is a variation on massage and touch that has its origins in **traditional Chinese medicine (TCM).** TCM states that *qi,* or *chi,* is the vital force of life, the energy of the body. If the energy is blocked or stagnated in any way, illness, pain, or other dysfunction can result. Energy travels on defined pathways throughout the body, called meridians, and on each meridian, a series of points corresponds to body function and various organs. Practitioners of TCM believe that by massaging or compressing a given point, the body energy to that corresponding organ or system can be restored or changed. When the energy flow is restored, healing can occur (Dossey, 1997; Elias & Ketcham, 1998; Gerber et al., 2001). Although nurses can learn a few select points to use with their clients, a comprehensive education program is desirable for the treatment of more complex health problems.

In nursing circles, one of the best-known methods of touch healing is **therapeutic touch (TT).** TT was designed by Dolores Krieger, PhD, RN, a professor of nursing at New York University. She documented a reproducible manner of touch, one in which the practitioner begins in a calm and centered state (called "centering") and holds thoughts of desiring to help or heal (called "intention"). TT has several steps in which the practitioner perceives the client's energy field and notes any areas of uneven activity, deficit, or increase. After observing and feeling the client's energy field, the practitioner can use techniques to modulate the energy and correct the deficiencies or abnormal areas. Krieger's seminal work in the field of human energy is well described in her many publications (Krieger, 1979, 1987, 1993, 2002). TT has been widely researched in the nursing field. Early studies documented pain relief, anxiety reduction, and wound healing; later work focused more on physiologic data (Easter, 1997; Krieger, 1990; Quinn, 1994; Sayre-Adams et al., 2001; Scheiber & Selby, 2000; Snyder & Lindquist, 2002).

Healing Touch (HT) is another energy-based touch healing modality. Whereas Krieger's work emphasizes a single sequence of energy modulation, HT combines a variety of techniques from a series of disciplines. This gives the practitioner an array of "tools" to use with clients. Practitioners are taught energetic diagnosis and treatment forms and the means for documenting the client's response and progress. These techniques are said to align and balance the human energy field, thereby enhancing the body's ability to heal itself. Proponents assert that HT can be useful for a variety of physical, mental, emotional, and spiritual disorders (Hover-Kramer et al., 2001; Shames & Hover-Kramer, 1997).

Nursing research on HT is expanding rapidly. Studies focusing on its use by nurses with clients experiencing chronic and acute pain, wound infections, cancer, human immunodeficiency virus infection, depression, fatigue, anxiety, and other health problems are being conducted or have been completed. Nurses also are investigating the phenomenologic implications of this modality, from both the client's and the provider's perspective. Of special note to nurses involved in women's health care are studies on HT with breast cancer clients and those recovering from abdominal hysterectomies (Healing Touch, 2001; Hover-Kramer et al., 2001).

TT and HT have been integrated in many health care facilities and institutions, and policies have been written and accepted to make these modalities part of inpatient care. As independent nursing interventions, they do not require a physician's order for the nurse to provide this service.

Mind-Body Healing

Use of the mind as a healing tool also is rooted in ancient teachings. The use of imagination, prayer, and meditation is found in numerous spiritual traditions dating back to the beginning of recorded history.

Guided imagery, the purposeful development of mental images while in a deep state of relaxation (Giedt, 1997), is used for relaxation, stress management, and enhancing immune function. Imagery allows or guides the normal flow of thoughts within the imagination. It can be likened to the sense of being worried, when mental pictures and thoughts of a dreaded event occur. Although there may not be a direct threat to the person at the time, the mind can induce feelings of fear with associated body symptoms such as tightening the chest or stomach or the onset of sweating. These symptoms are in response to a perception or a thought, but not always to a concurrent event. Imagery uses the power of the mind to induce positive images of healing, improve performance, and reduce anxiety. The mind will then influence the body to meet the image (Dossey et al., 2000; LeMaire, 2002; Snyder & Lindquist, 2002).

Proponents also state that a relaxed body and focused mind can bring about changes in perception and solutions to problems and heal emotional trauma. Imagery also has been used with clients with allergies, musculoskeletal pain, and acute injuries and in preoperative and postoperative situations. Cancer patients have used imagery to decrease the side effects of treatment. Nurses use guided imagery in private practice as well as in health care settings (Fig. 4-1). Imagery can assist relaxation, reduce anxiety, minimize the need for pain medications, and increase the client's ability to focus, while enhancing creativity. By using recall to enhance change, imagery also may alter emotional and biochemical processes (Dossey et al., 2000; Giedt, 1997; Hoffart & Pross-Keene, 1998).

One of the pioneers of imagery, O. Carl Simonton, MD, used imagery with his cancer patients to enhance their healing. For example, clients are asked to imagine the beams of radiation therapy hitting the cancer cells but leaving the healthy ones intact, or to envision a tumor mass shrinking. Simonton uses these methods in conjunction with other medical treatments, and his success has been well documented (Dossey, 1997).

Meditation, prayer, reflection, and **relaxation** are similar modalities, all creating an environment of inner quiet. These are ways of looking inside the self and connecting with inner wisdom and intuition. Although some religious traditions define prayer as a communication with God, others simply define it in terms of connecting with a divine or absolute power found within all beings. Prayer is said to be a speaking out, whereas meditation is a quiet listening. Reflection, then, is the evaluation and synthesis of the experience (Chilton, 1998; Dossey, 1997).

These techniques can aid in the relaxation response and decrease heart rate and blood pressure, thereby reducing stress, decreasing pain perception, and increasing self-understanding. This is thought to allow insight, cognitive awareness of body functioning, and an intuitive comprehension of what is needed for the individual healing process (Cassileth, 1998; Dossey, 1997; Snyder & Lindquist, 2002). The classic work of Benson and Proctor (1984) on the relaxation response indicated that physiologic function was enhanced when meditative and relaxing techniques were integrated into the subject's life. Stress-related illnesses decreased in severity, and the effects of chronic illness were reduced.

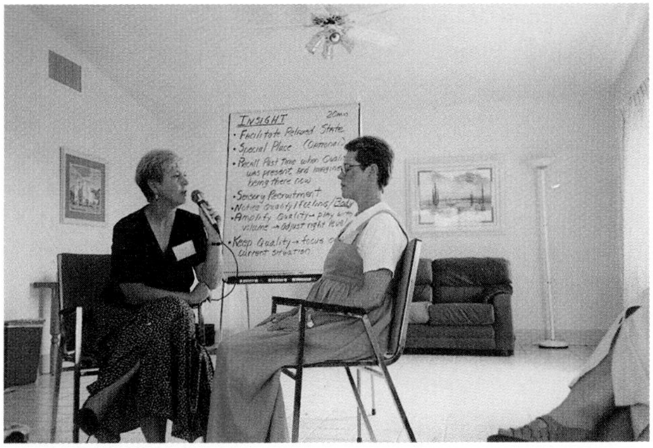
INSIGHT

FIG. 4-1 Nurse and client during guided imagery session. (Courtesy Nurses Certificate Program in Interactive Imagery, Foster City, CA.)

Biofeedback combines relaxation with consciously learning to regulate those body functions normally seen as automatic to improve health and decrease pain, blood pressure, and pulse rate. With specially designed equipment that can monitor heart rate, skin temperature, moisture, electrical conductivity, and muscle tension, clients are taught the means to reduce tension, induce relaxation, and isolate and exercise certain muscle groups. Biofeedback instruments provide immediate information to the client and show the progress made, thus enabling the client to reinforce the behaviors that brought about the desired change. For example, if a certain breathing technique induces a significant and desired change in heart rate and blood pressure, the client can immediately see the effects on the biofeedback instrumentation and feel the change within the body (Bray, 1998; Cassileth, 1998; Snyder & Lindquist, 2002).

Biofeedback has been used in a variety of settings for stress-related illness, as well as for systemic illnesses such as asthma. Treatment of disorders linked to muscle tension (headaches, temporomandibular joint disorders, hypertension) is especially effective and has been studied extensively (Bray, 1998; Cassileth, 1998; Gerber et al., 2001).

Biofeedback also can assist with muscle training. By enabling the client to focus on specific muscle groups, correct exercises can be learned with the help of biofeedback. After several sessions, the client is usually able to isolate and exercise the same muscle groups, even without the biofeedback equipment.

Alternative Pharmacologic Modalities

Some of the alternative therapies most frequently used by American consumers today are those involving alternatives to drug therapy. These modalities involve the use of herbs or other remedies outside the usual scope of pharmaceutic agents. Proper use of these therapies mandates additional education.

Herbs and other botanic substances were used for healing in many ancient civilizations. Although it is often considered a folk remedy, herbal medicine plays a significant role even today. Many of our current pharmacologic agents are derived from or originated in a plant-based model. Digitalis, for example, is a derivative of plants in the foxglove family, and atropine was first derived from the deadly nightshade. Recently herbal preparations have gained popularity, and several have been investigated for their medicinal qualities. St. John's wort has been identified as an antidepressant, and feverfew has been researched for its role in preventing migraines.

By definition, one is practicing herbal medicine if one uses a cup of mint tea to soothe an upset stomach. However, the science of herbal medicine is complex and precise. Herbs can vary in potency from day to day and season to season; whereas a small dose may be beneficial, a larger one can be hazardous. Herbal preparations are readily available to the public in a variety of settings, including health food stores and supermarkets. However, they can vary in concentration, and consumers should be advised to read all labels carefully for information about the actual herbal component of the selected preparation (Weed, 2001).

Herbs are classified according to their properties and effects. Most herbal medicine texts list the desired effect and the properties of the herb itself. Herbs can be delivered in whole form (dried and powdered), as a tea (steeped in water), as extracts and tinctures (small amounts dissolved in an alcohol base), in capsules or tablets, as concentrated "essential" oil, and in creams and salves.

Homeopathy is a system of healing founded by Samuel Hahnemann, a German physician, in the late 1700s. Hahnemann, also known for his work in pharmacology and toxicology, sought to find a more sensible and compassionate alternative to the medical practices of his day (for example, bloodletting with leeches and use of toxic laxatives). By experimenting with certain botanic agents, he confirmed Hippocrates' observation that small doses of the same agent that caused a disease would cure it. This also is the basis for modern immunologic medicine, wherein a small amount of a toxin, allergen, or virus stimulates the body to create immunity (Jonas, Jacobs, & Dossey, 1998; Skinner, 2001).

Homeopathic practitioners believe that each client is a unique individual, and care is directed to create and prescribe a remedy specific to that person. Although many standard remedies exist, practitioners often blend individual remedies based on the client's specific needs. Homeopathy also dictates that illness, as perceived on the physical level, is evidence of disturbances on other, deeper levels, and the remedies are thought to work through those other levels, from the most recent through the oldest, until full healing is achieved (Cassileth, 1998; Jonas et al., 1998; Skinner, 2001).

Combining herbal and energy medicine, TCM is experiencing a resurgence of popularity. It has been practiced for more than 3000 years and was one of the first methods of healing to be documented. TCM incorporates theories of energetic healing, often describing the energy flow as an excess or a deficiency. The goal of TCM is to restore total harmony on all levels, emotional, spiritual, and physical. Although acupressure is a discipline within TCM, traditional methods include **acupuncture** (the stimulation of specific points on the body with needles, herbs, or heat) and herbal treatments. Various movement forms such as *tai chi* and *qi gong* may be integrated into a program of TCM (Cassileth, 1998; Elias & Ketcham, 1998; Phalen, 1998).

Acupuncture is widely practiced in the United States for a variety of conditions and is showing promise in the areas of pain management (postoperative states, dental procedures, fibromyalgia, and myofascial pain) and nausea caused by pregnancy or chemotherapy. Research is continuing to determine its efficacy in other areas (National Institutes of Health, 1998).

Diet and Exercise

The current North American diet is changing; we have become a nation of "fast-food" eaters, quickly consuming meals that are high in fat and calories and often lacking in essential nutrients. Stress, lifestyle choices, and time constraints are most often cited as reasons for the lack of balanced food intake. Although there is no consistent agreement regarding actual intake and dietary structure, most will agree that reduction of saturated fats and calories and proportionate consumption of high-quality protein and complex carbohydrates are the keys to a balanced diet. Scores of weight-loss and food-management programs are available to the consumer, but not all provide the essential balance of nutrients (Martin & Jung, 2002; Northrup, 1998; Weil, 1998a, 1998b).

Adequate nutrition benefits the human system on all levels. These include but are not limited to normal organ development and functioning, appropriate metabolism, immune system response, optimal energy, reproductive function, functional repair of injury or tissue damage, appropriate emotional responses, and behavior (Dossey, 1997). Women seem especially sensitive to the lack of micronutrients and macronutrients in their diets, and deficiencies can manifest as hormonal changes or irregular menstrual periods, as well as affecting other endocrine functions (Martin & Jung, 2002; Northrup, 1998, 2001). Nurses should be aware that a diet history should be part of any care plan.

Citizens of our nation also lack the motivation for consistent exercise. Our lifestyle has become more sedentary, with hours spent in front of computers or television sets. Our children spend countless hours with video games. Current guidelines promote 60 minutes of some form of physical exercise daily to achieve the known benefits of improved cardiovascular health, decreased body fat, disease prevention, and increased sense of well-being. Exercise programs should be less outcome oriented and should focus more on daily progress. Weight-bearing exercise (especially walking) is extremely beneficial for women to prevent osteoporosis. Nursing interventions for the promotion of adequate physical exercise include providing motivation and support, working with the client to find an exercise form that suits the client's needs and ability, facilitating education regarding the numerous health benefits, and monitoring of the client's progress (Martin, 2002; Padden, 2002). Unlimited forms of exercise can be beneficial on a multitude of levels, including yoga, martial arts, aerobics, and weight and endurance training (Box 4-5, Fig. 4-2).

BOX 4-5 Yoga: An Example of Lifestyle Choice

With the increasing emphasis on diet and exercise programs, the practice of yoga can be used as an example of a lifestyle choice that meets a variety of needs, envisioning the client from a bio-psycho-social-spiritual perspective:

BIOLOGY

Yoga provides structured exercise that can increase strength, flexibility, and endurance. Postures or *asanas* focus on various body systems, are seen as corrective for certain disease states, and increase endorphin release. Although some definitions may be regionally different, yoga is practiced in a variety of forms, each presenting its own challenge and focus. *Hatha yoga* focuses on slowly and deliberately stretching within the asanas, lengthening and strengthening the various muscle groups. *Astanga yoga* promotes endurance with more difficult and athletic poses and stretches. *Vinyasa yoga* adds an aerobic component with more rapid progression with athletic postures. The postures are said to affect a variety of body functions, including balance, muscle tone, and coordination.

Yoga also incorporates controlled deep breathing or *pranayama* to energize and stimulate the body. This also is said to enhance cardiovascular functioning, stimulate blood flow, and reduce the effects of stress. Reduction in blood pressure has been noted.

Many practitioners adopt a vegetarian lifestyle, although that is not required. Practitioners state that the yoga lifestyle helps them to make healthier lifestyle choices, which may include goals of weight management and improved diet.

PSYCHOLOGY

Yoga seeks to relieve stress through the quieting of the mind and focused concentration. This meditative state is said to raise the level of consciousness beyond the daily mundane thought processes and bring inner peace. This, then, is a path to increased awareness.

Exercise has been shown to increase the release of endorphins, neurochemicals that can positively affect mood and mental state. This provides an increased sense of well-being, enhanced energy, and mental focus for other tasks.

SOCIAL

Yoga provides a community structure of other practitioners, offering common goals and experiences. Yoga comes for the Sanskrit word for "union," therefore bringing the practitioner from a fragmented state to one of unity of body, mind, and spirit. Yoga promotes a lifestyle of balance, harmony, unity, ethics, morals, and personal conduct.

SPIRITUALITY

Yoga promotes a form of meditation, focuses the flow of body energy, and connects the practitioner to the divine. This is said to promote inner peace and harmony. Yoga is congruent with a variety of spiritual practices and is not promoted as a religion.

Sources: Iyengar, B. (2001). *Yoga: The path to holistic health.* London: Dorling Kindersley; Martin, L., & Jung, P. (2002). *Taking charge of the change.* Albany, NY: Delmar; Mehta, M. (2001). *How to use yoga.* London: Anness Publishing Limited; Mehta, S., Mehta, M., & Mehta, S. (2001). *Yoga: The Iyengar way.* New York: Alfred A. Knopf.

Applications in Women's Health Care

Many women seek "natural" alternatives to invasive health care practices. Whether looking for natural childbirth or alternatives for menopause, women have been more open to complementary modalities and have more actively sought care from practitioners of holistic medicine. Research is ongoing, and significant strides are being made to open the doors to health care that encompasses the whole person while providing comprehensive health care (Collins, 2000; Northrup, 1998, 2001).

Pregnancy and Obstetric Care

Pregnancy is usually seen as a naturally occurring event, but highly technical medical practices have shifted the emphasis from a condition of health to one of potential disease. Although there is no disputing the advances in care of high risk obstetrics clients, most normal pregnancies can proceed safely with little or no intervention. Several commonly used alternative therapies can assist the expectant mother through gestation.

Nausea and vomiting of pregnancy can be a difficult problem. Although women with hyperemesis gravidarum must receive prompt and comprehensive care, the lesser nausea of the first trimester can be effectively treated with herbal teas. Herbs such as peppermint, spearmint, chamomile, and ginger can be used in teas and have been cited as possible remedies for "morning sickness." Other herbs, including fennel, hops, and wild yam, also have been named but are less accessible. Women may need to try several different herbal teas or alternate their use to achieve efficacy (Beal, 1998; Clark, 1999).

Certain homeopathic remedies also are noted to be effective for nausea. Many are available as over-the-counter products, or a skilled homeopath can construct an appropriate mixture based on the severity of the woman's symptoms (Beal, 1998; Clark, 1999).

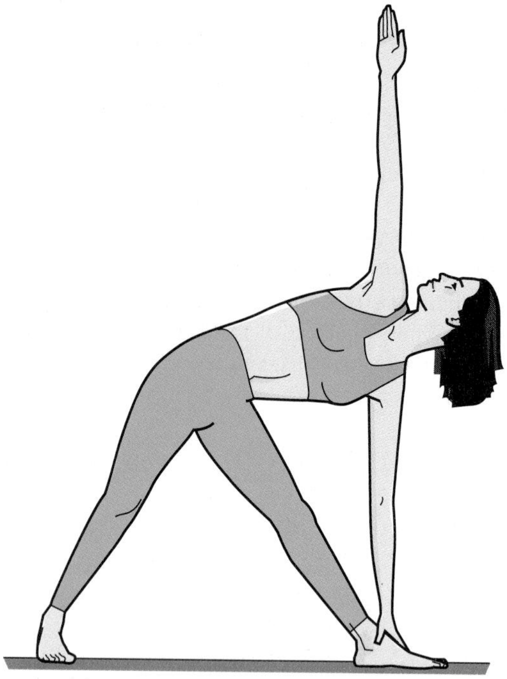

FIG. 4-2 Yoga Asana: Triangle Pose. Helpful for assisting digestion and for stretching and strengthening the spine; used also for dysmenorrhea and pelvic congestion.

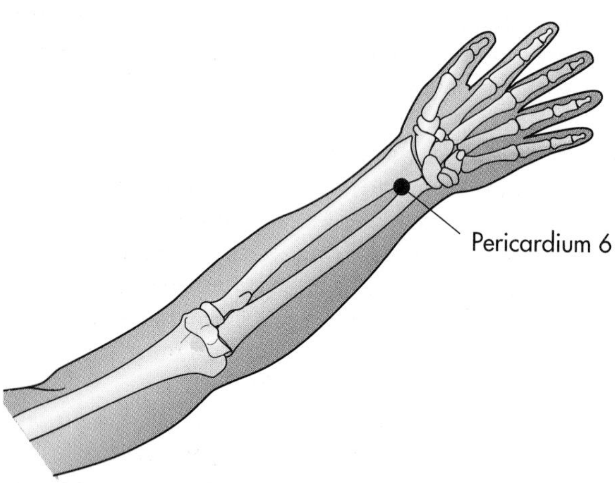
Pericardium 6

FIG. 4-3 Pericardium 6 (P6) acupressure/acupuncture point for nausea.

TCM also offers some alternatives in its herbal pharmacy, under the direction of a skilled practitioner. Certain acupressure or acupuncture points assist with the relief of nausea. One of these, pericardium 6 (P6), is a point that women can use for self-treatment. P6 is located two to three finger widths below the flexion crease of the wrist on the palmar side and between the flexor tendons (Fig. 4-3). By stimulating this point (with a fingertip or other blunt object), nausea can be relieved. Certain elasticized wristbands (Sea Bands, for example) use a bead or other firm object to stimulate the P6 point and can be worn continuously (Fig. 4-4). Several studies have shown that clients report a decrease in nausea when using the wrist bands on the appropriate point. This acupressure technique also has been studied in cases of nausea occurring with chemotherapy and after anesthesia (Carlsson, Axemo, & Bodin, 2000; Elias & Ketcham, 1998; Gentz, 2001; Norheim, Pedersen, & Fonnebo, 2001; O'Brien, Relyea, & Taerum, 1997).

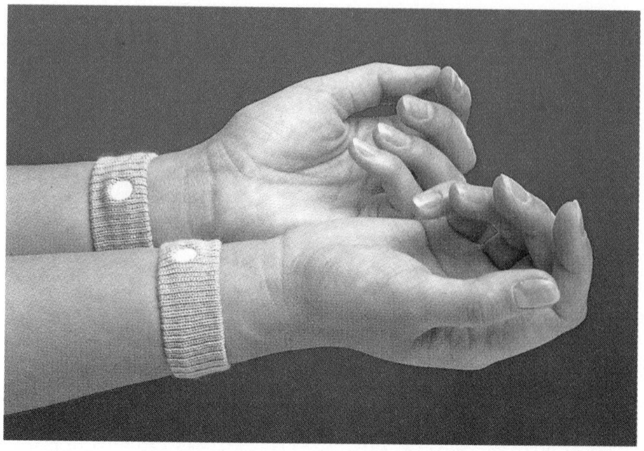

FIG. 4-4 Sea Bands used for stimulation of acupressure point P6. (Courtesy Sea Band International, Newport, RI.)

When appropriate acupressure alone does not relieve nausea or vomiting, acupuncture treatments may be more effective (see Research box). By using slender needles gently inserted into the specific points, licensed acupuncturists can treat not only the P6 point, but also various other points that govern the digestive process. Daily treatments often are required until the nausea subsides (Strong, 2001).

The management of labor pain long has been a nursing function. Prepared childbirth methods that use learned relaxation and imagery have been practiced since the 1950s. The Lamaze method was brought to the United States by Marjorie Karmel, an American woman who gave birth under the care of Fernand Lamaze, a French obstetrician, in Paris. Lamaze now encompasses more than labor management and includes a philosophic profile of holistic care. The Lamaze method encourages parents to take an active role in their pregnancy and obstetric care, to make informed choices, and to be guided by their inner wisdom. Techniques for stress reduction and pain management are taught in classes as life skills. Modalities such as imagery and progressive relaxation are emphasized along with communication skills and comfort measures (heat and cold, pressure points). The Lamaze method encourages realistic decision making and active participation on the part of the expectant parents (Lamaze International, 2000).

RESEARCH

Acupuncture for the Nausea and Vomiting of Early Pregnancy

Early pregnancy is often heralded by nausea and vomiting, which affects between 50% and 80% of all pregnant women. Women with nausea and vomiting can experience discomfort, loss of productivity and income, and nutritional deficits and dehydration. Women often try numerous strategies to alleviate their symptoms with limited success. As alternative therapies gain credence, evidence that nausea and vomiting of pregnancy may be improved with acupressure has been reported in a Cochrane Review. Interest has been spawned in the possible efficacy of acupuncture as a relief measure. Australian researchers designed a randomized controlled study of 593 women who were less than 14 weeks pregnant. Each woman was assigned to one of four groups: (1) traditional acupuncture (treatment points varied according to a traditional Chinese medicine diagnosis), (2) a single treatment point on the anterior forearm called "p6," (3) a sham treatment point near the p6 point, and (4) a control (no treatment) group. Outcome measures were nausea, vomiting, dry retching, and overall well-being; these were measured weekly. All groups showed improvement in symptoms and well-being scores over the 4-week trial. Traditional acupuncture showed the strongest and earliest improvement in nausea and dry retching, followed by the p6 group, when compared with the control group. The sham point group showed significant improvement by the third week of the trial. There were no significant differences between groups in the symptoms of vomiting.

IMPLICATIONS FOR PRACTICE

Nausea and vomiting of pregnancy is uncomfortable and can be distressing and debilitating. There is now some evidence that traditional acupuncture may offer some relief. The nurse can assist the patient in finding a reputable practitioner, if appropriate. More clinical trials are needed. As the body of research grows, health care providers can suggest a variety of beneficial therapies for their pregnant patients who are experiencing nausea and vomiting.

Smith, C., Crowther, C., & Beilby, J. (2002). Acupuncture to treat nausea and vomiting in early pregnancy: A randomized controlled trial. *Birth, 29*(1), 1-9.

Other methods, including the Bradley and Read methods, also are taught nationwide, although Lamaze still enjoys the greatest popularity and widest appeal (see also Chapter 18). Energetic healing modalities also are being used for labor management. Nurses practicing HT and TT have brought these modalities into the hospital setting. Krieger (1987) reported a study conducted with pregnant women and their partners and the use of TT in labor as an adjunct to the Lamaze method. Although pain control was not measured, couples using TT in addition to the Lamaze method reported a greater marital (relationship) satisfaction for their childbirth experience than did the control group. This small study points to the need for further research into pain management in laboring women. Healing touch (Fig. 4-5) also is used for labor care, but no studies have been published (Healing Touch, 2001; Hover-Kramer et al., 2001; Starn, 1998).

Massage techniques also are integrated into labor care. Studies have shown that therapeutic massage decreased labor time, hospital stay, and postpartum depression. Women receiving massage during pregnancy and labor had an increased positive outlook, reported less discomfort, and were less agitated than were those who did not receive massage (Gentz, 2001; Keenan, 2000).

Gynecology

Gynecologic complaints generate a large number of visits to health care practitioners. Menstrual cramps, irregular periods, pelvic pain, fibroids, and menopausal concerns make up the majority of episodic visits. Women in increasing numbers are seeking alternatives to standard surgical and pharmacologic treatments.

Menstrual cramping, or dysmenorrhea, affects a large number of women in all age groups. Various drug therapies, including nonsteroidal antiinflammatory agents, have been proposed over time with a measure of success; however, a vast number of alternatives can provide relief. Dietary changes, such as eliminating milk and dairy products and reducing the intake of complex carbohydrates and red meat, have been shown to decrease the incidence and severity of cramping. Dietary supplements, especially vitamin B_6 (100 mg per day), vitamin E (400 IU per day), and magnesium (up to 600 mg per day), are recommended. Certain herbal preparations, especially those containing cramp bark, white willow, red raspberry, and black cohosh, also may provide relief. Moderate aerobic exercise will stimulate blood flow and prevent congestion in the pelvic region. Visualization of healthy pelvic organs with guided imagery also can reduce pain and discomfort. Acupuncture has been shown to be useful as a complementary modality (Cassileth, 1998; NIH, 1998; Northrup, 1998, 2001) (see Chapter 7).

Irregular menstrual cycles and heavy menstrual flow are common problems. Often a result of hormonal imbalances, dysfunctional uterine bleeding may respond to synthetic hormone treatment. However, a significant number of women experience adverse effects that cause them to stop therapy. After other physiologic problems (thyroid dysfunction, bleeding disorders, diabetes, and other metabolic diseases) have been ruled out, treatment with human-identical hormones, especially progesterone, may be useful. Herbal therapy with black cohosh, red raspberry, and yarrow also is recommended. Increased soy in the diet also may provide some additional support (Martin & Jung, 2002; Northrup, 1998, 2001; Wetzel, 1998).

Premenstrual syndrome (PMS), or premenstrual dysphoria, is a common complaint. Some women experience

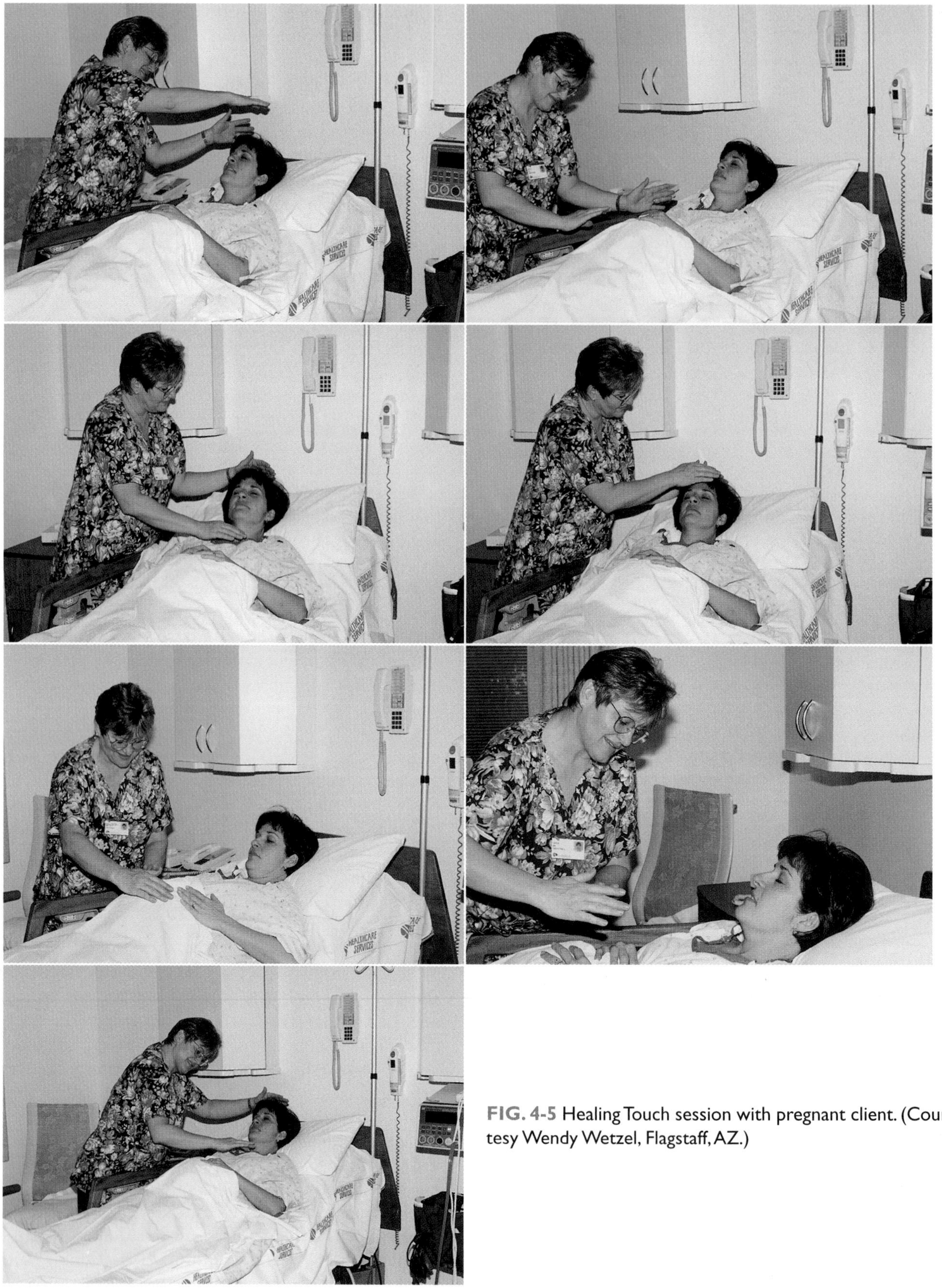

FIG. 4-5 Healing Touch session with pregnant client. (Courtesy Wendy Wetzel, Flagstaff, AZ.)

a variety of disturbing symptoms during the postovulatory period. These symptoms often are alleviated with the onset of menses but cause significant disability and discomfort while they exist. Various theories, including hormonal, emotional, and behavioral, have been proposed. Northrup (1998) suggested that PMS is a social condition brought about by years of shame regarding menstrual functioning; other authors proposed that environmental stressors and dietary habits are contributing factors. Suggested remedies include dietary changes; herbal treatments with evening primrose oil, dandelion, cramp bark, and valerian root; homeopathic remedies to treat the underlying imbalances; body work such as massage and energy healing; and acupuncture. Increasing attention has been paid to the role of hormones in PMS. Supplementation with "natural" or human-identical progesterone has been reported to provide some relief. Commercially prepared human-identical progesterone appeared on the pharmaceuticals market in 1998. Supplementation with this hormone is believed to provide the normal levels of progesterone in the luteal phase and to minimize, if not eliminate, the discomforts of PMS (Lee & Hanley, 1999; Northrup, 1998; Sauer, 1997; Wetzel, 1999; Wright & Morgenthaler, 1997).

As the number of menopausal women increases, so do the requests for "natural" hormone therapy. For almost 50 years, women have been offered only estrogens derived from the urine of pregnant horses (conjugated equine estrogens) and synthetic progestins. With the introduction of other botanically based formulas, there are more options than ever before. Although truly natural hormones may be difficult to obtain, certain plants (soy and yam, for example) have been found to have molecular components that are identical in structure and function to human hormones and can be used in these preparations. These offer a new horizon for menopausal treatment, often without the side effects of standard agents, but with similar benefits and actions (Northrup, 2001; Reiss & Zucker, 2002; Sauer, 1997; Taylor, 1997; Wetzel, 1998, 1999; Wright & Morgenthaler, 1997).

For women who cannot or choose not to take hormonal treatment for menopausal complaints, herbs and homeopathy offer some alternatives. With the increasing awareness and diagnosis of breast cancer, there is consensus that women with a history of breast cancer should not take hormone replacement until they have been in remission for several years. However, these women often need some support and treatment for their symptoms. Herbs such as black cohosh, chasteberry, motherwort, burdock, yam, valerian, and St. John's wort can provide symptomatic relief of hot flashes, night sweats, irritability, depression, and insomnia. A skilled herbalist can combine the ingredients into a mixture suited to the individual woman. Vitamin E oil can soothe atrophic vaginal tissues, and certain homeopathic

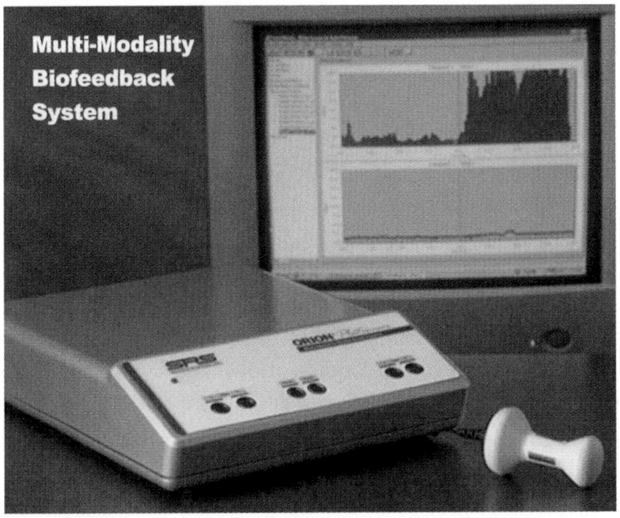
Multi-Modality
Biofeedback
System

FIG. 4-6 Biofeedback equipment used for pelvic floor training, showing typical display seen with pelvic floor contractions. Vaginal sensor is shown at lower right. (Courtesy SRS Medical Systems, Inc., Redmond, WA.)

remedies also can ease this time of transition. Chinese herbs such as dong quai and ginseng also may provide some essential relief (American College of Obstetricians and Gynecologists, 2001; Jonas et al., 1998; Martin & Jung, 2002; Northrup, 2001; Weed, 2001).

NURSE ALERT
Women should inform their health care providers that they are using herbal remedies; health care providers should inquire if women are using herbal remedies as part of their history taking.

Biofeedback is being integrated into women's health care as a noninvasive treatment for various forms of urinary incontinence (Fig. 4-6). Incontinence can be a disturbing problem, often compelling women to become homebound because of their loss of urine and the resulting embarrassment. Depending on the cause of the incontinence, biofeedback training can enhance the woman's ability to exercise the various muscles of the pelvic floor, thereby strengthening them and preventing urinary leakage. Biofeedback also can be used to strengthen pelvic floor muscles, weakened by childbirth, surgery, illness, or aging. These techniques also can be used for women with pelvic pain related to muscular weakness. Physical therapists and nurses are being trained in this technique, which provides a nonsurgical alternative for incontinence problems. Bladder training also offers a cost-effective means to solve an embarrassing dilemma. Women should be appropriately screened to determine the cause of incontinence and then referred to a trained therapist for the proper exercises and monitoring. Once considered an alternative therapy, biofeedback for urinary incontinence is now a covered expense under Medicare (Abdelghany et al., 2001; Continence Coalition, 2001; Hulme, 2000).

IMPLICATIONS FOR NURSING PRACTICE

With increased client awareness of health care models that are different from standard medical practice, the nurse is often the first to be consulted for her professional opinion and advice. Nurses can assist by being knowledgeable about current research, certification or licensure requirements, and professional organizations, and by fostering local networks of resources and practitioners. By maintaining an open and compassionate atmosphere, the nurse can determine the woman's level of knowledge about a given healing modality, as well as serve as a resource for concise and factual information.

At the intake interview, women should be asked if they are using any alternative or complementary modalities in their health plan. This also includes asking about the use of vitamins and over-the-counter remedies.

Beliefs and values can be explored by the nurse and the woman to determine her desires and value system. A congruent plan of care can then be formulated to integrate the woman's biopsychosocial and spiritual needs. By approaching the woman with a nonjudgmental attitude, the nurse can gain her trust and assist her in incorporating her desires for alternative and complementary healing into the overall plan of care.

Holistic nurses often are called on to guide clients through the healing process and may themselves be the care providers with certain modalities. In ever-increasing numbers, nurses are gaining the knowledge and skills to maintain independent practices in various modalities. In this role, they can provide nursing support and guidance along with their chosen modality, thus creating a more comprehensive program of wellness and healing.

KEY POINTS

- Integrative medicine combines modern technology with ancient healing practices and encompasses the whole of body, mind, and spirit.
- Alternative and complementary modalities address the whole client and seek to treat on a variety of levels.
- Although holistic research has been limited in the past, increasing efforts and governmental support are paving the way for more inquiries.
- Holistic nursing refers to a philosophic understanding and may integrate alternative and complementary therapies into nursing care.
- Holistic nurses recognize the importance of relationships within healing, as well as the necessity of self-care.
- A variety of alternative and complementary therapies are currently integrated into maternity and women's health care.
- Nurses are continuing to identify research opportunities to document the efficacy of integrative women's health care.

CRITICAL THINKING EXERCISES

1. Do an on-line search for resources for holistic health care, holistic medicine, and holistic nursing. What modalities did you find represented? What commonalities did you find in the websites? Did any sites list research studies or other means to verify the efficacy of a given modality? What organizations were listed? After reading the material you found, what impressions did you have? Were there any modalities or specialties you would like more information about? How can you obtain that information?
2. Visit a local health food store and observe the various types of vitamins, herbs, and supplements. Pay particular attention to those products marketed for menopausal women. What claims are made? What are the main ingredients? If possible, interview the store owner or the person in charge of the supplement department. What are their perceptions about women who use "natural" hormones and other nonpharmaceutic remedies for menopause?
3. Jacqueline is a new client in your clinic. She is 42 years old, still has regular periods, but is complaining of profound PMS symptoms. She is adamant about wanting only "natural treatment."
   - **a.** In taking her history, for what symptoms will you be alert?
   - **b.** What recommendations can you provide that are congruent with her needs and desires?
   - **c.** What social and spiritual factors might play a role in her PMS?
   - **d.** What are your reactions to her history and requests?

RESOURCES

The Academy for Guided Imagery
P.O. Box 2070
Mill Valley, CA 94942
800-726-2070
www.healthy.net/agi

American Holistic Nurses' Association
P.O. Box 2130
Flagstaff, AZ 86003-2130
800-278-AHNA
ahna.org

Healing Touch International, Inc.
12477 W. Cedar Drive, Suite 202
Lakewood, CO 80228
303-989-7982
www.healingtouch.net

Momentum98
3509 N. High Street
Columbus, OH 43214
800-533-4372
momentum98.com

National Center for Complementary and Alternative Medicine (NCCAM)
P.O. Box 8218
Silver Spring, MD 20907-8218
888-644-6226
altmed.od.nih.gov/nccam

Nurse Healers–Professional Associates International, Inc.
1211 Locust Street
Philadelphia, PA 19107
215-545-8079
www.therapeutictouch.org

Nurses Certificate Program in Interactive Imagery
Beyond Ordinary Nursing
P.O. Box 8177
Foster City, CA 94404
650-570-6157
members.aol.com/NCPII/NCPII.html

REFERENCES

Abdelghany, A. et al. (2001). Biofeedback and electrical stimulation therapy for treating urinary incontinence and voiding dysfunction: One center's experience. *Urologic Nursing, 21*(6), 401-404.

American College of Obstetricians and Gynecologists. (2001). *Use of botanicals for management of menopausal symptoms. ACOG Technical Bulletin 28.* Washington, DC: ACOG.

American Holistic Nurses' Association (AHNA). (2000). *Mission statement.* Flagstaff, AZ: AHNA.

Astin, J. (1998). Why patients use alternative medicine. *Journal of the American Medical Association, 278*, 1548-1553.

Beal, M. (1998). Women's use of complementary and alternative therapies in reproductive health care. *Journal of Nurse Midwifery, 43*(3), 224-234.

Benson, H., & Proctor, W. (1984). *Beyond the relaxation response.* New York: Putman/Berkley.

Bray D. (1998). Biofeedback. *Complementary Therapies in Nursing and Midwifery, 4*(1), 22-24.

Carlsson, C.P., Axemo, P., & Bodin, A. (2000). Manual acupuncture reduces hyperemesis gravidarum: A placebo-controlled, randomized, single-blind, crossover study. *Journal of Pain Symptom Management, 20*, 273-279.

Cassileth, B. (1998). *The alternative medicine handbook: The complete reference guide to alternative and complementary therapies.* New York: W.W. Norton.

Chilton, B. (1998). Recognizing spirituality. *Image: the Journal of Nursing Scholarship, 30*(4), 400-401.

Clark, C. (Ed.). (1999). *The encyclopedia of complementary health practice.* New York: Springer.

Collins, J. (2000). *What's your menopause type? The revolutionary program to restore balance and reduce discomforts of menopause.* Roseville, CA: Prima Publishing.

Continence coalition statement on ethical use of biofeedback and electrical stimulation for the treatment of incontinence. (2001). Society of Urologic Nurses and Associates. Available at www.suna.org.

Dossey, B. (Ed.). (1997). *Core curriculum for holistic nursing.* Gaithersburg, MD: Aspen.

Dossey, B. (2000). *Florence Nightingale: Mystic, visionary, healer.* Springhouse, PA: Springhouse.

Dossey, B. (1998). Holistic modalities and healing moments. *American Journal of Nursing, 98*(6), 44-47.

Dossey, B., Keegan, L., & Guzzetta, C. (2000). *Holistic nursing: A handbook for practice* (3rd ed.). Gaithersburg, MD: Aspen.

Easter, A. (1997). The state of research on the effects of therapeutic touch. *Journal of Holistic Nursing, 15*(2), 158-175.

Eisenberg, D. et al. (1998). Trends in alternative medicine use in the United States, 1990-1997. *Journal of the American Medical Association, 280*, 1569-1575.

Elias, J., & Ketcham, K. (1998). *The five elements of self-healing: Using Chinese medicine for maximum immunity, wellness, and health.* New York: Random House.

Ferguson, M. (1980). *The Aquarian conspiracy.* Los Angeles: J.P. Tarcher.

Frisch, N. et al. (2000). *AHNA standards of holistic nursing practice: Guides for caring and healing.* Gaithersburg, MD: Aspen.

Gentz, B. (2001). Alternative therapies for the management of pain in labor and delivery. *Clinical Obstetrics and Gynecology, 44*(4), 704-732.

Gerber, R., Tiller, W., & Cousens, G. (2001). *Vibrational medicine.* Rochester, VT: Inner Traditions.

Giedt, J. (1997). Guided imagery: A psychoneuroimmunological intervention in holistic nursing practice. *Journal of Holistic Nursing, 15*(2), 112-127.

Healing Touch. (2001). *The healing touch research survey.* Lakewood, CO: Healing Touch International.

Hoffart, M., & Pross-Keene, E. (1998). The benefits of visualization. *American Journal of Nursing, 98*(12), 44-47.

Hover-Kramer, D., Mentgen, J., & Scandrett-Hibdon, S. (2001). *Healing touch: A resource for health care professionals.* Albany, NY: Delmar.

Hulme, J.A. (2000). Research in geriatric urinary incontinence: Pelvic muscle force field. *Topics in Geriatric Rehabilitation, 16*(1), 10-21.

Iyengar, B.K.S. (2001). *Yoga: The path to holistic health.* London: Dorling Kindersley.

Jonas, W., Jacobs, J., & Dossey, L. (1998). *Healing with homeopathy: The doctor's guide.* New York: Warner Books.

Juhan, D. (1998). *Job's body: A handbook for bodywork.* Barrytown, NY: Barrytown Ltd.

Keegan, L., & Dossey, B.M. (1998). *Profiles of nurse healers.* Albany, NY: Delmar.

Keenan, P. (2000). Benefits of massage therapy and use of a doula during labor and childbirth. *Alternative Therapeutic Health Medicine, 6*(1), 66-74.

Krieger, D. (1993). *Accepting your power to heal: The personal practice of therapeutic touch.* Santa Fe, NM: Bear.

Krieger, D. (1987). *Living the therapeutic touch: Healing as a lifestyle.* New York: Dodd, Mead.

Krieger, D. (1979). *The therapeutic touch: How to use your hands to help or to heal.* Englewood Cliffs, NJ: Prentice-Hall.

Krieger, D. (1990). Therapeutic touch: Two decades of research, teaching and clinical practice. *Imprint, 37,* 83, 86-88.

Krieger, D. (2002). *Therapeutic touch as transpersonal healing.* New York: Lantern Books.

Lamaze International. (2000). *About Lamaze.* Internet document: www.lamaze.org/2000/about_lamaze.html.

Lee, J., & Hanley, J. (1999). *What your doctor may not tell you about pre-menopause.* New York: Warner Books.

LeMaire, B. (2002). Something extra. *Nurseweek, 3*(7), 10-12.

Martin, A. (2002). It's never too late: Seven steps toward good health. *Topics in Advanced Practice Nursing E-journal, 2*(1). Internet document: www.medscape.com/viewarticle/421471.

Martin, L., & Jung, P. (2002). *Taking charge of the change.* Albany, NY: Delmar.

Mehta, M. (2001). *How to use yoga.* London: Anness Publishing Ltd.

Mehta, S., Mehta, M., & Mehta, S. (2001). *Yoga: The Iyengar way.* New York: Alfred A. Knopf.

National Center for Complementary and Alternative Medicine (NCCAM). (2002). Internet document: nccam.nih.gov.

National Center for Complementary and Alternative Medicine (NCCAM)/Office of Alternative Medicine (OAM). (1999). Internet document: altmed.od.nih.gov/nccam.

National Institutes of Health. (1998). Acupuncture: NIH consensus development panel on acupuncture. *Journal of the American Medical Association, 280,* 1518-1524 [Abstract].

Norheim, A., Pedersen, E. J., & Fonnebo, V. (2001). Acupressure treatment of morning sickness in pregnancy: A randomized, double-blind, placebo-controlled study. *Scandinavian Journal of Primary Health Care, 19,* 43-47.

Northrup, C. (2001). *The wisdom of menopause.* New York: Bantam.

Northrup, C. (1998). *Women's bodies, women's wisdom.* New York: Bantam.

O'Brien, B., Relyea, M.J., & Taerum, T. (1997). Efficacy of P6 acupressure in the treatment of nausea and vomiting during pregnancy. *American Journal of Obstetrics and Gynecology, 176*(6), 1395-1397.

Oschman, J. (2000). *Energy medicine.* New York: Churchill Livingstone.

Padden, D. (2002). The role of the advanced practice nurse in the promotion of exercise and physical activity. *Topics in Advanced Practice Nursing E-journal, 2*(1). Internet document: www.medscape.com/viewarticle/421475.

Peters, D. et al. (2001). *Integrating complementary therapies in primary care: A practical guide for health practitioners.* New York: Churchill Livingstone.

Phalen, K. (1998). *Integrative medicine: Achieving wellness through the best of Eastern and Western medical practices.* Boston: Charles Tuttle.

Quinn, J. (1994). *Therapeutic touch: Healing through human energy fields, theory and research* [videotapes and study guide]. New York: National League for Nursing.

Reiss, U., & Zucker, M. (2002). *Natural hormone balance for women: Look younger, feel stronger, and live life with exuberance.* New York: Pocket Books.

Rogers, M. (1970). *The theoretical basis of nursing.* Philadelphia: F.A. Davis.

Sauer, M. (1997). Progesterone use in reproductive and gynecologic endocrinology: Current and future perspectives. *Contemporary Obstetrics and Gynecology, 42,* s4-s11.

Sayre-Adams, J. et al. (2001). *Therapeutic touch.* New York: Churchill-Livingstone.

Scheiber, B., & Selby, C. (Eds.). (2000). *Therapeutic touch.* New York: Prometheus Books.

Shames, K., & Hover-Kramer, D. (1997). *Energetic approaches to emotional healing: Expanding the art of counseling beyond words.* Albany, NY: Delmar.

Skinner, S. (2001). *An introduction to homeopathic medicine in primary care.* Gaithersburg, MD: Aspen.

Snyder, M., & Lindquist, R. (Eds.). (2002). *Complementary/alternative therapies in nursing* (4th ed.). New York: Springer.

Starn, J. (1998). Energy healing with women and children. *Journal of Obstetric, Gynecologic, and Neonatal Nursing, 27*(5), 576-584.

Strong, T. (2001). Alternative therapies of morning sickness. *Clinical Obstetrics and Gynecology, 44*(4), 653-660.

Taylor, M. (1997). Alternatives to conventional hormone replacement therapy. *Comprehensive Therapy, 23,* 514-532.

Weed, S. (2001). *The new menopausal years: The wise woman way.* Woodstock, NY: Ash Tree.

Weil, A. (1998a). *Health and healing.* Boston: Houghton Mifflin.

Weil, A. (1998b). *Natural health, natural medicine: A comprehensive manual for wellness and self-care.* Boston: Houghton Mifflin.

Wetzel, M., Eisenberg, D., & Kaptchuk, T. (1998). Courses involving complementary and alternative medicine at U.S. medical schools. *Journal of the American Medical Association, 280,* 784-787.

Wetzel, W. (1998). Human identical hormones: Real people, real problems, real solutions. *Nurse Practitioner Forum, 9*(4), 227-234.

Wetzel, W. (1999). Micronized progesterone: A new perspective for women's health care, a case study review. *Nurse Practitioner, 24*(5), 62-76.

World Health Organization. (2002). *Traditional medicine: Growing needs and potential, WHO Policy Perspectives on Medicine.* Geneva: WHO. Internet document: www.who.int/medicines/organization/trm/orgtrmmain.html

Wright, J., & Morgenthaler, J. (1997). *Natural hormone replacement.* Petaluma, CA: Smart.

CHAPTER 5

Jan Lamarche Zdanuk

Assessment and Health Promotion

http://evolve.elsevier.com/Lowdermilk/MatWmnHlth/

LEARNING OBJECTIVES

- Identify the structures and functions of the female reproductive system.
- Compare the menstrual cycle in relation to hormonal, ovarian, and endometrial response.
- Identify the four phases of the sexual response cycle.
- Analyze financial, cultural, and communication barriers that may affect a woman's decision to seek and follow through with health care.
- Investigate how the history and physical examination can be adapted for women with special needs.
- Compare the strategies for teaching safety and injury prevention during routine health examinations.
- Examine indications of abuse, appropriate screening, and referral to community agencies.
- Describe components of taking a woman's history and performing a physical examination.
- Identify the correct procedure for assisting with and collecting Papanicolaou smear specimens.
- Review client teaching of breast self-examination.
- Analyze conditions and characteristics that increase health risks for women across the life span.
- Evaluate programs of anticipatory guidance that promote health and prevention of disease.
- Outline health-screening schedules for women in the childbearing years.

Many women initially enter the health care system because of a gender-related concern such as vaginal infection, irregular menses, pregnancy, a desire for contraception, or an episodic illness such as a sinus infection. Once women are in the system, it is important for health care providers to recognize the need for health promotion and health maintenance and to offer these services across the life span of women.

This chapter reviews female anatomy and physiology including the menstrual cycle. Physical assessment and screening for disease prevention for women are presented. Barriers to seeking health care and an overview of conditions and circumstances that increase health risks across the life span are discussed. Anticipatory guidance suggestions including nutrition and stress management also are included.

FEMALE REPRODUCTIVE SYSTEM

The female reproductive system consists of external structures visible from the pubis to the perineum and internal structures located in the pelvic cavity. The external and internal female reproductive structures develop and mature in response to estrogen and progesterone, starting in fetal life and continuing through puberty and the childbearing years. Reproductive structures atrophy with age or in response to a decrease in ovarian hormone production. A complex nerve and blood supply supports the functions of these structures. The appearance of the external genitals varies greatly among women. Heredity, age, race, and the number of children a woman has borne determine the size, shape, and color of her external organs.

External Structures

The external genital organs, or *vulva*, include all structures visible externally from the pubis to the perineum: the mons pubis, labia majora, labia minora, clitoris, vestibular glands, vaginal vestibule, vaginal orifice, and urethral opening. The external genital organs are illustrated in Figure 5-1. The *mons pubis* is a fatty pad that lies over the anterior surface of the symphysis pubis. In the postpubertal female, the mons is covered with coarse curly hair. The *labia majora* are two rounded folds of fatty tissue covered with skin that extend downward and backward from the mons pubis. The labia are highly vascular structures that develop hair on the outer surfaces after puberty. They protect the inner vulvar structures. The *labia minora* are two flat, reddish folds of tissue visible when the labia majora

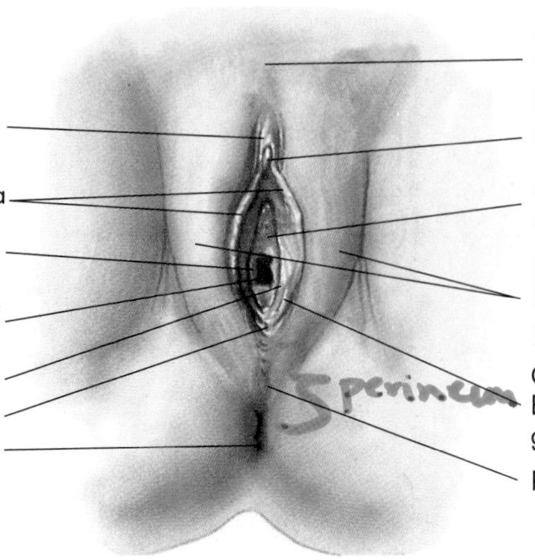
Mons pubis
(without
pubic hair)
Prepuce
Clitoris
Labia minora
Orifice
of urethra
Hymen
Labia majora
(without
pubic hair)
Orifice
of vagina
Vestibule
Opening of
Bartholin's
gland
Fourchette
Anus
Perineal body
perineum

FIG. 5-1 External female genitalia.

are separated. No hair follicles are in the labia minora, but many sebaceous follicles and a few sweat glands are present. The interior of the labia minora is composed of connective tissue and smooth muscle and supplied with extremely sensitive nerve endings. Anteriorly, the labia minora fuse to form the *prepuce* (hoodlike covering of the clitoris) and the *frenulum* (fold of tissue under the clitoris). The labia minora join to form a thin flat tissue called the *fourchette* underneath the vaginal opening at midline. The *clitoris* is located underneath the prepuce. It is a small structure composed of erectile tissue with numerous sensory nerve endings. During sexual arousal, the clitoris increases in size.

The vaginal *vestibule* is an almond-shaped area enclosed by the labia minora that contains openings to the urethra, Skene's glands, vagina, and Bartholin's glands. The urethra is not a reproductive organ but is considered here because of its location. It usually is found about 2.5 cm below the clitoris. Skene's glands are located on each side of the urethra and produce mucus, which aids in lubrication of the vagina. The vaginal opening is in the lower portion of the vestibule and varies in shape and size. The hymen, a connective tissue membrane, surrounds the vaginal opening. It can be perforated during strenuous exercise, insertion of tampons, masturbation, and vaginal intercourse. Bartholin's glands (see Fig. 5-1) lie under the constrictor muscles of the vagina and are located posteriorly on the sides of the vaginal opening, although the ductal openings are usually not visible. During sexual arousal, the glands secrete a clear mucus to lubricate the vaginal introitus.

The area between the fourchette and the anus is the **perineum,** a skin-covered muscular area that covers the pelvic structures. The perineum forms the base of the perineal body, a wedge-shaped mass that serves as an anchor for the muscles, fascia, and ligaments of the pelvis. The pelvic organs are supported by muscles and ligaments that form a sling.

Internal Structures

The internal structures include the vagina, uterus, uterine tubes, and ovaries. The vagina is a fibromuscular, collapsible tubular structure that extends from the vulva to the uterus and lies between the bladder and rectum. During the reproductive years, the mucosal lining is arranged in transverse folds called rugae. These rugae allow the vagina to expand during childbirth. Estrogen deprivation that occurs after childbirth, during lactation, and at menopause causes dryness and thinning of the vaginal walls and smoothing of the rugae. The vagina, particularly the lower segment, has few sensory nerve endings. Vaginal secretions are slightly acidic (pH 4 to 5) so that vaginal susceptibility to infections is reduced. The vagina serves as a passageway for menstrual flow, as a female organ of copulation, and as a part of the birth canal for vaginal childbirth. The uterine cervix projects into a blind vault at the upper end of the vagina. There are anterior, posterior, and lateral pockets called fornices that surround the cervix. The internal pelvic organs can be palpated through the thin walls of these fornices.

The *uterus* is a muscular organ shaped like an upside-down pear that sits midline in the pelvic cavity between the bladder and rectum above the vagina. Four pairs of ligaments support the uterus: the cardinal, uterosacral, round, and broad. Single anterior and posterior ligaments also support the uterus. The cul-de-sac of Douglas is a deep pouch, or recess, posterior to the cervix formed by the posterior ligament.

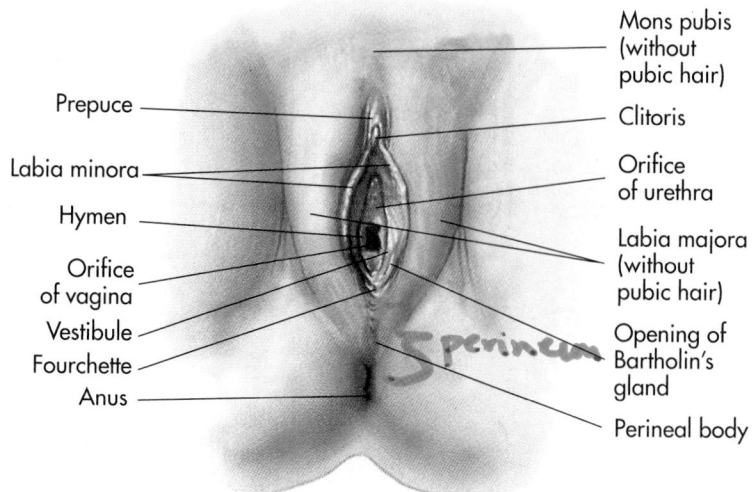

The uterus is divided into two major parts, an upper triangular portion called the corpus and a lower cylindric portion called the *cervix* (Fig. 5-2). The *fundus* is the dome-shaped top of the uterus and is the site at which the uterine tubes enter the uterus. The isthmus (lower uterine

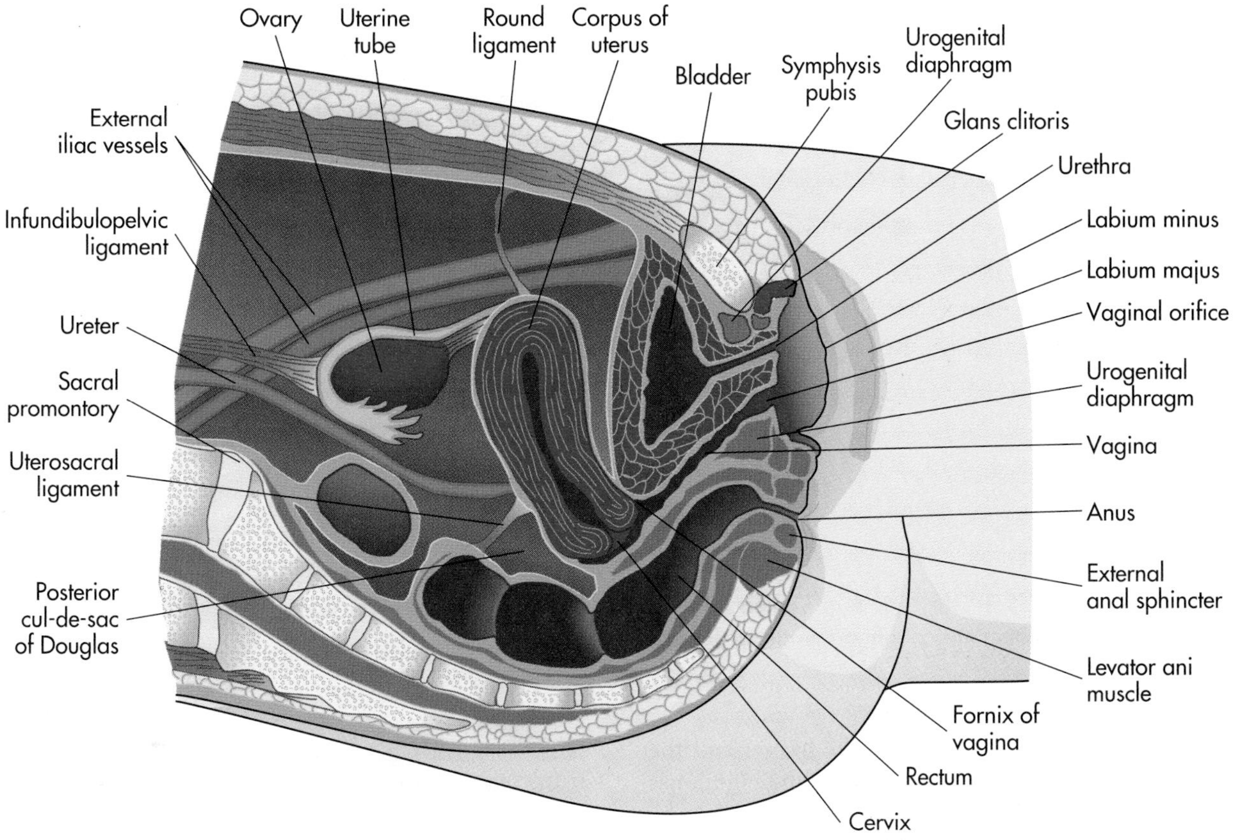
Ovary
Uterine tube
Round ligament
Corpus of uterus
Bladder
Symphysis pubis
Urogenital diaphragm
Glans clitoris
Urethra
Labium minus
Labium majus
Vaginal orifice
Urogenital diaphragm
Vagina
Anus
External anal sphincter
Levator ani muscle
Fornix of vagina
Rectum
Cervix
External iliac vessels
Infundibulopelvic ligament
Ureter
Sacral promontory
Uterosacral ligament
Posterior cul-de-sac of Douglas

FIG. 5-2 Midsagittal view of female pelvic organs with woman lying supine.

segment) is a short, constricted portion that separates the corpus from the cervix.

The uterus serves for reception, implantation, retention, and nutrition of the fertilized ovum and later of the fetus during pregnancy and for expulsion of the fetus during childbirth. It also is responsible for cyclic menstruation.

The uterine wall comprises three layers: the endometrium, the myometrium, and part of the peritoneum. The endometrium is a highly vascular lining made up of three layers, the outer two of which are shed during menstruation. The myometrium is made up of layers of smooth muscles that extend in three different directions (longitudinal, transverse, and oblique) (Fig. 5-3). Longitudinal fibers of the outer myometrial layer are found mostly in the fundus, and this arrangement assists in expelling the fetus during the birth process. The middle layer contains fibers from all three directions, which form a figure-eight pattern encircling large blood vessels. These fibers assist in ligating blood vessels after childbirth and control blood loss. Most of the circular fibers of the inner myometrial layer are around the site where the uterine tubes enter the uterus and around the internal cervical os (opening). These fibers help keep the cervix closed during pregnancy and prevent menstrual blood from flowing back into the uterine tubes during menstruation.

The cervix is made up of mostly fibrous connective tissues and elastic tissue, making it possible for the cervix to stretch during vaginal childbirth. The opening between the uterine cavity and the canal that connects the uterine cavity to the vagina (endocervical canal) is the internal os. The narrowed opening between the endocervix and the vagina is the external os, a small circular opening in women who have never been pregnant. The cervix feels firm (like the end of a nose) with a dimple in the center, which marks the external os.

The outer cervix is covered with a layer of squamous epithelium. The mucosa of the cervical canal is covered with columnar epithelium and contains numerous glands that secrete mucus in response to ovarian hormones. The **squamocolumnar junction,** where the two types of cells meet, is usually located just inside the cervical os. This junction also is called the *transformation zone,* the most common site for neoplastic changes; cells from this site are scraped for the Papanicolaou (Pap) test (see Fig. 5-14).

The *uterine tubes* (fallopian tubes) attach to the uterine fundus. The tubes are supported by the broad ligaments and range from 8 to 14 cm in length. The tubes are divided into four sections: the interstitial portion is closest to the uterus; the isthmus and the ampulla are the middle portions; and the infundibulum is closest to the ovary. The

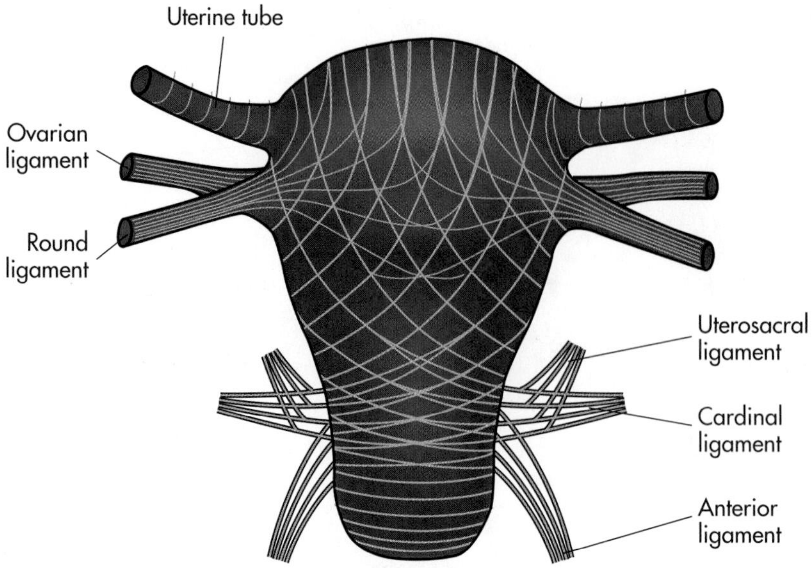
Uterine tube
Ovarian ligament
Round ligament
Uterosacral ligament
Cardinal ligament
Anterior ligament

FIG. 5-3 Schematic arrangement of directions of muscle fibers. Note that uterine muscle fibers are continuous with supportive ligaments of uterus.

uterine tubes form passages between the ovaries and the uterus for the passage of the ovum. The infundibulum has fimbriated ends, which pull the ovum into the tube. The ovum is pushed along the tubes to the uterus by rhythmic contractions of the muscles of the tubes and by the current that is produced by the movement of the cilia that line the tubes. The ovum is usually fertilized by the sperm in the ampulla portion of one of the tubes.

The *ovaries* are almond-shaped organs located on each side of the uterus below and behind the uterine tubes. During the reproductive years, they are approximately 3 cm long, 2 cm wide, and 1 cm thick; they diminish in size after menopause. Before menarche, each ovary has a smooth surface; after menarche, they become nodular because of repeated ruptures of follicles at ovulation. The two functions of the ovaries are ovulation and hormone production. **Ovulation** is the release of a mature ovum from the ovary at intervals (usually monthly). Estrogen, progesterone, and androgen are the hormones produced by the ovaries.

The Bony Pelvis

The bony pelvis serves three primary purposes: protection of the pelvic structures, accommodation of the growing fetus during pregnancy, and anchorage of the pelvic support structures. Two innominate (hip) bones (consisting of ilium, ischium, and pubis), the sacrum, and the coccyx make up the four bones of the pelvis (Fig. 5-4). Cartilage and ligaments form the symphysis pubis, sacrococcygeal joint, and two sacroiliac joints that separate the pelvic bones. The pelvis is divided into two parts: the false pelvis and the true pelvis (Fig. 5-5). The false pelvis is the upper portion above the pelvic brim or inlet. The true pelvis is the lower curved bony canal, which includes the inlet, the cavity, and the outlet through which the fetus passes during vaginal birth. The upper portion of the outlet is at the level of the ischial spines, and the lower portion is at the level of the ischial tuberosities and the pubic arch (see Fig. 5-4). Variations that occur in the size and shape of the pelvis are usually due to age, race, and sex. Pelvic ossification is complete at about age 20 years.

Breasts

The breasts are paired mammary glands located between the second and sixth ribs (Fig. 5-6). About two thirds of the breast overlies the pectoralis major muscle, between the sternum and midaxillary line, with an extension to the axilla referred to as the tail of Spence. The lower one third of the breast overlies the serratus anterior muscle. The breasts are attached to the muscles by connective tissue or fascia.

The breasts of healthy mature women are approximately equal in size and shape, but often are not absolutely symmetric. The size and shape vary depending on the woman's age, heredity, and nutrition. However, the contour should be smooth, with no retractions, dimpling, or masses. Estrogen stimulates growth of the breast by inducing fat deposition in the breasts, development of stromal tissue (i.e., increase in its amount and elasticity), and growth of the extensive ductile system. Estrogen also increases the vascularity of breast tissue.

Once ovulation begins in puberty, progesterone levels increase. The increase in progesterone causes maturation of mammary gland tissue, specifically the lobules and acinar

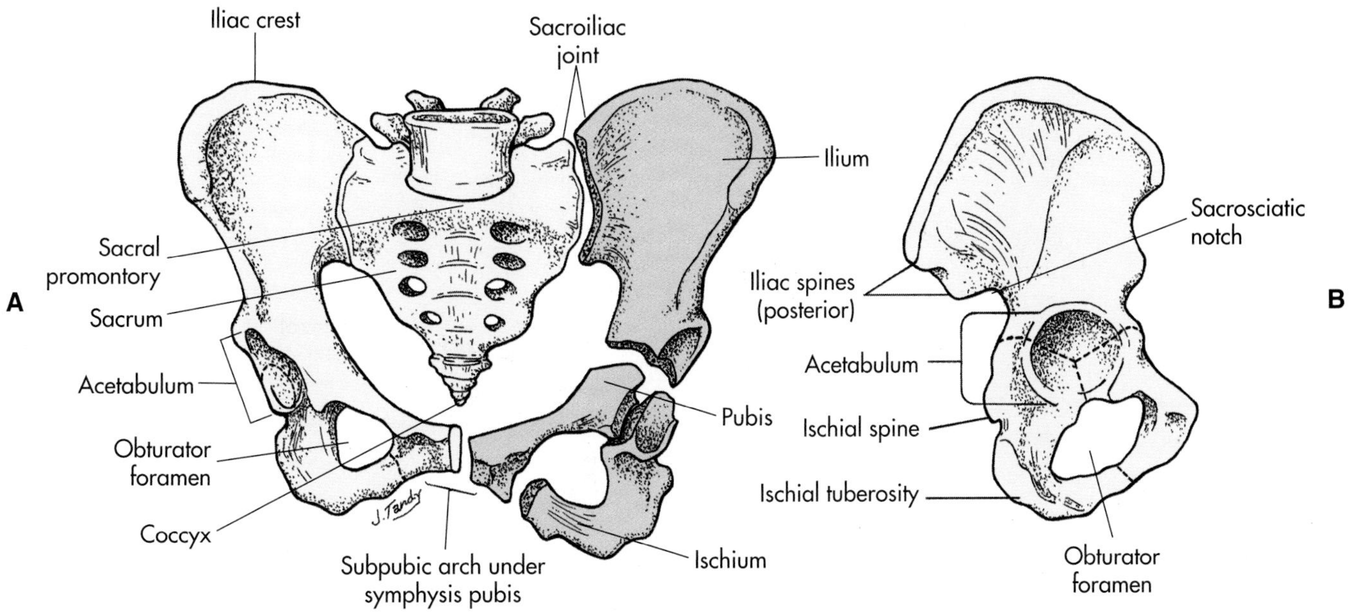
Iliac crest
Sacroiliac joint
Ilium
Sacral promontory
Sacrum
Acetabulum
Obturator foramen
Coccyx
Subpubic arch under symphysis pubis
Pubis
Ischium
A
Sacrosciatic notch
Iliac spines (posterior)
Acetabulum
Ischial spine
Ischial tuberosity
Obturator foramen
B

FIG. 5-4 Adult female pelvis. **A,** Anterior view. **B,** External view of innominate bone (fused).

structures. During adolescence, fat deposition and growth of fibrous tissue contribute to the increase in the gland's size. Full development of the breasts is not achieved until after the end of the first pregnancy or in the early period of lactation.

Each mammary gland comprises 15 to 20 lobes, which are divided into lobules. Lobules are clusters of acini. An *acinus* is a saclike terminal part of a compound gland emptying through a narrow lumen or duct. In discussions of mammary glands, the correct anatomic term (acinus) often is used interchangeably with the term alveolus. The acini are lined with epithelial cells that secrete colostrum and milk. Just below the epithelium is the myoepithelium (myo, or muscle), which contracts to expel milk from the acini.

The ducts from the clusters of acini that form the lobules merge to form larger ducts draining the lobes. Ducts from the lobes converge in a single nipple (mammary papilla) surrounded by an areola. Just as the ducts converge, they dilate to form common lactiferous sinuses, which also are called ampullae. The lactiferous sinuses serve as milk reservoirs. Many tiny lactiferous ducts drain the ampullae and exit in the nipple.

The glandular structures and ducts are surrounded by protective fatty tissue and are separated and supported by fibrous suspensory *Cooper's ligaments*. Cooper's ligaments provide support to the mammary glands while permitting their mobility on the chest wall (see Fig. 5-6). The round nipple is usually slightly elevated above the breast. On each breast, the nipple projects slightly upward and laterally. It contains 15 to 20 openings from lactiferous ducts. The nipple is surrounded by fibromuscular tissue and covered by wrinkled skin. Except during pregnancy and lactation, there is usually no discharge from the nipple.

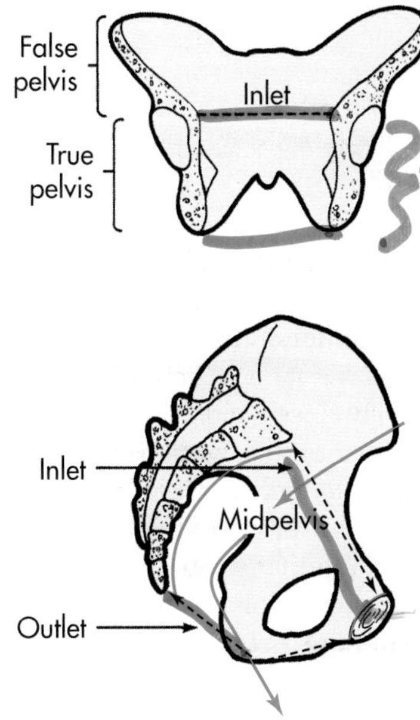
False pelvis
Inlet
A
True pelvis
Inlet
Midpelvis
B
Outlet

FIG. 5-5 Female pelvis. **A,** Cavity of false pelvis is shallow. **B,** Cavity of true pelvis is an irregularly curved canal (*arrows*).

The nipple and surrounding areola are usually more deeply pigmented than the skin of the breast. The rough appearance of the areola is caused by sebaceous glands, *Montgomery tubercles*, directly beneath the skin. These glands secrete a fatty substance, thought to lubricate the nipple. Smooth muscle fibers in the areola contract to

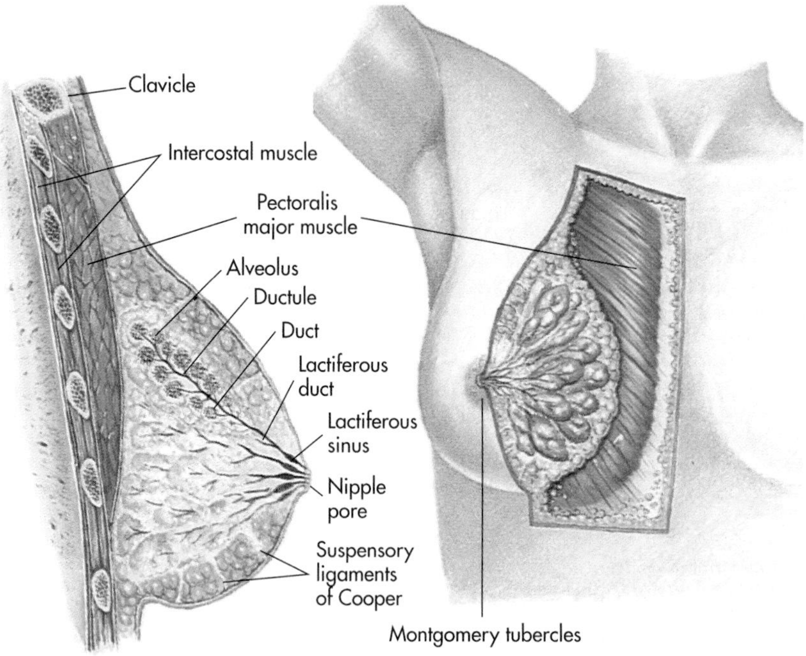
Clavicle
Intercostal muscle
Pectoralis major muscle
Alveolus
Ductule
Duct
Lactiferous duct
Lactiferous sinus
Nipple pore
Suspensory ligaments of Cooper
Montgomery tubercles

FIG. 5-6 Anatomy of the breast, showing position and major structures. (From Seidel, H., et al. [2003]. *Mosby's guide to physical examination* [5th ed.]. St. Louis: Mosby.)

stiffen the nipple to make it easier for the breastfeeding infant to grasp.

The vascular supply to the mammary gland is abundant. In the nonpregnant state, the skin does not have an obvious vascular pattern. The normal skin is smooth without tightness or shininess. The skin covering the breasts contains an extensive superficial lymphatic network that serves the entire chest wall and is continuous with the superficial lymphatics of the neck and abdomen. In the deeper portions of the breasts, the lymphatics form a rich network as well. The primary deep lymphatic pathway drains laterally toward the axillae.

Besides their function of lactation, breasts function as organs for sexual arousal in the mature adult.

The breasts change in size and nodularity in response to cyclic ovarian changes throughout reproductive life. Increasing levels of both estrogen and progesterone in the 3 to 4 days before menstruation increase the vascularity of the breasts, induce growth of the ducts and acini, and promote water retention. The epithelial cells lining the ducts proliferate in number, the ducts dilate, and the lobules distend. The acini become enlarged and secretory, and lipid (fat) is deposited within their epithelial cell lining. As a result, breast swelling, tenderness, and discomfort are common symptoms just before the onset of menstruation. After menstruation, cellular proliferation begins to regress; acini begin to decrease in size; and retained water is lost. After breasts have undergone changes numerous times in response to the ovarian cycle, the proliferation and involution (regression) are not uniform throughout the breast. In time, after repeated hormonal stimulation, small persistent areas of nodulations may develop. This normal physiologic change must be remembered when breast tissue is examined. Nodules may develop just before and during menstruation, when the breast is most active. The physiologic alterations in breast size and activity reach their minimal level about 5 to 7 days after menstruation stops. Therefore **breast self-examination (BSE)** (systematic palpation of breasts to detect signs of breast cancer or other changes) is best carried out during this phase of the menstrual cycle (see Teaching for Self-Care). Table 5-1 compares the variations in physical assessment related to age differences in women.

MENSTRUATION AND MENOPAUSE

Nurses should be knowledgeable about menarche, the endometrial cycle, the hypothalamic-pituitary cycle, the ovarian cycle, other cyclic changes, and the climacteric as they provide care for women across the life span.

Menarche and Puberty

Although young girls secrete small, rather constant amounts of estrogen, a marked increase occurs between ages 8 and 11 years. The term **menarche** denotes first menstruation. **Puberty** is a broader term that denotes the entire transitional stage between childhood and sexual maturity. Increasing amounts and variations in gonadotropin and estrogen secretion develop into a cyclic pattern at least a year before menarche. In North America, this occurs in most girls at about age 13 years.

TEACHING FOR SELF-CARE

Breast Self-Examination

1. The best time to do breast self-examination is after your period, when breasts are not tender or swollen. If you do not have regular periods or sometimes skip a month, do it on the same day every month.
2. Lie down and put a pillow under your right shoulder. Place your right arm behind your head (Fig. 1).
3. Use the finger pads of your three middle fingers on your left hand to feel for lumps or thickening. Your finger pads are the top third of each finger.
4. Press firmly enough to know how your breast feels. If you're not sure how hard to press, ask your health care provider, or try to copy the way your health care provider uses the finger pads during a breast examination. Learn what your breast feels like most of the time. A firm ridge in the lower curve of each breast is normal.
5. Move around the breast in a set way. You can choose either circles (Fig. 2, A), vertical lines (Fig. 2, B), or wedges (Fig. 2, C). Do it the same way every time. It will help you to make sure that you've gone over the entire breast area and to remember how your breast feels.
6. Gently compress the nipple between your thumb and forefinger and look for discharge.
7. Now examine your left breast using the finger pads of your right hand.
8. If you find any changes, see your health care provider right away.
9. You may want to check your breasts while standing in front of a mirror right after you do your breast self-examination each month. See if there are any changes in the way your breasts look: dimpling of the skin, changes in the nipple, or redness or swelling.
10. You may also want to do an extra breast self-examination while you're in the shower (Fig. 3). Your soapy hands will glide over the wet skin, making it easy to check how your breasts feel.
11. It is important to check the area between the breast and the underarm and the underarm itself. Also examine the area above the breast to the collarbone and to the shoulder.

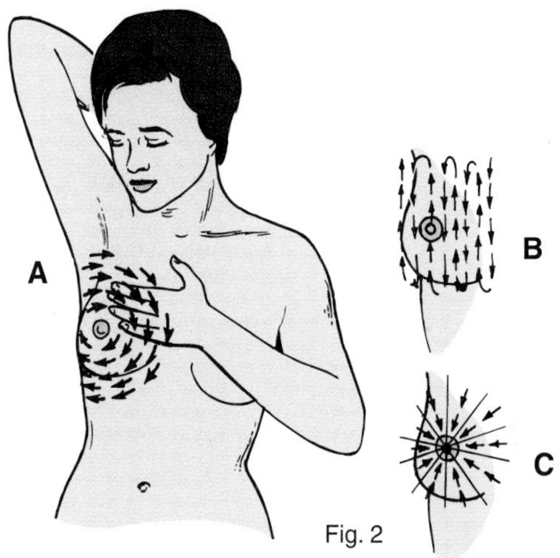
A
B
C
Fig. 2

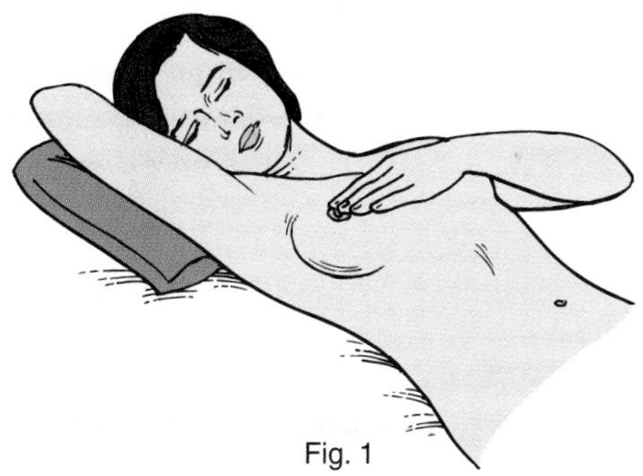
Fig. 1

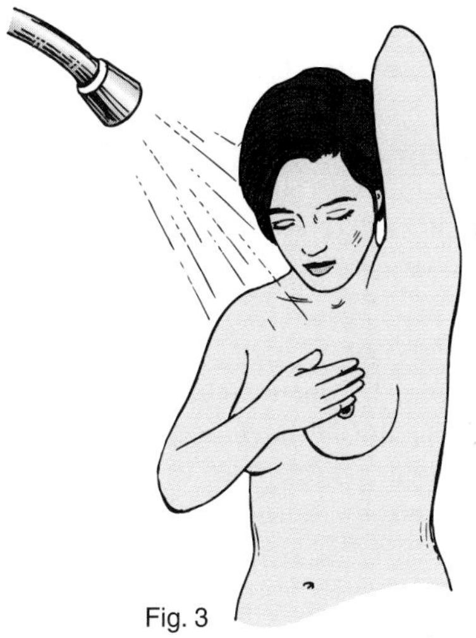
Fig. 3

Initially, periods are irregular, unpredictable, painless, and *anovulatory* (no ovum released from the ovary). After 1 or more years, a hypothalamic-pituitary rhythm develops, and the ovary produces adequate cyclic estrogen to make a mature ovum. *Ovulatory* (ovum released from ovary) periods tend to be regular, monitored by progesterone.

Although pregnancy can occur in exceptional cases of true precocious puberty, most pregnancies in young girls occur after the normally timed menarche. All young adolescents of both sexes would benefit from knowing that pregnancy can occur at any time after the onset of menses.

Menstrual Cycle

Menstruation is the periodic uterine bleeding that begins approximately 14 days after ovulation. It is controlled by a feedback system of three cycles: endometrial,

TABLE 5-1 **Female Reproductive Physical Assessment Across the Life Cycle**

	ADOLESCENT	ADULT	POSTMENOPAUSAL
Breasts	Tender when developing; buds appear; small, firm, one side may grow faster; areola diameter increases; nipples more erect	Grow to full shape in early adulthood; nipples and areolae become pinker and darker	Become stringy, irregular, pendulous, and nodular; borders less well delineated; may shrink, become flatter, elongated, and less elastic; ligaments weaken; nipples are positioned lower
Vagina	Vagina lengthens; epithelial layers thicken; secretions become acidic	Growth complete by age 20	Introitus constricts; vagina narrows, shortens, loses rugation; mucosa is pale, thin, and dry; walls may lose structural integrity
Uterus	Musculature and vasculature increase; lining thickens	Growth complete by age 20	Size decreases; endometrial lining thins
Ovaries	Increase in size and weight; menarche occurs between 8 and 16 years of age; ovulation occurs monthly	Growth complete by age 20	Size decreases to 1 to 2 cm; follicles disappear; surface convolutes; ovarian function ceases between 40 and 55 years of age
Labia majora	Become more prominent; hair develops	Growth complete by age 20	Labia become smaller and flatter; pubic hair sparse and gray
Labia minora	Become more vascular	Growth complete by age 20	Become shinier and dryer
Uterine tubes	Increase in size	Growth complete by age 20	Decrease in size

hypothalamic-pituitary, and ovarian. The average length of a menstrual cycle is 28 days, but variations are normal. The first day of bleeding is designated day 1 of the menstrual cycle, or menses (Fig. 5-7). The average duration of menstrual flow is 5 days (range, 3 to 6 days), and the average blood loss is 50 ml (range, 20 to 80 ml), but these vary greatly.

For about 50% of women, menstrual blood does not appear to clot. The menstrual blood clots within the uterus, but the clot usually liquefies before being discharged from the uterus. Uterine discharge includes mucus and epithelial cells in addition to blood.

The menstrual cycle is a complex interplay of events that occur simultaneously in the endometrium, hypothalamus and pituitary glands, and ovaries. The menstrual cycle prepares the uterus for pregnancy. When pregnancy does not occur, menstruation follows. The woman's age, physical and emotional status, and environment influence the regularity of her menstrual cycles.

Endometrial Cycle

The four phases of the **endometrial cycle** are (1) the menstrual phase, (2) the proliferative phase, (3) the secretory phase, and (4) the ischemic phase (see Fig. 5-7). During the menstrual phase, shedding of the functional two thirds of the endometrium (the compact and spongy layers) is initiated by periodic vasoconstriction in the upper layers of the endometrium. The basal layer is always retained, and regeneration begins near the end of the cycle from cells derived from the remaining glandular remnants or stromal cells in this layer.

The proliferative phase is a period of rapid growth lasting from about the fifth day to the time of ovulation. The endometrial surface is completely restored in approximately 4 days, or slightly before bleeding ceases. From this point on, an eightfold to tenfold thickening occurs, with a leveling off of growth at ovulation. The proliferative phase depends on estrogen stimulation derived from ovarian follicles.

The secretory phase extends from the day of ovulation to about 3 days before the next menstrual period. After ovulation, larger amounts of progesterone are produced. An edematous, vascular, functional endometrium becomes apparent.

At the end of the secretory phase, the fully matured secretory endometrium reaches the thickness of heavy, soft velvet. It becomes luxuriant with blood and glandular secretions, a suitable protective and nutritive bed for a fertilized ovum.

Implantation of the fertilized ovum generally occurs about 7 to 10 days after ovulation. If fertilization and implantation do not occur, the corpus luteum, which secretes estrogen and progesterone, regresses. With the rapid decrease in progesterone and estrogen levels, the spiral arteries

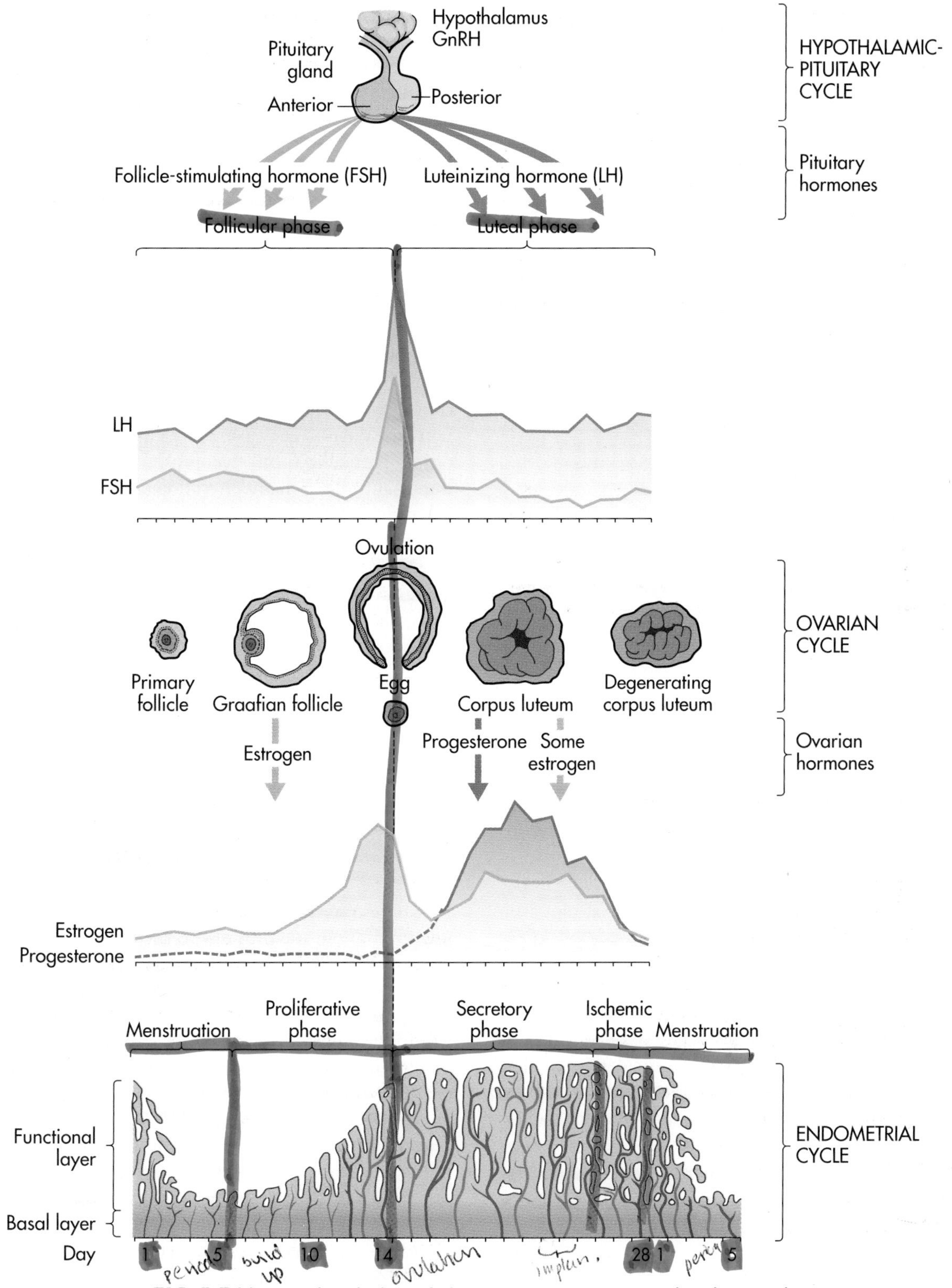
Hypothalamus
GnRH
Pituitary gland
Anterior
Posterior
HYPOTHALAMIC-PITUITARY CYCLE
Follicle-stimulating hormone (FSH)
Luteinizing hormone (LH)
Pituitary hormones
Follicular phase
Luteal phase
LH
FSH
Ovulation
Primary follicle
Graafian follicle
Egg
Corpus luteum
Degenerating corpus luteum
OVARIAN CYCLE
Estrogen
Progesterone
Some estrogen
Ovarian hormones
Estrogen
Progesterone
Menstruation
Proliferative phase
Secretory phase
Ischemic phase
Menstruation
Functional layer
Basal layer
ENDOMETRIAL CYCLE
Day
1
5
10
14
28
1
5

FIG. 5-7 Menstrual cycle: hypothalamic-pituitary, ovarian, and endometrial.

go into a spasm. During the ischemic phase, the blood supply to the functional endometrium is blocked, and necrosis develops. The functional layer separates from the basal layer, and menstrual bleeding begins, marking day 1 of the next cycle (see Fig. 5-7).

Hypothalamic-Pituitary Cycle

Toward the end of the normal menstrual cycle, blood levels of estrogen and progesterone decrease. Low blood levels of these ovarian hormones stimulate the hypothalamus to secrete gonadotropin-releasing hormone (GnRH).

In turn, GnRH stimulates anterior pituitary secretion of follicle-stimulating hormone (FSH). FSH stimulates development of ovarian graafian follicles and their production of estrogen. Estrogen levels begin to decrease, and hypothalamic GnRH triggers the anterior pituitary to release luteinizing hormone (LH). A marked surge of LH and a smaller peak of estrogen (day 12; see Fig. 5-7) precede the expulsion of the ovum from the graafian follicle by about 24 to 36 hours. LH peaks at about day 13 or 14 of a 28-day cycle. If fertilization and implantation of the ovum have not occurred by this time, regression of the corpus luteum follows. Levels of progesterone and estrogen decline, menstruation occurs, and the hypothalamus is once again stimulated to secrete GnRH. This process is called the **hypothalamic-pituitary cycle.**

Ovarian Cycle

The primitive graafian follicles contain immature oocytes (primordial ova). Before ovulation, from 1 to 30 follicles begin to mature in each ovary under the influence of FSH and estrogen. The preovulatory surge of LH affects a selected follicle. The oocyte matures, ovulation occurs, and the empty follicle begins its transformation to the corpus luteum. This follicular phase (preovulatory phase) (see Fig. 5-7) of the ovarian cycle varies in length from woman to woman. Almost all variations in ovarian cycle length are the result of variations in the length of the follicular phase. On rare occasions (i.e., 1 in 100 menstrual cycles), more than one follicle is selected, and more than one oocyte matures and undergoes ovulation.

After ovulation, estrogen levels decrease. For 90% of women, only a small amount of withdrawal bleeding occurs, so that it goes unnoticed. In 10% of women, there is sufficient bleeding for it to be visible, resulting in what is termed *midcycle bleeding*.

The luteal phase begins immediately after ovulation and ends with the start of menstruation. This postovulatory phase of the ovarian cycle usually requires 14 days (range, 13 to 15 days). The corpus luteum reaches its peak of functional activity 8 days after ovulation, secreting the steroids estrogen and progesterone. Coincident with this time of peak luteal functioning, the fertilized ovum is implanted in the endometrium. If no implantation occurs, the corpus luteum regresses, and steroid levels decrease. Two weeks after ovulation, if fertilization and implantation do not occur, the functional layer of the uterine endometrium is shed through menstruation.

Other Cyclic Changes

When the hypothalamic-pituitary-ovarian axis functions properly, other tissues undergo predictable responses. Before ovulation, the woman's basal body temperature (BBT) is often less than 37° C; after ovulation, with increasing progesterone levels, her BBT increases. Changes in the cervix and cervical mucus follow a generally predictable pattern. Preovulatory and postovulatory mucus is viscous (thick), so that sperm penetration is discouraged. At the time of ovulation, cervical mucus is thin and clear. It looks, feels, and stretches like egg white. This stretchable quality is termed *spinnbarkheit*. Some women have localized lower abdominal pain called *mittelschmerz* that coincides with ovulation.

Prostaglandins

Prostaglandins (PGs) are oxygenated fatty acids classified as hormones. The different kinds of PGs are distinguished by letters (PGE, PGF), numbers (PGE_2), and letters of the Greek alphabet ($PGF_{2\alpha}$).

Prostaglandins are produced in most organs of the body, including the uterus. Menstrual blood is a potent prostaglandin source. PGs are metabolized quickly by most tissues. They are biologically active in minute amounts in the cardiovascular, gastrointestinal, respiratory, urogenital, and nervous systems. They also exert a marked effect on metabolism, particularly on glycolysis. Prostaglandins play an important role in many physiologic, pathologic, and pharmacologic reactions. $PGF_{2\alpha}$, PGE_4, and PGE_2 are most commonly used in reproductive medicine.

Prostaglandins affect smooth muscle contractility and modulation of hormonal activity. Indirect evidence suggests that PGs have an effect on ovulation, fertility, changes in the cervix, and cervical mucus that affect receptivity to sperm, tubal and uterine motility, sloughing of endometrium (menstruation), onset of abortion (spontaneous and induced), and onset of labor (term and preterm).

After exerting their biologic actions, newly synthesized PGs are rapidly metabolized by tissues in such organs as the lungs, kidneys, and liver.

Prostaglandins may play a key role in ovulation. If PG levels do not increase along with the surge of LH, the ovum remains trapped within the graafian follicle. After ovulation, PGs may influence production of estrogen and progesterone by the corpus luteum.

The introduction of PGs into the vagina or into the uterine cavity (from ejaculated semen) increases the motility of uterine musculature, which may assist the transport of sperm through the uterus and into the oviduct.

Prostaglandins produced by the woman cause regression of the corpus luteum, regression of the endometrium, and sloughing of the endometrium, resulting in menstruation. PGs increase myometrial response to oxytocic stimulation, enhance uterine contractions, and cause cervical dilation. They may be a factor in the initiation of labor, the maintenance of labor, or both. They also may be involved in dysmenorrhea (see Chapter 7) and preeclampsia-eclampsia (see Chapter 30).

Climacteric and Menopause

The **climacteric** is a transitional phase during which ovarian function and hormone production decline. This phase spans the years from the onset of premenopausal ovarian decline to the postmenopausal time when symptoms stop. **Menopause** (from the Latin *mensis*, month, and

Greek *pausis*, to cease) refers only to the last menstrual period. Unlike menarche, however, menopause can be dated with certainty only 1 year after menstruation ceases. The average age at natural menopause is 51.4 years, with an age range of 35 to 60 years. **Perimenopause** is a period between 2 and 8 years before menopause, with an onset between the age of 39 and 51 years (Speroff et al., 1999).

SEXUAL RESPONSE

The hypothalamus and anterior pituitary gland in females regulate the production of FSH and LH. The target tissue for these hormones is the ovary, which produces ova and secretes estrogen and progesterone. A feedback mechanism between hormone secretion from the ovaries, hypothalamus, and anterior pituitary aids in the control of the production of sex cells and steroid sex hormone secretion.

Although the first outward appearance of maturing sexual development occurs at an earlier age in females, both females and males achieve physical maturity at approximately age 17 years; however, individual development varies greatly. Anatomic and reproductive differences notwithstanding, women and men are more alike than different in their physiologic response to sexual excitement and orgasm. For example, the glans clitoris and the glans penis are embryonic homologues. Little difference exists between female and male sexual response; the physical response is essentially the same whether stimulated by coitus, fantasy, or masturbation. Physiologically, according to Masters (1992), sexual response can be analyzed in terms of two processes: vasocongestion and myotonia.

Sexual stimulation results in increase in circulation to circumvaginal blood vessels (lubrication in the female), causing engorgement and distention of the genitals. Venous congestion is localized primarily in the genitals, but it also occurs to a lesser degree in the breasts and other parts of the body. Arousal is characterized by myotonia (increased muscular tension), resulting in voluntary and involuntary rhythmic contractions. Examples of sexually stimulated myotonia are pelvic thrusting, facial grimacing, and spasms of the hands and feet (carpopedal spasms).

The **sexual response cycle** is divided into four phases: excitement phase, plateau phase, orgasmic phase, and resolution phase. The four phases occur progressively with no sharp dividing line between any two phases. Specific body changes take place in sequence. The time, intensity, and duration for cyclic completion also vary for individuals and situations. Table 5-2 compares male and female body changes during each of the four phases of the sexual response cycle.

REASONS FOR ENTERING THE HEALTH CARE SYSTEM

Women's health assessment and screening focus on a systems evaluation, beginning with a careful history and physical examination. During the assessment and evaluation, the responsibilities for self-care, health promotion, and enhancement of wellness are emphasized. Nursing care includes assessment, planning, education, counseling, and referral as needed, as well as commendations for good self-care that the woman has practiced. This enables women to make informed decisions about their own health care.

Preconception Counseling and Care

Preconception health promotion provides women and their partners with information that is needed to make decisions about their reproductive future. Preconception counseling and care can be provided as part of routine health examinations such as premarital, employment, school, and family planning (Hobbins, 2001). Preconception counseling guides couples on how to avoid unintended pregnancies, how to identify and manage risk factors in their lives and their environment, and how to identify healthy behaviors that promote the well-being of the woman and her potential fetus.

The initiation of activities that promote healthy mothers and babies must occur before the period of critical fetal organ development, which is between 17 and 56 days after fertilization. By the end of the eighth week after conception and certainly by the end of the first trimester, any major structural anomalies in the fetus are already present. Because many women do not realize that they are pregnant and do not seek prenatal care until well into the first trimester, the rapidly growing fetus may be exposed to many types of intrauterine environmental hazards during this most vulnerable developmental phase. Thus preconception health care should occur well in advance of an actual pregnancy.

Preconception care is important for women who have had a problem with a previous pregnancy (e.g., miscarriage or preterm birth). Although causes are not always identifiable, in many cases, problems can be identified and treated and may not recur in subsequent pregnancies. Preconception care also is important to minimize fetal malformations. Many examples illustrate effects of maternal age or illnesses: conditions that produce anomalies in the fetus (teratogenic agents), such as drugs, viruses, chemicals; genetically inherited diseases; or conditions that might be harmful to the woman should a pregnancy occur. In many instances, counseling can allow behavior modification before damage is done, or a woman can make an informed decision about her willingness to accept potential hazards. The components of preconception care, such as health promotion, risk assessment, and interventions, are discussed in Chapter 17.

Pregnancy

A woman's entry into health care is often associated with pregnancy, either for diagnosis or for actual care. The possibility of pregnancy is realized most commonly when a woman is late with her menses. If she is pregnant, it is desirable for a woman to enter prenatal care within the

TABLE 5-2 **Four Phases of Sexual Response**

REACTIONS COMMON TO BOTH SEXES	FEMALE REACTIONS	MALE REACTIONS
Excitement Phase		
Heart rate and blood pressure increase. Nipples become erect. Myotonia begins.	Clitoris increases in diameter and swells. External genitals become congested and darken. Vaginal lubrication occurs; upper two thirds of vagina lengthen and extend. Cervix and uterus pull upward. Breast size increases.	Erection of the penis begins; penis increases in length and diameter. Scrotal skin becomes congested and thickens. Testes begin to increase in size and elevate toward the body.
Plateau Phase		
Heart rate and blood pressure continue to increase. Respirations increase. Myotonia becomes pronounced; grimacing occurs.	Clitoral head retracts under the clitoral hood. Lower one third of vagina becomes engorged. Skin color changes occur—red flush may be observed across breasts, abdomen, or other surfaces.	Head of penis may enlarge slightly. Scrotum continues to grow tense and thicken. Testes continue to elevate and enlarge. Preorgasmic emission of 2 or 3 drops of fluid appears on the head of the penis.
Orgasmic Phase		
Heart rate, blood pressure, and respirations increase to maximum levels. Involuntary muscle spasms occur. External rectal sphincter contracts.	Strong rhythmic contractions are felt in the clitoris, vagina, and uterus. Sensations of warmth spread through the pelvic area.	Testes elevate to maximum level. Point of "inevitability" occurs just before ejaculation and an awareness of fluid in the urethra. Rhythmic contractions occur in the penis. Ejaculation of semen occurs.
Resolution Phase		
Heart rate, blood pressure, and respirations return to normal. Nipple erection subsides. Myotonia subsides.	Engorgement in external genitalia and vagina resolves. Uterus descends to normal position. Cervix dips into seminal pool. Breast size decreases. Skin flush disappears.	Fifty percent of erection is lost immediately with ejaculation; penis gradually returns to normal size. Testes and scrotum return to normal size. Refractory period (time needed for erection to occur again) varies according to age and general physical condition.

BOX 5-1 **Major Goals of Prenatal Care**

- Define health status of mother and fetus.
- Determine the gestational age of the fetus, and monitor fetal development.
- Identify the woman at risk for complications, and minimize the risk whenever possible.
- Provide appropriate education and counseling.

first 12 weeks. This allows early pregnancy counseling, especially for the woman who has had no preconception care. Major goals of prenatal care are found in Box 5-1 and should be initiated at the first visit. Extensive discussion of pregnancy is found in Chapter 16.

Well-Woman Care

Current trends in the health care of women have expanded beyond a reproductive focus. A holistic approach to women's health care includes a woman's health needs throughout her lifetime. This view goes beyond simply her reproductive needs. This restructuring places women's health within the primary health care delivery system. Women's health assessment and screening focus on a multisystem evaluation emphasizing the maintenance and enhancement of wellness.

Support and reassurance begin with the woman's first contact with the health care team. It is often the nurse's responsibility in health promotion to coordinate the woman's care. A nurse often takes the history, orders diagnostic tests, interprets test results, makes referrals, and directs attention to the problems that require medical intervention and referral. Nurses who function in the expanded role as advanced practice nurses also can perform complete physical assessments, including the gynecologic examination.

Many women first enter the health care delivery system for a Pap smear or contraception. Visits to the nurse may be their only contact with the system unless they become ill. Some women postpone examination until a specific need arises, such as pregnancy, pain, abnormal bleeding, or vaginal discharge.

Health care needs vary with culture, religion, age, and personal differences. The changing responsibilities and roles of women, their socioeconomic status, and their personal lifestyles also contribute to differences in the health and behavior of women. Employment outside of the home, physical disability, inadequate or no health insurance, divorce, single parenthood, and sexual orientation also can affect women's ability to seek and receive health care in clinical settings. As women age, many continue to address their primary health care needs within their established gynecologic care setting; therefore well-women's health care should include a complete history, physical examination, and age-appropriate screening. In addition, health promotion must be included because it increases the levels of health and well-being and maximizes the health potential of all women.

Fertility Control and Infertility

As women become more informed about themselves and their health care, they are more willing to seek counseling and contraception appropriate to their varied and specific needs. Some women first enter the health care system to obtain such advice. More than half of the pregnancies in the United States each year are unintended, and the majority of these occur in the 10% of women who do not use birth control. Education is the key to encouraging women to make family planning choices based on preference and actual benefit-to-risk ratios. Providers can influence the user's motivation and ability to use the method correctly (see Chapter 9 for further discussion of contraception).

The concept of health promotion applies to contraception, as can be seen in Box 5-2. The nurse is in an ideal situation to influence women positively regarding the need for child spacing, methods of family planning that are consistent with religious and personal preferences, noncontraceptive benefits of certain methods, the appropriate use of methods selected, and the protection of future fertility when so desired.

Women also enter the health care system because of their desire to achieve a pregnancy. Approximately 15% of couples in the United States have some degree of infertility. Infertility can cause emotional pain for many couples, and the inability to produce an offspring sometimes results in feelings of failure and inordinate stress on the relationship. Significant amounts of time, money, and emotional investment can be used for testing and treatment in efforts to build a family.

BOX 5-2 Contraceptive Health Promotion

- Child spacing and quality maternity care improve perinatal outcomes and health in general of mother and children.
- Achieving desired family size enables a better sharing of all resources with attendant increases in education, health care, and other positive societal parameters.
- Contraceptives themselves may positively affect future health. For example, use of condoms may prevent acquisition of HIV infection; combined OCs may provide some protection against later development of cancer of ovary and endometrium; barrier methods decrease transmission of STIs, which can develop into pelvic inflammatory disease with resultant infertility or sterility and thus affect future childbearing capacity.

Infertility appears to be an ever-increasing problem. It is addressed more often in the media, and we may be seeing more couples trying to have babies because many have delayed starting their families until they are in their 30s or 40s, which allows more time to be exposed to situations negatively affecting fertility (including age-related infertility for the woman). In addition, sexually transmitted infections (STIs), which can predispose to decreased fertility, are becoming more common, and many women and men are in workplaces and home settings where they may be exposed to reproductive environmental hazards.

Steps toward prevention of infertility should be undertaken as part of ongoing routine health care, and such information is especially appropriate in preconception counseling. Primary care providers can undertake initial evaluation and counseling before couples are referred to specialists. For additional information about infertility, see Chapter 10.

Menstrual Problems

Irregularities or problems with the menstrual period are among the most common concerns of women and often cause them to seek help from the health care system. Common menstrual disorders include amenorrhea, dysmenorrhea, premenstrual syndrome, endometriosis, and menorrhagia or metrorrhagia. Simple explanation and counseling may handle the concern; however, history and examination must be completed, as well as laboratory or diagnostic tests, if indicated. Questions should never be considered inconsequential, and age-specific reading materials are recommended, especially for teenagers. Please see Chapter 7 for an in-depth discussion of menstrual problems.

Perimenopause

The body responds to this natural transition in a number of ways, most of which are due to the decrease in estrogen. Most women seeking health care during the perimenopausal period do so because of irregular bleeding. Others are concerned about vasomotor symptoms (hot flashes and flushes). Although fertility is greatly reduced during this period, women are urged to maintain some method of birth control because pregnancies still can occur. All women need to have factual information, the dispelling of myths, a thorough examination, and periodic health screenings thereafter. See Chapter 7 for discussion of perimenopause and menopause.

BARRIERS TO SEEKING HEALTH CARE

Financial Issues

The United States spends almost 15% of its gross domestic product on health, far more than any other industrialized nation in the world, yet major problems still exist. Employment-based financing of health insurance has resulted in a system in which one's health insurance is linked to a job, and the system is working well for fewer and fewer people, especially women. Fourteen percent of young women have no health insurance, and 5 million more have coverage so inadequate that it does not even include maternity care (National Women's Law Center, 2000).

In the United States, disparity among races and socioeconomic classes affects many facets of life, including health. With limited money and awareness, there is a lack of access to care, delay in seeking care, few prevention activities, and little accurate information about health and the health care system. Women use health services more often than do men but are more likely than men to have difficulty in financing the services; they are twice as often underinsured (i.e., have limited coverage with high-cost copayments or deductibles). Women make up the majority of Medicaid recipients; however, only 42% of poor women are eligible. Medicaid includes special benefits for pregnant women, but they are limited to treatment of pregnancy-related conditions and terminate 60 days after birth. Current questions abound regarding possible changes in the Medicaid coverage related to care for mother and child during the maternity cycle. More and more states are requiring their Medicaid recipients to enroll in managed care programs; whether this improves access and outcomes is yet to be determined.

Insurance coverage varies significantly by age, marital status, race, and ethnicity. Caucasians of all ages are more likely than African-Americans and other racial or ethnic groups to have private insurance. Caucasians possess insurance 2.5 times more often than Hispanics and 1.8 times more often than African-Americans. Single, separated, or divorced individuals are less likely to have insurance. Often unmarried teenagers, who are usually covered by their parents' medical insurance, do not have maternity coverage because policies have inclusion statements and cover only the employee or spouse.

Midwifery care has helped contain some health care costs, but reimbursement issues still exist in some areas. Nursing data must be identified and placed in a database to be included in public policy decisions; nursing variables such as client education and supportive care must become part of the national data-gathering system. Nurses should deal with the politics involved in cost-containment health care policies, because they, as knowledgeable experts, can provide solutions to many of the health care problems at a relatively low cost.

Parts of the health care delivery system remain in a state of flux. Great variation occurs depending on type and size of the system, source of payment for services, private versus public programs, availability of and accessibility to providers, individual preferences, and insurance coverage or ability to pay. The existing system continues to be oriented to treatment of acute or episodic conditions rather than the promotion of health and comprehensive care.

Cultural Issues

Although they are most significant, financial considerations are not the only barriers to obtaining high-quality health care. As our nation becomes more racially, ethnically, and culturally diverse, the health of minority groups becomes a major issue. A variety of reasons are given to explain some of the differences in accessing care when financial barriers are adjusted. Unfair treatment was described by women who experienced racial discrimination, or disrespectful, disillusioning, or discouraging encounters with community service providers such as social services and health care providers (Schulz, 2001). A lack of cross-cultural communication also presents problems. Desired health outcomes are best achieved when the health care provider has knowledge of and understanding about the culture, language, values, priorities, and health beliefs of those in minority groups. Conversely, members of the group should understand the health goals to be achieved and the methods proposed to do so. Language differences can produce profound barriers between women clients and those in the health care system. Even with a translator, information may be skewed in either direction.

Providers must consider culturally based differences that could affect the treatment of diverse groups of women, and the women themselves must share practices and beliefs that could influence their management responses or willingness to comply (Mattson, 2000a). For example, women in some cultures value privacy to such an extent that they are reluctant to disrobe and as a result avoid physical examination unless absolutely necessary. Other women rely on their husbands to make major decisions, including those affecting the woman's health. Religious beliefs may dictate a plan of care, as with birth control measures or blood transfusions. Some cultural groups prefer folk medicine, homeopathy, or prayer to traditional Western medicine, and others attempt combinations of some or all practices. In any event, it is incumbent on health care providers to value and appreciate their own and their client's various sources of information and beliefs about sickness and health. Even as there are increasing amounts of health information on the World Wide Web information in languages other than English is limited.

Gender Issues

Gender influences provider-client communication and may influence access to health care in general. The most obvious gender consideration is that between men and women. Researchers have reported significant male-female differences in receipt of major diagnostic and therapeutic interventions, especially with cardiac and kidney problems. Women tend to use primary care services more often than do men and, some believe, more effectively. The sex of the provider plays a role; studies have shown that female clients have Pap smears and mammograms more consistently if they are seen by female providers.

Sexual orientation may produce another barrier. Lesbian women have primary erotic attractions and relations with other women. Some lesbians may not disclose their orientation to health care providers because they feel they may be at risk for hostility, inadequate health care, or breach of confidentiality. In many health care settings, heterosexuality is assumed, and the setting may be one in which the woman does not feel welcome (magazines, brochures, and environment reflect heterosexual couples, or the health care provider shows discomfort interacting with the woman). Another problem is that lesbians themselves may hold beliefs that are incorrect, such as that they have immunity to human immunodeficiency virus (HIV), STIs, and certain cancers (e.g., cervical). The perceived lack of risk can result in lesbians avoiding medical care as well as in health care providers giving incorrect advice or not doing appropriate cancer screening for these women. Not all gynecologic cancers are related to sexual activity; lesbians who have never had children may be more at risk for breast, ovarian, and endometrial cancer. Their risk for heart disease, cancer of the lung, and colon cancer is not different from that of the heterosexual woman. To offset stereotypes, it is necessary for providers to develop an approach that does not assume that all clients are heterosexual (Stevens & Hall, 2001).

HEALTH RISKS IN THE CHILDBEARING YEARS

Maintaining optimal health is a goal for all women. Essential components of health maintenance are identification of unrecognized problems and potential risks and the education and health promotion needed to reduce them. This is especially important for women in their childbearing years, because conditions that increase a woman's health risks not only are of concern for her well-being but also are potentially associated with negative outcomes for both mother and baby in the event of a pregnancy. Prenatal care is an example of prevention that is practiced after conception; however, prevention and health maintenance are needed before pregnancy because many of the mother's risks can be identified and then eliminated or at least modified. An overview of conditions and circumstances that increase health risks in the childbearing years follows.

Age

Adolescence

As a girl progresses through development, she may be at risk for conditions that are age related. All teens undergo progressive growth of sexual characteristics and also undertake developmental tasks of adolescence, such as establishing identity, developing sexual preference, emancipating from family, and establishing career goals. Some of these situations can produce great stress for the adolescent, and the health care provider should treat her carefully. Female teenagers who enter the health care system usually do so for screening (Pap smears start at age 18 years or when the girl is sexually active) or because of a problem such as episodic illness or accidents. Gynecologic problems are often associated with menses (either bleeding irregularities or dysmenorrhea), vaginitis or leukorrhea, STIs, contraception, or pregnancy.

Many young women begin having sex in their mid to late teens; for those who do not, the likelihood of having intercourse increases steadily with age. A sexually active teen who does not use contraception has a 90% chance of pregnancy within 1 year (Alan Guttmacher Institute, 1998).

Teenage Pregnancy. Pregnancy in the teenager who is 16 years or younger often introduces additional stress into an already stressful developmental period. The emotional level of such teens is commonly characterized by impulsiveness and self-centered behavior, and they often place primary importance on the beliefs and actions of their peers. In attempts to establish a personal and independent identity, many teens do not realize the consequences of their behavior, and planning for the future is not part of their thinking processes.

Teenagers usually lack the financial resources to support a pregnancy and may not have the maturity to avoid teratogens or to have prenatal care and instruction or follow-up care. Children of teen mothers may be at risk for abuse or neglect because of the teen's inadequate knowledge of growth, development, and parenting. Implementation of specialized adolescent programs in schools, communities, and health care systems is demonstrating continued success in reducing the birth rate in teens, as evidenced by an overall 22% decline in teenage pregnancy between 1991 and 2000 (Hoyert et al., 2001).

Young and Middle Adulthood

Because women aged 20 to 40 years have need for contraception, pelvic and breast screening, and pregnancy care, they may prefer to use their gynecologic or obstetric provider as their primary care provider also. During these years, the woman may be "juggling" family, home, and career responsibilities, with resulting increases in stress-related conditions. Health maintenance includes not only pelvic and breast screening but also promotion of a healthy lifestyle, that is, good nutrition, regular exercise, no smoking, little or no alcohol consumption, sufficient rest, stress reduction, and referral for medical conditions and other specific problems. Common conditions requiring well-woman care include vaginitis, urinary tract infections, menstrual variations, obesity, sexual and relationship issues, and pregnancy.

Parenthood after Age 35 Years. The woman older than 35 years does not have a different physical response to a pregnancy, per se, but rather has had health status changes as a result of time and the aging process. These changes may be responsible for age-related pregnancy conditions. For example, a woman with type 2 diabetes may not have had expression of her diabetes at age 22 years, but may have full-blown disease at age 38 years. Other chronic or debilitating diseases or conditions increase in severity with time, and these, in turn, may predispose to increased risks during pregnancy. Of significance to women in this age group is the risk for certain genetic anomalies (e.g., Down syndrome), and the opportunity for genetic counseling should be available to all (see Research box and Chapter 3).

RESEARCH

Favorable Health Promotion Behaviors of Older Pregnant Women

It has been conventional to consider pregnancy in a woman over 35 years of age to be risky. Genetic abnormalities, early pregnancy loss, gestational diabetes, and pregnancy-induced hypertension increase in prevalence with age. There may be a lack of peer support for late-life pregnancy, as well as challenges caring for both young children and the women's own aging parents.

Nurse researchers set out to demonstrate the many positive attributes that the mature woman brings to her pregnancy and how nurses can maximize these strengths for healthy outcomes. They interviewed 50 women, ages 35-45, about their health concerns and health behaviors. Of the predominantly Caucasion, college-educated, and employed sample, 24% were primigravidas. Three fourths of the pregnancies were planned. Content analysis and coding revealed categories of maternal concern, including worries about fetal genetic problems, maternal pregnancy risk, and apprehension about postpartum maternal and family challenges. The overwhelming majority (86%) adopted health-promoting behaviors to enhance fetal and maternal health. Examples of these include adequate prenatal nutrition and intake of folic acid, strategies for adequate rest and weight control, early and consistent prenatal care, and avoidance of smoking, alcohol, and caffeine.

These older mothers were financially stable, enthusiastic about their pregnancies, and realistic. They were empowered to ask questions and seek a health care provider who would meet their individual needs. They were creative problem solvers and independently initiated positive changes.

IMPLICATIONS FOR PRACTICE

Nurses who recognize the strengths of the mature pregnant woman can collaborate with her for strategizing health behaviors that promote positive maternal and fetal outcomes. The nurse can provide educational resources, such as reputable websites and literature. Identifying conflicts and apprehensions about postpartum adaptation with the client can help her with problem solving. Lifestyle modifications during pregnancy can become permanent and enhance long-term health status.

Reference: Viau, P., Padula, C., & Eddy, B. (2002). An exploration of health concerns and health-promotion behaviors in pregnant women over age 35. *MCN American Journal of Maternal Child Nursing, 27*(6), 328-334.

Late Reproductive Age

Women of later reproductive age are often experiencing change and reordering of their personal priorities. Generally, the goals of education, career, marriage, and family have been achieved, and now the woman has increased time and opportunity for new interests and activities. Conversely, divorce rates are high at this age, and children leaving home may produce an "empty nest syndrome," resulting in increased levels of depression. Chronic diseases also become more apparent. Most problems for the well woman are associated with perimenopause (e.g., bleeding irregularities and vasomotor symptoms). Health maintenance screening continues to be of importance because some conditions such as breast disease or ovarian cancer occur more often during this stage.

Social-Cultural

Differences exist among people from different socioeconomic levels and ethnic groups with respect to risk for illness and distribution of disease and death. Some diseases are more common among people of selected ethnicity (e.g., sickle cell anemia in African-Americans, Tay-Sachs disease in Ashkenazi Jews, adult lactase deficiency in Chinese, β-thalassemia in Mediterranean peoples, and cystic fibrosis in northern Europeans). Cultural and religious influences also increase health risks because the woman and her family may have life and societal values and a view of health and illness that dictate practices different from those expected in the Judeo-Christian Western model. These may include food taboos, methods of hygiene, effects of climate, care-seeking behaviors, willingness to undergo screening and diagnostic procedures, and value conflicts.

Socioeconomic status affects birth outcomes. The rates of perinatal and maternal deaths, preterm births, and low-birth-weight babies are considerably higher in disadvantaged populations (Hoyert et al., 2001). Social consequences for poor women as single parents are great, because many mothers with few skills are caught in the bind of insufficient income to afford child care. These families generate fewer and fewer resources and increase their risks for health problems. Multiple roles for women in general produce overload, conflict, and stress, resulting in higher risks for psychologic illness.

Substance Use and Abuse

Use of illicit drugs and inappropriate use of prescription drugs continue to increase and are found in all ages, races, ethnic groups, and socioeconomic strata. Addiction to substances is seen as a biopsychosocial disease with several factors leading to risk. These include biogenetic predisposition, lack of resilience to stressful life experiences, and poor social support. Women are less likely than men to abuse drugs, but the rate in women is increasing significantly. Substance-abusing pregnant women create severe problems for themselves and their offspring, including interference with optimal growth and development and addiction. In many instances, the use of substances is identified through screening programs in prenatal clinics and obstetric units (see Chapter 35).

Smoking

Tobacco use is the leading cause of preventable death in the United States. Smoking is linked to cardiovascular heart disease, various types of cancers (especially lung and cervical), chronic lung disease, and negative pregnancy outcomes. Tobacco contains nicotine, which is an addictive substance that creates a physical and a psychologic dependence.

Smoking rates vary among women in different U.S. ethnic groups. Of the 22 million women smokers in the United States, Native American and Alaskan Native women have the highest rates of all ethnic groups. African-American and Caucasian women have the next highest rates, whereas Asian-American and Hispanic women have the lowest prevalence. Tobacco use among adolescents increased in the 1990s: 1.5 million adolescent girls in the United States smoke cigarettes (Surgeon General's Report on Women and Smoking, 2001).

Cigarette smoking impairs fertility in both women and men, may reduce the age for menopause, and increases the risk for osteoporosis after menopause. Passive, or secondhand, smoke (environmental tobacco smoke [ETS]) contains similar hazards and presents additional problems for the smoker, as well as harm for the nonsmoker. Smoking in pregnancy is known to cause a decrease in placental perfusion and is one cause of low birth weight in infants (American College of Obstetricians and Gynecologists, 1997).

Alcohol

Women aged 35 to 49 years have the highest rates of chronic alcoholism, but women aged 21 to 34 have the highest rates of specific alcohol-related problems. About one third of alcoholics are women, and many relate onset of their drinking problem to stressful events. Women who are problem drinkers are often depressed, have more motor vehicle injuries, and have a higher incidence of attempted suicide than do women in the general population. They also are at risk for alcohol-related liver damage. Early case finding and treatment are important in alcoholism for both the ill individual and for family members. See Chapter 35 for further discussion about alcohol use in women.

Prescription Drugs

Psychotherapeutic medications such as stimulants, sleeping pills, tranquilizers, and pain relievers are used by an estimated 2% of American women. Such medications can bring relief from undesirable conditions such as insomnia, anxiety, and pain, but because the medications have mind-altering capacity, misuse can produce psychologic and physical dependency in the same manner as do illicit drugs. Risk-to-benefit ratios should be considered when such medications are used for more than short periods.

Depression is the most common mental health problem in women. Many kinds of medications are used to treat depression. All of these psychotherapeutic drugs can have some effect on the fetus when taken during pregnancy and must be very carefully monitored (see Chapter 35).

Illicit Drugs

Illicit drugs are taken for unlawful purposes. When they are unprescribed, they are usually obtained on the street for the purpose of getting high or for their body-mind–altering characteristics. Almost any drug can be illegal if taken in excess, including alcohol and prescription medication. A brief list of illicit drugs follows in Box 5-3 (see Chapter 35 for further discussion of substance abuse).

Nutrition

Good nutrition is essential for optimal health. A well-balanced diet helps prevent illness and also is used to treat certain health problems. Conversely, poor eating habits, eating disorders, and obesity are linked to disease and debility.

Nutritional Deficiencies

Overt disease caused by lack of certain nutrients is rarely seen in the United States; however, insufficient amounts or imbalances of nutrients do pose problems for individuals and families. Overweight or underweight status, malabsorption,

BOX 5-3 Illicit Drugs

Amphetamines
Barbiturates
Club drugs
Cocaine
Depressants
Designer drugs
gamma-Hydroxybutyrate (GHB)
Hallucinogens
Heroin
Inhalants
Ketamine
Lysergic acid diethylamide (LSD)
Marijuana
Methamphetamines
Methylenedioxymethamphetamine (MDMA or Ecstasy)
Nitrous oxide
Phencyclidine (PCP)
Psychedelics
Flunitrazepam (Rohypnol)
Stimulants

Source: *Epidemiologic trends in drug abuse advance report.* (2000). Washington, DC: National Institute on Drug Abuse.

listlessness, fatigue, frequent colds and other minor infections, constipation, dull hair and thin nails, and dental caries are examples of problems that can be related to nutrition and indicate the need for further nutritional assessment. Poor nutrition, especially related to obesity and high fat and cholesterol intake, may lead to more serious conditions and is said to contribute to 4 of the 10 leading causes of death in the United States: diseases of the heart, malignant neoplasms, cerebrovascular diseases, and diabetes (Minino & Smith, 2001).

Obesity

During the past 20 years, there has been a dramatic increase in obesity in the United States. It is estimated that 25% of the women older than 20 years are obese (body mass index [BMI], 30 or higher), and 51% of the women older than 20 years are overweight (BMI, 25 to 25.9) (NCCDPHP, 2000). The BMI is defined as a measure of an adult's weight in relation to his or her height, specifically the adult's weight in kilograms divided by the square of his or her height in meters (Box 5-4 and Table 15-2).

Overweight and obesity are known risk factors for diabetes, heart disease, stroke, hypertension, gallbladder disease, osteoarthritis, sleep apnea, and some types of cancer (uterine, breast, colorectal, kidney, and gallbladder) (American Cancer Society, 2003). In addition, obesity is associated with high cholesterol, menstrual irregularities, hirsutism (excess body/facial hair), stress incontinence, depression, complications of pregnancy, increased surgical risk, and shortened life span (Surgeon General's Call to Action to Prevent and Decrease Overweight and Obesity, 2000). Pregnant women who are morbidly obese are at increased risk for hypertension, diabetes, gallbladder disease, postterm pregnancy, and musculoskeletal problems (de Groot, 1999).

BOX 5-4 Ideal Body Weight with Body Mass Index (BMI)

BMI ≤18.5, underweight
BMI 18.5 to 24.9, normal weight
BMI 25.0 to 29.9, overweight
BMI 30.0 to 34.5, obese
BMI 35.0 to 40, very obese

Source: Weiss, J., & Scott, L. (2001). Stalking the no. 1 killer of women: Detecting diabetes and heart diseases. *AWHONN Lifelines,* 5(5), 26-34.

Other Considerations

Other dietary extremes also can produce risk. For example, insufficient amounts of calcium can lead to osteoporosis, too much sodium can aggravate hypertension, and megadoses of vitamins can cause adverse effects in several body systems. Fad weight-loss programs and yo-yo dieting (repeated weight gain and weight loss) result in nutritional imbalances and, in some instances, medical problems. Such diets and programs are not appropriate for weight maintenance. Adolescent pregnancy produces special nutritional requirements because the metabolic needs of pregnancy are superimposed on the teen's own needs for growth and maturation at a time when eating habits are less than ideal.

Anorexia Nervosa. Some women have a distorted view of their bodies and, no matter what their weight, perceive themselves to be much too heavy. As a result, they undertake strict and severe diets and rigorous extreme exercise. This chronic eating disorder is known as anorexia nervosa. A coexisting depression usually accompanies anorexia. Women can carry this condition to the point of starvation, with resulting endocrine and metabolic abnormalities. If not corrected, significant complications of arrhythmias, amenorrhea, cardiomyopathy, and congestive heart failure occur and, in the extreme, can lead to death. The condition commonly begins during adolescence in young women who have some degree of personality disorder. They gradually lose weight over several months, have amenorrhea, and are abnormally concerned with body image. The condition requires both psychiatric and medical intervention.

Bulimia Nervosa. Bulimia refers to secret, uncontrolled binge eating alternating with methods to prevent weight gain: self-induced vomiting, laxatives or diuretics, strict diets, fasting, and rigorous exercise (Orbanic, 2001). During a binge episode, large numbers of calories are consumed, usually consisting of sweets and "junk foods." Binges occur at least twice per week. Bulimia usually begins in early adulthood (ages 18 to 25 years) and is found primarily in female clients. Complications can include dehydration and electrolyte imbalance, gastrointestinal abnormalities, and cardiac arrhythmias. Bulimia is somewhat similar to anorexia in that it is an eating disorder and usually involves some degree of depression. Unlike those with anorexia, individuals with bulimia may feel shame or disgust about their disorder and tend to seek help earlier.

Physical Fitness and Exercise

Exercise contributes to good health by reducing risks for a variety of conditions that are influenced by obesity and a sedentary lifestyle. It is effective in the prevention of cardiovascular disease and in the management of chronic conditions such as hypertension, arthritis, diabetes, respiratory disorders, and osteoporosis. Exercise also contributes to stress reduction and weight maintenance. Women report that engaging in regular exercise improves their body image and self-esteem and acts as a mood enhancer. Aerobic exercise produces cardiovascular involvement because increasing amounts of oxygen are delivered to working muscles. Anaerobic exercise, such as weight training, improves individual muscle mass without stress on the cardiovascular system. Because women are concerned about both cardiovascular and bone health, weight-bearing aerobic exercises such as walking, running, racket sports, and dancing are preferred. However, excessive or strenuous exercise can lead to hormonal imbalances, resulting in amenorrhea and its consequences. Physical injury also is a potential risk.

Stress

The modern woman faces increasing levels of stress and as a result is prone to a variety of stress-induced complaints and illness. Stress often occurs because of multiple roles in which coping with job and financial responsibilities conflicts with parenting and duties at home. To add to this burden, women are socialized to be caretakers, which is emotionally draining in itself. They also may find themselves in positions of minimal power that do not allow them to have control over their everyday environments. Some stress is normal and contributes to positive outcomes. Many women thrive in busy surroundings. However, excessive or high levels of ongoing stress trigger physical reactions in the body, such as rapid heart rate, elevated blood pressure, slowed digestion, release of additional neurotransmitters and hormones, muscle tenseness, and a weakened immune system. Consequently, constant stress can contribute to clinical illnesses such as flare-ups of arthritis or asthma, frequent colds or infections, gastrointestinal upsets, cardiovascular problems, and infertility. Box 5-5 lists symptoms that may be related to chronic or extreme stress. Psychologic signs such as anxiety, irritability, eating disorders, depression, insomnia, and substance abuse also have been associated with stress.

BOX 5-5 Stress Symptoms

PHYSICAL
- Perspiration/sweaty hands
- Increased heart rate
- Trembling
- Nervous tics
- Dryness of throat and mouth
- Tiring easily
- Urinating frequently
- Sleeping problems
- Diarrhea, indigestion, vomiting
- Butterflies in stomach
- Headaches
- Premenstrual tension
- Pain in the neck and lower back
- Loss of appetite or overeating
- Susceptibility to illness

BEHAVIOR
- Stuttering and other speech difficulties
- Crying for no apparent reason
- Acting impulsively
- Startling easily
- Laughing in a high-pitched and nervous tone of voice
- Grinding teeth
- Increasing smoking
- Increasing use of drugs and alcohol
- Being accident prone
- Losing appetite or overeating

PSYCHOLOGIC
- Feeling anxious
- Feeling scared
- Feeling irritable
- Feeling moody
- Low self-esteem
- Fear of failure
- Inability to concentrate
- Embarrassing easily
- Worrying about the future
- Preoccupation with thoughts or tasks
- Forgetfulness

Modified from The State University of New York Counseling Center. (2002). *Stress management.* Buffalo: University of Buffalo, The State University of New York.

Sexual Practices

Potential risks related to sexual activity are undesired pregnancy and STIs. The risks are particularly high for adolescents and young adults who engage in sexual intercourse at earlier and earlier ages (Hutchinson et al., 2001). Adolescents report many reasons for wanting to be sexually active, among which are peer pressure, desire to love and be loved, experimentation, enhancing self-esteem, and having fun. However, many teens do not have the decision-making or values-clarification skills needed to take this important step at a young age and lack the knowledge base regarding contraception and STIs. They also do not believe that becoming pregnant or getting an STI will happen to them.

Although some STIs can be cured with antibiotics, many can cause significant problems. Possible sequelae include infertility, ectopic pregnancy, neonatal morbidity and mortality, genital cancers, acquired immunodeficiency syndrome (AIDS), and even death (CDC, 2002). STIs are increasing rapidly and are in epidemic proportion. Choice of contraception has an impact on the risk of contracting an STI; however, no method of contraception offers complete protection. (See Chapter 8 for discussion of STIs and Chapter 9 for contraception.)

NURSE ALERT

A comprehensive sexual assessment should be integrated into all health histories (Peck, 2001).

Medical Conditions

Most women of reproductive age are relatively healthy. Heart disease; lung, breast, colon, and other nongynecologic cancers; chronic lung disease; and diabetes are all concerns for adult women, as they are among the leading causes of death in women (Box 5-6). Certain medical conditions present during pregnancy can have deleterious effects on both the woman and the fetus. Of particular concern are risks from all forms of diabetes, urinary tract disorders, thyroid disease, hypertensive disorders of pregnancy, cardiac disease, and seizure disorders. Effects on the fetus vary and include intrauterine growth restriction, macrosomia, anemia, prematurity, immaturity, and stillbirth. Effects on the woman also can be severe. These conditions are discussed in later chapters.

BOX 5-6 Leading Causes of Death in the United States from the 2000 Census Data

1. Diseases of the heart
2. Malignant neoplasms (cancer)
3. Cerebrovascular diseases (stroke)
4. Chronic lower respiratory diseases (chronic obstructive pulmonary disease [COPD])
5. Accidents
6. Diabetes mellitus
7. Influenza and pneumonia
8. Alzheimer's disease
9. Nephritis, nephrotic syndrome, and nephrosis
10. Septicemia

Source: Minino, A., & Smith, B. (2001). *Deaths: Preliminary data for 2000, National Vital Statistics Reports* (Vol. 49 no. 12). Hyattsville, MD: National Center for Health Statistics.

Gynecologic Conditions

Women are at risk for pelvic inflammatory disease, endometriosis, STIs and other vaginal infections, uterine fibroids, uterine deformities such as bicornuate uterus, ovarian cysts, and urinary incontinence related to pelvic relaxation throughout their reproductive years. These gynecologic conditions may contribute negatively to pregnancy by causing infertility, miscarriage, preterm labor, and fetal and neonatal problems. Gynecologic cancers also affect women's health, although the risk for most cancers is low in pregnancy. Risk factors depend on the type of cancer. The impact of developing a gynecologic problem or cancer on women and their families is shaped by a number of factors including the specific type of problem or cancer, the implications of the diagnosis for the woman and her family, and the timing of the occurrence in the woman's and the family's lives. These conditions are discussed in Chapters 7, 8, and 12.

Environmental and Workplace Hazards

Environmental hazards in the home, workplace, and community can contribute to poor health at all ages. Categories and examples of health-damaging hazards include the following: (1) pathogenic agents (viruses, bacteria, fungi, parasites); (2) natural and synthetic chemicals (natural toxins from animals, insects, and plants; consumer and industrial products such as pesticides and hydrocarbon gases; medical and diagnostic devices; tobacco; fuels; and drug and alcohol abuse); (3) radiation (radon, heat waves, sound waves); (4) food substances (added components that are not necessary for nutrition); and (5) physical objects (moving vehicles, machinery, weapons, water, and building materials).

Environmental hazards can affect fertility, fetal development, live birth, and the child's future mental and physical development. Children are at special risk for poisoning from lead found in paint and soil. Everyone is at risk from air pollutants, such as tobacco smoke, carbon monoxide, smog, suspended particles (dust, ash, and asbestos), and cleaning solvents; noise pollution; pesticides; chemical additives; and poor preparation of food. Workers also face safety and health risks caused by ergonomically poor workstations and stress. The lists could go on and on. It is important that risk assessments continue so that we may identify and understand environmental public health problems.

Violence Against Women

Violence against women is a major health care problem in the United States, affecting 2 to 4 million women each year and costing millions of dollars in annual medical costs. Women of all races and of all ethnic, educational, religious, and socioeconomic backgrounds are affected. Pregnancy is often a time when violence begins or escalates. The magnitude of the problem is far greater than the statistics indicate, because violent crimes against women are the most underreported data as a result of fear, lack of understanding, and stigma surrounding violent situations (Stringham, 1999).

Maternity and women's health nurses, by the very nature of their practice, are in a unique position to conduct case finding, provide sensitive care to women experiencing abusive situations, engage in prevention activities, and influence health care and public policy toward decreasing the violence. (For further discussion of violence against women, see Chapter 6.)

HEALTH ASSESSMENT

Profound changes in society and the family and in roles and expectations of women make maternity nursing and women's health care a challenging field. Current women's health trends have expanded beyond a reproductive focus to include a holistic approach to health care across the life span. This restructuring deemphasizes tertiary care and places women's health within the scope of primary care. Women's health assessment and screening focuses on a systems evaluation beginning with a careful history and physical examination. During the assessment and evaluation, the responsibility for self-care, health promotion, and enhancement of wellness is emphasized. Nursing is an interactive process that begins with establishing trust and a caring relationship, with the broader goal of enhancing and maintaining wellness. The nurse provides care that includes assessment, planning, education, counseling, and referral as needed, as well as commendations for good self-care that the woman has practiced. This enables women to make informed decisions about their own health care.

In a market-driven system such as managed care, specific guidelines may be provided for health screening by the insurer or managed care organization. A nurse often takes the history, orders diagnostic tests, interprets test results, makes referrals, coordinates care, and directs attention to problems requiring medical intervention. Advanced practice nurses who have specialized in women's health, such as nurse practitioners, clinical nurse specialists, and nurse midwives, perform complete physical examinations, including gynecologic examinations.

Culturally competent nursing care should be delivered with an awareness of cultural diversity while respecting the unique qualities of each woman. Such care cannot be provided in the absence of self-awareness. Nurses must acknowledge their own values, beliefs, and communication styles to understand what they contribute to cross-cultural communication (Mattson, 2000b).

Interview

The contact with the woman usually begins with an interview. This interview should be conducted in a private, comfortable, and relaxed setting (Fig. 5-8). The nurse is seated and makes sure the woman is comfortable. The woman is addressed by her title and name (e.g., Mrs. Gonzalez), and the nurse introduces herself or himself by using name and title. It is important to phrase questions in a sensitive and nonjudgmental manner. Body language should match verbal communication. The nurse is cognizant of a woman's vulnerability and assures her of strict confidentiality. For many women, fear, anxiety, and modesty make the examination a dreaded and stressful experience. Many women are uninformed, misguided by myths, or afraid they will appear ignorant by asking questions about sexual or reproductive functioning. The woman is assured that no question is irrelevant. The history begins with an open-ended question such as, "What brings you in to the office/clinic/hospital today? Anything else? Tell me about it."

Additional ways to get women to share information include the following:

- **Facilitation:** Using a word or posture that communicates interest; leaning forward; making eye contact; or saying "Mm-hmmm" or "Go on."
- **Reflection:** Repeating a word or phrase that a woman has used.
- **Clarification:** Asking the woman what is meant by a word or phrase.
- **Empathic responses:** Acknowledging the feelings of a woman by statements such as, "That must have been frightening."
- **Confrontation:** Identifying something about the woman's behavior or feelings not expressed verbally or apparently inconsistent with her history.
- **Interpretation:** Putting into words what you infer about the woman's feelings or about the meaning of her symptoms, events, or other matters.

Direct questions may be necessary to elicit specific details. These should be worded in language that is

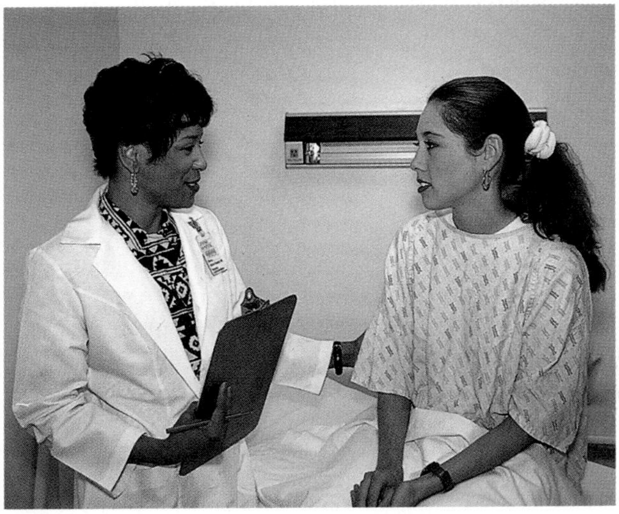

FIG. 5-8 Nurse interviews patient as part of annual physical examination. (From Potter, P., & Perry, A. (1997). *Fundamentals of nursing: concepts, process, and practice* (4th ed.). St. Louis: Mosby.)

understandable to the woman and expressed neutrally so that the woman will not be led into a specific response. The nurse asks about one item at a time and proceeds from the general to the specific (Seidel et al., 2003).

Cultural Considerations and Communication Variations

Recognizing signs and symptoms of disease and deciding when to seek treatment are influenced by cultural perceptions. Culture evolves over time and is a system of symbols that are learned, shared, and passed on through generations of a social group. Cultural competence in nursing is a complex combination of knowledge, attitudes, and skills mixed with personal attributes of flexibility, empathy, and language facility. It is more than simply acquiring knowledge about another ethnic group. It is essential that a nurse have respect for the rich and unique qualities that cultural diversity brings to individuals. In recognizing the value of these differences, the nurse can modify the plan of care to meet the needs of each woman. Trust that the woman is the expert on her life, culture, and experiences. If the nurse asks with respect and a genuine desire to learn, the client will tell the nurse how to care for her (Mattson, 2000a). The nurse communicates in an even-toned and nonjudgmental manner, keeps a calm facial expression, and recognizes that modifications may be necessary for the physical examination. In some cultures, it may be considered inappropriate for the woman to disrobe completely for the physical examination. In many cultures, a woman examiner is preferred.

Communication may be hindered by different beliefs even when the nurse and client speak the same language. Communication variations include the following (Mattson, 2000a):

- **Conversational style and pacing:** Silence may show respect or acknowledgment that the listener has heard. In cultures in which a direct "no" is considered rude, silence may mean no. Repetition or loudness may mean emphasis or anger.
- **Personal space:** Cultural conceptions of personal space differ, based on one's culture. Someone may be perceived as distant for backing off when approached or aggressive for standing too close.
- **Eye contact:** Eye contact varies among cultures from intense to fleeting. In an effort to refrain from invading personal space, avoiding direct eye contact may be a sign of respect.
- **Touch:** The norms about how people should touch each other vary among cultures. In some cultures, physical contact with the same sex (embracing, walking hand in hand) is more appropriate than that with an unrelated person of the opposite sex.
- **Time orientation:** In some cultures, involvement with people is more valued than being "on time." In other cultures, life is scheduled and paced according to clock time, which is valued over personal time.

Women with Special Needs

Women with Disabilities

Women with emotional or physical disorders have special needs. Women who have vision, hearing, emotional, or physical disabilities should be respected and involved in the assessment and physical examination to the full extent of their abilities. The nurse should communicate openly and directly with sensitivity. It is often helpful to learn about the disability directly from the woman while maintaining eye contact. Family and significant others should be relied on only when absolutely necessary. The assessment and physical examination can be adapted to each woman's individual needs.

Communication with a woman who is hearing impaired can be accomplished without difficulty. Most of these women read lips, write, or both; thus an interviewer who speaks and enunciates each word slowly and in full view may be easily understood. If a woman is not comfortable with lip reading, she may use an interpreter. In this case, it is important to continue to address the woman directly, avoiding the temptation to speak directly with the interpreter. The visually impaired woman needs to be oriented to the examination room and may have her guide dog with her. As with all clients, the visually impaired woman needs a full explanation of what the examination entails before proceeding. Before touching her, the nurse explains, "Now I am going to take your blood pressure. I am going to place the cuff on your right arm." The woman can be asked if she would like to touch each of the items that will be used in the examination to reduce her anxiety.

Many women with physical disabilities cannot comfortably lie in the lithotomy position for the pelvic examination. Several alternative positions may be used, including a lateral (side-lying) position, a V-shaped position, a diamond-shaped position, and an M-shaped position (Fig. 5-9). The woman can be asked what has worked best for her previously. If she has never had a pelvic examination, or has never had a comfortable pelvic examination, the nurse proceeds slowly by showing her a picture of various positions and asking her which one she prefers. The nurse's support and reassurance can help the woman to relax, which will make the examination go more smoothly. The woman is informed that she is in charge, and if the examination must stop for whatever reason, it can be scheduled again at a later date.

Abused Women

Nurses should screen all women entering the health care system for potential abuse. It is important to keep in mind the possibility that violence against this woman may have occurred. The risk for domestic violence increases during pregnancy and after separation or divorce. Many health care providers avoid questions about family violence because they are unaware of the extent of the problem; they find it difficult to ask about violence; or they feel helpless to assist the woman. Help for the woman may depend on

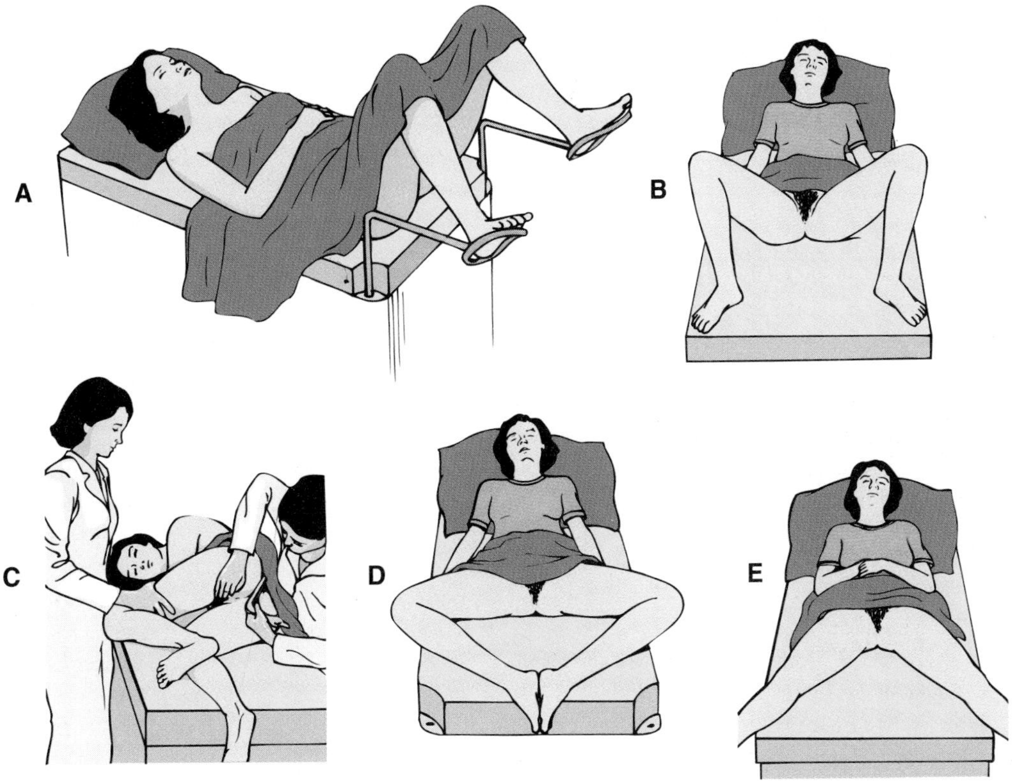
A
B
C
D
E

FIG. 5-9. Lithotomy and variable positions for women who have a disability. **A,** Lithotomy position. **B,** M-shaped position. **C,** Knee-chest position. **D,** Diamond-shaped position. **E,** V-shaped position.

the sensitivity with which the nurse screens for abuse, the discovery of abuse, and subsequent intervention. The nurse must be familiar with the laws governing abuse in the state in which she or he practices.

Pocket cards listing emergency numbers (abuse counseling, legal protection, and emergency shelter) may be available from the local police department, women's shelter, or an emergency department. It is helpful to have these on hand in the setting where screening is done. An abuse-assessment screen (Fig. 5-10) can be used as part of the interview or written history. If a male partner is present, he should be asked to leave the room because the woman may not disclose experiences of abuse in his presence, or he may try to answer questions for her to protect himself. The same procedure would apply for partners of lesbians, parents of teens, or adult children of older women.

Fear, guilt, and embarrassment may keep many women from giving information about family violence. Clues in the history and evidence of injuries on physical examination should give a high index of suspicion. The areas most commonly injured in women are the head, neck, chest, abdomen, breasts, and upper extremities. Burns and bruises in patterns resembling hands, belts, cords, or other weapons may be seen as well as multiple traumatic injuries. Attention should be given to women who repeatedly seek treatment for somatic complaints such as headaches; insomnia; choking sensation; hyperventilation; gastrointestinal symptoms; and pain in the chest, back, and pelvis. During pregnancy, the nurse should assess for injuries to the breasts, abdomen, and genitals. See Chapter 6 for further discussion of violence.

Adolescents (Aged 13 to 19 Years)

As a young woman matures, she should be asked the same questions that are included in any history. Particular attention should be paid to hints about risky behaviors, eating disorders, and depression. Do not assume that a teenager is not sexually active. After rapport has been established, it is best to talk to a teen with the parent (partner or friend) out of the room. Questions should be asked with sensitivity and in a gentle and nonjudgmental manner (Seidel et al., 2003).

A teen's first speculum examination is the most important because she will develop perceptions that will remain with her for future examinations. What the examination entails should be discussed with the teen while she is dressed. Models or illustrations can be used to show exactly what will happen. All of the necessary equipment should be assembled so that there are no interruptions. Pediatric specula that are 1- to 1.5-cm wide can be inserted

ABUSE ASSESSMENT SCREEN

1. Have you ever been emotionally or physically abused by your partner or someone important to you?

YES ☐ NO ☐

2. Within the last year, have you been hit, slapped, kicked, or otherwise physically hurt by someone?

YES ☐ NO ☐

If YES, by whom ______________________

Number of times ______________________

Mark the area of injury on body map.

3. Within the last year, has anyone forced you to have sexual activities?

YES ☐ NO ☐

If YES, by whom ______________________

Number of times ______________________

4. Are you afraid of your partner or anyone you listed above?

YES ☐ NO ☐

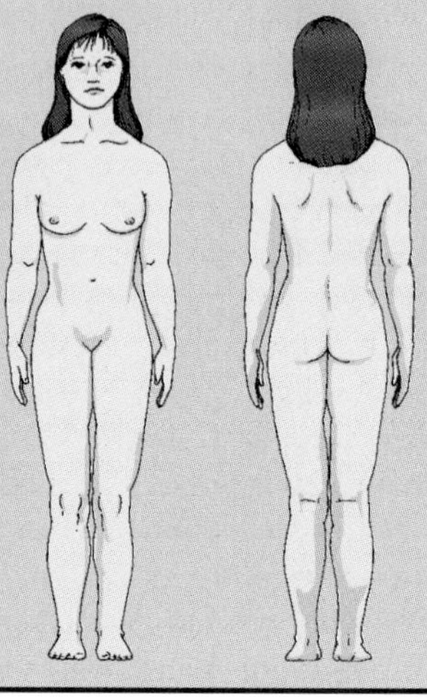

FIG. 5-10 Abuse assessment screen. (Modified from the Nursing Research Consortium on Violence and Abuse, 1991.)

with minimal discomfort. If the teen is sexually active, a small adult speculum may be used.

Injury prevention should be a part of the counseling at routine health examinations, with special attention to seat belts, helmets, firearms, recreational hazards, and sports involvement. The use of drugs and alcohol and the nonuse of seat belts contribute to motor vehicle injuries, accounting for the greatest proportion of accidental deaths in women (Hoyert et al., 2001). Contraceptive options, including use of condoms, should be addressed during visits.

To provide developmentally appropriate care, it is important to review the major tasks for women in this stage of life. Major tasks for teens include values assessment; education and work goal setting; formation of peer relationships that focus on love, commitment, and becoming comfortable with sexuality; and separation from parents. Individuality may be reflected in areas such as sexuality, politics, and career choices. Conflict exists between making and keeping commitments to keep options open. The teen is egocentric as she progresses rapidly through emotional and physical change. Her feelings of invulnerability may lead to serious misconceptions, such as that unprotected sexual intercourse will not lead to pregnancy.

Midlife and Older Women (Aged 50 Years and Older)

The assessment of women aged 50 and older presents unique challenges. Women may be experiencing major lifestyle changes, such as children leaving home, care for their aging parents, job retirement, divorce or death of a partner, aging changes, and health problems. The nurse has an opportunity to use reflection and empathy while listening and ensuring open and caring communication. It may be necessary to schedule a longer appointment time because older women have longer histories or have a need to talk. Some women may fail to report symptoms because they fear their complaints will be attributed to old age or they feel that they have lived with a chronic condition (e.g., incontinence, dyspareunia, decreased libido) for so long that nothing can be done. Women may choose to ignore a problem if they have symptoms that are life threatening (e.g., chest pain or a breast lump) because they traditionally put the needs of others first. As a result, the nurse should encourage the woman to express her concerns and fears and reassure her that her problems are important and will be addressed. Hormone therapy, diet, vitamin and calcium supplementation, daily aspirin, breast self-examination, mammogram, sigmoidoscopy, colonoscopy, updating immunizations, and need for exercise and sun protection should be discussed.

Sexual assessment continues to be important in women aged 50 and older. Unless directly asked, women may omit mention of sexual concerns. Questions asked with sensitivity may invite responses regarding changes in sexual desire or response or physical issues that challenge her sexual enjoyment. Open and reflective questions also affirm a woman's right to sexual enjoyment throughout the life span (Berg, 2001).

Women older than 50 years commonly experience menopause and have physical changes associated with decreased estrogen. A decrease in estrogen causes thinning of the mucosal tissue layers, resulting in a narrowing and a decrease in lubrication of the vagina. Estrogen also plays a role in the formation of bone matrix, and a decrease may lead to osteoporosis. Decreases in estrogen cause a relaxation of the ligaments and connective tissue, which affects the support of the bladder and uterus. Decreases in estrogen also affect the hypothalamus, causing hot flashes, which are disturbing to most women.

Physical changes can result in increased discomfort during the pelvic examination. It is important to be both gentle and thorough during the examination. A small adult speculum may be used to view the cervix. The uterus in a menopausal woman is small and firm, and the ovaries are nonpalpable. In postmenopausal women, the specimen from the vaginal pool may be useful to detect endometrial cells. A woman with palpable adnexal masses or vaginal bleeding after menopause needs immediate gynecologic referral.

A respectful and reassuring approach toward caring for women aged 50 and older will ensure their continued participation in seeking health care. Because the risk of breast, ovarian, uterine, cervical, and colon cancer increases with age, the nurse has the opportunity to educate women about the importance of preventive screening. It is the nurse's responsibility to ensure a positive health care experience that encourages future visits for prevention and chronic and acute care.

Advance directives can be introduced on any entry into a health care system. It is a good idea to have a formal statement in the medical record regarding a woman's wishes in the event of accident or illness regarding life-maintenance measures or organ donation. Most states have laws formalizing such statements in writing. The Durable Power of Attorney for Health Care can be used by a client to delegate decision-making authority to a trusted relative or friend.

Functional assessment is included as part of the history in women older than 70 years and those with disabilities. In the review of systems, the nurse should ask about self-care activities such as walking, getting to the bathroom, bathing, hair combing, dressing, and eating. Questions about driving, using public transportation or the telephone, hanging up clothes, buying groceries, taking medications, and meal preparation should be included.

History

At a woman's first visit, she is often expected to fill out a form with biographic and historic data before meeting with the examiner. This form aids the health care provider in completing the history. This medical history usually includes the following:

1. **Identifying data:** Name, age, race, living household preference, occupation, religion, culture, and ethnicity are obtained.
2. **Chief complaint(s):** A verbatim response to the question, "What problem or symptom brought you here today?" is recorded. If a lengthy list is recited, it may be necessary to tell the woman that her two complaints with the highest priority will be addressed today. To give all of her problems the full attention they deserve, a follow-up appointment in 1 to 2 weeks will be scheduled. Women are usually appreciative that the nurse is taking extra time and are agreeable to this.
3. **History of present illness:** A chronologic narrative that includes onset of the problem, the setting in which it developed, its manifestations, and any treatments received are noted. The woman's state of health before the onset of the present problem is determined. If the problem is of long standing, the reason for seeking attention at this time is elicited. The principal symptoms should be described as to the following:
   - Location
   - Quality
   - Quantity or severity
   - Timing (onset, duration, frequency)
   - Setting
   - Factors that aggravate or relieve
   - Associated manifestations
4. **Medical history:** Determine general state of health and strength:
   - Infectious diseases: measles, mumps, rubella, whooping cough, chickenpox, rheumatic fever, scarlet fever, diphtheria, polio, tuberculosis (TB), hepatitis
   - Chronic disease and system disorders: arthritis, cancer, diabetes, heart, lung, kidney, seizures, thyroid, stroke, ulcers
   - Adult injuries, accidents, illnesses, disabilities, hospitalizations, blood transfusions; note if the injury occurred on the job (workers' compensation) or if potential litigation is being considered
5. **Present health status:**
   - Allergies: medications, previous transfusion reactions, environmental allergies
   - Immunizations: diphtheria; pertussis; tetanus; polio; measles, mumps, rubella (MMR); hepatitis B; varicella; influenza; pneumococcal vaccine; last TB skin test

- Screening tests: Pap smear, mammogram, stool for occult blood, sigmoidoscopy/colonoscopy, chest radiograph, hematocrit, hemoglobin, rubella titer, urinalysis, cholesterol test; blood type/Rh; last eye examination; last dental examination
- Environmental/chemical hazards: home, school, work, and leisure setting; exposure to extreme heat/cold, noise, industrial toxins such as asbestos or lead, pesticides, diethylstilbestrol (DES), radiation exposure, cat feces, cigarette smoke
- Use of safety measures: seat belts, bicycle helmets, athletic protective devices, designated driver
- Exercise and leisure activities; stress-relieving activities
- Sleep patterns: length and quality
- Sexuality: Is she sexually active? With men, women, or both? Does she use condoms?
- Diet, including beverages: 24-hour dietary recall; brushes teeth 3 times daily; flosses daily
- Medications: name, dose, frequency, duration, reason for taking, and compliance with prescription medications; home remedies, over-the-counter drugs, vitamin and mineral or herbal supplements used over a 24-hour period
- Nicotine, alcohol, or recreational drugs: type, amount, frequency, duration, and reactions
- Caffeine: coffee, tea, cola, or chocolate intake

6. **Surgical history:** Type, date, reason, outcome, and any complications should be noted.
7. **Family history:** Information about age and health of family members may be presented in narrative or genogram: age, health/death of parents, siblings, spouse, children. Check for history of diabetes, heart disease, hypertension, stroke, respiratory, renal, thyroid, cancer, bleeding disorders, hepatitis, allergies, asthma, arthritis, TB, epilepsy, mental illness, human immunodeficiency virus (HIV), or other disorders.
8. **Social history:** Note birthplace, education, employment, marital status, living accommodations, children, persons at home, and hobbies. Does she enjoy what she is doing?
   - Screen for abuse: Has she ever been hit, kicked, slapped, or forced to have sex against her wishes? Verbally or emotionally abused? History of childhood sexual abuse? If yes, has she received counseling or does she need referral?
9. **Review of systems:** It is probable that all questions in each system will not be included every time a history is taken. Some questions regarding each system should be included in every history. The essential areas to be explored are listed in the following head-to-toe sequence. If a woman gives a positive response to a question about an essential area, more detailed questions should be asked.
   - **General:** weight change, fatigue, weakness, fever, chills, or night sweats
   - **Skin:** skin, hair, and nail changes; itching, bruising, bleeding, rashes, sores, lumps, or moles
   - **Lymph nodes:** enlargement, inflammation, pain, suppuration (pus), or drainage
   - **Head, eyes, ears, nose, and throat:**
     - **Head:** trauma, vertigo (dizziness), convulsive disorder, syncope (fainting), headache location, frequency, pain type, nausea/vomiting, or visual symptoms
     - **Eyes:** glasses, contact lenses, blurriness, tearing, itching, photophobia, diplopia, inflammation, trauma, cataracts, glaucoma, or acute visual loss
     - **Ears:** hearing loss, tinnitus (ringing), vertigo, discharge, pain, fullness, recurrent infections, or mastoiditis
     - **Nose/sinuses:** trauma, rhinitis, nasal discharge, epistaxis, obstruction, sneezing, itching, allergy, or smelling impairment
     - **Mouth/throat/neck:** hoarseness, voice changes, soreness, ulcers, bleeding gums, goiter, swelling, or enlarged nodes
   - **Breasts:** masses, pain, lumps, dimpling, nipple discharge, fibrocystic changes, or implants; BSE practice
   - **Respiratory:** shortness of breath, wheezing, cough, sputum, hemoptysis, pneumonia, pleurisy, asthma, bronchitis, emphysema, or TB; last chest radiograph
   - **Cardiac:** hypertension, rheumatic fever, murmurs, angina, palpitations, dyspnea, tachycardia, orthopnea, edema, chest pain, cough, cyanosis, cold extremities, ascites, intermittent claudication (leg pain caused by poor circulation to the leg muscles), phlebitis, or skin-color changes
   - **Gastrointestinal:** appetite, nausea, vomiting, indigestion, dysphagia, abdominal pain, ulcers, hematochezia (bleeding with stools), melena (black, tarry stools), bowel-habit changes, diarrhea, constipation, bowel-movement frequency, food intolerance, hemorrhoids, jaundice, or hepatitis; sigmoidoscopy, colonoscopy, barium enema, ultrasound
   - **Genitourinary:** frequency, hesitancy, urgency, polyuria, dysuria, hematuria, nocturia, incontinence, stones, infection, or urethral discharge; dysmenorrhea, intermenstrual bleeding, dyspareunia, discharge, sores, itching, sexually transmitted infections, gravidity (G), parity (P), problems in pregnancy, contraception, menopause, hot flashes, or sweats (may be included here or as part of endocrine)
   - **Vascular:** leg edema, claudication, varicose veins, thromboses, or emboli
   - **Endocrine:** heat/cold intolerance, dry skin, excessive sweating, polyuria, polydipsia, polyphagia, thyroid problems, diabetes, or secondary sex characteristic changes; age at menarche, length/flow of menses, last menstrual period (LMP), age at menopause, libido, or sexual concerns

- **Hematologic:** anemia, easy bruising, bleeding, petechiae, purpura, or transfusions
- **Musculoskeletal:** muscle weakness, pain, joint stiffness, scoliosis, lordosis, kyphosis, range-of-motion instability, redness, swelling, arthritis, or gout
- **Neurologic:** loss of sensation, numbness, tingling, tremors, weakness, vertigo, paralysis, fainting, twitching, blackouts, seizures, convulsions, loss of consciousness or memory
- **Psychiatric:** moodiness, depression, anxiety, obsessions, delusions, illusions, or hallucinations
- **Functional assessment:** should be done on women with disabilities and women 70 years of age and older (see previous discussion)

Physical Examination

In preparation for the physical examination, the woman is instructed on undressing and given a gown to wear during the examination. She is usually given the opportunity to undress privately. Some guidelines for assisting the Spanish-speaking woman during a physical examination are listed in the Guidelines/Guías box.

GUIDELINES/GUÍAS

Physical Examination

Take off all your clothes, please.
Quítese toda la ropa, por favor.

Put on the gown, please.
Póngase la bata, por favor.

I'm going to examine you.
Le voy a hacer un examen.

You will feel less discomfort if you relax.
Se sentirá mejor si relaja su cuerpo.

Lie down, please.
Acuéstese, por favor.

Put your feet in the stirrups.
Ponga sus pies en los estribos.

Open your legs, please.
Separa las piernas, por favor.

I'm going to take a sample from the lining of the cervix (Pap smear).
Voy a tomarle una muestra del cuello de la matriz para una prueba del cáncer; se llama la prueba "el pap."

We will test this sample for cancer.
Se le hara la prueba de cáncer.

It won't hurt.
Esto no le va a doler.

Everything looks fine.
Todo está bien.

You may get dressed.
Puede vestirse.

Objective data are recorded by system or location. A general statement of overall health status is a good way to start. Findings are described in detail.

- **General appearance:** age, race, sex, state of health, posture, height, weight, development, dress, hygiene, affect, alertness, orientation, cooperativeness, and communication skills
- **Vital signs:** temperature, pulse, respiration, blood pressure
- **Skin:** color; integrity; texture; hydration; temperature; edema; excessive perspiration; unusual odor; presence and description of lesions; hair texture and distribution; nail configuration, color, texture, condition, or presence of nail clubbing
- **Head:** size, shape, trauma, masses, scars, rashes, or scaling; facial symmetry; presence of edema or puffiness
- **Eyes:** pupil size, shape, reactivity, conjunctival injection, scleral icterus, fundal papilledema, hemorrhage, lids, extraocular movements, visual fields and acuity
- **Ears:** shape and symmetry, tenderness, discharge, external canal, and tympanic membranes; hearing–Weber should be midline (loudness of sound equal in both ears) and Rinne negative (no conductive or sensorineural hearing loss); should be able to hear whisper at 3 feet
- **Nose:** symmetry, tenderness, discharge, mucosa, turbinate inflammation, frontal or maxillary sinus tenderness; discrimination of odors
- **Mouth and throat:** hygiene, condition of teeth, dentures, appearance of lips, tongue, buccal and oral mucosa, erythema, edema, exudate, tonsillar enlargement, palate, uvula, gag reflex, ulcers
- **Neck:** mobility, masses, range of motion, trachea deviation, thyroid size, carotid bruits
- **Lymphatic:** cervical, intraclavicular, axillary, trochlear, or inguinal adenopathy; size, shape, tenderness, and consistency
- **Breasts:** skin changes, dimpling, symmetry, scars, tenderness, discharge or masses; characteristics of nipples and areolae
- **Heart:** rate, rhythm, murmurs, rubs, gallops, clicks, heaves, or precordial movements
- **Peripheral vascular:** jugular vein distention, bruits, edema, swelling, vein distention, Homans' sign, or tenderness of extremities
- **Lungs:** chest symmetry with respirations, wheezes, crackles, rhonchi, vocal fremitus, whispered pectoriloquy, percussion, and diaphragmatic excursion; breath sounds equal and clear bilaterally
- **Abdomen:** shape, scars, bowel sounds, consistency, tenderness, rebound, masses, guarding, organomegaly, liver span, percussion (tympany, shifting, dullness), costovertebral angle tenderness
- **Extremities:** edema, ulceration, tenderness, varicosities, erythema, tremor, or deformity
- **Genitourinary:** external genitalia, perineum, vaginal mucosa, cervix, inflammation, tenderness, discharge,

bleeding, ulcers, nodules, masses, internal vaginal support, bimanual, and rectovaginal; palpation of cervix, uterus, and adnexae

- **Rectal:** sphincter tone, masses, hemorrhoids, rectal wall contour, tenderness, and stool for occult blood
- **Musculoskeletal:** posture, symmetry of muscle mass, muscle atrophy, weakness, appearance of joints, tenderness or crepitus, joint range of motion, instability, redness, swelling, or spine deviation
- **Neurologic:** mental status, orientation, memory, mood, speech clarity and comprehension, cranial nerves II to XII, sensation, strength, deep tendon and superficial reflexes, gait, balance, and coordination with rapid alternating motions

Pelvic Examination

Many women are intimidated by the gynecologic portion of the physical examination. The nurse in this instance can take an advocacy approach that supports a partnership relationship between the woman and the care provider.

The woman is assisted into the lithotomy position (see Fig. 5-9, A) for the pelvic examination. When she is in the lithotomy position, the woman's hips and knees are flexed, with the buttocks at the edge of the table, and her feet are supported by heel or knee stirrups.

Some women prefer to keep their shoes or socks on, especially if the stirrups are not padded. Many women express feelings of vulnerability and strangeness when in the lithotomy position. During the procedure, the nurse assists the woman with relaxation techniques.

One method of helping the woman relax is to have her place her hands on her chest at about the level of the diaphragm, breathe deeply and slowly (in through her nose and out through her O-shaped mouth), concentrate on the rhythm of breathing, and relax all body muscles with each exhalation (Barkauskas et al., 2002). This breathing technique is particularly helpful for the adolescent or the woman whose introitus may be especially tight or for whom the experience may be new or may provoke tension. Some women relax when they are encouraged to become involved with the examination with a mirror placed so that they can view the area being examined. This type of participation helps with health teaching as well. Distraction is another technique that can be used effectively (e.g., placement of interesting pictures on the ceiling over the head of the table).

Many women find it distressing to attempt to converse in the lithotomy position. Most women appreciate an explanation of the procedure as it unfolds, as well as coaching for the types of sensations they may expect. Generally, however, women prefer not to have to respond to questions until they are again upright and at eye level with the examiner. Questioning during the procedure, especially if they cannot see their questioner's eyes, may make women tense.

External Inspection. The examiner sits at the foot of the table for the inspection of the external genitals and for the speculum examination. To facilitate open communication and to help the woman relax, the woman's head is raised on a pillow, and the drape is arranged so that eye-to-eye contact can be maintained. In good lighting, external genitals are inspected for sexual maturity, clitoris, labia, and perineum. After childbirth or other trauma, there may be healed scars.

External Palpation. The examiner proceeds with the examination by using palpation and inspection. The examiner wears gloves for this portion of the assessment. Before touching the woman, the examiner explains what is going to be done and what the woman should expect to feel (e.g., pressure). The examiner may touch the woman in a less sensitive area such as the inner thigh to alert her that the genital examination is beginning. This gesture may put the woman more at ease. The labia are spread apart to expose the structures in the vestibule: urinary meatus, Skene's glands, vaginal orifice, and Bartholin's glands (Fig. 5-11). To assess the Skene's glands, the examiner inserts one finger into the vagina and "milks" the area of the urethra. Any exudate from the urethra or the Skene's glands is cultured. Masses and erythema of either structure are assessed further. Ordinarily the openings to the Skene's glands are not visible; prominent openings may be seen if the glands are infected (e.g., with gonorrhea). During the examination, the examiner keeps in mind the data from the review of systems, such as history of burning on urination.

The vaginal orifice is examined. Hymenal tags are normal findings. With one finger still in the vagina, the examiner repositions the index finger near the posterior part of the orifice. With the thumb outside the posterior part of the labia majora, the examiner compresses the area of Bartholin's glands located at the 8 o'clock and 4 o'clock positions and looks for swelling, discharge, and pain.

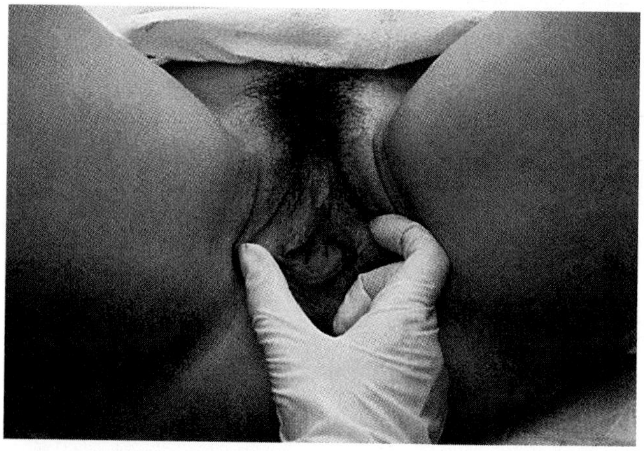

FIG. 5-11 External examination. Separation of the labia. (From Edge, V., & Miller, M. [1994]. *Women's health care*. St. Louis: Mosby.)

The support of the anterior and posterior vaginal wall is assessed. The examiner spreads the labia with the index and middle finger and asks the woman to strain down. Any bulge from the anterior wall (urethrocele or cystocele) or posterior wall (rectocele) is noted and compared with the history, such as difficulty to start the stream of urine or constipation.

The perineum (area between the vagina and anus) is assessed for scars from old lacerations or episiotomies, thinning, fistulas, masses, lesions, and inflammation. The anus is assessed for hemorrhoids, hemorrhoidal tags, and integrity of the anal sphincter. The anal area also is assessed for lesions, masses, abscesses, and tumors. If there is a history of STI, the examiner may want to obtain a culture specimen from the anal canal at this time. Throughout the genital examination, the examiner notes the odor. Odor may indicate infection or poor hygiene.

Vulvar Self-Examination. The pelvic examination provides a good opportunity for the practitioner to emphasize the need for regular **vulvar self-examination (VSE)** and to teach this procedure. Because there has been a dramatic increase in cancerous and precancerous conditions of the vulva in recent years, a VSE should be performed as an integral part of preventive health care by all women who are sexually active or aged 18 years or older, monthly between menses, or more frequently if there are symptoms or a history of serious vulvar disease. Most lesions, including malignancy, condyloma acuminatum (wartlike growth), and Bartholin's cysts, can be seen or palpated and are easily treated if diagnosed early.

The VSE can be performed by the practitioner and woman together, by using a mirror. A simple diagram of the anatomy of the vulva can be given to the woman, with instructions to perform the examination herself that evening to reinforce what she has learned. She does the examination in a sitting position with adequate lighting, holding a mirror in one hand and using the other hand to expose the tissues surrounding the vaginal introitus. She then systematically examines the mons pubis, clitoris, urethra, labia majora, perineum, and perianal area and palpates the vulva, noting any changes in appearance or abnormalities, such as ulcers, lumps, warts, and changes in pigmentation.

Internal Examination. A vaginal speculum consists of two blades and a handle. Speculums come in a variety of types and styles. A vaginal speculum is used to view the vaginal vault and cervix (see Procedure box). The speculum is gently placed into the vagina and inserted to the back of the vaginal vault. The blades are opened to reveal the cervix and are locked into the open position. The cervix is inspected for position and appearance of the os: color, lesions, bleeding, and discharge (Fig. 5-13). Cervical findings that are not within normal limits include ulcerations, masses, inflammation, and excessive protrusion into the vaginal vault. Anomalies, such as a cockscomb (a protrusion over the cervix that looks like a rooster's comb), a hooded or collared cervix (seen in DES daughters), or polyps, are noted.

Collection of Specimens. The collection of specimens for cytologic examination is an important part of the gynecologic examination. Infection can be diagnosed through examination of specimens collected during the

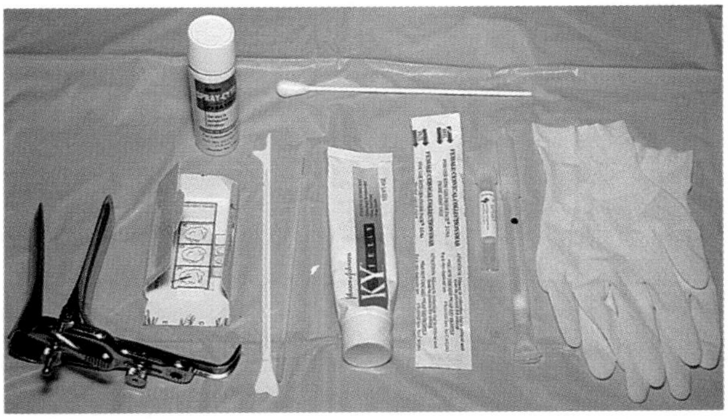

FIG. 5-12 Equipment used for pelvic examination. (Courtesy Michael S. Clement, MD, Mesa, AZ.)

PROCEDURE
Assisting with Pelvic Examination
(see Fig. 5-13)

- Wash hands. Assemble equipment (see Fig. 5-12).
- Ask woman to empty her bladder before the examination (obtain clean-catch urine specimen as needed).
- Assist with relaxation techniques. Have the woman place her hands on her chest at about the level of the diaphragm, breathe deeply and slowly (in through her nose and out through an O-shaped mouth), concentrate on the rhythm of breathing, and relax all body muscles with each exhalation (Barkauskas et al., 2002).
- Encourage the woman to become involved with the examination if she shows interest. For example, a mirror can be placed so that she can see the area being examined.
- Assess for and treat signs of problems such as supine hypotension.
- Warm the speculum in warm water if a prewarmed one is not available.
- Instruct the woman to bear down when the speculum is being inserted.
- Apply gloves and assist the examiner with collection of specimens for cytologic examination, such as a Pap test. After handling specimens, remove gloves and wash hands.
- Lubricate the examiner's fingers with water or water-soluble lubricant before bimanual examination.
- Assist the woman at completion of the examination to a sitting position and then a standing position.
- Provide tissues to wipe lubricant from perineum.
- Provide privacy for the woman while she is dressing.

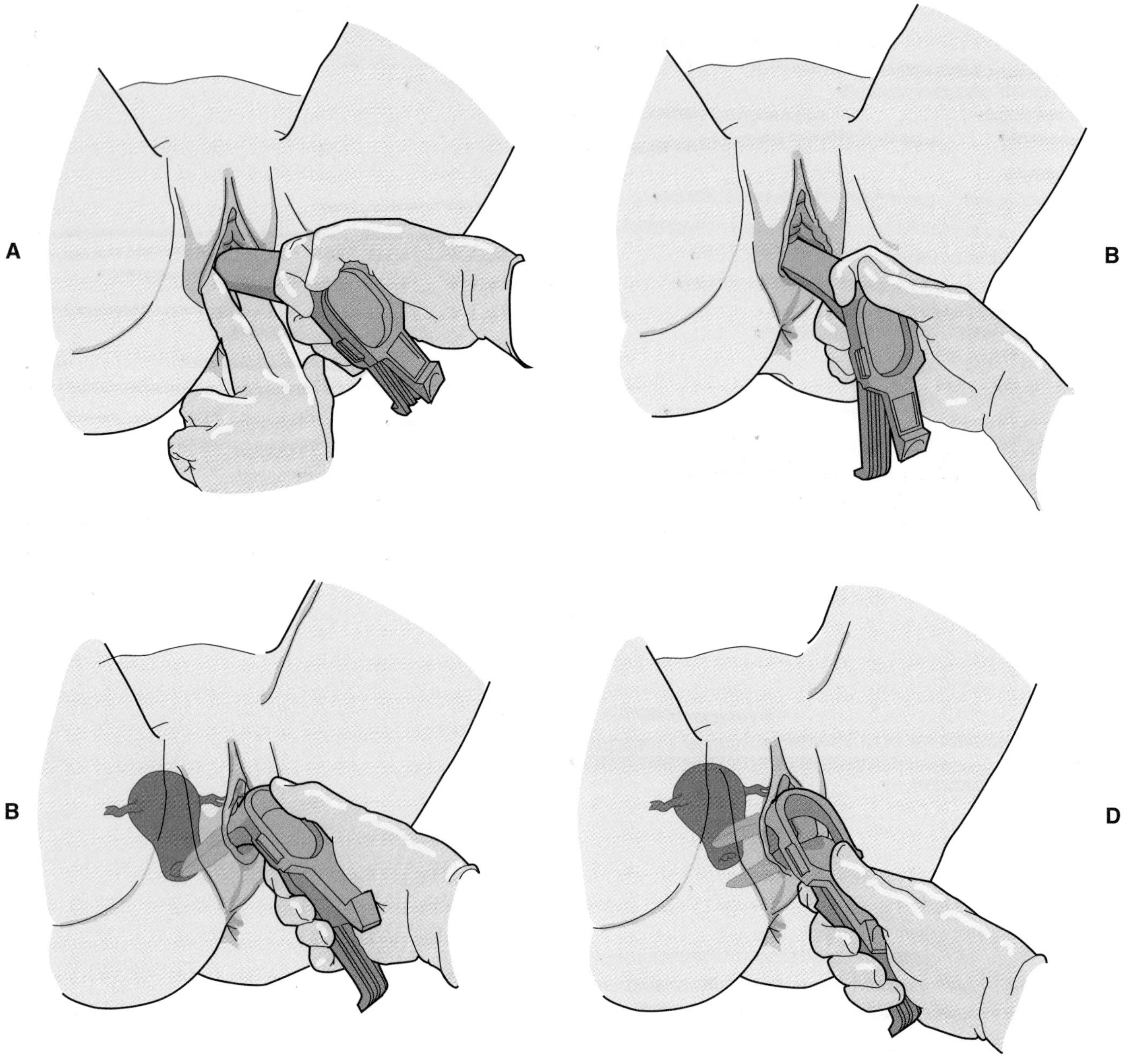
A
B
B
D

FIG. 5-13 Insertion of speculum for vaginal examination. **A,** Opening of the introitus. **B,** Oblique insertion of the speculum. **C,** Final insertion of the speculum. **D,** Opening of the speculum blades. (From Barkauskas, V., Baumann, L., & Darling-Fisher, C. [2002]. *Health and physical assessment* [3rd ed.]. St Louis: Mosby.)

pelvic examination. These infections include candidiasis, trichomoniasis, bacterial vaginosis, group B streptococcus, gonorrhea, chlamydia, and herpes simplex virus. Once the diagnoses have been made, treatment can be instituted.

Papanicolaou (Pap) Smear. Carcinogenic conditions, potential or actual, can be determined by examination of cells from the cervix collected during the pelvic examination (see Procedure box). This is termed a Pap smear (Fig. 5-14).

Vaginal Examination. After the specimens are obtained, the vagina is viewed when the speculum is rotated. The speculum blades are unlocked and partially closed. As the speculum is withdrawn, it is rotated, and the vaginal walls are inspected for color, lesions, rugae, fistulas, and bulging.

Bimanual Palpation. The examiner stands for this part of the examination. A small amount of lubricant is placed on the first and second fingers of the gloved hand for the

PROCEDURE
Papanicolaou Smear

In preparation, make sure the woman has not douched, used vaginal medications, or had sexual intercourse for 24 to 48 hours before the procedure. Reschedule the test if the woman is menstruating. Midcycle is the best time for test.

The woman is assisted into a lithotomy position. A speculum is inserted into the vagina.

Explain to the woman the purpose of the test and what sensations she will feel as the specimen is obtained (e.g., pressure but not pain).

The cytologic specimen is obtained before any digital examination of the vagina is made or endocervical bacteriologic specimens are taken with cotton swabbing of the cervix.

The Pap smear is obtained by using an endocervical sampling device (Cytobrush, Cervex-Brush, papette, or broom) (see Fig. 5-14). If the two-sample method of obtaining cells is used, the cytobrush is inserted into the canal and rotated 90 to 180 degrees, followed by a gentle smear of the entire transformation zone by using a spatula. Broom devices are inserted and rotated 360 degrees five times. They obtain endocervical and ectocervical samples at the same time. If the patient has had a hysterectomy, the vaginal cuff is sampled. Areas that appear abnormal on visualization will require colposcopy and biopsy. If using a one-slide technique, the spatula sample is smeared first. This is followed by applying the cytobrush sample (rolling the brush in the opposite direction from which it was obtained), which is less subject to drying artifact, and then the slide is sprayed with preservative within 5 seconds.

The ThinPrep Pap Test is an improved method of preserving cells that reduces blood, mucus, and inflammation. The Pap specimen is obtained in the manner described above, and the collection device (brush, spatula, or broom) is simply rinsed in a vial of preserving solution that is provided by the laboratory. The sealed vial with solution is sent off to the appropriate laboratory. A special processing device filters the contents, and a thin layer of cervical cells is deposited on a slide, which is then examined microscopically. Initial reports state that specimen adequacy is improved by 50%, and improved detection of low-grade and more severe lesions by 65%. The Autopap and Papnet tests are similar to the ThinPrep test (Huff, 2000).

Label the slides with the woman's name and site. Include on the form to accompany the slides the woman's name, age, parity, and chief complaint or reason for taking the cytologic specimens.

Send specimens to the pathology laboratory promptly for staining, evaluation, and a written report, with special reference to abnormal elements, including cancer cells.

Advise the woman that repeated smears may be necessary if the specimen is not adequate.

Instruct the woman concerning routine checkups for cervical and vaginal cancer. The American Cancer Society advises that women older than 18 years and those younger than 18 who are sexually active have the test at least every 3 years, but only after they have had three negative Pap tests a year apart. A pelvic examination is recommended every 3 years from age 20 to 40 and every 1 to 3 years thereafter.

Record the examination date on the woman's record.

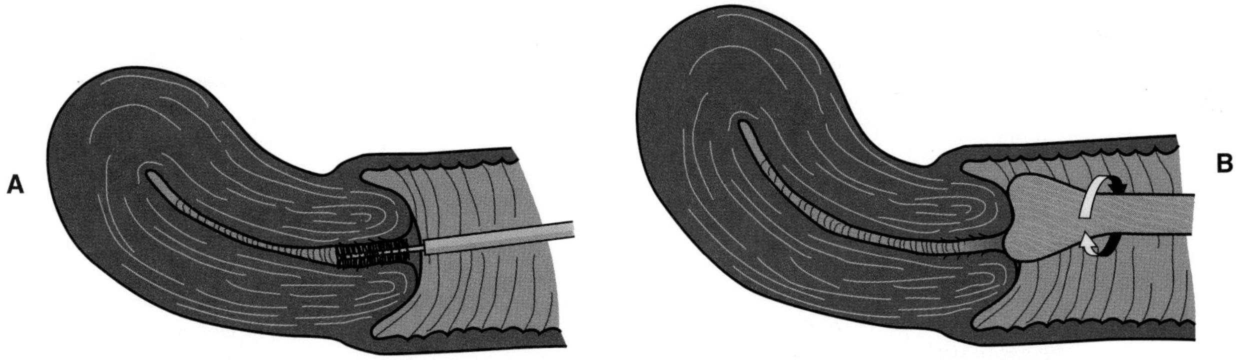
A
B

FIG. 5-14 Pap smear. **A,** Collecting cells from endocervix by using a cytobrush. **B,** Obtaining cells from the transformation zone using a wooden spatula. (From Stenchever, M., et al. [2001]. *Comprehensive gynecology* [4th ed.]. St. Louis: Mosby.)

internal examination. To avoid tissue trauma and contamination, the thumb is abducted and the ring and little fingers are flexed into the palm (Fig. 5-15).

The vagina is palpated for distensibility, lesions, and tenderness. The cervix is examined for position, shape, consistency, motility, and lesions. The fornix around the cervix is palpated.

The other hand is placed on the abdomen halfway between the umbilicus and symphysis pubis and exerts pressure downward toward the pelvic hand. Upward pressure from the pelvic hand traps reproductive structures for assessment by palpation. The uterus is assessed for position, size, shape, consistency, regularity, motility, masses, and tenderness.

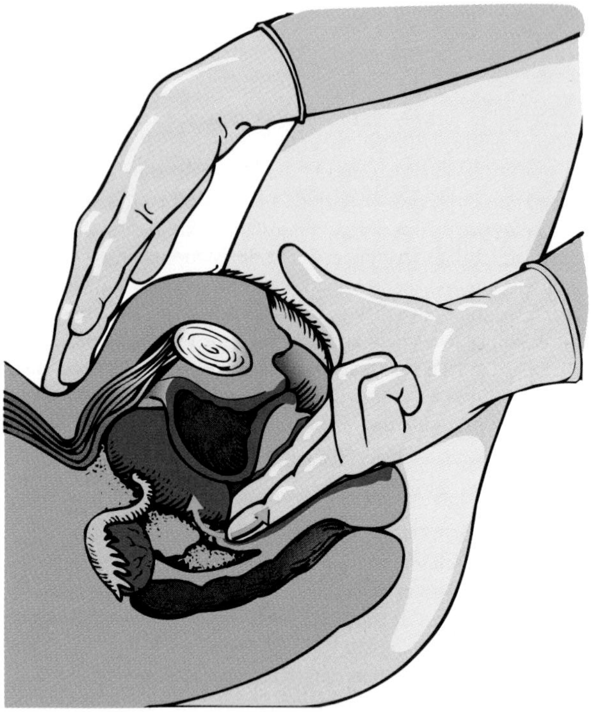

FIG. 5-15 Bimanual palpation of the uterus.

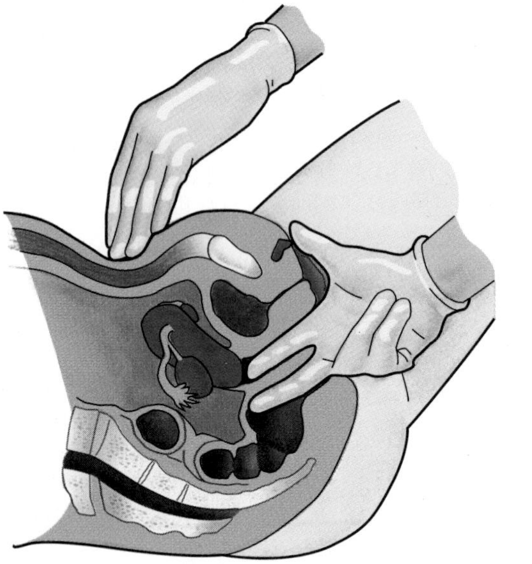

FIG. 5-16 Rectovaginal examination. (From Seidel, H., et al. [2003]. *Mosby's guide to physical examination* [5th ed.]. St. Louis: Mosby.)

With the abdominal hand moving to the right lower quadrant and the fingers of the pelvic hand in the right lateral fornix, the adnexa is assessed for position, size, tenderness, and masses. The examination is repeated on the woman's left side.

Just before the intravaginal fingers are withdrawn, the woman is asked to tighten her vagina around the fingers as much as she can. If the muscle response is weak, the woman is assessed for her knowledge about Kegel exercises.

Rectovaginal Palpation. To prevent contamination of the rectum from organisms in the vagina (such as *Neisseria gonorrhoeae*), it is necessary to change gloves, add fresh lubricant, and then reinsert the index finger into the vagina and the middle finger into the rectum (Fig. 5-16). Insertion is facilitated if the woman strains down. The maneuvers of the abdominovaginal examination are repeated. The rectovaginal examination permits assessment of the rectovaginal septum, the posterior surface of the uterus, and the region behind the cervix and the adnexa. The vaginal finger is removed and folded into the palm, leaving the middle finger free to rotate 360 degrees. The rectum is palpated for rectal tenderness and masses.

After the rectal examination, the woman is assisted into a sitting position, given tissues or wipes to cleanse herself, and given privacy to dress. The examiner returns after the woman is dressed to discuss findings and the plan of care.

Pelvic Examination during Pregnancy

The pelvic examination is done in the same way as it is during a routine examination on a nonpregnant woman. Pelvic measurements are completed, and uterine size is estimated. A Pap smear may be done initially, as well as collection of cytologic specimens to test for gonorrhea, chlamydia, human papillomavirus, herpes simplex virus, and group B streptococci. As the pregnancy progresses, the nurse will inspect the woman's abdomen, palpate fetal size and position, auscultate fetal heart tones, and measure fundal height at each visit.

While the pregnant woman is in lithotomy position, the nurse must watch for supine hypotension, caused by the weight of the abdomen pressing on the vena cava and aorta, causing a decrease in blood pressure. Symptoms of supine hypotension include pallor, dizziness, faintness, breathlessness, tachycardia, nausea, clammy skin, and sweating. The woman should be positioned on her side until symptoms resolve and vital signs stabilize. The vaginal examination can be done with the woman in lateral position.

Pelvic Examination after Hysterectomy

The pelvic examination is done much as it is done on a woman with a uterus, but only a plastic spatula is used for cell sampling during the Pap smear. The Pap smear may be done less frequently at the discretion of the clinician (e.g., every 2 to 3 years) (DiSaia & Creasman, 2002). Others suggest that if the hysterectomy was performed for benign disease, Pap testing may not be needed (Saraiya et al., 2001). Because of the epidemic of human papillomavirus, which causes vaginal intraepithelial neoplasia, sampling of the vaginal cuff and vaginal walls after hysterectomy is still recommended by most clinicians. Refer to Table 5-3 for suggested frequency of Pap smear screening after hysterectomy.

TABLE 5-3 **Pap Smear Screening after Hysterectomy**

CLIENT GROUP	SUGGESTED FREQUENCY
After hysterectomy for benign disease	Every 2 to 3 years if low cancer risk and previous test was negative; some clinicians suggest testing not needed at all
After hysterectomy for unknown reason, premalignant or malignant disease	Annually
Age 65 and older	Screening may be discontinued if three consecutive smears have been normal

Sources: DiSaia, P., & Creasman, W. (2002). *Clinical gynecologic oncology* (6th ed.). St. Louis: Mosby; National Women's Health Resource Center. (2001). Screening tests and women's health. *National Women's Health Report, 23*(6), 1-7; and Saraiya M. et al. (2001). Self-reported Papanicolaou smears and hysterectomies among women in the United States. *Obstetrics and Gynecology, 98*(2), 269-278.

Laboratory and Diagnostic Procedures

The following laboratory and diagnostic procedures are ordered at the discretion of the clinician, considering the client and family history: hemoglobin, fasting plasma glucose, total blood cholesterol, lipid profile, urinalysis, syphilis serology (VDRL or RPR) and other screening tests for sexually transmitted infections, mammogram, tuberculosis skin testing, hearing, visual acuity, electrocardiogram, chest radiograph, pulmonary function, fecal occult blood, flexible sigmoidoscopy, and bone mineral density (DEXA scan). Tests for HIV and drug screening may be offered with informed consent in high risk populations (National Women's Health Resource Center, 2001).

ANTICIPATORY GUIDANCE FOR HEALTH PROMOTION AND PREVENTION

Over the last several decades, women have made tremendous strides in education, careers, policy making, and overall participation in today's complex society. There have been costs for these advances, and although women are living longer, they may not be living better. As a result, the health care system must pay greater attention to the health consequences for women. In addition, women must be active participants in their own health promotion and illness prevention. **Health promotion** is the motivation to increase well-being and actualize health potential. **Health prevention** is the desire to avoid illness, detect it early, or maintain optimal functioning when illness is present.

Nurses have a major opportunity and responsibility to help women understand risk factors and to motivate them to adopt healthy lifestyles that prevent disease. Lifestyle factors that affect health over which the woman has some control include diet; tobacco, alcohol, and substance use; exercise; sunlight exposure; stress management; and sexual practices. Other influences, such as genetic and environmental factors, may be beyond the woman's control, although some opportunities for prevention exist (e.g., through environmental legislation activism or genetic counseling services).

Knowledge alone is not enough to bring about healthy behaviors. The woman must be convinced that she has some control over her life and that healthy life habits, including periodic health examinations, are a sound investment. She must believe in the efficacy of prevention, early detection, and therapy and in her ability to perform self-care practices, such as BSE. Many people believe that they have little control over their health, or they become immobilized by fear and anxiety in the face of life-threatening illnesses, such as cancer, so they delay seeking treatment. The nurse must explore the reality of each woman's perceptions about health behaviors and individualize teaching if it is to be effective. The model illustrated in Figure 5-17 incorporates the major aspects to be included when counseling women.

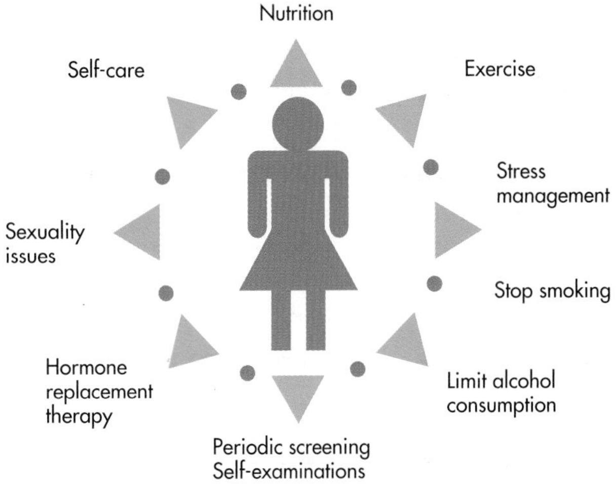
Nutrition
Self-care
Exercise
Stress management
Sexuality issues
Stop smoking
Hormone replacement therapy
Limit alcohol consumption
Periodic screening
Self-examinations

FIG. 5-17 Nursing care model for counseling women about self-care. (Courtesy University of North Carolina at Chapel Hill School of Nursing, Chapel Hill, NC.)

Nutrition

To maintain good nutrition, women should be counseled to include recommended servings from the major food categories of the Food Guide Pyramid (see Fig. 15-3). Recommended servings from the food groups also provide adequate vitamins, minerals, iron, and fiber. Fluid intake is not included in the Food Guide Pyramid, but individuals should be encouraged to drink at least four to six glasses of water every day in addition to other fluids such as juices. Coffee, tea, soft drinks, and alcoholic beverages should be used in moderation.

A class of organic substances called antioxidants is thought to be effective in helping to prevent cancer, heart disease, and stroke; however, more research is needed in this area. Vitamins C, E, and A; selenium (mineral); and a group known as carotenoids (pigment in fruit and vegetables such as orange in carrots) can be found in a diet containing fruits, vegetables, and whole grains. Foods such as almonds, avocados, mangos, spinach, broccoli, sweet potatoes, carrots, and cantaloupe are good sources of antioxidants.

Most women do not recognize the importance of calcium to health, and their diets are insufficient in calcium. Women who are unlikely to get enough calcium in the diet may need calcium supplements in the form of calcium carbonate, which contains more elemental calcium than do other preparations.

The diet can be assessed by using a standard assessment form—a 24-hour recall is adequate and quick—and then food likes and dislikes, including cultural variations and typical food portions and dietary habits should be discussed and incorporated into counseling.

Exercise

Physical activity and exercise counseling for persons of all ages should be undertaken at schools, work sites, and primary care settings. Specific recommendations include 30 to 60 minutes of moderate activity at least 3 times per week. Few Americans exercise this often, and physical activity decreases with age, especially during adolescence and early adulthood.

The nurse should stress the importance of daily exercise throughout life for weight management and health promotion, suggesting exercises that are enjoyable to the individual (Fig. 5-18 and Fig. 5-19). Many women who are sedentary during leisure time can profit from gradually increasing their physical activity. They may be encouraged to exercise with their children or in groups. Work-site fitness programs or community-based programs are increasing. Young women can be involved in physical education activities, games and group sports, and more active pursuits. Home maintenance, yard work, and gardening are other activities that promote health and a sense of well-being, especially for older adults. Attention to safety factors and wearing clothing and shoes appropriate to each activity are advised. Care should be taken not to aggravate existing conditions or create muscle and joint discomfort by an overly aggressive approach to exercise.

Kegel Exercises

Kegel exercises, or pelvic muscle exercises, were developed to strengthen the supportive pelvic floor muscles to control or reduce incontinent urine loss. These exercises also are beneficial during pregnancy and postpartum. They strengthen the muscles of the pelvic floor, providing support for the pelvic organs and control of the muscles surrounding the vagina and urethra.

The Association of Women's Health, Obstetric, and Neonatal Nurses conducted a research utilization project focused on continence for women (Sampselle et al., 1997). Educational strategies for teaching women how to perform Kegel exercises were compiled by nurse researchers involved in the project and are described in the Teaching for Self-Care box.

Stress Management

Because it is neither possible nor desirable to avoid all stress, women must learn how to manage stress. The nurse should assess each woman for signs of stress by using therapeutic communication skills to determine risk factors and the woman's ability to function.

Some women must be referred for counseling or other mental health therapy. Women are twice as likely as men

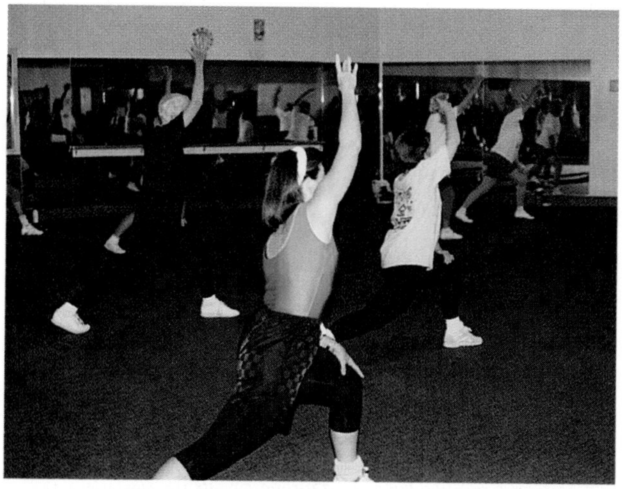

FIG. 5-18 Weight-bearing exercise may delay bone loss and increase bone mass. (Courtesy Jonas McCoy, Raleigh, NC.)

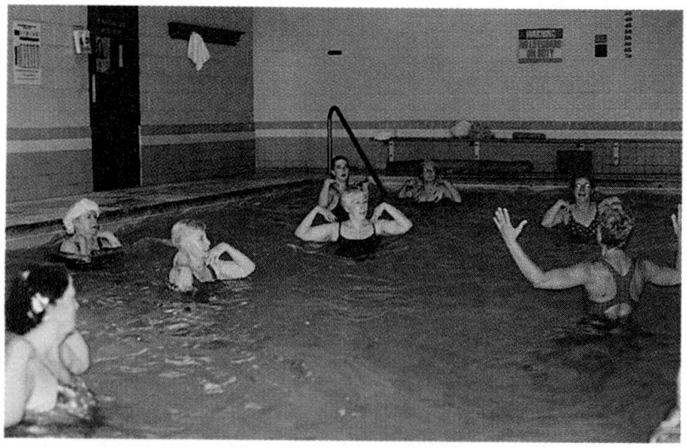

FIG. 5-19 Water aerobics improves cardiovascular function. (Courtesy Jonas McCoy, Raleigh, NC.)

to have depression, anxiety, or panic attacks (Japenga, 1998). Nurses must be alert to the symptoms of serious mental disorders, such as depression and anxiety, and make referrals to mental health practitioners when necessary. Women having major life changes, such as divorce and separation, bereavement, serious illness, and unemployment, also need special attention.

For many women, the nurse is able to provide comfort, reassurance, and advice concerning helping resources, such as support groups. Many centers offer support groups to help women prevent or manage stress. The nurse can help women become more aware of the relation between good nutrition, rest, relaxation, and exercise and diversion, and their ability to deal with stress. In the case of role overload, determining what needs immediate attention and what can wait is important. Practical advice includes having regular breaks, taking time for friends, developing interests outside of work or the home, setting realistic goals, and learning self-acceptance. Discussing how women can maintain meaningful relationships is important. Social support and good coping skills can improve a woman's self-esteem and give her a sense of mastery. Anticipatory guidance for developmental or expected situational crises can help her plan strategies for dealing with potentially stressful events.

The abundant literature on stress management interventions includes role-playing, relaxation techniques, biofeedback, meditation, desensitization, imagery, assertiveness training, yoga, diet, exercise, and weight control, techniques nurses can include in their repertoire of helping skills. Insufficient time prevents one-on-one assistance in many situations, but the more nurses know about these resources, the better able they are to intervene, counsel, and direct women to appropriate resources. Careful follow-up of all women experiencing difficulty in dealing with stress is important.

Substance Use Cessation

Women of all ages will receive substantial and immediate benefits from smoking cessation. This is not easy, however, and most people stop several times before they accomplish their goal. Many are never able to do so.

New approaches to increase cessation among smokers and to discourage smoking among young women–especially in adolescence and during pregnancy–are needed. Health care providers can have an impact on smoking behavior and should attempt to motivate smokers to stop (Box 5-7). Raising questions about social consequences–stained teeth, foul-smelling breath and clothes–is sometimes effective with young people.

TEACHING FOR SELF-CARE

Kegel Exercises

DESCRIPTION AND RATIONALE

Kegel exercise, or pelvic muscle exercise, is a technique used to strengthen the muscles that support the pelvic floor. This exercise involves regularly tightening (contracting) and relaxing the muscles that support the bladder and urethra. By strengthening these pelvic muscles, a woman can prevent or reduce accidental urine loss.

TECHNIQUE

The woman needs to learn how to target the muscles for training and how to contract them correctly. One suggestion for teaching is to have the woman pretend she is trying to prevent the passage of intestinal gas. Have her use this tightening motion on the muscles around her vagina and the upper pelvis. She should feel these muscles drawing inward and upward. Other suggested techniques are to have the woman pretend she is trying to stop the flow of urine in midstream or to have her think about how her vagina is able to contract around and move up the length of the penis during intercourse.

The woman should avoid straining or bearing-down motions while performing the exercise. She should be taught how bearing down feels by having her take a breath, hold it, and push down with her abdominal muscles as though she were trying to have a bowel movement. Then the woman can be taught how to avoid straining down by exhaling gently and keeping her mouth open each time she contracts her pelvic muscles.

SPECIFIC INSTRUCTIONS

1. Each contraction should be as intense as possible without contracting the abdomen, thighs, or buttocks.
2. Contractions should be held for at least 10 seconds. The woman may have to start with as little as 2 seconds per contraction until her muscles get stronger.
3. The woman should rest for 10 seconds or more between contractions so that the muscles have time to recover and each contraction can be as strong as the woman can make it.
4. The woman should feel the pulling up and over the three muscle layers so that the contraction reaches the highest level of her pelvis.

OTHER SUGGESTIONS FOR IMPLEMENTATION

1. At first the woman should set aside about 15 minutes a day to do the Kegel exercises.
2. The woman may want to put up reminders, such as notes on her bathroom mirror, her refrigerator, her TV, or a calendar, to do the exercises.
3. Guidelines for practicing Kegel exercises suggest performing between 30 and 80 contractions a day; however, positive results can be achieved with only 30 a day.
4. The best position for learning how to do Kegel exercises is to lie supine with the knees bent. Another position to use is on the hands and knees. Once the woman learns the proper technique, she can perform the exercises in other positions such as standing or sitting.

Sources: Sampselle, C. (2000). Behavioral interventions for urinary incontinence in women: Evidence for practice, *Journal of Midwifery and Women's Health, 45*(2), 94-103; Sampselle, C. et al. (1997). Continence for women: Evidence-based practice, *Journal of Obstretric, Gynecologic, and Neonatal Nursing 26*(4), 375-385.

Those who wish to stop smoking can be referred to a smoking-cessation program in which individualized methods can be implemented. At the very least, individuals should be guided to self-help materials available from the March of Dimes Birth Defects Foundation, the American Lung Association, and the American Cancer Society. During pregnancy, women seem to be highly motivated to stop or at least to limit smoking to 10 or fewer cigarettes a day. Insult to the fetus can be reduced or even avoided if this is done by the end of the first trimester.

Counseling women who appear to be drinking alcohol excessively or using drugs may include promoting strategies to increase self-esteem and teaching new coping skills to resist and maintain resistance to alcohol abuse and drug use. Appropriate referrals should be made, with the health care provider arranging the contact and then following up to be sure that appointments are kept. General referral to sources of support also should be provided. National groups that provide information and support for those who are chemically dependent are listed in the resources section at the end of the chapter. Many of these organizations have local branches or contacts that are listed in the telephone book.

Anticipatory guidance includes teaching about the health and safety risks of alcohol and mind-altering substances and discouraging drug experimentation among preteen and high school students, because the use of drugs at an early age tends to predict greater involvement later.

Safer Sexual Practices

Prevention of STIs is predicated on the reduction of high risk behaviors by educating toward a behavioral change. Behaviors of concern include multiple and casual sexual partners and unsafe sexual practices. Specific self-care measures for "safer sex" can be reviewed in Box 5-8. The abuse of alcohol and drugs also is a high risk behavior resulting in impaired judgment and thoughtless acts.

In addition to the prevention of STIs, women of childbearing years need information regarding contraception and family planning (see Chapter 9).

Health Screening Schedule

Periodic health screening includes history, physical examination, education, counseling, and selected diagnostic and laboratory tests. This regimen provides the basis for overall health promotion, prevention of illness, early diagnosis of problems, and referral for appropriate management. Such screening should be customized according to a woman's age and risk factors. In most instances, it is completed in health care offices, clinics, or hospitals; however, portions of the screening are now being carried out at events such as Community Health Fairs. An overview of health screening recommendations for women older than 18 years is provided in Table 5-4. Consistent with information provided earlier in this chapter, it is important for the nurse continually to

BOX 5-7 **Interventions for Smoking Cessation: The Four A's**

ASK

- What was her age when she started smoking? How many cigarettes does she smoke a day? When was her last cigarette? Has she tried to quit? Does she want to quit?

ASSESS

- What are her reasons for not being able to quit before, or what made her start again? Does she have anyone who can help her? Does anyone else smoke at home? Does she have friends or family who have quit successfully?

ADVISE

- Give her information about the effects of smoking on pregnancy and her fetus, on her own future health, and on the members of her household.

ASSIST

- Provide support; give self-help materials. Encourage her to set a quit date. Refer to a smoking cessation program or provide information about nicotine replacement products (not recommended during pregnancy) if she is interested. Teach and encourage use of stress reduction activities. Provide for follow-up with a phone call, letter, or clinic visit.

Source: American College of Obstetricians and Gynecologists. (1997). *Smoking and women's health. ACOG Technical Bulletin no. 240.* Washington, DC: ACOG.

BOX 5-8 **Safer Sex**

- Safer sex is possible only if there is no oral, genital, or rectal exchange of body fluids or if a person is in a long-term mutually monogamous relationship with an uninfected partner.
- Correct use of latex condoms, although greatly reducing risk, is not exclusively protective.

Sexual partners should be selected with great care.

- Partners should be asked about history of STIs.
- A new condom should be used for each act of sexual intercourse when a partner's infection status is unknown or if the partner is infected with HIV or another STI.
- Abstinence from sexual intercourse is encouraged for persons who are being treated for an STI or whose partners are being treated.

Source: Centers for Disease Control and Prevention. (2002). Sexually transmitted diseases treatment guidelines 2002. *MMWR, 51*(RR-6), 1-80.

TABLE 5-4 **Health Screening Recommendations for Women Aged 18 Years and Older**

INTERVENTION	RECOMMENDATION*
Physical Examination	
Blood pressure	Every visit, but at least every 2 years
Height and weight	Every visit, but at least every 2 years
Pelvic examination	Annually until age 70; recommended for any woman who has ever been sexually active
Breast examination	
Self-examination	Initiated/taught at time of first pelvic examination; done monthly at end of menses
Clinical examination†	Every 3 years, ages 20 to 39; annually after age 40
High risk	Annually after age 18 with history of premenopausal breast cancer in first-degree relative
Risk groups	At least annually:
Skin examination	Family history of skin cancer or increased exposure to sunlight after age 40; every 3 years between ages 20 to 40; monthly self-examinations also recommended
Oral cavity examination	Mouth lesion or exposure to tobacco or excessive alcohol
Laboratory/Diagnostic Tests	
Blood cholesterol (fasting lipoprotein analysis)	Every 5 years
High risk	More often per clinical judgment with potential for cardiac or lipid abnormalities
Papanicolaou smear†	Initially, 3 years after becoming sexually active but no later than age 21; yearly with conventional Pap test or every 2 years with liquid-based Pap tests. After age 30 and after three normal test results in a row, every 2 to 3 years; after age 70 and no abnormal test results in 10 years, screening may be stopped
Mammography‡	Annually over age 50 Annually over age 40 Every 1 to 2 years between ages 40 and 49 and annually thereafter
Colon cancer screening	Fecal occult blood test annually and flexible sigmoidoscopy every 5 years after age 50; more often if family history of colon cancer or polyps
Risk groups	
Fasting blood sugar	Annually with family history of diabetes, gestational diabetes, or significantly obese; every 3 to 5 years for all women older than 45 years of age
Hearing screen	Annually with exposure to excessive noise or when loss is suspected
Sexually transmitted infection screen	As needed with multiple sexual partners
Tuberculin skin test	Annually with exposure to persons with tuberculosis or in risk categories for close contact with the disease
Endometrial biopsy	At menopause for women at risk for endometrial cancer
Vision	Every 2 years between ages 40 and 64; annually after age 65
Bone mineral density testing	All women age 65 and older; younger women with risk for osteoporosis may need periodic screenings
Immunizations	
Tetanus-diphtheria	Booster is given every 10 years after primary series
Measles, mumps, rubella	Once if born after 1956 and no evidence of immunity
Hepatitis B	Primary series of three for all who are in risk categories
Influenza	Annually after age 65 or in risk categories, such as chronic diseases, immunosuppression, renal dysfunction

*Unless otherwise noted, the recommended intervention should be performed routinely every 1 to 3 years.

†Sources: American Cancer Society. (2003). *Cancer facts and figures 2003.* New York: American Cancer Society; Centers for Disease Control and Prevention. (2002). Sexually transmitted diseases treatment guidelines 2002. *MMWR, 51*(RR-6), 1-80; Expert Panel on Detection, Evaluation, and Treatment of High Blood Cholesterol in Adults. (2001). Executive summary of the third report of the national education program (NCEP) expert panel on detection, evaluation, and treatment of high blood cholesterol in adults (Adult treatment panel III). *Journal of the American Medical Association, 285*(19), 2486-2497; National Women's Health Resource Center. (2001). Screening tests and women's health. *National Women's Health Report, 23*(6), 1-7, U.S. Preventive Services Task Force. (1996). *Guide to clinical preventive services* (2nd ed.). Baltimore: Williams & Wilkins; U.S. Preventive Services Task Force. (2003). *Screening for cervical cancers. AHRQ Publication 03-535,* January, 2003. Rockville, MD: Agency for Healthcare Research and Quality.

‡Note: There is no consensus regarding mammograms for women between 40 and 49 years of age; thus various recommendations are listed. Women are urged to discuss circumstances with their health care provider.

educate and counsel on diet, exercise, cessation of smoking, alcohol moderation, help for drug abuse, and stress management.

Health Risk Prevention

Simple safety factors often are forgotten or perceived not to be important, yet injuries continue to have a major impact on the health status of all age groups. Being aware of hazards and implementing safety guidelines will reduce risks. The nurse should frequently reinforce the following common-sense concepts that will protect the individual:

- Wear seat belts at all times in a moving vehicle.
- Wear safety helmets when riding a motorcycle, bicycle, or inline skates.
- Follow driving "rules of the road."
- Place smoke alarms throughout the home and workplace.
- Avoid secondhand smoke.
- Reduce noise pollution or safeguard against hearing loss.
- Protect skin from ultraviolet light with the use of sunscreen and clothing.
- Handle and store firearms appropriately.
- Practice water safety.

Taking necessary precautions and avoiding dangerous situations is imperative.

Health Protection

Nurses can make a difference in stopping violence against women and preventing further injury. Educating women that abuse is a violation of their rights and facilitating their access to protective and legal services constitutes a first step. Encouraging health care institutions to implement appropriate domestic violence screening programs also is of great value (Gantt & Bickford, 1999). Other helpful measures for women to discourage their entry into abusive relationships include promoting assertiveness and self-defense courses; suggesting support and self-help groups that encourage positive self-regard, confidence, and empowerment; and recommending educational and skills development classes that will enhance independence and self-care.

Numerous national and local organizations provide information and assistance for women in abusive situations. Nurses and victims may find these resources helpful. National resources and hotlines are listed at the end of the chapter. All nurses who work in women's health care should become familiar with local services and legal options.

KEY POINTS

- Culture, religion, socioeconomic status, personal circumstances, the uniqueness of the individual, and stage of development are among the factors that influence a person's recognition of need for care and response to the health care system.
- The changing status and roles of women affect their health, needs, and ability to cope with problems.
- Assessment is more comprehensive and learning is enhanced in a safe environment in which the atmosphere is nonjudgmental and sensitive and the interaction is strictly confidential.
- Every woman is entitled to be respected and fully involved in the assessment and educational process.
- Preconception counseling allows identification and possible remediation of potentially harmful personal and social conditions, medical and psychologic conditions, environmental conditions, and barriers to care before conception.
- Conditions that increase a woman's health risks also increase risks for her offspring.
- Periodic health screening, including history, physical examination, and diagnostic and laboratory tests, provides the basis for overall health promotion, prevention of illness, early diagnosis of problems, and referral for management.
- Health promotion and prevention of illness assists women in actualizing health potential by increasing motivation, providing information, and incorporating recommendations for accessing specific resources.

CRITICAL THINKING EXERCISES

1. A 35-year-old woman, gravida 5, para 5, arrives in clinic for her 6-week postpartum check up. Her husband accompanies her and tells you that she is not sleeping or eating and is crying a lot. Besides neglecting herself and the newborn, she has abandoned her other childcare responsibilities.
   a. What is your initial impression and nursing diagnosis?
   b. What community resources are available for the woman and her family?
   c. Rank order the woman's immediate needs and develop a plan of care.

CRITICAL THINKING EXERCISES—cont'd

2. Analyze resources in your community for referring the following women. Then evaluate the resources in terms of access, confidentiality, cost, and follow-up services. Develop a resource file for each.
   a. A woman desiring tattoo removal.
   b. A lesbian woman who has just lost her partner to AIDS and is in need of counseling.
   c. A teenager with a BMI >30 desiring a fitness program.
   d. A woman who has just taken over full-time care of her 75-year-old mother-in-law who has senile dementia with psychoses.
   e. A 55-year-old woman who is menopausal with symptoms and wondering if she should take hormone replacement therapy.

RESOURCES

Alcoholics Anonymous (AA) World Services
475 Riverside Drive, 11th Floor
New York, NY 10115
212-870-3400
www.alcoholics-anonymous.org

Anorexia Nervosa and Related Eating Disorders, Inc.
www.anred.com

Cancer Information Service (CIS)
800-4-CANCER

Domestic Violence Hotline
800-799-SAFE
TDD line for the hearing impaired: 800-787-3224

Harvard Eating Disorders Center
356 Boylston St.
Boston, MA 02166
888-236-1188
www.hedc.org

Health Education for Mid-Life and Older Women
Food and Drug Administration
800-532-4440
www.fda.gov

HealthFinder
www.healthfinder.gov

Institute for Women's Policy Research
1707 L St., NW, Suite 750
Washington, DC 20036
202-785-5100
www.iwpr.org

Integration of Prevention Services into Reproductive Health Services
Centers for Disease Control and Prevention
770-488-5227
www.cdc.gov/nccdphp/drh

Mental Health Education Campaigns
Depression awareness: 800-421-4211
Anxiety disorders: 888-8-ANXIETY
Panic disorders: 800-64-PANIC

National Council of Women's Organizations
Women's Health
1126 16th St., NW, Suite 411
Washington, DC 20036
202-331-7343
womensorganizations.org/healthtopic_toc.cfm

National Organization for Women (NOW) Legal Defense and Education Fund
99 Hudson St.
New York, NY 10013-2871
212-925-6635

National Women's Health Information Center
The Office on Women's Health
Department of Health and Human Resources
800-994-9662
www.4woman.gov

National Women's Health Resource Center
120 Albany St., Suite 820
New Brunswick, NJ 08901
877-986-9472
www.healthywomen.org

New York Times on the Web
Women's Health
www.nytimes.com/specials/women/whome/index.html

Office of Minority Health Resource Center
P.O. Box 37337
Washington, DC 20013-7337
301-587-1938

Society for Women's Health Research
1828 L St., NW, Suite 625
Washington, DC 20036
202-223-8224
www.womens-health.org

REFERENCES

Alan Guttmacher Institute. (1998). *Risks and realities of early childbearing.* New York: The Institute.

American Cancer Society. (2003). *Cancer facts and figures 2003.* New York: American Cancer Society.

American College of Obstetricians and Gynecologists. (1999). *Good health before pregnancy: Preconception care.* Washington, DC: ACOG.

American College of Obstetricians and Gynecologists. (1997). *Smoking and women's health. ACOG Technical Bulletin no. 240.* Washington, DC: ACOG.

Barkauskas, V., Baumann, L., & Darling-Fisher, C. (2002). *Health and physical assessment* (3rd ed.). St. Louis: Mosby.

Berg, J. (2001). Dimensions of sexuality in the perimenopausal transition: A model for practice. *Journal of Obstetric, Gynecologic, and Neonatal Nursing, 30*(4), 421-428.

Centers for Disease Control and Prevention. (2002). Sexually transmitted diseases treatment guidelines 2002. *MMWR, 51*(RR-6), 1-80.

de Groot, L. (1999). High maternal body weight and pregnancy outcome. *Nutrition Review, 57*(2), 62.

DiSaia, P., & Creasman, W. (2002). *Clinical gynecologic oncology* (6th ed.). St. Louis: Mosby.

Edge, V., & Miller, M. (1994). *Women's health care.* St. Louis: Mosby.

Epidemiologic trends in drug abuse advance report. (2000). Washington, DC: National Institute on Drug Abuse.

Expert Panel on Detection, Evaluation, and Treatment of High Blood Cholesterol in Adults. (2001). Executive summary of the third report of the national education program (NCEP) expert panel on detection, evaluation, and treatment of high blood cholesterol in adults (Adult treatment panel III). *Journal of the American Medical Association, 285*(19), 2486-2497.

Gantt, L., & Bickford, A. (1999). Screening for domestic violence. *AWHONN Lifelines, 3*(2), 36-42.

Hobbins, D. (2001). Prepping for healthy moms and babies: Making the case for preconception care and counseling. *AWHONN Lifelines, 5*(4), 49-54.

Hoyert, D. et al. (2001). Annual summary of vital statistics. *Pediatrics, 108*(6), 1241-1255.

Huff, B. (2000). Screening for cervical cancer: It's time to check your technique. *AWHONN Lifelines, 4*(3), 53-55.

Hutchinson, M., Sosa, D., & Thompson A. (2001). Sexual protective strategies of late adolescent females: More than just condoms. *Journal of Obstetric, Gynecologic, and Neonatal Nursing, 30*(4), 429-438.

Japenga, A. (1998, Jan. 2). Depression: Are men hiding? *USA Weekend*, 20.

Masters, W. (1992). *Human sexuality* (4th ed.). New York: HarperCollins.

Mattson, S. (2000a). Striving for cultural competence: Providing care for the changing face of the US. *AWHONN Lifelines, 4*(3), 48-52.

Mattson, S. (2000b). Providing culturally competent care: Strategies and approaches for perinatal clients. *AWHONN Lifelines 4*(5), 37-39.

Minino, A., & Smith, B. (2001). *Deaths: Preliminary data for 2000, National Vital Statistics Reports* (Vol. 49, no. 12). Hyattsville, MD: National Center for Health Statistics.

National Center for Chronic Disease Prevention and Health Promotion. (2000). *U.S. obesity trends 1985 to 2000.* Atlanta: Centers for Disease Control and Prevention.

National Center for Health Statistics. (1998). *Health, United States, 1998.* Atlanta: Centers for Disease Control and Prevention.

National Women's Health Resource Center. (2001). Screening tests and women's health. *National Women's Health Report, 23*(6), 1-7.

National Women's Law Center. (2000). *Making the grade on women's health: A national and state-by-state report card.* Washington, DC: National Women's Law Center.

Orbanic, S. (2001). Understanding bulimia: Signs, symptoms, and the human experience. *American Journal of Nursing, 101*(3), 35-41.

Peck, S. (2001). The importance of the sexual health history in the primary care setting. *Journal of Obstetric, Gynecologic, and Neonatal Nursing, 30*(3), 269-274.

Sampselle, C. (2000). Behavioral interventions for urinary incontinence in women: Evidence for practice. *Journal of Midwifery and Women's Health, 45*(2), 94-103.

Sampselle, C. et al. (1997). Continence for women: Evidence-based practice. *Journal of Obstetric, Gynecologic, and Neonatal Nursing, 26*(4), 375-385.

Saraiya, M. et al. (2001). Self-reported Papanicolaou smears and hysterectomies among women in the United States. *Obstetrics and Gynecology, 98*(2), 269-278.

Schulz, A., et al. (2001). Social context, stressors and disparities in women's health. *Journal of the American Medical Women's Association, 56*(4), 143-150.

Seidel, H. et al. (2003). *Mosby's guide to physical examination* (5th ed.). St. Louis: Mosby.

Speroff L., Glass R., & Kase N. (1999). *Clinical gynecology, endocrinology, and infertility* (6th ed). Baltimore: Lippincott Williams & Wilkins.

Statistics related to overweight and obesity. (2000). NIH publication no. 96-4158. Washington, DC: National Institutes of Health.

Stenchever, M. et al. (2001). *Comprehensive gynecology* (4th ed.). St. Louis: Mosby.

Stevens, P., & Hall, J. (2001). Sexuality and safer sex: The issue of lesbians and bisexual women. *Journal of Obstetric, Gynecologic, and Neonatal Nursing, 30*(4), 439-447.

Stringham, P. (1999). Domestic violence. *Primary Care,* 26(2), 373-384.

Surgeon General's call to action to prevent and decrease overweight and obesity. (2000). Washington, DC: U.S. Government Printing Office, no. 017-001-00551-7.

Surgeon General's report on women and smoking. (2001). Washington, DC: U.S. Government Printing Office.

United States Preventive Services Task Force. (1996). *Guide to clinical preventive services* (2nd ed.). Baltimore: Williams & Wilkins.

The State University of New York Counseling Center. (2002). *Stress management.* Buffalo: University at Buffalo, The State University of New York.

Weiss, J., & Scott, L. (2001). Stalking the no. 1 killer of women: Detecting diabetes and heart diseases. *AWHONN Lifelines, 5*(5), 26-34.

CHAPTER 6

Kathleen K. Furniss

Violence Against Women

http://evolve.elsevier.com/Lowdermilk/MatWmnHlth/

LEARNING OBJECTIVES

- Describe the historic beliefs and practices that have perpetuated violence against women.
- Contrast the theoretic premises underlying the victimization of women.
- Examine the prevalence and effects of intimate partner violence.
- Explain the cycle of violence and its use in assessment and intervention for battered women.
- Develop a plan of care for a battered woman.
- Delineate behaviors associated with women who experienced sexual assault as children.
- Discuss the nursing care for a survivor of childhood sexual abuse.
- Review the dynamics of rape.
- Describe the rape-trauma syndrome.
- Develop a nursing plan of care for a woman in the acute phase of rape-trauma syndrome.
- Evaluate resources available to women experiencing abuse.

Violence against women is an epidemic that is not abating. A 2000 National Violence Against Women survey estimated that 25% of women worldwide have been victims of **intimate partner violence (IPV)** (Tjaden & Thoennes, 2000). Although there is no consensus on the definition of IPV, the National Violence Against Women survey definition will be used here: the actual or threatened physical or sexual or psychologic or emotional abuse by a spouse, ex-spouse, boyfriend, girlfriend, ex-boyfriend, ex-girlfriend, date, or cohabiting partner. IPV may include rape, physical assault, and stalking (Tjaden & Thoennes, 2000). The term often implies female victims and male perpetrators, as only 5% of IPV is committed against men (Gundersen, 2002).

IPV is a significant social problem and a major health and health care problem. It is estimated that 4.8 million women are victims of IPV annually (Tjaden & Thoennes, 2000). Health care setting surveys have found an annual prevalence of physical assault between 4% and 44% (Humphreys et al., 2001). Forty-five percent of abused women also report being forced into sexual activities (Campbell & Soeken, 1999). An average of three women a day are murdered by their intimate partners (Walton-Moss & Campbell, 2002). Women who are abused during pregnancy have a threefold increase in risk of being murdered (McFarlane et al., 2002). A *Healthy People 2010* objective is to decrease the rate of IPV to 4 per 1000 women older than 12 years (USDHHS, 2000).

In the United States, violence is the second leading cause of injuries to women in the 15- to 44-year-old age group (National Women's Health Information Center [NWHIC], 2002). In one study, women who had experienced abuse had a 50% to 70% increase in central nervous system (CNS), gynecologic, and anxiety-related problems (Campbell J., 2002). Women of all races, ethnicity, religions, and socioeconomic backgrounds are abused or at risk (NWHIC, 2002). In the United States, Caucasian women report less IPV than do non-Caucasians. Native American/Alaskan Native women report significantly more instances of IPV than do women of any other racial background; Asian women report significantly less IPV than do other racial groups (Tjaden & Thoennes, 2000). Reporting rates may not reflect the magnitude of the problem, as many women do not disclose violence because of fear, embarrassment, or not having been asked by those from whom they seek help.

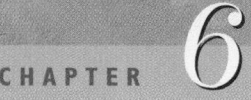

Maternity and women's health nurses, by the very nature of their practice, are in a unique position to identify and assist in the treatment of women experiencing any type of violence or sexual assault; to help prevent further harm through identification, treatment and education; and to influence public policy in decreasing violence. This chapter addresses battering, including battering of pregnant women; incest; sexual assault; and rape.

HISTORICAL PERSPECTIVE

Women have been treated inhumanely throughout history and often still are. In 2002, a woman from a middle-Eastern country was stoned to death, a punishment that was socially acceptable in her culture. Her crime was having been raped by a family member. Another woman was ordered to be raped by four men as punishment for a male cousin of hers who had been seeing a woman above his social class. Her relatives were prevented from rescuing her by armed officials, and she was ordered by the tribal jury to walk home naked after the group assault (Fisher, 2002).

In ancient Roman times, wives were divorced or killed by husbands for adultery, public drunkenness, or attending public games, whereas men could engage in these activities daily. In the 1700s, under English Common Law, the "rule of thumb" gave men permission to chastise their wives physically as long as the implement they used was no wider than their thumbs. This legacy carried over to the United States into the nineteenth century. After 1870, wife abuse became illegal in the United States (Gelles, 1995), although it did not cease to occur. Misogyny, patriarchy, devaluation of women, power imbalance, view of women as property, sex-role stereotyping, and acceptance of aggressive male behavior as appropriate all contributed and continue to contribute to the subordinate status of women in many of the world's societies.

The power imbalance and concept that family problems are private often kept women from disclosing abuse. There was little awareness and even less response from both medical professionals and the legal and justice systems to the plight of women in intimate relationships. As late as the 1960s, it was believed that violence in the family was rare and committed only by mentally ill or otherwise disturbed people. The women's movement of the 1970s first called attention to the inequality of women in all forms of interpersonal relationships; intolerance of violence then was manifested, and public sanctions against such behavior were initiated. Recognition of the extent of both female and male injustices, including incest, rape, and elder abuse, also increased at this time.

CONCEPTUAL PERSPECTIVES

Many attempts have been made to apply theoretic explanations to the causes and understanding of violence, none of which is conclusive. A brief summary of these is provided to assist in analyzing the persistent acts of violence against women.

Psychologic Perspective

Psychology, the study of individual behavior, places responsibility for all behavior, including aggression, on the individual. Early psychoanalytic theory postulated aggression as a basic instinctual drive leading to mastery and accomplishment and, in men, as a positive force that connotes boldness, forcefulness, energy, enterprise, and so on (Hanrahan et al., 1993). Psychoanalytic theory promotes gender-stereotypic expectations, and thus aggression in women is viewed negatively; aggressive women are labeled hostile and belligerent.

O'Leary (1993) proposed a continuum of aggression progressing from verbal aggression (yelling, name calling) to lesser forms of physical aggression (pushing, slapping) to true violent behavior (beating, punching) and to the extreme (murder). He contended that this model has implications for treatment as well as study, because empiric evidence indicates that the causes and the behaviors are different in each category on the continuum. Table 6-1 presents these differences.

Another psychologic stance is that abuse is committed by people who are mentally ill or deranged in some way and that the victims are innocent and defenseless (Gelles, 1997). This misconception perpetuates the notion that violence occurs among people who are not "normal." Mental illness accounts for only about 10% of all violence (Gelles, 1997). Some studies suggest that borderline and antisocial personality disorders are more prevalent in men who batter (Else et al., 1993). A mental health diagnosis of alcohol abuse is frequently found in abusers but should not be misconstrued as the cause of violence. There is evidence that alcohol may increase the risk of violent behavior, but only in some individuals in some situations and with some cultural or social influences (National Institute on Alcohol Abuse and Alcoholism, 1997).

There is no diagnostic profile of an abuser, but Box 6-1 provides some characteristics of men who batter that nurses can use to assess clients' relationships.

TABLE *6-1* **Causes of Aggression**

VERBAL AGGRESSION	PHYSICAL AGGRESSION	SEVERE PHYSICAL AGGRESSION
Need to control	Accept violence as a means of control	Personality disorder
Misuse of power	Modeling of physical aggression; abused as a child	Emotional lability
Jealousy	Alcohol abuse	Poor self-esteem
Marital discord		Aggressive personality styles

Modified from O'Leary, D. (1993). Through a psychological lens: Personality traits, personality disorders, and levels of violence. In R. Gelles & D. Loseke (Eds.), *Current controversies on family violence.* Newbury Park, CA: Sage.

Women with severe and persistent mental illness may be more vulnerable to being involved in controlling and violent relationships (Fishwick, 1995). However, numerous mental health problems (such as depression, psychophysiologic illnesses, substance abuse, eating disorders, and anxiety reactions) experienced by women with abusive partners are more likely to be consequences of long-term abuse rather than causes (Campbell, J. et al., 2002).

Sociologic Perspective

The social structure and conditions in Western society provide the basis for the prevailing attitudes toward violent behavior. The United States has a long history of using violence for social control reasons, as in wars and riots. Approval of violence in men is promoted in the double standard dictating that women are expected to be nonviolent, whereas men are expected to be aggressive; therefore, men's violence is treated with more leniency and less stigma, particularly in the justice system. The more a culture uses physical force for socially approved ends, the more the violence becomes generalized to other areas of social life (Hanrahan et al., 1993).

The structure of the family often sets the stage for violent behaviors: ascribed roles of family members, the amount of time spent together, the private nature of the family, the intensity of emotional involvement, and stress and conflict inherent in families (Gelles, 1997). Power and violence, or even the threat of physical force, serve to maintain the patriarchal view of woman's place in the home and in the rest of society. Gender inequality, in both economic opportunities and physical strength, serves to perpetuate the power imbalance in relationships; in essence, some women are still dependent on men both as providers and as protectors (Hanrahan et al., 1993).

Another family issue is the intergenerational transmission of violence; both perpetuators of violence and victims learn about violence in families of origin. Gelles (1995) stated that approximately 30% of abused children become abusers as adults, compared with 2% to 4% of nonabused children in the general population who become abusers as adults. Both lack of emotional support as children and awareness that people who love each other can be violent are prominent factors. Rynerson and Fishel (1993) found that childhood memories of more than 90% of the subjects (both men and women) in their study revealed a history of harsh physical punishment, ranging from spanking to being hit with closed fists and objects, as a means of discipline, and one third of the subjects observed violence between their parents.

Poverty and oppression are cited as being significant factors in violent behavior (Gelles, 1997; Hanrahan et al., 1993). Low income with its subsequent stress and limited resources adds to the potential for violence. Violent episodes are greater among unemployed people and those with low-prestige jobs (Gelles, 1997).

BOX *6-1* **Characteristics of a Potential Batterer**

- Low self-esteem
- Problems with abandonment, loss, helplessness, dependency, insecurity, and intimacy
- Inadequate verbal skills, especially difficulty expressing feelings
- Deficits in assertiveness
- Personality disorders frequently diagnosed
- Low frustration tolerance (loses temper easily)
- Higher incidence of growing up in an abusive or violent home
- Denies, minimizes, blames, and lies about own actions
- Violence is consistent with his view of himself and the world; it is an acceptable way of dealing with everyday life
- Inability to empathize with others
- Rigidity in male and female behaviors (sex-role stereotypes)
- Perception of self as "special" and deserving special attention for being the provider, protector
- Substance abuse problems are common
- Display of an unusual amount of jealousy (e.g., expects partner to spend all of her time with him or to keep him informed of her whereabouts)

Biologic Factors

A complete biologic perspective is beyond the scope of this chapter, but evidence indicates that neurobiologic and hormonal factors influence aggression in men. Studies using imaging technology indicate that aggressive behavior is associated with the limbic structures, temporal lobes, and frontal lobes of the brain (Garza-Trevino, 1994). Changes in structural functioning of the limbic system, such as occur with brain lesions, substance use, epilepsy, and head injuries, affect both emotional experience and behavior of the individual and thus may increase or decrease the potential for aggressive behavior (Harper-Jacques & Reimer, 1992).

Neurochemical factors also may play a role in aggressive behavior so that dysfunction or misregulation of certain neurotransmitters may result in aggression. Increased levels of both norepinephrine and L-dopa foster aggressive behavior. Reducing the levels of serotonin in animals causes aggressive behavior. The amino acid gamma-aminobutyric acid (GABA) inhibits aggressive behavior. The occurrence of violence in neurologic disorders also is reported, especially when violent reactions are out of proportion to the provoking events (Garza-Trevino, 1994).

In studies of animals, aggression is associated with abnormally high levels of testosterone. In reviewing the literature on the testosterone-aggression relation in men, studies often report conflicting results (Garza-Trevino, 1994). Solar et al. (2000) reported higher testosterone levels in abusive male subjects and suggest that heritability is an issue that warrants the inclusion of this variable in future studies of violent behavior.

Most research indicates that a combination of environmental and physical factors results in violence; in essence, aggressive behavior is an individual's response to his or her perception of the situation (Harper-Jacques & Reimer, 1992). No conclusive evidence in biologic theory, except perhaps in instances of neurologic damage, indicates that aggressive behavior cannot be controlled.

Feminist Perspective

The contemporary social view of violence is derived from feminist theory. This view, with the primary theme of male dominance and coercive control, enhances our understanding of all forms of violence against women, including wife battering, stranger and acquaintance rape, incest, and sexual harassment in the workplace. This gender and power perspective evolved from women's descriptions of their abusive experiences and from activists attempting to understand the victimization that occurred. In numerous cases, power and control tactics were central events leading to the violence (Renzetti et al., 2001). The power and control wheel developed by the Duluth, Minnesota, Domestic Abuse Intervention Project identifies the ways in which men exercise the power and control that underlie all types of intimate violence (Fig. 6-1).

Campbell and Fishwick (1993) discussed the concept of machismo, or compulsive masculinity, associated particularly with wife abuse. Machismo encompasses the traditional male values of "toughness" and aggression, and thus various authors characterize male identity as a preoccupation with physical strength, athletic prowess, demonstrations of daring and valor through aggression and violence, an inability to express emotions, treatment of women as commodities and conquest objects, and inability to be gentle toward and to cooperate with women. Men may say "I only hit her because I needed to keep her in line." This machismo framework is consistent with the feminist perspective on abuse.

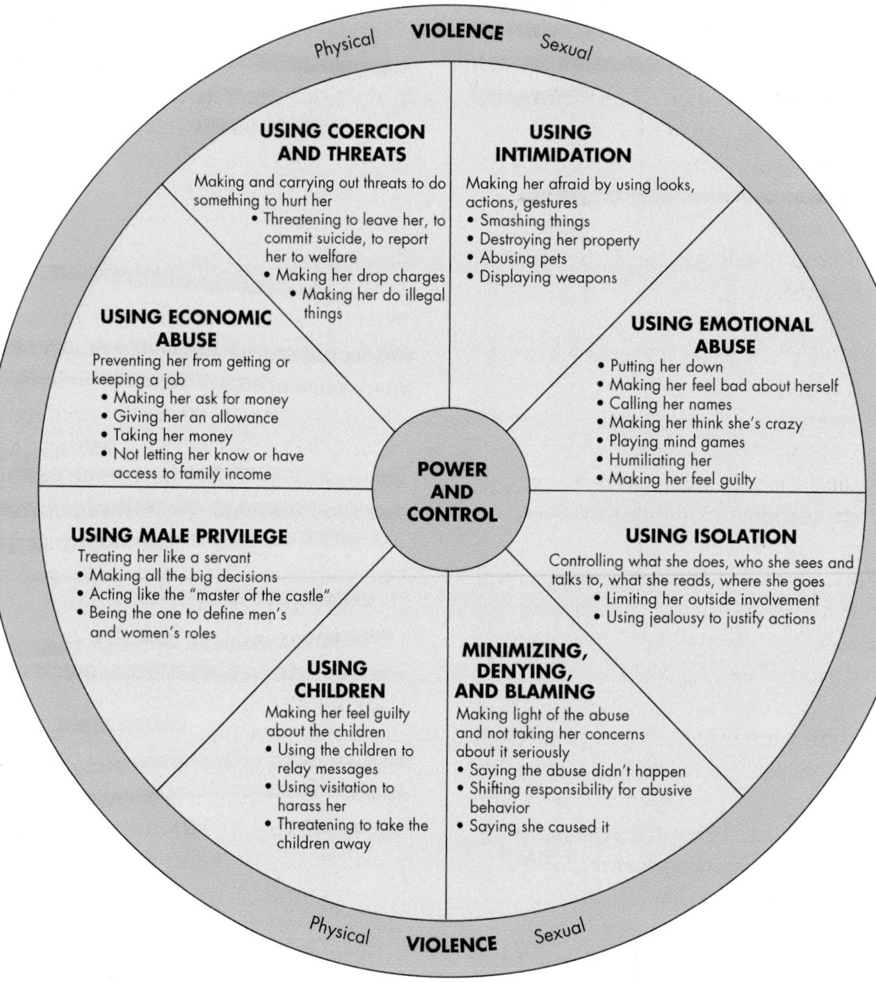
VIOLENCE
Physical
Sexual
USING COERCION AND THREATS
Making and carrying out threats to do something to hurt her
• Threatening to leave her, to commit suicide, to report her to welfare
• Making her drop charges
• Making her do illegal things
USING INTIMIDATION
Making her afraid by using looks, actions, gestures
• Smashing things
• Destroying her property
• Abusing pets
• Displaying weapons
USING ECONOMIC ABUSE
Preventing her from getting or keeping a job
• Making her ask for money
• Giving her an allowance
• Taking her money
• Not letting her know or have access to family income
USING EMOTIONAL ABUSE
• Putting her down
• Making her feel bad about herself
• Calling her names
• Making her think she's crazy
• Playing mind games
• Humiliating her
• Making her feel guilty
POWER AND CONTROL
USING MALE PRIVILEGE
Treating her like a servant
• Making all the big decisions
• Acting like the "master of the castle"
• Being the one to define men's and women's roles
USING ISOLATION
Controlling what she does, who she sees and talks to, what she reads, where she goes
• Limiting her outside involvement
• Using jealousy to justify actions
USING CHILDREN
Making her feel guilty about the children
• Using the children to relay messages
• Using visitation to harass her
• Threatening to take the children away
MINIMIZING, DENYING, AND BLAMING
Making light of the abuse and not taking her concerns about it seriously
• Saying the abuse didn't happen
• Shifting responsibility for abusive behavior
• Saying she caused it
Physical
VIOLENCE
Sexual

FIG. 6-1 Model of how power and control issues perpetuate battering. (From Duluth Domestic Abuse Intervention Project. (1986). *Power and control: Tactics of men who batter.* Duluth, MN: Author.)

Implications for Nursing

Theoretic frameworks assist the nurse to understand the dynamics and variables in the victimization of women. This knowledge is vital in dispelling myths that prevail among professionals and their clients. The more cognizant nurses become, the more information they can share with women, who ultimately make their own decisions about the quality of their lives and relationships.

CULTURAL CONSIDERATIONS

The objectification of women and power inequalities in human social arrangements support the abuse of women. These are especially apparent in any social or cultural system of oppression. Nurses must consider all forces that shape the client's identity: ethnicity, race, class, language, citizenship, religion, and culture, while recognizing that abuse is against the law and injurious to the health and well-being of women and children.

The cross-cultural meaning of violence is difficult to ascertain because cultures differ in their perceptions and definitions of abuse. Accurate data about the incidence and prevalence of violence in ethnic groups are lacking because they are infrequently represented in research studies and because violence seems to be underreported as a result of cultural norms (Counts et al., 1999). For example, groups that distrust police or immigration officials may not report abuse, as they fear the results. More than basic awareness of cultural influences on violence toward women is helpful to the nurse in being more sensitive to the needs of women whose cultural experiences differ from those of the nurse. Increasing the numbers of nurses from various ethnic groups will increase the opportunity to provide culturally appropriate care.

African-American Culture

The African-American culture supports unity among humans, nature, and the spiritual world, and social connectedness and relatedness as important norms. In men, traditional sex-role socialization tends to be lower (Campbell, D. et al., 2002). Despite advances of the last two decades, African-American men are more likely to be psychologically, socially, and economically oppressed and discriminated against. Violence may occur more frequently as a result of anger generated by environmental stresses and limited resources (Campbell, D. et al., 2002).

No valid evidence of greater violence seems to exist in this population, but women are more apt to report the violence. The devalued status of the female victim and racial stereotypes are barriers to African-Americans receiving help. Severity of abuse has been found to be less severe in African-American couples (Campbell & Parker, 1999).

Hispanic Culture

Hispanics in general are family oriented and have a strong family network in which unity, cooperation, respect, and loyalty are important. However, traditional families are very hierarchic, with authority often given to elderly people, parents, and men. Sex roles are clearly delineated. Religion plays an important role in most Hispanics' lives (Torres, 1993).

Hispanics typically seek health care from their families first, and thus women are sometimes not likely to report abuse or to seek assistance from professionals. They also are an oppressed group, and their access to health care may be limited. When women do come to the nurse's attention, the nurse must be conscious of not imposing his or her own values in learning how Hispanic women handle abusive situations. Both environmental and internal factors must be addressed in their health care (Torres, 1993). Hispanic women may be abused less in pregnancy than are other groups (Campbell & Parker, 1999).

Native American Culture

Empiric evidence about abuse in the Native American culture is lacking, but many believe that incest, sexual abuse, and domestic abuse may be the cultural norm rather than the exception, although this sounds offensive. Native American and Alaskan Native women report the highest rates of IPV in the United States; however, research is needed to determine whether the rate is higher in these women or the rate of reporting is higher (Tjaden & Thoennes, 2000).

Asian Women

Information on violence against Asian women is limited. The rate of reporting IPV may be low because of the Asian values that emphasize close family ties and discourage disclosure of abuse. Further research is recommended (Tjaden & Thoennes, 2000).

BATTERED WOMEN

Although IPV is the preferred term, *wife battering, spouse abuse*, and *domestic or family violence* are all terms that may be applied to a pattern of assaultive and coercive behaviors inflicted by a male partner in a marriage or other heterosexual, significant, intimate relationships. Relationship violence rarely consists of a single episode but is a pattern that may start with intimidation or threats (see Fig. 6-1) and progress to more aggressive physical and sexual acts resulting in injury to the woman. Common elements of battering are economic deprivation, sexual abuse, intimidation, isolation, and stalking and terrorizing victims and their children (NWHIC, 2002).

IPV often entraps a woman in a relationship with conflicting realities. One reality consists of the good aspects of the partner relationship and is supported by the partner and others. The second is the reality of the abuse, which the woman may not recognize or may minimize or deny (Landenburger, 1998). Both realities may elicit the woman's hopefulness that things will change.

Characteristics of Women in Abusive Relationships

Every segment of society is represented among abused women. Race, religion, social background, age, and educational level are not significant factors in differentiating women at risk. Poor and uneducated women tend to be disproportionately represented because they are seen in emergency departments (EDs), they are financially more dependent, they have fewer resources and support systems, and they may have fewer problem-solving skills.

Battered women may believe they are to blame for their situations because they are "not good enough, not efficient enough, not pretty enough." The woman may blame herself for bringing on the violent behavior in her relationship because she believes she must "try harder" to please the abuser. In many cases, a traumatic bonding with the man hinges on loyalty, fear, terror, and learned helplessness. Some women have low self-esteem and may have histories of domestic violence in their families of origin. They fear societal rejection if they discuss their problem openly. This fear is justified in many cases because society has stereotyped these women as masochistic, which was once believed to be the case with all women in abusive relationships; they were abused and stayed because they "liked" it. It is difficult for many people to comprehend why a woman would remain in a situation in which she is repeatedly beaten and injured (Berlinger, 1998).

Warren and Lanning (1992) found that strong, traditional feminine characteristics of nurturing, compassion, sympathy, and yielding were more apparent in women in abusive relationships, in contrast to the traits of assertiveness, independence, and willingness to take a stand in women who were in nonviolent relationships. They also found the former group to be more willing to tolerate control from others. Social isolation seems to be another characteristic of battered women, which may result from stigma, fear, or restrictions placed on them by their partners.

The **battered woman's syndrome** may be formally diagnosed in the fourth edition of the Diagnostic and Statistic Manual of Mental Disorders (DSM-IV) (American Psychiatric Association, 2000) as *posttraumatic stress disorder (PTSD),* provided that the symptoms meet the criteria. Table 6-2 compares the characteristics of PTSD with battered woman's syndrome and rape-trauma syndrome (discussed later in this chapter). Professionals making the diagnosis must guard against implying that the woman's problems are her issues alone.

TABLE 6-2 **Comparison of Characteristics of Posttraumatic Stress Syndrome, Battered Woman's Syndrome, and Rape-Trauma Syndrome**

POSTTRAUMATIC STRESS SYNDROME*	BATTERED WOMAN'S SYNDROME	RAPE-TRAUMA SYNDROME
1. The person experienced an event that involved or threatened death, a serious injury, or a threat to physical integrity of self or other.	Deliberate and repeated physical or sexual assault experienced by a woman at the hands of an intimate partner.	A violent, aggressive sexual assault on a woman without her consent from a stranger or someone she knows.
2. The person's response involved intense fear, helplessness, or horror.	The woman responds with terror, entrapment, and helplessness.	The woman responds with shock, terror, and humiliation.
3. The traumatic event is persistently reexperienced, such as through distressing recollections or dreams.	If the woman remains in the relationship, the repeated experience may be real rather than recalled.	The woman relives the scene and considers what she "should have done"; she experiences a range of emotions and may feel guilty.
4. Psychologic reactivity occurs on exposure to internal or external cues symbolic of the traumatic event.	The woman feels anxious and isolated (or alone) and reacts to any expression of anger or threat by cowering or attempting to placate the abuser.	Physical symptoms such as muscle tension, hyperventilation, and flushing may occur in response to reexperiencing the rape or when approached by men, especially strangers.
5. The person persistently avoids stimuli associated with the trauma; responses are numbed.	The woman attempts to avoid arousing the anger of the abuser and tries to please him; she exerts effort to control situations to avoid abuse.	The woman avoids situations in which she feels vulnerable; if in an intimate relationship, she may avoid intercourse.
6. The person has persistent symptoms of increased arousal, such as difficulty sleeping, hypervigilance, and exaggerated startle response.	The woman is alert to signs of increasing tension in the abuser during the tension-building stages; she withdraws from interaction.	The woman is afraid of being alone or in a crowd and of being attacked from behind; she takes extra precautions when going out and is suspicious.

*Modified from American Psychiatric Association. (2000). *Diagnostic and statistical manual of mental disorders* (4th ed. Text Revision). Washington, DC: American Psychiatric Association.

Myths About Battered Women

Many people have difficulty believing the tragedies inflicted on women and have even more trouble accepting that women stay in harmful relationships. Health professionals often become frustrated by women they see repeatedly who have numerous signs of abuse but seem unable to liberate themselves from the battering relationships. As with other human dynamics that are not easily explained, people tend to rationalize the woman's behaviors and justify their own noninvolvement. A number of misconceptions have emerged to account for this perceived self-destructive behavior. If these misconceptions are believed by nurses, they result in judgments (such as blaming the victim) or in unhelpful responses, rather than empathy and empowering women to take control over their lives. Empowering includes providing supportive empathy and information that can be lifesaving. Table 6-3 lists some myths and facts about abuse and battering.

Cycle of Violence: The Dynamics of Battering

Lenore Walker pioneered the cause of women as victims of violence in the United States when she published her research in her book, *The Battered Woman* (1979). By using the qualitative research method, she recorded results from interviews with 120 battered women.

Their accounts of the progress of the abuse were remarkably similar; the resulting pattern is now recognized as the cycle of violence. According to this concept, battering is neither random nor constant; rather, it occurs in repeated cycles (Fig. 6-2). A three-phase cyclic pattern in the battering behavior has been described as a period of increasing tension leading to the battery, which is then followed by a period of calm and remorse in which the male

TABLE 6-3 **Myths and Facts about Intimate Partner Violence**

MYTHS	FACTS
Battering occurs in a small percentage of the population.	One fourth of all women experience battering by an intimate partner.
Being pregnant protects the woman from battering.	From 4% to 8% of all women who are battered are battered during pregnancy.
	Battering frequently begins or escalates in frequency and intensity during pregnancy. Pregnancy may be the result of forced sex or of the man's control of contraception.
Battering occurs only in "problem" or lower-class families.	Intimate partner violence can occur in any family. Although lower-class families have a higher reported incidence of battering, it also occurs in middle- and upper-income families. Incidence is not really known because of the tendency of middle- and upper-income families to hide their battering.
Battered women like to be beaten and deliberately provoke the attack. They are masochistic.	Women are terrified of their assailants and go to great lengths to avoid a confrontation. In some cases, the woman may provoke her partner to release tension that, if left unchecked, might lead to a more severe beating and possible death.
Only men with psychologic problems abuse women.	Many batterers are successful professionals, including politicians, ministers, physicians, and lawyers. Research indicates that only a small number of abusers have psychologic problems.
Only people who come from abusive families end in abusive relationships.	Most battered women report that their partners were the first person to beat them.
Alcohol and drug abuse cause battering.	Although alcohol may be involved in abusive incidents, it is not the cause. Many batterers use alcohol as an excuse to batter and shift the blame to the alcohol.
Women would leave the relationship if the abuse were really that bad.	Those women who stay in the relationship do so out of fear and financial dependence. Shelters have long waiting lists.
Batterers and battered women cannot change.	Counseling may effectively help both batterers and battered women.

From Gelles, R. (1997). *Intimate violence in families* (3rd ed.). Thousand Oaks, CA: Sage; National Institute on Alcohol and Alcoholism. (1997). Alocohol violence and aggression. *Alcohol Alert, 38,* 1-6; National Women's Health Information Center. (2002). *Violence against women.* Available at www.4woman.gov/violence/index.cfm. Retrieved 8/14/02.

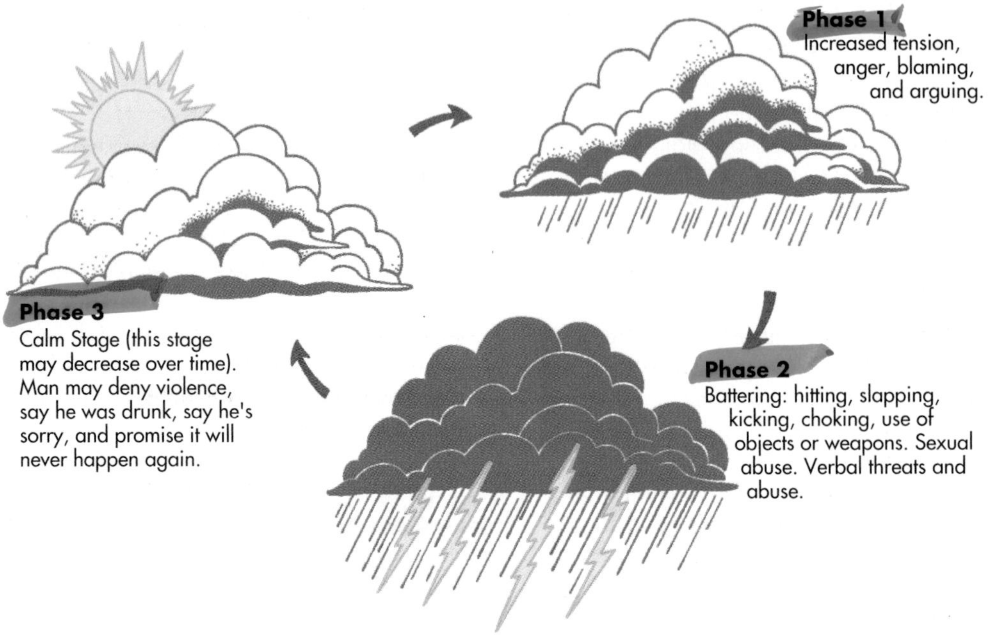
Phase 1
Increased tension, anger, blaming, and arguing.
Phase 2
Battering: hitting, slapping, kicking, choking, use of objects or weapons. Sexual abuse. Verbal threats and abuse.
Phase 3
Calm Stage (this stage may decrease over time). Man may deny violence, say he was drunk, say he's sorry, and promise it will never happen again.

FIG. 6-2 Cycle of violence. (From Helton, A. [1997]. *A protocol of care for the battered woman.* White Plains, NY: March of Dimes Birth Defects Foundation.)

partner displays kind, loving behavior and pleas for forgiveness. This "honeymoon" phase lasts until stress or other factors cause conflict and tension to mount again toward another episode of battering. Over time, the tension and battering phases last longer, and the calm phase becomes shorter, until there is no honeymoon phase (Walker, 1984).

Phase I: The Tension-Building State

Tension gradually escalates. The batterer expresses dissatisfaction and hostility without violent outbursts. He may be angered because the food is too cold, he cannot find his socks, or the children are unruly. The woman senses the danger and anxiously tries to placate him. These tactics work for a time but only reinforce the woman's unrealistic belief that she can control his violent behavior. Eventually, she can no longer control his anger, and she withdraws to cope. He senses this withdrawal and becomes angrier until the violent outburst occurs. The woman suppresses the knowledge of her mate's impending abuse.

Phase II: The Acute Battering Incident

The acute battering phase is characterized by the man's uncontrollable discharge of the tension that has been building for the purpose of "teaching her a lesson." The phase can last for hours to several days. The types of behaviors are slaps, punches to face and head, kicking, stomping, punching, choking, pushing, breaking of bones, burns from irons, and mutilation from knives and guns. The woman's injuries are usually to her face, buttocks, and hands and forearms, as she tries to protect herself. The woman denies to herself and others the severity of the damage and may not seek medical assistance even when it is needed.

Phase III: Kindness and Contrite, Loving Behavior

This "honeymoon" phase is characterized by the batterer feeling remorseful and apologizing profusely. He may try to help her, take her to the hospital, or shower her with gifts they may not be able to afford. He promises it will never happen again, and he may believe at that time that it will not. She desperately wants to believe him, and this behavior restores her hope that he will change. This stage is the positive reinforcement for remaining in the relationship. The woman denies the inevitable recurrence of the abuse. Not all abusive relationships follow these cycles, but many women recognize this pattern. See Box 6-2 for a poem by an unknown author that graphically illustrates the cycle of violence.

Battering During Pregnancy

Estimates of prevalence of battering in pregnancy vary, ranging from 4% to 8% (Martin et al., 2001). Most women abused before pregnancy will be abused during the pregnancy; the incidence may escalate. Abuse also may happen for the first time during pregnancy. Pregnant adolescents are abused at higher rates than are adult women, so they should be considered at high risk. McFarlane et al. (1999) reported on timing and severity of abuse before and during pregnancy in a group of Hispanic, African-American, and Caucasian women. They found that 51.9% of the women experienced abuse both the year before and during pregnancy. The timing and severity of the episodes were similar for the three groups.

Physical abuse is harmful not only to the mother; the risk of fetal injury is very high. Studies have demonstrated that battery during pregnancy also results in a higher rate of low-birth-weight newborns and maternal complications of depression, suicide, low weight gain, infections, bleeding, and anemia (McFarlane et al., 2002). In addition, the woman may smoke or use alcohol or other drugs as means of coping with IPV (Curry, 1998). These activities are significantly related to low-birth-weight infants (Humphreys et al., 2001).

Pregnancy is often a time of initial or increased battering episodes in violent relationships for a variety of reasons: (1) the biopsychosocial stresses of pregnancy may strain the relationship beyond the couple's ability to cope, and frustration is followed by violence; (2) the man may be jealous of the fetus, resenting the intrusion into the couple's relationship and the woman's displacement of attention; (3) the man may be angry at the unborn child or the woman; and (4) the beating may be the man's conscious or subconscious attempt to end the pregnancy. After birth, the mother may be so physically and emotionally drained that she may have difficulty bonding with her infant (Lindgren, 2001). She may be at risk of becoming an abusive mother whether or not she remains in the abusive relationship.

Physical and sexual abuse may predict poor health during pregnancy and the postpartum period. In one study, women who were abused reported an average of four medical symptoms, especially headaches, pain, and high levels of depression that did not abate during the postpartum period but did abate in the nonabused women (Leserman et al., 1999). Back pain, fainting, and seizures also have been reported. Gastrointestinal symptoms may occur from chronic stress, as may hypertension and chest pain. Gynecologic problems such as sexually transmitted infections (STIs), bleeding, infection, urinary tract infections, chronic pelvic pain, and genital trauma may result. Use of contraception may be hindered. Depression and PTSD are the most prevalent mental health sequelae, but substance abuse is common as a method of coping (Campbell, J. et al., 2002).

During pregnancy, the target body parts change during abusive episodes. Women report physical blows directed to the head, breasts, abdomen, and genitalia. Sexual assault is common. Physical and sexual assaults also increase the rate of miscarriages and preterm and stillborn infants. The battered woman should be treated as an obstetric client at high risk (Curry, 1998).

If the pregnant woman remains with her partner, she is at additional risk for repeated physical and psychologic trauma and even death (McFarlane et al., 2002). The potential for child abuse is great, especially if the batterer's anger is directed at the unborn child or if he is jealous of the fetus. If battering begins in pregnancy, it is likely to continue after the birth. This information is vital to share with the woman and other nurses involved in her care. Another factor in the health of both the mother and the newborn child is that the woman may expend energy on coping with the battering rather than on caring for the newborn child.

Pregnant women's difficulties may assist the nurse in identifying battering during pregnancy (see Research box). These include consumption of an inadequate diet including too little milk and milk products, lack of sleep, and minimal forms of self-relaxation; in essence, the battered pregnant woman may not take proper care of herself.

Battering and pregnancy in teenagers constitute a particularly difficult situation. Adolescents may be more trapped in the abusive relationship than are adult women because of their inexperience. Adolescents may ignore the violence because the jealous and controlling behavior is interpreted as love and devotion. Because pregnancy in young adolescent girls is frequently the result of sexual abuse, feelings about the pregnancy should be assessed.

BOX 6-2 I Got Flowers Today

I got flowers today. It wasn't my birthday or any other special day.
We had our first argument last night, and he said a lot of cruel things that really hurt me.
I know he is sorry and didn't mean the things he said because he sent me flowers today.
I got flowers today. It wasn't our anniversary or any other special day.
Last night he threw me into a wall and started to choke me. It seemed like a nightmare. I couldn't believe it was real. I woke up this morning sore and bruised all over.
I know he must be sorry because he sent me flowers today, and it wasn't Mother's Day or any other special day.
Last night he beat me up again, and it was much worse than all the other times. If I leave him, what will I do? How will I take care of my kids? What about money? I'm afraid of him and scared to leave.
But I know he must be sorry. Because he sent me flowers today.
I got flowers today. Today was a very special day.
It was the day of my funeral.
Last night he finally killed me. He beat me to death.
If only I had gathered enough courage and strength to leave him,
I would not have gotten flowers today.
—Author unknown

Teens report abuse from partners, former partners, and family members (Renker, 2002). Many who had been abused through the pregnancy also were abused after, and others who were not abused during pregnancy reported initial abuse after giving birth (Harrykissoon et al., 2002). Adolescents have been found to be at very high risk for abuse in the postpartum period.

Nurses must remember that although pregnancy is a time of risk for women owing to preeclampsia, diabetes, sepsis, coagulopathy, and other pregnancy-related disorders, IPV-related homicide may be the biggest risk facing pregnant women (Krulewich et al., 2001; McFarlane et al., 2002)

RESEARCH

Identifying Victims of Intimate Partner Violence Among Pregnant Women

Intimate partner violence (IPV) can affect women of any culture or socioeconomic status. Physical and emotional abuse inflicted by an intimate partner, as well as forced sexual relations, constitute IPV according to the American College of Obstetricians and Gynecologists (ACOG), who recommend routine screening and zero tolerance. The risk for IPV goes up during pregnancy, especially for adolescents, and is linked with low birth weight, maternal substance abuse, depression, anemia, reproductive tract infections, and preterm labor. However, only about one out of three women are screened during prenatal visits.

The purpose of this study was to determine if any clusters of characteristics found in the prenatal intake information were common to abused pregnant women. An established, valid screening tool for IPV, the Abuse Assessment Screen available from the March of Dimes, was administered when routine entry-to-care questions were asked. In a sample of 109 new prenatal intakes at a low-cost health clinic over a 6-month period, eight women were identified as victims of IPV. Analysis of their intake data revealed a profile of a young, single woman with a desired pregnancy, fearful of her partner, with self-reported depression, stress, and a history of childhood sexual abuse. The abused women in the study were likely to be without family or partner support but relied on friends for their support. Whether these findings on an entry-to-care interview with or without a positive score on an IPV screening tool are markers for increased risk of IPV needs further study.

IMPLICATIONS FOR PRACTICE

Knowledge of the characteristics common to abused women alert the nurse to the client who may need further screening. Because clients may not reveal IPV initially, screening for abuse should occur at the first visit, at each trimester, at delivery, postpartum, at all family planning and gynecologic visits, and at any time a red flag is raised. Identification and intervention in abuse can help break the escalating cycle of violence.

Reference: Anderson, B., Marshak, H., & Hebbler, D. (2002). Identifying intimate partner violence at entry to prenatal care: Clustering routine clinical information. *Journal of Midwifery & Women's Health, 47*(5), 353-359.

CARE MANAGEMENT

Care of the battered woman must begin with the nurse's self-assessment. An exploration of attitudes toward women in abusive situations, awareness of feelings that may result in judgmental communication, and knowledge about the many aspects of IPV are preparations for care.

Exactly what drives a woman to seek assistance is not clear. Women who belong to any of the following three groups are more likely to seek assistance: (1) women who are beaten frequently and severely; (2) those who have not experienced or witnessed family violence in their family of origin; and (3) those who see an alternative to life in an abusive relationship, specifically women with jobs. Sometimes women seek help after their children have been hurt or when their children start imitating the abuser's behavior.

Battered women may be reluctant to seek help for various reasons, including the need to avoid the stigma associated with the nature of the family violence; the fear that they will not be believed; the fear of reprisal from their husbands or partners; and in some states in which battering is a reportable crime, the desire to avoid involvement with police (see Legal Tip).

LEGAL TIP **Mandatory Reporting of Domestic Violence**

Domestic violence is considered a crime in all states but it varies between misdemeanor and felony offenses, the majority being misdemeanors. Forty states and the District of Columbia have laws that mandate reporting by health care providers in situations in which the woman has an injury that may be caused by a deadly weapon. Some states also require reports when there is a reason to believe that the woman's injury may have resulted from an illegal act or act of violence. California has the strongest reporting law. Colorado, New Mexico, and Kentucky mandate health provider reporting of injuries resulting from IPV to law enforcement or public welfare. Ohio mandates that IPV be documented in the medical record. Rhode Island requires that domestic violence injuries be reported for statistical purposes only. Texas mandates that IPV be documented and that clients be informed that IPV is against the law and offered shelter referral.

Because of the wide variation from state to state in mandatory reporting, nurses *must* be knowledgeable about the reporting requirements of the state in which they practice. Nurses can check the Family Violence Prevention Fund (2002) for a current listing and evaluation of reporting laws listed in the Resources section of this chapter, or they can call the local shelter for assistance.

Assessment and Nursing Diagnoses

Clients in women's health care settings are all at risk for abuse; therefore it is important that nurses assess all women entering the health care system for potential abuse (McFarlane et al., 2002). Health care providers are often the first and only contact that a severely isolated woman will make with someone outside the relationship. Failure to identify spousal abuse and to recognize the risk of serious injury or even death further endangers the lives of women and their children.

A suspected assaulted woman should be examined and interviewed in private, and she may feel safer and more comfortable with a female health care provider. When one is taking a psychosocial history, the following information provides clues to violence or potential for violence: how the woman and her partner resolve conflict; what happens when the woman's partner becomes angry; whether fighting occurs during disagreements; and when such fighting occurs, if it ever escalates to physical means. It may help the woman to disclose information if these events are normalized by the nurse stating, "Many people (families) have difficulty in expressing anger or dealing with conflict. What is that like for you and your partner?" The nurse listens for any evidence of power and control in the relationship. While inquiring about past trauma or injuries, the nurse also should ask directly if the woman has been injured by her husband or partner. At least the following questions should be asked: (1) Are you with a spouse or partner who threatens or physically hurts you?; (2) Within the past year or in this pregnancy has anyone hit, slapped, kicked, or otherwise hurt you?; and (3) Has anyone forced you to have sexual activities that made you uncomfortable? (ACOG, 2002). These questions give a woman permission to disclose sensitive information.

An assessment tool can be a part of the interview. It can be included in a written history (see Fig. 5-10), but women may be more open to disclosure when asked. Reports show an increase in the identification of victims of domestic violence when the nurse inquires at each visit whether a woman has been hit or threatened since her last visit (Walton-Moss & Campbell, 2002). Nurses should *never* ask about abuse with a partner present, as this may place the woman in danger. Other cues to abuse are delay in seeking medical assistance (hours or days), missed appointments, vague explanation of injuries, nonspecific somatic complaints, social isolation, lack of eye contact, a husband or partner who does not want to leave the client alone with the primary health care provider, and substance abuse.

In the United States, a pregnant woman is often accompanied by her husband to the antepartum appointment if the woman does not speak English and the husband does. Unless an interpreter is available, it is difficult to interview the woman alone; in addition, asking questions about abuse through an interpreter is more difficult unless the interpreter is a woman and can communicate the nurse's sensitivity and concern accurately. See the Guidelines/Guías box for descriptions of abusive relationships and how a woman can recognize whether she is in one.

GUIDELINES/GUÍAS

Recognizing Violence in a Relationship

ARE YOU IN A RELATIONSHIP IN WHICH YOU ARE . . .
¿TIENES UNA RELACIÓN CON TU PAREJA EN LA QUE ESTÁS . . .

afraid of your partner's temper?
con miedo de que él pierda control?

afraid to break up because your partner has threatened to hurt someone?
con miedo de dejarlo porque él te ha amenazado con pegar or lastimar a alguien?

constantly apologizing for or defending your partner's behavior?
constantemente disculpándote por su comportamiento o defendiéndolo?

afraid to disagree with your partner?
con miedo de contradecirle?

isolated from your family or friends?
aislada de otra gente, por ejemplo, tu familia o amigas?

embarrassed in front of others because of your partner's words or actions?
avergüenzada al frente de otros por las palabras o acciones de tu pareja?

intimidated by your partner and forced into having sex?
intimidada o forzada a tener relaciones sexuales con él?

depressed and jumpy?
deprimida y/o nerviosa?

A PERSON WHO IS VIOLENT IN A RELATIONSHIP OFTEN . . .
LA PERSONA QUE TIENE UN CARÁCTER VIOLENTO A MENUDO EN SU RELACIÓN . . .

has an explosive temper.
muestra un temperamento explosivo.

is possessive or jealous of his partner's time, friends, or family.
es posesivo y tiene celos de que su pareja pase tiempo con la familia o amigos.

constantly criticizes his partner's thoughts, feelings, or appearance.
siempre critica los sentimientos, ideas, y apariencia física de su pareja.

pinches, slaps, grabs, shoves, or throws things at his partner.
pellizca, abofetea, empuja, o lanza objetos que pueden lastimar a su pareja.

forces his partner into having sex.
fuerza a su pareja ha tener relaciones sexuales.

causes his partner to be afraid.
causa que su pareja le tenga miedo.

Because of the cycle of violence and the loving respite phase, denial is a coping mechanism often used by battered women. Abused women may deny the probability of impending abuse, severity of injury, future recurrence, and death. Women may be embarrassed about their abusive relationships and believe the abuse is caused by their inadequacies. By asking a woman directly about abuse, telling her that similar injuries are common in women who have been abused, and pointing out that she is not responsible for another's violent behavior, the nurse may help her disclose the violence she is experiencing. During pregnancy, the nurse should assess for abuse at each prenatal visit and on admission to labor, although it is not appropriate to ask questions during active labor. Assessment for abuse continues after birth, as abuse may begin then; well-baby clinics may be important settings for screening women for abuse (Martin et al., 2001).

During the physical examination, the nurse should observe for injuries to the face, breasts, abdomen, and buttocks. These injuries may be old or new and may range from minor bruising to serious injuries. Psychosocial-assessment findings may include anxiety, insomnia, self-directed abuse, depression, and drug or alcohol abuse (Coker et al., 2000). Other physical signs include fractures that require significant force or that would rarely occur by accident; multiple injuries at various stages of healing; and patterns left by whatever might inflict injury, such as teeth, utensils, fists, or hot objects.

Examples of potential nursing diagnoses for battered women include the following:

- *Hopelessness related to*
  - –prolonged exposure to physical, mental, social, and sexual abuse
- *Deficient knowledge related to*
  - –phenomenon of battering
  - –cycle of violence
  - –community resources
- *Ineffective individual and family coping related to*
  - –persistence of victim-abuser relationship
- *Injury related to*
  - –battering episode
- *Situational low self-esteem related to*
  - –continuing victim-abuser relationship

Expected Outcomes of Care

Expected outcomes for care should be formulated in collaboration with the woman. An overall outcome is to have the woman recognize the abuse she has experienced, to recognize that it is not her fault and is against the law, and to state all her options in making decisions about what actions to take. Specific expected outcomes are that the woman will do the following:

- Identify her areas of strength and develop goals for herself
- State her knowledge of alternatives, options, and choices; community resources (shelters, financial aid, child care, education, job or financial assistance); and roles of members of the health care team
- Express a feeling of empowerment and control
- Perceive herself as deserving of respect and not as "deserving" to be victimized
- Express measures to protect her children or, if she is pregnant, the fetus from abuse
- Formulate a plan for safety

Plan of Care and Interventions

A therapeutic relationship and skillful interviewing help women disclose and describe their abuse. Language is important when talking with women. For example, using the term *victim* connotes powerlessness and hopelessness (Ryan & King, 1998); a more empowering term is *survivor*. Women who have identified their abuse may appear passive, hostile, anxious, depressed, or hysterical because they may think they are at the mercy of the man's temper or may feel that he is "out of control." In addition, they may be embarrassed, afraid, angry, sad, and shocked. A tool developed by Holtz and Furniss (1993) provides the following framework for sensitive nursing interventions: the ABCDEs of caring for the abused woman:

- A is reassuring the woman that she is not *alone*. The isolation and denigration by the abuser keep her from knowing that others are in the same situation and that health care providers can help.
- B is expressing the *belief* that violence against the woman is not acceptable in any situation and that it is not her fault. This may be the first step in empowering her to think about self-protection and acceptable boundaries.
- C is *confidentiality*, particularly because the woman may believe that if the abuse is reported, the perpetrator will retaliate (and in reality, this may happen).
- D is *documentation* and includes the following: the woman's quoted statement, "My husband punched me," a clear statement by the client about the abuse. It should not include her subjective opinion, such as "I provoked the abusive behavior"; (2) accurate descriptions of injuries and a history of the first, worst, and most recent incident of violence may be included; and (3) with the woman's consent, evidence or photographs (Box 6-3).
- E is for *education*, especially about the cycle of violence, which it is likely to recur and escalate, and about options.
- S is for *safety*, the most significant part of the intervention to ensure that the woman has knowledge of the resources available to her and a plan of action should she stay with the battering partner. First, services and telephone numbers of a hotline and the battered women's shelter or other safe haven should be provided

by the nurse (see Resources at end of chapter). The woman can be offered a telephone to call the shelter if this is an option she chooses. If she chooses to go back to the abuser, a safety plan includes necessities for a quick escape: a bag packed with personal items for an overnight stay (can be hidden or left with a neighbor), money or a checkbook, an extra set of car keys, and any legal documents for identification. Legal options, such as those for restraining orders or arrest of the perpetrator, also are important aspects of the safety plan. A restraining order can be obtained 24 hours a day from the county court or police department. Shelters also can be helpful with assistance in obtaining orders of protection. If the woman chooses not to act in the middle of a violent episode, she may use the hotline or shelter for some counseling when the threat of harm is no longer present (Fishwick, 1998).

If the woman is pregnant, collaboration with maternity nurses who will be involved in her care during the pregnancy may be helpful. Each nurse can plan care that will point out the woman's strengths and increase her self-esteem. The husband or partner may attend prenatal visits and classes and is included in other ways if the woman chooses to stay with him. The first days after birth are particularly crucial because the mother is physically and emotionally vulnerable and usually tired, and the baby's crying may be intolerable to both the father and the mother. The danger of abuse to mother and child is acute during this time. Facilitating the woman's establishment of a support network of maternity and pediatric staff, community health nurses, and shelter and parental crisis center personnel is important during this crucial period (McFarlane et al., 1998). Referral to resources and provision for follow-up examination by health care providers also should be parts of the nursing intervention.

Many nurses become frustrated when a battered woman returns to a previously abusive situation. It is important to remember that many victims have been abused for a long time, which may make it difficult for them to seek and accept help. In addition to understanding the many reasons women stay in abusive relationships, recognizing that the most dangerous period for a battered woman is when she is in the process of leaving (Landenburger, 1998) may help nurses to be less judgmental about the woman's dilemma.

A woman may indicate her readiness to leave the relationship when she believes that she is capable of planning for herself, investing in herself, and recognizing that the abuse is part of a continuing pattern. She also needs to believe that she will have economic and other resources to "make it" on her own. Although shelters provide both, shelter stays are typically limited to 30 to 90 days, and therefore a long-term plan must be in place. Shelter staff assist women with this planning. Women in repeated abusive situations may have lost their ability to perceive the possibility of success and may have become very passive (Fishel & Rynerson, 1998). Nurses can be helpful in directing these women to sources of information, continuing to be expert listeners, and offering encouragement as women struggle in their decision-making process toward freedom and control in their lives.

BOX 6-3 **Documenting Abuse**

Documentation can be useful to women later in court should they choose to press charges or obtain child support, custody, or alimony. Write legibly. Medical records are most helpful if they do the following (Isaac & Enos, 2001):

- Contain photographs of visible injuries if any.
- Put the client's words in quotes, such as client states, "My husband hit me with a . . . ."
- Avoid phrases like *client claims* or *client alleges*, as these imply doubt about the woman's credibility. If the clinician's observations conflict with the woman's statement, the clinician should record the reason for the difference.
- Use medical terms and avoid legal terms such as perpetrator.
- Describe the person who hurt the woman in quotation marks (i.e., "my boyfriend").

Prevention

Nurses can make a difference in stopping the violence and preventing further injury. Educating women that abuse is a violation of their rights and facilitating their access to protective and legal services constitute a first step. Other helpful measures for women to discourage the risk of abusive relationships are promoting assertiveness and self-defense courses; suggesting support and self-help groups that encourage positive self-regard, confidence, and empowerment; and recommending educational and skills-development classes that will enhance independence or at least the ability to take care of oneself (Hadley et al., 1995). Classes for English Language Learning may be particularly helpful to immigrant women. Nurses can offer information on local classes.

Preventive education with children encourages and teaches them androgynous gender roles: both male and female persons are equal; both can be nurturing; and neither needs to dominate the other or to engage in violent behavior to have needs met. Helping children to gain problem-solving and conflict management skills may eliminate the need for violent solutions to life stresses. Encouraging schoolchildren to form and participate in Students Against Violence Everywhere (SAVE) groups, which is a nationwide pro-peace effort that promotes justice, respect, and love, gives them an appreciation for

Plan of Care **Battered Woman**

NURSING DIAGNOSIS Risk for self-directed violence related to history of battering by partner as evidenced by physical injuries

Expected Outcome *Woman will identify factors leading to cycle of violence and develop plan for safety.*

Nursing Interventions/*Rationales*

Provide opportunity to verbalize feelings in a nonthreatening atmosphere *to give emotional support.*

Be alert for cues indicative of battering *to provide database for interventions.*

Provide information on options available to battered women (e.g., shelters, legal assistance) *to provide information in developing a future plan for safety for herself and any children.*

Refer to social services and support groups *to give further information and share experiences.*

NURSING DIAGNOSIS Social isolation related to stigma of battering as evidenced by behaviors of withdrawal

Expected Outcome *Woman will demonstrate an increase in social contacts.*

Nursing Interventions/*Rationales*

Provide private opportunity to express feelings of aloneness *to initiate and maintain a therapeutic relationship.*

Support opportunities for social interaction *to increase feelings of self-worth and self-confidence.*

Encourage interaction with groups for socialization and support *to increase number of social contacts.*

NURSING DIAGNOSIS Ineffective family coping related to situational crisis

Expected Outcome *Family will identify feelings and the need for support during this situational crisis.*

Nursing Interventions/*Rationales*

Provide appropriate time and place for therapeutic communication *to promote trust and allow expression of feelings.*

Identify effective coping mechanisms *to provide the family with a foundation of familiar interventions.*

List support systems available *to assist the family to use outside resources.*

Refer the woman and family to counseling and social services *to provide ongoing support.*

these qualities in all facets of life. Adolescents benefit from discussion about sex roles, their relationships, and the consequences of the "macho" concept. School nurses can be instrumental in developing and implementing informational activities for adolescents (Walton-Moss & Campbell, 2002). Other means of prevention are to advocate against violence in all arenas and to participate actively in promoting legislation and policies toward stopping violent acts.

Evaluation

Evaluation of the care of the abused woman must be based on expected outcomes and must be in harmony with the choices the woman has made (see Plan of Care).

SEXUAL ABUSE

It is estimated that 3% to 27% of women and 2% to 16% of men have experienced childhood sexual abuse (Molnar et al., 2001). **Childhood sexual abuse** is defined as any type of sexual exploitation that involves (1) a child younger than 18 years at the time of the first molestation; (2) at least a 3-year age difference between the victim and perpetrator; and (3) a variety of behaviors between the victim and the perpetrator, which may include disrobing; nudity; masturbation; fondling; digital penetration; and anal, oral, or vaginal penetration (Urbanic, 1993). Childhood sexual abuse acts, according to law, are acts perpetrated by someone responsible for care of the child, such as the parents, boyfriends, stepfathers, grandparents, day-care providers, or babysitters. These childhood sexual abuse acts may include incest, which is any type of sexual exploitation between blood relatives or surrogate relatives before the victim reaches age 18 years. The peak abuse ages are from 7 to 12 years (Hunter, 1991). If a stranger commits sexual abuse, it is considered sexual assault.

Childhood sexual abuse continues over time and gradually escalates. The child is pressured by the adult to cooperate and maintain the relationship. The secrecy is maintained because of the child's domination by the adult, fear of punishment or of not being believed, shame, and rejection (Urbanic, 1993). This continuing victimization and accompanying feeling of helplessness, together with lack of confiding, lead to the long-term behavioral and relationship consequences seen in adult survivors of sexual assault (Molnar et al., 2001). Common psychopathologic consequences are dissociative identity disorder, borderline personality disorder, substance abuse, and generalized anxiety disorder. Although clients with these diagnoses may come to the attention of women's health nurses, women who experience symptoms of PTSD, sexual dysfunction, depression, anxiety, or substance abuse problems are more likely to be seen in obstetric and gynecologic practice. Female sexual abuse and assault victims appear to be the largest single group to experience PTSD (Silva et al., 1997).

Collaborative Care

Clients usually do not resent or object to being asked about their sexual abuse; they feel some relief because of the possibility of being relieved of the psychologic burden (Gallop et al., 1995).

The history obtained from an interview and review of medical records may reveal clues suggestive of sexual abuse. A history of dreams, flashbacks, or terror attacks may indicate PTSD (Silva et al., 1997). Hulme and Grove (1994) identified the most prominent symptoms:

- *Physical:* insomnia, sexual dysfunction, overeating, drug and alcohol abuse, severe headaches, and two or more major surgeries
- *Psychosocial:* depression, guilt, low self-esteem, inability to trust others, mood swings, suicidal thoughts, difficulty in relationships, confusion, extreme anger, and memory lapse

Clients also may exhibit feelings of self-blame, shame, body rejection, anxiety, fear, mistrust, and hatred. They may dislike physical examinations more than do other women.

Overall planning for the adult survivor of childhood sexual abuse must acknowledge that the survivor is able to recognize that the abuse occurred, to share her story, and to begin a healing process. Heritage (1998) stated that disclosing must be done whenever and however the survivor chooses, that it be done with someone she trusts, and that the survivor believes she can disclose without experiencing further alienation. Either verbal or nonverbal shock and horror reactions from the nurse are particularly devastating. Professional demeanor and professional empathy are essential.

Nursing Care

The survivor needs support on many different levels, and a women's health nurse may be the first person to whom she relates her story. Therapeutic communication skills and listening are initial interventions. Interventions may focus on empowering the victim to develop a sense of self-worth, mastery, competence, and control toward a resolution of the incest trauma.

Psychologic support is a necessary intervention when the survivor experiences flashbacks, learns to express feelings of anger without fear of losing control, and expresses needs without guilt. Consistently reinforcing that the adult was the responsible party is important (Urbanic, 1993).

Referral of incest survivors to appropriate support and recovery groups who assist each other in decreasing depression, anger, and guilt; reducing isolation; improving self-esteem; and developing effective coping mechanisms are effective interventions.

Prevention of child sexual abuse is an aspect of care that women's health nurses can consider in their practice. Mothers can be encouraged to teach their children about recognizing impermissible kinds of touching, fending off advances, and reporting abuse to a trusted adult. Safety instruction by parents has been found to increase the likelihood that children will disclose inappropriate treatment (Finkelhor et al., 1995). Adequate programs to assist abusers to recovery are essential in every community (Paradise, 2001).

Nurses must be aware that women who have been sexually abused may be very anxious and uncomfortable about being examined and being touched. Sensitivity, gentleness, patience, and tact are essential.

SEXUAL ASSAULT

Sexual assault is a broad term that encompasses a wide range of sexual victimization including rape and includes unwanted or uncomfortable touches, kisses, hugs, petting, intercourse, or other sexual acts (Kaplan et al., 2001). It consists of sexual contact with or without penetration but with force or physical coercion. **Rape** is an act of violence, is a legal and not a medical term, and, in its strictest sense, is forced sexual intercourse or the penile penetration of the female sex organ or labia without consent; it may or may not include the use of a weapon. **Molestation** consists of noncoital sexual activity between a child and adolescent or adult. **Statutory rape** involves penetration by a person who is 18 years or older of a person under the age of consent, which varies from state to state.

The key feature to establish rape is the absence of consent: threat or coercion implies the lack of consent. The victim who is mentally retarded, who is unconscious or otherwise physically unable to move, who has been drugged without her knowledge, or who is a minor (statutory rape) is not capable of giving consent. The court must prove absence of consent; thus the term alleged rape or alleged sexual assault is used in medical records.

More than 300,000 women are raped each year in the United States (NWHIC, 2002). Adolescents have the highest rates of rape and sexual assault. More than half of all rape victims are females younger than 25, and most perpetrators are acquaintances or a relative (Kaplan et al., 2001). Drugs often are involved in date rapes, and alcohol potentiates the effects. Date rape drugs (i.e., flunitrazepam and gamma-hydroxybutyrate) are often available at bars and clubs (Poirier, 2002). Signs indicating that a woman may have been drugged include no recall after taking a drink, feeling as if sex has occurred but not having any memory of the incident, feeling more intoxicated than a usual response to the amount of alcohol consumed, or feeling fuzzy on awakening (American College of Emergency Physicians [ACEP], 1999).

Elderly women also are victims. Gerophiles often seek employment in nursing homes and may be aggressive male residents or strangers who rape older women. Postassault examinations in this population may be traumatic, difficult, and uncomfortable, and more so if the victim is cognitively impaired or has dementia. This group may be neglected and not identified but are vulnerable (Burgess et al., 2000).

Many factors deter a woman from reporting the crime, so accurate statistics concerning psychosocial and demographic variables relating to rape are not available. It is estimated that one in every six women will be raped during her lifetime (Petter & Whitehill, 1998). Women do not report rape because of the associated stigma; embarrassment;

guilt that in some way they provoked the assault; fear of retribution from the rapist or his friends; dread of being humiliated and figuratively "raped" again by the criminal justice system publicity; and discouragement generated by the dismally small number of convictions. Fewer than one third of all rapes are reported (McConkey et al., 2001). Victims often fear the reactions of husbands, lovers, friends, family, and children and prefer to suffer alone.

The types of rape are reported as date or acquaintance rape, marital rape, gang rape, stranger rape, and psychic rape. *Acquaintance rape* involves persons who know one another, such as a classmate, neighbor, family member, or date; it is sexual assault that occurs when the trust of a relationship is violated, and one person is forced by another into sexual activity (Stuart & Laraia, 2001). Victims of date and acquaintance rape are most often between age 15 and 19 years.

Marital rape occurs partly because some men believe it is their right to engage in sex whenever they desire, regardless of the partner's desire or condition. It frequently occurs when there is physical abuse of the woman. Marital rape is particularly devastating to the woman because she is in a committed relationship and living with the partner (Stuart & Laraia, 2001). Most states now recognize marital rape as a legitimate, reportable crime.

Gang rape occurs when one woman is raped by two or more men. *Stranger rape* describes an unknown attacker actively seeking a woman who is vulnerable. This is the type of rape most feared by women (Aguilera, 1994).

Psychic rape occurs when one's personal dignity and self-respect are assaulted (Stuart & Laraia, 2001). *Sexual harassment*, although not classified as rape, is another form of using power and control tactics to victimize women sexually, particularly in workplaces.

Rape has the highest annual victim costs, much higher than those of other crimes, estimated at $86,464 per woman, including medical and psychologic care; losses in quality of life, productivity, and property damage; and others. To the victims, many of the highest costs are nonmonetary and include fear, pain, and suffering (ACEP, 1999).

Dynamics of Rape

Rape is not an act of lust or overzealous passion. Rape is a violent, aggressive assault on the victim's body and integrity. As one victim said, "No matter how terrible people think rape is, it's worse than they know. It's like a bomb going off at the center of your soul." Sexual assault is the use of power and control tactics and is often motivated by a desire to humiliate, defile, and dominate the victim (Stuart & Laraia, 2001).

The rapist has no regard for his victim's age, race, sexual attraction, or physical condition: 10-day-old infants as well as handicapped elderly women confined to wheelchairs have been sexually assaulted. Most rapes occur intraracially rather than interracially.

Victims of date and acquaintance rape may be less prone to recognize what is happening to them; the dynamics are different from those of stranger rape and may begin rather subtly. The rapist may begin contact by asking personal questions, invading personal space, and proceed to touching that is unwanted and uncomfortable. The woman may not be too alarmed by the perpetrator's actions, believing them to be normal and usual behavior. As she becomes less mindful of the uncomfortable behavior, she may find herself isolated, taken to an apartment, an isolated area in a car, or any place where the two are alone, which is where the forced act of sex frequently occurs.

Rape-Trauma Syndrome

To assess and provide care to a woman who experiences rape, the nurse must first understand the **rape-trauma syndrome.** This syndrome is characterized by extreme anxiety and stress, resulting in emotional and psychologic reactions and often somatic complaints in the woman. Burgess and Holmstrom, in their classic work (1986), defined three phases of the syndrome.

Acute Phase: Disorganization

The assault itself marks the beginning of this phase of rape-trauma syndrome, which can last for several days or up to 3 weeks. Reactions such as shock, denial, and disbelief are similar to those described by Kübler-Ross in the process of grief and dying. In addition, the rape survivor is embarrassed, degraded, fearful, angry, and vengeful, and she usually blames herself. She feels unclean and wants to bathe and douche, although that may destroy evidence. Her affect may change rapidly from crying to being calm and controlled. She relives the scene over and over in her mind and considers things she "should have done." Physiologically she may be uncomfortable, experiencing skeletal muscle pain or tension, gastrointestinal irritability, sighing respirations, hyperventilation, flushing, or a sense of feeling too hot or too cold.

Outward Adjustment Phase

During the adjustment phase, the survivor may appear to have resolved her crisis. She may return to a job or to maintaining a household, or both, but she is denying and suppressing her thoughts and feelings. She needs this time to regain some control in her life. She may move, change jobs, buy a weapon to protect herself, or install an alarm system in her home. She becomes less interested in discussing the rape. She may develop specific or generalized fears that restrict her activities.

Long-Term Process: Reorganization Phase

The third phase is reorganization. Denial and suppression cannot be maintained forever. Disclosing personal thoughts and feelings has a profound effect on improving health and reducing stress. As a rape survivor's suppression of feelings and emotions starts to deteriorate, she becomes depressed and anxious. Her own healthy spirit pressures her to discuss the rape with someone. Because she is losing her control of denial, her fears start to surface; she may be afraid to be alone or in a crowd or may fear being attacked from behind. Nightmares and eating disorders are common in these last two phases.

The recovery process may take years and can be difficult and painful. The victim has progressed through recovery when the physical distress and the constant memories of the rape have diminished. She no longer blames herself for what happened and can truly call herself a survivor.

Similar to the battered woman's syndrome, the rape-trauma syndrome may meet the criteria for PTSD and be formally diagnosed (see Table 6-2).

Collaborative Care

Nurses in women's health care and EDs are most likely to see rape victims in the acute phase. However, all women who manifest any of the signs of other phases should be assessed for posttraumatic experiences.

Facilities that treat rape victims vary in protocols and resources. In its 1992 guidelines, the Joint Commission on Accreditation of Healthcare Organizations (JCAHO) required EDs and ambulatory care departments to have protocols on physical assault; rape or sexual assault; and domestic abuse of elders, spouses, partners, and children. These protocols must address client consent, examination, and treatment guidelines and the health care facility's responsibility for collecting evidence, photographing injuries, and releasing evidence to law enforcement officials. In addition, the EDs and ambulatory care departments must provide to victims a referral list of community-based and private service agencies dealing with family violence. The nurse interacting with the sexual assault client should be guided by the particular treatment center's protocol (Box 6-4).

Many treatment centers have initiated the use of Sexual Assault Nurse Examiners (SANEs). An SANE is educated in the specialty of forensic nursing and is prepared to examine clients; recognize, collect, and preserve evidence; counsel the client; link the client with vital community

BOX *6-4* Adult Sexual Assault Protocol: Emergency Department

PURPOSE

To outline nursing care of sexual assault (rape and/or sexual offense) clients, which includes participation in the collection of forensic evidence and in the referral of clients for follow-up treatment.

Whenever possible, the sexual assault client will be cared for by a SANE (Sexual Assault Nurse Examiner) RN. These nurses have successfully completed a continuing education course in Forensic and Sexual Assault Evidence Collection. This course provides those nurses with the information and skills to care properly for clients after sexual assault by recognizing, collecting, and preserving evidence; interviewing the client; and linking the client to vital community resources for follow-up.

ASSESSMENT

1. Assess the client for any life-threatening injuries.
2. Assess the client's level of coping, coherence, and ability to control behavior.
3. Assess the client's priorities:
   - Is client seeking care for prevention of pregnancy or disease only?
   - Is client seeking forensic evidence collection?
   - Does the client want both?

     NOTE: Notify a SANE nurse to perform the examination if the client is seeking evidence collection for filing of police charges either at this time or in the future.
4. Assess the client's entire body for bruises, lacerations, and/or other skeletal or soft tissue injuries.
5. Initiate the collection of evidence using the sexual assault collection kit if client consents:
   - *If SANE nurse is available:*
     - SANE: Complete collection.
     - SANE: Examine the vagina and rectum to include the speculum examination.

       NOTE: A toluidine blue dye and colposcope may be used to collect evidence.
     - Physician performs the bimanual examination.
   - *If SANE nurse is not available:*
     - Primary nurse initiates collection with the exception of vaginal, rectal, and bimanual examinations.
     - Physician performs vaginal, rectal, and bimanual examinations.
6. Ask client whether or not those who are with the client know that the client has been sexually assaulted.

   NOTE: This information cannot be given to secondary victims without the client's permission.

SAFETY

7. Notify hospital police when a sexual assault client enters the emergency department.

   NOTE: Hospital police will complete a risk assessment of client safety.

CARE

8. Provide care for any physical injuries.
9. Provide for client privacy and nonjudgmental support.

Continued

BOX 6-4 Adult Sexual Assault Protocol: Emergency Department—cont'd

10. Protect client confidentiality by identifying the client as "7273" rather than by name or chief complaint.
11. Assign one nurse to the client for the duration of his or her stay and disposition of evidence collection.
12. Notify the sexual assault advocate office.
    NOTE: The client has the right to refuse an advocate. It is the policy of the emergency department to allow the advocate to offer services directly to the client unless the client expressly forbids it. Notify the advocate of any secondary victims who may have accompanied the client if the secondary victim is aware that the client has been sexually assaulted.
13. Reassure the client that he or she is safe.
14. Reassure the client that the incident is not his or her fault.
15. Prepare the client for the possibility that some questions asked may be embarrassing.
16. Obtain informed consent for the physical examination, to include photographs of injuries.
    NOTE: If the client permits the release of information to law enforcement agencies, explain to the victim that the evidence will be turned over to the appropriate jurisdiction for processing. If the client is unwilling to have law enforcement notified at this time, the client should mark "do not" on the release form. The client may later change this if he or she chooses to file charges or have law enforcement involved.
17. Collect the evidence as directed and in accordance with client consent.
    NOTE: All evidence should be marked with the client's identification. Any photographs taken should be labeled with the client's information and described in the nursing notes. These photographs should then be sealed in an envelope and secured per Department of Emergency Medicine policy. The evidence *must* remain in the possession of *one nurse* throughout the entire assessment procedure and treatment period, until it is released to a police agency.
18. Perform a urine test for pregnancy; the urine can also be tested for drugs if the client suspects that he or she was drugged.
19. Provide the opportunity for bathing and clean clothing after the examination.
20. Discuss and provide emergency contraception and prophylaxis against STIs, including HIV if desired.
21. Arrange for follow-up care per client preference for any medical and/or psychologic problems and/or injury.

CLIENT/SIGNIFICANT OTHER (SO) TEACHING

22. Explain to the client/SO:
    - All procedures and rationale
    - That feelings of anger, anxiety, and fear are normal
    - That options for medical, legal, and emotional counseling are available to both primary and secondary victims

      NOTE: Do not assume that a friend or SO is aware of the assault (see #6).
23. Inform client/SO of resources available:
    - Judicial system options (e.g., official police report, "blind" report)
    - Financial assistance
    - Other available resources:
        - Local rape crisis center
        - Mental health agency
        - Sites and phone numbers for HIV counseling and testing
        - Resource list of phone numbers (e.g., law enforcement)

DOCUMENTATION

24. Complete the forms for sexual assault evidence collection.
25. Attach forms to appropriate documents.
26. Seal the evidence kit as directed, and deliver it to a sworn law enforcement officer.
27. Seal all photographs in an envelope marked with client identification, and secure per Department of Emergency Medicine policy.
28. Document care rendered, teaching done, and client response and level of understanding on emergency department nursing record.

resources; follow up cases; and, if necessary, testify in court (Stermac & Stirpe, 2002). If SANE is not available in a particular facility, JCAHO member organizations must implement a plan for educating an appropriate staff member about identifying, treating, and referring abuse victims. Additional resources may include a social worker who is called when a woman who has been raped is admitted. A local rape crisis center may have volunteers on call who may help by providing emotional support; providing transportation; helping the woman interact with her family, friends, and various authorities; informing her of rape-trauma syndrome; and finding other resources for her as needed. Male volunteers may counsel male members of the victim's family and her male friends.

History

History taking is an important first step in care, and the client should be informed of all the steps involved in the rape examination and follow-up examination. Because rape is a crime, the first nurse to see the sexually assaulted client must consider the need to preserve evidence (see Legal Tip). However, the preservation of evidence should not overshadow a survivor's rights: to be treated as a human being with respect, courtesy, and dignity.

LEGAL TIP Collector of Evidence

Consent forms must be signed before evidence can be collected and released to the police and before photographs can be taken. If the victim is under 16 years of age, a pediatrician is notified. A parent or guardian is required to sign the consent forms. A children's protective service may need to be called to facilitate consent.

History includes a statement of the traumatic event. Box 6-5 lists information to be collected. The woman needs privacy but should not be left alone. She also needs assurance of confidentiality and may need a great deal of support and assistance in verbalizing the offender's acts. For example, giving the woman permission to describe the situation however she chooses and restating what the client has said (without minimizing) will show empathy. It is important to tell the woman that she is safe, that the incident is not her fault, and that she is not alone in what she has experienced. It also is important to obtain sexual, gynecologic, and obstetric histories (Petter & Whitehill, 1998) (see Chapter 5). Because determination of rape is made in court, the wording of the history should reflect the woman's report, and her exact words should be used as often as possible (Poirier, 2002).

BOX 6-5 Sexual Assault History Taking and Assessment

- Assess the client for life-threatening injuries.
- Assess the client's level of coping, coherency, and ability to control behavior.
- Assess the client's priorities:
  - Is the client seeking care for prevention of disease or pregnancy only?
  - Is the client seeking forensic evidence collection?
  - Does the client want both?
- Ask client to describe the event:
  - Time and place of the event.
  - Relationship to the assailant, if any.
  - Nature of suspected physical and sexual acts.
  - Time lapse between assault and current examination.
- Did the woman bathe, douche, or shower? Did she urinate or defecate?
- Ask client whether those who are with the client know that the client has been sexually assaulted.
- Ask the client if she can think of any other information that would help in her care, and inform her that it is safe and confidential to say whatever she needs to.
- Inspect the entire body for bruises, lacerations, and other injuries.
- Initiate collection of evidence using the sexual assault collection kit (or notify the Sexual Assault Nurse Examiner)

Physical Examination and Laboratory Tests

The nurse may assist with or, if trained, may perform the physical examination, which is conducted after the procedure is explained to the woman and consent is obtained. Preservation of the woman's dignity is of utmost importance during the examination. She remains clothed while her vital signs and blood pressure are determined, and her clothing is inspected for stains, tears, and foreign material. Clothing is handled only by the woman and may be collected and sealed in a bag to be checked for evidence. She is assisted to undress and is draped for the physical examination. A female attendant, rape counselor, or other person of her choice may remain with her during the examination. The physician or nurse practitioner informs her of every step of the procedure. Her body is inspected for bruises, swelling, scratches, lacerations, stab wounds, and body lice. A head-to-toe examination is performed. Many victims have injuries to other parts of their body, mostly involving head, face, and neck (Poirier, 2002). Special attention is given to the area assaulted, that is, pelvic structures and genitalia. External genitals, thighs, buttocks, and lower abdomen are assessed, and if there are injuries, photographs may be taken or drawings made. Pubic and scalp hair is combed for collection. Perianal, oral, and vaginal swabs are collected. If the victim scratched her attacker, her nails are scraped to obtain material that may aid in identification. Necessary equipment for the examination is usually packaged in standard rape kits, which should be available in most EDs.

A speculum examination is performed gently to detect tears or bruises and to collect appropriate specimens. Most victims have some type of genital injury, even if it is asymptomatic. The cervix is cultured for *Neisseria gonorrhoeae, Chlamydia* organisms, and herpes simplex virus, and vaginal fluid is aspirated for analysis. One slide is fixed and dried to be stained and examined for sperm. Fluid is evaluated for seminal contents, including acid phosphatase (an enzyme found in high concentrations in seminal fluid), p30 protein (specific to the prostate and indicates ejaculation), and seminal vesicle specific antigen and ABO antigens (McGregor et al., 2002). Cultures for gonorrhea and chlamydia may be obtained from any other sites of penetration or contact such as vagina, anus, and pharynx. Standard wet-mount slides and cultures also may be obtained to test for trichomoniasis. Colposcopy may be used to visualize small abrasions. Some care providers use a handheld magnifying glass. A bimanual pelvic examination is performed carefully to determine the size and position of the uterus and adnexa. If a pelvic mass is palpated, it may be caused by bleeding into the broad ligament. Internal pelvic assessment ends with a rectovaginal examination if the woman has given consent, and it is deemed necessary.

Sexual assault kits that are intended to facilitate collection of specimens, particularly if they are to be used as evidence should the woman decide to report the rape, give specific instructions on what specimens to collect from what body parts or articles of clothing and ways to preserve the evidence.

Laboratory tests may include a urine or serum pregnancy test and serum tests for syphilis, hepatitis B virus, and human immunodeficiency virus (CDC, 2002).

During the examination, the woman's emotional status is assessed, and findings are recorded: what reactions she exhibits to the assault; her orientation to time and place; and her attention span, affect, and verbal description and feelings about the assault. The availability of family or peer-support systems is assessed. She is asked about her plans to report or not to report the crime to the police.

After the physical examination, the woman should be allowed to shower and offered fresh clothes or a gown. She may be offered time to rest and to talk with the nurse, rape crisis counselor, family, or friends.

Nursing diagnoses for the rape victim during the immediate and later posttrauma periods include the following:

Immediate posttrauma period

- *Anxiety/fear related to*
  - –rape-trauma experience
  - –interactions with police and caregivers
  - –physical examination to assess injury and collect evidence
- *Acute pain related to*
  - –physical injury from rape
  - –examination
- *Disturbed body image related to*
  - –the rape
- *Rape-trauma syndrome related to*
  - –aftermath of being sexually assaulted
  - –feelings of being unclean and humiliation
  - –silent reaction of being unable to discuss the rape
- *Decisional conflict related to*
  - –discussing rape with family
  - –possible pregnancy

Later posttrauma period

- *Risk for infection with sexually transmitted infections related to*
  - –sexual assault by an assailant of unknown sexual history
- *Impaired social interaction related to*
  - –the rape

Immediate Care

Medical management includes (1) treating the physical injuries, including tetanus toxoid booster if indicated; (2) providing prophylactic antibiotic therapy for STIs (e.g., gonorrhea, syphilis); and (3) providing prophylaxis for pregnancy if the woman is not pregnant. If physical trauma is life threatening, appropriate intervention takes precedence over collecting evidence.

If the victim is at risk for pregnancy, emergency contraception should be discussed with her. Approximately 5% of women who are raped become pregnant (Holmes et al., 1996). Emergency contraception with progestin only or combined estrogen and progestin pills must be used within 72 hours of the sexual assault (American College of Obstetricians & Gynecologists, 2001) (see Table 9-2). The woman is told that the therapy might cause nausea and that she should expect withdrawal bleeding shortly after finishing the therapy. Antinausea therapy, such as prochlorperazine preparation (Compazine) or dimenhydrinate (Dramamine), may be prescribed to counter the side effects of estrogens. She is advised, before she takes the drug, about the possible teratogenic effects of estrogen in emergency contraception doses, if a pregnancy occurs. She should be advised that emergency contraception does not guarantee pregnancy prevention, and that she should repeat the pregnancy test if she has not had a menstrual period within 3 to 4 weeks. The woman is apprised of the availability of abortion or menstrual extraction as a backup measure. If the woman is pregnant at the time of the assault, she should be observed for several hours for uterine contractility.

The woman may be provided with prophylactic antibiotic therapy to prevent STIs, hepatitis B immunization if needed, and human immunodeficiency virus (HIV) prophylaxis (CDC, 2002).

Discharge

The woman is discharged with medications and printed instructions about their use, printed instructions for self-care, and names and telephone numbers of resource people if she requires assistance. Money as needed and transportation to wherever she is staying (an alternative place may be found for her) add to the woman's comfort and perception of being in control. A medical follow-up examination in the gynecology or pediatric clinic is scheduled in 1 to 2 weeks for repeated cultures for gonorrhea and other STIs; at 6 weeks for assessment of healing injuries; and at 6, 12, and 24 weeks for repeated serology tests for syphilis and HIV infection if initial test results were negative. The woman and her counselor determine whether there is a need for an additional medical or psychologic follow-up examination between the scheduled visits. The woman has a choice of site for follow-up testing. Some women choose to continue with the health care provider who first performed the examination; others prefer their primary health care provider; and still others need referral to a clinic in the area (city, state) in which they live.

Nurses must be aware that responses to rape are variable. Self-blame and humiliation may alternate with anger and fear. The patient needs to be reassured again before she leaves that her feelings are normal and that she is not alone. The initial care of a woman will affect her recovery and her decision to return for follow-up care. Nurses can assist clients through an examination that is as nontraumatic as possible, with kindness, skill, and empathy.

After Discharge

Because of the phases of recovery, telephone contact by the health care provider to whom the woman is referred is continued until the woman has no further need for such help. Education in prevention strategies is often offered by community agencies or rape-awareness groups (see Resources at end of chapter). The focus of the classes is usually on increasing women's awareness of situations that put them at high risk for rape or sexual assault. Other courses may teach self-defense methods or how to change personal behaviors to reduce the risk of being victimized, such as avoiding being alone in isolated places and being alert to unusual activities or persons in one's environment. Still other courses may focus on changing societal attitudes about rape. Nurses can play a role in preventive education by offering courses or participating in courses offered by community or health care groups. Nurses must be knowledgeable about the epidemiology of sexual assault, reporting requirements, services available in their community for victims, and should screen all women for a history of assault and any sequelae.

KEY POINTS

- Violence against women is a major social and health care problem in the United States, costing thousands of lives and billions of dollars in direct and indirect health care costs.
- Domestic violence includes physical, sexual, emotional, psychologic, and economic abuse.
- Nurses must increase awareness of their own beliefs and values regarding victimization of women to provide effective care.
- Theoretic frameworks—psychologic, sociologic, biologic, and feminist perspectives—provide the foundation for understanding the complexity of victimization of women.
- Cultural influences regarding violent behaviors and relationships sensitize the nurse to the special needs of women from various ethnic groups.
- Battering affects young, middle-aged, and older women of all races; all socioeconomic, educational, and religious groups; and pregnant women.
- All states have mandatory reporting of abuse of children and elderly people; some states have initiated mandatory reporting of wife abuse. Mandatory reporting may be helpful to some women who just are not comfortable making the call, whereas other women would prefer to have control over their own reporting choices.
- Rape is a legal term meaning a violent, aggressive sexual assault against one's will.
- Nurses in all professional areas should respond with sensitivity and caring to women who experience abuse and victimization.
- Women who have been physically or sexually assaulted as children or adults may find physical examinations difficult and anxiety producing and may have physical and emotional consequences resulting in poor health.

CRITICAL THINKING EXERCISES

1. An adolescent client, Terri, when screened for abuse, states that her partner is very caring and handsome, but he is very jealous and occasionally gets "tough." With some gentle probing, the nurse determines that extensive control and emotional abuse are occurring in the relationship. What would the nurse do with this information in relation to (1) the adolescent and (2) her mother, in the waiting room?
2. Ingrid, an admitted sex worker, is seen after a sexual assault but refuses to report the crime. She has no identification papers and speaks very little English. Describe the nurse's legal accountability and respect for the rights of a rape victim who chooses not to pursue legal action. Describe how the nurse would resolve the conflict.
3. Design a poster and brochure about victimization, for Muslim or Native American women, to be distributed at a women's health fair in your community.
4. Franki, a fellow nursing student, is occasionally late for class, sometimes unprepared, and often bruised and distracted. She states that the bruises are from the kids and the dog. She gets frequent calls from her husband and seems upset after talking to him. Describe how you would approach her with your concerns.

RESOURCES

Association of Women's Health, Obstetric, and Neonatal Nurses
2000 L St. NW
Washington, DC 20024
800-673-8499
Website offers an on-line continuing education program on domestic violence and a presentation for teaching.
www.awhonn.org

Center for Women Policy Studies
2000 P St. NW, Suite 508
Washington, DC 20036
202-872-1770
Publications and current federal legislation information.

Family Violence Prevention Fund
383 Rhode Island St., Suite 304
San Francisco, CA 94103-5133
415-252-8900
Resource for statistics, resources, and legal information.
www.fvpf.org; www.endabuse.org

The National Center on Women and Family Law
799 Broadway, Room 402
New York, NY 10003
212-674-8200
Provides legal information.

National Child Abuse Hotline
800-422-4453

National Coalition Against Domestic Violence
P.O. Box 34103
Washington, DC 20043-4301
202-638-8638
Site offers information and referrals.
www.ncadv.org

National Coalition Against Sexual Assault
912 North 2nd St.
Harrisburg, PA 17102
717-232-6771

National Domestic Violence/Abuse Hotline
800-799-SAFE
Many states have local coalitions against domestic violence.

National Organization for Women (NOW) Legal Defense and Education Fund
99 Hudson St.
New York, NY 10013-2871
212-925-6635

National Resource Center for Domestic Violence
800-537-2238

National Women's Health Information Center
The Office on Women's Health
Department of Health and Human Resources
800-994-9662
www.4woman.gov

No Safe Place
Companion website to PBS documentary offers articles, interviews, and study guides.
www.pbs.org/kued/nosafeplace

Rape Abuse and Incest National Network
Offers statistics, information, and a 24-hour hotline for referrals.
www.rainn.org

Violence against Women Office at the Department of Justice
810 Seventh St. NW
Washington, DC 20531
Department of Justice offers legal information and resources.
www.ojp.usdoj.gov/vawo

REFERENCES

Aguilera, D. (1994). *Crisis intervention: Theory and methodology* (7th ed.). St. Louis: Mosby.

American College of Emergency Physicians (ACEP). (1999). *Evaluation and management of the sexually assaulted or sexually abused patient.* Dallas: ACEP.

American College of Obstetricians and Gynecologists. (2001). *Emergency contraception. ACOG Practice Bulletin No. 25.* Washington, DC: ACOG.

American College of Obstetricians and Gynecologists. (2002). *Screening tools for domestic violence.* ACOG violence against women home page. http://www.acog.org. Retrieved 8/16/02.

American Psychiatric Association. (2000). *Diagnostic and statistical manual of mental disorders* (4th ed., rev.). Washington, DC: American Psychiatric Association.

Berlinger, J. (1998). Answers to questions about domestic violence: "Why don't you just leave him?" *Nursing, 28*(4), 34-39.

Burgess, A., Dowdell, E., & Brown, K. (2000). The elderly rape victim: stereotypes, perpetrators and implications for practice. *Journal of Emergency Nursing, 26*(5), 516-518.

Burgess, A., & Holmstrom, L. (1986). *Rape, crisis, and recovery.* West Newton, MA: Awab.

Campbell, D. et al. (2002). Intimate partner violence in African American women. *Online Journal of Issues in Nursing, 7*(1), 5.

Campbell, J., & Fishwick, N. (1993). Abuse of female partners. In J. Campbell & J. Humphreys (Eds.), *Nursing care of survivors of family violence.* St. Louis: Mosby.

Campbell, J. et al. (2002). Intimate partner violence and physical health consequences. *Archives of Internal Medicine, 162*(10), 1157-1163.

Campbell, J., & Parker, B. (1999). Clinical nursing research on battered women and their children: A review. In A. Hinshaw, S. Feetham, & J. Shaver (Eds.), *Handbook of clinical nursing research.* Thousand Oaks, CA: Sage.

Campbell, J., & Soeken, K. (1999). Forced sex and intimate partner violence: Effects on women's risk and women's health. *Journal of Interpersonal Violence, 5*, 1017-1035.

Centers for Disease Control. (2002). Sexually transmitted diseases treatment guidelines–2002. *MMWR, 51*(RR06), 1-80.

Coker, A. et al. (2000). Physical health consequences of physical and psychological intimate partner violence. *Archives of Family Medicine, 9*, 451-457.

Counts, D., Brown, J., & Campbell, J. (Eds.). (1999). *To have and to hit: Cultural perspectives on wife beating.* Urbana: University of Illinois Press.

Curry, M. (1998). The interrelationships between abuse, substance use, and psychosocial stress during pregnancy. *Journal of Obstetric, Gynecologic, and Neonatal Nursing, 27*(6), 692-699.

Else, L. et al. (1993). Personality characteristics of men who physically abuse women. *Hospital Commission on Psychiatry, 44*(1), 54-58.

Family Violence Prevention Fund (FVPF). (2002). *Preventing domestic violence: Clinical guidelines on routine screening.* San Francisco: FVPF. http://action.endabuse.org/fvpf/home/. Retrieved 6/01/02.

Finkelhor, D., Asdigian, N., & Dziuba-Leatherman, J. (1995). The effectiveness of victimization prevention instruction: An evaluation of children's responses to actual threats and assaults. *Child Abuse and Neglect, 19*, 141-153.

Fishel, A., & Rynerson, B. (1998). Domestic violence and family interdependence. *Aggression and Violent Behavior, 3*(3), 295-301.

Fisher, I. (2002). Doubt cast on charges that led to Pakistan rape. *New York Times,* July 12, 2002, Section A, p 8.

Fishwick, N. (1995). Getting to the heart of the matter: Nursing assessment and intervention with battered women in psychiatric mental health settings. *Journal of the American Psychiatric Nurses Association, 1*(2), 48.

Fishwick, N. (1998). Assessment of women for partner abuse. *Journal of Obstetric, Gynecologic, and Neonatal Nursing, 27*(6), 661-670.

Gallop, R. et al. (1995). The impact of childhood sexual abuse on the psychological well-being and practice of nurses. *Archives of Psychiatric Nursing, 9*(3), 137-145.

Garza-Trevino, E. (1994). Neurobiological factors in aggressive behavior. *Hospital Commission on Psychiatry, 45*(7), 690-699.

Gelles, R. (1997). *Intimate violence in families* (3rd ed.). Thousand Oaks, CA: Sage.

Gelles, R. (1995). *Contemporary families: A sociological view.* Thousand Oaks, CA: Sage.

Gunderson, L. (2002). Intimate partner violence: The need for primary prevention in the community. *Annals of Internal Medicine, 136*(8), 637-640.

Hadley, S. et al. (1995). Womankind: An innovative model of health care response to domestic abuse. *Women's Health Issues, 5*(4), 189-198.

Hanrahan, P., Campbell, J., & Ulrich, Y. (1993). Theories of violence. In J. Campbell & J. Humphreys (Eds.), *Nursing care of survivors of family violence.* St. Louis: Mosby.

Harper-Jacques, S., & Reimer, M. (1992). Aggressive behavior and the brain: A different perspective for the mental health nurse. *Archives of Psychiatric Nursing, 6*(5), 312-320.

Harrykissoon, S., Rickert, V., & Wiemann, C. (2002). Prevalence and patterns of intimate partner violence among adolescent mothers during the postpartum period. *Archives of Pediatric and Adolescent Medicine, 156*(4), 325-330.

Heritage, C. (1998). Working with childhood sexual abuse survivors during pregnancy, labor, and birth. *Journal of Obstetric, Gynecologic, and Neonatal Nursing, 27*(6), 671-676.

Holmes, M. et al. (1996). Rape-related treatment: Estimates and descriptive characteristics from a national sample of women. *American Journal of Obstetrics and Gynecology, 175*, 320-325.

Holtz, H., & Furniss, K. (1993). The health care provider's role in domestic violence. *Trends in Health Care Law and Ethics, 8*(2), 47-53.

Hulme, P., & Grove, S. (1994). Symptoms of female survivors of child sexual abuse. *Issues in Mental Health Nursing, 15*, 519-532.

Humphreys, J., Parker, B., & Campbell, J. (2001). Intimate partner violence against women. *Annual Review of Nursing Research, 19*, 275-306.

Hunter, J. (1991). A comparison of the psychological maladjustment of adult males and females sexually molested as children. *Journal of Interpersonal Violence, 6*(2), 205.

Isaac, N., & Enos, V. (2001). *Documenting domestic violence: How health care providers can help victims.* National Institute of Justice. http://www.ncjrs.org/txtfiles1/nij/188564.txt. Retrieved 5/14/02.

Kaplan, D. et al. (2001). Care of the adolescent sexual assault victim. *Pediatrics, 107*(6), 1476-1479.

Krulewich, C. et al. (2001). Hidden from view: Violent deaths among pregnant women in the District of Columbia, 1988-1996. *Journal of Nurse Midwifery and Women's Health, 46*(1), 4-9.

Landenberger, K. (1998). The dynamics of leaving and recovering from an abusive relationship. *Journal of Obstetric, Gynecologic, and Neonatal Nursing, 27*(6), 700-706.

Leserman, J., Stewart, J., & Dell, D. (1999). Sexual and physical abuse predicts poor health in pregnancy and postpartum. *Psychosomatic Medicine, 61*, 92.

Lindgren, K. (2001). Relationships among maternal fetal attachment, prenatal depression and health practices in pregnancy. *Research in Nursing & Health, 24*, 203-217.

Martin, S. et al. (2001). Physical abuse of women before, during, and after pregnancy. *Journal of the American Medical Association, 285*(12), 1581-1584.

McConkey, T., Sole, M., & Holcomb, L. (2001). Assessing the female sexual assault survivor. *Nurse Practitioner, 26*(7), 8-39.

McFarlane, J. et al. (2002). Abuse during pregnancy and femicide: Urgent implications for women's health. *Obstetrics and Gynecology, 100*(1), 27-35.

McFarlane, J. et al. (1999). Severity of abuse before and during pregnancy for African-American, Hispanic, and Anglo women. *Journal of Nurse Midwifery, 44*(2), 139-144.

McFarlane, J. et al. (1998). Safety behaviors of abused women after an intervention during pregnancy. *Journal of Obstetric, Gynecologic, and Neonatal Nursing, 27*(1), 64-69.

McGregor, M., Mont, J., & Myhr, T. (2002). Sexual assault forensic medical examination: Is evidence related to successful prosecution? *Annals of Emergency Medicine, 39*(6), 639-647.

Molnar, B., Buka, S., & Kessler, R. (2001). Child sexual abuse and subsequent psychopathology: Results from the national comorbidity survey. *American Journal of Public Health, 91*(5), 753-760.

National Institute on Alcohol Abuse and Alcoholism. (1997). Alcohol violence and aggression. *Alcohol Alert,* 38, 1-6.

National Women's Health Information Center. (2002). *Violence against women.* http://www.4woman.gov/violence/index.cfm. Retrieved 8/14/02.

O'Leary, D. (1993). Through a psychological lens: Personality traits, personality disorders, and levels of violence. In R. Gelles & D. Loseke (Eds.), *Current controversies on family violence.* Newbury Park, CA: Sage.

Paradise, J. (2001). Current concepts in preventing sexual abuse. *Current Opinion in Pediatrics, 13*(5), 402-407.

Petter, L., & Whitehill, D. (1998). Management of female sexual assault. *American Family Physician, 58*(4), 920-926, 929-930.

Phillips, D. (1998). Culture and systems of oppression in abused women's lives. *Journal of Obstetrics, Gynecology, and Neonatal Nursing, 27*(6), 678-683.

Poirier, M. (2002). Care of the female adolescent rape victim. *Pediatric Emergency Care, 18*(1), 53-59.

Renker, P. (2002). "Keep a blank face. I need to tell you what has been happening to me." Teens stories of abuse and violence before and during pregnancy. *MCN American Journal of Maternal and Child Nursing, 27*(2), 109-116.

Renzetti, C., Edleson, J., & Bergen, R. (2001). *The sourcebook on violence against women.* Thousand Oaks, CA: Sage.

Ryan, J., & King, M. (1998). Scanning for violence. *AWHONN Lifelines, 2*(3), 36-41.

Rynerson, B., & Fishel, A. (1993). Domestic violence prevention training: Participant characteristics and treatment outcomes. *Journal of Family Violence, 8*(3), 253-266.

Silva, C. et al. (1997). Symptoms of posttraumatic stress disorder in abused women in a primary care setting. *Journal of Women's Health, 6*(5), 543-552.

Soler, H., Vinayak, P., & Quadagno, D. (2000). Biosocial aspects of domestic violence. *Psychoneuroendocrinology, 25*(7), 721-739.

Stermac, L., & Stirpe, T. (2002). Efficacy of a 2-year-old sexual assault nurse examiner program in a Canadian hospital. *Journal of Emergency Nursing, 28*(1), 18-23.

Stuart G., & Laraia, M. (2001). *Principles and practice of psychiatric nursing* (7th ed.). St. Louis: Mosby.

Tjaden, P., & Thoennes, N. (2000). *Extent, nature and consequences of intimate partner violence: Findings from the national violence against women survey.* Washington, DC: U.S. Department of Justice.

Torres, S. (1993). Nursing care of low-income battered Hispanic pregnant women. *AWHONN Clinical Issues in Perinatal Women's Health Nursing, 4*(3), 416-423.

Urbanic, J. (1993). Intrafamilial sexual abuse. In J. Campbell & J. Humphreys (Eds.). *Nursing care of survivors of family violence.* St. Louis: Mosby.

U.S. Department of Health and Human Services (USDHHS). (2000). *Healthy people 2010: National health promotion and disease prevention objectives.* Washington, DC: USDHHS.

Walker, L. (1979). *The battered woman.* New York: Harper & Row.

Walker, L. (1984). *The battered woman syndrome* (vol. 6). New York: Springer.

Walton-Moss, B., & Campbell, J. (2002). Intimate partner violence: Implications for nursing. *Online Journal of Issues in Nursing, 7*(1), 6.

Warren, J., & Lanning, W. (1992). Sex role beliefs, control, and social isolation of battered women. *Journal of Family Violence, 7*(1), 1.

Campbell:

① Can you still get waxed when preg. or before deliv?

② Biofeedback

③ p. 158

CHAPTER 7

Catherine Ingram Fogel

Reproductive System Concerns

http://evolve.elsevier.com/Lowdermilk/MatWmnHlth/

LEARNING OBJECTIVES

- Differentiate signs and symptoms of common menstrual disorders.
- Develop a nursing plan of care for the woman with primary dysmenorrhea.
- Outline client teaching about premenstrual syndrome (PMS).
- Relate the pathophysiology of endometriosis to associated symptoms.
- Identify the health risks of perimenopausal women.
- Develop an assessment guide for perimenopausal women.
- Develop a nursing plan of care for the postmenopausal woman.
- Examine the risks and benefits of menopausal hormone therapy.
- Summarize client teaching strategies for prevention of osteoporosis.
- Evaluate the use of alternative therapies for menstrual disorders and menopausal symptoms.

Problems may occur at any point in the menstrual cycle. In addition, many factors, including anatomic abnormalities, physiologic imbalances, and lifestyle, can affect the menstrual cycle. Many women seek out nurses as advisors, counselors, and health care providers for information about menstrual cycle experiences, concerns, or disorders. If they are to meet their clients' needs, nurses must have accurate, up-to-date information. This chapter provides information on menstrual cycle experiences, including menarche and menopause, common menstrual disorders, and problems associated with menopause.

Knowledge of the normal parameters of menstruation is essential to the assessment of menstrual cycle experiences and disorders. The menstrual cycle is a result of a complex interplay among the reproductive, neurologic, and endocrine systems (Blackburn, 2003). The hypothalamus produces gonadotropin-releasing hormone (GnRH), which stimulates the pituitary gland to produce follicle-stimulating hormone (FSH) and luteinizing hormone (LH). In turn, FSH and LH stimulate the ovaries to produce first estrogen and then progesterone. In response to the hormones, the endometrium, or lining of the uterus, proliferates and then sheds. Chapter 5 provides additional information on the menstrual cycle and endocrine physiology.

Normal menstrual patterns are averages based on observations and reports from large groups of healthy women. When counseling an individual woman, remember that these values are averages only. Generally a woman's menstrual frequency stabilizes at 28 days within 1 to 2 years after puberty, with a range from 26 to 34 days (Blackburn, 2003). Although no woman's cycle is exactly the same length every month, the typical month-to-month variation in an individual's cycle is usually plus or minus 2 days. However, greater but still normal variations are noted frequently.

During her reproductive years, a woman may have more than one physiologic variation in her menstrual cycle. An understanding of the physiologic variations that occur in several age groups is essential knowledge for nurses. Menstrual cycle length is most irregular at the extremes of the reproductive years including the 2 years after menarche and the 5 years before menopause, when anovulatory cycles are most common. Irregular bleeding, both in length of cycle and amount, is the rule, rather than the exception, in early adolescence. It takes approximately 15 months for completion of the first 10 cycles and an average of 20 cycles before ovulation occurs regularly. Cycle lengths of 15 to 45 days are not unusual, and during the first 2 years after menarche, intervals of 3 to 6 months between menses can be normal.

Women's knowledge and understanding of the menstrual cycle may be limited and is often influenced by myths and misunderstandings. Women typically have menstrual cycles for about 40 years. Once the irregular nature of menses in the first 1 to 2 years after menarche subsides and a cyclic, predictable pattern of monthly bleeding is established, women may worry about any deviation from that pattern, or from what they have been told is normal for all menstruating women. A woman may be concerned about her ability to conceive and bear children or believe that she is not really a woman without monthly evidence. A symptom such as amenorrhea or excess menstrual bleeding can be a source of severe distress and concern for women. Sexual issues often are expressed and must be examined.

COMMON MENSTRUAL DISORDERS

Amenorrhea

Amenorrhea, the absence of menstrual flow, is a clinical symptom of a variety of disorders. Although these criteria for a clinical problem of amenorrhea are not universal, these circumstances should generally be evaluated: (1) the absence of both menarche and secondary sexual characteristics by age 14 years; (2) absence of menses by age 16 years, regardless of presence of normal growth and development (primary amenorrhea); or (3) a 3- to 6-month absence of menses after a period of menstruation (secondary amenorrhea) (Fogel, 1997; Harlow, 2000).

Although amenorrhea is not a disease, it is often the sign of one. Amenorrhea is most commonly a result of pregnancy. It may occur from any defect or interruption in the hypothalamic-pituitary-ovarian-uterine axis. It also may result from anatomic abnormalities, other endocrine disorders such as hypothyroidism or hyperthyroidism, chronic diseases such as type 1 diabetes, medications such as phenytoin (Dilantin), eating disorders, strenuous exercise, emotional stress, or oral contraceptive use.

Assessment of amenorrhea begins with a thorough history and physical examination. An important initial step, often overlooked, is to be sure that the woman is not pregnant. Specific components of the assessment process depend on a client's age–adolescent, young adult, or perimenopausal–and whether she has previously menstruated.

Hypogonadotropic Amenorrhea

Hypogonadotropic amenorrhea reflects a problem in the central hypothalamic-pituitary axis. In rare instances, a pituitary lesion or genetic inability to produce FSH and LH is at fault. Once pregnancy has been ruled out by a β-human chorionic gonadotropin (hCG) pregnancy test, diagnostic tests may include FSH level, thyroid-stimulating hormone (TSH) and prolactin levels, radiographic or computed tomography scan of the sella turcica, and a progestational challenge (Hall, 2002).

Hypogonadotropic amenorrhea often results from hypothalamic suppression as a result of stress (in the home, school, or workplace) or a sudden and severe weight loss, eating disorders, strenuous exercise, or mental illness (Parent-Stevens & Burns, 2000). Research on the interaction between nervous system or neurotransmitter functions and hormonal regulation throughout the body has demonstrated a biologic basis for the relation of stress to physiologic processes. Women who are more than 20% underweight for height or who have had rapid weight loss may report amenorrhea, as may women with eating disorders such as anorexia nervosa (Alexander, Shimp, & Smith, 2000; Parent-Stevens & Burns, 2000). Amenorrhea is one of the classic signs of anorexia nervosa, and the interrelatedness of disordered eating, amenorrhea, and premature osteoporosis has been described as the female athlete triad (Kleposki, 2002; Sabatini, 2001). A loss of calcium from the bone, comparable to that seen in postmenopausal women, may occur with this type of amenorrhea.

Exercise-associated amenorrhea can occur in women undergoing vigorous physical and athletic training (Sanborn, Horea, Siemers, & Dieringer, 2000) and is thought to be associated with many factors, including body composition (height, weight, and percentage of body fat); type, intensity, and frequency of exercise; nutritional status; and presence of emotional or physical stressors (Kleposki, 2002). Women who participate in sports emphasizing low body weight are at greatest risk, including the following (Sabatini, 2001):

- Sports in which performance is subjectively scored (e.g., dance, gymnastics)
- Endurance sports favoring participants with low body weight (e.g., distance running, cycling)
- Sports in which body contour–revealing clothing is worn for competition (e.g., swimming, diving, volleyball)
- Sports with weight categories for participation (e.g., rowing, martial arts)
- Sports in which prepubertal body shape favors success (e.g., gymnastics, figure skating).

Management. When amenorrhea is due to hypothalamic disturbances, the nurse is an ideal health professional to assist women because many of the causes are potentially reversible (e.g., stress, weight loss for nonorganic reasons). Counseling and education are primary interventions and appropriate nursing roles. When a stressor known to predispose a client to hypothalamic amenorrhea is identified, initial management involves addressing the stressor. Together the woman and nurse plan how the woman can decrease or discontinue medications known to affect menstruation, correct weight loss, deal more effectively with psychologic stress, address emotional distress, and alter exercise routine.

The nurse works with the woman to help her identify, cope with, and possibly resolve sources of stress in her life. Deep-breathing exercises and relaxation techniques are simple yet effective stress reduction measures. Referral for biofeedback or massage therapy also may be useful. In some instances, referrals for psychotherapy may be indicated.

If a woman's exercise program is thought to contribute to her amenorrhea, several options exist for management. She may decide to decrease the intensity or duration of her training if possible or to gain 2% to 3% in body weight. Coming to accept this alternative may be difficult for one who is committed to a strenuous exercise regimen, and the nurse and client may have several sessions before the woman elects to try exercise reduction. Many young female athletes may not understand the consequences of low bone density or osteoporosis; nurses can point out the connection between low bone density and stress fractures. The nurse and woman also should investigate other factors that may be contributing to the amenorrhea and develop plans for altering lifestyle and decreasing stress.

A daily calcium intake of 1200 to 1500 mg/day, accomplished by drinking 3 glasses of skim milk or taking a calcium supplement, is recommended for women with amenorrhea associated with the female athlete triad (West, 1998).

Dysmenorrhea

Dysmenorrhea, pain during or shortly before menstruation, is one of the most common gynecologic problems in women of all ages. Many adolescents have dysmenorrhea in the first 3 years after menarche. Young adult women ages 17 to 24 years are most likely to report painful menses. Dysmenorrhea improves in most women after a full-term pregnancy (Speroff, Glass, & Kase, 1999). Between 30% and 40% of women report some level of discomfort associated with menses, and 7% to 15% report severe dysmenorrhea (Parent-Stevens & Burns, 2000); however, the amount of disruption in women's lives is difficult to determine. It has been estimated that up to 10% of women with dysmenorrhea have severe enough pain to interfere with their functioning for 1 to 3 days a month. Menstrual problems, including dysmenorrhea, are more common in women who smoke and who are obese. Severe dysmenorrhea is also associated with early menarche, nulliparity, and stress (Stenchever et al., 2001). Traditionally dysmenorrhea is differentiated as primary or secondary. Symptoms usually begin with menstruation, although some women have discomfort several hours before onset of flow. The range and severity of symptoms are different from woman to woman and from cycle to cycle in the same woman. Symptoms of dysmenorrhea may last several hours or several days.

Pain is usually located in the suprapubic area or lower abdomen. Women describe the pain as either sharp, cramping, or gripping or as a steady dull ache; pain may radiate to the lower back or upper thighs.

Primary Dysmenorrhea

Primary dysmenorrhea, a condition associated with abnormally increased uterine activity, is due to myometrium contractions induced by prostaglandins in the second half of the menstrual cycle. During the luteal phase and subsequent menstrual flow, prostaglandin $F_{2\alpha}$ ($PGF_{2\alpha}$) is secreted. The uterine muscle of both normal and dysmenorrheic women is sensitive to prostaglandins; however, the amount of prostaglandin produced is the major differentiating factor (Speroff, Glass, & Kase, 1999). Excessive release of $PGF_{2\alpha}$ increases the amplitude and frequency of uterine contractions and causes vasospasm of the uterine arterioles, resulting in ischemia and cyclic lower abdominal cramps. Systemic responses to $PGF_{2\alpha}$ include backache, weakness, sweating, gastrointestinal symptoms (anorexia, nausea, vomiting, and diarrhea), and central nervous system symptoms (dizziness, syncope, headache, and poor concentration). Pain begins at the onset of menstrual flow and lasts from 8 to 48 hours. The release of most prostaglandins during menstruation occurs in the first 48 hours, which coincides with the greatest intensity of symptoms (Stenchever et al., 2001).

Primary dysmenorrhea is not caused by underlying pathology; rather it is the occurrence of a physiologic alteration in some women. Primary dysmenorrhea usually appears within 6 to 12 months after menarche when ovulation is established. Anovulatory bleeding, common in the few months or years after menarche, is painless. Because both estrogen and progesterone are necessary for primary dysmenorrhea to occur, it is experienced only with ovulatory cycles. This problem is most common in women in their late teens and early twenties; the incidence declines with age.

Management. Management of primary dysmenorrhea depends on the severity of the problem and an individual women's response to various treatments. Important components of nursing care are information and support. Because menstruation is so closely linked to reproduction and sexuality, menstrual problems such as dysmenorrhea can have a negative influence on sexuality and self-worth. Nurses can correct myths and misinformation about menstruation and dysmenorrhea by providing facts about what is normal. Nurses must support their clients' feelings of positive sexuality and self-worth.

Often more than one alternative for alleviating menstrual discomfort and dysmenorrhea can be offered. Women can then try options and decide which ones work best for them. Heat (heating pad or hot bath) minimizes cramping by increasing vasodilation and muscle relaxation and minimizing uterine ischemia. Massaging the lower back can reduce pain by relaxing paravertebral muscles and increasing pelvic blood supply. Soft rhythmic rubbing of the abdomen (effleurage) may be useful because it provides distraction and an alternative focal point. Guided imagery, progressive relaxation, hatha yoga, and meditation also have been used successfully to decrease menstrual discomfort.

Exercise has been found to help in relieving menstrual discomfort through increased vasodilation and subsequent decreased ischemia; release of endogenous opiates, specifically β-endorphins; suppression of prostaglandins; and shunting of blood flow away from the viscera, resulting in less pelvic congestion. Specific exercises that nurses can suggest to their clients include pelvic rock and heels-over-the-head yoga position.

In addition to maintaining good nutrition at all times, specific dietary changes may be helpful in decreasing some of the systemic symptoms associated with dysmenorrhea. Decreased salt and refined sugar intake 7 to 10 days before expected menses may reduce fluid retention. Increasing water intake may serve as a natural diuretic. Including natural diuretics, such as asparagus, cranberry juice, peaches, parsley, and watermelon in the diet may help reduce edema and related discomforts. Decreasing red meat intake also may help minimize dysmenorrheal symptoms. Some women with primary dysmenorrhea reported a decrease in symptoms when they switched from a high-fat to a low-fat diet.

Medications used to treat primary dysmenorrhea in women not desiring contraception include prostaglandin synthesis inhibitors, primarily nonsteroidal antiinflammatory drugs (NSAIDs) (Parent-Stevens & Burns, 2000) (Table 7-1). NSAIDS are effective if begun 2 to 3 days before menses or with the sign of first bleeding; this regimen decreases the possibility of a woman taking these drugs early in pregnancy (Speroff et al., 1999). Often if one NSAID is ineffective, a different one will be effective. All NSAIDs have potential gastrointestinal side effects, including nausea, vomiting, and indigestion. All women taking NSAIDs should be warned to report dark-colored stools, because this may be an indication of gastrointestinal bleeding. Women with a history of aspirin sensitivity or allergy should avoid all NSAIDs. Approximately 80% of dysmenorrheic women obtain relief with prostaglandin inhibitors.

TABLE *7-1* **Medications Used to Treat Dysmenorrhea**

DRUG	BRAND NAME AND STATUS	RECOMMENDED DOSAGE*	COMMON SIDE EFFECTS†
Diclofenac	Cataflam Rx	50 mg tid or 100 mg initially then 50 mg tid to 150 mg/day	Nausea, diarrhea, constipation, abdominal distress, dyspepsia, flatulence
Fenoprofen‡	Nalfon Rx	200-400 mg q6-8hr to 1200 mg/day	Nausea, diarrhea, constipation, abdominal distress, dyspepsia, flatulence
Ibuprofen	Motrin Rx	400-800 mg qid to 3200 mg/day	Nausea, dyspepsia, rash, pruritus
	Advil OTC, Nuprin OTC, Motrin IB OTC	200-400 mg q4-6hr to 1200 mg/day	
Ketoprofen	Orudis Rx	25-50 mg q6-8hr to 300 mg/day	Nausea, diarrhea, constipation, abdominal distress, dyspepsia, flatulence
	Orudis KT OTC	12.5 mg q6-8hr to 75 mg/day	
	Actron OTC		
Meclofenamate	Meclomen Rx	100 mg tid to 300 mg	
Mefenamic acid	Ponstel Rx	50 mg initially; then 250 mg q6-8hr to 1000 mg/day	
Naproxen	Naprosyn Rx	500 mg initially, then 250 mg q6-8hr to 1250 mg/day	See ibuprofen
Naproxen sodium	Anaprox Rx	550 mg initially, then 275 mg q6-8hr to 1375 mg/day 440 mg initially,	See ibuprofen
	Aleve OTC	then 220 mg q6-8hr to 660 mg/day	

Sources: Facts and Comparisons. (2002). *Loose-leaf drug information service.* St. Louis: Facts and Comparisons; Parent-Stevens, L., & Burns, E. (2000). Menstrual disorders. In M. Smith & L. Shimp (Eds.), *20 Common problems in women's health care.* New York: McGraw-Hill.

qid, Four times a day; *tid,* three times a day; *GI,* gastrointestinal; *OTC,* over the counter; *Rx,* prescription.

*Dosages are current recommendations and should be verified before use. Recommended dosages for over-the-counter preparations are generally less than recommendations for therapeutic dosages. PRN dosing is recommended by manufacturer; scheduled dosing may be more effective.

Oral contraceptive pills (OCPs) are a reasonable choice for women who want a contraceptive agent. The benefits of OCP use are attributed to decreased prostaglandin synthesis associated with an atrophic decidualized endometrium (Speroff et al., 1999). No single OCP has been shown to be superior to another for the relief of primary dysmenorrhea. Although generally prescribed on a 21-day cycle of hormones followed by 7 hormone-free days, OCPs can be used continuously in an attempt to produce amenorrhea if women have severe dysmenorrhea during withdrawal bleeding (Lipscomb & Ling, 1997). OCPs are a particularly good choice for therapy because they combine contraception with a positive impact on dysmenorrhea, menstrual flow, and menstrual irregularities. It should be remembered that OCPs have side effects and that women not needing or not wanting them may not wish to use them for dysmenorrhea. OCPs also may be contraindicated for some women. (See Chapter 9 for a complete discussion of OCPs.)

Over-the-counter (OTC) preparations that are indicated for primary dysmenorrhea include the same active ingredients (e.g., ibuprofen, naproxen sodium) as prescription preparations; however, the labeled recommended dose may be subtherapeutic. Preparations containing acetaminophen are even less effective because acetaminophen does not have the antiprostaglandin properties of NSAIDs.

If dysmenorrhea is not relieved by one of the NSAIDs, further investigation into the cause of the symptoms is necessary. Conditions associated with dysmenorrhea include müllerian duct anomalies, endometriosis, and pelvic inflammatory disease.

Herbal preparations have long been used for management of menstrual problems including dysmenorrhea (Table 7-2). Herbal medicines may be valuable in treating dysmenorrhea; however, it is essential that women understand that these therapies are not without potential toxicity and may cause drug interactions. It is important that women use herbal preparations from well-established companies.

NURSE ALERT

Nurses must routinely ask women about use of herbal and other alternative therapies and document their use.

Secondary Dysmenorrhea

Secondary dysmenorrhea is acquired menstrual pain that develops later in life than primary dysmenorrhea, typically after age 25 years. This condition is associated with pelvic pathology, such as adenomyosis, endometriosis, pelvic inflammatory disease, endometrial polyps, or submucous or interstitial myomas (fibroids). Women with secondary dysmenorrhea often have other symptoms that may suggest an underlying cause. For example, heavy menstrual flow with dysmenorrhea suggests a diagnosis of leiomyomata, adenomyosis, or endometrial polyps. Pain associated with endometriosis often begins a few days before menses, but can be present at ovulation and continue through the first days of menses or start after menstrual flow has begun. In contrast to primary dysmenorrhea, the pain of secondary dysmenorrhea is often characterized by dull, lower abdominal aching radiating to the back or thighs. Often women experience feelings of bloating or pelvic fullness. In addition to a physical examination with a careful pelvic examination, diagnosis may be assisted by ultrasound examination, dilation and curettage, endometrial biopsy, or laparoscopy. Treatment is directed toward removal of the underlying pathology. Many of the measures described for pain relief of primary dysmenorrhea also are helpful for women with secondary dysmenorrhea.

COMMENTS	CONTRAINDICATIONS
Enteric coated: immediate release	For all NSAIDs: do not give if client has hemophilia or bleeding ulcers; do not give if client has had an allergic or anaphylactic reaction to aspirin or another NSAID; do not give if client is taking anticoagulant medication
Use for mild to moderate pain only if other NSAIDS are not effective; take with meals; avoid alcohol	
If GI upset occurs, take with food, milk, or antacids; avoid alcoholic beverages. Do not take with aspirin	
See ibuprofen	
See ibuprofen	
Very potent and effective prostaglandin-synthesis inhibitor	
Antagonizes already formed prostaglandins	
Increased incidence of adverse GI side effects	
See ibuprofen	
See ibuprofen	

†Risk with all NSAIDs is gastrointestinal ulceration, possible bleeding, and prolonged bleeding time. Incidence of side effects is dose related. Reported incidence, 3% to 9%.
‡Unlabeled indications for use in treating dysmenorrhea.

TABLE 7-2 **Herbal Medicinals for Menstrual Disorders**

SYMPTOMS/ INDICATIONS	HERBAL	ACTION	ROUTE	DOSAGE	CONTRAINDICATIONS
Menstrual cramping	Black haw	Uterine antispasmodic; β_2-agonist activity	Oral	Decoction (2 tsp/8oz water) 3/day Tincture (1:5) 3-5 ml q3-4hr prn Capsules 500-1000 mg q3-4hr prn	NK
Premenstrual discomfort (anxiety, tension, depression), dysmenorrhea	Black cohosh root	Estrogen-like LH suppressant, binds to estrogen receptors	Oral	20-80 mg bid over 6-mo period	Pregnancy
Tension, breast pain	Bugleweed	Antigonadotropic, antithyrotropic, decreased prolactin levels	Oral	0.02-2 g	Thyroid disease
Mastodynia, premenstrual discomfort, menstrual cycle irregularities	Chaste tree fruit	Decreased prolactin levels	Oral	30-40 mg	NK
Menstrual cramping	Ginger	Antiinflammatory	Oral	1 g root (maximum 4 g) as tea, capsule	
Dysmenorrhea	Potentilla	Increased tonus and contraction frequency in uterus	Oral	Infusion: 0.1-0.3 g tid Tincture: (1:10, 25% ethanol) 0.5-3 ml tid	Pregnancy and lactation
Menorrhea and metrorrhagia	Shepard's purse	Increased uterine contractions	Oral	5-15 g	NK
Dysmenorrhea	Dong quai	Stimulate/relax uterus; anti-inflammatory; possibly analgesic activity	Oral	3.5-4.0 g/day	Phototoxicity Liver and renal damage in animal studies Abortifacient

Sources: Bascom, A. (2002). *Incorporating herbal medicine into clinical practice.* Philadelphia: F.A. Davis Company; Fugh-Berman, A., & Awang, D. (2001). Black cohosh. *Alternative Therapies in Women's Health, 39*(11), 81-85; Dog, L.. (2000). *An integrative approach to dysmenorrhea.* Corrales, NM: Integrative Medicine Education Association, LLC; Dog, L. (2001). *Endocrinology and women's issues.* Third Annual Conference on Clinical Relevance of Medicinal Herbs and Nutritional Supplements in the Management of Major Medical Problems, September 21-23, 2001; Schellenberg, R. (2001). Treatment for the premenstrual syndrome with *Agnus castus* fruit extract: Prospective, randomized, placebo controlled study. *British Medical Journal, 322,* 134-137; Stevinson, C., & Ernst, E. (2001). Complementary/alternative therapies for premenstrual

Premenstrual Syndrome

Premenstrual syndrome (PMS) is a complex, poorly understood condition that includes a number of cyclic symptoms occurring in the luteal phase of the menstrual cycle. Estimates of the number of women with some degree of problems related to their menstrual cycle range from 20% to 95%, with about 2% to 10% of women reporting some degree of disruption of their daily activities (Cronje & Studd, 2002; Lin & Thompson, 2001; Speroff et al., 1999). All age groups are affected, with women in their twenties and thirties most frequently reporting symptoms. Ovarian function is necessary for the condition to occur, as it does not occur before puberty, after menopause, or during pregnancy. The condition is not dependent on the presence of monthly menses, as women who have had a hysterectomy without bilateral salpingo-oophorectomy still can have cyclic symptoms.

It is difficult to establish a universal definition of PMS, as so many symptoms have been associated with the con-

ADVERSE REACTIONS	DRUG INTERACTIONS
NK	NK
Gastric irritation, CNS side effects at high doses	NK
Thyroid enlargement with prolonged high dose	Interferes with diagnostic radioactive isotopes
Itching, urticaria	Possible antagonism of dopaminergic antagonists
Gastric irritation	NK
NK	NK
Pregnancy	Coumarin components may increase risk of bleeding

syndrome: A systemic review of random controlled trials. *American Journal of Obstetrics and Gynecology, 185*, 227-235.
bid, Twice a day; *CNS*, central nervous system; *LH*, luteinizing hormone; *NK*, none known; *tid*, three times a day.

dition, and at least two different syndromes have been recognized: PMS and *premenstrual dysphoric disorder (PDD)*. PMS is a cluster of physical, psychologic, and behavioral symptoms (more than 100) beginning in the luteal phase of the menstrual cycle, occurring to such a degree that lifestyle or work is affected, and followed by a symptom-free period. Symptoms include fluid retention (abdominal bloating, pelvic fullness, edema of the lower extremities, breast tenderness, and weight gain); behavioral or emotional changes (depression, crying spells, irritability, panic attacks, and impaired ability to concentrate); premenstrual cravings (sweets, salt, increased appetite, and food binges); and headache, fatigue, and backache. PDD is a more severe variant of PMS in which women have marked irritability, dysphoria, mood lability, anxiety, fatigue, appetite changes, and a sense of feeling overwhelmed (Elliot, 2002).

A diagnosis of PMS is made only if the following criteria are met:

- Symptoms occur in the luteal phase and resolve within a few days of menses onset.
- Symptom-free period occurs in the follicular phase.
- Symptoms are recurrent.

The exact nature of PMS is widely debated, but there is general agreement that it is a distinct psychiatric and medical syndrome rather than an exacerbation of an underlying psychiatric disorder. It does not occur if there is no ovarian function. PMS is most likely not a single disorder but rather a collection of different problems. Speroff et al. (1999) suggested that PMS has a basic psychophysiologic origin tied to the menstrual cycle, primarily biologic but with a psychologic overlay. It also can be a learned response or a response in vulnerable individuals triggered by normal neuroendocrine and hormonal changes. Readers are encouraged to explore current feminist, medical, and social science literature for more information on PMS.

Management

There is little agreement on management. A careful, detailed history and daily log of symptoms and mood fluctuations spanning several cycles may give direction to a plan of management. Any changes that assist a woman with PMS to exert control over her life have a positive impact. For example, Morse (1999) found that women who participated in a peer support group had fewer negative PMS symptom reports and more positive perceptions of the menstrual cycle.

Education is an important component of the management of PMS. Nurses can advise women that self-help modalities often result in significant symptom improvement. Women have found a number of complementary and alternative therapies to be useful in managing the symptoms of PMS. Diet and exercise changes are a useful way to begin and provide symptom relief for some women. Nurses can suggest that clients not smoke and limit their consumption of refined sugar (less than 5 tbsp/day), salt (less than 3 g/day), red meat (up to 3 oz/day), alcohol (less than 1 oz/day), and caffeinated beverages. Clients can be encouraged to include whole grains, legumes, seeds, nuts, vegetables, fruits, and vegetable oils in their diet. Three small-to-moderate-sized meals and three small snacks a day that are rich in complex carbohydrates and fiber have been reported to improve symptoms (Jones, 2001). Use of natural diuretics (see section on dysmenorrhea management on p. 157) may help reduce fluid retention as well. Nutritional supplements may assist in symptom relief. Calcium (1000 to 1200 mg daily), magnesium (300 to 400 mg daily), and vitamin B_6 (100 to 150 mg daily) have been shown to be moderately effective in relieving symptoms, to have few side effects, and to be safe. Daily supplements of evening primrose oil are thought to be useful in relieving breast symptoms with minimal side effects. Regular exercise (aerobic exercise 3 to 4 times a week), especially in the luteal phase, is widely recommended for relief of PMS symptoms. A monthly program that varies in intensity and type of exercise according to PMS symptoms is best. Women who exercise regularly seem to have less premenstrual anxiety than do nonathletic women. It is thought that aerobic exercise increases β-endorphin levels to offset symptoms of depression and elevate mood.

Yoga, acupuncture, hypnosis, chiropractic therapy, and massage therapy have all been reported to have a beneficial effect on PMS. Herbal therapies have long been used to treat PMS; specific suggestions are found in Table 7-2.

Nurses can explain the relation between cyclic estrogen fluctuation and changes in serotonin levels, that serotonin is one of the brain chemicals that assist in coping with normal life stresses, and how the different management strategies recommended help maintain serotonin levels. Counseling, in the form of support groups or individual or couple counseling, may be helpful. Stress reduction techniques also may assist with symptom management (Baker, 1998).

If these strategies do not provide significant symptom relief in 1 to 2 months, medication is often begun. Many medications have been used in treatment of PMS, but no single medication alleviates all PMS symptoms. Medications often used in the treatment of PMS include diuretics, prostaglandin inhibitors (NSAIDs), progesterone, and OCPs. Fluoxetine (Sarafem or Prozac, 20 mg a day), a selective serotonin reuptake inhibitor (SSRI), is the only Food and Drug Administration (FDA)–approved agent for PMS. Use of this medication results in a decrease in emotional symptoms, especially depression (Jones, 2001; Lin & Thompson, 2001) (see Plan of Care).

Endometriosis

Endometriosis is characterized by the presence and growth of endometrial tissue outside of the uterus. The tissue may be implanted on the ovaries, cul-de-sac, uterine ligaments, rectovaginal septum, sigmoid colon, pelvic peritoneum, cervix, and inguinal area (Fig. 7-1). Endometrial lesions have been found in the vagina and surgical scars, as well as on the vulva, perineum, and bladder, and sites far from the pelvic area such as the thoracic cavity, gallbladder, and heart. A cystic lesion of endometriosis found in the ovary is sometimes described as a chocolate cyst because of the dark coloring of the contents of the cyst caused by the presence of old blood.

Endometrial tissue contains glands and stoma and responds to cyclic hormonal stimulation in the same way that the uterine endometrium does but often out of phase with it. During the proliferative and secretory phases of the cycle, the endometrial tissue grows. During or immediately after menstruation, the tissue bleeds, resulting in an

Plan of Care — Premenstrual Syndrome

NURSING DIAGNOSIS Pain related to cyclic breast changes as evidenced by client report

Expected Outcome *Client will report a decrease in the intensity of pain or discomfort after interventions.*

Nursing Interventions/*Rationales*

Assess timing and intensity of pain or discomfort *to validate relation to cyclic changes.*

Administer medications if prescribed *to minimize breast tenderness.*

Suggest that client wear a supportive bra *to minimize breast tenderness.*

NURSING DIAGNOSIS Situational low self-esteem related to cyclic hormonal changes as evidenced by client verbal report

Expected Outcome *Client will report increased number of feelings of self-worth.*

Nursing Interventions/*Rationales*

Provide therapeutic communication *to validate client feelings of depression and mood swings.*

Encourage client to limit caffeine and eat small, frequent meals *to lessen irritability aggravated by caffeine and hypoglycemia.*

Refer client to support groups *to encourage the sharing of experiences, feelings, and self-help tips.*

NURSING DIAGNOSIS Excess fluid volume related to cyclic hormonal influences as evidenced by weight gain before start of menstrual period

Expected Outcome *Client will report no significant changes in body weight before start of menstrual period.*

Nursing Interventions/*Rationales*

Encourage client to limit intake of salt- and sodium-containing foods *to decrease fluid retention.*

Administer diuretics as prescribed *to facilitate fluid excretion.*

Encourage consumption of natural diuretic foods *to encourage fluid excretion.*

NURSING DIAGNOSIS Anxiety related to anticipation of cyclical pain

Expected Outcome *Woman will report a decrease in anxiety level.*

Nursing Interventions/*Rationales*

Teach client to recognize anxiety *to prompt early preventive interventions.*

Identify relaxation techniques to decrease anxiety *to promote self-care.*

Encourage client to attend support groups *to encourage expression of feelings and self-help interventions.*

inflammatory response with subsequent fibrosis and adhesion to adjacent organs.

The overall incidence of endometriosis is about 5% to 10% in reproductive-age women, 25% to 35% in infertile women, and 28% in women with chronic pelvic pain (Speroff et al., 1999). Although the condition usually develops in the third or fourth decade of life, endometriosis has been found in adolescents, with disabling pelvic pain or abnormal vaginal bleeding. Additionally, endometriosis has been reported to occur in about 5% of postmenopausal women receiving menopausal hormone therapy (Nakad & Isaacson, 2002). At one time, endometriosis was believed to be more prevalent in Caucasion middle-class women; however, the condition appears equally in Caucasian, African-American, and Asian women (Nakad & Isaacson, 2002). Furthermore, endometriosis occurs across all socioeconomic levels. There appears to be a familial tendency to develop endometriosis; the incidence of severe endometriosis is higher (61.1%) in family groups than in nonfamily groups (23.8%) (Hadfield et al., 1997). Endometriosis may worsen with repeated cycles, or it may remain asymptomatic and undiagnosed, eventually disappearing after menopause. Endometriosis can occur in women who have been pregnant and may be a cause of secondary infertility (Speroff et al., 1999).

Several theories to account for the cause of endometriosis have been suggested, yet the etiology and pathology of this condition continue to be poorly understood. One of the most widely accepted, long-debated theories is transplantation or retrograde menstruation. According to this theory, endometrial tissue is refluxed through the uterine (fallopian) tubes during menstruation into the peritoneal cavity, where it implants on the ovaries and other organs. Retrograde menstruation has been documented in a number of surgical studies and is estimated to occur in 90% of menstruating women. For most women, endometrial tissue outside the uterus is destroyed before it can implant or seed in the peritoneal cavity or elsewhere. Perhaps endometriosis develops in only 10% to 15% of women because of differences in the functioning of an individual's immune system. It also may reflect differences in genetic makeup or environmental challenges (Speroff et al., 1999).

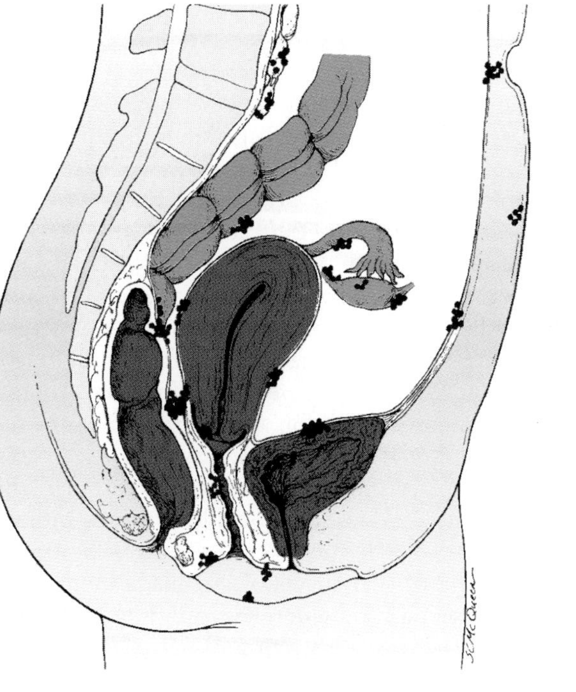

FIG. 7-1 Common sites of endometriosis. (From Stenchever, M. et al. [2001]. *Comprehensive gynecology* [4th ed.]. St. Louis: Mosby.)

Symptoms vary among women, from nonexistent to incapacitating. Severity of symptoms can change over time and may be disconnected from the extent of the disease. The major symptoms of endometriosis are dysmenorrhea and deep pelvic dyspareunia (painful intercourse). Women also have chronic noncyclic pelvic pain, pelvic heaviness, or pain radiating into the thighs. Many women report bowel symptoms such as diarrhea, pain with defecation, and constipation caused by avoiding defecation because of the pain. Less common symptoms include abnormal bleeding (hypermenorrhea, menorrhagia, or premenstrual staining) and pain during exercise as a result of adhesions.

Impaired fertility may result from adhesions around the uterus that pull the uterus into a fixed, retroverted position. Adhesions around the uterine tubes may block the fimbriated ends or prevent the spontaneous movement that carries the ovum to the uterus or blocks the fimbriated ends.

Management

Treatment is based on the severity of symptoms and the goals of the woman or couple. Women without pain who do not want to become pregnant need no treatment. In women with mild pain who may desire a future pregnancy, treatment may be limited to use of NSAIDs during menstruation (see earlier discussion of these medications).

Suppression of endogenous estrogen production and subsequent endometrial lesion growth is the cornerstone of management of the disease. Two main classes of drugs are used to suppress endogenous estrogen levels: GnRH agonists and androgen derivatives. GnRH-agonist therapy (leuprolide [Lupron], nafarelin [Synarel]) acts by suppressing pituitary gonadotropin secretion. FSH and LH stimulation of the ovary declines markedly, and ovarian function decreases significantly. A medically induced menopause develops, resulting in anovulation and amenorrhea. Shrinkage of already established endometrial tissue, significant pain relief, and an interruption in further lesion development follow. The hypoestrogenism results in hot flashes in almost all women. Trabecular bone loss is common, although most loss is reversible within 12 to 18 months after the medication is stopped. Leuprolide (3.75 mg intramuscular injection given once a month) or nafarelin (200 mg administered twice daily by nasal spray) are both effective and well tolerated. Both medications reduce endometrial lesions and pelvic pain associated with endometriosis and have post-treatment pregnancy rates similar to those of danazol therapy (Speroff et al., 1999). Common side effects of these drugs are those of natural menopause—hot flashes and vaginal dryness. Occasionally women report headaches and muscle aches. Treatment is usually limited to 6 months to minimize bone loss. Although unlikely, it is possible for a woman to become pregnant while taking a GnRH agonist. Because the potential teratogenicity of this drug is unclear, women should use a barrier contraceptive during treatment.

Danazol (Danocrine), a mildly androgenic synthetic steroid, suppresses FSH and LH secretion, thus producing anovulation and hypogonadotropinism, with resulting decreased secretion of estrogen and progesterone and regression of endometrial tissue. This medication was widely used to treat endometriosis in the 1970s and 1980s. Danazol side effects can cause a woman to discontinue the drug. Side effects include masculinizing traits in the woman (weight gain, edema, decreased breast size, oily skin, hirsutism, and deepening of the voice), all of which often disappear when treatment is discontinued. Other side effects are amenorrhea, hot flashes, vaginal dryness, insomnia, and decreased libido. Migraine headaches, dizziness, fatigue, and depression also are reported. Danazol treatment has been reported to affect lipids adversely, with a decrease in high-density lipoprotein (HDL) levels and an increase in low-density lipoprotein (LDL) levels. Danazol should never be prescribed when pregnancy is suspected, and contraception should be used with it because ovulation may not be suppressed. Danazol can produce pseudohermaphroditism in female fetuses. The medication is contraindicated in women with liver disease and should be used with caution in women with cardiac and renal disease. The recommended dosage is 200 to 400 mg/day for 3 to 6 months.

Women who have early symptomatic disease and can postpone pregnancy may be treated with continuous oral contraceptives that have a low estrogen-to-progestin ratio to shrink endometrial tissue. Any low-dose OCPs can be used if taken for 15 weeks followed by 1 week of withdrawal. This therapy is associated with minimal side effects and can be taken for extended periods (Nakad & Isaacson, 2002).

Surgical intervention is often needed for severe, acute, or incapacitating symptoms. Decisions regarding the extent and type of surgery are influenced by a woman's age, desire for children, and location of the disease. For women who do not want to preserve their ability to have children, the only definite cure is total abdominal hysterectomy with bilateral salpingo-oophorectomy (TAH with BSO). In women who are in their childbearing years and want children and in whom the disease does not prevent it, reproductive capacity should be retained through careful removal by surgery or laser therapy of all endometrial tissue possible and with retention of ovarian function (Nakad & Isaacson, 2002).

Regardless of the type of treatment, short of TAH with BSO, endometriosis reoccurs in approximately 40% of women; thus for many women, endometriosis is a chronic disease with conditions such as chronic pain or infertility. Counseling and education are critical components of nursing care for women with endometriosis. Women need an honest discussion of treatment options, with potential risks and benefits of each option reviewed. Because pelvic pain is a subjective, personal experience that can be frightening, support is important. Sexual dysfunction resulting from painful intercourse (dyspareunia) is common and may necessitate referral for counseling. Support groups for women with endometriosis may be found in some locations; Resolve, an organization for infertile couples, also may be helpful. The nursing care discussed in the section on dysmenorrhea is appropriate for managing chronic pelvic pain and dysmenorrhea in the woman with endometriosis (see Resources at the end of the chapter) (see Plan of Care).

Alterations in Cyclic Bleeding

Women often have changes in amount, duration, interval, or regularity of menstrual cycle bleeding. Often women worry about menstruation that is short, that is small in amount, or that occurs too frequently.

Dysfunctional Uterine Bleeding

Oligomenorrhea/Hypomenorrhea. The term **oligomenorrhea** often is used to describe decreased menstruation, either in amount, time, or both. However, oligomenorrhea more correctly refers to infrequent menstrual periods characterized by intervals of 40 to 45 days or longer, and **hypomenorrhea,** to scanty bleeding at normal intervals. The causes of oligomenorrhea are often abnormalities of hypothalamic, pituitary, or ovarian function. Oligomenorrhea also can be physiologic, or part of a woman's normal pattern for the first few years after menarche or for several years before menopause.

Treatment is aimed at reversing the underlying cause, if possible. Hormonal therapy using progestins, with or without estrogens, also may be used to prevent complications of unopposed estrogen production (endometrial hyperplasia or carcinoma) or of absent estrogen (vaginal dryness, hot flashes or flushes, osteoporosis).

Women with menstruation characterized by prolonged intervals between cycles need education and counseling. The cause of the condition and the rationale for a specific treatment should be discussed, as should advantages and disadvantages of hormonal therapy. If a woman chooses medical intervention, she should be provided with written instructions, taught how to take the medications, and made aware of side effects of any medications. Teaching and counseling should emphasize the importance of the woman keeping careful records of her vaginal bleeding.

One of the most common causes of scanty menstrual flow is OCPs. If a woman is considering OCPs for contraception, it is important that the nurse explain in advance that the use of OCPs can decrease menstrual flow by as

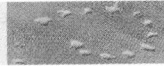

Plan of Care: Endometriosis

NURSING DIAGNOSIS Acute pain related to menstruation secondary to endometriosis

Expected Outcome *Client will verbalize a decrease in intensity and frequency of pain during each menstrual cycle.*

Nursing Interventions/Rationales

Assess location, type, and duration of pain and history of discomfort *to determine severity of dysmenorrhea.*

Administer analgesics *to assist with pain relief.*

Administer hormone altering medications if ordered *to suppress ovulation.*

Provide nonpharmacologic methods such as heat *to increase blood flow to the pelvic region.*

NURSING DIAGNOSIS Deficient knowledge related to unfamiliarity with treatment, as evidenced by client statements

Expected Outcome *Client will verbalize correct understanding of the use of self-care methods and prescribed therapies.*

Nursing Interventions/Rationales

Assess client's current understanding of the disorder and related therapies *to validate the accuracy of knowledge base.*

Give information to client regarding the disorder and treatment regimen *to empower the client to become a partner in her own care.*

NURSING DIAGNOSIS Situational low self-esteem related to infertility as evidenced by client's statements of decreased self-worth

Expected Outcome *Client will verbalize positive feelings of self-worth.*

Nursing Interventions/Rationales

Provide therapeutic communication *to validate feelings and provide support.*

Refer to support group *to enhance feelings of self-worth through group communication.*

NURSING DIAGNOSIS Anxiety related to possible invasive surgical procedure as evidenced by client's verbal report

Expected Outcome *Client will report a decreased number of anxious feelings.*

Nursing Interventions/Rationales

Provide opportunity to discuss feelings *to identify source of anxiety.*

Reinforce information provided *to keep expectations realistic and dispel myths or inaccuracies.*

Provide emotional support *to encourage verbalization of feelings.*

NURSING DIAGNOSIS Risk for injury related to disease progression

Expected Outcome *Woman will report any changes in health status to health care provider.*

Nursing Interventions/Rationales

Teach woman to report any changes in health status *to initiate prompt treatment.*

Review side effects of medications *to recognize possible rationales for changes in health status.*

Encourage ongoing communication with health care provider *to promote trust and comfort.*

much as two thirds. This effect is caused by the continuous action of the progestin component, which produces a decidualized endometrium with atrophic glands.

Hypomenorrhea also may be caused by structural abnormalities of the endometrium or uterus that result in partial destruction of the endometrium. These conditions include Asherman syndrome, in which adhesions resulting from curettage or infection obliterate the endometrial cavity, and congenital partial obstruction of the vagina.

Metrorrhagia. Metrorrhagia, or intermenstrual bleeding, refers to any episode of bleeding, whether spotting, menses, or hemorrhage, that occurs at a time other than the normal menses. *Mittlestaining*, a small amount of bleeding or spotting that occurs at the time of ovulation (14 days before onset of the next menses), is considered normal. The cause of mittlestaining is not known; however, its common occurrence can be documented by its repetition in the menstrual cycle.

Women taking OCPs may have midcycle bleeding or spotting. (See Chapter 9 for a discussion of the side effects of OCPs.) If the OCP does not sufficiently maintain a hypoplastic endometrium, the endometrium will begin to shed, usually in small amounts at a time, a process termed *breakthrough bleeding*. Breakthrough bleeding is most common in the first three cycles of OCPs. The reduced potency of OCPs (resulting in increased safety) has decreased the amount of available hormones, making it more important that blood levels be kept constant. Suggesting that women take their pill at exactly the same time each day may alleviate the problem. If the spotting continues, a different formulation of OCP that increases either the estrogen or progestin component of the pill can be tried.

Progestin-only contraceptive methods (oral and injectable) also may cause midcycle bleeding, especially in the first several cycles. Women should be advised of this and counseled to report continuation of breakthrough bleeding after the first three to six cycles to their health care provider.

Women with an intrauterine device (IUD) may have spotting between their periods and heavier menstrual flow.

The causes of intermenstrual bleeding are varied (Table 7-3). It is important that the nurse always consider the possibility that any woman who has not undergone menopause and who seeks care for intermenstrual bleeding is or recently has been pregnant.

Treatment of intermenstrual bleeding depends on the cause and may include reassurance and education concerning mittlestaining, observation of three menstrual cycles for presumed functional ovarian cyst, adjustment of an OCP, removal of foreign bodies, and treatment for vaginal infections. More complex treatment may consist of removal of polyps; evaluation and treatment of an

TABLE 7-3 **Causes of Intermenstrual Bleeding**

REPRODUCTIVE DISORDER	PREGNANCY PROBLEMS	INFECTIONS
Functional ovarian cyst	Pregnancy: implantation	Endometritis
Cervical erosion infection	Miscarriage	Sexually transmitted infections
Leiomyoma	Ectopic pregnancy	
Polyps, uterine or endocervix	Molar pregnancy	
Trauma	Retained placenta, miscarriage or induced abortion	
Foreign body	Retained placenta, birth	
Malignancy of reproductive tract		

abnormal Papanicolaou (Pap) smear, including colposcopy, biopsy, cautery, cryosurgery, or conization; and surgery, chemotherapy, or radiation treatment for malignancy. Important nursing roles include reassurance, counseling, education, and support.

Menorrhagia. **Menorrhagia (hypermenorrhea)** is defined as excessive menstrual bleeding, in either duration or amount. The causes of heavy menstrual bleeding are many, including hormonal disturbances, systemic disease, benign and malignant neoplasms, infection, and contraception (IUDs). A single episode of heavy bleeding may occur, or a woman may have regular flooding as a pattern in which she changes tampons or pads every few hours for several days.

NURSE ALERT

If the woman herself considers the amount or duration of bleeding to be excessive, the problem should be investigated.

Hemoglobin and hematocrit provide objective indicators to actual blood loss and should always be assessed.

A single episode of heavy bleeding may signal an early pregnancy loss. This type of bleeding is often thought to be a period that is heavier than usual, perhaps delayed, and is associated with abdominal pain or pelvic discomfort. When early pregnancy loss is suspected, a hematocrit and serum β-hCG pregnancy test should be done.

Infectious and inflammatory processes such as acute or chronic endometritis and salpingitis may cause heavy menstrual bleeding. Although rare, systemic diseases of nonreproductive origin such as blood dyscrasias, hypothyroidism, and lupus erythematosus also can cause hypermenorrhea. In obese women, anovulation caused by increased peripheral conversion of androstenedione to estrogen may develop and manifest as menorrhagia. Medications also may cause abnormal bleeding. Chemotherapy, anticoagulants, neuroleptics, and steroid hormone therapy all have been associated with excessive flow.

Uterine **leiomyoma** (fibroids or myomas) are a common cause of menorrhagia. Fibroids are benign tumors of the smooth muscle of the uterus, the etiology of which is unknown. Fibroids occur in one fourth of women of reproductive age; the incidence of fibroids is two to three times higher in African-American women than in Caucasian or Hispanic women (Friedman & Carlson, 2002). Fibroids are estrogen sensitive and commonly develop during the reproductive years and shrink after menopause. Fibroids are seen in 1% to 2% of pregnant women and can cause considerable discomfort as the uterus enlarges; furthermore, fetal palpation may be more difficult. The major symptoms associated with fibroids are menorrhagia and the physical effects produced by large myomas. Other uterine growths ranging from endometrial polyps to adenocarcinoma and endometrial cancer are common causes of heavy menstrual bleeding, as well as of intermenstrual bleeding.

Treatment for menorrhagia depends on the cause of the bleeding. If the bleeding is related to contraceptive method, the nurse provides factual information and reassurance and discusses other contraceptive options. If bleeding is related to presence of fibroids, the degree of disability and discomfort associated with the fibroids and the woman's plans for childbearing will influence treatment decisions. Treatment options include medical and surgical management. Most fibroids can be monitored by frequent examinations to judge growth, if any, and correction of anemia, if present. Women with metrorrhagia should be warned not to use aspirin because of its tendency to increase bleeding. Medical treatment is directed toward temporarily reducing symptoms, shrinking the myoma, and reducing its blood supply (Grabo et al., 1999). This reduction is often accomplished with the use of a GnRH agonist. If the woman wishes to retain childbearing potential, a myomectomy may be done. Myomectomy, or removal of the tumors only, is particularly difficult if multiple myomas must be removed. If the woman does not want to preserve her childbearing function, or if she has severe symptoms (severe anemia, severe pain, considerable disruption of lifestyle), hysterectomy or endometrial ablation (laser surgery or electrocoagulation) may be done (see Chapter 12).

Abnormal uterine bleeding (AUB) is any form of uterine bleeding that is irregular in amount, duration, or timing and not related to regular menstrual bleeding. Box 7-1 lists possible causes of AUB. Although often used inter-

BOX 7-1 Possible Causes of Abnormal Uterine Bleeding

ANOVULATION
- Hypothalamic dysfunction
- Polycystic ovary syndrome

PREGNANCY-RELATED CONDITIONS
- Threatened or spontaneous miscarriage
- Retained products of conception after elective abortion
- Ectopic pregnancy

LOWER REPRODUCTIVE TRACT INFECTIONS
- Chlamydial cervicitis
- Pelvic inflammatory disease

NEOPLASMS
- Endometrial hyperplasia
- Cancer of cervix and endometrium
- Endometrial polyps
- Hormonally active tumors (rare)
- Leiomyomata
- Vaginal tumors (rare)

TRAUMA
- Genital injury (accidental, coital trauma, sexual abuse)
- Foreign body
- Primary coagulation disorders

SYSTEMIC DISEASES
- Diabetes mellitus
- Thyroid dysfunction (hypothyroidism, hyperthyroidism)
- Severe organ disease (renal or liver failure)

IATROGENIC CAUSES
- Exogenous hormone use (oral contraceptives, menopausal hormone therapy)
- Medications with estrogenic activity
- Herbal preparation (ginseng)

Sources: ACNM Clinical Bulletin (2002). Clinical Bulletin No. 6. Abnormal and dysfunctional uterine bleeding. *Journal of Midwifery and Women's Health, 47*(3), 207-213; Hillard, P. (1999). Diagnosing and controlling abnormal uterine bleeding. *Contemporary Adolescent Gynecology 4*(1), 4-11; Kaunitz, A. (2002a). Abnormal uterine bleeding in the perimenopausal patient. *Contemporary Ob/GYN, April,* 69-88; Speroff, L., Glass, R., & Kase, N. (1999). *Clinical gynecologic endocrinology and infertility* (6th ed.). Baltimore: Lippincott Williams & Wilkins.

changeably, the terms AUB and dysfunctional uterine bleeding (DUB) are not synonymous. **Dysfunctional uterine bleeding** is a subset of AUB defined as "excessive uterine bleeding with no demonstrable organic cause, genital or extragenital" (Stenchever et al., 2001). DUB is most frequently caused by anovulation. When there is no LH surge, or if there is not sufficient progesterone produced by the corpus luteum to support the endometrium, it will begin to involute and shed. This most often occurs at the extremes of a woman's reproductive years–when the menstrual cycle is just becoming established at menarche or when it draws to a close at menopause. DUB also can be found with any condition that gives rise to chronic anovulation associated with continuous estrogen production. Such conditions include obesity, hyperthyroidism and hypothyroidism, polycystic ovarian syndrome, and any of the endocrine conditions discussed in the sections on amenorrhea and oligomenorrhea.

Women also may unknowingly use medications with an impact on the endometrium; for example, ginseng, an herbal root, has been associated with estrogen activity and abnormal bleeding. A diagnosis of DUB is made only after all other causes of abnormal menstrual bleeding have been ruled out (ACNM, 2002).

When uterine bleeding is severe and a woman's hemoglobin level is less than 8 g/100 ml (hematocrit of 23% or 24%), the woman may be hospitalized and given conjugated estrogens (Premarin), 25 to 40 mg intravenously every 4 to 6 hours or 2.5 mg orally every 6 hours (Hillard, 1999), until bleeding stops or slows significantly (up to three doses). If the bleeding has not stopped in 12 to 24 hours, dilation and curettage (D&C) may be done to control severe bleeding and hemorrhage. An endometrial biopsy may be collected at the same time to evaluate endometrial tissue or rule out endometrial cancer. After this treatment, oral conjugated estrogen, 2.5 mg to 3.75 mg, is given for 21 days. During the last 7 to 10 days of this estrogen regimen, progesterone (e.g., medroxyprogesterone [Provera], 10 mg PO) is added. Alternatively, a combined OCP is given for 21 days after intravenous therapy. Once the acute phase has passed, the woman is maintained on cyclic, low-dose OCPs for 3 to 6 months. Such long-term treatment will help prevent recurrence of the pattern of dysfunctional uterine bleeding and hemorrhage. If she wants contraception, she should continue to take OCPs. If the woman has no need for contraception, the treatment may be stopped to assess her bleeding pattern. If her menses does not resume, a progestin regimen (e.g., medroxyprogesterone, 10 mg/day for 10 days before the expected date of her menstrual period) may be prescribed after ruling out pregnancy. This is done to prevent persistent anovulation with chronic unopposed endogenous estrogen hyperstimulation of the endometrium, which can result in eventual atypical tissue changes.

If the recurrent, heavy bleeding is not controlled by hormonal therapy or D&C, ablation of the endometrium through laser treatment may be performed. Nursing roles include informing clients of their options, counseling and education as indicated, and referring to the appropriate specialists and health care services.

CARE MANAGEMENT

Assessment and Nursing Diagnoses

In addition to taking a careful menstrual, obstetric, sexual, and contraceptive history, the nurse should explore the woman's perceptions of her condition, cultural or ethnic influences, experiences with other caregivers, lifestyle, and patterns of coping. The amount of pain or bleeding and its effect on daily activities should be evaluated (see Guidelines/Guías). Home remedies and prescriptions to relieve discomfort are noted. A symptom diary, in which the woman records emotions, behaviors, physical symptoms, diet, and exercise and rest patterns, is a useful diagnostic tool.

Nursing diagnoses for women with menstrual disorders include the following:

- *Risk for ineffective individual or family coping related to*
  - –insufficient knowledge of the cause of the disorder
  - –emotional and physiologic effects of the disorder
- *Deficient knowledge related to*
  - –self-care
  - –available therapy for the disorder
- *Risk for disturbed body image related to*
  - –menstrual disorder
  - –sexual dysfunction
- *Risk for situational low self-esteem related to*
  - –others' perception of her discomfort
  - –inability to conceive
- *Acute pain related to*
  - –menstrual disorder

GUIDELINES/GUÍAS

Menstruation

At what age did you begin to menstruate?
¿A qué edad comenzó a menstruar?

When was your last menstrual cycle?
¿Cuándo fue su última menstruación?

Was it normal?
¿Fue normal?

Do you have pains with your period?
¿Tiene dolores con la menstruación?

How many days does your period last?
¿Por cuántos días sangra?

Is the flow light or heavy?
¿Sangra mucho o poco?

Expected Outcomes of Care

After data collection and review, mutual expected outcomes are established, and a plan of care is developed. The expected outcomes for the woman are that she will do the following:

- Verbalize understanding of reproductive anatomy, etiology of her disorder, medication regimen, and diary use.
- Verbalize her understanding and acceptance of her emotional and physical responses to her menstrual cycle.
- Develop personal goals that benefit her emotionally and physically.
- Choose appropriate therapeutic measures for her menstrual problems.
- Adapt successfully to the condition if cure is not possible.

Plan of Care and Interventions

During the history and diagnostic workup, the clinician's concern and acceptance of the woman's symptoms as valid are in themselves therapeutic. Data from the daily diary of emotional status, subjective feelings, and physical state are correlated with physiologic changes. If the woman has a partner, she and her partner should keep separate diaries that include how each perceives the other's responses day by day. Through the diaries, feelings are vented, problems are identified and clarified, insights occur, and possible solutions begin to develop. The clinician facilitates insights and suggests therapeutic options. The woman (couple) makes choices considered best for her (them).

Nurses should discuss the options available to women with menstrual disorders. Women must understand basic information about the anatomy and physiology, pathophysiology, psychologic impact, and treatment for the condition, including alternative therapies.

Support groups are an important resource. Nurses can use a local women's center or clinic to bring together women who want to learn more about their condition and support each other.

Evaluation

The nurse can be assured that care has been effective when the woman reports improvement in the quality of her life, skill in self-care, and a positive self-concept and body image.

MENOPAUSE

With the increasing life span of American women, most women can expect to live one third of their lives after their reproductive years. As women age, many experience transitions that present challenges such as changing health, work, or marital status that require adaptation. Nowhere is this more true than with the changes associated with menopause. In the United States, most women have menopause during their late forties and early fifties, with the median age being approximately 51 years (McAllister, 1998). The average age for the onset of the perimenopausal transition is 46 years;

95% of women experience the onset between ages 39 and 51. The average duration of the perimenopause is 5 years, with a range of 2 to 8 years for 95% of women (Speroff et al., 1999). Cigarette smoking and a history of short intermenstrual intervals seem to decrease the age at onset of menopause. However, the popular belief that an early menarche predisposes to a late menopause is not substantiated. Unlike menarche, the average age of menopause has remained about the same since the Middle Ages.

Perimenopause is the period that encompasses the transition from normal ovulatory cycles to cessation of menses and is marked by irregular menstrual cycles. Another term used to signal the period when a woman moves from the reproductive stage of life through the perimenopausal transition and menopause to the postmenopausal years is the **climacteric.** **Menopause** refers to the complete cessation of menses and is a single physiologic event said to occur when women have not had menstrual flow or spotting for 1 year and can be identified only in retrospect. **Surgical menopause** occurs with hysterectomy and bilateral oophorectomy. **Postmenopause** is the time after menopause.

Although all women have similar hormonal changes with menopause, the experience of each woman is influenced by her age, cultural background, health, type of menopause (spontaneous or surgical), childbearing desires, and relationships. Women may view menopause as a major change in their lives–either positive, such as freedom from troublesome dysmenorrhea or the need for contraception, or negative, such as feeling "old" or losing childbearing possibilities.

Perimenopausal = ↓ Prog

Physiologic Characteristics

Knowledge of the normal changes that occur during the perimenopause is essential to the assessment of menopausal experiences and problems. Natural menopause is a gradual process with progressive increases in anovulatory cycles and eventual cessation of menses. In the 2 to 8 years preceding menopause, subtle hormonal changes eventually lead to altered menstrual function and later to amenorrhea. When women are in their forties, anovulation occurs more often, menstrual cycles increase in length, and ovarian follicles become less sensitive to hormonal stimulation from FSH and LH. Because of these changes, a follicle is stimulated to the point that an ovum grows to maturity and is released in some months, and in other months, no ovulation takes place. Without ovulation and release of an ovum, progesterone is not produced by the corpus luteum. The lining continues to grow until it lacks a sufficient blood supply, at which point it will bleed. During this time, a woman's cycle will become more irregular. She may skip or miss periods; have shorter or lighter periods or longer, heavier periods; and have clotting. FSH levels become elevated, reflecting an attempt to stimulate a follicle to produce estrogen.

Physical Changes During the Perimenopausal Period

Bleeding

During the perimenopausal years, women may have longer menstrual periods that differ in the type of bleeding. They may have 2 to 3 days of spotting followed by 1 to 2 days of heavy bleeding, or they may have regular menses followed by 2 to 3 days of spotting. Such symptoms are characteristic of degenerating corpus luteum function. After menopause, women continue to have small amounts of circulating estrogen. Although the ovaries do not produce estrogen, androgens (androstenedione and testosterone) are produced for some time after menopause. Androgens produced by the adrenal glands are converted to estrone, a form of estrogen, in the liver and fat cells (Kendig & Sanford, 1998). With advanced age, the ovaries stop producing androstenedione, which further limits the amount of estrone in the body. Obese women are more likely to have dysfunctional uterine bleeding and endometrial hyperplasia because women with more body fat have higher estrone levels.

Genital Changes

The vagina and urethra are estrogen-sensitive tissues, and low levels of estrogen can cause atrophy of both. Age-related vaginal changes not affected by estrogen also occur. Through both processes, the vaginal membranes thin, hold less moisture, and lubricate more slowly. However, not all women have symptoms of genital atrophy. Women who are sexually active have less vaginal atrophy and fewer problems related to intercourse (Avioli et al., 1997). Thin women are more likely to have more symptoms related to reduced estrogen levels such as vaginal dryness because of lack of adipose tissue and thus stored estrogen. Additionally, vaginal pH increases, lactobacilli growth can be depressed, and other bacteria tend to multiply. This combination of factors can lead to vaginitis.

Dyspareunia (painful intercourse) can occur because the vagina becomes smaller, the vaginal walls become thinner and dryer, and lubrication during sexual stimulation takes longer (Levine, 1998) (see Guidelines/Guías). Intercourse

GUIDELINES/GUÍAS

Menopause: Vaginal Dryness

Lack of hormone production in menopause can make the vagina dry.
Falta de producción de hormonas durante la menopausia puede causar que se seque la vagina.

Do you have decreased vaginal lubrication?
¿Tiene disminución en la lubricación vaginal?

Is intercourse painful for you?
¿Le da dolor al tener relaciones sexuales?

You may need to use a lubricant with intercourse.
Puede que necesite usar un lubricante en sus relaciones sexuales.

becomes painful and may result in postcoital bleeding. Some women may decide to forego intercourse altogether.

In some women, the shrinking of the uterus, vulva, and distal portion of the urethra associated with aging leads to disturbing symptoms, including urinary frequency, dysuria, uterine prolapse, and stress incontinence. Vaginal relaxation with cystocele, rectocele, and uterine prolapse is not caused by reduced estrogen levels but may be a delayed result of childbearing or other cause of weakness of pelvic support structures. Urinary frequency sometimes occurs after menopause because the distal portion of the urethra, which has the same embryologic origin as the reproductive organs, shortens and shrinks. Irritants have easier access to the urinary tract with its shorter urethra and may cause frequency and urinary tract infections.

Urinary incontinence and uterine displacement are two other common age-related rather than menopause-related findings in the postmenopausal period. These conditions are discussed in Chapter 12.

Vasomotor Instability

During the past three decades, investigators have devoted significant attention to identifying ovarian, hypothalamic, and pituitary hormonal mechanisms that produce symptoms related to menopause. Two symptoms appear to increase in incidence as women progress through menopause: hot flashes and night sweats. Many of the other changes commonly associated with menopause, such as decrease in size of genital structures, skin changes, and changes in breast size, are more correctly attributed to aging.

Vasomotor instability in the form of hot flashes or flushes is a result of fluctuating estrogen levels and is the most common disturbance of the perimenopausal years, occurring in up to 75% of women having natural menopause and 90% of women who have a surgical menopause. Vasomotor instability occurs most frequently in the first 2 postmenopausal years; the number of episodes decreases over time. However, some women have hot flashes before menopause and continue to have them for 10 to 20 years afterward. During this time, women experience changeable vasodilation and vasoconstriction as a **hot flush** (visible red flush of skin and perspiration) or **hot flash** (sudden warm sensation in neck, head, and chest) and night sweats. These disturbances vary widely in severity, and only a minority of women seek health care for them. Hot flushes and flashes can occur often throughout the day and may continue for several months or years. For some women, hot flashes may be an infrequent, possibly pleasant, sensation of warmth; for others, they may be an intensely unpleasant sensation of heat or warmth that may occur 20 to 50 times a day, create intense anxiety, and significantly decrease quality of life. Surveys of midlife women have found that, in the absence of menopausal hormonal therapy, most affected women will have disturbances for 1 to 2 years, and 25%, up to 5 years (Speroff et al., 1999). Several factors can precipitate or aggravate an episode, including crowded or warm rooms, alcohol, hot drinks, spicy foods, proximity to a heat source, and stress.

Night sweats, characterized by profuse perspiration and heat radiating from the body during the night, are another form of vasomotor instability experienced by many women. Sleep may be interrupted nightly because nightclothes and bed linens may be soaked. Women may find that they are not able to go back to sleep. Other problems that may be associated with perimenopausal fluctuations of vasoconstriction or vascular spasms include dizziness, numbness and tingling in fingers and toes, and headaches.

Mood and Behavioral Responses

The tendency to associate hormonal changes with psychologic symptoms in midlife that has been prevalent in medical literature for decades and continues today was fueled by a belief that postmenopausal women have "estrogen deficiency." Contrary to this common belief, there is no concrete evidence that menopause has a deleterious effect on mental health of midlife women. Findings from the Massachusetts Women's Health Study documented that menopause is not associated with an increased risk for mental health problems. Furthermore, reviews of epidemiologic studies on menopause and depression found no causal association between menopause and depression (Sowers, 2000). Women with hot flashes and night sweats do report insomnia, fatigue from loss of sleep, and depressed mood. Women complain of feeling more emotionally labile, nervous, or agitated, with less control of their emotions. However, the interaction of psychologic, biologic, and sociocultural factors is so complex that it is difficult to determine whether a woman's reported mood shifts are the result of hormonal changes, normal aging, or cultural conditioning. Most likely a woman's psychologic makeup, cultural background, intercurrent stresses, and changing life roles and circumstances are more important than estrogen levels. Dealing with teenage children; having teenagers leave home; helping aging parents; becoming widowed or divorced; the onset of a major illness or disability (even death) in a spouse, relative, or friend; grieving for friends and family who are ill or dying; retirement; and financial insecurity are among the many stresses of women in their forties and fifties.

Cultural messages also influence individual women's perception of menopause. Women's experiences with menopause are not universal and vary among cultural groups. Most American women do not believe that menopause interferes with their quality of life (McAllister, 1998). Women do not find symptoms to be troublesome; however, they do report that symptoms are bothersome. Many women have accepted childbearing and child rearing as their major role in life, and the inability to bear children is a significant loss. Others see menopause as the first step to old age and associate it with a loss of attractiveness, physical ability, and energy. Western culture values youth and physical attractiveness; the wisdom gained from life experience is not valued, and the elderly have a loss of status, function, and role. No rituals give older women a special place and function. In cultures where postmenopausal women gain status, such as India, the Far East, and the South Pacific Islands, depression among menopausal women is not observed. Western women, however, may have little to compensate for their losses.

For other women, menopause is not a loss or a symbol of losses, but a relief. For some, menopause is a relief from the fear of pregnancy, the discomfort and bother of menstruation, and the inconveniences of contraception.

The ability to cope with any stress involves three factors: the person's perception or understanding of the event, support system, and coping mechanisms. Nurses counseling women in their perimenopausal years must therefore assess their understanding of perimenopausal changes, their perceptions of stressful experiences, their support systems, and their repertoire of coping skills.

Health Risks of Perimenopausal Women

Osteoporosis and coronary heart disease are the major health risks of perimenopausal women and are the focus of the following discussion.

Osteoporosis

Aging is associated with a progressive decrease in bone density in both men and women. **Osteoporosis** is a generalized, metabolic disease characterized by decreased bone mass and increased incidence of bone fractures. Normally there is a dynamic balance between bone formation (osteoblastic activity) and bone resorption (osteoclastic activity). Because one of the functions of estrogen is to stimulate the osteoblasts, the postmenopausal decrease in estrogen levels causes an imbalance between bone formation and resorption. Old bone deteriorates faster than new bone is formed, resulting in a slow thinning of the bones. Estrogen also is required for the conversion of vitamin D into calcitonin, which is essential in the absorption of calcium by the intestine. Reduced calcium absorption from the gut, in addition to the thinning of the bones, places postmenopausal women at risk for problems associated with osteoporosis.

Osteoporosis is a major health problem in the United States, affecting more than 25 million women older than 45 years (Garcini & Strong, 1999). Approximately 50% of American women have some degree of osteoporosis. One in two will have changes severe enough to predispose them to fractures. In the United States, the incidence of osteoporosis-related fractures has increased in the past 20 years. Among those who have a hip fracture, 12% to 20% die within 1 year after the fracture, and more than half are unable to return to independent living (Kendig & Sanford, 1998). Of these, the overwhelming majority are older women. During the first 5 to 6 years after menopause, women lose bone 6 times more rapidly than do men. By age 65 years, one third of women have had a vertebral fracture; by age 81 years, one third have had a hip fracture. By the time women reach age 80 years, they have lost 47% of their trabecular bone, concentrated in the vertebrae, pelvis and other flat bones, and the epiphyses. The most well-defined risk factor for osteoporosis is the loss of the protective effect of estrogen associated with cessation of ovarian function, particularly at menopause. Women at risk are likely to be Caucasian or Asian, small boned, and thin. Obese women have higher estrogen levels resulting from the conversion of androgens in adipose tissue; mechanical stress from extra weight also helps preserve bone mass. A family history of the disease is common. The influences of heredity, race, and sex may result in differences in peak bone mass.

Inadequate calcium intake is a risk factor, particularly during adolescence and into the third and fourth decade, when peak bone mass is attained (Speroff et al., 1999). An excessive caffeine intake increases calcium excretion, causing a systemic acidosis that stimulates bone resorption. Smoking is associated with earlier and greater bone loss and decreases estrogen production. Excessive alcohol intake interferes with calcium absorption and depresses bone formation. A greater phosphorus than calcium intake, which occurs with soft drink consumption, may be a risk factor. Other risk factors include steroid therapy and disorders such as hypogonadism and hyperthyroidism.

The first sign of osteoporosis is often loss of height resulting from vertebral fracture and collapse (Fig. 7-2). Back pain, especially in the lower back, may or may not be present. Later signs include "dowager's hump," in which the vertebrae can no longer support the upper body in an upright position, and fractured hip, in which the fracture often precedes a fall. Damage to the vertebrae usually precedes bone loss in the hip by an average of 10 years. Osteoporosis cannot be detected by radiographic examination until 30% to 50% of the bone mass has been lost;

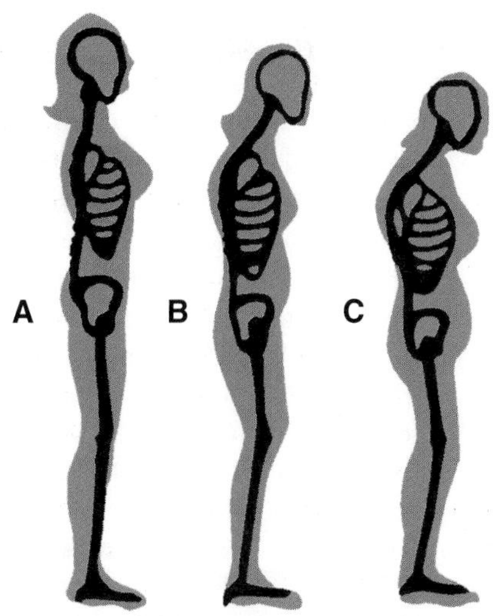
A
B
C

FIG. 7-2 Skeletal changes secondary to osteoporosis assessed by height and body shape at **A,** age 55 years; **B,** age 65 years; and **C,** age 75 years.

thus routine screening is not warranted. However, bone density testing is recommended by the National Osteoporosis Foundation for women at high risk for osteoporosis and for all women older than 65 years to assess fracture risk (National Osteoporosis Foundation, 2000). Medicare will pay for tests for high risk women. Insurance reimbursement varies for the tests, which cost about $700.

Coronary Heart Disease

A woman's risk of developing and dying of cardiovascular disease increases after menopause. Diseases of the heart are the leading cause of death for women in the United States. Known risk factors for coronary heart disease include obesity, cigarette smoking, elevated cholesterol and blood pressure levels, diabetes mellitus, family history of cardiac disease, alcohol abuse, and the effects of aging on the cardiovascular system (Keller, Fullerton, & Fleury, 1998; Speroff et al., 1999). Postmenopausal women are at risk for coronary artery disease because of changes in lipid metabolism: a decline in serum levels of HDL cholesterol and an increase in LDL levels.

These changes can be favorably reduced by diet and exercise (Halm & Penque, 1999). Estrogen has a favorable effect on circulating lipids, decreasing LDL and total cholesterol and increasing HDL, and has a direct antiatherosclerotic effect on arteries.

Menopausal Hormonal Therapy

Until recently, **menopausal hormonal therapy (MHT)**—more commonly known as **estrogen replacement therapy (ERT)** or **estrogen therapy (ET),** in which a woman takes only estrogen, or **hormonal replacement therapy (HRT),** in which she takes both estrogen and progestins—was widely prescribed for discomforts associated with the perimenopausal years, including hot flashes and vaginal and urinary tract atrophy. Further, MHT was aggressively used for both therapeutic and preventive management. At the same time, its use remained a highly controversial issue in women's health. Some authorities recommended MHT or ET for all women; these proponents viewed the perimenopause as a disease or deficiency state. Others insisted that the use of hormones was never indicated for menopausal symptoms. The middle-ground approach advocated the use of hormonal therapy for women who have specific discomforts (therapeutic management) and for women in certain high risk groups (preventive management). All that changed with research studies that challenged the long-held beliefs in the preventive and beneficial effects of MHT (Hulley et al., 1998; 2002; Kaunitz, 2002b; Writing Group for the Women's Health Initiative [WHI] Investigators, 2002) and documented increased risks for blood clots, heart attack, stroke, and invasive breast cancer with long-term use of the PremPro formulation (combined estrogen-progestin) of MHT.

These findings will change the way MHT is used in women without hysterectomies. Although the absolute risk for these adverse outcomes in an individual woman is very low, menopausal women should be aware of the most current research to make an informed decision regarding if, when, and for how long they use MHT.

Decision to Use Hormone Therapy

All women considering ET or MHT must understand that studies on MHT are ongoing, and there is still much to be learned. Nurses can provide information and counseling to assist women to make decisions regarding MHT use (see Research box). Important teaching points include (American College of Obstetricians and Gynecologists, 2002; American Health Consultants, 2002; Berg, 2002):

- For women taking MHT for short-term (1 to 3 years) relief of menopausal discomforts and who do not have increased risks for cardiovascular disease, the benefits may outweigh the risks. The decision to use HRT should be made between a woman and her health care provider.
- Women who are taking or considering MHT only for the prevention of cardiovascular disease should be counseled on other methods to reduce their risks of cardiovascular disease.
- Women who are taking MHT only for prevention of osteoporosis should be counseled regarding their personal risks and benefits for continuing the therapy and reassured that there are effective alternatives for long-term prevention. Bone density studies also may be indicated to determine the degree of risk in an individual woman.
- Women with a high risk for breast cancer or who have had breast cancer should be counseled against using MHT.
- Estrogen-only use by women who have had a hysterectomy continues to be studied.
- MHT may worsen myomas of the uterus and porphyria.
- Conjugated estrogens are associated with an increased incidence of gallbladder disease, and women with a known history of gallbladder disease should not use ET or MHT.
- When a woman decides to stop MHT, gradual withdrawal to prevent return of symptoms by rapid withdrawal of estrogen is advised (Warren & Kulak, 1999).

Nurses are encouraged to stay current with ongoing MHT research findings. At present the only type of MHT that may be contraindicated for menopausal women is the combined conjugated estrogen-medroxyprogesterone formulation. As other WHI data on MHT are analyzed, further clarification of the issues will be published. One easily accessible resource is the American College of Obstetricians and Gynecologists; this organization regularly produces national guidelines and standards of practice with midlife and menopausal women and will update recommendations as new information becomes available.

Side Effects

Side effects associated with estrogen use include headaches, nausea and vomiting, bloating, ankle and feet swelling, weight gain, breast soreness, brown spots on the skin, eye irritation with contact lenses, and depression.

RESEARCH

Factors Affecting Intent to Use Hormone Replacement Therapy for Menopause

As the cohort of menopausal women is growing, information about hormone replacement therapy (HRT) continues to evolve. Most dramatically, researchers halted clinical trials of the benefits of HRT because of increased health risks, including breast cancer and increased cardiovascular events. Still, women continue to experience menopause symptoms that may affect the quality of their life and wonder about the advisability of HRT for them.

Multiple factors affect women's decision to use HRT, according to retrospective urban studies. One nurse researcher developed a prospective study and surveyed 167 rural women from Wyoming and Nebraska, ages 39 to 58, most of whom were not experiencing menopausal symptoms. Variables measured included (1) attitude toward menopause; (2) knowledge about menopause; (3) perception of support for HRT from family, friends, and health care providers; and (4) self-efficacy, or perceived control, in adopting HRT. The investigator analyzed the effect of these independent variables on the dependent variable of clients' intent to use HRT in the future. Analysis showed that women's knowledge about menopause, perception of the support for HRT, and self-efficacy may be positive predictors of intent to use HRT. Self-efficacy was found to predict intent to use HRT more than any other variable. Attitudes about menopause were found to be mildly positive; knowledge about menopause physiology and risks of HRT was weak; and support for adoption of HRT was provided to some degree by the woman's support group, including her health care provider. Rural women tend to seek treatment only if their ability to function is affected. This study measured the theoretic future intent to take HRT, and the outcome may be different if menopausal symptoms occur and interfere with daily activities.

IMPLICATIONS FOR PRACTICE

This research and other studies underscore the need for nurses and other health care providers to educate midlife women about menopause and the risks and benefits of HRT and alternative therapies. The nurse can explore the woman's attitude about menopause as a normal event and encourage use of her support network as a way to assist her through the menopause transition.

Resource: Wilhelm, S. (2002). Factors affecting a woman's intent to adopt hormone replacement therapy for menopause. *Journal of Obstetric, Gynecologic, and Neonatal Nursing, 31*(6), 698-707.

The type of estrogen used for postmenopausal ET is much less potent than ethinyl estradiol used in OCPs and has fewer serious side effects. Side effects that occur with MHT or ET may disappear with a change in estrogen preparation or a decrease in the dose prescribed.

Treatment Guidelines

Although many women will discontinue use of MHT based on the current research findings, others will continue because they believe the benefits of the therapy in relieving their symptoms or preventing osteoporosis to outweigh the risks. Research in this important area continues; however, nurses who must counsel women about MHT must understand what is available and teach women who choose to continue MHT how to take the medications correctly. Thus the following discussion about the different regimens of MHT is included.

Many different estrogen preparations, natural and synthetic, and ways of administering them–oral tablets, topical creams, transdermal preparations, injectables, suppositories, and vaginal implants–exist (Table 7-4). However, most women today use either tablets or the transdermal patch.

Previous regimens of sequential MHT prescribed estrogen in combination with progesterone to simulate the normal menstrual cycle. This created a 5- to 6-day period at the end of the month when no hormones were taken and breakthrough bleeding occurred. This regimen was cumbersome to explain and difficult for women to follow; therefore a more convenient regimen of a continuous dose of estrogen (0.625 mg) on days 1 to 28 and intermittent progestins (2.5 mg medroxyprogesterone) on days 14 to 28 is the most commonly prescribed. Women usually do not have cyclical bleeding with this regimen and are less likely to have progestin side effects. An alternative regimen is continuous combined MHT with estrogen and progestin taken daily, but this regimen is no longer recommended.

The transdermal patch is applied once a week to a hairless area of skin. Any site on the trunk or upper arms provides adequate absorption. Sites should be rotated. The patches should not be placed on the breasts because of their sensitivity. Some women report minor skin irritation and reddening at the patch site. Generally transdermal estrogen offers the same relief of menopausal symptoms as the oral preparation. The transdermal method of delivery of estrogen does not have the same side effects such as breast tenderness and fluid retention. Oral progestin therapy can be used with transdermal ET. Combined estrogen-progestin transdermal patches also are available.

Alternative Therapies

Many complementary and alternative therapies are useful for relieving some of the changes associated with altered estrogen levels. Homeopathy, acupuncture, and herbs have been used successfully for menopausal problems such as heavy bleeding, hot flashes, irritability, and headaches (Box 7-2).

Homeopathy views menopausal symptoms as the body's efforts to heal itself from the hormonal changes it is experiencing. Examples of remedies commonly prescribed during menopause by homeopaths are sepia, made from the inky juice of the cuttlefish, to relieve symptoms

TABLE 7-4 **Oral and Transdermal Estrogen Equivalences, Vaginal Estrogen Creams, and Progestin Equivalences**

TRADE NAME	GENERIC NAME	DOSAGES	METHOD
Estrogen Equivalences			
Premarin	Conjugated estrogens	0.3 mg 0.625 mg 0.9 mg 1.25 mg 2.5 mg	Oral
Estrace	Micronized estradiol	0.5 mg 1.0 mg 2.0 mg	Oral
Estratab Menest	Esterified estrogens	0.3 mg 0.625 mg 1.25 mg 2.5 mg	Oral
Estratest	Esterified estrogens with methyltestosterone	0.635 mg esterified estrogen + 1.25 mg methyltestosterone 1.25 mg esterified estrogens + 2.5 mg methyltestosterone	Oral
Ortho-Est Ogen	Estropipate	0.625 mg 1.25 mg 2.5 mg	Oral
Estraderm	Transdermal estradiol	0.05 mg; 0.1 mg	Transdermal patch
Climera		0.05 mg; 0.1 mg	Release rates mg/24 hr
FemPatch		0.025 mg	
Esclim		0.025 mg; 0.0375 mg; 0.075 mg; 0.1 mg	
Vivelle		0.0375 mg; 0.05 mg; 0.075 mg; 0.1 mg	
Alora		0.05 mg; 0.075 mg; 0.1 mg	
Vaginal Estrogen Creams/Rings			
Premarin	Conjugated estrogens	0.625 mg/g	Vaginal
Estrace	Estadiol	0.1 mg/g	Vaginal
Ogen	Estropipate	1.5 mg/g	Vaginal
Dienestrol	Dienestrol	0.01%	Vaginal
Estring	Estradiol	2 mg	Vaginal
Progestin Equivalencies			
Provera	Medroxyprogesterone acetate	2.5 mg 5.0 mg 10 mg	Oral
Curretabs	Medroxyprogesterone	10 mg	Oral
Aygestin	Norethindrone acetate	5 mg	Oral
Micronor	Norethindrone	0.35 mg	Oral
Prometrium	Progesterone USP	200 mg	Oral
Combination Estrogen-Progestin			
Prempro	Conjugated estrogens Medroxyprogesterone acetate	0.625 mg 2.5 mg or 5 mg	Oral (1 combination tablet/day for 28 days)
Premphase	Conjugated estrogens Medroxyprogesterone acetate	0.625 mg 5 mg	Oral (14 days of estrogen only, then 14 days of both)
Combined Estrogen/Progestin			
CombiPatch	Estradiol/norethindone acetate (NETA)	0.05 mg estradiol/0.14 mg NETA or 0.05 mg estradiol/0.25 mg NETA	Transdermal (release rates mg/24 hr)

Source: Facts and Comparisons. (2002). *Loose-leaf drug information service.* St. Louis: Facts and Comparisons; CombiPatch package insert. Collegeville, PA, Rhone-Poulenc Rorer Pharmaceuticals, Inc.; Prometrium® capsule package insert (2001). Marietta, GA: Solvay Pharmaceuticals Inc.

BOX 7-2 **Alternatives to Hormonal Therapy for Menopausal Symptoms**

HOT FLASH/FLUSH

Vitamin E: 100-800 IU daily (≤100 IU in the presence of high blood pressure, diabetes, or rheumatic heart disease). Start with a low dose and increase over 6-8 weeks to 800 IU or less if symptoms improve.

Bioflavonoids (500 mg-1 g) combined with vitamin C. Dietary sources include wheat germ, whole grains, vegetable oils, soybeans, peanuts, spinach and other dark green leafy vegetables, and cold pressed oils.

Herbal therapy: see Table 7-5

Soy: 40 to 100 mg isoflavones or approximately 30 to 50 g soy protein

Vitamin B complex: 1 to 2 daily. Dietary sources include whole grains, wheat germ, yogurt, brewer's yeast, and milk.

Vitamin C

Acupuncture

Medications other than hormone replacement:
- Bellergal (can increase high blood pressure)
- Belladonna (side effects: dry mouth, rapid pulse, constipation)
- Clonidine (side effects: sleepiness, dry mouth, decreased blood pressure)

INSOMNIA

Herbal therapy:
- Valerian (natural tranquilizer)
- Peppermint, catnip, hops, passionflower
- Chamomile

HEADACHES

Herbal therapy:
- Natural diuretics (parsley)
- Chasteberry, peppermint oil, feverfew, royal jelly products

UROGENITAL SYMPTOMS

For vaginal dryness and itching:
- Vitamin E: 400-800 IU daily or vitamin E oil on the skin
- Evening primrose oil, aloe vera, slippery elm paste
- Witch hazel and glycerin (dip pads in mixture and apply to skin for itching)

NERVOUSNESS/IRRITABILITY

Vitamin B_6: 5 to 25 mg daily. Dietary sources include brewer's yeast, bran, wheat germ, organ meats, molasses, walnuts, peanuts, and brown rice.

Sources: ACOG Committee on Practice Bulletins & Taylor, M. (2001). Use of botanicals for management of menopausal symptoms. *ACOG Practice Bulletin No. 28, June 2001.* Accessed 10/11/02 at www.acog.org; Blumenthal, M. (Ed.). (1998). *The complete German Commission E monographs: Therapeutic guide to herbal medicines.* Austin, TX: The American Botanical Council; Israel, D., & Youngkin, E. (1997). Herbal therapies for perimenopausal and menopausal complaints. *Pharmacotherapy, 17*(5), 970-984; Lowdermilk, D., & Fogel, C. (1996). *Health care issues of midlife women.* Edwardsville, KS: Educational Software; Ramsey, L., Ross, B., & Fischer, R. (1999). Phytoestrogens and the management of menopause. *Advances for Nurse Practitioners, 7*(1), 27-30.

such as dry mouth, eyes, and vagina; nux vomica, derived from the poison nut, to relieve backaches, constipation, and frequent awakenings; and pulsatilla, made from the windflower, to relieve severe menstrual symptoms and hot flashes. Homeopathic remedies are subject to regulation by the U.S. FDA, although the FDA does not require proof of effectiveness (Beal, 1998).

Acupuncturists also treat hot flashes, but it is important that women evaluate their acupuncturists carefully. The American Association of Acupuncturists and Oriental Medicine will supply a list of acupuncturists in a given state (see Resources at end of chapter). Questions to ask are, "Is the acupuncturist certified by the National Commission for the Certification of Acupuncture? Is the acupuncturist certified in the state in which he or she practices? Does the acupuncturist carry malpractice insurance?"

Herbal therapy also has been used to treat menopausal discomforts (Table 7-5). Herbs can be ingested as teas or tinctures. Many herbal preparations also are available in capsule form. It is important that women understand mechanisms of action, contraindications, and potential side effects of each herb.

NURSE ALERT

Most herbal preparations have not undergone long-term testing for safety and efficacy. Benefits and risks are not completely known. Women should always consult with their health care provider before beginning herbal therapy.

In addition to resolving physical symptoms, herbs also are used to combat mood swings and depression. Ginseng has been claimed to be helpful in alleviating hot flashes, although research studies have not supported this assertion. Women should be advised against prolonged use of ginseng in high doses because it can increase blood pressure. Oriental herbal teas composed of licorice, ginseng, coptis, red raspberry leaf, and Chinese rhubarb may be of some help in relieving hot flashes.

Dong quai and black cohosh have been used to treat menopausal discomforts; both have been investigated for effectiveness, with varying results (Hirata, 1997; Liberman, 1998). Black cohosh has been used by Native Americans for a variety of problems, including gynecologic, and it was a major ingredient in Lydia Pinkham's Vegetable Compound, a well-known nineteenth-century patent medicine (Beal, 1998).

TABLE 7-5 **Herbals for Menopausal Symptoms**

SYMPTOM/INDICATION	HERB	ACTIONS	DOSE
Menopausal symptoms	Black cohosh*	Bind estrogen receptor, inhibits LH secretion and nonreceptor-mediated actions	Approved for 6-mo use. 20-80 mg bid
Premenstrual syndrome	Chaste tree fruit*	Alters FSH and LH levels; increases progesterone levels	30-40 mg extracts
Sleep disturbances, GI complaints, nervousness	Lemon balm	Tranquilizer/sedative	1.5-4.5 g herb as a tea
Memory deficits, impaired concentration	Ginkgo	Stimulates circulation and oxygen flow	120-240 mg in two to three doses
Fatigue, loss of concentration	Ginseng	Stimulant	1-2 g root as infusion in two to three doses
Anxiety, insomnia, nervousness	Passionflower	Tranquilizer/sedative	4-8 g herb as tea 2-3 times/day 30 min before sleep
Depression, anxiety	St. John's wort	Antidepressive	300 mg tid
Nervousness, insomnia	Valerian	Tranquilizer/sedative	2-3 g/day as infusion or extract, 1 or more times/day
"Women's discomforts"	Dong quai	Stimulate/relax uterus; anti-inflammatory; possibly analgesic activity	3.5-4.0 g/day 4.5 g tincture or extract

*Approved by Commission E specifically for treatment of menopausal symptoms.

Sources: Blumenthal, M. (ed.) (1998). *The complete German Commission E monographs: Therapeutic guide to herbal medicines.* Austin, TX: American Botanical Council; Gladstar, R. (1993). *Herbal healing for women.* New York: Simon & Schuster; Huntley, A. (2002). Complementary therapies for the relief of menopausal symptoms. *Focus on Alternative and Complementary Therapies,* 7(2), 121-125; Israel, D., & Youngkin, E. (1997). Herbal therapies for perimenopausal and menopausal complaints.

CONSIDERATIONS/ SIDE EFFECTS	CONTRAINDICATIONS
Additive hypotensive effects with antihypertensive agents	Pregnancy, lactation
GI side effects, headaches, dizziness, and bradycardia with high doses	
May inhibit prolactin secretion; may interfere with dopamine antagonist	Pregnancy, lactation
Pruritic rash, GI side effects	
No known side effects, no known drug interactions	NK
Side effects: allergic reactions, mild GI upset	Inhibits platelet-activating factor; not to be used with antithrombotic therapy
Side effects: insomnia, tachycardia, palpitations, hypertension, ginseng abuse syndrome reported with overuse	Do not take with vitamin C; avoid if diabetic; do not use if have cardiac problems
	May be associated with postmenopausal bleeding
NK side effects	NK
NK drug interactions	
Photosensitivity can occur	Contraindicated with MAO inhibitors or SSRIs
Allergic & GI side effects rare	NK
NK drug interactions with long-term use	
Headaches, restlessness, insomnia, cardiac dysfunction possible	
Phototoxicity	Pregnancy:
Liver and renal damage in animal studies; abortifacient	Coumarin components may increase risk of bleeding

Pharmacotherapy, 17(5), 970-984; Veet, L. (2000). *Women's health care clinical vignettes.* Philadelphia: Hanley & Belfus, Inc.

bid, Twice a day; *FSH,* follicle-stimulating hormone; *GI,* gastrointestinal; *LH,* luteinizing hormone; *MAO,* monoamine oxidase; *NK,* not known; *SSRI,* selective serotonin reuptake inhibitor; *tid,* three times a day.

Some plant foods contain **phytoestrogens** (isoflavones) and are capable of interacting with estrogen receptors in the body. These foods include wild yams, dandelion greens, cherries, alfalfa sprouts, black beans, and soybeans (Beal, 1998). Use of soy-rich foods as an alternative to traditional hormonal therapy for menopause has been studied, and beneficial effects on menopausal symptoms and on reducing cholesterol have been documented (Ramsay, Ross, & Fischer, 1999). However, more research is needed to better understand the potential effects of soy intake on prevention of osteoporosis and reducing risks of coronary heart disease (Lindsay & Claywell, 1998). For women who want to add soy to their diets, tofu, roasted soy nuts, and soy milk are good sources. Foods should be added gradually because some women have gastrointestinal discomfort from the high fiber content of these foods (National Women's Health Report, 1999).

Vitamin E is a popular alternative among women who do not take MHT. Women who take vitamin E regularly report relief from hot flushes, leg cramps, and loss of energy. Vitamin E is found in a variety of foods, including spinach, peanuts, wheat germ, vegetable oils, and soybeans, or may be taken as a supplement. Dosage varies widely, from 400 to 800 IU/day.

Layered clothing, ice packs, iced water, and fans may offer symptomatic relief from hot flashes (see Teaching for Self-Care box). Women can be counseled to avoid hot curries and other spicy foods. Reassurance that hot flashes will not last forever may be of comfort even if duration of the problem cannot be predicted accurately. Most women find that hot flashes disappear within 4 to 6 years after menopause.

Nurses should be aware of the availability of natural remedies for menopausal symptoms and be knowledgeable about the indications for complementary and alternative therapies so that clients can be counseled appropriately.

CARE MANAGEMENT

Assessment and Nursing Diagnoses

A thorough health history, physical examination, and laboratory tests are essential to distinguish pathologic conditions from the normal perimenopausal experiences. Personal or family history of breast or uterine cancer, hypertension, thrombophlebitis, liver or gallbladder disease, undiagnosed uterine bleeding, and other acute or chronic diseases are noted, as are hysterectomy and bilateral oophorectomy. Recent changes in menstrual history help identify the phase of the perimenopausal period the woman is experiencing, and risk factors for osteoporosis are identified. The woman's perception of this stage of life, ethnic and cultural factors, and knowledge and concerns about sexuality and care available are

TEACHING FOR SELF-CARE

Comfort Measures

HOT FLASHES/FLUSHES

During the day

- Wear layered clothing so you can take things off if you get warm.
- Avoid "triggers" that bring on a flash/flush; these include vigorous exercise on hot days, eating spicy foods, caffeine, hot beverages, and alcohol.
- Splash your face with cool water, drink iced water, or take a cool shower if you get warm.
- Try slow, deep breathing.

At night

- Sleep in cotton clothes, use cotton sheets, and keep room cool.
- Avoid heavy blankets that make you too warm at night.
- Keep a thermos of water by the bed.

INSOMNIA

- Avoid caffeine, alcohol, or tobacco in the evening.
- Avoid liquids after dinner.
- Exercise regularly but limit exercise to the daytime and early evening.
- Develop a bedtime routine.
- Establish a regular time to go to bed.
- Try drinking warm milk or having a hot bath.
- Use your bed only for sleeping or sexual activity; don't watch TV, read, etc.
- Encourage your body's circadian rhythm.
- If you can't sleep, get up and do something until you feel tired.
- Avoid naps during the day.
- Sprinkle lavender oil on the pillow.
- Drink chamomile tea (do not use if allergic to ragweed or chrysanthemums).

HEADACHES

- Try to avoid stress and get plenty of rest.
- Eat or drink foods that contain natural diuretics (parsley).

UROGENITAL SYMPTOMS

- Drink lots of water, and empty bladder frequently.
- Practice Kegel exercises daily.
- Wear cotton underwear and avoid wet bathing suits for a prolonged time.
- Use water-soluble lubricants for vaginal dryness.

NERVOUSNESS, IRRITABILITY

- Practice yoga or other meditation.
- Do relaxation or deep breathing exercises.
- Practice guided imagery.

Source: Lowdermilk, D., & Fogel, C. (1996). *Health care issues of midlife women.* Edwardsville, KS: Educational Software.

all recorded. The practices and remedies the woman has used for menopausal symptoms are assessed, including pharmacologic and alternative therapies.

Nursing diagnoses for perimenopausal women may include the following:

- *Deficient knowledge related to*
  - –menopause and its management
- *Readiness for enhanced family coping related to*
  - –receiving information about the condition, its management, and prognosis
  - –emotional support
- *Risk for pain related to*
  - –changing ovarian function
- *Risk for injury related to*
  - –osteoporosis
  - –heart disease
- *Risk for sexual dysfunction related to*
  - –changes associated with changing estrogen levels
- *Risk for situational low self-esteem related to*
  - –physical and emotional changes during the perimenopausal period

Expected Outcomes of Care

Planning requires knowledge of the perimenopausal period and great sensitivity. Informed consent regarding MHT, weight-bearing exercise, and calcium supplements is a major concern because treatment may involve expense, inconvenience, and side effects. Expected outcomes are stated in terms of client behaviors. The woman will do the following:

- Explain the physical changes associated with menopause.
- View the perimenopausal period as a normal developmental phase instead of a deficiency disease.
- Have no discomforts that interfere with daily activities.
- Develop no symptoms or signs of osteoporosis or experience only minimal effect.
- Experience a healthy perimenopausal transition.
- Report concerns about changes associated with menopause and treatment.

Plan of Care and Interventions

Most women know little about menopause, and old wives' tales and misinformation can cause anxiety. They need to know what to expect, why it happens, and what measures will help make them more comfortable. Women appreciate the opportunity to discuss what they are experiencing. They need to know that their discomforts have a normal physiologic basis and that other women experience similar discomforts.

Treatment must be individualized for the specific woman. Menopause clinics are needed where research on the effects of various treatments can be developed and evaluated and where care by the various specialty groups involved, such as endocrinology, radiology, psychosocial resources, exercise physiology, and nutrition, can be effectively coordinated. Women's support groups also are needed. Areas that need further discussion include sexuality, nutrition, exercise, and support.

Sexual Counseling

Sexuality is a lifelong behavior, and contrary to common stereotypes, sex does not end with menopause. Many women remain sexually active throughout their entire lives. However, women and their partners may change their expression of sexuality during and after menopause, depending on physical changes, changes in the partner, and cultural myths and messages. Some women report decreases in interest and desire. These decreases in sexuality with aging are influenced more by culture and attitudes than by nature and physiology (hormones). Although some women report that it takes longer to reach orgasm and that the orgasm is not so intense, the capacity for orgasm is not decreased. There is no way to prevent the inevitable aging process that the body undergoes. For people who see aging as loss, sexuality may become difficult to incorporate into what they perceive to be a less attractive identity. The fear of rejection may be present.

Changes in a male partner may influence whether he continues to want to engage in sexual activity. As men age, they, too, take longer to reach orgasm; erections take longer to occur and are less firm. Men may believe they are becoming impotent or ill and give up sexual activity, viewing it as too frustrating. Women may believe their partners are losing interest in them. Couples may need counseling to understand these changes.

The two most important influences on older women's sexual activity are the strength of a relationship and the physical condition of each partner. The lack of available male partners can have a negative effect on sexual expression for many midlife and older women. Women outlive men, and older widowed and divorced women frequently have fewer opportunities to develop relationships because they are less sought after. In counseling older women who do engage in intercourse, the nurse cannot assume that new or nonmonogamous partners are free of STIs and should inform clients of their risk for human immunodeficiency virus infection and other STIs and the need to use condoms.

Older lesbian women largely have been a silent group whose sexual needs and special social circumstances have not been acknowledged or recognized. Although lesbian women in midlife and in later years do not face the problem of a lack of available male partners, they are faced with negative attitudes accompanying being old, female, and lesbian–all of which can adversely affect sexuality and sexual expression.

As long as women are able to bear children, some accept intercourse as part of their responsibility as wives. When menopause frees them from this duty, they may choose to forego intercourse. For other women, libido may increase without the fuss of contraception, fear of pregnancy, or interruption from menses.

Nurses must give accurate information on matters such as appropriate contraception, sexuality, and the physiology of menopause and should offer support and nonjudgmental guidance. Women need advice about contraception, because ovulation may not cease for a year after the last menstrual cycle, and menopausal women can still become pregnant. The nurse's attitude toward sex and the older woman is important. Negative attitudes can reinforce the client's misgivings about maintaining an active and satisfying sex life. The nurse can reassure the woman grieving over lost youth and attractiveness that the desire for sex into old age is a natural one and that the body has the capacity for sexual satisfaction. Only minor adjustments may be required.

Muscle tone around the reproductive organs decreases after menopause. Kegel exercises strengthen these muscles, improve tone, and, if practiced regularly, help prevent prolapsed uterus and stress incontinence. This is a low-cost, effective, noninvasive intervention to control symptoms. However, symptoms return if exercises are discontinued.

K-Y lubricating jelly, Replens, and Astroglyde are examples of water-soluble lubricants that provide relief from painful intercourse. They may be applied directly to the vulva and the penis. Oil-based lubricants such as petroleum jelly (Vaseline) should not be used because they clog vaginal glands, which can then be sites for bacterial infection.

The nurse can refer couples to a counselor or physician for problems beyond the scope of nursing practice.

Prolonged hospitalization of an elderly partner may have a significant impact on the couple's sexual relationship. They may have difficulty renewing sexual activity when the separation is over and may need counseling or referral. In the event that a couple is admitted to a nursing home, the nurse should encourage placement of the couple together. With the aging of the American population and changing attitudes about the appropriateness of lifelong sexual expression, long-term care, extended care, and full-term care facilities are more receptive to providing opportunities for sexual activity between marital partners.

Nutrition

Obesity and osteoporosis are common health problems of midlife and older women. As women move out of their childbearing years, they may need to change their diets. Because metabolic rates decrease with age and many women exercise less, fewer calories are needed for weight maintenance as women age. In general, foods chosen should be high in nutrients, fiber, and calcium but moderate in calories and low in fat to allow adequate nutritional intake while maintaining body weight. Nurses can suggest that women substitute skim for whole milk or chicken without skin for steak. Foods high in calcium and low in phosphorus are recommended. Excessive protein should be avoided. Fat-free milk and yogurt are good sources of calcium and vitamin D. It is difficult to eat other foods that contain calcium (sesame seeds, spinach, greens, broccoli, and seaweed) in quantities sufficient to meet daily requirements. Women should avoid excessive intake of alcohol, soft drinks, and caffeinated coffee.

Calcium is an essential part of any therapeutic regimen for women with osteoporosis and those who want to prevent osteoporosis. The best source of calcium is food; however, calcium supplements are recommended when a woman's diet does not supply recommended amounts of calcium. Although calcium cannot reverse loss of bone mass or prevent fractures, calcium supplementation may retard the development of osteoporosis after menopause. Menopausal women without contraindications to calcium supplementation (history of kidney stones, kidney failure, hypercalcemia) should be encouraged to consume a diet that has 1200 to 1500 mg of calcium a day or to add an amount of calcium supplementation that will increase their daily intake to this level. Calcium supplements are best taken in divided doses and with meals because of the increase in acid secretions and extended time in the stomach. At least 8 ounces of water to increase solubility is recommended. Calcium supplements should not be taken with caffeinated beverages. Calcium is most commonly available as calcium carbonate, calcium lactate, and calcium phosphate. Some of the calcium preparations (e.g., some generic brands) on the market are useless because they do not dissolve; Tums are most soluble. A combination of vitamin D and calcium (1200 mg) may be recommended as a supplement because vitamin D aids in calcium absorption. Mineral supplements are not classified as drugs by the FDA and are therefore not regulated, making it difficult for consumers to know which product is best.

Exercise

All too often, midlife women are sedentary–the demands of family and work constraints increase, and energy levels decrease. Unfortunately little or no exercise predisposes women to weight gain and does not help prevent cardiac disease or osteoporosis. Exercise alone cannot prevent or reverse osteoporosis, but data indicate that weight-bearing exercise, such as walking and stair climbing 30 to 60 minutes a day, may delay bone loss and increase bone mass at any age (Fig. 7-3).

Water aerobics is excellent for cardiovascular fitness and is a good choice for older women who may be unable to engage in weight-bearing exercises. The nurse can help women plan an exercise program. Examples of exercises are available from the National Osteoporosis Foundation (Fig. 7-4).

Medications

In addition to calcium and exercise, estrogen therapy, calcitonin, alendronate sodium (Fosamax), risedronate sodium (Actonel), or raloxifene (Evista) can be offered to women with postmenopausal osteoporosis. Calcitonin reduces the rate of bone turnover and stabilizes bone mass in women with osteoporosis and may have some analgesic effects. Although calcitonin can reduce the incidence of spinal fractures, no data are available about the use of calcitonin to protect against hip fractures (McClung, 1999). Calcitonin may be used with women in whom estrogen is contraindicated or not tolerated. The medication is very safe; however, side effects of nausea, vomiting, and anorexia have been reported. The drug is expensive and must be administered parenterally, thus limiting its use (Box 7-3).

Alendronate sodium and risedronate sodium are approved by the FDA for the treatment of osteoporosis in postmenopausal women. The medications assist in delaying bone loss, increasing bone mass, and preventing fractures.

NURSE ALERT

Clients must take alendronate sodium and risedronate sodium on an empty stomach with 6 to 8 ounces of plain water only, at least 30 minutes before eating or drinking to improve absorption (McClung, 1999); remaining upright for this 30 minutes also is recommended.

Raloxifene is approved by the FDA for osteoporosis prevention in postmenopausal women only. This medication preserves the beneficial effects of estrogen, including protection against cardiovascular diseases and osteoporosis, without stimulating breast and uterine tissues. It is not effective in reducing hot flashes or flushes. The medication modestly increases bone density (McClung, 1999). Calcium supplements should be taken if dietary intake is inadequate.

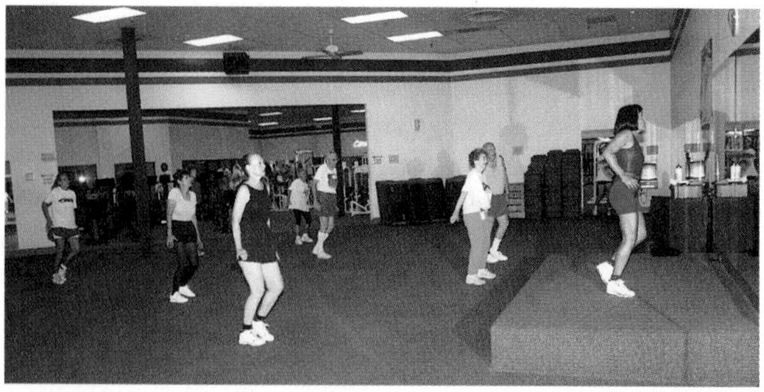

FIG. 7-3 Weight-bearing exercise is beneficial for the midlife woman. (Courtesy Jonas McCoy, Raleigh, NC).

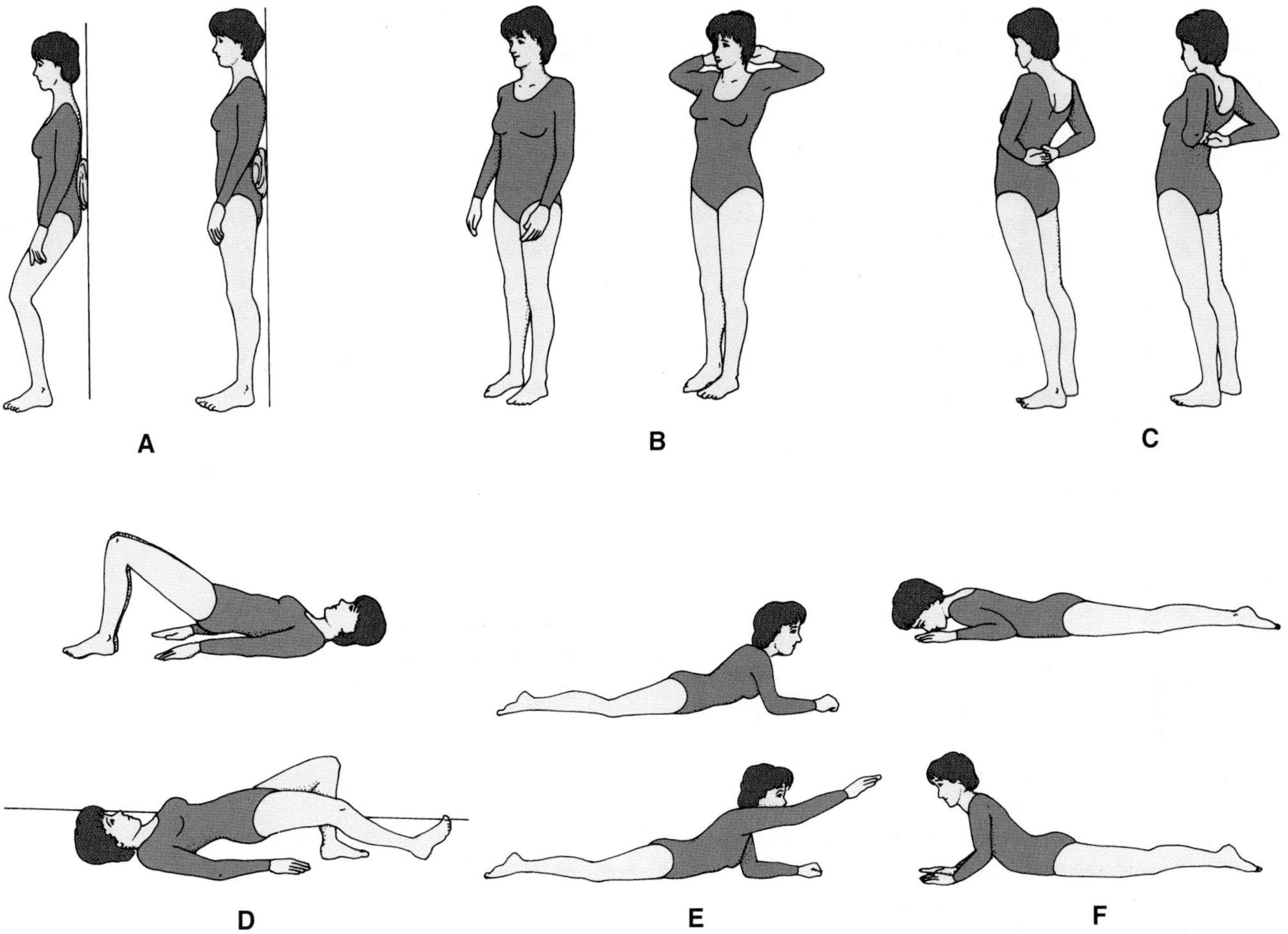
A
B
C
D
E
F

FIG. 7-4 **A,** Wall standing and pelvic tilt. **B,** Isometric posture correction. **C,** Standing back bend. **D,** The bridge. **E,** The elbow prop. **F,** Prone press-ups with deep breathing. (From *Boning Up On Osteoporosis*, courtesy the National Osteoporosis Foundation.)

BOX 7-3 Prevention of Osteoporosis

- Significant bone loss can be prevented by a well-balanced diet, including 200 to 400 IU of vitamin D and 1000 to 1200 mg of calcium a day, and regular weight-bearing exercise. Good sources of calcium are dairy products, fish, oysters, tofu, dark-green leafy vegetables, and whole wheat bread.
- Supplements of vitamin D and calcium can be taken, but the body cannot use them without the right balance of other vitamins and minerals.
- Eliminating environmental hazards in the home can decrease the risk of falls.
- Weight-bearing exercise 30 to 60 min/day may delay bone loss and increase bone mass.
- Raloxifene may be prescribed for prevention of osteoporosis in postmenopausal women.
- Alendronate sodium may be prescribed for women who already have osteoporosis to delay bone loss and increase bone mass.
- Estrogen therapy (ET) can be prescribed to prevent fractures from osteoporosis. The risks and benefits of ET used solely for osteoporosis prevention must be weighed on an individual basis with the health care provider.

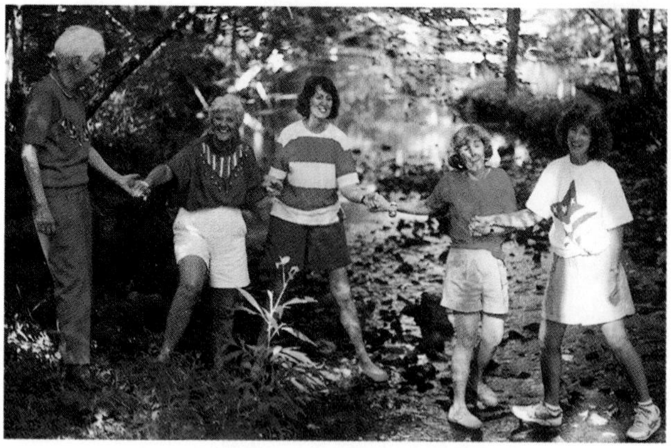

FIG. 7-5 Midlife women can develop a supportive network. (Courtesy Ed Lowdermilk, Chapel Hill, NC.)

Midlife Support Groups

Nurses should be familiar with local resources and direct women to classes that supply appropriate information and support. They can encourage women to develop a supportive network with other women with whom they can share their concerns (Fig. 7-5).

Women's centers and clinics may have support groups and classes for women who want to discuss menopause and other midlife events. If no group or class is available in the community, nurses should consider starting one.

Evaluation

The nurse can be reasonably assured that care was effective to the degree that the expected outcomes of care have been met.

KEY POINTS

- Menstrual disorders diminish the quality of life for affected women and their families.
- PMS, no longer considered a purely psychologic problem, is a disorder that begins in the luteal phase of the menstrual cycle and ends with the onset of menses.
- Endometriosis is characterized by secondary amenorrhea, dyspareunia, abnormal uterine bleeding, and infertility.
- The perimenopause is a normal developmental phase during which a woman passes from the reproductive to the nonreproductive stage.
- During the perimenopause, women seek care for symptoms that arise from bleeding irregularities, vasomotor instability, fatigue, genital changes, and changes related to sexuality.
- Alternative therapies are beneficial in relieving discomforts associated with menstrual disorders and menopause.
- Osteoporosis, a progressive loss of bone mass that results from decreasing levels of estrogen after menopause, can be prevented or minimized with lifestyle changes and medication
- Estrogen increases calcitonin levels to prevent bone resorption and maintain bone density.
- Sexuality and the ability for sexual expression continue after menopause.

CRITICAL THINKING EXERCISES

1. Prepare a presentation on the pros and cons of menopausal hormonal therapy. How would you counsel a 35-year-old woman who has had a hysterectomy? How would you counsel a 52-year-old woman who is having severe menopausal symptoms? How would you counsel a woman who is at high risk for osteoporosis?
2. Develop and present a session on self-help modalities for PMS symptoms. How would you evaluate the effectiveness of your presentation?
3. Review the literature for studies determining effectiveness of alternative therapies for menstrual problems. In a clinical conference, discuss therapies that have been shown to be beneficial, are likely to be beneficial, have unknown effects, or have effects that are likely not to be beneficial or may be harmful. Discuss how nurses can use this information in their clinical practices.

RESOURCES

American Association of Acupuncturists and Oriental Medicine Referrals
4101 Lake Boone Trail, Suite 201
Raleigh, NC 27607-6518
919-787-5181

American College of Obstetricians and Gynecologists
409 12th St.
Washington, DC 20024
800-762-2264
www.acog.org

Association of Women's Health, Obstetric, and Neonatal Nurses (AWHONN)
2000 L St., NW, Suite 740
Washington, DC 20036
800-673-8499 (United States)
800-245-0231 (Canada)
www.awhonn.org

Endometriosis Association
8585 North 76th Place
Milwaukee, WI 53223
414-355-2200
800-992-3636
www.ivf.com/endohtml.html

Food and Drug Administration (FDA)
Office of Consumer Affairs
Public Inquiries
5600 Fishers Lane (HFE-88)
Rockville, MD 20857
301-443-3170
www.fda.gov

National Osteoporosis Foundation
1150 17th St., Suite 500
Washington, DC 20036
800-223-9994
www.nof.org

National Women's Health Resource Center
120 Albany St., Suite 820
New Brunswick, NJ 08901
877-986-9472
www.healthywomen.org

Premenstrual Syndrome Action
P.O. Box 16292
Irvine, CA 92713
714-854-4407

Resolve, Inc. *(Impaired fertility)*
1310 Broadway, Dept. GM
Summerville, MA 02144-1713
617-623-0744
888-299-1585
www.resolve.org

The Jacob's Institute for Women's Health
409 12th St., SW
Washington, DC 20024

REFERENCES

Alexander, E., Shimp, L. & Smith, M. (2000). Obesity and eating disorders. In M. Smith & L. Shimp (Eds.), *20 common problems in women's health care.* New York: McGraw-Hill.

ACNM Clinical Bulletin (2002). Clinical Bulletin No. 6: Abnormal and dysfunctional uterine bleeding. *Journal of Midwifery and Women's Health, 47*(3), 207-213.

ACOG Committee on Practice Bulletins & Taylor, M. (2001). Use of botanicals for management of menopausal symptoms. *ACOG Practice Bulletin No. 28, June 2001.* http://www.acog.org. Retrieved 10/11/02.

American College of Obstetricians and Gynecologists. (2002). *Questions and answers on hormone replacement therapy.* Accessed 11/20/02 at www.acog.org.

American Health Consultants. (2002). Hormone replacement therapy: Review choices in light of new data. *Contraceptive Technology Update, 23*(9), 97-103.

Avioli, V. et al. (1997). *The postmenopausal health curriculum 101.* Chicago: Pramaton.

Baker, S. (1998). Menstruation and related problems and concerns. In E. Youngkin & M. Davis (Eds.), *Women's health.* Stamford, CT: Appleton & Lange.

Bascom, A. (2002). *Incorporating herbal medicine into clinical practice.* Philadelphia: F.A. Davis Company.

Beal, M. (1998). Women's use of complementary and alternative therapies in reproductive health. *Journal of Nurse Midwifery, 43*(3), 224-234.

Berg, E. (2002). When should HT be discontinued? *Journal Watch Women's health, 7*(9), 71.

Blackburn, S. (2003). *Maternal, fetal, & neonatal physiology: A clinical perspective* (3rd ed.). Philadelphia: Saunders.

Blumenthal, M. (Ed.). (1998). *The complete German commission E monographs: Therapeutic guide to herbal medicines.* Austin, TX: American Botanical Council.

Col, N. et al. (1997). Patient-specific decisions about hormone replacement therapy in postmenopausal women. *Journal of the American Medical Association, 277*(14), 1140-1147.

Cronje, W., & Studd, J. (2002). Premenstrual syndrome and premenstrual dysphoric disorder. *Primary Care, 29*(1), 1-12.

Dog, L. (2000). *An integrative approach to dysmenorrhea.* Corrales, NM: Integrative Medicine Education Association, LLC.

Dog, L. (2001). Conventional and alternative treatments for endometriosis. *Alternative Therapies, 7*(6), 50-56.

Dog, L. (2001). Endocrinology and women's issues. In *Third Annual Conference on Clinical Relevance of Medicinal Herbs and Nutritional Supplements in the Management of Major Medical Problems.* September 21-23, 2001.

Elliot, H. (2002). Premenstrual dysphoric disorder. *North Carolina Medical Journal, 63*(2), 72-75.

Facts and Comparisons. (2002). *Loose-leaf drug information service.* St. Louis: Facts and Comparisons.

Fogel, C. (1997). Endocrine causes of amenorrhea. *Primary Care Practice, 1*(5), 507-518.

Friedman, A., & Carlson, K. (2002). Uterine fibroids. In K. Carlson et al. (Ed.), *Primary care of women* (2nd ed.). St. Louis: Mosby.

Fugh-Berman, A., & Awang, D. (2001). Black cohosh. *Alternative Therapies in Women's Health, 39*(11), 81-85.

Garcini, F., & Strong, S. (1999). Care of the perimenopausal and postmenopausal woman. In M. Curtis & M. Hopkins (Eds.), *Glass's office gynecology* (5th ed.). Baltimore: Williams & Wilkins.

Gladstar, R. (1993). *Herbal healing for women.* New York: Simon & Schuster.

Grabo, T. et al. (1999). Uterine myomas: Treatment options. *Journal of Obstetric, Gynecologic and Neonatal Nursing, 28*(1), 23-31.

Hadfield, R. et al. (1997). Endometriosis in monozygotic twins. *Fertility and Sterility, 68*, 941-942.

Hall, J. (2002). Amenorrhea. In K. Carlson et al. (Eds.), *Primary care of women* (2nd ed.). St. Louis: Mosby.

Halm, M., & Penque, S. (1999). Heart disease in women. *American Journal of Nursing, 99*(4), 26-32.

Harlow, S. (2000). Menstruation and menstrual disorders. In M. Goldman & M. Hatch (Eds.), *Women and health.* San Diego: Academic Press.

Hillard, P. (1999). Diagnosing and controlling abnormal uterine bleeding. *Contemporary Adolescent Gynecology, 4*(1), 4-11.

Hirata, J. (1997). Does dong quai have estrogenic effects on postmenopausal women? A double-blind, placebo-controlled trial. *Fertility and Sterility, 68*(6), 981-986.

Hulley, S. et al. (1998). Randomized trial of estrogen plus progestin for secondary prevention of coronary heart disease in postmenopausal women: Heart and Estrogen/progestin Replacement Study (HERS) research group. *Journal of the American Medical Association, 280,* 605-513.

Hulley, S. et al. (2002). Noncardiovascular disease outcomes during 6.8 years of hormone therapy: Heart and Estrogen/progestin Replacement Study follow-up (HERS II). *Journal of the American Medical Association, 288*, 58-66.

Huntley, A. (2002). Complementary therapies for the relief of menopausal symptoms. *Focus on Alternative and Complementary Therapies, 7*(2), 121-125.

Israel, D., & Youngkin, E. (1997). Herbal therapies for perimenopausal and menopausal complaints. *Pharmacotherapy, 17*(5), 970-984.

Jones, C. (2001). Premenstrual dysphoric disorder. *Advances for Nurse Practitioners, (2001, March)*, 87-90.

Kaunitz, A. (2002a). Abnormal uterine bleeding in the perimenopausal patient. *Contemporary Obstetrics and Gynecology, (2001, April)*, 69-88.

Kaunitz, A. (2002b). Menopausal hormone therapy: Where do we go now? *Breast Journal, 8*(6), 329-337.

Keller, C., Fullerton, J., & Fleury, J. (1998). Primary and secondary strategies among older postmenopausal women. *Journal of Nurse Midwifery, 43*(4), 262-272.

Kendig, S., & Sanford, D. (1998). *Midlife and menopause: Celebrating women's health.* Washington, DC: AWHONN.

Kleposki, R. (2002). The female athlete triad: A terrible trio implications for primary care. *Journal of the American Academy of Nurse Practitioners, 14*(10), 26-31.

Levine, S. (1998). The sexual consequences of perimenopause and menopause. *Women's Health in Primary Care, 1*(6), 509-513.

Liberman, S. (1998). A review of effectiveness of *Cimicufuga nacemosa* (black cohosh) for the symptoms of menopause. *Journal of Women's Health, 7*(5), 525-529.

Lin, J., & Thompson, D. (2001). Treating premenstrual dysphoric disorder using serotonin agents. *Journal of Women's Health & Gender-Based Medicine, 10*(6), 745-750.

Lindsay, S., & Claywell, L. (1998). Considering soy: Its estrogenic effects may protect women. *AWHONN Lifelines, 2*(1), 41-44.

Lipscomb, G., & Ling, F. (1997). Chronic pelvic pain and dysmenorrhea. In S. Scott & S. McNeeley (Eds.), *Gynecology for the primary care provider.* Philadelphia: W.B. Saunders.

Lowdermilk, D., & Fogel, C. (1996). *Health care issues of midlife women.* Edwardsville, KS: Educational Software.

McAllister, M. (1998). Menopause: Providing comprehensive care for women in transition. *Primary Care Practice, 2*(3), 256-274.

McClung, B. (1999). Using osteoporosis management to reduce fractures in elderly women. *Nurse Practitioner, 24*(3), 26-42.

Morse, G. (1999). Positively reframing perceptions of the menstrual cycle among women with premenstrual syndrome. *Journal of Obstetric, Gynecologic, and Neonatal Nursing, 28*(2), 165-174.

Nakad, T., & Isaacson, K. (2002). Endometriosis. In K. Carlson et al. (Eds.), *Primary care of women* (2nd ed.). St. Louis: Mosby.

National Osteoporosis Foundation (NOF). (2000). *Physician's guide to osteoporosis.* Washington, DC: NOF.

National Women's Health Report. (1999). Fitness and nutrition after menopause. *National Women's Health Report, 21*(1), 7.

Parent-Stevens, L., & Burns, E. (2000). Menstrual disorders. In M. Smith & L. Shimp (Eds.), *20 Common problems in women's health care* (pp. 381-414). New York: McGraw-Hill.

Ramsay, L., Ross, B., & Fischer, R. (1999). Phytoestrogens and the management of menopause. *Advances for Nurse Practitioners, 7*(5), 26-30.

Sabatini, S. (2001). The female athlete triad. *American Journal of the Medical Sciences, 322*(4), 193-195.

Sanborn, C. et al. (2000). Disorders of eating and the female athlete triad. *Clinics in Sports Medicine, 19*(2), 199-213.

Schellenberg, R. (2001). Treatment for the premenstrual syndrome with *Agnus castus* fruit extract: Prospective, randomized, placebo controlled study. *British Medical Journal, 322,* 134-137.

Sowers, M. (2000). Menopause: Its epidemiology. In M. Goldman & M. Hatch, (Eds.), *Women & health.* San Diego: Academic Press.

Speroff, L., Glass, R., & Kase, N. (1999). *Clinical gynecologic endocrinology and infertility* (6th ed.). Baltimore: Lippincott Williams & Wilkins.

Stenchever, M. et al. (2001). *Comprehensive gynecology* (4th ed.). St. Louis: Mosby.

Stevinson, C., & Ernst, E. (2001). Complementary/alternative therapies for premenstrual syndrome: A systematic review of randomized controlled trials. *American Journal of Obstetrics and Gynecology, 185*, 227-235.

Veet, L (2000). *Women's health care clinical vignettes.* Philadelphia: Hanley & Belfus, Inc.

Warren, M., & Kulak, J. (1999). Benefits and drawbacks of hormone replacement therapy. *Women's Health in Primary Care, 2*(3), 21-33.

West, R. (1998). The female athlete: The triad of disordered eating, amenorrhea, and osteoporosis. *Sports Medicine, 26*(2), 63-71.

Writing Group for the Women's Health Initiative Investigators. (2002). Risks and benefits of estrogen plus progestin in health postmenopausal women: Principal results from the Women's Health Initiative randomized control trial. *Journal of the American Medical Association, 288*, 321-333.

CHAPTER 8

Catherine Ingram Fogel

Sexually Transmitted and Other Infections

http://evolve.elsevier.com/Lowdermilk/MatWmnHlth/

LEARNING OBJECTIVES

- Describe prevention of sexually transmitted infections in women.
- Differentiate signs, symptoms, diagnosis, and management of nonpregnant and pregnant women with bacterial sexually transmitted infections.
- Examine the care of nonpregnant and pregnant women with selected viral infections (human immunodeficiency virus; hepatitis A, B, C; human papillomavirus).
- Discuss the effect of group β streptococcus (GBS) on pregnancy and management of pregnant clients with GBS.
- Compare and contrast signs, symptoms, and management of selected vaginal infections in nonpregnant and pregnant women.
- Review principles of infection control for human immunodeficiency virus (HIV) and blood-borne pathogens.

Sexually transmitted diseases (STDs), or **sexually transmitted infections (STIs),** are infections or infectious disease syndromes primarily transmitted by close, intimate contact (Box 8-1). These terms, used interchangeably in this text, have replaced the older designation, *venereal disease*, which described primarily gonorrhea and syphilis. Caused by a wide spectrum of bacteria, viruses, protozoa, and ectoparasites (organisms that live on the outside of the body, such as a louse), STIs are a direct cause of tremendous human suffering, place heavy demands on health care services, and cost hundreds of millions of dollars to treat. The term *sexually transmitted disease* is not specific for any one disease; rather the term includes more than 25 infectious organisms that are transmitted through sexual activity and the dozens of clinical syndromes that they cause (Institute of Medicine, Committee on Prevention and Control of Sexually Transmitted Diseases, 1997). Despite the U.S. Surgeon General's targeting STIs as a priority for prevention and control efforts, STIs are among the most common health problems in the United States (Institute of Medicine, Committee on Prevention and Control of Sexually Transmitted Diseases, 1997). The Centers for Disease Control and Prevention (CDC) estimates that more than 15 million Americans are infected with STIs every year (Workowski, Levine, & Wasserheit, 2002). The most common STDs or STIs in women are chlamydia, human papillomavirus, gonorrhea, herpes simplex virus type 2, syphilis, and HIV infection; these are discussed in this chapter. Neonatal effects of STIs are discussed in Chapter 38.

PREVENTION

Preventing infection (primary prevention) is the most effective way of reducing the adverse consequences of STIs for women and for society. With the advent of serious and potentially lethal STIs that are not readily cured or are incurable, primary prevention becomes critical. Prompt diagnosis and treatment of current infections (secondary prevention) also can prevent personal complications and transmission to others.

Preventing the spread of STIs requires that women at risk for transmitting or acquiring infections change their behavior. A critical first step is for the nurse to include questions about a woman's sexual history, sexual risk behaviors, and drug-related risky behaviors as a part of her assessment (Box 8-2). When risk factors or risky behaviors are identified, the nurse has an opportunity to provide prevention counseling. Techniques that are effective in providing prevention counseling include using open-ended questions, using understandable language, and reassuring the woman that treatment will be provided regardless of consideration such as ability to pay, language spoken, or lifestyle (Centers for Disease Control and Prevention [CDC], 2002b). Prevention messages should include descriptions of specific actions to be taken to avoid acquiring or transmitting STIs (e.g., refrain from sexual activity if you have STI-related symptoms) and should be tailored to the individual woman, with attention given to her specific risk factors.

To be motivated to take preventive actions, a woman must believe that catching a disease will be serious for her and that she is at risk for infection. Unfortunately most individuals tend to underestimate their personal risk of infection in a given situation; thus many women may not perceive themselves as being at risk for contracting an STI, and telling them that they should carry condoms may not be well received. Although levels of awareness of STIs are generally high, widespread misconceptions or specific gaps in knowledge also exist. Therefore nurses have a responsibility to ensure that their clients have accurate, complete knowledge about transmission and symptoms of STIs and risky behaviors that place them at risk for contracting an infection (Hutchinson, 1999).

Primary preventive measures are individual activities aimed at deterring infection. Risk-free options include complete abstinence from sexual activities that transmit semen, blood, or other body fluids or that allow skin-to-skin contact (CDC, 2002b). Alternatively, involvement in a mutually monogamous relationship with an uninfected partner also eliminates risk of contracting STIs. When neither of these options is realistic for a woman, however, the nurse must focus on other, more feasible measures.

BOX 8-1 Sexually Transmitted Infections

BACTERIA
- Chlamydia
- Gonorrhea
- Syphilis
- Chancroid
- Lymphogranuloma venereum
- Genital mycoplasmas
- Group B streptococci

VIRUSES
- Human immunodeficiency virus
- Herpes simplex virus, types 1 and 2
- Cytomegalovirus
- Viral hepatitis A and B
- Human papillomavirus

PROTOZOA
- Trichomoniasis

PARASITES
- Pediculosis (may or may not be sexually transmitted)
- Scabies (may or may not be sexually transmitted)

Safer Sex Practices

An essential component of primary prevention is counseling women regarding safer sex practices, including knowledge of her partner, reduction of number of partners, low risk sex, and avoiding the exchange of body fluids.

No aspect of prevention is more important than knowing one's partner. Reducing the number of partners and avoiding partners who have had many previous sexual partners decreases a woman's chance of contracting an STI. Deciding not to have sexual contact with casual acquaintances also may be helpful. Discussing each new partner's previous sexual history and exposure to STIs will augment other efforts to reduce risk; however, sexual partners are not always truthful about their sexual history. Women must be cautioned that safer sex measures are al-

BOX 8-2 Assessing STI/HIV Risk Behaviors

SEXUAL RISK
- Are you sexually active now?
- If no, have you had sex in the past?*
- Ever had an oral, vaginal, or anal sexual experience with another person?
- With how many different people? 1? 2 or 3? 4 to 10? More than 10?
- Have your partners been men, women, both?
- Ever thought that a sex partner put you at risk for AIDS/STI (IV drug user, bisexual)?
- Ever had an STI (herpes, gonorrhea, genital warts, chlamydia)?
- Ever had sex against your will?
- What do you do to protect yourself from AIDS/STIs?
- Do you use male condoms? Female condoms? Other barriers?

DRUG USE–RELATED RISK
- Ever injected drugs using shared equipment, including street drugs, steroids?
- Ever had sex with a person who uses and shares?
- Ever had sex while stoned, high, or drunk, so that you can't remember the details?
- Ever exchanged sex for drugs, money, shelter?

BLOOD-RELATED RISKS
- Ever had a blood transfusion?
- Ever had sex with a person who had a blood transfusion?
- Ever had sex with a person with hemophilia?
- Ever received donor semen, egg, transplanted organ or tissue?
- Ever shared equipment for tattoo, body piercing?

OTHER
- Ever had a test for HIV?
- Ever worried about AIDS and would like to talk with someone about it?

Adapted from Hatcher, R. et al. (2003). *Contraceptive technology* (18th ed.). New York: Ardent Media, Inc.
*Risk of HIV infection not known to exist in humans until 1977.

ways advisable, even when partners insist otherwise. Critically important is whether male partners resist or accept wearing condoms. This is crucial when women are not sure about their partners' history. Women should be cautioned against making decisions about a partner's sexual and other behaviors based on appearances and unfounded assumptions such as the following (Hatcher et al., 2003):

- Single people have many partners and risky practices.
- Older people have few partners and infrequent sexual encounters.
- Sexually experienced people know how to practice safer sex.
- Married people are heterosexual, low risk, and monogamous.
- People who look healthy are healthy.
- People with good jobs do not use drugs.

Sexually active persons also may benefit from carefully examining a partner for lesions, sores, ulcerations, rashes, redness, discharge, swelling, and odor before initiating sexual activity.

Women should be taught low risk sexual practices and which sexual practices to avoid (Table 8-1). Sexual fantasizing is safe, as are caressing, hugging, body rubbing, and massage. Mutual masturbation is low risk as long as there is no contact with a partner's semen or vaginal secretions. All sexual activities when both partners are monogamous, trustworthy, and known to be free of disease (by testing) are safe.

TABLE 8-1 **Safer Sex Guidelines**

SAFEST	LOW RISK	POSSIBLY RISKY (POSSIBLE EXPOSURE)	HIGH RISK (UNSAFE)
Behavior			
Abstinence	Wet kissing*	Cunnilingus†	Unprotected anal intercourse
Self-masturbation	Vaginal intercourse with condom	Fellatio‡	Unprotected vaginal intercourse
Monogamous (both partners and no high risk activities)	Anal intercourse with condom	Mutual masturbation with skin breaks	Oral-anal contact
Hugging,* massage,* touching*	Urine contact with intact skin	Vaginal intercourse after anal contact without new condom	Any sex (fisting, rough vaginal or anal intercourse, rape) that causes tissue damage or bleeding
Dry kissing			Multiple sexual partners
Mutual masturbation§			Sharing sex toys, douche equipment
Drug abstinence			Sharing needles
Sexual fantasy			Blood contact, including menstrual blood
Erotic conversation, books, movies, video			
Erotic bathing, showering			
Eroticizing feet, fingers, buttocks, abdomen, ears			
Prevention			
Avoid high risk behaviors	Avoid exposure to potentially infected body fluids	Use dental dam or female condom with cunnilingus	Avoid exposure to potentially infected body fluids
	Consistent use of condom and spermicide	Use condom with fellatio	Use condom and spermicide consistently
	Avoid anal intercourse	Use latex gloves	Avoid anal penetration
			If anal penetration occurs, use condom with intercourse, latex glove with hand penetration
			Avoid oral-anal contact
			Do not share sex toys, needles, douching equipment
			If sharing needles, clean with bleach before and after use

Adapted from Centers for Disease Control and Prevention. (2002b). Sexually transmitted diseases treatment guidelines, 2002. *MMWR, 51*(RR-6), 1-82; Fogel, C. (2003). Sexuality. In E. Breslin & V. Lucas (Eds.), *AWHONN women's health nursing: Toward evidence-based practice*. Philadelphia: W.B. Saunders.
*Assumes no breaks in skin.
†Cunnilingus: oral stimulation of the female genitalia.
‡Fellatio: oral stimulation of the male genitalia.
§Assumes no contact with semen or vaginal secretions.

The physical barrier promoted for the prevention of sexual transmission of HIV and other STIs is the condom (male and female). Nurses can help motivate clients to use condoms by first discussing the subject with them. This gives women permission to discuss any concerns, misconceptions, or hesitations they may have about using condoms. The nurse may initiate a discussion of how to purchase and use a condom. Information to be discussed includes the importance of using latex or plastic male condoms rather than natural skin condoms for STI protection. The nurse should remind women to use a condom with every sexual encounter, to use each one only once, to use a condom with a current expiration date, and to handle it carefully to avoid damaging it with fingernails, teeth, or other sharp objects. Condoms should be stored away from high heat. Although it is not ideal, women may choose to safely carry condoms in wallets, shoes, or inside a bra. Women can be taught the differences between condoms: price ranges, sizes, and where they can be purchased. Explicit instructions for how to apply a male condom are included in Box 9-3.

The female condom—a lubricated polyurethane sheath with a ring on each end that is inserted into the vagina—has been shown in laboratory studies to be an effective mechanical barrier to viruses, including HIV. Although no clinical studies have been completed to evaluate the efficacy of female condoms in protecting against STIs, the CDC (2002b) states that, when used correctly and consistently, the female condom may substantially reduce STI risk and recommends the use when a male condom cannot be used properly. What is important and should be stressed by nurses is the consistent use of condoms for every act of sexual intimacy where there is the possibility of transmission of disease.

Recent evidence has shown that vaginal spermicides do not protect against certain STIs (e.g., chlamydia, cervical gonorrhea) and that frequent use of spermicides containing nonoxynol-9 has been associated with genital lesions and may increase HIV transmission (Wilkerson et al., 2002). Condoms lubricated with nonoxynol-9 are not recommended (CDC, 2002b).

A key issue in condom use as a preventive strategy is to stress to women that in sexual encounters, men must comply with a woman's suggestion or request that they use a condom. Moreover, condom use must be renegotiated with every sexual contact, and women must address the issue of control of sexual decision making every time they request a male partner to use a condom. Women may fear that their partner would be offended if a condom were introduced. Some women may fear rejection and abandonment, conflict, potential violence, or loss of economic support if they suggest the use of condoms to prevent STI transmission. For many individuals, condoms are symbols of extrarelationship activity. Introduction of a condom into a long-term relationship where one has not been used previously threatens the trust assumed in most long-term relationships.

Many women do not anticipate or prepare for sexual activity in advance; embarrassment or discomfort in purchasing condoms may prevent some women from using them. Cultural barriers also may impede the use of condoms; for example, Latino gender roles make it difficult for Latina women to suggest using condoms to a partner. Suggesting condom use implies that a woman is sexually active, that she is "available" for sex, and that she is "seeking" sex; these are messages that many women are uncomfortable conveying, given the prevailing mores of our country. In a society that commonly views a woman who carries a condom as overprepared, possibly oversexed, and willing to have sex with any man, expecting her to insist on the use of condoms in a sexual encounter is unrealistic.

Finally, women should be counseled to watch out for situations that make it hard to talk about and to practice safer sex. These include romantic times when condoms are not available and when alcohol or drugs make it impossible to make wise decisions about safer sex.

Certain sexual practices should be avoided to reduce one's risk of infection. Abstinence from any sexual activities that could result in exchange of infective body fluids will help decrease risk. Anal-genital intercourse, anal-oral contact, and anal-digital activity are high risk sexual behaviors and should be avoided. Sexual transmission occurs through direct skin or mucous membrane contact with infectious lesions or body fluids. Because mucosal linings are delicate and subject to considerable mechanical trauma during intercourse, small abrasions often may occur, facilitating entry of infectious agents into the bloodstream. The rectal epithelium is especially easy to traumatize with penetration. Sexual practices that increase the likelihood of tissue damage or bleeding, such as fisting (inserting a fist into the rectum), should be avoided. Deep kissing when lips, gums, or other tissues are raw or broken also should be avoided (Hatcher et al., 2003). Because enteric infections are transmitted by oral-fecal contact, avoiding oral-anal activities, "rimming" (licking the anal area), and digital-anal activities should reduce the likelihood of infection. Vaginal intercourse should never follow anal contact unless a condom has been used and then removed and replaced with a new condom.

Nurses must suggest strategies to enhance a woman's condom negotiation and communication skills. Suggesting that she talk with her partner about condom use at a time removed from sexual activity may make it easier to bring up the subject. Role playing possible partner reactions with a woman and her alternative responses can be helpful. Asking a woman who appears particularly uncomfortable to rehearse how she might approach the topic is useful, particularly when a woman fears her partner may be resistant. The nurse might suggest her client begin by saying, "I need to talk with you about something that is important to both of us. It's hard for me, and I feel embarrassed, but I think we need to talk about safer sex." If women are able to sort out their feelings and fears before talking with their partners, they may feel more comfortable and in control of the situation. Women can be reassured that it is natural to be uncomfortable and that the hardest part is getting started. Nurses should help their clients clarify what they will and will not do sexually because it will be easier to discuss their concerns with their partners if they have thought about what to say. Women can be reminded that their partner may need time to think about what they have said and that they must pay attention to their partner's response. If the partner seems to be having difficulty with the discussion, a woman may slow down and wait a while. She can be reminded that if her partner resists safer sex, she may wish to reconsider the relationship.

Women may delay seeking care for STIs because they fear social stigma, they have little access to health care services, they are asymptomatic, or they are unaware that they have an infection.

BACTERIAL SEXUALLY TRANSMITTED INFECTIONS

Chlamydia

Chlamydia trachomatis is the most common and fastest spreading STI in American women, with an estimated 3 million new cases each year (Walsh & Irwin, 2002). These infections are often silent and highly destructive; their sequelae and complications can be very serious. In women, chlamydial infections are difficult to diagnose; the symptoms, if present, are nonspecific, and the organism is expensive to culture.

Early identification of *C. trachomatis* is important because untreated infection often leads to acute salpingitis or pelvic inflammatory disease. Pelvic inflammatory disease is the most serious complication of chlamydial infections, and past chlamydial infections are associated with an increased risk of ectopic pregnancy and tubal factor infertility. Furthermore, chlamydial infection of the cervix causes inflammation, resulting in microscopic cervical ulcerations, and thus may increase the risk of acquiring HIV infection. More than half of infants born to mothers with chlamydia will develop conjunctivitis or pneumonia after perinatal exposure to the mother's infected cervix (Walsh & Irwin, 2002). Chlamydia is the most common infectious cause of ophthalmia neonatorum. Neonatal ocular prophylaxis with silver nitrate solution or antibiotic ointment does not prevent perinatal transmission from mother to infant, nor does it adequately treat chlamydial infection. Systemic treatment with erythromycin is recommended (CDC, 2002b).

Sexually active women younger than 20 years are 2 to 3 times as likely to become infected with chlamydia as are women between 20 and 29 years. Women older than 30 years have the lowest rate of infection. Risky behaviors, including multiple partners and nonuse of barrier methods of birth control, increase a woman's risk of chlamydial infection. Lower socioeconomic status may be a risk factor, especially with respect to treatment-seeking behaviors.

Screening and Diagnosis

In addition to obtaining information regarding the presence of risk factors, the nurse should inquire about the presence of any symptoms. The CDC (2002b) and U.S. Preventive Services Task Force (USPSTF, 2001a) strongly recommend screening of asymptomatic women at high risk in whom infection would otherwise go undetected. CDC guidelines recommend screening of sexually active adolescents, women between ages 20 and 25 years, women older than 25 years who do not use barrier contraceptives, and women older than 25 years with new or multiple partners. In addition, whenever possible, all women with two or more of the risk factors for chlamydia should be cultured. All pregnant women should have cervical cultures for chlamydia at the first prenatal visit. Repeated culturing late in the third trimester (36 weeks) should be carried out if the woman was positive previously or if she is younger than 25 years or has a new sex partner or multiple sex partners.

Although chlamydia infections are usually asymptomatic, some women may experience spotting or postcoital bleeding, mucoid or purulent cervical discharge, or dysuria. Bleeding results from inflammation and erosion of the cervical columnar epithelium. Women taking oral contraceptives also may have breakthrough bleeding.

Diagnosis of chlamydia is by culture (expensive and labor intensive), DNA probe (less expensive but less sensitivity), enzyme immunoassay (less expensive but less sensitivity), and nucleic acid amplification (expensive but about 90% sensitivity) (Rawlins, 2001). The chlamydial culture procedure requires collection of a sample that contains many epithelial cells. Endocervical (columnar) cells are required; cell scrapings provide better specimens, so the cervix should be swabbed with cotton or rayon swabs before collecting the specimen to remove mucus and discharge from the cervical os. Special culture media and proper handling of specimens are important, so the nurse should always know what is required in her individual practice site. Chlamydial culture testing is not always available, primarily because of expense.

Management

The CDC recommendations for treatment of urethral, cervical, and rectal chlamydial infections are doxycycline (100 mg orally twice a day for 7 days) or azithromycin (1 g orally in a single dose) (Table 8-2) (CDC, 2002b). Azithromycin is often prescribed when compliance may be a problem, because only one dose is needed; however, expense is a concern with this medication. If the woman is pregnant, erythromycin (500 mg orally 4 times a day for 7 days) or amoxicillin (500 mg orally 3 times a day for 7 days) is used. Women who have a chlamydial infection and also are infected with HIV should be treated with the same regimen as those who are not infected with HIV.

Because chlamydia is often asymptomatic, the woman should be cautioned to take all medication prescribed. All

TABLE 8-2 Sexually Transmitted Infections and Drug Therapies for Women

DISEASE	NONPREGNANT WOMEN (13-17 YR)	NONPREGNANT WOMEN (>18 YR)	PREGNANT WOMEN	LACTATING WOMEN*
Chlamydia	*Recommended:* Azithromycin, 1 g orally once or Doxycycline, 100 mg orally bid for 7 days *Alternatives:* Erythromycin or sulfamethoxazole/trimethoprim regimens or Levofloxacin, 500 mg orally for 7 days	*Recommended:* Azithromycin, 1 g orally once or Doxycycline, 100 mg orally bid for 7 days *Alternatives:* Erythromycin base, 500 mg orally qid for 7 days or Erythromycin ethylsuccinate, 800 mg orally qid for 7 days or Ofloxacin, 300 mg orally bid for 7 days or Levofloxacin, 500 mg orally for 7 days	*Recommended:* Erythromycin base, 500 mg orally qid for 7 days or Amoxicillin, 500 mg orally TID for 7 days *Alternatives:* Erythromycin base, 250 mg orally qid for 14 days or Erythromycin ethylsuccinate, 800 mg orally qid for 14 days or Erythromycin ethylsuccinate, 400 mg orally qid for 14 days or Azithromycin, 1 g orally once	*Recommended:* Erythromycin base, 500 mg orally qid for 7 days or Amoxicillin, 500 mg orally, tid for 7 days or *Alternatives:* Erythromycin base, 250 mg orally qid for 14 days or Erythromycin ethylsuccinate, 800 mg orally qid for 7 days or Erythromycin ethylsuccinate, 400 mg orally qid for 14 days Azithromycin, 1 g orally once
Gonorrhea	*Recommended:* Ceftriaxone, 125 mg IM once (Adolescents who weigh >45 kg can be treated with any regimen recommended for adults)	*Recommended:* Ceftriaxone, 125 mg IM once or Ciprofloxacin, 500 mg orally once or Ofloxacin, 400 mg orally once or Levofloxacin, 250 mg orally once PLUS† Azithromycin, 1 g orally once or Doxycycline, 100 mg orally bid for 7 days	*Recommended:* Ceftriaxone, 125 mg IM once If cephalosporin allergic, Spectinomycin, 2 g IM once PLUS† Erythromycin base, 500 mg orally qid for 7 days or Amoxicillin, 500 mg orally tid for 7 days	*Recommended:* Ceftriaxone, 125 mg IM once If cephalosporin allergic, Spectinomycin, 2 g IM once PLUS† Erythromycin base, 500 mg orally qid for 7 days or Amoxicillin 500 mg orally tid for 7 days
Syphilis	Primary, secondary, early latent disease: *Recommended:* Benzathine penicillin G, 2.4 million units IM once	Primary, secondary, early latent disease: *Recommended:* Benzathine penicillin G, 2.4 million units IM once	Primary, secondary, early latent disease: *Recommended:* Benzathine penicillin G, 2.4 million units IM once	Primary, secondary, early latent disease: *Recommended:* Benzathine penicillin G, 2.4 million units IM once (Some

Source: American Academy of Pediatrics Committee on Drugs. (2002). The transfer of drugs and other chemicals into human milk. *Pediatrics, 108*(3), 776-789; Centers for Disease Control and Prevention. (2002*b*). Sexually transmitted diseases treatment guidelines, 2002. *MMWR, 51*(RR-6), 1-82.
*These medications are usually compatible with breastfeeding.
†If chlamydial infection not ruled out, treatment is recommended.

TABLE 8-2 **Sexually Transmitted Infections and Drug Therapies for Women—cont'd**

DISEASE	NONPREGNANT WOMEN (13-17 YR)	NONPREGNANT WOMEN (>18 YR)	PREGNANT WOMEN	LACTATING WOMEN
Syphilis—cont'd	Late latent or unknown duration disease: *Recommended:* Benzathine penicillin G, 7.2 million units total, administered as three doses, 2.4 million units each, at 1-wk intervals Penicillin allergy: Doxycycline, 100 mg orally bid for 14 days or Tetracycline, 500 mg orally qid for 14 days	Late latent or unknown duration disease: *Recommended:* Benzathine penicillin G, 7.2 million units total, administered as three doses, 2.4 million units each, at 1-wk intervals Penicillin allergy: Doxycycline, 100 mg orally qid for 14 days or Tetracycline, 500 mg orally qid for 14 days	(Some experts recommend a second dose of benzathine penicillin, 2.4 million units, 1 wk later) Late latent or unknown duration disease: *Recommended:* Benzathine penicillin G, 7.2 million units total, administered as three doses, 2.4 million units each, at 1-wk intervals No proven alternatives to penicillin in pregnancy. Pregnant women who have a history of allergy to penicillin should be desensitized and treated with penicillin	experts recommend a second dose of benzathine penicillin, 2.4 million units, 1 wk later)
Human papillomavirus	Recommended for external genital warts: Client applied Podofilox, 0.5% solution, or gel to wart BID for 3 days followed by 4-day rest for ≤4 cycles or Imiquimod, 5% cream, at hs 3 times a week for ≤16 wk Provider applied: Cryotherapy with liquid nitrogen or cryoprobe or Podophyllin resin, 10%-25% in tincture of benzoin compound weekly (wash off in 1-4 hr). Repeat weekly as necessary	Recommended for external genital warts: Client applied Podofilox, 0.5% solution, or gel to wart bid for 3 days followed by 4-day rest for ≤4 cycles or Imiquimod, 5% cream, at hs 3 times a week for ≤16 wk Provider applied: Cryotherapy with liquid nitrogen or cryoprobe or Podophyllin resin, 10%-25% in tincture of benzoin compound weekly (wash off in 1-4 hr). Repeat weekly as necessary	Recommended for external genital warts: Provider applied: Cryotherapy with liquid nitrogen or cryoprobe or TCA or BCA 80%-90% weekly Imiquimod, podophyllin, and podofilox should not be used in pregnancy	Recommended for external genital warts: Provider applied: Cryotherapy with liquid nitrogen or cryoprobe or TCA or BCA 80%-90% weekly Imiquimod, podophyllin, and podofilox should not be used during lactation

Continued

TABLE 8-2 **Sexually Transmitted Infections and Drug Therapies for Women—cont'd**

DISEASE	NONPREGNANT WOMEN (13-17 YR)	NONPREGNANT WOMEN (>18 YR)	PREGNANT WOMEN	LACTATING WOMEN
Human papillomavirus—cont'd	or TCA or BCA, 80%-90% weekly	or TCA or BCA, 80%-90% weekly		
Genital herpes simplex virus (HSV type 1 or 2)	Primary infection: Acyclovir, 400 mg orally tid for 7-10 days or Acyclovir, 200 mg orally 5 times a day for 7-10 days or Famciclovir, 250 mg orally tid for 7-10 days or Valacyclovir, 1 g orally bid for 7-10 days Recurrent infection: Acyclovir, 400 mg orally tid for 5 days or Acyclovir, 200 mg orally 5 times a day for 5 days	Primary infection: Acyclovir, 400 mg orally tid for 7-10 days or Acyclovir, 200 mg orally 5 times a day for 7-10 days or Famciclovir, 250 mg orally tid for 7-10 days or Valacyclovir, 1 g orally bid for 7-10 days Recurrent infection: Acyclovir, 400 mg orally tid for 5 days or Acyclovir, 200 mg orally 5 times a day for 5 days	Safety of acyclovir use not established in pregnancy; may be used orally for first episode or severe recurrence	Safety of acyclovir use not established for lactating women; drug may be used with caution

exposed sexual partners should be treated. Woman treated with doxycycline or azithromycin do not need to be retested unless symptoms continue. Women treated with erythromycin may be retested 3 weeks after completing the medication, although the validity of this practice has not been established (CDC, 2002b).

Gonorrhea

Gonorrhea is probably the oldest communicable disease in the United States. An estimated 600,000 American men and women contract gonorrhea each year (CDC, 2002b). The incidence of drug-resistant cases of gonorrhea, in particular, penicillinase-producing *Neisseria gonorrhoeae* (PPNG), is increasing dramatically in the United States.

Gonorrhea is caused by the aerobic, gram-negative diplococci, *N. gonorrhoeae*. Gonorrhea is almost exclusively transmitted by the contact of sexual activity. The principal means of communication is genital-to-genital contact; however, it also is spread by oral-to-genital and anal-to-genital contact. There also is evidence that infection may spread in females from vagina to rectum. Gonorrhea also can be transmitted to the newborn in the form of ophthalmia neonatorum during birth by direct contact with gonococcal organisms in the cervix. Although the organism has been recovered from inanimate objects artificially inoculated with the bacteria, no evidence exists that natural transmission occurs this way (Schaffer, 1998).

Age is probably the most important risk factor associated with gonorrhea. The majority of those contracting gonorrhea are younger than 20 years. Traditionally the reported incidence of gonococcal disease has been higher in minority groups. Many of the apparent differences in infection rates can be explained by the disproportionate representation of African-Americans among the nation's poor and among inner city dwellers. Rates of gonorrhea are higher in urban areas than in rural areas, with even higher rates in the inner city. Adolescent girls have the highest rates of infection, and the incidence is higher in African-American adolescents than in Hispanic or Caucasian teens (Bonny & Biro, 1998). Sex workers and their partners, intravenous drug users, and crack cocaine users are considered groups at high risk.

TABLE 8-2 Sexually Transmitted Infections and Drug Therapies for Women—cont'd

DISEASE	NONPREGNANT WOMEN (13-17 YR)	NONPREGNANT WOMEN (>18 YR)	PREGNANT WOMEN	LACTATING WOMEN
Genital herpes—cont'd	or	or		
	Acyclovir, 800 mg orally tid for 5 days	Acyclovir, 800 mg orally tid for 5 days		
	or	or		
	Famciclovir, 125 mg orally bid for 5 days	Famciclovir, 125 mg orally bid for 5 days		
	or	or		
	Valacyclovir, 500 mg orally bid for 5 days	Valacyclovir, 500 mg orally bid for 5 days		
	Suppression therapy:	Suppression therapy:		
	Acyclovir, 400 mg orally bid	Acyclovir, 400 mg orally bid		
	or	or		
	Famciclovir, 250 mg orally bid	Famciclovir, 250 mg orally bid		
	or	or		
	Valacyclovir, 250 mg orally bid	Valacyclovir, 250 mg orally bid		
	or	or		
	Valacyclovir, 500 mg orally qd	Valacyclovir, 500 mg orally qd		
	or	or		
	Valacyclovir, 1000 mg orally qd	Valacyclovir, 1000 mg orally qd		

Other risk factors include early onset of sexual activity and multiple sexual partners.

Women are often asymptomatic, with one third of infections in adolescent women going unnoticed; when symptoms are present, they are often less specific than are the symptoms in men. Women may have a purulent endocervical discharge, but discharge is usually minimal or absent. Menstrual irregularities may be the presenting symptom, or women may complain of pain–chronic or acute severe pelvic or lower abdominal pain or longer, more painful menses. Infrequently, dysuria, vague abdominal pain, or low backache prompts a woman to seek care. Gonococcal rectal infection may occur in women after anal intercourse, with 10% to 30% of urogenital infections accompanied by rectal infection. Individuals with rectal gonorrhea may be completely asymptomatic or, conversely, have severe symptoms with profuse purulent anal discharge, rectal pain, and blood in the stool. Rectal itching, fullness, pressure, and pain also are common symptoms, as is diarrhea. A diffuse vaginitis with vulvitis is the most common form of gonococcal infection in prepubertal girls. There may be few signs of infection, or vaginal discharge, dysuria, and swollen, reddened labia may be present.

Gonococcal infections in pregnancy potentially affect both mother and infant. In women with cervical gonorrhea, salpingitis may develop in the first trimester. Perinatal complications of gonococcal infection include premature rupture of membranes, preterm birth, chorioamnionitis, neonatal sepsis, intrauterine growth restriction, and maternal postpartum sepsis. Amniotic infection syndrome manifested by placental, fetal, and umbilical cord inflammation after premature rupture of the membranes may result from gonorrheal infections during pregnancy. Ophthalmia neonatorum, the most common manifestation of neonatal gonococcal infections, is highly contagious, and if untreated, may lead to blindness of the newborn (see Chapter 26).

Screening and Diagnosis

Because gonococcal infections in women often are asymptomatic, the CDC recommends screening all women at risk for gonorrhea (CDC, 2002b). All pregnant women should be screened at the first prenatal visit, and infected women and those identified with risky behaviors rescreened at

36 weeks of gestation. Gonococcal infection cannot be diagnosed reliably by clinical signs and symptoms alone. Individuals may have "classic" symptoms, vague symptoms that may be attributed to a number of conditions, or no symptoms at all. Cultures with selective media are considered the gold standard for diagnosis of gonorrhea. Cultures should be obtained from the endocervix, rectum, and when indicated, the pharynx. Thayer-Martin cultures are recommended to diagnose gonorrhea in women. Any woman suspected of having gonorrhea should have a chlamydial culture and serologic test for syphilis if one has not been done in the past 2 months, because coinfection is common.

Management

Management of gonorrhea is straightforward, and the cure is usually rapid with appropriate antibiotic therapy (see Table 8-2). Single-dose efficacy is a major consideration in selecting an antibiotic regimen for women with gonorrhea. Another important consideration is the high percentage (45%) of women with coexisting chlamydial infections. The treatment of choice for uncomplicated urethral, endocervical, and rectal infections in pregnant and nonpregnant women is cefixime (400 mg orally once) or ceftriaxone (125 mg intramuscularly [IM] once). The CDC recommends concomitant treatment for chlamydia because coinfection is common (CDC, 2002b). All women with both gonorrhea and syphilis also should be treated for syphilis according to CDC guidelines (see discussion of syphilis in this chapter).

Gonorrhea is a highly communicable disease. Recent (past 30 days) sexual partners should be examined, cultured, and treated with appropriate regimens. Most treatment failures result from reinfection. The client must be informed of this, as well as of the consequences of reinfection in terms of chronicity, complications, and potential infertility. Women are counseled to use condoms. All clients with gonorrhea should be offered confidential counseling and testing for HIV infection.

Gonorrhea is a reportable communicable disease. Health care providers are legally responsible for reporting all cases to the health authorities, usually the local health department in the client's county of residence. Women should be informed that the case will be reported, told why, and informed of the possibility of being contacted by a health department epidemiologist.

Treatment failure after combined ceftriaxone/doxycycline therapy is rare; therefore follow-up culture (test of cure) is not essential. A more cost-effective approach is reexamination with a culture 1 to 2 months after treatment. This approach will detect both treatment failures and reinfections. Clients also should be counseled to return if symptoms persist after treatment.

Syphilis

Syphilis, one of the earliest described STIs, is caused by *Treponema pallidum*, a motile spirochete. Transmission is thought to be by entry in the subcutaneous tissue through microscopic abrasions that can occur during sexual intercourse. The disease also can be transmitted through kissing, biting, or oral-genital sex. Transplacental transmission may occur at any time during pregnancy; the degree of risk is related to the quantity of spirochetes in the maternal bloodstream.

The 2000 rate of primary and secondary syphilis was 2.2 per 100,000, the lowest rate ever reported in the United States (CDC, 2001a). Rates are highest among adolescents and women of color, and in southern states (Toney & Montero, 2001). Much of the increase in cases seen since 1990 is directly attributable to illicit drug use–particularly crack cocaine–and the exchange of sex for drugs and money.

Syphilis is a complex disease that can lead to serious systemic disease and even death when untreated. Infection manifests itself in distinct stages with different symptoms and clinical manifestations. *Primary* syphilis is characterized by a primary lesion, the chancre, that appears 5 to 90 days after infection; this lesion often begins as a painless papule at the site of inoculation and then erodes to form a nontender, shallow, indurated, clean ulcer several millimeters to centimeters in size (Fig. 8-1). *Secondary* syphilis

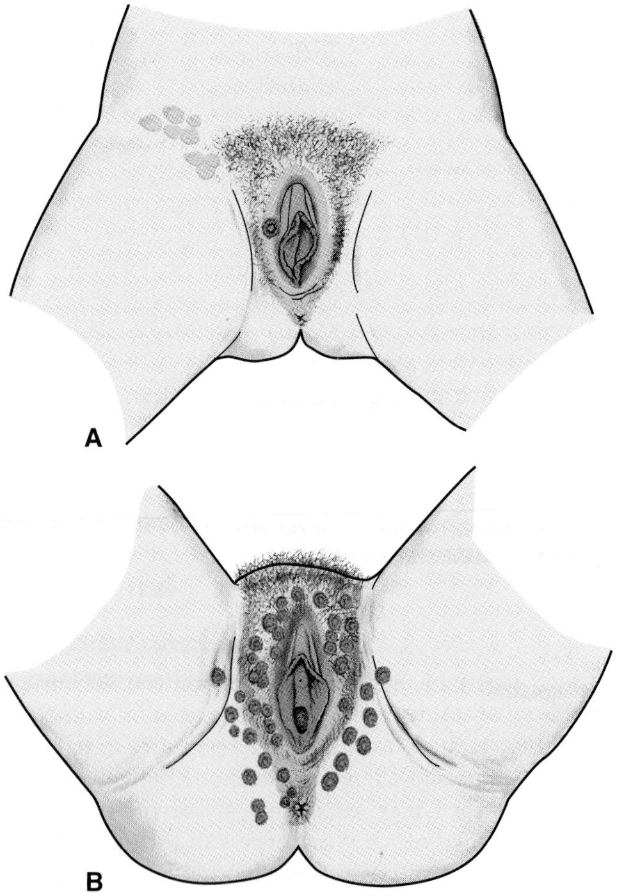
A
B

FIG. 8-1 Syphilis. **A,** Primary stage: chancre with inguinal adenopathy. **B,** Secondary stage: condylomata lata.

occurs 6 weeks to 6 months after the appearance of the chancre and is characterized by a widespread, symmetric maculopapular rash on the palms and soles and generalized lymphadenopathy. The infected individual also may experience fever, headache, and malaise.

Condylomata lata (broad, painless, pink-gray, wartlike infectious lesions) may develop on the vulva, perineum, or anus. If the woman is untreated, she enters a latent phase that is asymptomatic for the majority of individuals. If it is left untreated, tertiary syphilis will develop in about one third of these women. Neurologic, cardiovascular, musculoskeletal, or multiorgan system complications can develop in the third stage.

Screening and Diagnosis

All women who are diagnosed with another STI or with HIV should be screened for syphilis. All pregnant women should be screened for syphilis at the first prenatal visit and again in the late third trimester. Diagnosis is dependent on microscopic examination of primary and secondary lesion tissue and serology during latency and late infection. A test for antibodies may not be reactive in the presence of active infection because it takes time for the body's immune system to develop antibodies to any antigens. Up to one third of people in early primary syphilis may have nonreactive serologic tests. Two types of serologic tests are used: nontreponemal and treponemal. Nontreponemal antibody tests such as the VDRL (Venereal Disease Research Laboratories) or RPR (rapid plasma reagin) are used as screening tests. False-positive results are not unusual, particularly when conditions such as acute infection, autoimmune disorders, malignancy, pregnancy, and drug addiction exist and after immunization or vaccination. The treponemal tests, fluorescent treponemal antibody absorbed (FTA-ABS) and microhemagglutination assays for antibody to *T. pallidum* (MHA-TP), are used to confirm positive results. Test results in clients with early primary or incubating syphilis may be negative. Seroconversion usually takes place 6 to 8 weeks after exposure, so testing should be repeated in 1 to 2 months when a suggestive genital lesion exists.

Tests for concomitant STIs should be done (e.g., wet preps and cultures) and HIV testing offered if indicated.

Management

Penicillin is the preferred drug for treating clients with syphilis (see Table 8-2). It is the only proven therapy that has been widely used for clients with neurosyphilis, congenital syphilis, or syphilis during pregnancy. Intramuscular benzathine penicillin G (2.4 million units IM once) is used to treat primary, secondary, and early latent syphilis. Women with syphilis of longer than 1 year's duration (late latent or tertiary stages) require weekly treatment of 2.4 million units of benzathine penicillin G for 3 weeks. Although doxycycline, tetracycline, and erythromycin are alternative treatments for penicillin-allergic clients, both tetracycline and doxycycline are contraindicated in pregnancy, and erythromycin is unlikely to cure a fetal infection. Therefore pregnant women should, if necessary, receive skin testing and be treated with penicillin or be desensitized (CDC, 2002b). Specific protocols are recommended by the CDC.

NURSE ALERT

Clients treated for syphilis may experience a Jarisch-Herxheimer reaction. This acute febrile reaction is often accompanied by headache, myalgias, and arthralgias that develop within the first 24 hours of treatment. Women treated in the second half of pregnancy are at risk for preterm labor and birth if treatment precipitates this reaction. They should be advised to contact their health care provider if they notice any change in fetal movement or have any contractions.

Monthly follow-up is mandatory so that repeated treatment may be given if needed. The nurse should emphasize the necessity of long-term serologic testing even in the absence of symptoms. The woman should be advised to practice sexual abstinence until treatment is completed, all evidence of primary and secondary syphilis is gone, and serologic evidence of a cure is demonstrated. Women should be told to notify all partners who may have been exposed. They should be informed that the disease is reportable. Preventive measures should be discussed.

Pelvic Inflammatory Disease

Pelvic inflammatory disease (PID) is an infectious process that most commonly involves the uterine (fallopian) tubes (salpingitis), uterus (endometritis), and more rarely, the ovaries and peritoneal surfaces. Multiple organisms have been found to cause PID, and most cases are associated with more than one organism. In the past, the most common causative agent was thought to be *N. gonorrhoeae*; however, *C. trachomatis* is now estimated to cause half of all cases of PID. In addition to gonorrhea and chlamydia, a wide variety of anaerobic and aerobic bacteria are recognized to cause PID. PID encompasses a wide variety of pathologic processes; the infection can either be acute, subacute, or chronic and can have a wide range of symptoms.

Most PID results from ascending spread of microorganisms from the vagina and endocervix to the upper genital tract. This spread most frequently happens at the end of or just after menses following reception of an infectious agent. During the menstrual period, several factors facilitate the development of an infection: the cervical os is slightly open, the cervical mucus barrier is absent, and menstrual blood is an excellent medium for growth. PID also may develop after an abortion, pelvic surgery, or childbirth.

PID is the single most frequent serious infection encountered by women. Each year more than 1 million women in the United States have an episode of symptomatic PID (Institute of Medicine, Committee on Prevention and Control of Sexually Transmitted Diseases, 1997). Risk factors for acquiring PID are those associated with the risk of contracting an STI, including young age, multiple partners, high rate of new partners, and a history of STIs. Women who use intrauterine devices (IUDs) may be at increased risk for PID if they have more than one sexual partner or if the partner has other sexual partners, because they are at higher risk for acquiring an STI (World Health Organization, 2000). Most of this risk occurs in the first months after IUD insertion. PID tends to recur, with nearly one in five clients having recurrent PID (Bonny & Biro, 1998).

Women who have had PID are at increased risk for ectopic pregnancy, infertility, and chronic pelvic pain. After a single episode of PID, a woman's risk for ectopic pregnancy increases sevenfold compared with the risk for women who have never had PID. Other problems associated with PID include dyspareunia (painful intercourse), pyosalpinx (pus in the uterine tubes), tuboovarian abscess, and pelvic adhesions.

The symptoms of PID vary depending on whether the infection is acute, subacute, or chronic; however, pain is common to all clinical presentations. It may be dull, cramping, and intermittent (subacute) or severe, persistent, and incapacitating (acute). The woman with acute PID also may complain of intermenstrual bleeding. Physical examination reveals adnexal tenderness, with or without rebound, and exquisite tenderness with cervical movement (Chandelier sign). Pelvic tenderness is usually bilateral. There may or may not be a palpable adnexal swelling or thickening. A urethral or cervical discharge, often purulent, may be present. A fever of 39° C or above is characteristic. Significant laboratory data include an elevated white blood cell count and markedly elevated erythrocyte sedimentation rate. Fever and peritonitis are more characteristic of gonococcal PID than of PID caused by other organisms that are more likely to be "silent." Because PID caused by chlamydia is more commonly asymptomatic, it more often results in tubal obstruction from delayed diagnosis or inadequate treatment.

Subacute PID is far less dramatic, with a great variety in the severity and extent of symptoms. At times they are so mild and vague that the woman ignores them. Symptoms that suggest subacute PID are chronic lower abdominal pain, dyspareunia, menstrual irregularities, urinary discomfort, low-grade fever, low backache, and constipation. Abdominal examination usually reveals no rebound tenderness; there is slight adnexal tenderness with cervical movement, and cervical or urethral discharge may be present.

Screening and Diagnosis

A careful history is necessary to distinguish between PID and other conditions that cause abdominal pain, such as an ectopic pregnancy or appendicitis. A menstrual history is useful in establishing the relation of onset of pain to menses and in identifying any variations from normal in the cycle. Other relevant history includes recent pelvic surgery, birth, induced abortion, or dilation of the cervix; purulent vaginal discharge; irregular bleeding; and a longer, heavier menstrual period. A sexual history will assist in identifying possible increased risk for STI exposure. Symptoms of an STI in a woman's partner(s) also should be noted.

Vital signs are obtained, and a complete physical examination performed. CDC routine criteria for diagnosing PID include oral temperature greater than 38.3° C, abnormal cervical or vaginal discharge, elevated erythrocyte sedimentation rate, and laboratory documentation of cervical infection with *N. gonorrhoeae* or *C. trachomatis.* Physical findings of lower abdominal tenderness, bilateral adnexal tenderness, and cervical motion tenderness are important in making a clinical diagnosis of PID. Essential laboratory data are a complete blood count with differential and cervical cultures for gonorrhea and chlamydia.

Management

Perhaps the most important nursing intervention is prevention. Primary prevention would be education in avoiding acquisition of STIs, whereas secondary prevention involves preventing a lower genital tract infection from ascending to the upper genital tract. Instructing women in self-protective behaviors such as practicing safer sex and using barrier methods is critical. Women using hormonal contraception or the IUD and those who have chosen tubal ligation must be reminded to use a condom with intercourse when indicated. Also important is the detection of asymptomatic gonorrheal and chlamydial infections through routine screening of women who practice risky behaviors or have specific risk factors such as young age. Partner notification when an STI is diagnosed is essential to prevent reinfection.

When and if women with PID are hospitalized varies. The CDC recommends hospitalization in the following situations (CDC, 2002b):

- Surgical emergencies such as appendicitis cannot be excluded.
- The woman has a tuboovarian abscess.
- The woman is pregnant.
- Severe illness precludes outpatient management.
- The woman is unable to tolerate or follow an outpatient oral regimen.
- The woman has failed to respond to oral outpatient therapy.

Although many experts recommend that all women with PID be hospitalized so that parenteral antibiotic treatment can be done, the CDC does not.

Although treatment regimens vary with the infecting organism, a broad-spectrum antibiotic generally is used. Several antimicrobial regimens have proved to be effective, and no single therapeutic regimen of choice exists

(Table 8-3). The woman with acute PID should be on bed rest in a semi-Fowler's position. Comfort measures include analgesics for pain and all other nursing measures applicable to a client confined to bed. Few pelvic examinations should be done during the acute phase of the disease. During the recovery phase, the woman should restrict her activity and make every effort to get adequate rest and a nutritionally sound diet. Follow-up laboratory work after treatment should include endocervical cultures for a test of cure.

Health education is central to effective management of PID. Nurses should explain the nature of the disease to women and should encourage them to comply with all therapy and prevention recommendations, emphasizing the necessity of taking all medication, even if symptoms disappear. Any potential problems (such as lack of money for prescriptions or lack of transportation to return to the clinic for follow-up appointments) that would prevent a woman from completing a course of treatment should be identified and the importance of follow-up visits stressed. Women should be counseled to refrain from sexual intercourse until their treatment is completed. Contraceptive counseling should be provided, including barrier methods such as condoms, contraceptive sponge, or diaphragm. A woman with a history of PID should not choose an IUD as her contraceptive method.

The woman with PID may be acutely ill or have long-term discomfort. Either or both take an emotional toll. Pain in itself is debilitating and is compounded by the infectious process. The potential or actual loss of reproductive capabilities can be devastating and can adversely affect the woman's self-concept. Part of the nurse's role is to help the woman adjust her self-concept to fit reality and to accept alterations in a way that promotes health. Because PID is so closely tied to sexuality, body image, and self-concept, the woman diagnosed with it will need supportive care. Her feelings should be discussed and her partner(s) included when appropriate.

VIRAL SEXUALLY TRANSMITTED INFECTIONS

Human Papillomavirus

Human papillomavirus (HPV) infection, previously named genital or venereal warts, is a sexually transmitted infection that was first described in 25 A.D. and is now the most prevalent viral STI seen in ambulatory health care settings. HPV, a double-stranded DNA virus, has more than 40 known serotypes; more than 20 types can infect the genital tract. Most HPV infections are asymptomatic, subclinical, or unrecognized. The visible genital lesions are usually caused by HPV types 6 and 11. Other types (e.g., 16, 18, 31, 33, and 35) have the highest oncogenic potential, with types 16 and 18 associated with the highest mortality from cervical cancer (Thomas, 2001; Workowski et al., 2002). HPV types 31, 33, and 35 have

TABLE 8-3 **Treatment of Pelvic Inflammatory Disease**

	TREATMENT OF CHOICE	ALTERNATIVES
Parenteral regimen	Cefotetan, 2 g IV every 12 hr or Cefoxitin, 2 g IV every 6 hr PLUS Doxycycline, 100 mg IV or orally every 12 hr	Clindamycin, 900 mg IV every 8 hr PLUS Gentamycin, loading dose IV or IM (2 mg/kg of body weight), followed by maintenance dose (1.5 mg/kg) every 8 hr. Single daily dosing may be substituted
Oral regimen	Ofloxacin, 400 mg orally twice a day for 14 days or Levofloxacin, 500 mg orally, once a day for 14 days With or Without Metronidazole, 500 mg orally twice a day for 14 days	Ceftriaxone, 250 mg IM in a single dose or Cefoxitin, 2 g IM PLUS Probenecid, 1 g orally in a single dose, concurrently or Other parenteral third-generation cephalosporin PLUS Doxycycline, 100 mg orally twice a day for 14 days With or Without Metronidazole, 500 mg orally twice a day for 14 days

Source: Centers for Disease Control and Prevention. (2002b). Sexually transmitted diseases treatment guidelines 2002. *MMWR, 51*(RR-6), 1-82.

an intermediate oncogenic potential and are commonly associated with squamous cell carcinoma in situ (Canavan & Doshi, 2000).

Because health care providers are not required to report HPV infections, the true incidence of these infections is not known. An estimated 24 million Americans are infected with HPV, and as many as 1 million new infections occur yearly (CDC, 2002b). In addition to the general risk factors for STIs noted earlier, cigarette smoking and use of oral contraceptives for more than 5 years have been found to be risk factors for HPV.

In women, HPV lesions (also called condylomata acuminata) are most frequently seen in the posterior part of the introitus; however, lesions also are found on the buttocks, vulva, vagina, anus, and cervix (Fig. 8-2). Typically the lesions are small, 2 to 3 mm in diameter and 10 to 15 mm in height, soft, papillary swellings occurring singly or in clusters on the genital and anal-rectal region. Infections of long duration may appear as a cauliflower-like mass. In moist areas such as the vaginal introitus, the lesions may appear to have multiple, fine, fingerlike projections. Vaginal lesions are often multiple. Flat-topped papules, 1 to 4 mm in diameter, are seen most often on the cervix. Often these lesions are visualized only under magnification. Warts are usually flesh colored or slightly darker on Caucasian women, black on African-American women, and brownish on Asian women. Usually painless, the lesions also may be uncomfortable, particularly when very large, inflamed, or ulcerated. Chronic vaginal discharge, pruritis, or dyspareunia can occur.

HPV infections are thought to be more frequent in pregnant than in nonpregnant women, with an increase in incidence from the first trimester to the third. Furthermore, a significant proportion of preexisting HPV lesions enlarge greatly during pregnancy, a proliferation presumably resulting from the relative state of immunosuppression present during pregnancy. Lesions may become so large during pregnancy that they affect urination, defecation, mobility, and fetal descent, although birth by cesarean is rarely necessary (Thomas, 2001). Cesarean birth may be performed when extensive growths are present. Initial observation of large growths can be misleading, suggesting that the entire vagina is involved; however, all of the growth may derive from one stalk, and in such cases, it may be possible to push the large mass to the side, allowing the baby to pass through. HPV infection may be acquired by the neonate during birth; the frequency of such transmission is unknown. The preventive value of cesarean birth is unknown and is not recommended solely to prevent transmission of HPV infection to newborns.

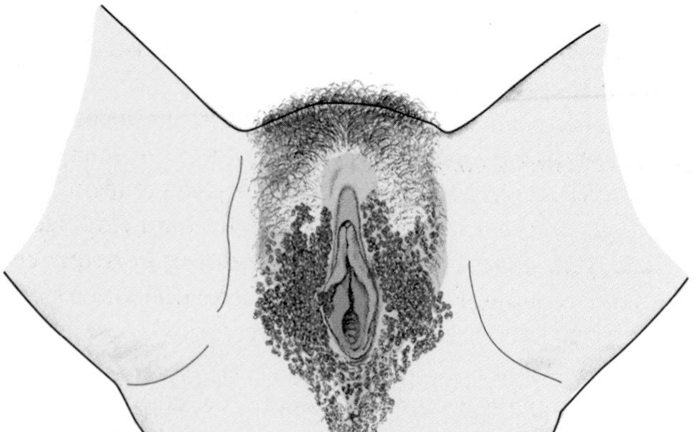

FIG. 8-2 Human papillomavirus infection. Genital warts or condylomata acuminata.

Screening and Diagnosis

A woman with HPV lesions may complain of symptoms such as a profuse, irritating vaginal discharge, itching, dyspareunia, or postcoital bleeding. She also may report "bumps" on her vulva or labia. History of a known exposure is important; however, because of the potentially long latency period and the possibility of subclinical infections in men, the lack of a history of known exposure cannot be used to exclude a diagnosis of HPV infection.

Physical inspection of the vulva, perineum, anus, vagina, and cervix is essential whenever HPV lesions are suspected or seen in one area. Because speculum examination of the vagina may block some lesions, it is important to rotate the speculum blades until all areas are visualized. When lesions are visible, the characteristic appearance previously described is considered diagnostic. However, in many instances, cervical lesions are not visible, and some vaginal or vulvar lesions also may be unobservable to the naked eye. Because of the potential spread of vulvar or vaginal lesions to the anus, gloves should be changed between vaginal and rectal examinations.

Diagnosis is made by colposcopy and direct visualization of the growths or by biopsy. It is imperative that women with vulvar HPV or who have partners with HPV have a cervical examination with a Papanicolaou (Pap) smear. Pap smears of the cervical transformation zone are used as a screening technique; however, because of false-negative results, a negative Pap smear does not indicate absence of disease. The severity of any cervical lesion reported on a Pap smear is best determined by colposcopy and biopsy. Vinegar solution may be used to highlight early or flat cervical lesions; however, it is important to note that a positive reaction also may be obtained with any inflammatory reaction, after sexual intercourse, and with vaginal trauma. DNA testing for high risk types of HPV also is recommended for Pap smears showing cervical abnormalities (Wright et al., 2002).

HPV lesions must be differentiated from molluscum contagiosum and condylomata lata. Molluscum contagiosum lesions are half-domed, smooth, flesh-colored to pearly white papules with depressed centers. Condylomata lata are a form of secondary syphilis and generally are flatter and wider than genital warts. A serologic test for syphilis would confirm the diagnosis of secondary syphilis.

Management

Treatment of genital warts is often difficult. No therapy has been shown to eradicate HPV. The goal of treatment therefore is removal of warts and relief of signs and symptoms, not the eradication of HPV (CDC, 2002b). The client often must make multiple office visits; frequently, many different treatment modalities will be used. Eradication of the virus is not considered conclusive even after there is no visible evidence of wart tissue because of the high incidence of recurrence.

Treatment of genital warts should be guided by preference of the woman, available resources, and experience of the health care provider. None of the treatments is superior to all other treatments, and no one treatment is ideal for all warts (CDC, 2002b). Available treatments are outlined in Table 8-2. Imiquimod, podophyllin, and podofilox should not be used during pregnancy. Because the lesions can proliferate and become friable during pregnancy, many experts recommend their removal by using cryotherapy or various surgical techniques during pregnancy (CDC, 2002b).

Women with discomfort associated with genital warts may find that bathing with an oatmeal solution and drying the area with a cool hair dryer will provide some relief. Keeping the area clean and dry will also decrease growth of the warts. Cotton underwear and loose-fitting clothes that decrease friction and irritation also may decrease discomfort. Women should be advised to maintain a healthy lifestyle to aid the immune system; women can be counseled regarding diet, rest, stress reduction, and exercise.

Client counseling is essential. Women must understand how the virus is transmitted, that no immunity is conferred with infection, and that reacquisition of the infection is likely with repeated contact. Women should know that their partners should be checked even if they are asymptomatic. Because HPV is highly contagious, the majority of women's partners will be infected and should be treated. All sexually active women with multiple partners or a history of HPV should be encouraged to use latex condoms and a vaginal spermicide for intercourse to decrease acquisition or transmission of condylomata.

Instructions for all medications and treatments must be detailed. Women should be informed before treatment of the possibility of posttreatment pain associated with specific therapies. The importance of thorough treatment of concurrent vaginitis or STI should be emphasized. The link between cervical cancer and HPV infections and the need for close follow-up should be discussed. Annual health examinations are recommended to assess disease recurrence and screening for cervical cancer. Women should be counseled to have regular Pap screening, as recommended for women without genital warts. The presence of genital warts is not an indication for a change in Pap smear test frequency or for cervical colposcopy (CDC, 2002b).

Women with HPV infection may radically alter their sexual practices both from fear of transmission to and from a partner and from genital discomfort associated with treatment, which may have a negative impact on their sexual relationships. Unless the partner accepts and understands the necessary precautions, it may be difficult for the woman to follow the treatment regimen. The nurse can offer to discuss feelings that the woman may have. When indicated, joint counseling can be suggested.

Herpes Simplex Virus

Unknown until the middle of the twentieth century, **herpes simplex virus (HSV)** infection is now widespread in the United States, especially in women. HSV infection results in painful recurrent genital ulcers and is caused by two different antigen subtypes of herpes simplex virus: herpes simplex virus 1 (HSV-1) and herpes simplex virus 2 (HSV-2). HSV-2 is usually transmitted sexually, and HSV-1, nonsexually. Although HSV-1 is more commonly associated with gingivostomatitis and oral labial ulcers (fever blisters) and HSV-2 with genital lesions, neither type is exclusively associated with the respective sites.

Although HSV infection is not a reportable disease, it is estimated that about one in five people in the United States are infected with genital herpes and that up to one million new infections occur each year (CDC, 2002b). Recurrent HSV infections are much more common. Most persons infected with HSV-2 have not been diagnosed, and most infections are transmitted by persons unaware that they are infected.

An initial HSV genital infection is characterized by multiple painful lesions, fever, chills, malaise, and severe dysuria and may last 2 to 3 weeks. Women generally have a more severe clinical course than do men. Women with primary genital herpes have many lesions that progress from macules to papules, then forming vesicles, pustules, and ulcers that crust and heal without scarring (Fig. 8-3). These ulcers are extremely tender, and primary infections may be bilateral. Women also may have itching, inguinal tenderness, and lymphadenopathy. Severe vulvar edema may develop, and women may have difficulty sitting. HSV cervicitis also is common with initial HSV-2 infections. The cervix may appear normal or be friable, reddened, ulcerated, or necrotic. A heavy, watery-to-purulent vaginal discharge is common. Extragenital lesions may be present because of autoinoculation. Urinary retention and dysuria may occur secondary to autonomic involvement of the sacral nerve root.

Women with recurrent episodes of HSV infections commonly have only local symptoms that are usually less severe than those associated with the initial infection. Systemic symptoms are usually absent, although the characteristic prodromal genital tingling is common. Recurrent lesions are unilateral, are less severe, and usually last 5 to

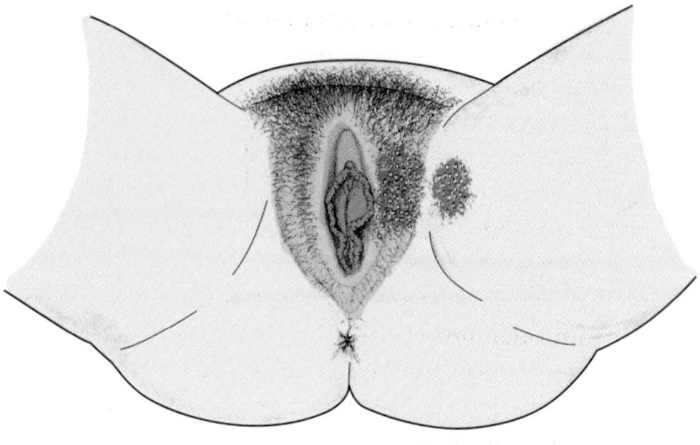

FIG. 8-3 Herpes genitalis.

7 days. Lesions begin as vesicles and progress rapidly to ulcers. Few women with recurrent disease have cervicitis.

During pregnancy, maternal infection with HSV-2 can have adverse effects on both the mother and fetus. Viremia occurs during the primary infection, and congenital infection is possible, though rare. Primary infections during the first trimester have been associated with increased miscarriage rates. The most severe complication of HSV infection is neonatal herpes, a potentially fatal or severely disabling disease occurring in 1 in 2000 to 1 in 10,000 live births. Most mothers of infants who contract neonatal herpes lack histories of clinically evident genital herpes. Risk of neonatal infection is highest among women with primary herpes infection who are near term and is low among women with recurrent herpes (CDC, 2002b). A 60% infant mortality rate is associated with infants who contract HSV infection, and about 50% of those who survive have serious neurologic damage (Corder-Mabe, 1998).

An association between cervical cancer and HSV-2 has been observed. It is theorized that genital herpes is a marker for high risk sexual behaviors that could transmit other STIs, including HPV (DiSaia & Creasman, 2002).

Screening and Diagnosis

A careful history provides much information when making a diagnosis of herpes. A history of exposure to an infected person is important, although infection from an asymptomatic individual is possible. A history of having viral symptoms such as malaise, headache, fever, or myalgia is suggestive. Local symptoms such as vulvar pain, dysuria, itching or burning at the site of infection, and painful genital lesions that heal spontaneously also are highly suggestive of HSV infections. The nurse should ask about a history of a primary infection, prodromal symptoms, vaginal discharge, and dyspareunia. Pregnant women should be asked whether they or their partner(s) have had genital lesions.

During the physical examination, the nurse should assess for inguinal and generalized lymphadenopathy and elevated temperature. The entire vulvar, perineal, vaginal, and cervical areas should be carefully inspected for vesicles or ulcerated or crusted areas. A speculum examination may be very difficult for the woman because of the extreme tenderness often associated with herpes infections. Any suggestive or recurrent lesions found during pregnancy should be cultured to verify HSV. Although a diagnosis of herpes infection may be suspected from the history and physical, it is confirmed by laboratory studies. A viral culture is obtained by swabbing exudate during the vesicular stage of the disease. In primary HSV infection, viral shedding is prolonged, and HSV is more easily isolated.

Management

Genital herpes is a chronic and recurring disease for which there is no known cure. Management is directed toward specific treatment during primary and recurrent infections, prevention, self-help measures, and psychologic support.

Systemic antiviral medications partially control the symptoms and signs of HSV infections when used for the primary or recurrent episodes or when used as daily suppressive therapy. However, these medications do not eradicate the infection, nor do they alter subsequent risk, frequency, or recurrences after the medication is stopped. Three antiviral medications provide clinical benefit: acyclovir, valacyclovir, and famciclovir. Treatment recommendations are given in Table 8-2. Safety and efficacy have been shown clearly in persons taking acyclovir daily for up to 3 years. The safety of acyclovir, valacyclovir, and famciclovir therapy during pregnancy has not been established; however, the first clinical episode of genital herpes during pregnancy may be treated with oral acyclovir. In the presence of severe maternal HSV infection, acyclovir IV is indicated (CDC, 2002b). Continued investigation of HSV therapy with these medications in pregnancy is needed.

Cleaning lesions twice a day with saline will help prevent secondary infection. Bacterial infection must be treated with appropriate antibiotics. Measures that may increase comfort for women when lesions are active include warm sitz baths with baking soda; keeping lesions dry by blowing the area dry with a hair dryer set on cool or patting dry with a soft towel; wearing cotton underwear and loose clothing; using drying aids such as hydrogen peroxide, Burow's solution, or oatmeal baths; applying cool, wet, black tea bags to lesions; and applying compresses with an infusion of cloves or peppermint oil and clove oil to lesions.

Oral analgesics such as aspirin or ibuprofen may be used to relieve pain and systemic symptoms associated with initial infections. Because the mucous membranes affected by herpes are extremely sensitive, any topical agents should be used with caution. Nonantiviral ointments, especially those containing cortisone, should be avoided. A thin layer of lidocaine ointment or an antiseptic spray may be applied to decrease discomfort, especially if walking is difficult.

A diet rich in vitamin C, B-complex vitamins, zinc, and calcium is thought to help prevent recurrences. The amino acid L-lysine has been used in doses of 750 to 1000 mg daily while lesions are active and 500 mg during asymptomatic periods. It is thought that L-lysine has an inhibitory effect on the multiplication of the HSV.

Counseling and education are critical components of the nursing care of women with herpes infections. Information regarding the etiology, signs and symptoms, transmission, and treatment should be provided. The nurse should explain that each woman is unique in her response to herpes and emphasize the variability of symptoms. Women should be helped to understand when viral shedding and thus transmission to a partner is most likely, and that they should refrain from sexual contact from the onset of prodrome until complete healing of lesions. Some authorities recommend consistent use of condoms for all persons with genital herpes. Condoms may not prevent transmission, particularly male-to-female transmission; however, this does not mean that the partners should avoid all intimacy. Women can be encouraged to maintain close contact with their partners while avoiding contact with lesions. Women should be taught how to look for herpetic lesions with a mirror and good light source and a wet cloth or finger covered with a finger cot to rub lightly over the labia. The nurse should ensure that women understand that when lesions are active, sharing intimate articles (e.g., washcloths, wet towel) that come into contact with the lesions should be avoided. Plain soap-and-water is all that is needed to clean hands that have come in contact with herpetic lesions; isolation is not necessary or appropriate.

The nurse should explain the role of precipitating factors in the reactivation of the latent virus and recurrent episodes. Stress, menstruation, trauma, febrile illnesses, chronic illness, and ultraviolet light have all been found to trigger genital herpes. Women may wish to keep a diary to identify stressors that seem to be associated with recurrent herpes attacks so that they can then avoid these stressors when possible. The role of exercise in reducing stress can be discussed. Referral for stress-reduction therapy, yoga, or meditation classes may be indicated. Avoiding excessive heat and sun and hot baths and using a lubricant during sexual intercourse to reduce friction also may be helpful. Women in their childbearing years should be counseled regarding the risk of herpes infection during pregnancy. They should be instructed to use condoms if there is any risk of contracting any STI from a sexual partner. If they are using acyclovir therapy, they should be counseled to use contraception because of the potential teratogenicity of acyclovir. Women who are breastfeeding should use acyclovir with caution because it concentrates in the milk.

Because neonatal HSV infection is such a devastating disease, prevention is critical. Current recommendations include carefully examining and questioning all women about symptoms at onset of labor (CDC, 2002b). If visible lesions are not present at onset of labor, vaginal birth is acceptable. Cesarean birth within 4 hours after labor begins or membranes rupture is recommended if visible lesions are present. Infants who are delivered through an infected vagina should be carefully observed and cultured (see Chapter 38). Some experts recommend presumptive treatment of infants who were exposed to HSV during birth. Because HSV infection may be associated with cervical dysplasia, women must be encouraged to have yearly Pap smears and gynecologic examinations.

The emotional impact of contracting herpes is considerable. Media publicity regarding this disease has made receiving a diagnosis of genital herpes a devastating experience. No cure is available, and most women will experience recurrences. At diagnosis, many emotions may surface–helplessness, anger, denial, guilt, anxiety, shame, or inadequacy. Women need the opportunity to discuss their feelings and help in learning to live with the disease. A woman can be encouraged to think of herself as a person who is not diseased but rather healthy and inconvenienced from time to time. Herpes can affect a woman's sexuality, her sexual practices, and her current and future relationships. She may need help in raising the issue with her partner or with future partners.

Viral Hepatitis

Five different viruses (hepatitis viruses A, B, C, D, and E) account for almost all cases of viral hepatitis in humans. Hepatitis viruses A, B, and C are discussed. Hepatitis D and E viruses, common among users of intravenous drugs and recipients of multiple blood transfusions, are not included in this discussion.

Hepatitis A

Hepatitis A virus (HAV) infection is acquired primarily through a fecal-oral route by ingestion of contaminated food, particularly milk, shellfish, or polluted water, or person-to-person contact. However, hepatitis A, like other enteric infections, can be transmitted during sexual activity. Women living in the western United States, Native Americans, Alaskan Natives, and children and employees in day care centers are at high risk.

HAV infection is characterized by flulike symptoms with malaise, fatigue, anorexia, nausea, pruritis, fever, and right upper quadrant pain. Serologic testing to detect the immunoglobulin M (IgM) antibody is done to confirm acute infections. The IgM antibody is detectable 5 to 10 days after exposure and can remain positive for up to 6 months. Because HAV infection is self-limited and does not result in chronic infection or chronic liver disease, treatment is usually supportive. Women who become dehydrated from nausea and vomiting or who have fulminating hepatitis A may need to be hospitalized. Medications that might cause liver damage or that are metabolized in the liver (e.g., acetaminophen, ethyl alcohol) should be avoided. A well-balanced diet is recommended. Immune globulin (gamma-globulin) or immune-specific globulin is indicated for any pregnant woman exposed to HAV to provide passive immunity through injected antibodies. All household contacts of the woman also should receive gamma-globulin. Vaccination is the most effective means of preventing HAV transmission; maintenance of "good personal hygeine" has not been successful in preventing HAV outbreaks (CDC, 2000a).

Hepatitis B

Hepatitis B virus (HBV) is the virus most threatening to the fetus and neonate. It is caused by a large DNA virus and is associated with three antigens and their antibodies: hepatitis B surface antigen (HBsAG), HBV antigen (HBeAG), HBV core antigen (HBcAG), antibody to HBsAG (anti-HBs), antibody to HBeAG (anti-HBe), and antibody to HBcAG (anti-HBc). Screening for active or chronic disease or disease immunity is based on testing for these antigens and their antibodies.

HBV infection can be transmitted parenterally, perinatally, and rarely, orally, as well as through intimate contact. It is 50 to 100 times more contagious than HIV. The hepatitis B carrier state affects 5% of the world's population, with higher percentages found in tropical areas and Southeast Asia. HBsAG has been found in blood, saliva, sweat, tears, vaginal secretions, and semen. Perinatal transmission does occur; however, the fetus is not at risk until it comes in contact with contaminated blood during birth. Infants born to mothers who are highly infectious (positive for both HBsAG and HBeAG) have a 10% to 90% chance of acquiring perinatal hepatitis B infection (Thomas, 2001). Approximately 90% of infected infants will become chronic carriers. HBV also has been transmitted by artificial insemination.

Factors considered to place a woman at risk for HBV are those associated with STI risk in general: history of multiple sexual partners, multiple STIs, and intravenous drug use; and behaviors that are associated with blood contact (e.g., work or treatment in a dialysis unit, history of multiple blood transfusions, public safety workers exposed to blood in the workplace, health care workers). Although HBV can be transmitted via blood transfusion, the incidence of such infections has decreased significantly since testing of blood for HBsAG became a routine procedure. Drug abusers who share needles are at risk, as are health care workers who are exposed to blood and needle sticks. In addition, women of Asian, Pacific Islander (Polynesian, Micronesian, and Melanesian), or Alaskan Eskimo descent and of Haitian or sub-Saharan Africa birth are considered to be at risk.

HBV infection is a disease of the liver and is often a silent infection. In the adult, the course of the infection can be fulminating, and the outcome, fatal. Symptoms of HBV infection are similar to those of hepatitis A: arthralgias, arthritis, lassitude, anorexia, nausea, vomiting, headache, fever, and mild abdominal pain. Later the woman may have clay-colored stools, dark urine, increased abdominal pain, and jaundice. Between 5% and 10% of individuals with HBV have persistence of HBsAG and become chronic hepatitis B carriers. Twenty-five percent of chronic carriers die of primary hepatocellular carcinoma or cirrhosis of the liver.

Screening and Diagnosis. All women at high risk for contracting HBV should be screened on a regular basis. Screening only individuals at high risk may not identify up to 50% of HBsAG-positive women; therefore current CDC guidelines recommend screening for the presence of HBsAG on all women at the first prenatal visit, regardless of whether they have been tested previously, and repeated later in pregnancy for women with high risk behaviors (CDC, 2002b).

Testing for HBV is complex. Clients with acute hepatitis B generally have detectable serum HBsAG levels in the late incubation phase of the disease, 2 to 5 weeks before symptoms appear. Anti-HBs with a negative HBsAG test signals immunity. Anti-HBs with a positive antigen denotes a chronic carrier state; during this time, the disease can be transmitted. During the recovery phase, the client may continue to be infectious even though HBsAG cannot be detected. This is called the "window phase" and is identified by anti-HBc in the absence of anti-Hbs. Women should be prepared for repeated testing because HBV screening tests also may be used to monitor the progression of the disease.

Components of the history to be obtained when hepatitis B is suspected include the inquiry about the symptoms of the disease and risk factors outlined earlier. Physical examination includes inspection of the skin for rashes, inspection of the skin and conjunctiva for jaundice, and palpation of the liver for enlargement and tenderness. Weight loss, fever, and general debilitation should be noted. If the HBsAG is positive, further laboratory studies may be ordered (anti-HBe, anti-HBc, serum glutamic-oxaloacetic transaminase [SGOT], alkaline phosphatase, and liver panel). If the HBsAG is negative in early pregnancy and the woman could be in the window phase or if high risk behaviors continue during pregnancy, a repeated HBsAG should be ordered in the third trimester.

Management. There is no specific treatment for hepatitis B. Recovery is usually spontaneous in 3 to 16 weeks. Pregnancies complicated by acute viral hepatitis are managed on an outpatient basis. Women should be advised to increase bed rest; eat a high-protein, low-fat diet; and increase their fluid intake. They should avoid medications metabolized in the liver, drugs, and alcohol. Pregnant women with a definite exposure to HBV should be given hepatitis B immune globulin and should begin the hepatitis B vaccine series within 14 days of the most recent contact to prevent infection (CDC, 2002b). Vaccination during pregnancy is not thought to pose risks to the fetus.

All nonimmune women at high or moderate risk of hepatitis should be informed of the availability of hepatitis B vaccine. Vaccination is recommended for all individuals who have had multiple sex partners within the past 6 months (CDC, 2002b). In addition, intravenous drug users, residents of correctional or long-term care facilities, persons seeking care for an STI, prostitutes, women whose partners are intravenous drug users or bisexual, and women whose occupation exposes them to high risk should be vaccinated. The vaccine is given in a series of three (four if rapid protection is needed) doses over a 6-month period, with the first two doses given at least 1 month apart. The vaccine is given in the deltoid muscle (CDC, 2002b).

Client education includes explaining the meaning of hepatitis B infection, including transmission, state of infectivity, and sequelae. The nurse also should explain the need for immunoprophylaxis for household members and sexual contacts. To decrease transmission of the virus, women with hepatitis B or who test positive for HBV should be advised to maintain a high level of personal hygiene (e.g., wash hands after using the toilet; carefully dispose of tampons, pads, bandages in plastic bags; do not share razor blades, toothbrushes, needles, manicure implements; have male partner use a condom if unvaccinated and without hepatitis; avoid sharing saliva through kissing, or sharing of silverware or dishes; wipe up blood spills immediately with soap and water). They should inform all health care providers of their carrier state. Postpartum women should be reassured that breastfeeding is not contraindicated if their infants received prophylaxis at birth and are currently on the immunization schedule.

Hepatitis C

Hepatitis C virus (HCV) infection, the most common blood-borne infection in the United States, has become an important health problem as increasing numbers of persons acquire the disease. Fourteen percent of the U.S. population is infected with HCV (Hunt, Carson, & Sharara, 1997). Because up to 70% of clients with HCV infection progress to chronic hepatitis, hepatitis C represents nearly 50% of chronic viral hepatitis. The most common risk factor for pregnant women is a history of injecting intravenous drugs. Other risk factors include STIs such as hepatitis B and HIV, multiple sexual partners, and a history of blood transfusions. Hepatitis C is readily transmitted through exposure to blood and much less efficiently through semen, saliva, or urine.

Most clients with hepatitis C are asymptomatic or have general flulike symptoms similar to hepatitis A. About 10% have fatigue, nausea, and anorexia (Hunt et al., 1997). HCV infection is confirmed by the presence of anti-C antibody during laboratory testing. Routine HCV testing is recommended for women who have ever injected drugs; women who received a blood transfusion prior to July 1992; children of HCV-positive women; health care, emergency, medical, and public safety workers; and women with chronic liver disease (CDC, 2002b).

Interferon alfa-2b is the main therapy for HCV infection, although effectiveness of this treatment varies. In addition, drug-abuse treatment is an important adjunct for many persons with HCV (CDC, 2002b). Currently there is no vaccine to prevent hepatitis C. Transmission of HCV through breastfeeding has not been reported.

Human Immunodeficiency Virus

Although HIV has traditionally been thought to be a homosexual or gay disease, heterosexual transmission is now the most common means of transmission in women. Furthermore, women are now the fastest-growing population of individuals with HIV infection and acquired immunodeficiency syndrome (AIDS). Between 1985 and 1997, the proportion of women with AIDS tripled. HIV/AIDS infections are seen disproportionately in women of color (African-American and Hispanic).

Transmission of HIV, a retrovirus, occurs primarily through exchange of body fluids (semen, blood, or less commonly, vaginal secretions). Severe depression of the cellular immune system associated with HIV infection characterizes AIDS. For both men and women, the most frequently reported opportunistic diseases are *Pneumocystis carinii* pneumonia (PCP), candida esophagitis, and wasting syndrome. Other viral infections such as HSV and cytomegalovirus infections seem to be more prevalent in women than men. PID may be more severe in HIV-infected women, and rates of HPV and cervical dysplasia may be higher. The clinical course of HPV infection in women with HIV infection is accelerated, and recurrence is more frequent.

Once HIV enters the body, seroconversion to HIV positivity usually occurs within 6 to 12 weeks. Although HIV seroconversion may be totally asymptomatic, it usually is accompanied by a viremic, influenza-like response. Symptoms include fever, headache, night sweats, malaise, generalized lymphadenopathy, myalgias, nausea, diarrhea, weight loss, sore throat, and rash.

Laboratory studies may reveal leukopenia, thrombocytopenia, anemia, and an elevated erythrocyte sedimentation rate. HIV has a strong affinity for surface-marker proteins on T lymphocytes. This affinity leads to significant T-cell destruction. Both clinical and epidemiologic studies have shown that declining CD4 levels are strongly associated with increased incidence of AIDS-related diseases and death in many different groups of HIV-infected persons.

Screening and Diagnosis

Screening, teaching, and counseling regarding HIV risk factors, indications for being tested, and testing are major roles for nurses caring for women today. A number of behaviors place women at risk for HIV infection, including intravenous drug use, high risk sexual partners, multiple sex partners, and a previous history of multiple STIs. HIV infection is usually diagnosed by using HIV-1 and HIV-2 antibody tests. Antibody testing is first done with a sensitive screening test such as the enzyme immunoassay (EIA). Reactive screening tests must be confirmed by an additional test, such as the Western blot or an immunofluorescence assay. If a positive antibody test is confirmed by a supplemental test, it means that a woman is infected with HIV and is capable of infecting others. HIV antibodies are detectable in at least 95% of clients within 3 months after infection. Although a negative antibody test usually indicates that a person is not infected, antibody tests cannot exclude recent infection. Because HIV antibody crosses the placenta, definite diagnosis of HIV in children younger than 18 months is based on laboratory evidence of HIV in blood or tissues by culture, nucleic acid, or antigen detection (CDC, 2002b).

CDC guidelines recommend offering HIV testing to all women whose behavior places them at risk for HIV infection (CDC, 2002b). It may be useful to allow women to self-select for HIV testing. On entry to the health care system, a woman can be handed written information about the risk factors for the AIDS virus and asked to inform the nurse if she believes she is at risk. She should be told that she does not have to say why she may be at risk, only that she thinks she might be.

Counseling for HIV Testing

Counseling before and after HIV testing is standard nursing practice today. It is a nursing responsibility to assess a woman's understanding of the information such a test would provide and to be sure the client thoroughly understands the emotional, legal, and medical implications of a positive or negative test before she is ready to take an HIV test. One's life is profoundly altered by knowledge of HIV seropositivity. A unique stigma associated with HIV infection can have a profound impact on the quality of life of those infected. This stigma extends to those who are asymptomatic but seropositive (see Research box).

Pregnant women should be counseled about their options and contraceptive counseling offered to HIV-positive women who do not desire pregnancy. HIV-infected women should be informed specifically about the risks for perinatal infection. Current evidence indicates that 15% to 25% of infants born to untreated HIV-infected women are infected with HIV; an additional 12% to 14% are infected when breastfeeding continues after age 1 year (CDC, 2002b).

All pregnant women should be offered voluntary counseling and HIV testing as early in pregnancy as possible (Allen et al., 2001; CDC, 2002b). This recommendation is essential because of the available treatments that can reduce the likelihood of perinatal transmission and maintain the health of the woman.

Perinatal transmission of HIV has decreased significantly in the past decade because of the prophylactic administration of antiretroviral prophylaxis (zidovudine [ZDV, AZT, Retrovir]) to pregnant women in the prenatal and perinatal period. Oral ZDV is initiated between 14 and 34 weeks of pregnancy and continued until labor. During labor, intravenous ZDV is administered. The newborn infant then receives oral ZDV for 6 weeks after birth. The transmission rate of HIV to the newborn with this protocol demonstrated a 66% decrease in the Pediatric AIDS Clinical Trials Group (PACTG protocol 076) in the early 1990s (Allen et al., 2001). The suspected means of protection for the fetus is preexposure prophylaxis. With this standard of care, rates of perinatal transmission to the fetus have been reported as low as 4% (Perinatal HIV Guidelines Working Group, 2001).

Other factors identified as potentially influencing perinatal transmission of HIV to the fetus include length of

RESEARCH

Disclosure Decisions by African-American Women with HIV

The stigma attached to being human immunodeficiency virus (HIV) positive is a very powerful force, especially in the southern United States. Negative attitudes toward HIV may mirror the underlying attitudes toward certain social groups, who are judged to display unacceptable behavior. Stigma is experienced both directly when one is shamed and vicariously when observing the shaming of another with similar circumstances. Stigma also flows laterally, reflecting poorly on the family and allies of the targeted person.

Low-income African-American women are already familiar with being marginalized, which is exacerbated by a diagnosis of HIV-positive status. To elucidate their coping strategies, nurse researchers analyzed themes from interviews with 48 women who were HIV positive. Data analysis revealed that the women carefully considered when and to whom to disclose their HIV status. The women were always calculating the risks and benefits of disclosure, trying to maximize the resources and support available to them and minimize the risk for censure and isolation that might occur to themselves and their families. A small group of very secretive women trusted no one with the information and suffered increasing isolation. An even smaller group of full disclosers informed all except their young children. The majority of women revealed their status on a "need to know" basis when they felt the support they would receive would outweigh the risk of disapproval or betrayal. Some women reported feeling "depersonalized" and stigmatized when they sought health care, especially in small town and rural settings.

IMPLICATIONS FOR PRACTICE

In this study, many women expressed relief and gratitude for finally being able to discuss their status. A therapeutic relationship with a nurse can neutralize negative societal pressures. The continuing challenge of educating the public about HIV is urgent as is the need to keep all health care workers updated.

Reference: Black, B., & Miles, M. (2002). Calculating the risks and benefits of disclosure in African American women who have HIV. *Journal of Obstetric, Gynecologic, and Neonatal Nursing, 31*(6), 688-697.

time membranes are ruptured before birth, mode of birth, duration of labor, especially prolonged second stage expulsion efforts, increased maternal viral load levels, and multiple births. Exposure to cervical and vaginal secretions is the likely mechanism of transmission to the newborn, rather than in utero exposure (Klirsfeld, 1998). Cesarean birth has been shown to be of undisputed benefit for preventing vertical transmission of HIV; however, complications after cesarean birth are more common in HIV-positive women than in uninfected women, and it is unknown whether postpartum morbidity is higher in HIV-infected than in uninfected women (Grubert et al., 1999; Perinatal HIV Guidelines Working Group, 2001). The American College of Obstetricians and Gynecologists (2001) issued recommendations on the use of cesarean birth as an intervention for prevention of HIV perinatal transmission.

Given the strong social stigma attached to HIV infection, nurses must consider the issue of confidentiality and documentation before providing counseling and offering HIV testing to clients.

LEGAL TIP HIV Testing

- If test results are placed in the woman's chart—the appropriate place for all health information—they are available to all who have access to the chart. The woman must be informed of this before testing. Informed consent must be obtained before an HIV test is performed. In some states, written consent is mandated.
- Counseling associated with HIV testing has two components: pretest and posttest counseling. During pretest counseling, nurses conduct a personalized risk assessment, explain the meaning of positive and negative test results, obtain informed consent for HIV testing, and help women develop a realistic plan for reducing risk and preventing infection. Posttest counseling includes informing the woman of the test results, reviewing the meaning of the results, and reinforcing infection prevention messages. All pretest and posttest counseling should be documented.

There is generally a 1-week to 3-week waiting period after testing for HIV, which can be a very anxious time for the woman. It is helpful if the nurse informs her that this time period between blood drawing and test results is routine. Test results, whatever they are, always must be communicated in person and women informed in advance that such is the procedure. Whenever possible, the person who provided the pretest counseling also should tell the woman her test results. Some women, when informed of negative results, may escalate their risk behaviors because of an equating of negativity with immunity. Others may believe that negative means "bad" and positive means "good." Women's reactions to a negative test should be explored, asking, "How do you feel?" HIV-negative result counseling sessions are another opportunity to provide education. Emphasis can be placed on ways in which a woman can remain HIV free. She should be reminded that if she has been exposed to HIV in the past 6 months, she should be retested, and that if she continues high risk behaviors, she should have ongoing testing.

In posttest counseling to an HIV-positive woman, privacy with no interruptions is essential. Adequate time for the counseling sessions also should be provided. The nurse should make sure that the woman understands what a positive test means and review the reliability of the test results. Safer sex guidelines should be reemphasized. Referral for appropriate medical evaluation and follow-up should be made, and the need or desire for psychosocial or psychiatric referrals should be assessed.

The importance of early medical evaluation so that a baseline assessment can be made and prophylactic medication begun should be stressed. If possible, the nurse should make a referral or appointment for the woman at the posttest counseling session.

As the number of HIV-infected women escalates, prevention, education, and counseling activities must be directed toward all women. It is very difficult to keep abreast of the ever-changing picture of AIDS. Important sources of information are listed in the Resources at the end of the chapter.

Management

During the initial contact with an HIV-infected woman, the nurse should establish what the woman knows about HIV infection and that she is being cared for by a medical practitioner or facility with expertise in caring for persons with HIV infections, including AIDS. Psychologic referral also may be indicated. Resources such as counseling for death and dying, suicide prevention, financial assistance, and legal advocacy may be appropriate. All women who are drug users should be referred to a substance-abuse program. A major focus of counseling is prevention of transmission of HIV to partners.

Nurses counseling seropositive women wishing contraceptive information may recommend oral contraceptives and latex condoms or tubal sterilization or vasectomy and latex condoms. The IUD is not an ideal choice for the HIV-infected woman because of increased risk of infection. Insertion in a woman who is immunocompromised should be avoided (World Health Organization, 2000). Female condoms or abstinence can be offered to women whose partners refuse to use condoms.

No cure is available for HIV infection. Rare and unusual diseases are characteristic of HIV infection. Opportunistic infections and concurrent diseases should be managed vigorously with treatment specific to the infection or disease. Discussion of the medical care of HIV-positive women and women with AIDS is beyond the scope of this chapter. The reader is referred to the Centers for Disease Control and Prevention AIDS hotlines and Internet websites for the current information and recommendations (see Resources at end of chapter).

Routine gynecologic care for HIV-positive women should include a pelvic examination every 6 months. Careful Pap screening is essential because of the greatly increased incidence of abnormal findings. In addition, HIV-positive women should be screened for syphilis, gonorrhea, chlamydia, and other vaginal infections.

Coinfection with syphilis is common in HIV-infected women, and unusual serologic responses have been documented among HIV-infected persons who have syphilis (CDC, 2002b). Because treatment failures with benzathine penicillin are common, follow-up and evaluation must be done at 3, 6, 9, 12, and 24 months after therapy. Furthermore, HIV infection increases susceptibility to neurosyphilis, which is difficult to differentiate clinically from HIV dementia.

VAGINAL INFECTIONS

Vaginal discharge and itching of the vulva and vagina are among the most frequent reasons a woman seeks help from a health care provider; more women complain of vaginal discharge than of any other gynecologic symptom. Vaginal discharge resulting from infection must be distinguished from normal secretions. Women who have adequate endogenous or exogenous estrogen will have vaginal secretions. Normal vaginal secretions, or leukorrhea, are clear to cloudy in appearance and may turn yellow after drying; the discharge is slightly slimy, is nonirritating, and has a mild, inoffensive odor. Normal vaginal secretions are acidic, with a pH range of 4 to 5. The amount of leukorrhea differs with phases of the menstrual cycle, with greater amounts occurring at ovulation and just before menses. Leukorrhea also is increased during pregnancy. Normal vaginal secretions contain lactobacilli and epithelial cells.

Vaginitis, or abnormal vaginal discharge, is an infection caused by a microorganism. The most common vaginal infections are bacterial vaginosis, candidiasis, and trichomoniasis. **Vulvovaginitis**, or inflammation of the vulva and vagina, may be caused by vaginal infection; copious leukorrhea, which can cause maceration of tissues; and chemical irritants, allergens, and foreign bodies, which may produce inflammatory reactions.

Bacterial Vaginosis

Bacterial vaginosis (BV), formerly called nonspecific vaginitis, *Haemophilus vaginitis*, or *Gardnerella*, is the most common type of vaginitis (Plourd, 1997). BV is associated with preterm labor and birth. The exact etiology of BV is unknown. It is a syndrome in which normal H_2O_2-producing lactobacilli are replaced with high concentrations of anaerobic bacteria (*Gardnerella* and *Mobiluncus*). With the proliferation of anaerobes, the level of vaginal amines is increased, and the normal acidic pH of the vagina is altered. Epithelial cells slough, and numerous bacteria attach to their surfaces (clue cells). When the amines are volatilized, the characteristic odor of BV occurs.

Screening and Diagnosis

A careful history may help distinguish BV from other vaginal infections if the woman is symptomatic. Women with previous occurrence of similar symptoms, diagnosis, and treatment should be queried, because women with BV often have been treated incorrectly because of misdiagnosis.

Most women with BV complain of a characteristic "fishy odor"; however, not all note it. The odor may be noticed by the woman or her partner after heterosexual intercourse because semen releases the vaginal amines. When present, the BV discharge is usually profuse; thin; and white, gray, or milky in appearance. Some women also may have mild irritation or pruritis.

Microscopic examination of vaginal secretions is always done (Table 8-4). Both normal saline and 10% potassium hydroxide smears should be made. The presence of clue cells (vaginal epithelial cells coated with bacteria) by wet smear is highly diagnostic because the phenomenon is specific to BV (USPSTF, 2001b). Vaginal secretions should be tested for pH and amine odor. Nitrazine paper is sensitive enough to detect a pH of 4.5 or greater. The fishy odor of BV will be released when KOH is added to vaginal secretions on the lip of the withdrawn speculum.

Management

Treatment of bacterial vaginosis with oral metronidazole (Flagyl) is most effective (CDC, 2002b). Table 8-5 outlines treatment guidelines.

TABLE 8-4 **Wet Smear Tests for Vaginal Infections**

INFECTION	TEST	POSITIVE FINDINGS
Trichomoniasis	Saline wet smear (vaginal secretions mixed with normal saline on a glass slide)	Presence of many white blood cell protozoa
Candidiasis	Potassium hydroxide (KOH) prep (vaginal secretions mixed with KOH on a glass slide)	Presence of hyphae and pseudohyphae (buds and branches of yeast cells)
Bacterial vaginosis	Normal saline smear	Presence of clue cells (vaginal epithelial cells coated with bacteria)
	Whiff test (vaginal secretions mixed with KOH)	Release of fishy odor

TABLE 8-5 **Vaginal Infections and Drug Therapies for Women**

DISEASE	NONPREGNANT WOMEN 13-17 YEARS OF AGE	NONPREGNANT WOMEN >18 YEARS OF AGE	PREGNANT WOMEN	LACTATING WOMEN
Bacterial vaginosis	*Recommended:* Metronidazole, 500 mg bid for 7 days (no alcohol) or Metronidazole gel 0.75%, 5 g per vagina bid for 7 days or Clindamycin cream 2%, 5 g per vagina for 7 days (less effective) or *Alternatives:* Metronidazole, 2 g orally once or Clindamycin, 300 mg orally bid for 7 days (less effective)	*Recommended:* Metronidazole, 500 mg bid for 7 days (no alcohol) or Metronidazole gel 0.75%, 5 g per vagina bid for 7 days or Clindamycin cream 2%, 5 g per vagina for 7 days (less effective) or *Alternatives:* Metronidazole, 2 g orally once or Clindamycin, 300 mg orally bid for 7 days (less effective)	High risk asymptomatic or symptomatic women *Recommended:* Metronidazole, 250 mg orally tid for 7 days *Alternatives:* Metronidazole, 2 g orally once or Clindamycin, 300 mg orally bid for 7 days Low risk symptomatic women *Recommended:* Metronidazole, 250 mg orally tid for 7 days *Alternatives:* Metronidazole, 2 g orally once or Clindamycin, 300 mg orally bid for 7 days or Metronidazole gel 0.75%, 5 g per vagina bid for 5 days	*Recommended:* Clindamycin cream
Trichomoniasis	*Recommended:* Metronidazole, 2 g orally once *Alternative:* Metronidazole, 500 mg bid for 7 days	*Recommended:* Metronidazole, 2 g orally once *Alternative:* Metronidazole, 500 mg bid for 7 days	*Recommended:* Metronidazole, 2 g orally once	Not recommended during lactation; stop lactation, treat, resume in 48 hr after drug completed
Candidiasis	Numerous over-the-counter topical intravaginal agents: butoconazole, clotrimazole, miconazole, tioconazole, terconazole; treatment with azole drugs more effective than nystatin Dose varies by agent from a single dose to 3 days to 7 to 14 days *Oral agent:* Fluconazole 150 mg oral tablet once	Numerous over-the-counter topical intravaginal agents: butoconazole, clotrimazole, miconazole, tioconazole, terconazole; treatment with azole drugs more effective than nystatin Dose varies by agent from a single dose to 3 days to 7 to 14 days *Oral agent:* Fluconazole 150 mg oral tablet once	Over-the-counter topical azole intravaginal agents: butoconazole, clotrimazole, miconazole, terconazole Use for 7 days Oral agents not recommended	Over-the-counter topical azole intravaginal agents: butoconazole, clotrimazole, miconazole, terconazole Use for 7 days

Source: Centers for Disease Control and Prevention. (2002b). Sexually transmitted diseases treatment guidelines 2002. *MMWR, 51*(RR-6), 1-82.

Metronidazole (Flagyl) is an antiprotozoal and antibacterial agent. Metronidazole was formerly contraindicated in the first trimester of pregnancy; however, because of the increased risk of preterm birth, current CDC guidelines recommend treatment of all asymptomatic pregnant women at high risk, as well as all symptomatic pregnant women (CDC, 2002). The medication is contraindicated if the woman is breastfeeding because high concentrations have been found in infants. If it is necessary to prescribe metronidazole for the lactating woman, she can suspend breastfeeding temporarily (pump and discard milk to maintain supply), and resume it 48 to 72 hours after taking the last dose. Metronidazole is contraindicated in clients with blood dyscrasia or central nervous system disease because in rare cases Flagyl may affect the hematopoietic or central nervous system.

Side effects of metronidazole are numerous, including sharp, unpleasant metallic taste in the mouth; furry tongue; central nervous system reactions; and urinary tract disturbances. When oral metronidazole is taken, the client is advised not to drink alcoholic beverages, or she will have the severe side effects of abdominal distress, nausea, vomiting, and headache. Gastrointestinal symptoms are common whether alcohol is consumed or not. Treatment of sexual partners is not recommended because sexual transmission of BV has not been proven (CDC, 2002b).

Candidiasis

Vulvovaginal candidiasis, or yeast infection, is the second most common type of vaginal infection in the United States. Although vaginal candidiasis infections are common in healthy women, those seen in women with HIV infection are often more severe and persistent. Genital candidiasis lesions may be painful, coalescing ulcerations necessitating continuous prophylactic therapy.

The most common organism is *Candida albicans*; it is estimated that 80% to 95% of the yeast infections in women are caused by this organism. However, in the past 10 years, the incidence of non–*C. albicans* infections has increased steadily. Women with chronic or recurrent infections often are infected with a higher percentage of non–*C. albicans* species than are women with their first infection or are those who have few recurrences.

Numerous factors have been identified as predisposing a woman to yeast infections, including antibiotic therapy, particularly broad-spectrum antibiotics such as ampicillin, tetracycline, cephalosporins, and metronidazole; diabetes, especially when uncontrolled; pregnancy; obesity; diets high in refined sugars or artificial sweeteners; use of corticosteroids and exogenous hormones; and immunosuppressed states. Clinical observations and research have suggested that tight-fitting clothing and underwear or pantyhose made of nonabsorbent materials create an environment in which a vaginal fungus can grow.

The most common symptom of yeast infections is vulvar and possibly vaginal pruritis. The itching may be mild or intense, interfere with rest and activities, and occur during or after intercourse. Some women report a feeling of dryness. Others may have painful urination as the urine flows over the vulva; this usually occurs in women who have excoriations resulting from scratching. Most often the discharge is thick, white, lumpy, and cottage cheese–like. The discharge may be found in patches on the vaginal walls, cervix, and labia. Commonly the vulva are red and swollen, as are the labial folds, vagina, and cervix. Although there is no characteristic odor with yeast infections, sometimes a yeasty or musty smell occurs.

Screening and Diagnosis

In addition to a careful history of the woman's symptoms, their onset, and course, the history is a valuable screening tool for identifying predisposing risk factors. Physical examination should include a thorough inspection of the vulva and vagina. A speculum examination is always done. Commonly saline and KOH wet smear and vaginal pH are obtained. Vaginal pH is normal with a yeast infection; if the pH is greater than 4.5, trichomoniasis or BV should be suspected. The characteristic pseudohyphae (bud or branching of a fungus) may be seen on a wet smear done with normal saline; however, they may be confused with other cells and artifacts.

Management

A number of antifungal preparations are available for the treatment of *C. albicans* (see Table 8-5). In 1990, many of these medications (e.g., miconazole [Monistat] and clotrimazole [Gyne-Lotrimin]) were made available as over-the-counter (OTC) agents. The first time a woman suspects that she may have a yeast infection, she should see a health care provider for confirmation of the diagnosis and treatment recommendation. If she has another infection, she may wish to purchase an OTC preparation and self-treat. If she elects to do this, she should always be counseled regarding seeking care for numerous recurrent or chronic yeast infections. If vaginal discharge is extremely thick and copious, vaginal debridement with a cotton swab followed by application of vaginal medication may be useful.

Women who have extensive irritation, swelling, and discomfort of the labia and vulva may find sitz baths helpful in decreasing inflammation and increasing comfort. Adding Aveeno powder to the bath also may increase the woman's comfort. Not wearing underpants to bed may help decrease symptoms and prevent recurrences. Completing the full course of treatment prescribed is essential to removing the pathogen, and women are instructed to continue medication even during menstruation. They should be counseled not to use tampons during menses because the medication will be absorbed by the tampon. If possible, intercourse is avoided during treatment; if this is not feasible, the woman's partner should use a condom to prevent introduction of more organisms. Suggested measures to prevent genital tract infections are outlined in the Teaching for Self-Care box.

Trichomoniasis

Trichomoniasis is almost always a sexually transmitted infection. It also is a common cause of vaginal infection (up to 25% of all vaginitis) and discharge and thus is discussed in this section.

Trichomoniasis is caused by *Trichomonas vaginalis*, an anaerobic one-celled protozoan with characteristic flagellae. Although trichomoniasis may be asymptomatic, commonly women have characteristically yellowish to greenish, frothy, mucopurulent, copious, malodorous discharge. Inflammation of the vulva, vagina, or both may be present, and the woman may complain of irritation and pruritis. Dysuria and dyspareunia are often present. Typically, the discharge worsens during and after menstruation. Often the cervix and vaginal walls will demonstrate the characteristic "strawberry spots" or tiny petechiae, and the cervix may bleed on contact. In severe infections, the vaginal walls, cervix, and occasionally the vulva may be acutely inflamed.

Screening and Diagnosis

In addition to obtaining a history of current symptoms, a careful sexual history should be obtained. Any history of similar symptoms in the past and treatment used should be noted. The nurse should determine whether the client's partner(s) were treated and if she has had subsequent relations with new partners.

A speculum examination is always done, even though it may be very uncomfortable for the woman; relaxation techniques and breathing exercises may help the woman with the procedure. Any of the classic signs may be present on physical examination. The typical one-celled flagellate trichomonads are easily distinguished on a normal saline wet prep. Trichomoniasis also may be identified on Pap smears. Because trichomoniasis is an STI, once diagnosis is confirmed, appropriate laboratory studies for other STIs should be carried out.

Management

The recommended treatment is metronidazole, 2 g orally in a single dose (CDC, 2002b) (see Table 8-5). Although the male partner is usually asymptomatic, it is recommended that he receive treatment also, because he often harbors the trichomonads in the urethra or prostate. It is important that nurses discuss the importance of partner treatment with their clients because if they are not treated, it is likely that the infection will recur.

Women with trichomoniasis need to understand the sexual transmission of this disease. The client must know that the organism may be present without symptoms being present, perhaps for several months, and that it is not possible to determine when she became infected. Women should be informed of the necessity for treating all sexual partners and helped with ways to raise the issue with their partner(s).

Group B Streptococcus

Group B streptococcus (GBS) may be considered a part of the normal vaginal flora in a woman who is not pregnant, and it is present in 9% to 23% of healthy pregnant women. GBS infection is associated with poor pregnancy outcomes (Guise, 2001). Furthermore, GBS infections are an important factor in neonatal morbidity and mortality, usually resulting from vertical transmission from the birth canal of the infected mother to the infant during birth (Lieu et al., 1998).

Risk factors for neonatal GBS infection include positive prenatal culture for GBS in the current pregnancy; preterm birth of less than 37 weeks of gestation; premature rupture of membranes for longer than 18 hours; intrapartum maternal fever higher than 38° C; and a positive history for early-onset neonatal GBS.

To decrease the risk of neonatal GBS infection, it is recommended that all women be screened at 35 to 37 weeks' gestation for GBS using a rectovaginal culture and intravenous antibiotic prophylaxis (IAP) be offered to all who test positive. If a culture is not available at onset of labor or if risk factor present, IAP is also offered. IAP is not recommended before a cesarean birth if labor or rupture of membranes has not occurred. The recommended treatment is penicillin G, 5 million units IV loading dose, and then 2.5 million units IV every 4 hours during labor. Ampicillin, 2 g loading dose IV, followed by 1 g IV every 4 hours, is an alternative therapy.

TEACHING FOR SELF-CARE

Prevention of Genital Tract Infections

- Practice genital hygiene.
- Choose underwear or hosiery with a cotton crotch.
- Avoid tight-fitting clothing (especially tight jeans).
- Select cloth car seat covers instead of vinyl.
- Limit time spent in damp exercise clothes (especially swimsuits, leotards, and tights).
- Limit exposure to bath salts or bubble bath.
- Avoid colored or scented toilet tissue.
- If sensitive, discontinue use of feminine hygiene deodorant sprays.
- Use condoms.
- Void before and after intercourse.
- Decrease dietary sugar.
- Drink yeast-active milk and eat yogurt (with lactobacilli).
- Do not douche.

EFFECTS OF SEXUALLY TRANSMITTED INFECTIONS ON PREGNANCY AND THE FETUS

Sexually transmitted infections in pregnancy are responsible for significant morbidity and mortality. Some consequences of maternal infection, such as infertility and sterility, last a lifetime. Congenitally acquired infection may affect a child's length and quality of life. Table 8-6 describes the effects of several common STIs on pregnancy and the fetus. It is difficult to predict these effects with certainty. Factors such as coinfection with other STIs and when in pregnancy the infection was treated can affect outcomes.

TORCH Infections

TORCH infections can affect a pregnant woman and her fetus. *T*oxoplasmosis, *o*ther infections (e.g., hepatitis), *r*ubella virus, *c*ytomegalovirus (CMV), and *h*erpes simplex virus, known collectively as TORCH infections, form a group of organisms capable of crossing the placenta and adversely affecting the development of the fetus. Generally, all TORCH infections produce influenza-like symptoms in the mother, but fetal and neonatal effects are more serious. TORCH infections and their maternal and fetal effects are shown in Table 8-7. Neonatal effects are discussed in Chapter 38.

Toxoplasmosis – Raw meat/kitty litter

Toxoplasmosis is a protozoan infection associated with the consumption of infested raw or undercooked meat and with poor handwashing after handling infected cat litter. Pregnant women with HIV antibodies are at higher risk because toxoplasmosis is a common accompanying opportunistic infection. The presence of toxoplasmosis can be determined through blood studies, although laboratory diagnosis is difficult. Women at risk for infection should have toxoplasmosis titers evaluated. Acute infection in pregnancy produces influenza-like symptoms and lymphadenopathy in some women but no symptoms in others. Miscarriage may occur.

The treatment of choice for toxoplasmosis is spiramycin, sulfadine, or a combination of pyrimethamine and sulfadiazine. Although pyrimethamine may be potentially harmful to the fetus, treatment of the parasitemia is essential (Lopez, Dietz, Wilson, Navin, & Jones, 2000).

Other Infections

The primary infection included in the category of other infections is hepatitis, which was discussed previously. Infections other than hepatitis also may be identified as "other" TORCH infections. These include GBS, varicella, and HIV.

Rubella

Rubella, also called German measles or 3-day measles, is a viral infection transmitted by droplets (such as from an infected person's sneeze). Rash, muscle aches, joint pain, and mild lymphedema are usually seen in the infected mother. Consequences for the fetus are much more serious and include miscarriage, congenital anomalies (referred to as congenital rubella syndrome), and death. Vaccination of

TABLE 8-6 **Pregnancy and Fetal Effects of Common Sexually Transmitted Infections**

INFECTION	PREGNANCY EFFECTS	FETAL EFFECTS
Chlamydia	Premature rupture of membranes Preterm labor	Preterm birth Conjunctivitis Pneumonia
Gonorrhea	Intraamniotic infection Preterm labor Premature rupture of membranes Postpartum endometritis Miscarriage	Preterm birth Sepsis Conjunctivitis
Group B streptococcus	Preterm labor Premature rupture of membranes Chorioamnionitis Postpartum sepsis Urinary tract infections	Preterm birth Early-onset sepsis
Herpes simplex	Rare: infection	Systemic infection
Human papillomavirus (HPV)	Dystocia from large lesions Excessive bleeding from lesions after birth trauma	Respiratory papillomatosis (rare)
Syphilis	Preterm labor Miscarriage	Preterm birth Stillbirth Congenital infection

Data from Cunningham, F. et al. (2001). *Williams obstetrics* (21st ed.). New York: McGraw-Hill; Gilbert, E., & Harmon, J. (2003). *Manual of high risk pregnancy and delivery* (3rd ed.). St. Louis: Mosby; Cowles, T., & Gonik, B. (2002). Perinatal infections. In A. Fanaroff & R. Martin (eds.), *Neonatal-perinatal medicine: Diseases of the fetus and infant* (7th ed). St. Louis: Mosby.

TABLE 8-7 **Maternal Infection: TORCH**

INFECTION	MATERNAL EFFECTS	FETAL EFFECTS	COUNSELING: PREVENTION, IDENTIFICATION, AND MANAGEMENT
Toxoplasmosis (protozoa)	Acute infection similar to influenza, lymphadenopathy Woman immune after first episode (except in immunocompromised clients)	With maternal acute infection, parasitemia Less likely to occur with maternal chronic infection Miscarriage likely with acute infection early in pregnancy	Use good handwashing technique Avoid eating raw meat and exposure to litter used by infected cats; if cats in house, have toxoplasma titer checked If titer is rising during early pregnancy, abortion may be considered an option
Other Hepatitis A (infectious hepatitis) (virus)	Miscarriage, cause of liver failure during pregnancy Fever, malaise, nausea, and abdominal discomfort	Exposure during first trimester, fetal anomalies, fetal or neonatal hepatitis, preterm birth, intrauterine fetal death	Usually spread by droplet or hand contact especially by culinary workers; gamma-globulin can be given as prophylaxis for hepatitis A; vaccine is available for populations at risk
Hepatitis B (serum hepatitis) (virus)	Symptoms variable: fever, rash, arthralgia, depressed appetite, dyspepsia, abdominal pain, generalized aching, malaise, weakness, jaundice, tender and enlarged liver	Infection occurs during birth Maternal vaccination during pregnancy presents no risk for fetus	Generally passed by contaminated needles, syringes, or blood transfusions or sexually; also can be transmitted orally (but incubation period is longer); hepatitis B immune globulin can be given prophylactically after exposure Hepatitis B vaccinations recommendations: universal infant immunizations, universal immunizations of previously unvaccinated adolescents age 11-12 yr, adolescents and adults at increased risk Populations at risk are women from Asia, Pacific Islands, Indochina, Haiti, South Africa, Alaska (women of Eskimo descent); other women at risk include health care providers, users of intravenous drugs, those sexually active with multiple partners or single partner with multiple risks

Source: Centers for Disease Control and Prevention. (2002b). Sexually transmitted diseases treatment guidelines 2002. *MMWR, 51*(RR-6), 1-82; Cowles, T., & Gonik, B. (2002). Perinatal infections. In A. Fanaroff & R. Martin (eds.), *Neonatal-perinatal medicine: Diseases of the fetus and infant* (7th ed.). St. Louis: Mosby.

Continued

TABLE 8-7 **Maternal Infection: TORCH—cont'd**

INFECTION	MATERNAL EFFECTS	FETAL EFFECTS	COUNSELING: PREVENTION, IDENTIFICATION, AND MANAGEMENT
Rubella (3-day German measles) (virus)	Joint pain, muscle aches, rash, fever, mild symptoms; suboccipital lymph nodes may be swollen; some photophobia Occasionally arthritis or encephalitis Miscarriage	Incidence of congenital anomalies: first trimester 50%-90% Exposure during first 2 mo: malformations of heart, eyes, ears, or brain; abnormal dermatoglyphics Exposure after fourth mo: hearing loss, psychomotor retardation, systemic infection, hepatosplenomegaly, intrauterine growth restriction, rash, heart disease, cataracts	Vaccination of pregnant women contraindicated; pregnancy should be prevented for 3 mo after vaccination; pregnant women nonreactive to hemagglutinin-inhibition antigen can be safely vaccinated after birth
Cytomegalovirus (CMV) (a herpesvirus)	Respiratory or sexually transmitted asymptomatic illness or mononucleosis-like syndrome, may have cervical discharge No immunity develops	Fetal death or severe, generalized disease: hemolytic anemia and jaundice, hydrocephaly or microcephaly, pneumonitis, hepatosplenomegaly, deafness, mental retardation	Virus may be reactivated and cause disease in utero or during birth in subsequent pregnancies; fetal infection may occur during passage through infected birth canal; disease is commonly progressive through infancy and childhood
Herpes genitalis (herpes simplex virus, type 2 [HSV-2])	Primary blisters, rash, fever, malaise, nausea, headache; pregnancy risks include miscarriage, preterm labor, stillbirths	Transmission occurs after rupture of membranes; congenital effects include skin lesions and scarring, IUGR, mental retardation, microcephaly Active HSV in first trimester, there is 20%-50% miscarriage/stillbirth rate	Risk of transmission is greatest during vaginal birth if woman has active lesions Acyclovir not recommended in pregnancy; treat symptomatically (see Table 8-2)

pregnant women is contraindicated because a rubella infection may develop after the live vaccine is administered. Rubella vaccine is given to women who are not immune as part of preconception counseling or in the postpartum period prior to discharge, with instructions to use contraception for at least 3 months after vaccination.

Cytomegalovirus

Maternal infection with CMV may begin as a mononucleosis-like syndrome. In most adults the onset of CMV infection is uncertain and asymptomatic; however, the disease may become a chronic persistent infection. Approximately 60% of the adult population have antibodies to CMV. This virus is primarily transmitted by close contacts but also has been isolated from semen, cervical and vaginal secretions, breast milk, placental tissue, urine, feces, and banked blood. Maternal CMV infection may be diagnosed by presence of CMV in urine or in serum, because many women have evidence of CMV infection. Women who show CMV infection in pregnancy (by positive viral titers) usually have chronic or recurrent infections (Cowles & Gonik, 2002).

Women at risk for infection include those who work in or have children in day care centers, institutions for the mentally retarded, or certain health care settings (such as nursery, dialysis, laboratory, and oncology).

In the United States, 1% to 2% of infants have congenital CMV infection. Fetal infection can cause microcephaly; eye, ear, and dental defects; and mental retardation. No treatment is available during pregnancy.

Herpes Simplex Virus[7]

The potential pregnancy effects of primary genital herpes infection include miscarriage, preterm labor, and intrauterine growth restriction. The main route of HSV transmission from mother to neonate is through an infected birth canal. The risk of maternal-infant transmission is greater during a primary HSV-2 infection than during a recurrent episode. Cesarean birth is not recommended for all mothers with HSV; only mothers with clinical evidence of active lesions during labor should have cesarean birth. Prenatal HSV cultures do not predict the presence of a live virus at time of birth. Cultures in women with HSV lesions at or near term may be done to determine the absence of the virus at time of birth and increase the likelihood of a vaginal birth (see Table 8-2 for treatment guidelines).

CARE MANAGEMENT

Women may delay seeking care for STIs and other infections because they fear social stigma, have little accessibility to health care services, are asymptomatic, or are unaware that they have an infection.

Assessment and Nursing Diagnoses

A comprehensive assessment focuses on lifestyle issues that are often personal or sensitive. A culturally sensitive, nonjudgmental approach is essential to facilitate accurate data collection. Specific areas to address are listed in Box 8-3. A history that is accurate, comprehensive, and specific is crucial to diagnosis.

History

Because many women are embarrassed or anxious, the history should be taken first, with the woman dressed. Information should be collected in a nonjudgmental manner, by using open-ended questions and avoiding assumptions of sexual preference. All partners should be referred to as partners and not by gender. A complete history is essential in identifying possible STIs. Factors that may influence the development and management of STIs in women include history of STI or PID, number of past or current sexual partners, and types of sexual activity. Women should be queried for specific lifestyle behaviors that place them at risk for STIs. Among these are intravenous drug use or partner intravenous drug use, smoking, alcohol use, inadequate or poor nutrition, and high levels of stress or fatigue.

Physical Examination

Before the actual physical examination is performed, the nurse should discuss the examination with the woman so she is prepared for it. A thorough assessment of symptoms including a comprehensive physical examination is essential to diagnosing STIs. Because the speculum usually is not lubricated before insertion into the vagina (cultures of vaginal secretions may have to be obtained), insertion may be more uncomfortable than usual. Women should be informed of this and reassured that every effort will be made to make the speculum examination as comfortable as possible.

Laboratory Tests

Appropriate laboratory studies will be suggested, in part, by the history and physical examination results. Bacterial STIs are easily determined from genital tract, urine, and blood studies. Viral agents also can be cultured, but less successfully. Because women often are infected with more than one STI simultaneously, and many are asymptomatic, additional laboratory studies may be done, including Pap smear, wet mounts, gonococcal culture, and VDRL or RPR test for syphilis. Cultures for HSV are obtained when indicated by history or physical examination. The woman should be offered the HIV-antibody test. When indicated, a complete blood count, sedimentation rate, urinalysis, or urine culture and sensitivity should be obtained.

BOX 8-3 Essential Areas of Assessment for a Woman at Risk for or Who Has a Sexually Transmitted Infection

CURRENT PROBLEM

What symptoms are present?
- Vaginal discharge
- Lesions
- Rash
- Dysuria
- Fever
- Itching, burning
- Dyspareunia
- Malaise

MEDICAL HISTORY

History of STIs
Allergies, especially to medications

MENSTRUAL HISTORY

Last menstrual period (possibility of pregnancy)

PERSONAL AND SOCIAL HISTORY

Sexual History
Sexual preference
Number of partners (past, present)
Types of sexual activity
Frequency of sexual activity

LIFESTYLE BEHAVIORS

Intravenous drug use (or use by partner)
Smoking
Alcohol use
Inadequate/poor nutrition
High levels of stress, fatigue

Nursing diagnoses are derived after carefully analyzing assessment findings, medical management, and health care provider directives. The following nursing diagnoses are representative of those used in a plan of care for women with STIs and other vaginal infections:

- *Anxiety/situational low self-esteem/disturbed body image related to*
  - –perceived effects on sexual relationships and family processes
  - –possible effects on pregnancy/fetus
  - –long-term sequelae of infection
- *Deficient knowledge related to*
  - –transmission/prevention of infection/reinfection
  - –safer sex behaviors
  - –management of infection
- *Acute pain/impaired tissue integrity related to*
  - –effects of infection process
  - –scratching (excoriation) of pruritic areas
  - –hygiene practices
- *Sexual dysfunction related to*
  - –effects of infection process
- *Social isolation and impaired social interaction related to*
  - –perceived effects on relationships with others if STI status is unknown

Expected Outcomes of Care

Care of the woman with an STI focuses on physical and psychologic needs. Avoidance of reinfection and harmful sequelae is critical. Measurable expected outcomes are mutually derived with the woman's input. Outcomes for the woman include that she will do the following:

- Be free of infection or, in the case of viral infection, have remission or stabilization of the infection.
- Identify and be able to discuss the etiology, management, and expected course of the infection and its prevention.
- Be able to identify her risky behaviors and discuss plans for decreasing her risk for infection.

Plan of Care and Interventions

The woman with an STI will need encouragement to seek care at the earliest stage of symptoms. Counseling women about STIs is essential for (1) preventing new infections or reinfection; (2) increasing compliance with treatment and follow-up; (3) providing support during treatment; and (4) assisting women in discussions with their partner(s). Women must be made aware of the serious potential consequences of STIs and the behaviors that increase the likelihood of infection.

The nurse must make sure that the woman understands what infection she has, how it is transmitted, and why it must be treated (see Teaching for Self-Care box). Women should be given a brief description of the infection in language that they can understand. This description should include modes of transmission, incubation period, symptoms, infectious period, and potential complications. Effective treatment of STIs necessitates careful, thorough explanation of the treatment regimen and follow-up procedures. Thorough, careful instructions about medications must be provided, both verbally and in writing. Side effects, benefits, and risks of the medication should be discussed. Unpleasant side effects or early relief of symptoms may discourage women from completing their medication course. Clients should be strongly urged to take all the medication and not stop even if their symptoms diminish or disappear in a few days. Comfort measures to decrease symptoms such as pain, itching, or nausea should be suggested. Providing written information is a useful strategy because this is a time of high anxiety for many women, and they may not be able to hear or remember what they were told. A number of booklets on STIs are available, or the nurse may wish to develop literature that is specific to the practice setting and clients.

In general, women will be advised to refrain from intercourse until all treatment is finished and a repeat culture, if appropriate, is done. After the infection is cured, women should be urged to continue using condoms to prevent repeat infections, especially if they have had one episode of PID or continue to have intercourse with new partners. Women may wish to avoid having sex with partners who have many other sexual partners. All women who have contracted an STI should be taught safer sex practices, if this has not been done already. Follow-up appointments should be made as needed.

Addressing the psychosocial component of STIs is essential. A woman may be afraid or embarrassed to tell her partner or to ask her partner to seek treatment. She may be embarrassed to admit her sexual practices, or she may be concerned about confidentiality. The nurse may need to help the woman deal with the impact of a diagnosis of an STI on a committed relationship, for the woman is now faced with the necessity of dealing with "uncertain monogamy."

TEACHING FOR SELF-CARE

Sexually Transmitted Infections

- Take your medication as directed.
- Use comfort measures for symptom relief as suggested by your health care provider.
- Keep your appointment for repeat cultures or checkups after your treatment to make sure your infection is cured.
- Inform your sexual partner(s) to be tested and treated, if necessary.
- Abstain from sexual intercourse until your treatment is completed or for as long as you are advised by your health care provider.
- Use safer sex practices when sexual intercourse is resumed.
- Call your health care provider immediately if you notice bumps, sores, rashes, or discharges.
- Keep all future appointments with your health care provider, even if things appear normal.

In many instances, sexual partners should be treated; thus the infected woman is asked to identify and notify all partners who might have been exposed. Often she will find this difficult to do. Empathizing with the client's feelings and suggesting specific ways of talking with partners will help decrease anxiety and assist in efforts to control infection. For example, the nurse might suggest that the woman say, "I care about you and I'm concerned about you. That's why I'm calling to tell you that I have a sexually transmitted infection. My clinician is _________ and she will be happy to talk with you if you would like." Offering literature and role playing situations with the client also may be of assistance. It is often helpful to remind the woman that although this is an embarrassing situation, most persons would rather know than not know that they have been exposed. Health professionals who take time to counsel their clients on how to talk with their partner(s) can improve compliance and case finding.

Interrupting the transmission of infection is crucial to STI control. For treatable and vaccine-preventable STIs, further transmission and reinfection can be prevented with referral of sex partners. Many STIs are reportable; all states require that the five traditional venereal diseases—gonorrhea, syphilis, chancroid, lymphogranuloma venereum, and granuloma inguinale—be reported to public health officials. Many other states require that other STIs such as chlamydial infections, genital herpes, and genital warts be reported. In addition, all states require that AIDS cases be reported; 35 states require that HIV infection be reported. The nurse is legally responsible for reporting all cases of those diseases identified as reportable and should know what the requirements are in the state in which she or he practices. The woman must be informed when a case will be reported and told why. Failure to inform the woman that the case will be reported is a serious breech of professional ethics. Confidentiality is a crucial issue for many clients. When an STI is reportable, women must be told that they may be contacted by a health department epidemiologist. They should be assured that the information reported to and collected by health authorities is not available to anyone without their permission. Every effort, within the limits of one's public health responsibilities, should be made to reassure clients (see Plan of Care).

Plan of Care: Sexually Transmitted Infections

NURSING DIAGNOSIS Ineffective health maintenance related to prevention of sexually transmitted infections evidenced by client positive diagnosis of sexually transmitted infection

Expected Outcome *Woman will verbalize which health practices directly led to positive diagnosis of a sexually transmitted infection.*

Nursing Interventions/*Rationales*

Inquire about woman's sexual history and sexual health practices *to provide database for current problem.*

Use therapeutic communication for private, nonjudgmental discussion *to facilitate learning and promote self-esteem.*

Provide emotional support *to indicate awareness of woman's feelings about this sensitive topic.*

Provide information about transmission of disease, including cause, symptoms, and treatment for both partners *to enhance woman's knowledge base and correct any misinformation.*

Discuss the use and importance of safe sexual practices *to raise woman's awareness and motivation to avoid future risk-taking behaviors.*

Instruct woman and sexual partner to complete medication regimen *to completely eradicate transmitted organism.*

NURSING DIAGNOSIS Impaired social interaction related to diagnosis of sexually transmitted disease as evidenced by client verbal report

Expected Outcome *Woman will report increased incidences of social interaction.*

Nursing Interventions/*Rationales*

Provide nonjudgmental, confidential therapeutic communication *to increase woman's feelings of self-worth.*

Refer to support groups *to provide group interaction, discussion, and information.*

NURSING DIAGNOSIS Impaired tissue integrity related to effects of disease process as evidenced by client report of itching and vaginal discharge

Expected Outcome *Woman's tissue integrity will be restored.*

Nursing Interventions/*Rationales*

Assess, monitor, and document characteristics of the damaged skin area, including color, lesions, drainage, and edema *to provide database.*

Instruct woman in correct genital hygiene practices *to prevent further infection of damaged tissues with other organisms.*

Provide warm soaks or sitz baths *to promote comfort, circulation, and healing.*

Administer prescribed medications *to promote comfort and eradication of organism.*

Provide written self-help materials and pamphlets *to prevent further skin integrity loss.*

Teach woman to perform self-vulvar examination to encourage participation in self-care.

NURSING DIAGNOSIS Anxiety related to diagnosis of STI

Expected Outcome *Woman will report decreased level of anxiety.*

Nursing Interventions/*Rationales*

Provide opportunity for therapeutic communication *to promote trust and expression of feelings.*

Assist woman to identify effective coping mechanisms *to decrease anxiety.*

Refer to support groups *to share feelings and common effective strategies.*

BOX 8-4 Standard Precautions

Medical history and examination cannot reliably identify all persons infected with HIV or other blood-borne pathogens. Standard Precautions should therefore be used consistently in the care of all persons. These precautions apply to blood, body fluids, and all secretions and excretions, except sweat, nonintact skin, and mucous membranes. Standard Precautions are recommended to reduce the risk of transmission of microorganisms from known and unknown sources of infection (Bolyard, E. et al., 1998; CDC, 2001b).

1. Prompt and thorough handwashing is recommended between client contacts. Hands and other skin surfaces should be washed immediately and thoroughly if contaminated with blood or other body fluids. Hands should be washed immediately after gloves are removed.
2. In addition to handwashing, all health care workers should routinely use appropriate barrier precautions to prevent skin and mucous membrane exposure when contact with blood or other body fluids of any person is anticipated. *Latex gloves* should be worn for touching blood and body fluids, mucous membranes, or nonintact skin of all persons; for handling items or surfaces soiled with blood or body fluids; and for performing venipuncture and other vascular access procedures. Gloves should be changed after contact with each client. *Masks and protective eyewear* or face shields should be worn during procedures that are likely to generate droplets of blood or other body fluids to prevent exposure of mucous membranes of the mouth, nose, and eyes. *Gowns or aprons* should be worn during procedures that are likely to generate splashes of blood or other body fluids.

   Leg coverings, boots, or shoe covers also can be worn to provide protection against splashes and may be recommended for certain procedures such as surgery.
3. All health care workers should take precautions to prevent injuries caused by needles, scalpels, and other sharp instruments or devices during procedures; when cleaning used instruments; during disposal of used needles; and when handling sharp instruments after procedures. *To prevent needle-stick injuries,* needles should not be recapped, purposely bent or broken by hand, removed from disposable syringes, or otherwise manipulated by hand. After they are used, disposable syringes and needles, scalpel blades, and other sharp items should be immediately placed in a puncture-resistant container for disposal; puncture-resistant containers should be located as close as is practical to the use area.
4. Although saliva has not been implicated in HIV transmission, to minimize the need for emergency mouth-to-mouth resuscitation, mouthpieces, resuscitation bags, or other ventilation devices should be available for use in areas in which the need for resuscitation is predictable.
5. Health care workers who have exudative lesions or weeping dermatitis should refrain from all direct client care and from handling client care equipment until the condition resolves.

PRECAUTIONS FOR INVASIVE PROCEDURES

An invasive procedure is surgical entry into tissues, cavities, or organs; or repair of major traumatic injuries (1) in an operating or birthing room, emergency department, or out-of-hospital setting, including both physicians' and dentists' offices; and (2) a vaginal or cesarean birth or other invasive obstetric procedure during which bleeding may occur. Standard Precautions, combined with the following precautions, should serve as minimum precautions for all such invasive procedures:

1. All health care workers who participate in invasive procedures must routinely use appropriate barrier precautions to prevent skin and mucous membrane contact with blood and other body fluids of all clients. Gloves and surgical masks must be worn for all invasive procedures. Protective eyewear or face shields should be worn for procedures that commonly result in the generation of droplets, splashing of blood or other body fluids, or the generation of bone chips. Gowns or aprons made of materials that provide an effective barrier should be worn during invasive procedures that are likely to result in the splashing of blood or other body fluids. All health care workers who perform or assist in vaginal or cesarean births should wear gloves and gowns when handling the placenta or the infant until blood and amniotic fluid have been removed from the infant's skin. Gloves should be worn during infant eye prophylaxis, care of the umbilical cord, circumcision site, parenteral procedures, diaper changes, contact with colostrum, and postpartum assessments.
2. If a glove is torn or a needle stick or other injury occurs, the glove should be removed and a new glove used as promptly as client safety permits; the needle or instrument involved in the incident also should be removed from the sterile field.
3. Any needle stick or other injury should be reported and appropriate treatment obtained as specified by the health care facility.

Management During Pregnancy

Treatment of specific STIs may be different for the pregnant woman and may even be different at different stages of pregnancy. Tables 8-2 and 8-5 describe treatment of common STIs and vaginal infections during pregnancy.

Infection Control

Infection-control measures are essential to protect care providers and to prevent nosocomial infection of clients, regardless of the infectious agent. The risk for occupational transmission varies with the disease. Even when the risk is low, as with HIV, the existence of any risk warrants reasonable precautions. Precautions against airborne disease transmission are available in all health care agencies. **Standard Precautions** (precautions to use in care of all persons for infection control) and additional precautions for labor and birth settings are listed in Box 8-4.

Evaluation

Evaluation is a continuous process. To be effective, evaluation is based on client-centered outcomes identified during the planning stage of nursing care. The nurse can be reasonably assured that care was effective to the extent that expected outcomes have been met.

KEY POINTS

- Safer sex practices are key STI-prevention strategies.
- HIV is transmitted through body fluids, primarily blood, semen, and vaginal secretions.
- HPV is the most common viral STI.
- Syphilis has reemerged as a common STI.
- Chlamydia is the most common STI in American women and the most common cause of PID.
- Viral hepatitis has several forms of transmission; HBV infections carry the greatest risk.
- Young, sexually active women who do not practice safer sex behaviors and have multiple partners are at greatest risk for STIs and HIV.
- STIs are responsible for substantial mortality and morbidity, great personal suffering, and heavy economic burden in the United States.
- STIs and vaginitis are biologic events for which all individuals have a right to expect objective, compassionate, and effective health care.
- Substance abuse can alter the body's immune system and possibly increase the risk for acquiring AIDS and associated conditions.
- Pregnancy confers no immunity against infection, and both mother and fetus must be considered when the pregnant woman contracts an infection.
- Because history and examination cannot reliably identify all persons with HIV or other blood-borne pathogens, blood and body-fluid precautions should be used consistently for everyone all the time.

CRITICAL THINKING EXERCISES

1. You are assigned to a clinic to take maternal histories at the first prenatal visit. A 16-year-old gives the following history. She has had unprotected intercourse with her boyfriend, who also has had sex with other girls in her class at school. She has missed one menstrual period, and her pregnancy test was positive.
   a. What risk factors are present, and what are the possible effects on the pregnancy?
   b. What interventions might be successful in working with this pregnant teen and why?
   c. Identify community resources that could be used in providing care.
2. You have been assigned to teach safe sex practices to a group of college freshmen during orientation week.
   a. Develop learning outcomes for the group
   b. Determine information that should be included
   c. Investigate sexual counseling resources on campus and the community and compose an annotated list to give to the group.
   d. Give presentation and collect evaluative data on how well learning outcomes were achieved.
3. Examine the pros and cons of mandatory HIV testing and prepare to debate the issue in a clinical conference.

RESOURCES

Centers for Disease Control and Prevention
1600 Clifton Rd NE
Atlanta, GA 30333
202-329-1819

www.cdc.gov: a site containing comprehensive data regarding the health of populations in the United States. The Centers for Disease Control and Prevention maintains the site, and provides the most up-to-date epidemiologic data available regarding HIV and AIDS in the United States.

National AIDS Hotline
800-342-2437 (English)
800-344-7432 (Spanish)
800-243-7889 (hearing-impaired)

National AIDS Information Clearing House
P.O. Box 6003
Rockville, MD 20850
800-458-5231 (English and Spanish)

National Sexually Transmitted Diseases Hotline
800-227-8922

Reliable and up-to-date information regarding HIV and AIDS epidemiology and treatment can be found at these websites:

www.hivinsite.ucsf.edu: A very informative site for health care professionals with a comprehensive AIDS knowledge base covering almost all HIV/AIDS-related issues.

www.hopkins-aids.edu: A comprehensive site including an epidemiology section. Maintained by the Johns Hopkins AIDS Service.

www.hivatis.org: A site dedicated to the most up-to-date recommendations for HIV and AIDS management. The Panel on Clinical Practices for Treatment of HIV Infection posts its latest recommendations on this site, maintained by the HIV/AIDS Treatment Information Service.

REFERENCES

Allen, D. et al. (2001). Revised recommendations for HIV screening of pregnant women. *MMWR, 50*(RR-19), 59-86.

American Academy of Pediatrics Committee on Drugs. (2002). The transfer of drugs and other chemicals into human milk. *Pediatrics, 108*(3), 776-789.

American College of Obstetricians and Gynecologists. (2001). ACOG committee opinion: Scheduled cesarean delivery and the prevention of vertical transmission of HIV infection. No. 234, May 2000. *International Journal of Gynaecology and Obstetrics, 73*(3), 279-281.

Bolyard, E. et al. (1998). Guidelines for infection control in health care personnel, 1998. *American Journal of Infection Control, 26*, 289-354.

Bonny, A., & Biro, F. (1998, Spring). Recognizing and treating STDs in the adolescent. *Contemporary Nurse Practitioner,* 15-18, 20-24.

Cavavan, T., & Doshi, N. (2000). Cervical cancer. *American Family Physician, 61,* 1369-1376.

Centers for Disease Control and Prevention. (1999). Prevention of hepatitis A through active or passive immunization: Recommendations of the Advisory Committee on Immunization Practice. *MMWR, 48*(RR-12), 1-37.

Centers for Disease Control and Prevention. (2001a). *Sexually transmitted disease surveillance, 2000.* http://www.cdc.gov/stc/stats.

Centers for Disease Control and Prevention. (2001b). Updated US Public Health Service guidelines for the management of occupational exposures to HBV, HCV, and HIV and recommendations for postexposure prophylaxis. *MMWR 50*(RR-11), 1-52.

Centers for Disease Control and Prevention. (2001c). Viral hepatitis C prevention and control. http://www.cdc.gov/ncidod/diseases/hepatitis/c/plan/HCV_infection.htm.

Centers for Disease Control and Prevention. (2002a). Prevention of perinatal group B streptococcal disease: Revised guidelines from CDC. *MMWR, 51*(RR-11), 1-23.

Centers for Disease Control and Prevention. (2002b). Sexually transmitted diseases treatment guidelines 2002. *MMWR, 51*(RR-6), 1-82.

Corder-Mabe, J. (1998). Complications of pregnancy. In E. Youngkin & M. Davis (Eds.), *Women's health care: A clinical guide* (2nd ed.). Stamford, CT: Appleton & Lange.

Cowles, T., & Gonik, B. (2002). Perinatal infections. In A. Fanaroff & R. Martin (Eds.), *Neonatal-perinatal medicine: Diseases of the fetus and infant* (7th ed.). St. Louis: Mosby.

Cunningham, F. et al. (2001). *Williams obstetrics* (21st ed.). New York: McGraw-Hill.

DiSaia, P., & Creasman, W. (2002). *Clinical gynecologic oncology* (6th ed.). St. Louis: Mosby.

Fogel, C. (2003). Sexuality. In E. Breslin & V. Lucas (Eds.), *AWHONN women's health nursing: Toward evidence-based practice.* Philadelphia: W.B. Saunders.

Gilbert, E., & Harmon, J. (2003). *Manual of high risk pregnancy and delivery* (3rd ed.). St. Louis: Mosby.

Grubert, T. et al (1999). Complications after cesarean section in HIV-1-infected women not taking antiretroviral treatment (Research letter). *Lancet, 354*(9190), 1612.

Guise, J. et al. (2001). Screening for bacterial vaginosis in pregnancy. *American Journal of Preventive Medicine, 20*(3S), 62-72.

Hatcher, R. et al. (2003). *Contraceptive technology* (18th ed.). New York: Ardent Media, Inc.

Hunt, C., Carson, K., & Sharara, A. (1997). Hepatitis C in pregnancy. *Obstetrics and Gynecology, 89*(5, pt 2), 883-890.

Hutchinson, M. (1999). Individual, family, and relationship predictors of young women's sexual risk perceptions. *Journal of Obstetric, Gynecologic, and Neonatal Nursing, 28*(1), 60-67.

Institute of Medicine, Committee on Prevention and Control of Sexually Transmitted Diseases. (1997). *The hidden epidemic: Confronting sexually transmitted diseases.* Washington, DC: National Academy of Sciences.

Klirsfeld, D. (1998). HIV disease and women. *Medical Clinics of North America, 82*(2), 335-357.

Lieu, T. et al. (1998). Neonatal group B streptococcal infection in a managed care population. *Obstetrics and Gynecology, 92* (1), 21-27.

Lopez, A. et al. (March 31, 2000). Preventing congenital toxoplasmosis. National Center for Infections Diseases. http://www.cdc.gov/epo/mmwr/preview/mmwthtml/rr4902a5.htm.

Perinatal HIV Guidelines Working Group. (2001). *Public Health Service Task Force recommendations for use of antiretroviral drugs in pregnant HIV-1-infected women for maternal health and interventions to reduce perinatal HIV-1 transmission in the United States.* [Online]. http://www.hivatis.org. Retrieved May 4, 2001.

Plourd, D. (1997). Practical guide to diagnosing and treating vaginitis. *Medscape Women's Health, 2*(1), 1-13.

Rawlins, S. (2001). Nonviral sexually transmitted infections. *Journal of Obstetric, Gynecologic, and Neonatal Nursing, 30*(3), 324-331.

Schaffer, S. (1998). Vaginitis and sexually transmitted diseases. In E. Youngkin & M. Davis (Eds.), *Women's health. A primary care clinical guide.* Stamford, CT: Appleton & Lange.

Thomas, D. (2001). Sexually transmitted viral infections: Epidemiology and treatment. *Journal of Obstetric, Gynecologic, and Neonatal Nursing, 30*(3), 316-323.

Toney, J., & Montero, J. (2000). Sexually transmitted diseases: Where do we go from here? *Infectious Medicine, 17*(2), 92-100, 127.

USPSTF. (2001a). Screening for chlamydial infection: Recommendations and rationale. *American Journal of Preventive Medicine, 20*(3S), 90-94.

USPSTF. (2001b). Screening for bacterial vaginosis in pregnancy: Recommendations and rationale. *American Journal of Nursing, 102*(8), 91-93.

Walsh, C., & Irwin, K. (2002). Combating the silent *Chlamydia* epidemic. *Contemporary OB/GYN,* 90-98.

Wilkerson, D. et al. (2002). Nonoxynol-9 spermicide for prevention of vaginally acquired HIV and other sexually transmitted infections: Systematic review and meta-analysis of randomised controlled trials including more than 5000 women. *Lancet Infectious Diseases, 2*(10), 613-617.

Workowski, K., Levine, W., & Wasserheit, J. (2002). U.S. Centers for Disease Control and Prevention guidelines for the treatment of sexually transmitted diseases: An opportunity to unify clinical and public health practice. *Annals of Internal Medicine, 137*(4), 255-262.

World Health Organization (WHO), Department of Reproductive Health and Research. (2000). *Improving access to quality care in family planning: Medical eligibility criteria for contraceptive use* (2nd ed). Geneva: WHO.

Wright, T. et al. (2002). 2002 consensus guidelines for the management of women with cervical cytology abnormalities. *Journal of the American Medical Association, 287*(16), 2120-2129.

CHAPTER 9

Sharon E. Lock

Contraception and Abortion

http://evolve.elsevier.com/Lowdermilk/MatWmnHlth/

LEARNING OBJECTIVES

- Compare the different methods of contraception.
- Identify the advantages and disadvantages of frequently used methods of contraception.
- Explain the common nursing interventions that facilitate contraceptive use.
- Examine the various ethical, legal, cultural, and religious considerations of fertility management.
- Describe the techniques used for medical and surgical interruption of pregnancy.
- Explain the various ethical and legal considerations of elective abortion.

CONTRACEPTION

Contraception is the voluntary prevention of pregnancy. Despite the large numbers of men and women who use contraception, more than half of the pregnancies every year are unintended in women 20 years and younger who live in the United States (U.S. Department of Health and Human Services, 2002). Those who use contraception may still be at risk for pregnancy simply because their choice of contraceptive method is not perfect or is used incorrectly. Providing adequate instruction about how to use a contraceptive method, when to use a backup method, and when to use emergency contraception could decrease the risk of unintended pregnancy (Hatcher et al., 2002). Couples choosing contraception also must be informed about protection against sexually transmitted infections (STIs). Nurses can be instrumental in assisting couples in their decision-making process.

CARE MANAGEMENT

A multidisciplinary approach may assist a woman in choosing and correctly using an appropriate contraceptive method. Nurses, nurse-midwives, nurse practitioners, and other advanced practice nurses and physicians have the knowledge and expertise to assist a woman in making decisions about contraception that will satisfy the woman's personal, social, cultural, and interpersonal needs.

Assessment and Nursing Diagnoses

The woman's knowledge about contraception and commitment to any particular method are determined. Data are required about the frequency of coitus, number of sexual partners, level of contraceptive involvement, and her or her partner's objections to any methods (see Guidelines/Guías). The woman's level of comfort and willingness to touch her genitals and cervical mucus are assessed. Myths are identified, and religious and cultural factors are determined. The woman's verbal and nonverbal responses to hearing about the various available methods are carefully noted. An individual's reproductive life plan must be considered. A history (including menstrual, contraceptive, and obstetric), physical examination (including pelvic examination), and laboratory tests are usually completed.

Informed consent is a vital component in the education of the client concerning contraception or sterilization. The nurse has the responsibility of documenting information provided and the understanding of that information by the client. Use of the acronym BRAIDED may be useful (see Legal Tip).

LEGAL TIP Informed Consent

B—Benefits: information about advantages and success rates

R—Risks: information about disadvantages and failure rates

A—Alternatives: information about other available methods

I—Inquiries: opportunity to ask questions

D—Decisions: opportunity to decide or to change mind

E—Explanations: information about method and how it is used

D—Documentation: information given and client's understanding

Nursing diagnoses reflect analysis of the assessment findings. Examples of nursing diagnoses that may emerge regarding contraception include those listed.

- *Decisional conflict related to*
  - –contraceptive alternatives
  - –partner's willingness to agree on contraceptive method
- *Fear related to*
  - –contraceptive method side effects
- *Risk for infection related to*
  - –unprotected sexual intercourse
  - –use of contraceptive method
  - –broken skin or mucous membrane after surgery or intrauterine device (IUD) insertion
- *Ineffective sexuality patterns related to*
  - –fear of pregnancy
- *Acute pain related to*
  - –postoperative recovery after sterilization
- *Risk for spiritual distress related to*
  - –discrepancy between religious or cultural beliefs and choice of contraception

Expected Outcomes of Care

Planning is a collaborative effort among the woman, her sexual partner (when appropriate), the primary health care provider, and the nurse. The expected outcomes are determined and stated in client-centered terms and may include that the woman or couple will do the following:

- Verbalize understanding about contraceptive methods
- Verbalize understanding of all information necessary to give informed consent
- State comfort and satisfaction with the chosen method
- Use the contraceptive method correctly and consistently
- Experience no adverse sequelae as a result of the chosen method of contraception
- Prevent unplanned pregnancy or plan a pregnancy

Plan of Care and Interventions

Unbiased client teaching is fundamental to initiating and maintaining any form of contraception. A care provider relationship based on trust is important for adherence by the client. The nurse counters myths with facts, clarifies misinformation, and fills in gaps of knowledge. The ideal contraceptive should be safe, easily available, economical, acceptable, simple to use, and promptly reversible. Although no method may ever achieve all these objectives, impressive progress has been made.

Contraceptive failure rate refers to the percentage of contraceptive users expected to have an accidental pregnancy during the first year, even when they use a method consistently and correctly. Contraceptive effectiveness varies from couple to couple (Box 9-1) and depends on both the properties of the method and the characteristics of the user (Hatcher et al., 2002). Failure rates decrease over time either because a user gains experience and uses a method more appropriately or because the less effective users stop using the method.

GUIDELINES/GUÍAS

Contraception

Do you plan to have more children?
¿Piensa tener más hijos?

Are you sexually active?
¿Está usted sexualmente activa?

Do you have many partners?
¿Tiene muchos compañeros?

Have you had many partners in the past?
¿He tenido muchos compañeros en el pasado?

Do you presently use contraception/birth control?
¿Usa actualmente anticonceptivos/control de nacimiento?

The Pill? Condoms? The diaphragm? The IUD?
¿La Píldora? ¿Los condones? ¿El diafragma? ¿El Dispositivo Intrauterino (DIU)?

Spermicides? The rhythm method? Implant (Depo-Provera) or injection?
¿Espermaticidas? ¿El método de ritmo? ¿El Implante o inyección?

How long have you used this method?
¿Por cuánto tiempo ha usado este método?

Do you like this method?
¿Le gusta este método?

Why did you stop using it?
¿Por qué dejó de usarlo?

Do you want to change to a different method?
¿Quiere cambiar a otro método?

Have you had a tubal ligation?
¿Le ataron los tubos?

Has he had a vasectomy?
¿Le hicieron a él vasectomía?

BOX 9-1 Factors Affecting Method Effectiveness

Frequency of intercourse
Motivation to prevent pregnancy
Understanding of how to use the method
Adherence to method
Provision of short-term or long-term protection
Likelihood of pregnancy for the individual woman
Consistent use of method

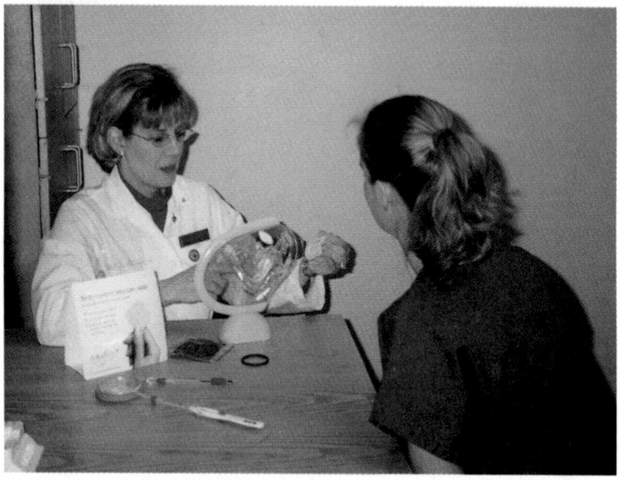

FIG. 9-1 Nurse counseling woman about contraceptive methods. (Courtesy Dee Lowdermillk, Chapel Hill, NC.)

Safety of a method depends on the woman's medical history. Barrier methods offer some protection from STIs, and oral contraceptives may reduce the incidence of ovarian and endometrial cancer but increase the risk of thromboembolic problems.

Methods of Contraception

The following discussion of contraceptive methods provides the nurse with information needed for client teaching. After implementing the appropriate teaching for contraceptive use, the nurse supervises return demonstrations and practice to assess client understanding (Fig. 9-1). The woman is given written instructions and telephone numbers for questions. If the woman has difficulty understanding written instructions, she (and her partner, if available) is offered graphic material and a telephone number to call as necessary or is offered an opportunity to return for further instruction.

Coitus Interruptus

Coitus interruptus (withdrawal) involves the male partner withdrawing the penis from the woman's vagina before he ejaculates. Although coitus interruptus has been criticized as being an ineffective method of contraception, it is a good choice for couples who do not have another contraceptive available (Hatcher et al., 2002). Effectiveness is similar to barrier methods and depends on the man's ability to withdraw his penis before ejaculation. The percentage of women who will experience an unintended pregnancy within the first year of typical use (failure rate) of withdrawal is about 19% (Trussell, 2003). Coitus interruptus does not protect against STIs or human immunodeficiency virus (HIV) infection.

Natural Family Planning and Fertility Awareness Methods

Natural family planning (NFP) provides contraception by using methods that rely on avoidance of intercourse during fertile periods. It is the only method of contraception acceptable to the Roman Catholic Church. **Fertility awareness methods (FAMs)** combine the charting of signs and symptoms of the menstrual cycle with the use of abstinence or other contraceptive methods during fertile periods. Techniques used to determine fertility include the calendar method, the cervical mucus ovulation-detection method, the basal body temperature (BBT) method, the postovulation method, and the symptothermal method (Hatcher et al., 2002).

Knowledge of the menstrual cycle is basic to the practice of NFP. To review, the human ovum can be fertilized no later than 16 to 24 hours after ovulation. Motile sperm have been recovered from the uterus and the oviducts as long as 7 days after coitus (Speroff et al., 1999). However, their ability to fertilize the ovum probably lasts no longer than 24 to 48 hours. Pregnancy is unlikely to occur if a couple abstains from intercourse for 4 days before and for 3 or 4 days after ovulation (fertile period). Unprotected intercourse on the other days of the cycle (safe period) should not result in pregnancy. However, couples may find it difficult to abstain from sexual intercourse for several days before and after ovulation. Women with irregular menstrual periods have the greatest risk of failure with this form of contraception; therefore, NFP methods are not recommended until regular menses have resumed postpartum (Hatcher et al., 2002). The typical failure rate for all fertility awareness methods is 25% during the first year of use (Trussell, 2003).

Ovulation usually occurs about 14 days before the onset of menstruation; therefore, variations in the length of menstrual cycles are usually a result of differences in the length of the preovulatory phase. The fertile period can be anticipated by the following:

- Calculating the time at which ovulation is likely to occur based on the lengths of previous menstrual cycles (calendar method)
- Recording the increase in basal body temperature, a result of the thermogenic effect of progesterone (BBT method)
- Recognizing the changes in cervical mucus at different phases of the menstrual cycle (ovulation-detection method)

- Using a combination of several methods (symptothermal method: cervical mucus and BBT changes)
- Using a predictor test for ovulation

Calendar Method. Practice of the **calendar method** (also called the *rhythm method*) is based on the number of days in each cycle counting from the first day of menses (Hatcher et al., 2002). With the calendar method, the fertile period is determined after accurately recording the lengths of menstrual cycles for 6 months. The beginning of the **fertile period** is estimated by subtracting 18 days from the length of the shortest cycle. The end of the fertile period is determined by subtracting 11 days from the length of the longest cycle. If the shortest cycle is 24 days and the longest cycle is 30 days, application of the formula is as follows:

Shortest cycle, 24 − 18 = 6th day
Longest cycle, 30 − 11 = 19th day

To avoid conception, the couple would abstain during the fertile period, days 6 through 19 of the menstrual cycle. If the woman has regular cycles of 28 days each, the formula indicates the fertile days to be as follows:

Shortest cycle, 28 − 18 = 10th day
Longest cycle, 28 − 11 = 17th day

To avoid pregnancy, the couple abstains from days 10 through 17 of the menstrual cycle because ovulation occurs on day 14 ± 2 days. A major drawback of the calendar method is that one is trying to predict future events with past data. The unpredictability of the menstrual cycle also is not taken into consideration. The calendar rhythm method is most useful as an adjunct to the basal body temperature or cervical mucus method.

Basal Body Temperature Method. The **BBT** is the lowest body temperature of a healthy person, taken immediately after waking and before getting out of bed. The BBT usually varies from 36.2° C to 36.3° C during menses and for about 5 to 7 days afterward (Fig. 9-2).

At about the time of ovulation, a slight decrease in temperature (approximately 0.05° C) may occur in some women, but others may have no decrease at all. After ovulation, in concert with the increasing progesterone levels of the early luteal phase of the cycle, the BBT increases slightly (approximately 0.4° C to 0.8° C) (Hatcher et al., 2002). The temperature remains on an elevated plateau until 2 to 4 days before menstruation, and then it decreases to the low levels recorded during the previous cycle, unless pregnancy has occurred, and the temperature remains elevated.

If ovulation fails to occur, this pattern of lower body temperature continues throughout the cycle. Infection, fatigue, less than 3 hours sleep per night, awakening late, and anxiety may cause temperature fluctuations, altering the expected pattern. If a new BBT thermometer is purchased, this fact is noted on the chart because the readings may vary slightly. Jet lag, alcohol taken the evening before, or sleeping in a heated waterbed also must be noted on the chart because each affects the BBT.

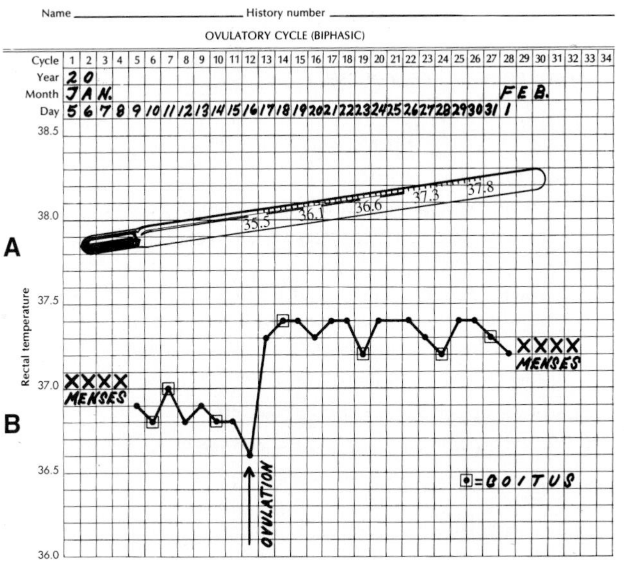
Name
History number
OVULATORY CYCLE (BIPHASIC)
Cycle
Year
Month
Day
JAN.
FEB.
Rectal temperature
38.5
38.0
37.5
37.0
36.5
36.0
A
B
35.5
36.1
36.6
37.3
37.8
MENSES
OVULATION
=COITUS

FIG. 9-2 **A,** Special thermometer for recording BBT, marked in tenths to enable person to read more easily. **B,** Basal temperature record shows decrease and sharp increase at time of ovulation. Biphasic curve indicates ovulatory cycle.

The decrease and subsequent increase in temperature are referred to as the thermal shift. When the entire month's temperatures are recorded on a graph, the pattern described is more apparent. It is more difficult to perceive day-to-day variations without the entire picture; therefore, the BBT alone is not a reliable method of predicting ovulation (Hatcher et al., 2002). To determine whether an increase in temperature is indeed the thermal shift, the woman must be aware of other signs of approaching ovulation while she continues to assess the BBT (see later discussion of symptothermal method for other indicators of ovulation).

Cervical Mucus Ovulation-Detection Method. The **cervical mucus ovulation-detection method** requires that the woman recognize and interpret the characteristic cyclic changes in the amount and consistency of cervical mucus (see Teaching for Self-Care box). Each woman has her own unique pattern of mucus changes. The cervical mucus that accompanies ovulation is necessary for viability and motility of sperm. Without adequate cervical mucus, coitus does not result in conception. To ensure an accurate assessment of changes, the cervical mucus should be free from semen, contraceptive gels or foams, and blood or discharge from vaginal infections for at least one full cycle. Other factors that create difficulty in identifying mucus changes include douches and vaginal deodorants, being in the sexually aroused state (which thins the mucus), and taking medications such as antihistamines, which dry the mucus.

Some women may find this method unacceptable if they are uncomfortable touching their genitals. Whether

TEACHING FOR SELF-CARE

Cervical Mucus Characteristics

SETTING THE STAGE

- Show charts of menstrual cycle along with changes in the cervical mucus.
- Have woman practice with raw egg white.
- Supply her with a BBT log and graph if she does not already have one.
- Explain that assessment of cervical mucus characteristics is best when mucus is not mixed with semen, contraceptive jellies or foams, or discharge from infections. Douching should not be done before assessment.

CONTENT RELATED TO CERVICAL MUCUS

- Explain to woman (couple) how cervical mucus changes throughout the menstrual cycle.
  a. Postmenstrual mucus: scant.
  b. Preovulation mucus: cloudy, yellow or white, sticky
  c. Ovulation mucus: clear, wet, sticky, slippery
  d. Postovulation fertile mucus: thick, cloudy, sticky
  e. Postovulation, postfertile mucus: scant
- Right before ovulation, the watery, thin, clear mucus becomes more abundant and thick (Fig. A). It feels like a lubricant and can be stretched 5+ cm between the thumb and forefinger; this is called spinnbarkheit (Fig. B). This indicates the period of maximal fertility. Sperm deposited in this type of mucus can survive until ovulation occurs.

ASSESSMENT TECHNIQUE

- Stress that good handwashing is imperative to begin and end all self-assessment.
- Start observation from last day of menstrual flow.
- Assess cervical mucus several times a day for several cycles. Mucus can be obtained from vaginal introitus; no need to reach into vagina to cervix.
- Record findings on the same record on which BBT is entered.

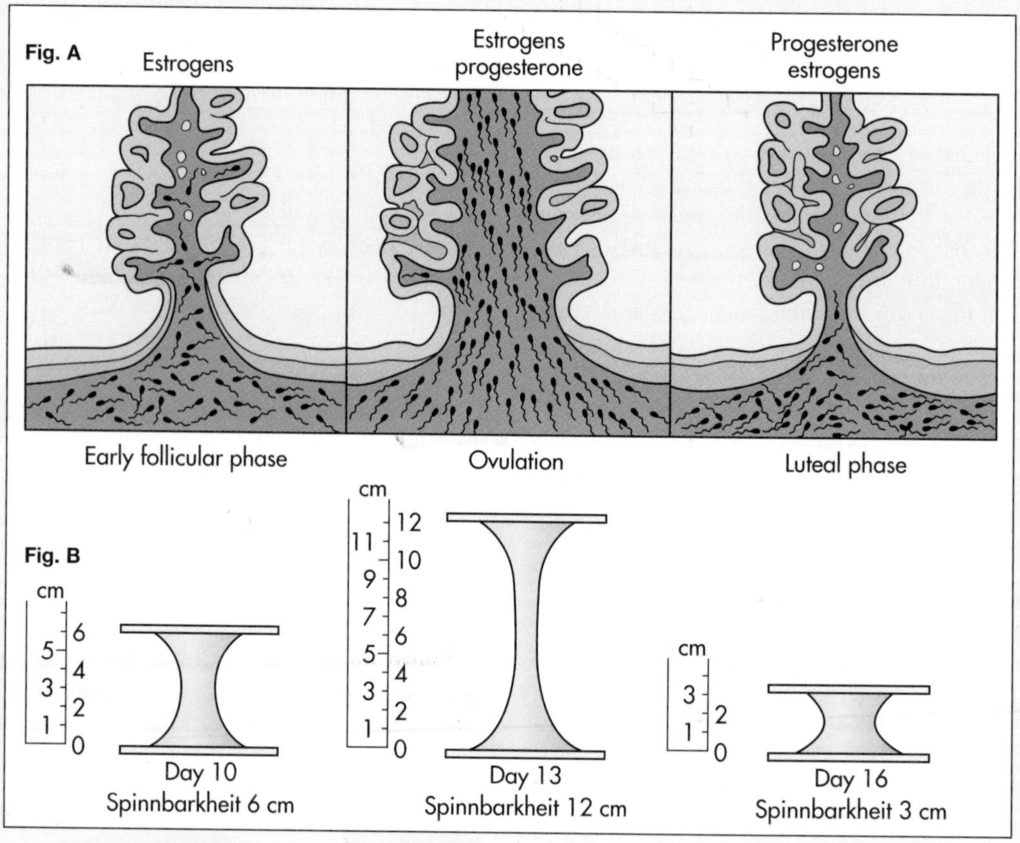
Fig. A
Estrogens
Estrogens progesterone
Progesterone estrogens
Early follicular phase
Ovulation
Luteal phase
Fig. B
cm
Day 10
Spinnbarkheit 6 cm
Day 13
Spinnbarkheit 12 cm
Day 16
Spinnbarkheit 3 cm

or not the individual wants to use this method for contraception, it is to the woman's advantage to learn to recognize mucus characteristics at ovulation. Self-evaluation of cervical mucus can be highly accurate and can be useful diagnostically for any of the following purposes:

- To alert the couple to the reestablishment of ovulation while breastfeeding and after discontinuation of oral contraception
- To note anovulatory cycles at any time and at the commencement of menopause
- To assist couples in planning a pregnancy

Symptothermal Method. The **symptothermal method** combines the BBT and cervical mucus methods with awareness of secondary, cycle phase–related symptoms. The woman gains fertility awareness as she learns the psychologic and physiologic symptoms that mark the phases of her cycle.

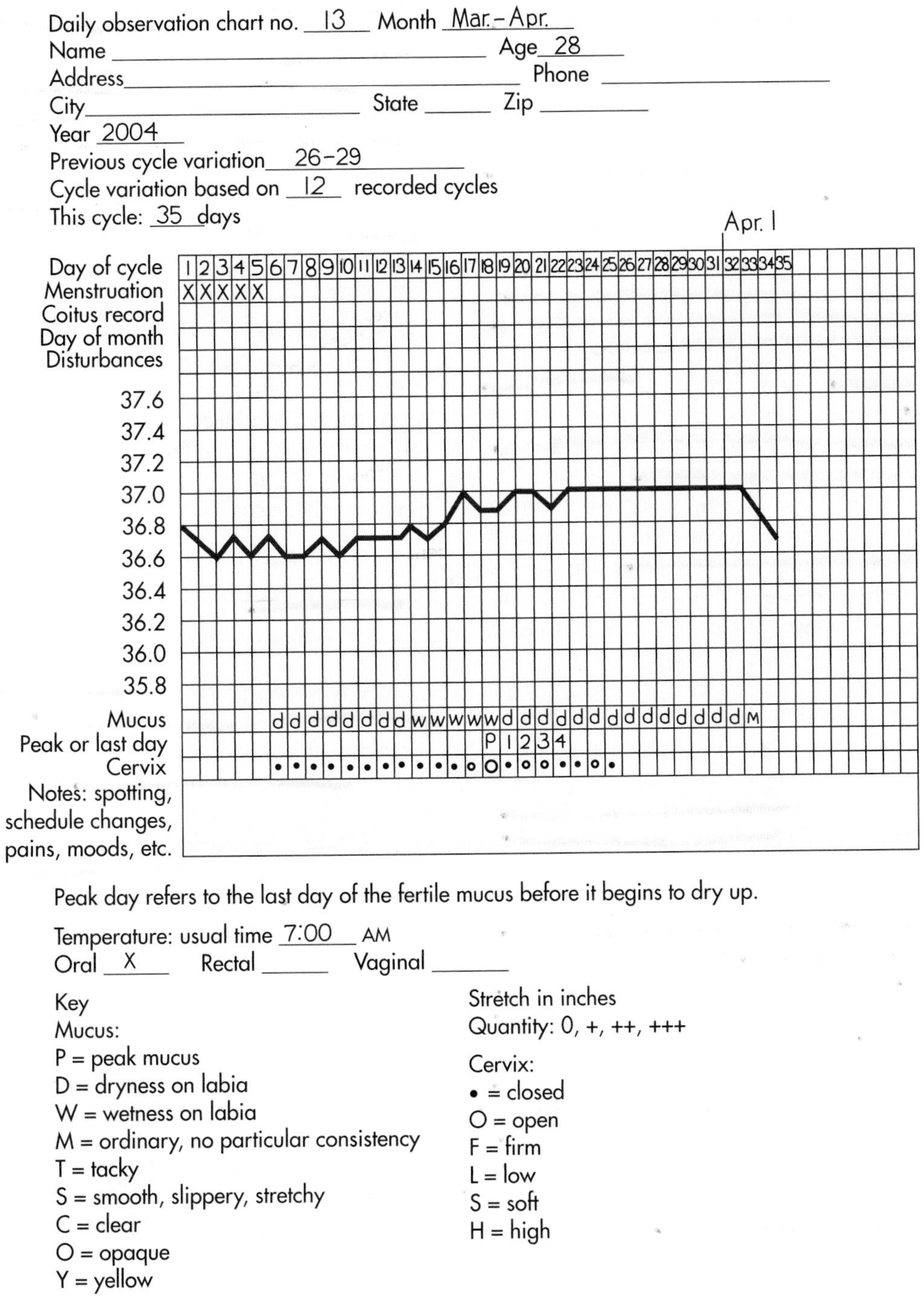
Daily observation chart no. 13 Month Mar.-Apr.
Name Age 28
Address Phone
City State Zip
Year 2004
Previous cycle variation 26-29
Cycle variation based on 12 recorded cycles
This cycle: 35 days
Apr. 1
Day of cycle
Menstruation
Coitus record
Day of month
Disturbances
37.6
37.4
37.2
37.0
36.8
36.6
36.4
36.2
36.0
35.8
Mucus
Peak or last day
Cervix
Notes: spotting, schedule changes, pains, moods, etc.
Peak day refers to the last day of the fertile mucus before it begins to dry up.
Temperature: usual time 7:00 AM
Oral X Rectal Vaginal
Key
Mucus:
P = peak mucus
D = dryness on labia
W = wetness on labia
M = ordinary, no particular consistency
T = tacky
S = smooth, slippery, stretchy
C = clear
O = opaque
Y = yellow
Stretch in inches
Quantity: 0, +, ++, +++
Cervix:
• = closed
O = open
F = firm
L = low
S = soft
H = high

FIG. 9-3 Example of a completed symptothermal chart.

Secondary symptoms include increased libido, midcycle spotting, mittelschmerz, pelvic fullness or tenderness, and vulvar fullness. The woman is taught to palpate the cervix to assess for changes indicating ovulation: the cervical os dilates slightly, the cervix softens and rises in the vagina, and cervical mucus is copious and slippery (Hatcher et al., 2002). The woman notes days on which coitus, changes in routine, illness, and so on have occurred (Fig. 9-3). Calendar calculations and cervical mucus changes are used to estimate the onset of the fertile period; changes in cervical mucus or the BBT are used to estimate its end.

Predictor Test for Ovulation. All of the preceding methods discussed are indicative of but do not prove the occurrence and exact timing of ovulation. The **predictor test for ovulation** is a major addition to the NFP and fertility-awareness methods to help women who want to plan the time of their pregnancies and those who are trying to conceive. The predictor test for ovulation detects the sudden surge of luteinizing hormone (LH) that occurs approximately 12 to 24 hours before ovulation. Unlike BBT, the test is not affected by illness, emotional upset, or physical activity. For home use, a test kit contains sufficient material for several days' testing during each cycle. A positive response indicative of an LH surge is noted by an easy-to-read color change. Directions for use of this home test kit vary with the manufacturer.

Marquette Method. The Marquette Method (MM) is a multiple indexed system of family planning that was developed through the Marquette University College of Nursing Institute for Natural Family Planning. The MM uses cervical monitoring along with the ClearPlan Easy Fertility Monitor (Unipath, Ltd, England). The ClearPlan Monitor is a handheld device that uses test strips to measure urinary metabolites of estrogen and LH. The monitor provides the user with "Low," "High," and "Peak" fertility readings. The MM incorporates the use of the monitor as an aid to learning NFP and fertility awareness. The MM is currently being tested for its effectiveness in helping couples avoid pregnancy at five different sites in the United States.

Barrier Methods

Barrier contraceptives have gained in popularity not only as a contraceptive method but also as a protective measure against the spread of STIs. Chemical barriers (spermicides) such as nonoxynol-9 may reduce the risk of some STIs (e.g., human papilloma virus) but are not effective against cervical chlamydia and gonorrhea or HIV infection (CDC, 2002). Male and female condoms provide a mechanical barrier to STIs and HIV (Hatcher et al., 2002).

Spermicides. A vaginal spermicide is a physical barrier to sperm penetration that also has a chemical action on sperm. Nonoxynol-9, the most commonly used spermicidal chemical in the United States, is a surfactant that destroys the sperm cell membrane; however, recent data suggest that frequent use of nonoxynol-9 may increase the transmission of HIV and can cause genital lesions (CDC, 2002; Stephenson, 2000). Intravaginal spermicides are marketed and sold without a prescription as aerosol foams, foaming tablets, suppositories, creams, films, sponges, and gels (Fig. 9-4). Preloaded, single-dose applicators small enough to be carried in a small purse are available. Effectiveness of spermicides depends on consistent and accurate use. The spermicide should be inserted into the vagina so that it makes contact with the cervix. Spermicide should be inserted no longer than 1 hour before sexual intercourse. Typical failure rate in the first year of spermicidal use alone is 29% (Hatcher, et al., 2002). Box 9-2 provides client teaching information about spermicide use. Women who are at high risk for HIV infection should not use spermicides with nonoxynol-9 (Hatcher et al., 2002).

Condoms. The male **condom** is a thin, stretchable sheath that covers the penis before genital contact (Fig. 9-5). Condoms are made of latex rubber, polyurethane, or natural membranes. In addition to providing a barrier for sperm, latex condoms also provide a barrier for STIs and HIV. Latex condoms will break down with oil-based lubricants and should be used only with water-based lubricants. A small percentage of condoms are made from the intestinal cecum of lambs (natural skin). Natural skin condoms do not provide the same protection against STIs and HIV infection. Unlike latex condoms, natural skin condoms contain small pores that could allow passage of viruses such as hepatitis B, herpes simplex, and HIV. More recently, condom manufacturers have begun using polyurethane, which is thinner and stronger than latex. Unlike latex condoms, polyurethane condoms can be used with oil-based lubricants (e.g., petroleum jelly, suntan oil) (Hatcher et al., 2002). Research is being conducted to determine the effectiveness of polyurethane condoms to protect against STIs and HIV.

NURSE ALERT
All clients should be questioned about the potential for latex allergy. Latex condom use is contraindicated for clients with latex sensitivity.

A functional difference in condom shape is the presence or absence of a sperm-reservoir tip. To enhance vaginal stimulation, some condoms are contoured and rippled or have ribbed or roughened surfaces. Thinner construction increases heat transmission and sensitivity; a variety of colors increase their acceptability and attractiveness (Hatcher et al., 2002). A wet jelly or dry powder lubricates some condoms. Condoms lubricated with nonoxynol-9 are no longer recommended for preventing STIs or HIV (CDC, 2002). Typical failure rate for first year of use of the male condom is 15% (Trussell, 2003).

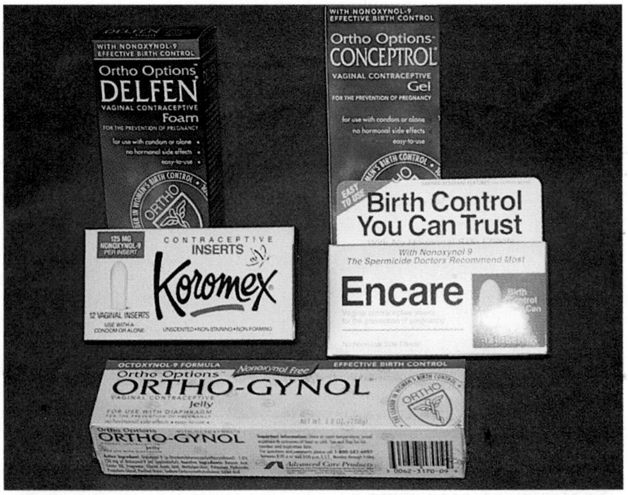
Ortho Options
DELFEN
Foam
Ortho Options
CONCEPTROL
Gel
Birth Control You Can Trust
Encare
CONTRACEPTIVE INSERTS
Koromex
ORTHO-GYNOL

FIG. 9-4 Spermicides. (Courtesy Marjorie Pyle, RNC, Life Circle, Costa Mesa, CA.)

To prevent unintended pregnancy and the spread of STIs, it is essential that condoms be used correctly. Instructions, such as those listed in Box 9-3, can be used for client teaching.

The vaginal sheath (female condom) is made of polyurethane and has flexible rings at both ends (see Fig. 9-5). The closed end of the pouch is inserted into the vagina and is anchored around the cervix, and the open ring covers the labia. The female condom can be inserted up to 8 hours before intercourse and is intended for one-time use. Both women and men report that intercourse with the sheath is generally as satisfying as intercourse without the sheath. It comes in one size and is available over the counter. Typical failure rate is 21% in the first year of use (Trussell, 2003).

Diaphragm. The vaginal **diaphragm** is a shallow, dome-shaped rubber device with a flexible rim that covers the cervix (see Fig. 9-5). Diaphragms are available in a wide range of diameters (50 to 95 mm) and differ in the inner construction of the circular rim. The types of rims are flat

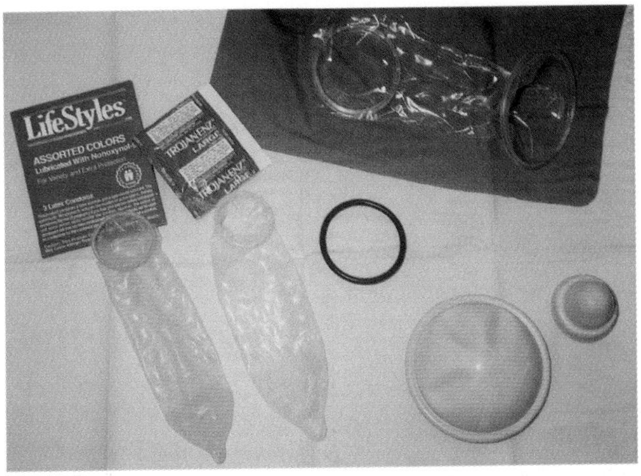
LifeStyles
ASSORTED COLORS
TROJAN-ENZ
LARGE

FIG. 9-5 Mechanical barriers. *Clockwise from top:* female condom, cervical cap, diaphragm, types of male condoms, vaginal ring (hormonal) *(center)*. (Courtesy Donna Rowe, University of North Carolina Student Health, Chapel Hill, NC.)

BOX 9-2 **Spermicides**

MODE OF ACTION

Spermicides provide a physical and chemical barrier that prevents viable sperm from entering the cervix. The effect is local, within the vagina. The spermicide is placed deeply into the vagina in contact with the cervix before each incidence of coitus.

FAILURE RATE

Typical failure, 29%

ADVANTAGES

- Easy to apply
- Safe
- Low cost
- Available without a prescription or previous medical examination
- Delicate vaginal mucosa is not harmed unless the woman is allergic to a particular preparation
- Aids in lubrication of the vagina
- Alternative for nursing mothers (does not interfere with lactation)
- Alternative for the premenopausal woman (to prevent masking symptoms of onset of the climacteric)
- Backup when the woman forgets her oral contraceptive
- Increases the effectiveness of condoms and other forms of contraception

STI PROTECTION

Spermicides containing nonoxynol-9 may decrease risk of some vaginal and cervical STIs but does not decrease risk of HIV infection, cervical chlamydia, or cervical gonorrhea. Must be used with condoms if protection from STIs is needed.

DISADVANTAGES

- Maximal spermicidal effectiveness lasts usually no longer than 1 hour.
- If intercourse is to be repeated, application of additional spermicide must precede it.
- Some users complain that it is messy and has an unpleasant fizz and taste.
- Allergic response or irritation of vaginal or penile tissue may occur.
- Possible decreased tactile sensation.
- Possible increase in STIs, including HIV.

NURSING CONSIDERATIONS/CLIENT TEACHING

- Can must be shaken to distribute foam spermicide before use.
- Tablets and suppositories take from 10 to 30 minutes to dissolve.
- Douching must be avoided for at least 6 hours after coitus.
- Encourage open communication between sexual partners to discuss intravaginal contraception.
- Provide opportunity to see and handle a variety of samples.
- Provide anatomic model to practice insertion into the vagina.

BOX 9-3 **Male Condoms**

MECHANISM OF ACTION

Sheath is applied over the erect penis before insertion or loss of preejaculatory drops of semen. Used correctly, condoms prevent sperm from entering the cervix. Spermicide-coated condoms cause ejaculated sperm to be immobilized rapidly, thus increasing contraceptive effectiveness.

FAILURE RATE

Typical users, 14%
Correct and consistent users, 3%

ADVANTAGES

- Safe.
- No side effects.
- Readily available.
- Premalignant changes in cervix can be prevented or ameliorated in women whose partners use condoms.
- Method of male nonsurgical contraception.

DISADVANTAGES

- Must interrupt lovemaking to apply sheath.
- Sensation may be altered.
- If used improperly, spillage of sperm can result in pregnancy.
- Condoms occasionally may tear during intercourse.

STI PROTECTION

If a condom is used throughout the act of intercourse and there is no unprotected contact with female genitals, a latex rubber condom, which is impermeable to viruses, can act as a protective measure against STIs.

NURSING CONSIDERATIONS

Teach man to do the following:

- Use a new condom (check expiration date) for each act of sexual intercourse or other acts between partners that involve contact with the penis.

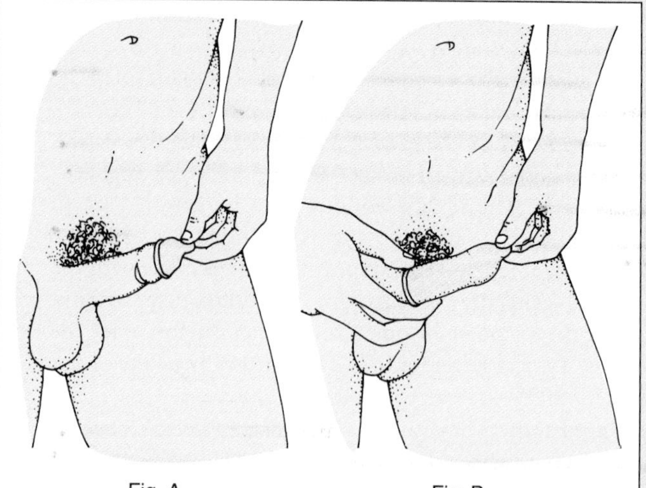

Fig. A Fig. B

- Place condom after penis is erect and before intimate contact.
- Place condom on head of penis (Fig. A) and unroll it all the way to the base (Fig. B).
- Leave an empty space at the tip (Fig. A); remove any air remaining in the tip by gently pressing air out toward the base of the penis.
- If a lubricant is desired, use water-based products such as K-Y lubricating jelly. Do not use petroleum-based products because they can cause the condom to break.
- After ejaculation, carefully withdraw the still-erect penis from the vagina, holding onto condom rim; remove and discard the condom.
- Store unused condoms in cool, dry place.
- Do not use condoms that are sticky, brittle, or obviously damaged.

spring, coil spring, arcing spring, and wide seal rim. The diaphragm is a mechanical barrier preventing the meeting of the sperm with the ovum.

The diaphragm should feel comfortable. It should be the largest size the woman can wear without being aware of its presence. Use of a spermicidal gel or cream with the diaphragm offers both mechanical and chemical barriers to pregnancy. The woman should use a backup method with the first few acts of intercourse with the diaphragm in case it is not used correctly (Hatcher et al., 2002). Typical failure rate of the diaphragm combined with spermicide is 16% in the first year of use. Effectiveness of the diaphragm is less when used without spermicide (Trussell, 2003). Women at high risk for HIV should avoid use of nonoxynol-9 spermicides with the diaphragm (Hatcher et al., 2002).

Nursing Considerations. The woman is informed that she needs an annual gynecologic examination to assess the fit of the diaphragm. The device should be replaced every 2 years and may need to be refitted after weight loss or weight gain, term birth, or second trimester abortion (Hatcher et al., 2002). Because various types of diaphragms are on the market, the nurse uses the package insert for teaching the woman how to use and care for the diaphragm (see Teaching for Self-Care box).

Except for occasional allergic responses to the diaphragm or spermicide, there are no side effects from a well-fitted device. The diaphragm can be inserted as long as 6 hours before intercourse, but spermicide must be inserted into the vagina each time intercourse is repeated (Hatcher et al., 2002). The diaphragm must be left in place for at least 6 hours after the last intercourse. The woman

TEACHING FOR SELF-CARE

Use and Care of the Diaphragm

POSITIONS FOR INSERTION OF DIAPHRAGM

Squatting

- Squatting is the most commonly used position, and most women find it satisfactory.

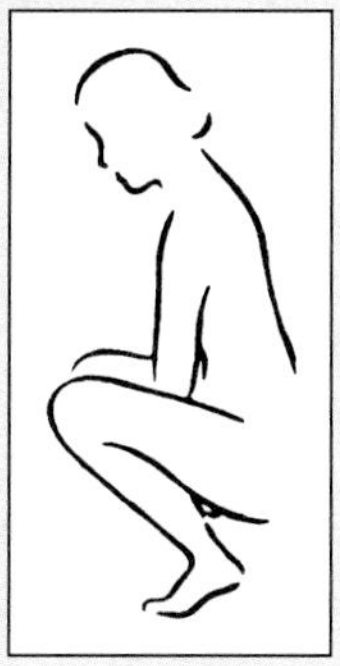

Leg-up Method

- Another position is to raise the left foot (if right hand is used for insertion) on a low stool and, while in a bending position, insert the diaphragm.

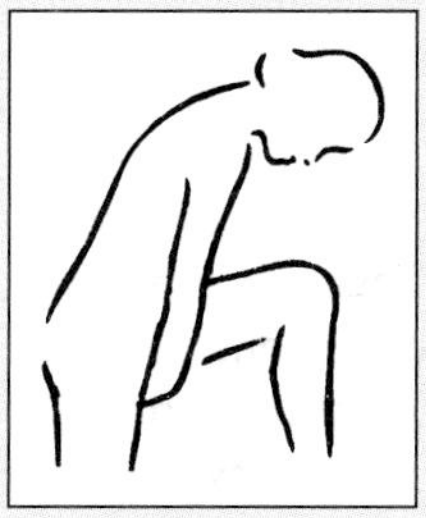

Chair Method

- Another practical method for diaphragm insertion is to sit far forward on the edge of a chair.

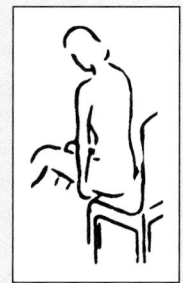

Reclining

- You may prefer to insert the diaphragm while in a semi-reclining position in bed.

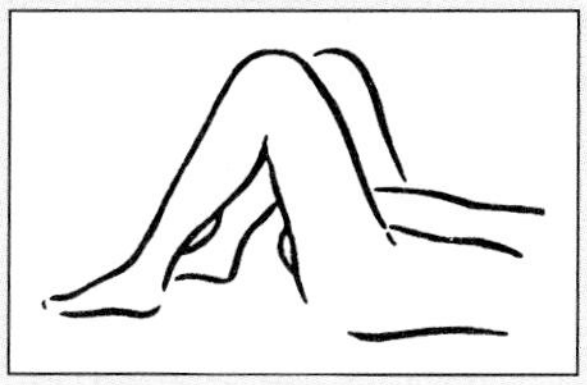

INSPECTION OF DIAPHRAGM

Your diaphragm must be inspected carefully before each use. The best way to do this is as follows:

- Hold the diaphragm up to a light source. Carefully stretch the diaphragm at the area of the rim, on all sides, to make sure there are no holes. Remember, it is possible to puncture the diaphragm with sharp fingernails.
- Another way to check for pinholes is carefully to fill the diaphragm with water. If there is any problem, it will be seen immediately.
- If your diaphragm is puckered, especially near the rim, this could mean thin spots.
- The diaphragm should not be used if you see any of these; consult your health care provider.

PREPARATION OF DIAPHRAGM

- Rinse off cornstarch. Your diaphragm must always be used with a spermicidal lubricant to be effective. Pregnancy cannot be prevented effectively by the diaphragm alone.
- Always empty your bladder before inserting the diaphragm. Place about 2 teaspoonfuls of contraceptive jelly or contraceptive cream on the side of the diaphragm that will rest against the cervix (or whichever way you have been instructed). Spread it around to coat the surface and the rim. This aids in insertion and offers a more complete seal. Many women also spread some jelly or cream on the other side of the diaphragm (Fig. A).

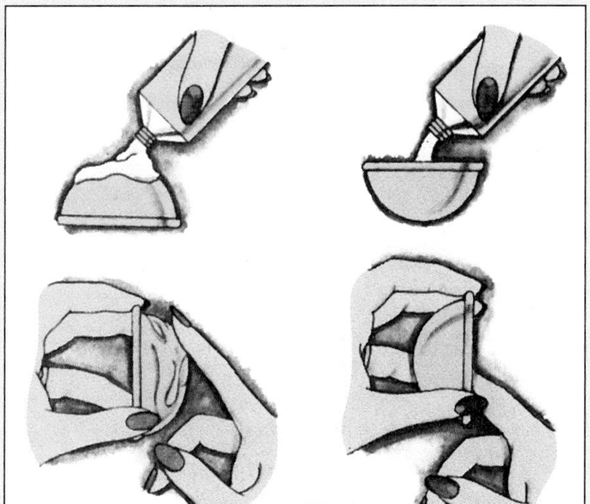

Fig. A

INSERTION OF DIAPHRAGM

- The diaphragm can be inserted as long as 6 hours before intercourse. Hold the diaphragm between your thumb and fingers. The dome can either be up or down, as directed by your health care provider. Place your index finger on the outer rim of the compressed diaphragm (Fig. B).
- Use the fingers of the other hand to spread the labia (lips of the vagina). This will assist in guiding the diaphragm into place.

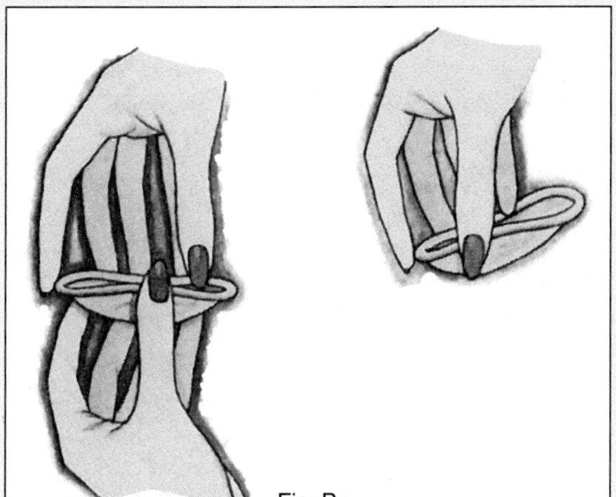

Fig. B

Continued

TEACHING FOR SELF-CARE

Use and Care of the Diaphragm—cont'd

- Insert the diaphragm into the vagina. Direct it inward and downward as far as it will go to the space behind and below the cervix (Fig. C).

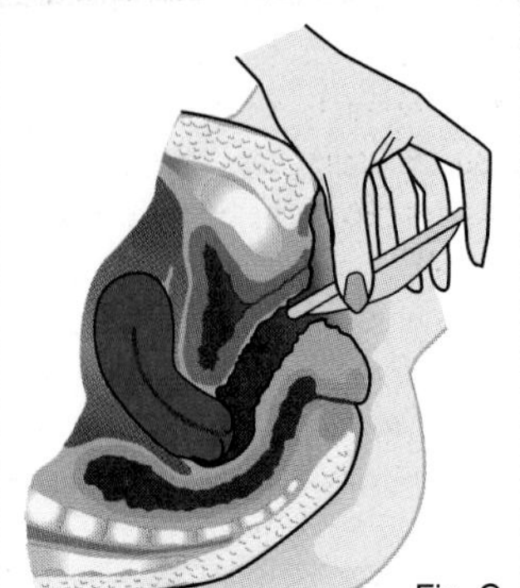

Fig. C

- Tuck the front of the rim of the diaphragm behind the pubic bone so that the rubber hugs the front wall of the vagina (Fig. D).

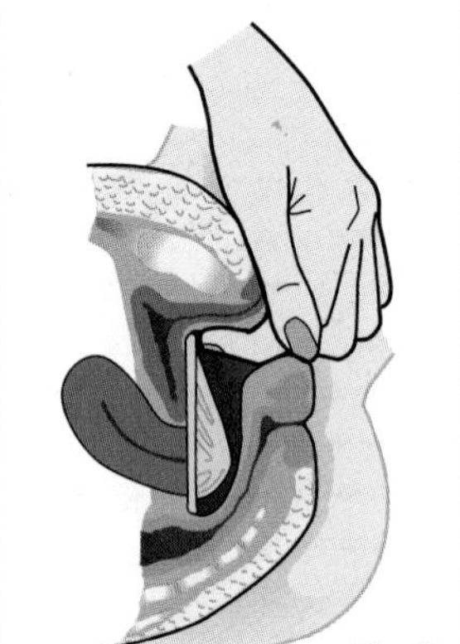

Fig. D

- Feel for your cervix through the diaphragm to be certain it is properly placed and securely covered by the rubber dome (Fig. E).

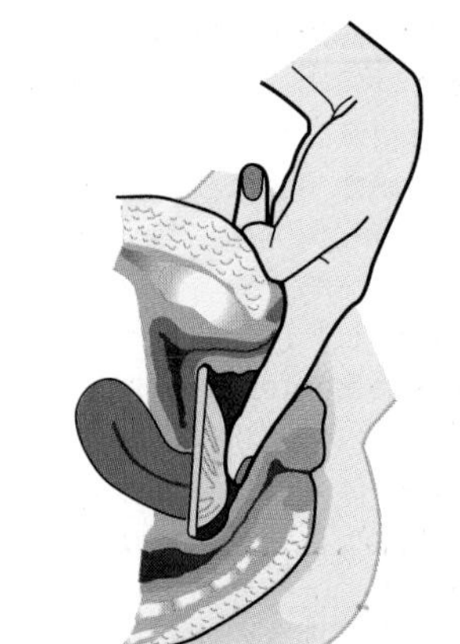

Fig. E

GENERAL INFORMATION

- Regardless of the time of the month, you must use your diaphragm every time intercourse takes place. Your diaphragm must be left in place for at least 6 hours after the last intercourse. If you remove your diaphragm before the 6-hour period, your chance of becoming pregnant could be greatly increased. If you have repeated acts of intercourse, you must add more spermicide for each act of intercourse.

REMOVAL OF DIAPHRAGM

- The only proper way to remove the diaphragm is to insert your forefinger up and over the top side of the diaphragm and slightly to the side.
- Next, turn the palm of your hand downward and backward, hooking the forefinger firmly on top of the inside of the upper rim of the diaphragm, breaking the suction.
- Pull the diaphragm down and out. This avoids the possibility of tearing the diaphragm with the fingernails. You should not remove the diaphragm by trying to catch the rim from below the dome (Fig. F).

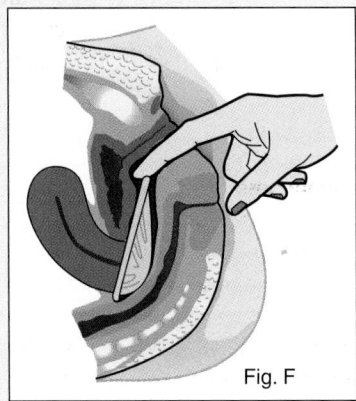

Fig. F

CARE OF DIAPHRAGM

- When using a vaginal diaphragm, avoid using oil-based products, such as certain body lubricants, mineral oil, baby oil, vaginal lubricants, or vaginitis preparations. These products can weaken the rubber.
- A little care means longer wear for your diaphragm. After each use, wash the diaphragm in warm water and mild soap. Do not use detergent soaps, cold-cream soaps, deodorant soaps, and soaps containing oil products, because they can weaken the rubber.
- After washing, dry the diaphragm thoroughly. All water and moisture should be removed with a towel. Then dust the diaphragm with cornstarch. Scented talc, body powder, baby powder, and the like should not be used because they can weaken the rubber.
- To clean the introducer (if one is used), wash with mild soap and warm water, rinse, and dry thoroughly.
- Place the diaphragm back in the plastic case for storage. Do not store it near a radiator or heat source or exposed to light for an extended period.

who engages in intercourse infrequently may choose this barrier method. The spermicide offers additional lubrication if it is needed. A decreased incidence of vaginitis, cervicitis (including cervicitis caused by *Chlamydia trachomatis* and *Neisseria gonorrhoeae*), and pelvic inflammatory disease has been reported among women who use contraceptive creams, foams, and gels with the diaphragm. A reduced risk of cervical dysplasia also has been reported among women who use a diaphragm (Hatcher et al., 2002).

Disadvantages of diaphragm use include the reluctance of some women to insert and remove the diaphragm. A cold diaphragm and a cold gel temporarily reduce vaginal response to sexual stimulation if insertion of the diaphragm occurs immediately before intercourse. Some women or couples object to the messiness of the spermicide. These annoyances of diaphragm use, along with failure to insert the device once foreplay has begun, are the most common reasons for failures of this method. Side effects may include irritation of tissues related to contact with spermicides. Urethritis and recurrent cystitis caused by upward pressure of the diaphragm rim against the urethra may be increased by the use of the contraceptive diaphragm (Hatcher et al., 2002). Diaphragms are contraindicated for women with pelvic relaxation (uterine prolapse) or a large cystocele. Women with a latex allergy should not use latex diaphragms.

Toxic shock syndrome (TSS), although reported in very small numbers, can occur in association with the use of the contraceptive diaphragm (Hatcher et al., 2002). The nurse should instruct the woman about ways to reduce her risk for TSS. These measures include prompt removal 6 to 8 hours after intercourse, not using the diaphragm during menses, and learning and watching for danger signs of TSS.

NURSE ALERT

The nurse should be alert for signs of TSS in women who use a diaphragm or cervical cap as a contraceptive method. The most common signs include fever of sudden onset greater than 38.4° C, hypotension (systolic less than 90 mm Hg or orthostatic dizziness), and a rash.

Cervical Cap. The cervical cap has a soft natural rubber dome with a firm but pliable rim (see Fig. 9-5). It fits snugly around the base of the cervix close to the junction of the cervix and vaginal fornices (Hatcher et al., 2002). The device is available in four sizes (22, 25, 28, and 31 mm). It is recommended that the cap remain in place no less than 8 hours and not more than 48 hours at a time. It is left in place at least 6 hours after the last act of intercourse. The seal provides a physical barrier to sperm; spermicide inside the cap adds a chemical barrier.

The extended period of wear is an added convenience for women who previously used the diaphragm. Instructions for the actual insertion and use of the cervical cap closely resemble the instructions for the use of the contraceptive diaphragm. Some of the differences are that the cervical cap can be inserted hours before sexual intercourse without a need for additional spermicide later; no additional spermicide is required for repeated acts of intercourse when the cap is used; and the cervical cap requires less spermicide than the diaphragm when initially inserted.

Some women are not good candidates for wearing the cervical cap. They include women with abnormal Papanicolaou (Pap) test results, women who cannot be fitted properly with the existing cap sizes, women who find the insertion and removal of the device too difficult, women with a history of TSS, women with vaginal or cervical infections (Hatcher et al., 2002), and women who have allergic responses to the latex cap or spermicide.

Nursing Considerations. The angle of the uterus, the vaginal muscle tone, and the shape of the cervix may interfere with the ease of fitting and use of the cervical cap. Correct fitting requires time, effort, and skill of both the woman and the clinician. The woman must check the cap's position before and after each act of intercourse. A repeated Pap smear should be done after 3 months of use because of increased risk of cervical dysplasia at 3 months. No increased risk of dysplasia is found at 1 year (Hatcher et al., 2002).

Although no link has been discovered between TSS and the use of the cervical cap, such an association is possible. The package insert recommends that another form of birth control be used during menstrual bleeding and for at least 6 weeks postpartum. The cap should be checked for proper fit after any gynecologic surgery or birth and after major weight losses or gains. Otherwise, the size should be checked at least once a year.

Strong client motivation is the most important criterion for successful cap use. Failure rate with typical use for parous women is 32% and for nulliparous women is 16% (Hatcher et al., 2002). The woman must be given the information available for this product, as presented previously. The nurse should assess the woman's understanding and skill in the use of the cervical cap (see Teaching for Self-Care box).

Contraceptive Sponge. The vaginal sponge was taken off the market in the United States in 1995 because of production problems of the manufacturer, and in 2002, the contraceptive sponge (Today sponge) was still unavailable in the United States because of manufacturing issues (Hatcher et al., 2002). Vaginal sponges continue to be available in other countries. The device is a small round polyurethane sponge that contains spermicide (e.g., nonoxynol-9, benzalkonium chloride, sodium chlorate). It is designed to fit over the cervix (one size fits all). The side that is placed next to the cervix is concave for better fit. The opposite side has a woven polyester loop to be used in removing the sponge.

The sponge should be moistened with water before it is inserted into the vagina to cover the cervix. It provides up to 24 hours of protection for numerous instances of sexual

TEACHING FOR SELF-CARE

Use of the Cervical Cap

- Push cap up into vagina until it covers cervix.

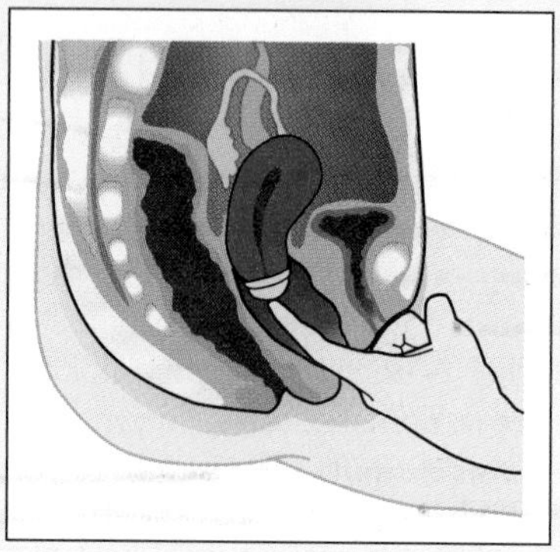

- Press rim against cervix to create a seal.

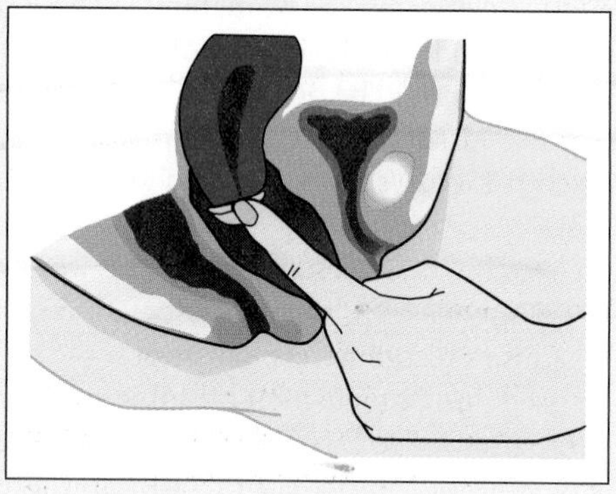

- To remove, push rim toward right or left hip to loosen from cervix, and then withdraw.

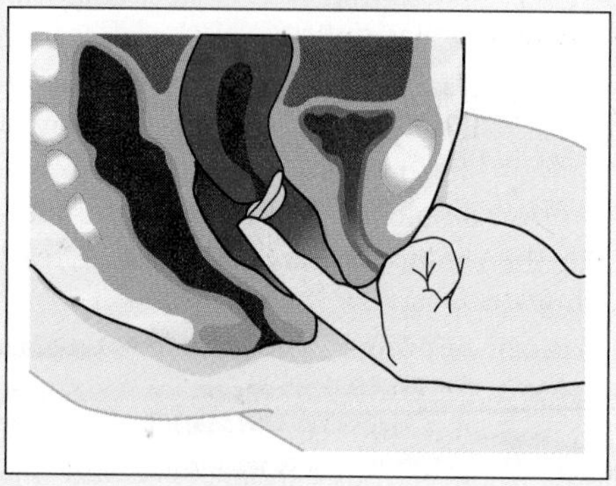

- The woman can assume several positions to insert the cervical cap. See the four positions shown for inserting the diaphragm.

intercourse. The sponge should be left in place for at least 6 hours after the last act of intercourse before its removal. Longer wearing time (greater than 24 to 30 hours) is not recommended because the woman may be at risk for TSS (Hatcher et al., 2002).

Hormonal Methods

More than 30 different contraceptive formulations are available in the United States today. General classes are described in Table 9-1. Because of the wide variety of preparations available, the woman and nurse must read the package insert for information about specific products prescribed. Formulations include combined estrogen-progestin medications and progestational agents. The formulations are administered orally, transdermally, vaginally, by implantation, or by injection.

Combined Estrogen-Progestin Contraceptives.

Oral Contraceptives. The normal menstrual cycle is maintained by a feedback mechanism. Follicle-stimulating hormone (FSH) and LH are secreted in response to fluctuating levels of ovarian estrogen and progesterone. Regular ingestion of combined oral contraceptive pills (COCs) suppresses the action of the hypothalamus and anterior pituitary, leading to inappropriate secretion of FSH and LH; therefore, follicles do not mature, and ovulation is inhibited.

Other contraceptive effects are induced by the combined steroids. Maturation of the endometrium is altered, making it a less favorable site for implantation. COCs also have a direct effect on the endometrium, so that from 1 to 4 days after the last COC is taken, the endometrium sloughs and bleeds as a result of hormone withdrawal. The **withdrawal bleeding** usually is less profuse than that of normal menstruation and may last only 2 to 3 days. Some women have no bleeding at all. The cervical mucus remains thick from the effect of the progestin.

Cervical mucus under the effect of progesterone does not provide as suitable an environment for sperm penetration as does the thin, watery mucus at ovulation (Hatcher et al., 2002). The possible effect, if any, of altered tubal and uterine motility induced by COCs is not clear. Typical failure rate is 8% in the first year of use (Trussell, 2003).

Monophasic pills provide fixed dosages of estrogen and progestin. Multiphasic pills (e.g., biphasic and triphasic oral contraceptives) alter the amount of progestin and sometimes the amount of estrogen within each cycle. These preparations reduce the total dosage of hormones in a single cycle without sacrificing contraceptive efficacy (Wallach & Grimes, 2000). To maintain adequate hormonal levels for contraception and enhance compliance, COCs should be taken at the same time each day.

Advantages. Because taking the pill does not relate directly to the sexual act, its acceptability may be increased. Improvement in sexual response may occur once the possibility of pregnancy is not an issue. For some women, it is convenient to know when to expect the next menstrual flow.

Evidence of noncontraceptive benefits of oral contraceptives is based on studies of high-dose pills (50 μg estrogen). Few data exist on noncontraceptive benefits of low-dose oral contraceptives (less than 35 μg estrogen)

TABLE 9-1 **Hormonal Contraception**

COMPOSITION	ROUTE OF ADMINISTRATION	DURATION OF EFFECT
Combination estrogen and progestin (synthetic estrogens and progestins in varying doses and formulations)	Oral	24 hours
	Transdermal patch	7 days
	Intramuscular injection	28 ± 5 days
	Vaginal ring insertion	3 weeks
Progestin only		
Norethindrone, norgestrel	Oral	24 hours
Medroxyprogesterone acetate	Intramuscular injection	3 months
Levonorgestrel	Subdermal implant	Up to 5 years
Progesterone	Intrauterine device	1 year

(Wallach & Grimes, 2000). The noncontraceptive health benefits of COCs include decreased menstrual blood loss and decreased iron-deficiency anemia, regulation of menorrhagia and irregular cycles, and reduced incidence of dysmenorrhea and premenstrual syndrome (PMS). Oral contraceptives also offer protection against endometrial cancer and ovarian cancer, reduce the incidence of benign breast disease, improve acne, protect against the development of functional ovarian cysts and salpingitis, and decrease the risk of ectopic pregnancy. Oral contraceptives are considered a safe option for nonsmoking women until menopause. Perimenopausal women can benefit from regular bleeding cycles, a regular hormonal pattern, and the noncontraceptive health benefits of oral contraceptives (Hatcher et al., 2002).

Women taking combined oral contraceptives are examined before the medication is prescribed and yearly thereafter. The examination includes medical and family history, weight, blood pressure, general physical and pelvic examinations, and screening cervical cytologic analysis (Pap smear). Consistent monitoring by the health care provider is valuable in the detection of non–contraception-related disorders as well, so that timely treatment can be initiated. Most health care providers assess the woman 3 months after beginning COCs to detect any complications.

Use of oral hormonal contraceptives is initiated on one of the first 7 days of the menstrual cycle (day 1 of the cycle is the first day of menses). Other women start their use after childbirth or abortion. With a "Sunday start," clients begin taking pills on the first Sunday after the start of their menstrual period. If contraceptives are to be started at any time other than during normal menses, or within 3 weeks after birth or abortion, another method of contraception should be used throughout the first week to avoid the risk of pregnancy (Wallach & Grimes, 2000). Taken exactly as directed, oral contraceptives prevent ovulation, and pregnancy cannot occur; the overall effectiveness rate is almost 100%. Almost all failures (i.e., pregnancy occurs) are caused by omission of one or more pills during the regimen. The typical failure rate of COCs due to omission is 8% (Trussell, 2003).

Disadvantages and Side Effects. Since hormonal contraceptives have come into use, the amount of estrogen and progestational agent contained in each tablet has been reduced considerably. This is important because adverse effects are, to a degree, dose related.

Women must be screened for conditions that present absolute or relative contraindications to oral contraceptive use. Contraindications for COC use include a history of thromboembolic disorders, cerebrovascular or coronary artery disease, breast cancer, estrogen-dependent tumors, pregnancy, impaired liver function, liver tumor, lactation less than 6 weeks postpartum, smoking if older than 35 years (more than 15 cigarettes per day), headaches with focal neurologic symptoms, surgery with prolonged immobilization or any surgery on the legs, hypertension (160/ 100), and diabetes mellitus (of more than 20 years' duration) with vascular disease (World Health Organization [WHO], 2000).

Certain side effects of COCs are attributable to estrogen, progestin, or both. Serious adverse effects documented with high doses of estrogen and progesterone include stroke, myocardial infarction, thromboembolism, hypertension, gallbladder disease, and liver tumors (Wallach & Grimes, 2000). Common side effects of estrogen excess include nausea, breast tenderness, fluid retention, and chloasma. Side effects of estrogen deficiency include early spotting (days 1 to 14), hypomenorrhea, nervousness, and atrophic vaginitis leading to painful intercourse (dyspareunia). Side effects of progestin excess include increased appetite, tiredness, depression, breast tenderness, vaginal yeast infection, oily skin and scalp, hirsutism, and postpill amenorrhea. Side effects of progestin deficiency include late spotting and breakthrough bleeding (days 15 to 21), heavy flow with clots, and decreased breast size. One of the most common side effects of combined COCs is bleeding irregularities (Wallach & Grimes, 2000).

In the presence of side effects, especially those that are bothersome to the woman, a different product, a different drug content, or another method of contraception may be required. The "right" product for a woman contains the lowest dose of hormones that prevents ovulation and that has the fewest and least harmful side effects. There is no way to predict the right dosage for any particular woman. Issues to consider in prescribing oral contraceptives include history of oral contraceptive use, side effects during past use, menstrual history, and drug interactions (Wallach & Grimes, 2000).

Large prospective studies have not shown a relation between oral contraceptive use and diabetes or glucose intolerance (Wallach & Grimes, 2000). The risks and benefits should be assessed before prescribing oral contraceptives for diabetic women. Because oral contraceptives are metabolized by the liver, the effectiveness of oral contraceptives is decreased when the following medications are taken simultaneously, because these drugs affect liver enzymes (Wallach & Grimes, 2000).

- Anticonvulsants (phenytoin sodium, carbamazepine, primidone, topiramate)
- Griseofulvin
- Rifampin

No strong pharmacokinetic evidence exists that shows a relation between broad-spectrum antibiotic use and altered hormonal levels among oral contraceptive users, although potential antibiotic interaction can occur (Wallach &

Flowchart for Missed *Active* Oral Contraceptive Pills

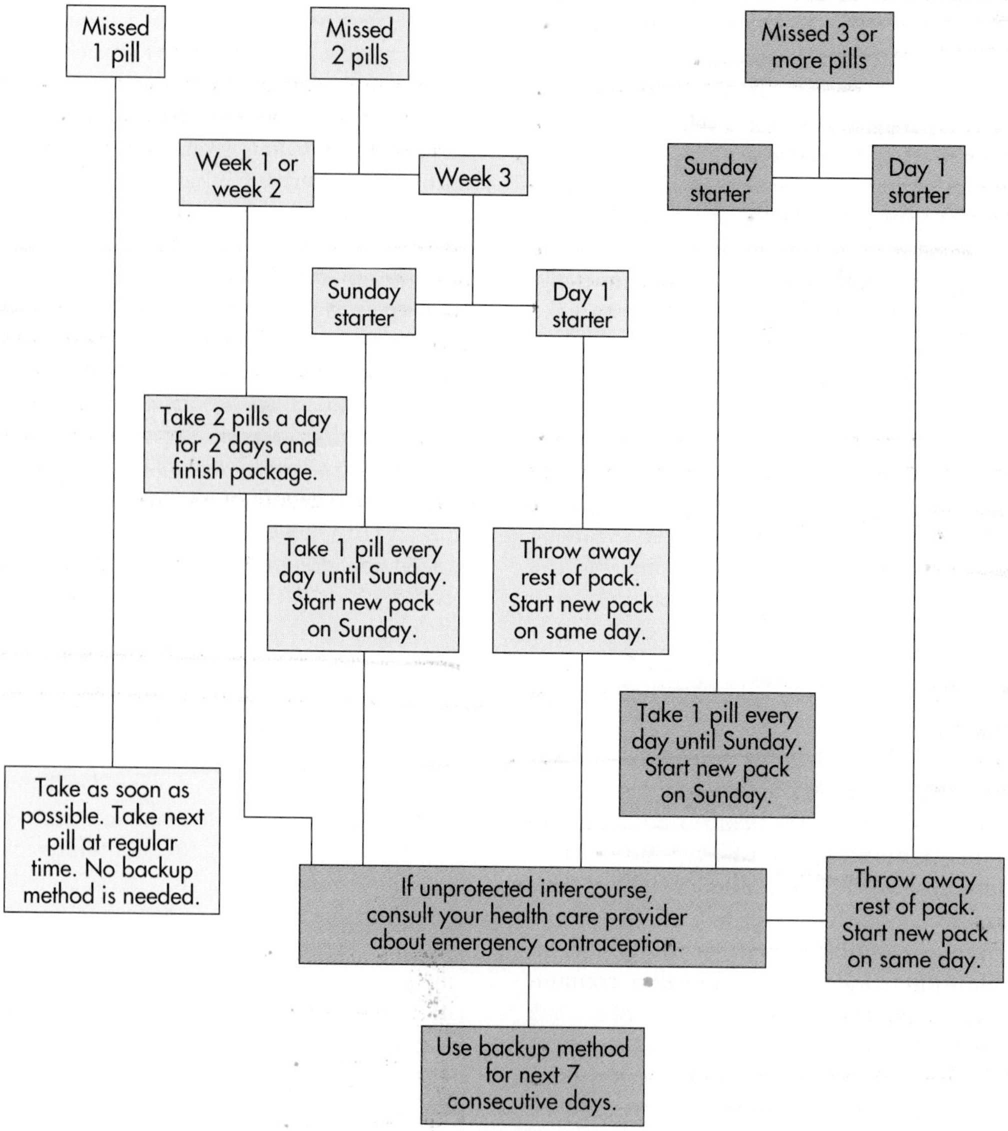
Missed 1 pill
Missed 2 pills
Missed 3 or more pills
Week 1 or week 2
Week 3
Sunday starter
Day 1 starter
Sunday starter
Day 1 starter
Take 2 pills a day for 2 days and finish package.
Take 1 pill every day until Sunday. Start new pack on Sunday.
Throw away rest of pack. Start new pack on same day.
Take 1 pill every day until Sunday. Start new pack on Sunday.
Take as soon as possible. Take next pill at regular time. No backup method is needed.
If unprotected intercourse, consult your health care provider about emergency contraception.
Throw away rest of pack. Start new pack on same day.
Use backup method for next 7 consecutive days.

FIG. 9-6 Flowchart for missed contraceptive pills. (Courtesy Patsy Huff, PharmD, Chapel Hill, NC.)

Grimes, 2000). The use of oral contraceptives may decrease the effectiveness of several medications (e.g., oral anticoagulants) (Goldzieher, 1998). Meta-analysis of studies on the incidence of breast cancer in COC users has not found a significant increase of breast cancer in women who use COCs (Grabrick et al., 2000).

After discontinuing oral contraception, return to fertility usually happens quickly, but fertility rates are slightly lower the first 3 to 12 months after discontinuation (Wallach & Grimes, 2000). Many women ovulate the next month after stopping oral contraceptives. Women who discontinue oral contraception for a planned pregnancy commonly ask whether they should wait before attempting to conceive. Studies indicate that these infants have no greater chance of being born with any type of birth defect than do infants born to women in the general population, even if conception occurred in the first month after the medication was discontinued (Wallach & Grimes, 2000). Little evidence suggests that oral contraceptives cause postpill amenorrhea. Amenorrhea after oral contraceptive use is probably related to the woman's menstrual cycle before taking the pill (Hatcher et al., 2002; Wallach & Grimes, 2000).

Nursing Considerations. Many different preparations of oral hormonal contraceptives are available. The nurse reviews the prescribing information in the package insert with the woman. Because of the wide variations, each woman must be clear about the unique dosage regimen for the preparation prescribed for her. Directions for care after missing one or two tablets also vary (Fig. 9-6).

Withdrawal bleeding tends to be short and scanty when some combination pills are taken. A woman may see no fresh blood at all. A drop of blood or a brown smudge on a tampon or the underwear counts as a menstrual period.

About 68% of women who start taking oral contraceptives are still taking them after 1 year (Trussell & Kowal, 2003). It therefore is important that nurses recommend that all women choosing to use oral contraceptives be provided with a second method of birth control and that women be instructed and comfortable with this backup method. Most women stop taking oral contraceptives for nonmedical reasons.

The nurse also reviews the signs of potential complications associated with the use of oral contraceptives (see Signs of Potential Complications box). Oral contraceptives do not protect a woman against STIs or HIV. A barrier method such as condoms and spermicide should be used for protection.

Combined Estrogen and Progestin Injection. The combined injectable contraception (e.g., Lunelle) contains 25 mg medroxyprogesterone acetate (DMPA) and 5 mg estradiol cypionate. The suspension is injected intramuscularly in the deltoid or gluteus maximus muscle every 28 ± 5 days. Typical failure rate in the first year of use is 3% (Trussell, 2003). Mechanism of action, contraindications, and side effects are similar to those of COCs (Hatcher et al., 2002).

Transdermal Contraceptive System. The contraceptive patch delivers continuous levels of norelgestromin (progesterone) and ethynyl estradiol. The patch can be applied to the lower abdomen, upper outer arm, buttock, or upper torso (except the breast). Application is on the same day once a week for 3 weeks, followed by a week without the patch. Withdrawal bleeding occurs during the "no patch" week. Mechanism of action, efficacy, contraindications, and side effects are similar to those of COCs (Speroff & Darney, 2001).

Vaginal Ring. The vaginal ring (made of ethylene vinyl acetate copolymer) delivers continuous levels of etonogestrel (progesterone) and ethynyl estradiol. One vaginal ring is worn for 3 weeks, followed by a week without the ring. Withdrawal bleeding occurs during the "no ring" week. The ring can be inserted by the woman and does not have to be fitted. Mechanism of action, efficacy, contraindications, and side effects are similar to those of COCs (Speroff & Darney, 2001).

Progestin-Only Contraception. Progestin-only methods impair fertility by inhibiting ovulation, thickening and decreasing the amount of cervical mucus, thinning the endometrium, and altering cilia in the uterine tubes (Hatcher et al., 2002; Wallach & Grimes, 2000).

Oral Progestins (Minipill). Failure rate of progestin-only pills for typical users is about 8% in the first year of use (Trussell, 2003). Effectiveness is increased if minipills are taken correctly. Because minipills contain such a low dose of progestin, the minipill must be taken at the same time every day (Wallach & Grimes, 2000). Users often complain of irregular vaginal bleeding.

Injectable Progestins. Depot medroxyprogesterone acetate (DMPA; Depo-Provera), 150 mg, is given intramuscularly in the deltoid or gluteus maximus muscle. A 21- to 23-gauge needle, 2.5 to 4 cm long, should be used. The injection site should not be massaged after administration because it could reduce the effectiveness of DMPA.

SIGNS OF POTENTIAL COMPLICATIONS

Oral Contraceptives (OCs)

Before OCs are prescribed and periodically throughout hormone therapy, alert the woman to stop taking the pill and to report any of the following symptoms to the health care provider immediately. The word *ACHES* helps in retention of this list:

- **A**—Abdominal pain may indicate a problem with the liver or gallbladder.
- **C**—Chest pain or shortness of breath may indicate possible clot problem within lungs or heart.
- **H**—Headaches (sudden or persistent) may be caused by cardiovascular accident or hypertension.
- **E**—Eye problems may indicate vascular accident or hypertension.
- **S**—Severe leg pain may indicate a thromboembolic process.

DMPA should be initiated during the first 5 days of the menstrual cycle and administered every 11 to 13 weeks (see Nurse Alert). Typical failure rate is 3% in the first year of use (Trussell, 2003).

NURSE ALERT
When administering an intramuscular injection of progestin (e.g., Depo-Provera), do not massage the site after the injection, because this action can hasten the absorption and shorten the period of effectiveness.

Advantages of DMPA include a contraceptive effectiveness comparable to that of combined oral contraceptives, long-lasting effects, the requirement of injections only 4 times a year, and lactation not likely to be impaired (Cunningham et al., 2001; Hatcher et al., 2002). Disadvantages are prolonged amenorrhea or uterine bleeding, increased risk of venous thrombosis and thromboembolism, and no protection against STIs (including HIV).

Implantable Progestins. The Norplant System consists of six flexible, nonbiodegradable polymeric silicone (Silastic) capsules. The Silastic capsules contain levonorgestrel, providing up to 5 years of contraception. Insertion and removal of the capsules are minor surgical procedures involving a local anesthetic, a small incision, and no sutures. The capsules are placed subdermally in the inner aspect of the upper arm. The progestin prevents some, but not all, ovulatory cycles and thickens cervical mucus. Other advantages include reversibility and long-term continuous contraception that is not related to coitus. Irregular menstrual bleeding is the most common side effect. Less common side effects include headaches, nervousness, nausea, skin changes, and vertigo. No STI protection is provided with the Norplant method, so condoms should be used for protection. The Norplant system is not available in the United States because of questions about effectiveness (Hatcher et al., 2002). A single rod implant is available in Europe and is expected to be available in the United States in 2003 (Speroff & Darney, 2001). A two-rod implant has been approved by the Food and Drug Administration, but it not yet on the market (Hatcher et al., 2002).

TABLE 9-2 **Dosages for Emergency Contraception**

DRUG	FIRST DOSE (WITHIN 72 HR)	SECOND DOSE (12 HR LATER)
Preven	2 light blue tablets	2 light blue tablets
Ovral	2 white tablets	2 white tablets
Ogestrel	2 white tablets	2 white tablets
Lo/Ovral	4 white tablets	4 white tablets
Low Ogestrel	4 white tablets	4 white tablets
Nordette	4 light orange tablets	4 light orange tablets
Levora	4 white tablets	4 white tablets
Levlen	4 light orange tablets	4 light orange tablets
Triphasil	4 yellow tablets	4 yellow tablets
Tri-Levlen	4 yellow tablets	4 yellow tablets
Trivora	4 pink tablets	4 pink tablets
Alesse	5 pink tablets	5 pink tablets
Levlite	5 pink tablets	5 pink tablets
Aviane	5 orange tablets	5 orange tablets
Ovrette*	20 yellow tablets	20 yellow tablets†
Plan B*	1 white tablet	1 white tablet

Source: American College of Obstetrics and Gynecology. (2001). *Emergency oral contraception. ACOG Practice Bulletin, No. 25.* Washington, DC: ACOG; Hatcher, R. et al. (2002). *A pocket guide to managing contraception.* Tiger, GA: Bridging the Gap Foundation.
*Contains only progestin.
†Take within 48 hours.

Emergency Contraception

Emergency contraception is used within 72 hours of unprotected intercourse to prevent pregnancy. The three methods available in the United States include high doses of oral progestins or COCs and insertion of the copper IUD (Hatcher et al., 2002). If taken before ovulation, emergency contraception prevents ovulation by inhibiting follicular development. If taken after ovulation occurs, there is little effect on ovarian hormone production or the endometrium. Recommended oral medication regimens with progestin only and estrogen-progestin pills for emergency contraception are presented in Table 9-2. Emergency contraception kits (Preven; Plan B) with the exact dosage and instructions for use also are available by prescription. Women with contraindications for estrogen use should use progestin-only emergency contraception. No medical contraindications for emergency contraception exist, except pregnancy and undiagnosed abnormal vaginal bleeding (ACOG, 2001; Hatcher et al., 2002). Emergency contraception is ineffective if the woman is pregnant. Pregnancy rates are reduced between 60% and 85% (Hatcher et al., 2002).

Oral contraception for emergency contraception can be offered to a woman who has had unprotected sexual intercourse and requests treatment within 72 hours of that event. To minimize the side effect of nausea that occurs with high doses of estrogen and progestin, the woman can be advised to take an over-the-counter antiemetic 1 hour before each dose. If the woman does not begin menstruation within 21 days after taking the pills, she should be evaluated for pregnancy (Hatcher et al., 2002).

Intrauterine devices containing copper (see later discussion) provide another emergency contraception option. The IUD should be inserted within 7 days of unprotected intercourse (Hatcher et al., 2002). This method is suggested only for women who wish to have the benefit of long-term contraception.

Contraceptive counseling should be provided to all women requesting emergency contraception, including a discussion of modification of risky sexual behaviors to prevent STIs and unwanted pregnancy (see Research box).

Intrauterine Devices

An **IUD** is a small, T-shaped device inserted into the uterine cavity. Medicated IUDs are loaded with either copper or a progestational agent (Fig. 9-7). These chemically active substances are released continuously (for example, copper-bearing devices for up to 10 years and progesterone devices for up to 5 years) (Hatcher et al., 2002). IUDs are impregnated with barium sulfate for radiopacity. The copper-bearing IUD damages sperm in transit to the uterine tubes, and few sperm reach the ovum, thus preventing fertilization (Hatcher et al., 2002).

The progesterone-bearing IUD causes progestin-related effects on cervical mucus and endometrial maturation (see Fig. 9-7). The effect of the progesterone IUD is primarily local, but there are some systemic effects, such as irregular menstrual bleeding. After 1 year of use, women usually experience amenorrhea or regular menses. The typical failure rate of the IUD ranges from 0.8% to 2.0% (Trussell, 2003).

The IUD offers constant contraception without the need to remember to take pills each day or engage in other manipulation before or between coital acts. If pregnancy can be excluded, an IUD may be placed at any time during the menstrual cycle. An IUD may be inserted immediately after childbirth or first trimester abortion (Hatcher et al., 2002; WHO, 2000). Contraceptive effects of the IUD are reversible. When pregnancy is desired, the IUD may be removed by the health care provider.

The progesterone IUD offers two important noncontraceptive progesterone-related advantages: less blood loss during menstruation and decreased primary dysmenorrhea. The average blood loss is increased with the copper IUD. IUD use is contraindicated in women with a history of pelvic inflammatory disease, known or suspected pregnancy, undiagnosed genital bleeding, suspected genital malignancy, or a distorted intrauterine cavity.

Disadvantages of IUD use include increased risk of pelvic inflammatory disease in the first 20 days after insertion, risk of bacterial vaginosis, and uterine perforation. The IUD offers no protection against STIs or HIV. The IUD is recommended primarily for women who want long-term contraception, who have had at least one child, and who are involved in stable monogamous relationships (Hatcher et al., 2002).

Nursing Considerations. The woman should be taught to check for the presence of the IUD thread after menstruation to rule out expulsion of the device. If pregnancy occurs with the IUD in place, the IUD should be removed immediately in the first trimester if the strings are visible. Later in pregnancy, ultrasound examination should be used to localize the IUD and to rule out placenta previa. IUD removal may not be recommended after the first trimester. Retention of the IUD during

RESEARCH

Emergency Contraception

Teenagers in the United States experience 1 million pregnancies and 500,000 live births a year, a rate about two to five times that of other developed nations. Teens are notoriously inconsistent contraceptive users for a variety of reasons, including lack of knowledge, ambivalence, poor self-esteem, and inability to negotiate condom use. Lack of understanding and ability to negotiate the health care system is also a factor. For the teen who has experienced unprotected intercourse, emergency contraception (EC) is a very useful second plan. Postcoital use is between 74% and 90% effective at preventing pregnancy. Barriers to its use are lack of knowledge about it, need for prescription, and lingering health care provider reluctance to prescribe it.

Two nurse-midwives surveyed 146 of their colleagues about their knowledge, attitudes, and policies regarding EC. Three-quarters of the respondents prescribed it only a few times a year or less. More than half had written material available for clients. About half would prescribe it for a client to have on hand, would not restrict the number of times used, and felt that repeated uses were safe. Two-thirds believed that EC does not discourage compliance with other contraceptives and would prescribe it even if a patient would continue a pregnancy. Up to 32% answered "unsure" to the questions, highlighting lingering unease with EC. Age over 52 years and graduation from midwifery school prior to 1982 were significant factors associated with infrequent recommended use of EC.

IMPLICATIONS FOR PRACTICE

The ideal contraception for adolescents would be safe, effective, freely available without examination or parental consent, confidential, free of side effects, and protective against sexually transmitted infections, and it would consider the lack of planning that is characteristic of this age. Routinely informing clients, especially teenagers, about the availability of EC as a safe and effective backup method, and facilitating its timely and confidential use, could be one of the best services a nurse can provide for young women.

Reference: Kettyle, E., & Klima, C. (2002). Adolescent emergency contraception: Attitudes and practices of certified nurse-midwives. *Journal of Midwifery & Women's Health, 47*(2), 68-73.

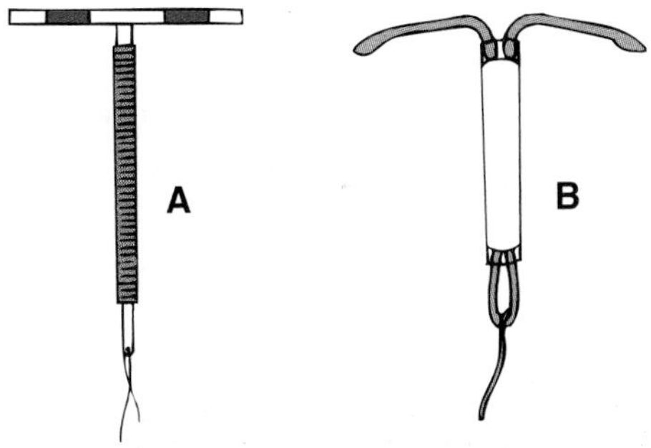
A
B

FIG. 9-7 Intrauterine devices (IUDs). **A,** Copper T380A. **B,** Levonorgestrel-releasing IUD.

pregnancy increases the risk of septic miscarriage and ectopic pregnancy (Hatcher et al., 2002). In some women who are allergic to copper, a rash develops, necessitating the removal of the copper-bearing IUD. Signs of potential complications to be taught to the woman are listed in the accompanying box.

Sterilization

Sterilization refers to surgical procedures intended to render the person infertile. Most procedures involve the occlusion of the passageways for the ova and sperm (Fig. 9-8). For the woman, the oviducts (uterine tubes) are occluded; for the man, the sperm ducts (vas deferens) are occluded. Only surgical removal of the ovaries (oophorectomy) or uterus (hysterectomy) or both will result in absolute sterility for the woman. All other sterilization procedures have a small but definite failure rate; that is, pregnancy may result.

Female Sterilization. Female sterilization **(bilateral tubal ligation [BTL])** may be done immediately after childbirth (within 24 to 48 hours), concomitant with abortion, or as an interval procedure (during any phase of the menstrual cycle). If sterilization is performed as an interval procedure, the health care provider must be certain that the woman is not pregnant. Half of all female sterilization procedures are performed immediately after a pregnancy (Hatcher et al., 2002). Sterilization procedures can be safely done on an outpatient basis. Failure rate for methods of female sterilization vary by the method and the woman's age, but the average is 0.5% (Trussell & Kowal, 2003).

Tubal Occlusion. A laparoscopic approach or a minilaparotomy may be used for tubal ligation (Fig. 9-9), tubal electrocoagulation, or the application of bands or clips. Electrocoagulation and ligation are considered to be permanent methods. Use of the bands or clips has the theoretic advantage of possible removal and return of tubal patency.

For the minilaparotomy, the woman is admitted the morning of surgery, having received nothing by mouth since midnight. Preoperative sedation is given. The procedure may be carried out with a local anesthetic, but a regional or general anesthetic also may be used. A small incision is made in the abdominal wall below the umbilicus. The woman may experience sensations of tugging, but no pain, and the operation is completed within 20 minutes. She may be discharged several hours later if she has recovered from anesthesia. Any abdominal discomfort usually can be controlled with a mild analgesic (e.g., acetaminophen). Within days the scar is almost invisible (see Teaching for Self-Care box). As with any surgery, there is always a possibility of complications of anesthesia, infection, hemorrhage, and trauma to other organs.

Tubal Reconstruction. Restoration of tubal continuity (reanastomosis) and function is technically feasible except after laparoscopic tubal electrocoagulation. Sterilization reversal, however, is costly, difficult (requiring microsurgery), and uncertain. The success rate varies with the extent of tubal destruction and removal. The loss of a segment of tube necessary for sperm capacitation and fertilization is probably the reason for low pregnancy rates.

SIGNS OF POTENTIAL COMPLICATIONS

Intrauterine Devices (IUDs)

Signs of potential complications related to IUDs can be remembered in the following manner (Hatcher et al., 2002):

P—Period late, abnormal spotting or bleeding
A—Abdominal pain, pain with intercourse
I—Infection exposure, abnormal vaginal discharge
N—Not feeling well, fever, or chills
S—String missing; shorter or longer

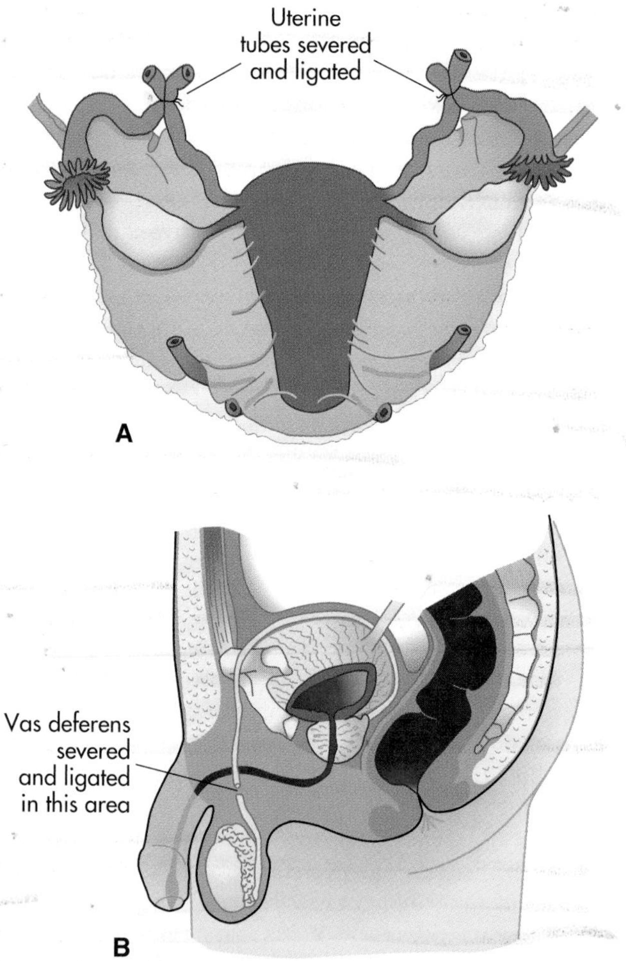
Uterine tubes severed and ligated
A
Vas deferens severed and ligated in this area
B

FIG. 9-8 Sterilization. **A,** Uterine tubes severed and ligated (tubal ligation). **B,** Sperm duct severed and ligated (vasectomy).

Male Sterilization. **Vasectomy** is the easiest and most commonly used operation for male sterilization. Vasectomy can be carried out with local anesthesia on an outpatient basis.

Small incisions are made into the anterior aspect of the scrotum above and lateral to each testis over the spermatic cord (see Fig. 9-8, *B*). Each vas deferens is identified and doubly ligated with fine, absorbable or nonabsorbable sutures, and then each vas deferens is severed between the ligatures. Occasionally the surgeon cauterizes the cut stumps of the sperm ducts. Many surgeons bury the cut ends into scrotal fascia to lessen the chance of reunion. Then the skin incisions are closed. Usually one suture is used for closure of each skin incision, and a dressing is applied (Hatcher et al., 2002).

The man is instructed in self-care to promote a safe return to routine activities. To reduce swelling and relieve discomfort, ice packs are applied to the scrotum intermittently for a few hours after surgery. A scrotal support may be applied to decrease discomfort. Moderate inactivity for about 2 days is advisable because of local scrotal tenderness. The skin suture can be removed 5 to 7 days after surgery. Sexual intercourse may be resumed as desired; however, sterility is not immediate. Some sperm will remain in the proximal portions of the sperm ducts after vasectomy. One week to several months are required to clear the ducts of sperm (i.e., after approximately 20 ejaculations); therefore, some form of contraception is needed until the sperm count in the ejaculate on two consecutive tests is down to zero (Hatcher et al., 2002).

Vasectomy has no effect on potency (ability to achieve and maintain erection) or volume of ejaculate. Endocrine production of testosterone continues so that secondary sex characteristics are not affected. Sperm production continues, but sperm are unable to leave the epididymis and are lysed by the immune system. Men occasionally may develop a hematoma, infection, or epididymitis (Hatcher et al., 2002). Less common are painful granulomas from accumulation of sperm.

Complications after bilateral vasectomy are uncommon and usually not serious. They include bleeding (usually external), suture reaction, and reaction to anesthetic agent. Failure rate for male sterilization is 0.15% (Trussell & Kowal, 2003).

Tubal Reconstruction. Microsurgery to reanastomose (restoration of tubal continuity) the sperm ducts can be accomplished successfully in more than 90% of cases (i.e., sperm in the ejaculate); however, the fertility rate is only about 50% (Hatcher et al., 2002). The rate of success decreases as the time since the procedure increases. The vasectomy may result in permanent changes in the testes that leave men unable to father children. The changes are those ordinarily seen only in the elderly (e.g., interstitial fibrosis [scar tissue between the seminiferous tubules]). In some men, antibodies develop against their own sperm (autoimmunization). The role of antisperm antibodies in fertility after vasectomy reversal has not been completely determined. Additional research is needed to explore a possible link between vasectomy and prostate cancer.

Laws and Regulations. All states have strict regulations for informed consent. Many states permit voluntary sterilization of any mature, rational woman without reference to her marital or pregnancy status. Although the partner's consent is not required by law, the woman is encouraged to discuss the situation with the partner, and health care providers may request the partner's consent. Sterilization of minors or mentally incompetent individuals is restricted by most states and often requires the approval of a board of eugenicists or other court-appointed individuals (see Legal Tip).

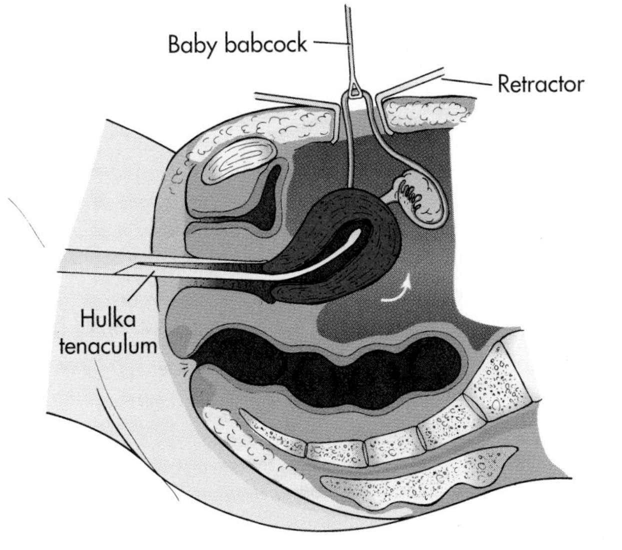
Baby babcock
Retractor
Hulka
tenaculum

FIG. 9-9 Use of minilaparotomy to gain access to uterine tubes for occlusion procedures. Tenaculum is used to lift uterus upward *(arrow)* toward incision.

TEACHING FOR SELF-CARE

What to Expect After Tubal Ligation

- You should expect no change in hormones and their influence.
- Your menstrual period will be about the same as before the sterilization.
- You may feel pain at ovulation.
- The ovum disintegrates within the abdominal cavity.
- It is highly unlikely that you will become pregnant.
- You should not have a change in sexual functioning; you may enjoy sexual relations more because you will not be concerned about becoming pregnant.
- Sterilization offers no protection against STIs; therefore, you may need to use condoms.

LEGAL TIP Sterilization

- If federal funds are used for sterilization, the person must be aged 21 years or older.
- Informed consent must include an explanation of the risks, benefits, and alternatives; a statement that describes sterilization as a permanent, irreversible method of birth control; and a statement that mandates a 30-day waiting period between giving consent and the sterilization.
- Informed consent must be in the person's native language, or a translator must be provided to read the consent form to the person.

Nursing Considerations. The nurse plays an important role in assisting people with decision making so that all requirements for informed consent are met. The nurse also provides information about alternatives to sterilization, such as contraception. The nurse acts as a "sounding board" for people who are exploring the possibility of choosing sterilization and their feelings about and motivation for this choice. The nurse records this information, which may be the basis for referral to a family-planning clinic, a psychiatric social worker, or another professional health care provider.

Information must be given about what is entailed in various procedures, how much discomfort or pain can be expected, and what type of care is needed. Many individuals fear sterilization procedures because of the imagined effect on their sex life. They need reassurance concerning the hormonal and psychologic basis for sexual function and that uterine tube occlusion or vasectomy has no biologic sequelae in terms of sexual adequacy (Hatcher et al., 2002).

Preoperative care includes health assessment, which includes a psychologic assessment, physical examination, and laboratory tests. The nurse assists with the health assessment, answers questions, and confirms the client's understanding of printed instructions (e.g., nothing by mouth after midnight). Ambivalence and extreme fear of the procedure are reported to the physician.

Postoperative care depends on the procedure performed (e.g., laparoscopy, laparotomy for tubal occlusion, or vasectomy). General care includes recovery after anesthesia, vital signs, fluid and electrolyte balance (intake and output, laboratory values), prevention of or early identification and treatment for infection or hemorrhage, control of discomfort, and assessment of emotional response to the procedure and recovery.

Discharge planning depends on the type of procedure performed. In general, the client is given written instructions about observing for and reporting symptoms and signs of complications, the type of recovery to be expected, and the date and time for a follow-up appointment.

Future Trends

Contraceptive options are more limited in the United States and Canada than in some other industrialized countries. Lack of funding for research, governmental regulations, conflicting values about contraception, and high costs of liability coverage for contraception have been cited as blocks to new and improved methods. Existing methods of contraception are being improved, however, and a variety of new methods are being developed.

Lower-dose COCs (10 to 15 μg of ethynyl estradiol) are available in Europe. In addition, female barrier methods are being tested. Male hormonal methods also are being investigated, including hormonal injections (testosterone), gonadotropin-releasing hormone antagonists, and contraceptive vaccines (Hatcher et al., 2002).

Plan of Care: Sexual Activity and Contraception

NURSING DIAGNOSIS Decisional conflict related to contraceptive alternatives

Expected Outcome *Client and partner will verbalize understanding of different methods of contraception and will choose the method best suited for their needs.*

Nursing Interventions/*Rationales*

Provide information regarding reliability, use, indications, contraindications, and side effects of different methods of contraception *to facilitate the decision-making process.*

Utilize privacy and therapeutic communication during discussion of sexual activity and methods of contraception *to provide clarification of information and client trust of caregiver.*

NURSING DIAGNOSIS Risk for infection related to ongoing sexual activity as evidenced by client history

Expected Outcome *Client and her partner will remain free of sexually transmitted infections.*

Nursing Interventions/*Rationales*

Provide information regarding safer sex practices, use of spermicides and barrier methods *to raise client awareness of methods to prevent infection.*

NURSING DIAGNOSIS Risk for ineffective health maintenance related to unfamiliarity with contraceptive method

Expected Outcome *Woman and partner will verbalize intent to utilize chosen contraception correctly.*

Nursing Interventions/*Rationales*

Review information given regarding use, reliability, and side effects of chosen contraceptive method *to ensure woman's and partner's understanding.*

Provide list of informational resources *to promote consistency of use of chosen method.*

Encourage ongoing effective communication with health care provider *to promote trust.*

Evaluation

The nurse can be reasonably assured that care was effective when the client-centered expected outcomes have been achieved: the woman and her partner learn about the various methods of contraception; the couple achieve pregnancy only when planned; and they have no adverse sequelae as a result of the chosen method of contraception (see Plan of Care).

ABORTION

Induced abortion is the purposeful interruption of a pregnancy before 20 weeks' gestation. (Spontaneous abortion [miscarriage] is discussed in Chapter 31.) If the abortion is performed at the woman's request, the term **elective abortion** is used; if performed for reasons of maternal or fetal health or disease, the term **therapeutic abortion** applies. Many factors contribute to a woman's decision to have an abortion. Indications include (1) preservation of the life or health of the mother, (2) genetic disorders of the fetus, (3) rape or incest, and (4) the pregnant woman's request. The control of birth, dealing as it does with human sexuality and the question of life and death, is one of the most emotional components of health care and has been the most controversial social issue in the last half of the twentieth century. Regulations exist to protect the mother from the complications of abortion.

The U.S. Supreme Court set aside previous antiabortion laws in January 1973, holding that first trimester abortion is permissible, inasmuch as the mortality rate from interruption of early gestation is less than the mortality rate after normal term birth; more than 90% of abortions are performed at this point in pregnancy. Second trimester abortion was left to the discretion of the individual states (Hatcher et al., 2002). Hospitals maintained by Catholics and some of those maintained by strict fundamentalists forbid abortion (and often sterilization), despite legal challenge (see Legal Tip).

LEGAL TIP Induced Abortion

It is important for nurses to know the laws regarding abortion in their state of practice before they offer abortion counseling or nursing care to a woman choosing an abortion. Many states enforce a mandatory delay or state-directed counseling before a woman may legally obtain an abortion.

Rates of biologic complications after abortions (e.g., ectopic pregnancy, infection, hemorrhage) tend to be low, especially if the woman aborts during the first trimester (Speroff & Darney, 1999). Psychologic sequelae of induced abortion are uncommon and may be related to circumstances and support systems surrounding the pregnant woman, such as the attitudes reflected by friends, family, and health care workers. It must be remembered that the woman facing an abortion is pregnant and may exhibit the emotional responses shared by all pregnant women, including postbirth depression (Williams, 2000).

Nurses often struggle with the same values and moral convictions as those of the pregnant woman. The conflicts and doubts of the nurse can be readily communicated to women who are already anxious and overly sensitive. Health care professionals need assistance to identify and come to terms with their own feelings. It is not uncommon for confusion to arise as beliefs are challenged by the reality of care. Nurses whose religious or moral beliefs do not support abortion have the right to refuse such an assignment. In reality, reassignment is usually an option, so that the abortion patient receives the needed care.

CARE MANAGEMENT

Assessment and Nursing Diagnoses

A thorough assessment is conducted through history, physical examination, and laboratory tests. The length of pregnancy and the condition of the woman must be determined to select the appropriate type of abortion procedure. An ultrasound examination should be performed before a second trimester abortion is done. If the woman is Rh negative, she is a candidate for prophylaxis against Rh isoimmunization. She should receive $Rh_0(D)$ immune globulin within 72 hours after the abortion if she is D negative and if Coombs' test results are negative (if the woman is unsensitized or isoimmunization has not developed) (Hatcher et al., 2002).

The woman's understanding of alternatives, the types of abortions, and expected recovery is assessed. Misinformation and gaps in knowledge are identified and corrected. The record is reviewed for the signed informed consent, and the client's understanding is verified. General preoperative, operative, and postoperative assessments are performed.

Analysis of data leads to identification of the appropriate nursing diagnoses for the woman undergoing elective abortion. Potential nursing diagnoses are listed.

- *Decisional conflict related to*
  - –value system
- *Fear related to*
  - –abortion procedure
  - –potential complications
  - –implications for future pregnancies
  - –what others might think
- *Anticipatory grieving related to*
  - –distress at loss or feelings of guilt
- *Risk for infection related to*
  - –effects of the procedure
  - –lack of understanding of preoperative and postoperative self-care
- *Acute pain related to*
  - –effects of the procedure or postoperative events

Expected Outcomes of Care

Planning is a collaborative effort among the woman, her sexual partner (as appropriate), the physician, and the nurse. Expected outcomes are established collaboratively, should be stated in client-centered terms, and may include that the woman will do the following:

- Verbalize understanding of the information necessary to give informed consent
- Undergo a successful procedure and uneventful recovery
- Continue to be satisfied with the decision for induced abortion, the procedure, and her experience with the health care team

Plan of Care and Interventions

Counseling about abortion includes help for the woman in identifying how she perceives the pregnancy, information about the choices available (i.e., having an abortion or carrying the pregnancy to term and then either keeping the infant or placing the baby for adoption), and information about the types of abortion procedures.

First Trimester Abortion

Methods for performing early elective abortion include vacuum aspiration and medical methods (mifepristone with misoprostol and methotrexate with misoprostol).

Vacuum Aspiration

Vacuum aspiration abortion is the most common procedure, with about 97% of all procedures being performed by suction curettage. Very early abortions (menstrual extraction, endometrial aspiration) can be done with a small flexible plastic cannula without cervical dilation or anesthesia. The insertion of a small **laminaria tent** (cone of dried seaweed that swells as it absorbs moisture and dilates the cervix) retained by a vaginal tampon for 4 to 24 hours will usually facilitate the purposeful interruption of a first trimester pregnancy of more than 8 weeks of gestation by dilating the cervix atraumatically (Hatcher et al., 2002). On removal of the moist, expanded laminaria tent, the cervix will have dilated 2 or 3 times its original diameter. Rarely will further mechanical dilation of the cervix be required. The insertion of an adequate-sized aspiration cannula (8.5 to 10.5 mm) is almost always possible. Cervical laceration and bleeding are reduced by the use of laminaria. A disadvantage is the delay necessary and the need for an additional visit to the physician's office or clinic. Prostaglandin gel also may be used to soften the cervix (Cunningham et al., 2001).

Aspiration abortion may be performed in the physician's office, the clinic, or the hospital. For the procedure, the vaginal area is cleansed (shaving is not necessary). The suction procedure for performing an early elective abortion (ideal time is 8 to 12 weeks after the last menstrual period) usually requires less than 5 minutes. During the procedure, the nurse or physician keeps the woman informed about what to expect next (e.g., menstrual-like cramping and sounds of the suction machine). The nurse assesses the woman's vital signs. The aspirated uterine contents must be carefully inspected to ascertain whether all fetal parts and adequate placental tissue have been evacuated. After the abortion, the woman rests on the operating table until she is ready to stand, and then she remains in the recovery area or waiting room for 1 to 3 hours for detection of excessive cramping or bleeding; then she is discharged. She may be discharged alone or in the company of a relative or friend, depending on the anesthetic used. If the procedure is done in the physician's office, preoperative sedation is usually not given, and local anesthesia is usually used.

Bleeding after the operation is normally about the equivalent of a heavy menstrual period, and cramps are rarely severe. Excessive vaginal bleeding and infection, such as endometritis or salpingitis, are the most common complications of induced abortion. Retained products of conception are the primary cause of vaginal bleeding. Evacuation of the uterus, uterine massage, and administration of oxytocin or methylergonovine (Methergine) may be necessary. Prophylactic antibiotics have been shown to decrease the risk of infection and should be considered (Hatcher et al., 2002).

Postabortal instructions differ among health care providers (e.g., tampons should not be used for at least 3 days or should be avoided for up to 3 weeks, and resumption of sexual intercourse may be permitted within 1 week or discouraged for 3 weeks). The woman may shower daily. Instruction is given to watch for excessive bleeding (i.e., more than one large pad per hour for 4 hours), cramps, or fever, and to avoid douches of any type. The woman may expect her menstrual period to resume 4 to 6 weeks after the day of the procedure. The nurse offers information about the birth control method the woman prefers, if this has not been done previously during the counseling interview that usually precedes the decision to have an abortion. The woman must be strongly encouraged to return for her follow-up visit so that complications can be detected and an acceptable contraceptive method prescribed. A pregnancy test also may be performed to determine if the pregnancy has been successfully terminated (Stenchever et al., 2001).

Mifepristone

Mifepristone (RU 486) can be used up to 9 weeks after conception. The effectiveness of mifepristone is inversely related to gestational age, as determined by β-human chorionic gonadotropin levels and the duration of amenorrhea (Hatcher et al., 2002). It is considered, however, to be an effective and safe method for termination of early pregnancy.

Uterine bleeding begins within 4 days of administration of the first dose. Usually a period of painless heavy bleeding is reported. Termination of pregnancy occurs for most women. When mifepristone is combined with administration of a prostaglandin agent (misoprostol) 36 to 48 hours later, the rate of abortion increases.

Supporters of this method believe that even with known disadvantages, mifepristone offers a reasonable alternative to surgical abortion, which carries the risk of anesthesia and surgical complications and infertility (Hatcher et al., 2002). Others have taken a strong stand against the use of mifepristone. Mifepristone was approved by the FDA for use in the United States in October 2000 but is not available for use. It is popular in France and other European countries and in China (Hatcher et al., 2002).

Methotrexate and Misoprostol

Methotrexate is a cytotoxic drug that causes early abortion by blocking folic acid in fetal cells so they cannot divide. There is no standard protocol, but up to 49 days of gestation, methotrexate can be given intramuscularly or orally, followed by vaginal placement of misoprostol (prostaglandin analogue). Women commonly have nausea, vomiting, and cramping after the misoprostol insertion. If abortion does not occur, an additional dose of misoprostol is given, or vacuum aspiration is performed (Carbonell et al., 1998; Hatcher et al. 2002).

Second Trimester Abortion

Second trimester abortion is associated with an increase of complications and costs. Dilation and evacuation, induction of uterine contractions, and major operations are methods used.

Dilation and Evacuation

Dilation and evacuation (D&E) can be performed at up to 20 weeks of gestation but is more appropriate between 13 and 16 weeks (Hatcher et al., 2002). The cervix requires more dilation because the products of conception are larger. Often laminaria are inserted several hours or several days before the procedure. Nursing care includes monitoring vital signs, providing emotional support, administering analgesics, and monitoring after the procedure. Disadvantages of D&E may be long-term harmful effects on the cervix.

Prostaglandins

The most common technique for medical termination in the second trimester is the administration of prostaglandins. Prostaglandins can be administered in suppository form, as a gel, or by intrauterine injection. Unpleasant side effects (e.g., nausea, vomiting, and diarrhea) usually occur. Repeated doses may be needed for expulsion of the products of conception.

Hypertonic and Uterotonic Agents

Hypertonic solutions (e.g., saline, urea) injected directly into the uterus and uterotonic agents (e.g., misoprostol and dinoprostone) account for fewer than 1% of all abortions because other methods are safer and easier to use.

Nursing Considerations

The woman will need help to explore the meaning of the various alternatives and consequences to herself and her significant others. It is often difficult for a woman to express her true feelings (e.g., what abortion means to her now and in the future and what support or regret her friends and peers may demonstrate). A calm, matter-of-fact approach on the part of the nurse can be helpful (e.g., "Yes, I know you are pregnant. I am here to help. Let's talk about alternatives."). Listening to what the woman has to say and encouraging her to speak are essential. Neutral responses such as "Oh," "Uh-huh," and "Umm" and nonverbal encouragement such as nodding, maintaining eye contact, and use of touch are helpful in setting an open, accepting environment. Clarifying, restating, and reflecting statements; open-ended questions; and feedback are communication techniques that can be used to maintain a realistic focus on the situation and bring the woman's problems into the open. Once a decision has been made, the woman must be assured of continued support. Information about what is entailed in various procedures, how much discomfort or pain can be expected, and what type of care is needed must be given. If family or friends cannot be involved, scheduling time for nursing personnel to give the necessary support is an essential component of the care plan.

After the abortion, studies have indicated that most women report relief, but some have temporary distress or mixed emotions. Guilt and anxiety may occur more with young women, women with poor social support, multiparous women, and women with a history of psychiatric illness. Women having second trimester abortions may have more emotional distress than do women having abortions in the first trimester (Williams, 2001). Women feeling pressure to have an abortion had symptoms of short-term grief in the study reported by Williams (2001). Because symptoms can vary among women who have had abortions, nurses must assess women for grief reactions and facilitate the grieving process through active listening and nonjudgmental support and care.

Evaluation

The nurse can be reasonably sure that care was effective when the expected outcomes have been met: the client understands all information necessary to give informed consent; the procedure is successful; recovery is uneventful; and the client continues to be satisfied with the decision for elective abortion, the procedure, and the experience with the health care team.

KEY POINTS

- A variety of contraceptive methods are available with various effectiveness rates, advantages, and disadvantages.
- Women and their partners should choose the contraceptive method or methods best suited to them.
- Effective contraceptives are available through both prescription and nonprescription sources.
- A variety of techniques are available to enhance the effectiveness of periodic abstinence in motivated couples who prefer this natural method.
- Hormonal contraception includes both precoital and postcoital prevention through various modalities and requires thorough client education.
- The barrier methods of diaphragm and cervical cap provide safe and effective contraception for women or couples motivated to use them consistently and correctly.
- Proper concurrent use of spermicides and latex condoms provides protection against STIs.
- Tubal ligations and vasectomies are permanent sterilization methods used by increasing numbers of women and men.
- Induced abortion performed in the first trimester is safer than an abortion performed in the second trimester.
- The most common complications of induced abortion include infection, retained products of conception, and excessive vaginal bleeding.
- Major psychologic sequelae of induced abortion are rare.

CRITICAL THINKING EXERCISES

1. You are interviewing a 45-year-old woman in the local health department family-planning clinic. She is seeking information about her risks of pregnancy at this time in her life.
   - **a.** What information will you need from her to respond?
   - **b.** How might you answer her question based on the answers you may receive in part a?
   - **c.** Assuming that contraceptive measures are necessary, what methods are appropriate for this client?
   - **d.** What further information may you need from this client to make a contraceptive recommendation?
   - **e.** What alterations would you make in a teaching plan for her, based on her age and previous experiences with contraception?
2. You are working in a health department clinic. A 16-year-old unmarried woman comes in requesting information about options for an unwanted pregnancy.
   - **a.** Examine your beliefs about teenage pregnancy. Explore your beliefs about options for an unwanted pregnancy. How might these beliefs affect your ability to provide information about options in a nonjudgmental manner?
   - **b.** What client information do you need to know before counseling a client about her options?
   - **c.** What information does the pregnant woman need to make a decision about her unwanted pregnancy?
   - **d.** What are the laws in your state related to abortion, informed consent, and treatment of minors?
   - **e.** Select one option for this hypothetic client and justify your choice.
   - **f.** Write a care plan addressing the physical and psychosocial needs of a client undergoing abortion.
3. Visit a clinic that provides family-planning services in your area.
   - **a.** Are there differences in fee schedules for women with and without insurance? Are local, state, or federal funds available?
   - **b.** Are the hours of service sufficient to meet the needs of clients? How long are typical waits to be seen during a scheduled appointment?
   - **c.** What is the nurse's role in the clinic? What other health care professionals are present, and what are their roles? Is there any collaboration among these care providers?
   - **d.** Make suggestions for changes in the way care is provided that increase efficacy and client satisfaction.

RESOURCES

American College of Obstetricians and Gynecologists
409 12th St. SW
Washington, DC 20024
800-762-2264
www.acog.com

American Fertility Foundation
2131 Magnolia Ave., Suite 201
Birmingham, AL 35256
205-251-9764

Emergency Contraception Hotline
P.O. Box 33344
Washington, DC 20033
888-668-2528
www.not-2-late.com

National Abortion Federation Consumer Hotline
1156 15th St. NW, Suite 700
Washington, DC 20005
800-772-9100

National Clearinghouse for Family Planning Information
P.O. Box 10716
Rockville, MD 20850
703-558-4990

National Women's Health Resource Center
120 Albany St., Suite 820
New Brunswick, NJ 08901
877-986-9472
www.healthywomen.org

Planned Parenthood Federation of America, Inc.
810 Seventh Ave.
New York, NY 10019
800-669-0156
www.plannedparenthood.org

REFERENCES

American College of Obstetricians and Gynecologists. (2001). *Emergency oral contraception: ACOG Practice Bulletin No. 25.* Washington, DC: ACOG.

Carbonell, J., et al. (1998). Oral methotrexate and vaginal misoprostol for early abortion. *Contraception, 57*(2), 83-88.

Centers for Disease Control and Prevention. (2002). Sexually transmitted disease treatment guidelines 2002. *MMWR, 51*(RR6), 1-80.

Cunningham, F. et al. (2001). *Williams obstetrics* (21st ed.). New York: McGraw- Hill.

Goldzieher, J.W. (1998). *Hormonal contraception: Pills, injections and implants* (4th ed.). Ontario: EMIS-CANADA.

Grabrick, D. et al. (2000). Risk of breast cancer with oral contraception use in women with a family history of breast cancer. *Journal of the American Medical Association, 284*(14), 1791-1798.

Hatcher, R. et al. (2002). *A pocket guide to managing contraception.* Tiger, GA: Bridging the Gap Foundation.

Speroff, L., & Darney, P. (2001). New methods. *Dialogues in Contraception, 7*(3), 1-4, 8.

Speroff, L., Glass, R., & Kase, N. (1999). *Clinical gynecologic endocrinology and infertility* (6th ed.). Baltimore, MD: Williams & Wilkins.

Stenchever, M. et al. (2001). *Comprehensive gynecology* (4th ed.). St. Louis: Mosby.

Stephenson. J. (2000). Widely used spermicide may increase, not decrease, risk of HIV transmission. *Journal of the American Medical Association, 284*(8), 949.

Trussell, J. (2003). Contraceptive efficacy. In R. Hatcher et al. (Eds.). *Contraceptive technology* (18th rev. ed.). New York: Ardent Media, Inc.

Trussell, J., & Kowal, D. (2003). The essentials of contraception. In R. Hatcher et al. (Eds.). *Contraceptive technology* (18th rev. ed.). New York: Ardent Media, Inc.

U.S. Department of Health and Human Services, Health Resources and Service Administration, Maternal and Child Health Bureau. (2002). *Women's Health USA 2002.* Rockville, MD: U.S. Department of Health and Human Services.

Wallach, M. & Grimes, D. (2000). *Modern oral contraception: Updates from The Contraceptive Report.* Totowa, NJ: Emron.

Williams, G. (2000). Grief after elective abortion: Exploring nursing interventions for another kind of perinatal loss. *AWHONN Lifelines, 4*(2), 37-40.

Williams, G. (2001). Short-term grief after an elective abortion. *Journal of Obstetric, Gynecologic, and Neonatal Nursing, 30*(2), 174-183.

World Health Organization. (2000). *Improving access to quality care in family planning: Medical eligibility criteria for contraceptive use* (2nd ed.). Geneva: World Health Organization.

CHAPTER 10

Christena Raines

Infertility

http://evolve.elsevier.com/Lowdermilk/MatWmnHlth/

LEARNING OBJECTIVES

- List common causes of infertility.
- Investigate the psychologic impact of infertility.
- Describe common diagnoses and treatments for infertility.
- Identify reproductive alternatives for infertile couples.
- Examine the various ethical and legal considerations of infertility.

This chapter addresses infertility, associated tests, and common therapies. The available alternatives and the psychosocial implications of infertility are discussed.

INCIDENCE

Infertility is a serious medical concern that affects quality of life and is a problem for about 10% of the reproductive-age population (ASRM, 2002). Infertility implies subfertility, a prolonged time to conceive, as opposed to sterility, which means inability to conceive. Normally a fertile couple has approximately a 20% chance of conception in each ovulatory cycle. Primary infertility applies to a woman who has never been pregnant; secondary infertility applies to a woman who has been pregnant in the past.

The prevalence of infertility is relatively stable among the overall population but increases with the age of the woman, particularly in those older than 40 years (Stenchever et al., 2001). Probable causes include the trend toward delaying pregnancy until later in life, when fertility decreases naturally and the prevalence of diseases such as endometriosis and ovulatory dysfunction increases. There is some controversy regarding whether there has been an increase in male infertility, or whether male infertility is being more readily identified because of improvements in diagnosis.

Diagnosis and treatment of infertility require considerable physical, emotional, and financial investment over an extended period. Men and women often perceive infertility differently, with women having more stress from tests and treatments, placing greater importance on having children, being more accepting of indicated treatments, and wanting children more than men (Stephen & Chandra, 1998).

In the United States, feelings connected with infertility are many and complex. The origins of some of these feelings are myths, superstitions, misinformation, or magical thinking about the causes of infertility. Other feelings arise from the need to undergo many tests and examinations and from a perception of being "different" from others. The attitude, sensitivity, and caring nature of those who are involved in the assessment of infertility lay the foundation for the clients' ability to cope with the subsequent therapy and management. Team members also must respect affected individuals' and couples' desires in choosing to stop treatment and to select other alternatives, such as adoption.

FACTORS ASSOCIATED WITH INFERTILITY

Many factors, both male and female, contribute to normal fertility. A normally developed reproductive tract in both the male and female partner is essential. Normal functioning of an intact hypothalamic-pituitary-gonadal axis supports gametogenesis–the formation of sperm and ova. The life span of the sperm and ovum is short. Although sperm remain viable in the female's reproductive tract for 48 hours or more, probably only a few retain fertilization potential for more than 24 hours. Ova remain viable for about 24 hours, but the optimal time for fertilization may be no more than 1 to 2 hours (Cunningham et al., 2001); thus timing of intercourse becomes critical.

The male must produce sperm that are normal, adequate in number, and motile. Accessory glands must provide secretions supportive to the sperm to form semen. The tube system to the urethra must be patent. Ejaculation must deposit semen around the cervix at the appropriate time of the female's menstrual cycle. After being deposited, sperm must undergo capacitation to prepare for fertilization, and then they migrate through the uterus to the ampulla of the uterine tube to fertilize a receptive normal ovum.

In the female, a graafian follicle must mature and release a healthy ovum able to be fertilized. The ovum must be drawn by the fimbria into a healthy, patent uterine tube and be fertilized within a few hours. The conceptus must migrate down the tube into a well-developed normal uterus. Implantation of the blastocyst must occur within 7 to 10 days in a hormone-prepared endometrium. The conceptus must develop normally, reach viability, and be born in good condition for extrauterine life.

An alteration in one or more of these structures, functions, or processes results in some degree of impaired fertility. Causes of impaired fertility are sometimes difficult to assign to either the male or female. In general a female factor such as ovulatory dysfunction or pelvic factor is responsible for infertility in about 50% of infertile couples (ASRM, 2002). A male factor (sperm and semen abnormalities) is responsible for infertility in about 35% of couples. Unexplained factors and unusual causes related to both partners are responsible for 15% of infertility (Session, 1998; Stenchever et al., 2001). Unexplained infertility and recurrent (habitual) miscarriage may be the result of aberrations of the immune system (e.g., antisperm antibodies, failure of implantation and growth of a blastocyst); however, these causes have not been proven (Carcio, 1998; Stenchever et al., 2001). Boxes 10-1 and 10-2 list factors affecting female and male infertility.

Infertility also may be caused by something as simple as poor timing or inadequate frequency of intercourse. The couple should be taught about the menstrual cycle and the way to detect ovulation (see Chapters 5 and 9).

Female Infertility

Congenital or Developmental Factors

Congenital factors rarely cause impaired fertility. If the woman has abnormal external genitals, surgical reconstruction of abnormal tissue and construction of a functional vagina may permit normal intercourse. However, if internal reproductive tract structures are absent, there is no hope for

---

BOX *10-1* Factors Affecting Female Fertility

CONGENITAL OR DEVELOPMENTAL FACTORS
- Abnormal external genitals
- Absence of internal reproductive structures

OVARIAN FACTORS
- Anovulation-primary
  - Pituitary or hypothalamic hormone disorder
  - Adrenal gland disorder
    - Congenital adrenal hyperplasia
- Anovulation-secondary
  - Disruption of hypothalamic-pituitary-ovarian axis
- Amenorrhea after discontinuing oral contraceptive pills
- Early menopause
- Increased prolactin levels

TUBAL/PERITONEAL FACTORS
- Tubal motility reduced
- Absence of fimbriated end of tube
- Absence of a tube
- Inflammation within the tube
- Tubal adhesions

UTERINE FACTORS
- Developmental anomalies
- Endometrial and myometrial tumors
- Asherman syndrome (uterine adhesions or scar tissue)

BOX *10-2* Factors Affecting Male Fertility

STRUCTURAL OR HORMONAL DISORDERS
- Undescended testes
- Hypospadias
- Varicocele
- Low testosterone levels
- Testicular damage caused by mumps

OTHER FACTORS
- Endocrine disorders
- Genetic disorders
- Psychologic disorders
- Sexually transmitted infections
- Exposure to workplace hazards such as radiation or toxic substances
- Exposure of scrotum to high temperatures

SUBSTANCE ABUSE
- Changes in sperm
  - Smoking, heroin, marijuana, amyl nitrate, butyl nitrate, ethyl chloride, methaqualone
  - Monoamine oxidase
- Decrease in sperm
  - Hypopituitarism
  - Debilitating or chronic disease
  - Trauma
  - Gonadotropic inadequacy
- Decrease in libido
  - Heroin, methadone, selective serotonin reuptake inhibitors, and barbiturates
- Impotence
  - Alcohol
  - Antihypertensive medications

OBSTRUCTIVE LESIONS OF THE EPIDIDYMIS AND VAS DEFERENS

NUTRITIONAL DEFICIENCIES

fertility. Vaginal and uterine anomalies and their surgical repair vary from individual to individual. If a functional uterus can be reconstructed, pregnancy may be possible.

Hormonal Factors

Anovulation may be primary or secondary. Primary anovulation may be caused by a pituitary or hypothalamic hormone disorder or an adrenal gland disorder such as congenital adrenal hyperplasia. It is usually seen in adolescents. Secondary anovulation, usually seen in young to midlife women, is relatively common and is caused by the disruption of the hypothalamic-pituitary-ovarian-axis. In amenorrheic states and instances of anovulatory cycles, hormone studies usually reveal the problem.

Although it is a relatively rare occurrence, amenorrhea after the discontinuation of oral contraceptives is seen more frequently in women with histories of menstrual dysfunction before initiation of contraceptive use. Because most clients resume menstruating within 6 months, the workup should be delayed until that time in the absence of other symptoms.

Occasionally, women experience menopause before they are 40 years old. In a vast majority of cases of early menopause, the ovaries do not respond to ovulation-inducing drugs.

Increased prolactin levels may cause anovulation and amenorrhea. Many drugs affect the secretion of prolactin, including phenothiazine, opiates, diazepam, reserpine, methyldopa, and tricyclic antidepressants. In general, these agents are thought to inhibit the release of prolactin-inhibiting factor from the hypothalamus. Stress also can inhibit the release of prolactin-inhibiting factor, thereby causing the release of excess prolactin. Physical stressors such as surgery, cranial lesions, or injury also may initiate this response. Another common cause of hyperprolactinemia is benign pituitary adenoma, which is diagnosed through sophisticated radiographic techniques or computed tomographic (CT) scan.

Tubal/Peritoneal Factors

The motility of the tube and its fimbriated end may be reduced or absent as a result of infections, adhesions, scarring, or tumors. Chlamydial infection negatively influences tubal function and impedes fertility (Thomas et al., 2000).

In rare instances, one tube may be congenitally absent. One tube may be relatively shorter than the other, which is often associated with an abnormally developed uterus.

Inflammation within the tube or involving the exterior of the tube or the fimbriated ends represents a major cause of impaired fertility. Tubal adhesions resulting from pelvic infections (e.g., ruptured appendix, sexually transmitted infections [STIs]) may impair fertility. When infection with purulent discharge heals, scar tissue adhesions form. In the process, the tube may be blocked anywhere along its length. It can be closed off at the fimbriated end, or it can be distorted and kinked by adhesions. Adhesions may permit the tiny sperm to pass through the tube but may prevent a fertilized egg from completing the journey into the intrauterine cavity. This results in an ectopic pregnancy that may completely destroy the tube. In other cases, adhesions of the tubes to the ovary or bowel may follow endometriosis (see Chapter 7). Endometriosis is more commonly seen in women who delay childbearing until they are older than 30 years. Women who have a first-degree relative with a history of endometriosis also have a slightly higher risk.

Uterine Factors

Abnormalities of the uterus are more common than might be expected. Minor developmental anomalies of the uterus are fairly common; major anomalies occur rarely. Hysterosalpingography may reveal double uteri or other anomalous congenital variations (Fig. 10-1). Endometrial and myometrial tumors (e.g., polyps or myomas) may also be revealed by x-ray studies of infertile women. These anomalies can affect implantation and maintenance of a pregnancy.

Asherman syndrome (uterine adhesions or scar tissue) is characterized by hypomenorrhea. The adhesions, which may partially or totally obliterate the uterine cavity, are sequelae to surgical interventions such as too vigorous curettage (scraping) after an abortion (elective or spontaneous). The hysteroscope is useful in the verification of intrauterine anomalies.

Endometritis (inflammation of the endometrium) may result from any of the causes of infection of the cervix or uterine tubes (e.g., *Chlamydia*). Women who have numerous sexual partners are more susceptible to endometrial infection than are women in monogamous relationships.

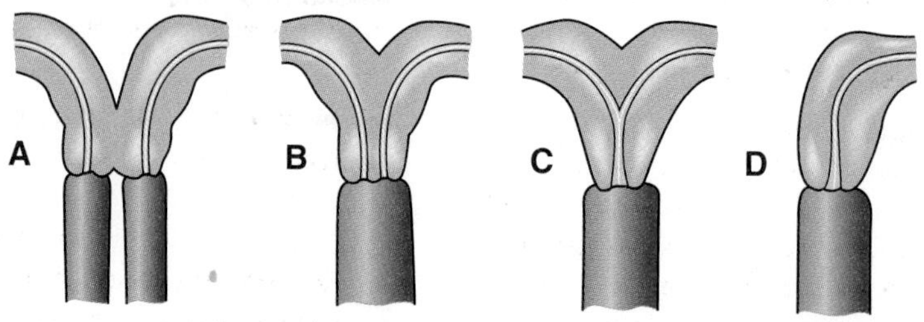
A
B
C
D

FIG. 10-1 Abnormal uterus. **A,** Complete bicornuate uterus with vagina divided by a septum. **B,** Complete bicornuate uterus with normal vagina. **C,** Partial bicornuate uterus with normal vagina. **D,** Unicornuate uterus.

Vaginal-Cervical Factors

Vaginal fluid is acidic (pH of 4 or less), whereas cervical mucus is normally alkaline (pH of 7 or more). Ejaculation should place the sperm at or near the cervical os. The alkalinity of cervical mucus helps support sperm and permits the ascending transportation of sperm around the time of ovulation.

Endocervical mucus normally obstructs or plugs the cervix, acting as a barrier against infection, until increasing estrogen levels cause the mucus to become clear, thin, and nutritionally supportive of sperm. This change occurs around the time of ovulation and lasts approximately 48 to 72 hours. The amount of cervical mucus and its characteristics are influenced by the hormone estrogen (see Teaching for Self-Care box, p. 224).

Vaginal-cervical infections (e.g., Trichomoniasis vaginitis) increase the acidity of the vaginal fluid and reduce the alkalinity of the cervical mucus. Thus vaginal infection often destroys or drastically reduces the number of viable motile sperm before they enter the cervical canal. The amount of mucus and its physical changes are influenced by the presence of blood, pathogenic bacteria, and irritants such as an intrauterine contraceptive device (IUD) or a tumor. Severe emotional stress, antibiotic therapy, and diseases such as diabetes mellitus alter the acidity of mucus.

Some infertile women develop sperm antibodies. The production of antibodies by one member of a species against something that is commonly found within that species is termed **isoimmunization.** Sperm may be immobilized within the cervical mucus, or they become incapable of migration into the uterus (see postcoital test, p. 255). A greater incidence of sperm agglutination occurs in women with otherwise unexplained impaired fertility; however, the true significance and reliability of tests for sperm immobilization or agglutination are uncertain.

Male Infertility

Male infertility can be caused by structural and hormonal disorders such as undescended testes, hypospadias, varicocele (varicose vein of the scrotum), and low testosterone levels, all of which can cause azoospermia (no sperm cells produced) or oligospermia (few sperm cells produced). Mumps, especially after adolescence, can result in permanent damage to the testes. Male infertility also may be caused by factors that also affect women, such as nutrition, endocrine disorders, genetic disorders, psychologic disorders, and STIs (ASRM, 2002; Bhasin et al., 1998; Hargreave & Ghosh, 1998). Exposure to hazards in the workplace such as radiation also can affect sperm production; exposure of the scrotum to high temperatures can both decrease and cause abnormal sperm production.

Substance abuse can be a major factor in male infertility. Alcohol consumption can cause erectile problems (impotence) (Kennedy, Griffin, & Frishman, 1999). In addition, cigarette smoking has been associated with abnormal sperm, a decreased number of sperm, and chromosome damage. The degree of abnormality is related to the number of cigarettes smoked per day (Giwercman & Bonde, 1998). Heroin and marijuana use may depress the number and motility of sperm and increase the percentage of abnormally formed sperm. Amyl nitrate, butyl nitrate, ethyl chloride, and methaqualone (used to prolong orgasm) cause changes in spermatogenesis. Heroin, methadone, selective serotonin reuptake inhibitors (SSRIs), and barbiturates decrease libido. Monoamine oxidase (MAO), an antidepressant, adversely affects spermatogenesis. In addition, some antihypertensives may cause impotence (Kennedy et al., 1998).

Male fertility declines slowly after age 40 years; however, no cessation of sperm production occurs analogous to menopause in women.

CARE MANAGEMENT

Assessment and Nursing Diagnoses

The nurse assists in the assessment by obtaining data relevant to fertility through interview and physical examination. The database must include information to identify whether infertility is primary or secondary. Religious, cultural, and ethnic data are noted (Box 10-3 and the Cultural Considerations box).

Some of the data needed to investigate impaired fertility are of a sensitive, personal nature. Obtaining these data may be viewed as an invasion of privacy. The tests and examinations are occasionally painful and intrusive and can take the romance out of lovemaking. A high level of motivation is needed to endure the investigation.

Many couples have already visited various physicians and have read extensively on the subject. Their previous experiences are recorded, and the depth and breadth of their knowledge base are explored.

Because multiple factors involving both partners are common, the investigation of impaired fertility is conducted systematically and simultaneously for both male and female partners. Both partners must be interested in the solution to the problem. The medical investigation requires time (3 to 4 months) and considerable financial expense (Box 10-4), and it causes emotional distress and strain on the couple's interpersonal relationship (Boivin et al., 2001).

Assessment of Female Infertility

Investigation of impaired fertility begins for the woman with a complete history and physical examination (Box 10-5). The history explores the duration of infertility and past obstetric events and contains a detailed sexual history. Medical and surgical conditions are evaluated. Exposure to reproductive hazards in the home (e.g., mutagens such as plastic-vinyl chlorides, teratogens such as alcohol, and emotional stresses) and workplace are explored.

A complete general physical examination is followed by a specific assessment of the reproductive tract. Evidence of endocrine system abnormalities is sought. Inadequate development of secondary sex characteristics (e.g., inappropriate distribution of body fat and hair) may point to problems with

BOX 10-3 Religious Considerations of Infertility

Civil laws and religious proscriptions about sex must always be kept in mind by the health care provider.

Conservative and reform Jewish couples are accepting of most infertility treatment; however, the Orthodox Jewish husband and wife may face infertility investigation and management problems because of religious laws that govern marital relations. For example, according to Jewish law, the Orthodox couple may not engage in marital relations during menstruation and through the following 7 "preparatory days." The wife then is immersed in a ritual bath (*Mikvah*) before relations can resume. Fertility problems can arise when the woman has a short cycle (i.e., a cycle of 24 days or fewer; when ovulation would occur on day 10 or earlier).

The Roman Catholic Church regards the embryo as a human being from the first moment of existence and regards as unacceptable technical procedures such as in vitro fertilization, therapeutic donor insemination, and freezing embryos.

Other religious groups may have ethical concerns about infertility tests and treatments. For example, most Protestant denominations and Muslims usually support infertility management as long as in vitro fertilization (IVF) is done with the husband's sperm, there is no reduction of fetuses, and insemination is done with the husband's sperm. These groups are less supportive of surrogacy and use of donor sperm and eggs. Christian Scientists do not permit surgical procedures or IVF but do permit insemination with husband and donor sperm.

Care providers should seek to understand the woman's spirituality and how it affects her perception of health care, especially in relation to infertility. Women may wish to seek infertility treatment but have questions about proposed diagnostic and therapeutic procedures because of religious proscriptions. These women are encouraged to consult their minister, rabbi, priest, or other spiritual leader for advice.

CULTURAL CONSIDERATIONS

Fertility/Infertility

Worldwide cultures continue to use symbols and rites that celebrate fertility. One fertility rite that persists today is the custom of throwing rice at the bride and groom. Other fertility symbols and rites include passing out of congratulatory cigars, candy, or pencils by a new father and baby showers held in anticipation of a child's birth.

In many cultures, the responsibility for infertility is usually attributed to the woman. A woman's inability to conceive may be due to her sins, to evil spirits, or to the fact that she is an inadequate person. The virility of a man in some cultures remains in question until he demonstrates his ability to reproduce by having at least one child (D'Avanzo & Geissler, 2003).

BOX 10-4 Insurance Coverage for Infertility

In 2001 only 14 states had mandated some form of insurance coverage for infertility (ASRM, 2002). These mandates included in vitro fertilization in some states, whereas others only covered some diagnostic tests. Some states require health maintenance organizations (HMOs) to cover some costs, whereas in others, HMOs are exempt. Clients need information about what they can expect from their insurers. The web site for the American Society for Reproductive Medicine (www.asrm.org) has more complete information.

the hypothalamic-pituitary-ovarian axis or genetic aberrations (e.g., polycystic ovarian syndrome, Turner syndrome).

A woman may have an abnormal uterus and tubes as a result of exposure to diethylstilbestrol (DES) in utero. Evidence of past infection of the genitourinary system is sought. Bimanual examination of internal organs may reveal lack of mobility of the uterus or abnormal contours of the uterus and adnexa. Laboratory data are assembled. Data from routine urine and blood tests are obtained along with other diagnostic tests.

Diagnostic Tests. Several examinations and tests for impaired fertility in the woman include the basic infertility survey, which involves evaluation of the cervix, uterus, tubes, and peritoneum; detection of ovulation; assessment of immunologic compatibility; and evaluation of psychogenic factors (Angard, 1999). The nurse can alleviate some of the anxiety associated with diagnostic testing by explaining to clients the timing and rationale for each test (Table 10-1). Test findings that are favorable to fertility are summarized in Box 10-6.

Couples should be cautioned that everything can be normal and conception still may not occur. Unexplained infertility accounts for 20% of cases (ARSM, 2002). In addition, even poor test results do not mean that pregnancy will not occur.

Detection of Ovulation. All infertile women should have ovulatory function assessed, because a history of monthly menstruation is inadequate to conclude that ovulation is occurring and is optimal for conception.

Documentation of time of ovulation is important in the investigation of impaired fertility. Direct proof of ovulation is pregnancy or the retrieval of an ovum from the uterine

BOX 10-5 Assessment of the Woman

HISTORY

1. Age
2. Duration of infertility: length of contraceptive and noncontraceptive exposure
3. Obstetric
   a. Number of pregnancies, miscarriages, and abortions
   b. Length of time required to initiate each pregnancy
   c. Complications of any pregnancy
   d. Duration of lactation
4. Gynecologic: detailed menstrual history, including age at onset, interruptions in regular menstruation, and any menstrual pain
5. Previous tests and therapy for infertility
6. Medical: general medical history, including chronic and hereditary disease (e.g., endocrine dysfunction); medications, including vitamins and over-the-counter medications; family history, especially of endocrine disorders; normal sexual development; any galactorrhea when not lactating
7. Surgical: especially abdominal or pelvic surgery
8. Sexual history: frequency of intercourse; number of lifetime sexual partners, previous history of STIs, types of sexual practices; pain or discomfort with intercourse; use of vaginal lubricants
9. Occupational and environmental exposure to chemicals or radiation; physical nature of occupation or hobbies; vacations and work habits
10. Personal: motivation for childbearing; attitude toward partner; reason for seeking advice regarding infertility at this time; support system available; amount of exercise; stress level; use of alcohol, recreational drugs, caffeine, or tobacco; weight changes

PHYSICAL EXAMINATION

1. General: complete physical examination
2. Genital tract: state of hymen (full penetration); clitoris; vaginal infection, including trichomoniasis and candidiasis; cervical tears, polyps, infection, patency of os, accessibility to insemination; uterus, including size and position, mobility; adnexae, tumors, evidence of endometriosis

LABORATORY DATA

1. *Chlamydia* test and gonorrhea culture; additional laboratory studies as indicated (e.g., urine test, complete blood cell count, serologic test for syphilis)
2. For women with irregular menstrual cycles or amenorrhea: serum prolactin level with tomographic radiographs of skull if prolactin level elevated, endometrial biopsy, FSH and LH determination. Other laboratory tests added as desired for a more complete diagnosis of endocrine problems: 17-ketosteroid assay test, 17-hydroxycorticosteroid test, glucose tolerance test
3. Rh factor and antibody titer tests—important in cases of ectopic pregnancy, abortion, and preterm birth problems
4. Sperm antibody agglutination studies: special laboratory procedure involves obtaining a fresh semen specimen from the man and a blood sample from the woman; sperm are incubated in the blood serum of the woman and checked at intervals for agglutination; the result is negative if no agglutinated sperm are found
5. Chromosome studies when indicated

tube. Several indirect or presumptive methods for detection of ovulation include assessment of basal body temperature (BBT) and cervical mucus characteristics (see Chapter 9), as well as endometrial biopsy and pelvic ultrasound examination. A serum progesterone level may be obtained in the latter half of the menstrual cycle as part of ovulation testing. These clinical tests more or less determine whether progesterone is secreted in significant amounts to accommodate implantation and maintain pregnancy. Occurrence of *mittelschmerz* and midcycle spotting provides unreliable presumptive evidence of ovulation.

Hormone Analysis. Hormone analysis is performed to assess endocrine function of the hypothalamic-pituitary-ovarian axis when menstrual cycles are absent or irregular. Determination of blood levels of prolactin, follicle-stimulating hormone (FSH), luteinizing hormone (LH), estradiol, progesterone, and the thyroid hormones may be necessary to diagnose the cause of irregular or absent menstrual cycles.

Ultrasonography. Abdominal or transvaginal ultrasound is used to assess pelvic structures (Fig. 10-2). This procedure is used to visualize pelvic tissues for a variety of reasons (e.g., to identify abnormalities such as fibroid tumors and ovarian cysts, to verify follicular development and maturity, and to assess thickness of the endometrium around the time of ovulation).

Timed Endometrial Biopsy. Endometrial biopsy is scheduled after ovulation, during the luteal phase of the menstrual cycle. Late in the menstrual cycle, 2 to 3 days before expected menses, a small cannula is introduced into the uterus, and a small portion of the endometrium is removed for histologic evaluation. To assess the response of the endometrium to progesterone production, the tissue is dated with respect to expected normal menstrual development. Tissue that is "out of phase" with expected development signifies either abnormal function of the corpus luteum or abnormal response of the endometrium.

TABLE 10-1 **Tests for Impaired Fertility**

TEST/EXAMINATION	TIMING (MENSTRUAL CYCLE DAYS)	RATIONALE
Hysterosalpingogram	7-10	Late follicular, early proliferative phase; will not disrupt a fertilized ovum; may open uterine tubes before time of ovulation
Postcoital test	1-2 days before ovulation	Ovulatory late proliferative phase; look for normal motile sperm in cervical mucus
Sperm immobilization antigen-antibody reaction	Variable, ovulation	Immunologic test to determine sperm and cervical mucus interaction
Assessment of cervical mucus	Variable, ovulation	Cervical mucus should have low viscosity, high spinnbarkeit
Ultrasound diagnosis of follicular collapse	Ovulation	Collapsed follicle is seen after ovulation
Serum assay of plasma progesterone	20-25	Midluteal midsecretory phase; check adequacy of corpus luteal production of progesterone
Basal body temperature	Chart entire cycle	Elevation occurs in response to progesterone, documents ovulation
Endometrial biopsy	21-27	Late luteal, late secretory phase; check endometrial response to progesterone and adequacy of luteal phase
Sperm penetration assay	After 2 days but ≤1 wk of abstinence	Evaluation of ability of sperm to penetrate an egg

BOX 10-6 **Summary of Findings Favorable to Fertility**

1. Follicular development, ovulation, and luteal development are supportive of pregnancy:
   a. BBT (presumptive evidence of ovulatory cycles) is biphasic, with temperature elevation that persists for 12 to 14 days before menstruation
   b. Cervical mucus characteristics change appropriately during phases of menstrual cycle
   c. Laparoscopic visualization of pelvic organs verifies follicular and luteal development
2. The luteal phase is supportive of pregnancy:
   a. Levels of plasma progesterone are adequate
   b. Findings from endometrial biopsy samples are consistent with day of cycle
3. Cervical factors are receptive to sperm during expected time of ovulation:
   a. Cervical os is open
   b. Cervical mucus is clear, watery, abundant, and slippery and demonstrates good spinnbarkeit and arborization (fern pattern)
   c. Cervical examination does not reveal lesions or infections
   d. Postcoital test findings are satisfactory (adequate number of live, motile, normal sperm present in cervical mucus)
   e. No immunity to sperm demonstrated
4. The uterus and uterine tubes are supportive of pregnancy:
   a. Uterine and tubal patency are documented by
      (1) Spillage of dye into peritoneal cavity
      (2) Outlines of uterine and tubal cavities of adequate size and shape, with no abnormalities
   b. Laparoscopic examination verifies normal development of internal genitals and absence of adhesions, infections, endometriosis, and other lesions
5. The male partner's reproductive structures are normal:
   a. No evidence of developmental anomalies of penis, testicular atrophy, or varicocele (varicose veins on the spermatic vein in the groin)
   b. No evidence of infection in prostate, seminal vesicles, and urethra
   c. Testes are >4 cm in largest diameter
6. Semen is supportive of pregnancy:
   a. Sperm (number per milliliter) are adequate in ejaculate
   b. Most sperm show normal morphology
   c. Most sperm are motile, forward moving
   d. No autoimmunity exists
   e. Seminal fluid is normal

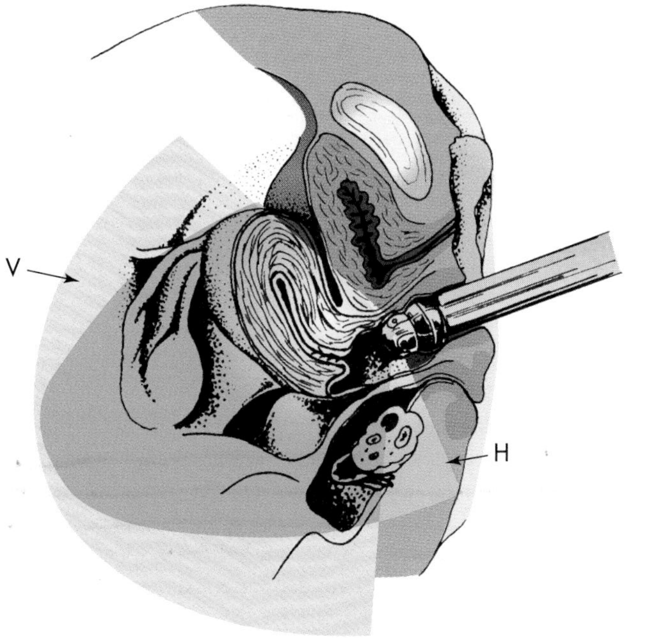
V
H

FIG. 10-2 Vaginal ultrasonography. Major scanning planes of transducer. *H*, Horizontal; *V*, vertical.

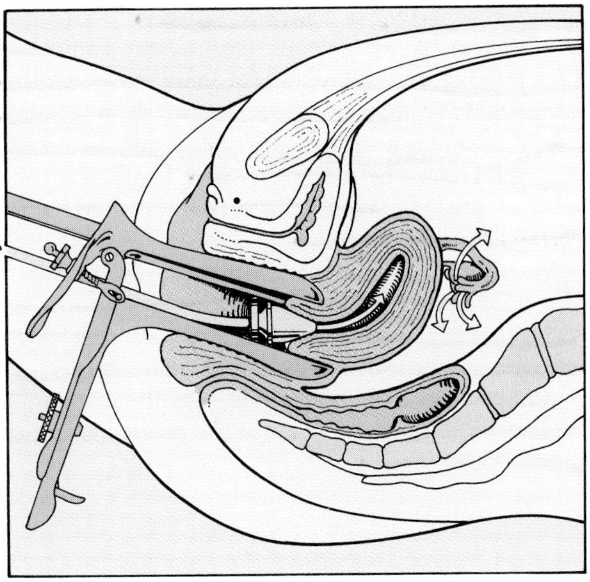

FIG. 10-3 Hysterosalpingography. Note that contrast medium flows through intrauterine cannula and out through the uterine tubes.

Findings favorable to fertility include endometrial tissue that shows no signs of tuberculosis, polyps, or inflammatory conditions and that reflects secretory changes normally seen in the presence of adequate luteal (progesterone) phase.

Hysterosalpingography. Radiographic (x-ray) film allows visualization of the uterine cavity and tubes after the instillation of radiopaque contrast material through the cervix (Fig. 10-3). It is possible to see abnormalities of the uterus such as congenital defects or defects produced by submucous myomas and endometrial polyps. Distortions of the uterine cavity or uterine tubes can be a result of current or past pelvic inflammatory disease (PID). Scar tissue and adhesions from inflammatory processes can immobilize the uterus and tubes, kink the tubes, and surround the ovaries.

Hysterosalpingography is scheduled 2 to 5 days after menstruation to avoid flushing a potential fertilized ovum out through a uterine tube into the peritoneal cavity. No open vessels exist at this time, and all menstrual debris has been discharged. This decreases the risk of embolism or of forcing menstrual debris out through the tubes into the peritoneal cavity.

Referred shoulder pain may occur during this procedure. The referred pain is indicative of subphrenic irritation from the contrast media if it is spilled out of the patent uterine tubes. The discomfort can be managed with position change and mild analgesics. Pain usually subsides within 12 to 14 hours. Women with blocked tubes may have cramping for up to 48 hours.

This procedure may be both therapeutic and diagnostic. The passage of contrast medium may clear tubes of mucous plugs, straighten kinked tubes, or break up adhesions within the tubes (caused by salpingitis). The procedure may stimulate cilia in the lining of the tubes to facilitate transport of the ovum. It also may aid healing as a result of the bacteriostatic effect of the iodine within the contrast medium.

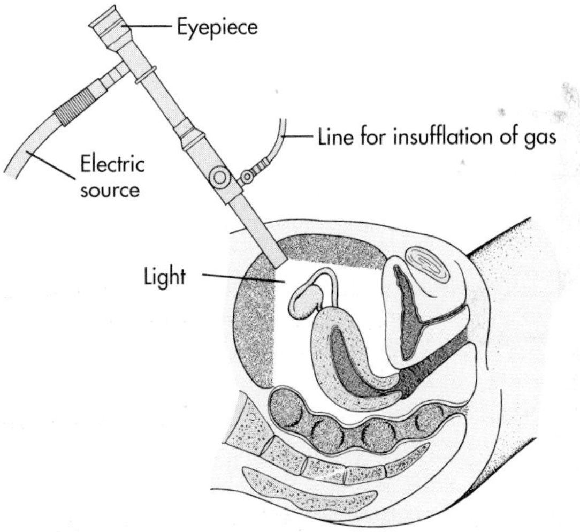
Eyepiece
Line for insufflation of gas
Electric source
Light

FIG. 10-4 Laparoscopy.

Laparoscopy. Laparoscopy is usually scheduled early in the menstrual cycle. During the procedure, a small endoscope is inserted through a small incision in the anterior abdominal wall. Cold fiberoptic light sources allow superior visualization of the internal pelvic structures (Fig. 10-4). The woman is usually admitted shortly before surgery, having taken nothing by mouth (NPO) for 8 hours. She voids before surgery. A general anesthetic is usually given, and the woman is placed in the lithotomy position. A needle is inserted, and carbon dioxide gas is pumped into the peritoneum to elevate the abdominal wall from the organs, thereby creating an empty space that permits visualization and exploration with the laparoscope. If tubal patency is being assessed, a cannula is used to instill a dye contrast medium through the cervix.

Visualization of the peritoneal cavity in infertile women may reveal endometriosis, pelvic adhesions, tubal occlusion, leiomyomas (fibroids), or polycystic ovaries. Fulguration (destruction of tissue by means of electricity) of small endometrial implants, lysis of adhesions, and taking ovarian biopsies are some of the procedures possible with a laparoscope.

After surgery, deflation of most gas is done by direct expression. Trocar and needle sites are closed with a single subcuticular absorbable suture or skin clip, and an adhesive bandage is applied. Postoperative recovery requires taking vital signs, assessing level of consciousness, preventing aspiration, monitoring intravenous fluids, and reassuring the client regarding referred shoulder discomfort. Discharge from the hospital usually occurs in 4 to 6 hours. Referred shoulder pain or subcostal discomfort usually lasts only 24 hours and is relieved with a mild analgesic. Severe pain may be relieved when the woman assumes a knee-chest position. The woman must be cautioned against heavy lifting or strenuous activity for 4 to 7 days, at which time she is usually asymptomatic.

Assessment of Male Infertility

The systematic investigation of infertility in the male client begins with a thorough history and physical examination (Box 10-7). Assessment of the male client proceeds in a manner similar to that of the female client, starting with noninvasive tests.

Semen Analysis. The basic test for male infertility is the **semen analysis.** A complete semen analysis, study of the effects of cervical mucus on sperm forward motility and survival, and evaluation of the sperm's ability to penetrate an ovum provide basic information. Sperm counts vary from day to day and are dependent on emotional and physical status and sexual activity; therefore a single analysis may be inconclusive (Hargreave & Ghosh, 1998). A minimum of two analyses must be performed several weeks apart to assess male fertility (Keye, 2000).

BOX *10-7* **Assessment of the Man**

HISTORY

1. Age
2. Fertility in this and other sexual relationships
3. Medical: General medical history, including infections (such as STIs, mononucleosis), mumps, orchitis after adolescence, chronic diseases, recent fever, medications, weight changes, undescended testes after age 3 mo, normal sexual development at puberty
4. Surgical: Herniorrhaphy, injuries to genitals, or other surgery in genital area
5. Occupational and environmental exposure to chemicals or radiation, physical nature of occupation and hobbies, vacations and work habits
6. Previous tests and therapy done for study of infertility, duration of infertility in this and previous relationships
7. Sex history in detail: libido, coital history (such as frequency and ability to ejaculate), adequacy of erection, number of lifetime sex partners, attitudes toward masturbation
8. Personal: Motivation for childbearing; attitude toward partner; support system available, reason for seeking advice regarding infertility at this time; amount of exercise and stress level; use of alcohol, recreational drugs, caffeine, tobacco, anabolic steroids

PHYSICAL EXAMINATION

1. General: Complete physical examination, with special attention given to physical condition and fat and hair distribution
2. Genital tract: Penis and urethra; scrotal size; position, size, and consistency of testes; epididymides and vasa deferentia; prostate size and consistency
3. Careful search for varicocele, with man in both supine and upright positions

LABORATORY DATA

1. Routine urine test, gonorrhea and *Chlamydia* tests; serologic test for syphilis
2. Complete semen analysis (see Box 10-8)
3. Additional laboratory studies as indicated
   a. Basic endocrine studies indicated in men with oligospermia or aspermia:
      (1) Serum FSH, LH, and testosterone levels
      (2) T_3, T_4, TSH
      (3) Test for sperm antibodies, autoimmunization: autoimmune antibodies (produced by the man against his own sperm) agglutinate or immobilize sperm in <5% of men who have infertility problems
      (4) 17-Hydroxycorticoids and 17-ketosteroids
      (5) Buccal smear and chromosome studies (e.g., Klinefelter syndrome, XXY sex chromosomes)
   b. Testicular biopsy where correct interpretation is available (may give a more accurate diagnosis and prognosis in cases of azoospermia and severe oligospermia), vasography if indicated and available

Semen is collected by ejaculation into a clean container or a plastic sheath that does not contain a spermicidal agent (Speroff, Glass, & Kase, 1999). The specimen is usually collected by masturbation after 2 to 5 days of abstinence from ejaculation. The semen is taken to the laboratory in a sealed container within 2 hours of ejaculation. Exposure to excessive heat or cold is avoided. Commonly accepted values for semen characteristics based on the World Health Organization criteria (1992) are given in Box 10-8.

Seminal deficiency may be attributable to one or more of a variety of factors. The male is assessed for these factors: hypopituitarism; nutritional deficiency; debilitating or chronic disease; trauma; exposure to environmental hazards such as radiation and toxic substances; use of tobacco, alcohol, and marijuana; gonadotropic inadequacy; and obstructive lesions of the epididymis and vas deferens. Congenital absence of the vas deferens can occur more frequently in men with the gene for cystic fibrosis. If this abnormality is found, genetic counseling would be helpful before any fertility treatments (Keye, 2000). Hormone analyses are done for testosterone, gonadotropin, FSH, and LH. The sperm penetration assay may be used to evaluate the ability of sperm to penetrate an egg. Because human oocytes are not readily available, hamster eggs have been used as a substitute to evaluate sperm penetration abilities (no actual fertilization occurs) (Hargreave & Ghosh, 1998). In addition, testicular biopsy may be warranted.

Ultrasonography. Scrotal ultrasound is used to examine the testes for presence of varicoceles and to identify abnormalities in the scrotum and spermatic cord. Transrectal ultrasound is used to evaluate the ejaculatory ducts, seminal vesicles, and the vas deferens (Zahalsky & Nagler, 2001).

BOX *10-8* **Semen Analysis**

- Liquefaction usually complete within 10 to 20 min
- Semen volume ≥ 2 ml
- Semen pH 7.2 to 8.0
- Sperm density 20 to 200 million /ml
- Total sperm count ≥40 million /ml
- Normal morphology ≥30% (normal oval)
- Motility (important consideration in sperm evaluation); percentage of forward-moving sperm estimated with respect to abnormally motile and nonmotile sperm ≥ 50%
- White cell count ≤ 1 million/ml
- Ovum penetration test (may be done if further evaluation necessary)

Note: These values are not absolute but are only relative to final evaluation of the couple as a single reproductive unit. Values also differ according to source used as a reference. These values are based on WHO, 1992.

Assessment of the Couple

Postcoital Test. The **postcoital test (PCT)** is one method used to test for adequacy of coital technique, cervical mucus, sperm, and degree of sperm penetration through cervical mucus. The test is performed within several hours after ejaculation of semen into the vagina. A specimen of cervical mucus is obtained from the cervical os and examined under a microscope. The quality of mucus and the number of forward-moving sperm are noted. A PCT with good mucus and motile sperm is associated with fertility (Hargreave & Ghosh, 1998).

Intercourse is synchronized with the expected time of ovulation (as determined from evaluation of BBT, cervical mucus changes, and usual length of menstrual cycle or use of LH detection kit to determine LH surge). It is performed only in the absence of vaginal infection. Couples may experience some difficulty abstaining from intercourse for 2 to 4 days before expected ovulation and then having intercourse with ejaculation on schedule. Sex on demand may strain the couple's interpersonal relationship. A problem may arise if the expected day of ovulation occurs when facilities or the physician is unavailable (such as over a weekend or holiday).

Nursing diagnoses are derived from the database. Examples of nursing diagnoses related to impaired fertility include the following:

- *Anxiety related to*
  –unknown outcome of diagnostic workup
- *Disturbed body image or self-esteem related to*
  –impaired fertility
- *Risk for ineffective individual/family coping related to*
  –methods used in the investigation of impaired fertility
  –alternatives to therapy: child-free living or adoption
- *Interrupted family processes related to*
  –unmet expectations for pregnancy
- *Acute pain related to*
  –effects of diagnostic tests (or surgery)
- *Sexual dysfunction related to*
  –loss of libido secondary to medically imposed restrictions
- *Deficient knowledge related to*
  –preconception risk factors
  –factors surrounding ovulation
  –factors surrounding fertility

Expected Outcomes of Care

Planning requires sensitivity to the couple's needs. Equipped with a knowledge of impaired fertility, the nurse can help develop a plan of care for the couple. The expected outcomes are phrased in client-centered terms and may include that the couple will do the following:

- Verbalize understanding of the anatomy and physiology of the reproductive system.
- Verbalize understanding of treatment for any abnormalities identified through various tests and examinations

(e.g., infections, blocked uterine tubes, sperm allergy, and varicocele) and be able to make an informed decision about treatment.
- Verbalize understanding of their potential to conceive.
- Resolve guilt feelings and not need to focus blame.
- Conceive or, failing to conceive, decide on an alternative acceptable to both of them (e.g., child-free living or adoption).
- Demonstrate acceptable methods for handling pressure they may feel from peers and relatives regarding their childless state.

Plan of Care and Interventions

Psychosocial

In the United States, feelings connected to impaired fertility are numerous and complex. The origins of some of these feelings are myths, superstitions, and misinformation about the causes of infertility. Other feelings arise from the need to undergo many tests and examinations and from being different from others.

Infertility is recognized as a major life stressor that can affect self-esteem; relations with the spouse, family, and friends; and careers. Couples often need assistance in separating their concepts of success and failure related to treatment for infertility from personal success and failure. Recognizing the significance of infertility as a loss and resolving these feelings are crucial to putting infertility into perspective, even if treatment is successful (Biovin et al., 2001; Klock, 2000).

Nurses can help couples express and discuss their feelings as honestly as possible. Ventilation may help couples to unburden themselves of negative feelings. Referral for mental health counseling may be beneficial.

Psychologic responses to a diagnosis of infertility may tax a couple's giving and receiving of physical and sexual closeness. The prescriptions and proscriptions for achieving conception may add tension to a couple's sexual functioning. Couples may report decreased desire for intercourse, orgasmic dysfunction, or midcycle erectile disorders.

To be able to deal comfortably with a couple's sexuality, nurses must be comfortable with their own sexuality so that they can better help couples understand why the private act of lovemaking must be shared with health care professionals. Nurses need up-to-date factual knowledge about human sexual practices and must be accepting of the preferences and activities of others without being judgmental, skilled in interviewing and in therapeutic use of self, sensitive to the nonverbal cues of others, and knowledgeable regarding each couple's sociocultural and religious tenets (Kennedy et al., 1998).

The woman or couple facing infertility exhibits behaviors of the grieving process that are associated with other types of loss (Table 10-2.) The loss of one's genetic continuity with the generations to come leads to a loss of self-esteem, to a sense of inadequacy as a woman or a man, to a loss of control over one's destiny, and to a reduced sense of self (Applegarth, 2000). Infertile individuals have impaired self-concept and greater dissatisfaction with their marriages (Newton, 2000). The investigative process leads to a loss of spontaneity and control over the couple's marital relationship and sometimes to a loss of control over progress toward career and life goals. All people do not have all the reactions described, nor can it be predicted how long any reaction will last for an individual.

The support systems of the couple with impaired fertility must be explored. This exploration should include persons available to assist, their relationship to the couple, their ages, their availability, and the available cultural or religious support.

If the couple conceives, nurses must be aware that the concerns and problems of the previously infertile couple may not be over. Many couples are overjoyed with the pregnancy; however, some are not. Some couples rearrange their lives, sense of self, and personal goals within their acceptance of their infertile state. The couple may feel that those who worked with them to identify and treat impaired fertility expect them to be happy with the pregnancy. The couple may be shocked to find that they feel resentment because the pregnancy, once a cherished dream, now necessitates another change in goals, aspirations, and identities. The normal ambivalence toward pregnancy may be perceived as reneging on the original choice to become parents. The couple might choose to abort the pregnancy at this time. Other couples worry about miscarriage. If the couple wishes to continue with the pregnancy, they will need the care other expectant couples need. The couple may need extra preparation for the realities of pregnancy, labor, and parenthood because they developed fantasies about childbearing when they thought it was beyond their reach. A history of impaired fertility is considered to be a risk factor for pregnancy. If the couple does not conceive, they are assessed regarding their desire to be referred for help with adoption, therapeutic intrauterine insemination, other reproductive alternatives, or choosing a child-free state. The couple may find a list of agencies, support groups, and other resources in their community helpful (see Resources at the end of the chapter).

Nonmedical

Simple changes in lifestyle may be effective in the treatment of subfertile men. Only water-soluble lubricants should be used during intercourse because many commonly used lubricants contain spermicides or have spermicidal properties. High scrotal temperatures may be caused by daily hot-tub bathing or saunas in which the testes are kept at temperatures too high for efficient spermatogenesis. It must be remembered that these conditions lead to only lessened fertility and should not be used as a means of contraception.

Treatment is available for women who have immunologic reactions to sperm. The use of condoms during genital intercourse for 6 to 12 months will reduce female antibody production in most women who have elevated antisperm antibody titers. After the serum reaction sub-

TABLE 10-2 **Nursing Actions in Response to Behavior Associated with Impaired Fertility**

BEHAVIORAL CHARACTERISTIC	NURSING ACTIONS
Surprise: Each person assumes she or he is fertile and that pregnancy is an option	Point out resemblance to grieving process—a normal, expected reaction to loss. Refer to support group*
	Prepare clients for length of time it may take to grieve and for types of feelings (psychologic, somatic) to expect
	Encourage and allow time to talk of past and present feelings of sexuality, self-image, and self-esteem
Denial: "It can't happen to me!"	Allow time for denial, because it gives the body and mind time to adjust a little at a time
	Do not feed into the client's denial; instead say, "It must be hard to believe such a devastating report"
Anger: Toward others (perhaps even the nurse) or themselves	Explain that the reaction to loss of control and to a feeling of helplessness is often anger, which can easily be projected onto another person. Anger is a natural feeling
	Allow time to express anger at losing sense of control over bodies and destinies
	A helpful approach may be, "It's OK to be angry . . . at those who are pregnant, at people who want abortions, at self, at mate, at caregivers, and so forth"
Bargaining: "If I get pregnant, I'll dedicate the child to God."	Accept bargaining statements without comment
Depression:	
Isolation: Personal	Allow time for both woman and man to talk about how it feels whenever a sight, event, or word serves as a reminder of own state of impaired fertility
	Develop role-playing situations to practice interactions with others under various circumstances to increase the couple's ability to cope and to solve problems (increases their self-confidence)
	The nurse may say, "You must feel so terribly alone sometimes"
Guilt or unworthiness	Allow time to identify feelings that may be related to earlier behaviors (such as abortion, premarital sex, contact with STIs)
Acceptance (resolution)	Couple or person comes to the realization that "unworthiness" and impaired fertility are unrelated
	Clients need to know that grief feelings are never laid away forever; they may be activated by special reminders (such as anniversaries)

*RESOLVE, Inc., 1310 Broadway, Somerville, MA 02144. www.resolve.org.

sides, condoms are used at all times except at the expected time of ovulation. Approximately one third of couples with this problem conceive by following this course of action.

Changes in nutrition and habits may increase fertility for both men and women. For example, a well-balanced diet, exercise, decreased alcohol intake, not smoking or abusing drugs, and stress management may be effective.

Medical

Pharmacologic therapy for female infertility is often directed at treating ovulatory dysfunction either by stimulating ovulation or by enhancing ovulation so that more oocytes mature. These medications include clomiphene citrate, human menopausal gonadotrophin (HMG), FSH, recombinant FSH (rFSH), and human chorionic gonadotrophin (hCG). Gonadotrophin-releasing hormone (GnRH) agonists, progesterone and bromocriptine (Parlodel) also are used (Angard, 1999; Leibowitz & Hoffman, 2000). Table 10-3 describes common medications used for treating female infertility. These medications are extremely potent and require daily monitoring with ovarian ultrasonography and monitoring of estradiol levels to prevent hyperstimulation (Angard, 1999). The prevalence of multiple pregnancy with the use of these medications is greater than 25%. When ovulation is caused either by hypothalamic-pituitary dysfunction or failure, or failure to respond to clomiphene, GnRH may be used. Thyroid-stimulating hormone (Synthroid) is indicated if the woman has hypothyroidism.

The woman who has low estrogen levels may be a candidate for conjugated estrogens and medroxyprogesterone. A hypoestrogenic condition may result from a high stress level or decreased percentage of body fat as a result of an eating disorder (e.g., anorexia nervosa) or excessive exercise. Hydroxyprogesterone supplementation with vaginal suppositories or intramuscular injection is used to treat luteal phase defects. The nurse may encounter other medications

TABLE 10-3 Medications Used in the Treatment of Infertility

DRUG	INDICATION	MECHANISM OF ACTION	DOSE	COMMON SIDE EFFECTS
Clomiphene citrate (Clomid, Serophene)	Ovulation induction, treatment of luteal-phase inadequacy	Thought to bind to estrogen receptors in the pituitary, blocking them from detecting estrogen	Tablets, starting with 50 mg/day for 5 days; may increase to 200 mg/day	Causes hypothalamus to release more GnRH, stimulating release of FSH and LH
Human menopausal gonadotropins (Pergonal)	Ovulation induction	Pergonal, LH and FSH in 1:1 ratio, direct stimulation of ovarian follicle	Intramuscular injections, dosage regimen variable	Ovarian enlargement, ovarian hyperstimulation, local irritation at injection site, multifetal gestations
Purified FSH (Metrodin)	Treatment of polycystic ovarian disease	Direct action on ovarian follicle	Intramuscular injections, dosage regimen variable	Ovarian enlargement, ovarian hyperstimulation, local irritation at injection site, multifetal gestations
Human chorionic gonadotropin (hCG) (Profasi)	Ovulation induction	Direct action on ovarian follicle to stimulate meiosis and rupture of the follicle	2000-10,000 units intramuscularly	Local irritation at injection site
Danazol (Danocrine)	Treatment of endometriosis	Combination of estrogen and androgen suppresses ovarian activity, eliminating stimulation to endometrial glands and stroma, with resultant shrinkage and disappearance	100-800 mg/day for 6 mo	Mild hirsutism, acne, edema and weight gain, increase of liver enzyme levels
GnRH agonists (Synarel, Lupron, Zoladex)	Treatment of endometriosis, uterine fibroids	Desensitization and downward regulation of GnRH receptors of pituitary, resulting in suppression of LH, FSH, and ovarian function	Synarel, 200 μg intranasally twice daily for 6 mo; Lupron, depot 375 mg every 28 days for 6 mo; Lupron, subcutaneously 0.1 mg daily for 6 mo	Synarel, nasal irritation, nosebleeds; Synarel and Lupron, hot flashes, vaginal dryness, myalgia and arthralgia, headaches, mild bone loss (usually reversible within 12-18 mo after treatment)
Progesterone (progesterone in oil, Progestoral)	Treatment of luteal-phase inadequacy	Direct stimulation of endometrium	Vaginal suppositories, 25-50 mg twice daily or 50 mg every night; rectal suppositories, 12.25 mg every 12 hr; progesterone capsules, 100 mg by mouth 3 times daily	Breast tenderness, local irritation, headaches

Adapted from Leibowitz, D. & Hoffman, J. (2000). Fertility drug therapies: Past, present and future. *Journal of Obstetric, Gynecologic, and Neonatal Nursing 29*(2), 201-210.

as well. In the presence of adrenal hyperplasia, prednisone, a glucocorticoid, is taken orally. Treatment of endometriosis may include danazol, progesterones, combined oral contraceptives, or GnRH agonists (Speroff et al., 1999; Stenchever et al., 2001) (Table 10-3). Infections are treated with appropriate antimicrobial formulations.

Drug therapy may be indicated for male infertility. Problems with the thyroid or adrenal glands are corrected with appropriate medications. Infections are identified and treated promptly with antimicrobials. FSH, HMG, and clomiphene may be used to stimulate spermatogenesis in men with hypogonadism (Leibowitz & Hoffman, 2000).

The primary care provider is responsible for informing clients fully about the prescribed medications. However, the nurse must be ready to answer clients' questions and to confirm their understanding of the drug, its administration, potential side effects, and expected outcomes. Because information varies with each drug, the nurse must consult the medication package inserts, pharmacology references, physician, and pharmacist as necessary.

Surgical

A number of surgical procedures can be used for problems causing female infertility. Ovarian tumors must be excised. Whenever possible, functional ovarian tissue is left intact. Scar tissue adhesions caused by chronic infections may cover much or all of the ovary. These adhesions usually necessitate surgery to free and expose the ovary so that ovulation can occur.

Hysterosalpingography is useful for identification of tubal obstruction and also for the release of blockage. During laparoscopy, delicate adhesions may be divided and removed, and endometrial implants may be destroyed by electrocoagulation or laser. Laparotomy and even microsurgery may be required to do extensive repair of the damaged tube. Prognosis is dependent on the degree to which tubal patency and function can be restored (Stenchever et al., 2001).

A woman with a relatively small uterus may become pregnant, but the uterus may be incapable of accommodating the enlarging fetus, and a miscarriage may result. In such cases, recurrent or habitual (three or more) miscarriages often occur. No medical therapy has been effective for the enlargement of an abnormally small uterus. Observation suggests that women who do become pregnant, but who miscarry, often abort at a later time with each successive pregnancy. Finally, after two or three pregnancy losses, they may give birth to a viable infant. Apparently actual growth of the uterus occurs with each pregnancy. Reconstructive surgery (e.g., the unification operation for bicornuate uterus) often improves a woman's ability to conceive and carry the fetus to term.

Surgical removal of tumors or fibroids involving the endometrium or uterus often improves the woman's chance of conceiving and maintaining the pregnancy to viability. Surgical treatment of uterine tumors or maldevelopment that results in successful pregnancy usually requires birth by cesarean surgery near term gestation. The uterus may rupture as a result of weakness of the area of surgical healing.

Radial chemocautery (destruction of tissue with chemicals) or thermocautery (destruction of tissue with heat, usually electrical) of the cervix, cryosurgery (destruction of tissue by application of extreme cold, usually liquid nitrogen), or conization (excision of a cone-shaped piece of tissue from the endocervix) is effective in eliminating chronic inflammation and infection. When the cervix has been deeply cauterized or frozen or when extensive conization has been performed, extreme limitation of mucus production by the cervix may result, so sperm migration may be difficult or impossible because of the absence of a mucus bridge from the vagina to the uterus. Therapeutic intrauterine insemination may be necessary to carry the sperm directly through the internal os of the cervix.

Surgical procedures also may be used for problems causing male infertility. Surgical repair of varicocele has been relatively successful in increasing sperm count but not fertility rates. A varicocele on the left side is found in a substantial number of subfertile men.

Microsurgery to reanastomose (restore tubal continuity) the sperm ducts can result in pregnancy rates greater than 50% (Speroff et al., 1999). The rate of success decreases as the time since the procedure increases.

Reproductive Alternatives

Although remarkable developments have occurred in reproductive medicine, **assisted reproductive therapies (ARTs)** account for less than 1% of all U.S. births (CDC, 2002) and less than 5% of infertility treatment (ASRM, 2002). They are associated with many ethical and legal issues (Box 10-9). The lack of information or misleading information about success rates and the risks and benefits of treatment alternatives prevents couples from making informed decisions. Nurses can provide information so that couples have an accurate understanding of their chances for a successful pregnancy and live birth. Nurses also can provide anticipatory guidance about the moral and ethical dilemmas regarding the use of ARTs. Some of the ARTs for treatment of infertility include in vitro fertilization-embryo transfer (IVF-ET), gamete intrafallopian transfer (GIFT), zygote intrafallopian transfer (ZIFT), ovum transfer (oocyte donation), embryo adoption, embryo hosting

BOX 10-9 Issues to Be Addressed by Infertile Couples Before Treatment

- Risks of multiple gestation
- Possible need for multifetal reduction
- Possible need for donor oocytes, sperm, or embryos or gestational carrier (surrogate mother)
- Freezing embryos for later use
- Possible risks of long-term effects of medications and treatment on women, children, and families

TABLE 10-4 **Assisted Reproductive Therapies (ARTs)**

PROCEDURE	DEFINITION	INDICATIONS
In vitro fertilization-embryo transfer (IVF-ET)	A woman's eggs are collected from her ovaries, fertilized in the laboratory with sperm, and transferred to her uterus after normal embryo development has occurred.	Tubal disease or blockage; severe male infertility; endometriosis; unexplained infertility; cervical factor; immunologic infertility
Gamete intrafallopian transfer (GIFT)	Oocytes are retrieved from the ovary, placed in a catheter with washed motile sperm, and immediately transferred into the fimbriated end of the uterine tube. Fertilization occurs in the uterine tube.	Same as for IVF-ET, except there must be normal tubal anatomy, patency, and absence of previous tubal disease in at least one uterine tube
IVF-ET and GIFT with donor sperm	This process is the same as described above except in cases where the husband's fertility is severely compromised and donor sperm can be used; if donor sperm are used, the wife must have indications for IVF and GIFT.	Severe male infertility; azoospermia; indications for IVF-ET or GIFT
Zygote intrafallopian transfer (ZIFT)	This process is similar to IVF-ET; after in vitro fertilization the ova are placed in one uterine tube during the zygote stage.	Same as for GIFT
Donor oocyte	Eggs are donated by an IVF procedure, and the donated eggs are inseminated. The embryos are transferred into the recipient's uterus, which is hormonally prepared with estrogen/progesterone therapy.	Early menopause; surgical removal of ovaries; congenitally absent ovaries; autosomal or sex-linked disorders; lack of fertilization in repeated IVF attempts because of subtle oocyte abnormalities or defects in oocyte/spermatozoa interaction
Donor embryo (embryo adoption)	A donated embryo is transferred to the uterus of an infertile woman at the appropriate time (normal or induced) of the menstrual cycle.	Infertility not resolved by less aggressive forms of therapy; absence of ovaries; male partner is azoospermic or is severely compromised
Gestational carrier (embryo host); surrogate mother	A couple undertakes an IVF cycle and the embryo(s) is transferred to another woman's uterus (the carrier) who has contracted with the couple to carry the baby to term. The carrier has no genetic investment in the child. Surrogate motherhood is a process by which a woman is inseminated with semen from the infertile woman's partner and then carries the baby until birth.	Congenital absence or surgical removal of uterus; a reproductively impaired uterus, myomas, uterine adhesions, or other congenital abnormalities; a medical condition that might be life-threatening during pregnancy, such as diabetes, immunologic problems, or severe heart, kidney, or liver disease
Therapeutic donor insemination (TDI)	Donor sperm are used to inseminate the female partner.	Male partner is azoospermic or has a very low sperm count; couple has a genetic defect; male partner has antisperm antibodies
Intracytoplasmic sperm injection	Selection of one sperm cell that is injected directly into the egg to achieve fertilization. Used with IVF.	Same as TDI
Assisted hatching	The zona pellucida is penetrated chemically or manually to create an opening for the dividing embryo to hatch and implant into uterine wall.	Recurrent miscarriages; to improve implantation rate in women with previously unsuccessful IVF attempts; advanced age

Data from American Society for Reproductive Medicine. (2002). *Frequently asked questions about infertility.* Accessed 10/1/02 at www.asrm.org; Angard, N. (1999). Diagnosis infertility. *AWHONN Lifelines 3*(3), 22-29; Kennedy, H., Griffin, M., & Frishman, G. (1998). Enabling conception and pregnancy. *Journal of Nurse Midwifery, 43*(3), 190-207; Stenchever, M. et al. (2001). *Comprehensive gynecology* (4th ed.). St. Louis: Mosby; Van Voorhis, B. et al. (1998). Cost effective treatment of the infertile couple. *Fertility and Sterility, 70*(6), 995-1005.

and surrogate parenting, and therapeutic donor insemination (TDI). Table 10-4 describes these procedures and the possible indications for the ARTs. Other options include intracytoplasmic sperm injection, assisted hatching, therapeutic donor insemination, adoption, and surrogate mothering.

In Vitro Fertilization-Embryo Transfer

In vitro fertilization-embryo transfer (IVF-ET) is a common approach for women with blocked or absent uterine tubes or with unexplained infertility and for men with very low sperm counts. About 97% of all ARTs use this procedure. Generally only three or fewer embryos are transferred, to minimize the risk of multiple pregnancy. When more than three embryos develop in the culture media, the extra embryos can be cryopreserved. If necessary, they can be thawed in a subsequent cycle for later uterine transfer.

LEGAL TIP Cryopreservation of Human Embryos
Couples who have excess embryos frozen for later transfer must be fully informed before consenting to the procedure, to make decisions regarding the disposal of embryos in the event of (1) death, (2) divorce, or (3) the decision that the couple no longer wants the embryos at a later time.

Success rates for pregnancy and for live births vary widely from center to center. Each couple's physical status and age factor into their individual chances for pregnancy as well as whether the embryos are fresh or frozen and donor or nondonor eggs (CDC, 2002) (Table 10-5). Costs vary by treatment and by region of the country: one cycle of IVF-ET averages $7800 but can be as high as $12,000 (ASRM, 2000).

Micromanipulation. *Micromanipulation* allows the handling of individual eggs and sperm through the use of specific instruments and controls. Techniques to improve fertilization, embryo growth, and genetic testing are improving at a rapid pace. **Intracytoplasmic sperm injection (ICSI)** is a technique that makes it possible to achieve fertilization or to correct abnormal fertilization by introducing sperm beneath the zona pellucida directly into the egg. Micromanipulation offers the opportunity to enhance the chances of fertilization in cases of a severe male factor; however, long-term risks and outcomes are unknown (Nudell & Lipshultz, 2001).

Micromanipulation also allows removal of a single cell from a multicellular embryo for genetic study, thus advancing the possibility of genetic diagnosis at the earliest stage of development (Carcio, 1998). Blastomere analysis results in characterization of specific genes of the genome, the complete set of genes on the chromosomes of the developing embryo. These scientific advances, although exciting, open up new ethical dilemmas. For example, the gene for cystic fibrosis is known. Couples who are both carriers of this recessive gene could have blastomere analysis performed before embryo transfer. Research on the

TABLE 10-5 **1999 Assisted Reproductive Technology Success Rates**

TYPE OF CYCLE	AGE OF WOMAN (YR) 35	35-37	38-40	41-42
Fresh embryos from nondonor eggs				
Number of cycles	29,682	15,291	12,848	5302
Percentage of cycles resulting in pregnancies	37.3	31.6	24.4	15.9
Percentage of cycles resulting in live births	32.2	26.2	18.5	9.7
Percentage of transfers resulting in live births	37.8	32.4	24.2	13.6
Average number of embryos transferred	3.0	3.3	3.5	3.7
Percentage of pregnancies with twins	32.6	28.6	22.7	14.0
Percentage of pregnancies with triplets or more	9.4	8.6	6.6	2.6
Percentage of live births having multiple infants	41.0	35.7	28.6	14.4
Frozen embryos from nondonor eggs				
Number of transfers	5615	2431	1670	513
Percentage of transfers resulting in live births	19.7	19.1	15.8	16.2
Average number embryos transferred	3.0	3.0	3.1	3.3

DONOR EGGS	ALL AGES COMBINED FRESH EMBRYOS	FROZEN EMBRYOS
Number of transfers	5844	2287
Percentage of transfers resulting in live births	41.6	23.5
Average number of embryos transferred	3.0	3.0

Source: Centers for Disease Control and Prevention. (2002). *1999 Assisted Reproductive Technology Success Rates. Results generated from SART/ASRM, CDC, and Resolve.* Accessed 10/1/02 at www.cdc.gov/nccdphp/drh.

manipulation of the genetic material of embryos before their implantation is ongoing, thus potentially making it possible to "correct" a defect before embryo transfer.

Gamete Intrafallopian Transfer

Gamete intrafallopian tube transfer (GIFT) is similar to IVF-ET. Ovulation is induced as in IVF-ET, and the oocytes are aspirated from follicles via laparoscopy (Fig. 10-5, *A*). Semen is collected before laparoscopy, and sperm are capacitated by the same technique used for IVF-ET. The ova and sperm are then transferred to one tube (Fig. 10-5, *B*), permitting natural fertilization and cleavage, with subsequent successful pregnancies possible. About 1% of all ARTs use this technique (CDC, 2002). GIFT requires women to have at least one normal uterine tube.

Zygote Intrafallopian Transfer

Zygote intrafallopian transfer (ZIFT) is similar to IVF-ET. In ZIFT, after in vitro fertilization, the ova are placed in the uterine tube during the zygote stage. ZIFT accounts for about 1% of all ART procedures (CDC, 2002).

Complications

Other than the established risks associated with laparoscopy and general anesthesia, few risks are associated with IVF-ET, GIFT, and ZIFT. The more common transvaginal needle aspiration requires only local or intravenous analgesia. Congenital anomalies occur no more frequently than among naturally conceived embryos. Ectopic pregnancies do occur more often, however, and these carry a significant maternal risk. No increase in maternal or perinatal complications occurs with TDI; the same frequencies of anomalies (about 5%) and obstetric complications (between 5% and 10%) that accompany natural insemination (through sexual intercourse) apply also to TDI.

Oocyte Donation

Women who have ovarian failure or oophorectomy, who have a genetic defect, or who fail to achieve pregnancy with their own oocytes may be eligible for the use of donor oocytes. **Oocyte donation** is usually done by women who are younger than 35 years and healthy, and who are recruited and paid to undergo ovarian stimulation and oocyte retrieval. The donor eggs are then fertilized in the laboratory with the male partner's sperm. The recipient woman undergoes hormonal stimulation to allow development of the uterine lining. Embryos are then transferred. The psychosocial issues are similar to those in therapeutic donor insemination. Historically the courts have upheld the gestational mother as the legal mother. It is expected that the egg donor will have no rights or responsibilities in relation to the offspring (see Research box).

On occasion, a couple decide that they do not want their frozen embryos, and they release these for "adoption" by other infertile couples. Infertility centers are struggling to develop guidelines and protocols to address the various legal and ethical issues associated with these procedures. Extensive medical testing of both partners is required as well (ARSM, 2002).

Therapeutic Donor Insemination

Therapeutic donor insemination (TDI), previously referred to as artificial insemination by donor, is used when the male partner has no sperm or a very low sperm count

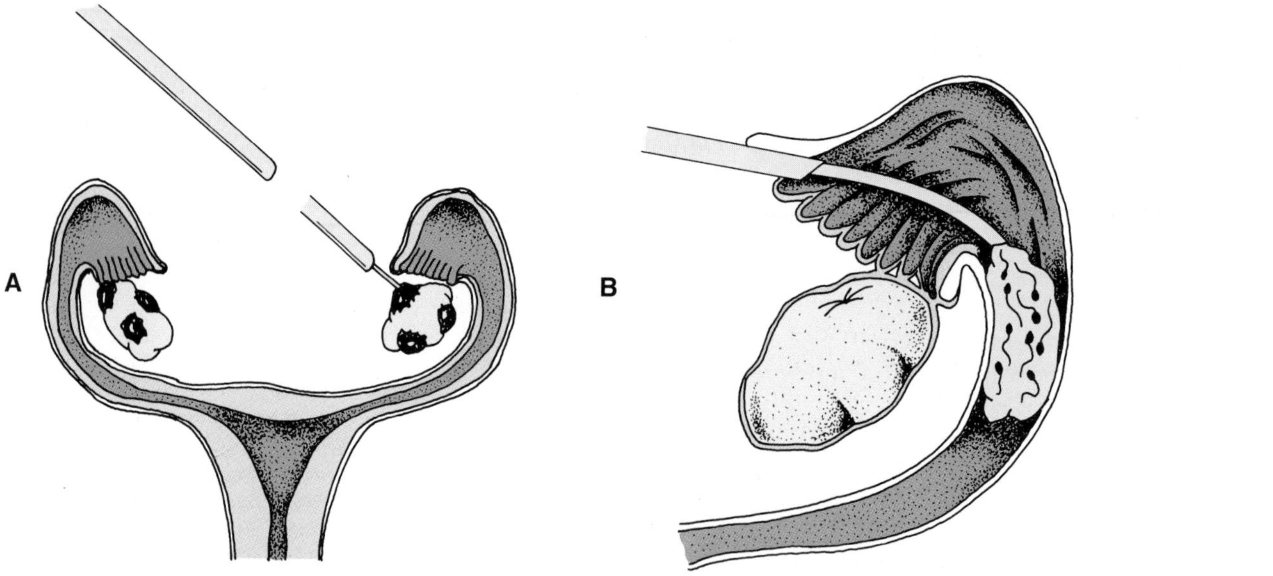
A
B

FIG. 10-5 Gamete intrafallopian transfer. **A,** Through laparoscopy, a ripe follicle is located and fluid containing the egg is removed. **B,** The sperm and egg are placed separately in the uterine tube, where fertilization occurs.

(less than 20 million motile sperm per milliliter), the couple has a genetic defect, or the male partner has antisperm antibodies. Couples need to be counseled extensively regarding the mutuality of their decision, their ability (particularly of the male partner) to grieve the loss of a biologic child, and long-term issues relating to parenting the child conceived through TDI (Biovin et al., 2001; Van Voorhis et al., 1998). Couples also must be aware of the legal status of TDI in their state.

In TDI, donor semen is subjected to laboratory testing to reduce the possibility of life-threatening illnesses for the recipient and her fetus, as well as for factors that could jeopardize the woman's future fertility or compromise the chance of the success of the procedure. Donor semen is tested for serology, serum hepatitis B antigen, *Neisseria gonorrhoeae, Chlamydia trachomatis,* cytomegalovirus antibodies, and human immunodeficiency virus (HIV) antibodies (Speroff et al., 1999; Yoshida, 1999).

The procedure is done in the physician's office or clinic, usually the day after the woman has an LH surge. The sperm are loaded into a catheter that is then inserted in the vagina, through the cervix, and placed high in the uterine cavity. The sperm are injected slowly, and the catheter is removed. The woman lies flat for a few minutes and then can get up and resume her usual activities (Stechever et al., 2001).

Assuming normal female fertility, intrauterine TDI at or about the time of ovulation has resulted in pregnancy in as many as 70% of cases. If pregnancy has not occurred within six cycles of well-timed insemination, further investigation of the female partner is warranted. The couple must know that there is no guarantee of pregnancy and that the miscarriage rate is approximately the same as in a control population.

Adoption

Couples may choose to build their family through **adoption** of children who are not their own biologically. With increased availability of birth control and abortion and increasing numbers of single mothers keeping their babies, however, the adoption of Caucasian infants is extremely limited. Minority infants and infants with special needs, older children, and foreign adoptions are other options.

Most adults assume that they will be able to have children of their own. The discovery that they are unable to do so is often accompanied by feelings of inferiority, doubts about masculinity or femininity, and feelings of guilt or blame in relation to the partner. These feelings and frustrations, combined with the anxiety of waiting for pregnancies, feelings of loss, and the endless medical procedures to investigate infertility create a unique situation for the adoptive couple preparing for parenthood (Salzer, 2000).

Couples who decide to adopt a child have decided that being a parent and having a child is more important than the actual process of birthing the child. The birth process is a very small aspect of having a baby and becoming a parent. So much emphasis is placed on being pregnant and having a child composed of one's own genetic makeup that the focus of the reason to have a child becomes cloudy. The question to be answered by couples who want to adopt is, "Do you want to have a baby, or do you want to become parents?"

Salzer (2000) describes five emotional stages that adoptive parents travel through as they make the decision to

RESEARCH

Children Conceived from Donor Eggs: To Tell or Not to Tell

Oocyte donation enables pregnancy and birth in situations of poor or absent ovarian function, intractable infertility, or serious inheritable diseases. Families that choose egg donation must discuss whether they plan to disclose to the resulting children their origin. Families make this decision based on multiple factors. To better understand their decision-making, two nurse researchers investigated 31 families (31 mothers and 27 fathers) who had children conceived from anonymous donor eggs. They measured family environment and social support using standardized questionnaires and then interviewed the families. Content analysis of the interview transcripts was followed by comparison of recurring themes identified. These themes were used to explain the rationale and worries that marked the decisions of the families in the study.

None of the parents thought disclosure would be easy. Disclosers (33) outnumbered nondisclosers (11) and undecideds (14). Compelling reasons to tell included medical reasons, the harmful effects of the child finding out elsewhere, and the harmful effect of secrecy. Nondisclosers felt no compelling reason to tell and wanted to preserve strong family ties. Concerns about disclosure included concern that the mother-child bond would be weakened; the child would someday seek out his or her genetic donor; and the child's relationship with siblings, extended family, or their community would be changed. Parents were also concerned about the irreversible nature of disclosure.

IMPLICATIONS FOR PRACTICE

Families in this study wanted to hear stories of how other parents made the decision to disclose and to obtain scripts of how to tell a child of their egg donor origins. Mothers wanted reassurance of their biologic contribution of pregnancy, birth, and breastfeeding. Written materials need to be developed for distribution by in vitro fertilization clinics. Parents can be encouraged to delay telling others until they have told the child. Referral for counseling may be indicated for parents who disagree about disclosure as well as for the child who has been told. Studies over time are needed to determine the effects of disclosure decisions on these families.

Reference: Hahn, S., & Craft-Rosenberg, M. (2002). The disclosure decisions of parents who conceive children using donor eggs. *Journal of Obstetric, Gynecologic, and Neonatal Nursing, 31*(3), 283-293.

adopt. These include (1) initial consideration of adoption as an option, (2) forming a decision as a couple, (3) soul searching (questioning personal beliefs, needs, and fears), (4) grieving over the unborn biologic child, and (5) gathering information. These stages do not always happen in a straightforward manner and are not mutually exclusive but are pieces of the path toward parenthood. Nurses should have information on options for adoption available for couples or refer to community resources for further assistance (see Resources section at the end of the chapter).

Surrogate Mothers

Surrogate motherhood can be achieved by two methods. The first is for the surrogate mother to be inseminated with semen from the infertile woman's partner and to carry the baby until the birth. The baby is then formally adopted by the infertile couple. A less common method is to retrieve an ovum from the infertile woman, fertilize it with her partner's sperm, and place it into the uterus of a surrogate, who becomes a gestational carrier. These newer interventions raise considerable legal and ethical issues that require extensive counseling of couples and the women who choose to become pregnant.

Preimplantation Genetic Diagnosis

Preimplantation genetic diagnosis (PGD) is a form of early genetic testing designed to eliminate embryos with serious genetic defects before implantation through one of the ARTs and to avoid future termination of pregnancy for genetic reasons (Fasouliotis & Schenker, 1999). In more than 20 worldwide centers, PGD is being used clinically. Experts caution that use of PGD could lead to "new" eugenics (Draper & Chadwick, 1999; King, 1999). Couples must be counseled about their options and choices as well as the implications of their choices when genetic analysis is considered (Jones, 2000).

Herbal Alternative Measures

Most herbal remedies have not been proven clinically to promote fertility or to be safe in early pregnancy and should be taken by the woman only as prescribed by a physician or nurse midwife who has expertise in herbology. Relaxation, stress management, and nutritional and exercise counseling have been reported to increase pregnancy rates in some women (Chez and Jonas, 1997). Herbal remedies that promote fertility in general include red clover flowers, nettle leaves, *dong quai,* and false unicorn root (Weed, 1986). Vitamin E, calcium, and magnesium may promote fertility and conception (Tiran & Mack, 2000). Herbs to avoid while trying to conceive include licorice root, yarrow, wormwood, ephedra, fennel, goldenseal, lavender, juniper, flaxseed, pennyroyal, passionflower, wild cherry, cascara, sage, thyme, and periwinkle (Kennedy et al., 1998).

Evaluation

Evaluation of the effectiveness of care of the couple with impaired fertility is based on the previously stated outcomes (see Plan of Care).

Plan of Care — Infertility

NURSING DIAGNOSIS Deficient knowledge related to lack of understanding of the reproductive process with regard to conception as evidenced by client questions

Expected Outcome *Client and partner will verbalize understanding of the components of the reproductive process, common problems leading to infertility, usual infertility testing, and the importance of completing testing in a timely manner.*

Nursing Interventions/*Rationales*

- Assess client's current level of understanding of the factors promoting conception *to identify gaps or misconceptions in knowledge base.*
- Provide information in a supportive manner regarding factors promoting conception including common factors leading to infertility of either partner *to raise client's awareness and promote trust in caregiver.*
- Identify and describe the basic infertility tests and the rationale for precise scheduling *to enhance completion of the diagnostic phase of the infertility workup.*

NURSING DIAGNOSIS Risk for ineffective individual/family coping related to inability to conceive as evidenced by client and partner statements

Expected Outcome *Client and partner will identify situational stressors and positive coping methods to deal with testing and unknown outcomes.*

Nursing Interventions/*Rationales*

- Provide opportunities through therapeutic communication to discuss feelings and concerns *to identify common feelings and perceived stressors.*
- Evaluate couple's support system, including support of each other during this process *to identify any barriers to effective coping.*
- Identify support groups and refer as needed *to enhance coping by sharing experiences with other couples experiencing similar problems.*

NURSING DIAGNOSIS Hopelessness related to inability to conceive as evidenced by woman's and partner's statements

Expected Outcome *Woman and partner will verbalize a realistic plan to decrease feelings of hopelessness.*

Nursing Interventions/*Rationales*

- Provide support for couple while grieving for loss of fertility *to allow couple to work through feelings.*
- Assess for behaviors indicating possible depression, anger, and frustration *to prevent impending crisis.*
- Refer to support groups *to promote a common bond with other couples during expression of feelings and concerns.*

KEY POINTS

- Infertility is the inability to conceive and carry a child to term gestation when the couple has chosen to do so.
- Infertility affects between 10% to 15% of otherwise healthy adults. Infertility increases as the woman ages, especially after age 40 years.
- In the United States, about 50% of infertility is related to female causes; 35% is related to male causes; and 10% to 15% of the causes are unexplained.
- Common etiologic factors of infertility include decreased sperm production, ovulation disorders, tubal occlusion, and endometriosis.
- The investigation of infertility is conducted systematically and simultaneously for both male and female partners.
- The couple's relationship dynamics, sexuality, and ability to cope with the psychologic and emotional effects caused by diagnostic procedures and treatment of infertility must be considered in the plan of care.
- Most infertility cases are treated with conventional medical and surgical therapies; less than 5% are treated with in vitro fertilization.
- Reproductive alternatives for family building include IVF-ET, GIFT, ZIFT, oocyte donation, embryo donation, TDI, surrogate motherhood, and adoption.

CRITICAL THINKING EXERCISES

1. You are assigned to a postpartum client whose chart states that she had conceived through IVF. Review her prenatal chart to identify what diagnostic tests she and her partner had and what treatments were done, including the one that produced the pregnancy. What risk factors did the couple have for infertility? What pregnancy complications were present? What if any complications did the newborn have? Interview the couple and ask them to share their thoughts and feelings about the diagnostic and treatment process, the pregnancy, and being parents. Compare their answers with what has been reported in the nursing literature.
2. Use two Internet websites for infertility to examine the information for couples concerning financial, ethical, and legal issues of in vitro fertilization, TDI, and adoption. Discuss the findings in clinical conference.

RESOURCES

American College of Obstetricians and Gynecologists
409 12th St., SW
Washington, DC 20024
800-762-2264
www.acog.org

American Fertility Foundation
2131 Magnolia Ave., Suite 201
Birmingham, AL 35256
205-251-9764

American Society for Reproductive Medicine
1209 Montgomery Hwy.
Birmingham, AL 35316
205-978-5000
www.asrm.org

Association of Reproductive Health Professionals
2401 Pennsylvania Ave. NW, Suite 350
Washington, DC 20037
202-466-3825
arhp.org

Infertility Resources
www.ihr.com/infertility/index.html

International Council on Infertility Information Dissemination
P.O. Box 6836
Arlington, VA 22206
703-379-9178
www.inciid.org

National Adoption Information Clearing House
330 C St. SW
Washington, DC 20447
888-251-0075
www.calib.com/naic

National Women's Health Resource Center
120 Albany St., Suite 820
New Brunswick, NJ 08901
877-986-9472
www.healthywomen.org

Resolve, Inc. *(Impaired fertility)*
1310 Broadway, Dept. GM
Summerville, MA 02144-1713
617-623-0744
888-299-1585
www.resolve.org

Internet Health Resources
www.ihr.com
This website is an infertility organization for consumers.

REFERENCES

American Society for Reproductive Medicine. (2002). *Frequently asked questions about infertility.* http://www.asrm.org. Retrieved 10/1/02.

Angard, N. (1999). Diagnosis infertility. *AWHONN Lifelines, 3*(3), 22-29.

Applegarth, L. (2000). Individual counseling and psychotherapy. In L. Burns & S. Covington (Eds.), *Infertility counseling: A comprehensive handbook for clinicians.* New York: Parthenon Publishing Group.

Bhasin, S. et al. (1998). The genetic basis of male infertility. *Endocrinology and Metabolism Clinics of North America, 27*(4), 783-805.

Boivin, J. et al. (2001). Guidelines for counseling in infertility: Outline version. *Human Reproduction, 16*(6), 1301-1304.

Carcio, H. (1998). *Management of the infertile woman.* Philadelphia: J.B. Lippincott.

Centers for Disease Control. (2002). *Results of joint SART/ASRM, CDC, and RESOLVE 1999 assisted reproductive technology success rate report.* http://www.cdc.gov/nccdphp/drh. Retrieved 10/1/02.

Chez, R., & Jonas, W. (1997). Complementary and alternative medicine, Part II: clinical studies in gynecology. *Obstetrics and Gynecology Survey, 52*(11), 709-716.

Cunningham, F. et al. (2001). *Williams obstetrics* (21st ed.). New York: McGraw-Hill.

D'Avanzo, C., & Geissler, E. (2003). *Mosby's pocket guide to cultural health assessment* (3rd ed.). St. Louis: Mosby.

Draper, H., & Chadwick, R. (1999). Beware! Preimplantation genetic diagnosis may solve some old problems but it raises new ones. *Journal of Medical Ethics, 25*, 114-120.

Fasouliotis, S., & Schenker, J. (1999). Social aspects in assisted reproduction. *Human Reproduction Update, 5*(1), 26-39.

Giwercman, A., & Bonde, J. (1998). Declining male fertility and environmental factors. *Endocrinology and Metabolism Clinics of North America, 27*(4), 807-830.

Hargreave, T., & Ghosh, C. (1998). Male fertility disorders. *Endocrinology and Metabolism Clinics of North America, 27*(4), 765-782.

Jones, S. (2000). Reproductive genetic technologies: Exploring ethical and policy implication. *AWHONN Lifelines, 4*(5), 33-36.

Kennedy, H., Griffin, M., & Frishman, G. (1998). Enabling conception and pregnancy. *Journal of Nurse Midwifery, 43*(3), 190-207.

Keye, W. (2000). Medical aspects of infertility for the counselor. In H. Burns & S. Covington (Eds.), *Infertility counseling: A comprehensive handbook for clinicians.* New York: Parthenon Publishing Group.

King, D. (1999). Preimplantation genetic diagnosis and the "new" genetics. *Journal of Medical Ethics, 25*, 176-182.

Klock, S. (2000). Psychosocial evaluation of the infertile patient. In H. Burns & S. Covington (Eds.), *Infertility counseling: A comprehensive handbook for clinicians.* New York: Parthenon Publishing Group.

Liebowitz, D., & Hoffman, J. (2000). Fertility drug therapies: Past present, and future. *Journal of Obstetric, Gynecologic, and Neonatal Nursing, 29*(2), 201-210.

Newton, C. (2000). Counseling the infertile couple. In H. Burns & S. Covington (Eds.), *Infertility counseling: A comprehensive handbook for clinicians.* New York: Parthenon Publishing Group.

Nudell, D., & Lipshultz, L. (2001). Is intracytoplasmic sperm injection safe? Current status and future concerns. *Current Urology Report, 2*(6), 423-431.

Salzer, L. (2000). Adoption after infertility. In H. Burns & S. Covington (Eds.), *Infertility counseling: A comprehensive handbook for clinicians.* New York: Parthenon Publishing Group.

Session, D. et al. (1998). Recent advances in infertility treatment. *Minnesota Medicine, 81*(10), 27-32.

Speroff, L., Glass, H., & Kase, G. (1999). *Clinical gynecologic endocrinology and infertility* (6th ed.). Philadelphia: Lippincott Williams & Wilkins.

Stenchever, M. et al. (2001). *Comprehensive gynecology* (4th ed.). St. Louis: Mosby.

Stephen, E., & Chandra, A. (1998). Updated projections of infertility in the United States, 1995-2025. *Fertility and Sterility, 70*(1), 30-34.

Thomas, K. et al. (2000). The value of *Chlamydia trachomatis* antibody testing as part of routine infertility investigations. *Human Reproduction, 15*(5), 1079-1082.

Tiran, D., & Mack, S. (2000). *Complementary therapies for pregnancy and childbirth.* Edinburgh: Bailliere Tindall.

Van Voorhis, B. et al. (1998). Cost-effective treatment of the infertile couple. *Fertility and Sterility, 70*(6), 995-1005.

Weed, S. (1986). *Wise woman herbal for the childbearing year.* Woodstock, NY: Ash Tree Publishing Co.

World Health Organization. (1992). *Laboratory manual for the examination of human semen and sperm-cervical mucus interaction.* Cambridge, UK: WHO.

Yoshida, T. (1999). Infertility update: Use of assisted reproductive technology. *Journal of the American Pharmacy Association, 39*(1), 65-72.

Zahalsky, M., & Nagler, H. (2001). Ultrasound and infertility: Diagnostic and therapeutic uses. *Current Urology Report, 2*(6), 437-442.

CHAPTER 11

Angela Sammarco

Problems of the Breast

http://evolve.elsevier.com/Lowdermilk/MatWmnHlth/

LEARNING OBJECTIVES

- Discuss the pathophysiology of selected benign and malignant breast disorders found in women.
- Explain the emotional effect of benign and malignant neoplasms.
- Design a nursing plan of care for the woman with a breast disorder.
- Evaluate treatment alternatives for women with breast cancer.
- Relate critical elements for teaching clients who have undergone medical-surgical management of benign or malignant neoplasms of the breast.

Approximately 50% of women have a breast problem at some point in their adult lives. The most common sign of a breast problem is a palpable mass. Most of these lumps are benign, although finding them may produce anxiety for the woman, who may fear she has cancer. Cancer of the breast is the most frequently diagnosed cancer in women in the United States (ACS, 2003). The development of breast cancer can have a far-reaching impact on the woman and her family. Beyond the obvious physiologic alterations, the woman also may experience threats to her self-concept and her ability to cope. The condition and its treatments can affect a woman's concept of herself as a sexual being. A woman's family also is challenged in the way it responds to her diagnosis. When breast cancer occurs during or after pregnancy, it adds to the complexity of both physical and emotional responses to childbearing.

Nurses have important roles in teaching women about early detection and treatment and in providing supportive care to clients and their families. This chapter presents information that will assist the nurse in providing care for women with benign breast conditions or breast cancer. Nursing care concepts related to early detection, treatment methods, and education are included. The ongoing investigations of new drug therapies to prevent breast cancer also are introduced.

BENIGN CONDITIONS OF THE BREAST

Fibrocystic Changes

The most common benign breast problem is **fibrocystic change,** found in varying degrees in healthy women's breasts. Fibrocystic changes are palpable thickenings in the breast usually associated with pain and tenderness. The pain and tenderness fluctuate with the menstrual cycle and can become progressively worse until menopause (Marchant, 1998).

Approximately 70% of fibrocystic changes are nonproliferative lesions; 26% are proliferative lesions without *atypia* (benign growing cells), and the rest are proliferative lesions with *atypical hyperplasia.* Women with a history of proliferative changes with hyperplasia have twice the risk of breast cancer, and women with atypical hyperplasia appear to have four times the risk (Marchant, 1998).

Etiology

No known etiologic agent is responsible for benign breast disease, although an imbalance of estrogen and progesterone may be responsible. One theory is that estrogen excess and progesterone deficiency in the luteal phase of the menstrual cycle may cause changes in breast tissue. Risk factors associated with benign breast disease include nulliparity, low parity, late menopause, and estrogen therapy. Research has shown no substantial association between smoking, alcohol or caffeine consumption, and risk of benign breast disease (Friedenreich et al., 2000).

Clinical Manifestations and Diagnosis

The usual clinical presentation of fibrocystic change is lumpiness in both breasts; however, single simple cysts also may occur. Symptoms usually develop about a week before menstruation begins and subside about a week after menstruation ends. They include dull, heavy pain and a sense of fullness and tenderness that increases in the premenstrual period (McCool et al., 1998). The woman with fibrocystic change may form cysts that manifest as painful enlarging lumps in her breasts. Cysts are common in premenopausal women who are not receiving estrogen therapy. The cysts are soft on palpation, well differentiated, and movable. Deeper cysts, especially aggregations of cysts, are indistinguishable by palpation from carcinomas, which are malignant growths that infiltrate surrounding tissue.

A first step in the workup of a breast lump is ultrasonography to determine if it is fluid filled or solid. Fluid-filled cysts are aspirated, and the woman is monitored on a routine basis for development of other cysts. If the lump is solid, mammography is obtained if the woman is older than 35 years. A fine-needle aspiration (FNA) is then performed, regardless of the woman's age, to determine the nature of the lump. In some cases, a core biopsy may be needed after FNA to harvest adequate amounts of tissue for pathologic examination (Stenchever et al., 2001).

Therapeutic Management

Treatment for fibrocystic changes is usually conservative, traditionally including diuretic administration and restriction of salt and fluid. Vitamin E supplements also have been recommended, although megadose therapy should be avoided. Even though no research support has been found, some advocate eliminating dimethylxanthines, such as caffeine. Some women report relief of symptoms by avoiding smoking and the consumption of alcohol (Marchant, 1998). Recommended pain-relief measures include taking analgesics or nonsteroidal antiinflammatory drugs (NSAIDs) such as ibuprofen, wearing a supportive bra, and applying heat to the breasts. Some women report relief while taking oral contraceptives, but others report worsening of symptoms.

It is important to stress that women may need to try several approaches for a number of months before improvement is noted. The recommended therapies are based on mostly anecdotal evidence; scientific validation of treatment strategies is lacking.

Surgical removal of nodules is attempted only in selected cases. In the presence of multiple nodules, the surgical approach involves multiple incisions and tissue manipulation and may not prevent the development of more nodules.

Fibroadenomas

The next most common benign condition of the breast is a **fibroadenoma.** Fibroadenomas occur in women from puberty through menopause. Masses are solid, encapsulated, nontender, and most often found in the upper outer quadrant of the breast.

The cause of fibroadenomas is unknown. Fibroadenomas are characterized by discrete, usually solitary lumps less than 3 cm in diameter. Occasionally the woman with a fibroadenoma will have tenderness in the tumor during the menstrual cycle. Fibroadenomas increase in size during pregnancy and shrink as the woman ages. Fibroadenomas do not increase in size in response to the menstrual cycle (in contrast to fibrocystic cysts). The mass tends to remain the same size or increase in size slowly over time (McCool et al., 1998).

Diagnosis is made by a review of the client history and physical examination. Mammography, ultrasonography, or magnetic resonance imaging (MRI) may be used to determine the type of lesion, and FNA may be used to determine the underlying disorder. Surgical excision may be necessary if the lump is suspicious or if the symptoms are severe. Fibroadenomas do not respond to either dietary changes or hormonal therapy. Periodic observation of masses by professional physical examination or mammography may be all that is necessary for those masses not requiring surgical intervention.

Lipomas

A **lipoma** is a soft tumor composed of fat and has discrete borders. The cause of lipoma is unknown. Lipomas are often found in women older than 45 years. They are usually located on the chest wall and breast. They are characterized as palpable soft masses that are mobile and nontender. Mammography can be used to make a diagnosis; biopsy usually is not needed. Lipomas can be surgically excised if removal is desired.

Nipple Discharge

Nipple discharge is a common occurrence that concerns many women. Although most nipple discharge is physiologic, each woman who has this problem must be evaluated carefully, because a small percentage will be found to have a serious endocrine disorder or malignancy. Bilateral serous discharge expressed during nipple stimulation can be considered a normal finding. Client education and reassurance are indicated (Marchant, 1998).

Another form of breast discharge not related to malignancy is galactorrhea. **Galactorrhea** manifests as a bilaterally spontaneous, milky, sticky discharge. It is a normal finding in pregnancy. It also may occur as the result of elevated prolactin levels. Increased prolactin levels may be a result of a thyroid disorder, pituitary tumor, coitus, eating, stress, trauma, or chest wall surgery. It is essential to have a complete medication history on each client. Oral con-

BOX *11-1* **Drugs Associated with Galactorrhea**

- Estrogens, including oral contraceptives
- Phenothiazines
- Cimetidine
- Methyldopa
- Opiates
- Antiemetics
- Long-term use of alcohol
- Marijuana

traceptives and neuroleptic drugs are known to precipitate galactorrhea in some women (Hawkins et al., 1997; Marchant, 1998). See Box 11-1 for other classes of drugs that may be associated with galactorrhea.

The optimal time to draw blood to determine a prolactin level is between 8 and 10 AM. Ideally, prolactin levels should not be determined directly after a breast examination, sexual activity, or exercise session. Other diagnostic tests that may be indicated include a microscopic analysis of the discharge from each breast, a thyroid profile, a pregnancy test, and a mammogram (Hawkins et al., 1997).

Mammary Duct Ectasia

Mammary duct ectasia is an inflammation of the ducts behind the nipple. The cause of mammary duct ectasia is unknown, although chronic inflammation and dilation of the lactiferous ducts has been suggested. It occurs most often in perimenopausal women and is characterized by a thick and sticky nipple discharge that is white, brown, green, or purple. Frequently the client will experience a burning pain, itching, or a palpable mass behind the nipple.

The workup includes a mammogram, aspiration of fluid, and culture of fluid. Duct ectasia is usually self-limiting, requiring only reassurance of the woman (Marchant, 1998). Development of an infection in the inflamed area requires antibiotic therapy, and incision and drainage is necessary if an abscess develops. Treatment also may include a local excision of the affected duct or ducts if the woman has no future plans to breastfeed.

Intraductal Papilloma

Intraductal papilloma is a rare, benign condition that develops in the terminal nipple ducts. The cause is unknown. It usually occurs in women between ages 30 and 50 years. Usually too small to be palpated (less than 0.5 cm), this papilloma has the characteristic sign of serous, serosanguineous, or bloody nipple discharge. The discharge is unilateral and spontaneous. After the possibility of malignancy is eliminated, the affected segments of the ducts and breasts are surgically excised (McCool et al., 1998).

Table 11-1 compares common manifestations of benign breast masses.

Macromastia and Micromastia

Macromastia, or breast hyperplasia, is a condition in which the woman has very large breasts. The size and weight of the breasts can cause chronic pain in the breast, back, neck, and shoulders, as well as significant disruption in psychosocial functioning and body image. Macromastia also can cause thoracic kyphosis, headache, paresthesia of the upper extremities, and shoulder grooving from brassiere straps. Macromastia is treated by reduction mammoplasty, in which the plastic surgeon removes breast tissue to reduce the size and weight of the breasts. Women who have had breast reduction surgery have significant improvement of preoperative signs and symptoms and their quality of life (Chadbourne et al., 2001). However, risks associated with the surgery include the potential to affect the woman's ability to breastfeed an infant in the future, infection, decreased nipple sensation, and scarring (Grassley, 2002). Breast reduction surgery is considered reconstructive surgery when done to relieve symptoms of macromastia and may be covered by health insurance policies. Women considering reduction mammoplasty should review their health insurance policies to determine exact coverage (Grassley, 2002).

Although it is not a breast disorder, **micromastia,** or having very small breasts, may negatively influence a woman's body image. Augmentation mammoplasty may be done to increase the size of the breasts. The plastic surgeon inserts implants filled with normal saline between the breast tissue and the chest wall. Silicone gel–filled implants are not available for breast augmentation done for cosmetic reasons (Arthur & Janssen, 2000) (see later discussion on

TABLE 11-1 **Comparison of Common Manifestations of Benign Breast Masses**

FIBROCYSTIC CHANGES	FIBROADENOMA	LIPOMA	INTRADUCTAL PAPILLOMA	MAMMARY DUCT ECTASIA
Multiple lumps	Single lump	Single lump	Single or multiple	Mass behind nipple
Nodular	Well delineated	Well delineated	Not well delineated	Not well delineated
Palpable	Palpable	Palpable	Nonpalpable	Palpable
Movable	Movable	Movable	Nonmobile	Nonmobile
Round, smooth	Round, lobular	Round, lobular	Small, ball-like	Irregular
Firm or soft	Firm	Soft	Firm or soft	Firm
Tenderness influenced by menstrual cycle	Usually asymptomatic	Nontender	Usually nontender	Painful, burning, itching
Bilateral	Unilateral	Unilateral	Unilateral	Unilateral
May or may not have nipple discharge	No nipple discharge	No nipple discharge	Serous or bloody nipple discharge	Thick, sticky nipple discharge

breast reconstruction). Breast augmentation surgery is considered cosmetic surgery and is usually not covered by health insurance policies. Breast implants do not last; most must be replaced in 10 to 15 years or sooner. About 25% of women who have breast implants will have them removed within 3 years of insertion because of complications (Zuckerman, 2002).

Care Management

Assessment should include a careful client history and physical examination. The history should focus on risk factors for breast diseases, events related to the breast mass, and health maintenance practices. Risk factors for breast cancer are discussed later in this chapter. Information related to the breast mass should include how, when, and by whom the mass was discovered. The interval between discovery and seeking care is crucial. Answers to these questions can give clues about breast self-examination (BSE) practice and access to care. The nurse should document the following client information: presence of pain, whether symptoms increase with menses, dietary habits, smoking habits, use of oral contraceptives, regular BSE, and the examination technique used. The woman's emotional status, including her stress level, fears, and concerns, and her ability to cope also should be assessed.

Physical examination may include assessment of the breasts for symmetry, masses (size, number, consistency, mobility), and nipple discharge.

Nursing actions might include the following:

- Demonstrate correct BSE technique (see Chapter 5).
- Discuss the intervals for and facets of breast screening, including professional examination and mammography (see Table 11-3). Women with breast implants may need special views of the breast and precautions taken not to rupture the implant during mammography.
- Provide written educational materials.
- Encourage the verbalization of fears and concerns about treatment and prognosis.
- Provide specific information regarding the woman's condition and treatment, including dietary changes, drug therapy, comfort measures, stress management, and surgery.
- Describe pain-relieving strategies in detail, and collaborate with the primary health care provider to ensure effective pain control.
- Encourage discussion of feelings about body image.
- Refer to a support group or stress management resource if needed to cope with long-term consequences of benign breast conditions.

MALIGNANT CONDITIONS OF THE BREAST

The United States has one of the highest rates of breast carcinoma in the world. In one in eight American women, breast cancer will develop in her lifetime. Statistics released from the American Cancer Society (2003) indicate that breast cancer incidence increased about 4% per year since 1980, and it leveled off in the 1990s to about 110 cases per 100,000 women. Increasing incidence may be related to better detection of early-stage breast cancer. The incidence of breast cancer is higher in Caucasian women than in African-American women, but the mortality rate for African-American women with breast cancer is higher. More African-American women are initially diagnosed with a later stage of breast cancer (Figs. 11-1 and 11-2) (American Cancer Society, 2003), even though they obtain clinical breast examinations and mammograms by a professional with a greater frequency than do Caucasian women (Lauver et al., 1999).

Incidence and Etiologies

Although the exact cause of breast cancer continues to elude investigators, certain factors that increase a woman's risk for developing a malignancy have been identified. These factors are listed in Box 11-2.

The most important predictor of risk for breast cancer is age. Each woman's risk of breast cancer increases as her age increases. Most of the other risk factors involve the effects of the menstrual-reproductive cycle (probably the effect of estrogen or progesterone) on the development of breast cancer. Fewer menstrual cycles and early childbearing appear to have a protective effect (McCool et al., 1998).

Although most breast cancers are not related to genetic factors, the identification of the BRCA1 and BRCA2 genes demonstrated the role of heredity and genetic mutations in this disease. Only about 5% of all breast cancers are attributed to heredity, but it is believed that mutations in the BRCA1 and BRCA2 genes are involved in 30% to 70% of all inherited cases of breast cancer (Nogueira & Appling, 2000).

Research has been ongoing to identify possible environmental factors that may represent significant risk for developing breast cancer. Some known and suspected

ETHICAL CONSIDERATIONS

The ability to test for BRCA1 and BRCA2 has generated heated ethical debate within the health care community. Testing is expensive (about $2500 for the first person in the family to be tested) and often not covered by insurance. Who should be tested and who should pay for it have not been addressed adequately. What to do when a positive result is discovered is not universally agreed on. Women and their families will most likely have increased anxiety after a positive finding. How often should screening be performed? Should prophylactic mastectomies be recommended? Will there be employment discrimination if this information is in a woman's medical record? Women requesting testing must be fully informed of the possible risks and benefits of testing before consenting to the procedure (Cummings, 2001; National Women's Health Resource Center, 2000).

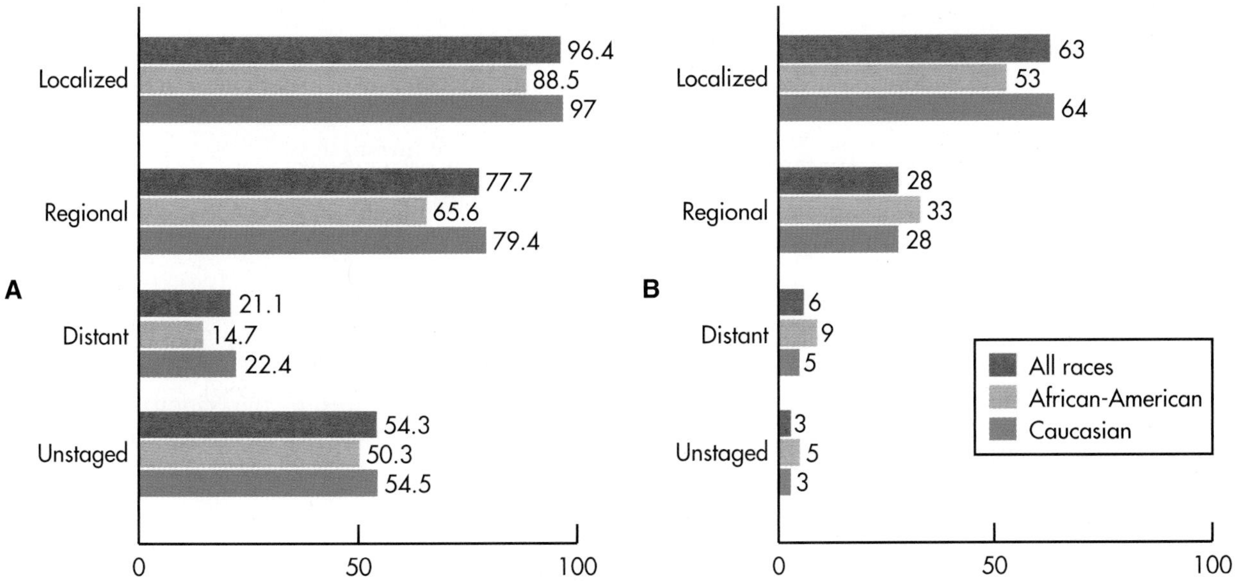
A
Localized
96.4
88.5
97
Regional
77.7
65.6
79.4
Distant
21.1
14.7
22.4
Unstaged
54.3
50.3
54.5
0
50
100
B
Localized
63
53
64
Regional
28
33
28
Distant
6
9
5
Unstaged
3
5
3
0
50
100
All races
African-American
Caucasian

* Survival rates are based on follow-up of patients through 1997.
American Cancer Society, Surveillance Research, 2001.
Data source: NCI Surveillance, Epidemiology, and End Results Program, 2001.

FIG. 11-1 Female breast cancer—United States, 1992-1997. **A,** Five-year survival rates by stage at diagnosis and race. **B,** Percentage diagnosed by stage and race. (Courtesy American Cancer Society.)

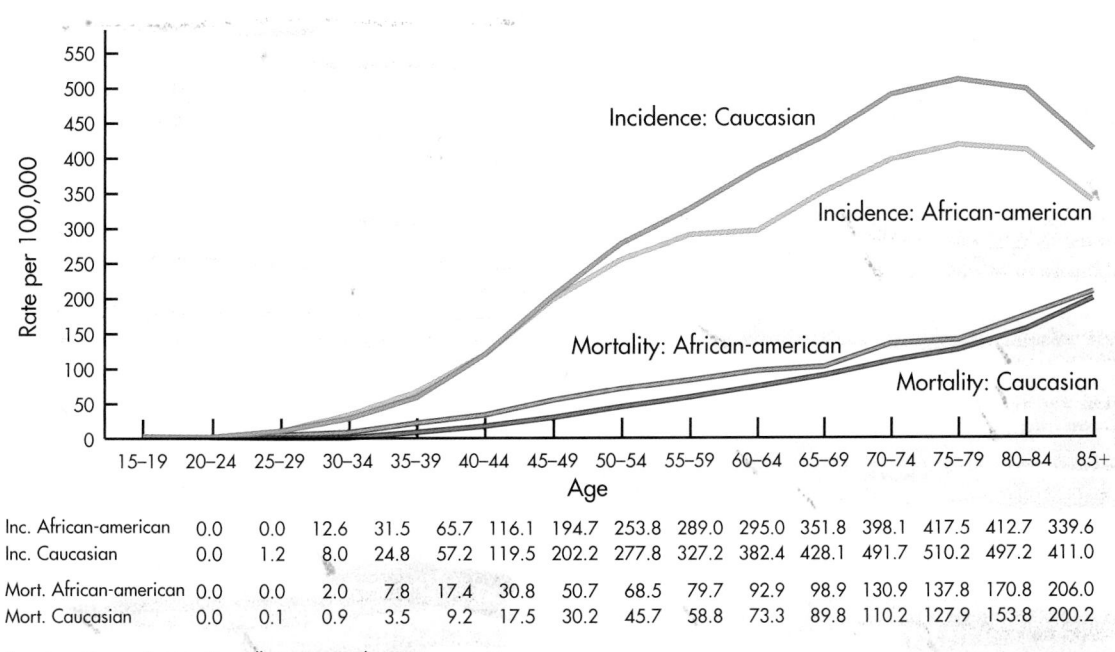

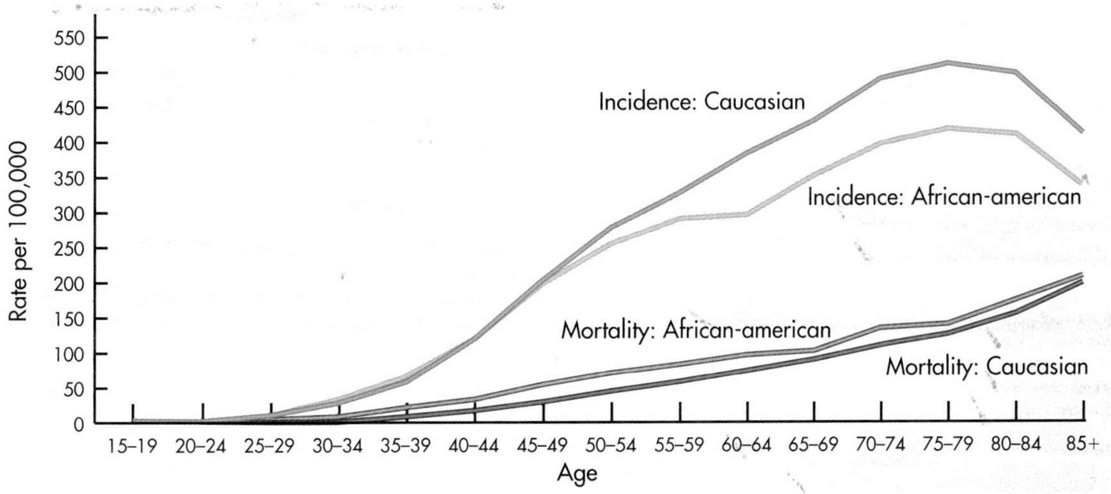
Rate per 100,000
550
500
450
400
350
300
250
200
150
100
50
0
Incidence: Caucasian
Incidence: African-american
Mortality: African-american
Mortality: Caucasian
15–19 20–24 25–29 30–34 35–39 40–44 45–49 50–54 55–59 60–64 65–69 70–74 75–79 80–84 85+
Age

	15–19	20–24	25–29	30–34	35–39	40–44	45–49	50–54	55–59	60–64	65–69	70–74	75–79	80–84	85+
Inc. African-american	0.0	0.0	12.6	31.5	65.7	116.1	194.7	253.8	289.0	295.0	351.8	398.1	417.5	412.7	339.6
Inc. Caucasian	0.0	1.2	8.0	24.8	57.2	119.5	202.2	277.8	327.2	382.4	428.1	491.7	510.2	497.2	411.0
Mort. African-american	0.0	0.0	2.0	7.8	17.4	30.8	50.7	68.5	79.7	92.9	98.9	130.9	137.8	170.8	206.0
Mort. Caucasian	0.0	0.1	0.9	3.5	9.2	17.5	30.2	45.7	58.8	73.3	89.8	110.2	127.9	153.8	200.2

American Cancer Society, Surveillance Research, 2001.
Data sources: NCI Surveillance, Epidemiology, and End Results Program, 2001, and National Center for Health Statistics, 2001.

FIG. 11-2 Female breast cancer age-specific incidence and mortality rates—Caucasian versus African-American women. (Courtesy American Cancer Society.)

environmental risk factors include exposure to organochlorine pesticides and other synthetic chemicals, hormonal factors (both exogenous and endogenous), diet, tobacco and alcohol use, radiation, and magnetic fields. Definitive links between pesticide or electromagnetic exposure and development of breast cancer have not been identified (Johnson-Thompson & Guthrie, 2000). Exposure to radiation has been observed to double breast cancer risk, particularly when exposure occurs during rapid breast formation, as in teenage years (McPherson et al., 2000).

A close correlation between the incidence of breast cancer and dietary fat intake has been observed, yet the actual relation between fat intake and breast cancer does not appear to be strong or consistent. A link between alcohol consumption and breast cancer incidence has been observed in some studies, but the association may be with other dietary factors rather than alcohol. No direct link between smoking and breast cancer has been identified (McPherson et al., 2000). In a long-term study of breast implant patients by the National Cancer Institute, silicone breast implants did not increase the risk of breast cancer (Nelson, 2000).

A comprehensive review of the research discussion about possible links between breast cancer and hormonal therapy revealed such a confounding range of variables that it has been impossible to draw definitive conclusions about hormonal replacement therapy and the risk of breast cancer. Observational data suggest that long-term use of estrogen replacement therapy (longer than 10 years) may slightly increase the risk, but the risk decreases after discontinuing use (Marsden, 2002). Clinical outcomes of the Women's Health Initiative randomized controlled trial to assess the risks and benefits of estrogen and progestin in healthy postmenopausal women were released in May 2002. The safety monitoring board recommended the trial be stopped because the overall health risks exceeded the benefits. These risks included 290 cases of breast cancer in the study group of about 8500 women (Writing Group for the Women's Health Initiative Investigators, 2002). Women considering hormonal replacement therapy should be cautious and consult with their health care providers to determine their suitability for hormonal therapy.

Information about breast cancer risks can be confusing, and women can overestimate or underestimate their risks. The Breast Cancer Risk Assessment Tool can be used by women and health professionals to calculate risk. This tool was developed and verified by the National Cancer Institute (NCI) to predict the risk of breast cancer in 5 years and over the lifetime (to age 90 years) of a woman. The risk factors used are listed in Box 11-3. The tool is available on the Internet at the NCI website (see Resources at end of chapter).

Risk factors help to identify fewer than 30% of women in whom breast cancer will eventually develop. Two problems prevent a clear understanding of the risk factors of breast cancer. One is the long latent period, 15 to 25 years, before the development of clinically recognizable carcinoma. The other is consideration of both the duration and the intensity of factors that may induce or promote cancer. Many risk factors are additive. Although the clinical applicability of risk factors has limits, women at increased risk should be screened at more frequent intervals (McCool et al., 1998).

Chemoprevention

Ongoing studies by the NCI and other groups are investigating the role of tamoxifen and raloxifene in the prevention of breast cancer (National Cancer Institute, 2002; Vogel et al., 2002). Raloxifene prevents osteoporosis without the possible increased cancer risks of estrogen replacement. This medication may be an ideal choice for the woman at high risk for both osteoporosis and breast cancer. Tamoxifen has already been shown to reduce the recurrence of breast cancer in women with prior breast malignancies. The current prevention studies are attempting to identify which women would most benefit from preventive tamoxifen administration. Although many women may want to start tamoxifen for breast cancer pre-

BOX 11-2 Risk Factors for Breast Cancer*

- Age
- Previous history of breast cancer
- Family history of breast cancer, especially a mother or sister (particularly significant if premenopausal)
- Previous history of ovarian, endometrial, colon, or thyroid cancer
- Early menarche (before age 12)
- Late menopause (after age 55)
- Nulliparity or first pregnancy after age 30
- Use of estrogen replacement therapy
- Obesity after menopause
- Previous history of benign breast disease with epithelial hyperplasia
- Race (Caucasian women have highest incidence)
- High socioeconomic status
- Sedentary lifestyle

*Risk factors are cumulative—the more risk factors present, the greater the likelihood of breast cancer occurring.

BOX 11-3 Risk Factors Included in the Breast Cancer Risk Assessment Tool

- Woman's age
- Number of first-degree relatives affected
- Age of woman at menarche
- Age of woman at first live birth
- Number of breast biopsies
- History of abnormal hyperplasia in biopsy specimens

vention, the risk of occasional serious side effects demands careful consideration before prescribing tamoxifen (Kissinger et al., 2002) (see later discussion).

Pathophysiology

Breast cancer occurs when there are genetic alterations in the deoxyribonucleic acid (DNA) of breast epithelial cells. Many types of breast cancer exist. Genetic alterations are found in the epithelial cells, compromising ductal or lobular tissue. These genetic abnormalities may have been inherited or may have developed spontaneously (Rosenzweig et al., 2000). Researchers are investigating which oncogenes (potentially cancer-inducing genes) may cause breast cancer or change its growth pattern and how the process can be stopped.

Breast cancer begins in the epithelial cells lining the mammary ducts of the breast. The rate of breast cancer growth depends on the effect of estrogen and progesterone. These cancers can be either invasive (infiltrating) or noninvasive (in situ). Invasive or infiltrating breast cancers can grow into the wall of the mammary duct and into the surrounding tissues. By far the most frequently occurring cancer of the breast is invasive ductal carcinoma. Ductal carcinoma originates in the lactiferous ducts and invades surrounding breast structures. The tumor is usually unilateral, not well delineated, solid, nonmobile, and nontender. Lobular carcinoma originates in the lobules of the breasts. It is usually bilateral and nonpalpable. Nipple carcinoma *(Paget's disease)* originates in the nipple. It usually occurs with invasive ductal carcinoma and can cause bleeding, oozing, and crusting of the nipple.

Breast cancer can invade surrounding tissues in such a way that the primary tumor can have tentacle-like projections. This invasive growth pattern can result in the irregular tumor border felt on palpation. As the tumor grows, fibrosis develops around it and can shorten Cooper's ligaments. When Cooper's ligaments are shortened, the result is the characteristic peau d'orange (orange skin) changes and edema associated with some breast cancers. If the breast cancer invades the lymphatic channels, tumors can develop in the regional lymph nodes, often occupying the axillary lymph nodes. The tumor may invade the outer layers of skin, creating ulcerations.

Metastasis results from seeding of the breast cancer cells into the blood and lymph systems, leading to tumor development in the bones, lungs, brain, and liver (Table 11-2).

Clinical Manifestations and Diagnosis

Breast cancer in its earliest form can be detected on a mammogram before it can be felt by the woman or her health care provider. It is estimated, however, that 90% of all breast lumps are detected by the woman. Of this 90%, only 20% to 25% are malignant. More than half of all lumps are discovered in the upper outer quadrant of the breast (Fig. 11-3). The most common initial symptom is a lump or thickening of the breast. The lump may feel hard and fixed or soft and spongy. It may have well-defined or irregular borders. It may be fixed to the skin, causing dimpling to occur. A bloody or clear nipple discharge also may be present.

Unilateral and spontaneous discharge (without nipple manipulation) is associated with mastitis, intraductal papilloma, and cancer. The discharge is usually intermittent and persistent and may be clear, serous, green-gray, purulent, serosanguineous, or sanguineous. Women with these findings need a complete diagnostic workup to determine the cause of their symptoms (Marchant, 1998; McCool et al., 1998).

As a general principle, any unilateral breast symptom (i.e., mass, discharge, pain, or itching) is a more ominous finding than a bilateral symptom. However, all findings must be carefully followed up to avoid missing a serious diagnosis such as cancer. Any delay in treatment may

TABLE *11-2* **Staging for Breast Cancer***

STAGE	DEFINITION
Stage 0	Carcinoma in situ (Tis-N0-M0)
Stage I	Tumor <2 cm with negative nodes (T1-N0-M0) (includes microinvasive T1, <0.1 cm)
Stage IIA	Tumor 0 to 2 cm with positive nodes (including micrometastasis N1, or <0.2 cm), or 2 to 5 cm with negative nodes (T0-N1, T1-N1, T2-N0, all M0)
Stage IIB	Tumor 2 to 5 cm with positive nodes or >5 cm with negative nodes (T2-N1, T3-N0, all M0)
Stage IIIA	No evidence of primary tumor or tumor <2 cm with involved fixed lymph nodes, or tumor >5 cm with involved movable or nonmovable nodes (T0-N2, T1-N2, T2-N2, T3-N1, T3-N2, all M0)
Stage IIIB	Tumor of any size with direct extension to chest wall or skin, with or without involved lymph nodes, or any size tumor with involved internal mammary lymph nodes (T4-any N, any T-N3, all M0)
Stage IV	Any distant metastasis (includes ipsilateral supraclavicular nodes) (all M1)

*Breast cancer is most frequently staged according to the *TNM classification system*, which evaluates the tumor size (*T*), involvement of regional lymph nodes (*N*), and distant spread of the disease or metastases (*M*).
From Crane-Okada, R. (2001). Breast cancers. In S. Otto (Ed.), *Oncology nursing* (4th ed). St. Louis: Mosby.

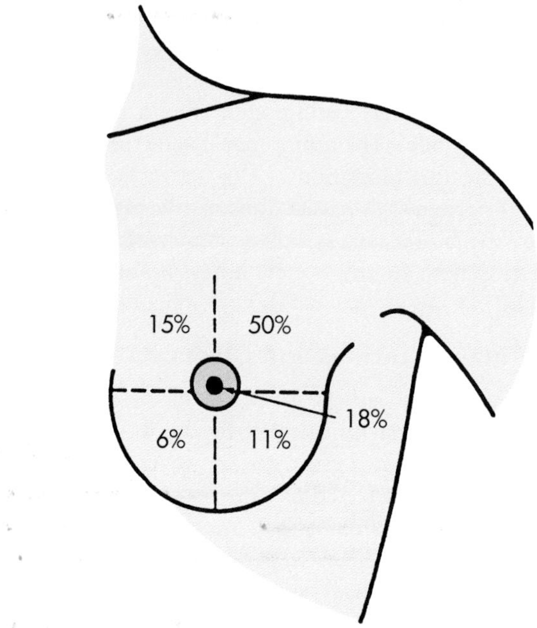
15%
50%
6%
11%
18%

FIG. 11-3 Relative location of malignant lesions of the breast. (Modified from DiSaia, P., & Creasman, W. [2002]. *Clinical gynecologic oncology* [6th ed.]. St. Louis: Mosby.)

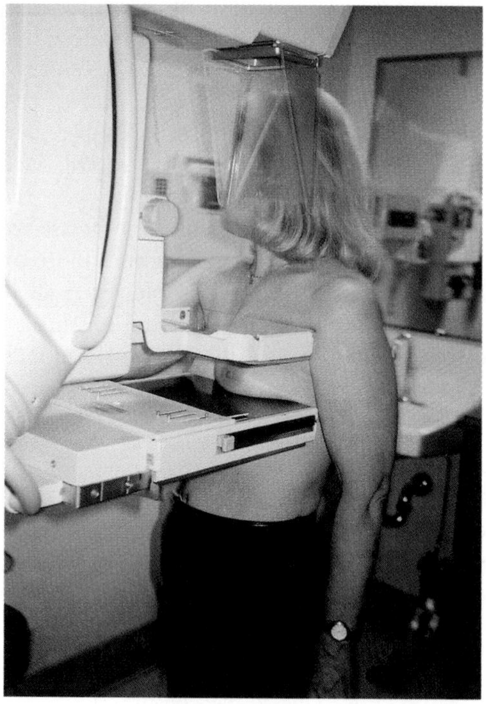

FIG. 11-4 Mammography. (Courtesy Shannon Perry, San Jose, CA.)

adversely affect the woman's subsequent prognosis and treatment options.

Early detection and diagnosis reduce the mortality rate because cancer is found when it is smaller, lesions are more localized, and there tends to be a lower percentage of positive nodes. Therefore it is imperative that protocols for assessment and diagnosis be established. In addition to regular BSE from midadolescence on, the use of clinical examination by a qualified health care provider and screening **mammography** (x-ray filming of the breast) (Fig. 11-4) may aid in the early detection of breast cancers. Table 11-3 lists the current recommendations of the American Cancer Society for breast cancer screening.

TABLE 11-3 **Screening Guidelines for Breast Cancer Detection in Asymptomatic Women Recommended by the American Cancer Society**

AGE (YR)	EXAMINATION	FREQUENCY
20-39	Breast self-examination (BSE)	Monthly
	Clinical breast examination	Every 3 yr
40 and older	BSE	Monthly
	Clinical breast examination	Yearly
	Mammography	Yearly

Source: American Cancer Society. (2003). *Cancer facts and figures, 2003.* New York: American Cancer Society.

Research suggests that the major barriers to screening behaviors are cost, lack of access to health care, and lack of availability of mammography services (Facione, 1999). Strategies that may be helpful to health care providers in improving screening for breast cancer include social marketing campaigns, provision of information about new affordable screening options, continuing education of providers, policies mandating insurance coverage, use of reminder systems in office practice, use of mobile vans and flexible clinic hours, and use of policies for free screenings and walk-in self-referrals (Gulitz et al., 1998).

Cultural factors may influence a woman's decision to participate in breast cancer screening. Knowledge of these factors and use of culturally sensitive tailored messages and materials that appeal to the unique concerns, beliefs, and reading abilities of target groups of underutilizers may assist the nurse in helping women overcome barriers to seeking care (see Cultural Considerations box).

In addition, it is important for a practitioner to assess a woman's BSE technique and frequency at the annual visit. Transillumination, thermography, and ultrasound breast imaging are being explored as methods to detect early breast carcinoma. Ultrasonography is useful in distinguishing between solid tumors and cysts; when combined with mammography, ultrasound examination is helpful in increasing detection of cancers in dense breast tissue (Cady et al., 1998; Jefferson, 1999).

When a suspicious mammogram is noted or a lump is detected, diagnosis is confirmed by FNA, core needle biopsy, or needle localization biopsy (Fig. 11-5). The latter

CULTURAL CONSIDERATIONS

Breast Screening Practices

Lower-income Hispanic women with less than a high school education were found to be more likely not to have participated in screening mammography. Reasons given by the women included fear of the test, misconceptions about cancer, embarrassment, and lack of knowledge (Fernandez et al., 1998). African-American women reported not participating in early breast cancer screening because breast cancer comes from chance, because getting it is determined by a higher being, because of fear of gynecologic examinations, because of doubting the value of early diagnosis and treatment, and because of not believing in vulnerability to cancer because no one in their family has had cancer (Barroso et al., 2000; Lawson, 1998). Both Hispanic and African-American women reported lack of available money to spend on health care, lack of insurance, and perceptions of being treated with prejudice by health care providers because of their race, age, income, or sexual orientation as reasons that they did not participate in breast cancer screening (Facione, 1999).

Chinese-American women were found to believe that they are not likely to get breast cancer and that getting cancer is related to bad luck. If they have symptoms of breast cancer, they are more likely to try Chinese medicine before Western medical treatments (Facione et al., 2000).

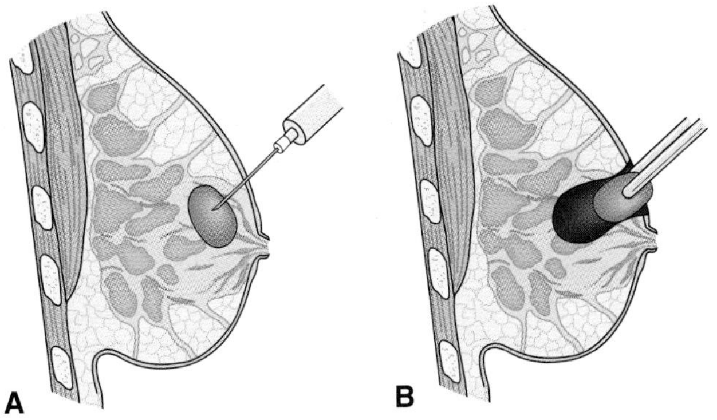
A
B

FIG. 11-5 Diagnosis. **A,** Needle aspiration. **B,** Open biopsy. (Redrawn from National Women's Health Resource Center. [1995]. Breast health. *National Women's Health Report, 13*[5], 3.)

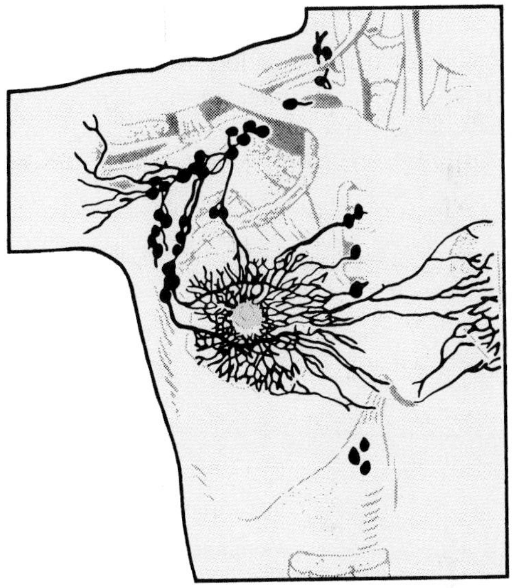

FIG. 11-6 Lymphatic spread of breast cancer.

procedure requires the collaborative efforts of both the radiologist and the surgeon. This often requires that the procedure take place in two different environments (radiology and surgery), so clients need specific information regarding procedures, duration, and outcomes.

Cytologic analysis of cells from aspirated breast tissue is extremely useful as an adjunct to the clinical evaluation of a palpable mass. If the mass remains after aspiration, it should be removed because there is a greater chance of cancer being present (Cady et al., 1998).

Laboratory diagnosis of breast cancer and possible cancer metastasis includes complete blood count, liver enzyme levels, serum calcium level, and alkaline phosphatase level. Elevated liver enzyme levels indicate possible liver metastasis, and increased serum calcium and alkaline phosphatase levels may indicate bone metastasis.

Prognosis

Major advances in the understanding of the biology of cancer have occurred in the past 10 years. Many studies now support the theory that breast cancer is a systemic disease, which means that micrometastasis could be present at the initial presentation with or without nodal involvement (Fiorica, 1997). The area in which affected lymph nodes are located also is prognostic. The closer the lymph nodes are to the shoulder joint, the worse is the prognosis. Nodal involvement and tumor size, however, remain the most significant prognostic criteria for long-term survival (Fig. 11-6).

Other biologic factors have been shown to be helpful in predicting response to therapy or survival. These biologic factors include estrogen receptor assay, progesterone receptor assay, tumor *ploidy* (the amount of DNA in a tumor cell compared with that in a normal cell), S-phase index or growth rate (the percentage of cells in the S phase of cellular division done by flow cytometric determinations of the S-phase fraction), and histologic or nuclear grade (Crane-Okada, 2001). Estrogen and progesterone receptors are proteins in the cell cytoplasm and surface of some breast cancer cells. When these receptors are present, they bind to estrogen or progesterone, and binding promotes growth of the cancer cell. A breast cancer can have estrogen or progesterone receptors (ERs, PRs) or both types. More than 60% of all breast cancers are ER positive, but only two of three tumors respond to antiestrogen therapy. Furthermore, 5% to 10% of ER-negative tumors respond to antiestrogen therapy. Seventy percent of PR-positive and 25% to 30% of PR-negative tumors respond to hormonal therapy (Rosenzweig et al., 2000).

Nuclear grade describes the degree of abnormalities present in the cancer cell tubules, nuclei morphology, and mitotic rates. Tumors with a high nuclear grade tend to have a large number of cells in mitosis and a high S-phase fraction. Tumors with a high S-phase fraction have a large number of cells in the synthesis phase of cell development. If a tumor has high numbers of cells in synthesis and preparing for mitosis and many cells in mitosis, it is growing at a fast rate, is considered aggressive, and carries a poor prognosis. Cancer cells possess altered DNA content. The DNA content of breast cancer cells is analyzed to predict prognosis. Cells with a greater degree of altered DNA content are termed *aneuploid.* High nuclear grade, high S-phase fraction, and aneuploid tumor cells are all indicators of high risk for relapse (Crane-Okada, 2001; Rosenzweig et al., 2000).

Therapeutic Management

Medical management of breast cancer includes surgery, breast reconstruction, radiation therapy, adjuvant hormone therapy, and chemotherapy.

Surgery

After a diagnosis of breast cancer is made, surgical treatment options are offered to the woman. The most frequently recommended surgical approaches for the treatment of breast cancer are lumpectomy and modified radical mastectomy (Fig. 11-7). **Lumpectomy** involves the removal of the breast tumor and a small amount of surrounding tissue, leaving the pectoralis major muscle intact. **Partial mastectomy** includes *tylectomy, wide excision,* and *quadrantectomy* or *segmental mastectomy* and involves removal of different amounts of tissue along with the tumor. Sampling of axillary lymph nodes is usually done through a separate incision at the time of these procedures, and surgery is usually followed by radiation therapy to the remaining breast tissue (Crane-Okada, 2001; DiSaia & Creasman, 2002). These procedures are used for the primary treatment of women with early-stage (I or II) breast cancer. Lumpectomy offers survival equivalent to that with modified radical mastectomy (DiSaia & Creasman, 2002).

Total mastectomy (also called *simple mastectomy)* is the removal of all breast tissue, nipple, and areola; the axillary

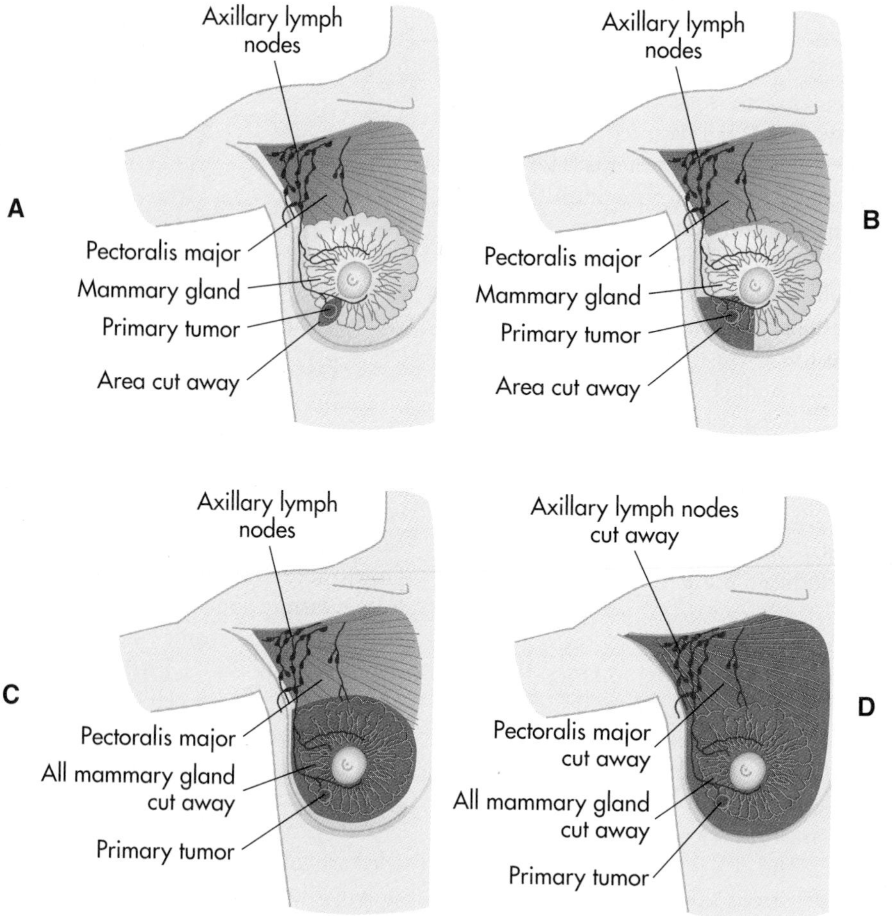
A
Axillary lymph nodes
Pectoralis major
Mammary gland
Primary tumor
Area cut away
B
Axillary lymph nodes
Pectoralis major
Mammary gland
Primary tumor
Area cut away
C
Axillary lymph nodes
Pectoralis major
All mammary gland cut away
Primary tumor
D
Axillary lymph nodes cut away
Pectoralis major cut away
All mammary gland cut away
Primary tumor

FIG. 11-7 Surgical alternatives for breast cancer. **A,** Lumpectomy. **B,** Partial mastectomy. **C,** Total (simple) mastectomy. **D,** Radical mastectomy.

nodes and pectoral muscles are not removed. **Modified radical mastectomy** is the removal of the entire breast and a sample of axillary lymph nodes, sparing the pectoral muscles. A **radical mastectomy,** although rarely performed, removes the entire breast, axillary nodes, and the pectoral muscles. Mastectomy is used for the treatment of early-stage breast cancer when the woman fits the criteria listed in Box 11-4. Women who are found to have metastatic breast cancer at the time of diagnosis usually do not have a mastectomy because it does not offer increased chances of survival. Women who have these surgeries experience cosmetic changes. Change in shape (because of lumpectomy) or loss of a breast results in a change in body image, which can cause significant alterations in perceptions of femininity and sexual image and interest (Fiorica, 1997).

Breast Reconstruction. The goals of surgical breast reconstruction are achievement of symmetry and preservation of body image (Fig. 11-8). Surgical reconstruction can be done immediately or at a later date. Immediate reconstruction at the time of mastectomy does not change survival rates or interfere with therapy or the treatment of recurrent disease (Hacker, 1998). It is important that women be aware of this information. Women choosing surgical reconstruction offer the following rationale for reconstructive surgery: the need to feel complete again, to avoid using an external prosthesis, to achieve symmetry, to decrease self-consciousness about appearance, and to enhance femininity (Fiorica, 1997).

Autologous flap reconstruction involves the use of the woman's own tissue to create a breast. Using the woman's own tissue results in a more natural shape. There are three types of autologous flaps: the latissimus dorsi flap, the transverse rectus abdominis myocutaneous (TRAM) flap, and the inferior gluteus free flap. The latissimus dorsi and TRAM flaps are the most common (Fig. 11-9). The latissimus flap consists of skin, fat, and muscle separated from the upper back, tunneled subcutaneously to an incision in the chest area, and attached to this area (Kroll, 1998). The TRAM flap consists of a portion of skin and fat harvested from the abdominal wall and used to reconstruct the chest area (Resnick & Belcher, 2002). When these flaps are used for reconstruction, they can be pedicled (attached to its blood supply) or free flaps (cut completely from the donor site); adequate blood supply to the reconstructed tissue is a major concern (Sandau, 2002). For this reason, plastic surgeons are careful not to offer this option to women who may be at high risk for complications. Women at high risk for complications include those with extensive, locally invasive breast cancers, extensive chest wall disease, metastatic breast cancer, diabetes mellitus, poorly controlled pulmonary disease, or hypertension (Fiorica, 1997). Women who smoke tobacco, are obese, or have had preoperative chemotherapy or radiation therapy also are at high risk for complications (Moran et al., 2000; Resnick & Belcher, 2002). After the reconstruction is done, postoperative care specific to the procedure focuses on monitoring the skin flap for signs of decreased capillary refill, hematoma, infection, and necrosis. Standard mastectomy activity restrictions and client education points also are followed.

BOX 11-4 Contraindications for Breast Conservation Treatment

- Presence of multiple tumors, especially in different parts of the breast
- Tumor removal alone would produce a cosmetically unacceptable result
- Previous breast radiation
- Pregnancy in the first or second trimester
- Persistent positive margins after reasonable surgery
- Possible history of collagen-vascular disease

Sources: DiSaia, P., & Creasman, W. (2002). *Clinical gynecologic oncology* (6th ed.). St. Louis: Mosby; Shuster, T. et al. (2000). Multidisciplinary care for patients with breast cancer. *Surgical Clinics of North America, 80*(2), 505-533.

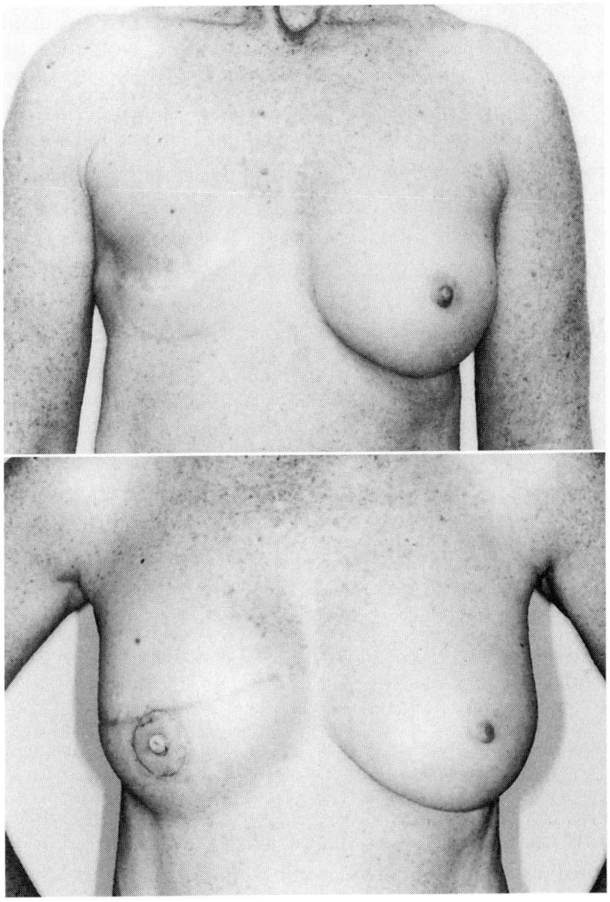

FIG. 11-8 Latissimus dorsi reconstruction after radical mastectomy.

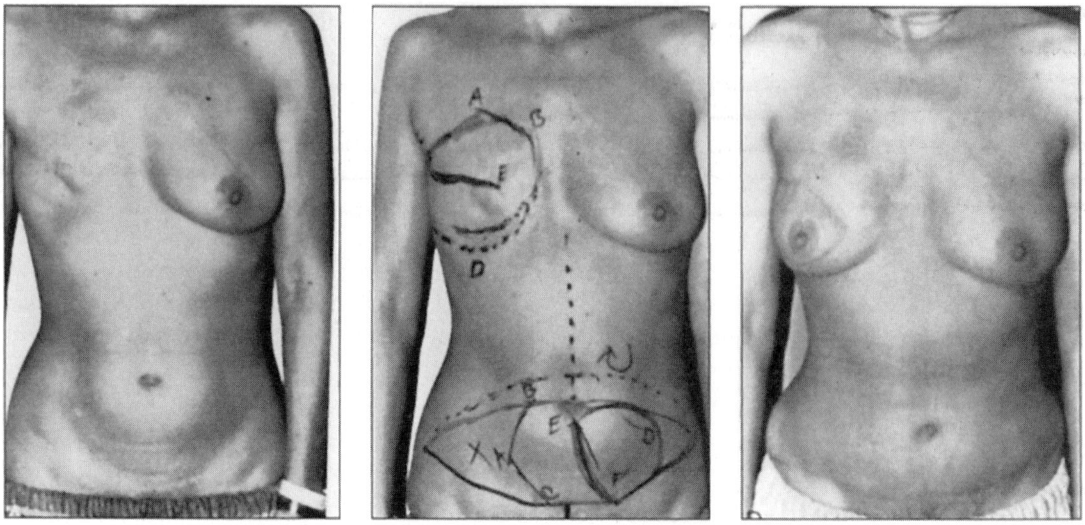

FIG. 11-9 Transverse rectus abdominis myocutaneous (TRAM) flap reconstruction. (From Harden, J., & Girard, N. [1994]. Breast reconstruction using an innovative flap procedure. *AORN Journal, 60*[2], 184-192.)

Another method of surgical reconstruction involves creating a breast mound with a saline-filled tissue expander implanted under the muscle or an autologous flap of the woman's own tissue. Breast reconstruction using implants is not a good option for women with inadequate skin coverage, changes in muscle innervation, or a large, pendulous contralateral breast. A tissue expander is placed under the chest tissue to stretch the surrounding tissue to create adequate space for the permanent implant. The tissue expander is slowly filled with saline, through an injection port, over a period of months, to stretch the skin gradually until the desired symmetry is attained (Resnick & Belcher, 2002). Ongoing emotional support is needed for women who choose this option because they often become impatient waiting for the implant to be totally filled or are self-conscious about the uneven appearance of their breasts. Use of cotton padding to equalize the appearance of the breasts may be helpful during this time. After each saline injection, the woman has mild discomfort, which is easily relieved with ibuprofen or naproxen. As with all implantation procedures, risks of surgical complications such as hematoma, infection, and delayed wound healing are possible, as well as the possibility of capsular contractions from, or leakage of, the implant (Resnick & Belcher, 2002).

The safety of silicone gel breast implants continues to be controversial. Since 1992, the U.S. Food and Drug Administration (FDA) has restricted use of silicone breast implants to women who are undergoing reconstruction after mastectomy, who have had severe breast injuries, who have birth defects that affect the breasts, who have a medical condition causing a severe breast abnormality, or who need to replace an existing implant (Zuckerman, 2002). Women interested in these implants should be informed of all the risks before making a decision (Resnick & Belcher, 2002).

After the woman has recovered from initial reconstructive surgery, she may choose to have nipple and areolar reconstruction. Nipple reconstruction is achieved by using an autologous skin graft to construct a nipple, either from tissue from the remaining nipple or from a donor site. Tiny flaps from the new breast itself also may be used. This outpatient procedure requires local anesthesia, intravenous sedation, or a combination of both, depending on how much sensation has returned to the breast. The procedure lasts about an hour and, 4 weeks later, tattooing may be used to create an areola and match the color of the natural nipple (Sandau, 2002).

Radiation

As mentioned, the conservative approach to treatment involves lumpectomy followed by radiation therapy as standard therapy for early stage breast cancer. Radiation to the breast destroys tumor cells remaining after manipulation and handling of the tumor during surgery. The total recommended radiation dose is 4500 to 5000 cGy over a 6- to 8-week period. A booster dose of up to 1000 cGy may be prescribed with the use of either implants or external beam irradiation (Shuster et al., 2000). The risk of local recurrence depends on several treatment factors such as extent of breast resection, tumor margins, technical details of radiation therapy, and the use of adjuvant systemic therapy. Although radiation after lumpectomy surgery is standard protocol, some large breast tumors may be irradiated before surgery to facilitate easier surgical removal. Side effects of radiation therapy include swelling and heaviness in the breast, sunburnlike skin changes in the treated area, and fatigue. Changes to the breast tissue and skin usually resolve in 6 to 12 months. The breast may become smaller and firmer after radiation therapy. Radiation therapy in the area of the axilla can cause lymphedema of the ipsilateral arm. Close medical follow-up is important after conservative surgery and radiation. Recommended guidelines include a breast physical examination every 4 to 6 months for 2 years, twice a year for 3 years, and then yearly. A mammogram is recommended 6 months after radiation and then annually (National Comprehensive Cancer Network, 2002).

Adjuvant Therapy

Chemotherapy administered soon after initial diagnosis and surgical removal of the tumor is referred to as **adjuvant chemotherapy.** The role of adjuvant chemotherapy in the treatment of breast cancer (chemotherapy and endocrine therapy) is either to eradicate or to impede the growth of micrometastatic (microscopic cell metastasis) disease. Often it is not possible to detect the presence of micrometastasis at the time of initial treatment, and when it is present, mutations can occur in the tumor cells. These mutations make tumor cells resistant to the effects of chemotherapeutic agents despite tumor sensitivity to drug therapy being greatest when the tumor burden is small. Consequently, the prediction cannot be made with confidence that all tumors of 1 cm or less can be cured with initial local and regional treatment. The early introduction of systemic adjuvant therapy, as determined by the estimated risk of tumor recurrence in certain subsets of women with node-negative disease, is a judicious course of treatment. Research findings suggest that adjuvant chemotherapy significantly reduces the risks for recurrence and mortality in patients with node-positive disease (Shuster et al., 2000).

Hormonal therapy. To determine whether a woman is a candidate for hormonal therapy, a receptor assay is done. After the entire tumor or a portion is removed by biopsy or excision, cancer cells are examined by a pathologist for ERs and PRs.

The presence of a receptor on the cell wall indicates that the woman is positive for that type of hormone receptor. If these receptors are present, the growth of the woman's breast cancer may be influenced by estrogen, progesterone, or both. It is unknown exactly how these hormones affect breast cancer growth. Some premenopausal women may undergo bilateral oophorectomy to decrease the supply of hormones available for tumor growth (Hacker, 1998; Shuster et al., 2000). This is done to decrease the odds of recurrence and increase length of survival. In addition to or instead of oophorectomy, medications may be given to stop tumor growth that is influenced by hormones.

Tamoxifen is an oral antiestrogen medication that mimics progesterone and estrogen. Tamoxifen attaches to the hormone receptors on cancer cells and prevents natural hormones from attaching to the receptors. When tamoxifen fits into the receptors, the cell is unable to grow. Research has demonstrated a clear benefit for use of tamoxifen in all age groups. Adjuvant hormonal therapy with tamoxifen is recommended for all women older than 50 years. In this age group, adjuvant tamoxifen therapy improves disease-free survival and, in some cases, length of survival. Use of hormonal therapy for 5 years in women younger than 50 years significantly reduces recurrence and mortality rates. Women treated with hormonal therapy should receive therapy for at least 5 years (DiSaia & Creasman, 2002). Use beyond 5 years in node-positive women remains an acceptable but controversial approach (Shuster et al., 2000). The side effects of hormonal therapy include hot flashes, nausea, vomiting, fluid retention, weight gain, and thrombocytopenia. Tamoxifen therapy also increases the risk of endometrial cancer and deep vein thrombosis (Fiorica, 1997; Pasacreta & McCorkle, 1998) (see Medication Guide box).

Chemotherapy. Chemotherapy drugs are most often given in combination regimens, which have been shown to improve or increase the disease-free survival time after therapy. The most common chemotherapy regimens used for adjuvant treatment of node-positive and node-negative tumors are the following:

CMF (cyclophosphamide, methotrexate, fluorouracil)
CAF (cyclophosphamide, doxorubicin, fluorouracil)
AC (doxorubicin, cyclophosphamide)
A → CMF (doxorubicin followed by CMF)
AC → T (doxorubicin, cyclophosphamide, followed by a taxene)
AT (doxorubicin and a taxene) (DiSaia & Creasman, 2002; Shuster et al., 2000)

MEDICATION GUIDE

Tamoxifen (Nolvadex)

ACTION ▪ Antiestrogenic effects; attaches to hormone receptors on cancer cells and prevents natural hormones from attaching to the receptors.

INDICATION ▪ For treatment of metastatic breast cancer; treatment of breast cancer in postmenopausal women after breast cancer surgery and radiation therapy; to reduce the incidence of breast cancer in women at high risk.

DOSAGE ▪ 20 to 40 mg orally, daily. Dosages greater than 20 mg should be given in divided doses (AM and PM).

ADVERSE REACTIONS ▪ Common side effects include hot flashes, nausea, vomiting, vaginal bleeding or discharge, menstrual irregularities, and rash. Hair loss is an uncommon effect. Serious side effects include deep vein thrombosis, increased risk of endometrial cancer, and stroke.

NURSING CONSIDERATIONS ▪ The medication may be taken on an empty stomach or with food. Missed doses should be taken as soon as possible, but taking two doses at once is not recommended. A barrier or nonhormonal form of contraception is recommended in premenopausal women because tamoxifen may be harmful to the fetus.

Adjuvant chemotherapy has been found to be most useful in premenopausal women who have breast cancer with positive nodes, regardless of hormone receptor status. It is postulated that younger women often have tumors with a higher S-phase fraction and proliferative rate, which makes the tumors more sensitive to chemotherapy (Hacker, 1998; Shuster et al., 2000). Additionally, research results have shown that adjuvant chemotherapy effectively decreases the risks for recurrence and mortality in women with node-positive disease, whether they are premenopausal or postmenopausal and regardless of their hormone receptor status. Numerous clinical trials have investigated the addition of tamoxifen with chemotherapy in various populations of patients with node-negative disease. Research findings showed significant improvement in survival and mortality with the use of adjuvant chemotherapy. Although research results indicated that adjuvant chemotherapy can be justified in all patients with stage I and II breast cancer, regardless of age, hormone receptor status, and nodal status, additional follow-up investigation is needed before any definite conclusions can be drawn regarding optimal management (Shuster et al., 2000).

Chemotherapy with multiple drug combinations is used in the treatment of recurrent and advanced breast cancer with positive results. Paclitaxel (Taxol) and docetaxel (Taxotere, a semisynthetic toxoid) offer first-line therapy for patients with locally advanced or metastatic breast cancer in whom anthracycline-based therapy (doxorubicin) has been unsuccessful or who have a recurrence during anthracycline-based therapy. Capecitabine (Xeloda), an oral chemical precursor of 5-fluorouracil, is given as a treatment for metastatic breast cancer unresponsive to paclitaxel and an anthracycline-containing regimen. It also is given if breast cancers are resistant to paclitaxel and further anthracycline therapy is contraindicated (Mrozek-Orlowski et al., 1999). Herceptin, another drug used in advanced breast cancer, is a recombinant, humanized monoclonal antibody. Herceptin is used for advanced tumors that demonstrate overexpression of the c-erB-2 gene (Goldhirsch et al., 1998). These chemotherapeutic agents provide additional treatment options for women with metastatic breast cancer.

Because chemotherapy drugs are designed to kill rapidly reproducing cells, normal body cells that rapidly reproduce (red and white blood cells, gastric mucosa, and hair) also can be affected during treatment. Thus chemotherapy can cause leukopenia, neutropenia, thrombocytopenia, anemia, gastrointestinal side effects (nausea, vomiting, anorexia, mucositis), and partial or full hair loss.

Chemotherapy treatments are usually given to ambulatory clients, once or twice per month. During the informed consent process, before the treatment is selected, the woman and her family members should be educated about the names of the medications, routes of administration, treatment schedule, timing and ordering of medications, length of time of administration, reimbursed and unreimbursed costs of therapy, potential side effects, management of side effects, possible changes in body image (e.g., full or partial hair loss), recovery time after treatment (necessitating lost work time), and need for a caregiver to transport the woman to treatment and care for her afterward. Depending on the medications used, the treatments may include intravenous, subcutaneous, and oral medications. Often a long-term central venous catheter is inserted when the women will be receiving chemotherapy for an extended period or when she will receive medications that may damage the vein. Presence of a central venous catheter, hair loss, loss of part or all of her breast, menopause, and possible infertility all have the potential to cause a change in body image and increase emotional distress for the woman with breast cancer.

Breast cancer treatment with chemotherapy, hormonal therapy, or a combination of the two often causes changes in reproductive function. The woman who has already been through menopause may have to cope with hair loss and other unpleasant side effects from chemotherapy and loss of part or all of her breast. The premenopausal woman may experience these changes along with symptoms of menopause and possible infertility. It is not known whether hormonal therapy to ease the effects of menopause is safe for women with breast cancer; therefore it is not recommended. For this reason, the nurse must use other measures to help the client cope with menopause (see Chapter 7). The young woman with breast cancer may become devastated by an early and abrupt menopause and the possibility of jeopardized reproductive function. These factors can seriously affect the quality of life of the young woman (Sammarco, 2001) (see Evidence-Based Practice box).

Women receiving chemotherapy and their partners must understand that chemotherapy is a *mutagen* and a *teratogen.* Any woman who is of childbearing age and receiving chemotherapy, even though no longer menstruating, must use birth control. Birth control pills are not recommended because they contain hormones that may assist in the growth of cancer. A birth control method must be chosen with the assistance of the gynecologist and the medical oncologist, and it must be used before chemotherapy begins and continue to be used until the medical oncologist and gynecologist believe it is safe to discontinue.

With the advance in monoclonal antibody technology, it is now possible to test for residual disease with a serum tumor marker, *CA 15-3,* if it is secreted by the client's tumor. From 75% to 80% of women with breast cancer secrete this tumor marker (Stearns et al., 1998). If the level of *CA 15-3* is elevated at the time of diagnosis, circulating levels of *CA 15-3* can be checked periodically through the treatment course to measure response. This technology is used to determine effectiveness of therapy for cancer without the need for second-look diagnostic surgery.

EVIDENCE-BASED PRACTICE

PSYCHOSOCIAL DISTRESS AND BREAST CANCER

Younger and older women with breast cancer have different needs, concerns, and quality-of-life issues in a context of psychosocial life stages that have changed significantly across generations since World War II. Younger women in whom breast cancer develops experience the demands of illness on top of juggling marriage, children, careers, and completion of education (Sammarco, 2001). Crucial issues that can profoundly affect their quality of life include physical and psychosocial effects of treatment, sexual dysfunction, early menopause, fear of recurrence, and disruption of marriage and family (Sammarco, 2001). Older women with breast cancer face the demands of illness on top of the challenges of aging. Older women are living longer, postponing retirement, and seeking to live more independent lifestyles (Sheehy, 1995), yet issues of limited function, development of chronic diseases, lack of support, and financial constraints serve to threaten their quality of life (Lickley, 1997).

Although older women with breast cancer tend to have less psychosocial distress than their younger counterparts (Ferrell et al., 1998), they tend to have inadequate social support, poorer communication with their physicians (Silliman et al., 1998), greater hesitation in seeking initial treatment, and they are more likely to assume a passive role in treatment decision making (Cameron & Horsburgh, 1998). Older women have more functional decline after treatment (Wyatt & Friedman, 1998), and their economic resources may determine how well they recover from breast cancer, because better resources enable them to select services that can hasten recovery (Silliman et al., 1997).

At each significant life stage, the unique emerging problems require specific supports that can decrease or prevent the resulting psychosocial distress (Schain, 1997). Nursing interventions must be developed to address the differences demonstrated by age and psychosocial life stage. Younger women will likely need thorough education, with particular emphasis on issues of sexual function, fertility, disease recurrence, and restoration of physical appearance. They need to understand how different types of therapies will affect the quality of their lives and the lives of their families (Schain, 1997). Older women will likely need thorough education about treatment and follow-up care issues, with particular attention to concerns about monetary costs and functional consequences of treatment in relation to expected benefits (Silliman et al., 1997). Health care providers may need to spend more time with older women during initial and follow-up visits and to encourage their greater participation in treatment decision making.

High-Dose Chemotherapy and Transplant. High-dose chemotherapy followed by *autologous bone marrow transplant (ABMT)* or *peripheral blood stem cell transplant (PSCT)* may be offered to women with breast cancer who have a high risk of relapse or metastatic disease (Crane-Okado, 2001). Although initial studies showed a favorable impact on disease-free survival in women who had metastatic disease, definitive analysis of the benefits or limitations of these treatments is not available (Hinterberger-Fischer & Hinterberger, 2001; Montemurro et al., 2000). PSCT may be preferred to ABMT because it seems to have lower morbidity and mortality and may cost less. Clinical trials are in progress to evaluate the effectiveness of these procedures.

CARE MANAGEMENT

Assessment and Nursing Diagnoses

The nurse takes a client history of symptoms, including timing of detection of lump, size, changes, location, nipple discharge, and breast symmetry.

In addition to taking a history and palpating the breast lump, a clinician should compare past and present mammographic findings with physical assessment findings. The mass should be described in terms of location (by using the clock-dial method), shape, size, consistency, and fixation to the surrounding tissues. Skin changes, such as dimpling, peau d'orange, increased vascularity, nipple retraction, or ulceration, may indicate advanced disease, so their presence should be recorded. Physical examination includes palpation of the infraclavicular, supraclavicular, and axillary lymph nodes. Pain and soreness in the affected breast and arm should be evaluated. Often a diagram of the breast is drawn, and findings are recorded in the client record. Psychosocial assessment should include not only the client's present emotional state but also the reaction of her family and significant others and history of handling crises. The nurse should determine what the diagnosis of cancer means to the woman and her family.

Nursing diagnoses for women with a diagnosis of breast cancer might include the following:

- *Fear/anxiety related to*
  - –diagnosis of breast cancer
  - –treatment choices
  - –choice of reconstructive procedure
- *Risk for decisional conflict related to*
  - –choices of and controversies about treatment options
- *Risk for sexual dysfunction related to*
  - –altered body image
  - –side effects of therapy
- *Risk for compromised/disabled family coping related to*
  - –diagnosis and prognosis
- *Anticipatory grieving related to*
  - –loss of breast or diagnosis of advanced cancer
- *Fatigue related to*
  - –cancer treatments
- *Acute pain related to*
  - –incision or metastatic cancer
- *Impaired skin integrity related to*
  - –surgery or radiation
- *Disturbed body image related to*
  - –loss of breast
  - –hair loss (chemotherapy)

Expected Outcomes of Care

Planning realistic outcomes in collaboration with the woman might include that the woman will do the following:

- Experience a reasonable level of anxiety related to diagnosis that does not interfere with use of healthy coping mechanisms.
- Elicit appropriate support from significant others.
- Choose among alternative treatment options and verbalize satisfaction with the decision-making process.
- Report satisfactory sexual functioning after surgery.
- Demonstrate necessary self-care techniques correctly.
- Accept a change in body image and demonstrate a positive self-concept.

Other expected outcomes include the following:

- The family will adapt to the diagnosis and provide appropriate support through all stages of treatment.
- The woman's skin will remain intact and will heal without complications.
- The woman will continue usual activities as tolerated during treatment.

Plan of Care and Interventions

Nursing actions that will best assist the woman in achieving her expected outcomes are selected, such as the following:

- Provide time to discuss the diagnosis, answer questions, and listen to concerns.
- Encourage ventilation of feelings by the woman and family in a nonjudgmental atmosphere.
- Offer information about support groups or individual therapy for the woman and the family members, including children.

Emotional Support After Diagnosis

When a woman is confronted with a diagnosis of cancer, she is confronted not only with possible major changes in appearance but also with the possibility of death. The emotional reaction to the diagnosis of cancer is always intense, and the many disruptions caused by the disease challenge the woman's and family's ability to cope. Disruptions may be caused by costs of treatment, loss of role function, lack of stress-relieving activities, spouse's or child's reaction to the diagnosis, change in body image and sexual function, disability, and pain. The woman may feel despair, fear, and shame. Sexuality issues related to breast cancer include a change in body image, changes in sexual function (such as decreased vaginal lubrication caused by hormonal therapy), and relational distress. It is the nurse's responsibility to discuss the influence of breast cancer on the woman's life and to assist the woman and her family in coping effectively with these changes. Some women find that after adjusting to the diagnosis of cancer, they have a greater appreciation of the experiences of daily life. They may feel encouraged to focus on what is most important and meaningful.

Clients and their families often undergo a period of distress after the diagnosis of cancer. It is difficult to accept the diagnosis of cancer when the woman may feel and look well. This period is characterized by anguish and shock followed by disbelief and denial. During this time, absorbing information and education can be difficult, and the nurse should be sensitive as to how this may affect decision-making abilities. Flexibility is the key to sensitive nursing care. As the woman and family begin to accept the diagnosis of breast cancer, more and more information can be shared, and care planning with full client participation can take place, including the following:

- Validate and reinforce accurate information processing by the woman and her family.
- Suggest approaches the woman might take to deal with the sexual concerns of her significant other.
- Discuss the application of alternative therapies to alleviate stress and promote healing, such as exercise, guided imagery, meditation, and progressive muscle relaxation (Kolcaba & Fox, 1999).
- Refer the woman to the American Cancer Society's Reach to Recovery program.
- Refer the woman to a cancer rehabilitation program, such as ENCORE, a program run by the YWCA.
- Assist in client decision-making and arrange for the woman to speak with breast cancer survivors who have chosen a variety of treatment options (Box 11-5).

The National Comprehensive Cancer Network (NCCN) and the American Cancer Society now provide specific, up-to-date recommendations on breast cancer treatments on the Internet (see Resources at end of the chapter). This is an invaluable resource for women to learn about scientifically tested treatment protocols for each stage of breast cancer (American Cancer Society, 2002).

BOX 11-5 Decision-Making Questions to Ask

1. What kind of breast cancer is it (invasive or noninvasive)?
2. What is the stage of the cancer (i.e., how extensive is the spread)?
3. Did the cancer test positive for hormone (estrogen)? (May be slower growing.)
4. What further tests are recommended?
5. What are the treatment options? (Pros and cons of each, including side effects.)
6. If surgery is recommended, what will the scar look like?
7. If a mastectomy is done, can breast reconstruction be done (at the time of surgery or later)?
8. How long will the client be in the hospital? What kind of postoperative care will the client need?
9. How long will treatment last if radiation or chemotherapy is recommended? What effects can the client expect from these treatments?
10. What community resources are available for support?

Source: National Women's Health Resource Center. (1999). Breast health. *National Women's Health Report, 17*(5), 1-11.

After assisting the woman with accepting the diagnosis and obtaining support, consider nursing care in the preoperative, postoperative, and convalescent period. The discussion that follows is pertinent to the care required by a woman who is having a modified radical mastectomy.

Preoperative Care

General preoperative teaching and care are given, including expectations regarding physical appearance, pain management, equipment to be used (e.g., intravenous therapy, drains), and emotional support. Some emotional support may be obtained by arranging for a visit from a member of an organization such as Reach for Recovery. The woman is reminded that when she awakens after surgery, her arm on the affected side will feel tight.

Immediate Postoperative Care

After recovery from anesthesia, the woman is returned to her room. Special precautions must be observed to prevent or to minimize lymphedema of the affected arm.

NURSE ALERT

When vital signs are taken, never apply the blood pressure cuff on the affected arm.

The affected arm is elevated with pillows above the level of the right atrium. Blood is not drawn from this arm, and this arm is not used for intravenous therapy. Early arm movement is encouraged. Any increase in the circumference of that arm is reported immediately.

Nursing care of the wound involves observation for signs of hemorrhage (dressing, drainage tubes, and Hemovac or Jackson-Pratt drainage reservoirs are emptied at least every 8 hours and more frequently as needed), shock, and infection. Dressings are reinforced as necessary. The woman is asked to turn (alternating between unaffected side and back), cough (while the nurse or the woman applies support to the chest), and deep breathe every 2 hours. Breath sounds are auscultated every 4 hours. Active range-of-motion (ROM) exercise of legs is encouraged. Parenteral fluids are given until adequate oral intake is possible. Emotional support is continued.

Care given during the immediate postoperative period is continued as necessary. Most women who undergo lumpectomy have surgery as ambulatory clients and return home a few hours after surgery. Women are discharged 24 to 48 hours after modified radical mastectomy. Because of the short time spent in the hospital, thorough teaching is important. It is best to do as much teaching as possible before surgery if the outcome is known. If this is not possible, discharge teaching should be done with the woman's caregiver present. This is to acknowledge the possibility that emotional stress or recovery from anesthesia may cause the woman to forget some of the discharge instructions. Printed information also should be provided for the woman and family to refer to at home.

Women who have had breast surgery are usually seen by their surgeon within 5 days of surgery. This follow-up visit is important because it allows the physician to assess the outcome of surgical treatment as well as to provide reinforcement of education and emotional support.

Mobility is a key subject to be addressed with women having breast surgery. Early ambulation is encouraged to improve circulation and ventilation and to prevent loss of calcium from bone. The psychologic benefits of early mobility include resumption of self-care and activities of daily living that serve to reinforce the woman's control over her life and help her move from a sick role to the role of breast cancer survivor.

Arm exercises are encouraged at least four times daily (Box 11-6). Exercise is increased as tolerated and is stopped at the point of pain. Initially the woman alternately clenches and extends her fingers and then progresses to wrist and elbow exercises, gradually abducting her arm and raising it to and over her head. She is encouraged to exercise by assisting with her care–washing her face, brushing her teeth, and eating with her hand and arm on the affected side. Physical therapy may be prescribed to improve strength and mobility of the affected arm.

BSE of the unaffected breast, bilateral axillae, and remaining breast in women who have had a lumpectomy is another key teaching subject. Written client education materials are available from the American Cancer Society and National Cancer Institute and should be shared with the woman and her family.

It is important to discuss the appearance of the woman's breast if dressings have not been removed before discharge. Some women may not want to view their surgical site, but it is important to give them the opportunity and to provide emotional support at that time. The woman should be encouraged to express her emotions and verbalize her feelings. The woman needs to know that it will take time to become accustomed to her change of appearance.

An option for restoration of body image is choosing an external prosthesis to replace the lost breast or portion of breast tissue. The external prosthesis is inserted into the brassiere. Women who choose to use a partial external prosthesis after lumpectomy or full external prosthesis after mastectomy need information about where to obtain prostheses and appropriate brassieres. Women need to be advised on how to submit the cost of the prosthesis to their insurance company. Volunteers of the American Cancer Society's Reach to Recovery program are able to provide this information, as well as a list of sources for prostheses and lingerie. They can offer helpful hints and suggestions for coping with prostheses and wearing apparel. Some women find that an external prosthesis does not restore body image and seek surgical reconstruction of the missing or disfigured breast (see previous discussion).

Discharge Planning and Follow-up Care

Before discharge, considerable time should be spent counseling the woman and her family about the aspects of self-care. These instructions are summarized in the Teaching for Self-Care box. Printed instructions should be given to the woman

BOX 11-6 Arm Exercises After Lymph Node Dissection

Check with your health care provider before performing these exercises. Perform exercises slowly to stretch the muscle gently. Repeat exercises several times a day with time to rest in between.

EXERCISE: CLIMBING THE WALL

1. Stand facing wall with toes close to wall.
2. Bend elbows and place palms of hands against wall at shoulder level.
3. Move both hands parallel to each other up the wall as far as possible until incisional pull or pain occurs.
4. Move both hands down to starting position either by sliding them back down or walking them back down.
5. Goal is to reach all the way up with arm in complete extension with elbow straight. Repeat several times.
6. Perform activities that use the same action: reaching top shelves, washing windows, blow-drying hair.

EXERCISE: ROPE PULL

1. Attach a 6-foot rope over a shower rod or a hook at the top of a door.
2. Grasp one end of the rope in each hand, and extend your arms to your sides. Pull down on one end while raising the other arm, raising arm as high as you can (on affected side to a point of incisional pull or pain). Reverse the exercise, with the raised arm being lowered and raising the lower arm.
3. Shorten rope over time until arm on affected side is raised almost directly overhead.

EXERCISE: ELBOW SPREAD

1. Clasp hands behind neck.
2. Raise elbows to chin level, holding head erect; move slowly and rest when incisional pull or pain occurs.
3. Gradually spread elbows apart; rest when pull or pain occurs. Repeat several times.

EXERCISE: ARM OVER HEAD

1. Lie down with your arms by your side.
2. Raise the arm on the surgery side straight up and reach over your head. Repeat several times.

TEACHING FOR SELF-CARE

After a Mastectomy

- Wash hands well before and after touching incision area or drains.
- Empty surgical drains twice a day and as needed, recording the date, time, drain site (if more than one drain is present), and amount of drainage in milliliters in diary you will take to each surgical checkup until your drains are removed. (Before discharge, you may receive a graduated container for emptying drains and measuring drainage.)
- Avoid driving, lifting more than 10 pounds, or reaching above your head until given permission by surgeon.
- Take medications for pain as soon as pain begins.
- Perform arm exercises as directed.
- Call physician if inflammation of incision or swelling of the incision or the arm occurs.
- Avoid tight clothing, tight jewelry, and other causes of decreased circulation in the affected arm.
- Until drains are removed, wear loose-fitting underwear (camisole or half-slip) and clothes, pinning surgical drains inside of clothing. (You will be taught how to do this safely.)
- After drains are removed and surgical sites are healing and still tender, wear a mastectomy bra or camisole with a cotton-filled, muslin temporary prosthesis. Temporary prostheses of this type are often available from Reach to Recovery.
- Avoid depilatory creams, strong deodorants, and shaving of affected chest area, axilla, and arm.
- Sponge bathe until drains are removed.
- Return to the surgeon's office for incision check, drain inspection, and possible drain removal as directed.
- Contact Reach to Recovery for assistance in obtaining external prosthesis and lingerie when dressings, drains, and staples are removed and wound is healing and nontender.
- Contact insurance company for information about coverage of prosthesis and wig if needed. Obtain prescriptions for prosthesis and wig to submit with receipts of purchase for these items to the insurance company. If insurance does not pay for these items, contact hospital or agency social worker or local American Cancer Society for assistance.
- Continue with monthly BSE of unaffected side and affected surgical site and axilla.
- Encourage mother, sisters, and daughters (if applicable) to learn and practice monthly BSE and to have annual professional breast examinations and mammography (if appropriate).
- Keep follow-up visits for professional examination, mammography, and testing to detect recurrent breast cancer.
- Expect decreased sensation and tingling at incision sites and in the affected arm for weeks to months after surgery.
- Resume sexual activities as desired.

and her family. A referral for home nursing care may be made if the woman needs assistance caring for her incision.

Teaching Needs for the Client and Family Undergoing Adjuvant Therapies

It is important that the woman and her family be given thorough instructions regarding side effects and avoidance of possible complications of adjuvant treatment. A common side effect of radiation therapy is skin irritation and breakdown. The woman should avoid using lotions, powders, or ointments on the skin at the radiation site unless instructed by the radiologist. The skin should be cleansed gently with mild soap and water, rinsed thoroughly, and patted dry. Skin markings that direct the placement of the radiation beam should not be removed. Soft, nonirritating clothing should be worn over the site,

Plan of Care — Woman After Breast Conserving Surgery and Axillary Node Dissection

NURSING DIAGNOSIS Acute pain related to surgical incision and surgical drains, as evidenced by client verbalizations

Expected Outcome *Woman will report minimal intensity and decreased number of painful episodes.*

Nursing Interventions/*Rationales*

Use pain scale to assess type and intensity of pain *to provide accurate database.*

Administer analgesics as ordered *to decrease perception of pain.*

Teach and reinforce use of relaxation techniques *to reduce anxiety and provide distraction that may decrease the perception of pain.*

Reposition woman with affected arm elevated *to promote comfort and lymphatic channel return.*

NURSING DIAGNOSIS Risk for infection related to disruption of skin integrity and removal of lymph nodes

Expected Outcome *Client will experience no clinical manifestations of infection.*

Nursing Interventions/*Rationales*

Assess clinical manifestations of infection at the incision and drain sites that may include redness, swelling, localized heat, fever, increasing pain, and foul-smelling drainage *to facilitate prompt treatment.*

Demonstrate the procedure for emptying and recording the amount of drainage from the Jackson-Pratt drain(s) *to provide information to the surgeon as to the appropriate removal time of drains. Drains are usually removed when 24 hours of drainage does not exceed 30 ml of fluid.*

Explain the need to avoid trauma or irritation to the affected arm *to reinforce to the woman that alterations in sensation and removal of some lymph nodes may affect ability to sense irritation or prevent infection.*

Reinforce to the woman the need to protect arm from injury and to avoid blood drawing or blood pressures to be taken on the affected arm *to avoid trauma and infection, because decreased sensation may be present as well as decreased lymphatic return.*

Explain the importance of reporting any clinical manifestations of infection to the caregiver as soon as possible *to provide identification and treatment of problem.*

NURSING DIAGNOSIS Disturbed body image related to loss of all or part of a breast as evidenced by client statements.

Expected Outcomes *Woman will report acceptance of herself as she is and regain a positive body image.*

Nursing Interventions/*Rationales*

Provide opportunity through therapeutic communication to express feelings about body image changes *to clarify and validate feelings.*

Provide information about breast prostheses and other cosmetic devices *to assist in maintaining an intact body image.*

Encourage woman to speak to physician about the possibility of breast reconstructive surgery *to provide additional resources for body image enhancement.*

Refer to support groups *to facilitate verbalization of feelings with women who have similar concerns.*

NURSING DIAGNOSIS Impaired physical mobility related to pain and tissue trauma

Expected Outcomes *The woman will return to her preoperative level of mobility*

Nursing Interventions/*Rationales*

Encourage woman to do hand, arm, and wrist exercises that can be performed in the immediate postoperative period *to enhance fluid return and prevent muscle atrophy.*

Encourage woman to perform activities of daily living as much as possible *to encourage woman to focus on her strengths rather than on her limitations.*

Teach woman exercises to be performed after the drains are removed *to promote range of motion in the arm that had the axillary nodes dissected.*

Teach woman to do exercises slowly and gently *to prevent injury and pain.*

Caution woman not to lift anything heavier than 10 pounds for 4 to 6 weeks *to avoid exerting strain on affected arm.*

and the skin should be protected from exposure to sun and heat.

Common side effects of chemotherapy include alopecia, fatigue, nausea, vomiting, mouth sores, and immunosuppression. The woman planning to receive chemotherapy that produces hair loss should be encouraged to obtain a wig matching her own hair color and style before beginning treatments so that she is prepared when hair loss begins. The American Cancer Society can assist the woman in obtaining a wig and head coverings designed for women experiencing hair loss from chemotherapy. The woman should be taught the importance of rest periods when fatigue occurs. The woman and her family will need to know that work and family schedules may need adjustment to accommodate needed rest. Nausea and vomiting should be reported to the physician and are treated with antiemetics. Mouth sores may be very painful, and the woman should be instructed to maintain good oral hygiene and avoid trauma to the oral mucosa. The mouth should be rinsed frequently with water or saline, and mouthwashes containing alcohol or glycerine should be avoided. Spicy or irritating foods should be avoided. Topical anesthetic medications may be prescribed by the physician. The woman with immunosuppression should be instructed to use frequent handwashing and avoid crowds and other large gatherings of people, especially during cold and flu season. She should be taught to avoid eating raw fruits and vegetables (low-bacteria diet) and maintain strict personal hygiene. The woman should be taught the signs and symptoms of infection and to report them to the physician immediately.

Evaluation

Evaluation is based on the client-centered expected outcomes. The nurse can be assured that care was effective to the extent that the goals for care have been achieved (see Plan of Care).

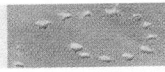

KEY POINTS

- The development of breast neoplasms, whether benign or malignant, can have a significant physical and emotional effect on the woman and her family.
- The risk of American women developing cancer of the breast is one in eight.
- An estimated 90% of all breast lumps are detected by the woman during BSE.
- Monthly BSE, routine screening mammography, and yearly breast examinations by practitioners are recommended for early detection of breast cancer.
- The modified radical mastectomy is the most common surgical procedure for breast cancer, although lumpectomy and radiation may be an alternative for stage I and II disease and tumors 4 cm or smaller.
- Adjuvant chemotherapy is most helpful to premenopausal women with breast cancer that has spread to the lymph nodes.
- Tamoxifen, along with other promising new drug therapies currently under investigation, may provide the first real hope for the prevention of breast cancer.
- The emotional diagnosis of breast cancer is always intense, and the many disruptions caused by the disease challenge the woman's and her family's ability to cope.

CRITICAL THINKING EXERCISES

1. Younger women with breast cancer are more vulnerable to psychosocial distress and poor emotional adjustment than are their older counterparts. What role demands of younger women are affected by this disease? What unique quality-of-life issues emerge as the younger woman's cancer is diagnosed and treated? What interventions would be most helpful in assisting the younger woman with breast cancer to maintain an acceptable quality of life?
2. You are assigned to a woman who is undergoing modified radical mastectomy followed by chemotherapy for breast cancer.
   a. What physical, psychosocial, spiritual, and socioeconomic needs may be exhibited by this woman? What might be the special needs of her family?
   b. What kind of effective support system is needed by the woman and her family undergoing treatment for breast cancer? What barriers to support may prevent the woman and her family from receiving adequate social support?
   c. Develop a plan of care for this woman and her family.
3. Assess the availability of breast cancer screening in your community. What services are provided? Are the programs accessible to multiethnic and lower socioeconomic populations? What kind of marketing strategies have been used to encourage women to use these services?

RESOURCES

American Cancer Society
1599 Clifton Rd., NE
Atlanta, GA 30329
800-ACS-2345
www.cancer.org

Breast Cancer Action
55 New Montgomery St., Suite 323
San Francisco, CA 94105
415-243-9301
www.bcaction.org

Food and Drug Administration (FDA)
Office of Consumer Affairs
Public Inquiries
5600 Fishers Lane (HFE-88)
Rockville, MD 20857
301-443-3170
www.fda.gov

National Alliance of Breast Cancer Organizations
9 East 37th St., 10th Floor
New York, NY 10016
800-719-0154
www.nabco.org

National Breast Cancer Coalition
P.O. Box 66373
Washington, DC 20035
202-296-7477
800-935-0434
www.natlbcc.org

National Cancer Institute Cancer Information Service
800-4-CANCER
www.nci.nih.gov

National Comprehensive Cancer Network
888-909-NCCN
www.nccn.org

National Women's Health Resource Center
120 Albany St., Suite 820
New Brunswick, NJ 08901
877-986-9472
www.healthywomen.org

Y-ME National Breast Cancer Organization
www.y-me.org

REFERENCES

American Cancer Society. (2002). Breast cancer information [on-line]. Available at www.cancer.org/bottomcancinfo.html. Accessed 6/15/02.

American Cancer Society. (2003). *Cancer facts and figures 2003.* New York: American Cancer Society.

Arthur, B., & Janssen, P. (2000). Silicone breast implants: What do we know about the long-term effects? *AWHONN Lifelines, 4*(5), 28-32.

Barroso, J. et al. (2000). Comparison between African-American and white women in their beliefs about breast cancer and their health locus of control. *Cancer Nursing, 23*(4), 268-276.

Cady, B. et al. (1998). Evaluation of common breast problems: Guidance for primary care providers. *CA: A Cancer Journal for Clinicians, 48*, 49-63.

Cameron, S., & Horsburgh, M. (1998). Comparing issues faced by younger and older women with breast cancer. *Canadian Oncology Nursing Journal, 8*(1), 40-44.

Chadbourne, E. et al. (2001). Clinical outcomes in reduction mammaplasty: A systematic review and meta-analysis of published studies. *Mayo Clinic Proceedings, 76*, 503-510.

Crane-Okada, R. (2001). Breast cancers. In S. Otto (Ed.), *Oncology nursing* (4th ed). St. Louis: Mosby.

Cummings, S. (2001). Weighing the risks: Genetic counseling for hereditary breast and ovarian cancer. *AWHONN Lifelines, 5*(3), 42-47.

DiSaia, P., & Creasman, W. (2002). *Clinical gynecologic oncology* (6th ed.). St. Louis: Mosby.

Facione, N. (1999). Breast cancer screening in relation to access to health services. *Oncology Nursing Forum, 26*(4), 689-696.

Facione, N. et al. (2000). Perceived risk and help-seeking behavior for breast cancer: A Chinese-American perspective. *Cancer Nursing, 23*(4), 258-267.

Fernandez, M., Tortolero-Luna, G., & Gold, R. (1998). Mammography and Pap test screening among low-income foreign-born Hispanic women in USA. *Cadernos de Saude Publica, 14*(suppl 3), 133-147.

Ferrell, B. et al. (1998). Quality of life in breast cancer survivors: Implications for developing support services. *Oncology Nursing Forum, 25*(5), 887-895.

Fiorica, J. (1997). Breast cancer. In P. Leppert & F. Howard (Eds.), *Primary care for women*. Philadelphia: Lippincott-Raven.

Friedenreich, C. et al. (2000). Risk factors for benign breast disease. *International Journal of Epidemiology, 29*, 637-644.

Furniss, K. (2000). Tomatoes, Pap smears and tea? Adopting behaviors that may prevent reproductive cancers and improve health. *Journal of Obstetric, Gynecologic, and Neonatal Nursing, 29*(6), 641-652.

Goldhirsch, A. et al. (1998). New treatments for breast cancer: Breakthroughs for patient care or just steps in the right direction? *Annals of Oncology, 9*, 973-976.

Grassley, B. (2002). Breast reduction surgery: What every woman needs to know. *AWHONN Lifelines, 6*(3), 244-249.

Gulitz, E., Bustillo-Hernandez, M., & Kent, E. (1998). Missed cancer screening opportunities among older women. *Cancer Practice, 6*(5), 289-295.

Hacker, N. (1998). Breast disease: A gynecologic perspective. In N. Hacker & J. Moore (Eds.), *Essentials of obstetrics and gynecology* (3rd ed.). Philadelphia: W.B. Saunders.

Harden, J., & Girard, N. (1994). Breast reconstruction using an innovative flap procedure. *AORN Journal, 60*(2), 184-192.

Hawkins, J., Roberto-Nichols, D., & Stanley-Haney, J. (1997). *Protocols for nurse practitioners in gynecologic settings* (6th ed.). New York: Tiresias Press.

Hinterberger-Fischer, M., & Hinterberger, T. (2001). Blood stem cell transplantation for breast cancer: New approaches using pre-peri-post-transplant immunotherapy. *Expert Opinion in Biologic Therapy, 1*(6), 1029-1048.

Jefferson, T. (1999). Ultrasound may markedly improve cancer detection in dense breasts. *Journal of the American Medical Association, 281*(4), 311-312.

Johnson-Thompson, M., & Guthrie, J. (2000). Ongoing research to identify environmental risk factors in breast carcinoma. *Cancer, 88*(5), 1224-1229.

Kissinger, L. et al. (2002). Chemoprevention of breast cancer: A summary of the evidence for the U.S. Preventive Services Task Force. *Annals of Internal Medicine, 137*(1), 59-69.

Kolcaba, K., & Fox, C. (1999). The effects of guided imagery on comfort of women with early stage breast cancer undergoing radiation therapy. *Oncology Nursing Forum, 26*(10), 72-76.

Kroll, S. (1998). Why autologous tissue? *Clinics in Plastic Surgery, 25*(2), 135-143.

Lauver, D. et al. (1999). Engagement in breast cancer screening behaviors. *Oncology Nursing Forum, 26*(3), 545-554.

Lawson, E. (1998). A narrative analysis: A black woman's perception of breast cancer risks and early breast cancer detection. *Cancer Nursing, 21*(6), 421-429.

Lickley, L. (1997). Primary breast cancer in the elderly. *Canadian Journal of Surgery, 40*(5), 341-351.

Marchant, D. (1998). Controversies in benign breast disease. *Surgical Oncology Clinics of North America, 7*(2), 285-298.

Marsden, J. (2002). Hormone-replacement therapy and breast cancer. *Lancet Oncology, 3*(5), 303-311.

McCool, W., Stone-Condry, M., & Bradford, H. (1998). Breast health care: A review. *Journal of Nurse Midwifery, 43*(6), 406-430.

McKeon, V. (1997). The Breast Cancer Prevention Trial: Evaluating tamoxifen's efficacy in preventing breast cancer. *Journal of Obstetric, Gynecologic, and Neonatal Nursing, 26*(1), 79-90.

McPherson, K., Steel, C., & Dixon, J. (2000). ABC of breast diseases: Breast cancer epidemiology, risk factors, and genetics. *British Medical Journal, 321*(9), 624-628.

Montemurro, F. et al. (2000). High dose chemotherapy with hematopoietic stem-cell transplantation for breast cancer: Current status, future trends. *Clinics in Breast Cancer, 1*(3), 197-209.

Moran, S. et al. (2000). TRAM flap breast reconstruction with expanders and implants. *AORN Journal, 71*(2), 354-362.

Mrozek-Orlowski, M., Frye, D., & Sanborn, H. (1999). Capecitabine: Nursing implications of a new oral chemotherapeutic agent. *Oncology Nursing Forum, 26*(4), 753-762.

National Cancer Institute. (2002). *Cancer trials information* [on-line]. Available at www.nci.nih.gov/clinicaltrials/. Accessed 5/22/02.

National Comprehensive Cancer Network. (2002). *Breast cancer treatment guidelines for patients* [on-line]. Available at www.nccn.org. Accessed 6/4/02.

National Women's Health Resource Center (1995). Breast health. *National Women's Health Report, 13*(5), 3.

National Women's Health Resource Center. (1999). Breast health. *National Women's Health Report, 17*(5), 1-11.

National Women's Health Resource Center. (2000). Genetic testing and women's health. *National Women's Health Report, 22*(6), 1-8.

Nelson, N. (2000). Silicone breast implants not linked to breast cancer risk. *Journal of the National Cancer Institute, 92*(21), 1714-1715.

Nogueira, S., & Appling, S. (2000). Breast cancer genetics, risks, and strategies. *Nursing Clinics of North America, 35*(3): 663-669.

Pasacreta, J., & McCorkle, R. (1998). Providing accurate information to women about tamoxifen therapy for breast cancer: Current indications, effects, and controversies. *Oncology Nursing Forum, 25*, 1577-1583.

Resnick, B., & Belcher, A. (2002). Breast reconstruction. *American Journal of Nursing, 102*(4), 26-33.

Rosenzweig, M., Rust, D., & Hoss, J. (2000). Prognostic information in breast cancer care: Helping patients utilize important information. *Clinical Journal of Oncology Nursing, 4*(6), 271-278.

Sammarco, A. (2001). Perceived social support, uncertainty, and quality of life of younger breast cancer survivors. *Cancer Nursing, 24*(3), 212-218.

Sandau, K. (2002). Free TRAM flap breast reconstruction. *American Journal of Nursing, 102*(4), 36-43.

Schain, W. (1997). Psychosocial issues and life-cycle concerns of women with breast cancer. *Cancer Prevention and Control, 1*(2), 122-132.

Sheehy, G. (1995). *New passages: Mapping your life across time*. New York: Random House.

Shuster, T. et al. (2000). Multidisciplinary care for patients with breast cancer. *Surgical Clinics of North America, 80*(2), 505-533.

Silliman, R. et al. (1998). Breast cancer care in older women: Sources of information, social support, and emotional health outcomes. *Cancer, 83*(4), 706-711.

Silliman, R. et al. (1997). The impact of age, marital status, and physician-patient interactions on the care of older women with breast carcinoma. *Cancer, 80*(7), 1326-1334.

Stearns, V., Yamauchi, H., & Hayes, D. (1998). Circulating tumor markers in breast cancer: Accepted utilities and novel prospects. *Breast Cancer Research and Treatment, 52*(13), 239-259.

Stenchever, M. et al. (2001). *Contemporary gynecology* (4th ed.). St. Louis: Mosby.

Vogel, V. et al. (2002). The study of tamoxifen and raloxifene: Preliminary enrollment data from a randomized breast cancer risk reduction trial. *Clinics in Breast Cancer, 3*(2), 153-159.

Writing Group for the Women's Health Initiative Investigators. (2002). Risks and benefits of estrogen plus progestin in healthy postmenopausal women: Principal results from the Women's Health Initiative randomized controlled trial. *Journal of the American Medical Association, 288*(3), 366-368.

Wyatt, G., & Friedman, L. (1998). Physical and psychosocial outcomes of midlife and older women following surgery and adjuvant therapy for breast cancer. *Oncology Nursing Forum, 25*(4), 761-768.

Zawacki, K., & Phillips, M. (2002). Cancer genetics and women's health. *Journal of Obstetric, Gynecologic, and Neonatal Nursing, 31*(2), 208-216.

Zuckerman, D. (2002). The breast cancer information gap. *RN, 65*(2), 39-41.

CHAPTER 12

Deitra Leonard Lowdermilk

Structural Disorders and Neoplasms of the Reproductive System

http://evolve.elsevier.com/Lowdermilk/MatWmnHlth/

LEARNING OBJECTIVES

- Describe the various structural disorders of the uterus and vagina.
- Discuss the pathophysiology of selected benign and malignant neoplasms of the female reproductive tract.
- Compare the common medical and surgical therapies for selected benign gynecologic conditions.
- Examine the emotional impact of benign and malignant neoplasms.
- Develop a nursing plan of care for a woman with endometrial cancer who has had a hysterectomy.
- Explain diagnostic procedures in client-centered terms.
- Differentiate treatments for preinvasive and invasive conditions.
- Investigate health-promoting behaviors that reduce cancer risk.
- Assess the impact of benign and malignant neoplasms on pregnancy.
- Discuss the development and sequelae of gestational trophoblastic neoplasia.
- Identify critical elements for teaching clients with selected benign or malignant neoplasms.

Women are at risk for structural disorders and neoplastic diseases of the reproductive system from the age of menarche through menopause and the older years. Problems may include structural disorders of the uterus and vagina related to pelvic relaxation and urinary incontinence. Benign neoplasms of the reproductive organs, such as fibroids and cysts, and malignant neoplasms of the reproductive system also may occur. Benign tumors usually do not endanger life, tend to grow slowly, and are not invasive. Malignant tumors (cancers) grow rapidly in a disorganized manner and invade surrounding tissues. The impact of the development of structural disorders and benign or malignant neoplasms can have far-reaching effects for the woman and her family. Beyond the obvious physiologic alterations, the woman also experiences threats to her self-concept and her ability to cope. A woman's concept of herself as a sexual being can be affected by the condition and its treatments. A woman's family also is challenged in the way it responds to her diagnosis. When cancer occurs with pregnancy, it adds to the complexity of both physical and emotional responses to childbearing.

Nurses have important roles in teaching women about early detection and treatment and in providing supportive care to women and their families. This chapter presents information that will assist the nurse in assessing and identifying problems associated with structural problems or benign or malignant reproductive neoplasms. Nursing care concepts related to early detection, treatment methods, and education are included.

STRUCTURAL DISORDERS OF THE UTERUS AND VAGINA

Alterations in Pelvic Support

Uterine Displacement and Prolapse

The round ligaments normally hold the uterus in anteversion, and the uterosacral ligaments pull the cervix backward and upward (see Fig. 5-2). **Uterine displacement** is a variation of this normal placement. The most common type of displacement is posterior displacement, or retroversion, in which the uterus is tilted posteriorly, and the cervix rotates anteriorly. Other variations include retroflexion and anteflexion (Fig. 12-1).

By 2 months postpartum, the ligaments should return to normal length, but in about one third of women, the uterus remains retroverted. This condition is rarely symptomatic, but conception may be difficult because the cervix points toward the anterior vaginal wall and away from the posterior fornix, where seminal fluid pools after coitus. If symptoms occur, they may include pelvic and low back pain, dyspareunia, and exaggeration of premenstrual symptoms.

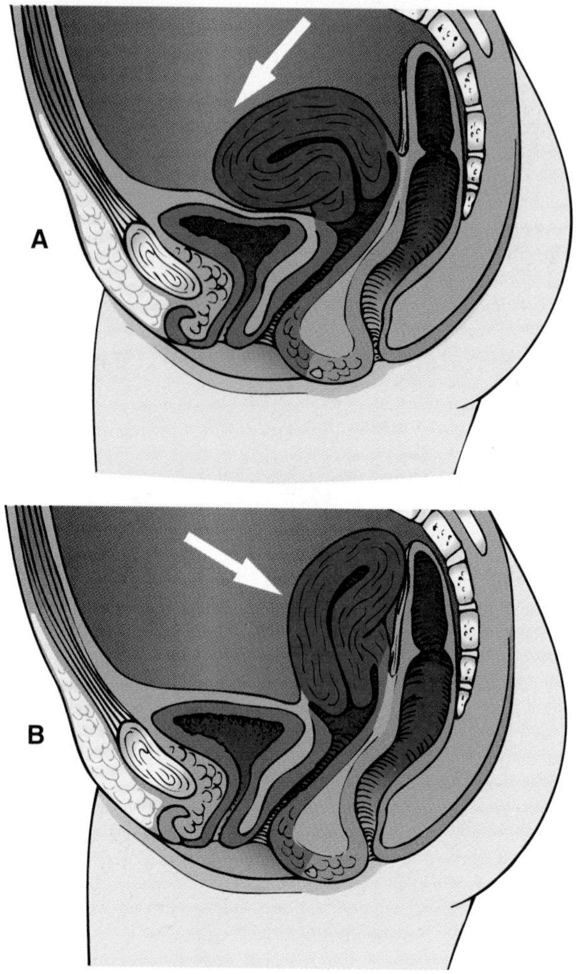
A
B

FIG. 12-1 Types of uterine displacement. **A,** Anterior displacement. **B,** Retroversion (backward displacement of the uterus).

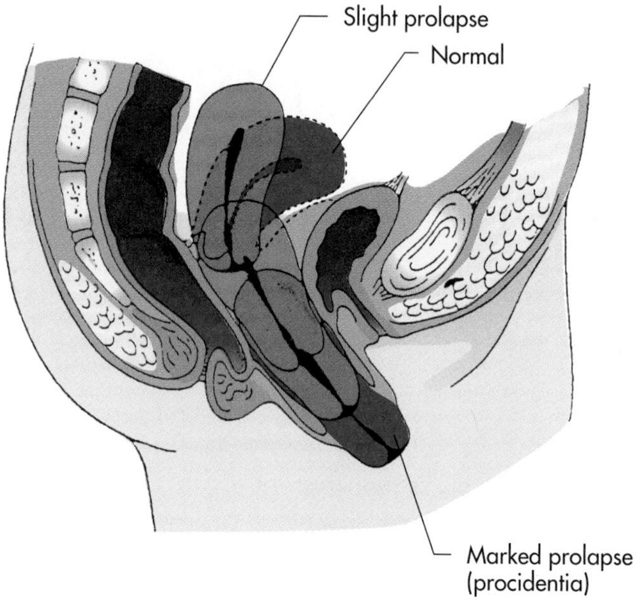
Slight prolapse
Normal
Marked prolapse
(procidentia)

FIG. 12-2 Prolapse of uterus.

Uterine prolapse is a more serious type of displacement. The degree of prolapse can vary from mild to complete. In complete prolapse, the cervix and body of the uterus protrude through the vagina, and the vagina is inverted (Fig. 12-2).

Uterine displacement and prolapse can be caused by congenital or acquired weakness of the pelvic support structures (often referred to as **pelvic relaxation**). In many cases, problems can be related to a delayed but direct result of childbearing. Although extensive damage may be noted and repaired shortly after birth, symptoms related to pelvic relaxation most often appear during the perimenopausal period, when the effects of ovarian hormones on pelvic tissues are lost, and atrophic changes begin. Pelvic trauma, stress and strain, and the aging process also are contributing factors. Other causes of pelvic relaxation include reproductive surgery and pelvic radiation.

Clinical Manifestations. Symptoms of pelvic relaxation generally relate to the structure involved: urethra, bladder, uterus, vagina, cul-de-sac, or rectum. The most common complaints are pulling and dragging sensations, pressure, protrusions, fatigue, and low backache. Symptoms may be worse after prolonged standing or deep penile penetration during intercourse. Urinary incontinence may be present.

Cystocele and Rectocele

Cystocele and rectocele almost always accompany uterine prolapse, causing the uterus to sag even farther backward and downward into the vagina. **Cystocele** (Fig. 12-3, *A*) is the protrusion of the bladder downward into the vagina that develops when supporting structures in the vesicovaginal septum are injured. Anterior wall relaxation gradually develops over time as a result of congenital defects of supports, childbearing, obesity, or advanced age. When the woman stands, the weakened anterior vaginal wall cannot support the weight of the urine in the bladder; the vesicovaginal septum is forced downward, the bladder is stretched, and its capacity is increased. With time the cystocele enlarges until it protrudes into the vagina. Complete emptying of the bladder is difficult because the cystocele sags below the bladder neck. **Rectocele** is the herniation of the anterior rectal wall through the relaxed or ruptured vaginal fascia and rectovaginal septum; it appears as a large bulge that may be seen through the relaxed introitus (Fig. 12-3, *B*).

Clinical Manifestations. Cystoceles and rectoceles often are asymptomatic. If symptoms of cystocele are present, they may include complaints of a bearing-down sensation or that "something is in my vagina." Other symptoms include urinary frequency, retention, and/or incontinence, and possible recurrent cystitis and urinary tract infections (UTIs). Pelvic examination will reveal a

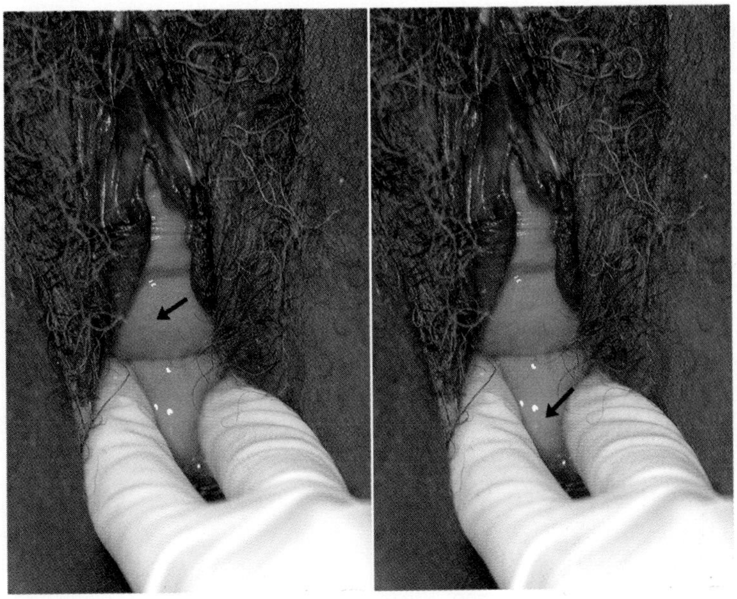
A
B

FIG. 12-3 **A,** Cystocele. **B,** Rectocele. (From Seidel, H. et al. [2003]. *Mosby's guide to physical examination* [5th ed.]. St. Louis: Mosby.)

bulging of the anterior wall of the vagina when the woman is asked to bear down. Unless the bladder neck and urethra are damaged, urinary continence is unaffected. Women with large cystoceles complain of having to push upward on the sagging anterior vaginal wall to be able to void.

Rectoceles may be small and produce few symptoms, but some are so large that they protrude outside of the vagina when the woman stands. Symptoms are absent when the woman is lying down. A rectocele causes a disturbance in bowel function, the sensation of "bearing down," or the sensation that the pelvic organs are falling out. With a very large rectocele, it may be difficult to have a bowel movement. Each time the woman strains during bowel evacuation, the feces are forced against the thinned rectovaginal wall, stretching it more. Some women facilitate evacuation by applying digital pressure vaginally to hold up the rectal pouch.

Urinary Incontinence

About 25% to 34% of women aged between 25 and 54 years have urinary incontinence (UI) (Thom, 1998). Although nulliparous women can have UI, the incidence is higher in women who have given birth, and it also increases with parity (Sampselle et al., 2000). Conditions that disturb urinary control include stress incontinence due to sudden increases in intraabdominal pressure (such as that due to sneezing or coughing); urge incontinence, caused by disorders of the bladder and urethra, such as urethritis and urethral stricture, trigonitis, and cystitis; neuropathies, such as multiple sclerosis, diabetic neuritis, and pathologic conditions of the spinal cord; and congenital and acquired urinary tract abnormalities.

Stress incontinence may follow injury to bladder neck structures. A sphincter mechanism at the bladder neck compresses the upper urethra, pulls it upward behind the symphysis, and forms an acute angle at the junction of the posterior urethral wall and the base of the bladder (Fig. 12-4). To empty the bladder, the sphincter complex relaxes, and the trigone contracts to open the internal urethral orifice and pull the contracting bladder wall upward, forcing urine out. The angle between the urethra and the base of the bladder is lost or increased if the supporting pubococcygeus muscle is injured; this change, coupled with urethrocele, causes incontinence. Urine spurts out when the woman is asked to bear down or cough in the lithotomy position.

Clinical Manifestations. Involuntary leaking of urine is the main sign. Episodes of leaking are common during coughing, laughing, and exercise.

Genital Fistulas

Genital **fistulas** are perforations between genital tract organs. Most occur between the bladder and the genital tract (e.g., vesicovaginal); between the urethra and the vagina (urethrovaginal); and between the rectum or sigmoid colon and the vagina (rectovaginal) (Fig. 12-5). Genital fistulas also may be a result of a congenital anomaly, gynecologic surgery, obstetric trauma, cancer, radiation therapy, gynecologic trauma, or infection (e.g., in the episiotomy).

Clinical Manifestations. Signs and symptoms of vaginal fistulas depend on the site but may include presence of urine, flatus, or feces in the vagina; odors of urine or feces in the vagina; and irritation of vaginal tissues.

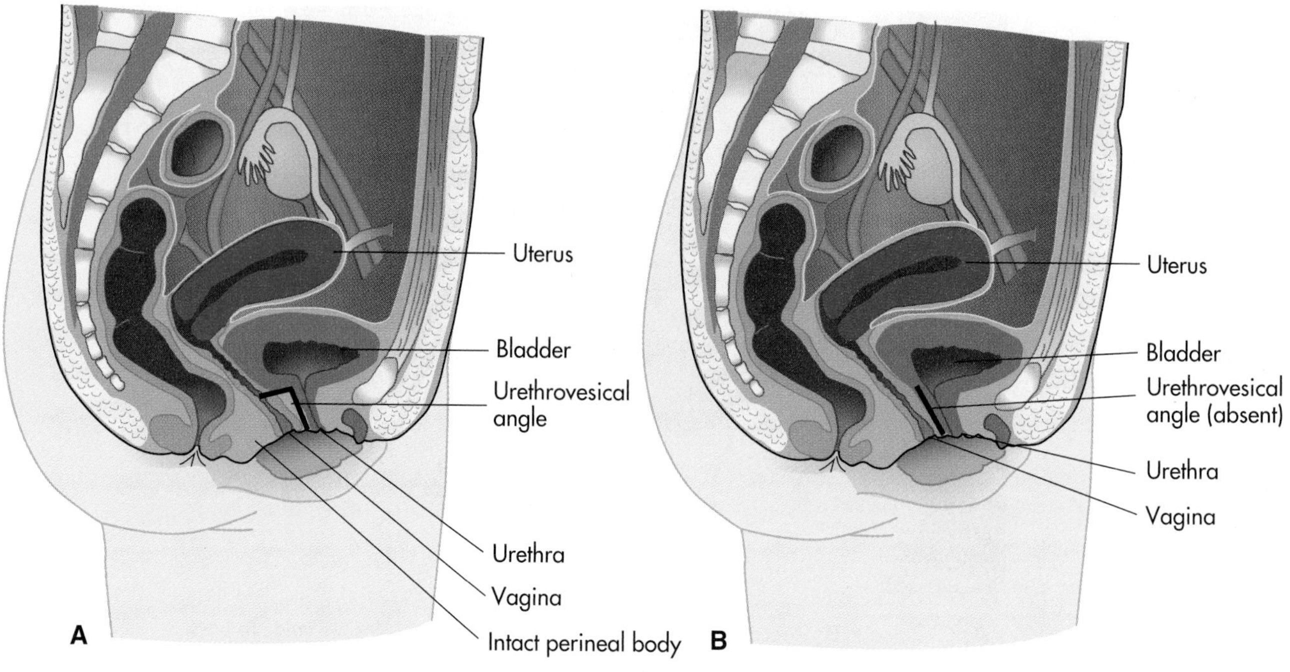

Uterus
Bladder
Urethrovesical angle
Urethra
Vagina
Intact perineal body
A
Uterus
Bladder
Urethrovesical angle (absent)
Urethra
Vagina
B

FIG. 12-4 Urethrovesical angle. **A,** Normal angle. **B,** Widening (absence) of angle.

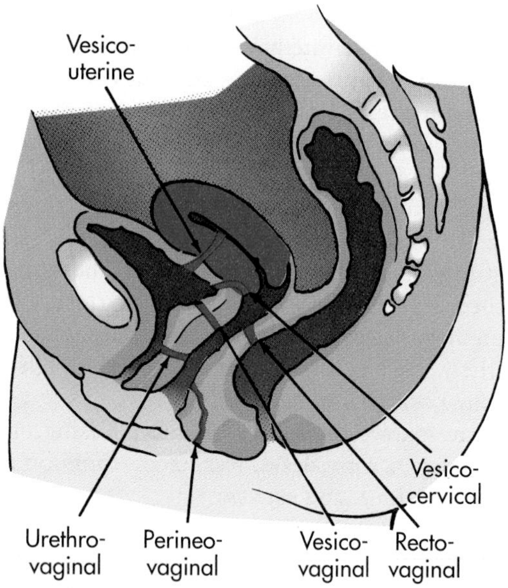

Vesico-uterine
Vesico-cervical
Urethro-vaginal
Perineo-vaginal
Vesico-vaginal
Recto-vaginal

FIG. 12-5 Types of fistulas that may develop in the vagina, uterus, or rectum. (From Phipps, W. et al. [2003]. *Medical-surgical nursing: Health and illness perspectives* [7th ed.]. St. Louis: Mosby.)

CARE MANAGEMENT

Assessment for problems related to structural disorders of the uterus and vagina focuses primarily on the genitourinary tract, the reproductive organs, bowel elimination, and psychosocial and sexual factors. A complete health history, a physical examination, and laboratory tests are done to support the appropriate medical diagnosis. The nurse must assess the woman's knowledge of the disorder, its management, and possible prognosis. Possible nursing diagnoses for structural problems of the uterus and vagina include the following:

- *Deficient knowledge related to*
  –causes of structural disorders and treatment options
- *Constipation or diarrhea related to*
  –anatomic changes
- *Acute pain related to*
  –relaxation of pelvic support or elimination difficulties
- *Ineffective coping related to*
  –changes in body image
- *Interrupted family processes or interpersonal relationships related to*
  –the woman's anatomic and functional changes
- *Risk for injury related to*
  –lack of skill in self-care procedures
  –lack of understanding of the reasons for the need to comply with therapy
- *Social isolation, spiritual distress, disturbed body image, or chronic low self-esteem related to*
  –changes in anatomy and function
- *Anxiety related to*
  –surgical procedure
  –prognosis

The health care team works together to treat the disorders related to alterations in pelvic support and to assist

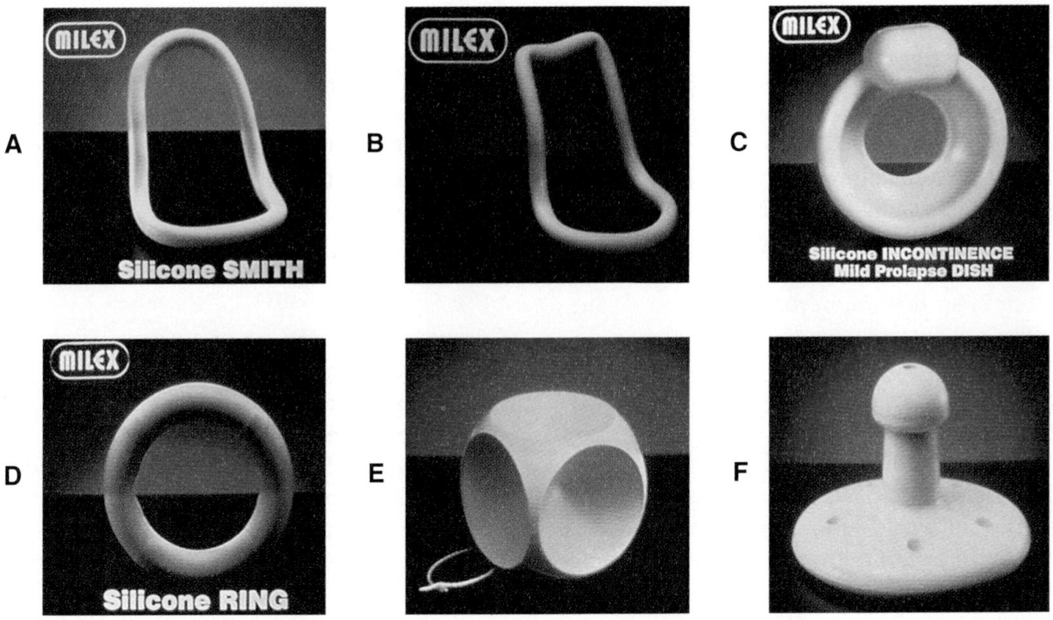
A
MILEX
Silicone SMITH
B
MILEX
C
MILEX
Silicone INCONTINENCE
Mild Prolapse DISH
D
MILEX
Silicone RING
E
F

FIG. 12-6 Examples of pessaries. **A**, Smith. **B**, Hodge without support. **C**, Incontinence dish without support. **D**, Ring without support. **E**, Cube. **F**, Gellhorn. (Courtesy Milex Products, Inc, Chicago, IL.)

the woman in management of her symptoms. In general, nurses working with these women can provide information and self-care education to prevent problems before they occur, to manage or reduce symptoms and promote comfort and hygiene if symptoms are already present, and to recognize when further intervention is needed. This information can be part of all postpartum discharge teaching or can be provided at postpartum follow-up visits in clinics or physician/midwife offices, during postpartum home visits, or during gynecologic health examinations. In addition, information on how to prevent or recognize problems can be a topic for workshops for women or health fairs in community settings.

Interventions for specific problems depend on the problem and the severity of the symptoms. If discomfort related to uterine displacement is a problem, several interventions can be implemented to treat uterine displacement. Kegel exercises (see p. 125) can be performed several times daily to increase muscle strength. A knee-chest position performed for a few minutes several times a day can correct a mildly retroverted uterus. A fitted **pessary** to support the uterus and hold it in the correct position (Fig. 12-6) may be inserted in the vagina. Usually a pessary is used only for a short time because it can lead to pressure necrosis and vaginitis. Good hygiene is important; some women can be taught to remove the pessary at night, cleanse it, and replace it in the morning. If the pessary is always left in place, regular douching with commercially prepared solutions or weak vinegar solutions (1 tablespoon to 1 quart of water) to remove increased secretions and keep the vaginal pH at 4 to 4.5 are suggested. After a period of treatment, most women are free of symptoms and do not require the pessary. Surgical correction is rarely indicated.

Treatment for uterine prolapse depends on the degree of prolapse. Pessaries may be useful in mild prolapse. Estrogen therapy also may be used in the older woman to improve tissue tone. If these conservative treatments do not correct the problem, or if there is a significant degree of prolapse, abdominal or vaginal hysterectomy (see p. 298) is usually recommended.

Treatment for a cystocele includes use of a vaginal pessary or surgical repair. Pessaries may not be effective. *Anterior repair (colporrhaphy)* is the usual surgical procedure and is usually done for large, symptomatic cystoceles. This involves a surgical shortening of pelvic muscles to provide better support for the bladder. An anterior repair is often combined with a vaginal hysterectomy.

Small rectoceles may not require treatment. The woman with mild symptoms may derive relief from a high-fiber diet and adequate fluid intake, stool softeners, or mild laxatives. Vaginal pessaries usually are not effective. Large rectoceles that are causing significant symptoms are usually repaired surgically. A *posterior repair (colporrhaphy)* is the usual procedure. This surgery is performed vaginally and involves shortening the pelvic muscles to provide better support for the rectum. Anterior and posterior repairs may be performed at the same time and with a vaginal hysterectomy.

Mild to moderate urinary incontinence can be significantly decreased or relieved in many women by bladder training and pelvic muscle (Kegel) exercises (Sampselle et al., 2000). Other management strategies include insertion of a bladder neck–support prosthesis, vaginal estrogen therapy, and surgery (National Women's Health Resource Center, 1999; Stenchever et al., 2001).

Management of genital fistulas depends on the location. Surgical repair is the usual treatment; however, it may not be successful.

Nursing care of the woman with a cystocele, rectocele, or fistula requires great sensitivity, because the woman's reactions are often intense. She may become withdrawn or hostile because of embarrassment caused by odors and soiling of her clothing that are beyond her control. She may have concerns about engaging in sexual activities because her partner is repelled by these problems. The nurse may tactfully suggest hygiene practices that reduce odor. Commercial deodorizing douches are available, or noncommercial solutions, such as chlorine solution (1 teaspoon of household chlorine bleach to 1 quart of water) may be used. The chlorine solution also is useful for external perineal irrigation. Sitz baths and thorough washing of the genitals with unscented, mild soap and warm water help. Sparse dusting with deodorizing powders can be useful. If a rectovaginal fistula is present, enemas given before leaving the house may provide temporary relief from oozing of fecal material until corrective surgery is performed. Irritated skin and tissues may benefit from use of the heat lamp or application of vitamin A&D ointment. Hygienic care is time consuming and may need to be repeated frequently throughout the day; protective pads or pants may need to be worn. All of these activities can be demoralizing to the woman and frustrating to her and her family. If surgical repair is performed, nursing care focuses on preventing infection and helping the woman avoid putting stress on the surgical site.

Many of the nurse's efforts with these problems are directed toward participating in a team effort to prepare the woman for surgery and self-care after discharge. Preoperative teaching involves the primary nurse, operating room nurse, surgeon, and anesthesiologist. Postoperatively, a nurse in the health promotion setting may be most aware of the woman's living circumstances, physical limitations, and social problems and therefore may be best suited to coordinate continuity of care after discharge.

BENIGN NEOPLASMS

Benign neoplasms include a variety of nonmalignant cysts and tumors of the ovaries, uterus, vulva, and other organs of the reproductive system.

Ovarian Cysts

Functional ovarian cysts (Fig. 12-7) are dependent on hormonal influences associated with the menstrual cycle. These cysts may be classified as follicular cysts, corpus luteum cysts, theca-lutein cysts, endometrial cysts, and polycystic ovarian syndrome. Other benign ovarian neoplasms include dermoid cysts and ovarian fibromas.

Follicular Cysts

Follicular cysts develop most commonly in normal ovaries of young women as a result of the mature graafian follicle failing to rupture or when an immature follicle does not reabsorb fluid after ovulation. A cyst is usually asymptomatic unless it ruptures, in which case, it causes severe pelvic pain. If the cyst does not rupture, it usually shrinks after two or three menstrual cycles.

Corpus Luteum Cysts

Corpus luteum cysts occur after ovulation and are possibly caused by an increased secretion of progesterone that results in an increase of fluid in the corpus luteum. Clinical manifestations associated with a corpus luteum cyst include pain, tenderness over the ovary, delayed menses, and irregular or prolonged menstrual flow. A rupture can cause intraperitoneal hemorrhage. Corpus luteum cysts usually disappear without treatment within one or two menstrual cycles.

Theca-lutein Cysts

Theca-lutein cysts are uncommon and in up to 50% of cases are associated with hydatidiform mole (see Chapter 31). Theca-lutein cysts develop as a result of prolonged stimulation of the ovaries by human chorionic gonadotrophin (hCG). They also may occur if the woman has taken ovulation induction drugs; if she is pregnant and a large placenta is present, such as in the presence of a multiple gestation; or if the woman has diabetes (Stenchever al., 2001). The cysts are almost always bilateral. A feeling of pelvic fullness may be noted by the woman if the ovary is enlarged, but most women are asymptomatic.

Polycystic Ovarian Syndrome

Polycystic ovarian syndrome (PCOS) occurs when an endocrine imbalance results in high levels of estrogen, testosterone, and luteinizing hormone (LH) and decreased secretion of follicle-stimulating hormone. This syndrome is associated with a variety of problems in the hypothalamic-pituitary-ovarian axis and with androgen-producing tumors. The condition can be transmitted as an X-linked dominant or autosomal dominant trait (Stein-Leventhal syndrome). Multiple follicular cysts develop on one or both ovaries and produce excess estrogen. The ovaries often double in size. Clinical manifestations include obesity, hirsutism (excessive hair growth), irregular menses or amenorrhea, and infertility. Impaired glucose tolerance and hyperinsulinemia occur in about 45% of women with PCOS (Stenchever et al., 2001).

Collaborative Care

A variety of interventions may be implemented for the woman with a functional cyst. If expectant management is the treatment, the woman is advised to keep appointments for pelvic examinations to monitor the changes in

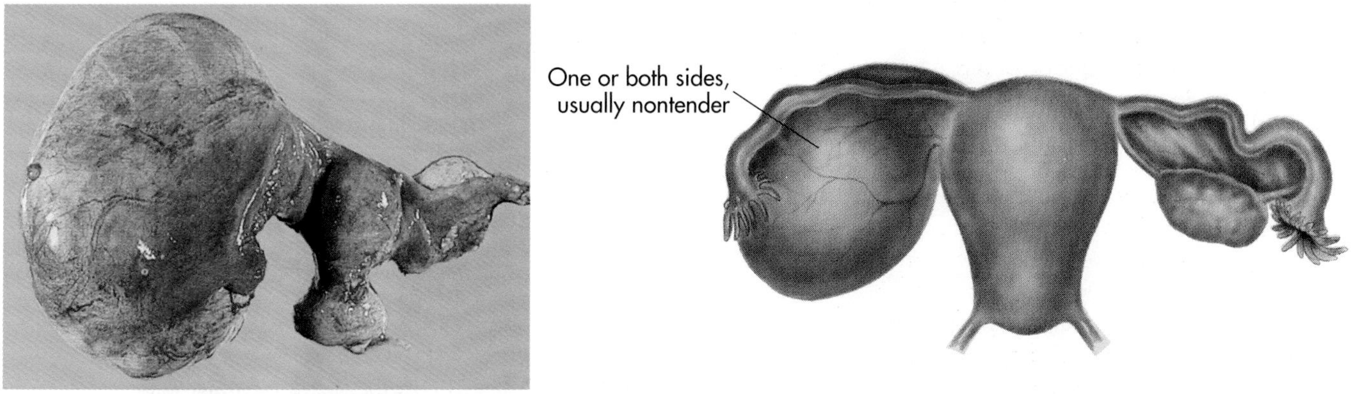
One or both sides,
usually nontender

FIG. 12-7 Ovarian cyst. (From Seidel, H. et al. [2003]. *Mosby's guide to physical examination* [5th ed.]. St. Louis: Mosby.)

size of the cyst (enlarging or shrinking). Pharmacologic interventions such as analgesics may be prescribed for pain management. Oral contraceptives may be ordered for several months for functional cysts to suppress ovulation. Large cysts (greater than 8 cm) or cysts that do not shrink may be removed surgically (cystectomy). Corpus lutein cysts are treated similarly. Theca-lutein cysts are usually managed conservatively (they usually regress) or by removal of the hydatidiform mole (Stenchever et al., 2001). The treatment for PCOS depends on what symptoms are of greatest concern to the woman. Oral contraceptives are the usual treatment if pregnancy is not desired because they inhibit LH and decrease testosterone levels. Gonadotropin-releasing hormone (GnRH) analogues may be used to treat hirsutism if oral contraceptives do not improve this condition. If pregnancy is desired, ovulation-inducing medications are given.

Nursing care focuses on educating the woman regarding treatment options and pain management with analgesics or comfort measures such as heat to the abdomen or relaxation techniques. If surgery is performed, the nurse provides preoperative and postoperative care. Discharge teaching includes signs of infection, postoperative incision care, the possibility of recurrence, and advice regarding follow-up appointments.

Other Benign Ovarian Cysts and Neoplasms

Two other ovarian neoplasms that need discussion include dermoid cysts and ovarian fibromas. **Dermoid cysts** are germ cell tumors, usually occurring in childhood. These cysts contain substances such as hair, teeth, sebaceous secretions, and bones. Unless the cyst is large enough to put pressure on other organs, it is usually asymptomatic. Dermoid cysts may develop bilaterally and are often attached to the ovary. Treatment is usually surgical removal.

Ovarian fibromas are solid ovarian neoplasms developing from connective tissue and most often occurring after menopause. Fibromas range in size from small nodules to large masses weighing more than 23 kg. Most fibromas are unilateral. They are usually asymptomatic, but if large enough, they may cause ascites, feelings of pelvic pressure, or abdominal enlargement. Treatment is usually surgical removal.

Nursing care of women treated for dermoid cysts and ovarian fibromas is similar to that described for functional ovarian cysts.

Uterine Polyps

Uterine polyps may be endometrial or cervical in origin. They are tumors that are on pedicles (stalks) arising from the mucosa (Fig. 12-8). The etiology is unknown, although they may develop in response to hormonal stimulus or be the result of inflammation. Polyps are the most common benign lesions of the cervix and endometrium that occur during the reproductive years. These polyps may be single or multiple. Endocervical polyps are most common in multiparous women older than 40 years. The woman may be asymptomatic or she may have premenstrual or postmenstrual bleeding or postcoital bleeding (Stenchever et al., 2001).

Collaborative Care

Clinical management of endometrial polyps is by surgical removal. Cervical polyps are usually removed as an office or clinic procedure without anesthesia. The polyp is grasped with a clamp and twisted or cut off. All polyps should be sent for pathologic examination. Endometrial sampling should be done to determine if other pathologic conditions are present (Stenchever et al., 2001).

Nursing care includes preparing the woman for what to expect during the removal procedure and encouraging relaxation and breathing exercises and providing support during the procedure. After the procedure, the woman is advised to avoid use of tampons, sexual intercourse, and douching for up to 1 week or until the site is healed. She is taught how to identify signs of infection and to notify

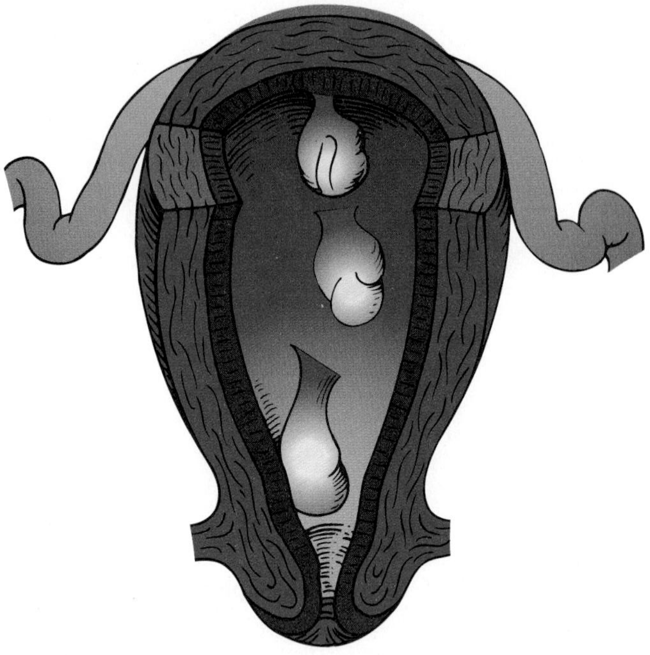

FIG. 12-8 Endometrial polyps.

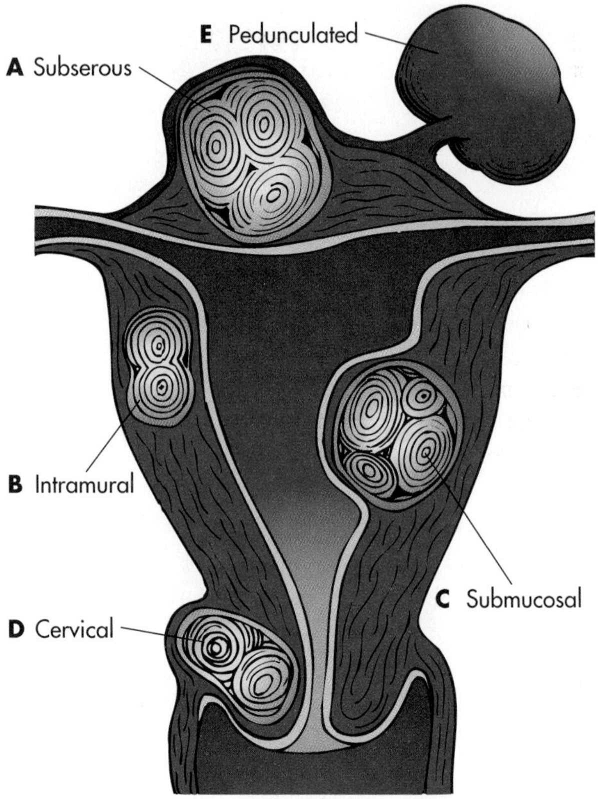
E Pedunculated
A Subserous
B Intramural
C Submucosal
D Cervical

FIG. 12-9 Types of leiomyomas. **A,** Subserous. **B,** Intramural. **C,** Submucosal. **D,** Cervical. **E,** Pedunculated.

her health care provider if she experiences heavy bleeding (more than one pad in 1 hour). Polyps rarely recur after removal (Stenchever et al., 2001).

Leiomyomas

Leiomyomas, also known as fibroid tumors, fibromas, myomas, or fibromyomas, are slow-growing benign tumors arising from the muscle tissue of the uterus (Stenchever et al., 2001). They are the most common benign tumors of the reproductive system, occurring most often after age 50 years. They tend to occur more often in African-American women and women who have never been pregnant (Stenchever et al., 2001). They rarely become malignant. Because their growth is influenced by ovarian hormones, these benign tumors can become quite large when the woman is taking birth control pills, is pregnant, or is receiving hormone therapy. They spontaneously shrink after menopause when circulating ovarian hormones are diminished (Grabo et al., 1999).

Clinical Manifestations and Diagnosis

The cause of leiomyomas remains unknown, although genetic factors may be involved in their development. Most of the tumors are found in the body of the uterus. Leiomyomas are classified according to the location in the uterine wall. *Subserous* leiomyomas develop beneath the peritoneal surface of the uterus and appear as small or large masses that protrude from the outer uterine surface (Fig. 12-9, *A*). *Intramural* leiomyomas are tumors that develop within the wall of the uterus (Fig. 12-9, *B*). *Submucosal* leiomyomas are the least common tumors, but often they cause the most symptoms. These tumors develop in the endometrium and protrude into the uterine cavity (Fig. 12-9, *C*). Leiomyomas also can develop in the cervix and on the broad ligaments (Fig. 12-9, *D*). They also can grow on pedicles or stalks (Fig. 12-9, *E*). Occasionally these break off the pedicle and attach to other tissues (become parasitic).

Most women are asymptomatic; abnormal uterine bleeding is the most common symptom of fibroids. If the tumor is very large, pelvic circulation may be compromised, and surrounding viscera may be displaced. A woman may complain of backache, low abdominal pressure, constipation, urinary incontinence, or dysmenorrhea (painful menstruation). Nausea and vomiting may occur if the tumor is obstructing the intestines. The woman also may notice an abdominal mass if the tumor is large. Anemia may be present if the woman has excessive bleeding (Grabo et al., 1999). Pedunculated tumors can twist and become necrotic, causing pain.

The tumors appear to be influenced by the presence of estrogen; during pregnancy, the tumors may produce complications such as preterm labor, miscarriage, or dystocia (difficult labor). The severity of the symptoms seems to be directly related to the size and location of the tumors.

CARE MANAGEMENT

Assessment and Nursing Diagnoses

Assessment should include a history of symptoms (which might include abnormal bleeding, abdominal pain, dysmenorrhea, pelvic fullness or heaviness, or problems with elimination) and a pelvic examination. Diagnosis is usually accomplished by a process of elimination. A pelvic examination usually identifies the presence of uterine enlargement. Pregnancy tests will rule out pregnancy as the cause of the symptoms. Laparoscopy may be used to differentiate ovarian masses from uterine masses. Ultrasound examination can differentiate between inflammatory masses or endometriosis and subserous fibroids.

Possible nursing diagnoses for a woman with a leiomyoma include the following:

- *Anxiety related to*
  - -uncertain diagnosis
  - -fear of malignancy
  - -potential surgical treatment
- *Pain related to*
  - -leiomyomas
- *Risk for sexual dysfunction related to*
  - -dyspareunia

Expected Outcomes of Care

Nursing diagnoses provide the direction for care. Expected outcomes are determined with the woman. Expected outcomes for the woman with a leiomyoma might include that the woman will do the following:

- Verbalize a decrease in anxiety related to the diagnosis and therapeutic regimen.
- Verbalize understanding of treatment options to make an informed decision.
- Report no compromise in sexual functioning as a result of the therapeutic intervention.

Plan of Care and Interventions

Knowledge of the medical-surgical management of leiomyomas is essential in planning nursing care. The knowledge enables the nurse to work collaboratively with other health care providers and to meet the woman's informational and emotional needs. Clinical management for benign tumors of the uterus depends on the severity of the symptoms, the age of the woman, and her desire to preserve childbearing potential.

Medical Management

If symptoms are mild, regular checkups may suffice to observe for growth or changes in size. Nonsteroidal anti-inflammatory drugs may be prescribed for pain; oral contraceptives inhibit ovulation and may relieve symptoms; and GnRH agonists such as leuprolide acetate (Lupron, Synarel) may be prescribed to reduce the size of the leiomyoma. Other medications used include medroxyprogesterone acetate (Depo-Provera), danazol (Danocrine), and mifepristone (RU486; Mifeprex) (Sharts-Hopko, 2001).

The woman who prefers medical treatment will need information about the different medications, their actions and side effects, and routes of administration.

NURSE ALERT

A woman who is receiving GnRH agonists to decrease the size of the fibroid must understand that regrowth will occur after the treatment is stopped.

She also must know that a small loss in bone mass and changes in lipid levels can occur; therefore long-term use is not recommended. Amenorrhea may occur; however, women who wish to avoid pregnancy should use a nonhormonal or barrier method of contraception (Grabo et al., 1999). A discussion of administration methods for GnRH agonists, including subcutaneous and intramuscular injections, intranasal administration, and subcutaneous implantation, will assist the woman in making a decision about her preferred method of administration.

Uterine Artery Embolization. Uterine artery embolization (UAE) is a treatment during which polyvinyl alcohol (PVA) pellets are injected into selected blood vessels to block the blood supply to the fibroid and cause shrinkage and resolution of symptoms (Todd, 2002). The procedure is done under local anesthesia and conscious sedation. An incision is made into the groin, and a catheter is threaded into the femoral artery to the uterine artery. An arteriogram identifies the vessels supplying the fibroid. Most fibroids are reduced in size by 50% within 3 months. Long-term effects of the procedure are unknown; temporary amenorrhea or early menopause can occur (Todd, 2002).

Preoperative teaching includes advising the woman not to drink alcohol or smoke and not to take aspirin or anticoagulant medications 24 hours before the procedure. The woman is told to expect cramping during injection of the PVA pellets. Explanations about what to expect postoperatively include that pelvic pain, fever, malaise, and nausea and vomiting may be caused by acute fibroid degeneration. Pain may be controlled with a patient-controlled analgesia pump. Nursing assessments include checking for bleeding in the groin, taking vital signs, assessing pain level, and checking the pedal pulse and neurovascular condition of the affected leg (Todd, 2002). Discharge teaching includes signs of possible complications and when to notify the physician, self-care instructions, and follow-up advice (see Teaching for Self-Care box). An ultrasound or magnetic resonance imaging (MRI) examination is usually done within 6 weeks after the UAE to determine the effectiveness of the procedure.

Surgical Management

Myomectomy. If the tumor is near the outer wall of the uterus, the uterine size no larger than that at 12 to 14 weeks of gestation, and symptoms are significant,

TEACHING FOR SELF-CARE

Home Care After Uterine Artery Embolization

- Take prescribed medications as ordered.
- Call your physician if you have any of the following symptoms:
  Bleeding
  Pain
  Swelling or hematoma at the puncture site
  Fever of 39° C
  Urinary retention
  Abnormal vaginal drainage (foul odor, brown color, tissue)
- Eat a normal diet including fluids and fiber.
- Do not use tampons, douche, or have vaginal intercourse for at least 4 weeks
- Avoid straining during bowel movements
- Keep your follow-up appointment

myomectomy (removal of the tumor) may be performed. Myomectomy can be performed through a laparoscopic or abdominal incision approach or vaginal (hysteroscopic) approach (American College of Obstetricians and Gynecologists, 2000; Stenchever et al., 2001). Myomectomy leaves the uterine muscle walls relatively intact, thereby preserving the uterus and allowing the possibility of future pregnancies. It is usually performed in the proliferative phase of the menstrual cycle to avoid interrupting a possible pregnancy. GnRH therapy may be given before surgery to reduce the size of the fibroid. Fibroids may recur after myomectomy; further treatment may be needed (Bieber & Macklin, 1998).

Laser Surgery. Laser surgery or electrocauterization can be used to destroy small fibroids through a laparoscopic (abdominal) or hysteroscopic (vaginal) approach. Hysteroscopic uterine *ablation* (vaporization of tissues) can be performed under local or general anesthesia, usually as an outpatient procedure. Medical therapy using GnRH agonists to control bleeding temporarily and to suppress endometrial tissue may be given for 8 to 12 weeks before surgery. Although the uterus remains in place, the vaporization process can cause scarring and adhesions in the uterine cavity and may affect future fertility (Grabo et al., 1999; NWHRC, 1999). Risks of the procedure include uterine perforation, cervical injury, and fluid overload (caused by the leaking into blood vessels of fluid used to expand the uterus during surgery). The woman may experience postoperative cramping and a slight vaginal discharge for a few days. Before discharge, the following information is given:

- The next menstrual period may be irregular.
- The physician should be called if the woman has heavy bleeding or signs of infection.
- Use of tampons or vaginal intercourse should be avoided for 2 weeks.

A

B

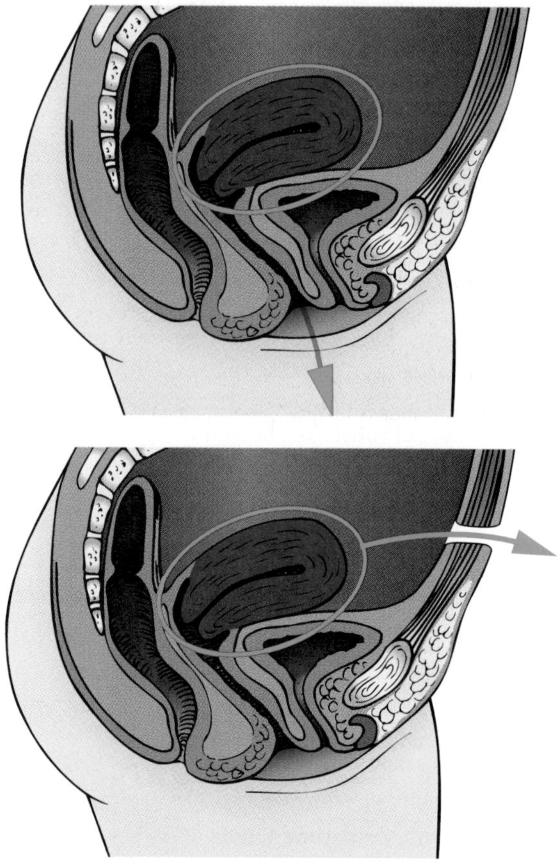

FIG. 12-10 Hysterectomy. **A,** Vaginal. **B,** Abdominal.

Hysterectomy. Hysterectomy (removal of the entire uterus) is the treatment of choice if bleeding is severe or if the fibroid is obstructing normal function of other organs. Fibroids are the most common reason for the 600,000 hysterectomies performed in the United States annually (Farquar & Steiner, 2002). An abdominal or vaginal surgical approach depends on the size and location of the tumors. For example, abdominal hysterectomy is usually performed for leiomyomas larger than a uterus would be at 12 to 14 weeks of gestation or for multiple leiomyomas. The uterus is removed through either a vertical or transverse incision. In some circumstances, the cervix may not be removed. Vaginal approaches can be used for smaller tumors. In both abdominal and vaginal approaches, the uterus is removed from the supporting ligaments (broad, round, and uterosacral). These ligaments are then attached to the vaginal cuff, allowing maintenance of normal depth of the vagina (Fig. 12-10). Alternatives to these procedures are the *laparoscopic assisted vaginal hysterectomy (LAVH)* and the laparoscopic supracervical hysterectomy (LSH). LVAH converts an abdominal procedure to a vaginal one by using a laparoscope in the abdomen to assist with removal of the uterus. LSH allows the cervix to remain. Both are associated with a quicker recovery and fewer postoperative complications,

BOX 12-1 **Questions for the Woman to Ask to Ensure Informed Consent**

Why is this procedure proposed for my condition/problem?
What are the risks/benefits of the proposed surgery?
Are there alternatives to this surgery? If so, what are the risks and benefits of these alternatives?
How many times have you performed this surgery?
How long will I be hospitalized? (or Can the procedure be done in an outpatient setting?) How long will it take to recover?
What types of anesthesia can be used?
What hospital and surgical procedures can I expect?
How will the surgery affect me (e.g., any changes in physical function, sexual function, or childbearing ability?)

Source: National Women's Health Resource Center. (1999). The woman's guide to preparing for surgery. *National Women's Health Report, 21*(5), 1-7; Wade, J., Pletsch, P., Morgan, S., & Menting, S. (2000). Hysterectomy: What do women need and want to know? *Journal of Obstetric, Gynecologic, and Neonatal Nursing, 29*(1), 33-42.

BOX 12-2 **Preoperative Procedures for Hysterectomy**

- Vaginal examination or physical examination
- Laboratory tests
  - Complete blood count, type, and crossmatch
  - Urinalysis
- Chest radiograph
- Electrocardiogram
- Teaching for postoperative routines
  - Turning, coughing, deep breathing
  - Passive and active leg exercises
  - Need for early ambulation
  - Pain relief options
- Nothing by mouth after midnight
- Enema if ordered
- Douche if ordered
- Abdominal: mons or perineal shave if ordered
- Removal of makeup, nail polish
- Removal of glasses, contact lenses, dentures, etc.
- Identification band in place
- Signed consent form in chart
- Have woman empty bladder immediately before surgery

and LSH may preserve bladder and sexual functioning (Falcone et al., 1999; Sharts-Hopko, 2001). More research is needed on these alternatives.

Preoperative Care. Assessments needed before surgery include the woman's knowledge of treatment options, her desire for future fertility if she is premenopausal, the benefits and risks of each procedure, preoperative and postoperative procedures (Boxes 12-1 and 12-2), and the recovery process (Wade et al., 2000). If the woman can demonstrate understanding of this information, she can make an informed decision about treatment and feel a sense of control over the surgical experience (Lindberg & Nolan, 2001). Resources on helping women to make decisions about treatment are listed at the end of this chapter.

Psychologic assessment is essential, particularly for a woman who is scheduled for a hysterectomy. Areas to be explored include the significance of the loss of the uterus for the woman, misconceptions about effects of surgery, and adequacy of her support system. Women who have not completed their childbearing, who believe that their self-concept is related to having a uterus (to be a complete woman), who feel that sexual functioning is related to having a uterus, or who have too little or too much anxiety about the surgery may be at risk for postoperative emotional reactions (Kim & Lee, 2001; Sharts-Hopko, 2001).

Postoperative Care. Postoperative assessments and care after myomectomy and abdominal hysterectomy are similar to those for other abdominal surgery (Box 12-3). Assessments specific to abdominal and vaginal hysterectomy include assessment for vaginal bleeding (one perineal pad saturated in less than 1 hour is excessive), urinary retention (especially after vaginal hysterectomy), perineal pain after vaginal hysterectomy, and psychologic assessments (depression is the most common emotional reaction) (Kjerulff et al., 2000).

Discharge Planning and Teaching. Discharge planning and teaching are similar for myomectomy and hysterectomy (see Teaching for Self-Care box). If a hysterectomy was performed, the woman is reminded that she will experience cessation of menses. If the woman is premenopausal, she will not experience menopause at this time unless her ovaries also were removed. In this case, there will be no reason for her to consider hormone replacement therapy. If the ovaries are removed, the woman will need the most current information on the risks and benefits of hormone replacement therapy (see Chapter 7). Other symptoms she may experience include pain, sleep disturbance, fatigue, anxiety, and depression. The level of severity of symptoms is influenced by physiologic, psychologic, and social factors (Kim & Lee, 2001). After laser surgery, the woman is instructed about the signs of infection, pain relief with analgesics or nonsteroidal antiinflammatory drugs, and resumption of normal activities within several days and informed that vaginal discharge is to be expected for 4 to 6 weeks. She should be reminded about the possible effects of ablation on her fertility, if appropriate. Vaginal intercourse may be uncomfortable at first. Use of water-soluble lubricants, relaxation exercises, and positions that control penile penetration may be beneficial (Katz, 2002). Preoperative education about sexual

BOX 12-3 Postoperative Care After Hysterectomy

- Monitor vital signs q15min until stable; then q4hr for 48 hr
- Maintain unobstructed airway
- Turn, cough, deep breathe q2hr for 24 hr
  Assist woman to splint incision with hands or pillow
- Incentive spirometry if ordered
- Leg exercises q2-4hr until ambulatory
  Assess Homans' sign
- Assess bleeding
  Abdominal: assess dressing or incision
  Vaginal: perineal pad count (one saturated pad in less than 1 hour is excessive; vaginal bleeding is usually minimal)
- Check laboratory values, especially hematocrit
- Assess lungs
- Assess bowel sounds and monitor bowel function
- Monitor intake and output
  Foley catheter may be in place for 24 hr after abdominal surgery
  After vaginal hysterectomy, urinary retention may be a problem because of manipulation of the urethra during surgery
- Assess abdominal incision or vagina for signs of infection
- Observe for signs of complications
  Abdominal hysterectomy: assess for signs of wound evisceration, pulmonary embolism, thrombophlebitis, pneumonia, bowel obstruction, bleeding (incisional or vaginal)
  Vaginal hysterectomy: assess for signs of urinary tract infection, urinary retention, wound infection, vaginal bleeding
- Pain relief
  Pharmacologic measures: Patient-controlled analgesia (PCA) or epidural narcotics may be ordered for the first 24 hr, followed by oral analgesics and nonsteroidal antiinflammatory drugs
  Nonpharmacologic measures: breathing and relaxation exercises, position changes, guided imagery, application of heat to the abdomen, and sitz baths or ice packs for the perineum; ambulation may relieve gas pains
- Psychologic assessments
  Assess for depression or other emotional reactions
  Assess support systems
  Assess sexual concerns

TEACHING FOR SELF-CARE

Self-Care After Myomectomy or Hysterectomy

- Eat foods high in protein, iron, and vitamin C to aid in tissue healing; include foods with high fiber content; and drink six to eight 8-oz glasses of water daily.
- Rest when tired; resume activities as comfort level permits. Avoid vigorous exercise and heavy lifting for 6 weeks. Avoid sitting for long periods. Resume driving when comfort allows or on advice from health care provider.
- Avoid tub baths, intercourse (vaginal rest), and douching until after the follow-up examination.
- When vaginal intercourse is resumed, use of water-soluble lubricants may decrease discomfort.
- Report the following symptoms to your health care provider: vaginal bleeding, gastrointestinal changes, persistent postoperative symptoms (cramping, distention, change in bowel habits), and signs of wound infection (redness, swelling, heat, or pain at incision site).
- Keep your follow-up appointment with your health care provider.

activity with the woman and her partner may prevent postoperative problems. The schedule for follow-up care depends on the procedure performed, but usually a postoperative visit is scheduled within a week. Papanicolaou (Pap) smear screening after total hysterectomy for a nonmalignant reason is no longer recommended (ACS, 2003); however, others suggest that a Pap smear be done every 2 to 3 years to assess for vaginal cancer (DiSaia & Creasman, 2002). General practice varies and includes Pap smear testing yearly; research is needed to determine if the 2003 recommendation is the best practice.

Evaluation

The nurse evaluates the care of the woman who has had treatment of uterine leiomyomas by using the outcome criteria.

Vulvar Neoplasms

Bartholin Cysts

Bartholin cysts are the most common benign lesions of the vulva. The cause is obstruction of the Bartholin duct, causing it to enlarge. Small cysts often are asymptomatic; however, large cysts or infected cysts cause symptoms such as vulvar pain, dyspareunia (painful intercourse), and a feeling of a mass in the vulvar area.

Collaborative Care. If the woman is asymptomatic, no treatment is necessary. If the cyst is symptomatic or infected, surgical incision and drainage may provide temporary relief. Cysts tend to recur; therefore a permanent opening for drainage may be recommended. This procedure is called *marsupialization* and is the formation of a new duct opening for drainage.

Nursing care after surgery includes teaching the woman about pain-relief measures such as sitz baths, heat lamps to the perineum, and use of analgesics. The woman is taught to assess the incision site for signs of healing and infection and to take antibiotics, if prescribed, for prevention of infection.

MALIGNANT NEOPLASMS

Malignant neoplasms of the reproductive system include cancers of the endometrium, cervix, ovary, vulva, vagina, and uterine tubes.

Cancer of the Endometrium

Incidence and Etiology

Endometrial cancer is the most common malignancy of the reproductive system (American Cancer Society [ACS], 2003). It is most commonly seen in perimenopausal and postmenopausal women between ages 50 and 65 years. Certain risk factors have been associated with the development of endometrial cancer, including obesity, nulliparity, infertility, late onset of menopause, diabetes mellitus, hypertension, and family history of ovarian or breast disease. There appears to be an increase in risk for endometrial cancer in families with hereditary nonpolyposis colorectal cancer (HNPCC) (Zawacki & Phillips, 2002). Hormone imbalance, however, seems to be the most significant risk factor. Numerous studies have correlated the use of exogenous estrogens (unopposed stimulation, i.e., absence of progesterone) in postmenopausal women with an increased incidence of uterine cancer. Tamoxifen taken by women for breast cancer also has been related to an increase in endometrial cancer (DiSaia & Creasman, 2002). Pregnancy and use of oral contraceptive pills appear to offer some protection (ACS, 2003). The incidence of endometrial cancer among Caucasian women is higher than that among African-American women; however, the mortality rates are almost twice as high in African-American women (Stenchever et al., 2001).

Endometrial cancer is slow growing and for that reason has a good prognosis if diagnosed at a localized stage. Most endometrial cancers are adenocarcinomas that develop from endometrial hyperplasia. The tumor usually develops in the fundus of the uterus and can spread directly to the myometrium and cervix, as well as to the reproductive organs. **Metastasis** (spread of cancer from its original site) is through the lymphatic system in the pelvis and through the blood to the liver, lungs, and brain.

CARE MANAGEMENT

Assessment and Nursing Diagnoses

Assessment includes a history of physical symptoms. The cardinal sign of endometrial cancer is abnormal uterine bleeding (e.g., postmenopausal bleeding and premenopausal recurrent metrorrhagia). Thirty percent of postmenopausal bleeding is caused by carcinoma. Late signs include a mucosanguineous vaginal discharge, low back pain, or low pelvic pain. A pelvic examination may reveal the presence of a uterine enlargement or mass.

NURSE ALERT

Women can be informed that they can identify their own risk for developing endometrial as well as ovarian, cervical, and breast cancers by filling out a confidential cancer risk assessment survey that is available on-line (see Resource list at the end of the chapter)

Histologic examination is used for diagnosis. A Pap smear of cellular material obtained by aspiration of the endocervix will identify only one third to one half of cases. Fractional curettage or endometrial biopsy yields the most accurate results. Fractional curettage involves scraping the endocervix and endometrium for histologic evaluation to determine the grade of neoplasm and its stage (extent). Perforation of the uterus is a possible complication of this procedure. Endometrial biopsy will identify about 90% of cases (DiSaia & Creasman, 2002). It is usually done on an outpatient basis under local anesthesia. A suction-type curette is used to remove tissue for sampling. It is recommended that women at risk for HNPCC have an annual biopsy beginning at age 35 years (Zawacki & Phillips, 2002). Other diagnostic tests that may be useful include hysteroscopy (examination of the uterus through an endoscope) and vaginal ultrasonography. Other tests may be done to determine the spread of cancer. These include liver function tests, renal function tests, chest x-ray, intravenous pyelography (IVP), barium enema, computed tomography (CT), bone scans, and biopsy of suggestive tissues. The International Federation of Gynecology and Obstetrics (FIGO) classification system is used to describe the stages of endometrial carcinoma (Table 12-1).

Possible nursing diagnoses that would apply to a woman with endometrial cancer include the following:

- *Deficient knowledge related to*
  - –the diagnosis, treatment, and prognosis
- *Decisional conflict related to*
  - –treatment options
- *Fear/anxiety related to*
  - –diagnosis of cancer, loss of uterus
- *Impaired skin integrity related to*
  - –surgery or radiation therapy
- *Acute or chronic pain related to*
  - –cancer
  - –surgical procedure
- *Disturbed body image related to*
  - –loss of uterus
- *Sexual dysfunction related to*
  - –anatomic and functional changes caused by cancer or its treatment

Expected Outcomes of Care

Planning for care of the woman with endometrial cancer depends on the stage of cancer and the treatment selected; however, some outcomes can be identified for the nursing diagnoses that have been established. Examples of expected outcome criteria are that the woman will do the following:

- Demonstrate understanding of her diagnosis of endometrial cancer, the treatments available, and her prognosis
- Make informed decisions about treatment options
- Describe a decrease in anxiety and fear
- Report that pain is reduced or manageable
- Experience no skin breakdown or infection related to treatment
- State that she understands the effects of cancer and treatment on her body image and that her concerns are reduced
- Report that she and her partner will be able to resume mutually satisfying sexual relations after treatment

Plan of Care and Interventions

Therapeutic Management

Collaborative efforts from various health disciplines are needed to work with the woman with endometrial cancer. All must have an understanding of the treatments that may be used.

TABLE 12-1 **FIGO Classification of Endometrial Carcinoma***

STAGE	DESCRIPTION
Ia G123	Tumor limited to endometrium
Ib G123	Invasion of less than half of the myometrium
Ic G123	Invasion of more than half of the myometrium
IIa G123	Endocervical glandular involvement only
IIb G123	Cervical stromal invasion
IIIa G123	Tumor invades serosa and/or adnexae and/or positive peritoneal cytology
IIIb G123	Vaginal metastases
IIIc G123	Metastases to pelvic and/or paraaortic lymph nodes
IVa G123	Tumor invasion of bladder and/or bowel mucosa
IVb	Distant metastases, including intraabdominal and/or inguinal lymph node
Histopathology: Degree of differentiation	
Cases of carcinoma of the corpus should be grouped according to the degree of differentiation of the adenocarcinoma as follows:	
GI = ≤5% of a nonsquamous or nonmorular solid growth pattern	
G2 = 6% to 50% of a nonsquamous or nonmorular solid growth pattern	
G3 = >50% of a nonsquamous or nonmorular solid growth pattern	

*Approved by FIGO, October 1988, Rio de Janeiro. From DiSaia, P., & Creasman, W. (2002). *Clinical gynecologic oncology* (6th ed.). St. Louis: Mosby.

For stage I adenocarcinoma of the endometrium, total abdominal hysterectomy (TAH) and bilateral salpingo-oophorectomy (BSO) are the usual treatments of choice. A radical hysterectomy (abdominal hysterectomy plus pelvic node dissection) usually is performed for stage II endometrial cancer. Removal of the upper third of the vagina and parametrium also may be done. Surgery may be combined with radiation therapy before or after surgery. External radiation therapy to the whole pelvis (see p. 312) usually is given when there is extensive uterine disease or metastasis outside the uterus (DiSaia & Creasman, 2002). Treatment is usually 4 to 5 days a week for 6 weeks as an outpatient. Internal radiation therapy (placement of an applicator loaded with a radiation source into the uterine cavity) also may be used (see p. 312). Treatment is usually 1 to 3 days for an inpatient but also may be given in an outpatient setting in a shorter time by using higher doses of radiation (DiSaia & Creasman, 2002). Radiation therapy may cause skin ulcerations, cystitis, enteritis, and delayed complications such as genital fistulas.

Chemotherapy is used to treat advanced and recurrent disease, although no effective treatment regimen has been established (Stenchever et al., 2001). Agents that have been somewhat effective include cisplatin, doxorubicin (Adriamycin), cyclophosphamide (Cytoxan), 5-fluorouracil (5-FU), vincristine (Oncovin), and paclitaxel (Taxol). Chemotherapy may cause hair loss, anemia, and bone marrow depression, as well as other side effects.

Progestational therapy–use of medroxyprogesterone (Depo-Provera) and megestrol (Megace)–may be effective for estrogen-dependent cancers. These drugs usually do not cause acute side effects. Tamoxifen (Tamofen) is an antiestrogen that is being investigated for its effectiveness against recurrent endometrial cancer. It may cause hot flashes and nausea and vomiting (DiSaia & Creasman, 2002; Stenchever et al., 2001).

Nursing Care

Nursing care is individualized to the woman and her specific situation and diagnosis. Interventions for the woman having surgery are directed by assessment of her perception of the anticipated surgery, her knowledge of what to expect after surgery, and any preoperative special procedures, such as cleansing enemas or douches. In today's practice of short hospital stays even for radical surgery, many of these preoperative procedures are performed at home before admission, so assessment of understanding becomes a critical nursing action (see Cultural Considerations box).

Preoperative Care. The nurse working with the woman preparing for a radical hysterectomy should explain any preoperative procedures to be done, as described on p. 299. Additional teaching is needed regarding possible postsurgical events (e.g., drainage tubes). The woman should be prepared to have a suprapubic drain that will remain in place for several days to a week.

Postoperative Care. Assessment of vital signs usually follows a postanesthesia protocol, gradually decreasing in frequency to 4 times a day. Intravenous fluids are maintained at a rate rapid enough to maintain hydration and electrolyte balance. Diet is gradually resumed as bowel sounds are heard and flatus is passed. A nasogastric tube may be in place to prevent distention. Intake and output are monitored.

Remind the woman to turn and take deep breaths, and give assistance as needed. Breath sounds are assessed, and any deviations from normal reported immediately. The most significant single cause of morbidity and prolonged hospitalization after major procedures is respiratory complications. Anesthesia and surgery alter breathing patterns and ability to cough. Atelectasis, pneumonia, and pulmonary embolus may occur.

Hemorrhage is always a possible complication after surgery. The wound drainage tube is emptied as needed or every 4 hours, and the amount and character of drainage is recorded. Drainage from any tube is assessed for bleeding. Vaginal drainage, if any, should be serosanguineous. Hematuria is noted and recorded. The primary health care provider is kept apprised of any deviations from normal expectations.

Paralytic ileus may occur after surgery in which the intestinal tract has been manipulated. Use of a nasogastric tube, limiting oral fluids, and early ambulation all support the return of gastrointestinal function. An enema or suppository may bring relief of flatus and stimulate the return of bowel function. Oral laxatives should not be given until lower bowel function has returned.

Sitting may result in pelvic congestion, so the high Fowler's position is avoided. Pelvic congestion is discouraged by avoiding use of the knee gatch (or pillow). Nursing measures such as massages, repositioning, fresh linen, regular perineal care, and emotional support are all helpful adjuncts to pharmacologic control of discomfort.

Discharge Planning and Teaching. Because the in-hospital convalescent period is generally short, close observation by the nurse and attention to detail are critical. Nursing actions appropriate to this period include monitoring for urinary retention after the catheter is removed, monitoring the woman's appetite and diet, monitoring bowel function, and encouraging progressive ambulation and self-care.

Estrogen replacement therapy, if prescribed, is usually started as soon as the woman can take oral fluids. The nurse can take this opportunity to remind the woman that she will no longer have menstrual periods (if she was premenopausal) and to encourage her to verbalize questions or concerns she may have about the risks and benefits of hormone replacement therapy after having a hysterectomy for endometrial cancer (Stenchever et al., 2001). If estrogen therapy is not given, the woman will need information on how to decrease her risk for osteoporosis (e.g., exercise and calcium), and how to combat menopausal symptoms (e.g., diet, herbal therapy, and water-based lubricants for vaginal dryness) (Otto, 2001).

Discharge planning and teaching is done throughout the preoperative and postoperative phases and culminates during the convalescent phase. Discharge teaching topics for the woman with a radical hysterectomy are similar to those for the woman who has had a hysterectomy for leiomyomas and can be found in the Teaching for Self-Care box on p. 300 (also see Plan of Care box).

Care for the woman who has had external or internal radiation therapy is the same as that described for the woman with cervical cancer (p. 312).

Nursing care for the woman undergoing chemotherapy will depend on the type of drug given. If alopecia is likely, the nurse can suggest wigs, scarves, or other kinds of head coverings. If the therapy affects the appetite or causes gastrointestinal side effects, suggestions such as those in Box 12-4 may be useful.

After discharge, the woman may require continued nursing care or monitoring of her physical status or advice for management of effects of treatment or the cancer. The family is likely to have to provide much of the woman's care. Nurses must identify what families see as their greatest need so that interventions are planned that best use the family's resources (Lowdermilk & Germino, 2000).

Psychologic care for the woman with endometrial cancer is essential. A women needs to be able to discuss her concerns about having cancer and the potential for recurrence. She may have fears of death; permanent disfigurement and change in functioning; altered feelings of self as a woman; concerns regarding her femininity, sexuality, and loss of reproductive capacity; and questions arising from things she has heard about posthysterectomy changes, radiation therapy, or chemotherapy. Significant others should be encouraged to express their questions and concerns as well. The woman may benefit from a referral to a community cancer support group.

Evaluation

The nursing care of a woman with endometrial cancer is evaluated by using the expected outcomes and measurable criteria to ascertain the degree to which the outcomes were met.

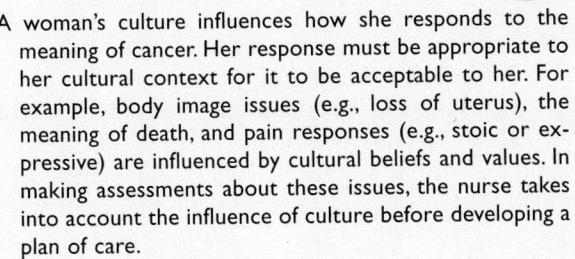

CULTURAL CONSIDERATIONS

Meaning of Cancer

A woman's culture influences how she responds to the meaning of cancer. Her response must be appropriate to her cultural context for it to be acceptable to her. For example, body image issues (e.g., loss of uterus), the meaning of death, and pain responses (e.g., stoic or expressive) are influenced by cultural beliefs and values. In making assessments about these issues, the nurse takes into account the influence of culture before developing a plan of care.

Plan of Care — Hysterectomy for Endometrial Cancer

NURSING DIAGNOSIS **Anxiety related to lack of understanding of diagnosis, treatment, and prognosis of endometrial cancer as evidenced by client questions and concerns**

Expected Outcome *Client will identify source of anxiety and verbalize understanding of diagnosis, effects of hysterectomy, and prognosis.*

Nursing Interventions/*Rationales*

Assess client's level of understanding of procedure and its effects *to correct any misunderstanding, provide clarification, and identify starting point for further information.*

Provide information about cancer of the endometrium, individualizing information to client's situation *to provide clarification concerning treatment regimen.*

Provide preoperative and postoperative teaching *to give anticipatory guidance and rationales for upcoming events.*

NURSING DIAGNOSIS **Fear related to diagnosis of endometrial cancer as evidenced by client questions and concerns**

Expected Outcomes *Client will be able to verbalize that fears have diminished after the procedure.*

Nursing Interventions/*Rationales*

Through therapeutic communication, encourage verbalization of fears *to provide clarification and validation of feelings.*

Encourage client to identify support system *to have resources readily available as needed.*

NURSING DIAGNOSIS **Acute pain related to surgical procedure as evidenced by client verbal and nonverbal behaviors**

Expected Outcome *Client will verbalize decrease in intensity and number of painful episodes after interventions.*

Nursing Interventions/*Rationales*

Assess the location and intensity of pain by using a pain scale *to use appropriate treatment.*

Administer prescribed analgesics *to decrease perception of pain.*

Use nonpharmacologic techniques such as distraction, relaxation, position changes, and heat *to decrease perception of pain.*

Monitor effectiveness of interventions *to modify interventions if needed.*

NURSING DIAGNOSIS **Risk for infection related to surgical incision and impaired skin integrity**

Expected Outcome *Client will experience no infection after the procedure.*

Nursing Interventions/*Rationales*

Assess for clinical manifestations of infection: fever, drainage, redness, swelling at the incision site *to provide prompt treatment.*

Encourage a diet high in protein, vitamin C, and calories *to promote wound healing.*

Teach client to maintain aseptic technique when performing dressing changes, such as good handwashing *to decrease chance of introducing microorganisms at the incision site.*

NURSING DIAGNOSIS **Disturbed body image related to loss of uterus as evidenced by client statements of fears or concerns**

Expected Outcome *Client will maintain a positive body image.*

Nursing Interventions/*Rationales*

Encourage expression of feelings through therapeutic communication *to provide clarification of and validity to feelings.*

Encourage client to share feelings with significant other *to obtain emotional support.*

Assist client to identify support systems *to be available in case of client need to ventilate feelings.*

NURSING DIAGNOSIS **Risk for sexual dysfunction related to perceived loss of femininity**

Expected Outcome *Client will resume usual sexual relationship with partner.*

Nursing Interventions/*Rationales*

Encourage verbalization of feelings related to sexuality *to provide clarification.*

Provide opportunity for role-playing *to alleviate fears about interactions with partner.*

Refer to sexual counselor *to provide in-depth intervention as needed.*

Cancer of the Ovary

Incidence and Etiology

Cancer of the ovary is the second most frequently occurring reproductive cancer and causes more deaths than any other female genital tract cancer (ACS, 2003). Because the symptoms of this type of cancer are vague and definitive screening tests do not exist, ovarian cancer is often diagnosed in an advanced stage. The 5-year survival rate for cancer diagnosed at a localized stage is about 95%; for all stages, the rate decreases to about 50%, and for advanced stages, the rate is less than 25% (ACS, 2003; DiSaia & Creasman, 2002). Malignant neoplasia of the ovaries occurs at all ages, including in infants and children. However, the greatest number of cases is found in women between ages 50 and 59 years.

Major histologic cell types occur in different age groups, with malignant germ cell tumors most common in women between 20 and 40 years of age and epithelial cancers occurring in the perimenopausal age groups. The spread of ovarian cancer is by direct extension to adjacent organs, but distal spread can occur through lymphatic spread to the liver and lungs.

The cause of ovarian cancer is unknown; however, a number of risk factors have been identified. These factors include nulliparity, infertility, previous breast cancer, and family history of ovarian or breast cancer. Although BRCA1 and BRCA2 mutations have been found in some families with a history of ovarian cancer, the disease in not inherited for most women (DiSaia & Creasman, 2002). Women of North American or northern European descent have the highest incidence of ovarian cancers. Genital

BOX 12-4 Nutritional Management for Common Problems Related to Gynecologic Cancer or Treatment

ALTERED TASTE
Perform mouth care after meals
Use extra seasoning
Use sauces and marinades for meats
Eat fish or chicken instead of red meat
Eat tart foods to stimulate taste buds

ANOREXIA
Eat with family, friends
Try new foods, recipes
Use smaller servings
Eat high-calorie snacks
Serve protein shakes
Exercise before meals to stimulate appetite
Eat when hungry

NAUSEA AND VOMITING
Drink clear liquids
Avoid carbonated fluids
Avoid sweet, rich, fatty foods
Eat cool foods rather than hot or warm foods
Eat small meals
Consume a high-calorie, high-protein diet
Eat toast, bland foods
Take antiemetics before meals

STOMATITIS: MILD TO MODERATE
Eat small meals
Eat soft, bland foods
Drink 3 L of fluids a day
Avoid citrus fruits, spicy foods
Avoid alcohol
Avoid very hot or very cold foods
Add nutritional supplements, as needed

SEVERE STOMATITIS
Eat liquid or pureed foods
Enteral or total parenteral nutrition may be needed

CONSTIPATION
Increase fiber (bran, fresh fruits and vegetables)
Increase fluid intake (3 L/day)
Eat natural laxative foods (prunes, apples)
Avoid cheese products

DIARRHEA
Avoid milk products
Avoid high-fiber, spicy foods
Eat foods high in potassium
Increase fluid intake (3 L/day); avoid caffeine and carbonated fluids
Add nutmeg to food to decrease gastric motility
Eat a high-protein, high-carbohydrate diet

POSTOPERATIVE RECOVERY
Eat food high in iron
Eat high-protein foods
Eat foods high in vitamin C, B complex, and K
Drink 6 to 8 glasses of fluids a day

From Lowdermilk, D. (1995). Home care of the patient with gynecologic cancer. *Journal of Obstetric, Gynecologic, and Neonatal Nursing, 24*(2), 159.

exposure to talc, a diet high in fat, lactose intolerance, and use of fertility drugs have been suggested as risk factors, but research findings are inconclusive (DiSaia & Creasman, 2002; Furniss, 2000). Pregnancy and use of oral contraceptives seem to have some protective benefits against ovarian cancer (ACS, 2003), whereas use of postmenopausal estrogen for more than 10 years may increase the risk (Rodriguez et al., 2001).

Clinical Manifestations and Diagnosis

Ovarian cancer has been called a silent disease because early warning symptoms that would send a woman to her health care provider are absent (e.g., no bleeding or other discharge and no pain). Vague lower abdominal discomfort and mild digestive complaints are the early symptoms for some. An ovary enlarged 5 cm or more than normal that is found during routine examination requires careful diagnostic workup. The accompanying increase in abdominal girth (caused by ovarian enlargement or ascites) is usually attributed to an increase in weight or a shift in weight that is seen commonly in women entering their middle years. Pelvic pain, anemia, and general weakness and malnutrition are signs of late-stage disease.

Early diagnosis of ovarian cancer is uncommon. Seventy percent of all women have metastasis outside of the pelvis at the time of diagnosis. Attempts at early detection have not proven to be reliable. Taking a family history is important because it may reveal cancer of the uterus or breast. Transvaginal ultrasound, CA-125 antigen (a tumor-associated antigen) testing, and frequent pelvic examinations have all been used without a great deal of success because these tumors grow quickly and painlessly. Transvaginal ultrasound and CA-125 screening currently are not recommended for routine screening in the general population but are recommended for women who are BRCA1 mutation carriers (Zawacki & Phillips, 2002). Routine pelvic examination continues to be the only practical screening method for detecting early disease, even though few cancers are detected in women without symptoms. Any ovarian enlargement should be considered highly suggestive and in need of further evaluation by laparoscopy or laparotomy. Responsibility for diagnosis rests with the pathologist. The size of the tumor is not indicative of the severity of disease. Clinical staging is done surgically and gives direction to treatment and prognosis (DiSaia & Creasman, 2002).

Therapeutic Management

Treatment is dictated by the stage of the disease at the time of initial diagnosis. Surgical removal of as much of the tumor as possible is the first step in therapy. This may involve just the removal of one ovary and tube or the radical excision of uterus, ovaries, tubes, and omentum. Cytoreductive surgery (the debulking of the poorly vascularized larger tumors) also is done. The smaller the volume of tumor remaining, the better the response to adjuvant therapy. Because about three fourths of women are in stage II, III, or IV disease at the time of diagnosis, surgical cure is not possible; therefore after tumor reduction surgery is performed, women with epithelial cell carcinoma will receive chemotherapy. Many institutions use a multiagent approach. Combinations of antineoplastic drugs such as cyclophosphamide (Cytoxan) and cisplatin or cisplatin and doxorubicin (Adriamycin) are common. Paclitaxel (Taxol) with cisplatin and other platinum drugs has become the first line of therapy in the United States. Combining immunotherapy with chemotherapy is being investigated (DiSaia & Creasman, 2002). Women being treated with chemotherapy are followed up closely with laboratory and radiologic tests and CA-125 levels to monitor their response to the therapy. Second-look surgery is a technique used to determine the response of the disease to chemotherapy and to determine whether treatment should be continued; however, this is no longer a widely used practice.

The efficacy of intraperitoneal installation with radioactive phosphorus (^{32}P) continues to be investigated. The role of radiation in treating advanced ovarian carcinoma is controversial. Radiation has been used as a palliative measure, and some women have had long-term survival after debulking surgery followed by radiation therapy (Stenchever et al., 2001). More research is needed regarding the role of radiation therapy in treatment of ovarian cancer.

Nursing Implications

The woman diagnosed with ovarian cancer has concerns similar to those described for the woman with endometrial and cervical cancer. Nursing interventions for the woman having surgery, chemotherapy, or external radiation therapy are described in other sections of this chapter.

Women with advanced ovarian cancer have a significant rate of recurrence. Follow-up for 5 years must be intensive. When a cure or remission cannot be achieved, palliative measures that alleviate symptoms of the progressing disease and provide comfort and maximal function are initiated. As the disease progresses, nutritional support, including enteral feedings and parenteral hyperalimentation, may be needed because of the effects of both the disease and the treatments on the gastrointestinal tract. The goal of nursing care is assisting the woman to maintain quality of life.

Because the period between a focus on cure and a focus on palliation is often prolonged, the woman with ovarian cancer is apt to experience most of the grief stages described by Kübler-Ross and to need support through each. After diagnosis, the woman often experiences denial and then anger. As treatment begins, she may "bargain" for a cure. If treatment is successful and death is forestalled by remission or cure, the process of adjustment to terminality ceases, and the woman again focuses on life and its challenges. When treatment fails to secure a cure or remission ends, the woman must turn again to the task of adjustment (see Legal Tip).

LEGAL TIP Advance Directives

Nurses who work with clients in hospitals with federal funding must know that because of the Patient Self-Determination Act, all clients must be asked if they have knowledge of Advance Directives and be provided with the information if desired. This is important to nurses working in gynecology-oncology settings, where decisions about living wills and no codes may be issues.

Family and friends also have diverse feelings. When grieving is prolonged, as it often is when the woman has cancer, the stress can be enormous and can interfere with other interpersonal relationships. If the woman is hospitalized, the environment may further intrude on relationships, limiting privacy and access to the woman and hindering opportunities for caring gestures. The nurse can assist the woman and her family to share their feelings with each other and help them to develop a support network (Lammers et al., 2000). Referral to a cancer support group may be useful.

Cancer of the Cervix

Incidence and Etiology

Cancer of the cervix is the third most common reproductive cancer. The accessible location of the cervix to both cell and tissue study and direct examination have led to a refinement of diagnostic techniques, contributing to improved management of these disorders. The incidence of invasive cancer has decreased by 50% over the last 25-year period, reducing mortality rates. However, the incidence of preinvasive cancer has increased, and more women in their twenties and thirties are being diagnosed with cervical neoplasia (ACS, 2003) (see Research box).

Cancer of the cervix begins as neoplastic changes in the cervical epithelium. Terms that have been used to describe these epithelial changes or preinvasive lesions include **dysplasia** and **cervical intraepithelial neoplasia (CIN).** Mild cervical dysplasia and CIN I refer to abnormal cellular proliferation in the lower one third of the epithelium; this dysplasia tends to be self-limiting and generally regresses

RESEARCH

Pap Test Abnormalities and Low-Income Youth

Abnormal Papanicolaou (Pap) tests have been increasing in adolescent females, ages 10 to 25 years of age, since the 1970s. Due to the exposure of endocervical cells on the developing cervix and increased unprotected sexual activity, adolescents may be more vulnerable to sexually transmitted infections (STIs) such as human papillomavirus (HPV), which is thought to cause most or all cervical dysplasias in young people. Although the American Cancer Society and some other groups recommend annual Pap tests for women over the age of 18 or women younger than 18 who are sexually active, there is controversy about routine Pap screening of adolescents for several reasons. Progression from cervical dysplasia to cervical cancer is usually slow and uncommon in young women, some studies suggest that HPV usually regresses spontaneously, and Pap tests and possible follow-up can be stressful for adolescents.

The purpose of this study was to describe the prevalence of cervical cell abnormalities found in Pap test results in low-income adolescent females. A multidisciplinary team led by a nurse researcher reviewed the 1996 Pap test reports of 5675 low-income females who were enrolled in a national job training program. Epithelial cell abnormalities suggesting further follow-up were found in 1 out of 20 students. Pap test results indicating dysplasia were found in 5.6%, or about 200 of the women. There were no significant differences in race, age, education, region of residence, public assistance, or drug use among the women with abnormal Pap tests. There also were no significant associations with positive tests for other bacterial STIs. Based on other studies that suggest that the true rate of HPV infections is 5 to 10 times higher than the Pap test findings, the researchers conclude that this sample may have an HPV infection rate of 25% to 50%.

IMPLICATIONS FOR PRACTICE

Pap tests alone or in combination with other tests can be an important screening tool for identifying cervical abnormalities. However, Pap screening is not universally agreed upon for screening adolescents. Nurses can use the results of this study to identify adolescents at risk and counsel them about options for screening for cervical abnormalities and for follow-up if needed. Educational literature needs to be developed and distributed to adolescents that describes the high rates of HPV in adolescents and its link to cervical cancer, prevention of HPV and other sexually transmitted infections, and the recommended screening and follow-up procedures available.

Reference: Halcon, L. et al. (2002). Pap test results among low-income youth: Prevalence of dysplasia and practice implications. *Journal of Obstetric, Gynecologic, and Neonatal Nursing, 31*(3), 294-304.

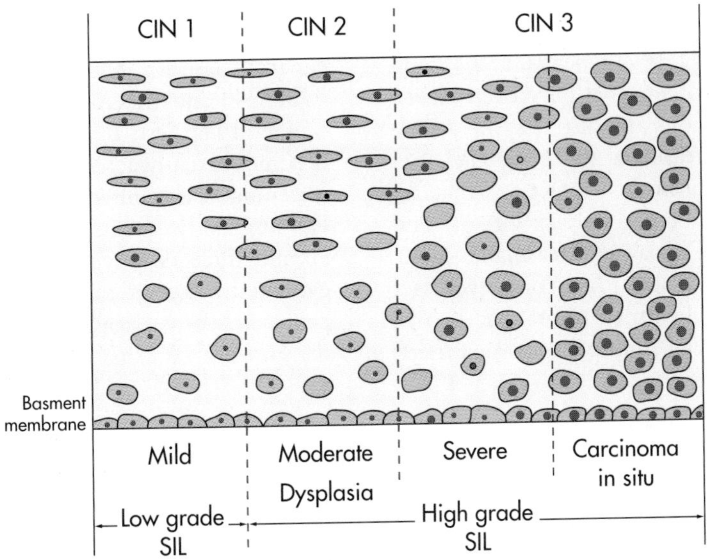
CIN 1
CIN 2
CIN 3
Basment membrane
Mild
Moderate
Dysplasia
Severe
Carcinoma in situ
Low grade SIL
High grade SIL

FIG. 12-11 Diagram of cervical epithelium showing progressive changes and various terminology.

to normal. Severe cervical dysplasia and CIN III involve the lower two thirds of the epithelium and often progress to carcinoma in situ. Carcinoma in situ (CIS) is diagnosed when the full thickness of epithelium shows abnormal cells (Fig. 12-11). Newer terms to describe neoplastic changes are low-grade and high-grade **squamous intraepithelial lesions (SILs);** however, CIN continues to be the most common term used in clinical practice.

Preinvasive lesions are limited to the cervix and usually originate in the squamocolumnar junction or

transformation zone (Fig. 12-12). Intensive study of the cervix and the cellular changes that take place has shown that most cervical tumors have a gradual onset rather than an explosive one. Preinvasive conditions may exist for years before the development of invasive disease. These preinvasive conditions are highly treatable in many cases.

Invasive carcinoma is the diagnosis when abnormal cells penetrate the basement membrane and invade the stroma. There are two types of invasive carcinoma of the cervix: microinvasive and invasive. Microinvasive carcinoma is defined as one or more lesions that penetrate no more than 3 mm into the stroma below the basement membrane with no areas of lymphatic or vascular invasion (DiSaia & Creasman, 2002). Invasive carcinoma describes invasion that goes beyond these parameters. The staging of invasive carcinoma extends from stage 0 (CIS) to stage IVb (distant metastasis or disease outside the true pelvis). A number of substages within each stage also exist. Clinical stages for cancer of the cervix are shown in Table 12-2.

Approximately 90% of cervical malignancies are squamous cell carcinomas; 10% are adenocarcinoma. Squamous cell carcinomas can spread by direct extension to the vaginal mucosa, pelvic wall, bowels, and bladder. Metastasis usually occurs in the pelvis, but it can occur to the lungs and brain through the lymphatic system.

The average age range for the occurrence of cervical cancer is 40 to 50 years; however, preinvasive conditions may exist for 10 to 15 years before the development of an invasive carcinoma. A strong link has been established between human papillomavirus (HPV) types 16 and 18 and cervical neoplasia. Eighteen other types have been associated with genital tract infections and also may be associated with CIN (DiSaia & Creasman, 2002; Stenchever et al., 2001). Other sexually transmitted infections that are identified as risk factors are herpes simplex virus II and possibly cytomegalovirus (DiSaia & Creasman, 2002). Other risk factors include early age at first coitus (younger than 20 years); multiple sexual partners (more than two); a sexual partner with a history of multiple sexual partners; and belonging to a lower socioeconomic group (ACS, 2003; DiSaia & Creasman, 2002; Reid, 2001; Stenchever et al., 2001). Other potential factors include use of oral contraceptives, cigarette smoking, and intrauterine exposure to diethylstilbestrol (DES). Vitamins A, C, E, and folate may be protective (Furniss, 2000).

The incidence of cervical cancer in the United States is highest in African-American and Hispanic women (ACS, 2003; DiSaia & Creasman, 2002). Factors that may influence cervical screening behaviors for these groups include lack of a health promotion or disease prevention perspective, lack of knowledge about Pap smears and availability of services, financial barriers, and failure of health care providers to recommend screening (Boyer et al., 2001). There also is a high rate of CIN in human immunodeficiency virus–positive women, suggesting that altered immune status is a risk factor.

Clinical Manifestations and Diagnosis

Preinvasive cancer of the cervix is often asymptomatic. Abnormal bleeding, especially postcoital bleeding, is the classic symptom of invasive cancer. Other late symptoms include rectal bleeding, hematuria, back pain, leg pain, and anemia. Diagnosis includes taking a history that includes menstrual and sexual activity information, particularly a history of sexually transmitted diseases and abnormal bleeding episodes (Adams, 2002). A pelvic examination usually will be normal except in late-stage cancer.

The single most reliable method to detect preinvasive cancer is the Pap test. The Pap test will detect 90% of early cervical changes. The U.S. Preventive Services Task Force (USPSTF) and the American Cancer Society (ACS) recommend Pap tests to begin about 3 years after a woman becomes sexually active but not later than age 21. Annual screening is recommended to age 30 (with conventional Pap test; every 2 years if liquid-based Pap tests). After age 30 and three negative Pap tests, screening may be done every 2 to 3 years in consultation with the health care provider. Women ages 65 to 70 with no abnormal tests in the previous 10 years may choose to stop screenings (ACS,

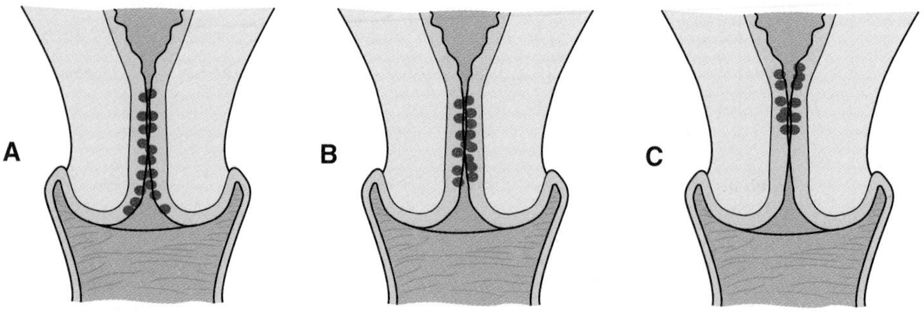
A
B
C

FIG. 12-12 Location of squamocolumnar junction according to age. The location where the endocervical glands meet the squamous epithelium becomes progressively higher with age. **A**, Puberty. **B**, Reproductive years. **C**, Postmenopausal. (From Willson, J., & Carrington, E. [1991]. *Obstetrics and gynecology*. St. Louis: Mosby.)

2003; USPSTF, 2003). Women in high risk categories should have more frequent Pap tests.

Pap test results in the past have been recorded by using several different classification systems. The reporting system most often used today is the Bethesda system, one that reports on gynecologic cytology as well as histology of cervical lesions (Table 12-3). Changes secondary to inflammation, treatment (e.g., radiation), and contraceptive devices can be reported, as well as changes caused by infections. Epithelial cell abnormalities are described in three categories: atypias, or atypical squamous cells of undetermined significance (ASCUS); low-grade SILs; and high-grade SILs. Low-grade SILs include cellular changes associated with HPV and mild dysplasia (CIN I). A finding of ASCUS is followed with repeated Pap tests every 4 to 6 months for 2 years until there have been three negative tests; if a second ASCUS is reported within 2 years, a colposcopy may be indicated. A finding of low-grade SIL is followed up with a repeated Pap test every 4 to 6 months; colposcopy and directed biopsy are indicated if repeated tests show abnormalities. High-grade SILs include lesions formerly described as moderate dysplasia (CIN II), severe dysplasia (CIN III), and CIS. Follow-up for a report of high-grade SIL includes colposcopy and directed biopsy (Centers for Disease Control and Prevention, 2002; DiSaia & Creasman, 2002).

HPV testing has been suggested as an alternative to these methods of follow-up for abnormal Pap results. A consensus conference sponsored by the American Society for Colposcopy and Cervical Pathology published guidelines for management of women with cervical cytology abnormalities. Repeated Pap testing, colposcopy, and DNA HPV tests are all safe and effective. However, if a Pap result shows ASCUS, DNA testing for high risk types of HPV is preferred, particularly if the Pap test was done by using liquid-based screening (Wright et al., 2002).

Colposcopy is the examination of the cervix with a stereoscopic binocular microscope that magnifies the view of the cervix. Usually a solution of 3% acetic acid is applied to the cervix for better visualization of the epithelium and to identify areas for biopsy. Colposcopy is not an invasive procedure and is usually well tolerated by the woman. However, the woman who is scheduled for colposcopy because of an abnormal Pap test may be anxious about the procedure and may need explanations or written information about what to expect during the procedure (Tomaino-Brunner et al., 1998).

Biopsy is the removal of cervical tissue for study, and several techniques can be used. An endocervical curettage is an effective diagnostic tool in about 90% of cases. It can be performed as an outpatient procedure with little or no anesthesia. It may be uncomfortable, and interventions to help the woman relax and cope with the pain may be needed.

Conization and loop electrosurgical excision procedure (LEEP) (p. 311) can be done as outpatient procedures, although neither is usually done unless the biopsy is positive or the results of the colposcopy are unsatisfactory. **Conization** involves removal of a cone of tissue

TABLE 12-2 **FIGO Classification of Cervical Carcinoma**

STAGE	DESCRIPTION
0	Carcinoma in situ, intraepithelial carcinoma
I	The carcinoma is strictly confined to the cervix (extension to the corpus should be disregarded)
Ia	Invasive cancer identified only microscopically; all gross lesions, even with superficial invasion, are stage Ib cancers. Invasion is limited to measured stromal invasion with maximum depth of 5.0 mm and no wider than 7.0 mm
Ia1	Measured invasion of stroma ≤3.0 mm in depth and no wider than 7.0 mm
Ia2	Measured invasion of stroma >3.0 mm and ≤5.0 mm and no wider than 7.0 mm. The depth of invasion should not be >5.0 mm taken from the base of the epithelium, surface or glandular, from which it originates. Vascular space involvement, venous or lymphatic, should not alter the staging
Ib	Clinical lesions confined to the cervix or preclinical lesions greater than stage Ia
Ib1	Clinical lesions ≤4.0 cm
Ib2	Clinical lesions >4.0 cm
II	Involvement of the vagina but not the lower third, or infiltration of the parametria but not out to the side wall
IIa	Involvement of the vagina, but no evidence of parametrial involvement
IIb	Infiltration of the parametria, but not out to the side wall
III	Involvement of the lower third of the vagina or extension to the pelvic side wall. All cases with a hydronephrosis or nonfunctioning kidney should be included, unless they are known to be attributable to other cause
IIIa	Involvement of the lower third of the vagina but not out to the pelvic side wall if the parametria are involved
IIIb	Extension onto the pelvic side wall and/or hydronephrosis or nonfunctional kidney
IV	Extension outside the reproductive tract
IVa	Involvement of the mucosa of the bladder or rectum
IVb	Distant metastasis or disease outside the true pelvis

From DiSaia, P., & Creasman, W. (2002). *Clinical gynecologic oncology* (6th ed.). St. Louis: Mosby.

TABLE 12-3 **Comparison of Bethesda System with Other Cytology Classification Systems**

DYSPLASIA/CIS	CIN	BETHESDA
Normal	Normal	Within normal limits
Benign atypia	Inflammatory atypia (organism)	Benign cellular changes
		Infection: specified
		Reactive changes:
		Inflammation
		Atrophy
		Radiation
		Squamous cell abnormalities
Atypical cells	Squamous atypia	ASCUS
Mild dysplasia	CIN I	Low-grade SIL: HPV, CIN I
Moderate dysplasia	CIN II	High-grade SIL
Severe (marked) dysplasia, Carcinoma in situ (CIS)	CIN III	CIN II, CIN III
Adenocarcinoma and CIS		Glandular cell abnormalities

From DiSaia, P., & Creasman, W. (2002). *Clinical gynecologic oncology* (6th ed.). St. Louis: Mosby.
CIN, Cervical intraepithelial neoplasia; *SIL*, squamous intraepithelial lesion; *ASCUS*, atypical squamous cells of undetermined significance; *HPV*, human papillomavirus.

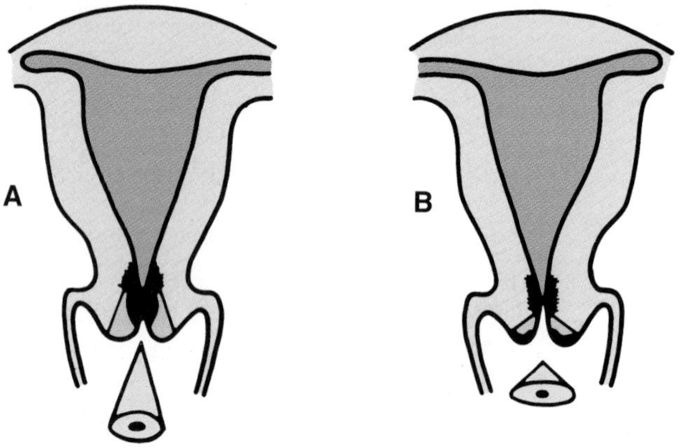

A
B

FIG. 12-13 A, Cone biopsy for endocervical disease. Limits of lesion were not seen colposcopically. **B,** Cone biopsy for cervical intraepithelial neoplasia of the exocervix. Limits of lesion were identified colposcopically. (From DiSaia, P., & Creasman, W. [2002]. *Clinical gynecologic oncology* [6th ed.]. St. Louis: Mosby.)

from the exocervix and endocervix (Fig. 12-13). It can be done as a cold knife procedure, a laser excision, or an electrosurgical excision (see discussion on p. 311). There are two advantages to a cone biopsy. It can be used (1) to establish the diagnosis and (2) to effect a cure. If CIS is diagnosed, and if the woman wishes to retain her childbearing capacity, conization removes the abnormal tissue; further treatment is unnecessary. The woman is monitored with Pap tests and colposcopy when indicated.

If invasive cancer is diagnosed, other diagnostic tests are done to assess the extent of spread (see previous discussion under endometrial cancer). Once the extent of the cancer is known, treatment begins.

CARE MANAGEMENT

Assessment and Nursing Diagnoses

For the woman diagnosed with invasive carcinoma of the cervix, pretherapy assessment includes physical, psychologic, and educational components, regardless of whether surgery or radiation is the method of treatment. Physical assessment includes a review of current medications, because medications for other medical problems may need to be continued. Skin is assessed to identify potential pressure points; respiratory and gastrointestinal status and state of nutrition are important factors to assess. Urinalysis and complete blood count also are commonly performed. An electrocardiogram and a chest x-ray examination may be done if use of a general anesthetic is anticipated for surgery or placement of internal applicators.

Psychologic assessment is important because frequently these women are emotionally distressed about the diagnosis and anticipated treatment (i.e., fear of being radioactive and fear of pain) and fear that family or significant others will become distant.

Educational assessment involves identifying the woman's current knowledge base regarding the diagnosis and proposed therapeutic regimen. Nursing diagnoses for the woman having surgery for cervical cancer are similar to those identified for the woman having a hysterectomy for endometrial cancer (p. 301). Nursing diagnoses that might arise from an assessment for the woman who is to have external or internal radiation therapy for treatment of cervical cancer include the following:

- *Deficient knowledge related to*
  - –treatment procedures
- *Fear/anxiety related to*
  - –diagnosis
  - –anticipated pain
  - –concerns about radioactivity
  - –the response of the significant other or family
- *Disturbed sensory perception related to*
  - –internal radiation therapy
  - –restricted contact with visitors and nursing staff
- *Risk for impaired skin integrity related to*
  - –external radiation exposure
  - –immobility and bed rest (internal radiation therapy)
- *Risk for injury related to*
  - –dislodgment of radiation source
- *Acute pain related to*
  - –internal applicators
- *Risk for sexual dysfunction related to*
  - –treatment or concerns of significant other

Expected Outcomes of Care

Mutually determined outcomes for the woman undergoing radiation therapy for cervical cancer related to the identified nursing diagnoses might include that the woman will do the following:

- Verbalize an understanding of the proposed treatment and accompanying procedures
- Verbalize her fears regarding diagnosis, treatment, and response of significant others and family
- Maintain contact with family and friends through short visits or by telephone if internal radiation therapy is done
- Remain free from skin breakdown
- Identify methods to maintain skin hygiene
- Remain on strict bed rest on her back to prevent dislodgment of the internal applicators if internal radiation therapy is done
- Verbalize control of pain
- Resume a satisfactory sexual relationship with her partner

Plan of Care and Interventions

Preinvasive Lesions

Once a diagnosis has been identified, a course of treatment is planned. For preinvasive lesions, several techniques are used. As stated earlier, because many preinvasive conditions are detected in younger women who may wish to continue childbearing, treatment is geared toward eradicating abnormal cells while attempting to preserve the structure of the cervix. The techniques currently available for preinvasive lesions are cryotherapy, laser therapy, and LEEP. Treatment for invasive cancer includes surgery, radiation therapy, and chemotherapy.

Cryosurgery. Cryosurgery uses a freezing technique that freezes abnormal cells, and when sloughing occurs, regeneration of tissue is normal. Side effects occurring after treatment are usually few and not of a serious nature. A profuse watery discharge can persist for 2 to 4 weeks. Follow-up examination and a Pap test are scheduled in 4 to 6 months. Endocervical cells are thought to regenerate, leaving a normal cervical canal in most instances. Spotting or cervical stenosis are rare complications. Surveillance with frequent Pap tests and colposcopic examination must continue indefinitely after this type of conservative therapy. Persistent abnormal cells require reevaluation, and plans are made for repeated cryosurgery or other therapy.

Laser Surgery. Laser surgery can eradicate most cases of CIN. This technique involves a laser mounted on a colposcope that allows precise direction of a beam of light (heat) to remove diseased tissue. For treatment of the cervix (relatively insensitive tissue), the woman may need no anesthesia. Some women complain of a burning or cramping sensation that is tolerable for most women. The cervix treated with CO_2 laser will show epithelial regrowth beginning by 2 days. The site is usually healed in 4 to 6 weeks. The original architecture of the cervix is preserved, and the squamocolumnar junction remains visible; however, there may be more damage to normal tissues than with other treatments. Women usually have less vaginal discharge than with cryosurgery, but there may be more discomfort after the procedure (Stenchever et al., 2001).

Electrosurgical Excision. The *LEEP* has become a standard treatment for cervical dysplasia in the United States. This procedure uses a wire loop electrode that can excise and cauterize with minimal tissue damage (Fig. 12-14). Healing is rapid, and there is only a mild discharge afterward. Possible complications include bleeding, cervical stenosis, infertility, and loss of cervical mucus (Stenchever et al., 2001).

Invasive Cancer of the Cervix

Once the cancer is staged, treatment is begun. Microinvasive cancer is usually treated with conization, but a hysterectomy is often done if childbearing is not desired. The choice of treatment for early-stage invasive cancer is by either surgery or radiation therapy because survival rates are comparable (American College of Obstetricians and Gynecologists, 2000; Stenchever et al., 2001). Locally advanced stages of cervical cancer usually are treated with radiation therapy, both external and internal. A radical hysterectomy is performed if the cancer has extended beyond the cervix but not to the pelvic wall.

Radical Hysterectomy. *Radical hysterectomy* involves removal of the uterus, tubes, ovaries, upper third of the vagina, entire uterosacral and uterovesical ligaments, and all of the parametrium on each side, along with pelvic node dissection encompassing the four major pelvic lymph node chains: ureteral, obturator, hypogastric, and iliac. Dissection serves to preserve the bladder, rectum, and ureters while removing as much of the remaining tissue of the pelvis as is feasible. Women with positive pelvic nodes usually receive postoperative whole pelvis irradiation, although there is little evidence that it alters the incidence of recurrence in the pelvic area (DiSaia & Creasman, 2002).

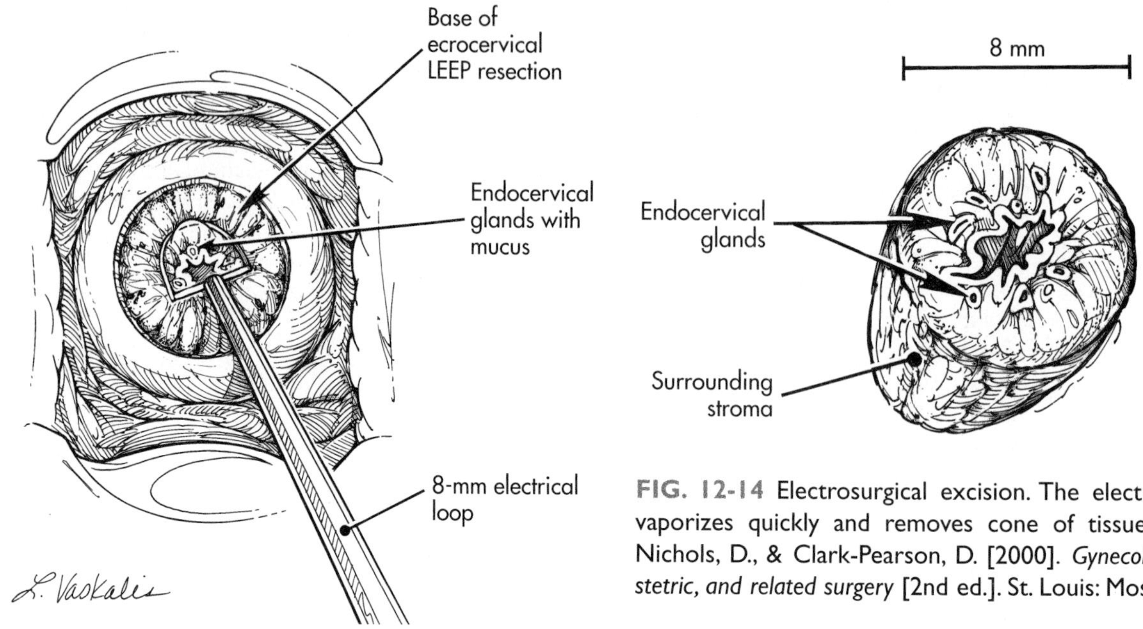
Base of
ecrocervical
LEEP resection
Endocervical
glands with
mucus
8-mm electrical
loop
L. Vaskalis
8 mm
Endocervical
glands
Surrounding
stroma

FIG. 12-14 Electrosurgical excision. The electric loop vaporizes quickly and removes cone of tissue. (From Nichols, D., & Clark-Pearson, D. [2000]. *Gynecologic, obstetric, and related surgery* [2nd ed.]. St. Louis: Mosby.)

Nursing Management. Nursing care for the woman having a radical hysterectomy was discussed in the previous section on endometrial cancer (p. 302).

Radiation Therapy. Radiation may be delivered by internal radium applications to the cervix or external radiation therapy that includes lymphatics of the pelvic side wall. In preparation for radiation therapy, the woman must maintain good nutritional status and a high-protein, high-vitamin, and high-calorie diet. Anemia, if present, should be corrected before the initiation of radiotherapy.

External irradiation and intracavitary radium therapy are used in various combinations for the best results and are tailored to each woman and her particular lesion. Megavoltage machines such as cobalt, linear accelerators, and the betatron have the distinct advantage of providing a more homogeneous dose to the pelvis. The hard, short rays of megavoltage pass through the skin without much absorption by the skin and therefore cause little dermal injury.

External radiation therapy and internal radiation therapy are given in various combinations. For example, external radiation may be given first to treat regional pelvic nodes and to shrink the tumor. External irradiation is usually an outpatient procedure given 5 days a week for 4 to 6 weeks. Internal radiation therapy consists of one or two intracavitary treatments at least 2 weeks apart (DiSaia & Creasman, 2002).

For internal radiation therapy, the woman may be treated in the hospital or in a special unit in an outpatient setting. If treatment is done in the hospital, the woman is taken to the operating room, and while she is under general anesthesia, a specially designed applicator is placed into her vagina and cervix. X-rays are taken to make sure the applicator is correctly placed. The woman is returned to her room, where the radioactive source is placed into the applicator (Fig. 12-15). The source remains in place

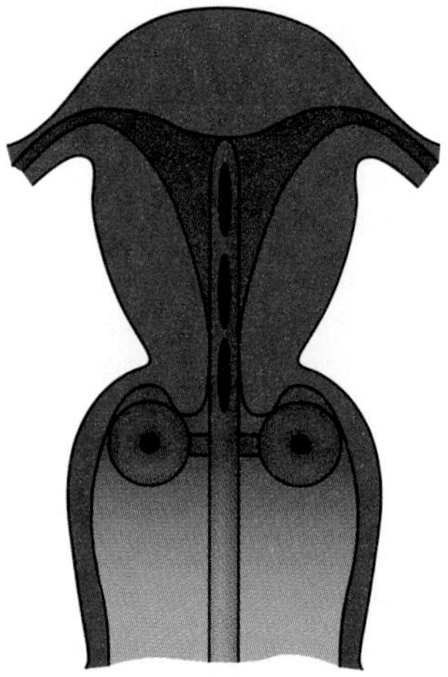

FIG. 12-15 Intracavitary implant. Applicator in place in uterus is loaded with radium source.

from 12 hours to 3 days. If treatment is in the outpatient setting, the applicator is inserted into the uterus in a treatment room; use of high-dose implants shortens the treatment time (DiSaia & Creasman, 2002).

In advanced carcinoma of the cervix, conventional intracavitary applicators are not applicable. Interstitial therapy uses a template to guide the transperineal insertion of a group of 18-gauge hollow steel needles into the lesion (Fig. 12-16). After the needles are placed, the iridium wires are inserted when the woman is returned to her room.

Nursing Management. Nursing actions for external and internal radiation differ, so they are discussed separately. Before external radiation therapy, the woman's anxiety may be so high that information given by the radiologist may not be processed. The nurse should reinforce or

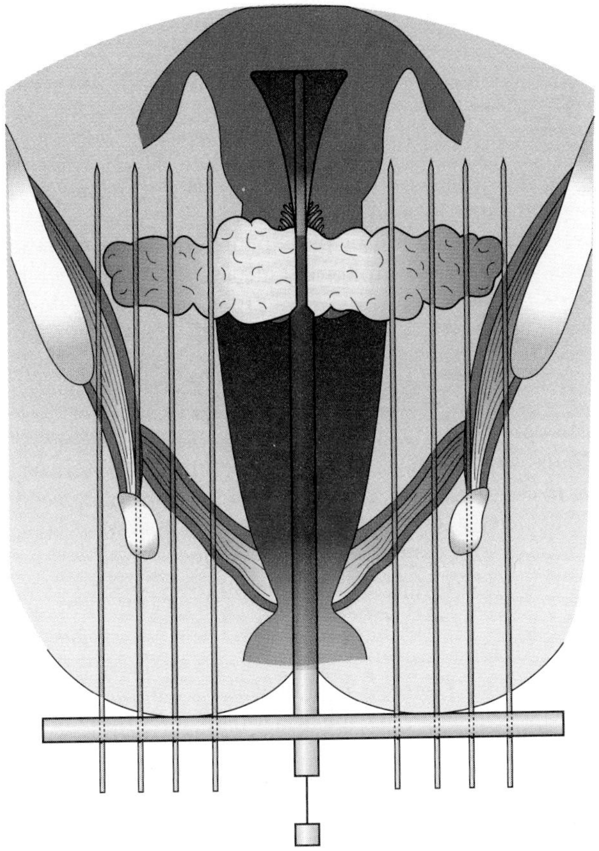

FIG. 12-16 Interstitial-intracavitary implant.

fill in gaps, especially related to the following: the equipment, which is similar to that used for x-ray examination except larger; the hyperbaric oxygen chamber, which may be used to increase cellular oxygen and thus make tumor cells more radiosensitive; the radiotherapist, who will be behind a shield, but still close by and in communication with her; the position she will be put in and asked to maintain for some minutes; and the therapy, which is painless.

During the course of the therapy, the woman is counseled regarding maintaining general good health. To maintain good skin care, the woman is taught to assess her skin often; avoid soaps, ointments, cosmetics, and deodorants if the axilla is being irradiated, and so on, because these may contain metals that would alter the dose she receives and could lead to skin breakdown; wear loose clothing over the area and cotton underwear (or no underwear); use an air mattress or cover the mattress with foam pads or sheepskin; avoid exposing the irradiated areas to temperature extremes; and especially avoid removing the markings made by the radiologist. If her skin becomes red or itchy, treat it with remedies recommended by the radiologist (e.g., aloe vera lotion or warm sitz baths). To treat skin that is broken or desquamating, the woman is shown how to use remedies prescribed by the radiologist (e.g., irrigation with equal parts peroxide and saline, application of antibiotic or lanolin ointment, exposure to air, and application

TEACHING FOR SELF-CARE

Care After External Radiation Therapy

- Avoid infection and report symptoms of infection to health care provider immediately.
- Maintain good nutrition and fluid intake.
- May experience effects of radiation for 10 to 14 days after last treatment.
- Expect signs of healing to occur in about 3 weeks.
- Maintain good skin and mouth care to support a sense of well-being and prevent infection.
- Report the following symptoms to health care provider:
  Continued gastrointestinal symptoms (nausea, vomiting, anorexia, diarrhea)
  Increasing skin irritation at the site of therapy (redness, swelling, pain, pruritis)
- Take medications as prescribed, and avoid any medications not prescribed or approved by health care provider.

of a loose dressing). Avoid the use of adhesive (or any) tape directly on the target area of skin (Stenchever et al., 2001).

NURSE ALERT
If a woman is receiving chemotherapy during radiation therapy, she is at a higher risk for developing a skin infection (Iwamoto, 2001).

To maintain good nutrition, the woman is reminded to maintain a daily record of weight; use high-protein supplements; eat small, attractive, appetizing meals that are more bland than spicy; and keep the environment light, airy, clean, and quiet (especially before and after meals). A dietitian consult may be needed to help the woman and her family plan to meet the woman's nutritional needs. If the woman is ill enough to be hospitalized, she may need total parenteral nutrition or tube feedings. Nausea interferes with adequate intake; therefore the woman may take antiemetics, as necessary. High daily fluid intake (2 to 3 L) should be suggested if not contraindicated. To increase her comfort, minimize infection, and promote adequate food intake, the woman is encouraged to perform frequent oral hygiene. Box 12-4 (p. 305) provides other suggestions for nutritional problems associated with radiation treatment.

The nurse explains, as necessary, the need for routine blood studies to monitor white blood cell count (to determine degree of immunosuppression). The woman and her family will need information about neutropenia, thrombocytopenia, and anemia and precautions to be taken. Because the woman is more vulnerable to infection, she is reminded of general measures to avoid infection (e.g., practice good hygiene, avoid people with infection, avoid large crowds, keep environment clean).

After the radiation treatment is completed, the woman needs information for self-care (see Teaching for Self Care box).

Internal radiation therapy may require hospitalization or be done in a special outpatient unit. Radiation safety officers determine the precautions to be observed in each situation. This discussion focuses on treatment in the hospital setting. Printed instruction sheets are usually available stating precautions to be followed for each type of radiation substance used. A precaution sign is placed on the door of the woman's room.

NURSE ALERT

Personnel who come in direct contact with anyone receiving radiation therapy should wear a film badge or other device to monitor the amount of exposure received.

Nurses must protect themselves from overexposure to radiation. Precautions include the following behaviors (Iwamato, 2001):

- Careful isolation techniques: wearing gloves while handling bodily fluids and observing good handwashing technique. These behaviors reflect knowledge that alpha and beta rays cannot pass through skin but may be in body fluids and excrement.
- Careful planning of nursing activity to limit time (to 30 minutes or less per 8 hours) spent in close proximity to the woman to avoid exposure to gamma rays, which can penetrate several inches of lead.

Exposure to radiation is controlled in three ways: distance, time, and shielding (with lead). For the woman with sealed radiotherapy, a movable lead screen can be placed between the area in which the therapeutic applicator is located and the personnel. The lead screen also is used to protect visitors from radiation. Increasing the distance from the source also decreases exposure (Iwamoto, 2001).

Familiarity with applicators is a must for all nurses working with people receiving radiotherapy so that if a "strange object" is found in the linen or on the floor, it is not touched. Today most hospital protocols include having a lead container and forceps in the room for use if a radioactive implant is dislodged.

The woman is prepared for insertion with the following care, which is accompanied by an explanation for each activity. To reduce the need for an enema or attention to bowel elimination for a few days, the gastrointestinal tract is usually prepared by using low-residue diet, enemas, and sometimes bowel sedation. The vaginal vault is usually prepared with an antiseptic douche, such as povidone-iodine.

An indwelling urinary bladder catheter is inserted, as ordered, to prevent urinary distention that could dislodge the applicator. Nothing is taken by mouth the night before the procedure in anticipation of general anesthesia. Preoperative medications may be ordered for the morning of the procedure. Deep-breathing exercises, range-of-motion exercises, and positioning are all demonstrated before the procedure to minimize the effects of immobilization afterward. An intravenous (IV) solution will probably be started before the procedure, and IV therapy may be continued if nausea prevents good oral intake of fluids. The woman is assured that pain will be managed.

Explanations about restricted visitation of personnel and visitors also are given in the preinsertion phase. Women are often encouraged to bring reading materials or other hobbies such as crossword puzzles to the hospital to combat the boredom that isolation imposes on them (Iwamoto, 2001).

The applicator is inserted in surgery with the woman under general anesthesia if necessary to facilitate vaginal examination and ease of placement. The usual postanesthesia recovery care follows, and she is returned to her room. The woman is positioned on her back. There the applicators are loaded with the radioactive substance.

A lead shield is placed next to the woman's pelvic area. Vital signs are monitored every 4 hours. Active range-of-motion and deep-breathing exercises are encouraged every 2 hours; the woman may not be permitted to turn from side to side, although log-rolling may be done occasionally to relieve back pressure. The head of the bed may or may not be elevated slightly (Iwamoto, 2001).

The woman's diet is changed from clear liquid to low residue, as ordered. Many women have difficulty eating while lying flat or even if the bed is elevated slightly. The nurse arranges the food so that it is easy to reach. Finger foods or liquids are generally more manageable. Parenteral or oral fluids are given, up to 3 L daily.

The urinary catheter remains in the bladder while the implant is in place. However, no perineal or catheter care is given. Intake and output are measured. The woman is given a partial bath, washing only above her waist. Massage is restricted to her shoulders and neck. Linen is changed only as absolutely necessary. Any linen or equipment used is retained in the room until therapy is complete to prevent loss of an applicator or seed. If vaginal or rectal bleeding or hematuria occurs, the physician is notified immediately.

Emotional support is provided by planning to be with the woman for short periods; encouraging her to verbalize concerns and needs; and encouraging family members, clergy, or others to visit for short periods daily or to communicate by telephone. Pregnant women and children are not permitted to visit.

Many women undergoing internal radiation treatment are given medication to prevent complications and to promote comfort during the procedure. Such medications might include antibiotics to prevent bladder infections, heparin injections to prevent thrombophlebitis, sedatives for relaxation, antiemetics for nausea, and narcotics for pain. The woman is considered radioactive during the time the internal sources are in place (Iwamoto, 2001).

After the radium is removed, the Foley catheter is removed, and the woman is assisted in getting out of bed the first time. She is usually discharged the same day. Discharge teaching can be found in the Teaching for Self-Care box. The woman and her family are reassured that she is not radioactive after the treatment.

Posttreatment complications range from those arising from immobilization, such as thrombophlebitis, pulmonary embolism, and pneumonia, to those arising from the treatment itself, such as hemorrhage, skin reactions (rashes or inflammation), diarrhea, cramping, dysuria, and vaginal stenosis. The woman is assessed for any of these complications before discharge.

The woman may experience altered patterns of sexuality related to treatment side effects. A decrease in vaginal secretions and sensation may occur, as well as vaginal stenosis. These can contribute to decreased sexual desire because pain and discomfort during intercourse can affect the desire to resume sexual activities. The nurse can initiate a discussion with the woman and her partner, offer information about the effects of radiation on the ability to have sexual intercourse, and offer suggestions for specific problems, such as using a water-based lubricant for vaginal dryness and using a vaginal dilator three times a week for a year or more. If necessary, the couple can be referred to other resources (Iwamoto, 2001; Wilmoth & Spinelli, 2000).

Complications of Radiation Therapy. Morbidity as a direct result from properly conducted therapy is usually minimal. Some of the morbidity seen may be caused by the uncontrolled tumor and not by the therapy. Acute treatment complications occurring during or shortly after therapy include irritation of the rectum, small bowel, and bladder; reactions in the skin folds; and mild bone marrow suppression. Dysuria and frequency may occur. Late complications, although not common, include genital fistulas and necrosis (Stenchever et al., 2001).

Chemoradiation. Chemoradiation also may improve survival for women with cervical cancer. This treatment includes weekly cisplatin therapy concurrent with the radiation therapy. Investigation of this mode of therapy continues (DiSaia & Creasman, 2002).

TEACHING FOR SELF-CARE

Care After Internal Radiation Therapy

- Eat three balanced meals a day, and increase fluid to 3 L daily.
- Rest when tired, and resume normal activities as comfort permits.
- Maintain good hygiene (e.g., daily showers and daily douches until discharge stops).
- Resume sexual intercourse in 7 to 10 days or as recommended by physician. Use vaginal dilator if needed for vaginal stenosis.
- Understand that sterility and cessation of menstruation usually occur with this procedure if you are premenopausal.
- Report any of the following to your health care provider: bleeding (vaginal, rectal, or in the urine), foul-smelling vaginal discharge, fever, abdominal distention, or pain.
- Take any prescribed medications as directed.
- Call your health care provider or clinic if there are concerns or problems.
- Plan follow-up visits to determine emotional as well as physical recovery.

Recurrent and Advanced Cancer of the Cervix

Approximately one third of women with invasive cervical cancer will have recurrent or persistent disease after therapy (Stenchever et al., 2001). Prognosis is discouraging, with a 1-year survival rate between 10% and 15% (DiSaia & Creasman, 2002). Irradiation of metastatic areas is commonly successful in providing local control and symptomatic relief. Irradiation for recurrent disease may be considered for women who were initially treated with surgery. Further radiation may not be effective for those women who were initially treated with radiation.

Pelvic Exenteration. The woman who has recurrence only within the pelvis may be considered for **pelvic exenteration** if a cure is thought to be possible. A total exenteration involves removal of the perineum, pelvic floor, levator muscles, and all reproductive organs. Additionally, pelvic lymph nodes, rectum, sigmoid colon, urinary bladder, and distal ureters are removed, and a colostomy and ileal conduit are constructed (Fig. 12-17, *A*). In very select cases, the procedure can be modified to either an anterior or a posterior exenteration. In anterior pelvic exenteration, all of the previously mentioned pelvic viscera are removed except the rectosigmoid, which is preserved. Urine is rerouted through an ileal conduit (Fig. 12-17, *B*). In the posterior pelvic exenteration procedure, all pelvic viscera with the exception of the bladder are removed. The feces are rerouted through a colostomy (Fig. 12-17, *C*). A neovagina (new vagina) may be constructed.

Women are carefully selected for this procedure; 5-year survival rates range from 20% to 62% (DiSaia & Creasman, 2002). Many of the complications that follow this surgery are those that follow any form of major surgery, for example, pulmonary embolism, pulmonary edema, myocardial infarction, and cerebrovascular accident. These complications are seen immediately after surgery. Infection originating in the pelvic cavity usually occurs later, if it occurs.

Nursing Management. Nursing care of the woman having a pelvic exenteration depends on what is removed. General preoperative considerations include assessments similar to those for a woman having a radical hysterectomy. Additionally, a thorough sexual assessment is needed because of the drastic changes involved. The woman needs information about the construction of a neovagina if that is an option. She will need to be assessed for stoma site selection and information about management of colostomy or ileal conduit if appropriate. Extensive preoperative bowel preparation is needed before surgery. Pain management is discussed, as is what to expect postoperatively (e.g., nasogastric tubes, arterial catheters). Significant others should be included in preoperative discussions when possible because their postoperative support is essential.

Postoperative care usually begins in an intensive care unit until the woman's condition is stable. She is monitored for signs of complications, including shock, hemorrhage, pulmonary embolus and other pulmonary complications, fluid and electrolyte imbalance, and urinary complications

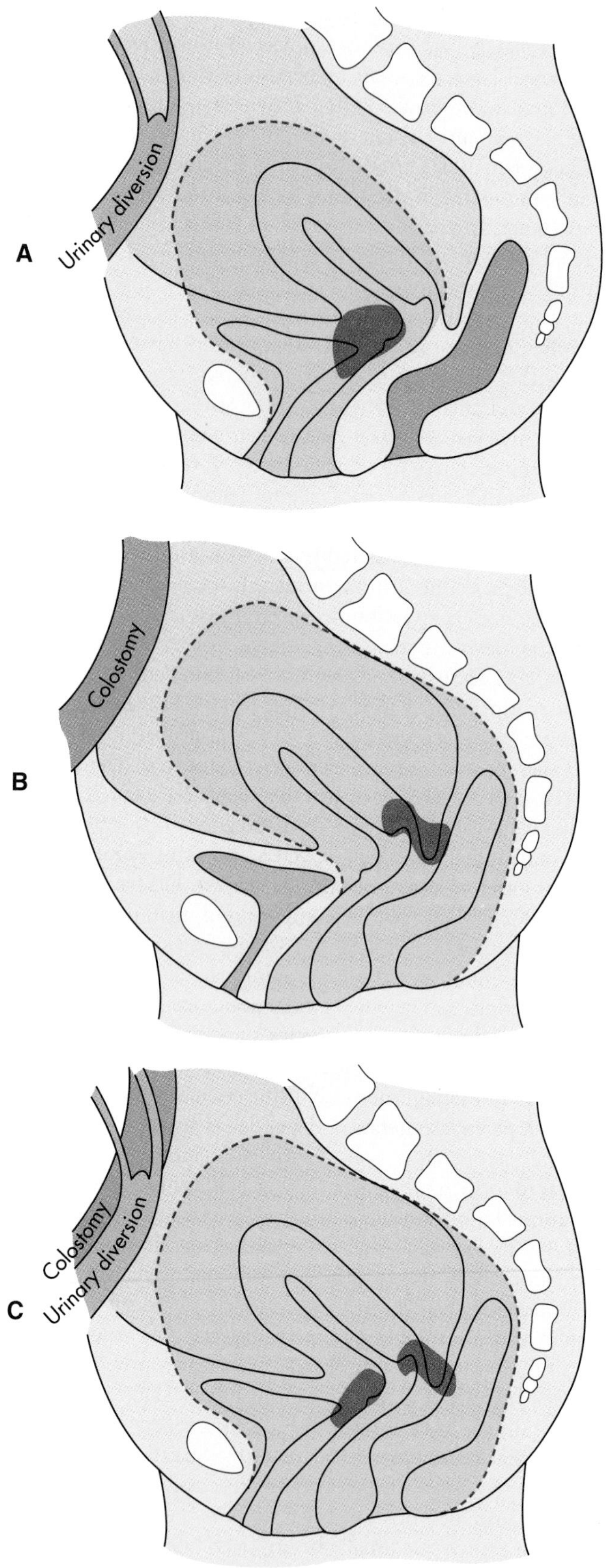
A
Urinary diversion
B
Colostomy
C
Colostomy
Urinary diversion

FIG. 12-17 Pelvic exenteration procedures. **A,** Anterior exenteration. **B,** Posterior exenteration. **C,** Total exenteration. (From DiSaia, P., & Morrow, C. [1973]. *California Medicine,* 118,13, Feb.)

(Otto, 2001). Nursing care continues after the woman is stabilized and moved back to her room. Wound care consists of irrigation with one-half normal saline, followed by drying of the area with either a hair dryer on cool setting or a heat lamp placed at least 12 inches from the perineal area. The woman is taught how to care for her colostomy or ileal conduit when she is able to begin self-care. Assessment for psychologic reactions is important. The woman will probably experience a grief reaction over her mutilated body. She may become depressed during the long convalescence.

The woman may be discharged to a long-term care facility or to her home. She will need assistance in her physical care for at least 6 months. Teaching needed for home care includes colostomy or ureterostomy care; dietary needs for healing; perineal care, including use of perineal pads to protect clothing from discharge; range-of-motion exercises and physical activities permitted by her health care provider; and signs of complication, especially infection and bowel obstruction (Otto, 2001).

Because the woman will have sexual disruption and the possibility of not being able to have vaginal intercourse (if the vagina is not reconstructed), counseling about sexual activity is needed. Usually even with a vaginal reconstruction, vaginal intercourse is not advised until healing has taken place, usually 12 to 18 months. Women with neovaginas may complain of decreased vaginal sensations, chronic discharge, or that the vagina is too short or too long. Women with colostomies or ureterostomies may worry about leakage or odors during sexual activities. Women may be concerned about their change in appearance. They may need counseling about alternative activities for sexual expression for themselves and their partners. The woman and her partner may need referral for further sexual counseling (Wilmoth & Spinelli, 2000).

Chemotherapy. Chemotherapy may be used in advanced cancer of the cervix to reduce tumor size before surgery or as adjuvant therapy for poor-prognosis tumors. In general, no long-term benefits are derived with chemotherapy, although cisplatin and 5-FU demonstrate the most effects. Chemotherapy is beneficial as a pain-relief method (DiSaia & Creasman, 2002). Chemotherapy in combination with radiation treatments is being evaluated as to whether there is improvement in the results of radiation therapy (Stenchever et al., 2001).

Evaluation

The nurse can be reasonably assured that care was effective to the extent that the expected outcomes of care for the woman who has had radiation therapy or other treatment have been achieved.

Cancer of the Vulva

Incidence and Etiology

Vulvar carcinoma accounts for about 5% of all female genital malignancies and is the fourth most commonly occurring gynecologic cancer. It appears most frequently in older women in their middle sixties to seventies; however, the incidence in women younger than 35 years has increased since 1980. The disease has been linked to the presence of condylomata acuminata (genital warts) caused by HPV (types 16, 18, 31, 33, 35, 51, and possibly others), but the exact relationship is unknown (DiSaia & Creasman, 2002).

By far the majority (90%) of vulvar carcinoma is squamous cell; other vulvar neoplasms are attributed to Paget's disease, adenocarcinoma of Bartholin glands, fibrosarcoma and melanoma, and basal cell carcinoma. Vulvar intraepithelial neoplasia (VIN) is the first neoplastic change. VIN progresses over time to CIS, and then to invasive cancer. Metastatic spread is by direct extension and lymphatic spread.

Prognosis depends on the size of the lesion and the tumor grade at the time of diagnosis. Fifty percent of women have symptoms for 2 to 16 months before seeking treatment. Fortunately, vulvar cancer grows slowly, extends slowly, and metastasizes fairly late. Even with a pattern of delayed diagnosis, survival rates are greater than 90% for all stages if nodes are negative. Survival rates plummet to less than 50%, however, if lymph node metastasis has occurred (DiSaia & Creasman, 2002).

Clinical Manifestations and Diagnosis

The most common site for vulvar lesions is on the labia majora. The vulvar lesion is usually asymptomatic until it is 1 to 2 cm in diameter. When it is symptomatic, women may complain of vulvar pruritis or burning or pain. Necrosis and infection of the lesion result in ulceration with bleeding or watery discharge.

VINs are usually multifocal in young women. Unifocal lesions are associated with invasive cancer and are more common in older women. Initially, growth is superficial but later extends into the urethra, vagina, and anus. In approximately 50% of late cases, superficial inguinal and femoral lymph nodes become involved.

Simple biopsy with histologic evaluation reveals the diagnosis. The areas of pathologic involvement are identified by staining the vulva with toluidine blue (1%), allowing an absorption time of 3 to 5 minutes, and then washing with acetic acid (2% to 3%); abnormal tissue retains the dye. Biopsy is necessary to rule out such conditions as sexually transmitted infections (e.g., chancroid, granuloma inguinale, syphilis), basal cell carcinoma, and CIS. In situ malignancies are initially small, red, white, or pigmented friable papules. In Paget's disease, the lesions are red, moist, and elevated. Melanomas appear as bluish-black, pigmented, or papillary lesions. Melanomas metastasize through the bloodstream and lymphatics.

Collaborative Care

Therapeutic Management. Treatment varies, depending on the extent of the disease. Laser surgery, cryosurgery, or electrosurgical excision may be used to treat VIN. A disadvantage to these treatments is that healing is slow, and the treated area is painful. A local wide excision may be performed for localized lesions or a simple **vulvectomy** (removal of vulva, labia majora and minora, and possibly the clitoris). A *skinning vulvectomy* (Fig. 12-18, *A*) is preferred to the simple vulvectomy because it is less disfiguring. It involves removal of the superficial vulvar skin without clitoral removal, followed by split-thickness skin grafts. The fat, muscle, and glands are preserved.

For invasive disease, a radical or modified radical vulvectomy is performed. These procedures involve the removal of the entire vulva, skin, clitoris, labia, subcutaneous tissues, and the inguinal and femoral nodes (Fig. 12-18, *B*). If these nodes are positive, pelvic lymphadenectomy or pelvic lymph node irradiation is done.

External radiation therapy can be used to shrink tumors before surgery, but it is not used as the primary treatment. Postoperative external radiation therapy may be used for women who are at risk for recurrence. Radiation treatment causes dermatitis and ulceration that are uncomfortable for the woman.

Chemotherapy has not been very effective as a treatment except for the topical application of 5-FU for VIN or CIS. This treatment is painful and not used often. Chemotherapy continues to be investigated in combination with radiation as an adjunct to surgery in advanced cancer of the vulva (Otto, 2001).

Nursing Management. Nursing care for the woman with vulvar cancer is similar to that for the woman with

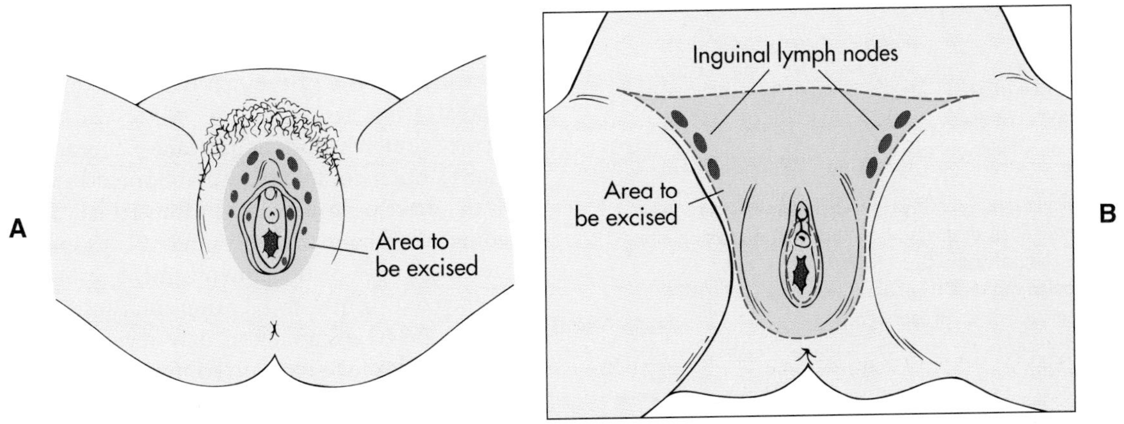
A
Area to be excised
Inguinal lymph nodes
Area to be excised
B

FIG. 12-18 Vulvectomy. **A,** Skinning vulvectomy. **B,** Radical vulvectomy.

other gynecologic malignancies. A history of symptoms and a physical examination should be done. An assessment of the woman's understanding of the surgical procedure and her emotional state also should be done. Possible nursing diagnoses include the following:

- *Risk for infection related to*
  –surgical incision
- *Sexual dysfunction related to*
  –vulvectomy
- *Disturbed body image related to*
  –loss of sexual organ
  –altered patterns of elimination as a result of surgery

Expected outcomes of care are based on the nursing diagnoses established, mutually determined, measurable, and stated in client-centered terms. A plan of care is developed based on the following outcomes that the woman will:

- Remain free of infection at the operative site
- Demonstrate positive adaptation to altered body image
- Maintain adequate elimination
- Discuss altered sexuality and, if desired, will identify alternative means to achieve sexual satisfaction

Interventions for the woman treated with laser therapy include applying topical steroids to the area, administering sitz baths and drying the area with a hair dryer, applying local anesthetics, or giving oral pain medication as needed. Women need to be informed that pain may get worse 3 to 4 days after the treatment.

A woman undergoing radical vulvectomy requires some special nursing actions in addition to the routine postoperative care given (see Teaching for Self-Care box). Additional nursing actions focused on the prevention of infection include the following:

- Irrigate the surgical site with a solution of half-strength normal saline or other recommended solution after each elimination.
- Dry the area thoroughly by using a hair dryer on cool setting or a heat lamp.
- Use a bed cradle or other means to lift bed covers and allow air to circulate around wound.
- Give stool softeners to decrease straining and disruption of the suture line.
- Note any change in color of the surgical site.
- Note any drainage or foul odor, and if present, notify primary health care provider.
- Perform catheter care as needed.
- Provide and instruct woman in the use of sitz baths.

The woman is at high risk for sexual dysfunction related to the effects of the surgery. Nursing actions that focus on minimizing these risks include the following:

- Encouraging verbalization of feelings
- Providing privacy for discussion
- Encouraging open communication between woman and partner
- Discussing when sexual activity can be safely resumed
- Discussing alternative methods to achieve sexual satisfaction
- Providing resources for counseling if necessary

With the expected outcomes of care set with the woman, evaluation is based on the complete or partial achievement of those outcomes.

TEACHING FOR SELF-CARE

Care After Radical Vulvectomy

- Avoid sexual activity for 4 to 6 weeks or as health care provider directs.
- Rest frequently.
- Avoid crossing legs, sitting, or standing for long periods.
- Avoid tight, constricting clothing, and wear cotton underwear.
- Keep perineal area clean and dry. Wash perineum with a solution of peroxide and water after each elimination, and pat dry.
- Report to your health care provider any swelling, redness, unusual tenderness, drainage, or foul odor of incision site.
- Report any temperature over 38.4° C.
- Eat a well-balanced diet to promote healing.
- Take all medications as prescribed.
- Elevate legs periodically to prevent pelvic congestion.
- Call your health care provider or clinic if there are concerns or problems.

Cancer of the Vagina

Vaginal carcinomas account for only 1% to 2% of gynecologic malignancy, with a peak incidence between 50 and 70 years of age. Most lesions are squamous cell carcinomas, and most are secondary carcinomas of the vagina rather than primary tumors. Vaginal intraepithelial neoplasia (VAIN) is uncommon, and clear-cell adenocarcinoma is even rarer. It is found primarily in young women (aged 15 to 30 years) and is related to intrauterine exposure to DES. Sarcoma botryoides (embryonal rhabdomyosarcoma) occurs in infants and children.

The etiology is unknown, but vaginal cancer may be caused by chronic vaginal irritation, vaginal trauma, and genital viruses. Women with VAIN often have had cancer or currently have cancer of another part of the genital tract (DiSaia & Creasman, 2002). Vaginal lesions, usually seen in the upper one third of the vagina, often extend into the bladder and rectum in late stages. Metastasis can occur early because of the rich lymphatic drainage in the vaginal area.

Some women with vaginal cancer are asymptomatic. Diagnosis often comes after an abnormal Pap test. Symptoms that have been associated with vaginal cancer include bleeding after coitus or examination, dyspareunia, and watery discharge. Bladder involvement results in urinary frequency or urgency; rectal extension causes painful defecation. A pelvic examination may reveal a single lesion, although multiple lesions are common.

Colposcopy examination and biopsy of Schiller-stained areas disclose the diagnosis. Therapy for vaginal cancer is directed by the extent of the lesion and the age and condition of the woman. Local excision is the preferred therapy for localized lesions. Topical application of 5-FU cream has been used with varying results. Laser surgery may be used to treat VAIN. Radical hysterectomy and removal of the upper vagina with dissection of the pelvic nodes or internal and external radiation are options for invasive cancer. Radiation therapy is the usual treatment of choice. If a vaginectomy is performed, sexual function will be lost without reconstructive surgery. Chemotherapy has not been effective in treatment of vaginal cancer, although studies are being conducted on the effectiveness of chemotherapy in combination with radiation. In early-stage cancer, 5-year survival rates approach 70% to 80%, with stage II survival rates in the 50% range (DiSaia & Creasman, 2002).

Nursing care for the woman with vaginal cancer is similar to that for other gynecologic cancers. Sexual counseling or referral may be needed.

Cancer of the Uterine Tubes

Primary carcinoma of the uterine (fallopian) tube (usually the distal one third) is rare (less than 1%), with a peak incidence between ages 50 and 60 years. The cause is unknown. Most women are asymptomatic in the early stages of tubal cancer. Vaginal bleeding is the most common symptom of tubal cancer, but clear vaginal discharge and lower abdominal pain also occur frequently. An enlarging unilateral pelvic mass or ascites may occur and are often misdiagnosed as ovarian carcinoma or endometrial carcinoma. Differential diagnosis of tubal cancer is usually made postoperatively. It is currently recommended that therapy guidelines parallel those established for ovarian carcinoma; therefore tumor-reducing surgery such as a total abdominal hysterectomy with bilateral salpingo-oophorectomy and omentectomy (removal of connective tissue covering the organs) is performed. Postoperative therapy consists of chemotherapy with cisplatin or other platinum-based drugs, sometimes followed by second-look surgery to determine whether further treatment is needed. Radiation therapy also may be used if the disease is limited to the tube, ovary, and uterus, although reports of its effectiveness vary (DiSaia & Creasman, 2002). Nursing care for the woman with uterine tube cancer is similar to that of the woman with ovarian cancer.

CANCER AND PREGNANCY

Cancer occurs with relative infrequency during the reproductive years. Approximately one of every 1000 pregnant women also will have cancer (Berman et al., 1999). These malignancies may be responsible for up to one third of maternal deaths. Although all forms of neoplasms have been documented in conjunction with pregnancy, the most frequently occurring types are breast cancer, cervical cancer, melanomas, ovarian cancer, leukemia and lymphomas, tubal cancers, and thyroid cancers. Bone, colorectal, vulvar, uterine, and vaginal cancers are rarely diagnosed during pregnancy. When pregnancy and cancer coincide, therapeutic issues are complex, and intense reactions occur in the woman, her family, and the health care team. Women are confronted with issues such as continuing or terminating the pregnancy. The selection and timing of therapies such as chemotherapy, radiation, and surgery are all affected by the pregnancy. Add to this the conflicting feelings the woman has (i.e., the joy of pregnancy versus the fear and anxiety associated with cancer), and the task of providing comprehensive care for the woman and her family presents a formidable challenge to the health care team. A brief discussion of the most frequent types of cancers that occur during pregnancy and the current therapies associated with them follows.

Cancer of the Breast

Approximately 2% to 3% of women are pregnant or lactating at the time of diagnosis of cancer of the breast (Copeland & Landon, 2002). Breast cancer complicates about one in 3000 pregnancies. The survival rate for women who are diagnosed with breast cancer while pregnant may be as low as 15% to 20% because the disease is generally in the advanced stages when first diagnosed (DiSaia & Creasman, 2002). Diagnosis is often delayed because breast engorgement may obscure the mass from palpation, and increased density of the tissue makes mammographic visualization more difficult. In addition, increased vascularity and lymphatic drainage in the breast of a pregnant woman may increase the speed of metastasis. Treatment is the same as for the nonpregnant woman, although surgery is usually the treatment of choice for breast cancer in pregnancy. If an invasive tumor is found, it must be determined whether the tissue is estrogen receptor (ER) positive or negative. ER-negative tumors spread more rapidly than ER-positive tumors and are more common in pregnancy.

Maternal-fetal management considers the gestational age of the fetus, extent of disease, the tumor growth potential, and the proposed treatment. Termination of the pregnancy in early stages of the disease appears to have no impact on survival. There is little evidence to suggest that pregnancy affects the malignant process. Therapeutic abortion may become an issue in the presence of advanced disease and may be deemed necessary to achieve effective palliation. Lumpectomy or partial mastectomy is the most commonly used surgical procedure, but radical mastectomy is tolerated well in these women. For advanced disease in the second or third trimester, alkylating agents, 5-FU, and vincristine are relatively safe for the fetus (DiSaia & Creasman, 2002). Chemotherapy may significantly improve the survival of these women. Radiation therapy is avoided if at all possible until after the birth, because even with careful shielding, the fetus may still receive sufficient radiation to produce detrimental effects.

There is no agreement about whether a postpartum woman with breast cancer should breastfeed, although many surgeons recommend formula feeding (Berman et al., 1999). There are theoretic concerns that if one of the oncogens for breast cancer is a virus, as many have postulated, the remaining breast may be contaminated, and the virus may be passed to the newborn, possibly acting as a latent inducer of breast carcinoma. Another reason is that lactation increases vascularity in the remaining breast, which may contain a neoplasm as well.

Breastfeeding after lumpectomy is possible, but the site of the incision may interrupt the milk ducts or prevent the nipple from extending during feeding (DiSaia & Creasman, 2002). Breastfeeding is contraindicated if the woman is receiving chemotherapy.

Pregnancy incidence after mastectomy is influenced by many factors, including prior treatment and duration of survival. About 7% of women will have one or more pregnancies within the first 5 years after mastectomy. In general, women with good prognoses (e.g., no positive nodes) are likely to be counseled to wait at least 3 years before attempting pregnancy (DiSaia & Creasman, 2002).

Cancer of the Cervix

The incidence of cervical cancer concurrent with pregnancy is reported to be 3% to 7%, or about one in 2000 pregnancies, making it the most common reproductive tract cancer associated with pregnancy (Copeland & Landon, 2002). Birth can be accomplished by either the vaginal or cesarean route; however, there is some concern regarding vaginal birth in the presence of invasive disease because the risk of hemorrhage and metastatic seeding from local trauma may be increased (DiSaia & Creasman, 2002).

The cancer itself does not harm the pregnancy: stage for stage, the outcome for the woman with cervical cancer is roughly the same as that for the nonpregnant woman (DiSaia & Creasman, 2002; Stenchever et al., 2001).

Cervical abnormalities are diagnosed during pregnancy with an abnormal Pap test. If the report suggests that the pregnant woman has a squamous intraepithelial lesion, a colposcopy, possibly with directed biopsy, is done. If invasive disease is not found, treatment is delayed until after the woman gives birth. Colposcopy is repeated in the third trimester and again postpartum. Cryosurgery has been performed with little effect on the pregnancy; however, conization is not advised during pregnancy unless necessary to rule out invasive cancer because it is associated with bleeding, miscarriage, and preterm birth.

The therapy of invasive carcinoma of the cervix during pregnancy is affected by many factors. The stage of the disease and the trimester in which the cancer is diagnosed are important. Equally important are the beliefs and desires of the woman and her family in terms of initiating therapy that can interrupt the pregnancy, as opposed to postponing the therapy until fetal viability is achieved. If the woman chooses not to continue the pregnancy, external radiation to the pelvis is done. Miscarriage usually occurs, and then internal radiation is done. If miscarriage does not occur, a modified radical hysterectomy may be performed. If the woman desires to continue the pregnancy, treatment of early-stage invasive cervical cancer can be delayed until fetal viability is reached, without harmful effects on the woman. Birth is usually by cesarean delivery, followed by radiation therapy (Copeland & Landon, 2002).

Leukemia

The average age for pregnant women with acute leukemia is 28 years; incidence during pregnancy is not specified, but the incidence in the general population in the United States is 10 in 100,000. Pregnancy seems to have no specific effect on the course of the disease, except that vigorous therapy is detrimental to early gestation. Preterm labor and postpartum hemorrhage are associated with acute leukemia (DiSaia & Creasman, 2002). Acute myelocytic leukemia (90% of cases) has a more fulminant course and requires immediate therapy; in the presence of chronic myelocytic leukemia, therapy can be delayed somewhat. Some pregnant women with the chronic form of the disease who had chemotherapy and radiation therapy directed at the spleen have given birth to apparently healthy infants. The decision to terminate the pregnancy rests with the woman and her family; however, prompt, aggressive therapy is always advisable if remission is to be achieved. Decisions may be influenced by the aggressiveness of the disease.

Hodgkin Disease

Hodgkin disease is a malignant lymphoma that affects many younger people and complicates about one in 6000 pregnancies. Younger women (younger than 40 years) have a better prognosis.

Pregnancy appears to have no effect on the disease and vice versa, other than those effects resulting from therapy. Radiation therapy of the nodes and multiagent chemotherapy result in about a 75% cure rate. Unless gestation is well into the third trimester, delay in initiating therapy should be minimal, which brings up the dilemma of therapeutic abortion. Radiation therapy to diseased areas above the diaphragm can be initiated during the third trimester with proper shielding of the fetus. Chemotherapy is strongly contraindicated during the first trimester and is relatively contraindicated in the second and third trimesters. Termination of the pregnancy during the course of the disease is not definitely indicated, although treatment is easier (DiSaia & Creasman, 2002).

Melanoma

Malignant melanoma may be one of the rare cancers that can be affected by pregnancy. This is suggested by reports in which pregnancy has been shown to induce or exacerbate a melanoma. These suggestions are based on changes that occur naturally during pregnancy and include hyperpigmentation, an increase in melanocyte-stimulating hormone (MSH), and increased production of estrogen. Estrogen receptors have been identified in about half of all melanomas (DiSaia & Creasman, 2002).

Although pregnancy has been implicated in the more rapid metastases to regional lymph nodes, stage for stage, there does not seem to be a significant difference in the survival of pregnant and nonpregnant women. As a result, most authorities recommend that women who have histories of malignant melanoma delay pregnancy for about 3 years after surgical excision, because this is the period of highest risk for recurrence (DiSaia & Creasman, 2002).

Diagnosis is established by biopsy. Therapy consists of radical local excision. For most other malignancies, the placenta is unexplainably resistant to invasion by maternal cancer. Although melanoma accounts for few cases of malignant disease during pregnancy, almost 50% of the placental metastases and almost 90% of fetal metastases occur from maternal melanoma (DiSaia & Creasman, 2002).

Thyroid Cancer

The incidence of thyroid cancer in pregnancy is not established. Normally the thyroid gland enlarges during pregnancy, and an asymptomatic nodular mass is a common finding. Diagnosis is usually by cytologic testing of fine-needle aspirate. Treatment is usually nonsurgical until after the birth. Thyroid suppression is the preferred treatment during pregnancy (DiSaia & Creasman, 2002).

Bone Tumors

Bone tumors are rare in pregnancy. Ewing sarcoma and osteogenic sarcoma and osteocystoma are the most common primary malignant bone tumors seen in pregnancy. Usually the areas involved are the clavicle, sternum, spine, humerus, and femur. A lump or mass, local pain, and disability are characteristic manifestations.

Osteogenic sarcoma affects areas of high bone turnover (especially during growth spurts); Ewing sarcoma is a rare condition that develops within bone marrow. Pregnancy does not affect and is not affected by the disease.

Surgical excision is usually well tolerated during pregnancy; adjuvant chemotherapy is delayed until after birth if the cancer is diagnosed near term. If the disease recurs, it usually does so within 3 years; therefore women are counseled to defer pregnancy during this time (DiSaia & Creasman, 2002).

Other Gynecologic Cancers

Cancer of the Vulva

The diagnosis of preinvasive (VIN) disease during pregnancy is rare. Therapy is postponed until the postpartum period. If invasive disease (a rare occurrence) is diagnosed during the first trimester, vulvectomy with bilateral groin dissection may be done after the fourteenth week. When it is diagnosed in the third trimester, local wide excision is done, deferring definitive surgery until after birth. Pregnancy does not alter the course of the disease.

After radical vulvectomy and bilateral inguinal lymphectomy, a woman who becomes pregnant again can carry the pregnancy to term and give birth vaginally. If vaginal stenosis is present and could impede birth, cesarean birth may be more appropriate.

Cancer of the Vagina

Except for clear-cell adenocarcinoma of DES-exposed women, cancer of the vagina is rare. If clear-cell adenocarcinoma of the cervix and vagina or sarcoma is found in the upper vagina, the preferred surgery is radical hysterectomy, upper vaginectomy, and bilateral pelvic lymphadenectomy, followed by chemotherapy. Radiation is usually not advocated during pregnancy. Pregnancy does not seem to affect the course of the disease or the prognosis.

Cancer of the Uterus

Endometrial carcinoma during pregnancy is very rare; only a few cases have been documented since 1900. Diagnosis was usually an incidental finding after therapeutic abortion or surgery, and the lesions were minimally or not invasive. Recommended therapy is total abdominal hysterectomy and bilateral salpingo-oophorectomy (TAH-BSO) and adjuvant radiotherapy (DiSaia & Creasman, 2002).

Cancer of the Uterine Tube

With a peak incidence between 50 and 55 years of age, concurrent pregnancy is only a remote possibility. Should it occur, the recommended therapy (TAH-BSO with postoperative radiotherapy or chemotherapy) is the same as that for the nonpregnant woman. Removal of the uterine tube is an alternative treatment (DiSaia & Creasman, 2002).

Cancer of the Ovary

Cancer of the ovary is the second most frequent reproductive cancer that occurs with pregnancy. Still, ovarian malignancy is relatively rare, being reported to occur in one per 10,000 to 25,000 births (DiSaia & Creasman, 2002).

Ovarian masses occur frequently during pregnancy. Because corpus luteum cysts account for a high percentage of these masses and because 99% of these resolve by the fourteenth week, any mass smaller than 5 cm may simply be observed until the end of the first trimester. Any mass larger than 5 cm, one that is growing, or one that does not resolve after the fourteenth week warrants further investigation. Abdominal palpation and ultrasound are the diagnostic tools of choice during pregnancy. However, in many cases, laparotomy is necessary to confirm the diagnosis. Laparotomy after 16 weeks of gestation has negligible fetal wastage associated with the procedure and is therefore considered safe.

An ovarian tumor may be first diagnosed at birth or after birth because the enlarged uterus obscured its presence. Definitive diagnosis is needed before treatment is selected. For stage I tumors, treatment includes conservative surgery (unilateral oophorectomy and salpingectomy) and use of chemotherapy. If diagnosis occurs in the second or third trimester, treatment choices are difficult to make. They include interrupting the pregnancy and starting chemotherapy immediately, preserving pregnancy and starting chemotherapy with the fetus in utero (controversial), or delaying chemotherapy until the fetus is more mature and early delivery is a low risk to the fetus (DiSaia & Creasman, 2002).

Cancer Therapy and Pregnancy

Decisions about the type and timing of therapy for cancer in the pregnant woman evoke moral and philosophic dilemmas, as well as complex medical judgments and intense emotional responses. The fetus is at risk with either chemotherapy or radiation therapy. The impact of cancer therapy on the fetus can include death, miscarriage, teratogenesis, alteration in growth and development, alterations in function, and genetic mutation. The long-term effects on the fetus are unknown. However, the long-term experiences of young women exposed to DES in utero make very real the possibility of long-term effects associated with cancer therapy. These theoretic dangers must be weighed against the potential detrimental effects to the mother if treatment is withheld (Blackwell et al., 2000).

Timing of therapy also is an important issue to discuss. Because most cancer therapy (except surgery) is geared toward having a differential and noxious effect on rapidly growing tissue, the fetus is most at risk during the first trimester, when organogenesis and rapid tissue growth occur. Surgery offers the least potential risk to the fetus; however, the risk of miscarriage and preterm labor may be increased.

Chemotherapy is avoided in the first trimester if at all possible. Although use of most chemotherapeutic agents has had isolated reports of fetal abnormalities, data on the agents used after the first trimester have recorded surprisingly few fetal abnormalities. The placenta may act as a barrier against the chemotherapeutic agents; therefore although risk still exists, the judicious use of chemotherapy after the first trimester can result in live births with few congenital abnormalities. Acute drug toxicities may occur if treatment has occurred just before birth. Breastfeeding by women who are taking cytotoxic drugs is not recommended because these drugs may be excreted in breast milk (Copeland & Landon, 2002).

Radiation therapy presents its own set of issues. During embryonic development, tissues are extremely radiosensitive. If cells are genetically altered or killed during this time, the child either will fail to survive or will be deformed. From a radiologic stance, there are three significant periods in embryonic development (DiSaia & Creasman, 2002):

1. Preimplantation: If irradiation does not destroy the fertilized egg, it probably does not affect it significantly.
2. Critical period of organogenesis: During this period, especially between days 18 and 38, the organism is most vulnerable; microcephaly, anencephaly, eye damage, growth restriction, spina bifida, and foot damage may occur.
3. After day 40: Large doses may still cause observable malformation and damage to the central nervous system.

ETHICAL CONSIDERATIONS

When a pregnant woman has cancer and her survival is contingent on treatment that will harm the fetus, the health care team must work with the woman and her significant others to make decisions about how to proceed with her care. If a one-client model of ethical decision making is used, the risk-benefit analysis is applied to the maternal-fetal unit. The pregnant woman decides what is best for her and the fetus. The woman may accept or refuse treatment. If a two-client model is used for decision making, more weight is given to fetal well-being, but the pregnant woman cannot be forced to accept harm to herself for the sake of the fetus. Thus she could elect to accept treatment.

Pregnancy After Cancer Treatment

If cancer therapy has not included the removal of the uterus, ovaries, or uterine (fallopian) tubes, there is a possibility that the woman may still be able to become pregnant. Although a woman's menstrual cycle may have resumed, pregnancy may be difficult to achieve. Therapy that has affected the pituitary or thyroid gland may make conception difficult. Radiation appears to have the most deleterious effects on the endocrine system. The use of chemotherapy may result in temporary or permanent sterility, depending on the drug, the dose, and the length of time since the therapy was completed. Alkylating agents are most commonly associated with infertility (DiSaia & Creasman, 2002).

Of growing concern is the increase in the number of childhood and adolescent cancer survivors. Long-term effects of therapy on fertility, including incidence of congenital anomalies, are not well known. The newly diagnosed client must be counseled on the potential effects of treatment on later reproductive function (Blackwell et al., 2000).

For recovery from the disease and treatment to be complete, a delay of at least 2 years from the end of therapy to conception is advised. An exception is the women who has had ovarian cancer, who is advised, because of a high incidence of a second primary tumor, to complete her childbearing as soon as possible (American College of Obstetricians and Gynecologists, 2000).

Before conception, a woman who has had cancer should have a complete physical examination to rule out complications that may place her or a fetus in jeopardy. Cardiac, pulmonary, hematologic, neurologic, renal, or gonadal function may be impaired. The woman and the potential father (if partnered) should be referred for reproductive and genetic counseling as well.

GESTATIONAL TROPHOBLASTIC DISEASE

Gestational trophoblastic disease (GTD) is a term that encompasses a spectrum of disorders arising from the placental trophoblast. It includes hydatidiform mole (see Chapter 31), invasive mole, and choriocarcinoma. **Gestational trophoblastic neoplasia (GTN)** refers to persistent trophoblastic tissue that is presumed to be malignant (DiSaia & Creasman, 2002).

Box 12-5 describes the clinical classifications of GTN. Before the middle 1950s, the prognoses of these neoplasias, especially end-stage choriocarcinoma, were dismal. Today, however, GTN is recognized as the most curable gynecologic malignancy. The reason for this change in thinking is related to several factors: a sensitive marker is produced by the tumor (hCG); the tumor is extremely sensitive to various chemotherapeutic agents; high risk factors in the disease process can be identified, allowing individualized therapy; and the aggressive use of multiple treatment methods is possible.

BOX 12-5 Classification of Gestational Trophoblastic Neoplasia

I. Nonmetastatic disease: no evidence of disease outside uterus
II. Metastatic disease: any disease outside uterus
   A. Good-prognosis metastatic disease
      1. Short duration (last pregnancy <4 months)
      2. Low pretreatment hCG titer (<100,000 IU/24 hr or <40,000 mIU/ml)
      3. No metastasis to brain or liver
      4. No significant prior chemotherapy
   B. Poor-prognosis metastatic disease
      1. Long duration (last pregnancy >4 mo)
      2. High pretreatment hCG titer (>100,000 IU/24 hr or >40,000 mIU/ml)
      3. Brain or liver metastasis
      4. Significant prior chemotherapy
      5. Term pregnancy

From DiSaia, P., & Creasman, W. (2002). *Clinical gynecologic oncology* (6th ed.). St. Louis: Mosby.

Malignant disease follows hydatidiform mole in about 50% of cases. Miscarriage or ectopic pregnancy precedes about 25% of cases, and normal pregnancy precedes another 25% of cases (DiSaia & Creasman, 2002). Metastasis occurs most often in the lungs, vagina, liver, and brain.

Continued bleeding after evacuation of a hydatidiform mole is usually the most suggestive symptom of GTN. Other clinical signs include abdominal pain and uterine and ovarian enlargement. Signs of metastasis include pulmonary symptoms (e.g., dyspnea, cough). The diagnosis is usually confirmed by increasing or plateauing hCG levels after evacuation of a molar pregnancy. Once diagnosis is confirmed, other clinical studies (e.g., CT scan of lungs and brain, chest x-ray, pelvic ultrasound, and liver scan) are done to determine the extent of the disease.

For women who wish to preserve their fertility, single-agent chemotherapy is chosen. Methotrexate has been the treatment of choice for years. High-dose methotrexate followed by folinic acid "rescue" within 24 hours also has shown excellent results and causes fewer toxic effects (DiSaia & Creasman, 2002). Dactinomycin also has been used with equally good results and is used for women with liver or renal disease, both of which are contraindications for methotrexate. Hysterectomy with adjuvant chemotherapy is often the choice of treatment for nonmetastatic tumors in women who have completed their childbearing.

Women who have metastasis are classified as having either a good or poor prognosis, depending on the absence or presence of brain or liver metastasis, unsuccessful prior chemotherapy, symptoms lasting longer than 4 months, and serum β-hCG levels greater than 40,000 mIU/ml. Treatment progresses from single-agent chemotherapy in the good-prognosis metastatic GTN to multiple-agent chemotherapy and multiple methods of treatment for the poor-prognosis group. Cure rates for the good-prognosis group are almost as positive as for those with nonmetastatic disease, both approaching 100% (DiSaia & Creasman, 2002).

Therapy is continued until negative hCG levels are obtained. Follow-up after successful chemotherapy is by serum hCG levels obtained every 2 weeks for 3 months, every month for 3 months, every other month for 6 months, and then every 6 months indefinitely. Physical examinations should be done at least yearly, and chest radiographs are done if indicated. Contraception is needed until the woman has been in remission for at least 6 months (DiSaia & Creasman, 2002). Oral contraceptives are preferred, but barrier methods are acceptable if oral contraceptives are contraindicated. During a subsequent pregnancy, pelvic ultrasonography is recommended because the woman is at higher risk to develop another molar pregnancy. Serum hCG levels should be obtained 6 weeks after the birth (DiSaia & Creasman, 2002).

KEY POINTS

- Gynecologic disorders diminish the quality of life for affected women and their families.
- Structural disorders of the uterus and vagina related to pelvic relaxation and urinary incontinence may be a delayed result of childbearing, but they may be seen in young or childless women.
- Bladder training and pelvic muscle exercises can significantly decrease or relieve mild to moderate urinary incontinence.
- The development of neoplasms, whether benign or malignant, can have a significant physical and emotional impact on the woman and her family.
- Abnormal uterine bleeding is the most common symptom of leiomyomas or fibroid tumors.
- Various alternatives to hysterectomy exist for structural and benign disorders of the uterus; women need to be informed about the risks and benefits to make an informed decision about treatment.
- Endometrial cancer is the most common reproductive system malignancy.
- Hysterectomy is the usual treatment for early-stage endometrial cancer.
- Infections such as human papillomavirus types 16 and 18 and possibly other types have been linked to subsequent cervical cancer.
- The squamocolumnar junction is an important landmark identified with neoplastic changes of the cervix.
- Preinvasive cancer of the cervix may be treated with techniques such as electrosurgical excision, cryotherapy, and laser therapy to save the structure of the cervix, particularly in women who desire to retain childbearing ability.
- External and internal radiation therapy in combination are as successful as surgery in treating early stages of cancer of the cervix.
- The Pap test will detect approximately 90% of early cervical dysplasias.
- Cancer of the ovary causes more deaths than any other female genital tract cancer.
- Nurses can control their exposure to radiation in three ways: by increasing the distance from the radiation source, by limiting the time of exposure, and by using lead shielding.
- Cancer is relatively infrequent during pregnancy, occurring about once in every 1000 pregnancies.
- Radiation or chemotherapy treatment of the pregnant woman who has cancer places the fetus at risk for death, miscarriage, teratogenesis, and alterations in growth and development.
- Gestational trophoblastic neoplasms are highly curable but require close monitoring of hCG levels after treatment.

CRITICAL THINKING EXERCISES

1. Prepare a one-page information sheet or chart on the various treatments for uterine fibroids, to be given out in gynecologic clinic for women who need information about alternatives. The information should be presented concisely, in understandable terms, and should include a description of the procedure and risks and benefits (e.g., safety and efficacy, effects on fertility, costs, recovery time).
2. For a clinical conference, prepare to debate the following issue related to cancer in pregnancy: A 34-year-old woman who is 18 weeks pregnant has advanced breast cancer. She is contemplating a therapeutic abortion so that she can receive chemotherapy and radiation.
   - **a.** Do you support the woman's right to make this decision for herself and the fetus, or do you support decision-making that gives consideration to fetal rights?
   - **b.** Would information about her stage of pregnancy and the effects of these treatments at different stages affect your decision to be for either choice?
   - **c.** What suggestions does the clinical group have for an Ethics Committee assigned to resolve this issue?
3. Develop a poster presentation on the risks and prevention of cervical cancer for Hispanic women.
   - **a.** Identify places in the community where the posters will be seen by your intended audience.
   - **b.** Use your knowledge of the effects of culture on health promotion and disease prevention behaviors in your poster design that will capture the attention of Hispanic women.
   - **c.** Suggest a plan for evaluating the impact of the posters on increasing knowledge about the risks of cervical cancer and on increasing cervical cancer screening in your community.

RESOURCES

American Cancer Society
1599 Clifton Rd. NE
Atlanta, GA 30329
800-ACS-2345
www.cancer.org

The Fibroid Treatment Collective
310-794-6645
www.fibroid.org

Gynecologic Cancer Foundation
www.wcn.org/gcf

Hysterectomy Educational Resource and Services (HERS)
422 Byrn Mawr Ave.
Bala Cynwyd, PA 19004
215-667-7757
www.ccon.com/hers

National Association for Continence
PO Box 8310
Spartanburg, SC 29305
800-252-3337
www.nafc.org

National Cancer Institute Cancer Information Service
800-4-CANCER
www.nci.nih.gov

National Cervical Cancer Coalition
www.nccc-online.org

National Ovarian Cancer Coalition
2335 East Atlantic Blvd., #401
Pompano Beach, FL 33062
888-682-7426
www.ovarian.org

National Women's Health Information Center
The Office on Women's Health
Department of Health and Human Resources
800-994-9662
www.4woman.gov

National Women's Health Resource Center
120 Albany St., Suite 820
New Brunswick, NJ 08901
877-986-9472
www.healthywomen.org

Women's Cancer Network
c/o Gynecologic Cancer Foundation
401 N. Michigan Ave
Chicago, IL 60611
312-644-6610
www.wcn.org

REFERENCES

Adams, K. (2002). Confronting cervical cancer: Screening is the key to stopping this killer. *AWHONN Lifelines, 6*(3), 216-222.

American Cancer Society. (2003). *Cancer facts and figures 2003.* New York: American Cancer Society.

Berman, M., DiSaia, P., & Brewster, W. (1999). Pelvic malignancies, gestational trophoblastic neoplasia, and non-pelvic malignancies. In R. Creasy & R. Resnick (Eds.), *Maternal-fetal medicine* (4th ed.). Philadelphia: W.B. Saunders.

Bieber, E., & Macklin, V. (Eds.). (1998). *Myomectomy*. Malden, MA: Blackwell Science.

Blackwell, D., Elam, S., & Blackwell, J. (2000). Cancer and pregnancy: A health care dilemma. *Journal of Obstetric, Gynecologic, and Neonatal Nursing, 29*(4), 405-412.

Boyer, L. et al. (2001). Hispanic women's perceptions regarding cervical cancer screening. *Journal of Obstetric, Gynecologic, and Neonatal Nursing, 30*(2), 240-245.

Centers for Disease Control and Prevention. (2002). Sexually transmitted diseases treatment guidelines 2002. *MMWR, 51*(RR-6), 1-80.

Copeland, L., & Landon, M. (2002). Malignant disease and pregnancy. In S. Gabbe, J. Niebyl, & J. Simpson (Eds.), *Obstetrics: Normal and problem pregnancies* (4th ed.). New York: Churchill Livingstone.

DiSaia, P., & Creasman, W. (2002). *Clinical gynecologic oncology* (6th ed.). St. Louis: Mosby.

Falcone, T., Paraiso, M., & Mascha, E. (1999). Prospective randomized clinical trial of laparoscopically assisted vaginal hysterectomy versus total abdominal hysterectomy. *American Journal of Obstetrics and Gynecology, 180*(4), 955-962.

Farquhar, C., & Steiner, C. (2002). Hysterectomy rates in the United States 1990-1997. *Obstetrics and Gynecology, 99*(2), 229-234.

Furniss, K. (2000). Tomatoes, Pap smears, and tea? Adopting behaviors that may prevent reproductive cancers and improve health. *Journal of Obstetric, Gynecologic, and Neonatal Nursing, 29*(6), 641-652.

Grabo, T. et al. (1999). Uterine myomas: Treatment options. *Journal of Obstetric, Gynecologic, and Neonatal Nursing, 28*(1), 23-31.

Iwamato, R. (2001). Radiation therapy. In S. Otto, *Oncology nursing* (4th ed.). St. Louis: Mosby.

Katz, A. (2002). Sexuality after hysterectomy. *Journal of Obstetric, Gynecologic, and Neonatal Nursing, 31*(3), 256-262.

Kim, K., & Lee, K. (2001). Symptom experience in women after hysterectomy. *Journal of Obstetric, Gynecologic, and Neonatal Nursing, 30*(5), 472-480.

Kjerulff, K. et al. (2000). Effectiveness of hysterectomy. *Obstetrics and Gynecology, 95*(3), 319-326.

Lammers, S. et al. (2000). Caring for women living with ovarian cancer: Recommendations for advanced practice nurses. *Journal of Obstetric, Gynecologic, and Neonatal Nursing, 29*(6), 567-573.

Lindberg, C., & Nolan, L. (2001). Women's decision making regarding hysterectomy. *Journal of Obstetric, Gynecologic, and Neonatal Nursing, 30*(6), 607-616.

Lowdermilk, D. (1995). Home care of the patient with gynecologic cancer. *Journal of Obstetric, Gynecologic, and Neonatal Nursing, 24*(2), 157-163.

Lowdermilk, D., & Germino, B. (2000). Helping women and their families cope with the impact of gynecologic cancer. *Journal of Obstetric, Gynecologic, and Neonatal Nursing, 29*(6), 653-660.

National Women's Health Resource Center. (1999). The woman's guide to preparing for surgery. *National Women's Health Report, 21*(5), 1-7.

National Women's Health Resource Center. (2000). Screening tests & women's health. *National Women's Health Report, 23*(6), 1-8.

Nichols, D., & Clark-Pearson, D. (2000). *Gynecologic, obstetric, and related surgery* (2nd ed.). St. Louis: Mosby.

Otto, S. (2001). Gynecologic cancers. In S. Otto, *Oncology nursing.* St. Louis: Mosby.

Phipps, W. et al. (2003). *Medical-surgical nursing: Health and illness perspectives* (7th ed.). St. Louis: Mosby.

Reid, J. (2001). Women's knowledge of Pap smears, risk factors, for cervical cancer, and cervical cancer. *Journal of Obstetric, Gynecologic, and Neonatal Nursing, 30*(3), 299-305.

Rodriguez, C. et al. (2001). Estrogen replacement therapy and ovarian cancer mortality in a large prospective study of U.S. women. *Journal of the American Medical Association, 285*(11), 1460-1465.

Sampselle, C. et al. (2000). Continence for women: A test of AWHONN's evidence-based protocol in clinical practice. *Journal of Obstetric, Gynecologic, and Neonatal Nursing, 29*(1), 18-26.

Sampselle, C. et al. (1997). Continence for women: Evidence-based practice. *Journal of Obstetric, Gynecologic, and Neonatal Nursing, 26*(4), 375-385.

Saraiya, M. et al. (2001). Self-reported Papanicolaou smears and hysterectomies among women in the United States. *Obstetrics and Gynecology, 98*(2), 269-278.

Seidel, H. et al. (2003). *Mosby's guide to physical examination* (5th ed.). St. Louis: Mosby.

Sharts-Hopko, N. (2001). Hysterectomy for nonmalignant conditions. *American Journal of Nursing, 101*(9), 32-40.

Stenchever, M. et al. (2001). *Comprehensive gynecology* (4th ed.). St. Louis: Mosby.

Thom, D. (1998). Variation in estimates of urinary incontinence prevalence in the community: Effects of differences in definition, population characteristics, and study type. *Journal of the American Geriatric Society, 46*(4), 473-480.

Todd, A. (2002). An alternative to hysterectomy. *RN, 65*(3), 30-35.

Tomaino-Brunner, C. et al. (1998). Can precolposcopy education increase knowledge and decrease anxiety? *Journal of Obstetric, Gynecologic, and Neonatal Nursing, 27*(6), 636-645.

U.S. Preventive Services Task Force. (2003). *Screening for cervical cancer.* AHRQ Publication No 03.575A, January 2003. Rockville, MD: Agency for Healthcare and Quality.

Wade, J. et al. (2000). Hysterectomy: What do women need and want to know? *Journal of Obstetric, Gynecologic, and Neonatal Nursing, 29*(1), 33-42.

Wilmoth, M., & Spinelli, A. (2000). Sexual implications of gynecologic cancer treatments. *Journal of Obstetric, Gynecologic, and Neonatal Nursing, 29*(4), 413-421.

Wright, T. et al. (2002). 2002 consensus guidelines for the management of women with cervical cytology abnormalities. *Journal of the American Medical Association, 287*(16), 2120-2129.

Zawacki, K., & Phillips, M. (2002). Cancer genetics and women's health. *Journal of Obstetric, Gynecologic, and Neonatal Nursing, 31*(2), 208-216.

CHAPTER 13

Shannon E. Perry

Conception and Fetal Development

http://evolve.elsevier.com/Lowdermilk/MatWmnHlth/

LEARNING OBJECTIVES

- Summarize the process of fertilization.
- Describe the development, structure, and functions of the placenta.
- Describe the composition and functions of the amniotic fluid.
- Identify three organs or tissues arising from each of the three primary germ layers.
- Summarize the significant changes in growth and development of the embryo and fetus.
- Identify the potential effects of teratogens during vulnerable periods of embryonic and fetal development.

This chapter presents an overview of the process of fertilization and the development of the normal embryo and fetus.

CONCEPTION

Conception, defined as the union of a single egg and sperm, marks the beginning of a pregnancy. Conception occurs not as an isolated event but as part of a sequential process. This sequential process includes **gamete** (egg and sperm) formation, ovulation (release of the egg), fertilization (union of the gametes), and implantation in the uterus.

Cell Division

Cells are reproduced by two different methods: mitosis and meiosis. In **mitosis,** body cells replicate to yield two cells with the same genetic makeup as the parent cell. First the cell makes a copy of its deoxyribonucleic acid (DNA), and then it divides, and each daughter cell receives one copy of the genetic material. Mitotic division facilitates growth and development or cell replacement.

Meiosis, the process by which germ cells divide and decrease their chromosomal number by half, produces gametes (eggs and sperm). Each homologous pair of chromosomes contains one chromosome received from the mother and one from the father; thus meiosis results in cells that contain one of each of the 23 pairs of chromosomes. Because these germ cells contain 23 single chromosomes, half of the genetic material of a normal somatic cell, they are termed *haploid.* This halving of the genetic material is accomplished by replicating the DNA once and then dividing twice. In mitosis, the DNA is replicated once and followed by a single cell division. When the female gamete (egg or ovum) and the male gamete (spermatozoon) unite to form the zygote, the diploid number of human chromosomes (46, or 23 pairs) is restored.

The process of DNA replication and cell division in meiosis allows different alleles for genes to be distributed at random by each parent and then rearranged on the paired chromosomes. The chromosomes then separate and proceed to different gametes. Many combinations of genes are possible on each chromosome because parents have genotypes derived from four different grandparents. This random mixing of alleles accounts for the variation of traits seen in the offspring of the same two parents.

Gametogenesis

When a male reaches puberty, his testes begin the process of **spermatogenesis.** The cells that undergo meiosis in the male are called *spermatocytes.* The primary spermatocyte, which undergoes the first meiotic division, contains the diploid number of chromosomes. The cell has already copied its DNA before division, so four alleles for each gene are present. The cell is still considered diploid because the copies are bound together (i.e., one allele plus its copy on each chromosome).

During the first meiotic division, two haploid secondary spermatocytes are formed. Each secondary spermatocyte contains 22 autosomes and one sex chromosome; one contains the X chromosome (plus its copy), and the other, the Y chromosome (plus its copy). During the second

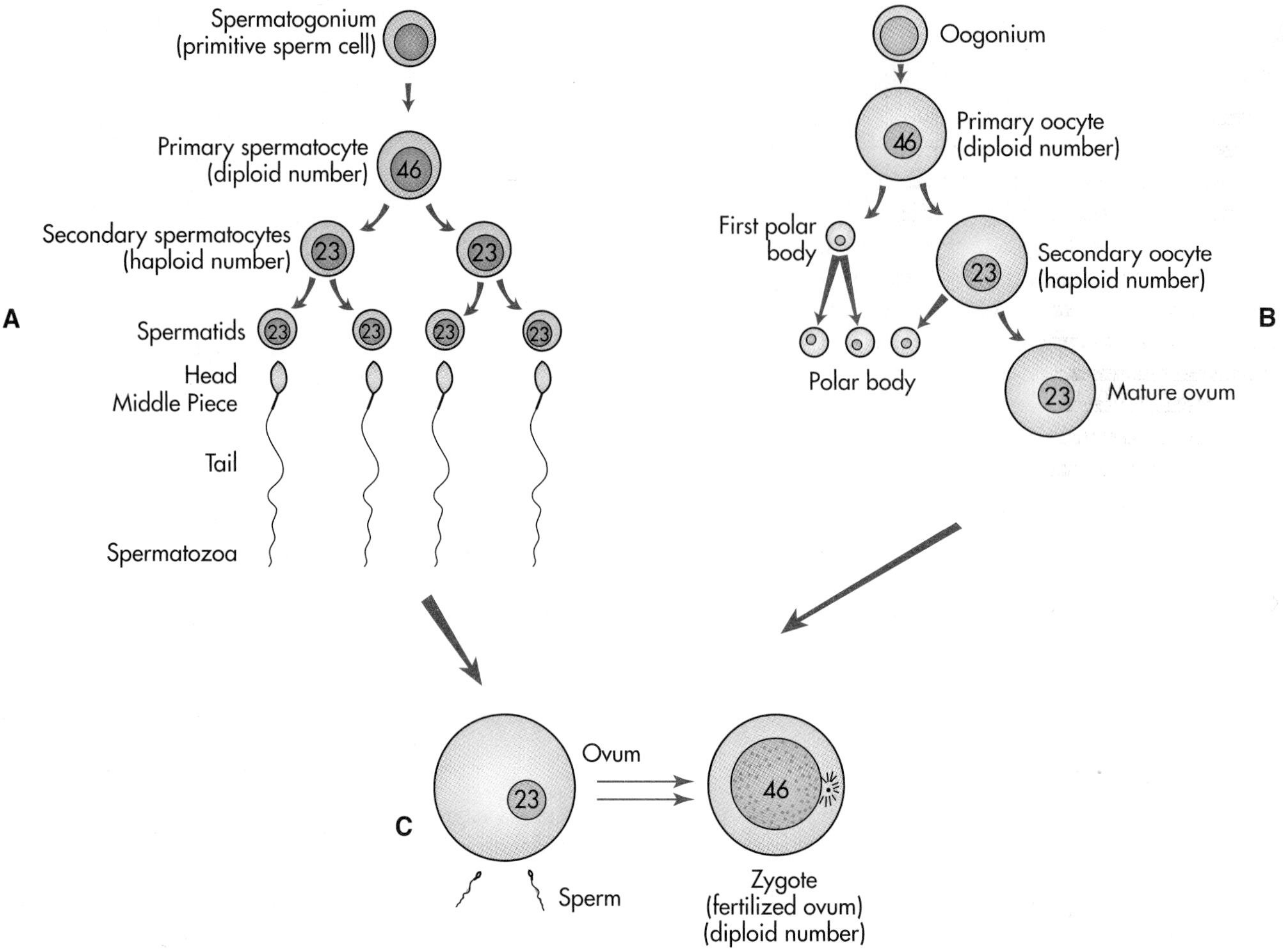
Spermatogonium
(primitive sperm cell)
Primary spermatocyte
(diploid number)
46
Secondary spermatocytes
(haploid number)
23
23
A
Spermatids
23
23
23
23
Head
Middle Piece
Tail
Spermatozoa
Oogonium
Primary oocyte
(diploid number)
46
First polar body
Secondary oocyte
(haploid number)
23
B
Polar body
23
Mature ovum
Ovum
23
C
46
Sperm
Zygote
(fertilized ovum)
(diploid number)

FIG. 13-1 **A,** Spermatogenesis. Gametogenesis of the male produces four mature gametes, the sperm. **B,** Oogenesis. Gametogenesis in the female produces one mature ovum and three polar bodies. Note the relative difference in overall size between the ovum and sperm. **C,** Fertilization results in the single-cell zygote and the restoration of the diploid number of chromosomes.

meiotic division, the male produces two gametes with an X chromosome and two gametes with a Y chromosome, all of which will develop into viable sperm (Fig. 13-1, *A*).

Oogenesis, the process of egg (ovum) formation, begins during fetal life in the female. All the cells that may undergo meiosis in a woman's lifetime are contained in her ovaries at birth. The majority of the estimated 2 million primary oocytes (the cells that undergo the first meiotic division) degenerate spontaneously. Only 400 to 500 ova will mature during the approximately 35 years of a woman's reproductive life. The primary oocytes begin the first meiotic division (i.e., they replicate their DNA) during fetal life but remain suspended at this stage until puberty (Fig. 13-1, *B*). Then usually monthly, one primary oocyte matures and completes the first meiotic division, yielding two unequal cells: the secondary oocyte and a small polar body. Both contain 22 autosomes and one X sex chromosome.

At ovulation the second meiotic division begins; however, the ovum does not complete the second meiotic division unless fertilization occurs. At fertilization, a second polar body and the **zygote** (the united egg and sperm) are produced (Fig. 13-1, *C*). The three polar bodies degenerate. If fertilization does not occur, the ovum also degenerates.

Ovum

Meiosis occurs in the female in the ovarian follicles and produces an egg, or ovum. Each month, one ovum matures with a host of surrounding supportive cells. At ovulation the ovum is released from the ruptured ovarian follicle. High estrogen levels increase the motility of the uterine tubes so their cilia are able to capture the ovum and propel it through the tube toward the uterine cavity. An ovum cannot move by itself.

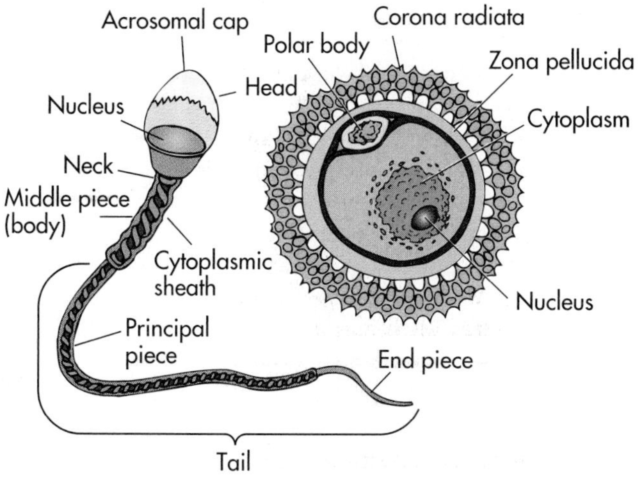
Acrosomal cap
Polar body
Corona radiata
Zona pellucida
Head
Nucleus
Cytoplasm
Neck
Middle piece (body)
Cytoplasmic sheath
Nucleus
Principal piece
End piece
Tail

FIG. 13-2 Sperm and ovum.

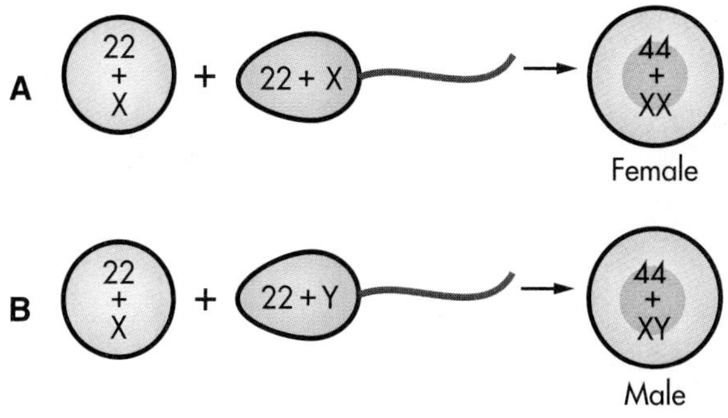
A
22 + X
+
22 + X
44 + XX
Female
B
22 + X
+
22 + Y
44 + XY
Male

FIG. 13-3 Fertilization. **A,** Ovum fertilized by X-bearing sperm to form female zygote. **B,** Ovum fertilized by Y-bearing sperm to form male zygote.

Two protective layers surround the ovum (Fig. 13-2). The inner layer is a thick, acellular layer, the *zona pellucida.* The outer layer, the *corona radiata,* is composed of elongated cells.

Ova are considered fertile for about 24 hours after ovulation. If unfertilized by a sperm, the ovum degenerates and is reabsorbed.

Sperm

Ejaculation during sexual intercourse normally propels about a teaspoon of semen, containing as many as 200 to 500 million sperm, into the vagina. The sperm swim propelled by the flagellar movement of their tails. Some sperm can reach the site of fertilization within 5 minutes, but average transit time is 4 to 6 hours. Sperm remain viable within the woman's reproductive system for an average of 2 to 3 days. Most sperm are lost in the vagina, within the cervical mucus, or in the endometrium, or they enter the uterine tube that contains no ovum.

As the sperm travel through the female reproductive tract, enzymes are produced to aid in their capacitation. *Capacitation* is a physiologic change that removes the protective coating from the heads of the sperm. Small perforations then form in the *acrosome* (a cap on the sperm) and allow enzymes (e.g., hyaluronidase) to escape (see Fig. 13-2). These enzymes are necessary for the sperm to penetrate the protective layers of the ovum before fertilization.

Fertilization

Fertilization takes place in the ampulla (outer third) of the uterine tube. When a sperm successfully penetrates the membrane surrounding the ovum, both sperm and ovum are enclosed within the membrane, and the membrane becomes impenetrable to other sperm; this process is termed the *zona reaction.* The second meiotic division of the secondary oocyte is then completed, and the ovum nucleus becomes the female pronucleus. The head of the sperm enlarges to become the male pronucleus, and the tail degenerates. The nuclei fuse, and the chromosomes combine, restoring the diploid number (46) (Fig. 13-3). Conception, the formation of the zygote, is now complete.

Mitotic cellular replication, called *cleavage,* begins as the zygote travels the length of the uterine tube into the uterus. This transit takes 3 to 4 days. Because the fertilized egg divides rapidly with no increase in size, successively smaller cells, *blastomeres,* are formed with each division. A 16-cell **morula,** a solid ball of cells, is produced within 3 days and is still surrounded by the protective zona pellucida (Fig. 13-4, *A*). Further development occurs as the morula floats freely within the uterus. Fluid passes through the zona pellucida into the intercellular spaces between the blastomeres, separating them into two parts, the trophoblast (which gives rise to the placenta) and the embryoblast (which gives rise to the embryo). A cavity forms within the cell mass as the spaces come together, forming a structure called the *blastocyst cavity.* When the cavity becomes recognizable, the whole structure of the developing embryo is known as the **blastocyst.** Stem cells are derived from the inner cell mass of the blastocyst (Box 13-1). The outer layer of cells surrounding the blastocyst cavity is the *trophoblast.*

Implantation

The zona pellucida degenerates, the trophoblast cells displace endometrial cells at the implantation site, and the blastocyst embeds in the endometrium, usually in the anterior or posterior fundal region. Between 6 and 10 days after conception, the trophoblast secretes enzymes that enable it to burrow into the endometrium until the entire blastocyst is covered. This is termed **implantation.** Endometrial blood vessels erode, and some women have slight implantation bleeding (slight spotting or bleeding during the time of the first missed menstrual period). **Chorionic villi,** fingerlike projections,

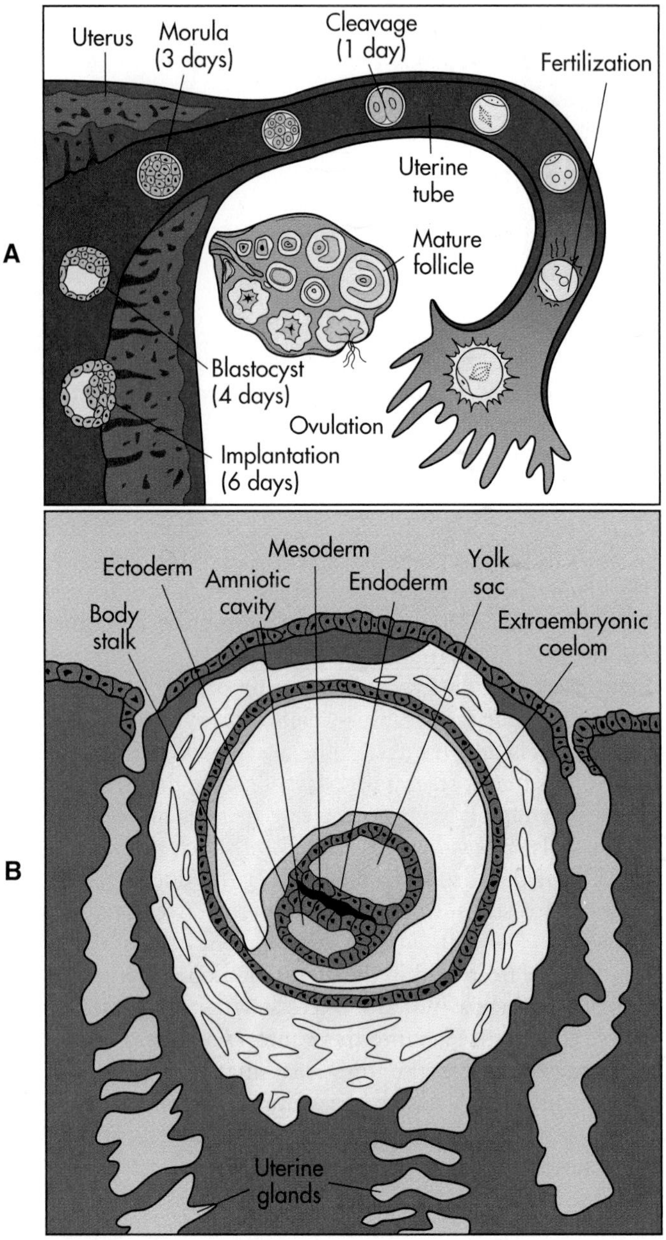
A
Uterus
Morula
(3 days)
Cleavage
(1 day)
Fertilization
Uterine
tube
Mature
follicle
Blastocyst
(4 days)
Ovulation
Implantation
(6 days)
B
Mesoderm
Yolk
sac
Ectoderm
Amniotic
cavity
Endoderm
Body
stalk
Extraembryonic
coelom
Uterine
glands

FIG. 13-4 First week of human development. **A,** Follicular development in the ovary, ovulation, fertilization, and transport of the early embryo down the uterine tube and into the uterus where implantation occurs. **B,** Blastocyst embedded in endometrium. Germ layers forming. (**A** from Carlson, B. [1994]. *Human embryology and developmental biology.* St. Louis: Mosby; **B** adapted from Langley, L., et al. [1980]. *Dynamic human anatomy and physiology* [5th ed.]. New York: McGraw-Hill.)

develop out of the trophoblast and extend into the blood-filled spaces of the endometrium. These villi obtain oxygen and nutrients from the maternal bloodstream and dispose of carbon dioxide and waste products into the maternal blood.

BOX 13-1 Stem Cells

Stem cells are able to divide for indefinite periods and can differentiate into the many different types of cells that make up an organism. Embryonic stem cells are derived from the blastocyst before it implants in the uterine wall. A zygote is described as totipotent because it has the potential to produce all the cells and tissues that compose an embryo and to support its in utero development. The term *pluripotent* is used to describe stem cells that generate cells derived from the three embryonic germ layers (endoderm, mesoderm, and ectoderm). The embryonic stem cell is pluripotent. Human stem cells were derived and maintained for the first time in 1998 by Thomson et al. by using blastocysts donated by couples undergoing in vitro fertilization. Potential uses of human embryonic stem cells include transplant therapy, in which tissues damaged by disease or injury are replaced or restored, as for example, in diabetes, Parkinson's disease, heart disease, and multiple sclerosis. Stem cell research engenders ethical concerns related to the source of human embryonic stem cells (embryos left over from in vitro fertilization and aborted fetuses). Currently federal support for research is restricted to existing cell lines.

From National Institutes of Health (2001). *Stem cells: Scientific progress and future research directions.* www.nih.gov/news/stemcell/scireport.htm. Accessed June 9, 2002.

After implantation, the endometrium is termed the *decidua.* The portion directly under the blastocyst, where the chorionic villi tap into the maternal blood vessels, is the **decidua basalis.** The portion covering the blastocyst is the *decidua capsularis,* and the portion lining the rest of the uterus is the *decidua vera* (Fig. 13-5).

EMBRYO AND FETUS

Pregnancy lasts approximately 10 lunar months, 9 calendar months, 40 weeks, or 280 days. Length of pregnancy is computed from the first day of the last menstrual period (LMP) until the day of birth. However, conception occurs approximately 2 weeks after the first day of the LMP; thus the postconception age of the fetus is 2 weeks less, for a total of 266 days or 38 weeks. Postconception age is used in the discussion of fetal development.

Intrauterine development is divided into three stages: ovum or preembryonic, embryo, and fetus (Fig. 13-6). The stage of the ovum lasts from conception until day 14. This period covers cellular replication, blastocyst formation, initial development of the embryonic membranes, and establishment of the primary germ layers.

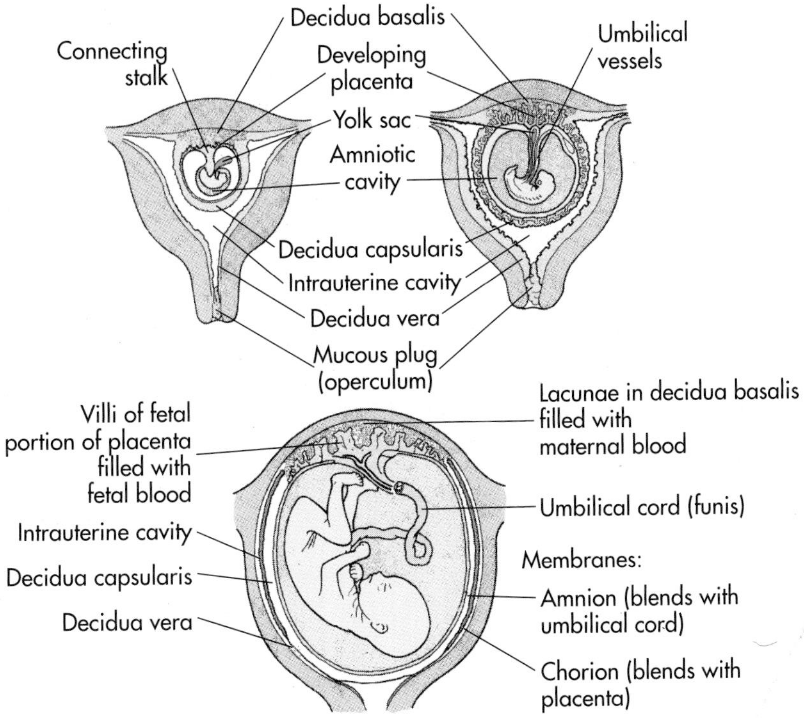
Decidua basalis
Connecting stalk
Developing placenta
Umbilical vessels
Yolk sac
Amniotic cavity
Decidua capsularis
Intrauterine cavity
Decidua vera
Mucous plug (operculum)
Villi of fetal portion of placenta filled with fetal blood
Lacunae in decidua basalis filled with maternal blood
Umbilical cord (funis)
Intrauterine cavity
Decidua capsularis
Decidua vera
Membranes:
Amnion (blends with umbilical cord)
Chorion (blends with placenta)

FIG. 13-5 Development of the fetal membranes. Note gradual obliteration of intrauterine cavity as decidua capsularis and deciduas vera meet. Also note thinning of uterine wall. Chorionic and amniotic membranes are in apposition to each other but may be peeled apart.

Primary Germ Layers

During the third week after conception, the embryonic disk differentiates into three primary germ layers: the ectoderm, the mesoderm, and the endoderm (or entoderm) (see Fig. 13-4, *B*). All tissues and organs of the embryo develop from these three layers.

The *ectoderm,* the upper layer of the embryonic disk, gives rise to the epidermis, the glands (anterior pituitary, cutaneous, and mammary), the nails and hair, the central and peripheral nervous systems, the lens of the eye, the tooth enamel, and the floor of the amniotic cavity.

The *mesoderm,* the middle layer, develops into the bones and teeth, the muscles (skeletal, smooth, and cardiac), the dermis and connective tissue, the cardiovascular system and spleen, and the urogenital system.

The *endoderm,* or lower layer, gives rise to the epithelium lining the respiratory tract and digestive tract, and the glandular cells of associated organs, including the oropharynx, liver and pancreas, urethra, bladder, and vagina. The endoderm forms the roof of the yolk sac.

Development of the Embryo

The stage of the **embryo** lasts from day 15 until approximately 8 weeks after conception or until the embryo measures 3 cm from crown to rump. This embryonic stage is the most critical time in the development of the organ systems and the main external features. Developing areas with rapid cell division are the most vulnerable to malformation caused by environmental **teratogens** (substances or exposure that causes abnormal development). At the end of the eighth week, all organ systems and external structures are present, and the embryo is unmistakably human (see Fig. 13-6).

Membranes

At the time of implantation, two **fetal membranes** that will surround the developing embryo begin to form. The *chorion* develops from the trophoblast and contains the chorionic villi on its surface. The villi burrow into the decidua basalis and increase in size and complexity as the vascular processes develop into the placenta. The chorion becomes the covering of the fetal side of the placenta. It contains the major umbilical blood vessels as they branch out over the surface of the placenta. As the embryo grows, the decidua capsularis stretches. The chorionic villi on this side atrophy and degenerate, leaving a smooth chorionic membrane.

The inner cell membrane, the *amnion,* develops from the interior cells of the blastocyst. The cavity that develops between this inner cell mass and the outer layer of cells (trophoblast) is the *amniotic cavity* (see Fig. 13-4, *B*). As it grows larger, the amnion forms on the side opposite the developing blastocyst (see Figs. 13-4 and 13-5). The

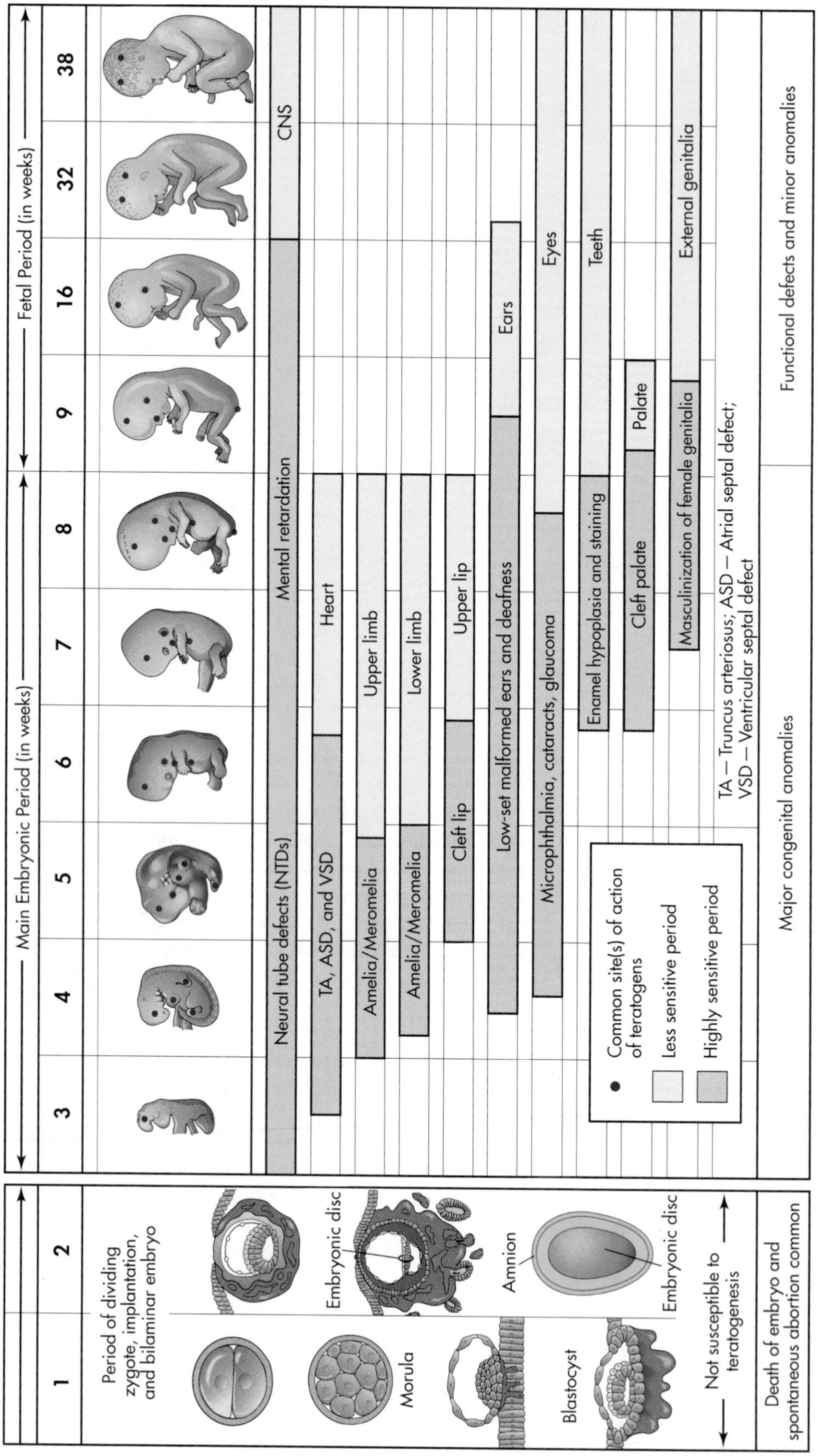

1
2
Period of dividing zygote, implantation, and bilaminar embryo
Morula
Blastocyst
Embryonic disc
Amnion
Embryonic disc
Not susceptible to teratogenesis
Death of embryo and spontaneous abortion common
Main Embryonic Period (in weeks)
Fetal Period (in weeks)
3
4
5
6
7
8
9
16
32
38
Neural tube defects (NTDs)
Mental retardation
CNS
TA, ASD, and VSD
Heart
Amelia/Meromelia
Upper limb
Amelia/Meromelia
Lower limb
Cleft lip
Upper lip
Low-set malformed ears and deafness
Ears
Microphthalmia, cataracts, glaucoma
Eyes
Enamel hypoplasia and staining
Teeth
Cleft palate
Palate
Masculinization of female genitalia
External genitalia
Common site(s) of action of teratogens
Less sensitive period
Highly sensitive period
TA – Truncus arteriosus; ASD – Atrial septal defect; VSD – Ventricular septal defect
Major congenital anomalies
Functional defects and minor anomalies

FIG. 13-6 Sensitive or critical periods in human development. Dark color denotes highly sensitive periods; light color indicates stages that are less sensitive to teratogens. (From Moore, K., & Persaud, T. [1998]. *Before we are born: Essentials of embryology and birth defects* [5th ed.]. Philadelphia: W.B. Saunders.)

developing embryo draws the amnion around itself, forming a fluid-filled sac. The amnion becomes the covering of the umbilical cord and covers the chorion on the fetal surface of the placenta. As the embryo grows larger, the amnion enlarges to accommodate the embryo/fetus and surrounding amniotic fluid. The amnion eventually comes in contact with the chorion surrounding the fetus.

Amniotic Fluid

The amniotic cavity initially derives its fluid by diffusion from the maternal blood. The amount of fluid increases weekly, and 800 to 1200 ml of transparent liquid is normally present at term. The amniotic fluid volume changes constantly. The fetus swallows fluid, and fluid flows into and out of the fetal lungs. The fetus urinates into the fluid, greatly increasing its volume.

Many functions are served by amniotic fluid for the embryo/fetus. **Amniotic fluid** helps maintain a constant body temperature. It serves as a source of oral fluid and a repository for waste. It cushions the fetus from trauma by blunting and dispersing outside forces. It allows freedom of movement for musculoskeletal development. The fluid keeps the embryo from tangling with the membranes, facilitating symmetric growth. If the embryo does become tangled with the membranes, amputations of extremities or other deformities can occur from constricting amniotic bands.

The volume of amniotic fluid is an important factor in assessing fetal well-being. Having less than 300 ml of amniotic fluid (*oligohydramnios*) is associated with fetal renal abnormalities. Having more than 2 L of amniotic fluid (*hydramnios*) is associated with gastrointestinal and other malformations.

Amniotic fluid contains albumin, urea, uric acid, creatinine, lecithin, sphingomyelin, bilirubin, fructose, fat, leukocytes, proteins, epithelial cells, enzymes, and lanugo hair. Study of fetal cells in amniotic fluid through amniocentesis yields much information about the fetus. Genetic studies (karyotyping) provide knowledge about the sex and the number and structure of chromosomes. Other studies, such as lecithin/sphingomyelin ratio, determine the health or maturity of the fetus (see Chapter 3).

Yolk Sac

When the amniotic cavity and amnion are forming, another blastocyst cavity forms on the other side of the developing embryonic disk (see Fig. 13-4, *B*). This cavity becomes surrounded by a membrane, forming the yolk sac. The yolk sac aids in transferring maternal nutrients and oxygen, which have diffused through the chorion, to the embryo. Blood vessels form to aid transport. Blood cells and plasma are manufactured in the yolk sac during the second and third weeks while uteroplacental circulation is being established and forming primitive blood cells until hematopoietic activity begins. At the end of the third week, the primitive heart begins to beat and circulate the blood through the embryo, connecting stalk, chorion, and yolk sac.

The folding in of the embryo during the fourth week results in incorporation of part of the yolk sac into the embryo's body as the primitive digestive system. Primordial germ cells arise in the yolk sac and move into the embryo. The shrinking remains of the yolk sac degenerate (see Fig. 13-5). By the fifth or sixth week, the remnant has separated from the embryo.

Umbilical Cord

By day 14 after conception, the embryonic disk, amniotic sac, and yolk sac are attached to the chorionic villi by the connecting stalk. During the third week, the blood vessels develop to supply the embryo with maternal nutrients and oxygen. During the fifth week, after the embryo has curved inward on itself from both ends, bringing the connecting stalk to the ventral side of the embryo, the connecting stalk becomes compressed from both sides by the amnion, forming the narrower umbilical cord (see Fig. 13-5). Two arteries carry blood from the embryo to the chorionic villi, and one vein returns blood to the embryo. Approximately 1% of umbilical cords contain only two vessels: one artery and one vein. This occurrence is sometimes associated with congenital malformations.

The cord rapidly increases in length. At term, the cord is 2 cm in diameter and ranges from 30 to 90 cm long (with an average of 55 cm). It twists spirally on itself and loops around the embryo/fetus. A true knot is rare, but false knots occur as folds or kinks in the cord and may jeopardize circulation to the fetus. Connective tissue called *Wharton's jelly* prevents compression of the blood vessels and ensures continued nourishment of the embryo/fetus. Compression can occur if the cord lies between the fetal head and the maternal pelvis or is twisted around the fetal body. When the cord is wrapped around the fetal neck, it is termed a **nuchal cord.**

Because the placenta develops from the chorionic villi, the umbilical cord is usually located centrally. A peripheral location is less common and is termed *battledore placenta*. The blood vessels are arrayed out from the center to all parts of the placenta.

Placenta

Structure. The placenta begins to form at implantation. During the third week after conception, the trophoblast cells of the chorionic villi continue to invade the decidua basalis. As the uterine capillaries are tapped, the endometrial spiral arteries fill with maternal blood. The chorionic villi grow into the spaces with two layers of cells: the outer syncytium and the inner cytotrophoblast. A third layer develops into anchoring septa, dividing the projecting decidua into separate areas called *cotyledons*. In each of the 15 to 20 cotyledons, the chorionic villi branch out, and a complex system of fetal blood vessels forms.

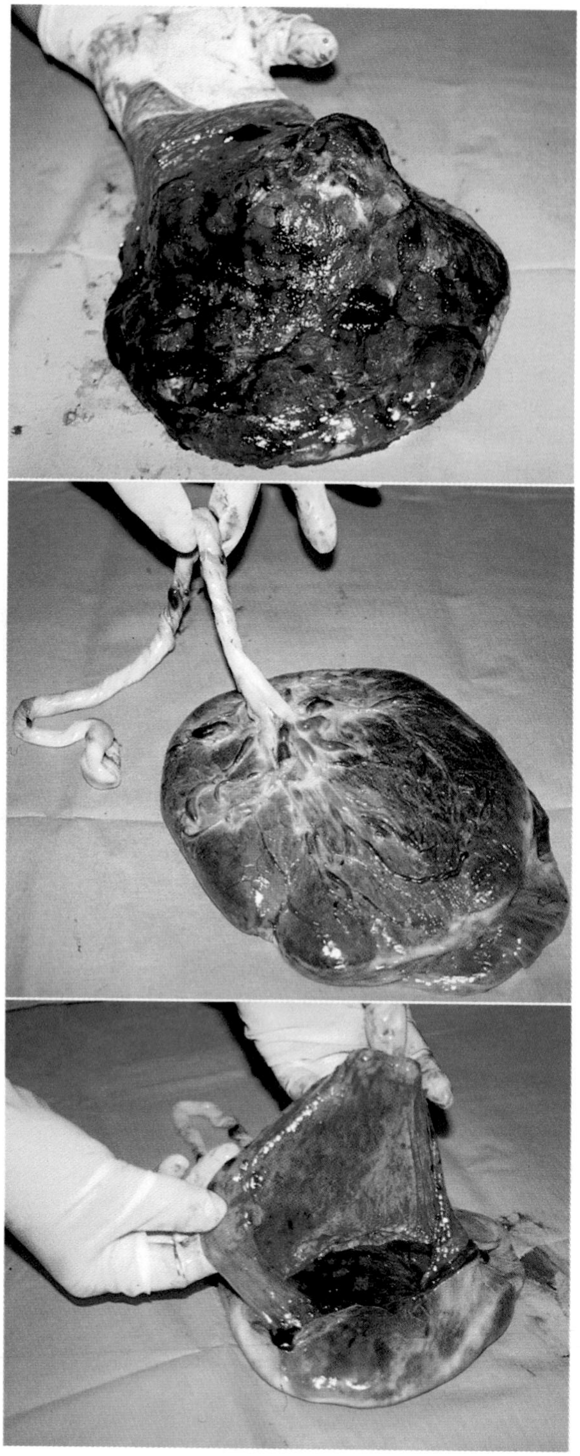
A
B
C

FIG. 13-7 Term placenta. **A,** Maternal (or uterine) surface, showing cotyledons and grooves. **B,** Fetal (or amniotic) surface, showing blood vessels running under amnion and converging to form umbilical vessels at attachment of umbilical cord. **C,** Amnion and smooth chorion are arranged to show that they are (1) fused and (2) continuous with margins of placenta. (Courtesy Marjorie Pyle, RNC, Lifecircle, Costa Mesa, CA.)

Each cotyledon is a functional unit. The whole structure is the **placenta** (Fig. 13-7).

The maternal-placental-embryonic circulation is in place by day 17, when the embryonic heart starts beating. By the end of the third week, embryonic blood is circulating between the embryo and the chorionic villi. In the intervillous spaces, maternal blood supplies oxygen and nutrients to the embryonic capillaries in the villi (Fig. 13-8). Waste products and carbon dioxide diffuse into the maternal blood.

The placenta functions as a means of metabolic exchange. Exchange is minimal at this time because the two cell layers of the villous membrane are too thick. Permeability increases as the cytotrophoblast thins and disappears; by the fifth month, only the single layer of syncytium is left between the maternal blood and the fetal capillaries. The syncytium is the functional layer of the placenta. By the eighth week, genetic testing may be done on a sample of chorionic villi by aspiration biopsy; however, limb defects have been associated with chorionic villus sampling done before 10 weeks. The structure of the placenta is complete by the twelfth week. The placenta continues to grow wider until 20 weeks, when it covers approximately half of the uterine surface. It then continues to grow thicker. The branching villi continue to develop within the body of the placenta, increasing the functional surface area.

Functions. One of the early functions of the placenta is as an endocrine gland that produces four hormones necessary to maintain the pregnancy and support the embryo and fetus. The hormones are produced in the syncytium.

The protein hormone **human chorionic gonadotropin (hCG)** can be detected in the maternal serum by 8 to 10 days after conception, shortly after implantation. This hormone is the basis for pregnancy tests. The hCG preserves the function of the ovarian corpus luteum, ensuring a continued supply of estrogen and progesterone needed to maintain the pregnancy. Miscarriage occurs if the corpus luteum stops functioning before the placenta is producing sufficient estrogen and progesterone. The amount of hCG reaches its maximal level at 50 to 70 days and then begins to decrease.

The other protein hormone produced by the placenta is **chorionic somatomammotropin,** or human placental lactogen (hPL). This substance is similar to a growth hormone and stimulates the maternal metabolism to supply nutrients needed for fetal growth. This hormone increases the resistance to insulin, facilitates glucose transport across the placental membrane, and stimulates breast development to prepare for lactation.

The placenta eventually produces more of the steroid hormone progesterone than the corpus luteum does during the first few months of pregnancy. Progesterone maintains the endometrium, decreases the contractility of the uterus, and stimulates maternal metabolism and development of breast alveoli.

By 7 weeks after fertilization, the placenta is producing most of the maternal estrogens, which are steroid hormones. The major estrogen secreted by the placenta is

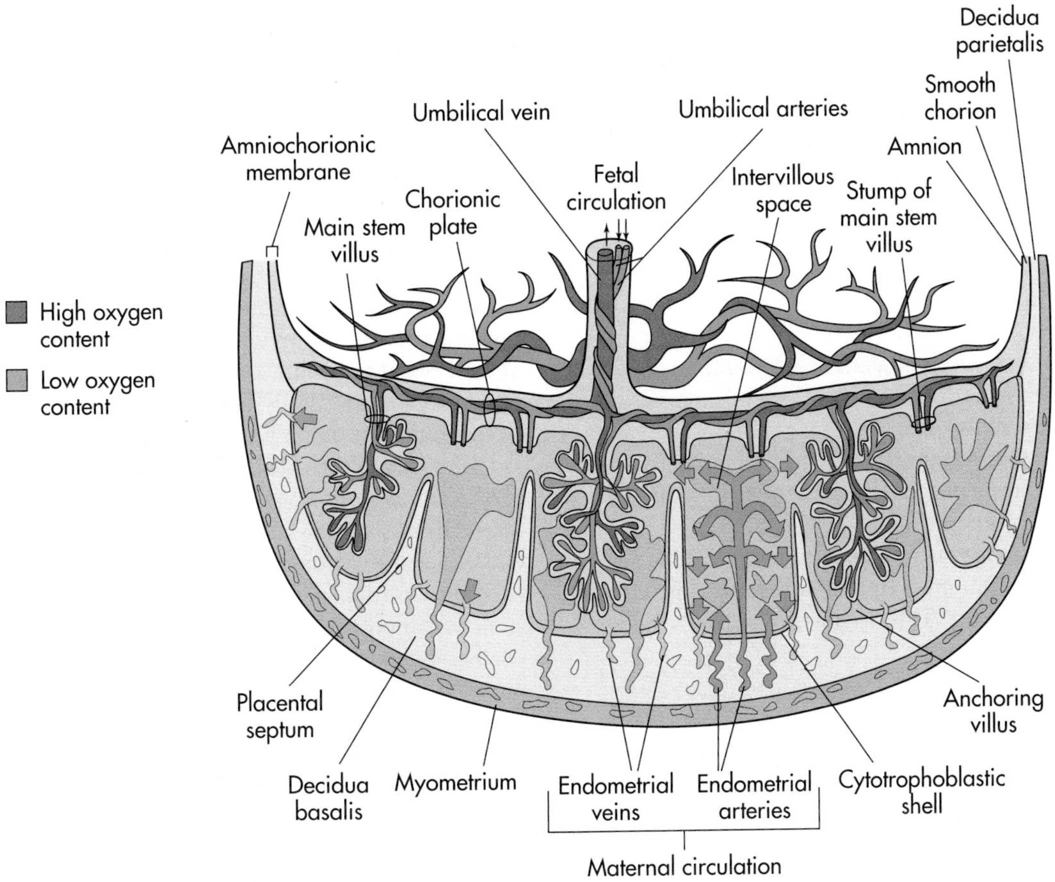
Decidua parietalis
Smooth chorion
Umbilical vein
Umbilical arteries
Amniochorionic membrane
Amnion
Fetal circulation
Intervillous space
Stump of main stem villus
Chorionic plate
Main stem villus
High oxygen content
Low oxygen content
Placental septum
Anchoring villus
Decidua basalis
Myometrium
Endometrial veins
Endometrial arteries
Cytotrophoblastic shell
Maternal circulation

FIG. 13-8 Schematic drawing of a transverse section through a term placenta, showing (1) the relation of the villous chorion (fetal part of placenta) to the decidua basalis (maternal part of placenta); (2) the fetal placental circulation; and (3) the maternal placental circulation. Maternal blood flows into the intervillous spaces in funnel-shaped spurts from the spiral arteries, and exchanges occur with the fetal blood as the maternal blood flows around the branch villi. The main exchange of material between the mother and the embryo or fetus occurs through the branch villi. The inflowing arterial blood pushes venous blood out of the intervillous space into the endometrial veins, which are scattered over the entire surface of the decidua basalis. Note that the umbilical arteries carry poorly oxygenated fetal blood (*blue*) to the placenta and that the umbilical vein carries oxygenated blood (*red*) to the fetus. Note that the cotyledons are separated from each other by placental septa, projections of the decidua basalis. Each cotyledon consists of two or more main stem villi and their many branches. In this drawing, only one stem villus is shown in each cotyledon, but the stumps of those that have been removed are indicated. (From Moore, K., & Persaud, T. [1998]. *Before we are born: Essentials of embryology and birth defects* [5th ed.]. Philadelphia: W.B. Saunders.)

estriol, whereas the ovaries produce mostly estradiol. Measuring estriol levels is a clinical assay for placental functioning. Estrogen stimulates uterine growth and uteroplacental blood flow. It causes a proliferation of the breast glandular tissue and stimulates myometrial contractility. Placental estrogen production increases greatly toward the end of pregnancy. One theory for the cause of the onset of labor is the decrease in circulating levels of progesterone and the increased levels of estrogen.

The metabolic functions of the placenta are respiration, nutrition, excretion, and storage. Oxygen diffuses from the maternal blood across the placental membrane into the fetal blood, and carbon dioxide diffuses in the opposite direction. In this way, the placenta functions as lungs for the fetus.

Carbohydrates, proteins, calcium, and iron are stored in the placenta for ready access to meet fetal needs. Water, inorganic salts, carbohydrates, proteins, fats, and vitamins pass from the maternal blood supply across the placental membrane into the fetal blood, supplying nutrition. Water and most electrolytes with a molecular weight less than 500 readily diffuse through the membrane. Hydrostatic and osmotic pressures aid the flow of water and some solutions. Facilitated and active transport assist in the transfer of glucose, amino acids, calcium, iron, and substances with higher molecular weight. Amino acids and calcium are transported against the concentration gradient between the maternal blood and fetal blood.

The fetal concentration of glucose is lower than the glucose level in the maternal blood because of its rapid metabolism by the fetus. This fetal requirement demands larger concentrations of glucose than simple diffusion can provide. Therefore maternal glucose moves into the fetal circulation by active transport.

Pinocytosis is a mechanism used for transferring large molecules, such as albumin and gamma globulins, across the placental membrane. This mechanism conveys the maternal immunoglobulins that provide early passive immunity to the fetus.

Metabolic waste products of the fetus cross the placental membrane from the fetal blood into the maternal blood, and the maternal kidneys then excrete them. Many viruses can cross the placental membrane and infect the fetus. Some bacteria and protozoa first infect the placenta and then infect the fetus. Drugs also can cross the placental membrane and may harm the fetus. Caffeine, alcohol, nicotine, carbon monoxide, and other toxic substances in cigarette smoke, as well as prescription and recreational drugs (such as cocaine and marijuana) readily cross the placenta (Box 13-2).

Although no direct link exists between the fetal blood in the vessels of the chorionic villi and the maternal blood in the intervillous spaces, only one cell layer separates them. Breaks occasionally occur in the placental membrane. Fetal erythrocytes then leak into the maternal circulation, and the mother may develop antibodies to the fetal red blood cells. This is often the way an Rh-negative mother becomes sensitized to the erythrocytes of her Rh-positive fetus. (See discussions of isoimmunization in Chapters 23 and 39.)

Although the placenta and fetus are living tissue transplants, they are not destroyed by the host mother (Silver & Branch, 1999). Either the placental hormones suppress the immunologic response, or the tissue evokes no response.

Placental function depends on the maternal blood pressure supplying circulation. Maternal arterial blood, under pressure in the small uterine spiral arteries, spurts into the intervillous spaces (see Fig. 13-8). As long as rich arterial blood continues to be supplied, pressure is exerted on the blood already in the intervillous spaces, pushing it toward drainage by the low-pressure uterine veins. At term gestation, 10% of the maternal cardiac output goes to the uterus.

If there is interference with the circulation to the placenta, the placenta cannot supply the embryo or fetus. Vasoconstriction, such as that caused by hypertension and cocaine use, diminishes uterine blood flow. Decreased maternal blood pressure or cardiac output also diminishes uterine blood flow.

When a woman lies on her back with the pressure of the uterus compressing the vena cava, blood return to the right atrium is diminished (see discussion of supine hypotension in Chapters 12 and 16; see Fig. 21-5). Excessive maternal exercise that diverts blood to the muscles away from the uterus compromises placental circulation. Optimal circulation is achieved when the woman is lying at rest on her side. Decreased uterine circulation may lead to intrauterine growth restriction of the fetus and to infants who are small for gestational age.

Braxton Hicks contractions appear to enhance the movement of blood through the intervillous spaces, aiding placental circulation. Prolonged contractions or too-short intervals between contractions during labor, however, reduce blood flow to the placenta.

BOX 13-2 **Developmentally Toxic Exposures in Humans**

Aminopterin
Androgens
Angiotensin-converting enzyme inhibitors
Carbamazepine
Cigarette smoking
Cocaine
Coumarin anticoagulants
Cytomegalovirus
Diethylstilbestrol
Ethanol (>1 drink/day)
Etretinate
Hyperthermia
Iodides
Ionizing radiation (>10 rads)
Isotretinoin
Lead
Lithium
Methimazole
Methyl mercury
Parvovirus B19
Penicillamine
Phenytoin
Radioiodine
Rubella
Syphilis
Tetracycline
Thalidomide
Toxoplasmosis
Trimethadione
Valproic acid
Varicella

Fetal Maturation

The stage of the **fetus** lasts from 9 weeks (when the fetus becomes recognizable as a human being) until the pregnancy ends. Changes during the fetal period are not so dramatic, because refinement of structure and function are taking place. The fetus is less vulnerable to teratogens, except for those affecting central nervous system functioning.

Viability refers to the capability of the fetus to survive outside the uterus. In the past, the earliest age at which fetal survival could be expected was 28 weeks after conception. With modern technology and advancements in maternal and neonatal care, viability is now possible at 20 weeks after conception (22 weeks after LMP, fetal weight of 500 g or more). The limitations on survival outside the uterus are based on central nervous system function and the oxygenation capability of the lungs.

Fetal Circulatory System

The cardiovascular system is the first organ system to function in the developing human. Blood vessel and blood cell formation begins in the third week and supplies the embryo with oxygen and nutrients from the mother. By the end of the third week, the tubular heart begins to beat, and the primitive cardiovascular system links the embryo, connecting stalk, chorion, and yolk sac. During the fourth and fifth weeks, the heart develops into a four-chambered organ. By the end of the embryonic stage, the heart is developmentally complete.

The fetal lungs do not function for respiratory gas exchange, so a special circulatory pathway, the **ductus arteriosus,** bypasses the lungs. Oxygen-rich blood from the placenta flows rapidly through the umbilical vein into the fetal abdomen (Fig. 13-9). When the umbilical vein

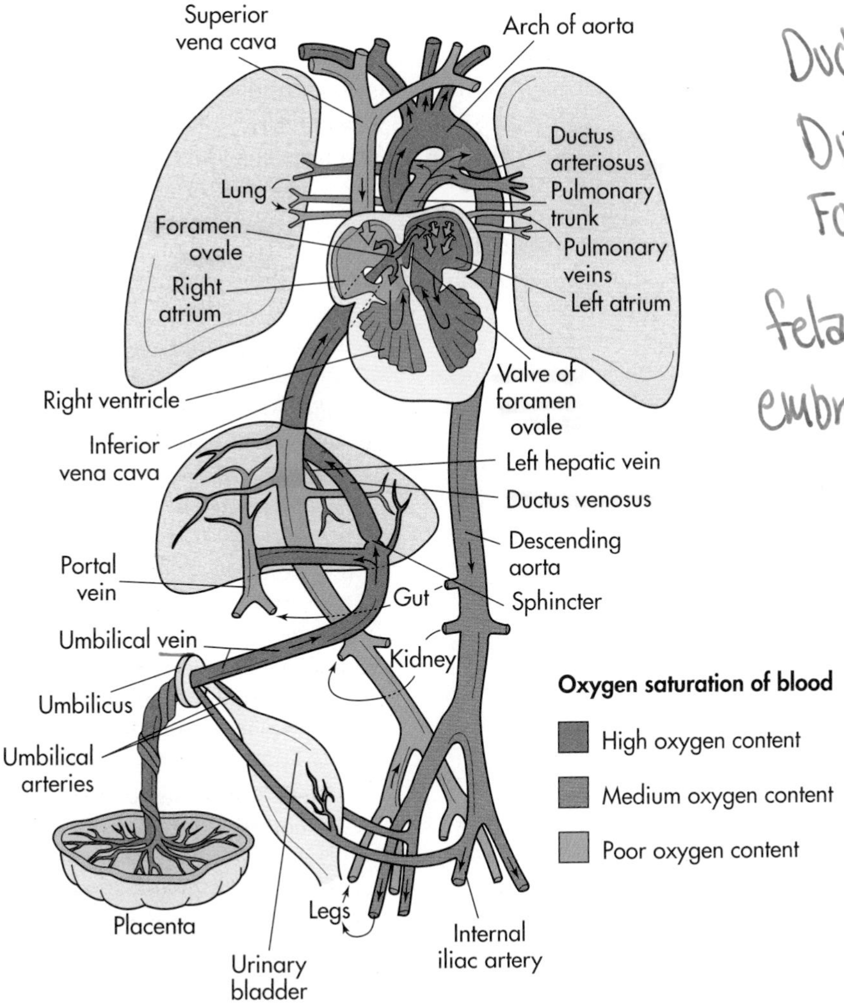
Superior vena cava
Arch of aorta
Ductus arteriosus
Lung
Pulmonary trunk
Foramen ovale
Pulmonary veins
Right atrium
Left atrium
Valve of foramen ovale
Right ventricle
Inferior vena cava
Left hepatic vein
Ductus venosus
Descending aorta
Portal vein
Gut
Sphincter
Umbilical vein
Kidney
Umbilicus
Umbilical arteries
Placenta
Legs
Urinary bladder
Internal iliac artery
Oxygen saturation of blood
High oxygen content
Medium oxygen content
Poor oxygen content

FIG. 13-9 Schematic illustration of the fetal circulation. The colors indicate the oxygen saturation of the blood, and the arrows show the course of the blood from the placenta to the heart. The organs are not drawn to scale. Observe that three shunts permit most of the blood to bypass the liver and lungs: (1) ductus venosus, (2) foramen ovale, and (3) ductus arteriosus. The poorly oxygenated blood returns to the placenta for oxygen and nutrients through the umbilical arteries. (From Moore, K., & Persaud, T. [1998]. *Before we are born: Essentials of embryology and birth defects* [5th ed.]. Philadelphia: W.B. Saunders.)

reaches the liver, it divides into two branches; one branch circulates some oxygenated blood through the liver. Most of the blood passes through the **ductus venosus** into the inferior vena cava. There it mixes with the deoxygenated blood from the fetal legs and abdomen on its way to the right atrium. Most of this blood passes straight through the right atrium and through the **foramen ovale,** an opening into the left atrium. There it mixes with the small amount of deoxygenated blood returning from the fetal lungs through the pulmonary veins.

The blood flows into the left ventricle and is squeezed out into the aorta, where the arteries supplying the heart, head, neck, and arms receive most of the oxygen-rich blood. This pattern of supplying the highest levels of oxygen and nutrients to the head, neck, and arms enhances the cephalocaudal (head-to-rump) development of the embryo/fetus.

Deoxygenated blood returning from the head and arms enters the right atrium through the superior vena cava. This blood is directed downward into the right ventricle, where it is squeezed into the pulmonary artery. A small amount of blood circulates through the resistant lung tissue, but the majority follows the path with less resistance through the ductus arteriosus into the aorta, distal to the point of exit of the arteries supplying the head and arms with oxygenated blood. The oxygen-poor blood flows through the abdominal aorta into the internal iliac arteries, where the umbilical arteries direct most of it back through the umbilical cord to the placenta. There the blood gives up its wastes and carbon dioxide in exchange for nutrients and oxygen. The blood remaining in the iliac arteries flows through the fetal abdomen and legs, ultimately returning through the inferior vena cava to the heart.

The following three special characteristics enable the fetus to obtain sufficient oxygen from the maternal blood:

- Fetal hemoglobin carries 20% to 30% more oxygen than maternal hemoglobin.
- The hemoglobin concentration of the fetus is about 50% greater than that of the mother.
- The fetal heart rate (FHR) is 110 to 160 beats/min, making the cardiac output per unit of body weight higher than that of an adult.

Hematopoietic System

Hematopoiesis, the formation of blood, occurs in the yolk sac (see Fig. 13-4, *B*) beginning in the third week. Hematopoietic stem cells seed the fetal liver during the fifth week, and hematopoiesis begins there during the sixth week. This accounts for the relatively large size of the liver between the seventh and ninth weeks. Stem cells seed the fetal bone marrow, spleen, thymus, and lymph nodes between weeks 8 and 11.

The antigenic factors that determine blood type are present in the erythrocytes soon after the sixth week. For this reason, the Rh-negative woman is at risk for isoimmunization in any pregnancy that lasts longer than 6 weeks after fertilization.

Gastrointestinal System

During the fourth week, the shape of the embryo changes from being almost straight to a C shape, as both ends fold toward the ventral surface. A portion of the yolk sac is incorporated into the body from head to tail as the primitive gut (digestive system).

The foregut produces the pharynx, part of the lower respiratory tract, the esophagus, the stomach, the first half of the duodenum, the liver, the pancreas, and the gallbladder. These structures evolve during the fifth and sixth weeks. The malformations that can occur in these areas are esophageal atresia, hypertrophic pyloric stenosis, duodenal stenosis or atresia, and biliary atresia.

The midgut becomes the distal half of the duodenum, jejunum and ileum, cecum and appendix, and proximal half of the colon. The midgut loop projects into the umbilical cord between weeks 5 and 10. A malformation (omphalocele) results if the midgut fails to return to the abdominal cavity, causing the intestines to protrude from the umbilicus. Meckel's diverticulum, the most common malformation of the midgut, occurs when a remnant of the yolk stalk that has failed to degenerate attaches to the ileum, leaving a blind sac.

The hindgut develops into the distal half of the colon, the rectum and parts of the anal canal, the urinary bladder, and the urethra. Anorectal malformations are the most common abnormalities of the digestive system.

The fetus swallows amniotic fluid beginning in the fifth month. Gastric emptying and intestinal peristalsis occur. Fetal nutrition and elimination needs are taken care of by the placenta. As the fetus nears term, fetal waste products accumulate in the intestines as dark green to black, tarry meconium. Normally, this substance is passed through the rectum within 24 hours of birth. Sometimes with a breech presentation or fetal hypoxia, meconium is passed in utero into the amniotic fluid. The failure to pass meconium after birth may indicate atresia somewhere in the digestive tract, an imperforate anus, or meconium ileus, in which a firm meconium plug blocks passage (seen in infants with cystic fibrosis).

The metabolic rate of the fetus is relatively low, but the infant has great growth and development needs. Beginning in week 9, the fetus synthesizes glycogen for storage in the liver. Between 26 and 30 weeks, the fetus begins to lay down stores of brown fat in preparation for extrauterine cold stress. Thermoregulation in the neonate requires increased metabolism and adequate oxygenation.

The gastrointestinal system is mature by 36 weeks. Digestive enzymes (except pancreatic amylase and lipase) are present in sufficient quantity to facilitate digestion; however, the neonate cannot digest starches or fats efficiently. Little saliva is produced.

Hepatic System

The liver and biliary tract develop from the foregut during the fourth week of gestation. Hematopoiesis begins during the sixth week and requires that the liver be large.

The embryonic liver is prominent, occupying most of the abdominal cavity. Bile, a constituent of meconium, begins to form in the twelfth week.

Glycogen is stored in the fetal liver beginning at week 9 or 10. At term, glycogen stores are twice those of the adult. Glycogen is the major source of energy for the fetus and neonate stressed by in utero hypoxia, extrauterine loss of the maternal glucose supply, the work of breathing, or cold stress.

Iron also is stored in the fetal liver. If the maternal intake is sufficient, the fetus can store enough iron to last for 5 months after birth.

During fetal life, the liver does not have to conjugate bilirubin for excretion because the unconjugated bilirubin is cleared by the placenta. Therefore the glucuronyl transferase enzyme needed for conjugation is present in the fetal liver in amounts less than those required after birth. This predisposes the neonate, especially the preterm infant, to hyperbilirubinemia.

Coagulation factors II, VII, IX, and X cannot be synthesized in the fetal liver because of the lack of vitamin K synthesis in the sterile fetal gut. This coagulation deficiency persists after birth for several days and is the rationale for the prophylactic administration of vitamin K to the newborn.

Respiratory System

The respiratory system begins development during embryonic life and continues through fetal life and into childhood until about 8 years of age. The development of the respiratory tract begins in week 4 and continues through week 17 with formation of the larynx, trachea, bronchi, and lung buds. Between 16 and 24 weeks, the bronchi and terminal bronchioles enlarge, and vascular structures and primitive alveoli are formed. Between 24 weeks and term birth, more alveoli form. Specialized alveolar cells, type I and type II cells, secrete pulmonary surfactants to line the interior of the alveoli. After 32 weeks, sufficient surfactant is present in developed alveoli to provide infants with a good chance of survival.

Pulmonary surfactants. The detection of the presence of pulmonary **surfactants,** surface-active phospholipids, in amniotic fluid has been used to determine the degree of fetal lung maturity, or the ability of the lungs to function after birth. Lecithin (L) is the most critical alveolar surfactant required for postnatal lung expansion. It is detectable at approximately 21 weeks and increases in amount after week 24. Another pulmonary phospholipid, sphingomyelin (S), remains constant in amount. Thus the measure of lecithin in relation to sphingomyelin, or the **L/S ratio,** is used to determine fetal lung maturity. When the L/S ratio reaches 2:1, the infant's lungs are considered to be mature. This occurs at approximately 35 weeks of gestation (Jobe, 1999).

Certain maternal conditions such as maternal hypertension, placental dysfunction, infection, or corticosteroid use cause decreased maternal blood flow and accelerate fetal lung maturity. This apparently is caused by the resulting fetal hypoxia, which stresses the fetus and increases the blood levels of corticosteroids that accelerate alveolar and surfactant development. Conditions such as gestational diabetes and chronic glomerulonephritis can retard fetal lung maturity.

Fetal respiratory movements have been seen on ultrasound examination as early as week 11. These fetal respiratory movements may aid in development of the chest wall muscles and regulate lung fluid volume. The fetal lungs produce fluid that expands the air spaces in the lungs. The fluid drains into the amniotic fluid or is swallowed by the fetus.

Before birth, secretion of lung fluid decreases. The normal birth process squeezes out approximately one third of the fluid. Infants of cesarean births do not benefit from this squeezing process; thus they may have more respiratory difficulty at birth. The fluid remaining in the lungs at birth is usually reabsorbed into the infant's bloodstream within 2 hours of birth.

Renal System

The kidneys form during the fifth week and begin to function approximately 4 weeks later. Urine is excreted into the amniotic fluid and forms a major part of the amniotic fluid volume. Oligohydramnios is indicative of renal dysfunction. Because the placenta acts as the organ of excretion and maintains fetal water and electrolyte balance, the fetus does not need functioning kidneys while in utero. At birth, however, the kidneys are required immediately for excretory and acid-base regulatory functions.

A fetal renal malformation can be diagnosed in utero. Corrective or palliative fetal surgery may treat the malformation successfully, or plans can be made for treatment immediately after birth.

At term, the fetus has fully developed kidneys. However, the glomerular filtration rate (GFR) is low, and the kidneys lack the ability to concentrate urine. This makes the newborn more susceptible to both overhydration and dehydration.

Most newborns void within 24 hours of birth. With the loss of the swallowed amniotic fluid and the metabolism of nutrients provided by the placenta, voidings for the first days of life are scanty until fluid intake increases.

Neurologic System

The nervous system originates from the ectoderm during the third week after fertilization. The open neural tube forms during the fourth week. It initially closes at what will be the junction of the brain and spinal cord, leaving both ends open. The embryo folds in on itself lengthwise at this time, forming a head fold in the neural tube at this junction. The cranial end of the neural tube closes, and then the caudal end closes. During week 5, different growth rates cause more flexures in the neural tube, delineating three brain areas: the forebrain, midbrain, and hindbrain.

The forebrain develops into the eyes (cranial nerve II) and cerebral hemispheres. The development of all areas of the cerebral cortex continues throughout fetal life and into childhood. The olfactory system (cranial nerve I) and thalamus also develop from the forebrain. Cranial nerves III and IV (oculomotor and trochlear) form from the midbrain. The hindbrain forms the medulla, the pons, the cerebellum, and the remainder of the cranial nerves. Brain waves can be recorded on an electroencephalogram by week 8.

The spinal cord develops from the long end of the neural tube. Another ectodermal structure, the neural crest, develops into the peripheral nervous system. By the eighth week, nerve fibers traverse throughout the body. By week 11 or 12, the fetus makes respiratory movements, moves all extremities, and changes position in utero. The fetus can suck his or her thumb and swim in the amniotic fluid pool, turn somersaults, and sometimes ties a knot in the umbilical cord. Box 13-3 describes the major types of fetal movements. Sometime between 16 and 20 weeks, when the movements are strong enough to be perceived by the mother as "the baby moving," quickening has occurred. The perception of movement occurs earlier in the multigravida than in the primigravida. The mother also becomes aware of the sleep and wake cycles of the fetus.

BOX 13-3 Major Types of Fetal Movements

General movements. These slow gross movements involve the whole body. Their duration is from several seconds to a minute.

Startle movements. These quick (less than 1 second), generalized movements always start in the limbs and may spread to the trunk and neck.

Hiccups. These are repetitive phasic contractions of the diaphragm. A bout may last several minutes.

Fetal breathing movements. These are paradoxical movements in which the thorax moves inward and the abdomen outward with each contraction of the diaphragm.

Isolated arm or leg movements. These movements of extremities occur without movement of the trunk.

Hand-face contact. This occurs any time the moving hand makes contact with the face or mouth.

Retroflexion of the head. This is a slow to jerky backward bending of the head.

Lateral rotation of the head. This involves isolated turning of the head from side to side.

Anteflexion of the head. This is a normally slow forward bending of the head.

Opening of the mouth. This isolated movement may be accompanied by protrusion of the tongue.

Yawn. The mouth is slowly opened and rapidly closed after a few seconds.

Sucking. This burst of rhythmical jaw movements is sometimes followed by swallowing. With this movement the fetus may be drinking amniotic fluid.

Stretch. This complex movement involves overextension of the spine, retroflexion of the head, and elevation of the arms.

From Carlson, B. (1994). *Human embryology and developmental biology*. St. Louis: Mosby.

Sensory Awareness. Purposeful movements of the fetus have been demonstrated in response to a firm touch transmitted through the mother's abdomen. Because it can feel, the fetus requires anesthesia when invasive procedures are done.

Fetuses respond to sound by 24 weeks. Different types of music evoke different movements. The fetus can be soothed by the sound of the mother's voice. Acoustic stimulation can be used to evoke a fetal heart rate response. The fetus becomes accustomed (i.e., habituates) to noises heard repeatedly. Hearing is fully developed at birth.

The fetus is able to distinguish taste. By the fifth month, when the fetus is swallowing amniotic fluid, a sweetener added to the fluid causes the fetus to swallow faster. The fetus also reacts to temperature changes. A cold solution placed into the amniotic fluid can cause fetal hiccups.

The fetus can see. Eyes have both rods and cones in the retina by the seventh month. A bright light shone on the mother's abdomen in late pregnancy causes abrupt fetal movements. During sleep time, rapid eye movements have been observed similar to those occurring in children and adults while dreaming (Cole, 1997).

At term, the fetal brain is approximately one fourth the size of an adult brain. Neurologic development continues. Stressors on the fetus and neonate (e.g., chronic poor nutrition or hypoxia, drugs, environmental toxins, trauma, disease) cause damage to the central nervous system long after the vulnerable embryonic time for malformations in other organ systems. Neurologic insult can result in cerebral palsy, neuromuscular impairment, mental retardation, and learning disabilities.

Endocrine System

The thyroid gland develops along with structures in the head and neck during the third and fourth weeks. The secretion of thyroxine begins during the eighth week. Maternal thyroxine does not readily cross the placenta; therefore the fetus that does not produce thyroid hormones will be born with congenital hypothyroidism. If untreated, hypothyroidism can result in severe mental retardation. Screening for hypothyroidism is typically included in the testing when screening for phenylketonuria (PKU) after birth.

The adrenal cortex is formed during the sixth week and produces hormones by the eighth or ninth week. As term approaches, the fetus produces more cortisol. This is believed to aid in initiation of labor by decreasing the maternal progesterone and stimulating production of prostaglandins.

The pancreas forms from the foregut during the fifth through eighth weeks. The islets of Langerhans develop during the twelfth week. Insulin is produced by week 20. In infants of mothers with uncontrolled diabetes, maternal hyperglycemia produces fetal hyperglycemia, stimulating hyperinsulinemia and islet cell hyperplasia. This results in a macrosomic (large) fetus. The hyperinsulinemia also blocks lung maturation, placing the neonate at risk for respiratory distress and hypoglycemia when the maternal glucose source is lost at birth. Control of the maternal glucose level before and during pregnancy minimizes problems for the fetus and infant.

Reproductive System

Sex differentiation begins in the embryo during the seventh week. Female and male external genitalia are indistinguishable until after the ninth week. Distinguishing characteristics appear around the ninth week and are fully differentiated by the twelfth week. When a Y chromosome is present, testes are formed. By the end of the embryonic period, testosterone is being secreted and causes formation of the male genitalia. By week 28, the testes begin descending into the scrotum. After birth, low levels of testosterone continue to be secreted until the pubertal surge.

The female, with two X chromosomes, forms ovaries and female external genitalia. By the sixteenth week, oogenesis has been established. At birth, the ovaries contain the female's lifetime supply of ova. Most female hormone production is delayed until puberty. However, the fetal endometrium responds to maternal hormones, and withdrawal bleeding or vaginal discharge (pseudomenstruation) may occur at birth when these hormones are lost. The high level of maternal estrogen also stimulates mammary engorgement and secretion of fluid ("witch's milk") in newborn infants of both sexes.

Musculoskeletal System

Bones and muscles develop from the mesoderm by the fourth week of embryonic development. At that time, the cardiac muscle is already beating. The mesoderm next to the neural tube forms the vertebral column and ribs. The parts of the vertebral column grow toward each other to enclose the developing spinal cord. Ossification, or bone formation, begins. If there is a defect in the bony fusion, various forms of spina bifida may occur. A large defect affecting several vertebrae may allow the membranes and spinal cord to pouch out from the back, producing neurologic deficits and skeletal deformity.

The flat bones of the skull develop during the embryonic period, and ossification continues throughout childhood. At birth, connective tissue sutures exist where the bones of the skull meet. The areas where more than two bones meet (called fontanels) are especially prominent. The sutures and fontanels allow the bones of the skull to mold or move during birth, enabling the head to pass through the birth canal.

The bones of the shoulders, arms, hips, and legs appear in the sixth week as a continuous skeleton with no joints. Differentiation occurs, producing separate bones and joints. Ossification will continue through childhood to allow growth. Beginning during the seventh week, muscles contract spontaneously. Arm and leg movements are visible on ultrasound examination, although the mother does not perceive them until sometime between 16 and 20 weeks.

Integumentary System

The epidermis begins as a single layer of cells derived from the ectoderm at 4 weeks. By the seventh week, there are two layers of cells. The cells of the superficial layer are sloughed and become mixed with the sebaceous gland secretions to form the white, cheesy vernix caseosa, the material that protects the skin of the fetus. The vernix is thick at 24 weeks but becomes scant by term.

The basal layer of the epidermis is the germinal layer, which replaces lost cells. Until 17 weeks, the skin is very thin and wrinkled, with blood vessels visible underneath. The skin thickens, and all layers are present at term. After 32 weeks, as subcutaneous fat is deposited under the dermis, the skin becomes less wrinkled and red in appearance.

By 16 weeks, the epidermal ridges are present on the palms of the hands, the fingers, the bottom of the feet, and the toes. These handprints and footprints are unique to that infant.

Hairs form from hair bulbs in the epidermis that project into the dermis. Cells in the hair bulb keratinize to form the hair shaft. As the cells at the base of the hair shaft proliferate, the hair grows to the surface of the epithelium. Very fine hairs, called *lanugo,* appear first at 12 weeks on the eyebrows and upper lip. By 20 weeks, they cover the entire body. At this time, the eyelashes, eyebrows, and scalp hair are beginning to grow. By 28 weeks, the scalp hair is longer than the lanugo, which thins and may disappear by term gestation.

Fingernails and toenails develop from thickened epidermis at the tips of the digits beginning during the tenth week. They grow slowly. Fingernails usually reach the fingertips by 32 weeks, and toenails reach the tips by 36 weeks.

Immunologic System

During the third trimester, albumin and globulin are present in the fetus. The only immunoglobulin that crosses the placenta, immunoglobulin G (IgG), provides passive acquired immunity to specific bacterial toxins. The fetus produces IgM immunoglobulins by the end of the first trimester. These are produced in response to blood group antigens, gram-negative enteric organisms, and some viruses. IgA immunoglobulins are not produced by the fetus; however, colostrum, the precursor to breast milk, contains large amounts of IgA and can provide passive immunity to the neonate who is breastfed.

The normal term neonate can fight infection but not so effectively as an older child. The preterm infant is at much greater risk for infection.

Table 13-1 summarizes embryonic and fetal development.

TABLE 13-1 Milestones in Human Development Before Birth Since Last Menstrual Period (LMP)

	4 WEEKS	8 WEEKS	12 WEEKS
EXTERNAL APPEARANCE	Body flexed, C-shaped; arm and leg buds present; head at right angles to body 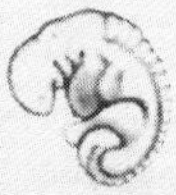	Body fairly well formed; nose flat, eyes far apart; digits well formed; head elevating; tail almost disappeared; eyes, ears, nose, and mouth recognizable 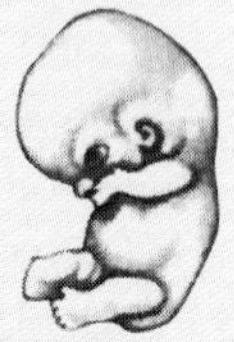	Nails appearing, resembling a human, head erect but disproportionately large, skin pink, delicate 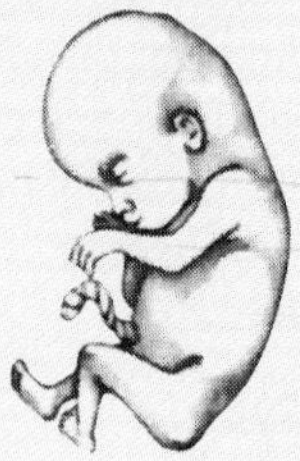
CROWN-TO-RUMP MEASUREMENT, WEIGHT	0.4-0.5 cm, 0.4 g	2.5-3 cm, 2 g	6-9 cm, 19 g
GASTROINTESTINAL SYSTEM	Stomach at midline and fusiform, conspicuous liver, esophagus short, intestine a short tube	Intestinal villi developing, small intestines coiling within umbilical cord; palatal folds present, liver very large	Bile secreted, palatal fusion complete, intestines withdrawn from cord and assume characteristic positions
MUSCULOSKELETAL SYSTEM	All somites present	First indication of ossification—occiput, mandible, and humerus; embryo capable of some movement, definitive muscles of trunk, limbs, and head well represented	Some bones well outlined, ossification spreading; upper cervical to lower sacral arches and bodies ossify; smooth muscle layers indicated in hollow viscera
CIRCULATORY SYSTEM	Heart developing; double chambers visible, beginning to beat; aortic arch and major veins completed	Main blood vessels assume final plan, enucleated red cells predominate in blood; heart beat detectable with sonography	Blood forming in marrow Heart beat audible by Doppler
RESPIRATORY SYSTEM	Primary lung buds appear	Pleural and pericardial cavities forming, branching bronchioles, nostrils closed by epithelial plugs	Lungs acquiring definite shape, vocal cords appear
RENAL SYSTEM	Rudimentary ureteral buds appear	Earliest secretory tubules differentiating, bladder-urethra separates from rectum	Kidney able to secrete urine, bladder expands as a sac
NERVOUS SYSTEM	Well-marked midbrain flexure, no hindbrain or cervical flexures, neural groove closed	Cerebral cortex begins to acquire typical cells; differentiation of cerebral cortex, meninges, ventricular foramina, cerebrospinal fluid circulation; spinal cord extends entire length of spine	Brain structural configuration roughly complete, cord showing cervical and lumbar enlargements, fourth ventricle foramina developed, sucking present
SENSORY ORGANS	Eye and ear appearing as optic vessel and otocyst	Primordial choroid plexuses develop, ventricles large relative to cortex, development progressing, eyes converging rapidly, internal car developing	Earliest taste buds indicated, characteristic organization of eye attained
GENITAL SYSTEM	Genital ridge appearing (fifth week)	Testes and ovaries distinguishable, external genitals sexless but beginning to differentiate	Sex recognizable, internal and external sex organs specific

TABLE 13-1 **Milestones in Human Development Before Birth Since Last Menstrual Period (LMP)—cont'd**

16 WEEKS	20 WEEKS	24 WEEKS
EXTERNAL APPEARANCE		
Head still dominant; face looks human; eyes, ears, and nose approaching typical appearance on gross examination; arm-leg ratio proportionate; scalp hair appears	Vernix caseosa and lanugo appear, legs lengthen considerably, sebaceous glands appear	Body lean but fairly well proportioned, skin red and wrinkled, vernix caseosa present, sweat glands forming
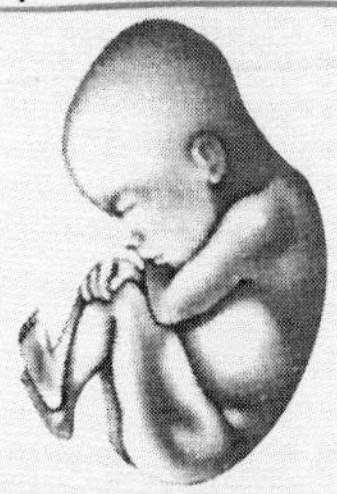	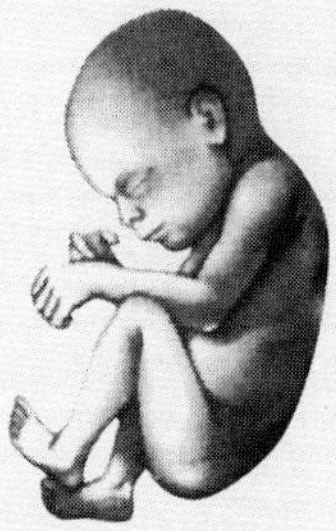	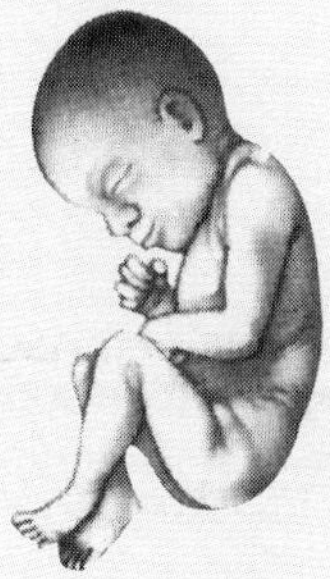
CROWN-TO-RUMP MEASUREMENT, WEIGHT		
11.5-13.5 cm, 100 g	16-18.5 cm, 300 g	23 cm, 600 g
GASTROINTESTINAL SYSTEM		
Meconium in bowel, some enzyme secretion, anus open	Enamel and dentine depositing, ascending colon recognizable	
MUSCULOSKELETAL SYSTEM		
Most bones distinctly indicated throughout body, joint cavities appear, muscular movements detectable	Sternum ossifies, fetal movements strong enough for mother to feel	
CIRCULATORY SYSTEM		
Heart muscle well-developed, blood formation active in spleen		Blood formation increases in bone marrow and decreases in liver
RESPIRATORY SYSTEM		
Elastic fibers appear in lungs, terminal and respiratory bronchioles appear	Nostrils reopen, primitive respiratory-like movements begin	Alveolar ducts and sacs present, lecithin begins to appear in amniotic fluid (weeks 26-27)
RENAL SYSTEM		
Kidney in position, attains typical shape and plan		
NERVOUS SYSTEM		
Cerebral lobes delineated, cerebellum assumes some prominence	Brain grossly formed; cord myelination begins; spinal cord ends at level of first sacral vertebra (S1)	Cerebral cortex layered typically, neuronal proliferation in cerebral cortex ends
SENSORY ORGANS		
General sense organs differentiated	Nose and ears ossifying	Ability to hear
GENITAL SYSTEM		
Testes in position for descent into scrotum, vagina open		Testes at inguinal ring in descent to scrotum

Continued

TABLE 13-1 **Milestones in Human Development Before Birth Since Last Menstrual Period (LMP)—cont'd**

	28 WEEKS	30-31 WEEKS	36 AND 40 WEEKS
EXTERNAL APPEARANCE	Lean body, less wrinkled and red; nails appear	Subcutaneous fat beginning to collect; more rounded appearance; skin pink and smooth; has assumed birth position	**36 Weeks** Skin pink, body rounded; general lanugo disappearing; body usually plump **40 Weeks** Skin smooth and pink; scant vernix caseosa; moderate to profuse hair; lanugo on shoulders and upper body only; nasal and alar cartilage apparent
CROWN-TO-RUMP MEASUREMENT; WEIGHT	27 cm; 1110 g	31 cm; 1800-2100 g	**36 Weeks** 35 cm; 2200-2900 g **40 Weeks** 40 cm; 3200+ g
MUSCULOSKELETAL SYSTEM	Astragalus (talus, ankle bone) ossifies; weak, fleeting movements, minimum tone	Middle fourth phalanges ossify; permanent teeth primordia seen; can turn head to side	**36 Weeks** Distal femoral ossification centers present; sustained, definite movements; fair tone; can turn and elevate head **40 Weeks** Active, sustained movement; good tone, may lift head
RESPIRATORY SYSTEM	Lecithin forming on alveolar surfaces	L/S ratio = 1.2:1	**36 Weeks** L/S ratio > 2:1 **40 Weeks** Pulmonary branching only two thirds complete
RENAL SYSTEM			**36 Weeks** Formation of new nephrons ceases
NERVOUS SYSTEM	Appearance of cerebral fissures, convolutions rapidly appearing; indefinite sleep-wake cycle; cry weak or absent; weak suck reflex		**36 Weeks** End of spinal cord at level of third lumbar vertebra (L3); definite sleep-wake cycle **40 Weeks** Myelination of brain begins; patterned sleep-wake cycle with alert periods; cries when hungry or uncomfortable; strong suck reflex
SENSORY ORGANS	Eyelids reopen; retinal layers completed, light receptive; pupils capable of reacting to light	Sense of taste present; aware of sounds outside mother's body	
GENITAL SYSTEM		Testes descending to scrotum	**40 Weeks** Testes in scrotum; labia majora well developed

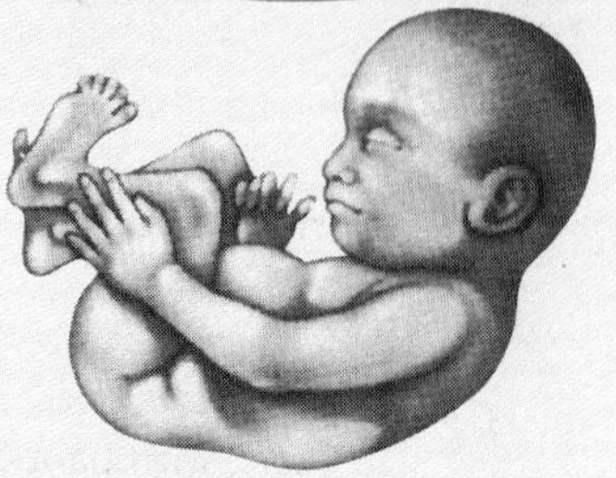

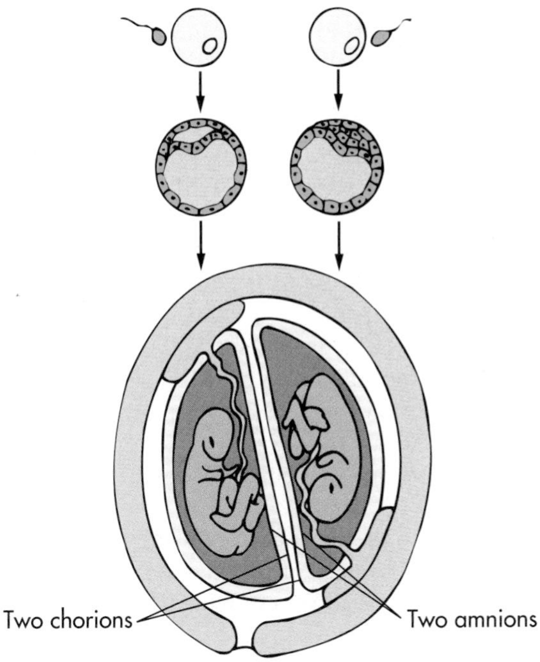
Two chorions
Two amnions

FIG. 13-10 Formation of dizygotic twins, with fertilization of two ova, two implantations, two placentas, two chorions, and two amnions.

Multifetal Pregnancy

Twins

When two mature ova are produced in one ovarian cycle, both have the potential to be fertilized by separate sperm. This results in two zygotes, or dizygotic twins (Fig. 13-10). There are always two amnions, two chorions, and two placentas, which may be fused. These dizygotic, or fraternal, twins may be the same sex or different sexes and are genetically no more alike than siblings born at different times. Dizygotic twinning occurs in families, more often among African-American women than among Caucasian women, and least often among Asian women. Dizygotic twinning increases in frequency with maternal age up to 35 years, with parity, and with the use of fertility drugs.

Identical twins, or monozygotic twins, develop from one fertilized ovum, which then divides (Fig. 13-11). They are the same sex and have the same genotype. If division occurs soon after fertilization, two embryos, two amnions, two chorions, and two placentas that may be fused will develop. Most often, division occurs between 4 and 8 days after fertilization, and there are two embryos, two amnions, one chorion, and one placenta. Rarely, division occurs after the eighth day after fertilization. In this case, there are two embryos within a common amnion and a common chorion

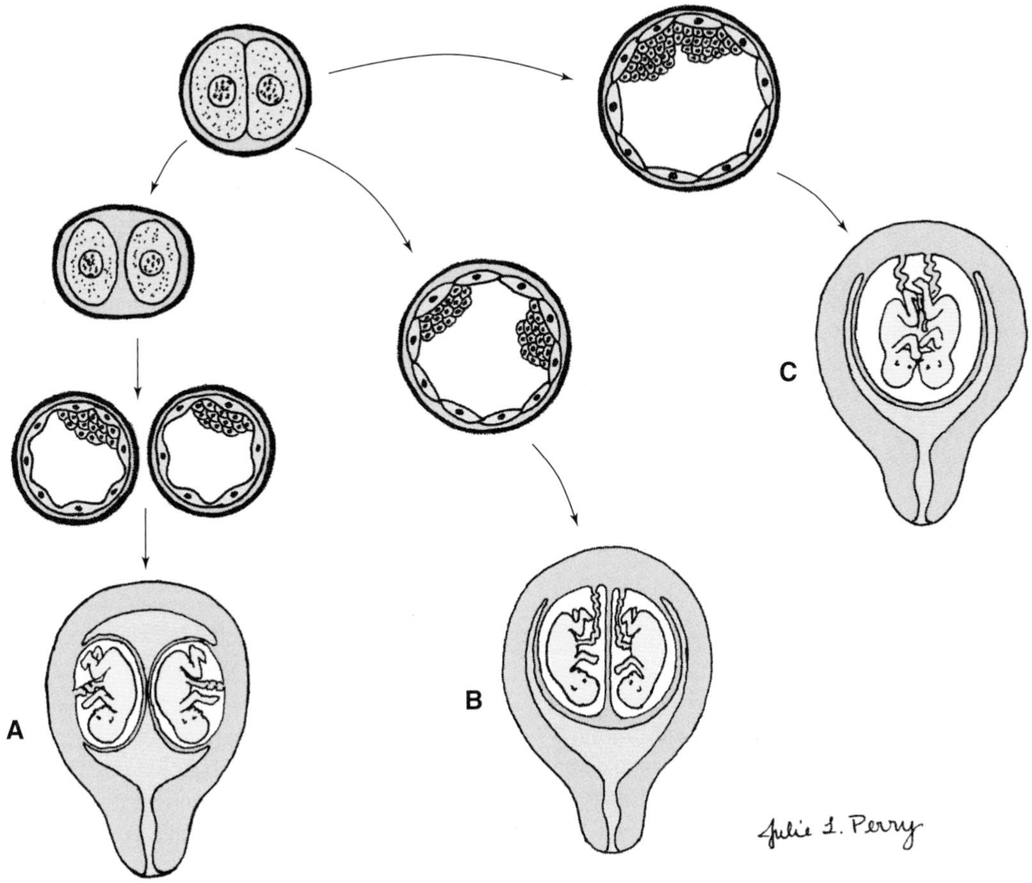
A
B
C
Julie L. Perry

FIG. 13-11 Formation of monozygotic twins. **A,** One fertilization: blastomeres separate, resulting in two implantations, two placentas, and two sets of membranes. **B,** One blastomere with two inner cell masses, one fused placenta, one chorion, and separate amnions. **C,** One blastomere with incomplete separation of cell mass, resulting in conjoined twins.

with one placenta. This often causes circulatory problems because the umbilical cords may tangle together, and one or both fetuses may die. If division occurs very late, cleavage may not be complete, and conjoined twins could result. Monozygotic twinning occurs in approximately four of 1000 births (Chitkara & Berkowitz, 2001). There is no association with race, heredity, maternal age, or parity. Fertility drugs increase the incidence of monozygotic twinning.

Other Multifetal Pregnancies

The occurrence of multifetal pregnancies with three or more fetuses has increased with the use of fertility drugs and in vitro fertilization. Triplets occur in approximately one of 7600 pregnancies. They can occur from the division of one zygote into two, with one of the two dividing again, producing identical triplets. Triplets also can be produced from two zygotes, one dividing into a set of identical twins, and the second zygote developing as a single fraternal sibling, or from three zygotes. Quadruplets, quintuplets, sextuplets, and so on, likewise have similar possible derivations.

Nongenetic Factors Influencing Development

Not all congenital disorders are inherited. *Congenital* means that the condition was present at birth. Some congenital malformations may be the result of teratogens. In contrast to other forms of developmental disabilities, disabilities caused by teratogens are theoretically totally preventable. Known human teratogens are drugs and chemicals, infections, exposure to radiation (Scialli, 1997), and certain maternal conditions such as diabetes and PKU (see Box 13-2). A teratogen has the greatest effect on the organs and parts of an embryo during its periods of rapid growth and differentiation. This occurs during the embryonic period, specifically from days 15 to 60. During the first 2 weeks of development, teratogens either have no effect or have effects so severe that they cause miscarriage. Brain growth and development continue during the fetal period, and teratogens can severely affect mental development throughout gestation.

In addition to the genetic makeup and the influence of teratogens, the adequacy of maternal nutrition influences development. The embryo and fetus must obtain the nutrients they need from the mother's diet; they cannot tap the maternal reserves. Malnutrition during pregnancy produces low-birth-weight newborns who are susceptible to infection. Malnutrition also affects brain development during the latter half of gestation and may result in learning disabilities in the child. Inadequate folic acid is associated with neural tube defects.

KEY POINTS

- Mitosis is the process by which body cells replicate for growth and development and cell replacement of the organism.
- Meiosis is the process by which gametes are formed for reproduction of the organism.
- Human gestation lasts approximately 280 days after the last menstrual period or 266 days after conception.
- Fertilization occurs in the uterine tube within 24 hours of ovulation. The zygote undergoes mitotic divisions, creating a 16-cell morula.
- Implantation begins 6 days after fertilization.
- The organ systems and external features develop during the embryonic period, that is, the third to the eighth week after fertilization.
- Refinement of structure and function occurs during the fetal period, and the fetus becomes capable of extrauterine survival.
- During critical periods in human development, the embryo and fetus are vulnerable to environmental teratogens.

CRITICAL THINKING EXERCISES

1. Sandra believes she is 8 weeks pregnant, but her obstetrician believes she is closer to 12 weeks of gestation. Sandra is scheduled for an ultrasound examination for dating. What fetal structures would be apparent on ultrasound if Sandra is 8 weeks pregnant? If she is 12 weeks pregnant? How long would the fetus be if she is 8 weeks pregnant? If she is 12 weeks pregnant? Would any structural anomalies be apparent at 8 weeks? At 12 weeks? Why is it important to date a pregnancy accurately?
2. Select five household chemicals used in your home. Identify the purpose of the chemicals and describe why they are hazardous to the reproductive health of women, men, and a developing embryo or fetus. List alternatives that can be substituted to accomplish the same purpose as the chemicals.

RESOURCES

American Academy of Pediatrics
141 Northwest Point Blvd.
Elk Grove, IL 60007-1098
847-228-5005
www.aap.org

Food and Drug Administration (FDA)
Office of Consumer Affairs
Public Inquiries
5600 Fishers Lane (HFE-88)
Rockville, MD 20857
301-443-3170
www.fda.gov

March of Dimes Birth Defects Foundation
National Foundation/March of Dimes
1275 Mamaroneck Ave.
White Plains, NY 10605
914-428-7100
888-663-4637 (MODIMES)
www.modimes.org

National Institute of Child Health and Human Development (NICHD)
National Institutes of Health
9000 Rockville Pike
Bldg. 31, Room 2A32
Bethesda, MD 20892
301-496-4000
www.nih.gov

JOURNALS

American Journal of Perinatology
Archives of Disease in Childhood: Fetal and Neonatal Edition
Early Human Development
Journal of Anatomy
Journal of Maternal-Fetal Medicine
Journal of Perinatology and Neonatology
Prenatal Diagnosis
Teratology

WEBSITES

Calculating Due Date
www3.health-center.com/family/pregnancy/fetal_developm/default.htm

Fetal Alcohol Syndrome Branch, Division of Birth Defects, Child Development, and Disability and Health, U.S. Centers for Disease Control and Prevention
www.cdc.gov/nceh/cddh/fashome.htm

National Institutes of Health
Stem cells
www.nih.gov/news/stemcell/scireport.htm

Visible Embryo
www.visembryo.com

REFERENCES

Carlson, B. (1994). *Human embryology and developmental biology.* St. Louis: Mosby.

Chitkara, U., & Berkowitz, R. (2002). Multiple gestation. In S. Gabbe, J. Niebyl, & J. Simpson (Eds.), *Obstetrics: Normal and problem pregnancies* (4th ed.). New York: Churchill Livingstone.

Cole, J. (1997). What can babies see at birth? *Mother Baby Journal, 2*(4), 45-47.

Jobe, A. (1999). Fetal lung development, tests for maturation, induction of maturation, and treatment. In R. Creasy & J. Resnik (Eds.), *Maternal-fetal medicine* (4th ed.). Philadelphia: W.B. Saunders.

Langley, L. et al. (1980). *Dynamic human anatomy and physiology* (5th ed.). New York: McGraw-Hill.

Moore, K., & Persaud, T. (1998). *Before we are born: Essentials of embryology and birth defects* (5th ed.). Philadelphia: W.B. Saunders.

National Institutes of Health (2001). *Stem cells: Scientific progress and future research directions.* www.nih.gov/news/stemcell/scireport.htm. Accessed June 9, 2002.

Scialli, A. (1997). Toxicology. *Contemporary Obstetrics and Gynecology, 42*(5), 15.

Silver, R., & Branch, D. (1999). The immunology of pregnancy. In R. Creasy & J. Resnik (Eds.), *Maternal-fetal medicine* (4th ed.). Philadelphia: W.B. Saunders.

Thomson, J. et al. (1998). Embryonic stem cell lines derived from human blastocysts. *Science, 282*, 1145-1147.

CHAPTER 14

Deitra Leonard Lowdermilk

Anatomy and Physiology of Pregnancy

http://evolve.elsevier.com/Lowdermilk/MatWmnHlth/

LEARNING OBJECTIVES

- Determine gravidity and parity by using the five- and four-digit systems.
- Describe the various types of pregnancy tests including the timing of tests and interpretation of results.
- Explain the expected maternal anatomic and physiologic adaptations to pregnancy for each body system.
- Differentiate among presumptive, probable, and positive signs of pregnancy.
- Compare normal adult laboratory values with values for pregnant women.
- Identify the maternal hormones produced during pregnancy, their target organs, and their major effects on pregnancy.
- Compare the characteristics of the abdomen, vulva, and cervix of the nullipara and multipara.

The goal of maternity care is a healthy pregnancy with a physically safe and emotionally satisfying outcome for mother, infant, and family. Consistent health supervision and surveillance are of utmost importance in achieving this outcome. However, many maternal adaptations are unfamiliar to pregnant women and their families. Helping the pregnant woman recognize the relation between her physical status and the plan for her care assists her in making decisions and encourages her to participate in her own care.

GRAVIDITY AND PARITY

An understanding of the following terms used to describe pregnancy and the pregnant woman is essential to the study of maternity care.

- **gravida:** a woman who is pregnant
- **gravidity:** pregnancy
- **multigravida:** a woman who has had two or more pregnancies
- **multipara:** a woman who has completed two or more pregnancies to the stage of fetal viability
- **nulligravida:** a woman who has never been pregnant
- **nullipara:** a woman who has not completed a pregnancy with a fetus or fetuses who have reached the stage of fetal viability
- **parity:** the number of pregnancies in which the fetus or fetuses have reached viability, not the number of fetuses (e.g., twins) born. Whether the fetus is born alive or is stillborn (fetus who shows no signs of life at birth) after viability is reached does not affect parity
- **postdate or postterm:** a pregnancy that goes beyond 42 weeks of gestation
- **preterm:** a pregnancy that has reached 20 weeks of gestation but before completion of 37 weeks of gestation
- **primigravida:** a woman who is pregnant for the first time
- **primipara:** a woman who has completed one pregnancy with a fetus or fetuses who have reached the stage of fetal viability
- **term:** a pregnancy from the beginning of week 38 of gestation to the end of week 42 of gestation
- **viability:** capacity to live outside the uterus; about 22 to 24 weeks since last menstrual period, or fetal weight greater than 500 g

Gravidity and parity information is obtained during history-taking interviews and may be recorded in client records in several ways. One abbreviation commonly used in maternity centers consists of five digits separated with hyphens. The first digit represents the total number of pregnancies, including the present one (gravidity); the second digit represents the total number of term births; the third indicates the number of preterm births; the fourth identifies the number of abortions (miscarriage or elective termination of pregnancy before viability); and the fifth is the number of children currently living. The acronym *GTPAL* (gravidity, term, preterm, abortions, living children) may be helpful in remembering

TABLE *14-1* **Gravidity and Parity Using Five-Digit (GTPAL) System**

CONDITION	GRAVIDITY PREGNANCIES	PARITY TERM BIRTHS	PARITY PRETERM BIRTHS	ABORTIONS/ MISCARRIAGES	LIVING CHILDREN
Jamilla is pregnant for the first time.	1	0	0	0	0
She carries the pregnancy to 35 weeks and the neonate survives.	1	0	1	0	1
She becomes pregnant again.	2	0	1	0	1
Her second pregnancy ends in miscarriage at 10 weeks.	2	0	1	1	1
During her third pregnancy, she gives birth at 38 weeks.	3	1	1	1	2

BOX *14-1* **Using TPAL to Define Parity**

T, term birth(s)
P, preterm birth(s)
A, abortion(s)/miscarriage(s)
L, living children

this system of notation. For example, if a woman pregnant only once with twins gives birth at week 35, and the babies survive, the abbreviation that represents this information is "1-0-1-0-2." During her next pregnancy, the abbreviation is "2-0-1-0-2." Additional examples are given in Table 14-1.

Others prefer a four-digit system. The first digit of the five-digit system, which signifies gravidity, is dropped. The acronym *TPAL* may be useful in remembering what the four digits stand for (Box 14-1).

PREGNANCY TESTS

Early detection of pregnancy allows early initiation of care. **Human chorionic gonadotropin (hCG)** is the earliest biochemical marker for pregnancy, and pregnancy tests are based on the recognition of hCG or a β subunit of hCG. Production of hCG begins as early as the day of implantation and can be detected in the blood as early as 6 to 11 days after conception if very sensitive tests are used (Buster & Carson, 2002), and in urine, about 26 days after conception (Cunningham et al., 2001). The level of hCG increases until it peaks at about 60 to 70 days of gestation and then declines until about 140 days of pregnancy. It remains stable until about 30 weeks and then gradually increases until term. Higher than normal levels of hCG may indicate ectopic pregnancy, abnormal gestation (e.g., fetus with Down syndrome), or multiple gestation; abnormally slow increase or a decrease in hCG levels may indicate impending miscarriage (Buster & Carson, 2002).

Serum and urine pregnancy tests are performed in clinics, offices, women's health centers, and laboratory settings, and urine pregnancy tests may be performed at home. Both serum and urine tests can provide accurate results. A 7- to 10-ml sample of venous blood is collected for serum testing. Most urine tests require a first-voided morning urine specimen because it contains levels of hCG approximately the same as those in serum. Random urine samples usually have lower levels. Urine tests are less expensive and provide more immediate results than do serum tests (Hatcher et al., 2002).

Many different pregnancy tests are available. The wide variety of tests precludes discussion of each; however, several categories of tests are described here. The nurse should read the manufacturer's directions for the test to be used.

Immunoassay or agglutination inhibition tests (AITs) depend on an antigen-antibody reaction between hCG and an antiserum. Usually the antiserum is mixed with urine, and hCG-coated particles (e.g., latex or blood cells) are added. If hCG is present in the urine, agglutination does not occur because the hCG neutralizes the hCG antibody, and the test is considered positive (Cunningham et al., 2001). Although immunologic tests are accurate from 4 to 10 days after a missed period, they are most appropriate for confirming a pregnancy at or after the sixth week of gestation (Hatcher et al., 2002).

Radioimmunoassay (RIA) pregnancy tests for the β-subunit of hCG in serum or urine samples use radioactively labeled markers and are usually performed in a laboratory. These tests are accurate with low hCG levels and can confirm pregnancy 1 week after conception (Hatcher et al., 2002).

Radioreceptor assay (RRA) is a serum test that measures the ability of a blood sample to inhibit the binding of radiolabeled hCG to receptors. The test is 90% to 95% accurate from 6 to 8 days after conception (Pagana & Pagana, 2003).

Enzyme-linked immunosorbent assay (ELISA) testing is the most popular method of testing for pregnancy. It uses a specific monoclonal antibody (anti-hCG) with enzymes

TEACHING FOR SELF-CARE

Home Pregnancy Testing

- Follow the manufacturer's instructions carefully. Do not omit steps.
- Review the manufacturer's list of foods, medications, and other substances that can affect the test results.
- Use a first-voided morning urine specimen.
- If the test done at the time of your missed period is negative, repeat the test in 1 week if you still have not had a period.
- If you have questions about the test, contact the manufacturer.
- Contact your health care provider for follow-up if the test is positive or if the test is negative and you still have not had a period.

to bond with hCG in urine. Depending on the specific test, levels of hCG as low as 5 to 50 mIU/ml can be detected as early as 4 days after implantation (Hatcher et al., 2002). As an office or home procedure, it requires minimal time and offers results in 5 minutes. A positive test is indicated by a simple color change reaction.

ELISA technology is the basis for most over-the-counter home pregnancy tests. With these one-step tests, the woman usually applies urine to a strip and reads the results. The test kits come with directions for collection of the specimen, the testing procedure, and reading of the results. Most manufacturers of the kits provide a toll-free telephone number to call if users have concerns and questions about test procedures or results (see Teaching for Self-Care box). The most common error in performing home pregnancy tests is performing the test too early in pregnancy (Hatcher et al., 2002).

Interpreting the results of pregnancy tests requires some judgment. The type of pregnancy test and its degree of sensitivity (ability to detect low levels of a substance) and specificity (ability to discern the absence of a substance) must be considered in conjunction with the woman's history. This includes the date of her last normal menstrual period (LNMP), her usual cycle length, and results of previous pregnancy tests. It is important to know if the woman is a substance abuser and what medications she is taking, because medications such as anticonvulsants and tranquilizers can cause false-positive results, whereas diuretics and promethazine can cause false-negative results (Pagana & Pagana, 2003). Improper collection of the specimen, hormone-producing tumors, and laboratory errors also may cause false results. Whenever there is any question, further evaluation or retesting may be appropriate.

ADAPTATIONS TO PREGNANCY

Maternal physiologic adaptations are attributed to the hormones of pregnancy and to mechanical pressures arising from the enlarging uterus and other tissues. These adaptations protect the woman's normal physiologic functioning, meet the metabolic demands pregnancy imposes on her body, and provide a nurturing environment for fetal development and growth. Although pregnancy is a normal phenomenon, problems can occur.

Signs of Pregnancy

Some of the physiologic adaptations are recognized as signs and symptoms of pregnancy. Three commonly used categories of **signs and symptoms of pregnancy** are **presumptive,** those changes felt by the woman (e.g., amenorrhea, fatigue, nausea and vomiting, breast changes); **probable,** those changes observed by an examiner (e.g., Hegar sign, ballottement, pregnancy tests); and **positive,** those signs that are attributed only to the presence of the fetus (e.g., hearing fetal heart tones, visualization of the fetus, and palpating fetal movements). Table 14-2 summarizes these signs of pregnancy in relation to when they might occur and other causes for their occurrence.

Reproductive System and Breasts

Uterus

Changes in Size, Shape, and Position. The phenomenal uterine growth in the first trimester is stimulated by high levels of estrogen and progesterone. Early uterine enlargement results from increased vascularity and dilation of blood vessels, hyperplasia (production of new muscle fibers and fibroelastic tissue) and hypertrophy (enlargement of preexisting muscle fibers and fibroelastic tissue), and development of the decidua. By 7 weeks of gestation, the uterus is the size of a large hen's egg; by 10 weeks of gestation, it is the size of an orange (twice its nonpregnant size); and by 12 weeks of gestation, it is the size of a grapefruit. After the third month, uterine enlargement is primarily the result of mechanical pressure of the growing fetus.

As the uterus enlarges, it also changes in shape and position. At conception the uterus is shaped like an upside-down pear. During the second trimester, as the muscular walls strengthen and become more elastic, the uterus becomes spherical or globular. Later, as the fetus lengthens, the uterus becomes larger and more ovoid and rises out of the pelvis into the abdominal cavity.

The pregnancy may "show" after the fourteenth week, although this depends to some degree on the woman's height and weight. Abdominal enlargement may be less apparent in the nullipara with good abdominal muscle tone (Fig. 14-1). Posture also influences the type and degree of abdominal enlargement that occurs. In normal pregnancies, the uterus enlarges at a predictable rate. As the uterus grows, it may be palpated above the symphysis pubis some time between the twelfth and fourteenth weeks of pregnancy (Fig. 14-2). The uterus rises gradually to the level of the umbilicus at 22 to 24 weeks of gestation and nearly reaches the xiphoid process at term. Between weeks 38 and 40, fundal height drops as the fetus begins to de-

TABLE 14-2 **Signs of Pregnancy**

TIME OF OCCURRENCE (GESTATIONAL AGE)	SIGN	OTHER POSSIBLE CAUSE
Presumptive Signs		
3-4 wk	Breast changes	Premenstrual changes, oral contraceptives
4 wk	Amenorrhea	Stress, vigorous exercise, early menopause, endocrine problems, malnutrition
4-14 wk	Nausea, vomiting	Gastrointestinal virus, food poisoning
6-12 wk	Urinary frequency	Infection, pelvic tumors
12 wk	Fatigue	Stress, illness
16-20 wk	Quickening	Gas, peristalsis
Probable Signs		
5 wk	Goodell sign	Pelvic congestion
6-8 wk	Chadwick sign	Pelvic congestion
6-12 wk	Hegar sign	Pelvic congestion
4-12 wk	Positive pregnancy test (serum)	Hydatidiform mole, choriocarcinoma
6-12 wk	Positive result to pregnancy test (urine)	False-positive results may be caused by pelvic infection, tumors
16 wk	Braxton Hicks contractions	Myomas, other tumors
16-28 wk	Ballottement	Tumors, cervical polyps
Positive Signs		
5-6 wk	Visualization of fetus by real-time ultrasound examination	No other causes
6 wk	Fetal heart tones detected by ultrasound examination	No other causes
16 wk	Visualization of fetus by radiographic study	No other causes
8-17 wk	Fetal heart tones detected by Doppler ultrasound stethoscope	No other causes
17-19 wk	Fetal heart tones detected by fetal stethoscope	No other causes
19-22 wk	Fetal movements palpated	No other causes
Late pregnancy	Fetal movements visible	No other causes

scend and engage in the pelvis **(lightening)** (see Fig. 14-2, *dashed line*). Generally, lightening occurs in the nullipara about 2 weeks before the onset of labor and at the start of labor in the multipara.

Uterine enlargement is determined by measuring fundal height, a measurement commonly used to estimate the duration of pregnancy. However, variation in the position of the fundus or the fetus, variations in the amount of amniotic fluid present, the presence of more than one fetus, maternal obesity, and variation in examiner techniques can reduce the accuracy of this estimation of the duration of pregnancy.

The uterus normally rotates to the right as it elevates, probably because of the presence of the rectosigmoid colon on the left side, but the extensive hypertrophy (enlargement) of the round ligaments keeps the uterus in the midline. Eventually the growing uterus touches the anterior abdominal wall and displaces the intestines to either side of the abdomen (Fig. 14-3). Whenever a pregnant woman is standing, most of her uterus rests against the anterior abdominal wall, and this contributes to altering her center of gravity.

At approximately 6 weeks of gestation, softening and compressibility of the lower uterine segment (the uterine isthmus) occur **(Hegar sign)** (Fig. 14-4). This results in exaggerated uterine anteflexion during the first 3 months of pregnancy. In this position, the uterine fundus presses on the urinary bladder, causing the woman to have urinary frequency.

Changes in Contractility. Soon after the fourth month of pregnancy, uterine contractions can be felt through the abdominal wall. These contractions are referred to as the **Braxton Hicks sign.** Braxton Hicks

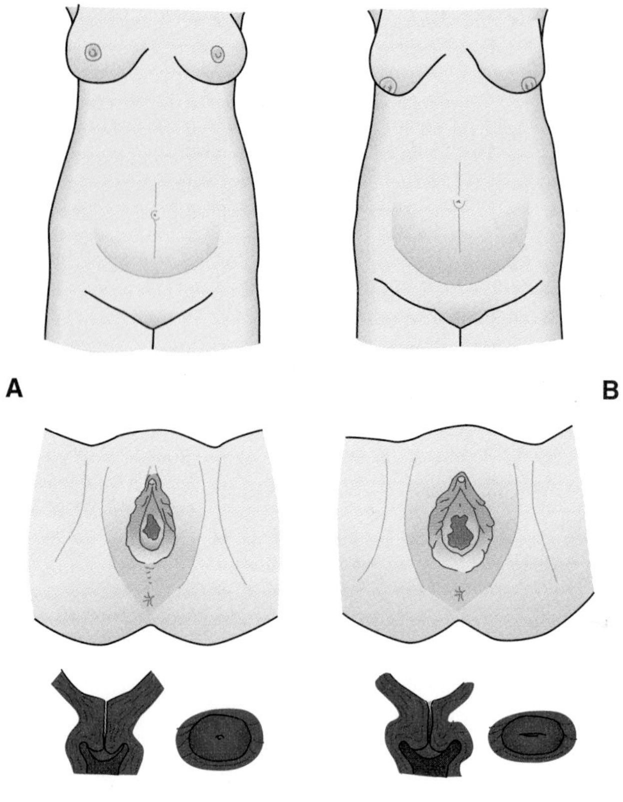
A
B

FIG. 14-1 Comparison of abdomen, vulva, and cervix in **A,** nullipara, and **B,** multipara, at the same stage of pregnancy.

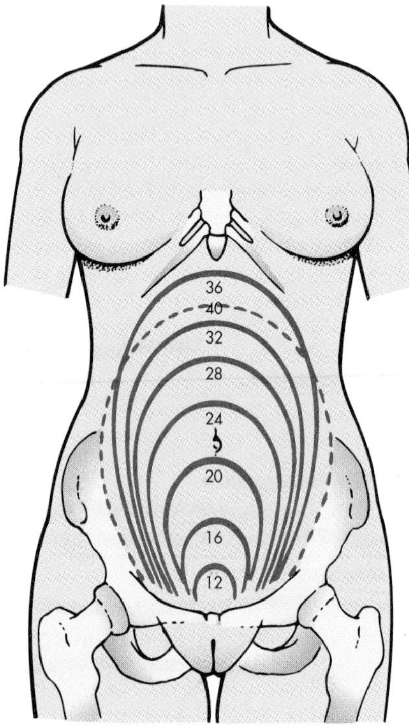
36
40
32
28
24
20
16
12

FIG. 14-2 Height of fundus by weeks of normal gestation with a single fetus. *Dashed line,* height after lightening. (From Seidel, H. et al. [2003]. *Mosby's guide to physical examination* [5th ed.]. St. Louis: Mosby.)

contractions are irregular, painless, and occur intermittently throughout pregnancy. These contractions facilitate uterine blood flow through the intervillous spaces of the placenta and thereby promote oxygen delivery to the fetus. Although Braxton Hicks contractions are not painful, some women complain that they are annoying. After the twenty-eighth week, these contractions become much more definite, but they usually cease with walking or exercise. Braxton Hicks contractions can be mistaken for true labor; however, they do not increase in intensity or frequency or cause cervical dilation.

Uteroplacental Blood Flow. Placental perfusion depends on the maternal blood flow to the uterus. Blood flow increases rapidly as the uterus increases in size. Although uterine blood flow increases twentyfold, the fetoplacental unit grows more rapidly. Consequently, more oxygen is extracted from the uterine blood during the latter part of pregnancy (Cunningham et al., 2001). In a normal term pregnancy, one sixth of the total maternal blood volume is within the uterine vascular system. The rate of blood flow through the uterus averages 500 ml/min, and oxygen consumption of the gravid uterus increases to meet fetal needs. A low maternal arterial pressure, contractions of the uterus, and maternal supine position are three factors known to decrease blood flow. Estrogen stimulation may increase uterine blood flow. Doppler ultrasound examination can be used to measure uterine blood flow velocity, especially in pregnancies at risk because of conditions associated with decreased placental perfusion such as hypertension, intrauterine growth restriction, diabetes mellitus, and multiple gestation (Trudinger, 1999). By using an ultrasound device or a fetal stethoscope, the health care provider may hear the **uterine souffle** (sound made by blood in the uterine arteries that is synchronous with the maternal pulse) or the **funic souffle** (sound made by blood rushing through the umbilical vessels and synchronous with the fetal heart rate).

Cervical Changes. A softening of the cervical tip called **Goodell sign** may be observed about the beginning of the sixth week in a normal, unscarred cervix. This sign is brought about by increased vascularity, slight hypertrophy, and hyperplasia (increase in number of cells) of the muscle and its collagen-rich connective tissue, which becomes loose, edematous, highly elastic, and increased in volume. The glands near the external os proliferate beneath the stratified squamous epithelium, giving the cervix the velvety appearance characteristic of pregnancy. **Friability** is increased and may cause slight bleeding after coitus with deep penetration or after vaginal examination. Pregnancy also can cause the squamocolumnar junction, the site for obtaining cells for cervical cancer screening, to be located away from the cervix. Because of all these changes, evaluation of abnormal Papanicolaou tests during pregnancy can be complicated. Careful assessment of all pregnant women is important, however, because about 3% of all cervical cancers are diagnosed during pregnancy (Berman, DiSaia, & Brewster, 1999).

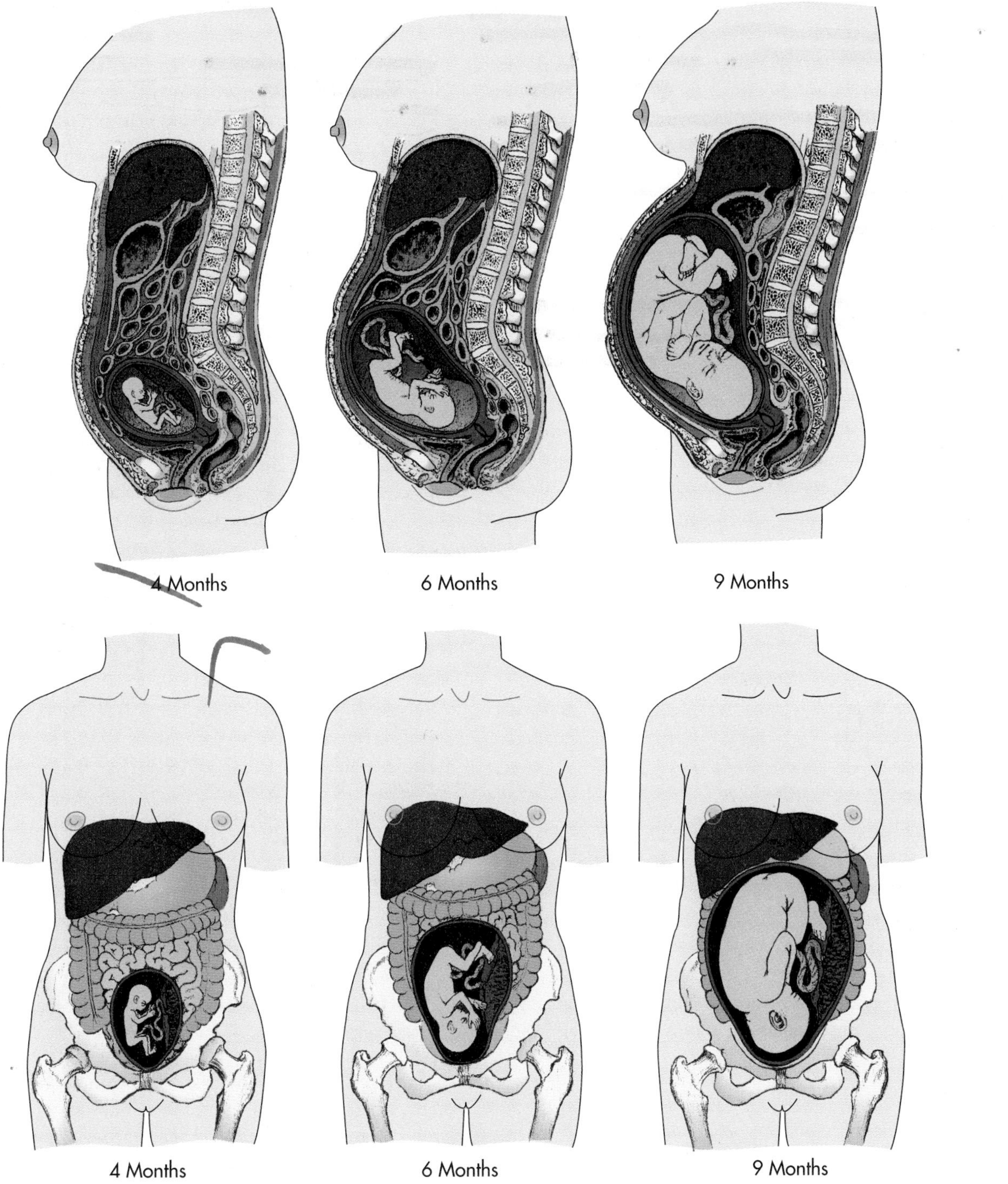
4 Months
6 Months
9 Months
4 Months
6 Months
9 Months

FIG. 14-3 Displacement of internal abdominal structures and diaphragm by the enlarging uterus at 4, 6, and 9 months of gestation.

The cervix of the nullipara is rounded. Lacerations of the cervix almost always occur during the birth process. With or without lacerations, however, after childbirth, the cervix becomes more oval in the horizontal plane, and the external os appears as a transverse slit (see Fig. 14-1).

Changes Related to the Presence of the Fetus. Passive movement of the unengaged fetus is called **ballottement** and can be identified generally between the sixteenth and eighteenth week. Ballottement is a technique of palpating a floating structure by bouncing it gently and feeling it rebound. In the technique used to palpate the fetus, the examiner places a finger in the vagina and taps gently upward, causing the fetus to rise. The fetus then sinks, and a gentle tap is felt on the finger (Fig. 14-5).

The first recognition of fetal movements, or "feeling life," by the multiparous woman may occur as early as the fourteenth to sixteenth week. The nulliparous woman may not notice these sensations until the eighteenth week or later. **Quickening** is commonly described as a flutter and is difficult to distinguish from peristalsis. Fetal movements gradually increase in intensity and frequency. The week when quickening occurs provides a tentative clue in dating the duration of gestation.

Vagina and Vulva

Pregnancy hormones prepare the vagina for stretching during labor and birth by causing the vaginal mucosa to thicken, the connective tissue to loosen, the smooth muscle to hypertrophy, and the vaginal vault to lengthen. Increased vascularity results in a violet-bluish color of the vaginal mucosa and cervix. The deepened color, termed the **Chadwick sign,** may be evident as early as the sixth week but is easily noted at the eighth week of pregnancy (Resnik, 1999).

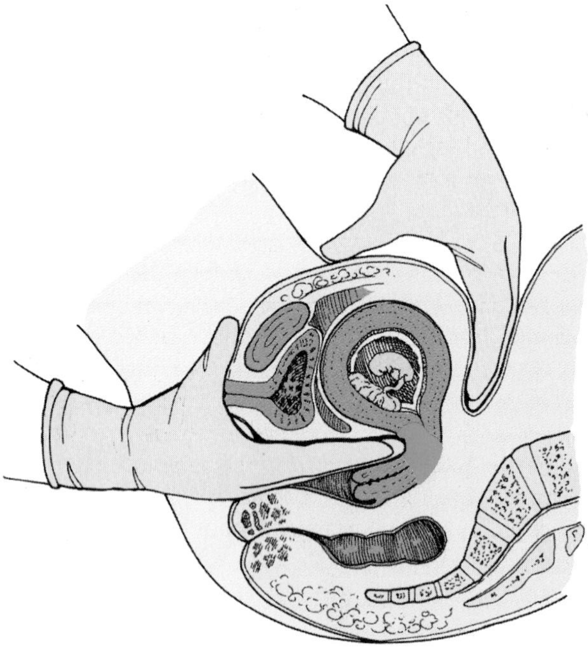

FIG. 14-4 Hegar sign. Bimanual examination for assessing compressibility and softening of isthmus (lower uterine segment) while the cervix is still firm.

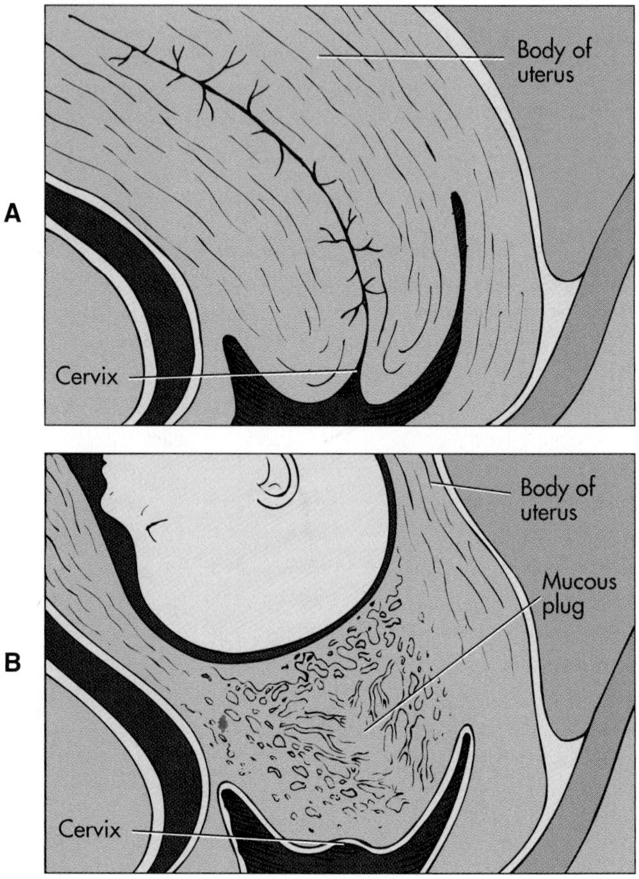

A
Body of uterus
Cervix
B
Body of uterus
Mucous plug
Cervix

FIG. 14-6 **A,** Cervix in nonpregnant woman. **B,** Cervix during pregnancy.

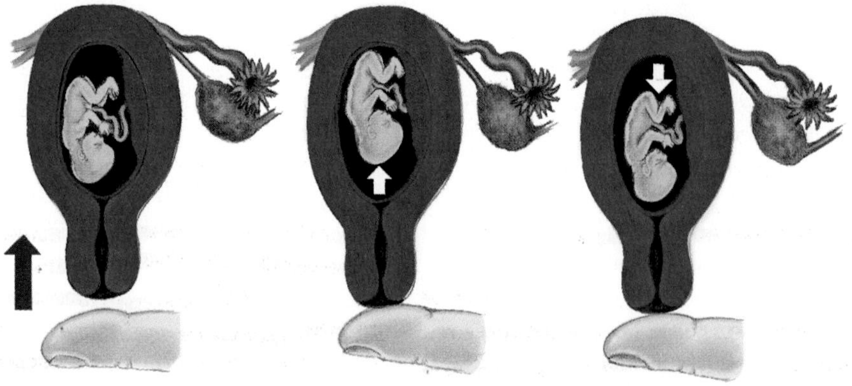

FIG. 14-5 Internal ballottement (18 weeks).

Leukorrhea is a white or slightly gray mucoid discharge with a faint musty odor. This copious mucoid fluid occurs in response to cervical stimulation by estrogen and progesterone. The fluid is whitish because of the presence of many exfoliated vaginal epithelial cells caused by the hyperplasia of normal pregnancy. This vaginal discharge is never pruritic or blood stained. Because of the progesterone effect, ferning usually does not occur in the dried cervical mucus smear, as it would in a smear of amniotic fluid. Instead, a beaded or cellular crystallizing pattern formed in the dried mucus is seen (Cunningham et al., 2001). The mucus fills the endocervical canal, resulting in the formation of the mucous plug **(operculum)** (Fig. 14-6). The operculum acts as a barrier against bacterial invasion during pregnancy.

During pregnancy, the pH of vaginal secretions is more acidic (ranging from about 3.5 to 6) because of increased production of lactic acid caused by *Lactobacillus acidophilus* action on glycogen in the vaginal epithelium, probably resulting from increased estrogen levels (Cunningham et al., 2001). While this acid environment provides more protection from some organisms, the pregnant woman is more vulnerable to other infections, especially yeast infections because the glycogen-rich environment is more susceptible to *Candida albicans* (Bennett & Brown, 1999).

The increased vascularity of the vagina and other pelvic viscera results in a marked increase in sensitivity. The increased sensitivity may lead to a high degree of sexual interest and arousal, especially during the second trimester of pregnancy. The increased congestion plus the relaxed walls of the blood vessels and the heavy uterus may result in edema and varicosities of the vulva. The edema and varicosities usually resolve during the postpartum period.

External structures of the perineum are enlarged during pregnancy because of an increase in vasculature, hypertrophy of the perineal body, and deposition of fat (Fig. 14-7). The labia majora of the nullipara approximate and obscure the vaginal introitus; those of the parous woman separate and gape after childbirth and perineal or vaginal injury. Figure 14-1 compares the perineum of the nullipara and the multipara in relation to the pregnant abdomen, vulva, and cervix.

Breasts

Fullness, heightened sensitivity, tingling, and heaviness of the breasts begin in the early weeks of gestation in response to increased levels of estrogen and progesterone. Breast sensitivity varies from mild tingling to sharp pain. Nipples and areolae become more pigmented, secondary pinkish areolae develop, extending beyond the primary areolae, and nipples become more erectile. Hypertrophy of the sebaceous (oil) glands embedded in the primary areolae, called **Montgomery's tubercles** (see Fig. 5-6), may be seen around the nipples. These sebaceous glands may have a protective role in that they keep the nipples lubricated for breastfeeding.

The richer blood supply causes the vessels beneath the skin to dilate. Once barely noticeable, the blood vessels become visible, often appearing in an intertwining blue network beneath the surface of the skin. Venous congestion in the breasts is more obvious in primigravidas. Striae gravidarum may appear at the outer aspects of the breasts.

During the second and third trimesters, growth of the mammary glands accounts for the progressive breast enlargement. The high levels of luteal and placental hormones in pregnancy promote proliferation of the lactiferous ducts

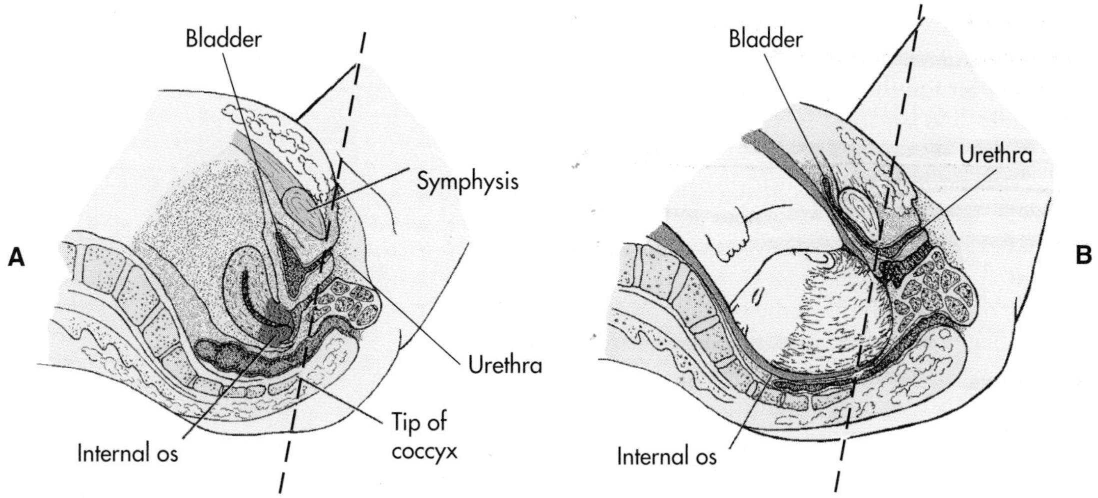
A
Bladder
Symphysis
Urethra
Tip of coccyx
Internal os
B
Bladder
Urethra
Internal os

FIG. 14-7 A, Pelvic floor in nonpregnant woman. **B,** Pelvic floor at end of pregnancy. Note marked hypertrophy and hyperplasia below *dotted line* joining tip of coccyx and inferior margin of symphysis. Note elongation of bladder and urethra as a result of compression. Fat deposits are increased.

and lobule-alveolar tissue, so that palpation of the breasts reveals a generalized, coarse nodularity. Glandular tissue displaces connective tissue, and as a result, the tissue becomes softer and looser.

Although development of the mammary glands is functionally complete by midpregnancy, lactation is inhibited until a decrease in estrogen level occurs after the birth. A thin, clear, viscous secretory material (precolostrum) can be found in the acini cells by the third month of gestation. **Colostrum,** the creamy, white-to-yellowish to orange premilk fluid, may be expressed from the nipples as early as 16 weeks of gestation (Lawrence, 1999). See Chapter 27 for discussion of lactation.

General Body Systems

Cardiovascular System

Maternal adjustments to pregnancy involve extensive changes in the cardiovascular system, both anatomic and physiologic. Cardiovascular adaptations protect the woman's normal physiologic functioning, meet the metabolic demands pregnancy imposes on her body, and provide for fetal developmental and growth needs.

Slight cardiac hypertrophy (enlargement) is probably secondary to the increased blood volume and cardiac output that occurs. The heart returns to its normal size after childbirth. As the diaphragm is displaced upward by the enlarging uterus, the heart is elevated upward and rotated forward to the left (Fig. 14-8). The apical impulse, a point of maximal intensity (PMI), is shifted upward and laterally about 1 to 1.5 cm. The degree of shift depends on the duration of pregnancy and the size and position of the uterus.

The changes in heart size and position and increases in blood volume and cardiac output contribute to auscultatory changes common in pregnancy. There is more audible splitting of S_1 and S_2, and S_3 may be readily heard after 20 weeks of gestation. Additionally, systolic and diastolic murmurs may be heard over the pulmonic area. These are transient and disappear shortly after the woman gives birth (Cunningham et al., 2001).

Between 14 and 20 weeks of gestation, the pulse increases about 10 to 15 beats/min, which then persists to term. Palpitations may occur. In twin gestations, the maternal heart rate increases significantly in the third trimester (Malone & D'Alton, 1999).

The cardiac rhythm may be disturbed. The pregnant woman may experience sinus arrhythmia, premature atrial contractions, and premature ventricular systole. In the healthy woman with no underlying heart disease, no therapy is needed; however, women with preexisting heart disease will need close medical and obstetric supervision during pregnancy (see Chapter 33).

Blood Pressure. Arterial blood pressure (brachial artery) is affected by age, activity level, presence of health problems, and circadian rhythm (Hermida et al., 2001). Additional factors must be considered during pregnancy. These factors include maternal anxiety, maternal position, and size and type of blood pressure apparatus.

Maternal anxiety can elevate readings. If an elevated reading is found, the woman is given time to rest, and the reading is repeated.

Maternal position affects readings. Brachial blood pressure is highest when the woman is sitting, lowest when she is lying in the lateral recumbent position, and intermediate when she is supine, except for some women who experience supine hypotensive syndrome (see discussion later). Therefore at each prenatal visit, the reading should be obtained in the same arm and with the woman in the same position. The position and arm used should be recorded along with the reading.

The proper-size cuff is absolutely necessary for accurate readings. The cuff should be 20% wider than the diameter of the arm around which it is wrapped, or about 12 to 14 cm for average-sized individuals and 18 to 20 cm for obese persons. Too small a cuff yields a false high reading; too large a cuff yields a false low reading. Caution also should be used when comparing auscultatory and oscillatory blood pressure readings, because discrepancies can occur (Shennan & Halligan, 1999).

In the first trimester, blood pressure usually remains the same as the prepregnancy level but then gradually decreases up to about 20 weeks of gestation. During the sec-

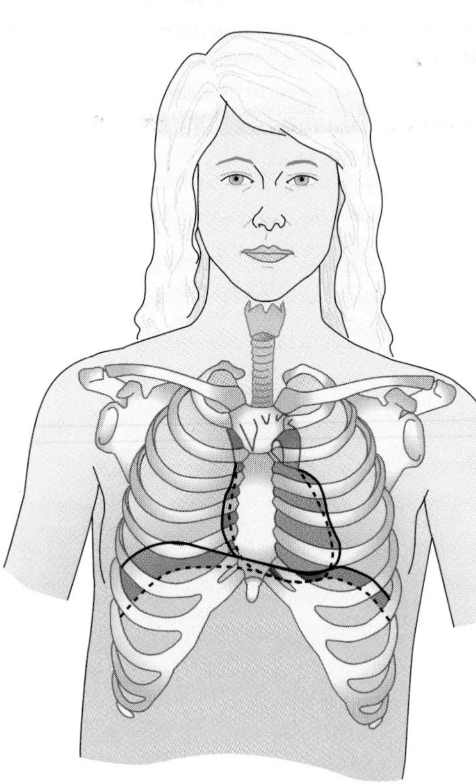

FIG. 14-8 Changes in position of heart, lungs, and thoracic cage in pregnancy. *Broken line,* nonpregnant; *solid line,* change that occurs in pregnancy.

ond trimester, both systolic and diastolic pressure decrease by about 5 to 10 mm Hg. After 20 weeks, the maternal blood pressure gradually increases and should return to the first-trimester levels by term (Cunningham, et al., 2001; Hermida, Ayala, & Iglesias, 2001).

Calculating the **mean arterial pressure (MAP)** (mean of the blood pressure in the arterial circulation) can increase the diagnostic value of the findings. Normal MAP readings in the nonpregnant woman are 86.4 mm Hg ± 7.5 mm Hg. MAP readings for a pregnant woman are slightly higher (Gonik, 1999). One way to calculate an MAP is illustrated in Box 14-2.

Some degree of compression of the vena cava occurs in all women who lie flat on their backs during the second half of pregnancy (see Fig. 21-5). Some women experience a decrease in their systolic blood pressure of more than 30 mm Hg. After 4 to 5 minutes, a reflex bradycardia is noted, cardiac output is reduced by half, and the woman feels faint. This condition is referred to as **supine hypotensive syndrome** (Cunningham et al., 2001).

Compression of the iliac veins and inferior vena cava by the uterus causes increased venous pressure and reduced blood flow in the legs (except when the woman is in the lateral position). These alterations contribute to the dependent edema, varicose veins in the legs and vulva, and hemorrhoids that develop in the latter part of term pregnancy (Fig. 14-9).

Blood Volume and Composition. The degree of blood volume expansion varies considerably. Blood volume increases by approximately 1500 ml, or 40% to 50% above nonpregnancy levels (Cunningham et al., 2001). This increase consists of 1000 ml plasma plus 450 ml red blood cells (RBCs). The blood volume starts to increase at about the tenth to twelfth week, peaks at about the thirty-second to thirty-fourth week, and then decreases slightly at the fortieth week. The increase in volume of a multiple gestation is greater than that for a pregnancy with a single fetus (Malone & D'Alton, 1999). Increased volume is a protective mechanism. It is essential for meeting the blood volume needs of the hypertrophied vascular system of the enlarged uterus, for adequately hydrating fetal and maternal tissues when the woman assumes an erect or supine position, and for providing a fluid reserve to compensate for blood loss during birth and the puerperium. Peripheral vasodilation maintains a normal blood pressure despite the increased blood volume in pregnancy.

During pregnancy there is an accelerated production of RBCs (normal, 4.2 to 5.4 million/mm^3). The percentage of increase depends on the amount of iron available. The RBC mass increases by about 20% to 30% (Monga, 1999).

Because the plasma increase exceeds the increase in RBC production, there is a decrease in normal hemoglobin values (12 to 16 g/dl blood) and hematocrit values (37% to 47%). This state of hemodilution is referred to as **physiologic anemia.** The decrease is more noticeable during the second trimester, when rapid expansion of blood volume takes place faster than RBC production. If the hemoglobin value decreases to 10 g/dl or less or if the hematocrit decreases to 35% or less, the woman is considered anemic.

The total white cell count increases during the second trimester and peaks during the third trimester. This increase is primarily in the granulocytes; the lymphocyte count stays about the same throughout pregnancy. See Table 14-3 for laboratory values during pregnancy.

Cardiac Output. Cardiac output increases from 30% to 50% over the nonpregnant rate by the thirty-second week of pregnancy; it declines to about a 20% increase at 40 weeks

BOX *14-2* **Calculation of Mean Arterial Pressure (MAP)**

Blood pressure: 106/70 mm Hg

Formula: $\frac{(\text{systolic}) + 2(\text{diastolic})}{3}$

$\frac{(106) + 2(70)}{3}$

$\frac{106 + 140}{3}$

246/3 = 82 mm Hg

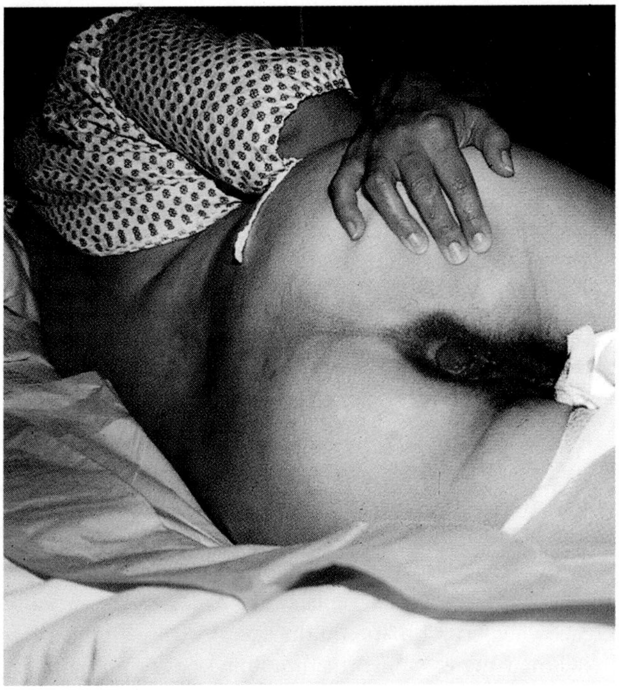

FIG. 14-9 Hemorrhoids. (Courtesy Marjorie Pyle, RNC, Lifecircle, Costa Mesa, CA.)

TABLE 14-3 Laboratory Values for Pregnant and Nonpregnant Women

VALUES	NONPREGNANT	PREGNANT
Hematologic		
Complete Blood Count (CBC)		
Hemoglobin, g/dl	12-16*	>11*
Hematocrit, PCV, %	37-47	>33*
Red blood cell (RBC) volume, per ml	1600	1500-1900
Plasma volume, per ml	2400	3700
RBC count, million/mm³	4.2-5.4	5.0-6.25
White blood cells, total per mm³	5000-10,000	5000-15,000
Neutophils, %	55-70	60-85
Lymphocytes, %	20-40	15-40
Erythrocyte sedimentation rate, mm/hr	20	Elevated in second and third trimesters
Mean corpuscular hemoglobin concentration (MCHC), g/dl packed RBCs	32-36	No change in hemoglobin concentration
Mean corpuscular hemoglobin (MCH), pg	27-31	No change per pg (less than 1 ng)
Mean corpuscular volume (MCV), μm³	80-95	No change per μm³
Blood Coagulation and Fibrinolytic Activity†		
Factor VII	65-140	Increase in pregnancy, return to normal in early puerperium; factor VIII increases during and immediately after birth
Factor VIII	55-145	
Factor IX	60-140	
Factor X	45-155	
Factor XI	65-135	Decrease in pregnancy
Factor XII	50-150	
Prothrombin time (PT), sec	11-12.5	Slight decrease in pregnancy
Partial thromboplastin time (PTT), sec	60-70	Slight decrease in pregnancy and decrease during second and third stage of labor (indicates clotting at placental site)
Bleeding time, min	1-9 (Ivy)	No appreciable change
Coagulation time, min	6-10 (Lee/White)	No appreciable change
Platelets, per mm³	150,000-400,000	No significant change until 3-5 days after birth and then a rapid increase (may predispose woman to thrombosis) and gradual return to normal
Fibrinolytic activity		Decreases in pregnancy and then abrupt return to normal (protection against thromboembolism)
Fibrinogen, mg/dl	200-400	Increased levels late in pregnancy
Mineral/Vitamin Concentrations		
Vitamin B_{12}, folic acid, ascorbic acid	Normal	Moderate decrease

From Gordon, M. (2002). Maternal physiology in pregnancy. In S. Gabbe, J. Niebyl, & J. Simpson (Eds.), *Obstetrics: Normal and problem pregnancies* (4th ed.). New York: Churchill Livingstone; Pagana, K., & Pagana, T. (2003). *Mosby's diagnostic and laboratory test reference* (6th ed). St. Louis: Mosby.
*At sea level. Permanent residents of higher levels (e.g., Denver) require higher levels of hemoglobin.
†Pregnancy represents a hypercoagulable state.

of gestation. This elevated cardiac output is largely a result of increased stroke volume and heart rate and occurs in response to increased tissue demands for oxygen (Monga, 1999). Cardiac output in late pregnancy is appreciably higher when the woman is in the lateral recumbent position than when she is supine. In the supine position, the large, heavy uterus often impedes venous return to the heart and affects blood pressure. Cardiac output increases with any exertion, such as labor and birth. Box 14-3 summarizes cardiovascular changes in pregnancy.

Circulation and Coagulation Times. The circulation time decreases slightly by week 32. It returns to near normal by near term. There is a greater tendency for blood to coagulate (clot) during pregnancy because of increases in various clotting factors (factors VII, VIII, IX, X, and fibrinogen). This, combined with the fact that fibri-

TABLE 14-3 **Laboratory Values for Pregnant and Nonpregnant Women—cont'd**

VALUES	NONPREGNANT	PREGNANT
Hematologic—cont'd		
Serum Proteins		
Total, g/dl	6.4-8.3	5.5-7.5
Albumin, g/dl	3.5-5.0	Slight increase
Globulin, total, g/dl	2.3-3.4	3.0-4.0
Blood Glucose		
Fasting, mg/dl	70-105	Decreases
2-hr postprandial, mg/dl	<140	<140 after a 100-g carbohydrate meal is considered normal
Acid-base Values in Arterial Blood		
Po_2, mm Hg	80-100	104-108 (increased)
Pco_2, mm Hg	35-45	27-32 (decreased)
Sodium bicarbonate (HCO_3), mEq/L	21-28	18-31 (decreased)
Blood pH	7.35-7.45	7.40-7.45 (slightly increased, more alkaline)
Hepatic		
Bilirubin, total, mg/dl	≤1	Unchanged
Serum cholesterol, mg/dl	120-200	Increases from 16 to 32 weeks of pregnancy; remains at this level until after birth
Serum alkaline phosphatase, U/L	30-120	Increases from week 12 of pregnancy to 6 weeks after birth
Serum albumin, g/dl	3.5-5.0	Slight increase
Renal		
Bladder capacity, ml	1300	1500
Renal plasma flow (RPF), ml/min	490-700	Increase by 25%-30%
Glomerular filtration rate (GFR), ml/min	88-128	Increase by 30%-50%
Nonprotein nitrogen (NPN), mg/dl	25-40	Decreases
Blood urea nitrogen (BUN), mg/dl	10-20	Decreases
Serum creatinine, mg/dl	0.5-1.1	Decreases
Serum uric acid, mg/dl	2.7-7.3	Decreases
Urine glucose	Negative	Present in 20% of pregnant women
Intravenous pyelogram (IVP)	Normal	Slight-to-moderate hydroureter and hydronephrosis; right kidney larger than left kidney

nolytic activity (the splitting up or the dissolving of a clot) is depressed during pregnancy and the postpartum period, provides a protective function to decrease the chance of bleeding but also makes the woman more vulnerable to thrombosis, especially after cesarean birth.

Respiratory System

Structural and ventilatory adaptations occur during pregnancy to provide for maternal and fetal needs. Maternal oxygen requirements increase in response to the acceleration in the metabolic rate and the need to add to the tissue mass in the uterus and breasts. In addition, the fetus requires oxygen and a way to eliminate carbon dioxide.

Elevated levels of estrogen cause the ligaments of the rib cage to relax, permitting increased chest expansion (see Fig. 14-8). The transverse diameter of the thoracic cage increases by about 2 cm, and the circumference increases by 6 cm (Cunningham et al., 2001). The costal angle increases, and the lower rib cage appears to flare out. The chest may not return to its prepregnant state after birth (Seidel et al., 2003).

BOX 14-3 Cardiovascular Changes in Pregnancy

Heart rate	Increases 10-15 beats/min
Blood pressure	Remains at prepregnancy levels in first trimester Slight decrease in second trimester Returns to prepregnancy levels in third trimester
Blood volume	Increases by 1500 ml or 40%-50% above prepregnancy level
Red blood cell mass	Increases 17%
Hemoglobin	Decreases
Hematocrit	Decreases
White blood cell count	Increases in second and third trimester
Cardiac output	Increases 30%-50%

The diaphragm is displaced by as much as 4 cm during pregnancy. As pregnancy advances, thoracic (costal) breathing replaces abdominal breathing, and it becomes less possible for the diaphragm to descend with inspiration. Thoracic breathing is accomplished primarily by the diaphragm rather than by the costal muscles (Swiet, 1999).

The upper respiratory tract becomes more vascular in response to elevated levels of estrogen. As the capillaries become engorged, edema and hyperemia develop within the nose, pharynx, larynx, trachea, and bronchi. This congestion within the tissues of the respiratory tract gives rise to several conditions commonly seen during pregnancy, including nasal and sinus stuffiness, epistaxis (nosebleed), changes in the voice, and a marked inflammatory response that can develop into a mild upper respiratory infection.

Increased vascularity of the upper respiratory tract also can cause the tympanic membranes and eustachian tubes to swell, giving rise to symptoms of impaired hearing, earaches, or a sense of fullness in the ears.

Pulmonary Function. Respiratory changes in pregnancy are related to the elevation of the diaphragm and to chest wall changes. Changes in the respiratory center result in a lowered threshold for carbon dioxide. The actions of progesterone and estrogen are presumed responsible for the increased sensitivity of the respiratory center to carbon dioxide. In addition, pregnant women become more aware of the need to breathe; some may even complain of dyspnea at rest, especially in the third trimester (Swiet, 1999) (see Box 14-4 for respiratory changes in pregnancy).

Although pulmonary function is not impaired by pregnancy, diseases of the respiratory tract may be more serious during this time (Cunningham et al., 2001). One important factor responsible for this may be the increased oxygen requirement.

BOX 14-4 Respiratory Changes in Pregnancy

Respiratory rate	Unchanged or slightly increased
Tidal volume	Increased 30%-40%
Vital capacity	Unchanged
Inspiratory capacity	Increased
Expiratory volume	Decreased
Total lung capacity	Unchanged to slightly decreased
Oxygen consumption	Increased 15%-20%

Basal Metabolism Rate. The basal metabolism rate (BMR) varies considerably in women at the beginning of and during pregnancy, although it usually increases by 15% to 20% at term (Worthington-Roberts & Williams, 1997). The BMR returns to nonpregnant levels by 5 to 6 days after birth. The elevation in BMR during pregnancy reflects increased oxygen demands of the uterine-placental-fetal unit and greater oxygen consumption because of increased maternal cardiac work (Chamberlain & Pipkin, 1998). Peripheral vasodilation and acceleration of sweat gland activity help dissipate the excess heat resulting from the increased BMR during pregnancy. Pregnant women may experience heat intolerance, which is annoying to some women. Lassitude and fatigability after only slight exertion are experienced by many women in early pregnancy. These feelings, along with a greater need for sleep, may persist and may be caused in part by the increased metabolic activity.

Acid-Base Balance. By about the tenth week of pregnancy, there is a decrease of about 5 mm Hg in the partial pressure of carbon dioxide (PCO_2). Progesterone may be responsible for increasing the sensitivity of the respiratory center receptors, so that tidal volume is increased, PCO_2 decreases, the base excess (HCO_3 or bicarbonate) decreases, and pH increases slightly. These alterations in acid-base balance indicate that pregnancy is a state of respiratory alkalosis compensated by mild metabolic acidosis (Chamberlain & Pipkin, 1998). These changes also facilitate the transport of CO_2 from the fetus and O_2 release from the mother to the fetus (see Table 14-3).

Renal System

The kidneys are responsible for maintaining electrolyte and acid-base balance, regulating extracellular fluid volume, excreting waste products, and conserving essential nutrients.

Anatomic Changes. Changes in renal structure during pregnancy result from hormonal activity (estrogen and progesterone), pressure from an enlarging uterus, and an increase in blood volume. As early as the tenth week of pregnancy, the renal pelves and the ureters dilate. Dilation of the ureters is more pronounced above the pelvic brim, in part because they are compressed between the uterus and the pelvic brim. In most women, the ureters below the pelvic brim are of normal size. The smooth-muscle walls of the ureters undergo hyperplasia, hypertrophy, and muscle tone relaxation. The ureters elongate, become tortuous, and form single or double curves. In the latter part of pregnancy, the renal pelvis and ureter are dilated more on the right side than on the left because the heavy uterus is displaced to the right by the sigmoid colon.

Because of these changes, a larger volume of urine is held in the pelves and ureters, and urine flow rate is slowed. The resulting urinary stasis or stagnation has the following consequences:

- A lag occurs between the time urine is formed and when it reaches the bladder. Therefore clearance test results may reflect substances contained in glomerular filtrate several hours before.
- Stagnated urine is an excellent medium for the growth of microorganisms. In addition, the urine of pregnant women contains more nutrients, including glucose, thereby increasing the pH (making the urine more alkaline). This makes pregnant women more susceptible to urinary tract infection.

Bladder irritability, nocturia, and urinary frequency and urgency (without dysuria) are commonly reported in early pregnancy. Near term, bladder symptoms may return, especially after lightening occurs.

Urinary frequency results initially from increased bladder sensitivity and later from compression of the bladder (see Fig. 14-7). In the second trimester, the bladder is pulled up out of the true pelvis into the abdomen. The urethra lengthens to 7.5 cm as the bladder is displaced upward. The pelvic congestion that occurs in pregnancy is reflected in hyperemia of the bladder and urethra. This increased vascularity causes the bladder mucosa to be traumatized and bleed easily. Bladder tone may decrease, which increases the bladder capacity to 1500 ml. At the same time, the bladder is compressed by the enlarging uterus, resulting in the urge to void even if the bladder contains only a small amount of urine.

Functional Changes. In normal pregnancy, renal function is altered considerably. Glomerular filtration rate (GFR) and renal plasma flow (RPF) increase early in pregnancy (Cunningham et al., 2001). These changes are caused by pregnancy hormones, an increase in blood volume, the woman's posture, physical activity, and nutritional intake. The woman's kidneys must manage the increased metabolic and circulatory demands of the maternal body and the excretion of fetal waste products. Renal function is most efficient when the woman lies in the lateral recumbent position and least efficient when the woman assumes a supine position. A side-lying position increases renal perfusion, which increases urinary output and decreases edema. When the pregnant woman is lying supine, the heavy uterus compresses the vena cava and the aorta, and cardiac output decreases. As a result, blood flow to the brain and heart is continued at the expense of other organs, including the kidneys and uterus.

Fluid and Electrolyte Balance. Selective renal tubular reabsorption maintains sodium and water balance regardless of changes in dietary intake and losses through sweat, vomitus, or diarrhea. From 500 to 900 mEq of sodium is normally retained during pregnancy to meet fetal needs. To prevent excessive sodium depletion, the maternal kidneys undergo a significant adaptation by increasing tubular reabsorption. Because of the need for increased maternal intravascular and extracellular fluid volume, additional sodium is needed to expand fluid volume and to maintain an isotonic state. As efficient as the renal system is, it can be overstressed by excessive dietary sodium intake or restriction or by use of diuretics. Severe hypovolemia and reduced placental perfusion are two consequences of using diuretics during pregnancy.

The capacity of the kidneys to excrete water during the early weeks of pregnancy is more efficient than it is later in pregnancy. As a result, some women feel thirsty in early pregnancy because of the greater amount of water loss. The pooling of fluid in the legs in the latter part of pregnancy decreases renal blood flow and GFR. This pooling of blood in the lower legs is sometimes referred to as *physiologic edema* or dependent edema and requires no treatment. The normal diuretic response to the water load is triggered when the woman lies down, preferably on her side, and the pooled fluid reenters general circulation.

Normally the kidney reabsorbs almost all of the glucose and other nutrients from the plasma filtrate. In pregnant women, however, tubular reabsorption of glucose is impaired, so that glucosuria occurs at varying times and to varying degrees. Normal values range from 0 to 20 mg/dl, meaning that during any day, the urine is sometimes positive and sometimes negative. In nonpregnant women, blood glucose levels must be at 160 to 180 mg/dl before glucose is "spilled" into the urine (not reabsorbed). During pregnancy, glucosuria occurs when maternal glucose levels are lower than 160 mg/dl. Why glucose, as well as other nutrients such as amino acids, is wasted during pregnancy is not understood, nor has the exact mechanism been discovered. Although glucosuria may be found in normal pregnancies (2+ levels may be seen with increased anxiety states), the possibility of diabetes mellitus and gestational diabetes must be kept in mind.

Proteinuria usually does not occur in normal pregnancy except during labor or after birth (Cunningham et al., 2001). However, the increased amount of amino acids that must be filtered may exceed the capacity of the renal tubules to absorb it, so that small amounts of protein are then lost in the urine. Values of trace to 1+ protein (dipstick assessment) or less than 300 mg per 24 hours are acceptable during pregnancy (Gordon, 2002). The amount of protein excreted is not an indication of the severity of renal disease, nor does an increase in protein excretion in a pregnant woman with known renal disease necessarily indicate a progression in her disease. However, a pregnant woman with hypertension and proteinuria must be carefully evaluated because she may be at greater risk for an adverse pregnancy outcome (see Table 14-3).

Integumentary System

Alterations in hormonal balance and mechanical stretching are responsible for several changes in the integumentary system during pregnancy. Hyperpigmentation is stimulated by the anterior pituitary hormone melanotropin, which is increased during pregnancy. Darkening of the nipples, areolae, axillae, and vulva occurs about the sixteenth week of gestation. Facial melasma, also called **chloasma** or mask of pregnancy, is a blotchy, brownish hyperpigmentation of the skin over the cheeks, nose, and forehead, especially in dark-complexioned pregnant women. Chloasma appears in 50% to 70% of pregnant women, beginning after the sixteenth week and increasing gradually until term. The sun intensifies this pigmentation in susceptible women. Chloasma caused by normal pregnancy usually fades after birth.

The **linea nigra** (Fig. 14-10) is a pigmented line extending from the symphysis pubis to the top of the fundus in the midline; this line is known as the *linea alba* before hormone-induced pigmentation. In primigravidas the extension of the linea nigra, beginning in the third month, keeps pace with the rising height of the fundus; in multigravidas, the entire line often appears earlier than the third month. Not all pregnant women develop linea nigra, and some women notice hair growth along the line with or without the change in pigmentation.

Striae gravidarum, or stretch marks (seen over lower abdomen in Fig. 14-11), which appear in 50% to 90% of pregnant women during the second half of pregnancy, may be caused by action of adrenocorticosteroids. Striae reflect separation within the underlying connective (collagen) tissue of the skin. These slightly depressed streaks tend to occur over areas of maximal stretch (i.e., abdomen, thighs, and breasts). The stretching sometimes causes a sensation that resembles itching. The tendency to develop striae may be familial. After birth they usually fade, although they never disappear completely. Color of striae varies depending on the pregnant woman's skin color. The striae appear pinkish on a woman with light skin and are lighter than surrounding skin in dark-skinned women. In the multipara, in addition to the striae of the present pregnancy, glistening silvery lines (in light-skinned women) or purplish lines (in dark-skinned women) are commonly seen. These represent the scars of striae from previous pregnancies.

Angiomas are commonly referred to as *vascular spiders.* They are tiny, star-shaped or branched, slightly raised and pulsating end-arterioles usually found on the neck, thorax, face, and arms. They occur as a result of elevated levels of circulating estrogen. The spiders are bluish in color and do not blanch with pressure. Vascular spiders appear during the second to the fifth month of pregnancy in 65% of Caucasian women and 10% of African-American women. The spiders usually disappear after birth.

Pinkish-red, diffuse mottling or well-defined blotches are seen over the palmar surfaces of the hands in about 60% of Caucasian women and 35% of African-American women during pregnancy (Cunningham et al., 2001). These color changes, called **palmar erythema,** are related primarily to increased estrogen levels.

NURSE ALERT

Because integumentary system changes vary greatly among women of different racial backgrounds, the color of a woman's skin should be noted along with any changes that may be attributed to pregnancy when performing physical assessments.

Some dermatologic conditions have been identified as unique to pregnancy or as having an increased incidence during pregnancy. Pruritis is a relatively common dermatologic symptom in pregnancy, with *cholestasis of pregnancy* being the most common cause of pruritic rash. Other

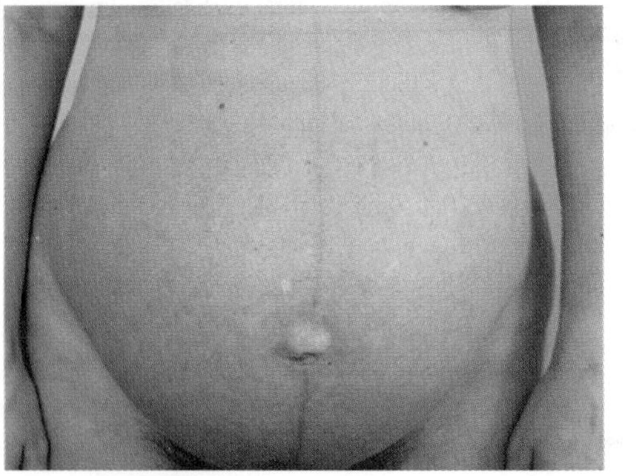

FIG. 14-10 Linea nigra. (From Seidel, H. et al. [2003]. *Mosby's guide to physical examination* [5th ed.]. St. Louis: Mosby.)

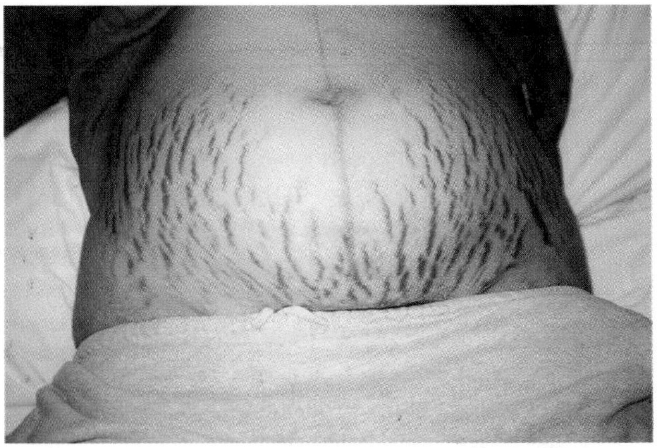

FIG. 14-11 Striae gravidarum and linea nigra in a dark-skinned person. (Courtesy Shannon Perry, San Jose, CA.)

forms are uncommon or rare (Cunningham et al., 2001) (Box 14-5). The goal of management is to relieve the itching. Topical steroids are the usual treatment, although systemic steroids may be needed. The problem usually resolves in the postpartum period (Stambuk & Colven, 2002). Preexisting skin diseases may complicate pregnancy or be improved.

NURSE ALERT

Women with severe acne taking isotretinoin (Accutane) should avoid pregnancy while receiving the treatment because it is teratogenic and is associated with major malformations.

Gum hypertrophy may occur. An **epulis** (gingival granuloma gravidarum) is a red, raised nodule on the gums that bleeds easily. This lesion may develop around the third month and usually continues to enlarge as pregnancy progresses. It is usually managed by avoiding trauma to the gums (e.g., using a soft toothbrush). An epulis usually regresses spontaneously after birth.

Nail growth may be accelerated. Some women may notice thinning and softening of the nails. Oily skin and acne vulgaris may occur during pregnancy. For some women, the skin clears and looks radiant. Hirsutism, the excessive growth of hair or growth of hair in unusual places, is commonly reported. An increase in fine hair growth may occur but tends to disappear after pregnancy; however, growth of coarse or bristly hair does not usually disappear.

Increased blood supply to the skin leads to increased perspiration. Women feel hotter during pregnancy, possibly related to a progesterone-induced increase in body temperature and the increased BMR.

BOX 14-5 **Frequency of Dermatologic Disorders of Pregnancy**

Cholestasis of pregnancy, 1%-2%
Pruritic urticarial papules and plaques of pregnancy, 0.25%-1%
Prurigo of pregnancy, 1:300 to 1:2400
Herpes gestationis, 1:10,000
Impetigo herpetiformis, rare

Reference: Cunningham, F. et al. (2001). *Williams obstetrics* (21st ed.). New York: McGraw-Hill.

Musculoskeletal System

The gradually changing body and increasing weight of the pregnant woman cause noticeable alterations in her posture (Fig. 14-12) and the way she walks. The great abdominal distention that gives the pelvis a forward tilt, decreased abdominal muscle tone, and increased weight bearing require a realignment of the spinal curvature late in pregnancy. The woman's center of gravity shifts forward. An increase in the normal lumbosacral curve (lordosis) develops, and a compensatory curvature in the cervicodorsal region (exaggerated anterior flexion of

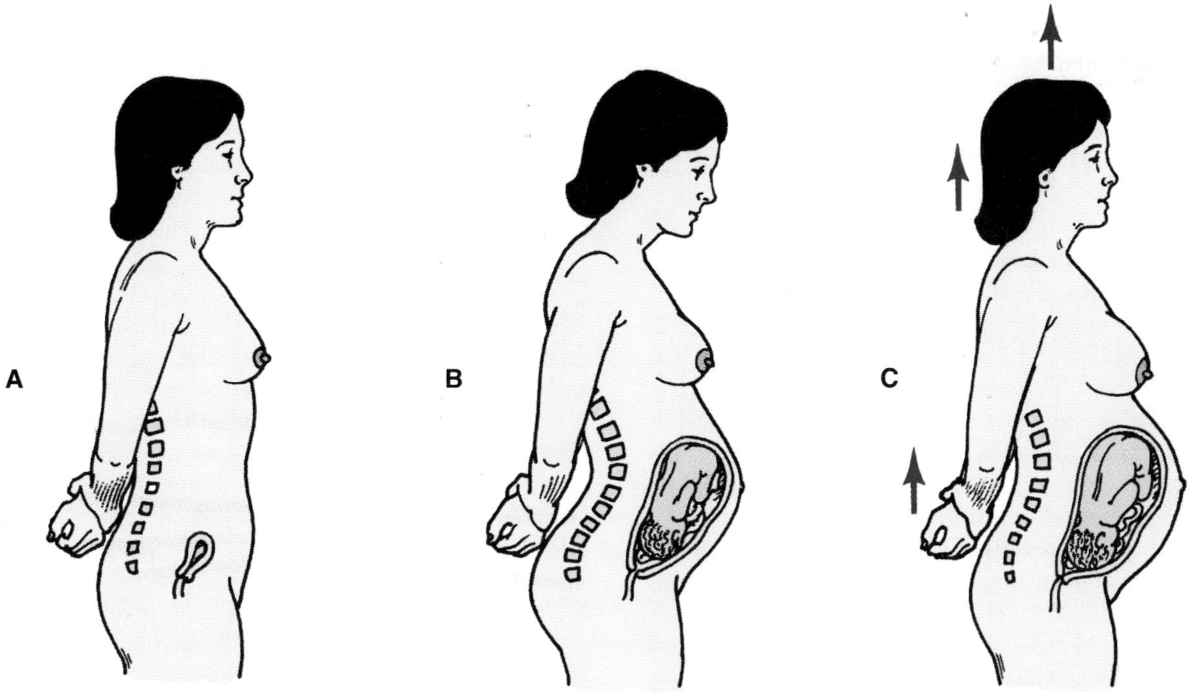
A
B
C

FIG. 14-12 Postural changes during pregnancy. **A,** Nonpregnant. **B,** Incorrect posture during pregnancy. **C,** Correct posture during pregnancy.

the head) develops to help her maintain her balance. Aching, numbness, and weakness of the upper extremities may result. Large breasts and a stoop-shouldered stance will further accentuate the lumbar and dorsal curves. Walking is more difficult, and the waddling gait of the pregnant woman, called "the proud walk of pregnancy" by Shakespeare, is well known. The ligamentous and muscular structures of the middle and lower spine may be severely stressed. These and related changes often cause musculoskeletal discomfort, especially in older women or those with a back disorder or a faulty sense of balance.

Slight relaxation and increased mobility of the pelvic joints are normal during pregnancy. They are secondary to the exaggerated elasticity and softening of connective and collagen tissue caused by increased circulating steroid sex hormones, especially estrogen. Relaxin, an ovarian hormone, assists in this relaxation and softening. These adaptations permit enlargement of pelvic dimensions to facilitate labor and birth. The degree of relaxation varies, but considerable separation of the symphysis pubis and the instability of the sacroiliac joints may cause pain and difficulty in walking. Obesity and multifetal pregnancy tend to increase the pelvic instability. Peripheral joint laxity also increases as pregnancy progresses, but the cause is not known (Cunningham et al., 2001).

The muscles of the abdominal wall stretch and ultimately lose some tone. During the third trimester, the rectus abdominis muscles may separate (Fig. 14-13), allowing abdominal contents to protrude at the midline. The umbilicus flattens or protrudes. After birth, the muscles gradually regain tone; however, separation of the muscles **(diastasis recti abdominis)** may persist.

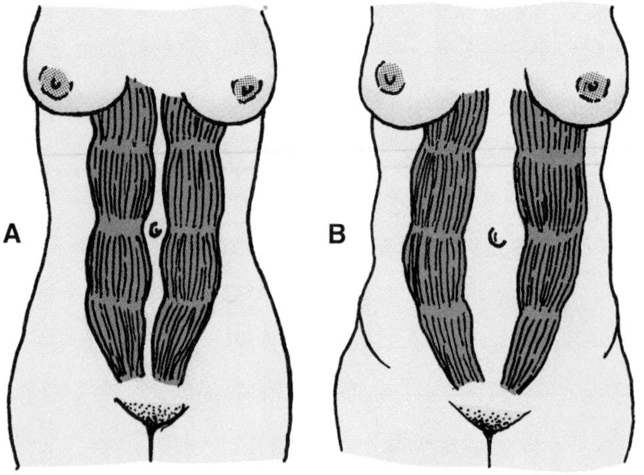
A
B

FIG. 14-13 Possible change in rectus abdominis muscles during pregnancy. **A,** Normal position in nonpregnant woman. **B,** Diastasis recti abdominis in pregnant woman.

Neurologic System

Little is known regarding specific alterations in function of the neurologic system during pregnancy, aside from hypothalamic-pituitary neurohormonal changes. Specific physiologic alterations resulting from pregnancy may cause the following neurologic or neuromuscular symptoms:

- Compression of pelvic nerves or vascular stasis caused by enlargement of the uterus may result in sensory changes in the legs.
- Dorsolumbar lordosis may cause pain because of traction on nerves or compression of nerve roots.
- Edema involving the peripheral nerves may result in **carpal tunnel syndrome** during the last trimester (Padua et al., 2001). The syndrome is characterized by paresthesia (abnormal sensation such as burning or tingling) and pain in the hand, radiating to the elbow. The sensations are caused by edema that compresses the median nerve beneath the carpal ligament of the wrist. Smoking and alcohol consumption can impair the microcirculation and may worsen the symptoms (Padua et al., 2001). The dominant hand is usually affected most, although as many as 80% of women experience symptoms in both hands. Symptoms usually regress after pregnancy. In some cases, surgical treatment may be necessary (Cunningham et al., 2001).
- Acroesthesia (numbness and tingling of the hands) is caused by the stoop-shouldered stance (see Fig. 14-12, *B*) assumed by some women during pregnancy. The condition is associated with traction on segments of the brachial plexus.
- Tension headache is common when anxiety or uncertainty complicates pregnancy. However, vision problems, sinusitis, or migraine also may be responsible for headaches.
- "Light-headedness," faintness, and even syncope (fainting) are common during early pregnancy. Vasomotor instability, postural hypotension, or hypoglycemia may be responsible.
- Hypocalcemia may cause neuromuscular problems such as muscle cramps or tetany.

Gastrointestinal System

Appetite. During pregnancy, the woman's appetite and food intake fluctuate. Early in pregnancy, some women have nausea with or without vomiting (*morning sickness*), possibly in response to increasing levels of hCG and altered carbohydrate metabolism (Gordon, 2002). Morning sickness or nausea and vomiting of pregnancy (NVP) appears at about 4 to 6 weeks of gestation and usually subsides by the end of the third month (first trimester) of pregnancy. Severity varies from mild distaste for certain foods to more severe vomiting. The condition may be triggered by the sight or odor of various foods. By the end of the second trimester, the appetite increases in response to increasing metabolic needs. Rarely does NVP have harmful effects on the embryo, fetus, or the woman; some beneficial effects may be that these pregnancies may be less likely to result in miscarriage, preterm labor, or intrauterine growth restriction (Furneaux et al., 2001). Whenever the vomiting is severe or persists beyond the first trimester, or when it is accompanied by fever, pain, or weight loss, further evaluation is necessary, and medical intervention is likely.

Women also may have changes in their sense of taste, leading to cravings and changes in dietary intake. Some women have nonfood cravings **(pica)**, such as for ice, clay, and laundry starch. Usually the subjects of these cravings, if consumed in moderation, are not harmful to the pregnancy if the woman has adequate nutrition with appropriate weight gain (Gordon, 2002).

Mouth. The gums become hyperemic, spongy, and swollen during pregnancy. They tend to bleed easily because the increasing levels of estrogen cause selective increased vascularity and connective tissue proliferation (a nonspecific gingivitis). Epulis (discussed in the section on the integumentary system) may develop at the gumline. Some pregnant women complain of **ptyalism** (excessive salivation), which may be caused by the decrease in unconscious swallowing by the woman when nauseated or from stimulation of salivary glands by eating starch (Cunningham et al., 2001).

Esophagus, Stomach, and Intestines. Herniation of the upper portion of the stomach (hiatal hernia) occurs after the seventh or eighth month of pregnancy in about 15% to 20% of pregnant women. This condition results from upward displacement of the stomach, which causes the hiatus of the diaphragm to widen. It occurs more often in multiparas and older or obese women.

Increased estrogen production causes decreased secretion of hydrochloric acid; therefore peptic ulcer formation or flare-up of existing peptic ulcers is uncommon during pregnancy and may improve (Winbery & Blaho, 2001).

Increased progesterone production causes decreased tone and motility of smooth muscles, resulting in esophageal regurgitation, slower emptying time of the stomach, and reverse peristalsis. As a result, the woman may experience "acid indigestion" or heartburn **(pyrosis).**

Iron is absorbed more readily in the small intestine in response to increased needs during pregnancy. Even when the woman is deficient in iron, it will continue to be absorbed in sufficient amounts for the fetus to have a normal hemoglobin level.

Increased progesterone (causing loss of muscle tone and decreased peristalsis) results in an increase in water absorption from the colon and may cause constipation. Constipation also may result from hypoperistalsis (sluggishness of the bowel), food choices, lack of fluids, iron supplementation, decreased activity level, abdominal distention by the pregnant uterus, and displacement and compression of the intestines. If the pregnant woman has hemorrhoids (see Fig. 14-9) and is constipated, the hemorrhoids may become everted or may bleed during straining at stool.

Gallbladder and Liver. The gallbladder is quite often distended because of its decreased muscle tone during pregnancy. Increased emptying time and thickening of bile caused by prolonged retention are typical changes. These features, together with slight hypercholesterolemia from increased progesterone levels, may account for the development of gallstones during pregnancy.

Hepatic function is difficult to appraise during pregnancy; however, only minor changes in liver function develop. Occasionally, intrahepatic cholestasis (retention and accumulation of bile in the liver, caused by factors within the liver) occurs late in pregnancy in response to placental steroids and may result in pruritus gravidarum (severe itching) with or without jaundice. These distressing symptoms subside soon after birth.

Abdominal Discomfort. Intraabdominal alterations that can cause discomfort include pelvic heaviness or pressure, round ligament tension, flatulence, distention and bowel cramping, and uterine contractions. In addition to displacement of intestines, pressure from the expanding uterus causes an increase in venous pressure in the pelvic organs. Although most abdominal discomfort is a consequence of normal maternal alterations, the health care provider must be constantly alert to the possibility of disorders such as bowel obstruction or an inflammatory process.

Appendicitis may be difficult to diagnose in pregnancy because the appendix is displaced upward and laterally, high and to the right, away from McBurney's point (Fig. 14-14).

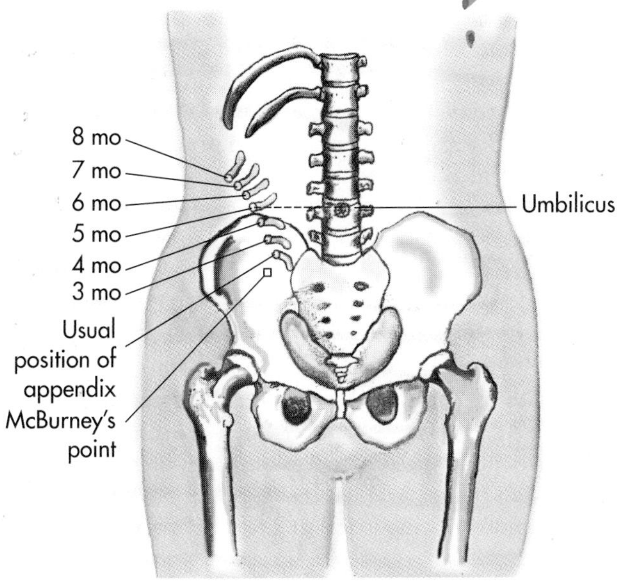
8 mo
7 mo
6 mo
5 mo
4 mo
3 mo
Usual position of appendix McBurney's point
Umbilicus

FIG. 14-14 Change in position of appendix in pregnancy. Note McBurney's point.

Endocrine System

Profound endocrine changes are essential for pregnancy maintenance, normal fetal growth, and postpartum recovery.

Pituitary and Placental Hormones. During pregnancy, the elevated levels of estrogen and progesterone (produced first by the corpus luteum in the ovary until about 14 weeks of gestation and then by the placenta) suppress secretion of follicle-stimulating hormone (FSH) and luteinizing hormone (LH) by the anterior pituitary. The maturation of a follicle and ovulation do not occur. Although the majority of women have amenorrhea (absence of menses), at least 20% have some slight, painless spotting during early gestation. Implantation bleeding and bleeding after intercourse related to cervical friability can occur. Most of the women experiencing slight gestational bleeding continue to term and have normal infants; however, all instances of bleeding should be reported and evaluated.

After implantation, the fertilized ovum and the chorionic villi produce hCG, which maintains the production by the corpus luteum of estrogen and progesterone until the placenta takes over production (Buster & Carson, 2002).

Progesterone is essential for maintaining pregnancy by relaxing smooth muscles, resulting in decreased uterine contractility and prevention of miscarriage. Progesterone and estrogen cause fat to deposit in subcutaneous tissues over the maternal abdomen, back, and upper thighs. This fat serves as an energy reserve for both pregnancy and lactation. Estrogen also promotes the enlargement of the genitals, uterus, and breasts and increases vascularity, causing vasodilation. Estrogen causes relaxation of pelvic ligaments and joints. It also alters metabolism of nutrients by interfering with folic acid metabolism, increasing the level of total body proteins, and promoting retention of sodium and water by kidney tubules. Estrogen may decrease secretion of hydrochloric acid and pepsin, which may be responsible for digestive upsets such as nausea.

Serum prolactin produced by the anterior pituitary begins to increase early in the first trimester and increases progressively to term. It is responsible for initial lactation; however, the high levels of estrogen and progesterone inhibit lactation by blocking the binding of prolactin to breast tissue until after birth (Guyton & Hall, 1997).

Oxytocin is produced by the posterior pituitary in increasing amounts as the fetus matures. This hormone can stimulate uterine contractions during pregnancy, but high levels of progesterone prevent contractions until near term. Oxytocin also stimulates the let-down or milk-ejection reflex after birth in response to the infant sucking at the mother's breast.

Human chorionic somatomammotropin (hCS), previously called human placental lactogen, produced by the placenta, acts as a growth hormone and contributes to breast development. It decreases the maternal metabolism of glucose and increases the amount of fatty acids for metabolic needs (Alsat et al., 1997; Guyton & Hall, 1997).

Thyroid Gland. During pregnancy, gland activity and hormone production increase. The increased activity is reflected in a moderate enlargement of the thyroid gland caused by hyperplasia of the glandular tissue and increased vascularity (Cunningham et al., 2001). Thyroxine-binding globulin (TBG) increases as a result of increased estrogen levels. This increase begins at about 20 weeks of gestation. The level of total (free and bound) thyroxine (T_4) increases between 6 and 9 weeks of gestation and plateaus at 18 weeks of gestation. Free thyroxine (T_4) and free triiodothyronine (T_3) return to nonpregnant levels after the first trimester. Despite these changes in hormone production, hyperthyroidism usually does not develop in the pregnant woman (Cunningham et al., 2001).

Parathyroid Gland. Parathyroid hormone controls calcium and magnesium metabolism. Pregnancy induces a slight hyperparathyroidism, a reflection of increased fetal requirements for calcium and vitamin D. The peak level of parathyroid hormone occurs between 15 and 35 weeks of gestation, when the needs for growth of the fetal skeleton are greatest. Levels return to normal after birth.

Pancreas. The fetus requires significant amounts of glucose for its growth and development. To meet its need for fuel, the fetus not only depletes the store of maternal glucose but also decreases the mother's ability to synthesize glucose by siphoning off her amino acids. Maternal blood glucose levels decrease. Maternal insulin does not cross the placenta to the fetus. As a result, in early pregnancy, the pancreas decreases its production of insulin.

As pregnancy continues, the placenta grows and produces progressively larger amounts of hormones (i.e., hCS, estrogen, and progesterone). Cortisol production by the adrenals also increases. Estrogen, progesterone, hCS, and cortisol collectively decrease the mother's ability to use insulin. Cortisol stimulates increased production of insulin but also increases the mother's peripheral resistance to insulin (i.e., the tissues cannot use the insulin). Decreasing the mother's ability to use her own insulin is a protective mechanism that ensures an ample supply of glucose for the needs of the fetoplacental unit. The result is an added demand for insulin by the mother that continues to increase at a steady rate until term. The normal beta cells of the islets of Langerhans in the pancreas can meet this demand for insulin.

Adrenal Glands. The adrenal glands change little during pregnancy. Secretion of aldosterone is increased, resulting in reabsorption of excess sodium from the renal tubules. Cortisol levels also are increased (Chamberlain & Pipkin, 1998).

KEY POINTS

- The biochemical, physiologic, and anatomic adaptations that occur during pregnancy are profound and revert to the nonpregnant state after birth and lactation.
- Maternal adaptations are attributed to the hormones of pregnancy and to mechanical pressures exerted by the enlarging uterus and other tissues.
- ELISA testing, with monoclonal antibody technology, is the most popular method of pregnancy testing and is the basis for most over-the-counter home pregnancy tests.
- Presumptive, probable, and positive signs of pregnancy aid in the diagnosis of pregnancy; only positive signs (identification of a fetal heartbeat, verification of fetal movements, and visualization of the fetus) can establish the diagnosis of pregnancy.
- Adaptations to pregnancy protect the woman's normal physiologic functioning, meet the metabolic demands pregnancy imposes, and provide for fetal development and growth needs.
- Although the pH of the pregnant woman's vaginal secretions is more acidic, she is more vulnerable to some vaginal infections, especially yeast infections.
- Increased vascularity and sensitivity of the vagina and other pelvic viscera may lead to a high degree of sexual interest and arousal.
- Some adaptations to pregnancy result in discomforts such as fatigue, urinary frequency, nausea, and breast sensitivity.
- As pregnancy progresses, balance and coordination are affected by changes in the woman's joints and her center of gravity.

CRITICAL THINKING EXERCISES

1. Interview three pregnant women (and partners, if present), one of whom is in the first trimester, one in the second trimester, and one in the third trimester. Ask the following questions:
   a. What changes in her body has she noticed?
   b. Which changes does she find pleasant?
   c. Which changes does she find uncomfortable or troublesome?
   d. What is her level of understanding of these changes?
   e. Has her partner expressed any feelings or opinions about these changes? If so, how have these feelings or opinions affected the woman?
   f. Use your findings to develop a teaching plan for each woman's specific concerns. Provide rationales for your choices of topics.
2. Go to a local pharmacy and get information on at least three different home pregnancy test kits. (The pharmacist may be able to provide product information.) Compare the directions for use, interpretation of test results, and the costs. Do any of the kits have directions in languages other than English? During a conference with others in your clinical group, discuss the pros and cons of using the different types of kits. Develop a poster presentation to guide women in decisions about use of home pregnancy tests for display in a family planning clinic.
3. During your experience in a prenatal clinic or physician-midwife office, observe one woman's care. Compare physical assessment and laboratory tests done with the expected findings for the weeks of pregnancy. What risk factors are present? Summarize your findings in a case study presentation during a clinical conference. Prepare a plan of care for any problems identified.

RESOURCES

Babyonline.com (source of information on pregnancy and baby care)
www.babyonline.com

Childbirth.org (source of links to other sites related to pregnancy and birth)
www.childbirth.org

New York Online Access to Health (consumer-level information site, includes information on tests, fetal development, postnatal topics, etc., in English and Spanish)
www.noah-health.org/english/pregnancy

Official site of the Perinatal Education Associates, Inc.
www.birthsource.com

Information on physiologic and emotional aspects of pregnancy
Alexian Brothers Medical Center
Elk Grove, IL
www.alexian.org/progserv/babies/babytoo.html

REFERENCES

Alsat, E. et al. (1997). Human placental growth hormone. *American Journal of Obstetrics and Gynecology, 177*(6), 526-534.

Bennett, V., & Brown, L. (1999). *Myles textbook for midwives* (13th ed.). Edinburgh: Churchill Livingstone.

Berman, M., DiSaia, P. & Brewster, W. (1999). Pelvic malignancies, gestational trophoblastic neoplasia, and nonpelvic malignancies. In R. Creasy & R. Resnik (Eds.), *Maternal-fetal medicine* (4th ed.). Philadelphia: W.B. Saunders.

Buster, J., & Carson, S. (2002). Endocrinology and diagnosis of pregnancy. In S. Gabbe, J. Niebyl, & J. Simpson (Eds.), *Obstetrics: Normal and problem pregnancies* (4th ed.). New York: Churchill Livingstone.

Chamberlain, G., & Pipkin, F. (Eds.). (1998). *Clinical physiology in obstetrics* (3rd ed.). Oxford: Blackwell Scientific.

Cunningham, F. et al. (2001). *Williams obstetrics* (21st ed.). New York: McGraw-Hill.

Furneaux, E., Langley-Evans, A., & Langley-Evans, S. (2001). Nausea and vomiting of pregnancy: Endocrine basis and contribution to pregnancy outcome. *Obstetrical and Gynecological Survey, 56*(12): 775-782.

Gonik, B. (1999). Intensive care monitoring of the critically ill pregnant patient. In R. Creasy & R. Resnik (Eds.), *Maternal-fetal medicine* (4th ed.). Philadelphia: W.B. Saunders.

Gordon, M. (2002). Maternal physiology in pregnancy. In S. Gabbe, J. Niebyl, & J. Simpson (Eds.), *Obstetrics: Normal and problem pregnancies* (4th ed.). New York: Churchill Livingstone.

Guyton, A., & Hall, J. (1997). *Human physiology and mechanism of disease* (6th ed.). Philadelphia: W.B. Saunders.

Hatcher, R. et al. (2002). *A pocket guide to managing contraception.* Tiger, GA: Bridging the Gap Foundation.

Hermida, R., Ayala, D., & Iglesias, M. (2001). Predictable blood pressure variability in healthy and complicated pregnancies. *Hypertension, 38*(3 Pt 2), 736-744.

Hermida, R. et al. (2001). Time-qualified reference values for ambulatory blood pressure monitoring in pregnancy. *Hypertension, 38*(3 Pt 2), 746-752.

Lawrence, R. (1999). *Breastfeeding: A guide for the medical profession* (5th ed.). St. Louis: Mosby.

Malone, F., & D'Alton, M. (1999). Multiple gestation: Clinical characteristics and management. In R. Creasy & R. Resnik (Eds.), *Maternal-fetal medicine* (4th ed.). Philadelphia: W.B. Saunders.

Monga, M. (1999). Maternal cardiovascular and renal adaptation to pregnancy. In R. Creasy & R. Resnik (Eds.), *Maternal-fetal medicine* (4th ed.). Philadelphia: W.B. Saunders.

Padua, L. et al. (2001). Symptoms and neurophysical picture of carpal tunnel syndrome in pregnancy. *Clinical Neurophysiology, 112*(10), 1946-1951.

Pagana, K., & Pagana, T. (2003). *Mosby's diagnostic and laboratory test reference* (6th ed.). St. Louis: Mosby.

Resnik, R. (1999). Anatomic alterations in the reproductive tract. In R. Creasy & R. Resnik (Eds.), *Maternal-fetal medicine* (4th ed.). Philadelphia: W.B. Saunders.

Seidel, H. et al. (2003). *Mosby's guide to physical examination* (5th ed.). St. Louis: Mosby.

Shennan, A., & Halligan, A. (1999). Measuring blood pressure in normal and hypertensive pregnancy. *Baillieres Best Practical Research in Clinical Obstetrics and Gynaecology, 13*(1), 1-26.

Stambuck, R., & Colven, R. (2002). Dermatologic disorders. In S. Gabbe, J. Niebyl, & J. Simpson (Eds.), *Obstetrics: Normal and problem pregnancies* (4th ed.). New York: Churchill Livingstone.

Swiet, M. (1999). Pulmonary disorders. In R. Creasy & R. Resnik (Eds.), *Maternal-fetal medicine* (4th ed.). Philadelphia: W.B. Saunders.

Trudinger, B. (1999). Doppler ultrasound assessment of blood flow. In R. Creasy & R. Resnik (Eds.), *Maternal-fetal medicine* (4th ed.). Philadelphia: W.B. Saunders.

Winbery, S., & Blaho, K. (2001). Dyspepsia in pregnancy. *Obstetrics and Gynecology Clinics of North America, 28*(2), 333-350.

Worthington-Roberts, B., & Williams, S. (1997). *Nutrition in pregnancy and lactation* (6th ed.). Dubuque, IA: Brown & Benchmark Publishers.

CHAPTER 15

Mary Courtney Moore

Maternal and Fetal Nutrition

http://evolve.elsevier.com/Lowdermilk/MatWmnHlth/

LEARNING OBJECTIVES

- Explain recommended maternal weight gain during pregnancy.
- State the recommended level of intake of energy sources, protein, and key vitamins and minerals during pregnancy and lactation.
- Give examples of the food sources that provide the nutrients required for optimal maternal nutrition during pregnancy and lactation.
- Examine the role of nutritional supplements during pregnancy.
- List five nutritional risk factors during pregnancy.
- Compare the dietary needs of adolescent and mature pregnant women.
- Analyze examples of eating patterns of two women from different ethnic or cultural backgrounds, and identify potential dietary problems.
- Assess nutritional status during pregnancy.

Nutrition is one of many factors that influence the outcome of pregnancy (Fig. 15-1). However, maternal nutritional status is an especially significant factor, both because it is potentially alterable and because good nutrition before and during pregnancy is an important preventive measure for a variety of problems. These problems include birth of **low-birth-weight (LBW;** birth weight of 2500 g or less) and preterm infants. Currently more than 20 developed nations report infant mortality rates lower than those in the United States, and LBW is a factor in 65% of infant deaths in the United States (Hoyert et al., 2001). It is essential that the importance of good nutrition be emphasized to all women of childbearing potential. Therefore the nurse must have a thorough understanding of nutrient needs before and during pregnancy, and nutrition assessment, intervention, and evaluation must be an integral part of the nursing care given to all pregnant women.

NUTRIENT NEEDS BEFORE CONCEPTION

The first trimester of pregnancy is a crucial one in terms of embryonic and fetal organ development. A healthful diet before conception is the best way to ensure that adequate nutrients are available for the developing fetus. Folate or folic acid intake is of particular concern in the periconceptual period. "Folate" is the form in which this vitamin is found naturally in foods, and "folic acid" is the form used in fortification of grain products and other foods and in vitamin supplements. **Neural tube defects,** or failures in closure of the neural tube, are more common in infants of women with poor folic acid intake. Proper closure of the neural tube is required for normal formation of the spinal cord, and the neural tube begins to close within the first month of gestation, often before the woman realizes that she is pregnant. It is estimated that the incidence of neural tube defects could be halved if all women had an adequate folate intake during the periconceptual period (Krishnaswamy & Madhavan Nair, 2001). All women capable of becoming pregnant are advised to consume 0.4 mg (400 μg) of folic acid daily in fortified foods (ready-to-eat cereals and enriched grain products) or supplements, in addition to a diet rich in folate-containing foods: green leafy vegetables, whole grains, and fruits (Box 15-1).

Both maternal and fetal risks in pregnancy are increased when the mother is significantly underweight or overweight when pregnancy begins. Ideally all women would achieve their desirable body weights before conception.

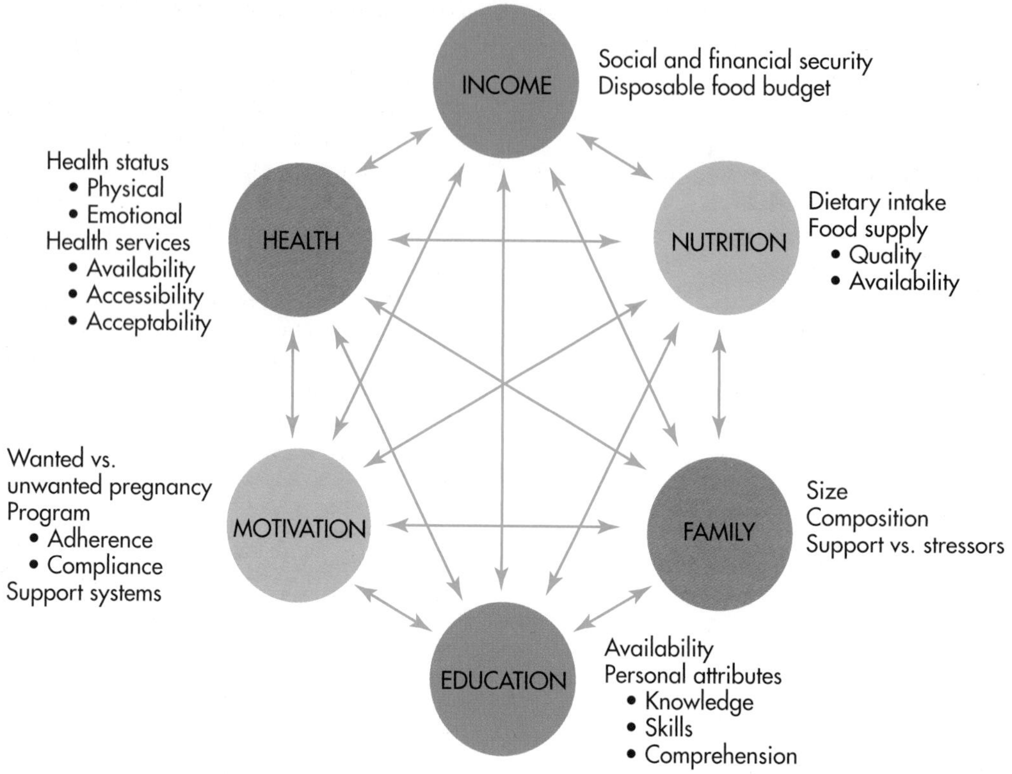
INCOME
Social and financial security
Disposable food budget
HEALTH
Health status
• Physical
• Emotional
Health services
• Availability
• Accessibility
• Acceptability
NUTRITION
Dietary intake
Food supply
• Quality
• Availability
MOTIVATION
Wanted vs. unwanted pregnancy
Program
• Adherence
• Compliance
Support systems
FAMILY
Size
Composition
Support vs. stressors
EDUCATION
Availability
Personal attributes
• Knowledge
• Skills
• Comprehension

FIG. 15-1 Web of influences that can affect outcome of pregnancy. (From Wardlaw, G., & Insel, P. [1993]. *Perspectives in nutrition* [2nd ed.]. St. Louis: Mosby.)

BOX *15-1* **Food Sources of Folate**

FOODS PROVIDING 500 μG OR MORE PER SERVING
Liver: Chicken, turkey, goose (3.5 oz)

FOODS PROVIDING 200 μG OR MORE PER SERVING
Liver: Lamb, beef, veal (3.5 oz)

FOODS PROVIDING 100 μG OR MORE PER SERVING
Legumes, cooked (½ cup)
Peas: Black-eye, chickpea (garbanzo)
Beans: Black, kidney, pinto, red, navy
Lentils
Vegetables (½ cup)
Asparagus
Spinach, cooked
Papaya (1 medium)
Breakfast cereal, ready-to-eat (½-1 cup)
Wheat germ (¼ cup)

FOODS PROVIDING 50 μG OR MORE PER SERVING
Vegetables (½ cup)
Broccoli
Beans: lima, baked, or pork and beans
Greens: collards or mustard, cooked
Spinach, raw
Fruits (½ cup)
Avocado
Orange or orange juice
Pasta, cooked (1 cup)
Rice, cooked (1 cup)

FOODS PROVIDING 20 μG OR MORE PER SERVING
Bread (1 slice)
Egg (1 large)
Corn (½ cup)

NUTRIENT NEEDS DURING PREGNANCY

Nutrient needs are determined, at least in part, by the stage of gestation, in that the amount of fetal growth varies during the different stages of pregnancy. During the first trimester, the synthesis of fetal tissues places relatively few demands on maternal nutrition; therefore during the first trimester when the embryo or fetus is very small, the needs are only slightly greater than those before pregnancy. In contrast, the last trimester is a period of noticeable fetal growth when most of the fetal stores of energy and minerals are deposited. Therefore as fetal growth progresses during the second and third trimesters, the pregnant woman's need for some nutrients increases greatly. Factors that contribute to the increase in nutrient needs include the following:

- The uterine-placental-fetal unit
- Maternal blood volume and constituents: During pregnancy the total blood volume increases by about 33% more than the normal volume. The plasma volume increases by 50% in women in their first pregnancies and more than this in multifetal pregnancies. Although red blood cell (RBC) production also is stimulated, the expansion of RBC mass is not so great as that of plasma volume.
- Maternal mammary development
- Metabolic needs: Basal metabolic rates, when expressed as kilocalories (kcal) per minute, are approximately 20% higher in pregnant women than in nonpregnant women. This increase includes the energy cost for tissue synthesis.

The Food and Nutrition Board of the National Academy of Sciences publishes recommendations for the people of the United States, the **Dietary Reference Intakes** or **DRIs.** The DRIs consist of **Recommended Dietary Allowances (RDAs)** and **Adequate Intakes (AIs),** as well as **Upper Limits (ULs),** guidelines for avoiding excessive intakes of nutrients that may be toxic if consumed in excess. RDAs for some nutrients have been available for many years, and they have been revised periodically. RDAs are recommendations for daily nutritional intakes that meet the needs of almost all (97% to 98%) of the healthy members of the population. AIs are similar to the RDAs and are believed to cover the needs for virtually all healthy individuals in a group, except that they deal with nutrients for which there are not enough data to be certain of their requirements. The RDAs and AIs include a wide variety of nutrients and food components, and they are divided into age, sex, and life-stage categories (e.g., infancy, pregnancy, and lactation). They can be used as goals in planning the diets of individuals (Table 15-1).

Energy Needs

Energy (kilocalories or kcal) needs are met by carbohydrate, fat, and protein in the diet. No specific recommendations exist for the amount of carbohydrate and fat in the

TABLE 15-1 **Recommendations for Daily Intakes of Selected Nutrients During Pregnancy and Lactation**

NUTRIENT (UNIT)	RECOMMENDATION FOR NONPREGNANT WOMAN	RECOMMENDATION FOR PREGNANCY*	RECOMMENDATION FOR LACTATION*	ROLE IN RELATION TO PREGNANCY AND LACTATION	FOOD SOURCES
Energy (kilocalories [kcal] or kilojoules [kJ]†)	Variable	First trimester, same as nonpregnant; second and third trimesters, nonpregnant + 300 kcal or 72 kJ	Nonpregnant + 500 kcal or 120 kJ	Growth of fetal and maternal tissues; milk production	Carbohydrate, fat, and protein
Protein (g)	50	60	65	Synthesis of the products of conception; growth of maternal tissue and expansion of blood volume; secretion of milk protein during lactation	Meats, eggs, cheese, yogurt, legumes (dry beans and peas, peanuts), nuts, grains

Recommendations are the Dietary Reference Intakes (RDA or AI, see text), where available. Sources: Food and Nutrition Board, National Academy of Sciences, Institute of Medicine. (1997). *Dietary reference intakes for calcium, phosphorus, magnesium, vitamin D, and fluoride* (1998); *Dietary reference intakes for thiamin, riboflavin, niacin, vitamin B_6, folate, vitamin B_{12}, pantothenic acid, biotin, and choline* (2000); *Dietary reference intakes for vitamin C, vitamin E, selenium, and carotenoids* (2001); *Dietary reference intakes for vitamin A, vitamin K, arsenic, boron, chromium, copper, iodine, iron, manganese, molybdenum, nickel, silicon, vanadium, and zinc.* Washington, DC: National Academy Press. Where DRIs are not available, the values are taken from Food and Nutrition Board, National Academy of Sciences, National Research Council. (1989). *Recommended dietary allowances* (10th ed.). Washington, DC: National Academy Press.

*When two values appear, separated by a diagonal slash, the first is for females younger than 19 years, and the second is for those 19 to 50 years of age.

†The international metric unit of energy measurement is the joule (J). 1 kcal = 4.184 kJ.

RBCs, Red blood cells.

Continued

TABLE 15-1 **Recommendations for Daily Intakes of Selected Nutrients During Pregnancy and Lactation—cont'd**

NUTRIENT (UNIT)	RECOMMENDATION FOR NONPREGNANT WOMAN	RECOMMENDATION FOR PREGNANCY*	RECOMMENDATION FOR LACTATION*	ROLE IN RELATION TO PREGNANCY AND LACTATION	FOOD SOURCES
Minerals					
Calcium (mg)	1300/1000	1300/1000	1300/1000	Fetal and infant skeleton and tooth formation; maintenance of maternal bone and tooth mineralization	Milk, cheese, yogurt, sardines or other fish eaten with bones left in, deep green leafy vegetables except spinach or Swiss chard, calcium-set tofu, baked beans, tortillas
Iron (mg)	15/18	27	10/9	Maternal hemoglobin formation, fetal liver iron storage	Liver, meats, whole grain or enriched breads and cereals, deep green leafy vegetables, legumes, dried fruits
Zinc (mg)	9/8	12/11	13/12	Component of numerous enzyme systems, possibly important in preventing congenital malformations	Liver, shellfish, meats, whole grains, milk
Iodine (μg)	150	220	290	Increased maternal metabolic rate	Iodized salt, seafood, milk and milk products, commercial yeast breads, rolls, and donuts
Magnesium (mg)	360/320	400/360	350/320	Involved in energy and protein metabolism, tissue growth, muscle action	Nuts, legumes, cocoa, meats, whole grains
Fat-soluble vitamins					
A (μg)	700	750/770	1200/1300	Essential for cell development, tooth bud formation, bone growth	Deep green leafy vegetables; dark yellow vegetables; and fruits, chili

TABLE 15-1 **Recommendations for Daily Intakes of Selected Nutrients During Pregnancy and Lactation—cont'd**

NUTRIENT (UNIT)	RECOMMENDATION FOR NONPREGNANT FEMALE	RECOMMENDATION FOR PREGNANCY*	RECOMMENDATION FOR LACTATION*	ROLE IN RELATION TO PREGNANCY AND LACTATION	FOOD SOURCES
A (μg)—cont'd					peppers, liver, fortified margarine and butter
D (μg)	5	5	5	Involved in absorption of calcium and phosphorus, improves mineralization	Fortified milk and margarine, egg yolk, butter, liver, seafood
E (mg)	15	15	19	Antioxidant (protects cell membranes from damage), especially important for preventing breakdown of RBCs	Vegetable oils, green leafy vegetables, whole grains, liver, nuts and seeds, cheese, fish
Water-soluble vitamins					
C (mg)	65/75	80/85	115/120	Tissue formation and integrity, formation of connective tissue, enhancement of iron absorption	Citrus fruits, strawberries, melons, broccoli, tomatoes, peppers, raw deep green leafy vegetables
Folate (μg)	400	600	500	Prevention of neural tube defects, support for increased maternal RBC formation	Fortified ready-to-eat cereals and other grain products, green leafy vegetables, oranges, broccoli, asparagus, artichokes, liver
B_6 or pyridoxine (mg)	1.2/1.3	1.9	2.0	Involved in protein metabolism	Meat, liver, deep green vegetables, whole grains
B_{12} (μg)	2.4	2.6	2.8	Production of nucleic acids and proteins, especially important in formation of RBC and neural functioning	Milk and milk products, egg, meat, liver, fortified soy milk

diet of the pregnant woman, but the intake of these nutrients should be adequate to support the recommended weight gain. Although protein can be used to supply energy, its primary role is to provide amino acids for the synthesis of new tissues (see discussion later in chapter). The RDA during the second and third trimesters of pregnancy is 300 kcal greater than the prepregnancy needs. Longitudinal assessment of weight gain during pregnancy is the best way to determine whether the kilocalorie intake is adequate; very underweight or active women may require more than the additional 300 kcal to sustain the desired rate of weight gain.

Weight Gain

The optimal weight gain during pregnancy is not known precisely. It is known, however, that the amount of weight gained by the mother during pregnancy has an important bearing on the course and outcome of the pregnancy. Although an adequate weight gain does not necessarily indicate that the diet is nutritionally adequate, it is associated with a reduced risk of giving birth to a **small-for-gestational age (SGA)** or preterm infant (Schieve et al., 2000).

The desirable weight gain during pregnancy varies among women. The primary factor to consider in making a weight gain recommendation is the appropriateness of the prepregnancy weight for the woman's height, that is, whether the woman's weight was normal before pregnancy, or whether she was underweight or overweight. Maternal and fetal risks in pregnancy are increased when the mother is significantly underweight or overweight before pregnancy and when weight gain during pregnancy is either too low or too high. Severely underweight women are more likely to have preterm labor and to give birth to LBW infants. Both normal-weight and underweight women with inadequate weight gain have an increased risk of giving birth to an infant with **intrauterine growth restriction (IUGR).** Greater-than-expected weight gain during pregnancy may occur for many reasons, including multiple gestation, edema, pregnancy-induced hypertension (PIH), and overeating. When obesity is present (either preexisting obesity or obesity that develops during pregnancy), there is an increased likelihood of macrosomia and fetopelvic disproportion; operative birth; emergency cesarean birth; postpartum hemorrhage; wound, genital tract, or urinary tract infection; birth trauma; and late fetal death (Nucci et al., 2001; Sebire et al., 2001). Obese women are more likely than normal-weight women to have PIH and gestational diabetes, and their risk of giving birth to a child with a major congenital defect is double that of normal-weight women.

A commonly used method of evaluating the appropriateness of weight for height is the **body mass index (BMI),** which is calculated by the following formula:

$$\text{BMI} = \frac{\text{Weight}}{\text{Height}^2}$$

where the weight is in kilograms and height is in meters. Thus for a woman who weighed 51 kg before pregnancy and is 1.57 m tall:

$$\text{BMI} = \frac{51}{(1.57)^2} = 20.7$$

Prepregnant BMI can be classified into the following categories: less than 19.8, underweight or low; 19.8 to 26.0, normal; 26.0 to 29.0, overweight or high; and greater than 29.0, obese (Institute of Medicine, 1992). Table 15-2 provides a simple way of estimating the BMI.

For women with single fetuses, current recommendations are that women with normal BMI should gain 11.5 to 16 kg during pregnancy (Fig. 15-2); underweight women should gain 12.5 to 18 kg; overweight women should gain 7 to 11.5 kg; and obese women should gain at least 7 kg (Institute of Medicine, 1992). Adolescents are encouraged to strive for weight gains at the upper end of the recommended range for their BMI, because it appears that the fetus and the still-growing mother compete for nutrients. The risk of mechanical complications at birth is reduced if the weight gain of short adult women (shorter than 157 cm or 5 feet 2 inches) is near the lower end of their recommended range. In twin gestations, gains of approximately 16 to 20 kg appear to be associated with the best outcomes (Ellings, Newman, & Bowers, 1998).

Pattern of Weight Gain

Weight gain should take place throughout pregnancy. The risk of giving birth to an SGA infant is greater when the weight gain early in pregnancy has been poor. The likelihood of preterm birth is greater when the gains during the last half of pregnancy have been inadequate. These risks exist even when the total gain for the pregnancy is in the recommended range.

The optimal rate of weight gain depends on the stage of pregnancy. During the first and second trimesters, growth takes place primarily in maternal tissues; during the third trimester, growth occurs primarily in fetal tissues. During the first trimester, the average total weight gain is only 1 to 2.5 kg; thereafter the recommended weight gain increases to approximately 0.4 kg per week for a woman of normal weight (see Fig. 15-2). The recommended weekly weight gain for overweight women during the second and third trimesters is 0.3 kg, and it is 0.5 kg for underweight women. The recommended caloric intake corresponds to this pattern of gain (see Table 15-1). There is no increment for the first trimester; an additional 300 kcal per day over the prepregnant intake is recommended during the second and third trimesters. The amount of food providing 300 kcal is not great. It can be provided by one additional serving from each of the following groups: milk, yogurt, or cheese (all skim milk products); fruits; vegetables; and bread, cereal, rice, or pasta.

The reasons for an inadequate weight gain (less than 1 kg per month for normal-weight women or less than 0.5 kg per

TABLE 15-2 **Body Mass Index**

BMI	HEIGHT IN INCHES 58	59	60	61	62	63	64	65	66	67	68	69	70	71	72	73	74	75	76
	BODY WEIGHT (POUNDS)																		
Normal																			
19	91	94	97	100	104	107	110	114	118	121	125	128	132	136	140	144	148	152	156
20	96	99	102	106	109	113	116	120	124	127	131	135	139	143	147	151	155	160	164
21	100	104	107	111	115	118	122	126	130	134	138	142	146	150	154	159	163	168	172
22	105	109	112	116	120	124	128	132	136	140	144	149	153	157	162	166	171	176	180
23	110	114	118	122	126	130	134	138	142	146	151	155	160	165	169	174	179	184	189
24	115	119	123	127	131	135	140	144	148	153	158	162	167	172	177	182	186	192	197
Overweight																			
25	119	124	128	132	136	141	145	150	155	159	164	169	174	179	184	189	194	200	205
26	124	128	133	137	142	146	151	156	161	166	171	176	181	186	191	197	202	208	213
27	129	133	138	143	147	152	157	162	167	172	177	182	188	196	199	204	210	216	221
28	134	138	143	148	153	158	163	168	173	178	184	189	195	200	206	212	218	224	230
29	138	143	148	153	158	163	169	174	179	185	190	196	202	208	213	219	225	232	238
Obese																			
30	143	148	153	158	164	169	174	180	186	191	197	203	209	215	221	227	233	240	246
31	148	153	158	164	169	175	180	186	192	198	203	209	216	222	228	235	241	248	254
32	153	158	163	169	175	180	186	192	198	204	210	216	222	229	235	242	249	256	263
33	158	163	168	174	180	186	192	198	204	211	216	223	229	236	242	250	256	264	271
34	162	168	174	180	186	191	197	204	210	217	223	230	236	243	250	257	264	272	279
35	167	173	179	185	191	197	204	210	216	223	230	236	243	250	258	265	272	279	287
36	172	178	184	190	196	203	209	216	223	230	236	243	250	257	265	272	280	287	295
37	177	183	189	195	202	208	215	222	229	236	243	250	257	265	272	280	287	295	304
38	181	188	194	201	207	214	221	228	235	242	249	257	264	272	279	288	295	303	312
39	186	193	199	206	213	220	227	234	241	249	256	263	271	279	287	295	303	311	320
Extreme Obesity																			
40	191	198	204	211	218	225	232	240	247	255	262	270	278	286	294	302	311	319	328
41	196	203	209	217	224	231	238	246	253	261	269	277	285	293	302	310	319	327	336
42	201	208	215	222	229	237	244	252	260	268	276	284	292	301	309	318	326	335	344
43	205	212	220	227	235	242	250	258	266	274	282	291	299	308	316	325	334	343	353
44	210	217	225	232	240	248	256	264	272	280	289	297	306	315	324	333	342	351	361
45	215	222	230	238	246	254	262	270	278	287	295	304	313	322	331	340	350	359	369
46	220	227	235	243	251	259	267	276	284	293	302	311	320	329	338	348	358	367	377
47	224	232	240	248	256	265	273	282	291	299	308	318	327	338	346	355	365	375	385
48	229	237	245	254	262	270	279	288	297	306	315	324	334	343	353	363	373	383	394
49	234	242	250	259	267	278	285	294	303	312	322	331	341	351	361	371	381	391	402
50	239	247	255	264	273	282	291	300	309	319	328	338	348	358	368	378	389	399	410
51	244	252	261	269	278	287	296	306	315	325	335	345	355	365	375	386	396	407	418
52	248	257	266	275	284	293	302	312	322	331	341	351	362	372	383	393	404	415	426
53	253	262	271	280	289	299	308	318	328	338	348	358	369	379	390	401	412	423	435
54	258	267	276	285	295	304	314	324	334	344	354	365	376	386	397	408	420	431	443

From the National Heart, Lung, and Blood Institute, Washington, D.C.
To use this table, find the appropriate height under the first row labeled "Height" and then find the weight closest to the person's weight on the rows below. The number in the first column is the BMI for that height and weight.

month for obese women during the last two trimesters) or excessive weight gain (more than 3 kg per month) should be thoroughly evaluated. Possible reasons for deviations from the expected rate of weight gain, besides inadequate or excessive dietary intake, include measurement or recording errors, differences in the weight of clothing, the time of day, and the accumulation of fluids. An exceptionally high gain is likely to result from the accumulation of fluids, and a gain of more than 3 kg in a month, especially after the twentieth week of gestation, often indicates the development of PIH.

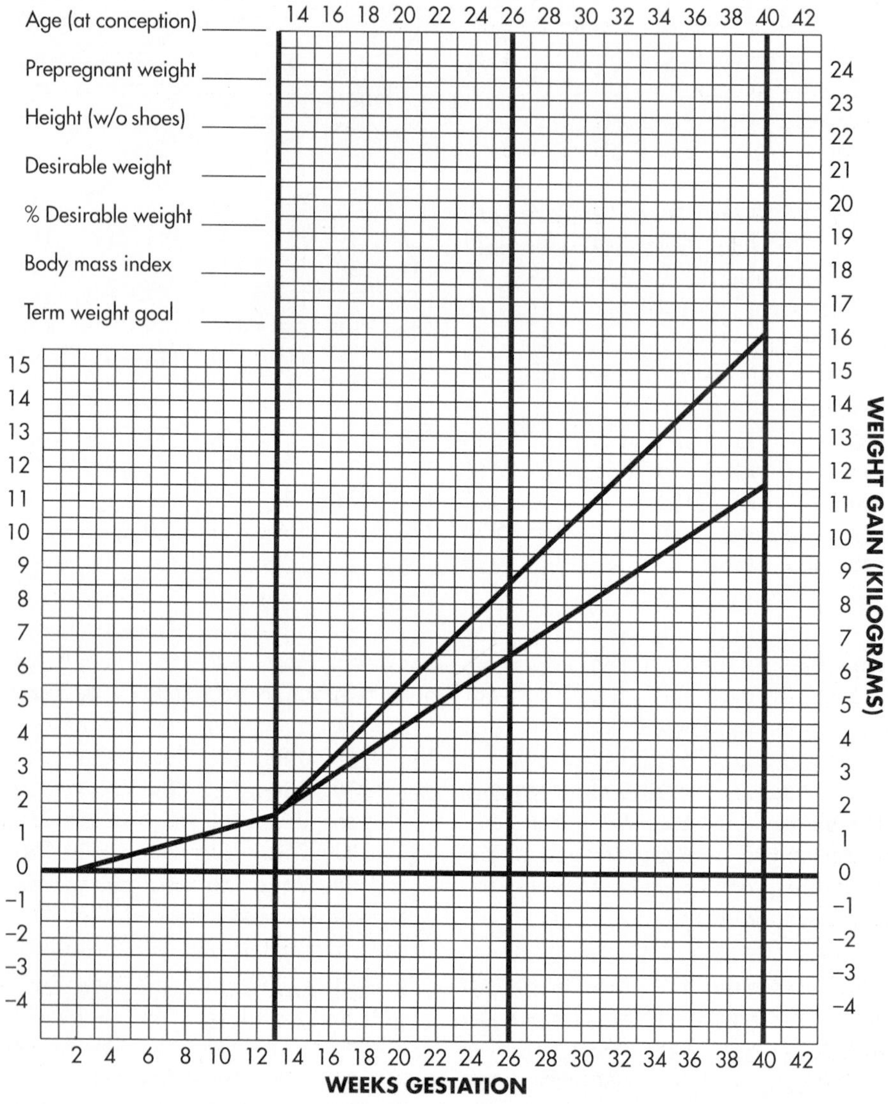
Age (at conception)
Prepregnant weight
Height (w/o shoes)
Desirable weight
% Desirable weight
Body mass index
Term weight goal
14 16 18 20 22 24 26 28 30 32 34 36 38 40 42
WEIGHT GAIN (KILOGRAMS)
2 4 6 8 10 12 14 16 18 20 22 24 26 28 30 32 34 36 38 40 42
WEEKS GESTATION

FIG. 15-2 Prenatal weight gain chart for plotting weight gain of normal weight women. *Note:* Young adolescents, African-American women, and smokers should aim for the upper end of the recommended range; short women (<157 cm or 5 feet 2 inches) should strive for gains at the lower end of the range.

Hazards of Restricting Adequate Weight Gain

An obsession with thinness and dieting pervades the North American culture. Figure-conscious women may find it difficult to make the transition from guarding against weight gain before pregnancy to valuing weight gain during pregnancy. In counseling these women, the nurse can emphasize the positive effects of good nutrition, as well as the adverse effects of maternal malnutrition (manifested by poor weight gain) on infant growth and development. This counseling includes information on the components of weight gain during pregnancy (Table 15-3) and the amount of this weight that will be lost after the birth. Because lactation can help to reduce maternal energy stores gradually, this also provides an opportunity to promote breastfeeding.

Pregnancy is not a time for a weight reduction diet. Even overweight or obese pregnant women need to gain at least enough weight to equal the weight of the products of conception (fetus, placenta, and amniotic fluid). If they limit their caloric intake to prevent weight gain, they also may excessively limit their intake of important nutrients. Moreover, dietary restriction results in the catabolism of fat stores, which in turn augments the production of ketones. The long-term effects of mild ketonemia during pregnancy are not known, but ketonuria has been found to be correlated with the occurrence of preterm labor. It should be stressed to obese women, and all pregnant women for that matter, that the quality of the weight gain is important, with emphasis placed on the consumption of nutrient-dense foods and the avoidance of empty-calorie foods.

Weight gain is important, but pregnancy is not an excuse for uncontrolled dietary indulgence. The old saying that the pregnant woman is "eating for two" should not be interpreted to mean that the food intake should be doubled. Instead the woman should place an emphasis on the quality of her food intake as she considers her needs and those of her fetus. Excessive weight gained during pregnancy may be difficult to lose after pregnancy, thus contributing to chronic overweight or obesity, an etiologic factor in a host of chronic diseases, including hypertension, diabetes mellitus, and arteriosclerotic heart disease. The woman who gains 18 kg or more is especially at risk.

Protein

Protein, with its essential constituent nitrogen, is the nutritional element basic to growth. An adequate protein intake is essential to meet increasing demands in pregnancy. These demands arise from the rapid growth of the fetus; enlargement of the uterus and its supporting structures, mammary glands, and placenta; increase in the maternal circulating blood volume and the subsequent demand for increased amounts of plasma protein to maintain colloidal osmotic pressure; and formation of amniotic fluid.

Milk, meat, eggs, and cheese are complete protein foods with a high biologic value. Legumes (dried beans and peas), whole grains, and nuts also are valuable sources of protein. In addition, these protein-rich foods are a source of other nutrients such as calcium, iron, and B vitamins; plant sources of protein often provide needed dietary fiber. The recommended daily food plan (Table 15-4) is a guide to the amounts of these foods that would supply the quantities of protein needed. The recommendations provide for only a modest increase in protein intake over the prepregnant levels in adult women. Protein intake in many people in the United States is relatively high, so many women may not need to increase their protein intake at all during pregnancy. Three servings of milk, yogurt, or cheese (four for adolescents) and two servings (5 to 6 ounces, 140 to 168 g) of meat, poultry, or fish would supply the recommended protein for the pregnant woman. Additional protein would be provided by vegetables and breads, cereals, rice, or pasta. Pregnant adolescents, women from impoverished backgrounds, and women adhering to unusual diets, such as a macrobiotic (highly restricted vegetarian) diet, are those whose protein intake is most likely to be inadequate. The use of high-protein supplements is not recommended, because they have been associated with an increased incidence of preterm births.

TABLE 15-3 **Tissues Contributing to Maternal Weight Gain at 40 Weeks of Gestation**

TISSUE	POUNDS
Fetus	7-8.5
Placenta	2-2.5
Amniotic fluid	2
Increase in uterine tissue	2
Breast tissue	1-4
Increased blood volume	4-5
Increased tissue fluid	3-5
Increased stores (fat)	4-6

Water

Essential during the exchange of nutrients and waste products across cell membranes, water is the main substance of cells, blood, lymph, amniotic fluid, and other vital body fluids. It also aids in maintaining body temperature. A good fluid intake promotes good bowel function, which is sometimes a problem during pregnancy. The recommended daily intake is about 6 to 8 glasses (1500 to 2000 ml) of fluid. Water, milk, and fruit juices are good sources. Dehydration may increase the risk of cramping, contractions, and preterm labor.

Women who consume more than 300 mg of caffeine daily (equivalent to about 500 to 750 ml of coffee) may be at increased risk of miscarriage and of giving birth to infants with IUGR. The ill effects of caffeine have been proposed to result from vasoconstriction of the blood vessels supplying the uterus or from interference with cell division in the developing fetus. Consequently, caffeine-containing products, including caffeinated coffee, tea, soft drinks, and cocoa beverages, should be avoided or consumed only in limited quantities.

Aspartame (Nutrasweet, Equal), acesulfame potassium (Sunett), and sucralose (Splenda), artificial sweeteners commonly used in low- or no-calorie beverages and low-calorie food products, have not been found to have adverse effects on the normal mother and fetus (Henkel, 1999). Aspartame, which contains phenylalanine, should be avoided by the mother with phenylketonuria (PKU), however.

Minerals and Vitamins

In general, the nutrient needs of pregnant women, with perhaps the exception of folate and iron, can be met through dietary sources. Counseling about the need for a varied diet rich in vitamins and minerals should be a part of the early prenatal care of every pregnant woman and should be reinforced throughout pregnancy. Supplements of certain nutrients (listed in the following discussion), however, are recommended whenever the woman's diet is

TABLE 15-4 **Daily Food Guide for Pregnancy and Lactation**

FOOD GROUP	SERVING SIZE	SUGGESTED NUMBER OF SERVINGS: NONPREGNANT, NONLACTATING WOMAN	PREGNANT WOMAN	LACTATING WOMAN
GRAIN PRODUCTS				
Include whole-grain and enriched breads, cereals, pasta, and rice.	1 slice bread; ½ bun, bagel, or English muffin; 1 oz ready-to-eat cereal; ½ c cooked grains	6-11	6-11	6-11
VEGETABLES				
Eat dark green leafy and deep yellow often. Eat dried beans and peas often; count ½ c cooked dried beans or peas as a serving of vegetables or 1 oz from meat group.	1 c raw leafy greens; ½ c of others	3-5	3-5	3-5
FRUITS				
Include citrus fruits, strawberries, or melons frequently.	1 medium apple, orange, banana, peach, etc; ½ c small or diced fruit; ¾ c juice	2-4	2-4	2-4
MILK AND MILK PRODUCTS	1 c milk or yogurt; 1½ oz cheese	2-3	3 or more	4 or more
MEAT, POULTRY, FISH, DRY BEANS, NUTS, AND EGGS				
Eat peanut butter or nuts rarely to avoid excessive fat intake. Limit egg intake to reduce cholesterol intake; trim fat from meat, and remove skin from poultry.	½ c cooked dried beans, 1 egg, or 1½ T peanut butter is equivalent to 1 oz of meat	Up to 6 oz total	Up to 6 oz total	Up to 6 oz total

c, Cup; *T*, tablespoon.

very poor or whenever significant nutritional risk factors are present. Nutritional risk factors in pregnancy are listed in Box 15-2.

Iron

Iron is needed both to allow transfer of adequate iron to the fetus and to permit expansion of the maternal RBC mass. Beginning in the latter part of the first trimester, the blood volume of the mother increases steadily, peaking at about 1500 ml more than that in the nonpregnant state. In twin gestations, the increase is at least 500 ml greater than that in pregnancies with single fetuses. Plasma volume increases more than RBC mass, with the difference between plasma and RBCs being greatest during the second trimester. The relative excess of plasma causes a modest decrease in the hemoglobin concentration and hematocrit, known as **physiologic anemia** of pregnancy. This is a normal adaptation during pregnancy.

However, poor iron nutriture, which can result in iron deficiency anemia, is relatively common among women in the childbearing years. It affects nearly one fifth of the pregnant women in industrialized countries. The maternal mortality rate is increased among anemic women, who are poorly prepared to tolerate hemorrhage at the time of birth. In addition, anemic women may have a greater likelihood of cardiac failure during labor, postpartum infections, and/or poor wound healing. The fetus also is affected by maternal anemia. The risk of preterm birth is about threefold greater in anemic women, and fetal iron stores also may be reduced by maternal anemia. In the United States, anemia is most common among adolescents, African-American women, and women of lower socioeconomic status (Siega-Riz et al., 2002; Swensen et al., 2001).

The Institute of Medicine (1992) recommended that all pregnant women receive a supplement of 30 mg of ferrous iron daily, starting by 12 weeks of gestation. (Iron supplements may be poorly tolerated during the nausea prevalent in the first trimester.) Some controversy exists about the value of iron supplementation in pregnancy (Haram et al., 2001; Mahomed, 2000; Scholl & Reilly, 2000). Although

BOX 15-2 Indicators of Nutritional Risk in Pregnancy

Adolescence
Frequent pregnancies: three within 2 years
Poor fetal outcome in a previous pregnancy
Poverty
Poor diet habits with resistance to change
Use of tobacco, alcohol, or drugs
Weight at conception under or over normal weight
Problems with weight gain
Any weight loss
Weight gain of <1 kg/mo after the first trimester
Weight gain of >1 kg/wk after the first trimester
Multifetal pregnancy
Low hemoglobin and/or hematocrit values

iron supplementation can improve maternal hematologic values, it is not clear that it improves pregnancy outcome. Nevertheless, some evidence suggests that maternal supplementation has beneficial effects on fetal iron stores, reducing the risk of anemia in the infant during the first year of life (Haram et al., 2001). If maternal iron-deficiency anemia is present (preferably diagnosed by measurement of serum ferritin, a storage form of iron), increased iron dosages (60 to 120 mg daily) are recommended. Certain foods taken with an iron supplement can promote or inhibit the absorption of iron from the supplement. See the Teaching for Self-Care box regarding iron supplementation. Even when a woman is taking an iron supplement, however, she also should include good food sources of iron in her daily diet (see Table 15-1).

Calcium

There is no increase in the DRI of calcium during pregnancy and lactation, in comparison to the recommendation for the nonpregnant woman (see Table 15-1). The DRI (1000 mg daily for women 19 years and older and 1300 mg for those younger than 19 years) appears to provide sufficient calcium for fetal bone and tooth development to proceed while maintaining maternal bone mass. Milk and yogurt are especially rich sources of calcium, providing approximately 300 mg per cup (240 ml). Nevertheless, many women do not consume these foods or do not consume adequate amounts to provide the recommended intakes of calcium. One problem that can interfere with milk consumption is **lactose intolerance**, which is the inability to digest milk sugar (lactose) because of the lack of the enzyme lactase in the small intestine. It is relatively common in adults, particularly African-Americans, Asians, Native Americans, and Inuits. Milk consumption may cause abdominal cramping, bloating, and diarrhea in such people, although many lactose-intolerant individuals can tolerate small amounts of milk without symptoms. Yogurt, sweet acidophilus

TEACHING FOR SELF-CARE

Iron Supplementation

- Vitamin C (in citrus fruits, tomatoes, melons, and strawberries) and heme iron (in meats) increase the absorption of iron supplement; therefore include these in the diet often.
- Bran, tea, coffee, milk, oxalates (in spinach and Swiss chard), and egg yolk decrease iron absorption. Avoid consuming them at the same time as the supplement.
- Iron is best absorbed if it is taken when the stomach is empty; that is, take it between meals with a beverage other than tea, coffee, or milk.
- Iron can be taken at bedtime if abdominal discomfort occurs when it is taken between meals.
- If an iron dose is missed, take it as soon as it is remembered if that is within 13 hours of the scheduled dose. Do not double up on the dose.
- Keep the supplement in a child-proof container and out of the reach of any children in the household.
- The iron may cause stools to be black or dark green.
- Constipation is common with iron supplementation. A diet high in fiber with adequate fluid intake is recommended.

milk, buttermilk, cheese, chocolate milk, and cocoa may be tolerated even when fresh fluid milk is not. Commercial products that contain lactase (e.g., Lactaid) are widely available, and many supermarkets stock lactase-treated milk. The lactase in these products hydrolyzes, or digests, the lactose in the milk, making it possible for lactose-intolerant people to drink milk.

In some cultures, it is uncommon for adults to drink milk. For example, Puerto Ricans and other Hispanic people may use it only as an additive in coffee. Pregnant women from these cultures may need to consume nondairy sources of calcium. Vegetarian diets also may be deficient in calcium (Box 15-3). If calcium intake appears low and the woman does not change her diet habits despite counseling, a supplement containing 600 mg of elemental calcium may be needed daily. Calcium supplements also may be recommended when a pregnant woman has leg cramps that are caused by an imbalance in the calcium-phosphorus ratio.

Sodium

During pregnancy, the need for sodium increases slightly, primarily because the body water is expanding (e.g., the expanding blood volume). Sodium is essential for maintaining body water balance. In the past, dietary sodium was routinely restricted in an effort to control the peripheral edema that commonly occurs during pregnancy. It is now recognized, however, that moderate peripheral edema is normal in pregnancy, occurring as a response to the fluid-retaining effects of elevated levels of estrogen. An excessive emphasis on sodium restriction also may make it difficult for pregnant women to achieve an adequate diet. Grain, milk, and meat products, which are good sources of

BOX 15-3 **Calcium Sources for Women Who Do Not Drink Milk**

Each of the following provides approximately the same amount of calcium as 1 cup of milk:

FISH
3-oz can of sardines
4½-oz can of salmon (if bones are eaten)

BEANS AND LEGUMES
3 c of cooked dried beans
2½ c of refried beans
2 c of baked beans with molasses
1 c of tofu (calcium added in processing)

GREENS
1 c of collards
1½ c of kale or turnip greens

BAKED PRODUCTS
3 pieces of cornbread
3 English muffins
4 slices of French toast
2 (7-inch diameter) waffles

FRUITS
11 dried figs
1⅛ c of orange juice with calcium added

SAUCES
3 oz of pesto sauce
5 oz of cheese sauce

the nutrients needed during pregnancy, are significant sources of sodium. In addition, sodium restriction may stress the adrenal glands and kidneys as they attempt to retain adequate sodium. In general, sodium restriction is necessary only if the woman has a medical condition such as renal or liver failure or hypertension.

Excessive intake of sodium is discouraged during pregnancy, just as it is in nonpregnant women, because it may contribute to abnormal fluid retention and edema. Table salt (sodium chloride) is the richest source of sodium. Most canned foods contain added salt, unless the label states otherwise. Large amounts of sodium also are found in many processed foods, including meats (e.g., smoked or cured meats, cold cuts, and corned beef), baked goods, mixes for casseroles or grain products, soups, and condiments. Products low in nutritive value and excessively high in sodium include pretzels, potato and other chips, pickles, catsup, prepared mustard, steak and Worcestershire sauces, some soft drinks, and bouillon. A moderate sodium intake can usually be achieved by salting food lightly during cooking, adding no additional salt at the table, and also by avoiding low-nutrient/high-sodium foods.

Zinc

Zinc is a constituent of numerous enzymes involved in major metabolic pathways. Zinc deficiency is associated with malformations of the central nervous system in infants. When large amounts of iron and folic acid are consumed, the absorption of zinc is inhibited, and the serum zinc levels are reduced as a result. Because iron and folic acid supplements are commonly prescribed during pregnancy, pregnant women should therefore be encouraged to consume good sources of zinc daily (see Table 15-1). Women with anemia who receive high-dose iron supplements also need supplements of zinc and copper (King, 2000).

Fluoride

There is no evidence that prenatal fluoride supplementation reduces the child's likelihood of tooth decay during the preschool years (Fluoride Recommendations Working Group, 2001). No increase in fluoride intake over the nonpregnant DRI is currently recommended during pregnancy.

Fat-Soluble Vitamins

Fat-soluble vitamins–A, D, E, and K–are stored in the body tissues; in the event of prolonged overdoses, these vitamins can reach toxic levels. Because of the high potential for toxicity, pregnant women are therefore advised to take fat-soluble vitamin supplements only as prescribed. Vitamins A and D deserve special mention, however.

Adequate intake of vitamin A is needed so that sufficient amounts of the vitamin can be stored in the fetus; however, dietary sources can readily supply sufficient amounts. Congenital malformations have occurred in infants of mothers who took excessive amounts of vitamin A during pregnancy, and thus supplements are not recommended for pregnant women (Institute of Medicine, 1992). Vitamin A analogues (e.g., isotretinoin [Accutane]), which are prescribed for the treatment of cystic acne, are a special concern. Isotretinoin use during early pregnancy has been associated with an increased incidence of heart malformations, facial abnormalities, cleft palate, hydrocephalus, and deafness and blindness in the infant, as well as an increased risk of miscarriage. Topical agents such as tretinoin (Retin-A) do not appear to enter the circulation in any substantial amounts, but their safety in pregnancy has not been confirmed.

Vitamin D plays an important role in the absorption and metabolism of calcium. The main food sources of this vitamin are enriched or fortified foods such as milk and ready-to-eat cereals. Vitamin D also is produced in the skin by the action of ultraviolet light (in sunlight). A severe deficiency may lead to neonatal hypocalcemia and tetany, as well as to hypoplasia of the tooth enamel. Women with lactose intolerance and those who do not include milk in their diet for any reason are at risk for vitamin D deficiency. Other risk factors for deficiency are dark skin, with African-American women being at high risk of deficiency; habitual use of clothing that covers most of the skin (e.g., Arab women with extensive body covering); and living in northern latitudes where sunlight exposure is limited, especially during the winter. Use of recommended amounts of sunscreen with an SPF rating of 15 reduces skin vitamin D production by as much as 99% (Scanlon, 2001), reinforcing the need for regular intake of fortified foods or a supplement.

Water-Soluble Vitamins

Body stores of water-soluble vitamins are much smaller than those of fat-soluble vitamins, and the water-soluble vitamins, in contrast to the fat-soluble ones, are readily excreted in the urine. Therefore good sources of these vitamins must be consumed frequently, and toxicity with overdose is less likely than it is in people taking fat-soluble vitamins.

Because of the increase in RBC production during pregnancy, as well as the nutritional requirements of the rapidly growing cells in the fetus and placenta, pregnant women should consume about 50% more folic acid than nonpregnant women, or about 0.6 mg (600 μg) daily. In the United States, all enriched grain products (which include most white breads, flour, and pasta) must contain folic acid at a level of 1.4 mg per kg flour. This level of fortification is designed to supply approximately 0.1 mg folic acid daily in the average American diet and has significantly increased folic acid consumption in the population as a whole (Boushey et al., 2001). All women of childbearing potential need careful counseling about including good sources of folate in their diets (see Box 15-1). Supplemental folic acid is usually prescribed to ensure that intake is adequate. Women who have borne a child with a neural tube defect are advised to consume 4 mg folic acid daily, and a supplement is required for them to achieve this level of intake.

Pyridoxine, or vitamin B_6, is involved in protein metabolism. Although levels of a pyridoxine-containing enzyme have been reported to be low in women with PIH, there is no evidence that supplementation prevents or eradicates the condition. No supplement is recommended routinely, but women with poor diets and those at nutritional risk (see Box 15-2) may need a supplement providing 2 mg/day (Institute of Medicine, 1992).

Vitamin C, or ascorbic acid, plays an important role in tissue formation and enhances the absorption of iron. The vitamin C needs of most women are readily met by a diet that includes at least one daily serving of citrus fruit or juice or another good source of the vitamin (see Table 15-1), but women who smoke need more. A supplement of 50 mg/day is recommended for women determined to be at nutritional risk (Institute of Medicine, 1992); however, if the mother should take excessive doses of this vitamin during pregnancy, vitamin C deficiency may develop in the infant after birth.

Multivitamin-Multimineral Supplements During Pregnancy

The consensus of the 1992 Institute of Medicine committee is that food can and should be the normal vehicle to meet the additional needs imposed by pregnancy, except for iron. Recall that a supplemental dose of 30 mg per day is recommended. In addition, the recommended folate intake may be difficult for some women to achieve. Some women habitually consume diets that are deficient in necessary nutrients and, for whatever reason, may be unable to change this intake. For these women, a multivitamin-multimineral supplement should be considered to ensure that they consume the RDA for most known vitamins and minerals. It is important that the pregnant woman understand that the use of a vitamin-mineral supplement does not lessen the need to consume a nutritious, well-balanced diet.

Pica and Food Cravings

Pica, which is the practice of consuming nonfood substances (e.g., clay, dirt, and laundry starch) or excessive amounts of foodstuffs low in nutritional value (e.g., ice or freezer frost, baking powder or soda, and cornstarch), often is influenced by the woman's cultural background (Fig. 15-3). In the United States, it appears to be most common among African-American women, women from rural areas, and women with a family history of pica. The regular and heavy consumption of low-nutrient products may cause more nutritious foods to be displaced from the diet, and the items consumed also may interfere with the absorption of nutrients, especially minerals. Women with pica have been found to have lower hemoglobin levels than do those without pica (Rainville, 1998). The possibility of pica must be considered when pregnant women are found to be anemic, and the nurse should provide counseling about the health risks associated with pica.

The existence of pica, as well as details of the types and amounts of products ingested, is likely to be discovered only by the sensitive interviewer who has developed a relationship of trust with the woman. It has been proposed that pica and **food cravings** (i.e., the urge to have ice cream, pickles, or pizza, for example) during pregnancy are caused by an innate drive to consume nutrients missing from the diet. However, research has not supported this hypothesis.

Adolescent Pregnancy Needs

Many adolescent females have diets that provide less than the recommended intakes of key nutrients, including energy, calcium, and iron. Pregnant adolescents and their infants are at increased risk of complications

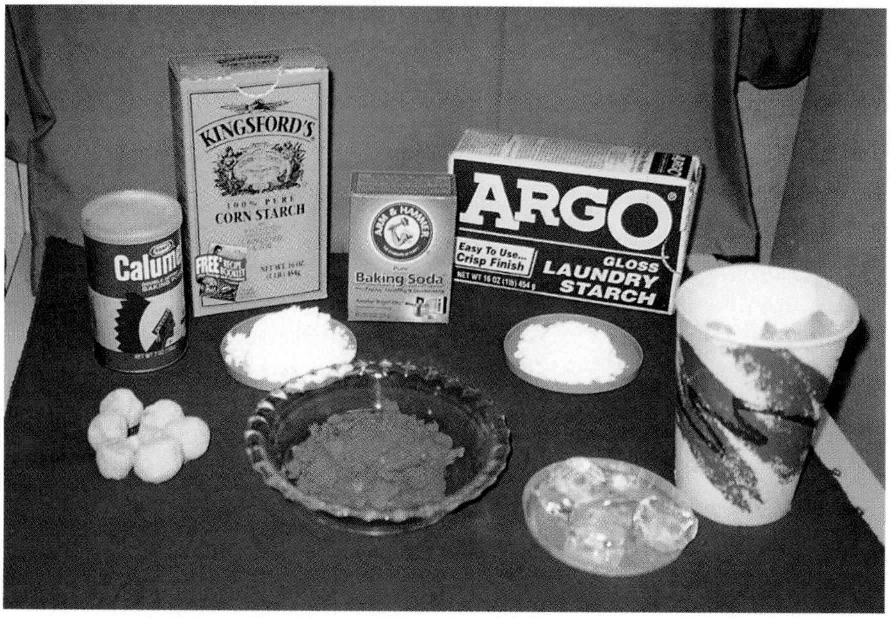
KINGSFORD'S
100% PURE CORN STARCH
Calum
Baking Soda
ARGO
Easy To Use... Crisp Finish
GLOSS LAUNDRY STARCH

FIG. 15-3 Nonfood substances consumed in pica: red clay from Georgia, Nzu from Eastern Nigeria, baking powder, corn starch, baking soda, laundry starch, and ice. Some individuals practice *poly-pica* (consuming more than one of these substances). (Courtesy Shannon Perry, San Jose, CA.)

during pregnancy and parturition. Growth of the pelvis is delayed in comparison to growth in stature, and this helps to explain why cephalopelvic disproportion and other mechanical problems associated with labor are common among young adolescents. Competition between the growing adolescent and the fetus for nutrients also may contribute to some of the poor outcomes apparent in teen pregnancies. Pregnant adolescents are encouraged to choose a weight-gain goal at the upper end of the range for their BMI (Institute of Medicine, 1992). The goal is to reduce the prevalence of LBW among infants of teen mothers. Adolescent pregnancy increases the woman's risk of obesity later in life (Gunderson et al., 2000; Hediger et al., 1997); thus the adolescent mother needs careful teaching regarding nutritional intake and physical activity to control body weight in the postpartum period.

Efforts to improve the nutritional health of pregnant adolescents focus on improving the nutrition knowledge, meal planning, and food preparation and selection skills of young women; promoting access to prenatal care; developing nutrition interventions and educational programs that are effective with adolescents; and striving to understand the factors that create barriers to change in the adolescent population.

Pregnancy-Induced Hypertension

The cause of PIH, or preeclampsia, is not known. There has been speculation that the poor intake of several nutrients, including calcium, magnesium, vitamin B_6, and protein, might foster its development, but there is no definite evidence that nutritional deficiencies are causes or that nutritional supplements can help prevent it. At present, a diet adequate in the recommended nutrients (see Table 15-1) appears to be the best means of reducing the risk of PIH.

Exercise During Pregnancy

Moderate exercise during pregnancy yields numerous benefits, including improving muscle tone, potentially shortening the course of labor, and promoting a sense of well-being. If no medical or obstetric problems contraindicate physical activity, pregnant women should obtain 30 minutes of moderate physical exercise on most, if not all, days of the week (American College of Obstetricians and Gynecologists, 2002). Two nutritional concepts are especially important for women who choose to exercise during pregnancy. First, a liberal amount of fluid should be consumed before, during, and after exercise because dehydration can trigger premature labor. Second, the calorie intake should be sufficient to meet the increased needs of pregnancy and the demands of exercise.

NUTRIENT NEEDS DURING LACTATION

Nutritional needs during lactation are similar in many ways to those during pregnancy (see Table 15-1). Needs for energy (calories), protein, calcium, iodine, zinc, the B vitamins (thiamin, riboflavin, niacin, pyridoxine, and vitamin B_{12}), and vitamin C remain greater than nonpregnant needs. The recommendations for some of these (e.g., vitamin C, zinc, and protein) are slightly to moderately higher than those during pregnancy (see Table 15-1). This allowance covers the amount of the nutrient released in the milk, as well as needs of the mother for tissue maintenance. In the case of iron and folic acid, the recommendation during lactation is lower than that during pregnancy. Both of these nutrients are essential for RBC formation and thus for maintaining the increase in the blood volume that occurs during pregnancy. With the decrease in maternal blood volume to nonpregnant levels after birth, maternal iron and folic acid needs also decrease. Many lactating women have a delay in the return of menses, and this also conserves blood cells and reduces iron and folic acid needs. It is especially important that the calcium intake be adequate; if it is not and the woman does not respond to diet counseling, a supplement of 600 mg of calcium per day may be needed.

The recommended energy intake is an increase of 500 kcal more than the woman's nonpregnant intake. The Institute of Medicine (1992) recommends that lactating women consume at least 1800 kcal per day, because it becomes difficult to obtain adequate nutrients for the maintenance of lactation at levels less than that. Because of the deposition of energy stores, the woman who has gained the optimal amount of weight during pregnancy is heavier after birth than at the beginning of pregnancy. As a result of the caloric demands of lactation, however, the lactating mother usually has a gradual but steady weight loss. Most women rapidly lose several pounds during the first month after birth, whether they breastfeed or not. After the first month, the average loss during lactation is 0.5 to 1.0 kg per month, and a woman who is overweight may be able to lose up to 2 kg without decreasing her milk supply (Institute of Medicine, 1992).

Fluid intake also must be adequate to maintain milk production, but the mother's level of thirst is the best guide to the right amount. There is no need to consume more fluids than those needed to satisfy thirst.

Smoking and alcohol and excessive caffeine intake should be avoided during lactation. Smoking not only may impair milk production, but it also exposes the infant to the risk of passive smoking. It is speculated that the infant's psychomotor development may be affected by maternal alcohol use, and alcoholic beverages (two drinks per day) may impair the milk ejection reflex. Coffee intake may lead to a reduced iron concentration in milk and consequently contribute to the development of anemia in the infant. The caffeine concentration in milk is only approximately 1% of the mother's plasma level, but caffeine seems to accumulate in the infant. Breastfed infants of mothers who drink large amounts of coffee or caffeine-containing soft drinks may be unusually active and wakeful.

CARE MANAGEMENT

During pregnancy, nutrition plays a key role in achieving an optimal outcome for the mother and her unborn baby. The motivation to learn about nutrition is usually greater during pregnancy because parents strive to "do what's right for the baby." Optimal nutrition cannot eliminate all the problems that may arise during pregnancy, but it does establish a good foundation for supporting the needs of the mother and her unborn baby.

Assessment and Nursing Diagnoses

Assessment is based on a **diet history** (a description of the woman's usual food and beverage intake and factors affecting her nutritional status, such as medications being taken and the adequacy of income to allow her to purchase the necessary foods) obtained from an interview and review of the woman's health records, physical examination, and laboratory results. Ideally a nutritional assessment is performed before conception so that any recommended changes in diet, lifestyle, and weight can be undertaken before the woman becomes pregnant.

Diet History

Obstetric and Gynecologic Effects on Nutrition. Nutritional reserves may be depleted in the multiparous woman or in the one who has had frequent pregnancies (especially three pregnancies within 2 years). A history of preterm birth or birth of an LBW or SGA infant may indicate inadequate dietary intake. PIH also may be a factor in poor maternal nutrition. Birth of a large-for-gestational age (LGA) infant may indicate the existence of maternal diabetes mellitus. Previous contraceptive methods also may affect reproductive health. Increased menstrual blood loss often occurs during the first 3 to 6 months after placement of an intrauterine contraceptive device; consequently the user may have low iron stores or even iron deficiency anemia. Oral contraceptive agents conversely are associated with decreased menstrual losses and increased iron stores; however, oral contraceptives may interfere with folic acid metabolism.

Medical History. Chronic maternal illnesses such as diabetes mellitus, renal disease, liver disease, cystic fibrosis or other malabsorptive disorders, seizure disorders and the use of anticonvulsant agents, hypertension, and PKU may affect a woman's nutritional status and dietary needs. In women with illnesses that have resulted in nutritional deficits or that require dietary treatment (e.g., diabetes mellitus or PKU), it is extremely important for nutritional care to be started and for the condition to be optimally controlled before conception. The registered dietitian can provide in-depth counseling for the woman who requires a therapeutic diet during pregnancy and lactation.

Usual Maternal Diet. The woman's usual food and beverage intake, the adequacy of her income and other resources to meet her nutritional needs, any dietary modifications, food allergies and intolerances, and all medications and nutrition supplements being taken, as well as pica and cultural dietary requirements, should be ascertained. In addition, the presence and severity of nutrition-related discomforts of pregnancy, such as morning sickness, constipation, and pyrosis (heartburn), should be determined. The nurse should be alert to any evidence of eating disorders such as anorexia nervosa, bulimia, and frequent and rigorous dieting before or during pregnancy.

The impact of food allergies and intolerances on nutritional status ranges from very important to almost nil. Lactose intolerance is of special concern in pregnant and lactating women because no other food group equals milk and milk products in terms of calcium content. If a woman has lactose intolerance, the interviewer should explore her intake of other calcium sources (see Box 15-3).

The assessment must include an evaluation of the woman's financial status and her knowledge of sound dietary practices. The quality of the diet improves with increasing socioeconomic status and educational level. Poor women may not have access to adequate refrigeration and cooking facilities and may find it difficult to obtain adequate nutritious food. The pregnancy rates are high among homeless women, and many such women cannot or do not take advantage of services such as food stamps.

Box 15-4 provides a simple tool for obtaining diet history information. When potential problems are identified, they should be followed up with a careful interview.

Physical Examination

Anthropometric (body) **measurements** provide short- and long-term information on a woman's nutritional status and are thus essential to the assessment. At a minimum, the woman's height and weight must be determined at the time of her first prenatal visit, and her weight should be measured at every subsequent visit (see earlier discussion of BMI).

A careful physical examination can reveal objective signs of malnutrition (Table 15-5). It is important to note, however, that some of these signs are nonspecific, and the physiologic changes of pregnancy may complicate the interpretation of physical findings. For example, lower-extremity edema often occurs when caloric and protein deficiencies are present, but it also may be a normal finding in the third trimester. The interpretation of physical findings is made easier by a thorough health history and by laboratory testing, if indicated.

Laboratory Testing

The only nutrition-related laboratory test necessary for most pregnant women is a hematocrit or hemoglobin measurement to screen for the presence of **anemia.** Because of the physiologic anemia of pregnancy, the reference values for hemoglobin and hematocrit must be adjusted during pregnancy. The lower limit of the normal range for hemoglobin during pregnancy is 11 g/dl in the first and third trimesters and 10.5 g/dl in the second trimester (compared with 12 g/dl in the nonpregnant state). The lower limit of the normal range for hematocrit is 33% during the first and third trimesters and 32% in the second trimester (compared with 36% in the nonpregnant state). Cutoff values for anemia are higher in women who smoke or live at high altitudes, because the decreased oxygen-carrying capacity of their RBCs causes them to produce more RBCs than other women (Institute of Medicine, 1992).

A woman's history or physical findings may indicate the need for additional testing, such as a complete blood cell count with a differential to identify megaloblastic or macrocytic anemia and the measurement of levels of specific vitamins or minerals believed to be lacking in the diet. The assessment gives a basis for making appropriate nursing diagnoses, such as the following:

- *Imbalanced nutrition: less than body requirements related to*
  - –inadequate information about nutritional needs and weight gain during pregnancy
  - –misperceptions regarding normal body changes during pregnancy and inappropriate fear of becoming fat
  - –inadequate income or skills in meal planning and preparation
- *Imbalanced nutrition: more than body requirements related to*
  - –excessive intake of energy (calories) or decrease in activity during pregnancy
  - –use of unnecessary dietary supplements, especially supplements of fat-soluble vitamins, protein (if diet is adequate in protein), and therapeutic amounts of iron (in the absence of iron-deficiency anemia)
- *Constipation related to*
  - –decrease in gastrointestinal (GI) motility because of elevated progesterone levels
  - –compression of intestines by enlarging uterus
  - –oral iron supplementation
- *Deficient knowledge related to*
  - –inadequate information regarding nutritional needs during pregnancy

Expected Outcomes of Care

An individualized nursing plan of care based on the nursing diagnoses should be developed in collaboration with the woman. For many women with uncomplicated pregnancies, the nurse can serve as the primary source of nutrition education during pregnancy. The registered dietitian, who has specialized training in diet evaluation and planning, nutritional needs during illness, and ethnic and cultural food patterns, as well as in translating nutrient needs into food patterns, frequently serves as a consultant. Pregnant women with serious nutritional problems, those with intervening illnesses such as diabetes (either preexisting or gestational), and any others requiring in-depth dietary

BOX 15-4 Food Intake Questionnaire

Which of the following did you eat or drink yesterday? If the way you ate yesterday wasn't the way you usually eat, choose a recent day that was typical for you.

FOOD OR DRINK	NUMBER OF SERVINGS	FOOD OR DRINK	NUMBER OF SERVINGS
Beer, wine, other alcoholic drinks		Orange or grapefruit juice	
Tea		Fruit juice other than orange or grapefruit	
Coffee		Soft drinks	
Fruit drink		Milk	
Water		Cereal with milk	
Cheese		Yogurt	
Macaroni and cheese		Pizza	
Other foods with cheese (such as lasagna, enchiladas, cheeseburgers)		Melon (such as watermelon, cantaloupe, honeydew)	
Orange or grapefruit		Berries (kind ___________)	
Bananas		Apples	
Peaches or apricots		Other fruit	
Green salad		Broccoli	
Spinach or greens		Green beans	
Green peas		Potatoes (other than fried)	
Sweet potatoes		Corn	
Carrots		Other vegetables	
Meat		Chicken or turkey	
Fish		Egg	
Peanut butter		Nuts	
Dried beans or peas		Hot dog	
Bacon or sausage		Cold cuts	
Bread		Roll	
Rice		Cereal	
Spaghetti or other pasta		Noodles	
Tortillas		Chips	
French fries		Cake	
Cookie		Donut or pastry	
Pie			

Are you often bothered by any of the following? (Circle all that apply.)
Nausea Vomiting Heartburn Constipation
Are you on a special diet? No____ Yes____ If yes, what kind?
Do you try to limit the amount or kind of food you eat to control your weight? No____ Yes____
Do you avoid any foods for health or religious reasons? No____ Yes____ If yes, what foods?
Do you take any prescribed drugs or medications? No____ Yes____
If yes, what are they?
Do you take any over-the-counter medications (such as aspirin, cold medicines, Tylenol)?
No____ Yes____ If yes, what are they?
Do you ever have trouble affording the food you need? No____ Yes____
Do you have any help getting the food you need? No____ Yes____ (Circle all that apply.)
Food stamps WIC School lunch or breakfast
Food from a food pantry, soup kitchen, or food bank

TABLE 15-5 **Physical Assessment of Nutritional Status**

SIGNS OF GOOD NUTRITION	SIGNS OF POOR NUTRITION
General Appearance	
Alert, responsive, energetic, good endurance	Listless, apathetic, cachectic, easily fatigued, looks tired
Muscles	
Well developed, firm, good tone, some fat under skin	Flaccid, poor tone, tender, "wasted" appearance
Gastrointestinal Function	
Good appetite and digestion, normal regular elimination, no palpable organs or masses	Anorexia, indigestion, constipation or diarrhea, liver or spleen enlargement
Cardiovascular Function	
Normal heart rate and rhythm, no murmurs, normal blood pressure for age	Rapid heart rate, enlarged heart, abnormal rhythm, elevated blood pressure
Hair	
Shiny, lustrous, firm, not easily plucked, healthy scalp	Stringy, dull, brittle, dry, thin and sparse, depigmented, can be easily plucked
Skin (General)	
Smooth, slightly moist, good color	Rough, dry, scaly, pale, pigmented, irritated, easily bruised, petechiae
Face and Neck	
Skin color uniform, smooth, pink, healthy appearance; no enlargement of thyroid gland; lips not chapped or swollen	Scaly, swollen, skin dark over cheeks and under eyes, lumpiness or flakiness of skin around nose and mouth; thyroid enlarged; lips swollen, angular lesions or fissures at corners of mouth
Oral Cavity	
Reddish pink mucous membranes and gums; no swelling or bleeding of gums; tongue healthy pink or deep reddish in appearance, not swollen or smooth, surface papillae present; teeth bright and clean, no cavities, no pain, no discoloration	Gums spongy, bleed easily, inflamed or receding; tongue swollen, scarlet and raw, magenta color, beefy, hyperemic and hypertrophic papillae, atrophic papillae; teeth with unfilled caries, absent teeth, worn surfaces, mottled
Eyes	
Bright, clear, shiny, no sores at corners of eyelids, membranes moist and healthy pink color, no prominent blood vessels or mound of tissue (Bitot's spots) on sclera, no fatigue circles beneath	Eye membranes pale, redness of membrane, dryness, signs of infection, redness and fissuring of eyelid corners, dryness of eye membrane, dull appearance of cornea, blue sclerae
Extremities	
No tenderness, weakness, or swelling; nails firm and pink	Edema, tender calves, tingling, weakness; nails spoon-shaped, brittle
Skeleton	
No malformations	Bowlegs, knock-knees, chest deformity at diaphragm, beaded ribs, prominent scapulas

counseling should be referred to the dietitian. The nurse, dietitian, physician, and nurse-midwife collaborate in helping the woman achieve nutrition-related expected outcomes. Some common nutrition-related outcomes require the woman to take the following actions:

- Achieve an appropriate weight gain during pregnancy—an appropriate goal for weight gain takes into account such factors as the woman's prepregnancy weight, whether she is overweight/obese or underweight, and whether the pregnancy is single or multifetal.

- Consume adequate nutrients from the diet and supplements to meet estimated needs.
- Cope successfully with the nutrition-related discomforts associated with pregnancy, such as pyrosis (heartburn), morning sickness, and constipation.
- Avoid or reduce potentially harmful practices such as smoking, alcohol consumption, and caffeine intake.
- Return to prepregnancy weight (or an appropriate weight for height) within 6 months of giving birth.

Plan of Care and Interventions

Nutritional care and teaching generally involve (1) acquainting the woman with the nutritional needs during pregnancy and the characteristics of an adequate diet, if necessary; (2) helping her to individualize her diet so that she achieves an adequate intake while conforming to her personal, cultural, financial, and health circumstances; (3) acquainting her with strategies for coping with the nutrition-related discomforts of pregnancy; (4) helping her use nutrition supplements appropriately; and (5) consulting with and making referrals to other professionals or services as indicated. Two programs that provide nutrition services are the food stamp program and the Special Supplemental Program for **Women, Infants, and Children (WIC),** which provides vouchers for selected foods to pregnant and lactating women, as well as infants and children at nutritional risk. WIC foods include eggs, cheese, milk, juice, and fortified cereals; these are chosen because they provide iron, protein, vitamin C, and other vitamins.

Adequate Dietary Intake

Diet teaching can take place in a one-on-one interview or in a group setting. In either case, teaching should emphasize the importance of choosing a varied diet composed of readily available foods (rather than specialized diet supplements). Good nutrition practices (and the avoidance of poor practices such as smoking and alcohol or drug use) are essential content for prenatal classes designed for women in early pregnancy (see Guidelines/Guías box).

The food pyramid (Fig. 15-4) can be used as a guide to making daily food choices during pregnancy and lactation, just as it is during other stages of the life cycle. The pyramid places the bread, cereal, rice, and pasta group at its base. This position was chosen to indicate that this group should serve as the basis for a healthy diet; six to eleven servings are recommended each day. Vegetables (three to five servings) and fruits (two to four servings) are just above the grains group. The milk, yogurt, and cheese group (two to three servings for nonpregnant adults, increasing to three to four servings for pregnant and lactating women) and the meat, poultry, fish, dried beans, eggs, and nuts group (two to three servings) form a narrow band near the top of the pyramid. At the apex are fats, oils, and sweets (not considered a food group), which are to be used sparingly. The importance of consuming adequate amounts from the milk, yogurt, and cheese group needs to be emphasized, especially for adolescents and women younger than 25 years who are still actively adding calcium to their skeletons; adolescents need at least 1 L of milk or the equivalent daily.

Pregnancy. The pregnant woman must understand what an adequate weight gain during pregnancy means, recognize the reasons for its importance, and be able to evaluate her own gain in terms of the desirable pattern (see Research box). Many women, particularly those who have worked hard to control their weight before pregnancy, may find it difficult to understand the reason the weight gain goal is so high when a newborn is so small. The nurse can explain that the maternal weight gain consists of increments in the weight of many tissues, not just the growing fetus (see Table 15-3).

Dietary overindulgence, conversely, which may result in excessive fat stores that persist after giving birth, should be discouraged. Nevertheless, it is best not to focus unduly on weight gain, which can result in feelings of stress and guilt in the woman who does not observe the preferred

GUIDELINES/GUÍAS

Diet and Nutrition

You need to gain weight
Usted necesita aumentar de peso.

You need to control your weight gain.
Usted necesita controlar su aumento de peso.

Eat nutritious foods.
Coma alimentos nutritivos.

Eat foods high in protein, calcium, vitamins, and iron.
Coma alimentos altos en proteínas, calcio, vitaminas, y hierro.

Eat a lot of fruits and vegetables.
Coma muchas frutas y vegetales.

Drink four glasses of milk a day.
Tome cuatro vasos de leche diariamente.

Drink low-fat instead of whole milk.
Tome la leche baja en grasa en lugar de la leche completa.

Avoid salty foods like sausage, hot dogs, and french fries.
Evite alimentos muy salados como salchichón, salchichas, y papitas fritas.

Avoid fried foods.
Evita las frituras.

Avoid caffeine.
Evita la cafeína.

There is caffeine in Coca-Cola, tea, and chocolate.
Hay cafeína en la Coca-Cola, té, y el chocolate.

Take prenatal vitamins.
Tome vitaminas prenatales.

pattern of gain. Teaching regarding weight gain during pregnancy is summarized in the Box 15-5.

Postpartum. The need for a varied diet consisting of a representation of foods from all the food groups continues throughout lactation. As mentioned previously, the lactating woman should be advised to consume at least 1800 kcal daily, and she should receive counseling if her diet appears to be inadequate in any nutrients. Special attention should be given to her zinc, vitamin B_6, and folic acid intake, because the recommendations for these remain higher than those for nonpregnant women (see Table 15-1). Sufficient calcium is needed to allow for both milk formation and

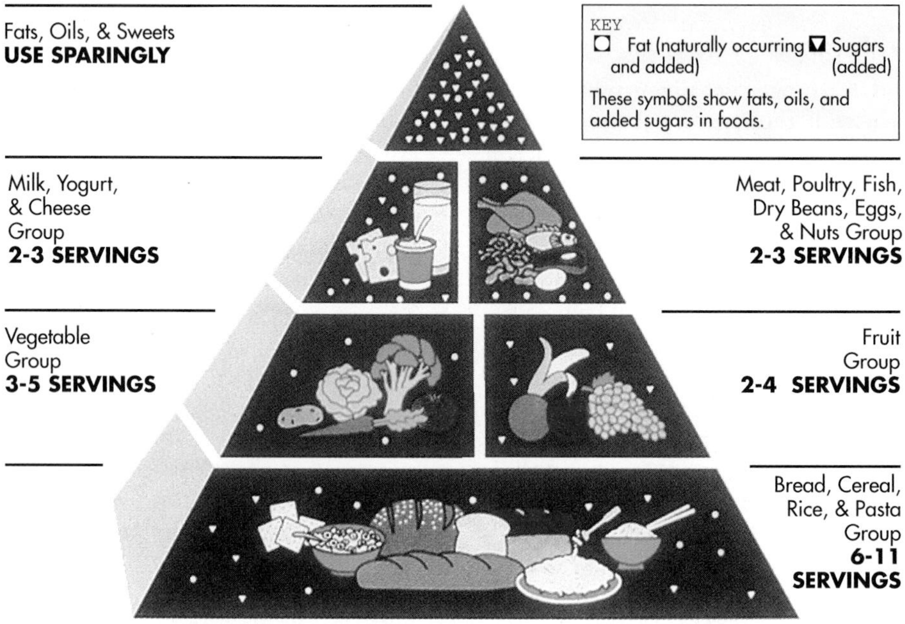
Fats, Oils, & Sweets
USE SPARINGLY
KEY
Fat (naturally occurring and added)
Sugars (added)
These symbols show fats, oils, and added sugars in foods.
Milk, Yogurt, & Cheese Group
2-3 SERVINGS
Meat, Poultry, Fish, Dry Beans, Eggs, & Nuts Group
2-3 SERVINGS
Vegetable Group
3-5 SERVINGS
Fruit Group
2-4 SERVINGS
Bread, Cereal, Rice, & Pasta Group
6-11 SERVINGS

FIG. 15-4 Food guide pyramid, a guide to daily food choices. (Courtesy U.S. Department of Agriculture, Washington, D.C.)

RESEARCH

Climbing the Food Pyramid: Pregnant Women's Dietary Knowledge and Practice

Nutritional intake during pregnancy has a direct affect on fetal well-being and birth outcome. Inadequate nutritional intake is associated with premature birth, low birth weight, and congenital anomalies, such as neural tube defects in the absence of adequate folic acid. Inadequate fluids (<8 glasses/day) put women at risk for oligohydramnios. Nutritional deficits for essential nutrients can occur with excessive intake. Excessive nutritional intake is linked with fetal macrosomia, leading to difficult birth, postpartum obesity, and neonatal hypoglycemia.

To describe what pregnant women know about nutrition in comparison to what they eat and how much weight they gain, a nurse researcher studied 109 pregnant women. The women were recruited from a free clinic run by a certified nurse-midwife for low-income women and a childbirth class composed of middle-class private physician clients. A questionnaire was used to test knowledge of the food groups and portions as listed in the Food Pyramid. The answers were compared with a 2-day diet recall that was analyzed for nutritianl content. Most of the women had poor nutritional knowledge, although women attending the free clinic had more accurate knowledge of nutrition attributed to the ongoing counseling of the nurse-midwife than the childbirth class women who got nutritional information only at their first physician visit. The clinic group tended to consume more bread, meat, and milk, and they had lower-quality protein than the childbirth class group. All the women needed more vitamin D, folate, calcium, iron, and phosphorus in their diets. Overweight women tended to gain more weight, while women with a low body mass index did not gain enough weight.

IMPLICATIONS FOR PRACTICE

Nurses can assess and counsel their clients throughout pregnancy about diet, emphasizing the Food Pyramid. Increasing fruits, vegetables, and water benefits all clients, especially pregnant women. Pregnancy can provide some women motivation to learn proper nutrition, which can lead to lasting lifetime improvement.

Reference: Fowles, E. (2002). Comparing pregnant women's nutritional knowledge to their actual diet intake. *MCN American Journal of Maternal Child Nursing, 27*(3), 171-177.

maintenance of maternal bone mass. It may be difficult for lactating women to consume enough of these nutrients without careful diet planning.

The woman who does not breastfeed will lose weight gradually if she consumes a balanced diet that provides slightly less than her daily energy expenditure. Lactating and nonlactating women should know that fat is the most concentrated source of calories in the diet (9 kcal/g versus 4 kcal/g in carbohydrates and proteins). Therefore the first step in weight reduction (or preventing excessive weight gain) is to evaluate the sources of fat in the diet and explore with the woman ways of reducing them. Even foods such as vegetables that are originally low in fat can become high in fat when fried or sautéed, served with excessive amounts of salad dressing, consumed with high-fat dips or sauces, or seasoned with butter or bacon drippings. A reasonable weight loss goal for nonlactating women is 0.5 to 1 kg per week; a loss of 1 kg per month is recommended for most lactating women.

Daily Food Guide and Menu Planning. The daily food plan (see Table 15-4 and Fig. 15-4) can be used as a guide for educating the woman about nutritional needs during pregnancy and lactation. This food plan is general enough to be used by women from a wide variety of cultures, including women following a vegetarian diet. One of the more helpful teaching strategies is to help the woman plan daily menus that follow the food plan and are affordable, are realistic in terms of preparation time, and are compatible with personal preferences and cultural practices. Information regarding cultural food patterns is provided later in this chapter.

Medical Nutrition Therapy. During pregnancy and lactation, the food plan for women receiving special medical nutrition therapy (therapeutic diets) may have to be modified. The registered dietitian can instruct these women about their diets and assist them in meal planning. However, the nurse should understand the basic principles of the diet and be able to reinforce the diet teaching.

The nurse should be especially aware of the dietary modifications necessary for women with diabetes mellitus (gestational or preexisting) because this disease is relatively common and because fetal deformity and death occur more often in pregnancies complicated by hyperglycemia or hypoglycemia. Every effort should be made to maintain blood glucose levels in the normal range throughout pregnancy. The food plan of the woman with diabetes usually includes four to six meals and snacks daily, with the daily carbohydrate intake distributed fairly evenly among the meals and snacks. The complex carbohydrates–fibers and starches–should be well represented in the diet. A diet plan with no more than approximately 40% of energy derived from carbohydrates has been used successfully in maintaining good blood glucose control during pregnancy. To maintain strict control of the blood glucose level, the pregnant woman with diabetes usually must monitor her own blood glucose daily (American Diabetes Association, 2002). Urine glucose and ketone measurements are not sensitive enough to detect hyperglycemia accurately and provide no information about hypoglycemia. The nurse must therefore teach the woman the way to monitor her own blood glucose level, unless she has already been doing this before pregnancy (see Chapter 32).

Counseling About Iron Supplementation. As mentioned earlier, the nutritional supplement most commonly needed during pregnancy is iron; however, a variety of dietary factors can affect the completeness of absorption of an iron supplement. Bran, milk, egg yolks, coffee, tea, or oxalate-containing vegetables such as spinach and Swiss chard consumed at the same time as iron will inhibit iron absorption. Conversely, iron absorption is promoted by a diet rich in vitamin C (e.g., citrus fruits or melons) or "heme iron" (found in red meats, fish, and poultry). Iron supplements are best absorbed on an empty stomach; thus they can be taken between meals with beverages other than milk, tea, or coffee. Some women have gastrointestinal discomfort when they take the supplement on an empty stomach; therefore a good time for them to take the supplement is just before bedtime. Constipation is common with iron supplementation. Iron supplements should be kept away from any children in the household because their ingestion could result in acute iron poisoning and even death. The Teaching for Self-Care box on p. 379 summarizes important points regarding iron supplementation.

Coping with Nutrition-Related Discomforts of Pregnancy

The most common nutrition-related discomforts of pregnancy are nausea and vomiting or "morning sickness," constipation, and pyrosis.

BOX 15-5 Weight Gain During Pregnancy

- Progressive weight gain during pregnancy is essential to ensure normal fetal growth and development and the deposition of maternal stores that promote successful lactation.
- Recommended weight gain during pregnancy is determined largely by prepregnancy weight for height: Normal-weight women, 11.5-16 kg; underweight women, 12.5-18 kg; overweight women, 7-11.5 kg.
- Weight gain should be achieved through a balanced diet of regular foods chosen from all the different food groups (see Table 15-4).
- The pattern of weight gain is important: approximately 0.4 kg per week during the second and third trimesters for normal-weight women; 0.5 kg per week for underweight women; and 0.3 kg per week for overweight women.

Nausea and Vomiting. Nausea and vomiting are most common during the first trimester. Most of the time the nausea and vomiting cause only mild to moderate problems nutritionally, although they may be a source of substantial discomfort. Antiemetic medications, vitamin B_6, and P6 acupressure may be effective in reducing the severity of nausea (Jewell & Young, 2000). In addition, the pregnant woman may find the following suggestions helpful in alleviating the problems:

- Eat dry, starchy foods such as dry toast, melba toast, or crackers on awakening in the morning and at other times when nausea occurs.
- Avoid consuming excessive amounts of fluids early in the day or when nauseated (but compensate by drinking fluids at other times).
- Eat small amounts frequently (every 2 to 3 hours) and avoid large meals that distend the stomach.
- Avoid skipping meals and thus becoming extremely hungry, which may worsen nausea. Have a snack such as cereal with milk, a small sandwich, or yogurt before bedtime.
- Avoid sudden movements. Get out of bed slowly.
- Decrease intake of fried and other fatty foods. Good choices are starches, such as pastas, rice, and breads, and low-fat protein foods (skinless broiled or baked poultry, cooked dried beans or peas, lean meats, and broiled or canned fish).
- Breathe fresh air to help relieve nausea. Keep the environment well ventilated (e.g., open a window), go for a walk outside, or decrease cooking odors by using an exhaust fan.
- Eat foods served at cool temperatures and foods that give off little aroma.
- Avoid brushing teeth immediately after eating.
- Try salty and tart foods (e.g., potato chips and lemonade) during periods of nausea.
- Try herbal teas such as those made with raspberry leaf or peppermint to decrease nausea.

Hyperemesis gravidarum, or severe and persistent vomiting causing weight loss, dehydration, and electrolyte abnormalities, occurs in up to approximately 1% of pregnant women. Intravenous fluid and electrolyte replacement is usually necessary for those women who lose 5% of their body weight. Often this is followed by improved tolerance to the oral intake of food; therapy then consists of the frequent consumption of small amounts of low-fat foods. Enteral tube feeding by means of small-bore nasogastric tubes has been successful in some women. Because the pulmonary aspiration of the feeding is a potential complication if vomiting occurs, antiemetic medications are sometimes administered in conjunction with the tube feedings. Tube feedings may be used to supplement oral intake, with the volume of the tube feeding gradually being decreased as oral intake improves. In some instances, total parenteral nutrition (balanced intravenous feedings of amino acids, carbohydrates, lipids, vitamins, and minerals) has been used to nourish women with hyperemesis gravidarum when their nutritional status has been severely impaired.

Constipation. Improved bowel function generally results from increasing the intake of fiber (e.g., wheat bran and whole wheat products, popcorn, and raw or lightly steamed vegetables) in the diet, because fiber helps to retain water within the stool, creating a bulky stool that stimulates intestinal peristalsis. The recommendation for adults for fiber is 25 to 35 g. An increase of approximately 15% would be optimal. An adequate fluid intake (at least 50 ml/kg/day) helps to hydrate the fiber and increase the bulk of the stool. Making a habit of regular exercise that uses large muscle groups (walking, swimming, cycling) also helps to stimulate bowel motility.

Pyrosis. **Pyrosis**, or heartburn, is usually caused by the reflux of gastric contents into the esophagus. This condition can be minimized by the consumption of small, frequent meals, rather than two or three larger meals daily. Because fluids further distend the stomach, they should not be consumed with foods. The woman needs to be sure to drink adequate amounts between meals, however. Avoiding spicy foods may help alleviate the problem. Lying down immediately after eating and wearing clothing that is tight across the abdomen can contribute to the problem of reflux.

Cultural Influences and Vegetarian Diets

Consideration of a woman's cultural food preferences enhances communication, providing a greater opportunity for compliance with the agreed-on pattern of intake. Women in most cultures are encouraged to eat a diet typical for them. The nurse needs to be aware of what constitutes a typical diet for each cultural or ethnic group; however, within one cultural group, several variations may occur. Thus careful exploration of individual preferences is needed. Although ethnic and cultural food beliefs may seem, at first glance, to conflict with the dietary instruction provided by physicians, nurses, and dietitians, it is often possible for the empathic health care provider to identify cultural beliefs that are congruent with the modern understanding of pregnancy and fetal development. Many cultural food practices have some merit, or the culture would not have survived. Food cravings during pregnancy are considered normal by many cultures, but the kinds of cravings often are culturally specific. In most cultures, women crave acceptable foods, such as chicken, fish, and greens among African-Americans. Cultural influences on food intake usually lessen if the woman and her family become more integrated into the dominant culture. Nutritional beliefs and the practices of selected cultural groups are summarized in Table 15-6.

Vegetarian diets represent another cultural effect on nutritional status. Foods basic to almost all **vegetarian diets** are vegetables, fruits, legumes, nuts, seeds, and grains, but with many variations. Semivegetarians, who are not truly vegetarians, include fish, poultry, eggs, and dairy products in their diets but do not eat beef or pork. Such a diet can be completely adequate for pregnant women. Another type

TABLE 15-6 **Popular Foods of Various Cultural and Ethnic Groups and Their Place in the Food Guide Pyramid**

CULTURAL OR ETHNIC GROUP OR EATING PATTERN	FOOD GROUPS					
	BREAD, CEREAL, RICE, AND PASTA	VEGETABLE	FRUIT	MILK, YOGURT, AND CHEESE	MEAT, POULTRY, FISH, DRY BEANS, EGGS, AND NUTS	FATS, OILS, AND SWEETS*
Mexican	Tortilla, 1 Taco shell, 1 Posole (corn soup), ½ c Sopa (rice soup), ½ c Rice, cooked, ½ c Postres (pastries), 1 med.†	Chayote (Mexican squash), ½ c Jicama (root vegetable) ½ c Nopales (cactus leaves), ½ c Tomato, 1 med. Corn, 1 small ear	Avocado, ¼ med. Mango, 1 med. Papaya, ½ c Plantano (cooking banana), 1 med. Zapote (sweet yellowish fruit), 1 med.	Queso blanco (white Mexican cheese), 1.5 oz Custard, 1 c Leche (milk), 1 c	Chorizo (sausage), 2-3 oz † Chicken or beef, 2-3 oz Beans, dry, cooked, ½ c	Lard, vegetable oil, butter Candy Fried pork rinds
African-American "Soul" Food and Southern-style cookery	Biscuit, 1 Cornbread, 1 oz piece Grits, rice, macaroni, or noodles, ½ c Hominy, ½ c Crackers, 2-4 Hush puppies, 1 small † Pound cake, 1 oz piece †	Collard, kale, mustard, turnip greens, cooked, ½ c Okra, snap or pole beans, turnips, potatoes, sweet potatoes, squash, corn, onions, ½ c Coleslaw, ½ c	Apple, banana, peach, mango, 1 med. Cantaloupe, ¼ med. Blackberries, ½ c Watermelon, ½ c Plums, 2 small Muscadines (grapes), ½ c	Buttermilk or milk, 1 c Ice cream, ice milk, or frozen yogurt, 1 c	Pork (cured ham and uncured cuts), chicken, beef, fish, 2-3 oz Peas or beans (black-eye, crowder, purple-hull, cream peas; lima, navy beans), ½ c	Bacon, fat back, pork neckbones, hog jowls, pigs feet, chitterlings, lard, shortening Fruit drinks (not 100% juice) Gelatin Jam, jelly Pies
Vegetarian	Bread, 1 slice Cereal, cooked or ready-to-eat, 1 oz or ½ c Rice, pasta, other grains, cooked, ½ c Bagel, ½	Vegetables, cooked or chopped raw, ½ c Vegetables, raw leafy, 1 c	Fruit, 1 med. piece Fruit, chopped raw, ½ c Juice, ¾ c Dried fruit, ¼ c	Milk or yogurt, 1 c Cheese, 1.5 oz Soy milk, calcium fortified, 1 c Frozen yogurt, 1 c	Cooked dry beans or peas, ½ c Tofu or tempeh, ½ c Nuts or seeds, ⅓ c Peanut butter, 2 tbsp Egg, 1, or egg whites, 2 Soy milk, 1 c‡	Candy Butter, margarine, cooking oil Salad dressing
Italian	Bread sticks, 2 Gnocchi (dumplings), ½ c Italian bread, 1 slice Linguine, ½ c Polenta (corn meal mush), ½ c Risotto (creamy rice dish), ½ c	Artichoke, ½ med. Eggplant, mushrooms, spinach, ½ c Marinara sauce, ½ c	Berries, ½ c Figs, 2 dried Grapefruit, ½ Pomegranate, 1	Gelato, ½ c Cheese, mozzarella, ⅕ oz Cheese, hard (Parmesan, Romano), ¼ c Cheese, ricotta, ½ c	Veal or beef, 2-3 oz Sausage, 2-3 oz † Luncheon meats, 2-3 oz† Lentils, ½ c Squid, 2-3 oz	Olives Olive oil Butter Italian ice Whipping cream Chocolate

c, Cup; *med.*, medium; *oz*, ounce; *tbsp*, tablespoon.
*Serving sizes vary; all should be used sparingly.
†High fat; use sparingly.
‡Can be placed in either the milk, yogurt, and cheese group or the meat, poultry, fish, dry beans, eggs, and nuts group

Continued

TABLE 15-6 **Popular Foods of Various Cultural and Ethnic Groups and Their Place in the Food Guide Pyramid—cont'd**

CULTURAL OR ETHNIC GROUP OR EATING PATTERN	FOOD GROUPS					
	BREAD, CEREAL, RICE, AND PASTA	VEGETABLE	FRUIT	MILK, YOGURT, AND CHEESE	MEAT, POULTRY, FISH, DRY BEANS, EGGS, AND NUTS	FATS, OILS, AND SWEETS*
Chinese	Rice or millet, ½ c Rice vermicelli (thin rice pasta), ½ c Cellophane noodles (bean thread), ½ c Rice congee (rice soup, ½ c Rice sticks (rice flour noodles), ½ c	Broccoli, pea pods, yard long beans, baby corn, bamboo shoots, straw mushrooms, bell peppers, eggplant, ½ c	Guava, lychee, persimmon, pummelo, ½ c Kumquat, 4 Star fruit, 1	Soy milk, 1 c Soy cheese, 1.5 oz	Pork, fish, or chicken, 2-3 oz Shrimp, crab, lobster, 2-3 oz Tofu (soybean curd), tempeh (fermented soy), ½ c	Peanut and sesame oil Oyster and hoisin sauce Soy sauce
Indian	Breads: roti (chapatti), 1; naan, ½; paratha, ½; batura, ½; puris, 1; dosa, ½; idli, 1 Rice or rice pilau, ½ c Pooha, upma, sabudana, ½ c	Bell peppers, bitter melon, cabbage, cauliflower, eggplant, green beans, methi (fenugreek leaves), okra, peas, potatoes, okra, saag, ½ c cooked or 1 c raw	Canteloupe, watermelon, pineapple, grapes, ½ c Mango, papaya, ½ Figs, ¼ c Fruit juices and nectar, ¾ c Dried fruit, ¼ c	Kadi, lassi, yogurt, 1 c Paneer, 4 cubes	Egg, 2 Chicken, lamb, seafood, 2-3 oz Nuts, ½ c Beans or lentils (dhal), cooked, ½ c	Ghee (clarified butter) or butter Oil Coconut
Native American	Bread, 1 slice Wild rice or oats, ½ c Popcorn, 1 c Tortilla, 1 Fry bread, 1 piece† Mush (cooked cereal), ½ c	Squash or rhubarb, ½ c Potato, 1 med. Corn, 1 med. ear Green leafy vegetables, 1 c raw or ½ c cooked	Berries or cherries, ½ c Plum, 2 small Apple or peach, 1	Cheese, 1.5 oz	Wild game (deer, rabbit, elk, beaver), lamb, salmon and other fish, clams, mussels, crab, duck or quail, 2-3 oz Nuts or sunflower seeds, ½ c	Honey Fish oil and animal fat Mayonnaise
Middle Eastern	Rice or bulgur, ½ c Bread, 1 slice Pita, ½	Peppers, tomatoes, cabbage, grape leaves, cucumbers, squash, ½ c cooked or 1 c raw	Apricots, 3 small Grapes and melon, ½ c Dried fruits, ¼ c	Yogurt, 1 c	Lamb, goat, fish, 2-3 oz Nuts or seeds, ½ c Dried beans, peas, lentils, cooked, ½ c	Olives Olive or vegetable oil Lamb fat Candy

of vegetarians, ovolactovegetarians, eat dairy products in addition to plant products. Iron and zinc intake may not be adequate in these women, but such diets can be otherwise nutritionally sound. Strict vegetarians, or vegans, consume only plant products. Because vitamin B_{12} is found only in foods of animal origin, this diet is therefore deficient in vitamin B_{12}. As a result, strict vegetarians should take a supplement or consume vitamin B_{12}-fortified foods (e.g., soy milk) regularly. Vitamin B_{12} deficiency can result in megaloblastic anemia, glossitis (inflamed red tongue), and neurologic deficits in the mother. Infants born to affected mothers are likely to have megaloblastic anemia and to exhibit neurodevelopmental delays. Iron, calcium, zinc, and vitamin B_6 intake also may be low in women on this diet, and some strict vegetarians have excessively low caloric intakes. The protein intake should be assessed especially carefully, because plant proteins tend to be "incomplete," in that they lack one or more amino acids required for growth and the maintenance of body tissues. However, the daily consumption of a variety of different plant proteins–grains, dried beans and peas, nuts, and seeds–helps to provide all of the essential amino acids.

Evaluation

It is essential to set concrete, measurable outcomes; evaluate the woman's progress toward these outcomes regularly; and revise the plan of care if the outcomes are not achieved. In evaluating the adequacy of nutritional intake during pregnancy, the woman's weight gain can be compared with standardized grids showing recommended patterns (see Fig. 15-2). These grids are based on mean data and do not always take into account factors such as ethnic or racial variations. To evaluate the adequacy of the woman's diet, compare her diet with the plan in Table 15-4. Again, it is essential that individual factors affecting nutritional needs and dietary intake be considered. Physical examination and laboratory testing (see section on assessment) can be used as a means of confirming that a woman's nutritional status is adequate. If an inadequate weight gain is found or nutritional deficits appear, it is essential that the nurse reassess the woman and her understanding of her nutritional needs, reinforce teaching as needed, make referrals as indicated, and continue to reevaluate her nutritional status regularly (see Plan of Care).

KEY POINTS

- A woman's nutritional status before, during, and after pregnancy contributes, to a significant degree, to her well-being and that of her developing fetus and newborn.
- Many physiologic changes occurring during pregnancy influence the need for additional nutrients and the efficiency with which the body uses them.
- Both the total maternal weight gain and the pattern of weight gain are important determinants of the outcome of pregnancy.
- The appropriateness of the mother's prepregnancy weight for height (BMI) is a major determinant of her recommended weight gain during pregnancy.
- Nutritional risk factors include adolescent pregnancy; bizarre or faddish food habits; abuse of nicotine, alcohol, or drugs; a low weight for height; and frequent pregnancies.
- Iron supplementation is usually recommended routinely during pregnancy, even though there is some controversy regarding its beneficial effects on successful outcome of pregnancy. Other supplements may be recommended when nutritional risk factors are present.
- The nurse and client are influenced by cultural and personal values and beliefs during nutrition counseling.
- Pregnancy complications that may be nutrition related include anemia, PIH, gestational diabetes, and intrauterine growth restriction.
- Dietary adaptation can be effective for some of the common discomforts of pregnancy, including nausea and vomiting, constipation, and heartburn.

Plan of Care: Nutrition During Pregnancy

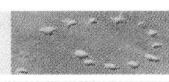

NURSING DIAGNOSIS Deficient knowledge related to nutritional requirements during pregnancy

Expected Outcomes *The woman will describe nutritional requirements and exhibit evidence of incorporating requirements into diet.*

Nursing Interventions/*Rationales*

Review basic nutritional requirements for a healthy diet by using recommended dietary guidelines and the food guide pyramid *to provide knowledge baseline for discussion.*

Discuss increased nutrient needs (calories, protein, minerals, vitamins) that occur as a result of being pregnant *to increase knowledge needed for altered dietary requirements.*

Discuss the relation between weight gain and fetal growth *to reinforce interdependence of fetus and mother.*

Calculate the appropriate total weight gain range during pregnancy using the woman's body mass index as a guide and discuss recommended rates of weight gain during the various trimesters of pregnancy *to provide concrete measures of dietary success.*

Review food preferences, cultural eating patterns or beliefs, and prepregnancy eating patterns *to enhance integration of new dietary needs.*

Discuss how to fit nutritional needs into usual dietary patterns and how to alter any identified nutritional deficits or excesses *to increase chances of success with dietary alterations.*

Discuss food aversions or cravings that may occur during pregnancy and strategies to deal with these if they are detrimental to fetus (e.g., pica) *to ensure well-being of fetus.*

Have woman keep a food diary delineating eating habits, dietary alterations, aversions, and cravings *to track eating habits and potential problem areas.*

NURSING DIAGNOSIS Imbalanced nutrition: more than body requirements related to excessive intake and/or inadequate activity levels.

Expected Outcomes *The woman's weekly weight gain will be reduced to the appropriate rate using her body mass index (BMI) and recommended weight gain ranges as guidelines.*

Nursing Interventions/*Rationales*

Review recent diet history (including food cravings) using a food diary, 24-hour recall, or food frequency approach *to ascertain food excesses contributing to excess weight gain.*

Review normal activity and exercise routines *to determine level of energy expenditure;* discuss eating patterns and reasons that lead to increased food intake (e.g., cultural beliefs or myths, increased stress, boredom) *to identify habits that contribute to excess weight gain.*

Review optimal weight gain guidelines and their rationale *to ensure that woman is knowledgeable about healthful weight gain rates.*

Set target weight gains for the remaining weeks of the pregnancy *to establish set goals.*

Discuss with the woman what changes can be made in diet, activity, and lifestyle *to enhance chances of meeting weight gain goals and dietary needs.* (Weight-reduction diets should be avoided, because they may deprive mother and fetus of needed nutrients and lead to ketonemia.)

NURSING DIAGNOSIS Imbalanced nutrition: less than body requirements related to inadequate intake of needed nutrients

Expected Outcomes *The woman's weekly weight gain will be increased to the appropriate rate using her BMI and recommended weight gain ranges as guidelines.*

Nursing Interventions/*Rationales*

Review recent diet history (including food aversions) using a food diary, 24-hour recall, or food frequency approach *to ascertain dietary inadequacies contributing to lack of sufficient weight gain.*

Review normal activity and exercise routines *to determine level of energy expenditure;* discuss eating patterns and reasons that lead to decreased food intake (e.g., morning sickness, pica, fear of becoming fat, stress, boredom) *to identify habits that contribute to inadequate weight gain.*

Review optimal weight gain guidelines and their rationale *to ensure that woman is knowledgeable about healthful weight gain rates.*

Set target weight gains for the remaining weeks of the pregnancy *to establish set goals.*

Review increased nutrient needs (calories, protein, minerals, vitamins) that occur as a result of being pregnant *to ensure woman is knowledgeable about altered dietary requirements.*

Review relation between weight gain and fetal growth *to reinforce that adequate weight gain is needed to promote fetal well-being.*

Discuss with woman what changes can be made in diet, activity, and lifestyle *to enhance chances of meeting set weight gain goals and nutrient needs of mother and fetus.*

If woman has fear of being fat, if symptoms of an eating disorder are evident, or if problems in adjusting to a changing body image surface, refer woman to the appropriate mental health professional for evaluation, *because intensive treatment and follow-up may be required to ensure fetal health.*

NURSING DIAGNOSIS Nausea related to physiologic alterations of the first trimester of pregnancy

Expected Outcomes *Nausea will not be so severe that it interferes with adequate nutrient intake or substantially reduces quality of life.*

Nursing Interventions/*Rationales*

Assess state of hydration *to ensure that the patient does not have fluid volume deficit* and assess pattern of weight gain during pregnancy *to ensure that nausea is not causing inadequate energy intake.*

Review the nausea history (i.e., frequency of episodes of nausea, the likelihood of nausea progressing to vomiting, factors precipitating or associated with nausea, and any relief measures that the patient has tried) *to determine the severity of the problem and to begin to identify effective and ineffective measures for coping with nausea.*

Review measures for prevention or relief of morning sickness *to ensure that the woman is knowledgeable about measures that are often effective in alleviating morning sickness.*

Discuss with the woman what relief measures she will try *to determine whether she understands how to implement the measures.*

CRITICAL THINKING EXERCISES

1. Interview an adolescent who is pregnant. Determine her usual dietary intake, and estimate the amount of her dietary energy, calcium, and sodium intake. Determine her teaching needs and help her devise a balanced diet plan. Take into account her usual eating habits (e.g., frequency of eating at fast food restaurants, purchase of food in the school cafeteria, and snacking patterns).

2. A community health nurse conducts a series of classes for young women at a prenatal clinic in an inner city. She has asked you to discuss appropriate weight gain during pregnancy but also to explain the health risks associated with obesity and therefore the need for weight control after pregnancy. Devise a teaching plan for this group. Include recommendations for appropriate types and amounts of physical activity during and after pregnancy.

RESOURCES

American Botanical Council
P.O. Box 144345
Austin, TX 78714-4345
512-926-4900
www.herbalgram.org

American Diabetes Association
Diabetes Information Service Center
1660 Duke St.
Alexandria, VA 22314
800-342-2383
www.diabetes.org

American Dietetic Association
216 West Jackson Blvd., Suite 800
Chicago, IL 60606-6995
www.eatright.org

American Medical Association
Department of Foods and Nutrition
515 North State St.
Chicago, IL 60610
www.ama-assn.org

Anorexia Nervosa and Related Eating Disorders, Inc.
www.anred.com

Body Mass Index Calculator
National Heart, Lung, and Blood Institute Information Center
P.O. Box 30105
Bethesda, MD 20824-0105
301-592-8573
www.nhlbisupport.com/bmi

Center for Food Safety and Applied Nutrition
Food and Drug Administration
200 C St., SW
Washington, DC 20250
202-720-2791
www.usda.gov/usda.htm

Food and Nutrition Board
Institute of Medicine
2101 Constitution Ave., NW
Washington, DC 20418
202-334-1732
www.iom.edu
E-mail: fnb@nas.edu

The Food Guide Pyramid
www.nal.usda.gov/fnic/Fpyr/pyramid.html

March of Dimes Birth Defects Foundation
1275 Mamaroneck Ave.
White Plains, NY 10605
914-428-7100
www.modimes.org

National Dairy Council
6300 N. River Rd.
Rosemont, IL 60018
www.nutritionexplorations.org

Nutritional content of foods:
www.nal.usda.gov/fnic/foodcomp

Office of Dietary Supplements
National Institutes of Health
31 Center Dr., Room 1829
Bethesda, MD 20892-2086
301-435-2920
www.odp.od.nih.gov/ods

RDAs according to age and sex
www.nal.usda.gov/fnic/dga/rda/htm

Society of Nutrition Education
1001 Connecticut Ave., NW, Suite 529
Washington, DC 20036-5528
202-452-8534
www.sne.org
E-mail: info@sne.org

Special Supplemental Nutrition Program for Women, Infants, and Children (WIC)
Food and Consumer Service
3101 Park Center Dr., Room 819
Alexandria, VA 22302
703-305-2286
www.usda.gov/fns/wic.html

U.S. Department of Agriculture
Food and Nutrition Information Center
14th and Independence Ave., SW
Washington, DC 20250
202-720-2791
www.usda.gov/usda.htm

REFERENCES

American College of Obstetricians and Gynecologists. (2002). ACOG Committee opinion: exercise during pregnancy and the postpartum period. Number 267. *Obstetrics and Gynecology, 99*(1), 171-173.

American Diabetes Association. (2002). Position statement: Gestational diabetes mellitus. *Diabetes Care, 25,* S94-S96.

Boushey, C., Edmonds, W., & Welshimer, K. (2001). Estimates of the effects of folic-acid fortification and folic-acid bioavailability for women. *Nutrition, 17*(10), 873-879.

Ellings, J., Newman, R., & Bowers, N. (1998). Prenatal care and multiple pregnancy. *Journal of Obstetric, Gynecologic, and Neonatal Nursing, 27*(4), 457-465.

Fluoride Recommendations Work Group. (2001). Recommendations for using fluoride to prevent and control dental caries in the United States. *MMWR, 50* (RR-14), 1-42.

Food and Nutrition Board, Institute of Medicine. (1997). *Dietary reference intakes for calcium, phosphorus, magnesium, vitamin D, and fluoride.* Washington, DC: National Academy Press.

Food and Nutrition Board, Institute of Medicine. (1998). *Dietary reference intakes for thiamine, riboflavin, niacin, vitamin B_6, folate, vitamin B_{12}, pantothenic acid, biotin, and choline.* Washington, DC: National Academy Press.

Food and Nutrition Board, Institute of Medicine. (2000). *Dietary reference intakes for vitamin C, vitamin E, selenium, and carotenoids.* Washington, DC: National Academy Press.

Food and Nutrition Board, Institute of Medicine. (2001). *Dietary reference intakes for vitamin A, vitamin K, arsenic, boron, chromium, copper, iodine, iron, manganese, molybdenum, nickel, silicon, vanadium, and zinc.* Washington, DC: National Academy Press.

Food and Nutrition Board, National Academy of Science, National Research Council. (1989). *Recommended dietary allowances* (10th ed.). Washington, DC: National Academy Press.

Gunderson, E., Abrams, B., & Selvin, S. (2000). The relative importance of gestational gain and maternal characteristics associated with the risk of becoming overweight after pregnancy. *International Journal of Obesity and Related Metabolic Disorders, 24*(12), 1660-1668.

Haram, K., Nilsen, S., & Schall, J. (2001). Iron supplementation in pregnancy: Evidence and controversies. *Acta Obstetrica et Gynecologica Scandinavica, 80,* 683-688.

Hediger, M., Scholl, T., & Schall, J. (1997). Implications of the Camden Study of adolescent pregnancy: Interactions among maternal growth, nutritional status, and body composition. *Annals of the New York Academy of Medicine, 817,* 281-291.

Henkel, J. (1999). Sugar substitutes: Americans opt for sweetness and lite. *FDA Consumer, 33*(6), 12-16.

Hoyert, D. et al. (2001). Annual summary of vital statistics: 2000. *Pediatrics, 108*(6), 1241-1255.

Institute of Medicine. (1992). *Nutrition during pregnancy and lactation: An implementation guide.* Washington, DC: National Academy Press.

Jewell, D., & Young, G. (2002). Interventions for nausea and vomiting in early pregnancy (Cochrane Review). *The Cochrane Library,* Issue 4. Oxford: Update Software.

King, J. (2000). Determinants of maternal zinc status during pregnancy. *American Journal of Clinical Nutrition,* 71(5 Suppl), 1334S-1343S.

Krishnaswamy, K., & Madhavan Nair, K. (2001). Importance of folate in human nutrition. *British Journal of Nutrition, 85*(Suppl 2), S115-S124.

Mahomed, K. (2002). Iron supplementation in pregnancy (Cochrane Review). *The Cochrane Library,* Issue 4. Oxford: Update Software.

Nucci, L. et al. (2001). Nutritional status of pregnant women: Prevalence and associated pregnancy outcomes. *Revista de saude publica, 35*(6), 502-507.

Rainville, A. (1998). Pica practices of pregnant women are associated with lower maternal hemoglobin level at delivery. *Journal of the American Dietetic Association, 98*(3), 293-295.

Scanlon, K. (Ed.) (2001). *Final report of the vitamin D expert panel.* Atlanta: Centers for Disease Control and Prevention.

Schieve, L. et al. (2000). Prepregnancy body mass index and pregnancy weight gain: Associations with preterm delivery: The NMIHS Collaborative Study Group. *Obstetrics and Gynecology, 96*(2), 194-200.

Scholl, T., & Reilly, T. (2000). Anemia, iron and pregnancy outcome. *Journal of Nutrition, 130*(25 Suppl), 443S-447S.

Sebire, N. et al. (2001). Maternal obesity and pregnancy outcome: A study of 287,213 pregnancies in London. *International Journal of Obesity and Related Metabolic Disorders, 25*(8), 1175-1182.

Siega-Riz, A., & Savitz, D. (2001). What are pregnant women eating? Nutrient and food group differences by race. *American Journal of Obstetrics and Gynecology, 186*(3), 480-486.

Swensen, A., Harnack, L., & Ross, J. (2001). Nutritional assessment of pregnant women enrolled in the Special Supplemental Program for women, infants, and children (WIC). *Journal of the American Dietetic Association, 101*(8), 903-908.

U.S. Department of Agriculture. (1992). *The food guide pyramid.* Hyattsville, MD: U.S. Department of Agriculture.

Wardlaw, G., & Insel, P. (1993). *Perspectives in nutrition* (2nd ed.). St. Louis: Mosby.

Worthington-Roberts, B., & Williams, S. (1997). *Nutrition in pregnancy and lactation* (6th ed.). Dubuque, IA: Brown and Benchmark.

CHAPTER 16

Rebecca Burdette Saunders

Nursing Care During Pregnancy

http://evolve.elsevier.com/Lowdermilk/MatWmnHlth/

LEARNING OBJECTIVES

- Describe the process of confirming pregnancy and estimating the date of birth.
- Summarize the physical, psychosocial, and behavioral changes that usually occur as the mother and other family members adapt to pregnancy.
- Discuss the benefits of prenatal care and problems of accessibility for some women.
- Outline the patterns of health care used to assess maternal and fetal health status at the initial and follow-up visits during pregnancy.
- Identify the typical nursing assessments, diagnoses, interventions, and methods of evaluation in providing care for the pregnant woman.
- Discuss education needed by pregnant women to understand physical discomforts related to pregnancy and to recognize signs and symptoms of potential complications.
- Examine the impact of culture, age, parity, and number of fetuses on the response of the family to the pregnancy and on the prenatal care provided.

The prenatal period is a time of physical and psychologic preparation for birth and parenthood. Becoming a parent is considered one of the maturational milestones of adult life, and as such, it is a time of intense learning for both parents and those close to them. The prenatal period provides a unique opportunity for nurses and other members of the health care team to influence family health. During this period, essentially healthy women seek regular care and guidance. The nurse's health promotion interventions can affect the well-being of the woman, her unborn child, and the rest of her family for many years.

Regular prenatal visits, ideally beginning soon after the first missed menstrual period, offer opportunities to ensure the health of the expectant mother and her infant. Prenatal health care permits diagnosis and treatment of maternal disorders that may have preexisted or may develop during the pregnancy. Care is designed to monitor the growth and development of the fetus and to identify abnormalities that may interfere with the course of normal labor. Education and support for self-care and parenting can be provided.

Pregnancy spans 9 months, but health care providers seldom use the familiar calendar to discuss the duration of pregnancy or gestational age of the fetus. Instead, they use the concept of lunar months, which last 28 days, or 4 weeks. Normal pregnancy, then, lasts about 10 lunar months, which is the same as 40 weeks or 280 days. Health care providers also refer to early, middle, and late pregnancy as **trimesters.** The first trimester lasts from weeks 1 through 13; the second, from weeks 14 through 26; and the third, from weeks 27 through 40. A pregnancy is considered at **term** if it advances to 38 to 40 weeks. The focus of this chapter is on meeting the health needs of the expectant family over the course of pregnancy, which is known as the **prenatal period.**

DIAGNOSIS OF PREGNANCY

Women may suspect pregnancy when they miss a menstrual period. Many women come to the first prenatal visit after a positive home pregnancy test; however, the clinical diagnosis of pregnancy before the second missed period may be difficult in some women. Physical variations, lack of relaxation, obesity, or tumors, for example, may confound even the experienced examiner. Accuracy is important, however, because emotional, social, medical, or legal consequences of an inaccurate diagnosis, either positive or negative, can be extremely serious. A correct date for the *last (normal) menstrual period (LMP* or *LNMP)* and for the date of intercourse and a basal body temperature (BBT) record may be of great value in the accurate diagnosis of pregnancy (see Chapter 9).

Signs and Symptoms

Great variability is possible in the subjective and objective symptoms of pregnancy; therefore the diagnosis of pregnancy may be uncertain for a time. Many of the indicators of pregnancy are clinically useful in the diagnosis of pregnancy, and they are classified as presumptive, probable, or positive.

Presumptive indicators of pregnancy include subjective symptoms and objective signs. Subjective symptoms are reported by the woman and may include amenorrhea, nausea and vomiting **(morning sickness),** breast tenderness, urinary frequency, and fatigue. **Quickening,** the mother's first perception of fetal movement, may be noted between weeks 16 and 20. Objective signs that may be validated by the examiner include elevation of BBT, breast and abdominal enlargement, and changes in the uterus and vagina. Other visible changes occur in the skin, such as striae gravidarum, deeper pigmentation of the areola, chloasma (mask of pregnancy), and linea nigra (pigmented line on the abdomen) (see Chapter 14).

The presumptive indicators of pregnancy can be caused by conditions other than gestation. For example, amenorrhea may be caused by illness or excessive exercise; fatigue may signify anemia or infection; a tumor may cause enlargement of the abdomen; and nausea or vomiting may be caused by a gastrointestinal upset or food allergy. Therefore these signs alone are not reliable for diagnosis.

Probable indicators of pregnancy are detected by an examiner and are related mainly to physical changes in the uterus. Objective signs include uterine enlargement, Braxton Hicks contractions, uterine souffle, ballottement, and a positive pregnancy test. When combined with presumptive signs and symptoms, they strongly suggest pregnancy, but they are not conclusive. For example, uterine enlargement may be due to the presence of tumors; unusual bowel sounds may be misinterpreted; or positive results on a pregnancy test may be due to a malignant tumor that secretes the hormone human chorionic gonadotropin (hCG).

The **positive indicators** of pregnancy are directly attributed to the fetus and include the presence of a fetal heartbeat distinct from that of the mother, fetal movement felt by someone other than the mother, and visualization of the fetus with a technique such as ultrasound examination. The fetal heartbeat can be detected as early as 6 weeks of gestation with Doppler techniques, but ultrasound examination becomes 100% reliable only at 8 to 9 weeks of gestation. However, the fetal heartbeat usually cannot be detected with a stethoscope until weeks 16 to 20. An experienced examiner may palpate fetal movements with increasing reliability after 20 to 24 weeks.

Estimating Date of Birth

After the diagnosis of pregnancy, the woman's first question usually concerns when she will give birth. This date has traditionally been termed the estimated date of confinement (EDC), although estimated date of delivery (EDD) also has been used (Katz et al., 2001). To promote a more positive perception of both pregnancy and birth, however, the term **estimated date of birth** (EDB) is now used. Because the precise date of conception generally is unknown, several formulas have been suggested for calculating the EDB. None of these guides is infallible, but Nägele's rule is reasonably accurate and is usually used.

Nägele's rule is as follows: After determining the first day of the LMP, subtract 3 calendar months, add 7 days and 1 year; or alternatively, add 7 days to the LMP and count forward 9 calendar months. Box 16-1 demonstrates use of Nägele's rule.

Nägele's rule assumes that the woman has a 28-day menstrual cycle and that pregnancy occurred on the fourteenth day. An adjustment is in order if the woman's cycle is longer or shorter than 28 days. With the use of Nägele's rule, only about 5% of pregnant women give birth spontaneously on the EDB (Katz et al., 2001). Most women give birth during the period extending from 7 days before to 7 days after the EDB.

BOX 16-1 Use of Nägele's Rule

July 10, 2003, is the first day of the last menstrual period.

	7	10	2002
	−3	+7	
EDB =	4	17	2003

The estimated date of birth is April 17, 2004.

ADAPTATION TO PREGNANCY

Pregnancy affects all family members, and each family member must adapt to the pregnancy and interpret its meaning in light of his or her own needs. This process of family adaptation to pregnancy takes place within a cultural environment influenced by societal trends. Dramatic changes have occurred in Western society in recent years, and the nurse must be prepared to support single-parent families, reconstituted families, dual-career families, and alternative families, as well as traditional families, in the childbirth experience (Blackwell & Blackwell, 1999).

Much of the investigation of family dynamics in pregnancy by scholars in the United States and Canada has been done with Caucasian, middle-class nuclear families, and findings may not apply to families who do not fit the traditional American model. Terms such as spouse, husband, and wife, for example, are used consistently in family literature but may not fit the configuration of a given family in the nurse's care. Adaptation of terms is appropriate to avoid embarrassment to the nurse and offense to the family. Additional research is needed on a variety of families to determine if study findings generated in traditional families are applicable to others.

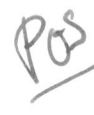

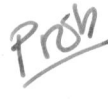

Maternal Adaptation

Women of all ages use the months of pregnancy to adapt to the maternal role, a complex process of social and cognitive learning. Early in pregnancy, nothing seems to be happening, and a woman may spend much time sleeping. With the perception of fetal movement in the second trimester, the woman turns her attention inward to her pregnancy and to relationships with her mother and other women who have been or who are pregnant.

Pregnancy is a maturational milestone that can be stressful but also rewarding as the woman prepares for a new level of caring and responsibility. Her self-concept changes in readiness for parenthood as she prepares for her new role. She moves gradually from being self-contained and independent to being committed to a lifelong concern for another human being. This growth requires mastery of certain developmental tasks: accepting the pregnancy, identifying with the role of mother, reordering the relationships between herself and her mother and between herself and her partner, establishing a relationship with the unborn child, and preparing for the birth experience (Lederman, 1996). The partner's emotional support is an important factor in the successful accomplishment of these developmental tasks. Single women with limited support may have difficulty making this adaptation.

Accepting the Pregnancy

The first step in adapting to the maternal role is accepting the idea of pregnancy and assimilating the pregnant state into the woman's way of life. Mercer (1995) described this process as cognitive restructuring and credited Reva Rubin (1984) as the nurse theorist who pioneered our understanding of maternal role attainment. The work of these scholars and of Lederman (1996) and others should be studied for a deeper understanding of the complex psychosocial processes that affect behaviors of pregnant women.

The degree of acceptance is reflected in the woman's emotional responses. Many women are dismayed initially at finding themselves pregnant, especially if the pregnancy is unintended. However, research shows that even 25% of women with contraceptive failures, thus having pregnancies classified as unintended, are happy or very happy to be pregnant (Sable, 1999). Eventual acceptance of pregnancy parallels the growing acceptance of the reality of a child. Nonacceptance of the pregnancy, however, should not be equated with rejection of the child, for a woman may dislike being pregnant but feel love for the child to be born.

Women who are happy and pleased about their pregnancy often view it as biologic fulfillment and part of their life plan. They have high self-esteem and tend to be confident about outcomes for themselves, their babies, and other family members. Despite a general feeling of well-being, many women are surprised to experience **emotional lability,** that is, rapid and unpredictable changes in mood. These swings in emotions and increased sensitivity to others are disconcerting to the expectant mother and those around her. Increased irritability, explosions of tears and anger, and feelings of great joy and cheerfulness alternate, apparently with little or no provocation.

Profound hormonal changes that are part of the maternal response to pregnancy may be responsible for mood changes, much as they are before menstruation or during menopause. Other reasons such as concerns about finances and changed lifestyle contribute to this seemingly erratic behavior.

Pregnant women are affected emotionally by changes that occur in the physical contours and functions of their bodies. During the first trimester, body shape changes little, but by the second trimester, obvious bulging of the abdomen, thickening of the waist, and enlargement of the breasts proclaim the state of pregnancy. A feeling develops of an overall increase in the size of her body and of occupying more space.

The woman's attitude about her body is influenced by her values and personality traits. This attitude often changes as pregnancy progresses. A positive body image usually is expressed during the first trimester. As the pregnancy advances, however, the feelings become more negative. For most women, the feeling of liking or not liking their bodies in the pregnant state is temporary and does not cause permanent changes in their self-perceptions.

Most women have ambivalent feelings during pregnancy whether the pregnancy was intended or not. **Ambivalence,** having conflicting feelings simultaneously, is considered a normal response for people preparing for a new role. During pregnancy, women may, for example, feel great pleasure that they are fulfilling a lifelong dream, but they also may feel great regret that life as they now know it is ending.

Even women who are pleased to be pregnant may experience feelings of hostility toward the pregnancy or unborn child from time to time. Such incidents as a partner's chance remark about the attractiveness of a slim, nonpregnant woman or news of a colleague's promotion can give rise to ambivalent feelings. Body sensations, feelings of dependence, or the realization of the responsibilities of child care also can generate such feelings.

Intense feelings of ambivalence that persist through the third trimester may indicate an unresolved conflict with the motherhood role (Mercer, 1995). After the birth of a healthy child, memories of these ambivalent feelings usually are dismissed. If the child is born with a defect, however, a woman may look back at the times when she did not want the pregnancy and feel intensely guilty. She may believe that her ambivalence caused the birth defect. She then will need assurance that her feelings were not responsible for the problem.

Identifying with the Mother Role

The process of identifying with the mother role begins early in each woman's life when she is being mothered as a child. Her social group's perception of what constitutes the feminine role can subsequently influence her toward choosing between motherhood or a career, being married or single, being independent rather than interdependent, or being able to manage multiple roles. Practice roles, such as playing with dolls, baby-sitting, and taking care of siblings, may increase her understanding of what being a mother entails.

Many women have always wanted a baby, liked children, and looked forward to motherhood. Their high motivation to become a parent promotes acceptance of pregnancy and eventual prenatal and parental adaptation. Other women apparently have not considered in any detail what motherhood means to them. During pregnancy, conflicts such as not wanting the pregnancy and child-related or career-related decisions must be resolved.

Reordering Personal Relationships

Close relationships of the pregnant woman undergo change during pregnancy as she prepares emotionally for the new role of mother. As family members learn their new roles, periods of tension and conflict may occur. An understanding of the typical patterns of adjustment can help the nurse to reassure the pregnant woman and explore issues related to social support. Promoting effective communication patterns between the expectant mother and her own mother and between the expectant mother and her partner are common nursing interventions provided during the prenatal visits.

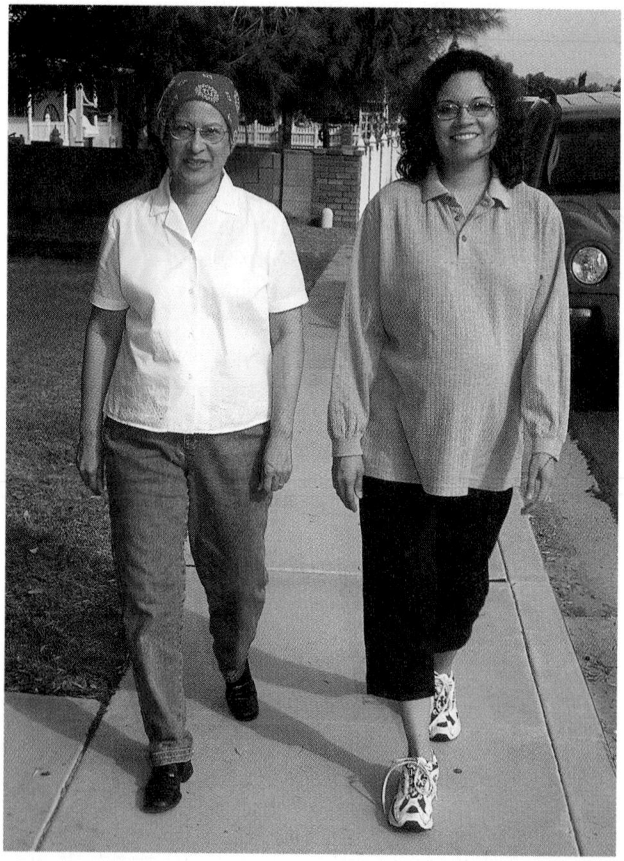

FIG. 16-1 A pregnant woman and her mother enjoying their walk together. (Courtesy Michael S. Clement, MD, Mesa, AZ.)

The woman's own relationship with her mother is significant in adaptation to pregnancy and motherhood. Important components in the pregnant woman's relationship with her mother are the mother's availability (past and present), her reactions to the daughter's pregnancy, respect for her daughter's autonomy, and the willingness to reminisce (Mercer, 1995).

The mother's reaction to the daughter's pregnancy signifies her acceptance of the grandchild and of her daughter. If the mother is supportive, the daughter has an opportunity to discuss pregnancy and labor and her feelings of joy or ambivalence with a knowledgeable and accepting woman (Fig. 16-1). Rubin (1975) noted that if the pregnant woman's mother is not pleased with the pregnancy, the daughter begins to have doubts about her self-worth and the eventual acceptance of her child by others. Mothers who respect their daughters' autonomy promote their feelings of self-confidence.

Reminiscing about the pregnant woman's early childhood and sharing the prospective grandmother's account of her childbirth experience help the daughter to anticipate and prepare for labor and birth. Hearing about themselves as young children makes pregnant women feel loved and wanted. They draw closer to their parents and begin to feel that, despite the errors they might make in their own mothering experiences, they will continue to be loved by their children.

Although the woman's relationship with her mother is significant in considering her adaptation in pregnancy, the most important person to the pregnant woman is usually the father of her child. The support and concern of a partner during pregnancy have positive consequences for a woman's desire to carry out the pregnancy (Kroelinger & Oths, 2000), and she has fewer emotional and physical symptoms, fewer labor and childbirth complications, and an easier postpartum adjustment. Women express two major needs within this relationship during pregnancy: feeling loved and valued and having the child accepted by the partner.

The marital or committed relationship is not static but evolves over time. The addition of a child changes forever the nature of the bond between partners. Couples grow closer during pregnancy, and pregnancy has a maturing effect on the partners' relationship as they assume new roles and discover new aspects of one another. Partners who trust and support each other are able to share mutual-dependency needs (Mercer, 1995).

Sexual expression during pregnancy is highly individual. The sexual relationship is affected by physical, emotional, and interactional factors, including myths about sex during pregnancy, sexual dysfunction, and physical changes in the woman. Myths about body functions and fantasies about the influence of the fetus as a third party in lovemaking are commonly expressed. An individual may also inaccurately attribute anomalies, mental retardation, and other injuries to the fetus and mother to sexual relations during pregnancy. Some couples fear that the woman's genitals will be drastically changed by the birth process. Couples may not express their concerns to the health care provider because of embarrassment or because they do not want to appear foolish. Unless nurses overcome their reluctance to incorporate sexuality counseling, couples often do not receive the information and support that they desire (Alteneder & Hartzell, 1997).

As pregnancy progresses, changes in body shape, body image, and levels of discomfort influence both partners' desire for sexual expression. During the first trimester, the woman's sexual desire may decrease, especially if she has breast tenderness, nausea, fatigue, or sleepiness. As she progresses into the second trimester, however, her sense of well-being combined with the increased pelvic congestion that occurs at this time may increase her desire for sexual release. In the third trimester, somatic complaints and physical bulkiness may increase her physical discomfort and again diminish her interest in sex.

Partners need to feel free to discuss their sexual responses during pregnancy. Their sensitivity to each other and willingness to share concerns can strengthen their sexual relationship. Partners who do not understand the rapid physiologic and emotional changes of pregnancy can become confused by the other's behavior. By talking to each other about the changes they are experiencing, couples can define problems and then offer the needed support. Nurses can facilitate communication between partners by talking to expectant couples about possible changes in feelings and behaviors they may experience as pregnancy progresses (Alteneder & Hartzel, 1997).

Establishing Relationship with Fetus

Emotional **attachment,** feelings of being tied by affection or love, begins during the prenatal period as women use fantasizing and daydreaming to prepare themselves for motherhood (Rubin, 1975). They think of themselves as mothers and imagine maternal qualities they would like to possess. Expectant parents desire to be warm, loving, and close to their child. They try to anticipate changes that the child will bring in their lives and wonder how they will react to noise, disorder, reduced freedom, and caregiving activities. The mother-child relationship progresses through pregnancy as a developmental process that unfolds in three phases.

In phase 1 the woman accepts the biologic fact of pregnancy. She needs to be able to state, "I am pregnant" and incorporate the idea of a child into her body and self-image. The woman's thoughts center around herself and the reality of her pregnancy. The child is viewed as part of herself, not a separate and unique person.

In phase 2 the woman accepts the growing fetus as distinct from herself, usually accomplished by the fifth month. She can now say, "I am going to have a baby." This differentiation of the child from the woman's self permits the beginning of the mother-child relationship that involves not only caring but also responsibility. Attachment by a mother to her child is enhanced by experiencing a planned pregnancy, and it increases when ultrasound examination and quickening confirm the reality of the fetus (Smith, 1998).

With acceptance of the reality of the child (hearing the heartbeat and feeling the child move) and an overall feeling of well-being, the woman enters a quiet period and becomes more introspective. A fantasy child becomes precious to the woman. As the woman seems to withdraw and to concentrate her interest on the unborn child, her partner sometimes feels left out. If there are children in the family, they may become more demanding in their efforts to redirect the mother's attention to themselves.

During phase 3 of the attachment process, the woman prepares realistically for the birth and parenting of the child. She expresses the thought, "I am going to be a mother," and defines the nature and characteristics of the child. She may, for example, speculate about the child's sex and personality traits based on patterns of fetal activity.

Although the mother alone experiences the child within, both parents and siblings believe the unborn child responds in a very individualized, personal manner. Family members may interact a great deal with the unborn child by talking to the fetus and stroking the mother's abdomen, especially when the fetus shifts position (Fig. 16-2).

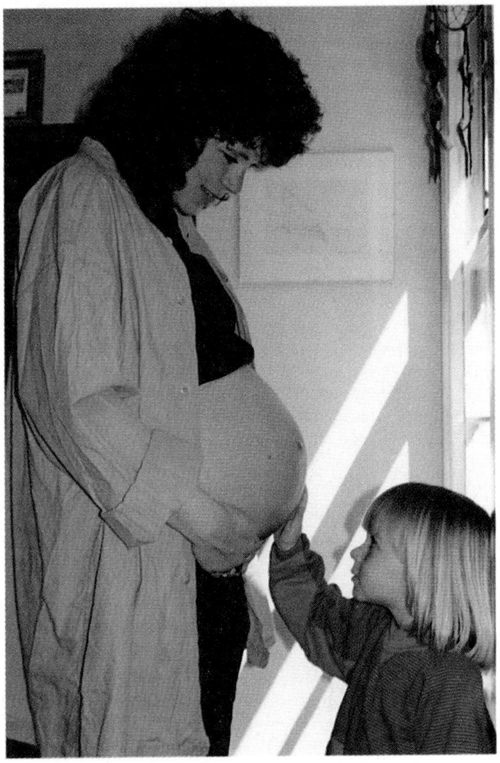

FIG. 16-2 Sibling feeling movement of fetus. (Courtesy Kim Molloy, Knoxville, IA.)

Women in all trimesters of pregnancy fantasize about their fetuses. Such fantasies may be useful in facilitating healthy behaviors in families (Sorenson & Schuelke, 1999). The content of fantasies may be either positive or negative; they change over time. Knowledge of the fantasies can be used to facilitate anticipatory guidance (Sorenson & Schuelke, 1999). More research is necessary to help nurses understand the factors that promote early attachment.

Preparing for Childbirth

Many women actively prepare for birth by reading books, viewing films, attending parenting classes, and talking to other women. They seek the best caregiver possible for advice, monitoring, and caring. The multipara has her own history of labor and birth, which influences her approach to preparation for this childbirth experience.

Anxiety can arise from concern about a safe passage for herself and her child during the birth process (Mercer, 1995; Rubin, 1975). This concern may not be expressed overtly, but cues are given as the nurse listens to plans women make for care of the new baby and other children in case "anything should happen." These feelings persist despite statistical evidence about the safe outcome of pregnancy for mothers and their infants. Many women fear the pain of childbirth or mutilation because they do not understand anatomy and the birth process. Education by the nurse can alleviate many of these fears. Women also express concern over what behaviors are appropriate during the birth process and whether caregivers will accept them and their actions. The best preparation for labor is "a healthy sense of the realistic–an awareness of work, pain, and risk balanced by a sense of excitement and expectation of the final reward" (Lederman, 1996) (see Chapter 17).

Toward the end of the third trimester, breathing is difficult, and fetal movements become vigorous enough to disturb the woman's sleep. Backaches, frequency and urgency of urination, constipation, and varicose veins can become troublesome. The bulkiness and awkwardness of her body interfere with the woman's ability to care for other children, perform routine work-related duties, and assume a comfortable position for sleep and rest. By this time, most women become impatient for labor to begin, whether the birth is anticipated with joy, dread, or a mixture of both. A strong desire to see the end of pregnancy, to be over and done with it, makes women at this stage ready to move on to childbirth.

Paternal Adaptation

The father's beliefs and feelings about the ideal mother and father and his cultural expectation of appropriate behavior during pregnancy affect his response to his partner's need for him. One man may engage in nurturing behavior. Another may feel lonely and alienated as the woman becomes physically and emotionally engrossed in the unborn child. He may seek comfort and understanding outside the home or become interested in a new hobby or involved with his work. Some men view pregnancy as proof of their masculinity and their dominant role. To others, pregnancy has no meaning in terms of responsibility to either mother or child. However, for most men, pregnancy can be a time of preparation for the parental role with intense learning.

Accepting the Pregnancy

The ways fathers adjust to the parental role is the subject of considerable research (Diemer, 1997). In older societies the man enacted the ritual **couvade;** that is, he behaved in specific ways and respected taboos associated with pregnancy and giving birth so the man's new status was recognized and endorsed. His behavior acknowledged his psychosocial and biologic relationship to the mother and child. Changing cultural and professional attitudes have encouraged fathers' participation in the birth experience in the past 30 years (Draper, 1997).

A man's readiness for fatherhood may be reflected in the way he views the couple's relative financial security and the stability of the couple relationship and in the way he deals with the realization that the upcoming birth marks the end of the childless period. Many men express concern for the family's economic security. Today, most young married women are employed outside the home but have a period of unemployment for childbearing and child care. The length of unemployment is determined by the couple's economic status, the policies of the woman's employer, and the couple's value system. Some men compensate for anticipated needs by keeping their current jobs even though they had planned a change, by working overtime, or by taking on extra work. Some men acquire new or additional insurance at this time.

The man's emotional responses to becoming a father, his concerns, and his informational needs change during the course of pregnancy. Phases of the developmental pattern become apparent. May (1982) described three phases characterizing the developmental tasks experienced by the expectant father: the announcement phase, the moratorium phase, and the focusing phase.

The *announcement phase* may last from a few hours to a few weeks. The developmental task is to accept the biologic fact of pregnancy. Men react to the confirmation of pregnancy with joy or dismay, depending on whether the pregnancy is desired or unplanned or unwanted. Ambivalence in the early stages of pregnancy is common.

If pregnancy is unplanned or unwanted, some men find the alterations in life plans and lifestyles difficult to accept. Some men engage in extramarital affairs for the first time during their partner's pregnancy. Others batter their wives for the first time or escalate the frequency of battering episodes (Martin et al., 2001). Chapter 6 provides detailed information about violence against women with guidance on assessment and intervention.

The second phase, the *moratorium phase*, is the period when he adjusts to the reality of pregnancy. The developmental task is to accept the pregnancy. Men appear to put conscious thought of the pregnancy aside for a time. They become more introspective and engage in many discussions about their philosophy of life, religion, childbearing, and childrearing practices and their relationships with family members and friends. Depending on the man's readiness for the pregnancy, this phase may be relatively short or persist until the last trimester.

The third phase, called the *focusing phase*, begins in the last trimester and is characterized by the father's active involvement in both the pregnancy and his relationship with his child. The developmental task is to negotiate with his partner the role he is to play in labor and to prepare for parenthood. In this phase the man concentrates on his experience of the pregnancy and begins to think of himself as a father.

May (1980, 1982) also determined that men are involved in pregnancy in a variety of ways. She described three styles of involvement in the pregnancy exhibited by men during their wives' first pregnancy: the observer style, the expressive style, and the instrumental style. All styles are common, and no single pattern is considered "normal."

The *observer* style is exhibited by those fathers who are happy about the pregnancy and supportive of their wives. However, because of cultural values or shyness, they avoid involvement in activities such as parent education classes, decisions about breastfeeding, or the choice of professional care. Other fathers who are ambivalent about pregnancy and the role of father need time to adjust to the idea of pregnancy and fatherhood. Some men cope by becoming involved in careers and resisting their wives' attempts to involve them in preparations for the coming child.

Men who show the *expressive* style display a strong emotional response to pregnancy and a desire to be a full partner in the project (Fig. 16-3). These men are aware of their partner's needs for support. They experience the same emotional lability and ambivalence as experienced by pregnant women. Some expectant fathers report having nausea and other gastrointestinal complaints, fatigue, and other physical discomforts. Known as the **couvade syndrome,** the phenomenon of men's experiencing pregnancy-like symptoms has been explored by scholars in several disciplines, including nursing.

Further investigation is needed to determine whether the basis of men's experience is primarily physiologic or psychologic.

The *instrumental* style is adopted by men who see tasks they can perform in their role as manager of the pregnancy. They ask questions; are interested in the role of labor coach; and plan for photographs during pregnancy, birth, and the neonatal period. They feel responsible for the outcome of pregnancy and are protective and supportive of their wives.

These three styles of involvement provide examples of the different ways men can experience pregnancy. Each man needs to feel free to define his unique role in pregnancy, just as the woman does. Because of cultural conditioning, personality, or a different supportive style, however, not all men are able or willing to attend childbirth classes or act as labor coaches. More research is needed to determine whether similar styles of involvement occur in the partners of multiparous women, in men from various cultural groups, and in same-sex partners, and what the effects on the relationship are when the partners' expectations do not coincide.

Identifying with Father Role

Each man brings to pregnancy attitudes that affect the way in which he adjusts to the pregnancy and parental role. His memories of the fathering he received from his own father, the experiences he has had with child care, and the perceptions of the male and father roles within his social group will guide his selection of the tasks and responsibilities he will assume. Some men are highly motivated to nurture and love a child. They may be excited and pleased about the anticipated role of father. Others may be more detached or even hostile to the idea of fatherhood.

Reordering Personal Relationships

The partner's main role in pregnancy is to nurture and respond to the pregnant woman's feelings of vulnerability. The partner also must deal with the reality of the pregnancy. The partner's support indicates involvement in the pregnancy and preparation for attachment to the child.

Some aspects of a partner's behavior may indicate rivalry, and it may be especially evident during sexual activity. For example, men may protest that fetal movements

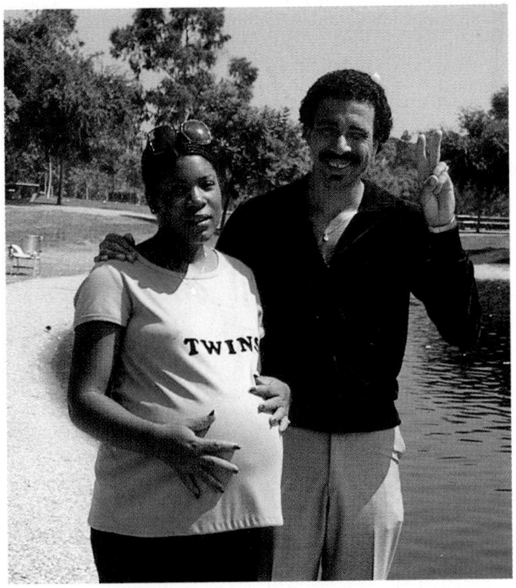
TWIN

FIG. 16-3 Prospective mother and father walk together. Women respond positively to their partner's interest and concern. (Courtesy Marjorie Pyle, RNC, Lifecircle, Costa Mesa, CA.)

prevent sexual gratification or that they are being watched by the fetus during sexual activity. However, feelings of rivalry may be unconscious and not verbalized, but expressed in subtle behaviors.

The woman's increased introspection may cause her partner to feel uneasy as she becomes preoccupied with thoughts of the child and of her motherhood, with her growing dependence on her physician or midwife, and with her reevaluation of the couple's relationship. Couples who are told early in the pregnancy that ambivalence, anxiety, and increased tensions are common experiences for expectant couples then can devote energy to managing the changes. Perinatal educators are in an especially favorable position to incorporate needs of prospective fathers as well as mothers in their class plans (Diemer, 1997) (see Chapter 17).

Deciding on the infant's feeding method is of concern when the partners' preferences differ or one partner has intense opinions about a method. The recognized benefits and disadvantages of one method over another appear to be irrelevant. Some partners insist that the woman breastfeed; others are adamantly opposed to breastfeeding. If one partner refuses to voice an opinion, the other may experience uneasiness or uncertainty (Pavill, 2002).

Establishing Relationship with Fetus

The father-child attachment can be as strong as the mother-child relationship, and fathers can be as competent as mothers in nurturing their infants. The father-child attachment also begins during pregnancy. A father may rub or kiss the maternal abdomen, try to listen, talk, or sing to the fetus, or play with the fetus as he notes movement.

Men prepare for fatherhood in many of the same ways as women do for motherhood–by reading and by fantasizing about the baby. Daydreaming about their role as father is common in the last weeks before the birth; men rarely describe their thoughts unless they are reassured that such daydreams are normal. They may adjust work commitments or plan vacations so that they can spend time with their new family.

Nurses can help fathers identify concerns and prepare for the reality of a baby by asking questions such as the following:

- What do you expect the baby to look and act like?
- What do you think being a father will be like?
- Have you thought about the baby's crying? Changing diapers? Burping the baby? Being awakened at night? Sharing your partner with the baby?

The father may not wish to answer such questions when he is asked but may need time to think them through or discuss them with his partner.

As the birth date approaches, men have more questions about fetal and newborn behaviors. Some men are shocked or amazed at the smallness of clothes and furniture for the baby. If an expectant father can imagine only an older child and has difficulty visualizing or talking about an infant, this situation must be explored. The nurse can tell the father about the unborn child's ability to respond to light, sound, and touch and encourage him to feel and talk to the fetus. A tour of a newborn nursery may be welcomed.

Some men become involved by picking the child's name and anticipating the child's sex, if it is not already known. Some couples select the name of the child as early as the first month of pregnancy. Family tradition, religious customs, and the continuation of the parent's name or names of relatives or friends are important in the selection process. Calling the unborn child by name helps to confirm the reality of pregnancy and promote attachment.

Parents may occasionally show or voice disappointment over the sex of the child. The parents may experience grief and a sense of loss at birth as they release their fantasized image of the child and begin to accept the real child. These negative responses toward a normal, healthy baby may be difficult for nurses to understand; however, most such responses are temporary. Providing an accepting environment for parental reactions facilitates the parent's ability to move beyond disappointment to acceptance.

Preparing for Childbirth

The days and weeks immediately before the expected day of birth are characterized by anticipation and anxiety. Boredom and restlessness are common as the couple focuses on the birth process; however, during the last 2 months of pregnancy, many expectant fathers experience a surge of creative energy at home and on the job. They may become dissatisfied with their present living space. If possible, they tend to act on the need to alter the environment (remodeling, painting, etc.). This activity may be overt evidence of their sharing in the childbearing experience. They are able to channel the anxiety and other feelings experienced during the final weeks before birth into productive activities. This behavior earns recognition and compliments from friends, relatives, and their partners.

The man's anxieties also may be expressed by his refusal to think about the birth, disinterest in planning for other activities during his partner's labor, or excessive sleeping. The expectant mother may become concerned about possibly being deserted physically or emotionally at a time when she is feeling most vulnerable.

Major concerns for the man are getting the woman to a medical facility in time for the birth and not appearing ignorant. Many men want to be able to recognize labor and determine when it is appropriate to leave for the hospital or call the physician or midwife. They may fantasize different situations and plan what they will do in response to them, or they may rehearse taking various routes to the hospital, timing each route at different times of the day.

Some prospective fathers have questions about the labor suite's furniture, nursing staff, and location, as well as the availability of the physician and anesthesiologist. Others want to know what is expected of them when their partners are in labor. The man also may have fears concerning safe passage of his partner and the mutilation or death of his partner and child. While he harbors these fears, he cannot help his mate deal with her own unspoken or overt apprehension.

With the exception of childbirth preparation classes, a man has few opportunities to learn ways to be an involved and active partner in this rite of passage into parenthood. The tensions and apprehensions of the unprepared, unsupportive father are readily transmitted to the mother and may increase her fears. His own self-doubts and fear of inadequacy may be realized if he is not supported. Self-confidence comes from achieving realistic goals and earning the approval of others.

The same fears, questions, and concerns may affect birth partners who are not the biologic fathers. Birth partners need to be kept informed, supported, and included in all activities in which the mother desires their participation. The nurse can do much to promote pregnancy and birth as a family experience.

Sibling Adaptation

Sharing the spotlight with a new brother or sister may be the first major crisis for a child. The older child often experiences a sense of loss or feels jealous at being "replaced" by the new sibling. Some of the factors that influence the child's response are age, the parents' attitudes, the role of the father, the length of separation from the mother, the hospital's visitation policy, and the way the child has been prepared for the change.

A mother with other children must devote time and effort to reorganizing her relationships with existing children. She needs to prepare siblings for the birth of the child (see Fig. 17-4 and Box 17-4) and begin the process of role transition in the family by including the children in the pregnancy and being sympathetic to older children's concerns about losing their places in the family hierarchy. No child willingly gives up a familiar position.

Siblings' responses to pregnancy vary with their age and dependency needs. The 1-year-old infant seems largely unaware of the process, but the 2-year-old child notices the change in his or her mother's appearance and may comment that "Mommy's fat." The toddlers' need for sameness in the environment makes the children aware of any change. They may exhibit more clinging behavior and revert to dependent behaviors in toilet training or eating.

By age 3 or 4 years, children like to be told the story of their own beginning and accept its being compared with the present pregnancy. They like to listen to the fetal heartbeat and feel the baby moving in utero (see Fig. 16-2). Sometimes they worry about how the baby is being fed and what it wears.

School-age children take a more clinical interest in their mother's pregnancy. They may want to know in more detail, "How did the baby get in there?" and "How will it get out?" Children in this age group notice pregnant women in stores, churches, and schools and sometimes seem shy if they need to approach a pregnant woman directly. On the whole, they look forward to the new baby, see themselves as "mothers" or "fathers," and enjoy buying baby supplies and readying a place for the baby. Because they still think in concrete terms and base judgments on the here and now, they respond positively to their mother's current good health.

Early and middle adolescents preoccupied with the establishment of their own sexual identity may have difficulty accepting the overwhelming evidence of the sexual activity of their parents. They reason that if they are too young for such activity, certainly their parents are too old. They seem to take on a critical parental role and may ask, "What will people think?" or "How can you let yourself get so fat?" Many pregnant women with teenage children will confess that the attitudes of their teenagers are the most difficult aspect of their current pregnancy.

Late adolescents do not appear to be unduly disturbed. They are busy making plans for their own lives and realize that they soon will be gone from home. Parents usually report they are comforting and act more as other adults than as children.

Grandparent Adaptation

Every pregnancy affects all family relationships. For expectant grandparents, a first pregnancy in a child is undeniable evidence that they are growing older. Many think of a grandparent as old, white-haired, and becoming feeble of mind and body; however, some people face grandparenthood while still in their 30s or 40s. A mother-to-be announcing her pregnancy to her mother may be greeted by a negative response, indicating that she is not ready to be a grandmother. Daughter and mother both may be startled and hurt by the response.

Some expectant grandparents not only are nonsupportive but also use subtle means to decrease the self-esteem of the young parents-to-be. Mothers may talk about their terrible pregnancies; fathers may discuss the endless cost of rearing children; and mothers-in-law may complain that their sons are neglecting them because their concern is now directed toward the pregnant daughters-in-law.

However, most grandparents are delighted at the prospect of a new baby in the family. It reawakens the feelings of their own youth, the excitement of giving birth, and their delight in the behavior of the parents-to-be when they were infants. They set up a memory store of the child's first smiles, first words, and first steps, which they can use later for "claiming" the newborn as a member of the family. Their and the parents' satisfaction comes with the realization that the continuity between past and present is guaranteed.

In addition, the grandparent is the historian who transmits the family history, a resource person who shares knowledge based on experience; a role model; and a support person. The grandparent's presence and support can

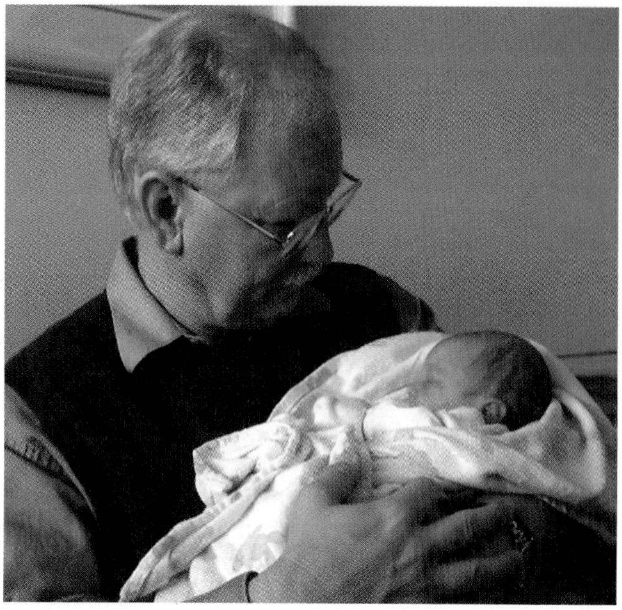

FIG. 16-4 Grandfather getting to know his grandson. (Courtesy Sharon Johnson, Petaluma, CA.)

strengthen family systems by widening the circle of support and nurturance (Fig. 16-4). Other sources of information cannot replace the unique contribution of the grandparents. The parent in turn acts as a negotiator in establishing the grandparent-grandchild relationship.

Many women report that their pregnancies bridged the final gap between them and their own mothers. The estrangement that began in adolescence disappears as the now-pregnant daughter experiences joys, concerns, and anxieties similar to those felt by her mother before her.

Expectant grandparenthood also can represent a maturational milestone for the parent of an expectant parent. To be truly family oriented, maternity care must include the grandparent in the implementation of the nursing process with the whole childbearing family. A class for grandparents is one method of incorporating the grandparents into the family system and encouraging communication between the generations.

Grandparents' anxieties and concerns and their relationships with expectant parents and grandchildren should be discussed during courses for expectant parents. The expectant parents may use this opportunity to begin to resolve conflicts and perceived differences with their parents, a task that can also enhance their ability to relate to their own children.

CARE MANAGEMENT

The purpose of prenatal care is to identify existing risk factors and other deviations from normal so that pregnancy outcomes may be enhanced (Johnson & Niebyl, 2002). Major emphasis is placed on preventive aspects of care, primarily to motivate the pregnant woman to practice optimal self-care and to report unusual changes early so that problems can be minimized or prevented. If health behaviors must be modified in early pregnancy, nurses need to understand psychosocial factors that may have influence on the woman (Walker, Cooney, & Riggs, 1999). In holistic care, nurses provide information and guidance about not only the physical changes but also the psychosocial impact of pregnancy on the woman and members of her family. The goals of prenatal nursing care, therefore, are to foster a safe birth for the infant and to promote satisfaction of the mother and family with the pregnancy and birth experience.

Advances have been made in the number of women in the United States who receive adequate prenatal care, currently at 83% (HRSA, 2002). Although prenatal care is sought routinely by women of middle or high socioeconomic status, women living in poverty or who lack health insurance may not be able to use public medical services or gain access to private care. Lack of culturally sensitive care providers and barriers in communication due to differences in language also interfere with access to care (Shaffer, 2002). Likewise, immigrant women who come from cultures in which prenatal care is not emphasized may not know to seek routine prenatal care. Birth outcomes in these populations are thus less positive, with higher rates of maternal and fetal or newborn complications. Problems with low birth weight (LBW; less than 2500 g) and infant mortality have in particular been associated with lack of adequate prenatal care. Outcomes for these women can be improved with enhanced prenatal services (Shaffer, 2002; Stankaitis & Hollander, 2002).

Barriers to obtaining health care during pregnancy include lack of transportation, unpleasant clinic facilities or procedures, inconvenient clinic hours, and personal attitudes (Braveman et al., 2000; Chandler, 2002; Mikhail & Curry, 1999). Much effort has been focused on finding ways to improve access and quality of care to ensure that all women and infants have the best opportunity for the most positive outcomes. The availability and accessibility to prenatal care may be improved by the increasing use of advanced practice nurses in collaborative practice with physicians (Mvula & Miller, 1998). The effectiveness of a regular schedule of home visiting by nurses during pregnancy also has been validated (Chestnut, 1998).

The current model for provision of prenatal care has been used for more than a century. The initial visit usually occurs in the first trimester, with monthly visits through week 28 of pregnancy. Thereafter, visits are scheduled every 2 weeks until week 36, and then every week until birth. This model is currently being questioned, and in some practices, there is a growing tendency to have fewer visits with women who are at low risk for complications (Villar et al., 2002). Health care providers are challenged to create a system of prenatal care that has minimal barriers and a focus on individualized care (Fuller & Gallagher, 1999).

In recent years the concept of preconception care has been recognized as an important contributor to good outcomes of pregnancy. If women can be taught about the benefits of nutrition, the importance of folic acid intake, avoidance of smoking and abuse of substances, avoidance of sexually transmitted infections (STIs) and other health hazards, a healthier pregnancy may be planned. Likewise, women who have health problems related to chronic diseases such as diabetes mellitus can be counseled regarding their special needs. This area of nursing care is not well developed, and the opportunities for health promotion services are evident.

Prenatal care is ideally a multidisciplinary activity in which nurses work with physicians or midwives, nutritionists, social workers, and others. Collaboration among these individuals is necessary to provide holistic care. The case management model, which makes use of care maps and critical pathways, is one system that promotes comprehensive care with limited overlap in services. To emphasize the nursing role, care management here is organized around the central elements of the nursing process: assessment, nursing diagnoses, expected outcomes, plan of care and interventions, and evaluation.

Assessment and Nursing Diagnoses

Once the presence of pregnancy has been confirmed and the woman's desire to continue the pregnancy has been validated, prenatal care is begun. The assessment process begins at the initial prenatal visit and is continued throughout the pregnancy. Assessment techniques include the interview, physical examination, and laboratory tests. Because the initial visit and follow-up visits are distinctly different in content and process, they are described separately.

Initial Visit

The pregnant woman and family members who may be present should be told that the first prenatal visit is more lengthy and detailed than are future visits. The initial evaluation includes a comprehensive health history emphasizing the current pregnancy, previous pregnancies, the family, a psychosocial profile, a physical assessment, diagnostic testing, and an overall risk assessment. A prenatal history form (Fig. 16-5) is the best way to document information obtained. To be useful in communicating with other care providers, entries on the form should be made with attention to neatness and clarity.

Interview. The therapeutic relationship between the nurse and the woman is established during the initial assessment interview. It is a time for planned, purposeful communication that focuses on specific content. The data collected are of two types: the woman's subjective appraisal of her health status and the nurse's objective observations. During the interview the nurse observes the woman's affect, posture, body language, skin color, and other physical and emotional signs.

Often the pregnant woman is accompanied by one or more family members. The nurse needs to build a relationship with these people as part of the social context of the client. With her permission, those accompanying the woman can be included in the initial prenatal interview, and the observations and information about the woman's family form part of the database (Fig. 16-6 on p. 412). For example, if the woman is accompanied by small children, the nurse can ask about her plans for child care during the time of labor and birth. Special needs are noted at this time (e.g., wheelchair access, assistance in getting on and off the examining table, and cognitive deficits).

Reason for Seeking Care. Although pregnant women are scheduled for "routine" prenatal visits, they often come to the health care provider seeking information or reassurance about a particular concern. When the client is asked a broad, open-ended question such as, "How have you been feeling?", she may reveal problems that could otherwise be overlooked. The woman's chief concerns should be recorded in her own words to alert other personnel to the priority of needs as identified by her. At the initial visit, the desire for information about what is normal in the course of pregnancy is typical (see Guidelines/Guías box on p. 412).

Current Pregnancy. The presumptive signs of pregnancy may be of great concern to the woman. A review of symptoms she is experiencing and how she is coping with them helps to establish a database to develop a plan of care. Some early teaching may be provided at this time.

Obstetric-Gynecologic History. Data are gathered on the woman's age at menarche, menstrual history, and contraceptive history; the nature of any infertility or gynecologic conditions; her history of any STIs; her sexual history; and a detailed history of all her pregnancies, including the present pregnancy, and their outcomes. The date of the last Papanicolaou test and the result are noted. The date of her LMP is obtained to establish the EDB. (See the Guidelines/Guías box on p. 412 for questions that may be used with Spanish-speaking women.)

Medical History. The medical history includes those medical or surgical conditions that may affect the pregnancy or that may be affected by the pregnancy. For example, a pregnant woman who has diabetes or epilepsy requires special care. Because most women are anxious during the initial interview, the nurse's reference to cues, such as a MedicAlert bracelet, prompts the woman to explain allergies, chronic diseases, or medications being taken (e.g., cortisone, insulin, or anticonvulsants).

The nature of previous surgical procedures also should be described. If a woman has undergone uterine surgery or extensive repair of the pelvic floor, a cesarean birth may be necessary; appendectomy rules out appendicitis as a cause of right lower quadrant pain in pregnancy; and spinal surgery may contraindicate the use of spinal or epidural anesthesia. Any injury involving the pelvis is noted.

Patient Addressograph

Date ____________________

Name ____
Last First Middle

ID # ______________________ Hospital of delivery ______________________

Newborn's physician ______________________ Referred by ______________________

Final EDD ______________ | Primary provider group ______________________

Birth date Month Day Year	Age	Race	Marital status S M W D SEP	Address:
Occupation ☐ Homemaker ☐ Outside work ☐ Student	Type of work		Education (last grade completed)	Zip: Phone: (H) (O) Insurance Carrier/Medicaid #
Husband/father of baby:		Phone:		Emergency contact: Phone:

Total preg	Full term	Premature	AB, induced	AB, spontaneous	Ectopics	Multiple births	Living

Menstrual History

LMP ☐ Definite ☐ Approximate (month known) Menses monthly ☐ Yes ☐ No Frequency: Q ____ days Menarche ____ (age onset)
☐ Unknown ☐ Normal amount/duration Prior menses ________ Date On BCP at concept. ☐ Yes ☐ No hCG + ___/___/___
☐ Final ______

Past Pregnancies (last six)

Date/month/year	GA weeks	Length of labor	Birth weight	Sex M/F	Type delivery	Anes.	Place of delivery	Preterm labor yes/no	Comments/complications

Past Medical History

	O Neg + Pos	Detail positive remarks Include data and treatment
1. Diabetes		
2. Hypertension		
3. Heart disease		
4. Autoimmune disorder		
5. Kidney disease/UTI		
6. Neurologic/epilepsy		
7. Psychiatric		
8. Hepatitis/liver disease		
9. Varicosities/phlebitis		
10. Thyroid dysfunction		
11. Trauma/domestic violence		
12. History of blood tranfus.		

	AMT/day Prepreg	AMT/day Preg	# Years use
13. Tobacco			
14. Alcohol			
15. Street drugs			

	O Neg + Pos	Detail positive remarks Include data & treatment
16. D (Rh) sensitized		
17. Pulmonary (TB, asthma)		
18. Allergies (drugs)		
19. Breast		
20. Gyn surgery		
21. Operations/hospitalizations (year and reason)		
22. Anesthetic complications		
23. History of abnormal PAP		
24. Uterine anomaly/DES		
25. Infertility		
26. Relevant family history		
27. Other		

Comments: ____

The American College of Obstetricians and Gynecologists, 409 12th Street, SW, PO Box 96920, Washington, DC 20090-6920

ACOG ANTEPARTUM RECORD (FORM A)

FIG. 16-5 Prenatal history form. (From American College of Obstetricians and Gynecologists. [1997]. *Antepartum record.* Washington, DC: ACOG. To order this publication, please call 1-800-762-2264, ext. 199).

Often women who have chronic or handicapping conditions forget to mention them during the initial assessment because they have become so adapted to them. Special shoes or a limp may indicate the existence of a pelvic structural defect, which is an important consideration in pregnant women. The nurse who observes these special characteristics and inquires about them sensitively can obtain individualized data that will provide the basis for a comprehensive nursing care plan. Observations are vital components of the interview process because they prompt

Patient Addressograph

Symptoms since LMP

Genetic Screening/Teratology Counseling
includes patient, baby's father, or anyone in either family with:

	Yes	No		Yes	No
1. Patient's age ≥35 years			12. Mental retardation/autism		
			If yes, was person tested for fragile X?		
2. Thalassemia (Italian, Greek, Mediterranean, or Asian background): MCV <80			13. Other inherited genetic or chromosomal disorder		
3. Neural tube defect (meningomyelocele, spina bifida, or anencephaly)			14. Maternal metabolic disorder (e.g., insulin-dependent diabetes, PKU)		
4. Congenital heart defect					
5. Down syndrome			15. Patient or baby's father had a child with birth defects not listed above		
6. Tay-Sachs (e.g., Jewish, Cajun, French-Canadian)					
7. Sickle cell disease or trait (African)			16. Recurrent pregnancy loss, or a stillbirth		
8. Hemophilia			17. Medications/street drugs/alcohol since last menstrual period		
9. Muscular dystrophy					
10. Cystic fibrosis			If yes, agent(s):		
11. Huntington chorea			18. Any other		

Comments/counseling: ______

Infection History	Yes	No		Yes	No
1. High risk hepatitis B/immunized?			4. Rash or viral illness since last menstrual period		
2. Live with someone with TB or exposed to TB			5. History of STD, GC, chlamydia, HPV, syphilis		
3. Patient or partner has history of genital herpes			6. Other (see comments)		

Comments: ______

Interviewer's signature: ______

Initial Physical Examination

Date ____/____/____ Prepregnancy weight ______ Height ______ BP ______

1. HEENT	☐ Normal	☐ Abnormal	12. Vulva	☐ Normal	☐ Condyloma	☐ Lesions
2. Fundi	☐ Normal	☐ Abnormal	13. Vagina	☐ Normal	☐ Inflammation	☐ Discharge
3. Teeth	☐ Normal	☐ Abnormal	14. Cervix	☐ Normal	☐ Inflammation	☐ Lesions
4. Thyroid	☐ Normal	☐ Abnormal	15. Uterus size	____ Weeks		☐ Fibroids
5. Breasts	☐ Normal	☐ Abnormal	16. Adnexa	☐ Normal	☐ Mass	
6. Lungs	☐ Normal	☐ Abnormal	17. Rectum	☐ Normal	☐ Abnormal	
7. Heart	☐ Normal	☐ Abnormal	18. Diagonal conjugate	☐ Reached	☐ No	____ cm
8. Abdomen	☐ Normal	☐ Abnormal	19. Spines	☐ Average	☐ Prominent	☐ Blunt
9. Extremities	☐ Normal	☐ Abnormal	20. Sacrum	☐ Concave	☐ Straight	☐ Anterior
10. Skin	☐ Normal	☐ Abnormal	21. Subpubic arch	☐ Normal	☐ Wide	☐ Narrow
11. Lymph nodes	☐ Normal	☐ Abnormal	22. Gynecoid pelvic type	☐ Yes	☐ No	

Comments (Number and explain abnormals): ______

Exam by: ______

ACOG ANTEPARTUM RECORD (FORM B)

Continued

FIG. 16-5, cont'd For legend see opposite page.

the nurse and woman to focus on the specific needs of the woman and her family.

Nutritional History. The woman's nutritional history is an important component of the prenatal history because her nutritional status has a direct effect on the growth and development of the fetus. A dietary assessment can reveal special diet practices, food allergies, eating behaviors, and other factors related to her nutritional status. Pregnant women are usually motivated to learn about good nutrition and respond well to nutritional advice generated by this assessment.

Patient Addressograph

Name ______________________________
Last First Middle

Drug allergy:	
Religious/cultural considerations ________	Anesthesia consult planned ☐ Yes ☐ No

Problems/plans	Medication List	Start date	Stop date
1.	1.		
2.	2.		
3.	3.		

EDD Confirmation		18-20-Week EDD Update	
Initial EDD:		Quickening	__/__/__+22 wks = __/__/__
LMP	__/__/__ = EDD __/__/__	Fundal ht. at umbil.	__/__/__+20 wks = __/__/__
Initial exam	__/__/__= ___ wks = EDD __/__/__	FHT w/fetoscope	__/__/__+20 wks = __/__/__
Ultrasound	__/__/__= ___ wks = EDD __/__/__	Ultrasound	__/__/__= ___ wks = __/__/__
Initial EDD	__/__/__ Initialed by ______	Final EDD	__/__/__ Initialed by ______

Visit date (year)	Weeks gest. (best est.)	Fundal height (cm)	Presentation	FHR	Fetal movement	Preterm labor Signs/symptoms: +=Present O=Absent	Cervix exam (dil./eff./sta.)	Blood pressure	Edema	Weight	Urine (glucose/albumin)	Next appointment	Provider (initials)

Comments:

Problems: ______________________________

Comments: ______________________________

ACOG ANTEPARTUM RECORD (FORM C)

FIG. 16-5, cont'd For legend see page 408.

History of Drug Use. A woman's past and present use of legal (over-the-counter [OTC], prescription, and herbal drugs; caffeine; alcohol; nicotine) and illegal (marijuana, cocaine, heroin) drugs must be assessed because many substances cross the placenta and may therefore harm the developing fetus. Periodic urine toxicology screening tests are often recommended during the pregnancies of women who have a history of illegal drug use. Results of such tests have been used for criminal prosecution, which results in a breach in client-provider relationship and in ethical responsibilities to the client (Foley, 2002).

Family History. The family history provides information about the woman's immediate family, including parents, siblings, and children. These data help identify familial or genetic disorders or conditions that could affect the present health status of the woman or her fetus.

Social and Experiential History. Situational factors such as the family's ethnic and cultural background and socioeconomic status are assessed while the history is obtained. The following information may be obtained in several encounters. The woman's perception of this pregnancy is explored by asking her such questions as the following: Is this pregnancy planned or not, wanted or not? Is the woman pleased, displeased, accepting, or nonaccepting? What problems related to finances, career, or living accommodations may arise as a result of the pregnancy? The family support system is determined by asking her such questions as the following: What primary support is available to her? Are changes needed to promote adequate support? What are the existing relationships among the mother, father/partner, siblings, and in-laws? What preparations are being made for her care and that of dependent family members during labor and for the care of the infant after birth? Is financial, educational, or other support needed from the community? What are the woman's ideas about childbearing, her expectations of the infant's behavior, and her outlook on life and the female role?

Other such questions that should be asked include the following: What does the woman think it will be like to

Patient Addressograph

Laboratory and Education

Initial Labs	Date	Result	Reviewed
Blood type	__/__/__	A B AB O	
D (Rh) type	__/__/__		
Antibody screen	__/__/__		
HCT/HGB	__/__/__	___% ___ g/dl	
Pap test	__/__/__	Normal/Abnormal/__	
Rubella	__/__/__		
VDRL	__/__/__		
Urine culture/screen	__/__/__		
HBsAg	__/__/__		
HIV counseling/testing	__/__/__	☐ Pos. ☐ Neg. ☐ Declined	
Optional Labs	**Date**	**Result**	
HGB Electrophoresis	__/__/__	AA AS SS AC SC AF ↑A_2	
PPD	__/__/__		
Chlamydia	__/__/__		
GC	__/__/__		
Tay-Sachs	__/__/__		
Other			
8-18-Week Labs (When indicated/elected)	**Date**	**Result**	
Ultrasound	__/__/__		
MSAFP/multiple markers	__/__/__		
Amnio/CVS	__/__/__		
Karyotype	__/__/__	46, XX or 46, XY/other	
Amniotic fluid (AFP)	__/__/__	Normal __ Abnormal __	
24-28-Week Labs (When indicated)	**Date**	**Result**	
HCT/HGB	__/__/__	___% ___ g/dl	
Diabetes screen	__/__/__	1 hour _____	
GTT (If screen abnormal)	__/__/__	__ FBS __ 1 hour __ 2 hour __ 3 hour	
D (Rh) antibody screen	__/__/__		
D Immune globulin (RhIG) given (28 wks)	__/__/__	Signature _____	
32-36-Week Labs (When indicated)	**Date**	**Result**	
HCT/HGB (recommended)	__/__/__	___% ___ g/dl	
Ultrasound	__/__/__		
VDRL	__/__/__		
GC	__/__/__		
Chlamydia	__/__/__		
Group B Strep (35-37 wks)	__/__/__		

Comments/Additional Labs

Plans/Education (Counseled ☐)

- ☐ Anesthesia plans _____
- ☐ Toxoplasmosis precautions (cats/raw meat) _____
- ☐ Childbirth classes _____
- ☐ Physical/sexual activity _____
- ☐ Labor signs _____
- ☐ Nutrition counseling _____
- ☐ Breast or bottle feeding _____
- ☐ Newborn car seat _____
- ☐ Postpartum birth control _____
- ☐ Environmental/work hazards _____
- ☐ Tubal sterilization _____
- ☐ VBAC counseling _____
- ☐ Circumcision _____
- ☐ Travel _____
- ☐ Lifestyle, tobacco, alcohol _____

Requests _____

Tubal Sterilization Consent signed	Date	Initials
	__/__/__	_____

ACOG ANTEPARTUM RECORD (FORM D)

AA 128 2345/10987

Provider signature (as required) _____

FIG. 16-5, cont'd For legend see page 408.

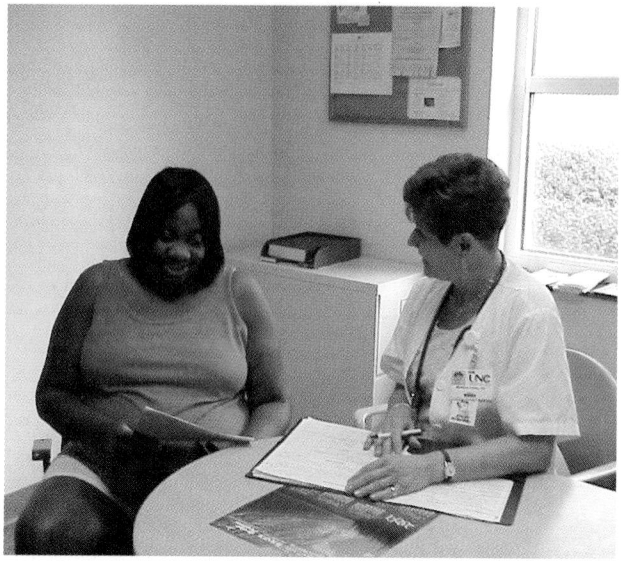

FIG. 16-6 Prenatal interview. (Courtesy Dee Lowdermilk, Chapel Hill, NC.)

GUIDELINES/GUÍAS

Prenatal Interview

Have you had a pregnancy test?
¿Se ha hecho la prueba de embarazo?

When was your last menstrual cycle?
¿Cuándo fue su última regla?

Have you been pregnant before?
¿Estuvo embarazada antes?

How many times?
¿Cuántas veces?

How many children do you have?
¿Cuántos hijos tiene usted?

Have you ever had a miscarriage?
¿Ha tenido un aborto natural?

Have you ever had a therapeutic abortion?
¿Ha tenido un aborto provocado?

Have you ever had a stillborn?
¿Ha tenido un niño que nació muerto?

Have you ever had a cesarean?
¿Ha tenido una cesárea?

Have you had any problems with past pregnancies?
¿Ha tenido algún problema en sus embarazos previos?

Do you take drugs? Prescription medicine?
¿Usa drogas? ¿Medicina recetada?

If so, which type of medicine do you use and for what?
¿Cuál medicina usa y para qué?

Do you drink alcohol? Do you smoke?
¿Toma licor o bebidas alcohólicas? ¿Fuma?

ETHICAL CONSIDERATIONS

Nurses may have ethical concerns if pregnant women are not informed of the possibility of random urine testing for presence of drugs. The other side of this concern is the unborn child and whether the mother has a duty not to harm him or her.

have a baby in the home? How is her life going to change by having a baby? What plans does having a baby interrupt? During interviews throughout the pregnancy the nurse should remain alert to the appearance of potential parenting problems, such as depression, lack of family support, and inadequate living conditions. The nurse needs to assess the woman's attitude toward health care, particularly during childbearing, her expectations of health care providers, and her view of the relationship between herself and the nurse.

Coping mechanisms and patterns of interacting also are identified. Early in the pregnancy the nurse should determine the woman's knowledge of pregnancy; maternal changes; fetal growth; self-care; and care of the newborn, including feeding. Asking about attitudes toward unmedicated or medicated childbirth and about her knowledge of the availability of parenting skills classes is important. Before planning for nursing care, the nurse needs information about the woman's decision-making abilities and living habits (e.g., exercise, sleep, diet, diversional interests, personal hygiene, clothing). Common stressors during childbearing include the baby's welfare, labor and birth process, behaviors of the newborn, woman's relationship with the baby's father, changes in body image, and physical symptoms.

Attitudes concerning the range of acceptable sexual behavior during pregnancy also should be explored by asking questions such as the following: What has your family (partner, friends) told you about sex during pregnancy? The woman's sexual self-concept is given more emphasis by asking questions such as the following: How do you feel about the changes in your appearance? How does your partner feel about your body now? How do you feel about wearing maternity clothes?

All women should be assessed for a history or risk of physical abuse, particularly because the likelihood of abuse increases during pregnancy. (See Chapter 6 for detailed information.) Although visual cues from the woman's appearance or behavior may sometimes suggest the possibility of abuse, no one profile of battered women exists. Identification of abuse and immediate clinical intervention that includes information about safety can result in behaviors that may prevent future abuse and increase the safety and well-being of the woman and her infant (McFarlane et al., 1998).

Review of Systems. During this portion of the interview, the woman is asked to identify and describe preexisting or concurrent problems with any of the body systems, and her mental status is assessed. The woman is questioned about physical symptoms she has experienced, such as shortness of breath or pain. Pregnancy affects and is affected by all body systems; therefore information on the present status of the body systems is important in planning care. For each sign or symptom described, the following additional data should be obtained: body location, quality, quantity, chronology, aggravating or alleviating factors, and associated manifestations (onset, character, course) (Seidel et al., 2003).

Physical Examination. The initial physical examination provides the baseline for assessing subsequent changes. The examiner should determine the woman's needs for basic information regarding reproductive anatomy and provide this information, along with a demonstration of the equipment that may be used and an explanation of the procedure itself. The interaction requires an unhurried, sensitive, and gentle approach with a matter-of-fact attitude.

The physical examination begins with assessment of vital signs including blood pressure (BP), height, and weight. The bladder should be empty before pelvic examination. This may be the opportunity to collect a specimen to test for protein, glucose, leukocytes, or other tests.

Each examiner develops a routine for proceeding with the physical examination; most choose the head-to-toe progression. Heart and breath sounds are evaluated, and extremities are examined. Distribution, amount, and quality of body hair is of particular importance because the findings reflect nutritional status, endocrine function, and attention to hygiene. The thyroid gland is assessed carefully. The height of the fundus is noted if the first examination is done after the first trimester of pregnancy. The typical basic examination is usually completed without much discomfort for the healthy woman. During the examination, the examiner needs to remain alert to the woman's cues that give direction to the remainder of the assessment and that indicate imminent untoward response such as **supine hypotension,** low blood pressure that occurs while the woman is lying on her back, causing feelings of faintness. See Chapter 5 for a detailed description of the physical examination.

Whenever a pelvic examination is performed, the tone of the pelvic musculature and the need for the woman's knowledge of Kegel exercises are assessed. Particular attention is paid to the size of the uterus because this is an indication of the duration of gestation. The nurse present during the examination can coach the woman in breathing and relaxation techniques at this time, as needed. One vaginal examination during pregnancy is recommended, but another is usually not done unless medically indicated (Bergsjo & Villar, 1997).

Laboratory Tests. The laboratory data yielded by the analysis of the specimens obtained during the examination provide important information concerning the symptoms of pregnancy and the woman's health status. Such information is used for making nursing and medical diagnoses.

Specimens are collected at the initial visit so that the cause of any abnormal findings can be treated (Table 16-1). Blood is drawn for a variety of tests: RPR (rapid plasma reagent)/VDRL (Venereal Disease Research Laboratory) test for syphilis; complete blood cell count (CBC) with hematocrit, hemoglobin, and differential values; tests for blood type and Rh factor; antibody screen (Kell, Duffy, rubella, toxoplasmosis, and anti-Rh); and measurement of the folacin level, when indicated. The woman is tested for hepatitis B surface antigen (HBsAG) and hepatitis B surface antibody (HBsAB), if she has not received hepatitis B vaccine. A sickle cell screen is recommended for women of African, Asian, or Middle Eastern descent, and testing for antibody to the human immunodeficiency virus (HIV) is strongly recommended for all pregnant women (Barron, 2001) (Box 16-2). Urine is tested for glucose (diabetes), protein (pregnancy-induced hypertension [PIH]), and nitrites and leukocytes (urinary tract infection); culture and sensitivity tests are ordered as necessary. A Tine or purified protein derivative (PPD) tuberculin test may be administered to assess exposure to tuberculosis. During the pelvic examination, cervical and vaginal smears may be obtained for cytologic studies and for diagnosis of infection (e.g., *Chlamydia*, gonorrhea).

The finding of risk factors during pregnancy may indicate the need to repeat some tests at other times. For example, exposure to tuberculosis or an STI would necessitate repeat testing. STIs are common in pregnancy and may have negative effects on mother and fetus. Careful assessment and screening are essential.

Follow-Up Visits

Monthly visits are scheduled routinely during the first and second trimesters, although additional appointments may be made as the need arises. During the third trimester, however, the possibility for complications increases, and closer monitoring is warranted. Starting with week 28, maternity visits are scheduled every 2 weeks until week 36, and then every week until birth, unless the health care provider individualizes the schedule. Individual needs and risks of the pregnant woman may warrant visits more or less often. The pattern of interviewing the woman first and then assessing physical changes and performing laboratory tests is maintained.

Interview. Follow-up visits are less intensive than the initial prenatal visit. At each of these follow-up visits, the woman is asked to summarize relevant events that have occurred since the previous visit. She is asked about her general emotional and physiologic well-being, complaints or problems, or questions she may have. Personal and family needs also are identified and explored.

TABLE 16-1 **Laboratory Tests in Prenatal Period**

LABORATORY TEST	PURPOSE
Hemoglobin/hematocrit/WBC, differential	Detects anemia/detects infection
Hemoglobin electrophoresis	Identifies women with hemoglobinopathies (e.g., sickle cell anemia, thalassemia)
Blood type, Rh, and irregular antibody	Identifies those fetuses at risk for developing erythroblastosis fetalis or hyperbilirubinemia in neonatal period
Rubella titer	Determines immunity to rubella
Tuberculin skin testing; chest film after 20 weeks' gestation in women with reactive tuberculin tests	Screens for exposure to tuberculosis
Urinalysis, including microscopic examination of urinary sediment; pH, specific gravity, color, glucose, albumin, protein, RBCs, WBCs, casts, acetone; hCG	Identifies women with unsuspected diabetes mellitus, renal disease, hypertensive disease of pregnancy; infection; occult hematuria
Urine culture	Identifies women with asymptomatic bacteriuria
Renal function tests: BUN, creatinine, electrolytes, creatinine clearance, total protein excretion	Evaluates level of possible renal compromise in women with a history of diabetes, hypertension, or renal disease
Pap test	Screens for cervical intraepithelial neoplasia, herpes simplex type 2, and HPV
Vaginal or rectal smear for *Neisseria gonorrhoeae, Chlamydia,* HPV, GBS	Screens high-risk population for asymptomatic infection. GBS done at 35-37 wk
RPR/VDRL/FTA-ABS	Identifies women with untreated syphilis
HIV* antibody, hepatitis B surface antigen, toxoplasmosis	Screens for infection
1-hr glucose tolerance	Screens for gestational diabetes; done at initial visit for women with risk factors; done at 24-28 weeks for all pregnant women
3-hr glucose tolerance	Screens for diabetes in women with elevated glucose level after 1-hr test; must have two elevated readings for diagnosis
Cardiac evaluation: ECG, chest x-ray film, and echocardiogram	Evaluates cardiac function in women with a history of hypertension or cardiac disease

BUN, Blood urea nitrogen; *ECG,* electrocardiogram; *FTA-ABS,* fluorescent treponemal antibody absorption test; *GBS,* group B streptococcus; *hCG,* human chorionic gonadotropin; *HIV,* human immunodeficiency virus; *HPV,* human papillomavirus; *RBCs,* red blood cells; *RPR,* rapid plasma reagin; *VDRL,* Venereal Disease Research Laboratory; *WBC,* white blood cell.
*With client permission.

BOX 16-2 **HIV Screening**

Pregnant women are ethically obligated to seek reasonable care during pregnancy and to avoid causing harm to the fetus. Maternity nurses should be advocates for the fetus but not at the expense of the pregnant woman.

The incidence of perinatal transmission from an HIV-positive mother to her fetus ranges from 25% to 35%. Zidovudine decreases perinatal transmission and the risk of infant death (Brocklehurst & Volmink, 2002). Elective cesarean birth significantly reduces the risk of transmission from the mother to child (Brocklehurst, 2002). Thus testing has the potential to identify HIV-positive women who can then be treated. Health care providers have an obligation to ensure that pregnant women are well informed about HIV symptoms, testing, and methods of decreasing maternal-fetal transmission. However, mandatory HIV screening involves ethical issues related to privacy invasion, discrimination, social stigma, and reproductive risks to the pregnant woman. Although some professional groups advocate mandatory testing, the Association of Women's Health, Obstetric, and Neonatal Nurses (AWHONN) does not support either mandatory or universal HIV testing of pregnant women because these models do not have the same standards of confidentiality and counseling that are present with voluntary, confidential testing with counseling (AWHONN, 1999).

Because the woman's emotional state affects her and her family's general well-being, the emotional adjustment for all is assessed at each visit. Because emotional changes are expected during pregnancy, the nurse logically asks whether the woman has had any mood swings; reactions to changes in her body image, bad dreams, or worries. The reactions of family members to the pregnancy and the woman's progression through the developmental tasks of pregnancy also are assessed and recorded.

During the third trimester, current family situations and their effect on the woman are assessed (e.g., siblings' and grandparents' responses to the pregnancy and the coming child). In addition, the following questions are addressed:

- What anticipatory planning is in progress concerning new parenting responsibilities, sibling rivalry, recuperation from pregnancy and birth, and fertility management?
- What successes or frustrations with diet, rest and relaxation, sexuality, and emotional support is the woman experiencing?
- What is the woman's understanding of her family's needs in relation to the pregnancy and the unborn child?
- How well prepared are the parents for coping with an emergency? That is, does the woman know the warning signs (e.g., bleeding, abdominal pain, signs of preeclampsia), understand what they represent, and know how and to whom to report them?
- Does the woman know the signs of preterm and term labor?
- What is the woman's understanding of the labor process and expectations of herself and others during labor? Does she know what to bring to the hospital or birthing center?
- If she is having a home birth, have all the necessary supplies been obtained?
- What plans have the woman and her family made for labor?
- What anxieties are the woman or her family experiencing regarding labor or the unborn child?
- What does the woman wish to know about the control of discomfort during labor?
- Is the woman (and her partner or support person) planning to attend any parent education classes?
- Does the woman have questions about fetal development and methods to assess fetal well-being?

A review of the woman's body systems is appropriate at each visit, and any suggestive signs or symptoms are assessed in depth. Discomforts reflecting adaptations to pregnancy are identified. Special inquiries are made about possible infections (e.g., genitourinary tract, respiratory tract). The woman's knowledge of and success with self-care measures are assessed, as well as outcomes of prescribed therapy.

GUIDELINES/GUÍAS

Prenatal Physical Assessment

Get up on the scale, please.
Súbase a la báscula/la pesa, por favor.

I need a urine sample.
Necesito una muestra de orina.

Go to the bathroom, please.
Vaya al baño, por favor.

I need to take your blood pressure.
Necesito tomarle la presión arterial.

I am going to listen to the baby's heartbeat.
Voy a escuchar el latido del corazón del bebé.

The doctor is going to examine you.
El doctor le va hacer un examen.

Don't be afraid.
No tenga miedo.

Lie down, please.
Acuéstese, por favor.

Open your legs, please.
Separe las piernas, por favor.

Relax.
Relájese/cálmese.

Go to the laboratory for a blood test.
Vaya al laboratorio para un análisis de sangre.

Go to this office for your ultrasound.
Vaya a esta oficina para que le hagan el sonograma.

Physical Examination. Reevaluation is a constant aspect of a pregnant woman's care (see the Guidelines/Guías box for phrases in Spanish for prenatal physical assessment). Each woman reacts differently to pregnancy. As a result, careful monitoring of the pregnancy and her reactions to care is vital. The database is updated at each time of contact with the pregnant woman. Physiologic changes are documented as the pregnancy progresses and reviewed for possible deviations from normal progress.

At each visit, physical parameters are measured. Ideally, BP is taken by using the same arm at every visit, with the woman sitting. Her weight is determined, and the appropriateness of the weight gain is evaluated. Urine may be checked by dipstick, and the presence and degree of edema are noted. For examination of the abdomen, the woman lies on her back with her arms by her side and head supported by a pillow. The bladder should be empty. Abdominal inspection is followed by measurement of the height of the fundus. While the woman lies on her back, the nurse should be alert for the occurrence of supine hypotension (see Emergency box). When a woman is lying in this position, the weight of

EMERGENCY

Supine Hypotension

SIGNS/SYMPTOMS

Pallor
Dizziness, faintness, breathlessness
Tachycardia
Nausea
Clammy (damp, cool) skin; sweating

INTERVENTIONS

Position woman on her side until her signs/symptoms subside and vital signs stabilize within normal limits (WNL).

abdominal contents may compress the vena cava and aorta, causing a decrease in BP and a feeling of faintness.

The findings revealed during the interview and physical examination reflect the status of maternal adaptations. When any of the findings is suspicious, an in-depth examination is performed. For example, careful interpretation of BP is important in the risk factor analysis of all pregnant women. BP is evaluated on the basis of absolute values and the length of gestation and is interpreted in the light of modifying factors.

An absolute systolic BP of 140 mm Hg or more and a diastolic BP of 90 mm Hg or more suggest the presence of hypertension (Helewa et al., 1997). Although the BP of 140/90 is an excellent point of reference, further investigation is needed. An increase in the systolic BP of 30 mm Hg or more than the baseline pressure or in the diastolic BP of 15 mm Hg more than the baseline pressure also is a significant finding, regardless of the absolute values. Gilbert and Harmon (2003) suggested that an increase of 20 mm Hg or more in the mean arterial pressure (MAP) also is an important indicator of hypertension (see Box 14-2).

While completing the prenatal assessments, the nurse always keeps in mind that an increase in BP could indicate the onset of PIH or preeclampsia. Investigations by Caritis et al. (1998) indicated that an absolute value MAP greater than 80 in nulliparous women may be predictive of preeclampsia and more severe complications. See Chapter 30 for an in-depth discussion of problems associated with hypertension.

The pregnant woman is monitored continuously for a range of signs and symptoms that indicate potential complications in addition to hypertension. For example, persistent and excessive vomiting and ketonuria may indicate the development of hyperemesis gravidarum. Uterine cramping and vaginal bleeding are signs of threatened miscarriage. Chills and fever are symptoms of infection. Discharge from the vagina may be amniotic fluid or may be associated with infection (see Signs of Potential Complications box).

Fetal Assessment. Toward the end of the first trimester, before the uterus is an abdominal organ, the fetal heart tones (FHTs) can be heard with an ultrasound fetoscope or an ultrasound stethoscope. To hear the FHTs, place the instrument in the midline, just above the symphysis pubis, and apply firm pressure. The woman and her family should be offered the opportunity to listen to the FHTs. The health status of the fetus is assessed at each visit for the remainder of the pregnancy.

Fundal Height. During the second trimester, the uterus becomes an abdominal organ. The **fundal height,** measurement of the height of the uterus above the symphysis pubis, is used as one indicator of fetal growth. The measurement also provides a gross estimate of the duration of pregnancy. In addition, it may aid in the identification of high risk factors. A stable or decreased fundal height may indicate the presence of intrauterine growth restriction (IUGR); an excessive increase could indicate the presence of **multifetal** gestation (more than one fetus) or hydramnios.

A paper tape typically is used to measure fundal height. To increase the reliability of the measurement, the same person examines the pregnant woman at each of her prenatal visits, but often this is not possible. All clinicians who examine a particular pregnant woman should be consistent in their measurement technique. Ideally, a protocol should be established for the health care setting in which the measurement technique is explicitly set forth, and the woman's position on the examining table, the measuring device, and method of measurement used are specified. Conditions under which the measurements are taken also can be described in the woman's records, including whether the bladder was empty and whether the uterus was relaxed or contracted at the time of measurement.

Various positions for measuring fundal height have been described. The woman can be supine, have her head elevated, have her knees flexed, or have both her head elevated and knees flexed. Measurements obtained with the woman in the various positions differ, making it even more important to standardize the fundal height measurement technique. The bladder must be empty before the measurement is taken. As much as 3-cm variation is possible if the bladder is full (Cunningham et al., 2001).

Placement of the tape measure also can vary. The tape can be placed in the middle of the woman's abdomen, and the measurement made from the upper border of the symphysis pubis to the upper border of the fundus with the tape measure held in contact with the skin for the entire length of the uterus (Fig. 16-7, *A*). In another measurement technique, the upper curve of the fundus is not included in the measurement. Instead, one end of the tape measure is held at the upper border of the symphysis pubis with one hand, and the other hand is placed at the upper border of the fundus. The tape is placed between the middle and index fingers of the other hand, and the point where these fingers intercept the tape measure is taken as the measurement (Fig. 16-7, *B*).

During the second and third trimesters (weeks 18 to 30), the height of the fundus in centimeters is approximately

SIGNS OF POTENTIAL COMPLICATIONS
First, Second, and Third Trimesters

FIRST TRIMESTER Signs/Symptoms	Possible Causes
Severe vomiting	Hyperemesis gravidarum
Chills, fever	Infection
Burning on urination	Infection
Diarrhea	Infection
Abdominal cramping; vaginal bleeding	Miscarriage, ectopic pregnancy

SECOND AND THIRD TRIMESTERS Signs/Symptoms	Possible Causes
Persistent, severe vomiting	Hyperemesis gravidarum, hypertension, pregnancy-induced hypertension (PIH)
Sudden discharge of fluid from vagina before 37 wk	Premature rupture of membranes (PROM)
Vaginal bleeding, severe abdominal pain	Miscarriage, placenta previa, abruptio placentae
Chills, fever, burning on urination, diarrhea	Infection
Severe backache or flank pain	Kidney infection or stones; preterm labor
Change in fetal movements: absence of fetal movements after quickening, any unusual change in pattern or amount	Fetal jeopardy or intrauterine fetal death
Uterine contractions; pressure; cramping before 37 wk	Preterm labor
Visual disturbances: blurring, double vision, or spots	Hypertensive conditions, PIH
Swelling of face or fingers and over sacrum	Hypertensive conditions, PIH
Headaches: severe, frequent, or continuous	Hypertensive conditions, PIH
Muscular irritability or convulsions	Hypertensive conditions, PIH
Epigastric or abdominal pain (perceived as severe stomachache)	Hypertensive conditions, PIH, abruptio placentae
Glycosuria, positive glucose tolerance test reaction	Gestational diabetes mellitus

A

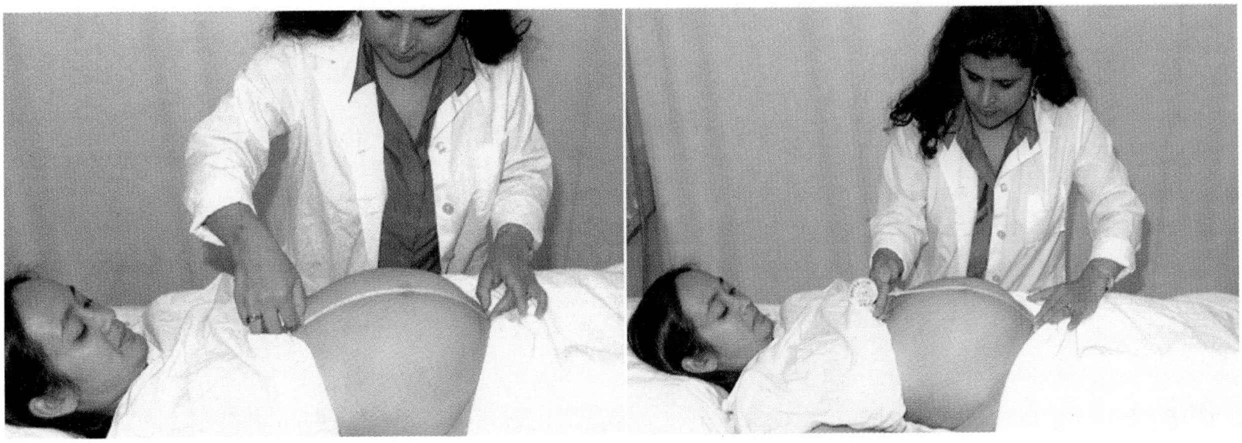

B

FIG. 16-7 Measurement of fundal height from symphysis that (**A**) includes the upper curve of the fundus and (**B**) does not include the upper curve of the fundus. Note position of hands and measuring tape. (Courtesy Chris Rozales, San Francisco, CA.)

the same as the number of weeks of gestation, if the woman's bladder is empty at the time of measurement (Cunningham et al., 2001).

Gestational Age. In an uncomplicated pregnancy, fetal gestational age is estimated after the duration of pregnancy and the EDB are determined. Fetal gestational age is determined from the menstrual history, contraceptive history, pregnancy test result, and the following findings obtained during the clinical evaluation:

- First uterine evaluation: date, size
- Fetal heart (FH) first heard: date, method (Doppler stethoscope, fetoscope)
- Date of quickening
- Current fundal height, estimated fetal weight (EFW)

- Current week of gestation by history of LMP and/or ultrasound examination
- Ultrasound examination: date, week of gestation, biparietal diameter (BPD)
- Reliability of dates

Quickening ("feeling of life") refers to the mother's first perception of fetal movement. It usually occurs between weeks 16 and 20 of gestation and is initially experienced as a fluttering sensation. The mother's report should be recorded.

Routine use of ultrasound examination, also called a **sonogram,** in early pregnancy has been recommended, and many health care providers have equipment readily available in the office. This procedure may be used to establish the duration of pregnancy if the woman cannot give a precise date for her LMP or if the size of the uterus does not correspond to the EDB calculated with Nägele's rule. Ultrasound examination also provides information about the well-being of the fetus; however, the routine use of ultrasound has not been found to improve clinical outcomes substantially (Bricker & Neilson, 2002). The debate continues about whether the expense justifies routine use of ultrasound examination early in pregnancy, but nurses who have been adequately taught to perform the ultrasound examination have a valuable opportunity to provide both education and support (Huffman & Sandelowski, 1997).

Health Status. The assessment of fetal health status includes consideration of fetal movement. The mother is instructed to note the extent and timing of fetal movements and to report immediately if the pattern changes or if movement ceases. Regular movement has been found to be a reliable indicator of fetal health.

The FHR is checked on routine visits once it has been heard (Fig. 16-8). Early in the second trimester, the heartbeat may be heard with the Doppler stethoscope (Fig. 16-8, *B*). To detect the heartbeat before the fetus can be palpated by Leopold's maneuvers (see Fig. 27-5), the scope is moved around the abdomen until the heartbeat is heard. Each nurse develops a set pattern for searching the abdomen for the heartbeat; for example, starting first in the midline about 2 to 3 cm above the symphysis, then mov-

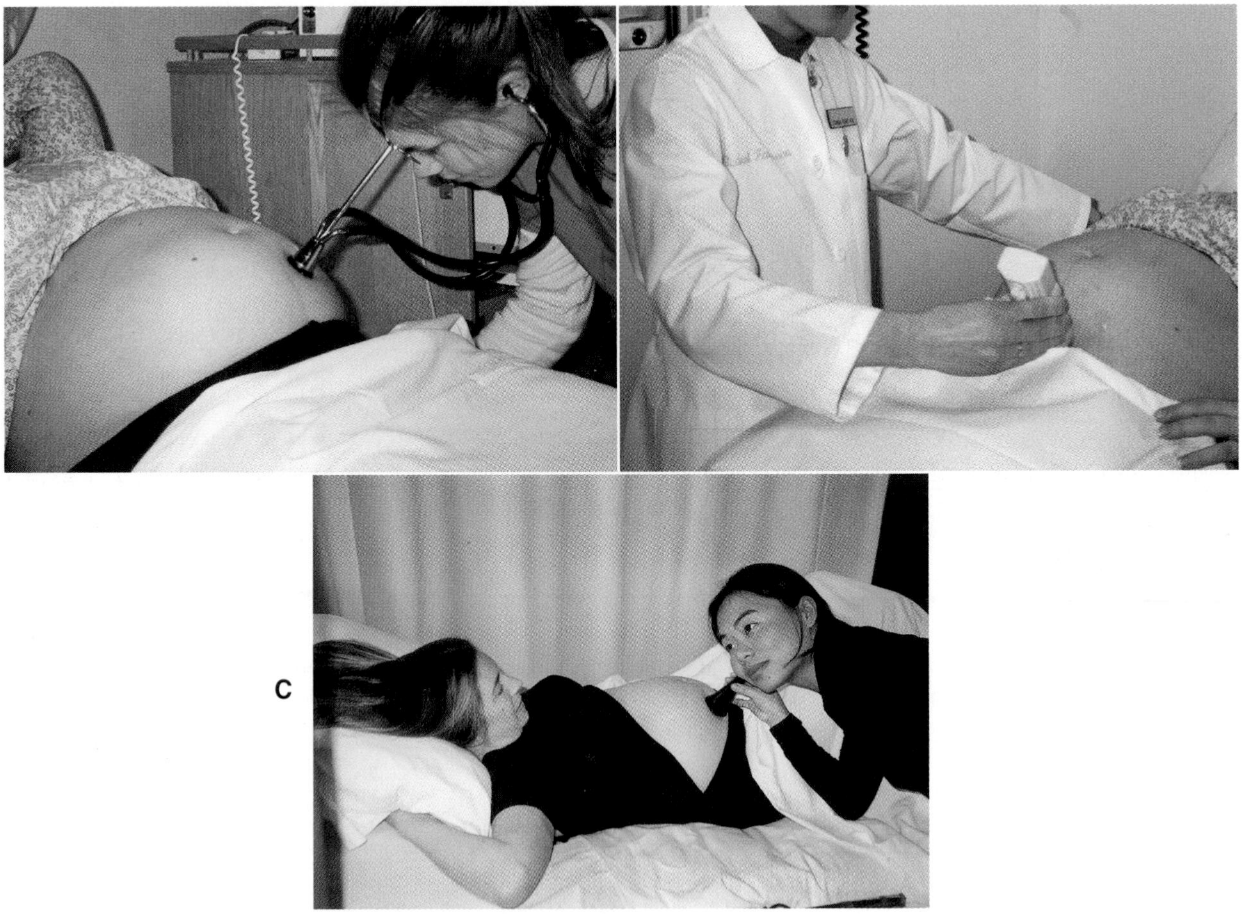

A

B

C

FIG. 16-8 Detecting fetal heart rate. **A,** Fetoscope (18 to 20 wk). NOTE: Hands should not touch fetoscope while nurse is listening. **B,** Doppler ultrasound stethoscope (12 wk). **C,** Pinard fetoscope. (**A** and **B,** Courtesy Dee Lowdermilk, Chapel Hill, NC. **C,** Courtesy Shannon Perry, San Jose, CA.)

ing to the left lower quadrant, and so on. The heartbeat is counted, and the quality and rhythm noted. Later in the second trimester, the FHR can be determined with the fetoscope or Pinard fetoscope (Fig. 16-8, *A* and *C*). A normal rate and rhythm are other good indicators of fetal health. Once the heartbeat is noted, its absence is cause for immediate investigation.

Fetal health status is investigated intensively if any maternal or fetal complications arise (e.g., maternal hypertension, intrauterine growth restriction, premature rupture of membranes [PROM], irregular or absent FHR, or absence of fetal movements after quickening). Careful, precise, and concise recording of client responses and laboratory results contributes to the continuous supervision vital to ensuring the well-being of the mother and fetus.

Laboratory Tests. The number of routine laboratory tests done during follow-up visits in pregnancy is limited. A clean-catch urine specimen is obtained to test for glucose, protein, nitrites, and leukocytes at each visit. Urine specimens for culture and sensitivity, as well as blood samples, are obtained only if signs and symptoms warrant.

The multiple-marker, or triple-screen, blood test is recommended (Graves, Miller, & Sellers, 2002). Done between 16 and 18 weeks' gestation, it measures the maternal serum level of α-fetoprotein (MSAFP), hCG, and unconjugated estriol, whose levels are combined to yield one value. Low levels may be associated with Down syndrome and other chromosomal abnormalities (Cunningham et al., 2001).

Other blood tests are repeated as necessary: RPR/VDRL test for syphilis; CBC with hematocrit, hemoglobin, and differential values; antibody screen (Kell, Duffy, rubella, toxoplasmosis, anti-Rh, HIV; sickle cell; and level of folacin when indicated). Cervical and vaginal smears are repeated as necessary.

If not done earlier in pregnancy, a glucose screen is performed in women older than 25 years. A glucose challenge is usually done between 24 and 28 weeks' gestation. Group B streptococcus (GBS) testing is done between 35 and 37 weeks' gestation; cultures collected earlier will not accurately predict GBS status at time of birth (Box 16-3).

Other Tests. Other diagnostic tests are available to assess the health status of both the pregnant woman and the fetus. Ultrasonography, for example, may be performed to determine the status of the pregnancy and to confirm gestational age of the fetus. Amniocentesis, a procedure used to obtain amniotic fluid for analysis, may be needed to evaluate the fetus for genetic disorders or gestational maturity. These and other tests that are used to determine health risks for the mother and infant are described in Chapter 29.

After obtaining information through the assessment process, the data are analyzed to identify deviations from the norm and unique needs of the pregnant woman and her family. Although comprehensive health care requires collaboration among professionals from several disciplines, nurses are in an excellent position to formulate diagnoses that can be used to guide independent interventions. The following are examples of the nursing diagnoses that may be appropriate in the prenatal period.

- *Anxiety related to*
  - –physical discomforts of pregnancy
  - –ambivalent and labile emotions
  - –changes in family dynamics
  - –fetal well-being
  - –ability to manage anticipated labor
- *Interrupted family processes related to*
  - –changing roles and responsibilities
  - –inadequate understanding of physical and emotional changes in pregnancy
- *Imbalanced nutrition: less than body requirements related to*
  - –morning sickness
  - –fatigue
- *Disturbed body image related to*
  - –anatomic and physiologic changes of pregnancy
  - –changes in the couple relationship
- *Disturbed sleep pattern related to*
  - –discomforts of late pregnancy
  - –anxiety about approaching labor

Expected Outcomes of Care

The plan of nursing care for women and their families during pregnancy is given direction by the diagnoses that have been formulated during prenatal visits. Individualized plans that are developed mutually with the pregnant woman are more likely to result in desirable outcomes than are those developed by the nurse for the woman. Measured outcomes of prenatal care include not only physical outcomes but also developmental and psychosocial outcomes.

The following are examples of outcomes that may be expected. The pregnant woman will achieve the following:

- Indicate decreased anxiety about the health of her fetus and herself
- Describe improved family dynamics
- Show appropriate weight gain patterns
- Report increasing acceptance of changes in body image
- Demonstrate knowledge for self-care
- Ask for clarification of information about pregnancy and birth

BOX 16-3 Risk Factors Indicating Need for GBS Prophylaxis

Previous infant with a group B streptococcus infection
GBS bacteriuria during this pregnancy
Membranes ruptured or onset of labor before 37 wk of gestation

Data from Himmelberger, S. (2002). Preventing group B strep in newborns. *AWHONN Lifelines, 6*(4), 339-342.

- Report signs and symptoms of complications
- Describe appropriate measures taken to relieve physical discomforts
- Develop a realistic birth plan

Plan of Care and Interventions

The nurse-client relationship is critical in setting the tone for further interaction. The techniques of listening with an attentive expression, touching, and using eye contact have their place, as does recognizing the woman's feelings and her right to express these feelings. The interaction may occur in various formal or informal settings. The clinic, home visits, or telephone conversations all provide opportunities for contact and can be used effectively for this purpose.

Sometimes women repeatedly seek information about a particular problem. At other times, the woman may be hesitant to broach another underlying problem. The nurse must be perceptive in identifying such unvoiced needs and can help the woman by asking for a client-generated solution and a subsequent report of its effectiveness.

In supporting a client, the nurse must remember that both the nurse and the woman are contributing to the relationship. The nurse has to accept the woman's responses as a factor in trying to be of help. An example of one nurse-client relationship is as follows:

> Frances had been very forthright in saying that this pregnancy was unplanned but had countered this observation with comments such as, "All things happen for the best," and "Children bring their own love." Over time, as our relationship developed to one of mutual trust, she complained increasingly of her fear of pain, of hating to wear maternity clothes, and of having to give up helping the family. Finally I ventured to say, "Sometimes when a pregnancy is unplanned, women resent it and are angry about it." Her relief was evident. She said, "Oh, you don't know how angry I've been." As a result, the whole tenor of support being offered changed, and the plan was adjusted to meet her real needs.

The nurse also must accept that the woman must be a willing partner in a purely voluntary relationship. As such, the relationship can be refused or terminated at any time by the pregnant woman or her family.

Supportive care involves developing, augmenting, or changing the mechanisms used by women and their families in coping with stress. The nurse tries to promote active participation by the people in the solution of their own problems. The nurse can help a woman gather pertinent information, explore options, decide on a course of action, and assume responsibility for the outcomes. These outcomes may include living with a problem as it is, easing the effects of a problem so that it can be accepted more readily, or eliminating the problem by effecting change.

At other times a successful outcome can be documented readily. For example, a woman who early in her pregnancy had predicted a severe depressive state in the postbirth period was elated when such a state did not materialize. She remarked to the nurse who had provided support during the pregnancy and birth, "You're the best nerve medicine I've ever had!"

Care Paths

Better coordination of prenatal care services for childbearing families is emphasized in current health care systems. However, a large number of health care professionals are involved in care of the expectant mother, and unintentional gaps or overlaps in care may occur. Care paths are used to improve the consistency of care and to reduce costs (Simon, Heaps, & Chodroff, 1997). Although the Care Path on p. 421 focuses only on prenatal education, it is one example of the type of form that might be developed to guide health care providers in carrying out the appropriate assessments and interventions in a timely way. Use of care paths also may contribute to improved satisfaction of families with the prenatal care provided, and members of the health care team may function more efficiently and effectively.

Education About Maternal and Fetal Changes

Expectant parents are typically curious about the growth and development of the fetus and the consequent changes that occur in the mother's body. Mothers in particular are sometimes more tolerant of the discomforts related to the continuing pregnancy if they understand the underlying causes. Commercial literature that describes the fetal and maternal changes is often available and can be used in explaining changes as they occur. The nurse's familiarity with any reading material given to families is essential to effective client education.

Education for Self-Care

The expectant mother needs information about many subjects. The nurse who is observant, listens, and knows typical concerns of expectant parents can anticipate questions that will be asked and prompt mothers and partners to discuss what is on their minds. Many times, printed literature can be given to supplement the individualized teaching the nurse provides, and women often avidly read books and pamphlets related to their own experience. When nurses read the literature before they distribute it, they have an opportunity to point out areas that may not correspond with local health care practices. Clients who receive conflicting advice or instruction are likely to grow increasingly frustrated with members of the health care team and the care provided. Several topics that may cause concerns in pregnant women are discussed in the following sections.

Nutrition

Good nutrition is important in the maintenance of maternal health during pregnancy and the provision of adequate nutrients for embryonic and fetal development. The nourishment the fetus receives from its mother influences health in later life (Campbell-Brown & Hytten, 1998).

Care Path Prenatal Care Pathway

PRENATAL EDUCATION CLINICAL PATHWAY

INITIAL VISIT AND ORIENTATION: ______ SOCIAL SERVICE: ______ DIETICIAN: ______

I. EARLY PREGNANCY (WEEKS 1-20) (initial and date after education given)

Fetal growth and development	______	Testing: Labs / Ultrasound	______
Maternal changes	______	Possible Complications:	
		a. Threatened miscarriage	______
Lifestyle: exercise/stress/nutrition	______	b. Diabetes	______
Drugs, OTC, tobacco, alcohol	______	c. ______	______
STIs	______		
		Introduction to breastfeeding	______
Psycho/social adjustments:	______		
FOB involved/accepts	______	Acceptance	______
Baby for adoption	______	and childbirth preparation	______
		Dietary follow-up	______

II. MIDPREGNANCY (WEEKS 21-27) (initial and date after education given)

Fetal growth and development	______	Breast or bottle feeding	______
Maternal changes	______	Birth plan initiated	______
Daily fetal movement	______	Childbirth preparation	______
Possible complications:			______
a. Preterm labor prevention	______	Dietary follow-up	______
b. PIH symptoms	______		
c. ______	______		

III. LATE PREGNANCY (WEEKS 28-40) (initial and date after education given)

Fetal growth and development	______	Childbirth preparation:	
Fetal evaluation:		S/S of labor; labor process	______
Daily movement ______	NSTs ______	Pain management: natural childbirth, meds, epidural	______
Kick counts ______	BPPs ______	Cesarean; VBAC	______
		Birth plan complete	______
Maternal changes	______	Review hospital policies	______
Possible complications:		Parenting preparation:	
a. Preterm labor prevention	______	Pediatrician ______	Childcare ______
b. PIH symptoms	______	Siblings ______	Immunizations ______
c. ______	______	Car seat/safety ______	
Breastfeeding preparation:		Postpartum:	
Nipple assessment	______	PP care/check-up	______
		Emotional changes	______
Dietary follow-up	______	BC options	______
		Safer sex/STIs	______

Signature: ______________ ______________ ______________

BC, Birth control; *BPP*, biophysical profile; *FOB*, father of baby; *NST*, nonstress test; *OTC*, over the counter; *PIH*, pregnancy-induced hypertension; *PP*, postpartum; *S/S*, signs and symptoms; *STI*, sexually transmitted infection; *VBAC*, vaginal birth after cesarean.

Assessing a woman's nutritional status and providing information on nutrition are part of the nurse's responsibilities in providing prenatal care. In some settings, a registered dietitian conducts classes for pregnant women on the topics of nutritional status and nutrition during pregnancy or interviews them to assess their knowledge of these topics. Nurses can refer women to a registered dietitian if a need is revealed during the nursing assessment. (For detailed information concerning maternal and fetal nutritional needs and related nursing care, see Chapter 15).

Personal Hygiene

During pregnancy, the sebaceous (sweat) glands are highly active because of hormonal influences, and women often perspire freely. They may be reassured that the increase is normal and that their previous patterns of perspiration will return after the postpartum period. Washing the body regularly is basic to good personal hygiene. Baths and warm showers can be therapeutic because they relax tense, tired muscles; help counter insomnia; and make the pregnant woman feel fresh. Tub bathing is permitted even in late pregnancy because little water enters the vagina unless under pressure. However, late in pregnancy, when the woman's center of gravity lowers, she is at risk for falling. Tub bathing is contraindicated after rupture of the membranes.

Prevention of Urinary Tract Infections

Because of dramatic changes that occur in the renal system during pregnancy (see Chapter 14), urinary tract infections are common, but they may be asymptomatic. Women should be instructed to inform their health care provider if blood or pain occurs with urination. These infections pose a risk to the mother and fetus; thus the prevention or early treatment of these infections is essential (Polivka, Nickel, & Wilkins, 1997).

The nurse can assess the woman's understanding and use of good handwashing techniques before and after urinating and whether she knows to wipe from front to back. Soft, absorbent toilet tissue, preferably white and unscented, should be used; harsh, scented, or printed toilet paper may cause irritation. Bubble bath or other bath oils should be avoided because these may irritate the urethra. Women should wear underpants and panty hose with a cotton crotch and avoid wearing tight-fitting slacks or jeans for long periods; anything that allows a buildup of heat and moisture in the genital area may foster the growth of bacteria.

Some women do not consume enough fluid and food. After discovering her food preferences, the nurse should advise the woman to drink at least 2 L (eight glasses) of liquid a day to maintain an adequate fluid intake that ensures frequent urination. Pregnant women should not limit fluids in an effort to reduce the frequency of urination. Women need to know that if urine looks dark (concentrated), they must increase their fluid intake. Vitamin C makes the urinary tract less hospitable to bacteria by lowering the pH. The consumption of yogurt and acidophilus milk also may help prevent urinary tract and vaginal infections. Although cranberry juice is often recommended, that sold to consumers is too dilute to lower the pH of urine.

The nurse should review healthy urination practices with the woman. Women should be told not to ignore the urge to urinate because holding urine lengthens the time bacteria are in the bladder and allows them to multiply. Women should plan ahead when they are faced with situations that may normally require them to delay urination (e.g., a long car ride). They always should urinate before going to bed at night. Bacteria can be introduced during intercourse; therefore, women are advised to urinate before and after intercourse, and then drink a large glass of water to promote additional urination.

Kegel Exercises

Kegel exercises, deliberate contraction and relaxation of the pubococcygeus muscle, strengthen the muscles around the reproductive organs and improve muscle tone. Many women are not aware of the muscles of the pelvic floor until it is pointed out that these are the muscles used during urination and sexual intercourse that can be consciously controlled. The muscles of the pelvic floor encircle the vaginal outlet, and they need to be exercised, because an exercised muscle can then stretch and contract readily at the time of birth. Practice of pelvic muscle exercises during pregnancy also results in fewer complaints of urinary incontinence in late pregnancy and postpartum (Sampselle et al, 1998).

Several ways of performing Kegel exercises have been described. The method that is suggested by nurse researchers involved in a research utilization project for continence in women is described in the Teaching for Self-Care box in Chapter 5. The nurse can be reasonably assured that the teaching has been effective if the woman reports an increased ability to control urine flow and greater muscular control during sexual intercourse.

Preparation for Breastfeeding

Pregnant women are usually eager to discuss their plans for feeding the newborn. Breast milk is the food of choice, in part because breastfeeding is associated with a decreased incidence of perinatal morbidity and mortality. The American Academy of Pediatrics recommends breastfeeding for at least a year. However, a deep-seated aversion to breastfeeding on the part of the mother or partner, the mother's need for certain medications, and certain medical complications, such as active tuberculosis, newly diagnosed breast cancer, and hepatitis C, are contraindications to breastfeeding (Lawrence, 1999). Although hepatitis B antigen has not been shown to be transmitted through breast milk, as an added precaution, it is recommended that infants born to HBsAg-positive women receive the hepatitis B vaccine and hepatitis B immune globulin (HBIg) immediately after birth. Women who are HIV positive are discouraged from nursing because the risk of HIV transmission outweighs the risk of the infant dying from another cause (Lawrence, 1999).

Skinner et al. (1997) reported that a woman's decision about the method of infant feeding is made before pregnancy; thus the education of women of childbearing age about the benefits of breastfeeding is essential. The pregnant woman and her partner are encouraged to decide which method of feeding is suitable for them; however, the benefits of breastfeeding should be emphasized. Once the couple has been given information about the advantages and disadvantages of bottle feeding and breastfeeding, they can make an informed choice. Health care providers support their decisions and provide any needed assistance.

Women with inverted nipples need special consideration if they are planning to breastfeed. The **pinch test** is done to determine whether the nipple is everted or inverted (Fig. 16-9). The nurse shows the woman the way to perform the pinch test. It involves having the woman place her thumb and forefinger on her areola and gently press inward. This action will cause her nipple either to stand erect or to invert. Most nipples will stand erect.

Exercises to break the adhesions that cause the nipple to invert do not work and may precipitate uterine contractions (Lawrence, 1999). The use of **breast shells,** small plastic devices that fit over the nipple, is suggested for women who have flat or inverted nipples (Fig. 16-10). Breast shells work by exerting a continuous, gentle pressure around the areola that pushes the nipple through a central opening in the inner shield. Breast shells should be worn for 1 to 2 hours daily during the last trimester of pregnancy. They should be worn for gradually increasing lengths of time (Lawrence, 1999). Breast stimulation is contraindicated in women at risk for preterm labor; therefore the decision to suggest the use of breast shells to women with flat or inverted nipples must be made judiciously. Continuous support and guidance must be given to the woman as part of the nursing plan of care.

The woman is taught to cleanse the nipples with warm water to keep the ducts from being blocked with dried colostrum. Soap, ointments, alcohol, and tinctures should not be applied because they remove protective oils that keep the nipples supple. The use of these substances may cause the nipples to crack during early lactation (Lawrence, 1999).

The woman who plans to breastfeed should purchase a nursing bra that will accommodate her increased breast size during the last few months of pregnancy and during lactation. If her breasts are very heavy, or if the woman feels uncomfortable with the weight unsupported, the bra can be worn day and night.

Dental Care

Dental care during pregnancy is especially important because nausea during pregnancy may lead to poor oral hygiene, allowing dental caries to develop. A fluoride toothpaste should be used daily. Inflammation and infection of the gingival and periodontal tissues may occur (Carl, Roux, & Matacale, 2000). There is some evidence linking periodontal infections and preterm birth and LBW (Jared et al., 1999).

Because calcium and phosphorus in the teeth are fixed in enamel, the old adage "for every child a tooth" is not true. There is no scientific evidence to support the belief that filling teeth or even dental extraction involving the administration of local or nitrous oxide-oxygen anesthesia precipitates miscarriage or premature labor. Antibacterial therapy should be considered for sepsis, however, especially in pregnant women who have had rheumatic heart disease or

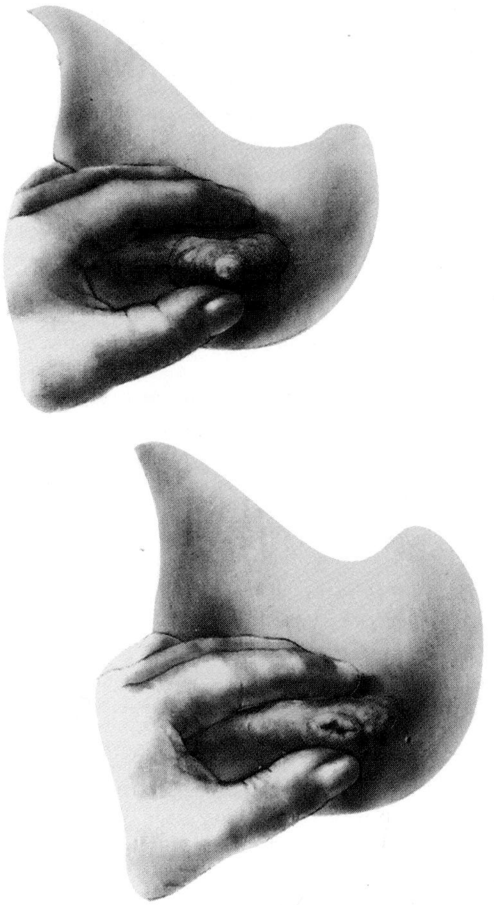
A

B

FIG. 16-9 A, Normal nipple everts with gentle pressure. **B,** Inverted nipple inverts with gentle pressure. (Modified from Lawrence, R. [1999]. *Breastfeeding: A guide for the medical profession* [5th ed.]. St. Louis: Mosby.)

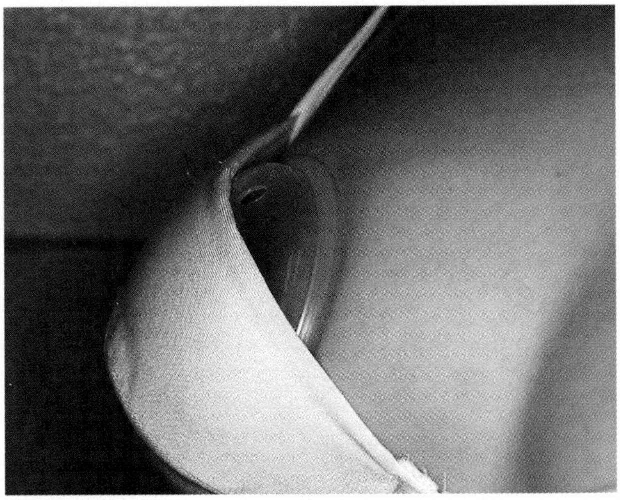

FIG. 16-10 Breast shell in place inside bra to evert nipple. (Courtesy Michael S. Clement, MD, Mesa, AZ.)

TEACHING FOR SELF-CARE

Exercise Tips For Pregnant Women

Consult your health care provider when you know or suspect you are pregnant. Discuss your medical and obstetric history, your current exercise regimen, and the exercises you would like to continue throughout pregnancy.

Seek help in determining an exercise routine that is well within your limit of tolerance, especially if you have not been exercising regularly.

Consider decreasing weight-bearing exercises (jogging, running) and concentrating on non–weight-bearing activities such as swimming, cycling, or stretching. If you are a runner, starting in your seventh month, you may wish to walk instead.

Avoid risky activities such as surfing, mountain climbing, skydiving, and racquetball because such activities that require precise balance and coordination may be dangerous. Avoid activities that require holding your breath and bearing down (Valsalva maneuver). Jerky, bouncy motions also should be avoided.

Exercise regularly at least three times a week, as long as you are healthy, to improve muscle tone and increase or maintain your stamina. Exercising sporadically may put undue strain on your muscles. Limit activity to shorter intervals. Exercise for 10 to 15 minutes, rest for 2 to 3 minutes, then exercise for another 10 to 15 minutes.

Decrease your exercise level as your pregnancy progresses. The normal alterations of advancing pregnancy, such as decreased cardiac reserve and increased respiratory effort, may produce physiologic stress if you exercise strenuously for a long time.

Take your pulse every 10 to 15 minutes while you are exercising. If it is more than 140 beats/min, slow down until it returns to a maximum of 90 beats/min. You should be able to converse easily while exercising. If you cannot, you need to slow down.

Avoid becoming overheated for extended periods. It is best not to exercise for more than 35 minutes, especially in hot, humid weather. As your body temperature rises, the heat is transmitted to your fetus. Prolonged or repeated elevation of fetal temperature may result in birth defects, especially during the first 3 months. Your temperature should not exceed 38° C.

Avoid the use of hot tubs and saunas.

Warm-up and stretching exercises prepare your joints for more strenuous exercise and lessen the likelihood of strain or injury to your joints. After the fourth month of gestation, you should not perform exercises flat on your back.

A cool-down period of mild activity involving your legs after an exercise period will help bring your respiration, heart, and metabolic rates back to normal and prevent the pooling of blood in the exercised muscles.

Rest for 10 minutes after exercising, lying on your side. As the uterus grows, it puts pressure on a major vein in your abdomen, which carries blood to your heart. Lying on your side removes the pressure and promotes return circulation from your extremities and muscles to your heart, thereby increasing blood flow to your placenta and fetus. You should rise gradually from the floor to prevent dizziness or fainting (orthostatic hypotension).

Drink two or three 8-oz glasses of water after you exercise to replace the body fluids lost through perspiration. While exercising, drink water whenever you feel the need.

Increase your caloric intake to replace the calories burned during exercise and provide the extra energy needs of pregnancy. (Pregnancy alone requires an additional 300 kcal/day.) Choose such high-protein foods as fish, milk, cheese, eggs, or meat.

Take your time. This is not the time to be competitive or train for activities requiring speed or long endurance.

Wear a supportive bra. Your increased breast weight may cause changes in posture and put pressure on the ulnar nerve.

Wear supportive shoes. As your uterus grows, your center of gravity shifts and you compensate for this by arching your back. These natural changes may make you feel off balance and more likely to fall.

Stop exercising immediately if you experience shortness of breath, dizziness, numbness, tingling, pain of any kind, more than four uterine contractions per hour, decreased fetal activity, or vaginal bleeding, and consult your health care provider.

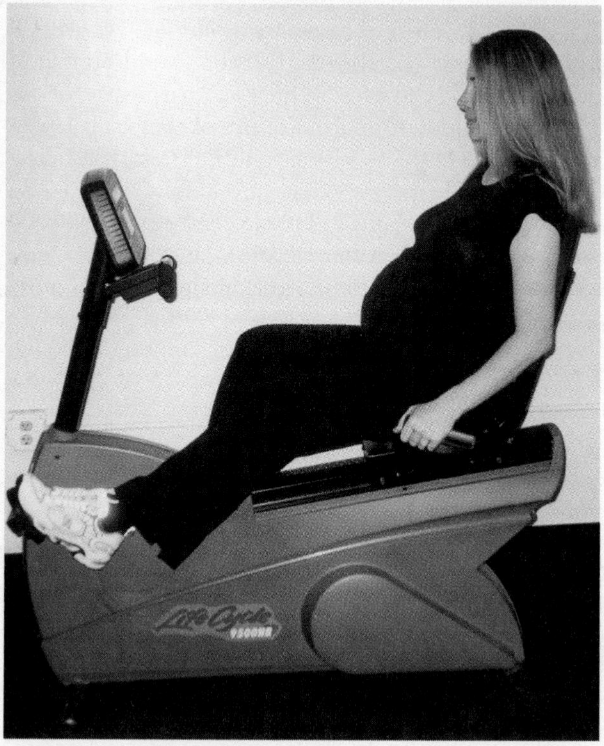
Life Cycle
9500HR

Riding a recumbent bicycle provides exercise while supplying back support. (Courtesy Shannon Perry, San Jose, CA.)

Sources: American College of Obstetricians and Gynecologists. (1994). *Exercise during pregnancy and the postpartum period. Technical Bulletin No. 189.* Washington, DC: ACOG; Artal, R., & Subak-Sharpe, G. (1998). *Pregnancy & exercise.* New York: Delacorte Press; Fishbein, E., & Phillips, M. (1990). How safe is exercise during pregnancy? *Journal of Obstetric, Gynecologic, and Neonatal Nursing, 19*(1), 45-49; Kramer, M. (2001). Regular aerobic exercise during pregnancy (Cochrane Review). *The Cochrane Library,* Issue 1. Oxford: Update Software; Pivarnik, J. (1994). Maternal exercise during pregnancy. *Sports Medicine 18,* 215-217.

nephritis. Emergency dental surgery is not contraindicated during pregnancy. However, the risks and benefits of dental surgery must be explained. If dental treatment is necessary, the woman will be most comfortable during the second trimester (Carl, Roux, & Matacale, 2000).

Physical Activity

Physical activity promotes a feeling of well-being in the pregnant woman. It improves circulation, promotes relaxation and rest, and counteracts boredom, as it does in the nonpregnant woman. Detailed exercise tips for pregnancy are presented in the Teaching for Self-Care box. Exercises that help relieve the low back pain that often arises during the second trimester because of the increased weight of the fetus are demonstrated in Fig. 16-11.

Posture and Body Mechanics

Skeletal and musculature changes in pregnancy may predispose the woman to backache and possible injury. As pregnancy progresses, the pregnant woman's center of gravity changes, pelvic joints soften and relax, and stress is placed on abdominal musculature. Poor posture and body mechanics contribute to the discomfort and potential for injury. To minimize these problems, women can acquire a kinesthetic sense for good body posture (Fig. 16-12). Strategies to prevent or relieve backache are presented in the Teaching for Self-Care box.

Rest and Relaxation

The pregnant woman is encouraged to plan regular rest periods, particularly as pregnancy advances. The side-lying position is recommended because it promotes uterine perfusion and fetoplacental oxygenation by eliminating pressure on the ascending vena cava and descending aorta,

TEACHING FOR SELF-CARE

Posture and Body Mechanics

TO PREVENT OR RELIEVE BACKACHE

Do pelvic tilt:

- Pelvic tilt (rock) on hands and knees (see Fig. 16-11, *A*) and while sitting in straight-back chair.
- Pelvic tilt (rock) in standing position against a wall, or lying on floor (see Fig. 16-11, *B* and *C*).
- Perform abdominal muscle contractions during pelvic tilt while standing, lying, or sitting to help strengthen rectus abdominis muscle (see Fig. 16-11, *D*).
- Use good body mechanics.
- Use leg muscles to reach objects on or near floor. Bend at the knees, not the back. Knees are bent to lower body to squatting position. Feet are kept 12 to 18 inches apart to provide a solid base to maintain balance (see Fig. 16-12, *A*).
- Lift with the legs. To lift heavy object (e.g., young child), one foot is placed slightly in front of the other and kept flat as woman lowers herself onto one knee. She lifts the weight holding it close to her body and never higher than the chest. To stand up or sit down, one leg is placed slightly behind the other as she raises or lowers herself (see Fig. 16-12, *B*).

TO RESTRICT THE LUMBAR CURVE

For prolonged standing (e.g., ironing, employment), place one foot on low footstool or box; change positions often.

Move car seat forward so that knees are bent and higher than hips. If needed, use a small pillow to support low back area.

Sit in chairs low enough to allow both feet to be placed on floor, preferably with knees higher than hips.

TO PREVENT ROUND LIGAMENT PAIN AND STRAIN ON ABDOMINAL MUSCLES

Implement suggestions given in Table 16-2.

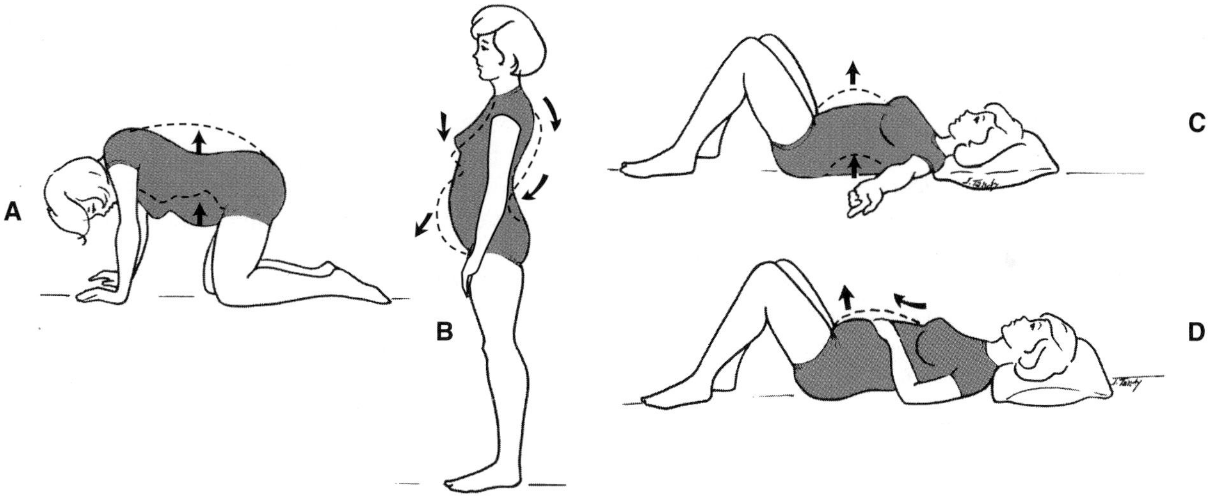
A
B
C
D

FIG. 16-11 Exercises. **A** to **C,** Pelvic rocking relieves low backache (excellent for relief of menstrual cramps as well). **D,** Abdominal breathing aids relaxation and lifts abdominal wall off uterus.

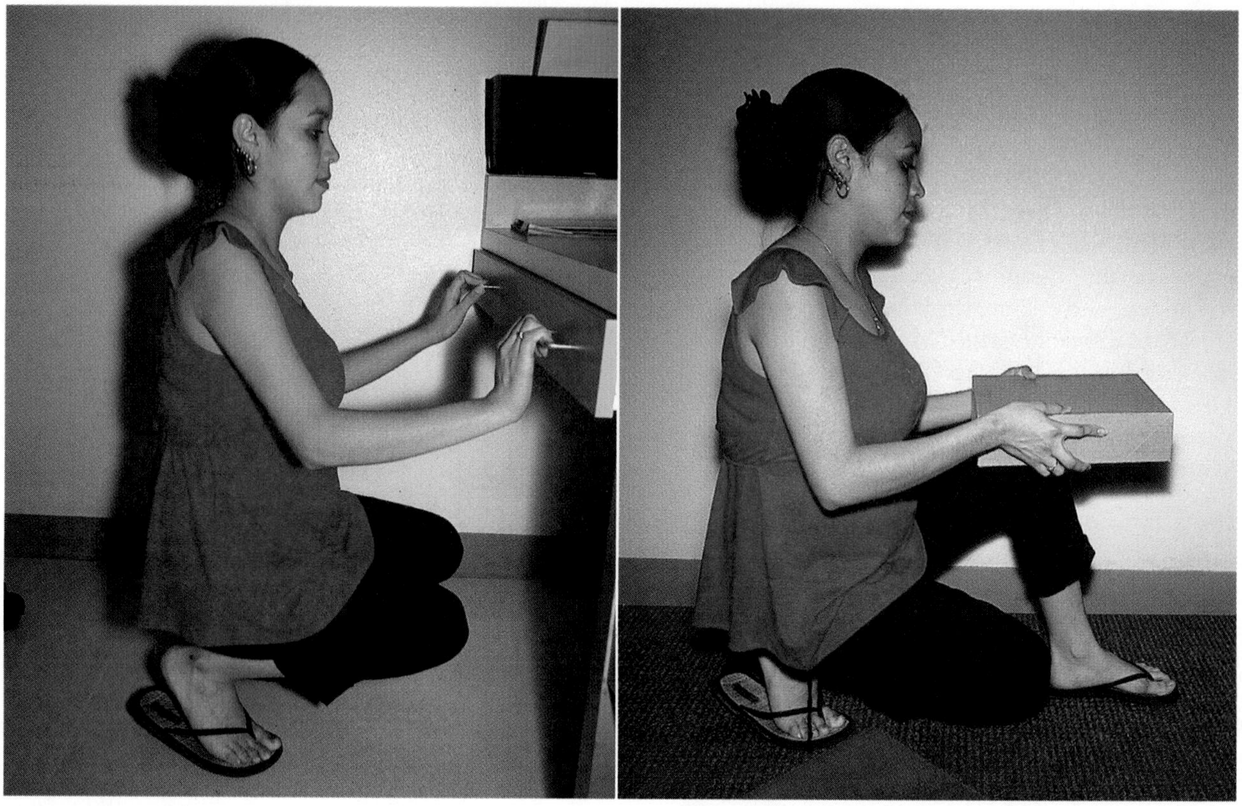
A
B

FIG. 16-12 Correct body mechanics. **A,** Squatting. **B,** Lifting. (Courtesy Michael S. Clement, MD, Mesa, AZ.)

which can lead to supine hypotension (Fig. 16-13). The mother also should be shown the way to rise slowly from a side-lying position to prevent placing strain on the back and to minimize the orthostatic hypotension caused by changes in position common in the latter part of pregnancy. To stretch and rest back muscles at home or work, the nurse can show the woman the way to do the following exercises:

Stand behind a chair. Support and balance self by using the back of the chair (Fig. 16-14). Squat for 30 seconds; stand for 15 seconds. Repeat six times, several times per day, as needed. Then, while sitting in a chair, lower head to knees for 30 seconds. Raise head. Repeat six times, several times per day, as needed.

Conscious relaxation is the process of releasing tension from the mind and body through deliberate effort and practice. The ability to relax consciously and intentionally can be beneficial for the following reasons:

- To relieve the normal discomforts related to pregnancy
- To reduce stress and therefore diminish pain perception during the childbearing cycle
- To heighten self-awareness and trust in one's own ability to control responses and functions
- To help cope with stress in everyday life situations, whether the woman is pregnant or not

The techniques for conscious relaxation are numerous and varied. The guidelines given in Box 16-4 can be used by anyone.

Employment

Employment of pregnant women usually has no adverse effects on pregnancy outcomes. Job discrimination that is based strictly on pregnancy is illegal. However, some job environments pose potential risk to the fetus (e.g., dry-cleaning plants, chemistry laboratories, parking garages). Work activities that depend on a good sense of balance should be discouraged, however, especially during the latter half of pregnancy. Excessive fatigue is usually the deciding factor in the termination of employment; strategies to assess fatigue thoroughly have been suggested by Pugh et al. (1999). Strategies to improve safety during pregnancy are described in the Teaching for Self-Care Box.

Women with sedentary jobs need to walk around at intervals to counter the usual sluggish circulation in the legs that can cause varices and thrombophlebitis to develop. They should neither sit nor stand in one position for long periods, and they should avoid crossing their legs at the knees because these activities foster such conditions. Standing for long periods also increases the risk of preterm labor. The pregnant woman's chair should provide ade-

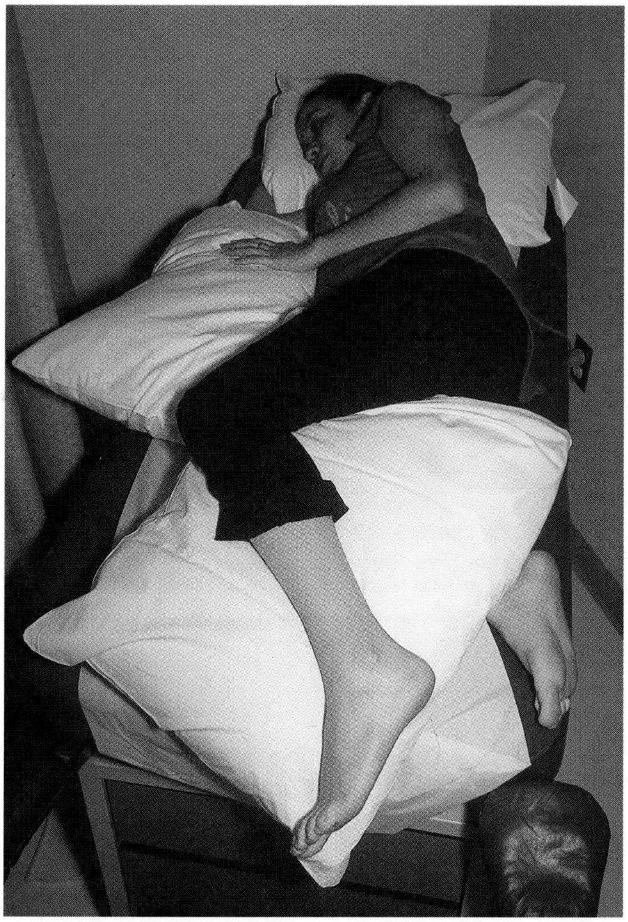

FIG. 16-13 Side-lying position for rest and relaxation. Some women prefer to support upper part of leg with pillows. (Courtesy Michael S. Clement, MD, Mesa, AZ.)

quate back support. Use of a footstool can prevent pressure on veins, relieve strain on varicosities, and minimize swelling of feet.

Clothing

Some women continue to wear their usual clothes during pregnancy as long as they fit and feel comfortable. If maternity clothing is needed, outfits may be purchased new or found at thrift shops or garage sales in good condition because they rarely wear out. Comfortable, loose clothing is best. Tight bras and belts, stretch pants, garters, tight-top knee socks, panty girdles, and other constrictive clothing should be avoided because tight clothing over the perineum encourages vaginitis and miliaria (heat rash), and impaired circulation in the legs can cause varicosities.

Maternity bras are constructed to accommodate the increased breast weight, chest circumference, and the size of breast tail tissue (under the arm). These bras also have drop-flaps over the nipples to facilitate breastfeeding. A good bra can help prevent neckache and backache.

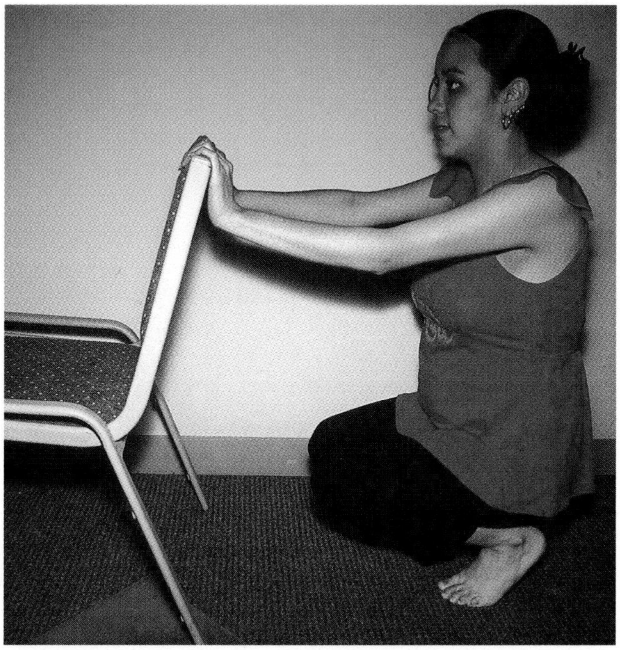

FIG. 16-14 Squatting for muscle relaxation and strengthening and for keeping leg and hip joints flexible. (Courtesy Michael S. Clement, MD, Mesa, AZ.)

BOX 16-4 Conscious Relaxation Tips

Preparation: Loosen clothing, assume a comfortable sitting or side-lying position with all parts of body well supported with pillows. The use of soothing music is optional.

Beginning: Allow self to feel warm and comfortable. Inhale and exhale slowly, and imagine peaceful relaxation coming over each part of the body, starting with the neck and working down to the toes. People who learn conscious relaxation often speak of feeling relaxed even if some discomfort is present.

Maintenance: Use imagery (fantasy or daydream) to maintain the state of relaxation. Using *active imagery,* imagine yourself moving or doing some activity and experiencing its sensations. Using *passive imagery,* imagine yourself watching a scene, such as a lovely sunset.

Awakening: Return to the wakeful state gradually. Slowly begin to take in stimuli from the surrounding environment.

Further retention and development of the skill: Practice regularly for some periods each day, for example, at the same hour for 10 to 15 minutes each day, to feel refreshed, revitalized, and invigorated.

Elastic hose give considerable comfort and promote greater venous emptying in women with large varicose veins. Ideally, support stockings should be put on before the woman gets out of bed in the morning. Figure 16-15 demonstrates a position for resting the legs and reducing swelling and varicosities.

TEACHING FOR SELF-CARE

Safety During Pregnancy

Changes in the body due to pregnancy include relaxation of joints, alteration to center of gravity, faintness, and discomforts. Problems with coordination and balance are common. Therefore the woman should follow these guidelines:

- Use good body mechanics.
- Use safety features on tools/vehicles (safety seat belts, shoulder harnesses, headrests, goggles, helmets) as specified.
- Avoid activities requiring coordination, balance, and concentration.
- Take rest periods; reschedule daily activities to meet rest and relaxation needs.

Embryonic and fetal development is vulnerable to environmental teratogens. Many potentially dangerous chemicals are present in the home, yard, and workplace: cleaning agents, paints, sprays, herbicides, and pesticides. The soil and water supply may be unsafe. Therefore the woman should follow these guidelines:

- Read all labels for ingredients and proper use of product.
- Ensure adequate ventilation with clean air.
- Dispose of wastes appropriately.
- Wear gloves when handling chemicals.
- Change job assignments or workplace as necessary.
- Avoid high altitudes (not in pressurized aircraft), which could jeopardize oxygen intake.

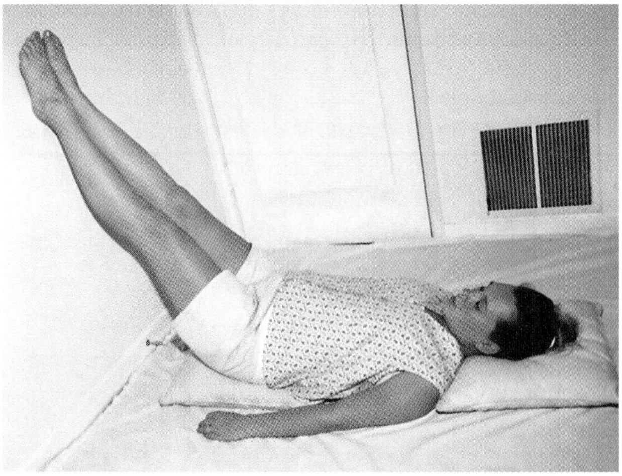

FIG. 16-15 Position for resting legs and for reducing edema and varicosities. Encourage woman with vulvar varicosities to include pillow under her hips. (Courtesy Dale Ikuta, San Jose, CA.)

Comfortable shoes that provide firm support and promote good posture and balance also are advisable. Very high heels and platform shoes are not recommended because of the woman's changed center of gravity, which can cause her to lose her balance. In addition, in the third trimester, the woman's pelvis tilts forward, and her lumbar curve increases. The resulting leg aches and cramps are aggravated by nonsupportive shoes (Fig. 16-16).

Travel

Travel is not contraindicated in low risk pregnant women, but those with high risk pregnancies are advised to avoid long-distance travel after fetal viability has been reached to

A

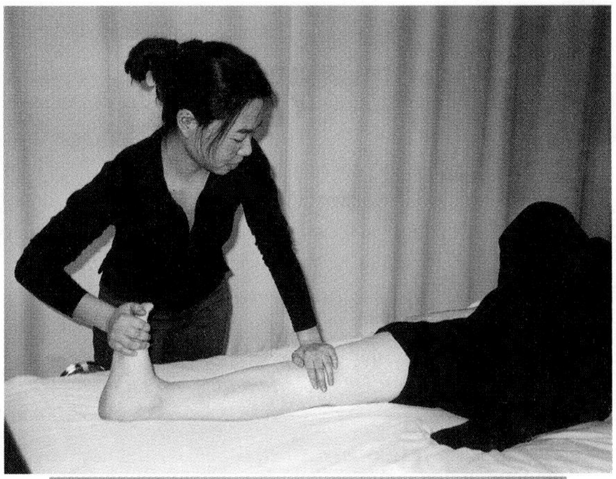

B

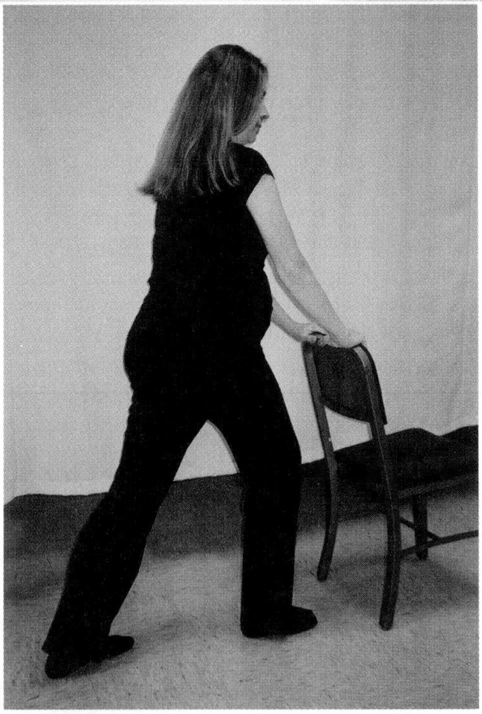

FIG. 16-16 Relief of muscle spasm (leg cramps). **A,** Another person dorsiflexes foot with knee extended. **B,** Woman stands and leans forward, thereby dorsiflexing foot of affected leg. (Courtesy Shannon Perry, San Jose, CA.)

avert possible economic and psychologic consequences of giving birth to a preterm infant far from home. Travel to areas where medical care is poor, water is untreated, or malaria is prevalent should be avoided if possible. Women who contemplate foreign travel should be aware that many health insurance carriers do not cover a birth in a foreign setting or even hospitalization for preterm labor.

Pregnant women who travel for long distances should schedule periods of activity and rest. While sitting, the woman can practice deep breathing, foot circling, and alternately contracting and relaxing different muscle groups. She should avoid becoming fatigued. Although travel in itself is not a cause of adverse outcomes such as miscarriage or preterm labor, certain precautions are recommended while traveling in a car. A woman who does not wear automobile restraints risks injury to herself and her fetus.

Maternal death as a result of injury is the most common cause of fetal death. The next most common cause is placental separation that occurs because body contours change in reaction to the force of a collision. The uterus as a muscular organ can adapt its shape to that of the body, but the placenta is not resilient. At the impact of collision, placental separation can occur. A combination lap belt and shoulder harness is the most effective automobile restraint, and both should be used (Fig. 16-17). The lap belt should be worn low across the pelvic bones and as snug as is comfortable. The shoulder harness should be worn above the gravid uterus and below the neck to prevent chafing. The pregnant woman should sit upright. The headrest should be used to prevent a whiplash injury.

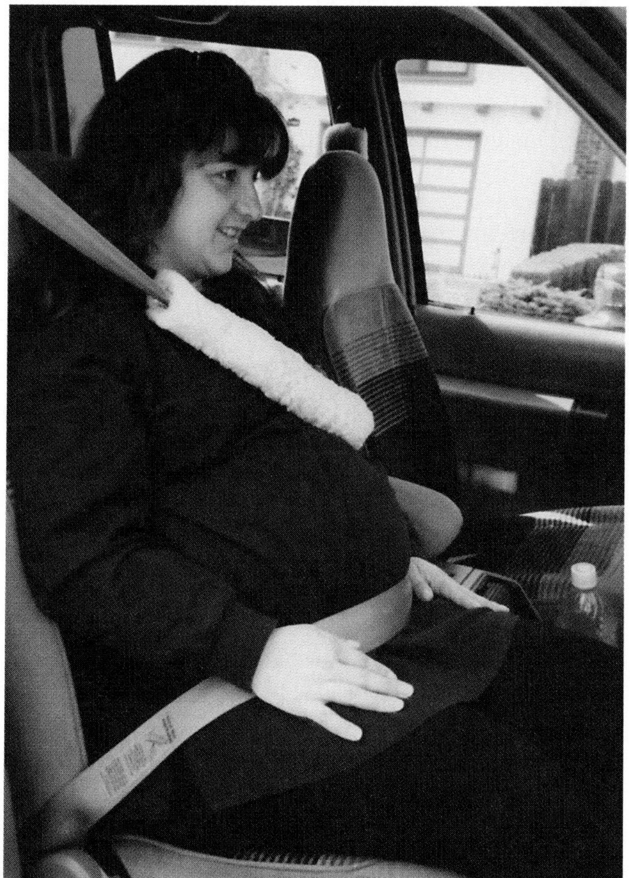

FIG. 16-17 Proper use of seat belt and headrest. (Courtesy Tammie McGee, Millbrae, CA.)

Pregnant women traveling in high-altitude regions have lowered oxygen levels that may cause fetal hypoxia, especially if the pregnant woman is anemic. However, the current information on this condition is limited, and recommendations are not standardized.

Airline travel in large commercial jets usually poses little risk to the pregnant woman, but policies vary from airline to airline. The pregnant woman is advised to inquire about restrictions or recommendations from her carrier (Cunningham et al., 2001). Metal detectors used at airport security checkpoints are not harmful to the fetus. The 8% humidity at which the cabins of commercial airlines are maintained may result in some water loss; hydration (with water) should therefore be maintained under these conditions. Sitting in the cramped seat of an airliner for prolonged periods may increase the risk of superficial and deep thrombophlebitis; thus a pregnant woman is encouraged to take a 15-minute walk around the aircraft during each hour of travel to minimize this risk.

Medications

Although much has been learned in recent years about fetal drug toxicity (see Box 13-2), the possible teratogenicity of many medications, both prescription and OTC, is still unknown. This fact is especially true for new medications and combinations of drugs. Moreover, certain subclinical errors or deficiencies in intermediate metabolism in the fetus may cause an otherwise harmless drug to be converted into a hazardous one. The greatest danger of drug-caused developmental defects in the fetus extends from the time of fertilization through the first trimester, a time when the woman may not realize she is pregnant. Self-treatment must be discouraged. The use of all drugs, including OTC medications, herbs, and vitamins, should be limited and a careful record kept of all therapeutic agents used.

Immunizations

Some concern has been raised over the safety of various immunization practices during pregnancy (Cunningham et al., 2001). Immunization with live or attenuated live viruses is contraindicated during pregnancy because of its potential teratogenicity. Live-virus vaccines include those for measles (rubeola and rubella), chickenpox, and mumps, as well as the Sabin (oral) poliomyelitis vaccine (no longer used in the United States). Vaccines consisting of killed viruses may be used. Those that may be administered during pregnancy include tetanus, diphtheria, recombinant hepatitis B, and rabies vaccines.

Alcohol, Cigarette Smoke, and Other Substances

A safe level of alcohol consumption during pregnancy has not yet been established. Although the consumption of occasional alcoholic beverages may not be harmful to the mother or her developing embryo or fetus, complete abstinence is strongly advised. Maternal alcoholism is associated with high rates of miscarriage and fetal alcohol syndrome; the risk for miscarriage in the first trimester is dose related (three or more drinks per day). Growing evidence indicates that the pattern of drinking (frequency, timing, and duration), especially in the first trimester, is more predictive of fetal damage than is the amount (Wagner et al., 1998). Considerably less alcohol use is reported among pregnant women than in nonpregnant women, but a high prevalence of some alcohol use among pregnant women still exists. Such a finding underscores the need for more systematic public health efforts to educate women about the hazards of alcohol consumption in pregnancy (Ebrahim et al., 1998).

All pregnant women who smoke should be strongly encouraged to quit or at least cut down. Pregnant women should be told about the negative effects of even secondhand smoke on the fetus and encouraged to avoid such environments (ACOG, 1997). Nurse-managed interventions hold promise for helping pregnant smokers quit (Gebauer et al., 1998; Kilby, 1997). Better still are efforts focused on preventing girls and women from beginning to smoke (Johnson, 1998) (see Research box).

Most studies of human pregnancy have revealed no association between caffeine consumption and birth defects or LBW (Cunningham et al., 2001). Because other effects are unknown, however, pregnant women are advised to limit their caffeine intake.

Any drug or environmental agent that enters the pregnant woman's bloodstream has the potential to cross the placenta and harm the fetus. Marijuana, heroin, and cocaine are common examples of such substances. Although the problem of substance abuse in pregnancy is considered a major public health concern, comprehensive care of drug-addicted women improves maternal and neonatal outcomes (see Chapters 35 and 38).

Normal Discomforts

Pregnant women are confronted with symptoms that would be considered abnormal in the nonpregnant state. Much of the prenatal care requested by women pregnant for the first time is prompted by the need for explanations of the causes of the discomforts and for advice on ways to relieve the discomforts. The discomforts of the first trimester are fairly specific. Information about the physiology and prevention of and self-care for discomforts experienced during the three trimesters is given in Table 16-2. Box 16-5 on p. 435 lists alternative and complementary therapies and why they might be used in pregnancy (see Figs. 4-2 and 4-3). Nurses can do much to allay a first-time mother's anxiety about such symptoms by telling her about them in advance, using terminology that the woman (or couple) can understand. Women who understand the physical discomforts of pregnancy are less apt to become overly anxious about their health. In addition, under-

Text continues on p. 435.

RESEARCH

Kicking the Habit During Pregnancy: Factors in Successful Smoking Cessation

Smoking is hazardous to women's health by increasing the incidence of cancer of the lung, oropharynx, bladder, and cervix, and increasing the incidence of lung and heart disease. It is harmful to women's reproductive function, causing infertility, miscarriage, fetal anomalies, preterm births, placenta previa, fetal and neonatal deaths, and sudden infant death syndrome. It is also the primary preventable risk factor for low birth weight in the United States.

If the smoking behavior of pregnant women can be more fully understood, interventions can be targeted to where they will do the most good. Researchers conducted a retrospective study of 5288 new mothers in the United States and compared sociodemographic data of smokers and nonsmokers during pregnancy to identify factors associated with smoking cessation. Nearly 1 in 20 women reported smoking at the beginning of their pregnancy. Risk factors for smoking included being a Caucasian, being young, being not currently married, and having less than a high school education. The smokers who attempted to quit during their pregnancy tended to be Hispanic, had a higher education, were above poverty income, and had a shorter duration of smoking. Successful quitters tended to be Hispanic and women who had smoked for less than 10 years.

IMPLICATIONS FOR PRACTICE

Longer smoking duration had the strongest association with unattempted and unsuccessful smoking cessation, leading to the conclusion that more research is needed on the physiologic and psychologic effects of smoking. Another area for future research is to study the protective effect attributed to the Hispanic culture to see if it can be duplicated in other groups. Women's health nurses can urge girls and women to not smoke or quit before pregnancy. Nurse policy makers can use this study to target interventions for groups that would gain the most benefit. Clinic-based smoking cessation materials and interventions are available from the Public Health Service and the National Cancer Institute, but future materials may need to incorporate age, ethnicity, income, and education level.

Reference: Yu, S., Park, C., & Schwalberg, R. (2002). Factors associated with smoking cessation among U.S. pregnant women. *Maternal and Child Health Journal, 6*(2), 89-97.

TABLE 16-2 Discomforts Related to Pregnancy

DISCOMFORT	PHYSIOLOGY	EDUCATION FOR SELF-CARE
FIRST TRIMESTER		
Breast changes, new sensation: pain, tingling, tenderness	Hypertrophy of mammary glandular tissue and increased vascularization, pigmentation, and size and prominence of nipples and areolae caused by hormonal stimulation	Wear supportive maternity bras with pads to absorb discharge, may be worn at night; wash with warm water and keep dry; breast tenderness may interfere with sexual expression/foreplay but is temporary
Urgency and frequency of urination	Vascular engorgement and altered bladder function caused by hormones; bladder capacity reduced by enlarging uterus and fetal presenting part	Empty bladder regularly; perform Kegel exercises; limit fluid intake before bedtime; wear perineal pad; report pain or burning sensation to primary health care provider
Languor and malaise; fatigue (early pregnancy, most commonly)	Unexplained; may be caused by increasing levels of estrogen, progesterone, and hCG or by elevated BBT; psychologic response to pregnancy and its required physical/psychologic adaptations	Rest as needed; eat well-balanced diet to prevent anemia
Nausea and vomiting, morning sickness—occurs in 50%-75% of pregnant women; starts between first and second missed periods and lasts until about fourth missed period; may occur any time during day; fathers also may have symptoms	Cause unknown; may result from hormonal changes, possibly hCG; may be partly emotional, reflecting pride in, ambivalence about, or rejection of pregnant state	Avoid empty or overloaded stomach; maintain good posture—give stomach ample room; stop smoking; eat dry carbohydrate on awakening; remain in bed until feeling subsides, or alternate dry carbohydrate 1 hr with fluids such as hot herbal decaffeinated tea, milk, or clear coffee the next hour until feeling subsides; eat five to six small meals per day; avoid fried, odorous, spicy, greasy, or gas-forming foods; consult primary health care provider if intractable vomiting occurs
Ptyalism (excessive salivation) may occur starting 2 to 3 weeks after first missed period	Possibly caused by elevated estrogen levels; may be related to reluctance to swallow because of nausea	Use astringent mouth wash, chew gum, eat hard candy as comfort measures
Gingivitis and **epulis** (hyperemia, hypertrophy, bleeding, tenderness of the gums); condition will disappear spontaneously 1 to 2 months after birth	Increased vascularity and proliferation of connective tissue from estrogen stimulation	Eat well-balanced diet with adequate protein and fresh fruits and vegetables; brush teeth gently and observe good dental hygiene; avoid infection; see dentist
Nasal stuffiness; epistaxis (nosebleed)	Hyperemia of mucous membranes related to high estrogen levels	Use humidifier; avoid trauma; normal saline nose drops or spray may be used
Leukorrhea: often noted throughout pregnancy	Hormonally stimulated cervix becomes hypertrophic and hyperactive, producing abundant amount of mucus	Not preventable; do not douche; wear perineal pads; perform hygienic practices such as wiping front to back; report to primary health care provider if accompanied by pruritus, foul odor, or change in character or color
Psychosocial dynamics, mood swings, mixed feelings	Hormonal and metabolic adaptations; feelings about female role, sexuality, timing of pregnancy, and resultant changes in life and life-style	Participate in pregnancy support group; communicate concerns to partner, family, and others; request referral for supportive services if needed (financial assistance)

hCG, Human chorionic gonadotropin; *BBT*, basal body temperature; *PIH*, pregnancy-induced hypertension.

Continued

	SECOND TRIMESTER	
DISCOMFORT	**PHYSIOLOGY**	**EDUCATION FOR SELF-CARE**
Pigmentation deepens, acne, oily skin	Melanocyte-stimulating hormone (from anterior pituitary)	Not preventable; usually resolves during puerperium
Spider nevi (angiomas) appear over neck, thorax, face, and arms during second or third trimester	Focal networks of dilated arterioles (end arteries) from increased concentration of estrogens	Not preventable; they fade slowly during late puerperium; rarely disappear completely
Palmar erythema occurs in 50% of pregnant women; may accompany spider nevi	Diffuse reddish mottling over palms and suffused skin over thenar eminencies and fingertips; may be caused by genetic predisposition or hyperestrogenism	Not preventable; condition will fade within 1 wk after giving birth
Pruritus (noninflammatory)	Unknown cause; various types as follows: nonpapular; closely aggregated pruritic papules	Keep fingernails short and clean; contact primary health care provider for diagnosis of cause
	Increased excretory function of skin and stretching of skin possible factors	Not preventable; symptomatic; Keri baths; mild sedation
		Distraction; tepid baths with sodium bicarbonate or oatmeal added to water; lotions and oils; change of soaps or reduction in use of soap; loose clothing
Palpitations	Unknown; should not be accompanied by persistent cardiac irregularity	Not preventable; contact primary health care provider if accompanied by symptoms of cardiac decompensation
Supine hypotension (vena cava syndrome) and bradycardia	Induced by pressure of gravid uterus on ascending vena cava when woman is supine; reduces uteroplacental and renal perfusion	Side-lying position or semisitting posture, with knees slightly flexed (see supine hypotension, pp. 415-416)
Faintness and, rarely, syncope (orthostatic hypotension) may persist throughout pregnancy	Vasomotor lability or postural hypotension from hormones; in late pregnancy may be caused by venous stasis in lower extremities	Moderate exercise, deep breathing, vigorous leg movement; avoid sudden changes in position* and warm crowded areas; move slowly and deliberately; keep environment cool; avoid hypoglycemia by eating 5 to 6 small meals per day; wear elastic hose; sit as necessary; if symptoms are serious, contact primary health care provider
Food cravings	Cause unknown; craving influenced by culture or geographic area	Not preventable; satisfy craving unless it interferes with well-balanced diet; report unusual cravings to primary health care provider
Heartburn (pyrosis or acid indigestion): burning sensation, occasionally with burping and regurgitation of a little sour-tasting fluid	Progesterone slows gastrointestinal (GI) tract motility and digestion, reverses peristalsis, relaxes cardiac sphincter, and delays emptying time of stomach; stomach displaced upward and compressed by enlarging uterus	Limit or avoid gas-producing or fatty foods and large meals; maintain good posture; sip milk for temporary relief; hot herbal tea; primary health care provider may prescribe antacid between meals; contact primary health care provider for persistent symptoms
Constipation	GI tract motility slowed because of progesterone, resulting in increased resorption of water and drying of	Drink six glasses of water per day; include roughage in diet; moderate exercise; maintain regular schedule

*Caution woman to rise slowly and sit on edge of bed or to assume hands-and-knee posture before rising and to get up slowly after sitting or squatting.

SECOND TRIMESTER—cont'd		
DISCOMFORT	**PHYSIOLOGY**	**EDUCATION FOR SELF-CARE**
Constipation—cont'd	stool; intestines compressed by enlarging uterus; predisposition to constipation because of oral iron supplementation	for bowel movements; use relaxation techniques and deep breathing; do not take stool softener, laxatives, mineral oil, other drugs, or enemas without first consulting primary health care provider
Flatulence with bloating and belching	Reduced GI motility because of hormones, allowing time for bacterial action that produces gas; swallowing air	Chew foods slowly and thoroughly; avoid gas-producing foods, fatty foods, large meals; exercise; maintain regular bowel habits
Varicose veins (varicosities): may be associated with aching legs and tenderness; may be present in legs and vulva; hemorrhoids are varicosities in perianal area	Hereditary predisposition; relaxation of smooth muscle walls of veins because of hormones causing tortuous dilated veins in legs and pelvic vasocongestion; condition aggravated by enlarging uterus, gravity, and bearing down for bowel movements; thrombi from leg varices rare but may occur in hemorrhoids	Avoid obesity, lengthy standing or sitting, constrictive clothing, and constipation and bearing down with bowel movements; moderate exercises; rest with legs and hips elevated (see Fig. 16-15); wear support stocking; thrombosed hemorrhoid may be evacuated; relieve swelling and pain with warm sitz baths, local application of astringent compresses
Leukorrhea: often noted throughout pregnancy	Hormonally stimulated cervix becomes hypertrophic and hyperactive, producing abundant amount of mucus	Not preventable; do not douche; maintain good hygiene; wear perineal pads; report to primary health care provider if accompanied by pruritus, foul odor, or change in character or color
Headaches (through week 26)	Emotional tension (more common than vascular migraine headache); eye strain (refractory errors); vascular engorgement and congestion of sinuses resulting from hormone stimulation	Conscious relaxation; contact primary health care provider for constant "splitting" headache, to assess for PIH
Carpal tunnel syndrome (involves thumb, second, and third fingers, lateral side of little finger)	Compression of median nerve resulting from changes in surrounding tissues; pain, numbness, tingling, burning; loss of skilled movements (typing); dropping of objects	Not preventable; elevate affected arms; splinting of affected hand may help; regressive after pregnancy; surgery is curative
Periodic numbness, tingling of fingers (acrodysesthesia) occurs in 5% of pregnant women	Brachial plexus traction syndrome resulting from drooping of shoulders during pregnancy (occurs especially at night and early morning)	Maintain good posture; wear supportive maternity bra; condition will disappear if lifting and carrying baby does not aggravate it
Round ligament pain (tenderness)	Stretching of ligament caused by enlarging uterus	Not preventable; rest, maintain good body mechanics to avoid overstretching ligament; relieve cramping by squatting or bringing knees to chest, sometimes heat helps
Joint pain, backache, and pelvic pressure; hypermobility of joints	Relaxation of symphyseal and sacroiliac joints because of hormones, resulting in unstable pelvis; exaggerated lumbar and cervicothoracic curves caused by change in center of gravity resulting from enlarging abdomen	Maintain good posture and body mechanics; avoid fatigue; wear low-heeled shoes; abdominal supports may be useful; conscious relaxation; sleep on firm mattress; apply local heat or ice; get back rubs; do pelvic tilt exercises; rest; condition will disappear 6 to 8 wk after birth

Continued

TABLE 16-2 **Discomforts Related to Pregnancy—cont'd**

DISCOMFORT	PHYSIOLOGY	EDUCATION FOR SELF-CARE
	THIRD TRIMESTER	
Shortness of breath and dyspnea occur in 60% of pregnant women	Expansion of diaphragm limited by enlarging uterus; diaphragm is elevated about 4 cm; some relief after lightening	Good posture; sleep with extra pillows; avoid overloading stomach; stop smoking; contact health care provider if symptoms worsen to rule out anemia, emphysema, and asthma
Insomnia (later weeks of pregnancy)	Fetal movements, muscle cramping, urinary frequency, shortness of breath, or other discomforts	Reassurance; conscious relaxation; back massage or **effleurage;** support of body parts with pillows; warm milk or warm shower before retiring
Psychosocial responses: mood swings, mixed feelings, increased anxiety	Hormonal and metabolic adaptations; feelings about impending labor, birth, and parenthood	Reassurance and support from significant other and nurse; improved communication with partner, family, and others
Urinary frequency and urgency return	Vascular engorgement and altered bladder function caused by hormones; bladder capacity reduced by enlarging uterus and fetal presenting part	Empty bladder regularly, Kegel exercises; limit fluid intake before bedtime; reassurance; wear perineal pad; contact health care provider for pain or burning sensation
Perineal discomfort and pressure	Pressure from enlarging uterus, especially when standing or walking; multifetal gestation	Rest, conscious relaxation, and good posture; contact health care provider for assessment and treatment if pain is present
Braxton Hicks contractions	Intensification of uterine contractions in preparation for work of labor	Reassurance; rest; change of position; practice breathing techniques when contractions are bothersome; effleurage
Leg cramps (gastrocnemius spasm), especially when reclining	Compression of nerves supplying lower extremities because of enlarging uterus; reduced level of diffusible serum calcium or elevation of serum phosphorus; aggravating factors: fatigue, poor peripheral circulation, pointing toes when stretching legs or when walking, drinking more than 1 L (1 qt) of milk per day	Check for Homan's sign; if negative, use massage and heat over affected muscle; dorsiflex foot until spasm relaxes (see Fig. 16-16, *A*); stand on cold surface; oral supplementation with calcium carbonate or calcium lactate tablets; aluminum hydroxide gel, 30 ml, with each meal removes phosphorus by absorbing it (consult primary healthcare provider before taking these remedies)
Ankle edema (nonpitting) to lower extremities	Edema aggravated by prolonged standing, sitting, poor posture, lack of exercise, constrictive clothing, or by hot weather	Ample fluid intake for natural diuretic effect; put on support stockings before arising; rest periodically with legs and hips elevated (see Fig. 16-15), exercise moderately; contact health care provider if generalized edema develops; *diuretics are contraindicated*

standing the rationale for treatment promotes their participation in their care. Interventions should be individualized with attention given to the woman's lifestyle and culture.

NURSE ALERT
Although complementary and alternative therapies may benefit the woman during pregnancy, some practices should be avoided because they may cause miscarriage or preterm labor (Beal, 1998). It is important to ask the woman what therapies she may be using.

Recognizing Potential Complications

One of the most important responsibilities of care providers is to alert the pregnant woman to signs and symptoms that indicate a potential complication of pregnancy. The woman needs to know how to report such warning signs. When one is stressed by a disturbing symptom, it is difficult to remember specifics. Therefore the pregnant woman and her family can be reassured if they receive and use a printed form listing the signs and symptoms that warrant an investigation and the telephone numbers to call in an emergency.

The nurse must answer questions honestly as they arise during pregnancy. Pregnant women often have difficulty deciding when to report signs and symptoms. The mother is encouraged to refer to the printed list of potential complications and to listen to her body. If she senses that something is wrong, she should call her care provider. Several signs and symptoms must be discussed more extensively. These include vaginal bleeding, alteration in fetal movements, symptoms of PIH, rupture of membranes, and preterm labor (see Signs of Potential Complications box on p. 417).

Recognizing Preterm Labor

Teaching each expectant mother to recognize preterm labor is necessary for early diagnosis and treatment. Preterm labor occurs after the twentieth week but before the thirty-seventh week of pregnancy and consists of uterine contractions that, if untreated, cause the cervix to open earlier than normal and results in preterm birth.

Although the exact etiology of preterm labor is unknown, it is assumed to have multiple causes. An increased incidence of preterm birth is associated with sociodemographic factors such as poverty, low educational level, lack of social support, smoking, domestic violence, and stress (Moore & Freda, 1998), and the rate is almost twice as high in the African-American population as in Caucasians (March of Dimes, 1997). The pathology associated with preterm labor also is far from clear, but it has recently been conceptualized as having either, or sometimes both, intrinsic and extrinsic pathways (Abrahams & Katz, 2002). Intrinsic pathways are in effect when no known or detectable factors precede the onset of preterm labor; this type is called idiopathic and may result from neural, hormonal, or fetal signals that are not well understood. Extrinsic pathways are associated with overt and clinically detectable changes that occur within the uterus itself, such as infection, distortion of the uterine size or shape, cervical anomalies, and separation of the placenta. Changes within these pathways are thought to be in effect for some time before overt clinical symptoms occur; thus preterm labor is considered the end stage of events already established.

If a woman knows the warning signs and symptoms of preterm labor and seeks care early enough, prevention of preterm birth may be possible. Warning signs and symptoms of preterm labor are given in the Teaching for Self-Care box. Moore et al. (1998) demonstrated that nursing telephone support to at-risk women can result in a significant decrease in LBW and preterm births in African-American women. This study and others demonstrate the power of nursing care, nursing support, and client education in the care of women at highest risk for preterm birth. Figure 16-18 shows the possible locations of symptoms in the body.

BOX 16-5 Complementary and Alternative Therapies Used in Pregnancy

MORNING SICKNESS AND HYPEREMESIS
- Acupuncture
- Acupressure (see Figs. 4-2 and 4-3)
- Shiatzu
- Herbal remedies*
  - Peppermint
  - Spearmint
  - Ginger root
  - Raspberry leaf
  - Fennel
  - Chamomile
  - Hops
- Meadowsweet
  - Wild yam root

RELAXATION AND MUSCLE-ACHE RELIEF
- Yoga
- Biofeedback
- Reflexology
- Therapeutic touch

From Beal, M. (1998). Women's use of complementary and alternative therapies in reproductive health. *Journal of Nurse Midwifery, 43*(3), 224-233; and Schirmer, G. (1998). *Herbal medicine.* Bedford, TX: MED2000 Inc.

*Some herbs can cause miscarriage, preterm labor, or fetal or maternal injury. Pregnant women should discuss use with pregnancy health care provider, as well as an expert qualified in the use of the herb.

Sexual Counseling

Sexual counseling of expectant couples includes countering misinformation, providing reassurance of normality, and suggesting alternative behaviors. The uniqueness of each couple is considered within a biopsychosocial framework (see the Teaching for Self-Care box on p. 437). Nurses can

TEACHING FOR SELF-CARE

How to Recognize Preterm Labor

Because the onset of preterm labor is subtle and often hard to recognize, it is important to know how to feel your abdomen for uterine contractions. You can feel for contractions in the following way. While lying down, place your fingertips on the top of your uterus. A contraction is the periodic tightening or hardening of your uterus. If your uterus is contracting, you will actually feel your abdomen get tight or hard and then feel it relax or soften when the contraction is over.

If you think you are having any of the other signs and symptoms of preterm labor, empty your bladder, drink three to four glasses of water for hydration, lie down tilted toward your side, and place a pillow at your back for support.

Check for contractions for 1 hour. To tell how often contractions are occurring, check the minutes that elapse from the beginning of one contraction to the beginning of the next.

It is *not normal* to have frequent uterine contractions (every 10 minutes or more often for 1 hour).

Contractions of labor are regular, frequent, and hard. They also may be felt as a tightening of the abdomen or a backache. This type of contraction causes the cervix to efface and dilate.

Call your doctor, nurse-midwife, clinic, or labor and birth unit, or go to the hospital if any of the following signs occur:

- You have uterine contractions every 10 minutes or more often for 1 hour or
- You have any of the other signs and symptoms for 1 hour or
- You have any bloody spotting or leaking of fluid from your vagina

It is often difficult to identify preterm labor. Accurate diagnosis requires assessment by the health care provider, usually in the hospital or clinic.

Post these instructions where they can be seen by everyone in the family.

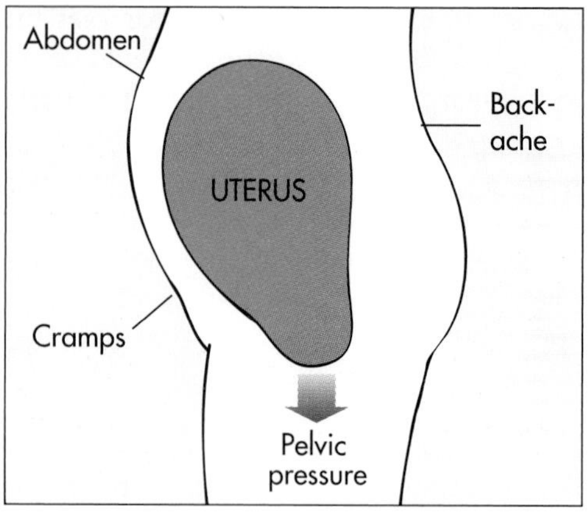
Abdomen
Back-
ache
UTERUS
Cramps
Pelvic
pressure

FIG. 16-18 Symptoms of preterm labor.

initiate discussion about sexual adjustments that must be made during pregnancy, but they themselves need a sound knowledge base about the physical, social, and emotional responses to sex during pregnancy. Not all maternity nurses are comfortable dealing with the sexual concerns of their clients; therefore those nurses who are aware of their personal strengths and limitations in dealing with sexual content are better prepared to make referrals if necessary.

Many women merely need permission to be sexually active during pregnancy. Many other women, however, need to be given information about the physiologic changes that occur during pregnancy and have the myths dispelled that are associated with sex during pregnancy. Such tasks are within the purview of the nurse and should be an integral component of the health care rendered (Alteneder & Hartzell, 1997).

Some couples need to be referred for sex therapy or family therapy. Couples with long-standing problems with sexual dysfunction that are intensified by pregnancy are candidates for sex therapy. Whenever a sexual problem is a symptom of a more serious relationship problem, the couple would benefit from family therapy.

Using the History

The couple's sexual history provides a basis for counseling, but history taking also is an ongoing process. The couple's receptivity to changes in attitudes, body image, partner relationships, and physical status are relevant topics throughout pregnancy. Whenever changes occur, unexpected problems may require intervention. The history reveals the woman's knowledge of female anatomy and physiology and her attitudes about sex during pregnancy, as well as her perceptions of the pregnancy, the health status of the couple, and the quality of their relationship. An understanding of the couple's subjective experience provides the direction and focus for sexual counseling.

Countering Misinformation

Many myths and much of the misinformation related to sex and pregnancy are masked by seemingly unrelated issues. For example, a discussion about the baby's ability to hear and see in utero may be prompted by questions about the baby being an observer of lovemaking. The counselor must be extremely sensitive to the questions behind such questions when counseling in this highly charged emotional area.

Suggesting Alternative Behaviors

Research has not demonstrated conclusively that coitus and orgasm are contraindicated at any time during pregnancy for the obstetrically and medically healthy woman (Cunningham et al., 2001). However, a history of more than one miscarriage; a threatened miscarriage in the first trimester; impending miscarriage in the second trimester;

TEACHING FOR SELF-CARE

Sexuality in Pregnancy

- Be aware that maternal physiologic changes, such as breast enlargement, nausea, fatigue, abdominal changes, perineal enlargement, leukorrhea, pelvic vasocongestion, and orgasmic responses, may affect sexuality and sexual expression.
- Discuss responses to pregnancy with your partner.
- Keep in mind that cultural prescriptions (dos) and proscriptions (don'ts) may affect your responses.
- Although your libido may be depressed during the first trimester, it often increases during the second and third trimesters.
- Discuss and explore with your partner:
  - Alternative behaviors (e.g., mutual masturbation, foot massage, cuddling)
  - Alternative positions (e.g., female superior, side-lying) for sexual intercourse
- Intercourse is safe as long as it is not uncomfortable. There is no correlation between intercourse and miscarriage, but observe the following precautions:
  - Abstain from intercourse if you experience uterine cramping or vaginal bleeding; report event to your caregiver as soon as possible.
  - Abstain from intercourse (or any activity that results in orgasm) if you have a history of cervical incompetence, until the problem is corrected.
- Continue to use "safer sex" behaviors. Women at risk for acquiring or conveying STIs are encouraged to use condoms during sexual intercourse throughout pregnancy.

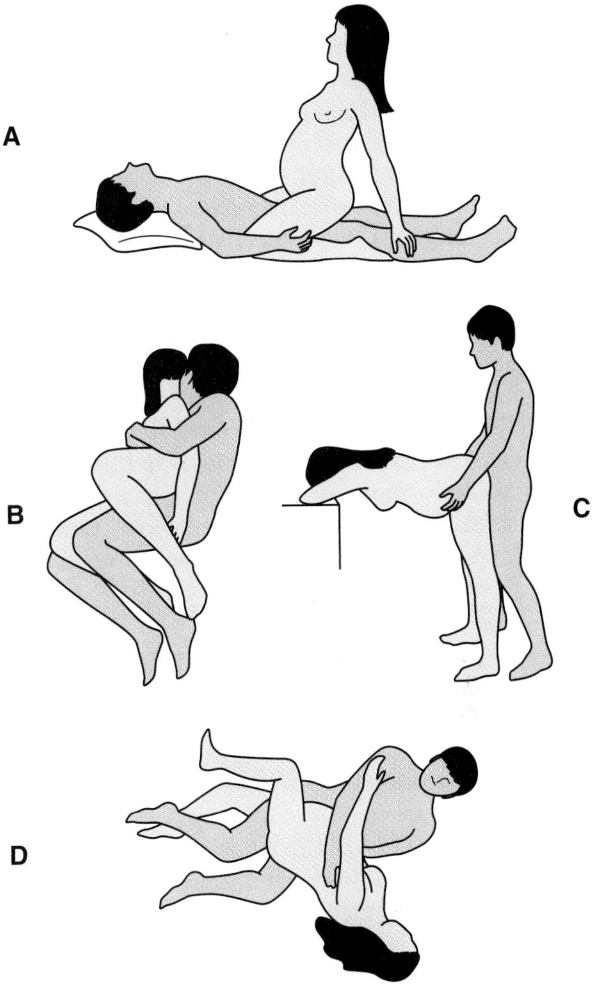
A
B
C
D

FIG. 16-19 Positions for sexual intercourse during pregnancy. **A,** Female superior. **B,** Side by side. **C,** Rear entry. **D,** Side lying, facing each other.

and PROM, bleeding, or abdominal pain during the third trimester warrant caution when it comes to coitus and orgasm.

Solitary and mutual masturbation and oral-genital intercourse may be used by couples as alternatives to penile-vaginal intercourse. Partners who enjoy cunnilingus (oral stimulation of the clitoris or vagina) may feel "turned off" by the normal increase in the amount and odor of vaginal discharge during pregnancy. Couples who practice cunnilingus should be cautioned against the blowing of air into the vagina, particularly during the last few weeks of pregnancy when the cervix may be slightly open. An air embolism can occur if air is forced between the uterine wall and the fetal membranes and enters the maternal vascular system through the placenta.

Showing the woman or couple pictures of possible variations of coital position often is helpful (Fig. 16-19). The female-superior, side-by-side, rear-entry, and side-lying positions are possible alternative positions to the traditional male-superior position. The woman astride (superior position) allows her to control the angle and depth of penile penetration, as well as to protect her breasts and abdomen. The side-by-side position or any position that places less pressure on the pregnant abdomen and requires less energy may be preferred during the third trimester.

Multiparous women sometimes have significant breast tenderness in the first trimester. A coital position that avoids direct pressure on the woman's breasts and decreased breast fondling during love play can be recommended to such couples. The woman also should be reassured that this condition is normal and temporary.

Some women complain of lower abdominal cramping and backache after orgasm during the first and third trimesters. A back rub can often relieve some of the discomfort and provide a pleasant experience. A tonic uterine contraction, often lasting up to a minute, replaces the rhythmic contractions of orgasm during the third trimester. Changes in the FHR without fetal distress also have been reported.

The objective of "safer sex" is to provide prophylaxis against the acquisition and transmission of STIs (e.g., herpes simplex virus [HSV], HIV). Because these diseases may be transmitted to the woman and her fetus, the use of condoms is recommended throughout pregnancy if the woman is at risk for acquiring an STI.

Well-informed nurses who are comfortable with their own sexuality and the sexual counseling needs of expectant couples can offer information and advice in this valuable but often neglected area. They can establish an open environment in which couples can feel free to introduce their concerns about sexual adjustment and seek support and guidance. This intervention is as important for lesbian women and their partners as it is for women partnered with men.

Psychosocial Support

Esteem, affection, trust, concern, consideration of cultural and religious responses, and listening are all components of the emotional support given to the pregnant woman and her family. The woman's satisfaction with her relationships and support, her feeling of competence, and her sense of being in control are important issues to be addressed in the third trimester. A discussion of fetal responses to stimuli, such as sound, light, maternal posture, and tension, as well as patterns of sleeping and waking, can be helpful. Also discussed are emotional tensions that can arise in relation to the childbirth experience, such as those stemming from fear of pain, loss of control, and possible birth of the infant before reaching the hospital; anxieties about the recognized responsibilities and tasks of parenthood; parental concerns about the safety of the mother and unborn child; parental concerns about siblings and their acceptance of the new baby; parental concerns about social and economic responsibilities; and parental concerns arising from conflicts in cultural, religious, or personal value systems.

The father's or partner's commitment to the pregnancy, the couple's relationship, and their concerns about sexuality and sexual expression can emerge as issues for many expectant parents. Validation, feedback, and social comparison characterize the support given.

Providing the prospective mother and father with an opportunity to discuss their concerns and validating the

Plan of Care: Discomforts of Pregnancy and Warning Signs

FIRST TRIMESTER

NURSING DIAGNOSIS Anxiety related to deficient knowledge about schedule of prenatal visits throughout pregnancy as evidenced by woman's questions and concerns

Expected Outcomes *Woman will verbalize correct appointment schedule for the duration of the pregnancy and feelings of being "in control."*

Nursing Interventions/*Rationales*

Provide information regarding schedule of visits, tests, and other assessments and interventions that will be provided throughout the pregnancy *to empower client to function in collaboration with the caregiver and diminish anxiety.*

Allow woman time to describe level of anxiety *to establish basis for care.*

Provide information to woman regarding prenatal classes and labor area tours *to decrease feelings of anxiety about the unknown.*

NURSING DIAGNOSIS Imbalanced nutrition: less than body requirements, related to nausea and vomiting as evidenced by woman's report and weight loss

Expected Outcomes *Woman will gain 1 to 2.5 kg during the first trimester.*

Nursing Interventions/*Rationales*

Verify prepregnant weight *to plan a diet realistic according to individual woman's nutritional needs.*

Obtain diet history *to identify current meal patterns and foods that may be implicated in nausea.*

Advise woman to consume small frequent meals and avoid having empty stomach *to avoid further nausea episodes.*

Suggest that woman eat a simple carbohydrate such as dry crackers before arising in the morning *to avoid empty stomach and decrease incidence of nausea and vomiting.*

Advise woman to call health care provider if vomiting is persistent and severe *to identify possible incidence of hyperemesis gravidarum.*

NURSING DIAGNOSIS Fatigue related to hormonal changes in the first trimester as evidenced by woman's complaints

Expected Outcomes *Woman will report a decreased number of episodes of fatigue.*

Nursing Interventions/*Rationales*

Rest as needed *to avoid increasing feeling of fatigue.*

Eat a well-balanced diet *to meet increased metabolic demands and avoid anemia.*

Discuss the use of support systems to help with household responsibilities *to decrease workload at home and decrease fatigue.*

Reinforce to woman the transitory nature of first trimester fatigue *to provide emotional support.*

Explore with the woman a variety of techniques to prioritize roles *to decrease family expectations.*

SECOND TRIMESTER

NURSING DIAGNOSIS Constipation related to progesterone influence on GI tract as evidenced by woman's report of altered patterns of elimination

Expected Outcomes *Woman will report a return to normal bowel elimination pattern following implementation of interventions.*

Nursing Interventions/*Rationales*

Provide information to woman regarding pregnancy-related causes: progesterone slowing gastrointestinal motility, growing uterus compressing intestines, and influence of iron supplementation *to provide basic information for self-care during pregnancy.*

Assist woman to plan a diet that will promote regular bowel movements, such as increasing amount of oral fluid intake to at least six glasses of water a day, increasing the amount of fiber in daily diet, and to maintain moderate exercise *to promote self-care.*

Reinforce for woman that she should not take any laxatives, stool softeners, or enemas without first consulting the health care provider *to prevent any injuries to woman or fetus.*

normality of their responses can meet their needs to varying degrees. Nurses also must recognize that men feel more vulnerable during their partner's pregnancy. Female partners also may have these feelings. Anticipatory guidance and health promotion strategies can help partners cope with their concerns. Nursing intervention may help them to deal with such concerns either directly through counseling or indirectly through the education of the mothers. Health care providers can stimulate and encourage open dialogue between the couple.

Evaluation

Evaluation of the effectiveness of care of the woman during pregnancy is based on the previously stated outcomes. More effort is needed in evaluating outcomes of nursing care during the prenatal period. A formal systematic follow-up on quality of care is not common but should be developed and incorporated in all settings (see Plan of Care).

VARIATIONS IN PRENATAL CARE

The course of prenatal care described thus far may seem to suggest that the experiences of childbearing women are similar and that nursing interventions are uniformly consistent across all populations. Although typical patterns of response to pregnancy are easily recognized and many aspects of prenatal care indeed are consistent, pregnant women enter the health care system with individual concerns and needs. The nurse's ability to assess unique needs and to tailor interventions to the individual is the hallmark of expertise in providing care. Variations that influence prenatal care include culture, age, and number of fetuses.

Cultural Influences

Prenatal care as we know it is a phenomenon of Western medicine. In the American biomedical model of care, women are encouraged to seek prenatal care as early as possible in their pregnancy by visiting a physician, nurse-

Plan of Care — Discomforts of Pregnancy and Warning Signs—cont'd

NURSING DIAGNOSIS Anxiety related to deficient knowledge about course of first pregnancy as evidenced by woman's questions regarding possible complications of second and third trimesters

Expected Outcomes *Woman will correctly list signs of potential complications that can occur during the second and third trimesters and exhibit no overt signs of stress.*

Nursing Interventions/*Rationales*

Provide information concerning the potential complications or warning signs that can occur during the second and third trimesters, including possible causes of signs and the importance of calling the health care provider immediately *to ensure identification and treatment of problems in a timely manner.*

Provide a written list of complications *to have a reference list for emergencies.*

THIRD TRIMESTER

NURSING DIAGNOSIS Fear related to deficient knowledge regarding onset of labor and the processes of labor related to inexperience as evidenced by woman's questions and statement of concerns

Expected Outcomes *Woman will verbalize basic understanding of signs of labor onset, when to call the health care provider, identify resources for childbirth education, and express increasing confidence in readiness to cope with labor.*

Nursing Interventions/*Rationales*

Provide information regarding signs of labor onset, when to call the health care provider, and give written information regarding local childbirth education classes *to empower and promote self-care.*

Promote ongoing effective communication with health care provider *to promote trust and decrease fear of unknown.*

Provide the woman with decision-making opportunities *to promote effective coping.*

Provide opportunity for woman to verbalize fears regarding childbirth *to assist in decreasing fear through discussion.*

NURSING DIAGNOSIS Disturbed sleep pattern related to discomforts/insomnia of third trimester as evidenced by woman's report of inadequate rest

Expected Outcomes *Woman will report an improvement of quality and quantity of rest and sleep.*

Nursing Interventions/*Rationales*

Assess current sleep pattern and review need for increased requirement during pregnancy *to identify need for change in sleep patterns.*

Suggest change of position to side-lying with pillows between legs or to sleep in semi-Fowler's position *to increase support and decrease any problems with dyspnea or heartburn.*

Reinforce the possibility of the use of various sleep aides such as relaxation techniques, reading, and decreased activity before bedtime *to decrease the possibility of anxiety or physical discomforts before bedtime.*

NURSING DIAGNOSIS Ineffective sexuality patterns related to changes in comfort level and fatigue

Expected Outcome *Woman will verbalize feelings regarding changes in sexual desire.*

Nursing Interventions/*Rationales*

Assess couple's usual sexuality patterns *to determine how patterns have been altered by pregnancy.*

Provide information regarding expected changes in sexual patterns during pregnancy *to correct any misconceptions.*

Allow the couple to express feelings in a nonjudgmental atmosphere *to promote trust.*

Refer couple for counseling as appropriate *to assist the couple to cope with sexuality pattern changes.*

Suggest alternative sexual positions *to decrease pressure on enlarging abdomen of woman and increase sexual comfort and satisfaction of couple.*

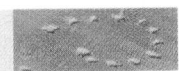

midwife, office, or clinic. Such visits are usually routine and follow a systematic sequence, with the initial visit followed by monthly, then semimonthly, and then weekly visits. Monitoring weight and BP; testing blood and urine; teaching specific information about diet, rest, and activity; and preparing for childbirth are common components of prenatal care. This model not only is unfamiliar but also seems strange to many groups. Different models for providing prenatal care for women throughout the world are being explored (Chalmers, Mangiaterra, & Porter, 2001).

Many cultural variations are found in prenatal care. Even if the prenatal care described is familiar to a woman, some practices may conflict with the beliefs and practices of a subculture group to which she belongs. Because of these and other factors, such as lack of money, lack of transportation, and language barriers, women from many such groups do not participate in the prenatal care system (Shaffer, 2002). Such behavior may be misinterpreted by nurses as uncaring, lazy, or ignorant.

A concern for modesty also is a deterrent to many women's seeking prenatal care. For some women, exposing body parts, especially to a man, is considered a major violation of their modesty. For many women, invasive procedures, such as a vaginal examination, may be so threatening that they cannot be discussed, even with their own husbands; thus many women prefer a female to a male health care provider. Too often, health care providers assume women lose this modesty during pregnancy and labor, but actually most women value and appreciate efforts to maintain their modesty.

For numerous cultural groups, a physician is deemed appropriate only in times of illness, and because pregnancy is considered a normal process and the woman is in a state of health, the services of a physician are considered inappropriate. Even if what are considered problems with pregnancy by standards of Western medicine do develop, they may not be perceived as problems by members of other cultural groups.

Although pregnancy is considered normal by many, certain practices are expected of women of all cultures to ensure a good outcome. **Cultural prescriptions** tell women what to do, and **cultural proscriptions** establish taboos. The purposes of these practices are to prevent maternal illness resulting from a pregnancy-induced imbalanced state and to protect the vulnerable fetus. Prescriptions and proscriptions regulate the woman's emotional response, clothing, activity and rest, sexual activity, and dietary practices. Exploration of the woman's beliefs, perceptions of the meaning of childbearing, and health care practices may help health care providers foster her self-actualization, promote attainment of the maternal role, and positively influence her relationship with her spouse.

To provide culturally sensitive care, the nurse must be knowledgeable about practices and customs, although it is not possible to know all there is to know about every culture and subculture or the many lifestyles that exist. When exploring cultural beliefs and practices related to childbearing, the nurse can support and nurture those beliefs that promote physical or emotional adaptation. However, if potentially harmful beliefs or activities are identified, the nurse should carefully provide education and propose modifications.

Emotional Response

Virtually all cultures emphasize the importance of maintaining a socially harmonious and agreeable environment for a pregnant woman. An absence of stress is important in ensuring a successful outcome for the mother and baby. Harmony with other people must be fostered, and visits from extended family members may be required to demonstrate pleasant and noncontroversial relationships. If discord exists in a relationship, it is usually dealt with in culturally prescribed ways.

Besides proscriptions regarding food, other proscriptions involve forms of magic. For example, some Mexicans believe that pregnant women should not witness an eclipse of the moon because it may cause a cleft palate in the infant. They also believe that exposure to an earthquake may precipitate preterm birth, miscarriage, or even a breech presentation. In some cultures, a pregnant woman must not ridicule someone with an affliction for fear her child might be born with the same handicap. A mother should not hate a person lest her child resemble that person, and dental work should not be done because it may cause a baby to have a "harelip." A widely held folk belief in some cultures is that the pregnant woman should refrain from raising her arms above her head, because such movement ties knots in the umbilical cord and may cause it to wrap around the baby's neck. Another belief is that placing a knife under the bed of a laboring woman will "cut" her pain.

Clothing

Although most cultural groups do not prescribe specific clothing to be worn during pregnancy, modesty is an expectation of many. Some Mexican women of the Southwest wear a cord beneath the breasts and knotted over the umbilicus. This cord, called a muñeco, is thought to prevent morning sickness and ensure a safe birth. Amulets, medals, and beads also may be worn to ward off evil spirits.

Physical Activity and Rest

Norms that regulate the physical activity of mothers during pregnancy vary tremendously. Many groups, including Native Americans and some Asian groups, encourage women to be active, to walk, and to engage in normal, although not strenuous, activities to ensure that the baby is healthy and not too large. Conversely, other groups such as Filipinos believe that any activity is dangerous, and others willingly take over the work of the pregnant woman. Some Filipinos believe that this inactivity protects the mother and child. The mother is encouraged simply to produce the succeeding generation. If health care providers do not know of this belief, they could misinterpret this behavior as laziness or noncompliance with the desired prenatal health care regimen. It is important for the nurse to find out the way each pregnant woman views activity and rest.

Sexual Activity

In most cultures, sexual activity is not prohibited until the end of pregnancy. Some Latinos view sexual activity as necessary to keep the birth canal lubricated. Conversely, some Vietnamese may have definite proscriptions against sexual intercourse, requiring abstinence throughout the pregnancy because it is thought that sexual intercourse may harm the mother and fetus.

Diet

Nutritional information given by Western health care providers also may be a source of conflict for many cultural groups, but such a conflict commonly is not known by health care providers unless they understand the dietary beliefs and practices of the people for whom they are caring. For example, Muslims have strict regulations regarding preparation of food, and if meat cannot be prepared as prescribed, they may omit meats from their diets. Many cultures permit pregnant women to eat only warm foods.

Age Differences

The age of the childbearing couple may have a significant influence on their physical and psychosocial adaptation to pregnancy. Normal developmental processes that occur in both very young and older mothers are interrupted by pregnancy and require a different type of adaptation to pregnancy than that of the woman of typical childbearing age. Although the individuality of each pregnant woman is recognized, special needs of expectant mothers 15 years of age or younger or those 35 years of age or older are summarized.

Adolescents

Teenage pregnancy is a worldwide problem (Cherry, Dillon, & Rugh, 2001). About one million adolescents, 4 of every 10 girls, in the United States become pregnant each year. Most of the pregnancies are unintended, and nearly 40% end in abortion. Nevertheless, adolescents are responsible for almost 500,000 births in the United States annually. African-American adolescents currently have the highest birth rate, whereas the rate for Hispanic adolescents is second highest (Hoyert et al., 2001). Of girls who become pregnant, one in six will have a repeat pregnancy within 1 year. Most of these young women are unmarried, and many are not ready for the emotional, psychologic, and financial responsibilities of parenthood.

Despite these alarming statistics and the fact that the United States has the highest adolescent birth rate in the industrialized world, the birth rate for adolescents has steadily declined since 1991 (Hoyert et al., 2001). Concentrated national efforts have generated a host of adolescent pregnancy–prevention programs that have had varying degrees of success (Ford et al., 2002). Characteristics of programs that make a difference are those that have sustained commitment to adolescents over a long time, involve the parents and other adults in the community, promote abstinence and personal responsibility, and assist adolescents to develop a clear strategy for reaching future goals such as a college education or a career.

When adolescents do become pregnant and decide to give birth, they are much less likely than older women to receive adequate prenatal care, with many receiving no care at all (Ford et al., 2002). These young women also are more likely to smoke and less likely to gain adequate weight during pregnancy. As a result of these and other factors, babies born to adolescents are at greatly increased risk of LBW, of serious and long-term disability, and of dying during the first year of life.

Delayed entry into prenatal care may be the result of late recognition of pregnancy, denial of pregnancy, or confusion about the available services. Such a delay in care may leave an inadequate time before birth to attend to correctable problems. The very young pregnant adolescent is at higher risk for each of the confounding variables associated with poor pregnancy outcomes (e.g., socioeconomic factors) and for those conditions associated with a first pregnancy regardless of age (e.g., PIH). However, when prenatal care is initiated early and consistently, and confounding variables are controlled, very young pregnant adolescents are at no greater risk (nor are their infants) for an adverse outcome than are older pregnant women. The role of the nurse in reducing the risks and consequences of adolescent pregnancy is thus twofold: first, to encourage early and continued prenatal care and, second, to refer the adolescent, if necessary, for appropriate social support services, which can help reverse the effects of a negative socioeconomic environment (Fig. 16-20) (see Plan of Care).

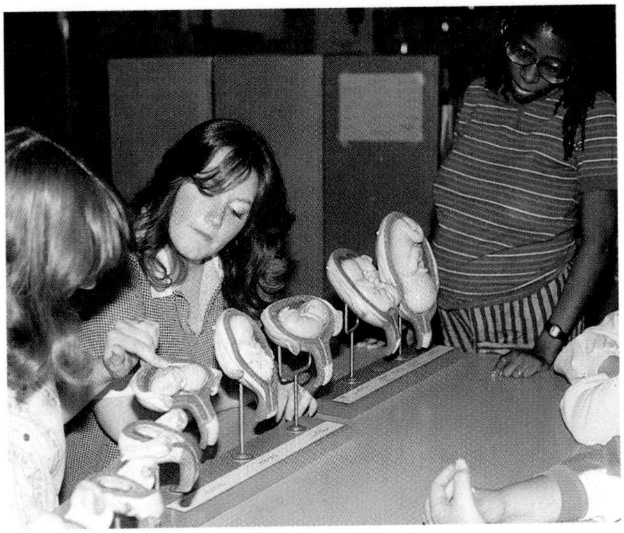

FIG. 16-20 Pregnant adolescents reviewing fetal development. (Courtesy Marjorie Pyle, RNC, Lifecircle, Costa Mesa, CA.)

Plan of Care Adolescent Pregnancy

NURSING DIAGNOSIS Imbalanced nutrition: less than body requirements related to intake insufficient to meet metabolic needs of fetus and adolescent client

Expected Outcomes *Client will gain weight as prescribed by age, take prenatal vitamins/iron as prescribed, and maintain normal hematocrit and hemoglobin.*

Nursing Interventions/*Rationales*

Assess current diet history/intake *to determine prescriptions for additions or changes in present dietary pattern.*

Compare prepregnancy weight with current weight *to determine if pattern is consistent with appropriate fetal growth and development.*

Provide information concerning food prescriptions for appropriate weight gain, considering preferences for "fast food" and peer influences *to correct any misconceptions and increase chances for compliance with diet.*

Include client's immediate family or support system during instruction *to ensure that person preparing family meals receives information.*

NURSING DIAGNOSIS Risk for injury, maternal or fetal, related to inadequate prenatal care and screening

Expected Outcomes *Client will experience uncomplicated pregnancy and deliver a healthy fetus at term.*

Nursing Interventions/*Rationales*

Provide information, using therapeutic communication and confidentiality *to establish relationship and build trust.*

Discuss importance of ongoing prenatal care and possible risks to adolescent client and fetus *to reinforce that ongoing assessment is crucial to health and well-being of client and fetus, even if client feels well. The adolescent client is more at risk for certain complications that may be avoided or managed early if prenatal visits are maintained.*

Discuss risks of alcohol, tobacco, and recreational drug use during pregnancy *to minimize risks to client and fetus, because adolescent client has a higher abuse rate than the rest of the pregnant population.*

Assess for evidence of sexually transmitted infection (STI) and provide information regarding safer sexual practice *to minimize risk to client and fetus, because adolescent is more at risk for STIs.*

Screen for pregnancy-induced hypertension (PIH) on an ongoing basis *to minimize risk, because adolescent population is more at risk for PIH.*

NURSING DIAGNOSIS Social isolation related to body-image changes of pregnant adolescent as evidenced by client statements and concerns

Expected Outcomes *Client will identify support systems and report decreased feelings of social isolation.*

Nursing Interventions/*Rationales*

Establish a therapeutic relationship *to listen objectively and establish trust.*

Discuss with client changes in relationships that have occurred as a result of the pregnancy *to determine extent of isolation from family, peers, and father of the baby.*

Provide referrals and resources appropriate for developmental stage of client *to give information for client support.*

Provide information regarding parenting classes, breastfeeding classes, and childbirth-preparation classes *to give further information and group support, which lessens social isolation.*

NURSING DIAGNOSIS Interrupted family processes related to adolescent pregnancy

Expected Outcome *Client will reestablish relationship with her mother and father of baby.*

Nursing Interventions/*Rationales*

Encourage communication with mother *in order to clarify roles and relationships related to birth of infant.*

Encourage communication with father of baby (if she desires continued contact) *to ascertain level of support to be expected of father of baby.*

Refer to support group *to learn more effective ways of problem-solving and reduce conflict within the family.*

NURSING DIAGNOSIS Disturbed body image related to situational crisis of pregnancy

Expected Outcome *Pregnant adolescent will verbalize positive comments regarding her body image during the pregnancy.*

Nursing Interventions/*Rationales*

Assess pregnant adolescent's perception of self related to pregnancy *to provide basis for further interventions.*

Give information regarding expected body changes occurring during pregnancy *to provide a realistic view of these temporary changes.*

Provide opportunity to discuss personal feelings and concerns *to promote trust and support.*

NURSING DIAGNOSIS Risk for impaired parenting related to immaturity and lack of experience in new role of adolescent mother

Expected Outcome *Parents will demonstrate parenting roles with confidence.*

Nursing Interventions/*Rationales*

Provide information on growth and development *to enhance knowledge so that adolescent mother can have basis for caring for her infant.*

Refer to parenting classes *to enhance knowledge and obtain support for providing appropriate care to newborn and infant.*

Initiate discussion of child care *to assist adolescent in problem solving for future needs.*

Assess parenting abilities of adolescent mother and father *to provide baseline for education.*

Provide information on parenting classes that are appropriate for parents' developmental stage *to give opportunity to share common feelings and concerns.*

Assist parents to identify pertinent support systems *to give assistance with parenting as needed.*

Women Older than 35 Years of Age

Two groups of older parents have emerged in the population of women having a child late in their childbearing years. One group consists of women who have many children or who have an additional child during the menopausal period. The other group consists of relative newcomers to maternity care. These are women who have deliberately delayed childbearing until their late 30s or early 40s.

Older Multiparous Women. Multiparous women may have never used contraceptives because of personal choice or lack of knowledge concerning contraceptives. They also may be women who have used contraceptives successfully during the childbearing years, but as menopause approaches, they may cease menstruating regularly or stop using contraceptives and consequently become pregnant. The older multiparous woman may feel that pregnancy separates her from her peer group and that her age is a hindrance to close associations with young mothers. Other parents welcome the unexpected infant as evidence of continuing maternal and paternal roles.

Older Primiparous Women. The number of first-time pregnancies in women between the ages of 35 and 40 years has increased significantly over the past three decades (Tough et al., 2002). Seeing women in their late 30s or 40s during their first pregnancy is no longer unusual for health care providers. Reasons for delaying pregnancy include a desire to obtain advanced education, career priorities, and better contraceptive measures. Women who are infertile do not delay pregnancy deliberately but may have a delayed one.

These women choose parenthood as opposed to a child-free lifestyle. They often are successfully established in a career and a lifestyle with a partner that includes time for self-attention, the establishment of a home with accumulated possessions, and freedom to travel. When asked the reason they chose pregnancy later in life, many reply, ". . . because time is running out."

The dilemma of choice includes the recognition that being a parent will have positive and negative consequences. Couples should discuss the consequences of childbearing and child rearing before committing themselves to this lifelong venture. Partners in this group seem to share the preparation for parenthood, planning for a family-centered birth, and desire to be loving and competent parents; however, the reality of child care may prove difficult for such parents.

First-time mothers older than 35 years select the "right time" for pregnancy; this time is influenced by their awareness of the increasing possibility of infertility or of genetic defects in the infants of older women. Such women seek information about pregnancy from books and friends. They actively try to prevent fetal disorders and are careful in searching for the best possible maternity care. They identify sources of stress in their lives. They have concerns about having enough energy and stamina to meet the demands of parenting and their new roles and relationships.

If older women become pregnant after treatment for infertility, they may suddenly have negative or ambivalent feelings about the pregnancy. They may experience a multifetal pregnancy that may create emotional and physical problems. Adjusting to parenting two or more infants requires adaptability and additional resources.

During pregnancy, parents explore the possibilities and responsibilities of changing identities and new roles. They must prepare a safe and nurturing environment during pregnancy and after birth. They must integrate the child into an established family system and negotiate new roles (parent roles, sibling roles, grandparent roles) for family members.

Adverse perinatal outcomes are more common in older primiparas than in younger women, even when they receive good prenatal care. Tough et al. (2002) reported that women 35 years and older are more likely than are younger primiparas to have LBW infants, premature birth, and multiple births. The occurrence of these complications is quite stressful for the new parents, and nursing interventions that provide information and psychosocial support are needed, as well as care for physical needs. In uncomplicated pregnancies, older mothers have significantly less fear of helplessness and loss of control in labor than do younger women (Stark, 1997). Age and education are thought to balance the concerns of older mothers related to age.

Multifetal Pregnancy

When the pregnancy involves more than one fetus, both the mother and fetuses are at increased risk for adverse outcomes. The maternal blood volume is increased, resulting in an increased strain on the maternal cardiovascular system. Anemia often develops because of a greater demand for iron by the fetuses. Marked uterine distention and increased pressure on the adjacent viscera and pelvic vasculature and diastasis of the two rectus abdominis muscles (see Fig. 14-13) may occur. Placenta previa develops more commonly in multifetal pregnancies because of the large size or placement of the placentas (Cunningham et al., 2001). Premature separation of the placenta may occur before the second and any subsequent fetuses are born.

Twin pregnancies often end in prematurity. Spontaneous rupture of membranes before term is common. Congenital malformations are twice as common in monozygotic twins as in singletons, although there is no increase in the incidence of congenital anomalies in dizygotic twins. In addition, two-vessel cords–that is, cords with a vein and a single umbilical artery instead of two–occur more often in twins than in singletons, but this abnormality is most common in monozygotic twins. The most serious problem for the fetus is the local shunting of blood between placentas (twin-to-twin transfusion), causing the recipient twin to be larger and the donor twin to be small, pallid, dehydrated, malnourished, and hypovolemic. However, congenital heart failure may develop in the larger twin during the first 24 hours after birth.

The clinical diagnosis of multifetal pregnancy is accurate in about 90% of cases. The likelihood of a multifetal pregnancy is increased if any one or a combination of the following factors is noted during a careful assessment:

- History of dizygous twins in the female lineage
- Use of fertility drugs
- More rapid uterine growth for the number of weeks of gestation
- Hydramnios
- Palpation of more than the expected number of small or large parts
- Asynchronous fetal heartbeats or more than one fetal electrocardiographic tracing
- Ultrasonographic evidence of more than one fetus

The diagnosis of multifetal pregnancy can come as a shock to many expectant parents, and they may need additional support and education to help them cope with the changes they face. The mother needs nutrition counseling so that she gains more weight than that needed for a singleton birth, counseling that maternal adaptations will probably be more uncomfortable, and information about the possibility of a preterm birth.

If the presence of more than three fetuses is diagnosed, the parents may receive counseling regarding selective reduction of the pregnancies to reduce the incidence of premature birth and improve the opportunities for growth to term gestation for the remaining infants (Berkowitz, 1998). This situation poses an ethical dilemma for many couples, especially those who have worked hard to overcome problems with infertility and harbor strong values regarding right to life. Nurse-initiated discussion to identify what resources could help the couple (e.g., a minister, priest, or mental health counselor) can make the decision-making process somewhat less traumatic.

The prenatal care given women with multifetal pregnancies includes changes in the pattern of care and modifications in other aspects such as the amount of weight gained and the nutritional intake observed. The prenatal visits of these women are scheduled at least every 2 weeks in the second trimester and weekly thereafter. In twin gestations, the recommended weight gain is 16 to 20 kg. Iron and vitamin supplementation is desirable. Attempts are made to prevent preeclampsia and eclampsia, which occur more commonly during multifetal pregnancies, and vaginitis; if these conditions cannot be prevented, they are treated.

The considerable uterine distention involved can cause the backache commonly experienced by pregnant women to be even worse. Elastic stockings or maternity tights may be worn to control leg varicosities. If risk factors such as premature dilation of the cervix or bleeding are present, abstinence from orgasm and nipple stimulation during the last trimester is recommended to help avert preterm labor. Frequent ultrasound examinations and heart rate monitoring will occur. Some practitioners recommend bed rest beginning at 20 weeks in women carrying multiple fetuses to prevent preterm labor. Other practitioners question the value of prolonged bed rest. If bed rest is recommended, the mother assumes a lateral position to promote increased placental perfusion. If birth is delayed until after the thirty-sixth week, the risk of morbidity and mortality decreases for the neonates.

Multiple newborns will likely place a strain on finances, space, workload, and the woman's and family's coping capability. Lifestyle changes may be necessary. Parents will need assistance in making realistic plans for the care of the babies (e.g., whether to breastfeed and whether to raise them as "alike" or as separate persons). Parents should be referred to national organizations such as Parents of Twins, Mothers of Multiples, and the La Leche League for further support (see Resources at end of chapter).

KEY POINTS

- The prenatal period is a period of significant psychosocial adaptation for all members of the expectant family as they anticipate changes in roles and responsibilities.
- Prenatal care is common among women of middle and high socioeconomic status, but women living in poverty or those who lack health insurance may not be able to use public medical services or gain access to private care.
- Prenatal care is ideally a multidisciplinary activity that fosters a safe birth and promotes satisfaction of the woman and family with the pregnancy and birth experience.
- Important components of the initial prenatal visit include an in-depth interview to determine the presence of potential complications, a comprehensive physical examination, and selected laboratory tests.
- Follow-up visits are shorter than the initial visit but are important for monitoring the health of the mother and fetus and providing anticipatory guidance as needed.
- Individualized care may be implemented through the assessment process, the formulation of nursing diagnoses, and planning mutually derived outcomes with the woman and her family when appropriate; evaluation of care is an ongoing process.
- The nurse has an important role in teaching the pregnant woman and her family about the physical changes and discomforts of pregnancy and self-care measures that can be implemented.
- Each woman needs to know how to recognize and report preterm labor and other warning signs and symptoms.
- Culture, age, parity, and multiple pregnancy may have a significant impact on the course and outcome of the pregnancy.

CRITICAL THINKING EXERCISES

1. Role play a situation in which the nurse is providing care for a woman whose pregnancy is well advanced. She has come to the clinic with her husband for her first prenatal visit. During the interview, the nurse begins to suspect that the woman is experiencing physical abuse, and she wants to talk to her privately. The husband objects and wants to remain in the examination room. What goals does the nurse want to achieve? What strategies might she use to achieve those goals?
2. Roxanne is in a successful business career, but at age 33, unintentionally becomes pregnant. She has missed three prior appointments and becomes agitated if she has to wait. The nurse notices that now in her seventh month of pregnancy, Roxanne continues to wear her usual business attire, which appears uncomfortable. Discuss possible causes of Roxanne's behavior and the nurse's role in making additional assessments.
3. Sue is a single 15-year-old who is 6 months pregnant and attending high school. Her infant is due during the winter break, and she intends to return to classes when school resumes. She lives with her mother and four younger siblings. Her mother is employed and has told Sue that, although she may continue to live at home, she is "on her own" otherwise. Identify resources in the community that the nurse can discuss with Sue.

RESOURCES

Baby Center (source for expectant parents)
www.babycenter.com

Babyonline.com (source of articles on pregnancy and baby care)
www.babyonline.com

Childbirth Graphics
P.O. Box 21207
Waco, TX 76702
800-229-3366
www.childbirthgraphics.com

Childbirth.org (source of links to other sites related to pregnancy and birth)
www.childbirth.org

COPE (Coping with the Overall Pregnancy/Parenting Experience)
37 Clarendon St.
Boston, MA 02116
617-357-5588

Healthy Mothers, Healthy Babies Coalition
409 12th St., SW
Washington, DC 20024
202-863-2458

Lesbian Mother's Support Society
www.lesbian.org/lesbian-moms

National Center for Complementary and Alternative Medicine (NCCAM) Clearinghouse
P.O. Box 7923
Gaithersburg, MD 20898
nccam.nih.gov

National Organization of Fathers of Twins Clubs, Inc.
www.nofotc.org

National Organization of Mothers of Twins Clubs, Inc.
P.O. Box 23188
Albuquerque, NM 87192
505-275-0955

National Organization on Adolescent Pregnancy, Parenting, and Prevention
2401 Pennsylvania Ave., Suite 350
Washington, DC 20037
202-293-8370

Parenthood After Thirty
451 Vermont
Berkeley, CA 94707
415-524-6635

Sex Information and Education Council of the United States (provides publications [e.g., "Sexual relations in pregnancy and postpartum"] and teaching aids)
130 W. 42nd St., Suite 350
New York, NY 10036
www.siecus.org

REFERENCES

Abrahams, C., & Katz, M. (2002). A perspective on the diagnosis of preterm labor. *Journal of Perinatal and Neonatal Nursing, 16*(1), 1-11.

Alteneder, R., & Hartzell, D. (1997). Addressing couples' sexuality concerns during the childbearing period: Use of the PLISSIT model. *Journal of Obstetric, Gynecologic, and Neonatal Nursing, 26*, 651-658.

American College of Obstetricians and Gynecologists. (1994). *Exercise during pregnancy and the postpartum period. Technical Bulletin No. 189.* Washington, DC: ACOG.

American College of Obstetricians and Gynecologists. (1997). *Smoking and women's health. Technical Bulletin No. 240,* Washington, DC: ACOG.

Artal, R., & Subak-Sharpe, G. (1998). *Pregnancy & exercise.* New York: Delacorte Press.

Association of Women's Health, Obstetric, and Neonatal Nurses. (1999). *HIV testing and disclosure for pregnant women and newborns.* Policy Position Statement. Washington, DC: AWHONN.

Barron, M. (2001). Antenatal care. In K. Simpson & P. Creehan (Eds.), *Perinatal nursing* (2nd ed.). Philadelphia: Lippincott.

Beal, M. (1998). Women's use of complementary and alternative therapies in reproductive health. *Journal of Nurse Midwifery, 43*(3), 224-233.

Bergsjo, P., & Villar, J. (1997). Scientific basis for the content of routine antenatal care. *Acta Obstetrica et Gynecologica Scandinavica, 76,* 15-25.

Berkowitz, R. (1998). Ethical issues involving multifetal pregnancies. *Mt Sinai Journal of Medicine, 65,* 185-190.

Blackwell, D., & Blackwell, J. (1999). Building alternative families. *AWHONN Lifelines, 3*(5), 45-48.

Braveman, P. et al. (2000). Barriers to timely prenatal care among women with insurance: The importance of prepregnancy factors. *Obstetrics and Gynecology, 95,* 874-880.

Bricker, L., & Neilson, J. (2002). Routine Doppler ultrasound in pregnancy (Cochrane Review). *The Cochrane Library,* Issue 3. Oxford: Update Software.

Brocklehurst, P. (2002). Interventions for reducing the risk of mother-to-child transmission of HIV infection (Cochrane Review). *The Cochrane Library,* Issue 3. Oxford: Update Software.

Brocklehurst, P., & Volmink, J. (2002). Antiretrovirals for reducing the risk of mother-to-child transmission of HIV infection (Cochrane Review). *The Cochrane Library,* Issue 3. Oxford: Update Software.

Campbell-Brown, M., & Hytten, F. (1998). Nutrition. In G. Chamberlain & F. Broughton-Pipkin (Eds.), *Clinical physiology in obstetrics* (3rd ed.). Oxford: Blackwell Science.

Caritis, S. et al. (1998). Predictors of preeclampsia in women at high risk. *American Journal of Obstetrics and Gynecology, 179,* 946-951.

Carl, D., Roux, G., & Matacale, R. (2000). Exploring dental hygiene and perinatal outcomes: Oral health implications for pregnancy and early childhood. *AWHONN Lifelines, 4*(1), 22-27.

Chalmers, B., Mangiaterra, V., & Porter, R. (2001). WHO principles of prenatal care: The essential antenatal, perinatal, and postpartum care course. *Birth, 28*(3), 202-207.

Chandler, D. (2002). Late entry into prenatal care in a rural setting. *Journal of Midwifery and Women's Health, 47*(1), 28-34.

Cherry, A., Dillon, M., & Rugh, D. (2001). *Teenage pregnancy: A global view.* Westport: Greenwood Press.

Chestnut, M. (1998). *High risk perinatal home care manual.* Philadelphia: Lippincott.

Cunningham, F. et al. (2001). *Williams obstetrics* (21st ed.). New York: McGraw-Hill.

Diemer, G. (1997). Expectant fathers: Influence of perinatal education on stress, coping, and spousal relations. *Research in Nursing and Health, 20,* 281-293.

Draper, J. (1997). Whose welfare in the labour room? A discussion of the increasing trend of fathers' birth attendance. *Midwifery, 13,* 132-138.

Ebrahim, S. et al. (1998). Alcohol consumption by pregnant women in the United States during 1988-1995. *Obstetrics and Gynecology, 92,* 187-192.

Fishbein, E., & Phillips, M. (1990). How safe is exercise during pregnancy? *Journal of Obstetric, Gynecologic, and Neonatal Nursing, 19*(1), 45-49.

Foley, E. (2002). Drug screening and criminal prosecution of pregnant women. *Journal of Obstetric, Gynecologic, and Neonatal Nursing, 33*(2), 133-137.

Ford, K. et al. (2002). Effects of a prenatal care intervention for adolescent mothers on birth weight, repeat pregnancy, and educational outcomes at one year postpartum. *Journal of Perinatal Education, 11*(1), 35-38.

Fuller, C., & Gallagher, R. (1999). What's happening: Perceived benefits and barriers of prenatal care in low income women. *Journal of the American Academy of Nurse Practitioners, 11*(12), 527-531.

Gebauer, C. et al. (1998). A nurse-managed smoking cessation intervention during pregnancy. *Journal of Obstetric, Gynecologic, and Neonatal Nursing, 27,* 47-53.

Gilbert, E., & Harmon, J. (2003). *Manual of high risk pregnancy & delivery* (3rd ed.). St. Louis: Mosby.

Graves, J., Miller, E., & Sellers, A. (2002). Maternal serum triple analyte screening in pregnancy. *American Family Physician, 65*(5), 915-920.

Health Resources and Services Administration (HRSA). (2002). *Women's health USA, 2002.* Washington, DC: U.S. Department of Health and Human Services.

Helewa, M. et al. (1997). Report of the Canadian Hypertension Society Consensus Conference: Definitions, evaluation, and classification of hypertensive disorders in pregnancy. *Canadian Medical Association Journal, 157,* 715-725.

Himmelberger, S. (2002). Preventing group B strep in newborns. *AWHONN Lifelines, 6*(4), 339-342.

Hoyert, D. et al. (2001). Annual summary of vital statistics: 2000. *Pediatrics, 108*(6), 1241-1255.

Huffman, C., & Sandelowski, M. (1997). The nurse-technology relationship: The case of ultrasonography. *Journal of Obstetric, Gynecologic, and Neonatal Nursing, 26,* 673-682.

Hypertension Society Consensus Conference: Definitions, evaluation and classification of hypertensive disorders in pregnancy. *Canadian Medical Association Journal, 157,* 715-725.

Jared, J.H. et al. (1999). Perioperative peridontal disease and low birth weight: A critical link? *Access, 13*(3), 32, 34-37.

Johnson, C. (1998). Reducing smoking among women. *AWHONN Lifelines, 2*(5), 16.

Johnson, T., & Niebyl, J. (2002). Preconception and prenatal care: Part of the continuum. In S. Gabbe, J. Niebyl, & J. Simpson (Eds.), *Obstetrics: Normal and problem pregnancies* (4th ed.). New York: Churchill Livingstone.

Katz, V. et al. (2001). Why we should eliminate the due date: A truth in jest. *Obstetrics and Gynecology, 98*(6), 1127-1129.

Kilby, J. (1997). A smoking cessation plan for pregnant women. *Journal of Obstetric, Gynecologic, and Neonatal Nursing, 26,* 397-402.

Kramer, M. (2001). Regular aerobic exercise during pregnancy (Cochrane Review). *The Cochrane Library,* Issue 1. Oxford: Update Software.

Kroelinger, C., & Oths, K. (2000). Partner support and pregnancy wantedness. *Birth, 27*(2), 112-119.

Lawrence, R. (1999). *Breastfeeding: A guide for the medical profession* (5th ed.). St. Louis: Mosby.

Lederman, R. (1996). *Psychosocial adaptation in pregnancy* (2nd ed.). New York: Springer.

March of Dimes. (1997). *Stat book.* White Plains, NY: March of Dimes Birth Defects Foundation.

Martin, S. et al. (2001). Physical abuse of women before, during, and after pregnancy. *Journal of the American Medical Association, 285*(12), 1581-1584.

May, K. (1980). A typology of detachment and involvement styles adopted during pregnancy by first-time expectant fathers. *Western Journal of Nursing Research, 2*, 445-453.

May, K. (1982). Three phases of father involvement in pregnancy. *Nursing Research, 31*, 337-342.

McFarlane, J. et al. (1998). Safety behaviors of abused women after an intervention during pregnancy. *Journal of Obstetric, Gynecologic, and Neonatal Nursing, 27*, 64-69.

Mercer, R. (1995). *Becoming a mother.* New York: Springer.

Mikhail, B., & Curry, M. (1999). Perceived impediments to prenatal care among low-income women. *Western Journal of Nursing Research, 21*(3), 335-355.

Moore, M., & Freda, M. (1998). Reducing preterm and low birthweight births: Still a nursing challenge. *MCN American Journal of Maternal Child Nursing, 23*, 200-208.

Moore, M. et al. (1998). A randomized trial of nurse intervention to reduce preterm and low birthweight births. *Obstetrics and Gynecology, 91*, 656-661.

Mvula, M., & Miller, J. (1998). A comparative evaluation of collaborative prenatal care. *Obstetrics and Gynecology, 91*, 169-173.

Pavill, B. (2002). Fathers and breastfeeding: Consider these ways to get dad involved. *AWHONN Lifelines, 6*(4), 324-331.

Pivarnik, J. (1994). Maternal exercise during pregnancy. *Sports Medicine, 18*, 215-217.

Polivka, B., Nickel, J., & Wilkins, J. (1997). Urinary tract infection during pregnancy. *Journal of Obstetric, Gynecologic, and Neonatal Nursing, 26*, 405-413.

Pugh, L. et al. (1999). Clinical approaches in the assessment of childbearing fatigue. *Journal of Obstetric, Gynecologic, and Neonatal Nursing, 28*(1), 74-80.

Rubin, R. (1975). Maternal tasks in pregnancy. *Maternal Child Nursing Journal, 4*, 143-153.

Rubin, R. (1984). *Maternal identity and the maternal experience.* New York: Springer.

Sable, M. (1999). Pregnancy intentions may not be a useful measure for research on maternal and child health outcomes. *Family Planning Perspectives, 31*(5), 249-250.

Sampselle, C. et al. (1998). Effect of pelvic muscle exercise on transient incontinence during pregnancy and after birth. *Obstetrics and Gynecology, 91*, 406-412.

Schirmer, G. (1998). *Herbal medicine.* Bedford, TX: MED2000, Inc.

Seidel, H. et al. (2003). *Mosby's guide to physical examination* (5th ed.). St. Louis: Mosby.

Shaffer, C. (2002). Factors influencing the access to prenatal care by Hispanic pregnant women. *Journal of the American Academy of Nurse Practitioners, 14*(2), 93-98.

Simon, N., Heaps, K., & Chodroff, C. (1997). Improving the processes of care and outcomes in obstetrics/gynecology. *Joint Commission Journal of Quality Improvement, 23*, 485-497.

Skinner, J. et al. (1997). Transitions in infant feeding during the first year of life. *Journal of the American College of Nutrition, 16*, 209-215.

Smith, M. (1998). Professional issues: Maternal-fetal attachment. *British Journal of Midwifery, 6*, 188-192.

Sorenson, D., & Schuelke, P. (1999). Fantasies of the unborn among pregnant women. *MCN American Journal of Maternal Child Nursing, 24*(2), 92-97.

Stankaitis, J., & Hollander, H. (2002). Toward improving birth outcomes in Medicaid managed care. *Journal of Clinical Outcomes Management, 9*(3), 135-139.

Stark, M. (1997). Psychosocial adjustment during pregnancy: The experience of mature gravidas. *Journal of Obstetric, Gynecologic, and Neonatal Nursing, 26*, 206-211.

Tough, S. et al. (2002). Delayed childbearing and its impact on population rate changes in lower birth weight, multiple birth, and preterm delivery. *Pediatrics, 109*(3), 399-403.

Villar, J. et al. (2002). Patterns of routine antenatal care for low-risk pregnancy. *The Cochrane Library*, Issue 4. Oxford: Update Software.

Wagner, C. et al. (1998). The impact of prenatal drug exposure on the neonate. *Obstetrics and Gynecology Clinic of North America, 25*, 169-194.

Walker, L., Cooney, A., & Riggs, M. (1999). Psychosocial and demographic factors related to health behaviors in the 1st trimester. *Journal of Obstetric, Gynecologic, and Neonatal Nursing, 28*(6), 606-614.

Yu, S., Park, C., & Schwalberg, R. (2002). Factors associated with smoking cessation among U.S. pregnant women. *Maternal and Child Health Journal, 6*(2), 89-97.

CHAPTER 17

Sharron S. Humenick

Childbirth and Perinatal Education

http://evolve.elsevier.com/Lowdermilk/MatWmnHlth/

LEARNING OBJECTIVES

- Explain the importance of preconception care.
- Identify the purpose of childbirth education.
- Describe the role and benefits of a doula.
- Contrast the different choices of care providers.
- Differentiate four birth settings.
- Compare methods of education for childbirth.

The goal of childbirth and perinatal education is to assist individuals and their family members to make informed, safe decisions about pregnancy, birth, and early parenthood. It also is to assist them to comprehend the long-lasting potential that empowering birth experiences have in the lives of women and that early experiences have on the development of children and the family. The perinatal education program is an expansion of the earlier childbirth education movement that originally offered a set of classes in the third trimester of pregnancy to prepare parents for birth. Today perinatal education programs consist of a menu of class series and activities from preconception through the early months of parenting.

PRECONCEPTION EDUCATION AND CARE

Parents welcome children best when they consciously prepare their own bodies, minds, and spirits for pregnancy and birth and think of conception as a deep commitment between themselves and the baby. Even when pregnancy is unplanned, parents can create a healthy, nurturing environment for their unborn child (aTLC, 2001). **Preconception education** and care are designed to foster conscious conception and health maintenance and to promote healthy behaviors for the health of the woman and her potential fetus and foster risk management as needed.

Traditionally women who intended to become pregnant did so without specific preconception planning with a health care provider. Health care providers today promote preconception care as an important component of perinatal services. Thus many perinatal education programs offer preconception and early pregnancy classes as part of their program series. Once a family has decided to have a baby, ideally, the next decisions involve preparing to conceive and choosing a health care provider based on competence, care philosophy, and associated birth-site choices. Related choices for the family follow, including desired birth experiences and plans for infant feeding and infant care. However, to reach women most in need of preconception education, nurses in roles that interact with young women may need to reach out creatively beyond the offices of traditional care providers. School nurses and college health service nurses can arrange to be guest lecturers in appropriate high school and college classes. Community health nurses can develop displays for community health fairs or offer programs through day care centers where they would encounter young women who may conceive again. Nurses in family planning agencies can be alert to reaching out with preconception education to women who may become pregnant, intentionally or unintentionally.

The period of greatest danger from intrauterine environmental hazards for the developing fetus is between 17 and 56 days after fertilization. By the end of the eighth week after conception and certainly by the end of the first trimester, any major structural anomalies in the fetus are already present. Because many women do not realize that they are pregnant, do not have their pregnancy confirmed, or do not seek prenatal care until well into the first trimester, the rapidly growing fetus may be exposed to many intrauterine environmental hazards during this vulnerable developmental phase.

Preconception and early pregnancy education, therefore, fosters behaviors in potential parents to:

- Establish lifestyle behaviors to maintain optimal health (e.g., eating a healthy diet including sources of folic acid; getting enough rest and exercise; and avoiding alcohol use, smoking, and other drugs).

- Prepare psychologically for pregnancy and the responsibilities that come with parenthood and build a support system to sustain the new family throughout the perinatal year.
- Identify, minimize, or treat risk factors before conception (e.g., medical conditions such as diabetes mellitus, substance abuse, use of medications for chronic illness, or infections, including those sexually transmitted).
- Screen for health hazards in the workplace or home.
- Obtain, when warranted, genetic counseling to identify carriers of inherited diseases (i.e., Tay-Sachs disease, sickle-cell disease, or thalassemia).
- Compare the quality and philosophic bases of the perinatal care options available.

The components of general preconception education such as health promotion, risk assessment, and interventions, are outlined in Box 17-1.

The provision of education is an essential component of contemporary maternity services to enable parents to be true participants in their care and agents in achieving desired birth outcomes. The context of health care can be challenging for consumers as well as health professionals. In childbirth, an emphasis by some on the use of technology versus an emphasis on health promotion and disease prevention by others are frequently contradictory (Roberts, 2000). Perinatal educators can assist aspiring or newly expectant parents to choose knowledgeably between preferred models of prenatal care (i.e., a midwifery model [natural oriented] versus a medical [intervention oriented] model). Development and understanding of their own philosophy and desires will enable expectant parents to choose compatible care providers and the place of giving birth. These early decisions will strongly influence the remaining choices in their perinatal experiences. In many communities, preconception or early pregnancy classes emphasize health-promoting behavior as well as choices of care. For example, an adequate maternal intake of folic acid (400 μg/day) decreases the risk of having a child with a neural tube defect (NTD). For those women who have had a previous pregnancy affected by NTD, an intake of 400 μg/day of folic acid from 1 month before conception through the first trimester is recommended (AAP, 1999). All health-promoting education should be provided in a context that emphasizes how well designed a healthy body is to adapt to the changes that accompany pregnancy. Without this context of health, routine care and testing for risks may contribute to a mindset of families that pregnancy is a pathologic as opposed to a healthy mind-body-spirit event (Strong, 2002).

Individualized education, as an aspect of early perinatal education, is especially important for women who have had a problem with a previous pregnancy (i.e., miscarriage or preterm birth) (Lamb, 2002). Preconception care also may minimize fetal malformations through identification and treatment of problems. Women with insulin-dependent diabetes mellitus who maintain excellent control of blood sugar at the time of conception could reduce the risk for congenital anomalies (malformations) in the fetus (Herman & Charron-Prochownik, 2000). Women who have systemic lupus erythematosus are at high risk for miscarriage or preterm labor; planning a pregnancy during a remission period can increase the chances of a healthy pregnancy.

BOX 17-1 Components of Preconception Care

HEALTH PROMOTION: GENERAL TEACHING

- Nutrition
  - Healthy diet, including folic acid
  - Optimal weight
- Exercise and rest
- Avoidance of substance abuse (tobacco, alcohol, "recreational" drugs)
- Use of safer sex practices
- Attending to family and social needs

RISK FACTOR ASSESSMENT

- Medical history
  - Immune status (e.g., rubella)
  - Family history (e.g., genetic disorders)
  - Illnesses (e.g., infections)
  - Current use of medication (prescription, nonprescription, herbal)
- Reproductive history
  - Contraceptive
  - Obstetric
- Psychosocial history
  - Spouse/partner and family situation, including domestic violence
  - Availability of family or other support systems
  - Readiness for pregnancy (e.g., age, life goals, stress)
- Financial resources
- Environmental (home, workplace) conditions
  - Safety hazards
  - Toxic chemicals
  - Radiation

INTERVENTIONS AS INDICATED

- Anticipatory guidance/teaching
- Treatment of medical conditions and results
  - Medications
  - Cessation/reduction in substance use/abuse
  - Immunizations (e.g., rubella, hepatitis)
- Nutrition, diet, and weight management
- Exercise
- Referral for genetic counseling
- Referral to and use of
  - Family planning services
  - Family and social needs management

(A preconception assessment that identifies areas to be explored is provided in Box 17-2.)

Demographic information such as age and race also are important in early care. Women younger than 15 or older than 35 years are at a higher risk for negative outcomes than are women aged 16 to 34 years. Some ethnic groups have special risks; for example, African-Americans and Southeast Asians are at risk for sickle cell disease, and people of Jewish descent are at risk for Tay-Sachs disease. Once care is established, parents have additional decisions to make including the use and frequency of ultrasound examination and amniocentesis, if recommended.

Prenatal Support and Partner Relationships

Prenatal social support is linked to positive birth outcomes, whereas prenatal stress and depression are linked to negative birth outcomes, including low-birth-weight or preterm infants (DaCosta, 2000; Dole, 2001). Thus early perinatal or preconception education includes helping the woman and the couple build a strong social support network to carry them through the perinatal year and beyond. Pregnancy is a time when the partner relationship can be strengthened or stressed. Pregnancy, birth, and parenthood are major developmental tasks that slowly move the partners to becoming a family of three or more. In addition to the physical changes during pregnancy, the pregnant woman and her partner face significant emotional, social, and cognitive changes. Expectant fathers or male partners often have weight gain and nausea. They may be concerned about finances, their role as a father, sexuality, and the child's effect on the couple's relationship. Fathers or partners often worry about their role during childbirth classes and labor and birth, as well as the safety of their partner and baby during the birth. Female partners may have the same concerns, although research on lesbian partners is lacking. Both the pregnant woman and her partner need an assessment of the symptoms and changes they are experiencing and their individual coping styles.

BOX 17-2 Preconception Assessment

INTERVIEW

- Lifestyle
  - Nutrition
  - Exercise, rest
  - Substance use: alcohol, tobacco, cocaine, other
  - Occupation
  - Psychosocial: stress, anxiety, depression; support from partner, family, friends; domestic violence
  - Financial resources
- Immunization status
  - *Rubella*
  - Hepatitis B
  - Toxoplasmosis (not universal)
- Medications
  - Over-the-counter, nonprescription (e.g., aspirin)
  - Herbal remedies
  - Prescription
  - Medical conditions: review of systems
  - Hypertension, cardiovascular disease
  - Seizure disorders
  - Diabetes mellitus
  - Renal disease
  - Autoimmune disorders (e.g., lupus, rheumatoid arthritis)
  - Tuberculosis, asthma, allergies
- Reproductive system
  - Fertility problems, endometriosis
  - Contraceptive history
  - Obstetric history (e.g., prior pregnancies, miscarriages, child with a disorder)
  - Abnormal Pap smear results
  - Sexually transmitted infections (STIs)
  - Sexual practices
- Family history, including father of baby
  - Medical conditions
  - Genetic conditions (e.g., sickle cell disease, Tay-Sachs disease, cystic fibrosis, bleeding disorders, phenylketonuria [PKU])
  - Birth defects
- Treatment history
  - Previous abdominal reproductive surgery
  - Trauma
  - Previous blood transfusion(s)
- Environmental history
  - Work exposures
  - Home exposures

PHYSICAL EXAMINATION

- General medical with emphasis on
  - Thyroid gland
  - Breasts
  - Pelvic structures

LABORATORY STUDIES

- General: CBC, urinalysis, blood type and Rh, rubella titer, STIs (e.g., syphilis, gonorrhea, *Chlamydia*), hepatitis B surface antigen, Pap smear, and cervical culture
- Depending on risk:
  - PPD
  - HIV
  - Toxicology screen
  - Thalassemia

CBC, Complete blood count; *PPD*, purified protein derivative test (for tuberculosis); *HIV*, human immunodeficiency virus.

Helping couples in educational programs acknowledges the many changes they are experiencing; teaching exercises and skills to keep the lines of communication open may enhance the couple's relationship and pregnancy outcome.

THE ROLE OF THE NURSE AS A PRECONCEPTION AND EARLY PREGNANCY EDUCATOR

If a couple is planning a pregnancy, the perinatal educator or the primary health care provider may assist them in the timing of conception after implementing lifestyle recommendations for their health. These recommendations could include diet and weight management, physical conditioning, immunizations, and genetic counseling. Fostering normal adaptations to an ever-changing physiology should be a focus of a preconception curriculum or plan of care. Preventive measures are suggested throughout this text for infection, nutrition, substance abuse, and other health-related concerns. Recommendations can be reinforced with videotapes or audiotapes, illustrations, and printed teaching aids (Nichols & Humenick, 2000a). Teaching stress reduction through relaxation (Humenick, Schrock, & Libresco, 2000), guided imagery (Steffes, 2000), moderate exercise (Smith, 2000), and rest also is useful in promoting behaviors appropriate for early pregnancy. Expectant fathers may not yet have established a source of heath care as adults; they too can be encouraged to have a physical examination and to care for their own health. Selected aspects of health education and health screening for expectant fathers are woven into some perinatal education classes (Polomeno, 1998).

Approximately 8% to 10% of birth defects occur as a result of environmental factors and may be amenable to educational awareness (Pletsch, 1990). Families can be taught that cleanliness, ventilation, adherence to manufacturer's directions for use and disposal of materials, use of protective gear to shield against known and unknown hazards, and avoidance of exposure to radiation are examples of strategies to reduce risk. In some instances, safer materials can be substituted for potentially hazardous ones. For example, most household cleaning needs can be met with baking soda, table salt, distilled white vinegar, lemon juice, trisodium phosphate (TSP, which does not emit fumes), a plunger, and some common sense. These substances can be used to clean drains, wash windows, degrease, prevent mold and mildew, disinfect, and scour. Nurses must be alert to conditions in the workplace that may affect the reproductive health of workers and their partners. As private citizens, nurses should become involved in professional and political organizations to promote and support legislation to control pollution of the environment. Nurses can teach about alternative ways to clean the home and care for yards and gardens to reduce exposure to potentially harmful substances.

Evaluation of short-term results of environmental consciousness is possible only when observing outcomes in large populations. The birth of a healthy baby with no apparent disorder or disease, the uncomplicated recovery of the new mother, continued fertility, and demonstration of a lifestyle that supports good reproductive health are some expected outcomes when preconception and pregnancy care are effective. Long-term effects may not be known for many years or generations.

Perinatal Care Choices

The Coalition to Improve Maternity Services (CIMS), a group of more than 50 nursing and maternity care–oriented organizations, produced a document to assist women in selecting their perinatal care. After some explanation of choices, women are encouraged to ask potential care providers the following questions:

- Who can be with me during labor and birth?
- What happens during a normal labor and birth in your setting?
- How do you allow for differences in culture and beliefs?
- Can I walk and move around during labor? What position do you suggest for birth?
- How do you make sure everything goes smoothly when my nurse, doctor, midwife, or agency work with each other?
- What things do you normally do to a woman in labor?
- How do you help mothers stay as comfortable as they can be? Besides drugs, how do you help mothers relieve the pain of labor?
- What if my baby is born early or has special problems?
- Do you circumcise babies?
- How do you help mothers who want to breastfeed?

The entire document can be obtained at www.motherfriendly.org. By using a related CIMS questionnaire provided by Hotelling (2001), hospitals and birthing centers can apply to CIMS to be designated Mother Friendly, and such ratings can be passed on to expectant parents.

CHILDBIRTH EDUCATION

Childbirth, when one is prepared and well supported, presents to women a unique and powerful opportunity to find their core strength in a manner that forever changes their self-perception. Additionally, it can offer women an experience in trusting their body wisdom in a way that may alter how they respond throughout life to health challenges. "It takes a well-informed, scientifically based, and articulate childbirth educator to teach consumer-oriented childbirth classes today" (Nichols & Humenick, 2000b).

Prior participation in the pregnancy and birth of others or in care of younger siblings or relatives is increasingly uncommon, given the small size of many American families. As a result, many individuals facing parenthood have little information about what to expect and do not have the skills necessary to deal effectively with pregnancy, childbirth, or parenthood. Childbirth or perinatal education classes can fill this void.

Professional nurses are prepared by their education and practice to participate in aspects of perinatal education, particularly the immediate situation-based teaching needed in clinical settings. Certified childbirth education is an interdisciplinary, postprofessional specialty made up largely of nurses joined by physical therapists, social workers, psychologists, and others who have taken course work to prepare them for this role. This specialized education and certification is especially important for the nurse teaching group classes or offering instruction for individuals where a more complex approach is needed and involves exploration of feelings and adjustment of expectations.

History

Women have always shared information about and assisted each other in childbirth. Until the late nineteenth century, childbirth was a family and social event in which women gave birth at home, often with the help of a midwife and a group of friends. The Industrial Revolution, with attendant urban crowding and associated health problems, led to higher rates of maternal and infant death from puerperal fever, sepsis, and infant diarrhea (Wertz & Wertz, 1979). The associated changes of male domination of obstetrics, drugs, and medication for pain and infection control in birth, as well as the weakened family bonds consequent to industrialization, moved childbirth from being "women's work" and controlled by nature into the hospital (Lindell, 1988).

Despite these changes, women sought to have some choice in the management of birth. During the late nineteenth century, women organized the National Twilight Sleep Association to promote the use of the new technique of giving morphine and scopolamine to control labor pain. However, by the early twentieth century, most women had accepted centralized and routine birth practices over which they had little or no control in the belief that childbirth would be safer for themselves and their babies. Not until the mid-twentieth century did women (energized by the consumer rights movement, women's movement, and increased availability of certified nurse-midwives) begin to question the rigid policies, the preemption by the medical profession, and the regimentation of birth. The childbirth education movement began in the 1950s and grew until prepared childbirth classes are now recommended for all expectant parents by most caregivers and by *Healthy People 2010* (USDHHS, 2000).

Early Methods of Childbirth Education

An English physician, Grantly Dick-Read, published two books in which he theorized that pain in childbirth is socially conditioned and caused by a fear-tension-pain syndrome. His first book, *Natural Childbirth,* was published in 1933. Dick-Read's second book, *Childbirth without Fear,* was published in the United States in 1944. The work of Dick-Read became the foundation for organized programs of preparation for childbirth and teacher training throughout the United States, Canada, Great Britain, and South Africa. In 1960 the nurses and others prepared through such programs established the International Childbirth Education Association (ICEA). The **Grantly Dick-Read method,** referred to as *Childbirth without Fear,* initially recommended deep abdominal breathing during early first-stage contractions, shallow breathing for later first stage, and sustained pushing with breath holding (Dick-Read, 1987). Women were taught to relax different muscle groups through the entire body, consciously and progressively, until a high degree of skill at relaxation was achieved. Consequently a woman was taught to relax completely between contractions and keep all muscles except the uterus relaxed during contractions.

During the 1960s the **Lamaze method,** originally known as the **psychoprophylactic method (PPM),** gained popularity in the United States. PPM offered new perspectives on preparation for childbirth by emphasizing control by using the mind. Marjorie Karmel introduced PPM to the United States in her book *Thank You, Dr. Lamaze,* which was published in the United States in 1959. PPM combined controlled muscular relaxation and breathing techniques. Active relaxation has been an integral part of the Lamaze method. The woman was taught to contract specific muscle groups (neuromuscular control) while relaxing the remainder of her body. She thus learned to relax the uninvolved muscles in her body while her uterus contracted. Instead of tensing during uterine contractions, women were conditioned to respond with relaxation and breathing patterns. In 1960 the American Society for Psychoprophylaxis in Obstetrics (ASPO) was formed in New York and became a national organization to promote use of the Lamaze method and prepare teachers of the method (Lamaze, 1999b). It continues to be an active organization, known since 1998 as Lamaze International.

A third, early advocate of prepared childbirth was the Denver obstetrician, Robert Bradley, who published *Husband-Coached Childbirth* in 1965. He advocated what he called true "natural" childbirth, without any form of anesthesia or analgesia and with a husband-coach and breathing techniques for labor. The American Academy of Husband-Coached Childbirth (AAHCC) was founded to make the **Bradley method** available and to prepare teachers. This method of partner-coached childbirth used breath control, abdominal breathing, and general body relaxation. Working in harmony with the body was emphasized (Bradley, 1965). Bradley's technique emphasizes environmental variables such as darkness, solitude, and quiet to make childbirth a more natural experience. Women using the Bradley method often appear to be sleeping during labor because they are in such a deep state of mental relaxation.

Current Practices

In 1994, under the leadership of Lamaze International, a summit meeting of maternity organizations was held, which in 1996 became the Coalition to Improve Maternity Services (CIMS). The group drafted standards for normal birth entitled the Mother Friendly Childbirth Initiative (MFCI). This document was ratified by Lamaze International, La Leche League, Birth Works, the American Academy of Husband-Coached Childbirth, the American College of Nurse Midwives (ACNM), The Association of Women's Health, Obstetrical, and Neonatal Nurses (AWHONN), ICEA, Midwife Alliance of North America (MANA), and Physicians for Midwifery Care, to name a few of the more than 50 early endorsers.

CIMS adopted the Lamaze International (1999a) philosophy of birth as follows:

- Birth is normal, natural, and healthy.
- The experience of birth profoundly affects women and their families.
- Women's inner wisdom guides them through birth.
- Women's confidence and ability to give birth is either enhanced or diminished by the care provider and place of birth.
- Women have a right to give birth free from routine medical interventions.
- Birth can safely take place in birth centers and homes.
- Childbirth education empowers women to make informed choices in health care, to assume responsibility for their health, and to trust their inner wisdom.

This philosophy has become an ideal for many childbirth education organizations in the United States. It fits closely with the principles of Perinatal Care put forth by the World Health Organization (WHO, 1998), which state that care for normal pregnancy and birth should be removed from control of doctors, based on the use of appropriate technology (as opposed to overuse), evidence based, regionalized, multidisciplinary, holistic, family centered, culturally appropriate, involve women in decision making, and should respect the privacy, dignity, and confidentiality of women.

The perinatal educator has ready access to the evidence basis for effective care in pregnancy and childbirth through *Cochrane Reviews* (Enkin et. al., 2001) (see Chapter 1). How the childbirth educator uses this evidence in education programs depends on the population who attend classes and the practices in the community. Expectant parents cannot and should not be taught to manage all details of medical interventions that are listed. Expectant parents can, however, ask their care providers if they are familiar with this database and use it to discontinue routines that have been found to be useless or harmful. In the role as advocate, the childbirth educator can let families know that items on the list of ineffective or harmful care routines might affect their choice of care provision. These include routine or liberal episiotomy for birth, routine restriction of mother-infant contact including nursery care, routine supplements of water or formula for breastfeeding babies, and samples of formula for breastfeeding mothers.

Childbirth Education Outcomes

Researchers studying childbirth education outcomes have not adopted a standard set of operational definitions of childbirth education; thus research outcomes on the influence of childbirth education on birth itself have been conflicting. The research on other benefits of childbirth education has been more consistent (see Evidence-Based Practice box).

EVIDENCE-BASED PRACTICE

THERAPEUTIC EFFECTS OF CHILDBIRTH EDUCATION

Over many decades, confidence building, birth satisfaction, and family relationships have consistently been shown as positive childbirth education outcomes. In a review of studies between 1995 and 2001, Koehn (2002) found that the three studies that investigated health promotion all found positive changes in selected health behaviors among class attendees. Examples were communication with partner, relaxation, interpersonal support, and health responsibility. A frequent finding across 12 studies was more prenatal confidence in ability to cope with birth at the end of the class. Findings on birth experiences were mixed. These finding are similar to those of a decade ago that found that childbirth education "promotes positive attitudes towards labor and delivery and fosters early maternal-infant attachment" (Lindell, 1988). A 1990 study of 800 women in England found that information and a feeling of control were important components of women's satisfaction with the birth and their subsequent emotional well-being (Hetherington, 1990). No consistent changes are related to childbirth education and physiologic components such as effects on length of labor, use of anesthesia or analgesia; and obstetric intervention (Hetherington, 1990; Lindell, 1988; Slager-Earnest, Hoffman, & Beckman, 1987). Jones (1983), in a meta-analysis of 58 studies published between 1960 and 1981, examined the effects of childbirth education. The following clinically significant effect sizes were found: 0.40 on maternal fear and anxiety, 0.48 on women's self-esteem, 0.39 on the mother's relationship with her infant, 0.37 on marital relationships, and 0.30 on reduced medical interventions. In summary, the effects of childbirth education consistently have been shown to be in birth satisfaction, building confidence, and building relationships. Physiologic measures and use of interventions by birth attendants are less consistently demonstrated to be influenced by educating expectant parents.

CLINICAL APPLICATION

The perinatal period is a transitional time in which the health and strength of women, infants, and families can be fostered by childbirth and perinatal education. Perinatal education programs are an important part of a perinatal care package. Classes should be made available in a format appropriate to women of different economic, cultural, and social backgrounds. The role of the labor nurse includes actively supporting rather than being antagonistic toward birth plans of informed mothers, and family participation regardless of the types of classes the family attended.

Many researchers have treated childbirth education as a direct influence on the birth without considering the mediating influence of care providers' philosophy and the usual type of care. Humenick (2000b) suggested that researchers use a model to evaluate childbirth education such as the Interactive Quality Health Education Model (Mitchell, Ferketich, & Jennings, 1998).

Education Strategies

Childbirth classes focus on preparing families intellectually, emotionally, and physically for childbirth and promoting wellness and improved lifestyle behaviors during the childbearing years. Because of the multicultural composition of the North American population, great diversity exists in attitudes, expectations, and behaviors judged appropriate during pregnancy and early parenthood. No one approach can meet all needs. For example, classes for new immigrants are particularly effective when taught in class members' primary language. For classes to be meaningful, childbirth educators must understand the value systems in other cultures and their influences on issues such as nutrition, early prenatal care, maternal weight gain, and infant feeding practices. Educators must establish rapport, be understood, and build on cultural practices, reinforcing the positive and promoting change only if a practice is directly harmful (Davis-Floyd & Sargent, 1997).

Most childbirth education classes are attended by the pregnant woman and her partner, although a friend, teenage daughter, or parent may be the selected support person, or more than one support person may attend classes. Where family-centered care is practiced, other family members may be present for the birth. When there has been prior birth trauma, healing these issues during pregnancy may promote a more satisfying labor and assist people to become more attuned parents (aTLC, 2002; Gardner, 2002).

Nichols (2000) identified theoretic frameworks that have been used for childbirth education including Adaptation Theory (Roy, 1999), Crisis Theory (Aguilera, 1998), Competence Model (Nichols, 1992), Health Education Model (Engleman & Forbes, 1986), and Self-Care Theory (Orem, 1995). Using a theoretic framework assists the childbirth educator to organize facts into sets of meaningful and related concepts, which, for the expectant parents, increases their understanding, problem solving, and decision making related to these facts.

OPTIONS FOR CARE

Based on their stated philosophy, CIMS identified the following principles for mother-friendly services. These principles give expectant parents an idea of what they have a right to expect in their perinatal care and may influence how they make choices when interacting with the health care system throughout their lives.

Mother-friendly services should do the following:

- Promote birth as a normal, natural, and healthy process.
- Empower a woman to develop confidence in her ability to give birth and care for her baby.
- Give the woman autonomy to make informed choices about the care she and her baby receive.
- Do no harm by applying only medically necessary interventions.
- Take responsibility for the quality of care provided, based on the needs of the mother and child.

Birth Plan

Some expectant parents develop a birth plan to identify their options and set priorities. The birth plan is a natural evolution of the contemporary wellness-oriented lifestyle in which clients assume a level of responsibility for their own health. For some, beginning this approach to perinatal care will influence their approach to health care throughout their lives. The birth plan is a tool with which parents can explore their childbirth options and choose those that are most important to them. Many parents already indicate some of their preferences by the type of health care provider and birth setting (hospital, freestanding birth center, or home) they have chosen. Some pregnant women enlist the services of a health care provider only after an interview and a tour of the birth facility. Others do not give conscious thought to the conduct of their pregnancies, the labor and birth process, recovery, and early parenthood. These women may need help with decision making.

After the confirmation of pregnancy, couples tend to be focused on the reality of their situation and their emotional responses. It is useful for the nurse in early classes or a prenatal care setting, however, to initiate a discussion of choices and birth planning during the first and second prenatal visits. Some maternity clinics provide printed material describing available options and giving answers to commonly asked questions, and tours of the birth setting are offered by almost all birthing facilities. The nurse can provide couples with pertinent information so that they can make informed decisions, alerting them to various options for care and the advantages and consequences of each.

The birth plan also can serve as a means of open communication between the pregnant woman and her partner and between the couple and health care providers. An early introduction to the idea of a birth plan allows the couple time to think about events or situations that could make their childbearing experience more meaningful and those they would prefer to avoid. The nurse-client discussion of the birth plan should take place in an accepting atmosphere in which women can see themselves as unique and yet normal. The nurse should assess clients' readiness to learn and avoid overloading them with information. Some health care providers provide birth plan templates. A discussion of the printed template can assist the couples to start thinking about, discussing, and identifying what is important to them. However, some options may be appropriate only for low risk women. The options of women with a high risk pregnancy or those in whom complications develop during labor may be more limited. Berg, Lundgren, & Lindmark (in press) found that for women with complications during pregnancy, the use of a birth plan appeared to intensify their negative feelings related to being more vulnerable.

Topics for birth plan discussion and decision making may include any or all of the following:

- Partner's participation: Attend prenatal visits? Childbirth and parent education classes? Present during labor? During birth? During cesarean birth?
- Birth setting: Hospital delivery room or birthing room (if available)? A birthing center? Home?
- Labor management: Walk around during labor? Use a rocking chair? Use a shower? Use a jacuzzi, if available? Intermittent versus continuous use of an electronic fetal monitor? Have music or dimmed lighting? Have older children or other people present? Is telemetry monitoring available? Consider stimulation of labor? Consider medication–what kind?
- Birth: Positions–side lying? On hands and knees, kneeling, or squatting? Use a birthing bed? Or delivery table? Will you be photographing, videotaping, or recording any of the labor or birth? Who would you like to be present–partner, older siblings, other family members, or friends? What do you know about the use of forceps? Episiotomies? Will your partner want to cut the umbilical cord?
- Immediately after birth: Do you want to hold the baby right away? Breastfeed immediately?
- Postpartum care: What kind of care do you anticipate–labor, delivery, recovery, postpartum room; mother-baby coupling? How long does your insurance company provide coverage for you to stay? Would you like to attend self-care classes or prefer to get such information from videotapes? On which subjects?

Care Provider Choices

The nurse can provide information about the different types of health care providers and in general the kind of care to expect from each type.

Physicians

Physicians (obstetricians and family practice physicians) attend about 93% of births in the United States and Canada, although this number has decreased slightly over the last decade as births attended by midwives increased to 7% (Ventura et al., 1998). Physicians see low and high risk clients. Care often includes pharmacologic and medical management of problems and the use of technologic procedures such as ultrasound examination and amniocentesis. Family practice physicians may need backup by obstetricians if a specialist is needed for a problem such as a cesarean birth. Most physicians manage births in a hospital setting.

Nurse-Midwives

Nurse-midwives are registered nurses with additional education and training in the care of obstetric clients. Throughout history, midwives have held a holistic view of childbirth (Capitulo, 1998). They provide care for about 7% of the births in the United States and Canada (Ventura et al., 1998). Certified nurse-midwives may practice with physicians or independently with an arrangement for physician backup. They usually see low risk obstetric clients. Care in a midwifery model is noninterventional in orientation, and the woman and family are usually encouraged to be active participants in the care. Nurse-midwives must refer clients to physicians for complications. Most nurse-midwife births are managed in hospital settings or birth centers; a few may be managed in home settings.

Direct-Entry Midwives

Direct-entry midwives (also called certified professional midwives) are trained through self-study, apprenticeship, midwifery schools, or universities as a profession distinct from nursing. Their certification process is administered by the American College of Nurse Midwives. They manage approximately 1% of births in the United States and Canada (Ventura et al., 1998). They refer to physicians the clients in whom problems develop. A majority (61%) of births attended by these midwives take place in the home setting.

Doulas

Whereas the caregivers discussed previously provide medical and health supervision, manage the birth, and provide immediate and later postpartal and infant care, the doula provides a support service. A **doula** is professionally trained to provide labor support, including physical, emotional, and informational support, to women and their partners during labor and birth. The doula does not become involved with clinical tasks (Doulas of North America, 1999a, 1999b, 1999c). Some childbirth educators serve in the doula role for those who attend their classes.

A doula typically meets with the woman and her husband or partner before labor. At this meeting, she ascertains the woman's expectations and desires for the birth experience. With this information as her guide during labor and birth, the doula focuses her efforts on assisting the woman to achieve her goals. Doulas work collaboratively with other health care providers and the husband or other supportive individuals, but their primary goal is assisting the woman. This approach has a number of positive outcomes.

Klaus and Kennell (1997) examined outcomes in 11 studies of doulas. Each study randomly assigned expectant mothers to either regular support or regular support plus a doula. Doulas provided continuous support, including praise, encouragement, reassurance, comfort measures, physical contact, and explanations regarding progress of labor. Labor outcomes for the doula-assisted group included shorter labor, less medication for pain relief, fewer operative vaginal deliveries, and in several studies, a lower rate of cesarean births. Six weeks after the birth, the doula-assisted group had a higher proportion of women breastfeeding, and they had greater self-esteem and lower rates of depression, regarded their infants more positively, and were more confident of their ability to provide effective infant care. When a doula was present, fathers provided more personal support to their partners. The authors concluded that although the presence of the father is important to both the father and the woman, the doula's presence is a significant factor in a positive outcome. Today many couples, no matter which type of childbirth classes they take, also employ a doula for the labor support.

In a study comparing Lamaze preparation alone with doula instruction and support during the labor, Manning-Orenstein (1998) found that doula-supported women "were significantly less rejecting and significantly less helpless than mothers who used the Lamaze method with no doula." Four months after giving birth, they had more positive moods, had higher self-esteem, and rated their infants as less fussy. This suggests that childbirth education without good support in labor is not enough.

Doulas may be found through community contacts, other health care providers, or childbirth educators; a number of organizations offer information or referral services (see Resources at end of chapter). It is important that the expectant mother be comfortable with the doula who will be attending her. See Box 17-3 for a list of questions to ask.

Although the doula role originally developed as an assistant during labor, some women need assistance during the postpartum period. There are small but growing numbers of postnatal doulas, who provide assistance to the new mother as she develops competence with infant care, feeding, and other maternal tasks.

BOX 17-3 Questions to Ask When Choosing a Doula

To discover the specific training, experience, and services offered by anyone who provides labor support, potential clients, nursing supervisors, physicians, midwives, and others should ask the following questions of that person:

- What training have you had?
- Tell me about your experience with birth, personally and as a doula.
- What is your philosophy about childbirth and supporting women and their partners through labor?
- May we meet to discuss our birth plans and the role you will play in supporting me through childbirth?
- May we call you with questions or concerns before and after the birth?
- When do you try to join women in labor? Do you come to our home or meet us at the hospital?
- Do you meet with us after the birth to review the labor and answer questions?
- Do you work with one or more backup doulas for times when you are not available? May we meet them?
- What is your fee?

From Simkin, P., & Way, K. (1998). *DONA position paper: The doula's contributions to modern maternity care.* Seattle: Doulas of North America.

BIRTH SETTING CHOICES

An important choice of the expectant couple that is presented in early perinatal education is the birth setting. With careful thought, the concept of natural, family, or woman-centered maternity care can be implemented in any setting. The three primary options for birth settings today are the hospital, birth center, and home. Women consider several factors in choosing a setting for childbirth, including the preference of their health care provider, characteristics of the birthing unit, and preference of their third-party payer. Approximately 99% of all births in the United States take place in a hospital setting (Ventura et al., 1998). However, the types of labor and birth services available in hospitals vary greatly, from the traditional labor and delivery rooms with separate postpartum and newborn units to in-hospital birthing centers where all or almost all care takes place in a single unit.

Labor, Delivery, Recovery, and Postpartum (Birthing) Rooms

Labor, delivery, recovery (LDR) and **labor, delivery, recovery, postpartum (LDRP)** rooms offer families a comfortable, private space for childbirth. Women are admitted to LDR units, labor and give birth, and spend the first 1 to 2 hours there for immediate postpartum recovery and for having time with their families to bond with their newborns (Fig. 17-1, *A*). After this period of recovery, the mothers and newborns are transferred to a postpartum unit and nursery or mother-baby unit for the duration of their stay. Care is provided by different nursing staff (e.g., labor and delivery nurses, postpartum nurses, nursery nurses). In some hospitals, the same nurse provides care for both mothers and newborns.

In LDRP units, total care is provided from admission for labor through postpartum discharge in the same room, usually by the same nursing staff. The woman and her family may stay in this unit for 6 to 48 hours after giving birth. The units are furnished similar to LDR units but have accommodations for family members to stay overnight (Fig. 17-1, *B*).

Both units are equipped with fetal monitors, emergency resuscitation equipment for both mother and newborn, and heated cribs or warming units for the newborn. Often this equipment is out of sight in cabinets or closets when it is not being used (Fig. 17-2).

Birth Centers

Freestanding **birth centers** are usually built in locations separate from the hospital but may be located in close proximity in case the transfer of the woman or newborn is needed. These birth centers are intended to offer families an alternative to home or hospital birth, providing a third choice that is a safe and cost-effective compromise. Nurse-midwives or physicians who also have privileges at the local hospital usually staff the centers. Clients are evaluated carefully as a measure to ensure that only women who are at low risk for complications are included for care. This is a requirement of the commission for standards for freestanding birth centers.

Birth centers typically have homelike accommodations, including perhaps a double bed for the couple and a crib for the newborn (see Fig. 17-2). Emergency equipment is available but ideally stored out of view. Many centers have an early-labor lounge or a living room, and a small kitchen may be available. The family is admitted to the birth center for labor and birth and will remain there until discharge, often within 6 hours of the birth.

Other services provided by free-standing birth centers include those necessary for safe management during the childbearing cycle. In addition, attendance at childbirth and parenting classes is often required of all clients. Prenatal supervision of the woman, whose nutritional and health status must be good and who must be experiencing a low risk pregnancy, begins in the first trimester. Clients are ideally presented with situations that may require transfer to a hospital and must agree to abide by those guidelines. Expectant families develop birth plans (see section on Birth Plans).

Birth centers as well as a hospital with a comprehensive birthing program may have resources such as a lending library for parents, reference files on related topics, recycled maternity clothes and baby clothes and equipment, and supplies and reference materials for childbirth educators. The centers also may have referral files for community resources that offer services related to childbirth and early parenting, including support groups (such as for single parents, postbirth support group, and parents of twins), genetic counseling, women's issues, and consumer action.

A

B

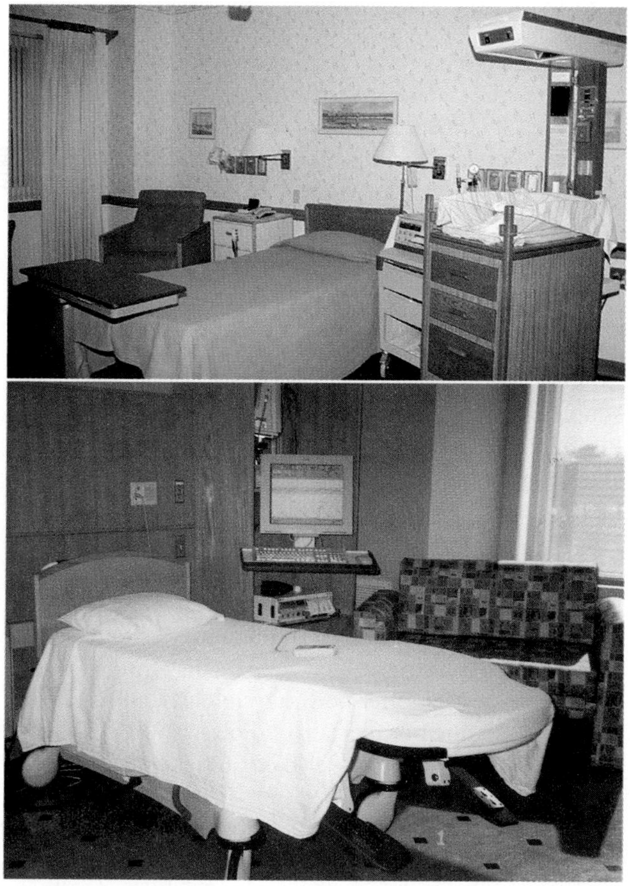

FIG. 17-1 **A,** LDR unit. **B,** LDRP unit. (**A,** Courtesy Marjorie Pyle, RNC, Lifecircle, Costa Mesa, CA. **B,** Courtesy Dee Lowdermilk, Chapel Hill, NC.)

A

B

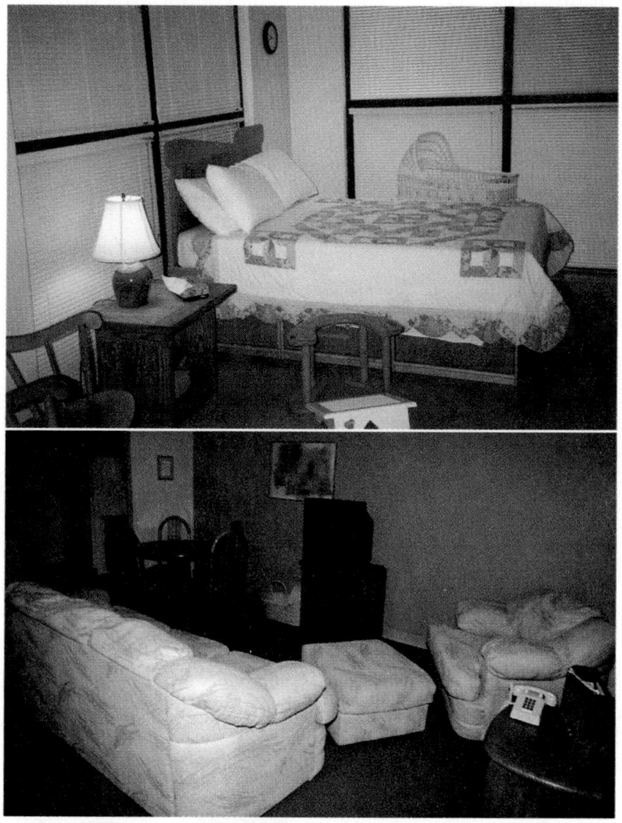

FIG. 17-2 Birth center. **A,** Note double bed, baby crib, and birthing stool. (Courtesy Dee Lowdermilk, Chapel Hill, NC.) **B,** Lounge and kitchen. (Courtesy Michael S. Clement, MD, Mesa, AZ. Photo location: Bethany Birth Center, Phoenix, AZ)

When births occur in a birth center or a home setting, they should be located close to a major hospital so that quick transfer to that institution is possible when necessary. Ambulance service and emergency procedures must be readily available. Fees vary with the services provided but typically are less than or equal to those charged by local hospitals. Some centers base fees on the ability of the family to pay (reduced-fee sliding scale). Several third-party payers, Medicaid, and TRICARE/CHAMPUS (the armed services insurance) recognize and reimburse these centers; however, clients should check with their health care payers regarding reimbursement for prenatal care and birth in a birth center.

Home Birth

Home birth has always been popular in certain countries such as Sweden and the Netherlands. In developing countries, hospitals or adequate lying-in facilities are often unavailable to most pregnant women, and home birth is a necessity. In North America, home births account for less than 1% of births (Ventura et al., 1998). National groups supporting home birth are the Home Oriented Maternity Experience (HOME) and the National Association of Parents for Safe Alternatives in Childbirth (NAPSAC). These groups work to foster more humane childbearing practices at all levels, integrating the alternatives for childbirth to meet the needs of the total population.

Many studies have documented the safety of home births. For example, Schlenzka (1999) examined 816,000 California births in 1989 through 1990. After comparing both low risk and high risk births outside and inside the hospital, he found that each approach produced the same perinatal mortality outcomes for both high and low risk births. He additionally noted that the out-of-the-hospital approach shows significant advantage with respect to lower maternity care costs as well as reduced mortality and morbidity from unnecessary cesareans and other obstetric interventions, and significant benefits from avoiding negative long-term consequences from unnecessary obstetric interventions and procedures. Similarly, Jewell (2000) reported a meta-analysis of observational studies that suggested that planned home birth may be safe, with fewer interventions than planned hospital births. Thus although home births are considered countercultural by many in the United States, there is no evidence basis to discourage couples who desire a carefully planned out-of-the-hospital birth. Many of the services and precautions related to birth centers apply to home birth as well.

Advantages

One advantage of home birth is that the family is in control of the experience. Another is that the birth may be more physiologically natural in familiar surroundings. The mother may be more relaxed than she would be in the hospital environment. Care providers who participate in home births tend to be more support oriented and less intervention oriented. The family can assist in and be a part of the happy event, and contact with the newborn is immediate and sustained. In addition, home birth may be less expensive than a hospital confinement. Serious infection may be less likely, assuming strict aseptic principles are followed, because people generally are relatively immune to their own home bacteria.

Disadvantages

Although some physicians, nurse-midwives, and nurses support home births that use good medical and emergency backup systems, many fear this practice as exposing the mother and fetus to unnecessary danger. Thus home births are not widely accepted by the North American medical community, making it difficult for a family to find a qualified health care provider to give prenatal care and attend the birth. In some communities, backup emergency care by a physician in a hospital may be difficult to arrange in advance.

Factors Increasing the Safety of Home Birth

Most health care providers agree that if home birth is the woman's choice, certain criteria promote a safe experience. The woman must be comfortable with her decision to have her baby at home. She should be in good health. Home birth is not indicated for women with diabetes, heart disease, or preeclampsia. A drive to the hospital (if needed) should ideally take no more than 10 to 15 minutes. A well-trained care provider with adequate medical supplies and resuscitation equipment should attend the woman.

COMPONENTS OF PERINATAL PROGRAMS

In addition to preparing families for childbirth, childbirth educators promote many aspects of perinatal wellness. Pregnancy is a time of personal growth, during which most couples are open to making changes in lifestyle and habits. Information on infant care, feeding, and stimulation and couple and family adjustments also is incorporated into many prenatal classes (see Guidelines/Guías box). A variety of approaches to perinatal education beyond preparation for birth have evolved as educators attempt to meet learning and support needs of expectant parents and to capitalize on the openness to learning they exhibit (see Research box). For example, prenatal and new-mother weekly exercise classes can offer both physiologic and social support for a mixture of expectant and new mothers who may even elect to stay supportively connected between weekly classes with e-mail.

Refresher classes for parents with children review coping techniques for labor and birth. In areas with sufficient population, there may be classes designed specifically for pregnant adolescents and their partners or parents (Podgurski, 2000) or classes designed for groups with special learning needs, such as first-time mothers over 35 years

GUIDELINES/GUÍAS

Childbirth Education: General Advice

Go to childbirth education classes.
Vaya a clases prenatales.

Do preparatory exercises for labor.
Haga ejercicios preparatorios para el parto.

Avoid strenuous exercise.
Evite los ejercicios fuertes.

Sexual activity is normal during pregnancy.
La actividad sexual es normal durante el embarazo.

It is not harmful to your baby.
No hará daño a su bebé.

You may experience an increase or a decrease in your sexual interest.
Usted puede experimentar un aumento o una disminuación de su interés sexual.

Rest as much as possible.
Descanse mucho.

Try to sleep 8 hours a night.
Trate de dormir ocho horas cada noche.

Don't smoke.
No fume.

Don't drink alcoholic beverages.
No tome bebidas alcohólicas.

Don't take any medications without consulting your doctor.
No tome ninguna medicina sin consultar a su doctor.

of age, single women, adoptive parents, and parents of multiples.

Pain Management

Before birth, fear of pain in labor is a key issue and a reason many give for attending childbirth education classes. Numerous studies show that women who have received childbirth preparation later report no less pain but do report greater ability to cope with the pain during labor and birth and increased birth satisfaction than unprepared women. Thus although pain management strategies are an essential component of childbirth education, pain eradication is not the primary source of birth satisfaction. Control in childbirth, meaning participation in decision making, has been repeatedly found to be the primary source of birth satisfaction (Nichols & Gennaro, 2000). The advantages and disadvantages of pain medication and techniques for coping with labor are covered in detail in Chapter 19.

Childbirth Preparation

Childbearing couples are taught to recognize labor's start, what to expect, and when to start using coping skills such as relaxation, slow breathing, and other nonpharmacologic strategies. The concept of coaching a woman in labor by "calling the plays" has been replaced by the concept of supporting a woman who knows how to give birth and benefits from support and encouragement. Supportive techniques include reassurance, massage, pressure on the palms or soles of the feet, applications of heat or cold, breathing patterns, and focusing of attention. Additional techniques to increase coping and decrease the distress from labor pain include vocalization or "sounding" to relieve tension, subdued lighting, warm water for showers or bathing during labor, and aromatherapy (Marks, 2000).

RESEARCH

Concerns of Expectant Parents

As expectant parents imagine life after the baby comes, many psychosocial and practical concerns arise. Relationships will change, lifestyles will be altered, and the newborn's needs will call for skills and wisdom. Preexisting problems, such as poor relationships with spouse or mother or prior losses, can put a woman at risk for postpartum depression. Studies of expectant fathers have found that their concerns about role changes, parenting ability, and marital relationship needs were unmet in traditional childbirth education. Addressing these issues prenatally can be beneficial to the smooth transition to the demanding, rewarding new role as a parent.

To determine the concerns of expectant parents, an Australian team of researchers gave a checklist of items identifying interpersonal, intrapersonal, parental competency, and infant care concerns to 201 women and 182 men of low to middle income status. Most were attending childbirth classes during the third trimester of their first pregnancy. The items were rated according to the extent the item was a concern. Responses to the items did not differ much between the fathers and mothers. Both were concerned with the responsibility of being a good enough parent and the struggle to cope. Men were more concerned about their partner being bored or resentful at home (Australian women can have up to a 6-month maternity leave), the effect of parenthood on their own work and family leisure, and financial concerns. They were twice as likely to worry a lot about diapers and about how their relationship with their own parents would change. Women were worried about whether they would have difficulty feeding and settling the baby, their own physical attractiveness, loneliness, and feeling close to the baby.

IMPLICATIONS FOR PRACTICE

This study provides some issues of concern that the childbirth educator needs to consider addressing with first-time expectant parents. A discussion format that might be appropriate for childbirth classes is one that was described in this study. After completing the checklist, the expectant parents separated into women's and men's groups to discuss their answers. Later, they shared their answers with their partners for further discussion. Follow-up in the postpartum period to see if these concerns were adequately addressed prenatally could also be implemented.

Reference: Matthey, S. et al. (2002). Postpartum issues for expectant mothers and fathers. *Journal of Obstetric, Gynecologic, and Neonatal Nursing, 31*(4), 428-434.

Relaxation

Relaxation is a technique promoted by virtually all childbirth education organizations. Learning relaxation in childbirth education classes can help couples with the stresses of pregnancy, childbirth, and adjustment to parenting and can be a form of stress management throughout life (Fig. 17-3). The research is clear that relaxation skill is the most effective nonpharmacologic strategy for coping with the stress of labor (Humenick, Schrock, & Libresco, 2000). Relaxation is ideally combined with activity such as walking, slow dancing, rocking, and position changes that help the baby rotate through the pelvis.

Approaches to relaxation can include neuromuscular relaxation, autogenic training, meditation, imagery, hypnosis, or touch relaxation. Women vary unpredictably in their relaxation technique preferences during labor, so it is useful to teach them a variety of approaches. For effective teaching, varied relaxation techniques should be incorporated across class sessions, with a new one introduced each week and collectively practiced during the week. When couples work together in class to learn relaxation, they also increase communication skills. For example, by using massage with a light touch to encourage relaxation, they can learn to give each other positive reinforcement and enhance their sense of being a team.

Imagery and visualization also are taught in classes during preparation for birth. Although research on their use is scant, clinical reports suggest that imagery and visualization can be used to produce a sense of well-being during pregnancy as well as assist with cervical dilation and decrease the experience of pain and tension during labor. Imagery involves techniques such as imagining a walk through a restful garden or breathing in light, energy, and healing color and breathing out worries and tension (Hoffart & Pross-Keene, 1998; Steffes, 2000).

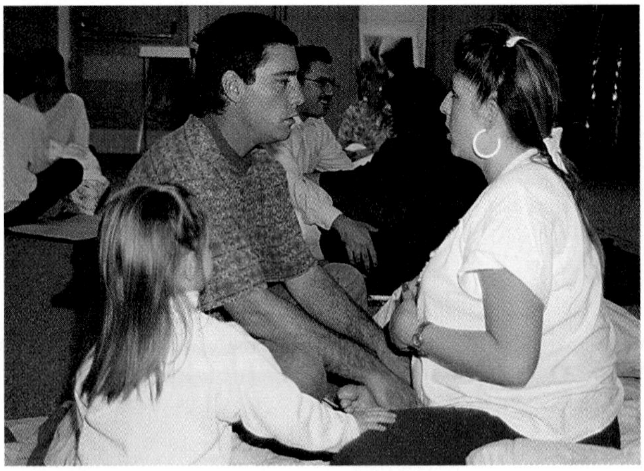

FIG. 17-3 Childbirth class: learning relaxation with the whole family. (Courtesy Marjorie Pyle, RNC, Lifecircle, Costa Mesa, CA.)

A variety of skills taught in childbirth classes augment relaxation during the pregnancy and as well as in labor. All can be taught as lifetime skills useful to the couple and used to teach their children to cope with the stresses of life.

Paced Breathing

Paced breathing is a visible technique and thus is frequently used in the media to characterize childbirth preparation. Relaxed individuals automatically slow their breathing, and conversely, slowing one's breathing serves to increase one's relaxation. During labor, nursing support includes guiding couples in the application of breathing and relaxation methods and adapting methods to their particular needs. This approach is useful to help people of all ages through a number of painful situations and thus is a valuable skill for clients to learn and for nurses to be able to teach (see Box 19-21).

Biofeedback

The use of observation in class (informal biofeedback) helps couples develop awareness of their bodies and learn strategies to change their responses to stress. In other words, if the woman responds to pain during a contraction or any other situation with tightening muscles, frowning, moaning, or breath holding, her partner can use verbal and touch feedback to help her relax. During preparation for birth, formal biofeedback (which uses machines prenatally to detect skin temperature, blood flow, or muscle tension) has been studied and also can prepare women to perfect their relaxation response. With information from biofeedback machines, women have been shown to develop progressively more relaxed states. However, the skilled childbirth educator can check relaxation responses, provide feedback during class practice sessions, and teach the partner to do the same. Thus biofeedback *machines* per se are not routinely needed for childbirth classes, but weekly feedback on relaxation progress is important (DiFranco, 2000).

Therapeutic Touch, Music, and Acupressure

Therapeutic touch involves energy fields around the body and can be taught in class for use during labor to decrease anxiety and pain and to increase relaxation. Therapeutic touch requires a subjective, intuitive approach and may be taught by having the partners first experience their own energy field between their palms. They then learn the phases of centering, assessing differences of energy flow across the body, unruffling the field, and directing energy (usually over the uterus or back) to restore harmony (Marks, 2000).

Music promotes relaxation and has been known for centuries to be generally therapeutic. Research supports the use of music for enhancing relaxation at any time and for reducing pain responses during childbirth (Wiand,

1997). Couples who use music as a strategy often integrate it with other techniques during labor.

Acupressure, which consists of applying pressure to various pressure points, has been correlated with relief of dizziness, headaches, back pain, nausea, and leg cramps, as well as labor pain (Koehn, 2000; Steele, V. et al., 2001).

Cesarean Birth

Education regarding cesarean birth is threefold in nature. The first component is helping expectant parents know what they can do to avoid the necessity of a cesarean birth. Cesarean birth rates vary widely by care provider and care setting. Cesarean births are more common in women who choose epidurals, in part because the powers of the mother's muscles do not effectively assist the infant in rotation through the pelvis; in part because if given early, epidurals prolong labor; and in part because the mother has less urge to push. In a setting where nursing labor support is low and care provider rate of cesarean birth is high, women should be aware that their chances of a cesarean birth are increased. Expectant parents can be encouraged to inquire about the cesarean rates of both their care provider and their planned birth site. Healthy mothers also can be encouraged to refrain from being admitted to the hospital before they are in active labor (can no longer walk and talk through contractions), because the longer their hospitalization, the greater the tendency for them and their care providers to become impatient with their progress and resort to cesareans. Recently there has been a move by some care providers to offer and expectant parents to request elective cesarean births. Throughout a perinatal program, the risks involved for both mothers and fetus should be well described. All women should be encouraged to attempt a vaginal birth, with the exception of those who have a history of classic vertical or unknown uterine incisions or those with medical contraindications (Spiegelberg, 2002).

In the second approach, the effort can be to prevent the need for a subsequent cesarean or preparing for it when it is inevitable or highly likely. Women with prior cesarean births can be informed on how to obtain access to their medical records to understand the reason it occurred and the implications for a subsequent birth. In many communities, there are Vaginal Birth After Cesarean (VBAC) support groups and special childbirth classes for those attempting a VBAC. Similarly, in larger communities, there are special classes for women who know they will need a cesarean birth.

The third educational aspect is to prepare all mothers for the differences in postpartum recovery for women after a cesarean birth. Their hospital stay will be longer, their need for assistance at home will be greater, and they may need extra support to establish breastfeeding comfortably.

Sibling Classes

Many perinatal education programs include classes that can be attended by siblings whether or not their parents intend for siblings to attend the birth. Siblings experience transitions when a new baby enters the family. Parents need to know about sibling regression and ways to help older children adapt to a new brother or sister. Sibling classes that offer a tour of the birthing unit, show a birth film, and help the children talk about the changes that are apt to occur, such as Mommy being busy with the baby, offer valuable interventions (Fig. 17-4; Box 17-4). When siblings are being prepared to attend the birth, it is important that plans be made to have an adult present whose sole focus is on meeting the needs of the sibling.

Grandparent Classes

Grandparents benefit from classes that help them learn strategies for assisting the couple's transition to parenthood (Polomeno, 1999a, 2000). Grandparents can be a valuable asset, especially if they help with household chores and the care of any older siblings and provide social support. Grandparents may need to be cautioned about taking over caring for the baby themselves instead of allowing the new parents time to develop parenting skills, criticizing the parents' care taking, questioning whether the baby is being adequately breastfed, or other activities that would undermine new parents' adjustment. Grandparents also can benefit by learning about child-rearing practices that have changed since they had infants, including infant stimulation and breastfeeding support.

Parenting

During the perinatal period, parents can be assisted to develop a general approach to parenting that will foster resilience in their child throughout childhood. Corwin (1999) describes an integration of childbirth preparation with parenting. Effective parenting is an art that can be learned, so making parents aware of resources about children's developmental stages, temperament, and individuality will help

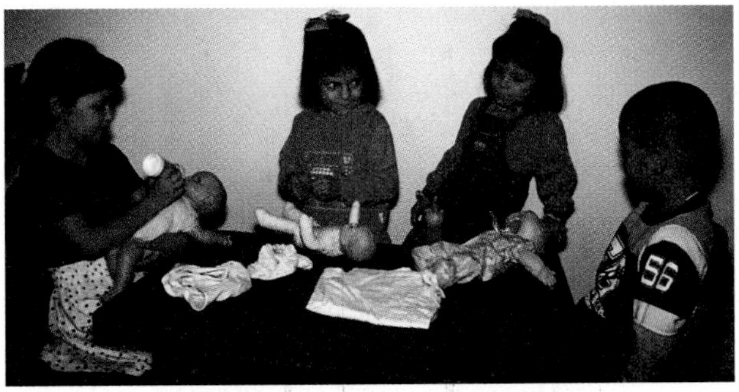

FIG. 17-4 Sibling class of preschoolers learning infant care by using dolls. (Courtesy Michael S. Clement, MD, Mesa, AZ.)

BOX 17-4 Tips for Sibling Preparation

PRENATAL

1. Adjust the timing and content of information about an anticipated infant to the age and understanding of the older child.
2. Take your child on a prenatal visit. Let the child listen to the fetal heartbeat and feel the baby move.
3. Involve the child in preparations for the baby, such as helping decorate the baby's room.
4. Move the child to a bed (if still sleeping in a crib) at least 2 months before the baby is due.
5. Read books, show videos, or take child to sibling preparation classes, including a hospital tour.
6. Answer your child's questions about the coming birth, what babies are like, and any other questions.
7. Take your child to the homes of friends who have babies so that the child has realistic expectations of what babies are like.

DURING THE HOSPITAL STAY

1. Have someone bring the child to the hospital to visit you and the baby (unless you plan to have the child attend the birth).
2. Do not force interactions between the child and the baby. Often the child will be more interested in seeing you and being reassured of your love.
3. Help the child explore the infant by showing how and where to touch the baby.
4. Give the child a gift (from you or from you, the father, and the baby).

GOING HOME

1. Leave the child at home with a relative or babysitter.
2. Have someone else carry the baby from the car so that you can hug the child first.

ADJUSTMENT AFTER THE BABY IS HOME

1. Arrange for a special time with the child alone with each parent.
2. Do not exclude the child during infant feeding times. The child can sit with you and the baby and feed a doll or drink juice or milk with you or sit quietly with a game.
3. Prepare small gifts for the child so that when the baby gets gifts, the sibling will not feel left out. The child also can help open the baby gifts.
4. Praise the child for acting age appropriately (so that being a baby does not seem better than being older).

parents make informed decisions and serve as advocates of the child's well-being. Parents also can be taught to carry the baby in the arms or in a sling through the day to provide the near-constant movement that optimizes brain development as well as the touch, safety, and comfort essential to secure bonding (aTLC, 2001).

Childbearing couples who have grown up in large families or have had exposure to infants from babysitting or careers in nursing, early childhood education, or medicine may already be aware of the 24-7 care and feeding needs of a newborn. Many couples, however, are surprised by the needs of an infant in the first 2 months, no matter how much others have told them. They also may be surprised at their own response to fatigue after several weeks of lacking uninterrupted sleep. Bringing in parents of a recent newborn to a childbirth class to describe their early parenting experiences is an effective way to help expectant parents envision the task ahead. Informing parents that the newborn's stomach is roughly the size of a walnut can help them understand why the typical infant initially needs to eat 8 to 10 times a day.

Many communities have support or new parents' groups that are helpful to couples making the transition to parenthood. Besides the routine mother-baby classes after birth, some organizations have begun to offer father-baby classes in which new fathers spend time with their babies learning about babies' unique characteristics and the basics of infant care. Childbirth educators also have an opportunity with new families to introduce issues such as the effect of disposable diapers on the environment.

Breastfeeding

The American Academy of Pediatrics has joined the call by many other nursing and breastfeeding organizations for infants to be exclusively breastfed for 6 months and breastfed for a year or longer, based on the long list of benefits to mother and child (AAP, 1997). Now childbirth educators no longer present breastfeeding as a choice without important consequences. The prenatal breastfeeding presentation to expectant couples should refrain from being overly detailed with problem-solving techniques lest the parents be overwhelmed and left with the impression that breastfeeding is too complex and fraught with problems. The focus is to present basic information so that breastfeeding is portrayed as both desirable and readily achievable. The information presented prenatally in classes should be designed to do the following:

"*Motivate:* ensure that pregnant mothers and their immediate supporters know why breastfeeding is a desirable, worthwhile effort, and minimize their barriers to breastfeeding

Explicate: provide a basic overview of breastfeeding to expectant parents

Initiate: educate parents on basic techniques and the optimal characteristics of postpartum care for the launching of breastfeeding

Maintain: educate parents on the techniques to promote lactation and the available resources to assist them in making the adjustments commonly needed in early weeks of breastfeeding, and

Sustain: introduce families to strategies to develop the environment and support system that will encourage mothers to sustain breastfeeding through the first year and beyond" (Humenick, 2000a). It is not helpful, before birth, to review a long list of potential problems and solutions. Rather it is important to make certain that a good source of 24-hour-a-day support is available, including hotlines, friends, family, literature, and professionals. For example, in some communities, the postpartum staff will take calls in the night from mothers who recently gave birth at their hospital.

Infant Stimulation and Massage

Many parents do not know about their infant's capabilities to see and hear in the early weeks of life. It is helpful for parents to realize that the senses are the primary source of information for babies during the first 6 months of life. Infant massage is one technique that expectant parents can learn to soothe and comfort the infant, promote relaxation and less irritability and crying, and provide a mechanism for positive interaction between parents and infants. Giving the father this role in relating to the infant may prevent some fathers from inadvertently sabotaging breastfeeding by pressuring the mother to let him feed the baby.

Couple Sexuality

The role of the childbirth educator in sexuality is to promote the couple's understanding of the sexual changes of pregnancy and the postpartum period and to facilitate their choices for meeting sexual needs during this time. Wilkerson and Shrock (2000) identified the following summary of what couples need to learn from class discussions:

- Information and basic understanding about the process of human sexual response and the effect of pregnancy on this response,
- Reassurance regarding the safety of sexual activities,
- Awareness of their own needs, likes, and dislikes,
- How to maintain a loving relationship,
- Creative ways to improve their sexual relationship,
- Effective communication skills to make their needs known to each other, and
- How to provide each other feedback.

To hold class discussions on this subject, the childbirth educator must be aware of his or her own values and attitudes regarding human sexuality. He or she also must develop an adequate knowledge base about sexuality in general and the changes during the perinatal year. The pregnancy, postpartum resumption, and challenges related to breastfeeding bring an ever-changing set of sexual adjustments during the perinatal year (Polomeno, 1999a, 1999b, 1999c). Finally, he or she must develop skills and methods for integrating this content into childbirth classes.

Family Adjustments to Parenthood

Couples making the transition to parenthood experience challenges that can threaten the quality and stability of their relationships and the health of family members. The movement in health care systems to be involved in strengthening marriage and family life is already under way, and the focus of perinatal education can be expanded to include helping parents create stronger, more stable relationships that will improve the physical and psychologic health of children and adults throughout their lives (Hawkins et al., 2002). The addition of a baby brings change to all members of the family. The workload increases significantly as parents add the demands of the new infant to their other responsibilities. Childbirth educators help expectant parents anticipate these changes. One example involves working through the family workload exercise, in which parents project the way they will divide their responsibilities after birth. Stainton et al. (1999), in the study of four cultures, found that both new fathers and mothers were highly focused on their own needs and cautioned that family-centered support could miss these needs if not alert to that potential.

If both partners work outside the home, a discussion about negotiating maternity and paternity leaves and plans for returning to work is important. Couples who do not have family or friends available for childcare must find competent child care providers. Discussions on the way to select licensed child care providers and federal and state guidelines regarding rights to maternity and paternity leaves are important. Couples also need information about the intensity and length of emotional and physiologic recovery from childbirth and the demands of adapting to parenthood. This knowledge should lead to more realistic planning for household help during the early days or weeks and more appropriate expectations of when women are typically ready to return to work. An understanding of the impact on breastfeeding of returning to work may result in some couples arranging to prolong the mother's time at home.

In summary, pregnancy is a time when expectant parents expect change in their lives and are open to many types of education. This education can enhance their health and coping in pregnancy, childbirth, and early parenting. It also can influence how they relate to health professionals over a lifetime, how the parents problem solve with each other, and how they launch their new family. It is an opportunity for nurses to engage in meaningful health promotion and the building of resilience in families.

KEY POINTS

- Preconception care stresses healthy behavior that promotes the health of the woman and her fetus.
- Childbirth education should be available to all pregnant women and their families in a culturally sensitive format.
- Childbirth education teaches tuning into the body's inner wisdom and coping strategies that enhance coping during labor and birth.
- Stress and pain management strategies are valuable family tools throughout life.
- Childbirth education strives to promote healthier pregnancies and family lifestyles.
- Childbirth education strives to support and strengthen the couple and family relationships.
- Active support during labor and birth, directed toward achieving the woman's goals, promotes personal satisfaction and adaptation to the maternal role.

CRITICAL THINKING EXERCISES

1. Role play a situation in which the nurse moderates a discussion with a woman and her partner, in which she wants a home birth, and he doubts the safety of the services available.
2. Develop an outline for a class for couples seeking information before conception about planning a pregnancy.
3. Prepare an explanation of the short- and long-term benefits to the mother of having a natural childbirth.

RESOURCES

Alliance for Transforming the Lives of Children (aTLC)
901 Preston Avenue, Suite 400
Charlottesville, VA 22903-4491
888-574-7580 x3922 or 434-977-8550
www.atlc.org

American Academy of Husband-Coached Childbirth (AAHCC)
P.O. Box 5224
Sherman Oaks, CA 91413-5224
818-788-6662 or 800-422-4783
www.bradleybirth.com

American College of Nurse-Midwives (ACNM)
1522 K Street NW, Suite 1120
Washington, DC 20005
202-347-5445
www.acnm.org

Association of Labor Assistants and Childbirth Educators (ALACE)
P.O. Box 382724
Cambridge, MA 02238
617-441-2500
E-mail: alacehq@aol.com

Center for Study of Multiple Births
333 E. Superior, #463-5
Chicago, IL 60611
312-266-9093

Cesarean Awareness Network, International
1304 Kingsdale Avenue
Redondo Beach, CA 90278
310-542-6400 Fax: 310-542-5368
www.childbirth.org/section/ICAN

Coalition to Improve Maternity Services (CIMS)
P.O. Box 2346
Ponte Vedra Beach, FL 32004
888-282-CIMS or 904-285-2120
www.motherfriendly.org

Doulas of North America (DONA)
44 Brooks Road
Plymouth, MA 02360
206-324-5440
www.dona.com

International Association of Parents and Professionals for Safe Alternatives in Childbirth (NAPSAC)
Route 1
Maple Hill, MO 63764
313-238-2010
www.social.com

International Board of Certified Lactation Consultants Examiners (IBLCE)
P.O. Box 2348
Falls Church, VA 22042-0348
www.iblce.org

International Childbirth Education Association (ICEA)
P.O. Box 20048
Minneapolis, MN 55420
612-854-8660 Fax: 612-854-8772
www.icea.org

Johnson and Johnson Pediatrics Institute
Grandview Road
Skillman, NJ 08558
877-JNJ-LINK
www.jnjpediatricinstitute.com

LaLeche League International
1400 North Meacham Road
P.O. Box 4079
Schaumburg, IL 60168
800-525-3243
www.lalecheleague.org

Lamaze International
(aka: ASPO/Lamaze)
1200 19th Street, NW
Suite 300
Washington, DC 20036-2422
202-857-1128 Fax: 202-223-4579
800-368-4404
www.lamaze-childbirth.com

Midwife Alliance of North America (MANA)
309 Main Street
Concord, NH 03301
316-283-4543

National Association of Childbearing Centers
Route 1, Box 1
Perkiomenville, PA 18074
215-234-8068

National Association of Postpartum Care Services
P.O. Box 1012
Edmonds, WA 98020
800-45-DOULA

National Center for Education in Maternal and Child Health
2000 15th Street North, Suite 701
Arlington, VA 22201
703-524-7802

Polymorph Films, Inc.
95 Chapel Street
Newton, MA 02158
617-965-9335

Sex Information and Educational Council of the United States (SIECUS)
130 West 42nd Street, Suite 350
New York, NY 10036
212-819-9770 Fax: 212-819-9776
www.siecus.org

Vida Health Communications
6 Bigelow Street
Cambridge, MA 02139
617-864-4334

REFERENCES

Aguilera, D. (1998). *Crisis intervention: Theory and methodology*. St. Louis: Mosby.

American Academy of Pediatrics (1997). Breastfeeding and the use of human milk (policy statement RE9729). *Pediatrics, 100*(6), 1035-1039.

American Academy of Pediatrics (1999). Folic acid for the prevention of neural tube defects. *Pediatrics, 104*(2), 325-327.

aTLC (The Alliance for Transforming the Lives of Children) (2001). A blueprint for transforming the lives of children. *Journal of Perinatal Education, 10*(4), iv-50. [On-line]. Available URL: www.atlc.org.

Berg, M., Lundgren, I., & Lindmark, G. (in press). Childbirth experience in women at high risk: Is it improved by use of a birth plan? *Journal of Perinatal Education, 12*(2).

Bradley, R. (1965). *Husband-coached childbirth*. New York: HarperCollins.

Capitulo, K. (1998). The rise, fall, and rise of nurse-midwifery in America. *MCN American Journal of Maternal Child Nursing, 23*(6), 314-321.

Corwin, A. (1999). Integrating preparation for parenting into childbirth education: Part II, a study. *Journal of Perinatal Education, 8*(1), 22-28.

Da Costa, D. (2000). A prospective study on the influence of stress, social support and coping on birth outcomes and depressive symptomology during pregnancy and the postpartum. *Dissertation Abstracts International: Section B: the Sciences & Engineering, 60*(8-B), 4213.

Davis-Floyd, R., & Sargent, C. (1997). *Childbirth and authoritative knowledge: Cross-cultural perspectives*. Berkeley: University of California Press.

Dick-Read, G. (1987). *Childbirth without fear* (5th ed.). New York: Harper & Collins.

DiFranco, J.T. (2000). Biofeedback. In F. Nichols & S. Humenick. *Childbirth education: Practice, research, and theory* (2nd ed.) (pp. 200-212). Philadelphia: W.B. Saunders.

Dole, N. (2001). Psychosocial risks for preterm birth. *Dissertation Abstracts International: Section B: the Sciences & Engineering, 62* (3-B), 1348.

Doulas of North America (1999a). *Do I need a doula?* [On-line]. Available URL: www.dona.com.faq.html.

Doulas of North America (1999b). *Doulas of North America position paper: The doula's contribution to modern maternity care* [On-line]. Available URL: www.dona.com/positionpapers.html.

Doulas of North America (1999c). *Mission statement* [On-line]. Available URL www.dona.com/mission.html.

Engleman, S., & Forbes, J. (1986). Economic aspects of health education. *Social Science Medicine, 22,* 443.

Enkin, M. et al. (2001). Effective care in pregnancy and childbirth: A synopsis. *Birth, 28*(1), 41-51.

Gardner, P. (2003). Previous traumatic birth: An impetus for requested cesarean birth. *Journal of Perinatal Education, 12*(1), 1-50.

Hawkins, A. et al. (2002) Integrating marriage education into perinatal education. *Journal of Perinatal Education, 11*(4), 1-10.

Herman, W., & Charron-Prochownik, D. (2000). Preconception counseling: An opportunity not to be missed. *Clinical Diabetes, 18*(3), 122-126.

Hetherington, S. (1990). A controlled study of the effect of prepared childbirth classes on obstetric outcome. *Birth, 17*(2), 86-90.

Hoffart, M., & Pross-Keene, E. (1998). The benefits of visualization. *American Journal of Nursing, 98*(12), 44-47.

Hotelling, B. (2001). A call to action and a challenge to use a standard to measure mother-friendly birth classes. *Journal of Perinatal Education, 10*(3), 27-31.

Humenick, S. (2000a). Prenatal preparation for breastfeeding. In F. Nichols & S. Humenick (Eds.), *Childbirth education: Practice, research and theory* (2nd ed.). Philadelphia: W.B. Saunders.

Humenick, S. (2000b). Program evaluation. In F. Nichols & S. Humenick (Eds.), *Childbirth education: Practice, research and theory* (2nd ed.). Philadelphia: W.B. Saunders.

Humenick, S., Schrock, P., & Libresco, M. (2000). Relaxation. In F. Nichols & S. Humenick (Eds.), *Childbirth education: Practice, research and theory* (2nd ed.). Philadelphia: W.B. Saunders.

Jewell, O. (2000). *Home versus hospital birth.* Copenhagen: The Nordic Cochrane Centre, Rigshospitalet, Blegdamsveu 9, Dept. 7112.

Jones, L. (1983). *A meta-analytic study of the effects of childbirth education research from 1960 to 1981.* Unpublished doctoral dissertation, Texas A & M University.

Klaus, M., & Kennell, J. (1997). The doula: An essential ingredient of childbirth rediscovered. *Acta Paediatricia, 86*, 1034-1036.

Koehn, M. (2000). Acupuncture and acupressure. In F. Nichols & S. Humenick (Eds.), *Childbirth education: Practice, research and theory* (2nd ed.). Philadelphia: W.B. Saunders.

Koehn, M. (2002). Childbirth education outcomes: An integrated review of literature. *Journal of Perinatal Education, 11*(3), 10-19.

Lamaze International. (1999a). *About Lamaze International, Inc.* [On-line]. Available URL: www.lamazechildbirth.com/fact_sheet.html.

Lamaze International. (1999b). *Lamaze certified childbirth educator (LCCE) program* [On-line]. Available URL: www.lamazechildbirth.com.

Lamb, E. (2002). The impact of previous perinatal loss on subsequent pregnancy and parenting. *Journal of Perinatal Education, 11*(2), 33-40.

Lindell, S. (1988). Education for childbirth: A time for change. *Journal of Obstetric, Gynecologic, and Neonatal Nursing, 17*(2), 108-112.

Manning-Orenstein, G. (1998). A birth intervention: The therapeutic effects of doula support versus Lamaze preparation on first-time mothers' working models of caregiving. *Alternative Therapies in Health and Medicine, 4*(4), 73-81.

Marks, G. (2000). Alternative therapies. In F. Nichols & S. Humenick (Eds.), *Childbirth education: Practice, research and theory* (2nd ed.). Philadelphia: W.B. Saunders.

Matthey, S. et al. (2002). Postpartum issues for expectant mothers and fathers. *Journal of Obstetric, Gynecologic, and Neonatal Nursing, 31*(4), 428-434.

Mitchell, P., Ferketich, S., & Jennings, B. (1998). Quality health outcomes model. *Image: Journal of Nursing Scholarship, 301*(1), 43-46.

Nichols, F. (1992). The psychological effects of prepared childbirth on single adolescent mothers. *Journal of Perinatal Education, 1*(1), 541-549.

Nichols, F. (2000). The content. In F. Nichols & S. Humenick (Eds.), *Childbirth education: Practice, research and theory* (pp. 575-592). Philadelphia: W.B. Saunders.

Nichols, F., & Gennaro, S. (2000). The childbirth experience. In F. Nichols & S. Humenick (Eds.), *Childbirth education: Practice, research and theory* (2nd ed.). Philadelphia: W.B. Saunders.

Nichols, F., & Humenick, S. (2000a). Appendices A-Organizations, B-Audiovisuals & C-Selected Publications. In F. Nichols & S. Humenick (Eds.), *Childbirth education: Practice, research and theory* (2nd ed.). Philadelphia: W.B. Saunders.

Nichols, F., & Humenick, S. (2000b). Preface. *Childbirth education: Practice, research and theory* (2nd ed.). Philadelphia: W.B. Saunders.

Orem, D. (1995). *Nursing: Concepts of practice.* New York: McGraw-Hill.

Pletsch, P. (1990). Birth defect prevention: Nursing interventions. *Journal of Obstetric, Gynecologic, and Neonatal Nursing, 19*(6), 482-488.

Podgurski, M. (2002). Childbirth education for teens. In F. Nichols & S. Humenick (Eds.), *Childbirth education: Practice, research and theory* (2nd ed.). Philadelphia: W.B. Saunders.

Polomeno, V. (1998) An exemplary service: Health promotion for expectant fathers: Part II. Practical considerations. *Journal of Perinatal Education, 7*(2) 27-36.

Polomeno, V. (1999a). Perinatal education and grandparents: Creating an interdependent family environment. *Journal of Perinatal Education, 8*(3), 1-11.

Polomeno, V. (1999b). An independent study continuing education program: Sex and breastfeeding: An educational perspective. *Journal of Perinatal Education, 8*(1), 30-39.

Polomeno, V. (1999c). Sex and babies: Pregnant couples' postnatal sexual concerns. *Journal of Perinatal Education, 8*(4), 9-18.

Polomeno, V. (2000). Evaluation of a pilot project: Preparenthood and pregrandparenthood education. *Journal of Perinatal Education, 9*(2), 27-38.

Roberts, J. (2000). Foreward. In F. Nichols & S. Humenick (Eds.), *Childbirth education: Practice, research and theory* (2nd ed.). Philadelphia: W.B. Saunders.

Roy, C. (1999). *An introduction to nursing: An adaptation model* (2nd ed.). Englewood Cliffs, NJ: Prentice Hall.

Schlenzka, P. (1999). Safety of alternative approaches to childbirth. *Dissertation Abstracts International* (Accession number AAG 9924602.). Palo Alto, CA: Stanford University.

Simkin, P., & Way, K. (1998). *DONA position paper: The doula's contributions to modern maternity care.* Seattle: Doulas of North America.

Slager-Earnest, S.E., Hoffman, S.J., & Beckman, C.J. (1987). Effects of a specialized prenatal adolescent program on maternal and infant outcomes. *Journal of Obstetric, Gynecologic, and Neonatal Nursing, 16*(6), 422-429.

Smith, S. (2000). Exercise. In F. Nichols & S. Humenick (Eds.), *Childbirth education: Practice, research and theory* (2nd ed.). Philadelphia: W.B. Saunders.

Stainton, C. et al. (1999). The needs of postbirth parents: An international, multi-site study. *Journal of Perinatal Education, 8*(3), 21-29.

Steele, V. et al. (2001). Effect of acupressure by Sea-Bands on nausea and vomiting of pregnancy. *Journal of Obstetric, Gynecologic, and Neonatal Nursing, 30*(1), 61-70.

Steffes, S. (2000). Relaxation: Imagery. In F. Nichols & S. Humenick (Eds.), *Childbirth education: Practice, research and theory* (2nd ed.). Philadelphia: W.B. Saunders.

Strong, T. (2002). *Expecting trouble: The myth of prenatal care in America.* New York: New York University Press.

USDHHS (2000). *Healthy People 2010: Conference edition.* Volume II. Washington, DC: US Government Printing Office.

Ventura, S. et al. (1998). Advance report of final natality statistics, 1996. *Monthly Vital Statistics Report, 46*(11 suppl), 1-99.
Wertz, R., & Wertz, D. (1979). *Lying in: A history of childbirth in America*. New York: Schoder.
Wiand, N. (1997). Relaxation levels achieved by Lamaze-trained pregnant women listening to music and ocean sound tapes. *Journal of Perinatal Education, 6(*4), 1-8.
Wilkerson, N., & Shrock, P. (2000). Sexuality and the perinatal period. In F. Nichols & S. Humenick (Eds.), *Childbirth education: Practice, research and theory* (2nd ed.). Philadelphia: W.B. Saunders.
World Health Organization (1998). *Workshop on perinatal care proceedings. Venice, 16-18 April 1998.* Geneva: WHO.

CHAPTER 18

Deitra Leonard Lowdermilk

Labor and Birth Processes

http://evolve.elsevier.com/Lowdermilk/MatWmnHlth/

LEARNING OBJECTIVES

- Explain the five factors that affect the labor process.
- Describe the anatomic structure of the bony pelvis.
- Recognize the normal measurements of the diameters of the pelvic inlet, cavity, and outlet.
- Explain the significance of the size and position of the fetal head during labor and birth.
- Summarize the cardinal movements of the mechanism of labor for a vertex presentation.
- Assess the maternal anatomic and physiologic adaptations to labor.
- Describe fetal adaptations to labor.

During late pregnancy, the woman and fetus prepare for the labor process. The fetus has grown and developed in preparation for extrauterine life. The woman has undergone various physiologic adaptations during pregnancy that prepare her for birth and motherhood. Labor and birth represent the end of pregnancy, the beginning of extrauterine life for the newborn, and a change in the lives of the family. This chapter discusses the factors affecting labor, the process involved, the normal progression of events, and the adaptations made by both the woman and fetus.

FACTORS AFFECTING LABOR

At least five factors affect the process of labor and birth. These are easily remembered as the five Ps: passenger (fetus and placenta), passageway (birth canal), powers (contractions), position of the mother, and psychologic response. The first four factors are presented here as the basis of understanding the physiologic process of labor. The fifth factor is discussed in Chapter 19. Other factors that may be a part of the woman's labor experience may be important as well. VandeVusse (1999) identified external forces including place of birth, preparation, type of provider (especially nurses), and procedures. Physiology (sensations) was identified as an internal force. These factors are discussed generally in Chapter 21 as they relate to nursing care during labor. Further research investigating essential forces of labor is recommended.

Passenger

The way the passenger, or fetus, moves through the birth canal is determined by several interacting factors: the size of the fetal head, fetal presentation, fetal lie, fetal attitude, and fetal position. Because the placenta also must pass through the birth canal, it can be considered a passenger along with the fetus; however, the placenta rarely impedes the process of labor in normal vaginal birth, except in cases of placenta previa.

Size of the Fetal Head

Because of its size and relative rigidity, the fetal head has a major effect on the birth process. The fetal skull is composed of two parietal bones, two temporal bones, the frontal bone, and the occipital bone (Fig. 18-1, *A*). These bones are united by membranous sutures: the sagittal, lambdoidal, coronal, and frontal (Fig. 18-1, *B*). Membrane-filled spaces called **fontanels** are located where the sutures intersect. During labor, after rupture of membranes, palpation of fontanels and sutures during vaginal examination reveals fetal presentation, position, and attitude.

The two most important fontanels are the anterior and posterior ones (see Fig. 18-1, *B*). The larger of these, the anterior fontanel, is diamond shaped, about 3 cm by 2 cm, and lies at the junction of the sagittal, coronal, and frontal sutures. It closes by 18 months after birth. The posterior fontanel lies at the junction of the sutures of the two parietal bones and the one occipital bone, is triangular, and is about 1 cm by 2 cm. It closes 6 to 8 weeks after birth.

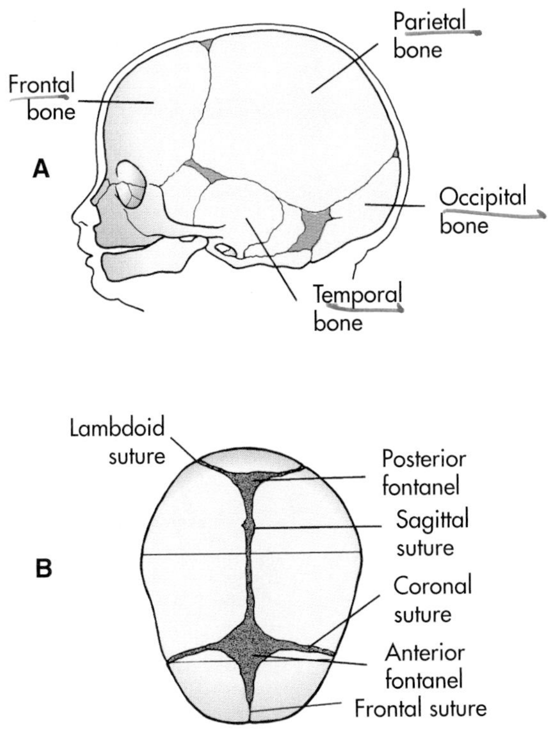
Parietal bone
Frontal bone
A
Occipital bone
Temporal bone
Lambdoid suture
Posterior fontanel
Sagittal suture
B
Coronal suture
Anterior fontanel
Frontal suture

FIG. 18-1 Fetal head at term. **A,** Bones. **B,** Sutures and fontanels.

Sutures and fontanels make the skull flexible to accommodate the infant brain, which continues to grow for some time after birth. Because the bones are not firmly united, however, slight overlapping of the bones, or **molding** of the shape of the head, occurs during labor. This capacity of the bones to slide over one another also permits adaptation to the various diameters of the maternal pelvis. Molding can be extensive, but the heads of most newborns assume their normal shape within 3 days after birth.

Although the size of the fetal shoulders may affect passage, their position can be altered relatively easily during labor, so that one shoulder may occupy a lower level than the other. This creates a shoulder diameter that is smaller than the skull, facilitating passage through the birth canal. The circumference of the fetal hips is usually small enough not to create problems.

Fetal Presentation

Presentation refers to the part of the fetus that enters the pelvic inlet first and leads through the birth canal during labor at term. The three main presentations are **cephalic presentation** (head first), occurring in 96% of births (Fig. 18-2); **breech presentation** (buttocks or feet first), occurring in 3% of births (Fig. 18-3, *A–C*); and **shoulder presentation,** seen in 1% of births (Fig. 18-3, *D*). **Presenting part** refers to that part of the fetal body first felt by the examining finger during a vaginal examination. In a cephalic presentation, the presenting part is usually the occiput; in a breech presentation, it is the sacrum; in the shoulder presentation, it is the scapula. When the presenting part is the occiput, the presentation is noted as **vertex** (see Fig. 18-2). Factors that determine the presenting part include fetal lie, fetal attitude, and extension or flexion of the fetal head.

Fetal Lie

Lie is the relation of the long axis (spine) of the fetus to the long axis (spine) of the mother. The two primary lies are *longitudinal,* or vertical, in which the long axis of the fetus is parallel with the long axis of the mother (see Fig. 18-2); and *transverse,* horizontal, or oblique, in which the long axis of the fetus is at a right angle diagonal to the long axis of the mother (see Fig. 18-3, *D*). Longitudinal lies are either cephalic or breech presentations, depending on the fetal structure that first enters the mother's pelvis. Vaginal birth cannot occur when the fetus stays in a transverse lie. An oblique lie, one in which the long axis of the fetus is lying at an angle to the long axis of the mother, is less common and usually converts to a longitudinal or transverse lie during labor (Cunningham et al., 2001).

Fetal Attitude

Attitude is the relation of the fetal body parts to each other. The fetus assumes a characteristic posture (attitude) in utero partly because of the mode of fetal growth and partly because of the way the fetus conforms to the shape of the uterine cavity. Normally the back of the fetus is rounded so that the chin is flexed on the chest, the thighs are flexed on the abdomen, and the legs are flexed at the knees. The arms are crossed over the thorax, and the umbilical cord lies between the arms and the legs. This attitude is termed **general flexion** (see Fig. 18-2).

Deviations from the normal attitude may cause difficulties in childbirth. For example, in a cephalic presentation, the fetal head may be extended or flexed in a manner that presents a head diameter that exceeds the limits of the maternal pelvis, leading to prolonged labor, forceps- or vacuum-assisted birth, or cesarean birth.

Certain critical diameters of the fetal head are usually measured. The **biparietal diameter,** which is about 9.25 cm at term, is the largest transverse diameter and an important indicator of fetal head size (Fig. 18-4, *B*). In a well-flexed cephalic presentation, the biparietal diameter will be the widest part of the head entering the pelvic inlet. Of the several anteroposterior diameters, the smallest and the most critical one is the **suboccipitobregmatic diameter,** (about 9.5 cm at term). When the head is in complete flexion, this diameter allows the fetal head to pass through the true pelvis easily (Fig. 18-4, *A*; Fig. 18-5, *A*). As the head is more extended, the anteroposterior diameter widens, and the head may not be able to enter the true pelvis (see Fig. 18-5).

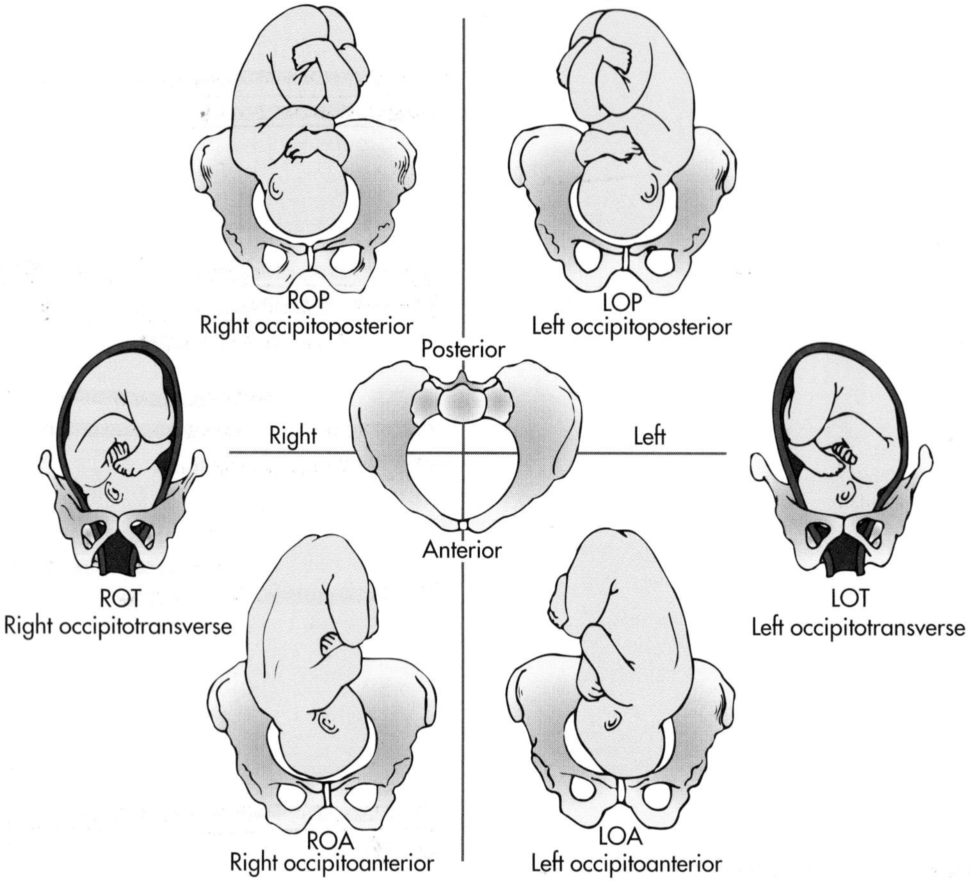
ROP
Right occipitoposterior
LOP
Left occipitoposterior
Posterior
Right
Left
Anterior
ROT
Right occipitotransverse
LOT
Left occipitotransverse
ROA
Right occipitoanterior
LOA
Left occipitoanterior
Lie: Longitudinal or vertical
Presentation: Vertex
Reference point: Occiput
Attitude: Complete flexion

FIG. 18-2 Examples of fetal vertex (occiput) presentations in relation to front, back, or side of maternal pelvis.

Fetal Position

The presentation or presenting part indicates that portion of the fetus that overlies the pelvic inlet. **Position** is the relation of the presenting part (occiput, sacrum, mentum [chin], or sinciput [deflexed vertex]) to the four quadrants of the mother's pelvis (see Fig. 18-2). Position is denoted by a three-letter abbreviation. The first letter of the abbreviation denotes the location of the presenting part in the right (R) or left (L) side of the mother's pelvis. The middle letter stands for the specific presenting part of the fetus (O for occiput, S for sacrum, M for mentum [chin], and Sc for scapula [shoulder]). The third letter stands for the location of the presenting part in relation to the anterior (A), posterior (P), or transverse (T) portion of the maternal pelvis. For example, ROA means that the occiput is the presenting part and is located in the right anterior quadrant of the maternal pelvis (see Fig. 18-2). LSP means that the sacrum is the presenting part and is located in the left posterior quadrant of the maternal pelvis (see Fig. 18-3).

Station is the relation of the presenting part of the fetus to an imaginary line drawn between the maternal ischial spines and is a measure of the degree of descent of the presenting part of the fetus through the birth canal. The placement of the presenting part is measured in centimeters above or below the ischial spines (Fig. 18-6). For example, when the lowermost portion of the presenting part is 1 cm above the spines, it is noted as being minus (−) 1. At the level of the spines, the station is referred to as 0 (zero). When the presenting part is 1 cm below the spines, the station is said to be plus (+) 1. Birth is imminent when the presenting part is at +4 to +5 cm. The station of the presenting part should be determined when

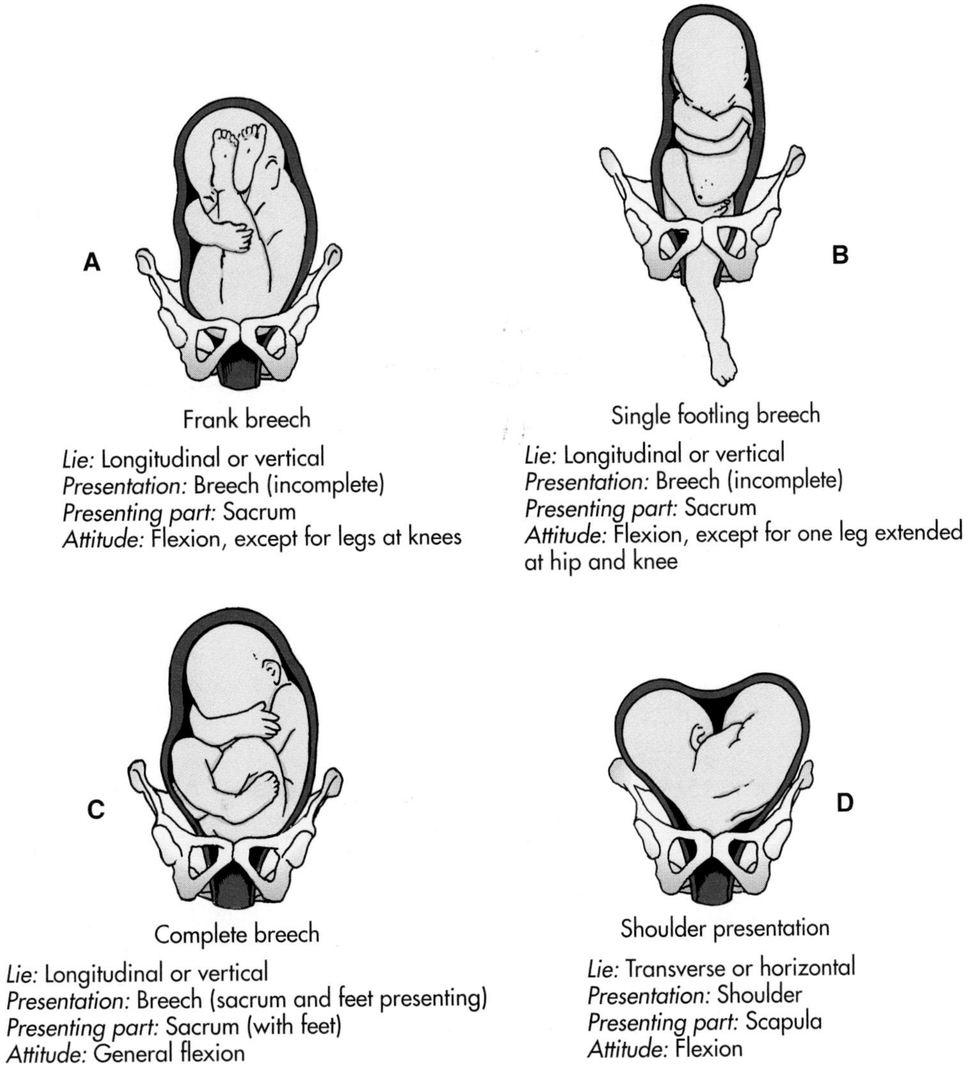
A
Frank breech
Lie: Longitudinal or vertical
Presentation: Breech (incomplete)
Presenting part: Sacrum
Attitude: Flexion, except for legs at knees
B
Single footling breech
Lie: Longitudinal or vertical
Presentation: Breech (incomplete)
Presenting part: Sacrum
Attitude: Flexion, except for one leg extended at hip and knee
C
Complete breech
Lie: Longitudinal or vertical
Presentation: Breech (sacrum and feet presenting)
Presenting part: Sacrum (with feet)
Attitude: General flexion
D
Shoulder presentation
Lie: Transverse or horizontal
Presentation: Shoulder
Presenting part: Scapula
Attitude: Flexion

FIG. 18-3 Fetal presentations. **A–C,** Breech (sacral) presentation. **D,** Shoulder presentation.

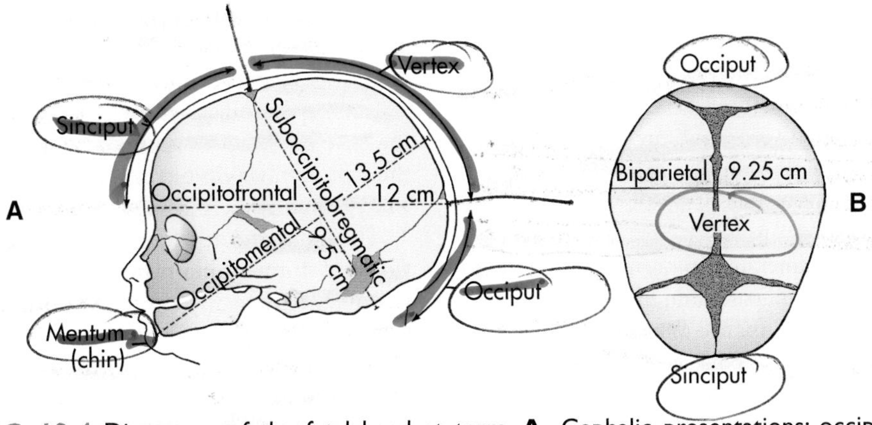
A
Vertex
Sinciput
Suboccipitobregmatic
13.5 cm
Occipitofrontal
12 cm
Occipitomental
9.5 cm
Occiput
Mentum
(chin)
B
Occiput
Biparietal
9.25 cm
Vertex
Sinciput

FIG. 18-4 Diameters of the fetal head at term. **A,** Cephalic presentations: occiput, vertex, and sinciput; and cephalic diameters: suboccipitobregmatic, occipitofrontal, and occipitomental. **B,** Biparietal diameter.

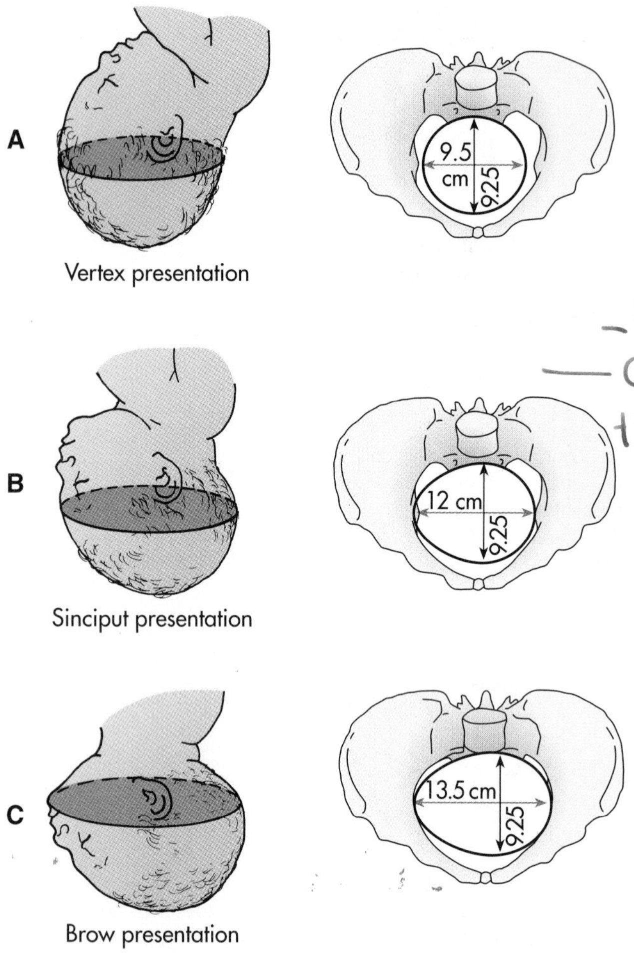
A
9.5
cm
9.25
Vertex presentation
B
12 cm
9.25
Sinciput presentation
C
13.5 cm
9.25
Brow presentation

FIG. 18-5 Head entering pelvis. Biparietal diameter is indicated with shading (9.25 cm). **A,** Suboccipitobregmatic diameter: complete flexion of head on chest so that smallest diameter enters. **B,** Occipitofrontal diameter: moderate extension (military attitude) so that large diameter enters. **C,** Occipitomental diameter: marked extension (deflection), so that the largest diameter, which is too large to permit head to enter pelvis, is presenting

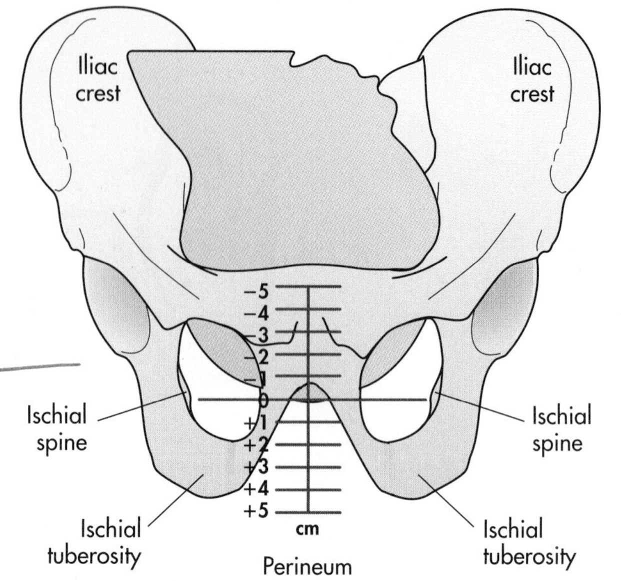
Iliac
crest
Iliac
crest
-5
-4
-3
-2
-1
0
+1
+2
+3
+4
+5
cm
Ischial
spine
Ischial
spine
Ischial
tuberosity
Ischial
tuberosity
Perineum

FIG. 18-6 Stations of presenting part, or degree of descent. The lowermost portion of the presenting part is at the level of the ischial spines, station 0.

labor begins so that the rate of descent of the fetus during labor can be accurately determined.

Engagement is the term used to indicate that the largest transverse diameter of the presenting part (usually the biparietal diameter) has passed through the maternal pelvic brim or inlet into the true pelvis and usually corresponds to station 0. Engagement often occurs in the weeks just before labor begins in nulliparas and may occur before labor or during labor in multiparas. Engagement can be determined by abdominal or vaginal examination.

Passageway

The passageway, or birth canal, is composed of the mother's rigid bony pelvis and the soft tissues of the cervix, pelvic floor, vagina, and introitus (the external opening to the vagina). Although the soft tissues, particularly the muscular layers of the pelvic floor, contribute to vaginal birth of the fetus, the maternal pelvis plays a far greater role in the labor process because the fetus must successfully accommodate itself to this relatively rigid passageway. Therefore the size and shape of the pelvis must be determined before childbirth begins.

Bony Pelvis

The anatomy of the bony pelvis is described in Chapter 5. The following discussion focuses on the importance of pelvic configurations as they relate to the labor process. (It may be helpful to refer to Fig. 5-4).

The bony pelvis is formed by the fusion of the ilium, ischium, pubis, and sacral bones. The four pelvic joints are the symphysis pubis, the right and left sacroiliac joints, and the sacrococcygeal joint (Fig. 18-7, *A*). The bony pelvis is separated by the brim, or inlet, into two parts: the false pelvis and the true pelvis. The false pelvis is the part above the brim and plays no part in childbearing. The true pelvis, the part involved in birth, is divided into three planes: the inlet, or brim; the midpelvis, or cavity; and the outlet.

The pelvic inlet, which is the upper border of the true pelvis, is formed anteriorly by the upper margins of the pubic bone, laterally by the iliopectineal lines along the innominate bones, and posteriorly by the anterior, upper margin of the sacrum and the sacral promontory.

The pelvic cavity, or midpelvis, is a curved passage with a short anterior wall and a much longer concave posterior wall. It is bounded by the posterior aspect of the symphysis pubis, the ischium, a portion of the ilium, the sacrum, and the coccyx.

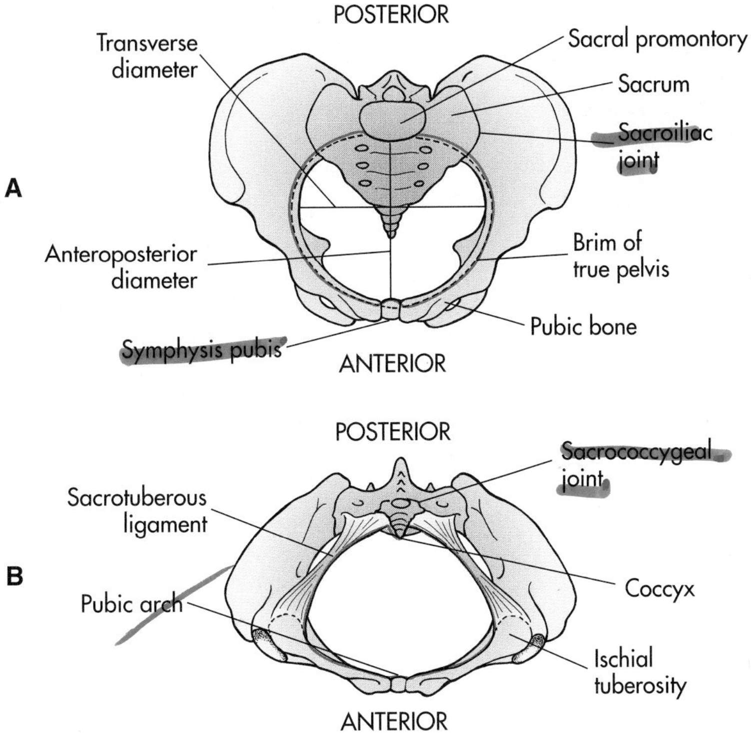
A
POSTERIOR
Transverse diameter
Sacral promontory
Sacrum
Sacroiliac joint
Anteroposterior diameter
Brim of true pelvis
Pubic bone
Symphysis pubis
ANTERIOR
B
POSTERIOR
Sacrococcygeal joint
Sacrotuberous ligament
Coccyx
Pubic arch
Ischial tuberosity
ANTERIOR

FIG. 18-7 Female pelvis. **A,** Pelvic brim above. **B,** Pelvic outlet from below.

The pelvic outlet is the lower border of the true pelvis. Viewed from below, it is ovoid, somewhat diamond shaped, bounded by the pubic arch anteriorly, the ischial tuberosities laterally, and the tip of the coccyx posteriorly (Fig. 18-7, *B*). In the latter part of pregnancy, the coccyx is movable (unless it has been broken in a fall during skiing or skating, for example, and has fused to the sacrum during healing).

The pelvic canal varies in size and shape at various levels. The diameters at the plane of the pelvic inlet, midpelvis, and outlet, plus the axis of the birth canal (Fig. 18-8), determine whether vaginal birth is possible and the manner by which the fetus may pass down the birth canal.

The subpubic angle, which determines the type of pubic arch, together with the length of the pubic rami and the intertuberous diameter, is of great importance. Because the fetus must first pass beneath the pubic arch, a narrow subpubic angle will be less accommodating than a rounded wide arch. The method of measurement of the subpubic arch is shown in Figure 18-9. A summary of obstetric measurements is given in Table 18-1.

The four basic types of pelvis are classified as follows:

1. Gynecoid (the classic female type)
2. Android (resembling the male pelvis)
3. Anthropoid (resembling the pelvis of anthropoid apes)
4. Platypelloid (the flat pelvis).

The **gynecoid** pelvis is the most common, with major gynecoid pelvic features present in 50% of all women. Anthropoid and android features are less common, and platypelloid pelvic features are the least common. Mixed types of pelves are more common than are pure types (Cunningham et al., 2001). Examples of pelvic variations and their effects on mode of birth are given in Table 18-2.

Assessment of the bony pelvis can be performed during the first prenatal evaluation and need not be repeated if the pelvis is of adequate size and suitable shape. In the third trimester of pregnancy, the examination of the bony pelvis may be more thorough and the results more accurate because there is relaxation and increased mobility of the pelvic joints and ligaments due to hormonal influences. Widening of the joint of the symphysis pubis and the resulting instability may cause pain in any or all of the pelvic joints.

Because the examiner does not have direct access to the bony structures and because the bones are covered with varying amounts of soft tissue, estimates of size and shape are approximate. Precise bony pelvis measurements can be determined by use of computed tomography, ultrasound, or x-ray films. However, radiographic examination is rarely done during pregnancy because the x-rays may damage the developing fetus.

Soft Tissues

The soft tissues of the passageway include the distensible lower uterine segment, cervix, pelvic floor muscles, vagina, and introitus. Before labor begins, the uterus is

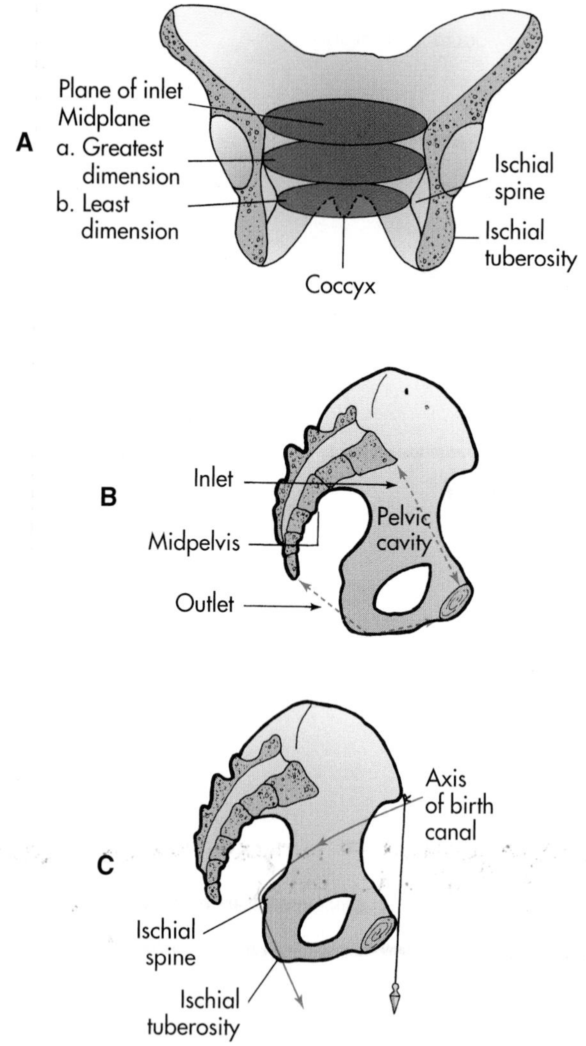
A
Plane of inlet
Midplane
a. Greatest dimension
b. Least dimension
Ischial spine
Ischial tuberosity
Coccyx
B
Inlet
Midpelvis
Outlet
Pelvic cavity
C
Axis of birth canal
Ischial spine
Ischial tuberosity

FIG. 18-8 Pelvic cavity. **A,** Inlet and midplane. Outlet now shown. **B,** Cavity of true pelvis. **C,** Note curve of sacrum and axis of birth canal.

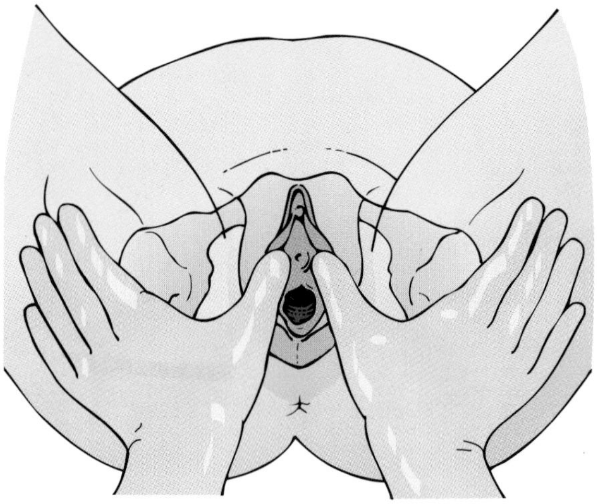

FIG. 18-9 Estimation of angle of subpubic arch. With both thumbs, examiner externally traces descending rami down to tuberosities. (From Barkauskas, V., Baumann, L., & Darling-Fisher, C. [2002]. *Health and physical assessment* [3rd ed.]. St. Louis: Mosby.)

composed of the uterine body (corpus) and cervix (neck). After labor has begun, uterine contractions cause the uterine body to have a thick and muscular upper segment and a thin-walled, passive, muscular lower segment. A physiologic retraction ring separates the two segments (Fig. 18-10). The lower uterine segment gradually distends to accommodate the intrauterine contents as the wall of the upper segment thickens and its accommodating capacity is reduced. The contractions of the uterine body thus exert downward pressure on the fetus, pushing it against the cervix.

The cervix effaces (thins) and dilates (opens) sufficiently to allow the first fetal portion to descend into the vagina. As the fetus descends, the cervix is actually drawn upward and over this first portion.

The pelvic floor is a muscular layer that separates the pelvic cavity above from the perineal space below. This structure helps the fetus rotate anteriorly as it passes through the birth canal. As noted earlier, the soft tissues of the vagina develop throughout pregnancy until at term the vagina can dilate to accommodate the fetus and permit passage of the fetus to the external world.

Powers

Involuntary and voluntary powers combine to expel the fetus and the placenta from the uterus. Involuntary uterine contractions, called the *primary powers,* signal the beginning of labor. Once the cervix has dilated, voluntary bearing-down efforts by the woman, called the *secondary powers,* augment the force of the involuntary contractions.

Primary Powers

The involuntary contractions originate at certain pacemaker points in the thickened muscle layers of the upper uterine segment. From the pacemaker points, contractions move downward over the uterus in waves, separated by short rest periods. Terms used to describe these involuntary contractions include *frequency* (the time from the beginning of one contraction to the beginning of the next), *duration* (length of contraction), and *intensity* (strength of contraction).

The primary powers are responsible for the effacement and dilation of the cervix and descent of the fetus. **Effacement** of the cervix means the shortening and thinning of the cervix during the first stage of labor. The cervix, normally 2 to 3 cm long and about 1 cm thick, is obliterated or "taken up" by a shortening of the uterine muscle bundles during the thinning of the lower uterine segment that occurs in advancing labor. Only a thin edge of the cervix can be palpated when effacement is complete. Effacement

TABLE 18-1 **Obstetric Measurements**

PLANE	DIAMETER	MEASUREMENTS
Inlet (superior strait) Conjugates Diagonal Obstetric: measurement that determines whether presenting part can engage or enter superior strait True (vera) (anteroposterior)	 12.5-13 cm 1.5-2 cm less than diagonal (radiographic) ≥11 cm (12.5) (radiographic)	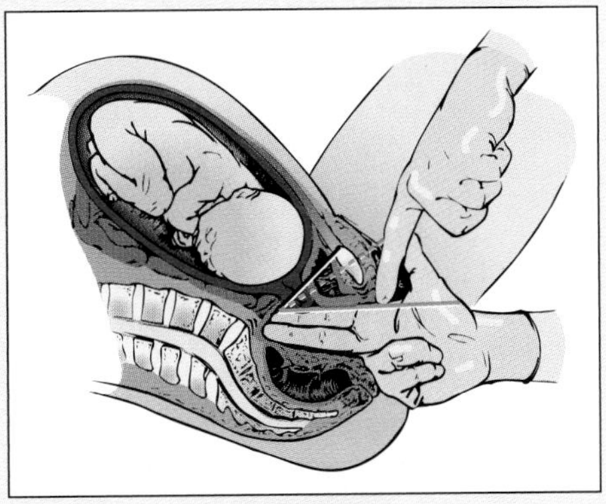 Length of diagonal conjugate (solid colored line), obstetric conjugate (broken colored line), and true conjugate (black line)*
Midplane Transverse diameter (interspinous diameter) The midplane of the pelvis normally is its largest plane and the one of greatest diameter	10.5 cm	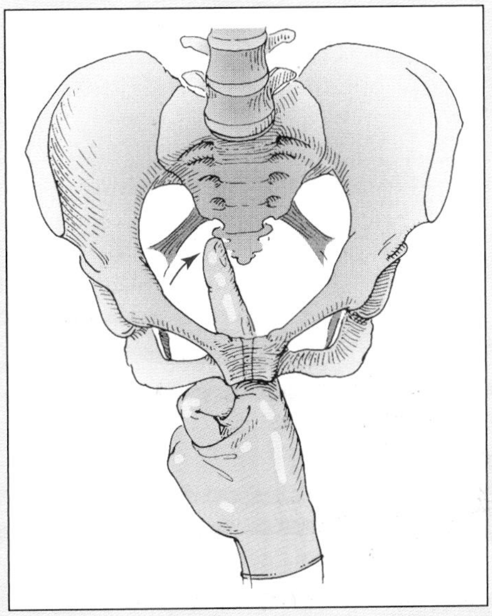 Measurement of interspinous diameter*
Outlet Transverse diameter (intertuberous diameter) (biischial) The outlet presents the smallest plane of the pelvic canal	≥8 cm	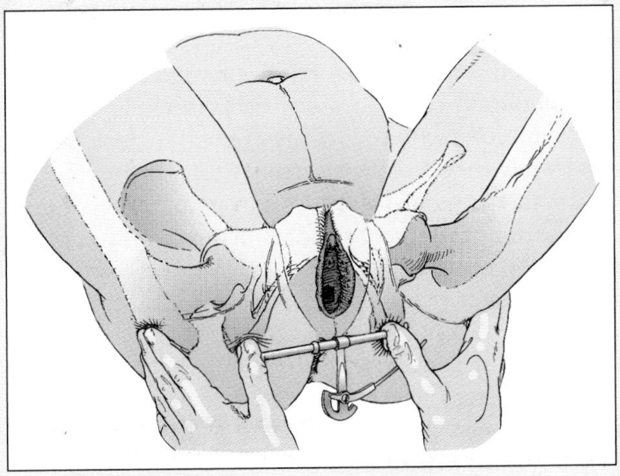 Use of Thom's pelvimeter to measure intertuberous diameter*

*From Seidel, H. et al. (2003). *Mosby's guide to physical examination* (5th ed.). St. Louis: Mosby.

TABLE 18-2 **Comparison of Pelvic Types**

	GYNECOID (50% OF WOMEN)	ANDROID (23% OF WOMEN)	ANTHROPOID (24% OF WOMEN)	PLATYPELLOID (3% OF WOMEN)
Brim	Slightly ovoid or transversely rounded Round	Heart shaped, angulated Heart	Oval, wider anteroposteriorly Oval	Flattened anteroposteriorly, wide transversely Flat
Depth	Moderate	Deep	Deep	Shallow
Side walls	Straight	Convergent	Straight	Straight
Ischial spines	Blunt, somewhat widely separated	Prominent, narrow interspinous diameter	Prominent, often with narrow interspinous diameter	Blunted, widely separated
Sacrum	Deep, curved	Slightly curved, terminal portion often beaked	Slightly curved	Slightly curved
Subpubic arch	Wide	Narrow	Narrow	Wide
Usual mode of birth	Vaginal Spontaneous Occipitoanterior position	Cesarean Vaginal Difficult with forceps	Vaginal Forceps/spontaneous occipitoposterior or occipitoanterior position	Vaginal spontaneous

generally is advanced in first-time term pregnancy before more than slight dilation occurs. In subsequent pregnancies, effacement and dilation of the cervix tend to progress together. Degree of effacement is expressed in percentages from 0 to 100% (e.g., a cervix is 50% effaced) (Fig. 18-11, *A-C*).

Dilation of the cervix is the enlargement or widening of the cervical opening and the cervical canal that occurs once labor has begun. The diameter of the cervix increases from less than 1 cm to full dilation (approximately 10 cm) to allow birth of a term fetus. When the cervix is fully dilated (and completely retracted), it can no longer be palpated (Fig. 18-11, *D*). Full cervical dilation marks the end of the first stage of labor.

Dilation of the cervix occurs by the drawing upward of the musculofibrous components of the cervix, caused by strong uterine contractions. Pressure exerted by the amniotic fluid while the membranes are intact or by the force applied by the presenting part also can promote cervical dilation. Scarring of the cervix as a result of prior infection or surgery may slow cervical dilation.

In the first and second stages of labor, increased intrauterine pressure caused by contractions exerts pressure on the descending fetus and the cervix. When the presenting part of the fetus reaches the perineal floor, mechanical stretching of the cervix occurs. Stretch receptors in the posterior vagina cause release of endogenous oxytocin that triggers the maternal urge to bear down, or the **Ferguson reflex.**

Uterine contractions are usually independent of external forces. For example, laboring women who are paraplegic will have normal but painless uterine contractions (Cunningham et al., 2001). Uterine contractions may decrease temporarily in frequency and intensity if narcotic analgesic medication or epidural analgesia is given early in labor (Alexander et al., 1998). The exact relation between prolonged labor and epidural analgesia continues to be investigated (Fontaine & Adam, 2000; Zhang, Klebanoff, & DerSimonian, 1999).

Secondary Powers

As soon as the presenting part reaches the pelvic floor, the contractions change in character and become expulsive. The laboring woman experiences an involuntary urge to push. She uses secondary powers (bearing-down efforts) to aid in expulsion of the fetus as she contracts her diaphragm and abdominal muscles and pushes. These bearing-down efforts result in increased intraabdominal pressure that compresses the uterus on all sides and adds to the power of the expulsive forces.

The secondary powers have no effect on cervical dilation, but they are of considerable importance in the expulsion of the infant from the uterus and vagina after the cervix is fully dilated. Studies have shown that pushing in the second stage is more effective and the woman is less fatigued when she begins to push only after she has the urge to do so rather than beginning to push when she is fully dilated without an urge to do so (Roberts, 2002; Roberts & Woolley, 1996).

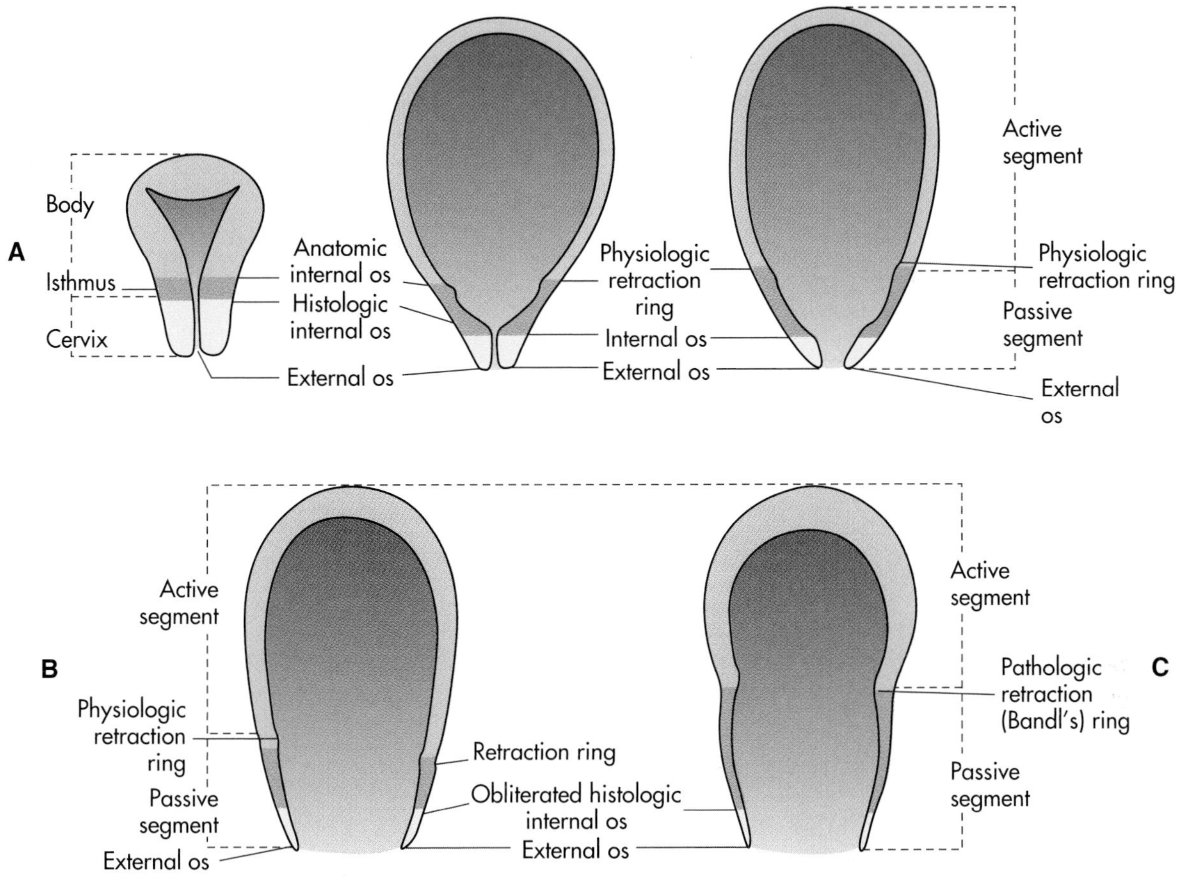
A
Body
Isthmus
Cervix
Anatomic internal os
Histologic internal os
External os
Physiologic retraction ring
Internal os
External os
Active segment
Physiologic retraction ring
Passive segment
External os
B
Active segment
Physiologic retraction ring
Passive segment
External os
Retraction ring
Obliterated histologic internal os
External os
C
Active segment
Pathologic retraction (Bandl's) ring
Passive segment

FIG. 18-10 **A,** Uterus in normal labor in early first stage, and **B,** in second stage. Passive segment is derived from lower uterine segment (isthmus) and cervix, and physiologic retraction ring is derived from anatomic internal os. **C,** Uterus in abnormal labor in second-stage dystocia. Pathologic retraction (Bandl's) ring that forms under abnormal conditions develops from the physiologic ring.

When and how a woman pushes in the second stage is a much-debated topic. Studies have investigated the effects of spontaneous bearing-down efforts, directed pushing, delayed pushing, **Valsalva** (closed glottis and prolonged bearing down) pushing, and open glottis pushing (Hansen, Clark, & Foster, 2002; Mayberry et al., 1999b; Petrou, Coyle, & Fraser, 2000; Sampselle, 1999). Although no significant differences have been found in the duration of second-stage labor, adverse consequences have been reported. Fetal hypoxia and subsequent acidosis have been associated with prolonged breath holding and forceful pushing efforts (Mayberry et al., 1999a). Perineal tears have been associated with directed pushing (Sampselle & Hines, 1999). Continued study is needed to determine the effectiveness and appropriateness of strategies used by nurses to teach pushing techniques, the suitability and effectiveness of various pushing techniques related to nonreassuring fetal heart patterns, and the standards for length of pushing in terms of maternal and fetal outcomes (Minato, 2000/2001).

Position of the Laboring Woman

Position affects the woman's anatomic and physiologic adaptations to labor. Frequent changes in position relieve fatigue, increase comfort, and improve circulation (Gupta & Nikodem, 2001). Therefore a laboring woman should be encouraged to find positions that are most comfortable to her (Fig. 18-12, *A*) (see Research box).

An upright position (walking, sitting, kneeling, or squatting) offers a number of advantages. Gravity can promote the descent of the fetus. Uterine contractions are generally stronger and more efficient in effacing and dilating the cervix, resulting in shorter labor (Gupta & Nikodem, 2001; Shermer & Raines, 1997; Simkin & Ancheta, 2000).

An upright position also is beneficial to the mother's cardiac output, which normally increases during labor as uterine contractions return blood to the vascular bed. The increased cardiac output improves blood flow to the uteroplacental unit and the maternal kidneys. Cardiac output is compromised if the descending aorta and ascending vena cava are compressed during labor.

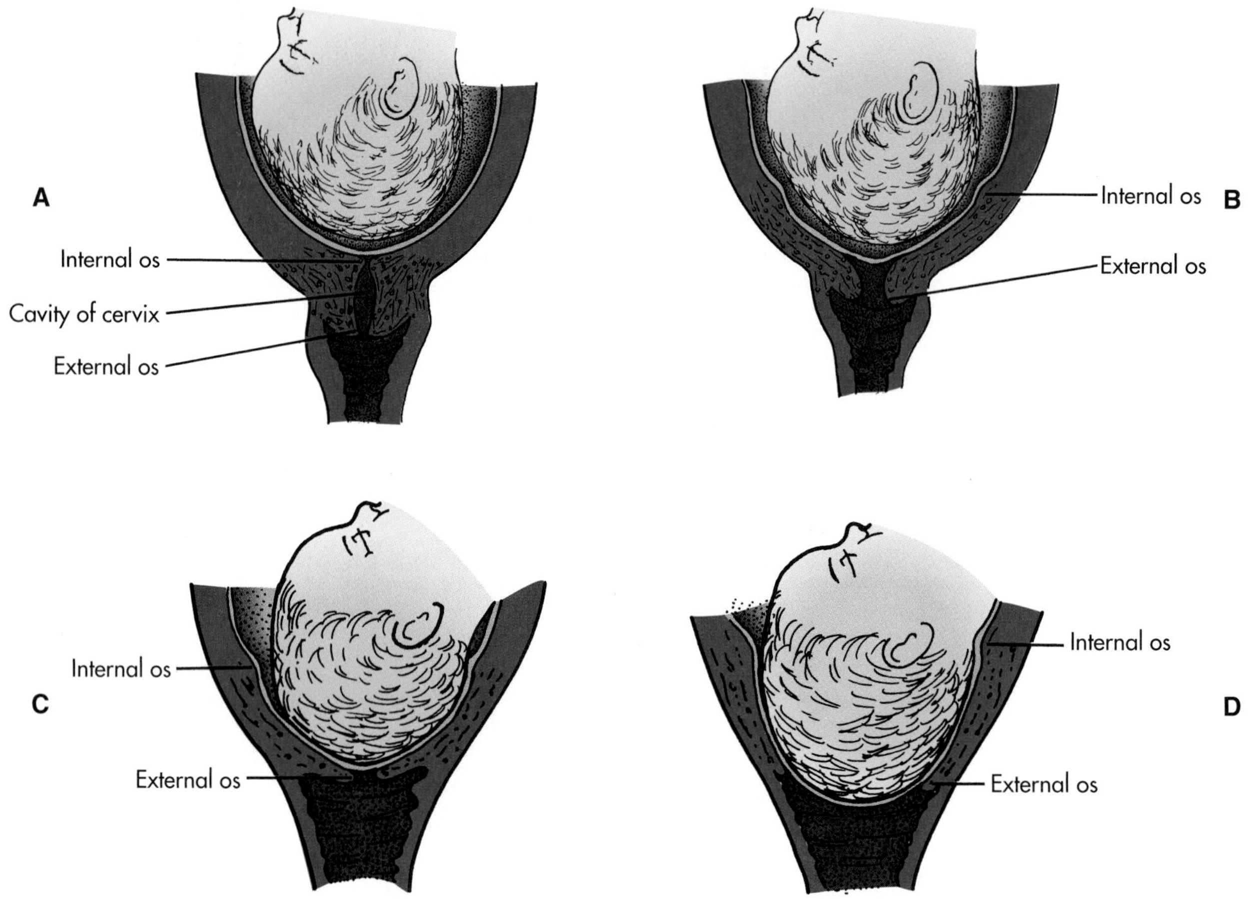
A
Internal os
Cavity of cervix
External os
Internal os
B
External os
Internal os
C
External os
Internal os
D
External os

FIG. 18-11 Cervical effacement and dilation. Note how cervix is drawn up around presenting part (internal os). Membranes are intact, and head is not well applied to cervix. **A,** Before labor. **B,** Early effacement. **C,** Complete effacement (100%). Head is well applied to cervix. **D,** Complete dilation (10 cm). Cranial bones overlap somewhat, and membranes are still intact.

Compression of these major vessels may result in supine hypotension that decreases placental perfusion. With the woman in an upright position, pressure on the maternal vessels is reduced, and compression is prevented. If the woman wishes to lie down, a lateral position is suggested (Cunningham et al., 2001).

The "all fours" position (hands and knees) may be used to relieve backache if the fetus is in an occipitoposterior position and may assist in anterior rotation of the fetus and in cases of shoulder dystocia (Hofmeyr & Kulier, 2000; Simkin & Ancheta, 2000).

Positioning for second-stage labor (Fig. 18-12, *B*) may be determined by the woman's preference, but it is constrained by the condition of the woman or fetus, the environment, and the health care provider's confidence in assisting in a birth in a specific position (Simkin & Ancheta, 2000). The predominant position in the United States in physician-attended births is the lithotomy position. Alternative positions and position changes are more commonly practiced by nurse-midwives (Hanson, 1998).

A woman who pushes in a semirecumbent position needs adequate body support to push effectively because her weight will be on her sacrum, moving the coccyx forward and causing a reduction in the pelvic outlet. In a sitting or squatting position, abdominal muscles work in greater synchrony with uterine contractions during bearing-down efforts. Kneeling or squatting moves the uterus forward and aligns the fetus with the pelvic inlet and can facilitate the second stage of labor by increasing the pelvic outlet (Simkin & Ancheta, 2000).

The lateral position can be used by the woman to help rotate a fetus that is in a posterior position. It also can be used when there is a need for less force to be used during bearing down, such as when there is a need to control the speed of a precipitate birth (Simkin & Ancheta, 2000).

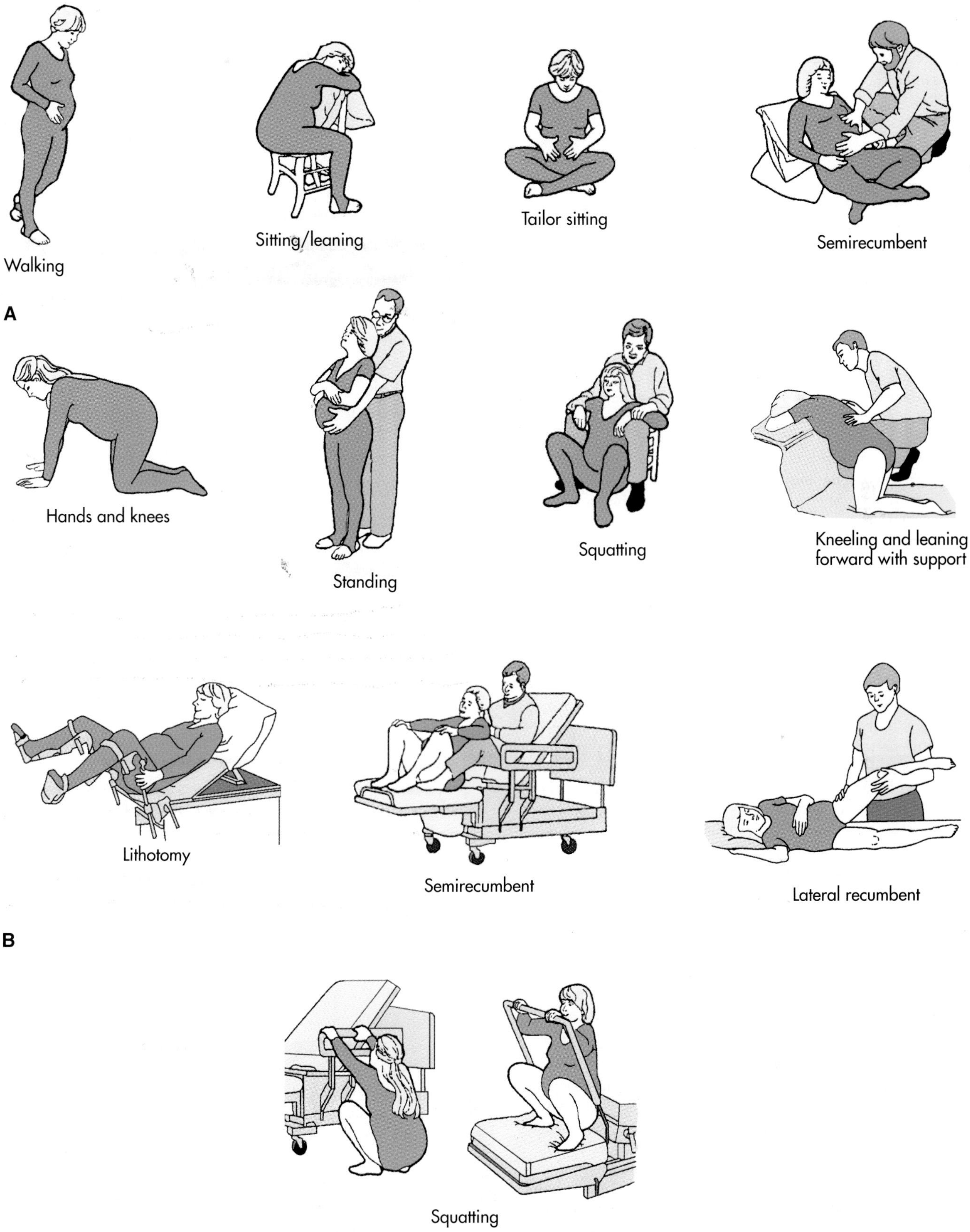
Walking
Sitting/leaning
Tailor sitting
Semirecumbent
A
Hands and knees
Standing
Squatting
Kneeling and leaning forward with support
Lithotomy
Semirecumbent
Lateral recumbent
B
Squatting

FIG. 18-12 Positions for labor and birth. **A,** Positions for labor. **B,** Positions for birth.

No evidence exists that any of these positions suggested for second-stage labor increases the need for use of operative techniques (e.g., forceps- or vacuum-assisted birth, cesarean birth, episiotomy) or causes perineal trauma. No evidence has been found that use of any of these positions adversely affects the newborn (Mayberry et al., 2000).

RESEARCH

Perineal Tearing and Episiotomy During Vaginal Birth

An unwelcome consequence of vaginal birth is perineal tearing and episiotomies. Perineal injury can lead to pain, bleeding, scarring, dyspareunia (painful intercourse), infection, urinary or fecal incontinence, and interference with establishment of breastfeeding. Evidence about the association between birth position and perineal outcomes is inconclusive, although there is some evidence to suggest that an upright position is more favorable than the supine position for reducing perineal trauma.

To provide guidance for practice, an Australian research team examined the possible association of birth positions and types of childbirth clinician on perineal outcomes. A retrospective analysis of data from 2891 normal, vaginal births was performed. The independent variables were birth position (lateral, all fours, kneeling, standing, squatting, and semirecumbent) and type of clinician ("accoucheurs"-midwives or obstetricians); the dependent variable was the perineal outcome (intact, tear with suture, or episiotomy).

Analysis revealed that the nonrecumbent positions used by midwives resulted in fewer episiotomies but more tears. The lateral (side-lying) position had the highest rate of intact perineum (66.6%). Squatting had the worst tearing, including third-degree tears, especially in primiparous women. Semirecumbent positions had the worst perineal profile. The semirecumbent position was the preferred position of obstetricians, whose episiotomy rate (26%) was five times higher than the midwives' rate. Obstetricians had a tear-requiring-suture rate of 42% compared with the midwives' rate of 36%. The obstetricians' rate for assisting with birth over an intact perineum was 32%, while the midwives' rate was 56%. Student midwives had the highest rate of births over an intact perineum at 63%.

Other factors found to be associated with increased tear and episiotomy rates were high infant birth weight, older age of mother, low parity, and longer duration of second-stage labor.

IMPLICATIONS FOR PRACTICE

The medical literature is clear in recommending minimal perineal trauma during childbirth. Midwives in the United States put great value on perineal management during labor and birth, and their practices can be used by other clinicians. Intrapartal nurses can advocate for laboring women to have input into decisions about birth positions and can participate in research that studies the effectiveness of perineal care techniques used to decrease perineal trauma.

Reference: Shorten, A., Donsante, J., & Shorten, B. (2002). Birth position, accoucheur, and perineal outcomes: Informing women about choices for vaginal birth. *Birth, 29*(1), 18-27.

PROCESS OF LABOR

Labor is the process of moving the fetus, placenta, and membranes out of the uterus and through the birth canal. Various changes take place in the woman's reproductive system in the days and weeks before labor begins. Labor itself can be discussed in terms of the mechanisms involved in the process and the stages the woman moves through.

Signs Preceding Labor

In first-time pregnancies, the uterus sinks downward and forward about 2 weeks before term, when the fetus's presenting part (usually the fetal head) descends into the true pelvis. This settling is called **lightening,** or "dropping," and usually happens gradually. After lightening, women feel less congested and breathe more easily, but usually more bladder pressure results from this shift and consequently a return of urinary frequency. In a multiparous pregnancy, lightening may not take place until after uterine contractions are established and true labor is in progress.

The woman may complain of persistent low backache and sacroiliac distress as a result of relaxation of the pelvic joints. She may identify strong, frequent, but irregular uterine (Braxton Hicks) contractions.

The vaginal mucus becomes more profuse in response to the extreme congestion of the vaginal mucous membranes. Brownish or blood-tinged cervical mucus may be passed **(bloody show).** The cervix becomes soft (ripens), partially effaced, and may begin to dilate. The membranes may rupture spontaneously.

Other phenomena are common in the days preceding labor: (1) loss of 0.5 to 1.5 kg in weight, caused by water loss resulting from electrolyte shifts that in turn are produced by changes in estrogen and progesterone levels; and (2) a surge of energy. Women speak of having a burst of energy that they often use to clean the house and put everything in order. Less commonly, some women have diarrhea, nausea, vomiting, and indigestion (Varney, 1997). Box 18-1 lists signs that may precede labor.

BOX 18-1 Signs Preceding Labor

- Lightening
- Return of urinary frequency
- Backache
- Stronger Braxton Hicks contractions
- Weight loss 0.5-1.5 kg
- Surge of energy
- Increased vaginal discharge; bloody show
- Cervical ripening
- Membranes may rupture

Onset of Labor

The onset of true labor cannot be ascribed to a single cause. Many factors, including changes in the maternal uterus, cervix, and pituitary gland, are involved. Hormones produced by the normal fetal hypothalamus, pituitary, and adrenal cortex probably contribute to the onset of labor. Progressive uterine distention, increasing intrauterine pressure, and aging of the placenta seem to be associated with increasing myometrial irritability. This is a result of increased concentrations of estrogen and prostaglandins, as well as decreasing progesterone levels. The mutually coordinated effects of these factors result in the occurrence of strong, regular, rhythmic uterine contractions. The outcome of these factors working together is normally the birth of the fetus and the expulsion of the placenta; however, how certain alterations trigger others and how proper checks and balances are maintained is not known.

Fetal fibronectin is a protein found in plasma and cervicovaginal secretions of pregnant women before the onset of labor. Assessment for the presence of fetal fibronectin is being used to predict the likelihood of preterm labor in women who are at increased risk for this complication. (Coleman et al., 1998; Goldenberg et al., 2000). The value of detection of fetal fibronectin in management of women with preterm labor has yet to be determined.

Stages of Labor

Labor is considered "normal" when the woman is at or near term, no complications exist, a single fetus presents by vertex, and labor is completed within 18 hours. The course of normal labor, which is remarkably constant, consists of (1) regular progression of uterine contractions, (2) effacement and progressive dilation of the cervix, and (3) progress in descent of the presenting part. Four stages of labor are recognized. These stages are discussed in greater detail, along with nursing care for the laboring woman and family, in Chapter 21.

The **first stage of labor** is considered to last from the onset of regular uterine contractions to full dilation of the cervix. Commonly the onset of labor is difficult to establish because the woman may be admitted to the labor unit just before birth, and the beginning of labor may be only an estimate. The first stage is much longer than the second and third combined. Great variability is the rule, however, depending on the factors discussed previously in this chapter. Full dilation may occur in less than 1 hour in some multiparous pregnancies. In first-time pregnancy, complete dilation of the cervix can take up to 20 hours. Variations may reflect differences in the patient population (e.g., risk status, age) or in clinical management of the labor and birth (Albers, 1999).

The first stage of labor has been divided into three phases: a latent phase, an active phase, and a transition phase. During the *latent phase*, there is more progress in effacement of the cervix and little increase in descent. During the *active phase* and the *transition phase*, there is more rapid dilation of the cervix and increased rate of descent of the presenting part.

The **second stage of labor** lasts from the time the cervix is fully dilated to the birth of the fetus. The second stage takes an average of 20 minutes for a multiparous woman and 50 minutes for a nulliparous woman. Labor of up to 2 hours has been considered within the normal range for the second stage, but there can be significant variations. For example, a woman who has received epidural analgesia may take up to 3 hours (Zhang et al., 2000). Ethnicity may shorten the length of the second stage labor for African-American and Puerto Rican women (Diegmann, Andrews, & Niemczura, 2000).

Simkin and Ancheta (2000) describe the latent and active phases of second-stage labor. The latent phase is a period that begins about the time of complete dilation of the uterus when the contractions are weak or not noticeable and the woman is not feeling the urge to push, is resting, or is exerting only small bearing-down efforts with contractions. The active phase is a period when contractions resume, the woman is making strong bearing-down efforts, and the fetal station is advancing.

The **third stage of labor** lasts from the birth of the fetus until the placenta is delivered. The placenta normally separates with the third or fourth strong uterine contraction after the infant has been born. After it has separated, the placenta can be delivered with the next uterine contraction. The duration of the third stage may be as short as 3 to 5 minutes, although up to 1 hour is considered within normal limits. The risk of hemorrhage increases as the length of the third stage increases (Cunningham et al., 2001).

The **fourth stage of labor** arbitrarily lasts about 2 hours after delivery of the placenta. It is the period of immediate recovery, when homeostasis is reestablished. It is an important period of observation for complications, such as abnormal bleeding (see Chapter 37).

Mechanism of Labor

As already discussed, the female pelvis has varied contours and diameters at different levels, and the presenting part of the passenger is large in proportion to the passage. Therefore for vaginal birth to occur, the fetus must adapt to the birth canal during the descent. The turns and other adjustments necessary in the human birth process are termed the **mechanism of labor** (Fig. 18-13). The seven cardinal movements of the mechanism of labor that occur in a vertex presentation are engagement, descent, flexion, internal rotation, extension, external rotation (restitution), and finally birth by expulsion. Although these movements are discussed separately, in actuality, a combination of movements occurs simultaneously. For example, engagement involves both descent and flexion.

Engagement

When the biparietal diameter of the head passes the pelvic inlet, the head is said to be engaged in the pelvic inlet (Fig. 18-13, *A*). In most nulliparous pregnancies,

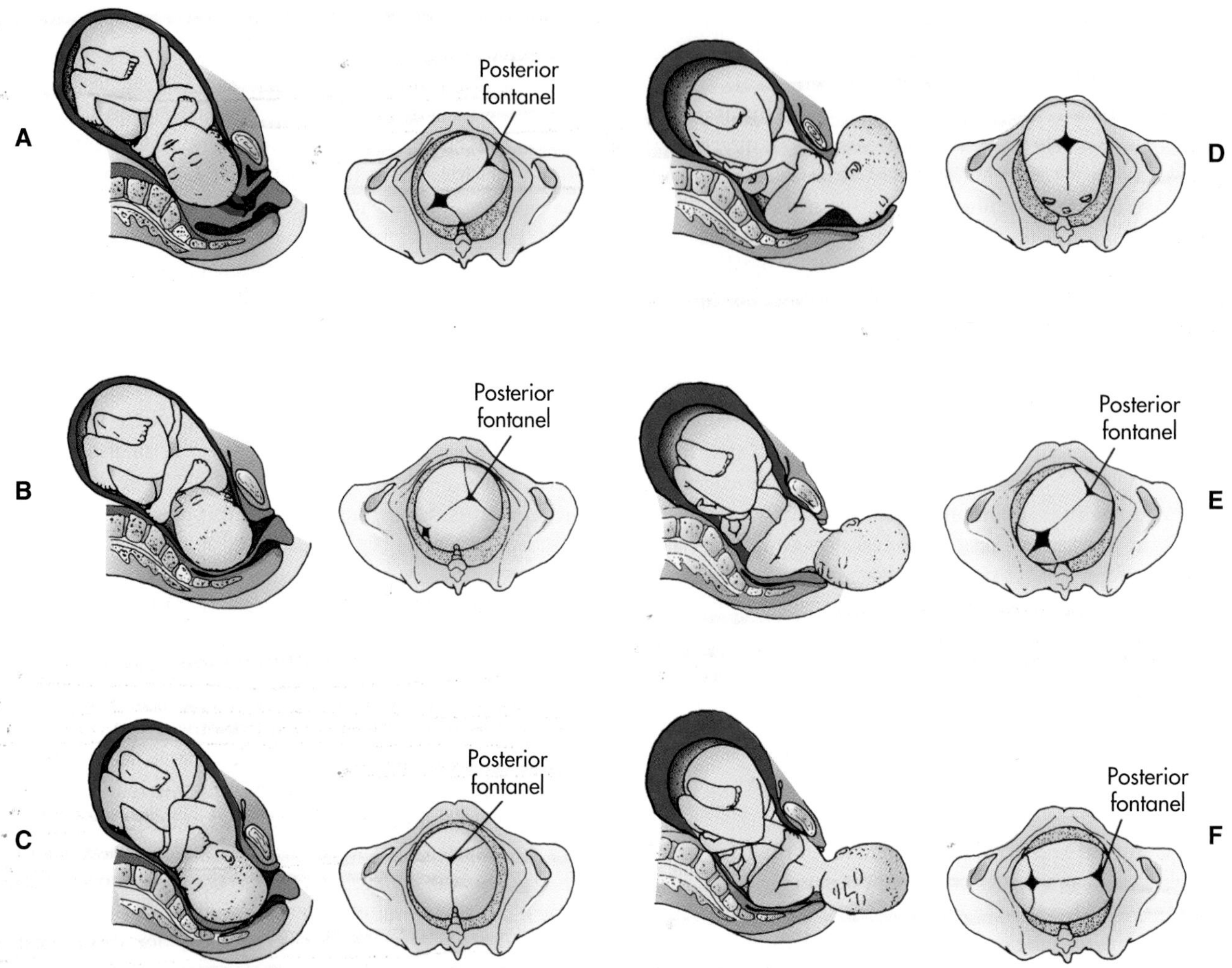
A
B
C
D
E
F
Posterior fontanel
Posterior fontanel
Posterior fontanel
Posterior fontanel
Posterior fontanel

FIG. 18-13 Cardinal movements of the mechanism of labor. Left occipitoanterior (LOA) position. **A,** Engagement and descent. **B,** Flexion. **C,** Internal rotation to occipitoanterior position (OA). **D,** Extension. **E,** External rotation beginning (restitution). **F,** External rotation.

this occurs before the onset of active labor because the firmer abdominal muscles direct the presenting part into the pelvis. In multiparous pregnancies, in which the abdominal musculature is more relaxed, the head often remains freely movable above the pelvic brim until labor is established.

Asynclitism. The head usually engages in the pelvis in a synclitic position, one that is parallel to the anteroposterior plane of the pelvis. Frequently **asynclitism** occurs (the head is deflected anteriorly or posteriorly in the pelvis), which can facilitate descent because the head is being positioned to accommodate to the pelvic cavity (Fig. 18-14). Extreme asynclitism can cause cephalopelvic disproportion, even in a normal-size pelvis, because the head is positioned so that it cannot descend.

Descent

Descent refers to the progress of the presenting part through the pelvis. Descent depends on at least four forces: (1) pressure exerted by the amniotic fluid, (2) direct pressure exerted by the contracting fundus on the fetus, (3) force of the contraction of the maternal diaphragm and abdominal muscles in the second stage of labor, and (4) extension and straightening of the fetal body. The effects of these forces are modified by the size and shape of the maternal pelvic planes and the size of the fetal head and its capacity to mold.

The degree of descent is measured by the station of the presenting part (see Fig. 18-6). As mentioned, little descent occurs during the latent phase of the first stage of labor. Descent accelerates in the active phase when the cervix has dilated to 5 to 7 cm. It is especially apparent when the membranes have ruptured.

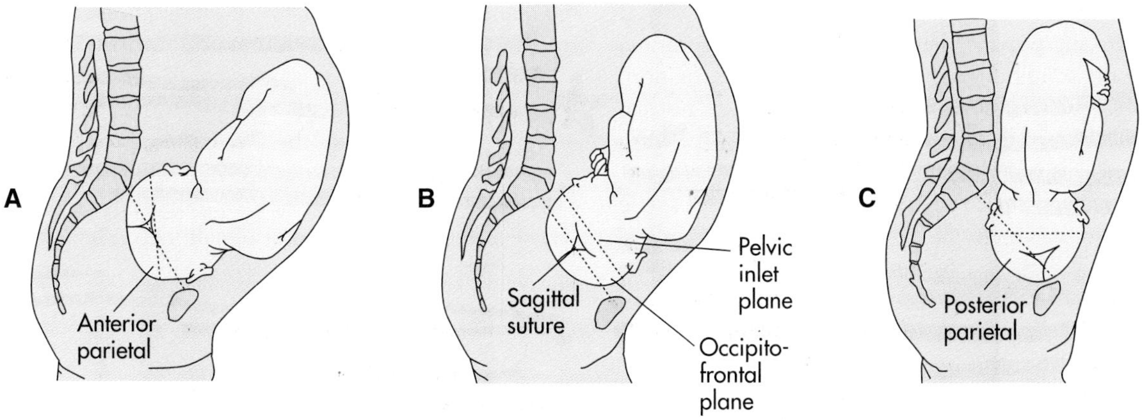
A
Anterior parietal
B
Sagittal suture
Pelvic inlet plane
Occipito-frontal plane
C
Posterior parietal

FIG. 18-14 Synclitism and asynclitism. **A,** Anterior asynclitism. **B,** Normal synclitism. **C,** Posterior asynclitism.

In a first-time pregnancy, descent is usually slow but steady; in subsequent pregnancies descent may be rapid. Progress in descent of the presenting part is determined by abdominal palpation (Leopold maneuvers) and vaginal examination until the presenting part can be seen at the introitus.

Flexion

As soon as the descending head meets resistance from the cervix, pelvic wall, or pelvic floor, it normally flexes, so that the chin is brought into closer contact with the fetal chest (see Fig. 18-13, *B*). Flexion permits the smaller suboccipitobregmatic diameter (9.5 cm) rather than the larger diameters to present to the outlet.

Internal Rotation

The maternal pelvic inlet is widest in the transverse diameter; therefore the fetal head passes the inlet into the true pelvis in the occipitotransverse position. The outlet is widest in the anteroposterior diameter, however; therefore for the fetus to exit, the head must rotate. Internal rotation begins at the level of the ischial spines but is not completed until the presenting part reaches the lower pelvis. As the occiput rotates anteriorly, the face rotates posteriorly. With each contraction, the fetal head is guided by the bony pelvis and the muscles of the pelvic floor. Eventually the occiput will be in the midline beneath the pubic arch. The head is almost always rotated by the time it reaches the pelvic floor (see Fig. 18-13, *C*). Both the levator ani muscles and the bony pelvis are important for achieving anterior rotation. A previous childbirth injury or regional anesthesia may compromise the function of the levator sling.

Extension

When the fetal head reaches the perineum for birth, it is deflected anteriorly by the perineum. The occiput passes under the lower border of the symphysis pubis first, and then the head emerges by extension: first the occiput, then the face, and finally the chin (see Fig. 18-13, *D*).

Restitution and External Rotation

After the head is born, it rotates briefly to the position it occupied when it was engaged in the inlet. This movement is referred to as restitution (see Fig. 18-13, *E*). The 45-degree turn realigns the infant's head with her or his back and shoulders. The head can then be seen to rotate further. This external rotation occurs as the shoulders engage and descend in maneuvers similar to those of the head (see Fig. 18-13, *F*). As noted earlier, the anterior shoulder descends first. When it reaches the outlet, it rotates to the midline and is delivered from under the pubic arch. The posterior shoulder is guided over the perineum until it is free of the vaginal introitus.

Expulsion

After birth of the shoulders, the head and shoulders are lifted up toward the mother's pubic bone and the trunk of the baby is born by flexing it laterally in the direction of the symphysis pubis. When the baby has completely emerged, birth is complete, and the second stage of labor ends.

PHYSIOLOGIC ADAPTATION TO LABOR

In addition to the maternal and fetal anatomic adaptations that occur during birth, physiologic adaptations must occur. Accurate assessment of the laboring woman and fetus requires knowledge of these expected adaptations.

Fetal Adaptation

Several important physiologic adaptations occur in the fetus. These changes occur in fetal heart rate (FHR), fetal circulation, respiratory movements, and other behaviors.

Fetal Heart Rate

FHR monitoring provides reliable and predictive information about the condition of the fetus related to oxygenation. The average FHR at term is 140 beats/min. The normal range is 110 to 160 beats/min. Earlier in gestation, the FHR is higher, with an average of approximately 160 beats/min at 20 weeks of gestation. The rate decreases progressively as the maturing fetus reaches term. However, temporary accelerations and slight early decelerations of the FHR can be expected in response to spontaneous fetal movement, vaginal examination, fundal pressure, uterine contractions, abdominal palpation, and fetal head compression. Stresses to the uterofetoplacental unit result in characteristic FHR patterns (see Chapter 20 for further discussion).

Fetal Circulation

Fetal circulation can be affected by many factors, including maternal position, uterine contractions, blood pressure, and umbilical cord blood flow. Uterine contractions during labor tend to decrease circulation through the spiral arterioles and subsequent perfusion through the intervillous space. Most healthy fetuses are well able to compensate for this stress and exposure to increased pressure while moving passively through the birth canal during labor. Usually umbilical cord blood flow is undisturbed by uterine contractions or fetal position (Uçkar & Townsend, 1999).

Fetal Respiration

Certain changes stimulate chemoreceptors in the aorta and carotid bodies to prepare the fetus for initiating respirations immediately after birth (Rosenberg, 2002; Uçkar & Townsend, 1999). These changes include the following:

- Fetal lung fluid is cleared from the air passages during labor and (vaginal) birth.
- Fetal oxygen pressure (Po_2) decreases.
- Arterial carbon dioxide pressure (Pco_2) increases.
- Arterial pH decreases.
- Bicarbonate level decreases.
- Fetal respiratory movements decrease during labor.

Maternal Adaptation

As the woman progresses through the stages of labor, various body system adaptations cause the woman to exhibit both objective and subjective symptoms (Box 18-2).

Cardiovascular Changes

During each contraction, 400 ml of blood is emptied from the uterus into the maternal vascular system. This increases cardiac output by about 10% to 15% in the first stage and by about 30% to 50% in the second stage. The heart rate increases slightly.

Changes in the woman's blood pressure also occur. Blood flow, which is reduced in the uterine artery by contractions, is redirected to peripheral vessels. As a result, peripheral resistance increases, and blood pressure increases (Chamberlain & Pipkin, 1998). During the first stage of labor, uterine contractions cause systolic readings to increase by about 10 mm Hg; assessing blood pressure between contractions therefore provides more accurate readings (Varney, 1997). During the second stage, contractions may cause systolic pressures to increase by 30 mm Hg and diastolic readings to increase by 25 mm Hg, with both systolic and diastolic pressures remaining somewhat elevated even between contractions. Therefore the woman already at risk for hypertension is at increased risk for complications such as cerebral hemorrhage.

Supine hypotension (see Fig. 21-5) occurs when the ascending vena cava and descending aorta are compressed. The laboring woman is at greater risk for supine hypotension if the uterus is particularly large because of multifetal pregnancy, hydramnios, or obesity or if the woman is dehydrated or hypovolemic. In addition, anxiety and pain, as well as some medications, can cause hypotension.

The woman should be discouraged from using the **Valsalva maneuver** (holding one's breath and tightening abdominal muscles) for pushing during the second stage. This activity increases intrathoracic pressure, reduces venous return, and increases venous pressure. The cardiac output and blood pressure increase and the pulse slows temporarily. During the Valsalva maneuver, fetal hypoxia may occur. The process is reversed when the woman takes a breath.

The white blood cell (WBC) count can increase (Pagana & Pagana, 2002). Although the mechanism leading to this increase in WBCs is unknown, it may be secondary to physical or emotional stress or to tissue trauma. Labor is strenuous, and physical exercise alone can increase the WBC count.

Some peripheral vascular changes occur, perhaps in response to cervical dilation or to compression of maternal

BOX 18-2 Maternal Physiologic Changes During Labor

Cardiac output increases 10%-15% in first stage; 30%-50% in second stage.
Heart rate increases slightly in first and second stages.
Systolic blood pressure increases during uterine contractions in first stage; systolic and diastolic pressures increase during uterine contractions in second stage.
White blood cell count increases.
Respiratory rate increases.
Temperature may be slightly elevated.
Proteinuria 1+ may occur.
Gastric motility and absorption of solid food is decreased; nausea and vomiting may occur during transition to second-stage labor.
Blood glucose level decreases.

vessels by the fetus passing through the birth canal. Flushed cheeks, hot or cold feet, and eversion of hemorrhoids may result.

Respiratory Changes

Increased physical activity with greater oxygen consumption is reflected in an increase in the respiratory rate. Hyperventilation may cause respiratory alkalosis (an increase in pH), hypoxia, and hypocapnia (decrease in carbon dioxide). In the unmedicated woman in the second stage, oxygen consumption almost doubles. Anxiety also increases oxygen consumption.

Renal Changes

During labor, spontaneous voiding may be difficult for various reasons: tissue edema caused by pressure from the presenting part, discomfort, analgesia, and embarrassment. Proteinuria of 1+ is a normal finding because it can occur in response to the breakdown of muscle tissue from the physical work of labor.

Integumentary Changes

The integumentary system changes are evident, especially in the great distensibility (stretching) in the area of the vaginal introitus. The degree of distensibility varies with the individual. Despite this ability to stretch, even in the absence of episiotomy or lacerations, minute tears in the skin around the vaginal introitus do occur.

Musculoskeletal Changes

The musculoskeletal system is stressed during labor. Diaphoresis, fatigue, proteinuria (+1), and possibly an increased temperature accompany the marked increase in muscle activity. Backache and joint ache (unrelated to fetal position) occur as a result of increased joint laxity at term. The labor process itself and the woman's pointing her toes can cause leg cramps.

Neurologic Changes

Sensorial changes occur as the woman moves through phases of the first stage of labor and as she moves from one stage to the next. Initially she may be euphoric. Euphoria gives way to increased seriousness, then to amnesia between contractions during the second stage, and finally to elation or fatigue after giving birth. Endogenous endorphins (a morphinelike chemical produced naturally by the body) raise the pain threshold and produce sedation. In addition, physiologic anesthesia of perineal tissues, caused by pressure of the presenting part, decreases perception of pain.

Gastrointestinal Changes

During labor, gastrointestinal motility and absorption of solid foods are decreased, and stomach-emptying time is slowed. Nausea and vomiting of undigested food eaten after onset of labor are common. Nausea and belching also occur as a reflex response to full cervical dilation. The woman may state that diarrhea accompanied the onset of labor, or the nurse may palpate the presence of hard or impacted stool in the rectum.

Endocrine Changes

The onset of labor may be triggered by decreasing levels of progesterone and increasing levels of estrogen, prostaglandins, and oxytocin. Metabolism increases, and blood glucose levels may decrease with the work of labor.

Accurate assessment of the mother and fetus during labor and birth depends on knowledge of these expected adaptations so that appropriate interventions can be implemented.

KEY POINTS

- Labor and birth are affected by the five Ps: passenger, passageway, powers, position of the woman, and psychologic responses.
- Because of its size and relative rigidity, the fetal head is a major factor in determining the course of birth.
- The diameters at the plane of the pelvic inlet, midpelvis, and outlet, plus the axis of the birth canal, determine whether vaginal birth is possible and the manner in which the fetus passes down the birth canal.
- Involuntary uterine contractions act to expel the fetus and placenta during the first stage of labor; these are augmented by voluntary bearing-down efforts during the second stage.
- The first stage of labor lasts from the time dilation begins to the time when the cervix is fully dilated. The second stage of labor lasts from the time of full dilation to the birth of the infant. The third stage of labor lasts from the infant's birth to the expulsion of the placenta. The fourth stage is the first 2 hours after birth.
- The cardinal movements of the mechanism of labor are engagement, descent, flexion, internal rotation, extension, restitution and external rotation, and expulsion of the infant.
- Although the events precipitating the onset of labor are unknown, many factors, including changes in the maternal uterus, cervix, and pituitary gland, are thought to be involved.
- A healthy fetus with an adequate uterofetoplacental circulation will be able to compensate for the stress of uterine contractions.
- As the woman progresses through labor, various body systems adapt to the birth process.

CRITICAL THINKING EXERCISES

1. You have been asked by the staff at the community health center to prepare a childbirth class on the signs that precede labor for a group of Spanish-speaking nulliparas.
   a. Identify essential content to be covered, and describe how you would collect data about the group's knowledge and educational levels (e.g., through an interpreter).
   b. Plan a 10-minute class, including appropriate audiovisuals. Discuss the plan with your faculty.
   c. Give the class, and ask the women and the staff at the health center to evaluate it.
2. Interview three women who have given birth within the last 18 hours.
   a. Ask them to identify factors (forces) that had an impact on their labor.
   b. Compare these with the factors described in the chapter.
   c. Discuss your findings in a clinical conference. Suggest how you can use this information in providing labor care.
3. During your clinical experience in the labor and birth unit, identify nursing interventions (especially selection of positions and pushing techniques) that affected the progress of labor either negatively or positively.
   a. Ask the nurses for their rationale for implementing these interventions, and then use nursing research to identify those evidence-based interventions that could have been used.
   b. Discuss in clinical conference ways to share this information with the nurses in the labor and birth unit.

RESOURCES

Alexian Brothers Medical Center
Elk Grove, IL
Information on stages of labor and other labor and birth topics
847-437-5500
www.alexian.org/progserv/babies/babytoo.html

Baby Center
Source for expectant parents
www.babycenter.com/pregnancy

Childbirth Organization
Source of links to other sites related to labor and birth
www.childbirth.org

Childbirth Graphics
P.O. Box 21207
Waco, TX 76702
800-229-3366
www.childbirthgraphics.com

REFERENCES

Albers, L. (1999). The duration of labor in healthy women. *Journal of Perinatology, 19*(2), 114-119.

Alexander, J. et al. (1998). The course of labor with and without epidural analgesia. *American Journal of Obstetrics and Gynecology, 718*(3), 516-520.

Barkauskas, V., Baumann, L., & Darling-Fisher, C. (2002). *Health and physical assessment* (3rd ed.). St. Louis: Mosby.

Chamberlain, G., & Pipkin, F. (1998). *Clinical physiology in obstetrics* (3rd ed.). Oxford: Blackwell Scientific.

Coleman, M. et al. (1998). Fetal fibronectin detection in preterm labor: Evaluation of a prototype bedside dipstick technique and cervical assessment. *American Journal of Obstetrics and Gynecology, 179*(6), 1553-1558.

Cunningham, F. et al. (2001). *Williams obstetrics* (21st ed.). New York: McGraw-Hill.

Diegmann, E., Andrews, C., & Niemczura, C. (2000). The length of the second stage of labor in uncomplicated, nulliparous African American and Puerto Rican women. *Journal of Midwifery and Women's Health, 45*(1) 67-71.

Fontaine, P., & Adam, P. (2000). Intrathecal narcotics are associated with prolonged second-stage labor and increased oxytocin use. *Journal of Family Practrice, 49*(6), 515-520.

Goldenberg, R. et al. (2000). The preterm prediction study: Sequential cervical length and fetal fibronectin testing for the prediction of spontaneous preterm birth, National Institute of Child Health and Human Development Maternal-Fetal Medicine Units Network. *American Journal of Obstetrics and Gynecology, 182*(3), 636-643.

Gupta, J., & Nikodem, V. (2001). Woman's position during second stage of labor (Cochrane Review). *The Cochrane Library*, Issue 2. Oxford: Update Software.

Hansen, S., Clark, S., & Foster, J. (2002). Active pushing versus passive fetal descent in the second stage of labor: A randomized controlled trial. *Obstetrics and Gynecology, 99*(1), 29-34.

Hanson, L. (1998). Second-stage pushing in nurse-midwifery practices, Part 2: Factors affecting use. *Journal of Nurse Midwifery, 43*(5), 326-330.

Hofmeyr, G., & Kulier, R. (2000). Hands/knees posture in later pregnancy or labour for fetal malposition (lateral or posterior) (Cochrane Review). *The Cochrane Library*, Issue 2. Oxford: Update Software.

Mayberry, L. et al. (1999a). Maternal fatigue: Implications of second stage labor nursing care. *Journal of Obstetric, Gynecologic, and Neonatal Nursing, 28*(2), 175-181.

Mayberry, L. et al. (1999b). Use of delayed pushing with epidural anesthesia: Findings from a randomized, controlled trial. *Journal of Perinatology, 19*(1), 26-30.

Mayberry, L. et al. (2000). *AWHONN Symposium: Second-stage labor management: Promotion of evidence-based practice and a collaborative approach to patient care.* Washington, DC: Association of Women's Health, Obstetrics, and Neonatal Nurses.

Minato, J. (2000/2001). Is it time to push? Examining rest in second-stage labor. *AWHONN Lifelines, 4*(6), 20-23.

Pagana, K., & Pagana, T. (2002). *Mosby's manual of diagnostic and laboratory tests* (2nd ed.). St. Louis: Mosby.

Petrou, S., Coyle, D., & Fraser, W. (2000). Cost-effectiveness of a delayed pushing policy for patients with epidural anesthesia: The PEOPLE (Pushing Early or Pushing Late with Epidural) Study Group. *American Journal of Obstetrics and Gynecology, 182*(5), 1158-1164.

Roberts J. (2002). The "push" for evidence: Management of the second stage. *Journal of Midwifery and Women's Health, 47*(1), 2-15.

Roberts, J., & Woolley, D. (1996). A second look at the second stage of labor. *Journal of Obstetric, Gynecologic, and Neonatal Nursing, 25*(5), 415-423.

Rosenberg, A. (2002). The neonate. In S. Gabbe, J. Niebyl, & J. Simpson (Eds.), *Obstetrics: Normal and problem pregnancies* (4th ed.). New York: Churchill Livingstone

Sampselle, C. (1999). Spontaneous pushing during birth. *Journal of Nurse Midwifery, 44*(1), 36-39.

Sampselle, C., & Hines, S. (1999). Spontaneous pushing during birth: Relationship to perineal outcomes. *Journal of Nurse Midwifery, 44*(1), 36-39.

Seidel, H. et al. (2003). *Mosby's guide to physical examination* (5th ed.). St. Louis: Mosby.

Shermer, R., & Raines, D. (1997). Positioning during the second stage of labor: Moving back to basics. *Journal of Obstetric, Gynecologic, and Neonatal Nursing, 26*(6), 727-734.

Simkin, P., & Ancheta, R. (2000). *The labor progress handbook: Early interventions to prevent and treat dystocia.* Oxford: Blackwell Science Ltd.

Uçkar, E., & Townsend, N. (1999). Fetal adaptation. In L. Mandeville & N. Troiano (Eds.), *AWHONN's high-risk and critical care intrapartum nursing* (2nd ed). Philadelphia: Lippincott.

VandeVusse, L. (1999). The essential forces of labor revisited: 13 Ps reported in women's birth stories. *MCN American Journal of Maternal Child Nursing, 24*(4), 176-184.

Varney, H. (1997). *Varney's midwifery* (3rd ed.). Sudbury, MA: Jones & Bartlett.

Zhang, J., Klebanoff, M., & DerSimonian, R. (1999). Epidural analgesia in association with duration of labor and mode of delivery: a quantitative review. *American Journal of Obstetrics and Gynecology, 180*(4), 970-977.

CHAPTER 19

Karen A. Piotrowski

Management of Discomfort

http://evolve.elsevier.com/Lowdermilk/MatWmnHlth/

LEARNING OBJECTIVES

- Compare the various childbirth preparation methods.
- Describe breathing and relaxation techniques used for each stage of labor.
- Identify nonpharmacologic strategies to enhance relaxation and decrease discomfort during labor.
- Discuss the types of analgesia and anesthesia used during labor.
- Compare pharmacologic methods used to relieve discomfort in different stages of labor and for different methods of birth.
- Discuss the use of naloxone (Narcan).
- Apply the nursing process to the management of the discomfort of a woman in labor.
- Describe the nursing responsibilities appropriate for a woman receiving analgesia or anesthesia during labor.

Pain is an unpleasant, complex, highly individualized phenomenon with both sensory and emotional components. Pregnant women commonly worry about the pain they will experience during labor and birth and about how they will react to and deal with that pain. Many physiologic, psychosocial, and environmental factors influence the nature and degree of pain of a woman in labor and the manner in which she will respond to and cope with the pain (Lowe, 2002). A variety of nonpharmacologic and pharmacologic methods can help the woman cope with the discomfort of labor. The methods selected depend on the situation, availability, and the preferences of both the woman and her primary health care provider.

DISCOMFORT DURING LABOR AND BIRTH

Neurologic Origins

The pain and discomfort of labor have two origins, visceral and somatic (Lowe, 2002). During the first stage of labor, uterine contractions cause cervical dilation and effacement. Uterine ischemia (decreased blood flow and therefore local oxygen deficit) results from compression of the arteries supplying the myometrium during uterine contractions. Pain impulses during the first stage of labor are transmitted via the T11 to T12 spinal nerve segment and accessory lower thoracic and upper lumbar sympathetic nerves. These nerves originate in the uterine body and cervix.

The pain from cervical changes, distention of the lower uterine segment, and uterine ischemia that predominates during the first stage of labor is **visceral pain.** It is located over the lower portion of the abdomen. **Referred pain** occurs when the pain that originates in the uterus radiates to the abdominal wall, lumbosacral area of the back, iliac crests, gluteal area, and down the thighs. The woman usually has discomfort only during contractions and is free of pain between contractions, although some women have continuous contraction-related low back pain, even in the interval between contractions (Lowe, 2002).

During the second stage of labor, the woman has **somatic pain,** which is often described as intense, sharp, burning, and well localized. Pain results from stretching and distention of perineal tissues and the pelvic floor to allow passage of the fetus, from distention and traction on the peritoneum and uterocervical supports during contractions, and from lacerations of soft tissue (e.g., cervix, vagina, perineum). Discomfort also can be produced by expulsive forces or by pressure exerted by the presenting part on the bladder, bowel, or other sensitive pelvic structures. Pain impulses during the second stage of labor are transmitted via the pudendal nerve through S2 to S4 spinal nerve segments and the parasympathetic system (Lowe, 2002).

Pain during the third stage of labor and the afterpains of the early postpartum period are uterine, similar to that experienced early in the first stage of labor. Areas of discomfort during labor are shown in Fig. 19-1.

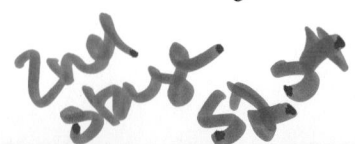

Perception of Pain

Although the pain threshold is remarkably similar in all persons regardless of gender, social, ethnic, or cultural differences, these differences play a definite role in the person's perception of and behavioral responses to pain. The effects of factors such as culture, counterstimuli, and distraction in coping with pain are not fully understood. The meaning of pain and the verbal and nonverbal expressions given to pain are apparently learned from interactions within the primary social group. Cultural influences may impose unrealistic expectations. For instance, Asian women typically believe it shameful to scream or show pain, and they avoid verbal expression (Weber, 1996).

Expression of Pain

Pain results in physiologic effects and sensory and emotional (affective) responses. During childbirth, pain gives rise to identifiable physiologic effects. Sympathetic nervous system activity is stimulated in response to intensifying pain, resulting in increased catecholamine levels. Blood pressure and heart rate increase. Maternal respiratory patterns change in response to an increase in oxygen consumption. Hyperventilation, sometimes accompanied by respiratory alkalosis, can occur as pain intensifies. Pallor and diaphoresis may be seen. Gastric acidity increases, and nausea and vomiting are common in the active phase of labor. Placental perfusion may decrease, and uterine activity may diminish, potentially prolonging labor and affecting fetal well-being.

The sensory quality of visceral and somatic pain has been described as prickling, stabbing, burning, bursting, aching, heavy, pulling, throbbing, sharp, shooting, stinging, or cramping. The emotional (affective) quality of pain has been described as tiring, exhausting, annoying, sickening, and nauseating (Lowe, 2002).

Certain emotional (affective) expressions of suffering are often seen. Such changes include increasing anxiety with lessened perceptual field, writhing, crying, groaning, gesturing (hand clenching and wringing), and excessive muscular excitability throughout the body. Cultural expression of pain may vary. For example, Native American women may endure pain quietly, whereas Hispanic women may endure pain stoically, because it is expected and esteemed, but consider it acceptable to cry out (Villarruel, 1995).

Factors Influencing Pain Response

Each woman's pain during childbirth is unique and is influenced by a variety of physiologic, psychosocial, and environmental factors.

Physiologic Factors

A variety of physiologic factors can affect the intensity of pain experienced by women during childbirth. Women with a history of dysmenorrhea may experience increased pain during childbirth as a result of higher prostaglandin levels. Back pain associated with menstruation also may increase the likelihood of contraction-related low back pain. Upright positions, when assumed during labor, seem to result in decreased pain and an overall increase in comfort when compared with the supine position. Women also report that being able to move freely to find a position of comfort is an important factor in reducing

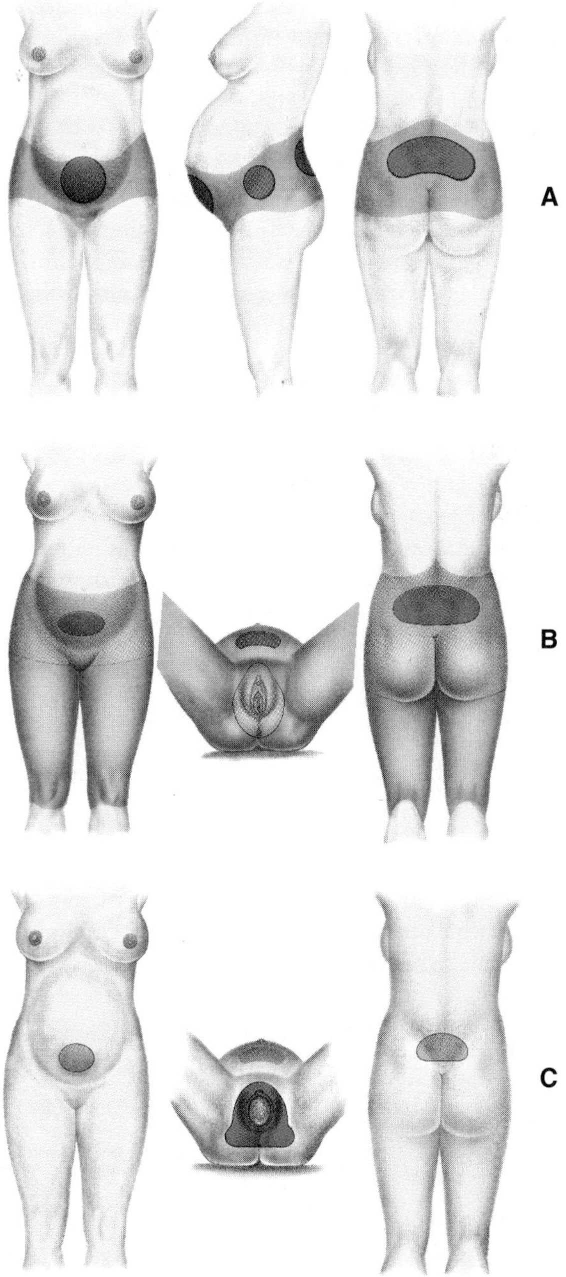
A
B
C

FIG. 19-1 Discomfort during labor. **A,** Distribution of labor pain during first stage. **B,** Distribution of labor pain during transition and early phase of second stage. **C,** Distribution of pain during late second stage and actual birth. (*Gray areas,* mild discomfort; *light-colored areas,* moderate discomfort; *dark areas,* intense discomfort).

pain and muscle tension and maintaining control during labor. Finally, the relation of fetal size to the dimensions of the maternal pelvis may influence pain intensity (Lowe, 2002; Simkin & O'Hara, 2002).

Endorphins are endogenous opioids secreted by the pituitary gland that act on the central and peripheral nervous systems to reduce pain. Beta-endorphin is the most potent of the endorphins. The physiologic role of endorphins is not completely understood. It is thought that endorphin levels increase during pregnancy and birth in humans. Higher endorphin levels may increase the ability of women in labor to tolerate acute pain and may reduce their irritability and anxiety. Levels of beta-endorphins are higher when a woman experiences a spontaneous, natural childbirth (Righard, 2001).

Culture

The obstetric population reflects the increasingly multicultural nature of U.S. society. As nurses care for women and families from a variety of cultural backgrounds, they must have knowledge and understanding of how culture mediates pain (Lee & Essoka, 1998; Mattson, 2000). An understanding of the beliefs, values, expectations, and practices of various cultures will narrow the cultural gap and help the nurse to assess the laboring woman's pain experience more accurately and to provide culturally sensitive care by using appropriate pain relief measures (see Cultural Considerations box; see Table 21-2). The nurse must take care not to have cultural blindness, an inability to see other courses of action, which may lead to cultural clashes, resulting in less than optimal care and less than satisfied women of a different culture from that of the nurse (Weber, 1996). It is important for the nurse to recognize that although a woman's behavior in response to pain may vary according to her cultural background, it may not accurately reflect the intensity of the pain she is experiencing. The nurse must assess the woman for the physiologic effects of pain and must listen to the words the woman uses to describe the sensory and affective qualities of her pain (Lowe, 2002).

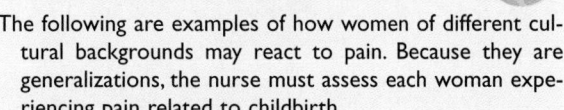

> **CULTURAL CONSIDERATIONS**
>
> **Some Cultural Responses to Pain**
>
> The following are examples of how women of different cultural backgrounds may react to pain. Because they are generalizations, the nurse must assess each woman experiencing pain related to childbirth.
>
> Chinese women may not exhibit reactions to pain, although it is acceptable to exhibit pain during childbirth. They consider it impolite to accept something when it is first offered; therefore pain interventions must be offered more than once. Acupuncture may be used for pain relief.
>
> Arab or Middle Eastern women may be vocal in response to labor pain. They may prefer medication for pain relief.
>
> Japanese women may be stoic in response to labor pain, but they may request medication when pain becomes severe.
>
> Southeast Asian women may endure severe pain before requesting relief.
>
> Hispanic women may be stoic until late in labor, when they may become vocal and request pain relief.
>
> Native American women may use medications or remedies made from indigenous plants. They are often stoic in response to labor pain.
>
> African-American women may express pain openly. Use of medication for pain relief varies.

Anxiety

Anxiety is commonly associated with increased pain during labor. Mild anxiety is considered normal for a woman during labor and birth; however, excessive anxiety and fear increase catecholamine secretion, resulting in more pelvic pain stimuli reaching the brain; this in turn magnifies pain perception (Lowe, 2002). As anxiety heightens, muscle tension increases, the effectiveness of uterine contractions decreases, and discomfort intensifies; a cycle of increased fear and anxiety begins. Ultimately this cycle will slow the progress of labor. The woman's "self-efficacy" or confidence in her ability to cope with pain will be diminished, potentially resulting in reduced effectiveness of pain relief measures being used.

Previous Experience

Previous experience with pain and childbirth may affect a woman's description of her pain and her ability to cope with the pain. Childbirth, for a healthy young adult woman, may be her first experience with significant pain, and as a result, she may not have developed effective pain coping strategies. She may describe the intensity of even early labor pain as pain "as bad as it can be." Sensory pain for nulliparous women is often greater than that for multiparous women during early labor (dilation less than 5 cm) because their reproductive tract structures are less supple. During the transition phase of the first stage of labor and during the second stage of labor, multiparous women may experience greater sensory pain than nulliparous women because their more supple tissue increases the speed of fetal descent and thereby intensifies pain. The firmer tissue of nulliparous women results in a slower more gradual descent. Affective pain is usually greater for nulliparous women throughout the first stage of labor but decreases for both nulliparous and multiparous women during the second stage of labor (Lowe, 2002).

The nature of previous childbirth experiences also may affect a woman's responses to pain. For women who have had a difficult and painful previous birth experience, anxiety and fear from this past experience may lead to an increased perception of pain. Conversely, a woman who has experienced a labor and birth in which the degree of pain matched expectations and her coping skills were successful may have decreased anxiety. However, if those previously successful coping skills no longer work because of a more difficult labor, anxiety will increase.

Women with a history of substance abuse have as much pain during labor as other women. Although it is usually unnecessary to withhold pain medications, close monitoring for complications associated with each substance is part of the nursing assessment. For example, opioid antagonists or opioid agonist-antagonists should be avoided for women with a history of opioid abuse because abstinence syndrome (withdrawal) may be precipitated in the woman and her newborn (Hawkins, Chestnut, & Gibbs, 2002).

Pain is a personal response in each individual. As pain is experienced, people develop various coping mechanisms to deal with it. Emotional tension from anxiety and fear may increase pain and perception of pain during labor. Pain, or the possibility of pain, can induce fear, in which anxiety borders on panic. Fatigue and sleep deprivation magnify pain. Parity may affect labor pain because nulliparous women often have longer labors and thus greater fatigue, causing a vicious cycle of increased pain, fatigue, reduced ability to cope, and a more likely use of pharmacologic support.

Childbirth Preparation

Even particularly intense pain stimuli can, at times, be ignored. This is possible because certain nerve cell groupings within the spinal cord, brainstem, and cerebral cortex have the ability to modulate the pain impulse through a blocking mechanism. This **gate-control theory** of pain helps explain the way hypnosis and the pain relief techniques taught in childbirth preparation classes work to relieve the pain of labor. According to this theory, pain sensations travel along sensory nerve pathways to the brain, but only a limited number of sensations, or messages, can travel through these nerve pathways at one time. Distraction techniques such as massage or stroking, music, focal points, and imagery reduce or completely block the capacity of nerve pathways to transmit pain. These distractions are thought to work by closing down a hypothetic gate in the spinal cord, thus preventing pain signals from reaching the brain. The perception of pain is thereby diminished.

In addition, when the laboring woman engages in neuromuscular and motor activity, activity within the spinal cord itself further modifies the transmission of pain. Cognitive work involving concentration on breathing and relaxation requires selective and directed cortical activity that activates and closes the gating mechanism as well. As labor intensifies, more complex cognitive techniques are required to maintain effectiveness. The gate-control theory underscores the need for a supportive birth setting that allows the laboring woman to relax and use various higher mental activities.

Comfort

Although the predominant medical approach to labor is that it is painful, and the pain must be removed, an alternative view is that labor is a natural process, and women can have comfort and transcend the discomfort or pain to reach the joyful outcome of birth. Having needs and desires met engenders a feeling of comfort. Comfort may be viewed as strengthening (Schuiling & Sampselle, 1999). This represents a paradigm shift in the interpretation of pain in labor. The most helpful interventions in enhancing comfort are a caring nursing approach and supportive presence.

Support

A critical issue for the nurse is how support can make a difference in the pain of the woman during labor and birth. The pain and the management of this pain belong to the woman having the pain; the nurse must engage in a cooperative effort to provide whatever external tools the woman requires to manage her pain. These tools include both nonpharmacologic and pharmacologic interventions. A woman's satisfaction with her childbirth experience is primarily influenced by the attitudes and behaviors of her caregivers, including the caregivers' ability to communicate and to be helpful, supportive, accepting, and kind. In addition, satisfaction is influenced by the degree to which she was able to stay in control of her labor and to participate in decision making regarding her labor, including the pain relief measures to be used (Hodnett, 2002).

The presence of a person (e.g., doula, partner, family member, friend, nurse) who provides continuous physical, emotional, and psychologic support of the woman in labor is a beneficial form of care. Continuous support significantly relieves pain, improves outcomes, decreases interventions (e.g., use of pharmacologic pain relief measures) and complication rates (e.g., cesarean births) associated with labor, and enhances overall maternal satisfaction (Enkin et al., 2000; Righard, 2001; Simkin & O'Hara, 2002). The Hawthorne effect may in part explain the positive benefit of continuous support during labor and birth. According to this effect, the woman in labor will perform better when receiving special attention and encouragement from a support person (Nichols & Humenick, 2000).

Environment

According to Lowe (2002), environment should be viewed in terms of the persons present (e.g., how they communicate, their philosophy of care, practice policies, and quality of support) and the physical space in which the labor occurs. The quality of the environment can influence a woman's ability to cope with the pain of labor. Women prefer to be cared for by familiar caregivers in a comfortable, homelike setting (Hodnett, 2002). An environment should be safe and private, allowing a woman to feel free to be herself as she tries out different comfort measures. Stimuli including light, noise, and temperature should be adjusted according to the woman's preferences. There should be space for movement, and equipment should be readily available for a variety of nonpharmacologic pain relief measures such as birth balls, comfortable chairs, tubs, and showers. The familiarity of the environment can be enhanced by bringing items from home such as pillows, objects for a focal point, music, and videos.

NONPHARMACOLOGIC MANAGEMENT OF DISCOMFORT

The alleviation of pain is important. Commonly it is not the amount of pain the woman has but whether the pain meets her expectations and whether she meets her goals for herself in coping with the pain that influences her perception of the birth experience as "good" or "bad." The observant nurse looks for clues to the woman's desired level of control in the management of pain and its relief.

Nonpharmacologic measures are often simple, safe, and relatively inexpensive. They provide the woman with a sense of control over her childbirth as she makes choices about the measures that are best for her. She should be encouraged to write a birth plan that lists her preferences for pain relief measures. Using these measures requires the woman's active participation and support from her partner and caregivers.

The woman who chooses to deal with childbirth pain by using nonpharmacologic methods needs care and support from nurses and other care providers who are skilled in pain management. Many of the nonpharmacologic methods for relief of discomfort are taught in different types of prenatal preparation classes, or the woman or couple may have read various books and magazine articles on the subject in advance. Many of these methods require practice for best results (e.g., hypnosis, patterned breathing and controlled relaxation techniques, biofeedback), although the nurse may use some of them successfully without the woman or couple having prior knowledge (e.g., slow paced breathing, massage and touch, effleurage, counterpressure). Women should be encouraged to try a variety of methods and to seek alternatives, including pharmacologic methods, if the measure being used is no longer effective (Box 19-1).

BOX 19-1 Nonpharmacologic Strategies to Encourage Relaxation and Relieve Pain

CUTANEOUS STIMULATION STRATEGIES
Counterpressure*
Effleurage (light massage)*
Therapeutic touch and massage*
Walking*
Rocking*
Changing positions*
Application of heat or cold*
Transcutaneous electrical nerve stimulation
Acupressure
Water therapy (hydrotherapy)
Intradermal water block

SENSORY STIMULATION STRATEGIES
Aromatherapy
Breathing techniques*
Music*
Imagery*
Use of focal points*

COGNITIVE STRATEGIES
Childbirth education*
Hypnosis
Biofeedback

*Forms of care likely to be beneficial (Enkin et al., 2000).

Childbirth Preparation Methods

Most health care providers recommend or offer childbirth preparation classes to expectant parents. The major methods taught in the United States are the Dick-Read method, or natural childbirth method; the Lamaze method, or psychoprophylactic method (PPM); and the Bradley method, or husband-coached childbirth. These methods are discussed in more detail in Chapter 17.

Relaxing and Breathing Techniques

Focusing and Relaxation

By reducing tension and stress, focusing and relaxation techniques allow a woman in labor to rest and to conserve energy for the task of giving birth. Attention-focusing and distraction techniques are forms of care likely to be beneficial in relieving labor pain (Enkin et al., 2000). Some women bring a favorite object such as a photograph or stuffed animal to the labor room and focus their attention on this object during contractions. Others choose to fix their attention on some object in the labor room. As the contraction begins, they focus on their chosen object and perform a breathing technique to reduce their perception of pain.

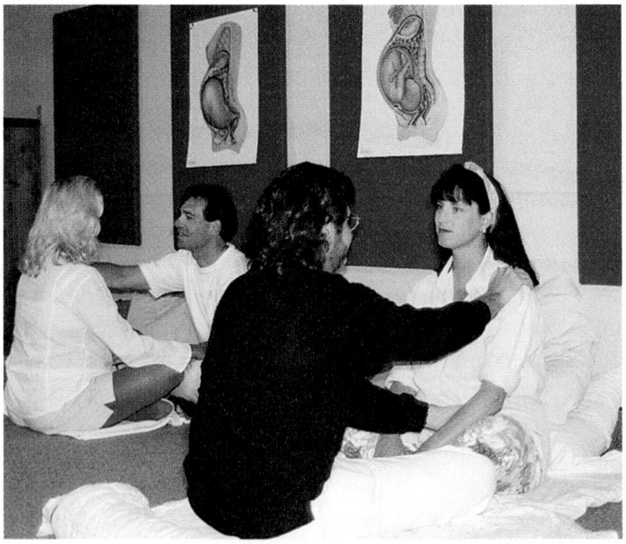

FIG. 19-2 Expectant parents learning relaxation techniques. (Courtesy Marjorie Pyle, RNC, Lifecircle, Costa Mesa, CA.)

With imagery, the woman focuses her attention on a pleasant scene, a place where she feels relaxed, or an activity she enjoys. She can imagine walking through a restful garden or breathing in light, energy, and healing color and breathing out worries and tension. Choosing the subject for the imagery and practicing the technique during pregnancy will enhance effectiveness during labor (Hoffart & Pross-Keene, 1998). These techniques, coupled with feedback relaxation, help the woman work with her contractions rather than against them. The support person monitors this process, telling the woman when to begin the breathing techniques (Fig. 19-2).

During childbirth preparation classes (e.g., Lamaze), the coach can learn how to palpate a woman's body to detect tense and contracted muscles. The woman then learns how to relax the tense muscle in response to the gentle stroking of the muscle by the coach (Fig. 19-3). In a common feedback mechanism, the woman and her coach say the word "relax" at the onset of each contraction and throughout it as needed. With practice, the coach can effectively use support, feedback, and touch to facilitate the woman's relaxation and thereby reduce tension and stress and enhance the progress of labor (Nichols & Humenick, 2000). The nurse can assist the woman by providing a quiet environment and offering cues as needed.

Breathing Techniques

Different approaches to childbirth preparation stress varying breathing techniques to provide distraction, thereby reducing the perception of pain and helping the woman maintain control throughout contractions. In the first stage of labor, such breathing techniques can promote relaxation of the abdominal muscles and thereby increase the size of the abdominal cavity. This lessens discomfort generated by friction between the uterus and abdominal wall during contractions. Because the muscles of the genital area also become more relaxed, they do not interfere with fetal descent. In the second stage, breathing is used to increase abdominal pressure and thereby assist in expelling the fetus. Breathing also can be used to relax the pudendal muscles to prevent precipitate expulsion of the fetal head.

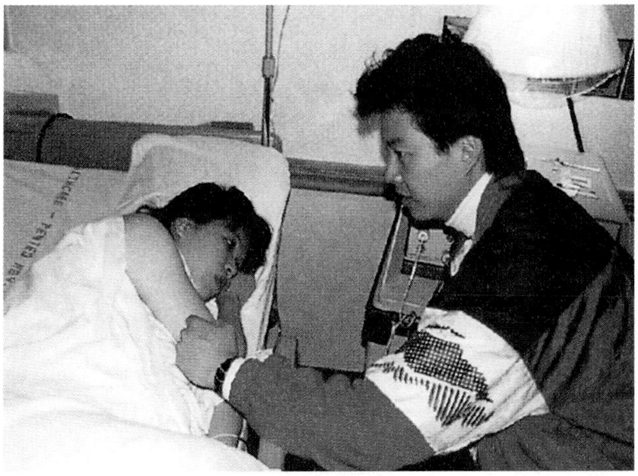

FIG. 19-2 Laboring woman using focusing and breathing techniques during a uterine contraction with coaching from her partner. (Courtesy Marjorie Pyle, RNC, Lifecircle, Costa Mesa, CA.)

For couples who have prepared for labor by practicing relaxing and breathing techniques, occasional reminders may be all that are necessary to help them along. For those who have had no preparation, instruction in simple breathing and relaxation can be given early in labor and often is surprisingly successful. Motivation is high, and readiness to learn is enhanced by the reality of labor.

There are various breathing techniques for controlling pain during contractions (Box 19-2). The nurse needs to ascertain what, if any, techniques the laboring couple knows before giving them instruction. Simple patterns are more easily learned. Paced breathing is the technique most associated with prepared childbirth. The Lamaze method uses slow-paced, modified-paced, and patterned-paced breathing techniques with the understanding that each labor is different and that couples need to adapt breathing techniques to their individual labor experience.

All patterns begin with a routine deep relaxing cleansing breath to "greet the contraction" and end with another deep breath exhaled to "gently blow the contraction away." In general, slow-paced breathing, at approximately half the woman's normal breathing rate, is initiated when the woman can no longer walk or talk through contractions. She should continue to use this technique for as long as it is effective in reducing the perception of pain and maintaining control. As contractions increase in frequency and intensity, the woman often needs to change to a more complex breathing technique, which is shallower and approximately twice her normal rate of breathing. This modified-paced pattern requires more concentration and therefore, blocks more painful stimuli than the simpler slow-paced breathing pattern (Nichols & Humenick, 2000; Shapiro et al., 1997).

The most difficult time to maintain control during contractions comes when the cervix dilates from 8 cm to 10 cm. This phase is the *transition phase* of the first stage of labor. Even for the woman who has prepared for labor, concentration on breathing techniques is difficult to maintain. The patterned-paced breathing technique is used during this phase. It may be the 4:1 pattern: breath, breath, breath, breath, blow (as though gently blowing out a candle). This ratio may be increased to 6:1 or 8:1. An undesirable side effect of this type of breathing is **hyperventilation.** The woman and her support person must be aware of and watch for symptoms of the resultant respiratory alkalosis: light-headedness, dizziness, tingling of the fingers, or circumoral numbness. Respiratory alkalosis may be eliminated by having the woman breathe into a paper bag held tightly around the mouth and nose. This enables her to rebreathe carbon dioxide and replace

BOX 19-2 Breathing Techniques

CLEANSING BREATH
Relaxed breath in through nose and out mouth. Used at the beginning and end of each contraction.

SLOW-PACED BREATHING (APPROXIMATELY 6 TO 9 BREATHS PER MINUTE)
Not less than half normal breathing rate (no. breaths/min divided by 2)
IN-2-3-4/OUT-2-3-4/IN-2-3-4/OUT-2-3-4 …

MODIFIED-PACED BREATHING (APPROXIMATELY 32 TO 40 BREATHS PER MINUTE)
Not more than twice normal breathing rate (no. breaths/min times 2)
IN-OUT/IN-OUT/IN-OUT/IN-OUT …
For more flexibility and variety, the woman may combine the slow and modified breathing by using the slow breathing for beginnings and ends of contractions and modified breathing for more intense peaks. This technique conserves energy, lessens fatigue, and decreases the chance of hypoventilation.

PATTERNED-PACED BREATHING (SAME RATE AS MODIFIED)
Enhances concentration

a. 3:1 Patterned breathing
IN-OUT/IN-OUT/IN-OUT/IN-BLOW
(repeat through contraction)

b. Patterned breathing
IN-OUT/IN-OUT/IN-OUT/IN-OUT/IN-BLOW
(repeat through contraction)
You may do any pattern desired, although ratios of 5:1 or higher tend to be very tiring. Some people like to do patterned breathing to a tune ("Yankee Doodle," "Old McDonald"), to a repeated phrase ("I think I can, I think I can"), or in a pyramid pattern such as 1:1, 2:1, 3:1, 4:1, 5:1—5:1, 4:1, 3:1, 2:1, 1:1.

c. *Coach call:* May be used when the woman needs more distraction and concentration (e.g., during transition). The woman's coach signals the breathing ratio with his or her fingers or by verbal cues, changing the ratio after each "IN-BLOW."
Example:
IN-OUT/IN-OUT/IN-BLOW
IN-OUT/IN-OUT/IN-OUT/IN-OUT/IN-BLOW
IN-OUT/IN-BLOW

From Shapiro, H. et al. (1997). *The Lamaze ready reference guide for labor and birth* (2nd ed.). Washington, DC: Chapter ASPO/Lamaze.

the bicarbonate ion. The woman also can breathe into her cupped hands if no bag is available. Maintaining a breathing rate that is no more than twice the normal rate will lessen chances of hyperventilation. The partner can help the woman maintain her breathing rate with visual, tactile, or auditory cues (Nichols & Humenick, 2000; Shapiro et al., 1997).

As the fetal head reaches the pelvic floor, the woman may feel the urge to push and may automatically begin to exert downward pressure by contracting her abdominal muscles. Nurses guide couples in the application of breathing and relaxation methods during labor, adapting methods to their particular needs, and using pushing techniques for birth that avoid a Valsalva response (Sampselle, 1999). Such techniques often involve moaning or other noises as women push without holding their breath.

The woman can control the urge to push by taking panting breaths or by slowly exhaling through pursed lips. This type of breathing can be used to overcome the urge to push when the cervix is not fully prepared (e.g., less than 8 cm dilated, not retracting) and to facilitate a slow birth of the fetal head.

Effleurage and Counterpressure

Effleurage (light massage) and counterpressure have brought relief to many women during the first stage of labor. The gate-control theory may supply the reason for the effectiveness of these measures. **Effleurage** is light stroking, usually of the abdomen, in rhythm with breathing during contractions. It is used to distract the woman from contraction pain. Often the presence of monitor belts makes it difficult to perform effleurage on the abdomen; thus a thigh or the chest may be used. As labor progresses, hyperesthesia may make effleurage uncomfortable and thus less effective.

Counterpressure is steady pressure applied by a support person to the sacral area with the fist or heel of the hand. This technique helps the woman cope with the sensations of internal pressure and pain in the lower back. It is especially helpful when back pain is caused by pressure of the occiput against spinal nerves when the fetal head is in a posterior position. Counterpressure lifts the occiput off these nerves, thereby providing pain relief. Although not scientifically evaluated, pressure also may be applied bilaterally to the hips or knees to reduce low back pain (Simkin & Ancheta, 2000). The support person will need to be relieved occasionally because application of counterpressure is hard work.

Music

Music, taped or live, enhances relaxation during labor, thereby reducing stress, anxiety, and the perception of pain. It can be used to promote relaxation in early labor and to stimulate movement as labor progresses. Women should be taught about the effectiveness of using music during labor for relaxation and for reduction of the perception of pain. They should be encouraged to prepare their musical preferences in advance and bring their tape or compact disc player to the hospital or birthing center. Use of a headset or earphones may increase the effectiveness of the music because other sounds will be shut out. Live music provided at the bedside by a support person may also be very helpful in transmitting energy that decreases tension and elevates mood (Gentz, 2001). A study of Lamaze-trained women suggested that women who listened to ocean waves and Baroque and New Age music demonstrated an improvement in relaxation responses when compared with women who used only progressive relaxation techniques (Wiand, 1997). Changing the tempo of the music to coincide with the rate and rhythm of each breathing technique may facilitate proper pacing (Gentz, 2001; Nichols & Humenick, 2000).

Water (Hydrotherapy) Therapy

Bathing, showering, and jet hydrotherapy (whirlpool baths) with warm water (e.g., at or below body temperature) are nonpharmacologic measures that can be used to promote comfort and relaxation during labor (Fig. 19-4). Sitting in a tub of water up to the shoulders or lower for 1 to 2 hours has several immediate benefits. Buoyancy in the water results in general body relaxation and temporary relief from discomfort and pain. This reduces the woman's anxiety and enhances a feeling of well-being. Catecholamine production decreases. This triggers an increase in the levels of oxytocin (to stimulate uterine contractions) and endorphins (to reduce pain perception). In addition, the bubbles and gentle lapping of the water stimulate the nipples, also triggering an increase in oxytocin production; this has not been observed to cause uterine hyperstimulation. The cervix has often been observed to dilate 2 to 3 cm in 30 minutes of whirlpool therapy. In addition, it promotes diuresis and a decrease in blood pressure (Simkin, 1995). Whirlpool baths in labor also have been found to have positive effects on analgesia requirements, instrumentation rates, condition of the perineum, and personal satisfaction with labor (Simkin & O'Hara, 2002).

If the woman is having "back labor" as the result of an occiput posterior or transverse position, she is encouraged to assume the hands-and-knees or the side-lying position in the tub. Because these positions decrease pain and increase relaxation and production of oxytocin, the fetus can then rotate spontaneously to the occiput anterior position. Less effort is required when changing positions in water.

In some settings, jet hydrotherapy should be approved by the woman's primary health care provider. The woman's vital signs must be within normal limits, and she should be in the active phase of the first stage of labor (e.g., cervix at least 5 cm dilated). If she is in the latent phase, her contractions could slow (Mackey, 2001).

Fetal heart rate (FHR) monitoring is done by Doppler device, fetoscope, or wireless external monitor device (see Fig. 19-4, *C*). Placement of internal electrodes is contraindicated for jet hydrotherapy. The woman's membranes may be intact or ruptured. If they are ruptured, the fluid must be clear or only lightly stained with meconium (Mackey, 2001).

There is no limit to the time women can stay in the bath, and often women are encouraged to stay in it as long as desired. However, most women use jet hydrotherapy for

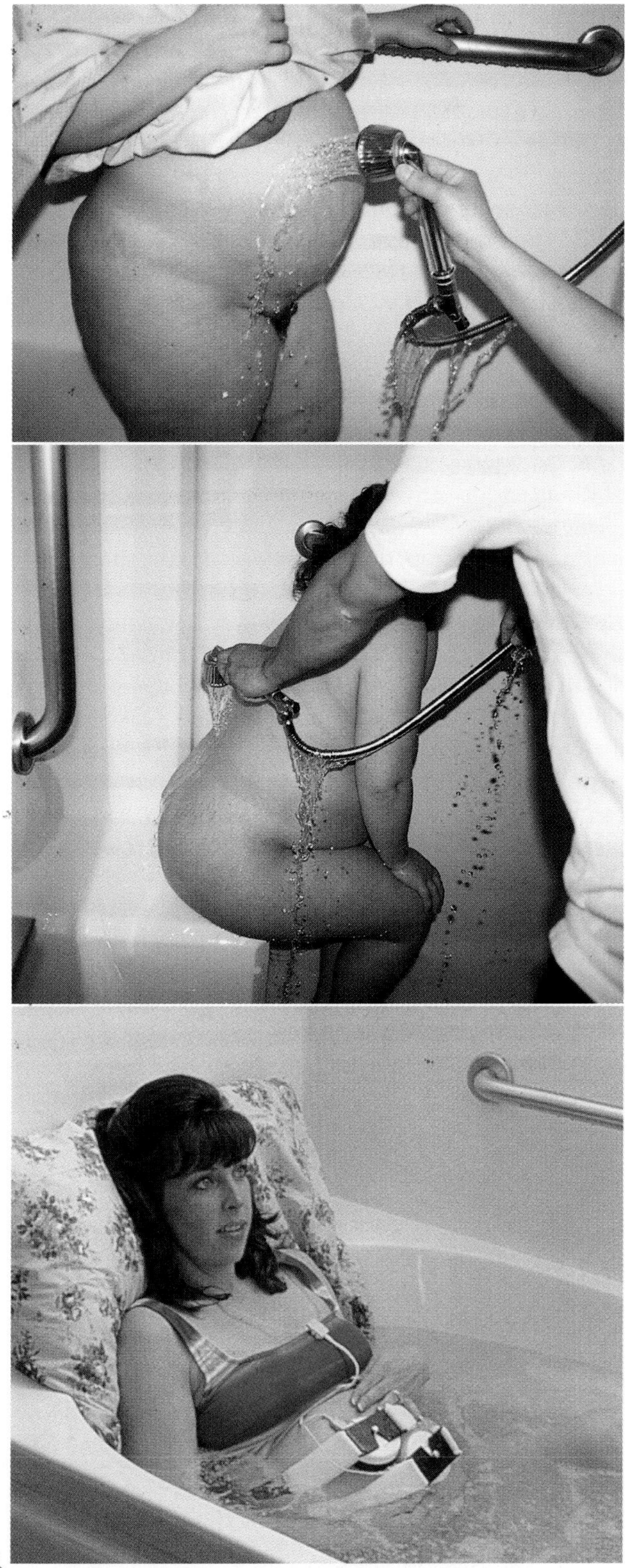

A

B

C

FIG. 19-4 Water therapy during labor. **A,** Use of shower during labor. **B,** Woman experiencing back labor relaxes as partner sprays warm water on her back. **C,** Laboring woman relaxes in jacuzzi. Note that fetal monitoring can continue during time in the jacuzzi. (**A, B,** Courtesy Marjorie Pyle, RNC, Lifecircle, Costa Mesa, CA. **C,** Courtesy Spacelabs Medical, Redmond, WA.)

30 to 60 minutes at a time. During the bath, if the woman's temperature and the FHR increase, if the labor process becomes less effective (e.g., slows or becomes too intense), or if relief of pain is reduced, the woman can come out of the bath and return at a later time. Repeated baths with occasional breaks may be more effective in relieving pain in long labors than unlimited amounts of time in the water. Fluids to maintain hydration and a cool face cloth for comfort are offered during the bath (Mackey, 2001; Simkin & O'Hara, 2002).

Transcutaneous Electrical Nerve Stimulation

Transcutaneous electrical nerve stimulation (TENS) involves the placing of two pairs of flat electrodes on either side of the woman's thoracic and sacral spine (Fig. 19-5). These electrodes provide continuous low-intensity electrical impulses or stimuli from a battery-operated device. During a contraction, the woman increases the stimulation from low to high intensity by turning control knobs on the device. High intensity should be maintained for at least 1 minute to facilitate release of endorphins. Women describe the resulting sensation as a tingling or buzzing and the pain relief as good or very good. TENS is most useful for lower back pain during the early first stage of labor. Using TENS poses no risk to the mother or fetus, and it is credited with reducing or eliminating the need for analgesia and with increasing the woman's perception of control over the experience. It may be effective because of the placebo effect; that is, confidence in the effectiveness of TENS may stimulate the release of endogenous opiates (endorphins) in the woman's body and thus alleviate the discomfort (Gentz, 2001; Scott et al., 1999). TENS is now considered a form of care with insufficient quality data to recommend its use (Enkin et al., 2000). The nurse assists the woman in using TENS by explaining the device and its use, by carefully placing and securing the electrodes, and by closely evaluating its effectiveness.

Acupressure

Acupressure techniques can be used in pregnancy, labor, and postpartum to relieve pain and other discomforts. Pressure, heat, or cold is applied to acupuncture points called *tsubos*. These points have an increased density of neuroreceptors and increased electrical conductivity. The effectiveness of acupressure has been attributed to the gate-control theory of pain and an increase in endorphin levels (Tiran & Mack, 2000). Acupressure is best applied over the skin without using lubricants. Pressure is usually applied with the heel of the hand, fist, or pads of the thumbs and fingers (Fig. 19-6). Tennis balls or other devices also may be used to apply pressure. Pressure is applied with contractions initially and then continuously as labor progresses to the transition phase at the end of the first stage of labor. Synchronized breathing by the caregiver and the woman is suggested for greater effectiveness. Acupressure points are found on the neck, shoulders, wrists, lower back including sacral points, hips, below the kneecaps, ankles, nails on the small toes, and soles of the feet.

Application of Heat and Cold

Warmed blankets, warm compresses, heated rice bags, a warm bath or shower, or a moist heating pad can enhance relaxation and reduce pain during labor. Heat relieves muscle ischemia and increases blood flow to the area of discomfort. Heat application is effective for back pain caused by a posterior presentation or general backache from fatigue (Simkin, 1995).

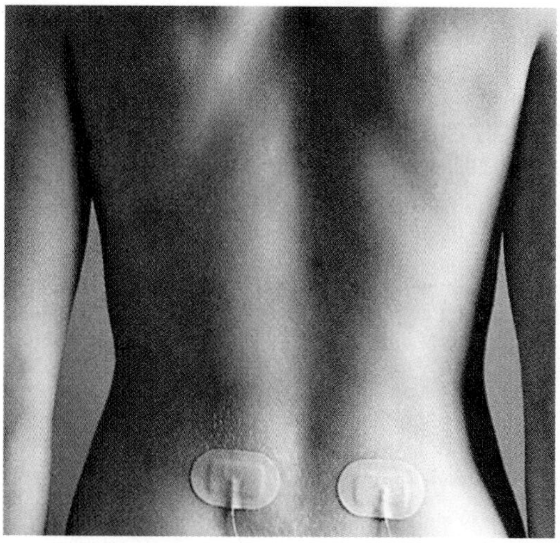

FIG. 19-5 Placement of transcutaneous electrical nerve stimulation electrodes on back for relief of labor pain.

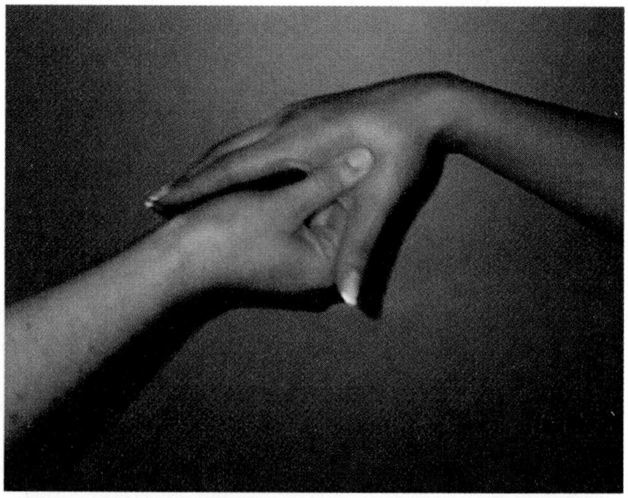

FIG. 19-6 Ho-Ku acupressure point (back of hand where thumb and index finger come together) used to enhance uterine contractions without increasing pain. (From Dickason, E., Silverman, B., & Kaplan, J. [1998]. *Maternal-infant nursing care* [3rd ed.]. St. Louis: Mosby.)

Cold application such as cool cloths or ice packs may be effective in increasing comfort when the woman feels warm and may be applied to areas of pain. Cooling relieves pain by reducing the muscle temperature and relieving muscle spasms (Simkin, 1995).

Heat and cold may be used alternately for a greater effect. Neither heat nor cold should be applied over ischemic or anesthetized areas because tissues can be damaged.

Touch and Massage

Touch and massage have been an integral part of the traditional care process for women in labor. They are likely to be beneficial in relieving labor pain (Enkin et al., 2000).

Touch can be as simple as holding the woman's hand, stroking her body, and embracing her. When using touch to communicate caring, reassurance, and concern, it is important that the woman's preferences for touch (e.g., who can touch her, where they can touch her, and how they can touch her) and responses to touch be determined (Simkin & O'Hara, 2002). Touch also can involve very specialized techniques that require manipulation of the human energy field. Therapeutic touch (TT) uses the concept of energy fields within the body called *prana*. Prana are thought to be deficient in some people who are in pain. TT uses laying-on of hands by a specially trained person to redirect energy fields associated with pain (Schieber & Selby, 2000). Research has demonstrated effectiveness of TT to enhance relaxation, reduce anxiety, and relieve pain (Nichols & Humenick, 2000); however, little is known about the use or effectiveness of TT for relieving labor pain.

Healing touch (HT) is another energy-based healing modality. Whereas TT emphasizes a single sequence of energy modulation, HT combines a variety of techniques from a series of disciplines. This gives the practitioner an array of "tools" to use with clients. Practitioners are taught energetic diagnosis and treatment forms and the means of documenting the client's response and progress. These techniques are said to align and balance the human energy field, thereby enhancing the body's ability to heal itself. HT has been used in labor management, but no studies have been published about its effectiveness (Hover-Kramer et al., 2001) (see Fig. 4-4).

Head, hand, back, and foot massage may be very effective in reducing tension and enhancing comfort. Hand and foot massage may be especially relaxing in advanced labor when hyperesthesia limits a woman's tolerance for touch on other parts of her body. The woman and her partner should be encouraged to experiment with different types of massage during pregnancy to determine what might feel best and be most relaxing during labor.

Hypnosis

Hypnosis, although not commonly used for pain management in the United States, is associated with shorter labors and less analgesia (Tiran & Mack, 2000). Hypnosis techniques used for labor and birth place an emphasis on enhancing relaxation and diminishing fear, anxiety, and perception of pain. The woman may be given direct suggestions about pain relief or indirect suggestions that she is experiencing diminished sensations. The woman receives posthypnotic suggestions, such as, "You will be able to push the baby out easily," to increase her confidence. To be successful, the woman must be educated regarding hypnosis and practice the techniques during the prenatal period (Gentz, 2001).

Biofeedback

Biofeedback may provide another relaxation technique that can be used for labor. Biofeedback is based on the theory that if a person can recognize physical signals, certain internal physiologic events can be changed (i.e., whatever signs the woman has that are associated with her pain). During the prenatal period, the woman must be educated to become aware of her body and its responses and how to relax for biofeedback to be effective. The woman must learn how to use thinking and mental processes (e.g., focusing) to control body responses and functions. Informational biofeedback helps couples develop awareness of their bodies and use strategies to change their responses to stress. If the woman responds to pain during a contraction with tightening of muscles, frowning, moaning, and breath holding, her partner uses verbal and touch feedback to help her relax. Formal biofeedback, which uses machines to detect skin temperature, blood flow, or muscle tension, also can prepare women to intensify their relaxation responses (Gentz, 2001; Snyder & Lindquist, 2000).

Aromatherapy

Aromatherapy uses oils distilled from plants, flowers, herbs, and trees to promote health and well-being and treat illnesses. The use of herbal teas and vapors is reported to have good effects in pregnancy and labor for some women (Tiran & Mack, 2000). Lavender, clary sage, and bergamot promote relaxation and can be used by adding a few drops to a warm bath, to warm water used for soaking compresses that can be applied to the body, to an aromatherapy lamp to vaporize a room, or to oil for a back massage (Tiran & Mack, 2000).

NURSE ALERT

Caution: Never apply the essential oils used for aromatherapy in full strength directly to the skin. Most oils should be diluted in a vegetable oil base before use. In addition, essential oils vary in terms of safe use during pregnancy (Gentz, 2001).

Intradermal Water Block

An intradermal water block involves the injection of small amounts of sterile water (e.g., 0.05 to 0.1 ml) by using a fine needle (e.g., 25 gauge) into four locations on the lower back to relieve back pain. It may be effective in early labor and in an effort to delay the initiation of pharmacologic pain relief measures. Stinging will occur for about 20 to 30 seconds after injection, but back pain will be relieved for approximately 45 minutes to 2 hours. Effectiveness of this method may be related to the mechanisms of counterirritation (i.e., reducing localized pain in one area by irritating the skin in an area nearby), gate control, or an increase in the level of endogenous opioids (endorphins). When the effect wears off, the treatment can be repeated, or another method of pain relief can be used (Gentz, 2001; Simkin & O'Hara, 2002).

PHARMACOLOGIC MANAGEMENT OF DISCOMFORT

Pharmacologic measures for pain management should be implemented before pain becomes so severe that catecholamines increase and labor is prolonged. Pharmacologic and nonpharmacologic measures, when used together, increase the level of pain relief and create a more positive labor experience for the woman and her family. Nonpharmacologic measures can be used for relaxation and for pain relief, especially in early labor. Pharmacologic measures can be implemented as labor becomes more active and discomfort and pain intensify. Less pharmacologic intervention often is required because nonpharmacologic measures enhance relaxation and potentiate the analgesic's effect (Faucher & Brucker, 2000).

Sedatives

Sedatives such as barbiturates relieve anxiety and induce sleep. They should be used only in prodromal or early latent labor and in the absence of pain. If the woman is feeling pain, sedatives given without an analgesic may increase apprehension and cause the woman to become hyperactive and disoriented. Undesirable side effects include respiratory and vasomotor depression affecting the woman and newborn. These effects are increased if a barbiturate is administered with another central nervous system (CNS) depressant such as an opioid analgesic. Because of these disadvantages, barbiturates are seldom used (Faucher & Brucker, 2000; Scott et al., 1999). Instead of a barbiturate, morphine, an opioid-agonist analgesic, can be used during prodromal labor to achieve the dual effect of sedation and analgesia. Morphine is seldom used in active labor because it is longer acting than other opioid analgesics and causes greater CNS depression, especially related to respiratory function (Hawkins et al., 2002). Administered intramuscularly, morphine's onset of action is 10 to 30 minutes, but the onset of action is rapid when it is administered intravenously. The duration of morphine's effect for both routes is 4 to 5 hours. Because morphine releases histamine, it should be avoided or used cautiously in women with asthma (Lehne, 2001).

Analgesia and Anesthesia

The use of analgesia and anesthesia was not generally accepted as part of obstetric management until Queen Victoria used chloroform during the birth of her son in 1853. Since then, much study has gone into the development of pharmacologic measures for controlling discomfort during the birth period. The goal of researchers is to develop methods that will provide adequate pain relief to women without increasing maternal or fetal risk or affecting the progress of labor.

Nursing management of obstetric analgesia and anesthesia combines the nurse's expertise in maternity care with a knowledge and understanding of anatomy and physiology and of medications and their therapeutic effects, adverse reactions, and methods of administration.

Anesthesia encompasses analgesia, amnesia, relaxation, and reflex activity. Anesthesia abolishes pain perception by interrupting the nerve impulses to the brain. The loss of sensation may be partial or complete, sometimes with the loss of consciousness.

The term **analgesia** refers to the alleviation of the sensation of pain or the raising of the threshold for pain perception without loss of consciousness.

The type of analgesic or anesthetic chosen is determined in part by the stage of labor of the woman and by the method of birth planned (Box 19-3).

Systemic Analgesia

Systemic analgesia remains the major pharmacologic method for relieving the pain of labor when personnel trained in regional analgesia (e.g., epidural analgesia) are not available (Bricker & Lavender, 2002; Caton et al., 2002; Scott et al., 1999). It is a form of care with a trade-off between beneficial and adverse effects (Enkin et al., 2000). Systemic analgesics cross the maternal blood-brain barrier to provide central analgesic effects. They also cross through the placenta. Once transferred to the fetus, analgesics cross the fetal blood-brain barrier more readily than the maternal blood-brain barrier. The duration of action also will be longer because the systemic analgesics used during labor have a significantly longer half-life in the fetus and newborn. Effects on the fetus and newborn can be profound (e.g., respiratory depression, decreased alertness, delayed sucking), depending on the characteristics of the specific systemic analgesic used, the dosage given, and the route and timing of administration. Intravenous (IV) administration is preferred to intramuscular (IM) administration because the medication's onset of action is faster and more predictable; as a result, a higher level of pain relief usually occurs. IV patient-controlled analgesia (PCA) is now available for use during labor. With this method, the woman self-administers small doses of an opioid analgesic by using a pump programmed for dose and frequency. Overall, a lower total amount of analgesic is used, and maternal satisfaction is high (Bricker & Lavender, 2002). Classifications of analgesic drugs used to relieve the pain of childbirth include opioid (narcotic) agonists and opioid (narcotic) agonist-antagonists. Co-drugs such as tranquilizers (ataractics), antiemetics, and benzodiazepines can be used to potentiate the analgesic effect of opioids and reduce adverse reactions such as nausea and vomiting.

Opioid (Narcotic) Agonist Analgesics. Opioid agonist analgesics such as meperidine (Demerol) and fentanyl (Sublimaze) are especially effective for relieving severe, persistent, or recurrent pain. They have no amnesic effect but create a feeling of well-being or euphoria. These analgesics decrease gastric emptying and increase nausea and vomiting. Bladder and bowel elimination can be inhibited. Because heart rate (e.g., bradycardia, tachycardia), blood pressure (e.g., hypotension), and respiratory effort (e.g., depression) can be adversely affected, opioid analgesics should be used cautiously in women with respiratory and cardiovascular disorders. Safety precautions should be taken because sedation and dizziness can occur after administration, increasing the risk for injury. Research findings suggest that women who receive opioids for their labor pain have less effective pain relief and are less satisfied with their pain management method than women whose pain is managed by using epidural analgesia. Conversely, opioid use is associated with shorter labors, less oxytocin augmentation, and fewer instrumental vaginal births (e.g., forceps-assisted, or vacuum-assisted birth) when compared with epidural analgesia (Bricker & Lavender, 2001; Caton et al., 2002; Leighton & Halpern, 2002).

Meperidine is the most commonly used opioid agonist analgesic for women in labor throughout the world (Scott et al., 1999). It overcomes inhibitory factors in labor and may even relax the cervix. After IV injection, the onset of action is rapid (30 to 60 seconds), the peak effect is reached in 5 to 7 minutes, and the duration of action is approximately 2 to 4 hours. The onset of action begins in 10 to 15 minutes after an IM injection of meperidine; the peak is reached in 30 to 50 minutes; and the duration of action is 2 to 4 hours. Ideally, birth should occur less than 1 hour or more than 4 hours after administration so that neonatal CNS depression resulting from meperidine is minimized. Because tachycardia is a possible adverse reaction, meperidine is used cautiously in women with cardiac disease (Bricker & Lavender, 2002; Faucher & Brucker, 2000; Hawkins et al., 2002; Lehne, 2001) (see Medication Guide).

Fentanyl is a potent, short-acting opioid agonist analgesic (see Medication Guide). Onset of the medication action after IV injection occurs within 2 minutes; the action peaks in 3 to 5 minutes; and the duration of action is about 30 to 60 minutes. Onset of the medication action occurs in 7 to 8 minutes after IM injection, reaches its peak effect in 20 to 30 minutes, and lasts for 1 to 2 hours. More frequent dosing is required with fentanyl because of its shorter duration of action. Additive CNS and respiratory depression occurs if fentanyl is given with alcohol, antihistamines, antidepressants, or sedative-hypnotics. Fentanyl is commonly used alone or in combination with a local anesthetic agent for induction of spinal nerve block analgesia (Faucher & Brucker, 2000; Lehne, 2001) (see Medication Guide).

Opioid (Narcotic) Agonist-Antagonist Analgesics. An agonist is an agent that activates or stimulates a receptor to act; an antagonist is an agent that blocks a receptor or a medication designed to activate a receptor. **Opioid agonist-antagonist analgesics** such as butorphanol (Stadol) and nalbuphine (Nubain), in the doses used during labor, provide adequate analgesia without causing significant respiratory depression in the mother or neonate. They are less likely to cause nausea and vomiting when compared with meperidine, but sedation may be as great or greater. Both IM and IV routes of administration are used. This classification of opioid analgesics is not suitable for women with an opioid dependence because the antagonist activity could precipitate withdrawal symptoms (abstinence syndrome) in both the mother and her newborn (Hawkins et al., 2002;

BOX *19-3* **Pharmacologic Control of Discomfort by Stage of Labor and Method of Birth**

FIRST STAGE
- Systemic analgesia
  - Opioid agonist analgesics
  - Opioid agonist-antagonist analgesics, co-drugs
- Epidural (block) analgesia
- Combined spinal epidural (CSE) analgesia
- Paracervical block (rarely used)
- Nitrous oxide

SECOND STAGE
- Nerve block analgesia/anesthesia
  - Local infiltration anesthesia
  - Pudendal block
  - Spinal (block) anesthesia
  - Epidural (block) analgesia
  - Combined spinal-epidural (CSE) analgesia
- Nitrous oxide

VAGINAL BIRTH
- Local infiltration anesthesia
- Pudendal block
- Epidural (block) analgesia/anesthesia
- Spinal (block) anesthesia
- Combined spinal-epidural (CSE) analgesia/anesthesia
- Nitrous oxide

CESAREAN BIRTH
- Spinal (block) anesthesia
- Epidural (block) anesthesia
- General anesthesia

MEDICATION GUIDE
Opioid Analgesics for Labor

Meperidine (Demerol)

ACTION ▪ Opioid agonist analgesic; stimulates mu and kappa opioid receptors to decrease transmission of pain impulses
INDICATION ▪ Labor pain; postoperative pain after cesarean birth
DOSAGE AND ROUTE ▪ 25 mg IV; 50-75 mg IM/SC. May repeat in 1-3 hr; use of co-drugs may potentiate analgesic effect and decrease nausea and vomiting.
ADVERSE EFFECTS ▪ Nausea and vomiting, sedation, confusion, drowsiness, tachycardia or bradycardia, hypotension, dry mouth, pruritis, urinary retention, respiratory depression (woman and newborn), decreased fetal heart rate (FHR) variability, decreased uterine activity if given in early labor
NURSING CONSIDERATIONS ▪ Assess FHR and uterine activity; observe for respiratory depression; if birth occurs within 1-4 hr of dose, observe newborn for respiratory depression; have naloxone available as antidote; keep side rails up; continue use of nonpharmacologic pain relief measures

Butorphanol Tartrate (Stadol)

ACTION ▪ Mixed agonist-antagonist analgesic; stimulates kappa opioid receptor and blocks mu opioid receptor
INDICATION ▪ Labor pain; postoperative pain after cesarean birth
DOSAGE AND ROUTE ▪ 1 mg IV q3-4 hr; 2 mg IM q3-4 hr
ADVERSE EFFECTS ▪ Confusion, sedation, sweating; transient sinusoidal-like FHR rhythm; less respiratory depression, nausea and vomiting
NURSING CONSIDERATIONS ▪ See meperidine; may precipitate withdrawal symptoms in opioid-dependent women and their newborns

Nalbuphine (Nubain)

ACTION ▪ Mixed agonist-antagonist analgesic; stimulates kappa opioid receptor and blocks mu opioid receptor
INDICATION ▪ Labor pain; postoperative pain after cesarean birth
DOSAGE AND ROUTE ▪ 10 mg IV; 10-20 mg IM q3-6 hr
ADVERSE EFFECTS ▪ See butorphanol
NURSING CONSIDERATIONS ▪ See butorphanol

MEDICATION GUIDE
Fentanyl (Sublimaze) and Sufentanil (Sufenta)

ACTION ▪ Opioid analgesics, rapid action with short duration (1-2 hr IM; ½-1 hr IV)
INDICATION ▪ For epidural or intrathecal analgesia, alone or in combination with a local anesthetic
DOSAGE AND ROUTE ▪ Fentanyl—IM 50 to 100 μg; IV 25 to 50 μg. Epidural—fentanyl, 1 to 2 μg with 0.125% bupivacaine at rate of 8 to 10 ml/hr; sufentanil, 1 μg with 0.125% bupivacaine at rate of 10 ml/hr.
ADVERSE EFFECTS ▪ Dizziness, drowsiness, allergic reactions, rash, pruritus, respiratory depression, nausea and vomiting, urinary retention
NURSING CONSIDERATIONS ▪ Assess for respiratory depression; naloxone should be available as antidote

MEDICATION GUIDE
Naloxone (Narcan)

ACTION ▪ Opioid antagonist
INDICATION ▪ Reverses opioid-induced respiratory depression in woman or newborn; may be used to reverse pruritis from epidural opioids
DOSAGE AND ROUTE ▪ Adult, 0.1-0.2 mg IV q2-3 min until adequate reversal; repeat q1-2 hr if needed. Newborn, 0.01 mg/kg IV, IM, SC q2-3 min until adequate reversal; repeat q1-2 hr if needed.
ADVERSE EFFECTS ▪ Maternal hypotension and hypertension, tachycardia, nausea and vomiting, sweating, and tremulousness
NURSING CONSIDERATIONS ▪ Woman should delay breastfeeding until medication is out of system; do not give if woman is opioid dependent—may cause abrupt withdrawal; if given to woman for reversal of respiratory depression due to opioid analgesic, pain will return suddenly

Lehne, 2001) (see Medication Guide and Signs of Potential Complications box).

Co-Drugs. Medications such as **ataractics** (tranquilizers) can be used to augment or potentiate the desirable effects but few of the undesirable effects of the opioid analgesics. Ataractics such as the phenothiazines (e.g., promethazine [Phenergan], hydroxyzine [Vistaril]) do not relieve pain but decrease anxiety and apprehension, increase sedation, and potentiate opioid analgesic effects. This potentiation effect causes the two drugs to work together more effectively, so the opioid dose can be reduced. In addition, ataractics can be used to reduce the nausea and vomiting that often accompany opioid use. Metoclopramide (Reglan) is an antiemetic that also can be used for this purpose. Benzodiazepines (e.g., diazepam [Valium], lorazepam [Ativan]), when given with an opioid analgesic, seem to enhance pain relief and reduce nausea and vomiting, although the increased sedation experienced may be unacceptable to women in labor (Bricker & Lavender, 2002; Lehne, 2001). Although data are limited, fetal or neonatal problems appear infrequently when women are given therapeutic doses of these co-drugs.

Opioid (Narcotic) Antagonists. Opioids such as meperidine and fentanyl can cause excessive CNS depres-

SIGNS OF **POTENTIAL COMPLICATIONS**

Maternal Opioid Abstinence Syndrome (Opioid/Narcotic Withdrawal)

- Yawning, rhinorrhea (runny nose), sweating, lacrimation (tearing), mydriasis (dilation of pupils)
- Anorexia
- Irritability, restlessness, generalized anxiety
- Tremor
- Chills and hot flashes
- Piloerection ("gooseflesh")
- Violent sneezing
- Weakness, fatigue, and drowsiness
- Nausea and vomiting
- Diarrhea, abdominal cramps
- Bone and muscle pain, muscle spasm, kicking movements

sion in the mother, the newborn, or both. Today's practice of giving lower doses of opioids intravenously has reduced the incidence and severity of opioid-induced CNS depression. **Opioid antagonists** such as naloxone (Narcan) can promptly reverse the CNS depressant effects, especially respiratory depression. In addition, the antagonist counters the effect of the stress-induced levels of endorphins. An opioid antagonist is especially valuable if labor is more rapid than expected, and birth is anticipated when the opioid is at its peak effect. The antagonist may be given through the woman's IV line, or it can be administered intramuscularly (see Medication Guide). The woman should be told that the pain that was relieved with the use of the opioid analgesic will return with the administration of the opioid antagonist. Some authorities believe that unless maternal CNS depression is severe enough to affect her well-being and that of her fetus, the woman should not receive naloxone just before birth in an attempt to prevent neonatal CNS depression. Placental transfer of naloxone is unpredictable; the newborn may not require treatment with an opioid antagonist; and the sudden return of severe pain could have adverse physiologic and psychologic effects on the mother (Hawkins et al., 2002; Lehne, 2001).

NURSE ALERT
An opioid antagonist must be administered cautiously to an opioid-dependent woman because it may precipitate abstinence syndrome (withdrawal symptoms) in both the mother and her newborn (see Signs of Potential Complications).

An opioid antagonist can be given to the newborn as one part of the treatment for **neonatal narcosis,** which is a state of CNS depression in the newborn produced by an opioid. Prophylactic administration of naloxone is controversial. Affected infants may exhibit respiratory depression, hypotonia, lethargy, and a delay in temperature regulation. Risk for hypoxia, hypercarbia, and acidosis increases if neonatal narcosis is not treated promptly. Treatment involves ventilation, administration of oxygen, and gentle stimulation. Naloxone is administered, if still required, to reverse CNS depression. More than one dose of naloxone may be required because its half-life is shorter than the half-life of opioids. Alterations in neurologic and behavioral responses may be evident in the newborn for as long as 2 to 4 days after birth. Meperidine may be present in the neonate's urine for up to 3 weeks. Some depression of attention and social responsiveness can be evident for up to 6 weeks after birth. The significance of these neurobehavioral changes is unknown (Hawkins et al., 2002; Lehne, 2001)

Nerve Block Analgesia and Anesthesia

A variety of local anesthetic agents are used in obstetrics to produce regional analgesia (some pain relief and motor block) and anesthesia (complete pain relief and motor block). Most of these agents are related chemically to cocaine and end with the suffix "-caine." This helps to identify a local anesthetic.

The principal pharmacologic effect of local anesthetics is the temporary interruption of the conduction of nerve impulses, notably pain. Examples of common agents given in 0.125% to 1% solutions are bupivacaine, chloroprocaine, lidocaine, ropivacaine, and tetracaine. The solution strength of the local anesthetic agent and the amount used will depend on the type of nerve block being performed.

Rarely people are sensitive (allergic) to one or more local anesthetics. Such a reaction may include respiratory depression, hypotension, and other serious adverse effects. Epinephrine, antihistamines, oxygen, and supportive measures should reverse these effects. Sensitivity may be identified by administering minute amounts of the drug to be used to test for an allergic reaction.

Local Perineal Infiltration Anesthesia. Local perineal infiltration anesthesia is commonly used when an episiotomy is to be performed and when time or the fetal head position does not permit a pudendal block to be administered (Scott et al., 1999). Rapid anesthesia is produced by injecting approximately 10 to 20 ml of 1% lidocaine or 2% chloroprocaine into the skin and then subcutaneously into the region to be anesthetized. Epinephrine often is added to the solution to localize and intensify the effect of the anesthesia in a region and to prevent excessive bleeding and systemic absorption by constricting local blood vessels (Lehne, 2001). Repeated injection will prolong the anesthesia as long as needed.

Pudendal Nerve Block. Pudendal nerve block is useful for the second stage of labor, episiotomy, and birth. Although it does not relieve the pain from uterine contractions, it does relieve pain in the lower vagina, vulva, and perineum (Fig. 19-7, *A*). A pudendal nerve block must be administered 10 to 20 minutes before perineal anesthesia is needed.

The pudendal nerve traverses the sacrosciatic notch just medial to the tip of the ischial spine on each side.

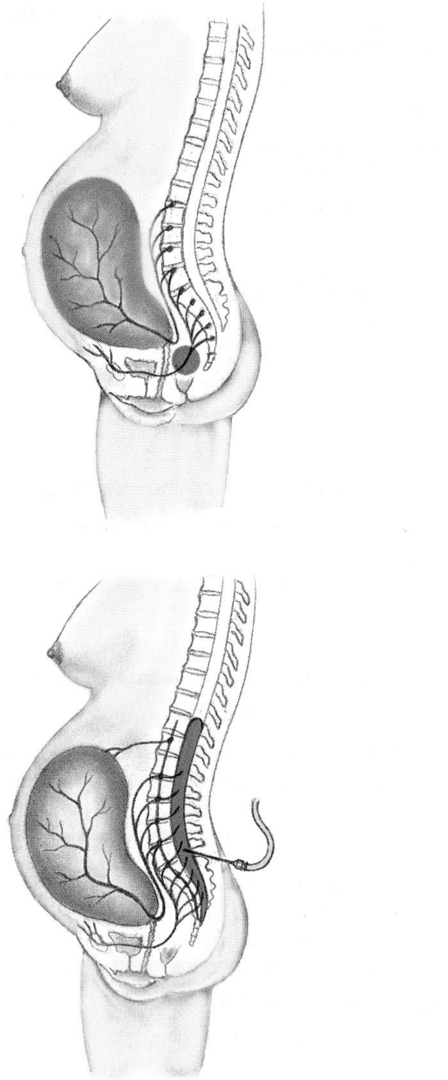
A
B

FIG. 19-7 Pain pathways and sites of pharmacologic nerve blocks. **A,** Pudendal nerve block; suitable during second and third stages of labor and for repair of episiotomy and lacerations. **B,** Epidural block; suitable for all stages of labor and types of birth and for repair of episiotomy and lacerations.

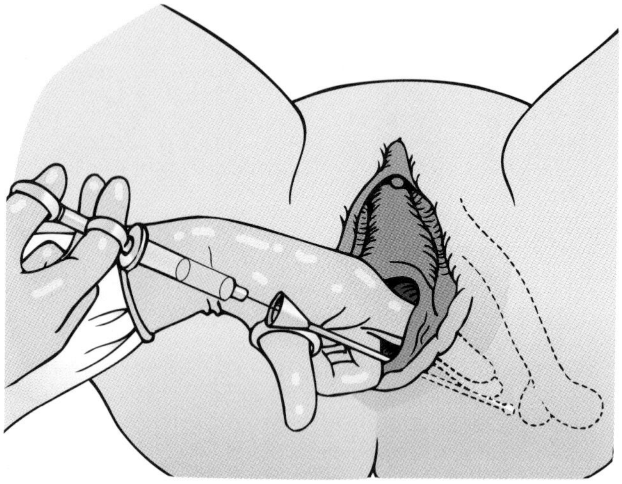

FIG. 19-8 Pudendal nerve block. Use of needle guide (Iowa trumpet) and Luer-Lok syringe to inject medication.

Injection of an anesthetic solution at or near these points anesthetizes the pudendal nerves peripherally (Fig. 19-8). The transvaginal approach is generally used because it is less painful for the woman, has a higher rate of success in blocking pain, and tends to cause fewer fetal complications (Chestnut, 1999). Pudendal block does not change maternal hemodynamic or respiratory functions, vital signs, or the FHR. However, the bearing-down reflex is lessened or lost completely.

If all branches of the pudendal nerve are anesthetized, analgesia is sufficient for a spontaneous vaginal birth, an outlet (low) forceps-assisted birth, or a vacuum-assisted birth. A pudendal block does not provide analgesia for uterine exploration or the manual removal of the placenta (Scott et al., 1999).

Spinal Anesthesia (Block). In **spinal anesthesia (block),** an anesthetic solution containing a local anesthetic alone or in combination with fentanyl is injected through the third, fourth, or fifth lumbar interspace into the subarachnoid space (Fig. 19-9), where the anesthetic solution mixes with cerebrospinal fluid (CSF). This technique is commonly used for cesarean births. Low spinal anesthesia (block) may be used for vaginal birth, but it is not suitable for labor. Spinal anesthesia (block) used for cesarean birth provides anesthesia from the nipple (T6) to the feet. If it is used for vaginal birth, the anesthesia level is from the hips (T10) to the feet (Fig. 19-9, *C*).

For spinal anesthesia (block), the woman is sitting or lying on her side (e.g., modified Sims position) with back curved to widen the intervertebral space to facilitate insertion of a small-gauge spinal needle and injection of the anesthetic solution. The nurse supports the woman because she must remain still during the placement of the spinal needle. The insertion is made between contractions. After the anesthetic solution has been injected, the woman may be positioned upright to allow the heavier (hyperbaric) anesthetic solution to flow downward to obtain the lower level of anesthesia suitable for a vaginal birth. She may be positioned supine with head and shoulders slightly elevated and the uterus displaced with a wedge under one of her hips to obtain the higher level of anesthesia desired for cesarean birth. The anesthetic effect usually begins 1 to 2 minutes after the anesthetic solution is injected and lasts 1 to 3 hours, depending on the type of agent used (Chestnut, 1999; Hawkins et al., 2002) (Fig. 19-10).

Marked hypotension, impaired placental perfusion, and an ineffective breathing pattern may occur during spinal

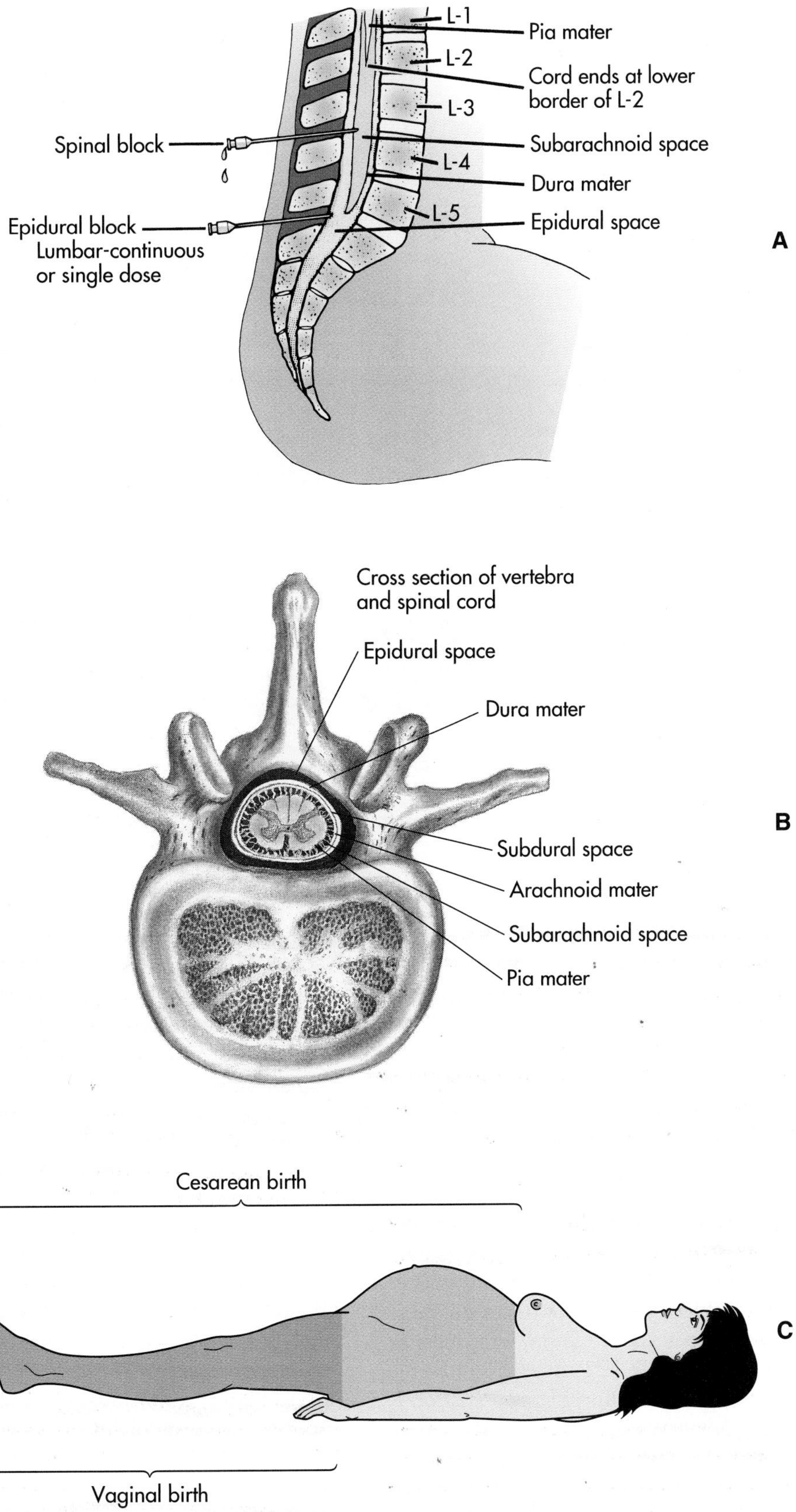
L-1
Pia mater
L-2
Cord ends at lower border of L-2
L-3
Spinal block
Subarachnoid space
L-4
Dura mater
L-5
Epidural block
Lumbar-continuous or single dose
Epidural space
A
Cross section of vertebra and spinal cord
Epidural space
Dura mater
Subdural space
Arachnoid mater
Subarachnoid space
Pia mater
B
Cesarean birth
C
Vaginal birth

FIG. 19-9 **A,** Membranes and spaces of spinal cord and levels of sacral, lumbar, and thoracic nerves. **B,** Cross section of vertebra and spinal cord. **C,** Level of anesthesia necessary for cesarean birth and for vaginal births.

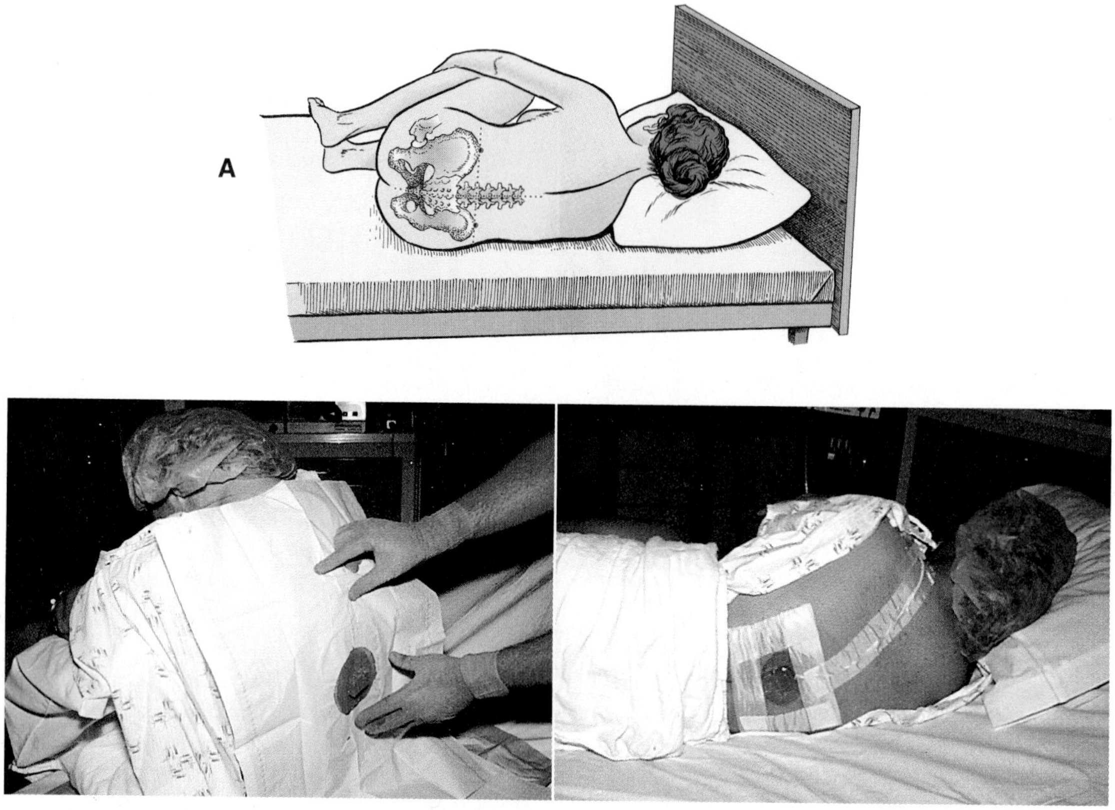
A
B
C

FIG. 19-10 Position for spinal and epidural blocks. **A,** Lateral position. **B,** Upright position. **C,** Catheter is taped to woman's back with port segment located near her shoulder. (**B** and **C**, Courtesy Michael S. Clement, MD, Mesa, AZ.)

anesthesia. Before induction of the spinal anesthetic (block), the woman's fluid balance is assessed, and IV fluid usually is administered to decrease the potential for hypotension caused by sympathetic blockade (i.e., vasodilation with pooling of blood in the lower extremities decreases cardiac output). After induction of the anesthetic, maternal blood pressure, pulse, and respirations and FHR and pattern must be checked and documented every 5 to 10 minutes. If signs of serious maternal hypotension or fetal distress develop, emergency care must be given (see Emergency box).

Because the woman is unable to sense her contractions, she must be instructed when to bear down during a vaginal birth. If the birth occurs in a delivery room (rather than a labor-delivery-recovery room), the woman will need assistance in the transfer to a recovery bed after expulsion of the placenta.

Advantages of spinal anesthesia include ease of administration and absence of fetal hypoxia with maintenance of normotension. Maternal consciousness is maintained, excellent muscular relaxation is achieved, and blood loss is not excessive.

Disadvantages of spinal anesthesia include medication reactions (e.g., allergy), hypotension, and an ineffective breathing pattern; cardiopulmonary resuscitation may be needed. When a spinal anesthetic is given, the need for operative birth (e.g., episiotomy, forceps-assisted birth, vacuum-assisted birth) tends to increase because voluntary expulsive efforts are reduced or eliminated. After birth, the incidence of bladder and uterine atony, as well as postspinal headache, is higher.

Leakage of CSF from the site of puncture of the dura mater (membranous covering of the spinal cord) is thought to be the major causative factor in postdural puncture headache (PDPH). Presumably postural changes cause the diminished volume of CSF to exert traction on pain-sensitive CNS structures. Characteristically, assuming an upright position triggers or intensifies the headache, whereas assuming a supine position achieves relief in 30 minutes or less (Govenar, 2000). The resulting headache and auditory (e.g., tinnitus) and visual (e.g., blurred vision, photophobia) problems begin within 2 days of the puncture and may persist for days or weeks.

The likelihood of headache after dural puncture can be reduced, however, if the anesthesiologist uses a small-gauge spinal needle and avoids making multiple punctures of the meninges. Positioning the woman flat in bed (with only a small, flat pillow for her head) for at least 8 hours after spinal anesthesia also has been recommended to pre-

EMERGENCY

Maternal Hypotension with Decreased Placental Perfusion

SIGNS/SYMPTOMS

- Maternal hypotension (20% decrease from preblock baseline level or <100 mm Hg systolic)
- Fetal bradycardia
- Decreased beat-to-beat FHR variability

INTERVENTIONS

- Turn woman to lateral position or place pillow or wedge under hip (see Fig. 21-5) to deflect uterus.
- Maintain IV infusion at rate specified, or increase prn per hospital protocol.
- Administer oxygen by face mask at 10-12 L/min or per protocol.
- Elevate the woman's legs.
- Notify the primary health care provider/anesthesiologist/nurse anesthetist.
- Administer IV vasopressor (e.g., ephedrine 5-10 mg) per protocol if above measures are ineffective.
- Remain with woman; continue to monitor maternal blood pressure and FHR every 5 minutes until her condition is stable or per primary health care provider's order.

vent headache, but no definitive evidence shows that this measure is effective. Positioning the woman on her abdomen, a difficult if not impossible position after a cesarean birth, is thought to decrease the loss of CSF through the puncture site. Hydration has been claimed to be of value in preventing and treating headache, but no compelling evidence supports its use (Cunningham et al., 2001). Initial treatment for a postdural puncture headache usually includes oral analgesics, bed rest in a quiet dimly lit or dark room, caffeine, and increased fluid intake (Govenar, 2000; Hawkins et al., 2002).

An autologous **epidural blood patch** is the most rapid, reliable, and beneficial relief measure for PDPH. The woman's blood (i.e., 10 to 20 ml) is injected slowly into the lumbar epidural space, creating a clot that patches the tear or hole in the dura mater around the spinal cord. It is considered if the headache does not resolve spontaneously or after use of more conservative, noninvasive techniques (Govenar, 2000; Scott et al., 1999) (Fig. 19-11).

After the blood-patch procedure, the woman should be observed for alteration of vital signs, pallor, clammy skin, and leakage of CSF. A bandage and cold pack are placed on the puncture site, and the woman rests in bed for approximately 1 hour. Discharge instructions include resting in bed for 24 to 48 hours, applying cold packs to the site as needed for comfort, avoiding analgesics that affect platelet aggregation (e.g, nonsteroidal antiinflammatory drugs [NSAIDs]) for 2 days, drinking plenty of fluids, and observing for signs of infection at the site and for neurologic symptoms such as pain, numbness and tingling in

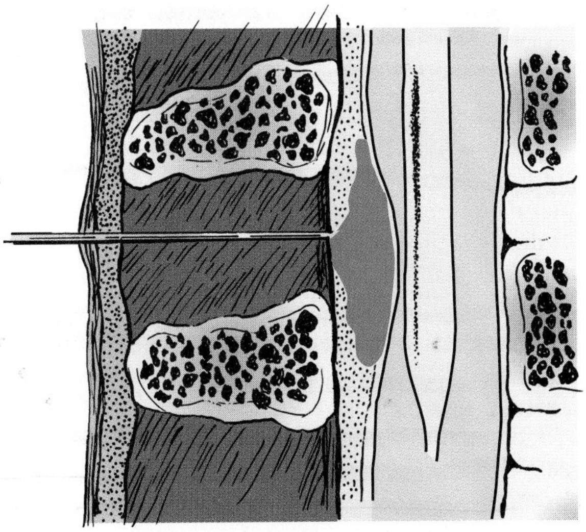

FIG. 19-11 Blood-patch therapy for spinal headache.

legs, and difficulty with walking or elimination. The woman should be cautioned to avoid lifting, straining at stool, coughing, tub bathing, or swimming for at least 2 days (Govenar, 2000; Hawkins et al., 2002).

Epidural anesthesia/analgesia (block). Relief from the pain of uterine contractions and birth (vaginal and cesarean) can be relieved by injecting a suitable local anesthetic agent (e.g., bupivacaine, ropivacaine), an opioid analgesic (e.g., fentanyl, sufentanil), or both into the epidural (peridural) space. Injection is made between the fourth and fifth lumbar vertebrae for a lumbar epidural block (see Figs. 19-7, *B*, and 19-9, *A*) and through the sacral hiatus for a caudal epidural block. Depending on the type and amount of medication(s) used, an anesthetic or analgesic effect will occur with varying degrees of motor impairment.

Lumbar Epidural Anesthesia/Analgesia. **Lumbar epidural anesthesia/analgesia (block)** is the most effective pharmacologic pain relief method for labor currently available. As a result, it is the most commonly used method for relieving pain during labor in the United States. More than half of the women giving birth each year choose epidural analgesia (Lieberman & O'Donoghue, 2002). For relieving the discomfort of labor and vaginal birth, a block from T10 to S5 is required. For cesarean birth, a block from at least T8 to S1 is essential. The diffusion of epidural anesthesia depends on the location of the catheter tip, the dose and volume of the anesthetic agent used, and the woman's position (e.g., horizontal or head-up position) (Cunningham et al., 2001).

For the induction of a lumbar epidural block, the woman is positioned as for a spinal block. She may sit with her back curved or she may assume a modified Sims position with her shoulders parallel, legs slightly flexed, and back arched (see Fig. 19-10).

After the epidural has been started, the woman is positioned preferably on her side so that the uterus does not compress the ascending vena cava and descending aorta, which can impair venous return, reduce cardiac output and blood pressure, and decrease placental perfusion. Her position should be alternated from side to side every hour. Upright positions and ambulation may be encouraged, depending on the degree of motor impairment. Oxygen should be available if hypotension occurs despite maintenance of hydration with IV fluid and displacement of the uterus to the side. Ephedrine (a vasopressor used to increase maternal blood pressure) and increased IV fluid infusion may be needed (see Emergency box). The FHR, pattern, and progress in labor must be monitored carefully because the woman in labor may not be aware of changes in the strength of the uterine contractions or the descent of the presenting part.

Several methods can be used for an epidural block. An intermittent block is achieved by using repeated injections of anesthetic solution; it is the least common method. The most commonly used method is the continuous block, achieved by using a pump to infuse the anesthetic solution through an indwelling plastic catheter. Patient-controlled epidural analgesia (PCEA) is the newest method; it uses an indwelling catheter and a programmed pump that allows the woman to control the dosing. The advantages of an epidural block are numerous: the woman remains alert and able to participate, good relaxation is achieved, airway reflexes remain intact, only partial motor paralysis develops, gastric emptying is not delayed, and blood loss is not excessive. Fetal complications are rare but may occur in the event of rapid absorption of the medication or marked maternal hypotension. The dose, volume, and type of medication(s) used can be modified to allow the woman to push, to assume upright positions and to walk, to produce perineal anesthesia, and to permit forceps-assisted, vacuum-assisted, or cesarean birth if required (Cunningham et al., 2001).

The disadvantages of epidural block also are numerous. The woman's ability to move freely is limited, related to the use of an intravenous infusion and electronic monitoring, orthostatic hypotension and dizziness, sedation, and weakness of the legs. CNS effects such as excitation, bizarre behavior, tinnitus, disorientation, paresthesia, and convulsions can occur if a solution containing a local anesthetic agent is accidentally injected into a blood vessel. Respiratory arrest can occur if the relatively high dosage used with an epidural block is accidentally injected into the subarachnoid space. Women who receive an epidural have a higher rate of fever (i.e., intrapartum temperature of 38° C or higher), especially when labor lasts longer that 12 hours; the temperature elevation most likely is related to thermoregulatory changes, although infection cannot be ruled out. The elevation in temperature can result in fetal tachycardia and neonatal workup for sepsis, whether or not signs of infection are present. Hypotension as a result of sympathetic blockade can be an outcome of an epidural block (see Emergency Box). Urinary retention and stress incontinence can occur in the immediate postpartum period. This temporary difficulty in urinary elimination could be related not only to the effects of the epidural block but also to the increased duration of labor and need for instrumental birth associated with the block (Leiberman & O'Donoghue, 2002). Pruritus (itching) is a side effect associated with the use of an opioid, especially fentanyl. A relation between epidural analgesia and longer second-stage labor, increased incidence of fetal malposition, use of oxytocin, and forceps-assisted or vacuum-assisted birth has been documented. Current research findings have been unable to demonstrate a significant increase in cesarean birth associated with epidural analgesia (Howell, 2001; Lieberman & O'Donoghue, 2002). Occasionally a PDPH can occur after accidental perforation of the dura mater during the administration of the epidural block. Because a larger needle is used for an epidural block, the risk for severe headache is high as a result of greater CSF loss (Hawkins et al., 2002). For some women, the epidural block is not effective, and a second form of analgesia is required to establish effective pain relief. When women progress rapidly in labor, pain relief may not be obtained before birth occurs.

Caudal Epidural Block. A **caudal epidural block** is rarely used today for several reasons. A higher dose of a local anesthetic agent is required because the sacral canal must be filled first for the anesthetic solution to reach the required level in the epidural space. Another disadvantage of a caudal block relates to its greater effect on pelvic floor muscles compared with a lumbar epidural block. The muscles are more insensitive and relaxed, thereby inhibiting adequate bearing-down efforts and interfering with the resistance required by the fetal head to rotate to an occiput anterior position. More motor function in the lower extremities also is lost. A rare but serious complication is accidental injection of the anesthetic solution into the fetal head because of its close proximity to the sacral hiatus (Hawkins et al., 2002).

Walking Epidural Analgesia. Using opioids such as fentanyl and sufentanil to potentiate the effects of local anesthetic agents has resulted in the ability to reduce the amount of the local anesthetic used and thereby reduce motor blockade. Opioids also can be used alone, eliminating the effect of a local anesthetic altogether. A combined *spinal-epidural (CSE)* technique is another approach that can be used to achieve a walking epidural. There is a high concentration of opioid receptors along the pain pathway in the spinal cord, in the brainstem, and in the thalamus. Because these receptors are highly sensitive to opioids, a small quantity of an opioid-agonist analgesic produces marked pain relief lasting for several hours. The opioid is injected into the subarachnoid space for rapid activation of the opioid receptors. Pain transmission is blocked without compromising motor ability. A catheter is left in place in the epidural space to extend the duration of the analgesia by using a lower dose of a local anesthetic agent. Although women can walk, they often choose not to do so because of sedation and fatigue, abnormal sensations perceived in their legs, weakness of the legs, and a feeling of insecurity. Often health care providers are reluctant to encourage or assist women to ambulate for fear of injury (Mayberry, Clemmens, & De, 2002). The CSE may be associated with fetal bradycardia, necessitating close assessment of FHR and pattern (Lieberman & O'-Donoghue, 2002).

Epidural and Intrathecal Opioids. The use of epidural or intrathecal opioids without the addition of a local anesthetic agent during labor has several advantages. Opioids administered in this manner do not cause maternal hypotension or affect vital signs. The woman feels contractions but not pain. Her ability to bear down during the second stage of labor is preserved because the pushing reflex is not lost, and her motor power remains intact.

Fentanyl, sufentanil, or preservative-free morphine may be used. Fentanyl and sufentanil produce short-acting analgesia (i.e., 1.5 to 3.5 hours), and morphine may provide pain relief for 4 to 7 hours. Morphine may be combined with fentanyl or sufentanil. The short-acting opioids are often used with multiparous women, and the morphine may be used with nulliparous women or women with a history of long labor (Manning, 1996). For most women, intrathecal opioids do not provide adequate analgesia for second-stage labor pain, episiotomy, or birth (Cunningham et al., 2001). Pudendal nerve blocks or local perineal infiltration anesthesia may be necessary.

A more common indication for the administration of epidural or intrathecal analgesics is the relief of postoperative pain. For example, women who give birth by cesarean can receive fentanyl or morphine through a catheter. The catheter may then be removed, and the women are usually free of pain for 24 hours. Occasionally the catheter is left in place in the epidural space in case another dose is needed.

Women receiving epidurally administered morphine after the cesarean birth are up soon after surgery with surprising ease and are able to care for their babies. The early ambulation and freedom from pain afforded also facilitate bladder emptying, enhance peristalsis, and prevent clot formation in the lower extremities (e.g. thrombophlebitis). To those women who have had a previous cesarean birth and have had the usual postoperative pain, the effects of this approach seem miraculous. However, the mother may not understand why she may have pain after the opioid effect wears off.

Side effects of opioids administered by the epidural and intrathecal routes include nausea, vomiting, pruritus, urinary retention, and delayed respiratory depression. These side effects are more common when morphine is administered. Antiemetics, antipruritics, and opioid antagonists are used to relieve these symptoms. For example, naloxone (Narcan), promethazine (Phenergan), or metoclopramide (Reglan) may be administered. Hospital protocols should provide specific instructions for the treatment of these side effects. Use of epidural opioids is not without risks. Respiratory depression is a serious concern; for this reason, the woman's respiratory rate should be assessed and documented every hour for 24 hours, or as designated by hospital protocol. Naloxone should be readily available for use if the respiratory rate decreases to less than 10 breaths per minute or if the oxygen saturation rate decreases to less than 89%. Administration of oxygen by face mask also may be initiated, and the anesthesiologist should be notified.

Contraindications to Subarachnoid and Epidural Blocks. Some contraindications to epidural analgesia apply equally to caudal and subarachnoid blocks (Scott et al., 1999):

- Antepartum hemorrhage. Acute hypovolemia leads to increased sympathetic tone to maintain the blood pressure. Any anesthetic technique that blocks the sympathetic fibers can produce significant hypotension that can endanger the mother and baby.
- Anticoagulant therapy or bleeding disorder. If a woman is receiving anticoagulant therapy or has a bleeding disorder, injury to a blood vessel may cause the formation of a hematoma that may compress the cauda equina or the spinal cord and lead to serious CNS complications.
- Infection at the injection site. Infection can be spread through the peridural or subarachnoid spaces if the needle traverses an infected area.
- Allergy to the anesthetic drug.

Epidural Block Effects on Neonate. Debate persists concerning the effects of epidural anesthesia and analgesia on the newborn's neurobehavioral responses. Findings from studies that examine associations between neurobehavioral outcome and epidural block are far from consistent. For example, studies comparing the neonatal neurobehavioral scores for infants born to mothers who did and mothers who did not receive epidural analgesia either have shown little or no difference in the scores or have shown that the infants of mothers who received epidural anesthesia did not score as well on neurobehavioral tests. In one research study, infants exposed to an epidural block tended to have less muscle tone but were better able to orient and habituate to sound when compared with infants whose mother received opioids during labor (Lieberman & O'Donoghue, 2002).

Paracervical (Uterosacral) Nerve Block. Paracervical nerve block can be used during the first stage of labor effectively to relieve pain resulting from uterine contractions and cervical dilation. A diluted local anesthetic solution (e.g., lidocaine without epinephrine is preferred) is injected into the cervical mucosa. The duration of the effect is relatively short (i.e., up to 2 hours) depending on the anesthetic used; therefore the block must be repeated in long labors. It cannot be used during the second stage of labor.

Although commonly used in the 1960s and early 1970s, it is rarely used today because of its association with fetal bradycardia. Although the bradycardia is transient, with a duration of 3 to 30 minutes, it can lead to fetal acidosis and even death. Fetal bradycardia occurs as a result of a combination of mechanisms including a high concentration of local anesthetic in the fetus (i.e., accidental direct injection into the fetus; indirect diffusion across uterine artery), vasoconstriction of the uterine artery by the anesthetic agent, or increased uterine activity by accidental injection of the anesthetic agent into the uterine muscle. Maternal complications, although rare, can include cardiotoxicity or neurotoxicity (i.e., accidental direct injection of anesthetic agent into a blood vessel), infection (e.g., abscess formation), hematoma formation, and nerve damage (e.g., sacral plexus injury). Because of the potential for adverse reactions, paracervical nerve block should be used only when maternal and fetal well-being is established (Hawkins et al., 2002; Rosen, 2002a).

Nitrous Oxide for Analgesia

Nitrous oxide mixed with oxygen can be inhaled in a low concentration (50% or less) to reduce but not eliminate pain during the first and second stages of labor. At the lower doses used for analgesia, the woman remains awake, and the danger of aspiration is avoided because the laryngeal reflexes are unaffected. It can be used in combination with other nonpharmacologic and pharmacologic measures for pain relief.

A face mask or mouthpiece is used to self-administer the gas. The woman should place the mask over her mouth and nose or insert the mouthpiece 30 seconds before the onset of a contraction (if regular) or as soon as a contraction begins (if irregular). When she inhales, a valve opens, and the gas is released. She should continue to inhale the gas slowly and deeply until the contraction starts to subside. When inhalation stops, the valve closes. Onset of action is 50 seconds; therefore beginning the inhalation process 30 seconds before the onset of a contraction provides the best pain relief. During the interval between contractions, the woman should remove the device and breathe normally (Rosen, 2002b).

Most women who use nitrous oxide obtain adequate pain relief and are satisfied with the method. The nurse should observe the woman for nausea and vomiting, drowsiness, dizziness, hazy memory, and loss of consciousness. Loss of consciousness is more likely to occur if opioids are used with the nitrous oxide. The use of nitrous oxide does not appear to depress uterine contractions or cause adverse reactions in the fetus and newborn (Rosen, 2002b).

Nitrous oxide for pain relief during labor is more readily available in Canada and European countries than in the United States (Caton et al., 2002).

General Anesthesia

General anesthesia rarely is used for uncomplicated vaginal birth and is infrequently used for cesarean birth. It may be necessary if there is a contraindication to a spinal or epidural block or if indications necessitate rapid birth (vaginal or cesarean) without sufficient time to perform a block. In addition, being awake and aware during major surgery may be unacceptable for some women having a cesarean birth.

If general anesthesia is being considered, the nurse gives the woman nothing by mouth and ensures that an IV infusion is in place. If time allows, the nurse premedicates the woman with a nonparticulate (clear) oral antacid (e.g., sodium citrate, Bicitra, Alka-Seltzer) to neutralize the acidic contents of the stomach. Aspiration of highly acidic gastric contents will damage lung tissue. Some anesthesiologists and physicians also order the administration of a histamine (H_2)-receptor blocker such as cimetidine (Tagamet) to decrease the production of gastric acid and metoclopramide (Reglan) to increase gastric emptying (Hawkins et al., 2002; Scott et al., 1999). Before the anesthesia is given, a wedge should be placed under one of the woman's hips to displace the uterus. Uterine displacement prevents aortocaval compression, which interferes with placental perfusion.

Thiopental, a short-acting barbiturate, is administered IV to render the woman unconscious, and then succinylcholine, a muscle relaxer, is administered to facilitate passage of an endotracheal tube. Sometimes the nurse is asked to assist with applying cricoid pressure before intubation as the woman begins to lose consciousness. This maneuver blocks the esophagus and prevents aspiration should the woman vomit or regurgitate (Fig. 19-12). Pressure is released once the endotracheal tube is securely in place.

After the woman is intubated, nitrous oxide and oxygen in a 50:50 mixture are administered. A low concentration of a volatile halogenated agent (e.g., isoflurane) also may be administered to increase pain relief and to reduce maternal awareness and recall (Hawkins et al., 2002). In higher concentrations, isoflurane or methoxyflurane relaxes the uterus quickly and facilitates intrauterine manipulation, version, and extraction. However, at higher concentrations, these agents cross the placenta readily and can produce narcosis in the fetus and could reduce uterine tone after birth, increasing the risk for hemorrhage.

Priorities for recovery room care are to maintain an open airway and cardiopulmonary function and to prevent postpartum hemorrhage. Routine postpartum care is organized to facilitate parent-child attachment as soon as possible and to answer the mother's questions. When appropriate, the nurse assesses the mother's readiness to see the baby, as well as her response to the anesthesia and to the event that necessitated general anesthesia (e.g., emergency cesarean birth when vaginal birth was anticipated).

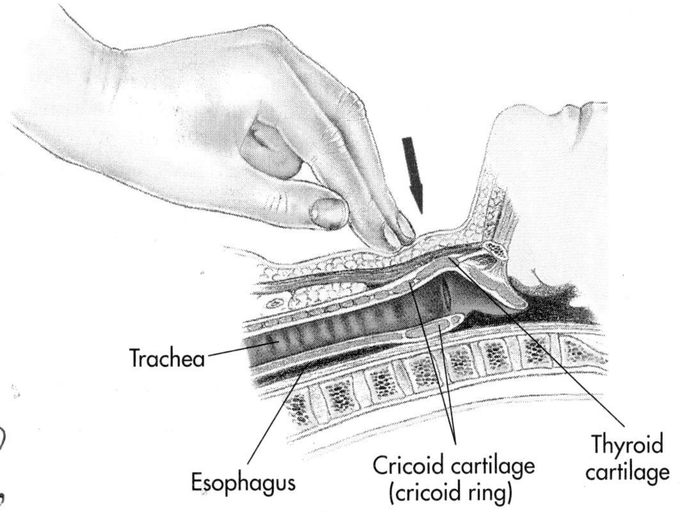
Trachea
Esophagus
Cricoid cartilage
(cricoid ring)
Thyroid
cartilage

FIG. 19-12 Technique of applying pressure on cricoid cartilage to occlude esophagus to prevent pulmonary aspiration of gastric contents during induction of general anesthesia.

CARE MANAGEMENT

The choice of pain relief depends on a combination of factors, including the woman's special needs and wishes, the availability of the desired method(s), the knowledge and expertise in nonpharmacologic and pharmacologic methods of the health care providers involved in the woman's care, and the phase and stage of labor. The nurse is responsible for maintaining continuous maternal and fetal assessment, establishing mutual goals with the woman (and her family), formulating nursing diagnoses, planning and implementing nursing care, and evaluating the effects of care. It is essential for the nurse to document carefully all aspects of care management.

Assessment and Nursing Diagnoses

The assessment of the woman, her fetus, and her labor is a joint effort of the nurse and the primary health care providers, who consult with the woman regarding their findings and recommendations. The needs of each woman are different, and many factors must be considered before deciding whether nonpharmacologic methods, pharmacologic methods, or a combination of both will be used to manage labor pain. It is critical that the nurse take note of all pain characteristics including location, intensity, quality, frequency, duration, and effectiveness of relief measures. The nurse should never assume that because a woman is in labor, her pain must be uterine in origin. Because pain is a subjective phenomenon, the nurse must listen to the woman's description of her pain. One self-assessment tool that can be used is a visual analogue scale (VAS). The VAS allows the woman to indicate on a line how severe or intense she perceives her pain to be from "no pain" to "pain as bad as it could possibly be." The McGill Pain Questionnaire provides a more complete picture of the pain experience because the woman is able to describe the sensory and emotional/affective dimensions of her pain and not just intensity (Lowe, 2002). Self-assessment is recommended to ensure that pain management is based on the subjective nature of the woman's pain rather than just on the nurse's judgment. It is not unusual for a nurse to over- or underestimate the pain being experienced by his or her client. Baker et al. (2001) found that midwives consistently underestimated pain intensity that women described as severe. When there are major cultural differences between the health care provider and the client, inaccurate interpretation of pain intensity often occurs (Lowe, 2002) (see Guidelines/Guías box).

History

The woman's prenatal record is read and relevant information identified. This includes the woman's parity, estimated date of birth, and complications and medications during pregnancy. If the woman has a history of allergies, this is noted, and a warning is displayed in a prominent place. A history of smoking and neurologic and spinal disorders also is noted.

Interview

Interview data consist of the time of the woman's last meal and the type of food and fluid consumed; the nature of any existing respiratory condition (e.g., cold, allergy); and unusual reactions (e.g., allergy) to medications, cleansing agents, or tape. The woman is asked whether she attended childbirth preparation classes. The extent of her preparation and her preferences for management of discomfort including a birth plan are reviewed. Her knowledge of the options for the

GUIDELINES/GUÍAS

Pain Management

Do you want to get up and walk?
¿Desea levantarse y caminar?

Do you want pain medication?
¿Quiere medicina para el dolor?

I am going to give you the pain medicine in an injection.
Le voy a dar la medicina para el dolor en una inyección.

I am going to give you the pain medicine through an IV.
Le voy a dar la medicina para el dolor por medio del suero.

This is a pain reliever called Demerol/Stadol/Nubain.
Este es una medicina para aliviar el dolor que se llama Demerol/Stadol/Nubain.

The effects of this medicine are relatively short.
Los efectos de esta medicina son relativamente cortos.

The epidural is a stronger method of pain relief.
La anestesia espinal es un método más fuerte para aliviar el dolor.

You should not be able to feel the contraction pain.
No debe de sentir los dolores de las contracciónes.

management of discomfort also is assessed. Information on the woman's perception of discomfort and her expressed need for medication is added to the database. Relevant events that have occurred since the woman's last contact with her primary health care provider also are reviewed (e.g., infections, diarrhea, a change in fetal movement patterns). If verbal and physical signs indicate the existence of substance abuse (e.g., opioids, alcohol), the nurse should ask the woman to identify the type of substance used, the last time it was taken, and the method of administration.

Physical Examination

The character and status of the labor and fetal response are assessed during a physical examination. The nurse evaluates the woman's hydration status by assessing intake and output measurements, the moistness of the mucous membranes, skin turgor, and concentration of urine. Bladder distention is noted. Any evidence of skin infection near sites of possible needle insertion is recorded and reported. Signs of apprehension such as fist clenching and restlessness also are noted.

If the woman is in labor, the status of maternal vital signs, FHR and pattern, uterine contractions, amniotic membranes and fluid, cervical effacement and dilation, and fetal descent is determined. The anticipated time until birth is estimated if possible. The length of labor and degree of fatigue are other important considerations. If pharmacologic methods are to be used, the type of analgesia or anesthesia chosen will vary depending on the status of the maternal-fetal unit, the progress of labor, and the method of birth planned (see Box 19-3).

Laboratory Tests

The results of laboratory tests are reviewed to determine whether the woman is experiencing anemia (hemoglobin and hematocrit), a coagulopathy or bleeding disorder (prothrombin time and platelet count), or infection (white blood cell count and differential).

Signs of Potential Problems

Any medication can cause a minor or severe allergic reaction. As part of the assessment for such allergic reactions, the nurse should monitor the woman's vital signs, respiratory status, cardiovascular status, integument, and platelet and white blood cell count. The woman is observed for side effects of drug therapy, especially drowsiness. Minor reactions can consist of a rash, rhinitis, fever, asthma, or pruritus. Management of the less acute allergic response is not an emergency (Lehne, 2001).

Severe reactions may occur suddenly and lead to shock. The most dramatic form of anaphylaxis is sudden severe bronchospasm, vasospasm, severe hypotension, and death. Signs of anaphylaxis are largely caused by contraction of smooth muscles and may begin with irritability, extreme weakness, nausea, and vomiting. This may lead to dyspnea, cyanosis, convulsions, and cardiac arrest. An acute allergic reaction (anaphylaxis) must be diagnosed and treated immediately. Treatment usually consists of 1:1000 epinephrine injected subcutaneously or intramuscularly, followed by parenteral administration of antihistamines. Supportive care is given to alleviate the symptoms; the type of care is determined by the rapidly assessed cardiovascular and respiratory response of the woman to the primary interventions (Lehne, 2001). Cardiopulmonary resuscitation may be necessary. The nurse also must be alert for changes in fetal well-being; nonreassuring changes in FHR and pattern should be noted and reported to the primary health care provider.

Nursing Diagnoses

The following nursing diagnoses are relevant in the management of discomfort during labor and birth:

- *Acute pain related to*
  –processes of labor and birth
- *Risk for ineffective tissue perfusion related to*
  –effects of analgesia or anesthesia
  –maternal position
- *Hypothermia related to*
  –effects of analgesia or anesthesia
- *Situational low self-esteem related to*
  –negative perception of the woman's (or her family's) behavior
- *Fear related to deficient knowledge of*
  –procedure for epidural analgesia
  –expected sensation during spinal anesthesia
- *Risk for maternal injury related to*
  –effects of analgesia and anesthesia on sensation and motor control

Expected Outcomes of Care

The expected outcomes of nursing care in the management of the discomfort of labor and birth include the following:

- The woman will promptly report the characteristics of her pain and discomfort.
- The woman will verbalize understanding of her needs and rights with regard to pain relief management that uses a variety of nonpharmacologic and pharmacologic methods reflecting her preferences.
- The woman will have adequate pain relief without adding maternal risk (e.g., through the use of appropriate nonpharmacologic methods and appropriate medication, including the appropriate dose, timing, and route of administration).
- Fetus will maintain well-being, and the newborn will adjust to extrauterine life.

Plan of Care and Interventions

A plan of care is developed for each woman to address her particular clinical and nursing problems. The nurse collaborates with the primary health care provider and laboring woman in selecting those aspects of care relevant to the woman and her family.

Nonpharmacologic Interventions

The nurse supports and assists the woman as she uses nonpharmacologic interventions for pain relief and relaxation. During labor, the nurse should ask the woman how she feels to evaluate the effectiveness of the specific pain management techniques used. Appropriate interventions can then be planned or continued for effective care, such as trying other nonpharmacologic methods or combining nonpharmacologic methods with medications (see Plan of Care on p. 514).

The woman's perception of her behavior during labor is of utmost importance. If she planned a nonmedicated birth but then needs and accepts medication, her self-esteem may falter. Verbal and nonverbal acceptance of her behavior is given as necessary by the nurse and reinforced by discussion and reassurance after birth. Providing explanations about the fetal response to maternal discomfort, the effects of maternal stress and fatigue on the progress of labor, and the medication itself is a supportive measure. The woman also may experience anxiety and stress related to anticipated or actual pain. Stress can cause increased maternal catecholamine production. Increased levels of catecholamines have been linked to dysfunctional labor and fetal and neonatal distress and illness. Nurses must be able to implement strategies aimed at reducing this stress (Hodnett, 2002; Lowe, 2002).

Informed Consent

The primary health care provider and anesthesia care provider are responsible for informing women of the alternative methods of pharmacologic pain relief available in the hospital. A description of the various anesthetic techniques and what they entail is essential to informed consent, even if the woman has received information about analgesia and anesthesia earlier in her pregnancy. The discussion of pain management options ideally should take place in the third trimester so the woman has time to consider alternatives. Nurses play a part in the informed consent by clarifying and describing procedures or by acting as the woman's advocate and asking the primary health care provider for further explanations. The procedure and its advantages and disadvantages must be thoroughly explained.

LEGAL TIP Informed Consent for Anesthetic

The woman receives (in an understandable manner), the following:

- Explanation of alternative methods of anesthesia and analgesia available
- Description of anesthetic and procedure for administration
- Description of the benefits, discomforts, risks, and consequences for the mother and the fetus
- Explanation of how complications can be treated
- Information that the anesthetic is not always effective
- Indication that the woman may withdraw consent at any time
- Opportunity to have any question answered
- Opportunity to have components of the consent explained in the woman's own words

Consent form will

- Be written or explained in the woman's primary language
- Have the woman's signature
- Have the date of consent
- Carry the signature of anesthetic care provider, certifying that the woman has received and appears to understand the explanation

Timing of Administration

It is often the nurse who notifies the primary health care provider that the woman is in need of pharmacologic measures to relieve her discomfort. Orders are often written for the administration of pain medication as needed by the woman and based on the nurse's clinical judgment. Generally, pharmacologic measures for pain relief are not implemented until labor has advanced to the active phase of the first stage of labor and the cervix is dilated approximately 4 to 5 cm to avoid suppressing the progress of labor (see Box 19-3). Conversely, nonpharmacologic measures can be used to relieve pain in early labor while relieving stress and enhancing progress.

Preparation for Procedures

The nurse reviews the methods of pain relief available to the woman (or validates her choices) and clarifies information as necessary. The procedure and what will be asked of the woman (e.g., to maintain flexed position during insertion of epidural needle) must be explained. The woman also can benefit from knowing the way that the medication is to be given, the interval before the medication takes effect, and the expected pain relief from the medication. Skin-preparation measures are described, and the nurse explains the need for emptying the bladder before the analgesic or anesthetic is administered and the reason for keeping the bladder empty. When an indwelling catheter is to be threaded into the epidural space, the woman should be told that she may have a momentary twinge down her leg, hip, or back, and that this feeling is not a sign of injury.

Administration of Medication

Accurate monitoring of the progress of labor forms the basis for the nurse's judgment that a woman needs pharmacologic control of discomfort. Knowledge of the medications used during childbirth is essential. The most effective route of administration is selected for each woman; then the medication is prepared and administered correctly.

Intravenous Route. The preferred route of administration of medications such as meperidine, fentanyl, or nalbuphine is through IV tubing, administered into the port nearest the woman while the infusion of the IV solution is stopped. The medication is given slowly in small doses at the beginning of a contraction and over the period of three to five consecutive contractions. Because uterine blood vessels are constricted during contractions, the medication stays within the maternal vascular system for several seconds before the uterine blood vessels reopen. The IV infusion is then restarted slowly to prevent a bolus of medication from being administered. With this method of injection, along with smaller but more frequent dosing, the amount of medication crossing the placenta to the fetus is reduced. With decreased placental transfer and more frequent dosing, the mother's degree of pain relief is maximized, even with the smaller analgesic dose. The IV route is associated with the following advantages:

- The onset of pain relief is more predictable.
- Pain relief is obtained with small doses of the drug.
- The duration of effect is more predictable.

Intramuscular Route. IM injections of analgesics, although still used, are not the preferred route for administration for women in labor. Identified disadvantages of the IM route include the following:

- The onset of pain relief is delayed.
- Higher doses of medication are required.
- Medication from muscle tissue is released at an unpredictable rate and is available for transfer across the placenta to the fetus.

IM injections given in the upper arm (deltoid muscle) seem to result in more rapid absorption and higher blood levels of the medication (Bricker & Lavender, 2002). If regional anesthesia is planned later in labor, the autonomic blockade from the regional (e.g., epidural) anesthesia increases blood flow to the gluteal region and accelerates absorption of medication that may be sequestered there. The maternal plasma level of the medication necessary to bring pain relief usually is reached 45 minutes after IM injection, followed by a decline in plasma levels. The maternal medications levels (after IM injections) also are unequal because of uneven distribution (maternal uptake) and metabolism. The advantage of using the IM route is quick administration.

Spinal Nerve Blocks. An intravenous infusion is usually established before the induction of spinal nerve blocks (e.g., epidural, subarachnoid). Anesthesia protocols often include the prophylactic administration of IV fluid before epidural and spinal anesthesia for blood volume expansion to prevent maternal hypotension. However, routine preloading with IV fluids before epidural analgesia is a form of care with a trade-off between beneficial and adverse effects (Enkin et al., 2000).

Lactated Ringer's or normal saline solutions are commonly used infusion solutions. Infusion solutions without dextrose are preferred, especially when the solution must be infused rapidly (e.g., to treat dehydration or to maintain blood pressure) because solutions containing dextrose rapidly increase maternal blood glucose levels. The fetus responds to high blood glucose levels by increasing insulin production; neonatal hypoglycemia may result. In addition, dextrose changes the osmotic pressure so that fluid is excreted from the kidneys more rapidly.

Because spinal nerve blocks can reduce bladder sensation, resulting in difficulty voiding, the woman should empty her bladder before the induction of the block and should be encouraged to void at least every 2 hours thereafter. The nurse should palpate for bladder distention and measure urinary output to ensure that the bladder is being completely emptied. A distended bladder can inhibit uterine contractions and fetal descent, resulting in a slowing of the progress of labor. The status of the maternal-fetal unit and the progress of labor must be established before the block is performed. The nurse or the woman's partner must assist the woman to assume and maintain the correct position for induction of epidural and spinal anesthesia (see Fig. 19-11).

Safety and General Care

After administration of a spinal nerve block, the woman is protected from injury by raising the side rails and placing a call bell within easy reach when the nurse is not in attendance. Oxygen and suction should be readily available at the bedside. The nurse must make sure there is no prolonged pressure on an anesthetized part (e.g., lying on one side with weight on one leg, tight linen on feet). If stirrups are used for birth, the nurse should pad them, adjust both stirrups to the same level and angle, place both of the woman's legs into them simultaneously while avoiding putting pressure on the popliteal angle, and apply restraints without restricting circulation.

Depending on the level of motor blockade, the woman should be assisted to remain as mobile as possible. When in bed, her position should be alternated from side to side every hour to ensure adequate distribution of the anesthetic solution and to maintain circulation to the uterus and placenta. Assisting the woman to assume upright positions such as sitting (e.g., modified throne position in which the woman sits on the bed with the bottom part lowered to place her feet below her body), tug-of-war position (woman tugs on towel or sheet that is tied to the bar on the bed or held by the nurse), and squatting by using the head of the bed for support will facilitate fetal descent and enhance bearing-down efforts (Gilder et al., 2002). Ambulation also should be encouraged if the woman has received a "walking" epidural. Upright positions are very important in the prevention of operative births (e.g., forceps-assisted or vacuum-assisted birth). To prevent injury, the nurse must assess the level motor of function (e.g., three unassisted steps with accompaniment, stand and close eyes noting the degree of unsteadiness, ability to flex legs or rise from a supine position), level of sensation in legs (e.g., degree of numbness), and level of sedation before the woman is assisted out of bed and periodically thereafter (Mayberry, Clemmens, & De, 2002). The woman should sit on the side of the bed before standing to determine if orthostatic hypotension occurs. If she is not dizzy or lightheaded, then she can stand at the side of the bed and finally walk.

Health care providers should recognize that the second stage of labor is often prolonged in women who use epidural analgesia for pain management. Research evidence indicates that as long as the well-being of the maternal-fetal unit is established, a period of "laboring down" to allow the fetus to descend and rotate with uterine contractions and the use of open-glottis pushing techniques when the fetus has reached a 1+ station and is rotating to an anterior position are the best approaches to use for the management of second-stage labor (Mayberry et al., 2002) (see Chapter 21 for a full discussion of second stage labor management).

The nurse monitors and records the woman's response to nonpharmacologic pain relief methods and to medication(s). This includes the degree of pain relief, the level of apprehension, the return of sensations and perception of pain, and allergic or adverse reactions (e.g., hypotension, respiratory depression, hypothermia, fever, pruritus, nausea and vomiting). The nurse continues to monitor maternal vital signs, blood pressure, the strength and frequency of uterine contractions, changes in the cervix and station of the presenting part, the presence and quality of the bearing-down reflex, bladder filling, and state of hydration. Determining the fetal response after administration of analgesia or anesthesia is vital. The woman is asked if she (or the family) has any questions. The nurse also assesses the woman's and her family's understanding of the need for ensuring her safety (e.g., keeping side rails up, calling for assistance as needed).

The time that elapses between the administration of an opioid and the baby's birth is documented. Medications given to the newborn to reverse opioid effects are recorded. After birth, the woman who has had spinal, epidural, or general anesthesia is assessed for return of sensory and motor function in addition to the usual postpartum assessments.

Anesthesia in the Obese Woman

Obesity is defined as an excess of body fat causing weight to be greater than 20% more than ideal weight. Research findings indicate that women who are obese before pregnancy have an increased risk for cesarean birth when compared with women who are not obese (Crane et al., 1997; Hood & Dewan, 1993).

Maternal physiologic changes are the product of hormonal influences and mechanical effects. In obese women, the weight of fat tissue and the added metabolic demands this involves also affect maternal physiology (Endler, 1990). Both pregnancy and obesity cause blood volume and cardiac output to increase, and in the latter case, they expand in proportion to the amount of fat tissue. During labor and vaginal birth, and in the immediate postpartum period, blood values and cardiac output in obese women can reach levels 80% greater than prelabor values. The enlarged uterus and abdominal fat mass also further increase the possibility of aortocaval compression.

The respiratory system also is stressed in obese pregnant women (Endler, 1990), and the pulmonary function of an obese laboring woman is in a precarious state; therefore the woman's oxygenation must be carefully monitored during birth and the immediate postpartum period. Monitoring by pulse oximeter has been suggested.

The gastric emptying time is delayed; the tone of the cardiac sphincter is decreased; and the gastric contents are hyperacidic in all pregnant women. The obese woman also is more likely to have a hiatal hernia and a marked increase in intragastric pressure and volume; therefore these women are at great risk for regurgitation and aspiration (Endler, 1990).

Management of the obese woman during labor should focus on efforts to minimize oxygen consumption and maximize pulmonary function. Epidural analgesia administered during the first stage of labor can bring about a decreased demand on the metabolic and respiratory systems and improved oxygenation. This is because pain causes the catecholamine levels to increase, which in turn causes cardiac output to increase. Effective epidural analgesia retards this increase in catecholamine levels.

Intravenous opioids may be used during the first stage of labor; however, the doses and the effects must be monitored carefully because obese women are extremely sensitive to the respiratory depressant effects of opioids (Endler, 1990). An epidural block during the second stage

Plan of Care: Nonpharmacologic Management of Discomfort

NURSING DIAGNOSIS Anxiety related to lack of confidence in ability to cope effectively with pain during labor

Expected Outcome *Woman will express decrease in anxiety and experience satisfaction with her labor and birth performance.*

Nursing Interventions/*Rationales*

Assess whether woman and significant other have attended childbirth classes, her knowledge of labor process, and her current level of anxiety *to plan supportive strategies.*

Encourage support person to remain with woman in labor *to provide support and increase probability of response to comfort measures.*

Teach or review nonpharmacologic techniques available to decrease anxiety and pain during labor (e.g., focusing and feedback, breathing techniques, effleurage, and sacral pressure) *to enhance chances of success in using techniques.*

Explore other techniques that the woman or significant other may have learned in childbirth classes (e.g., hypnosis, yoga, acupressure, biofeedback, therapeutic touch, aromatherapy, imaging, music) *to provide largest repertoire of coping strategies.*

Explore use of hydrotherapy if ordered by physician and if woman meets use criteria (i.e., vital signs within normal limits [WNL], cervix 4 to 5 cm dilated, active phase of first stage labor) *to aid relaxation and stimulate production of natural oxytocin.*

Explore use of transcutaneous nerve stimulation per physician order *to provide an increased perception of control over pain and an increase in release of endogenous opiates.*

Assist woman to change positions and to use pillows *to reduce stiffness, aid circulation, and promote comfort.*

Assess bladder for distention and encourage voiding often *to avoid bladder distention and subsequent discomfort.*

Encourage rest between contractions *to minimize fatigue.*

Keep woman and significant other informed about progress *to allay anxiety.*

Guide couple through the labor stages and phases, helping them use and modify comfort techniques that are appropriate to each phase *to ensure greatest effectiveness of techniques employed.*

Support couple if pharmacologic measures are required to increase pain relief explaining safety and effectiveness *to reduce anxiety and maintain self-esteem and sense of control over labor process.*

NURSING DIAGNOSIS Health-seeking behavior (labor) related to desire for a healthy outcome of labor and birth

Expected Outcome *Woman will participate in care planning for labor.*

Nursing Interventions/*Rationales*

Discuss woman's birth plan and knowledge about the birth process *to collect data for plan of care.*

Provide information about the labor process *to correct any misconceptions.*

Inform woman about her labor status and fetus's well-being *to promote comfort and confidence.*

Discuss rationales for all interventions *to incorporate woman into plan of care.*

Incorporate nonpharmacologic interventions into plan of care *to increase woman's sense of control during labor.*

Provide emotional support and ongoing positive feedback *to enhance positive coping mechanisms.*

of labor provides complete pain relief and also supports cardiovascular function.

An epidural block is preferred to general anesthesia in the obese woman who must give birth by cesarean. Problems associated with general anesthesia in obese women include potential difficulties during intubation, a hypertensive effect of laryngoscopy and intubation, and aspiration and pulmonary complications. A spinal block may be used if there is insufficient time to induce an epidural block. Uterine displacement to prevent aortocaval compression is more difficult to achieve in the obese woman in the supine position needed for cesarean birth. If the woman is extremely obese, a wedge may not be able to elevate one hip enough to prevent compression. In this case, it may be necessary to lift the abdominal fat pad off the abdomen manually until the peritoneal cavity has been entered (Endler, 1990).

Maternal Hypothermia After Analgesia and Anesthesia

Hypothermia is defined as a core body temperature of less than 35° C. During labor and immediately after the birth, women are predisposed to hypothermia because of the combination of the vasodilation that normally occurs during pregnancy and the effects of the analgesia and anesthesia.

Opioids, barbiturates, tranquilizers, and antiemetics are thought to affect thermoregulation by increasing vasodilation and radiant loss; general anesthetic agents are thought to do so by depressing thermoregulation; and epidural and spinal anesthesia are thought to do so by inducing peripheral dilation (Buggy & Bardiner, 1995). During labor, during vaginal or cesarean birth, or immediately after birth, women may have shivering, hypotension, and respiratory distress. The hypothermia may result in cardiovascular, pulmonary, circulatory, hematologic, neurologic, or renal complications (Buggy & Bardiner, 1995). The nurse can minimize these complications by making sure that the birthing areas are warm, wet drapes and towels are removed, women are covered with warm blankets after birth, and hypothermia is recognized early. Explaining these effects to the woman and her support people will help allay concerns.

Evaluation

Evaluation of the effectiveness of care of the woman needing management of discomfort during labor and birth is based on the previously stated outcomes (see Plan of Care).

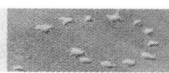

KEY POINTS

- The expected outcome of preparation for childbirth and parenting is "education for choice."
- Nonpharmacologic pain and stress management strategies are valuable for managing labor discomfort alone or in combination with pharmacologic methods.
- The gate-control theory of pain and the stress response are the bases for many of the nonpharmacologic methods of pain relief.
- The type of analgesic or anesthetic to be used is determined in part by the stage of labor and the method of birth.
- Opioid effects can be potentiated with ataractics.
- Naloxone (Narcan) is an opioid antagonist that can reverse opioid effects, especially respiratory depression.
- Pharmacologic control of discomfort during labor requires collaboration among the health care providers and the laboring woman.
- The nurse must understand medications, their expected effects, their potential adverse reactions, and their methods of administration.
- Maintenance of maternal fluid balance is essential during spinal and epidural nerve blocks.
- Maternal analgesia or anesthesia potentially affects neonatal neurobehavioral response.
- The use of opioid agonist-antagonist analgesics in women with preexisting opioid dependence may cause symptoms of abstinence syndrome (opioid withdrawal).
- General anesthesia is rarely used for vaginal birth but may be used for cesarean birth or whenever rapid anesthesia is needed in an emergency childbirth situation.

CRITICAL THINKING EXERCISES

1. During a prenatal visit, a pregnant woman (1-0-0-0-0) at 28 weeks of gestation tells her nurse midwife, "Most of my friends had epidurals for their labors, but I am not sure if that approach is right for me—I don't like the thought of having something stuck into my back—what if I become paralyzed? They tell me that the pain of labor is so terrible that I really have no other choice and would be crazy not to take advantage of something that will give me a pain-free labor." Describe the approach that the nurse midwife should take in helping this woman make an informed decision about pain relief during labor that is right for her.
2. The nurse manager of the labor and birth unit where you work asks you to develop a protocol for the use of nonpharmacologic and complementary (alternative) methods to relieve discomfort and to enhance progress during labor. She emphasizes that the protocol you develop should be evidence based. Create a protocol that includes at least six nonpharmacologic and complementary approaches. Describe the process you would use to facilitate the changes required to implement the protocols you developed.

RESOURCES

Academy for Guided Imagery, Inc.
P.O. Box 2070
Mill Valley, CA 94942
800-726-2070
www.healthy.net/agi

American Academy of Husband-Coached Childbirth (The Bradley Method of Natural Childbirth)
P.O. Box 5224
Sherman Oaks, CA 91413
800-422-4784
www.bradleybirth.com

Birthworks, Inc.
P.O. Box 2045
Medford, NJ 08055
888-862-4784
www.birthworks.org

Childbirth and Postpartum Professional Association (CAPPA)
310 Sweet Ivy Lane
Lawrenceville, GA 30043
888-548-3672
www.childbirthprofessional.com

Cutting Edge Press
Source for information and equipment regarding childbirth support measures by Polly Perez
www.childbirth.org/CEP.html

Healing Touch International, Inc.
12477 W. Cedar Drive, Suite 202
Lakewood, CO 80228
303-989-7982
www.healingtouch.net

RESOURCES—cont'd

HypnoBirthing Institute
P.O. Box 810
Epsom, NH 03234
603-798-3286
www.hypnobirthing.com

Lamaze International
2025 M Street, Suite 800
Washington, DC 20036-3309
800-368-4404
www.lamaze.org

Maternity Center Association
281 Park Avenue South, 5th floor
New York, NY 10010
212-777-5000
www.maternitywise.org

Read Natural Childbirth Foundation
P.O. Box 150956
San Rafael, CA 94915
415-456-8462

Touch Research Institutes
University of Miami School of Medicine (located at Mailman Center for Child Development)
1601 N.W. 12th Avenue, 7th Floor, Suite 7037
Miami, FL 33101
305-243-6781
www.miami.edu/touch-research/home.html

REFERENCES

Baker, A. et al. (2001). Perceptions of labour pain by mothers and their attending midwives. *Journal of Advanced Nursing, 35*(2), 171-179.

Bricker, L., & Lavender, T. (2002). Parenteral opioids for labor pain relief: A systematic review. *American Journal of Obstetrics and Gynecology, 186*(5), S94-S109.

Buggy, D., & Bardiner, J. (1995). The space blanket and shivering during extradural anesthesia in labour. *Acta Anaesthesiologica Scandinavica, 39*(4), 551-553.

Caton D. et al. (2002). The nature and management of labor pain: Executive summary. *American Journal of Obstetrics and Gynecology, 186*(5), S1-S15.

Chestnut, D. (1999). Alternative regional anesthetic techniques: Paracervical block, lumbar sympathetic block, pudendal block and perineal infiltration. In D. Chestnut (Ed.), *Obstetrics anesthesia: Principles and practice* (2nd ed.). St. Louis: Mosby.

Crane, S. et al. (1997). Association between prepregnancy obesity and the risk of cesarean delivery. *Obstetrics and Gynecology, 89*(2), 2001.

Cunningham, F. et al. (2001). *Williams obstetrics* (21st ed.). New York: McGraw-Hill.

Dickason E., Silverman, B., & Kaplan, J. (1998). *Maternal-infant nursing care* (3rd ed.). St. Louis: Mosby.

Endler, G. (1990). The risk of anesthesia in obese patients. *Journal of Perinatology, 10*(2), 175-179.

Enkin, M. et al. (2000). *A guide to effective care in pregnancy and childbirth* (3rd ed.). Oxford, NY: Oxford University Press.

Faucher, M., & Brucker, M. (2000). Intrapartum pain: Pharmacologic management. *Journal of Obstetric, Gynecologic, and Neonatal Nursing, 29*(2), 169-180.

Gentz, B. (2001). Alternative therapies for the management of pain in labor and delivery. *Clinical Obstetrics and Gynecology, 44*(4), 704-732.

Gilder, K. et al. (2002). Maternal positions in labor with epidural analgesia: Results from a multi-site survey. *AWHONN Lifelines, 6*(1), 40-45.

Govenar, J. (2000). Handling headache after dural puncture. *RN, 63*(12), 26-31.

Hawkins, J., Chestnut, D., & Gibbs, C. (2002). Obstetric anesthesia. In S. Gabbe, J. Niebyl, & J. Simpson (Eds.), *Obstetrics: Normal and problem pregnancies* (4th ed.)(pp. 431-472). Philadelphia: Churchill Livingstone.

Hodnett, E. (2002). Pain and women's satisfaction with the experience of childbirth: A systematic review. *American Journal of Obstetrics and Gynecology, 186*(5), S160-S172.

Hoffart, M., & Pross-Keene, E. (1998). The benefits of visualization. *American Journal of Nursing, 98*(12), 44-47.

Hood, D., & Dewan, D. (1993). Anesthetic and obstetric outcome in morbidly obese parturients. *Anesthesiology, 79*(6), 1210-1218.

Hover-Kramer, D. et al. (2001). *Healing touch: A resource for health care professionals*. Albany, NY: Delmar.

Howell, C. (2001). Epidural vs. nonepidural analgesia for pain relief in labour (Cochrane Review). *The Cochrane Library*, Issue 2, Oxford: Update Software.

Lee, M., & Essoka, G. (1998). Continuing education: Patient's perception of pain: Comparison between Korean-American and Euro-American obstetric patients. *Journal of Cultural Diversity, 5*(1), 29-40.

Lehne, R. (2001). *Pharmacology for nursing care* (4th ed.). Philadelphia: W.B. Saunders.

Leighton, B., & Halpern, S. (2002). The effects of epidural analgesia on labor, maternal, and neonatal outcomes: A systematic review. *American Journal of Obstetrics and Gynecology, 186*(5), S69-S77.

Lieberman, E., & O'Donoghue, C. (2002). Unintended effects of epidural anesthesia during labor: A systematic review. *American Journal of Obstetrics and Gynecology, 186*(5), S31-S68.

Lowe, N. (2002). The nature of labor pain. *American Journal of Obstetrics and Gynecology, 186*(5), S16-S24.

Mackey, M. (2001). Use of water in labor and birth. *Clinical Obstetrics and Gynecology, 44*(4), 733-749.

Manning, J. (1996). Intrathecal narcotics: New approach for labor anesthesia. *Journal of Obstetric, Gynecologic, and Neonatal Nursing, 25*(3), 221-224.

Mattson, S. (2000). Striving for cultural competence: Providing care for the changing face of the U.S. *AWHONN Lifelines, 4*(3), 48-52.

Mayberry, L., Clemmens, D., & De, A. (2002). Epidural analgesia side effects, co-interventions, and care of women during childbirth: A systematic review. *American Journal of Obstetrics and Gynecology, 186*(5), S81-S93.

Nichols, F., & Humenick, S. (2000). *Childbirth education: Practice, research, and theory* (2nd ed.). Philadephia: W.B. Saunders.

Righard, L. (2001). Making childbirth a normal process. *Birth, 28*(1), 1-4.

Rosen, M. (2002a). Paracervical block for labor analgesia: A brief historical review. *American Journal of Obstetrics and Gynecology, 186*(5), S127-S130.

Rosen, M. (2002b). Nitrous oxide for relief of labor pain: A systematic review. *American Journal of Obstetrics and Gynecology, 186*(5), S110-S126.

Sampselle, C. (1999). Spontaneous pushing during birth. *Journal of Nurse Midwifery, 44*(1), 36-39.

Scheiber, B., & Selby, C. (Eds.) (2000). *Therapeutic touch.* New York: Prometheus Books.

Schuiling, K., & Sampselle, C. (1999). Comfort in labor and midwifery art. *Image: Journal of Nursing Scholarship, 31*(1), 77-81.

Scott, J. et al. (Eds.) (1999). *Danforth's obstetrics and gynecology* (8th ed.). Philadelphia: Lippincott Williams & Wilkins.

Shapiro, H. et al. (1997). *The Lamaze ready reference guide for labor and birth* (2nd ed.). Washington, DC: Chapter ASPO/Lamaze.

Simkin, P. (1995). Reducing pain and enhancing progress in labor: A guide to nonpharmacologic methods of maternity caregivers. *Birth, 22*(3), 161-171.

Simkin, P., & Ancheta, R. (2000). *The labor progress handbook: Early interventions to prevent and treat dystocia.* Malden, MA: Blackwell Science, Inc.

Simkin, P., & O'Hara, M. (2002). Nonpharmacologic relief of pain during labor: Systematic reviews of five methods. *American Journal of Obstetrics and Gynecology, 186*(5), S131-S159.

Snyder, M., & Lindquist, R. (Eds.) (2000). *Complementary/alternative therapies in nursing* (4th ed). New York: Springer.

Tiran, D., & Mack, S. (2000). *Complementary therapies for pregnancy and childbirth* (2nd ed.). Edinburgh: Bailliere-Tindall.

Villarruel, A. (1995). Mexican-American cultural meanings, expressions, self-care and dependent-care actions associated with experiences of pain. *Research in Nursing and Health, 18*, 427-436.

Weber, S. (1996). Cultural aspects of pain in childbearing women. *Journal of Obstetric, Gynecologic, and Neonatal Nursing, 25*(1), 67-72.

Wiand, N. (1997). Relaxation levels achieved by Lamaze-trained pregnant women listening to music and ocean sound tapes. *Journal of Perinatal Education, 6*(4), 1-8.

CHAPTER 20

Susan Martin Tucker

Fetal Assessment During Labor

http://evolve.elsevier.com/Lowdermilk/MatWmnHlth/

LEARNING OBJECTIVES

- Identify typical signs of nonreassuring fetal heart rate (FHR) patterns.
- Compare FHR monitoring done by intermittent auscultation (IA) with external and internal electronic methods.
- Explain the baseline FHR and evaluate periodic changes.
- Describe nursing measures that can be used to maintain FHR patterns within normal limits.
- Differentiate among the nursing interventions used for managing specific FHR patterns, including tachycardia and bradycardia; increased and decreased variability; and late and variable decelerations.
- Review the application of the monitor.
- Review the documentation of the monitoring process necessary during labor.

The ability to assess the fetus by auscultation of fetal heart tones was initially described more than 300 years ago. With the advent of the fetoscope and stethoscope after the turn of the twentieth century, the listener could hear clearly enough to count the fetal heart rate (FHR). When electronic FHR monitoring made its debut for clinical use in the early 1970s, it was anticipated that its use would effect a decrease in cerebral palsy and be more sensitive than stethoscopic auscultation in predicting and preventing fetal compromise (Simpson & Knox, 2000). Although neither of these possibilities has been realized, electronic fetal monitoring (EFM) is a useful tool for visualizing FHR patterns on a monitor screen or printed tracing.

Pregnant women should be informed about the equipment and procedures used and the risks, benefits, and limitations of intermittent auscultation (IA) and EFM. This chapter discusses the basis for fetal monitoring, the types of monitoring, and nursing assessment and management of nonreassuring fetal status.

BASIS FOR MONITORING

Fetal Response

Because labor is a period of physiologic stress for the fetus, frequent monitoring of fetal status is part of the nursing care during labor. The fetal oxygen supply must be maintained during labor to prevent fetal compromise and to promote newborn health after birth. The fetal oxygen supply can decrease in a number of ways:

1. Reduction of blood flow through the maternal vessels as a result of maternal hypertension (chronic hypertension or pregnancy-induced hypertension), hypotension (caused by supine maternal position, hemorrhage, or epidural analgesia or anesthesia), or hypovolemia (caused by hemorrhage)
2. Reduction of the oxygen content in the maternal blood as a result of hemorrhage or severe anemia
3. Alterations in fetal circulation, occurring with compression of the umbilical cord (transient: during uterine contractions [UCs]; or prolonged, resulting from cord prolapse), placental separation or complete abruption, or head compression (head compression causes increased intracranial pressure and vagal nerve stimulation with an accompanying decrease in the FHR)
4. Reduction in blood flow to the intervillous space in the placenta secondary to uterine hypertonus (generally caused by excessive exogenous oxytocin) or secondary to deterioration of the placental vasculature associated with maternal disorders such as hypertension or diabetes mellitus

Fetal well-being during labor can be measured by the response of the FHR to UCs. In general, **reassuring FHR patterns** are characterized by the following:

- A baseline FHR in the normal range of 110 to 160 beats/min with no periodic changes and a moderate baseline variability
- Accelerations with fetal movement

A normal uterine activity pattern in labor is characterized by contractions occurring every 2 to 5 minutes and lasting less than 90 seconds; such contractions are moderate to strong in intensity, as evidenced by palpation, or intensity is less than 100 mm Hg, as measured by an intrauterine pressure catheter (IUPC); 30 seconds or more should elapse between the end of one contraction and the beginning of the next contraction; between contractions, uterine relaxation should be detected by palpation or by an average intrauterine pressure of 15 mm Hg or less.

Fetal Compromise

The goals of intrapartum FHR monitoring are to identify and differentiate the reassuring patterns from the nonreassuring patterns, which can be indicative of fetal compromise.

Nonreassuring FHR patterns are those associated with fetal **hypoxemia,** which is a deficiency of oxygen in the arterial blood. If uncorrected, hypoxemia can deteriorate to severe fetal **hypoxia,** which is an inadequate supply of oxygen at the cellular level. Nonreassuring FHR patterns include the following:

- Progressive increase or decrease in baseline rate
- Tachycardia of 160 beats/min or more
- Progressive decrease in baseline variability
- Severe variable decelerations (FHR less than 60 beats/min lasting longer than 30 to 60 seconds, with rising baseline, decreasing variability, or slow return to baseline)
- Late decelerations of any magnitude, especially those that are repetitive and uncorrectable
- Absence of FHR variability
- Prolonged deceleration (greater than 60 to 90 seconds)
- Severe bradycardia (less than 70 beats/min)

The nurse's role is to assess continually whether the FHR pattern is reassuring, which reflects adequate fetal oxygenation. When the pattern is nonreassuring, the nurse must discriminate between those patterns that indicate mild fetal hypoxemia and other nonreassuring patterns that indicate severe fetal hypoxia. The nursing interventions to be taken when encountering nonreassuring patterns are described in detail in this chapter.

MONITORING TECHNIQUES

The ideal method of fetal assessment during labor continues to be debated. Results from multiple research studies indicate that both intermittent auscultation of the FHR and electronic FHR monitoring are associated with similar fetal outcomes (American College of Obstetricians and Gynecologists, 1995; Feinstein, Sprague, & Trepanier, 2000; Thacker, Stroup, & Chang, 2001). Although intermittent auscultation is a high-touch, low-technology method of assessing fetal status during labor that places fewer restrictions on maternal activity, more than 80% of laboring women in the United States are monitored electronically for at least part of their labor (Albers, 2001).

Intermittent Auscultation

Intermittent auscultation (IA) uses listening to fetal heart sounds at periodic intervals to assess the FHR. IA of the fetal heart can be performed with a Leff scope, a DeLee-Hillis fetoscope, or an ultrasound device. If a Leff scope is used, the domed side should be opened to the connective tubing to the earpieces. The domed side is then applied to the maternal abdomen. The fetoscope is applied over the listener's head because bone conduction amplifies the fetal heart sounds for counting. The ultrasound device transmits ultrahigh-frequency sound waves reflecting movement of the fetal heart and converts these sounds into an electronic signal that can be counted (Fig. 20-1).

One procedure for performing auscultation is as follows:

1. Perform Leopold maneuvers (see p. 562) by palpating the maternal abdomen to identify fetal presentation and position.
2. Place the listening device over the area of maximal intensity and clarity of the fetal heart sounds to obtain the clearest and loudest sound, which is easiest to count.
3. Palpate the abdomen for the absence of uterine activity to be able to count the FHR between contractions.
4. Count the maternal radial pulse at the same time as listening to the FHR to differentiate it from the fetal rate.
5. Count the FHR for 30 to 60 seconds between contractions to identify the baseline rate. This rate can be assessed only during the absence of uterine activity.
6. Auscultate the FHR during a contraction and for 30 seconds after the end of the contraction to identify any increases or decreases in FHR in response to the contraction.

By using IA, the nurse can assess the FHR baseline rate, rhythm, and increases and decreases from baseline (Feinstein, 2000). The method and frequency of fetal surveillance during labor will vary depending on maternal-fetal risk factors and the preference of the facility. In the

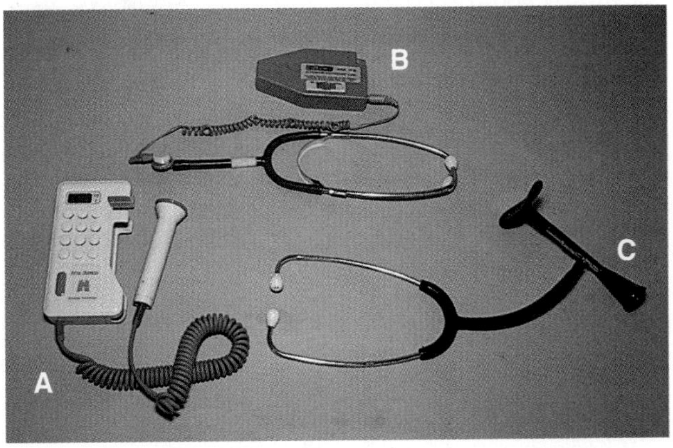

A
B
C

FIG. 20-1 **A,** Ultrasound fetoscope. **B,** Ultrasound stethoscope. **C,** DeLee-Hillis fetoscope. (Courtesy Michael S. Clement, MD, Mesa, AZ.)

absence of risk factors, one recommended practice is to auscultate the FHR as follows (Feinstein et al., 2000):

- First stage
  - Latent phase: every 60 minutes
  - Active phase: every 30 minutes
- Second stage
  - Every 15 minutes

If risk factors are present, the FHR is auscultated as follows:

- First stage
  - Latent phase: every 30 minutes
  - Active phase: every 15 minutes
- Second stage
  - Every 5 minutes

In addition, the FHR is assessed before and after ambulation, rupture of membranes, administration of medications and anesthesia, and more frequently when nonreassuring FHR patterns are heard (AWHONN, 1997; Tucker, 2000).

NURSE ALERT

When the FHR is auscultated and documented, it is inappropriate to use the descriptive terms associated with EFM because most of the terms are visual descriptions of the patterns produced on the monitor tracing. Terms that are numerically defined, however, such as bradycardia and tachycardia, can be used.

Every effort should be made to use the method of fetal assessment the woman desires, if possible. However, auscultation of the FHR in accordance with the frequency guidelines just given may be difficult in today's busy labor and birth units. When used as the primary method of fetal assessment, auscultation requires a one-to-one nurse-to-client staffing ratio. If acuity and census change so that auscultation standards are no longer met, the nurse must inform the physician or nurse-midwife that continuous EFM will be used until staffing can be arranged to meet the standards.

The woman can become anxious if the examiner cannot readily count the fetal heartbeats. It often takes time for the inexperienced listener to locate the heartbeat and find the area of maximal intensity. To allay the mother's concerns, she can be told that the nurse is "finding the spot where the sounds are loudest." If it takes considerable time to locate the fetal heartbeats, the examiner can reassure the mother by offering her an opportunity to listen to them, too. If the examiner cannot locate the fetal heartbeat, assistance should be requested. In some cases, ultrasound can be used to help locate the fetal heartbeat. Seeing the FHR on the ultrasound screen will be reassuring to the mother if there was initial difficulty in locating the best area for auscultation.

When using IA, uterine activity is assessed by palpation. The examiner should keep his or her hand placed over the fundus before, during, and after contractions. The contraction intensity is usually described as mild, moderate, or strong. The contraction duration is measured in seconds, from the beginning to the end of the contraction. The frequency of contractions is measured in minutes, from the beginning of one contraction to the beginning of the next contraction. The examiner should keep his or her hand on the fundus after the contraction is over to evaluate uterine resting tone or relaxation between contractions. Resting tone between contractions is usually described as soft or relaxed (Goodwin, 2000).

Accurate and complete documentation of fetal status and uterine activity is especially important when IA and palpation are being used because no paper tracing record of these assessments is provided as is by continuous EFM. Labor flow records or computer charting systems that prompt notations of all assessments are useful for ensuring such comprehensive documentation.

Auscultation and palpation require the nurse to obtain the fetal heart rate and uterine activity manually and to document this at the appropriate intervals on the woman's medical record. In contrast, a continuous recording of the FHR and uterine activity is independent of the medical record and can be viewed by multiple care providers concurrently and retrospectively (Chez, Harvey, & Harvey, 2000).

Electronic Fetal Monitoring

The purpose of electronic FHR monitoring is the ongoing assessment of fetal oxygenation. FHR tracings are analyzed for characteristic patterns that signify specific hypoxic and nonhypoxic events (King & Parer, 2000; Parer & King, 2000). These characteristic FHR patterns are associated with fetal and maternal physiologic processes and have been identified for many years, but some variations in descriptions, definitions, and interpretations have limited the study of the validity and effectiveness of electronic FHR monitoring. In 1995 a research-planning workshop was held to develop research guidelines for EFM interpretation. Experts in the field participated, including those in medicine, nursing, epidemiology, basic science, and the general public. The first document to be published by the group was a proposed nomenclature system for EFM interpretation. This document presented standardized definitions for FHR monitoring (National Institute of Child Health and Human Development Research Planning Workshop, 1997). These definitions are being tested for reliability and accuracy and will be refined based on results of the tests.

Some effect on current clinical practice is likely. For that reason, this chapter includes the new definitions and discussion of the current systems of interpretation of EFM. Practitioners who continue to use the established terminology during this period of transition should continue to use guidelines developed by the Association of Women's Health, Obstetric, and Neonatal

TABLE 20-1 **External and Internal Modes of Monitoring**

EXTERNAL MODE	INTERNAL MODE
FHR	
Ultrasound transducer: High-frequency sound waves reflect mechanical action of the fetal heart. Noninvasive. Does not require rupture of membranes or cervical dilation. Used during both the antepartum and intrapartum periods.	*Spiral electrode:* This electrode converts the fetal ECG as obtained from the presenting part to the FHR via a cardiotachometer. This method can be used only when membranes are ruptured and the cervix is sufficiently dilated during the intrapartum period. Electrode penetrates into fetal presenting part by 1.5 mm and must be attached securely to ensure a good signal.
Uterine Activity	
Tocotransducer: This instrument monitors frequency and duration of contractions by means of pressure-sensing device applied to the maternal abdomen. Used during both the antepartum and intrapartum periods.	*Intrauterine pressure catheter (IUPC):* This instrument monitors the frequency, duration, and intensity of contractions. The two types of IUPCs are a fluid-filled system and a solid catheter. Both measure intrauterine pressure at the catheter tip and convert the pressure into millimeters of mercury on the uterine activity panel of the strip chart. Both can be used only when membranes are ruptured and the cervix is sufficiently dilated during the intrapartum period.

Nurses (AWHONN, 1997, 1998) and the American College of Obstetricians and Gynecologists (1995). Practitioners who wish to use the new terminology should communicate with other health care providers about the use of the new terminology instead of established definitions (Harvey, 1997). They also will need to make changes in their practice as the definitions are refined through testing. All perinatal health care providers must keep abreast of the new developments in EFM technology and knowledge to ensure the best possible outcomes for mothers and newborns.

The two modes of **electronic fetal monitoring** include the external mode, which uses external transducers placed on the maternal abdomen to assess FHR and uterine activity, and the internal mode, which uses a **spiral electrode** applied to the fetal presenting part to assess the FHR and an **intrauterine pressure catheter** to assess uterine activity and pressure. The differences between the external and internal modes of EFM are summarized in Table 20-1.

External Monitoring

Separate transducers are used to monitor the FHR and UCs (Fig. 20-2). The **ultrasound transducer** works by reflecting high-frequency sound waves off a moving interface: in this case, the fetal heart and valves; therefore short-term variability and beat-to-beat changes in the FHR cannot be assessed accurately by this method. It is sometimes difficult to reproduce a continuous and precise record of the FHR because of artifacts introduced by fetal and maternal movement. The FHR is printed on specially formatted monitor paper. The standard paper speed is 3 cm/min. Once the area of maximal intensity of the FHR has been located, conductive gel is applied to the surface of the ultrasound transducer, and the transducer is then positioned over this area.

The **tocotransducer** (tocodynamometer) measures uterine activity transabdominally. The device is placed over the fundus above the umbilicus. UCs or fetal movements depress a pressure-sensitive surface on the side next to the abdomen. The tocotransducer can measure and record the frequency, regularity, and approximate duration of UCs but not their intensity. This method is especially valuable for measuring uterine activity during the first stage of labor in women with intact membranes or for antepartum testing. Because the tocotransducer of most electronic fetal monitors is designed for assessing uterine activity in the term pregnancy, it may not be sensitive enough to detect preterm uterine activity. When monitoring the woman in preterm labor, remember that the fundus may be located below the level of the umbilicus. The nurse may need to rely on the woman to indicate when uterine activity is occurring and to use palpation as an additional way of assessing contraction frequency.

The external transducer is easily applied by the nurse, but it must be repositioned as the woman or fetus changes position (see Fig. 20-2, *B*). The woman is asked to assume a semisitting position or lateral position. The equipment is removed periodically to wash the applicator sites and to give back rubs. Use of an external transducer confines the woman to bed. Portable telemetry monitors allow observation of the FHR and uterine contraction patterns by means of centrally located electronic display stations. These portable units permit the woman to walk around

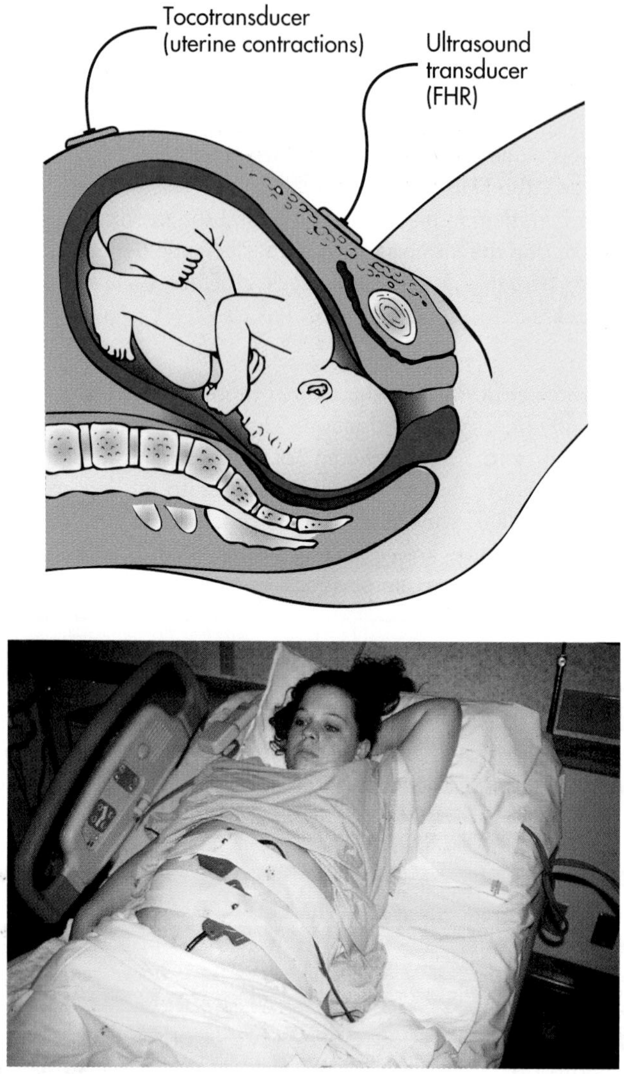
A
Tocotransducer
(uterine contractions)
Ultrasound
transducer
(FHR)
B

FIG. 20-2 **A,** External noninvasive fetal monitoring with tocotransducer and ultrasound transducer. **B,** Ultrasound transducer is placed below umbilicus, over the area where fetal heart rate is best heard, and tocotransducer is placed on uterine fundus. (Courtesy Marjorie Pyle, RNC, Lifecircle, Costa Mesa, CA.)

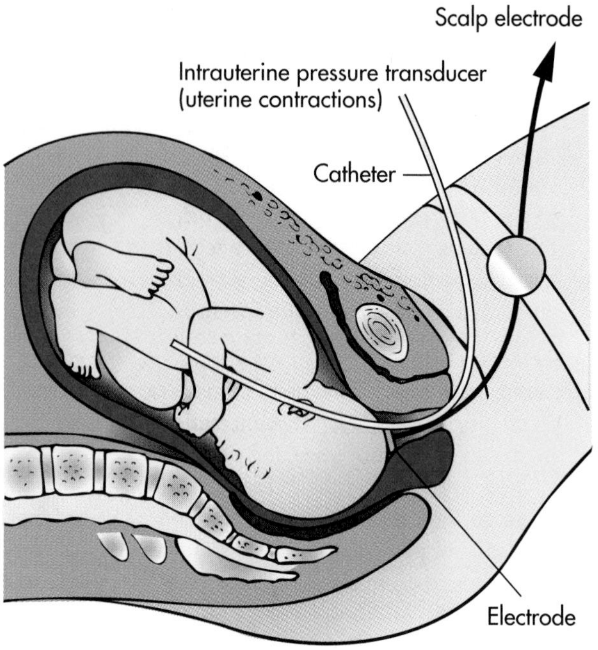
Scalp electrode
Intrauterine pressure transducer
(uterine contractions)
Catheter
Electrode

FIG. 20-3 Diagrammatic representation of internal invasive fetal monitoring with intrauterine pressure catheter and spiral electrode in place (membranes ruptured and cervix dilated).

during electronic monitoring. Other monitoring equipment can be used when the woman is submerged in water (see Fig. 19-4).

Internal Monitoring

The technique of continuous internal monitoring provides an accurate appraisal of fetal well-being during labor (Fig. 20-3). For this type of monitoring, the membranes must be ruptured, the cervix sufficiently dilated, and the presenting part low enough to allow placement of the electrode. A small **spiral electrode** attached to the presenting part shows a continuous FHR on the fetal monitor strip.

Internal monitoring of the FHR may be implemented without internal monitoring of uterine activity. To monitor uterine activity, a solid or fluid-filled IUPC is introduced into the uterine cavity. A solid catheter has a pressure-sensitive tip that measures changes in intrauterine pressure. A catheter filled with sterile water also can be used. As the catheter is compressed during a contraction, pressure is placed on the pressure transducer or strain gauge; this pressure is then converted into a pressure reading in millimeters of mercury. The average pressure during a contraction ranges from 50 to 85 mm Hg. The IUPC can measure the frequency, duration, and intensity of UCs.

The FHR and uterine activity (UA) are displayed on the monitor paper with the FHR in the upper section and UA in the lower section. Figure 20-4 contrasts the internal and external modes of electronic monitoring. Note that each small square represents 10 seconds; each larger box of six squares equals 1 minute (when paper is moving through the monitor at 3 cm/min).

FETAL HEART RATE PATTERNS

Baseline Fetal Heart Rate

The intrinsic rhythmicity of the fetal heart, the central nervous system (CNS), and the fetal autonomic nervous system control the FHR. An increase in sympathetic response results in acceleration of the FHR, whereas an augmenta-

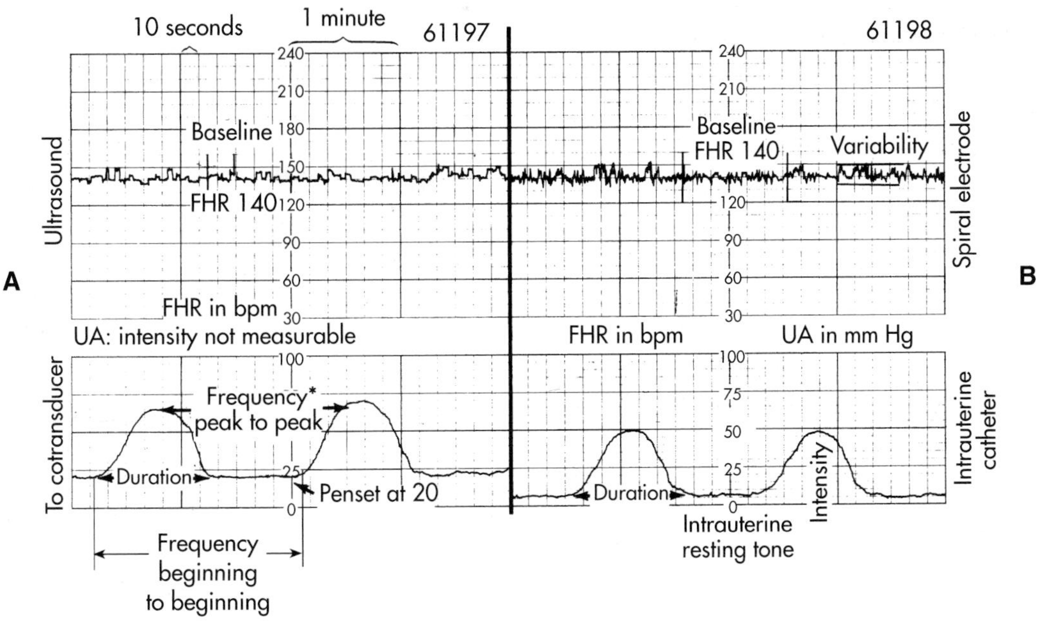
10 seconds
1 minute
61197
61198
Ultrasound
Baseline
FHR 140
FHR in bpm
UA: intensity not measurable
To cotransducer
Frequency*
peak to peak
Duration
Penset at 20
Frequency
beginning
to beginning
A
Baseline
FHR 140
Variability
Spiral electrode
B
FHR in bpm
UA in mm Hg
Intrauterine catheter
Duration
Intensity
Intrauterine
resting tone

FIG. 20-4 Display of fetal heart rate and uterine activity on monitor paper. **A,** External mode with ultrasound and tocotransducer as signal source. **B,** Internal mode with spiral electrode and intrauterine catheter as signal source. Frequency of contractions is measured from the beginning of one contraction to the beginning of the next. Peak-to-peak measurement is sometimes used when electronic uterine activity monitoring is done. (From Tucker, S. [2000]. *Pocket guide to fetal monitoring and assessment* [4th ed.]. St. Louis: Mosby.)

tion in parasympathetic response produces a slowing of the FHR. Usually a balanced increase of sympathetic and parasympathetic response occurs during contractions, with no observable change in the baseline FHR.

Baseline fetal heart rate is the average rate during a 10-minute segment that excludes periodic or episodic changes, periods of marked variability, and segments of the baseline that differ by more than 25 beats/min (National Institute, 1997). The normal range at term is 110 to 160 beats/min.

Variability of the FHR can be described as irregular fluctuations in the baseline FHR of two cycles per minute or greater (National Institute, 1997). Variability has been described as short term (beat to beat) or long term (rhythmic waves or cycles from baseline). The current definition for research does not distinguish between short-term and long-term variability because in actual practice, they are viewed together (National Institute, 1997); however, this definition does identify four ranges of variability as seen in Figure 20-5. These are based on visualization of the amplitude of the FHR in the peak-to-trough segment in beats per minute and include the following:

- Absent or undetected variability
- Minimal variability (greater than undetected but not more than 5 beats/min)

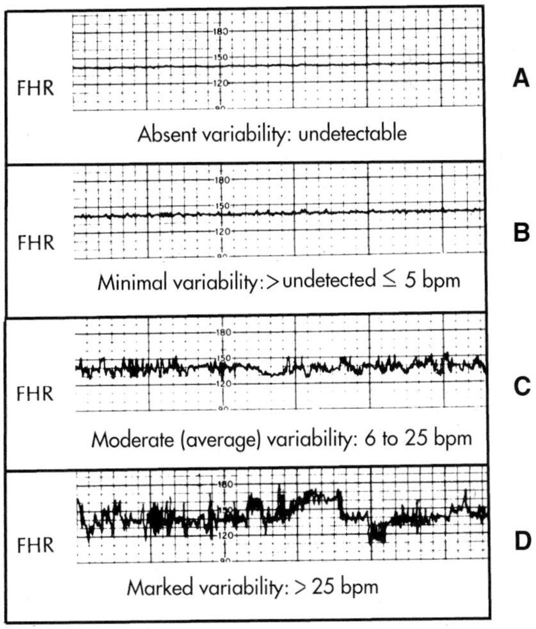
FHR
Absent variability: undetectable
A
FHR
Minimal variability: > undetected ≤ 5 bpm
B
FHR
Moderate (average) variability: 6 to 25 bpm
C
FHR
Marked variability: > 25 bpm
D

FIG. 20-5 Fetal heart rate variability. **A,** Absent or undetected. **B,** Minimal. **C,** Moderate. **D,** Marked. (Modified from Tucker, S. [2000]. *Pocket guide to fetal monitoring and assessment* [4th ed.]. St. Louis: Mosby.)

- Moderate variability (6 to 25 beats/min)
- Marked variability (greater than 25 beats/min)

In many facilities, short-term and long-term variability continue to be used to describe the FHR fluctuations.

Absence of or undetected variability is considered nonreassuring. Diminished variability can result from fetal hypoxemia and acidosis, as well as from certain drugs that depress the CNS, including analgesics, narcotics (meperidine [Demerol]), barbiturates (secobarbital [Seconal] and pentobarbital [Nembutal]), tranquilizers (diazepam [Valium]), ataractics (promethazine [Phenergan]), and general anesthetics. In addition, a temporary decrease in variability can occur when the fetus is in a sleep state. These sleep states do not usually last longer

TABLE 20-2 **Increased and Decreased Variability**

INCREASED VARIABILITY	DECREASED VARIABILITY
Cause	
Early mild hypoxemia Fetal stimulation by the following: Uterine palpation Uterine contractions Fetal activity Maternal activity Illicit drugs (e.g., cocaine and methamphetamines)	Hypoxia/acidosis Central nervous system (CNS) depressants Analgesics/narcotics Meperidine (Demerol) Alphaprodine (Nisentil) Morphine Pentazocine (Talwin) Barbiturates Secobarbital (Seconal) Pentobarbital (Nembutal) Amobarbital (Amytal) Tranquilizers Diazepam (Valium) Ataractics Promethazine (Phenergan) Propiomazine (Largon) Hydroxyzine (Vistaril) Promazine (Sparine) Parasympatholytics Atropine General anesthetics Prematurity: <24 wk Fetal sleep cycles Congenital abnormalities Fetal cardiac dysrhythmias
Clinical Significance	
Significance of marked variability not known; increased variability from a previous average variability is earliest fetal heart rate (FHR) sign of mild hypoxemia	Benign when associated with periodic fetal sleep states, which last 20 to 30 min; if caused by drugs, variability usually increases as drugs are excreted Decreased variability is not reassuring and is considered a sign of fetal stress *unless* it has an identifiable temporary (e.g., fetal sleep) or correctable cause Decreased variability associated with uncorrectable late decelerations indicates presence of fetal acidosis and can result in low Apgar scores
Nursing Intervention	
Observe FHR tracing carefully for any nonreassuring patterns, including decreasing variability and late decelerations; if using external mode of monitoring, consider using internal mode (spiral electrode) for a more accurate tracing	Dependent on cause; intervention not warranted if associated with fetal sleep states or temporarily associated with CNS depressants; consider performing external stimulation or scalp stimulation during a vaginal examination to elicit an acceleration of FHR or return to average variability; consider application of spiral electrode; assist health care provider with fetal oxygen saturation monitoring if ordered; prepare for birth if so indicated by the primary health care provider

than 30 minutes. Table 20-2 contrasts key differences between increased and decreased variability.

A sinusoidal pattern, a regular smooth, undulating wavelike pattern, is not included in the current research definition of FHR variability. This uncommon pattern occurs when fetal hypoxia results from Rh isoimmunization or fetal anemia.

Tachycardia is a baseline FHR greater than 160 beats/min for a duration of 10 minutes or longer. It can be considered an early sign of fetal hypoxemia, especially when associated with late decelerations and minimal or absent variability. Fetal tachycardia can result from maternal or fetal infection, such as prolonged rupture of membranes with amnionitis; from maternal hyperthyroidism or fetal anemia; or in response to drugs such as atropine, hydroxyzine (Vistaril), terbutaline, or illicit drugs such as cocaine or methamphetamines.

Bradycardia is a baseline FHR less than 110 beats/min for a duration of 10 minutes or longer. (Bradycardia should be distinguished from prolonged deceleration patterns, which are periodic changes described later in this chapter.) It can be considered a later sign of fetal hypoxia and is known to occur before fetal death. Bradycardia can result from placental transfer of drugs such as anesthetics, prolonged compression of the umbilical cord, maternal hypothermia, and maternal hypotension. Maternal supine hypotension syndrome, caused by the weight and pressure of the gravid uterus on the vena cava, decreases the return of blood flow to the maternal heart, which then reduces maternal cardiac output and blood pressure. These responses in the mother subsequently result in a decrease in the FHR and fetal bradycardia. Table 20-3 contrasts tachycardia with bradycardia.

Changes in Fetal Heart Rate

Changes in FHR from the baseline are categorized as periodic or episodic. **Periodic changes** are those that occur with UCs. **Episodic changes** (nonperiodic changes) are those that are not associated with UCs. These patterns include accelerations and decelerations (National Institute, 1997).

TABLE *20-3* **Tachycardia and Bradycardia**

	TACHYCARDIA	BRADYCARDIA
Definition	FHR >160 beats/min lasting >10 min	FHR <110 beats/min lasting >10 min
Cause	Early fetal hypoxemia Maternal fever Parasympatholytic drugs (atropine, hydroxyzine) β-Sympathomimetic drugs (ritodrine, isoxsuprine) Intraamniotic infection Maternal hyperthyroidism Fetal anemia Fetal heart failure Fetal cardiac dysrhythmias Illicit drugs (cocaine, methamphetamines)	Late fetal hypoxemia/hypoxia β-Adrenergic blocking drugs (propranolol; anesthetics for epidural, spinal, caudal, and pudendal blocks) Maternal hypotension Prolonged umbilical cord compression Fetal congenital heart block Maternal hypothermia Prolonged maternal hypoglycemia
Clinical Significance	Persistent tachycardia in absence of periodic changes does not appear serious in terms of neonatal outcome (especially true if tachycardia is associated with maternal fever); tachycardia is a nonreassuring sign when associated with late decelerations, severe variable decelerations, or absence of variability.	Bradycardia with moderate variability and absence of periodic changes is not a sign of fetal compromise if FHR remains >80 beats/min; bradycardia caused by hypoxia is a nonreassuring sign when associated with loss of variability and late decelerations.
Nursing Intervention	Dependent on cause; reduce maternal fever with antipyretics as ordered and cooling measures; oxygen at 8 to 10 L/min by face mask may be of some value; carry out health care provider's orders based on alleviating cause.	Dependent on cause; intervention not warranted in fetus with heart block diagnosed by ECG; oxygen at 8 to 10 L/min by face mask may be of some value; carry out health care provider's orders based on alleviating cause. Scalp stimulation may be performed to determine whether the fetus has the ability to compensate physiologically for stress (FHR will accelerate).

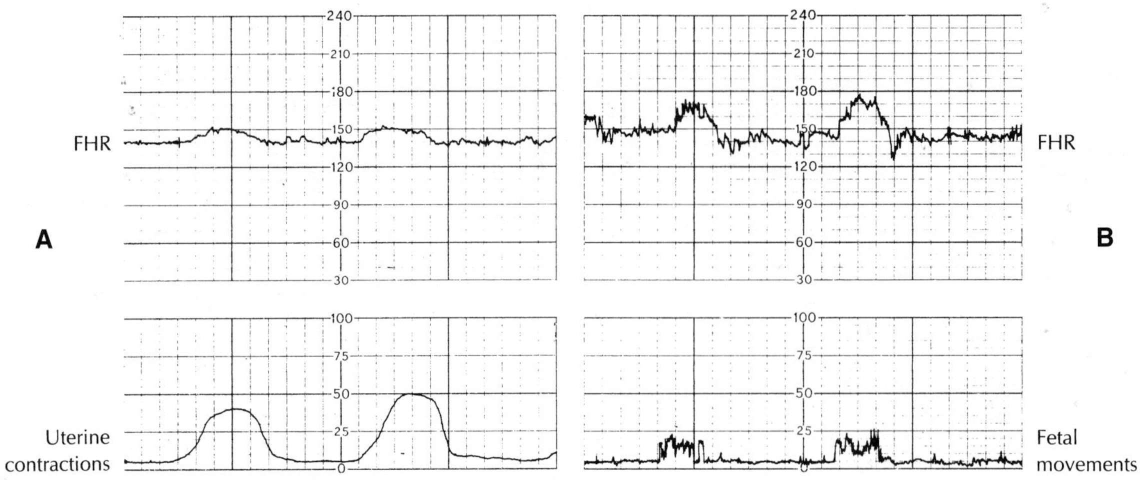

240
210
180
150
120
90
60
30
FHR
A
B
100
75
50
25
0
Uterine contractions
Fetal movements

FIG. 20-6 **A,** Acceleration of fetal heart rate (FHR) with uterine contractions. **B,** Acceleration of FHR movement. (From Tucker, S. [2000]. *Pocket guide to fetal monitoring and assessment* [4th ed.]. St. Louis: Mosby.)

Accelerations

Acceleration of the FHR is defined as a visually apparent abrupt increase in FHR above the baseline rate. The increase is 15 beats/min or greater and lasts 15 seconds or more, with the return to baseline less than 2 minutes from the beginning of the acceleration. In preterm gestations, the definition of an acceleration is a peak of 10 beats/min or more above baseline for at least 10 seconds. Acceleration of the FHR for more than 10 minutes is considered a change in baseline rate.

Accelerations can be periodic or episodic. Periodic accelerations are caused by dominance of the sympathetic nervous response and are usually encountered with breech presentations (Fig. 20-6, *A*). Pressure of the contraction applied to the fetal buttocks results in accelerations, whereas pressure applied to the head results in decelerations. Accelerations may occur, however, during the second stage of labor in cephalic presentations. Episodic accelerations (Fig. 20-6, *B*) of the FHR occur during fetal movement and are indications of fetal well-being.

Decelerations

A **deceleration** (caused by dominance of parasympathetic response) may be benign or nonreassuring. Three types of decelerations are encountered during labor: *early, late,* and *variable*. FHR decelerations are described by their visual relation to the onset and end of a contraction and by their shape.

Early Decelerations. *Early deceleration* of the FHR is a visually apparent gradual decrease and return to baseline FHR in response to **fetal head compression.** It is a normal and benign finding (Fig. 20-7, *A*) (National Institute, 1997). The deceleration generally starts before the peak of the uterine contraction (UC) and returns to the baseline at the same time as the UC returns to its baseline. Early decelerations may also occur during UCs, during vaginal examinations, as a result of fundal pressure, and during placement of the internal mode of fetal monitoring. When present, they usually occur during the first stage of labor when the cervix is dilated 4 to 7 cm. Early decelerations sometimes are seen during the second stage when the woman is pushing.

Because early decelerations are considered to be benign, interventions are not necessary. The value of identifying early decelerations is so that they can be distinguished from late or variable decelerations, which can be nonreassuring and for which interventions are appropriate. The different characteristics of accelerations of the FHR and early decelerations are contrasted in Table 20-4.

Late Decelerations. Uteroplacental insufficiency causes late decelerations. *Late deceleration* of the FHR is a visually apparent gradual decrease in and return to baseline FHR associated with UCs (National Institute, 1997). The deceleration begins after the contraction has started, and the lowest point of the deceleration occurs after the peak of the contraction. The deceleration usually does not return to baseline until after the contraction is over (Fig. 20-7, *B*).

Persistent and repetitive late decelerations usually indicate the presence of fetal hypoxemia stemming from insufficient placental perfusion. They can be associated with fetal hypoxemia progressing to hypoxia and acidemia progressing to acidosis. They should be considered an ominous sign when they are uncorrectable, especially if they are associated with decreased variability and tachycardia. Late decelerations caused by the maternal supine hypotension syndrome are usually correctable when the woman turns on her side to displace the weight

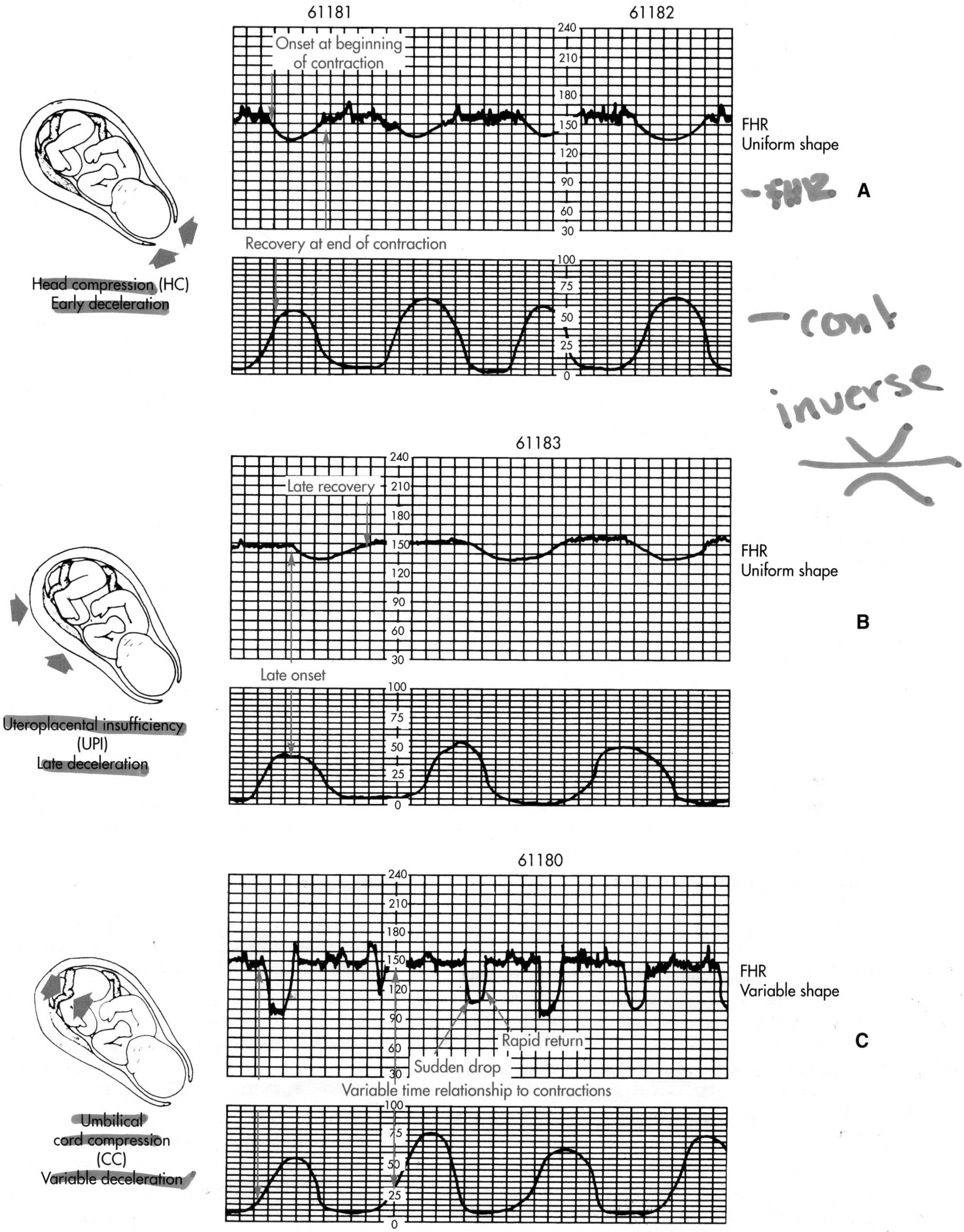
61181
61182
Onset at beginning of contraction
Recovery at end of contraction
240
210
180
150
120
90
60
30
100
75
50
25
0
FHR
Uniform shape
A
Head compression (HC)
Early deceleration
61183
Late recovery
Late onset
FHR
Uniform shape
B
Uteroplacental insufficiency
(UPI)
Late deceleration
61180
Rapid return
Sudden drop
Variable time relationship to contractions
FHR
Variable shape
C
Umbilical
cord compression
(CC)
Variable deceleration

FIG. 20-7 Decelerations patterns. **A,** Early decelerations caused by head compression. **B,** Late decelerations caused by uteroplacental insufficiency. **C,** Variable decelerations caused by cord compression. (From Tucker, S. [2000]. *Pocket guide to fetal monitoring and assessment* [4th ed.]. St. Louis: Mosby.)

TABLE 20-4 **Accelerations and Early Decelerations**

	ACCELERATION	EARLY DECELERATION
Description	Transitory increase of fetal heart rate (FHR) above baseline (see Fig. 20-6)	Transitory decrease of FHR below baseline concurrent with uterine contractions (see Fig. 20-7, *A*)
Shape	May resemble shape of uterine contraction or be spikelike	Uniform shape; mirror image of uterine contraction
Onset	Onset to peak (30 sec; often precedes or occurs simultaneous with uterine contraction)	Early in contraction phase before peak of contraction
Recovery	Less than 2 min from onset	By end of contraction as uterine pressure returns to its resting tone
Amplitude	Usually 15 beats/min above baseline	Usually proportional to amplitude of contraction; rarely decelerates to <100 beats/min
Baseline	Usually associated with average baseline variability	Usually associated with average baseline variability
Occurrence	Variable; may be repetitive with each contraction	Repetitious (occurs with each contraction); usually occurs between 4- and 7-cm dilation and in second stage of labor
Cause	Spontaneous fetal movement Vaginal examination Electrode application Breech presentation Occiput posterior position Uterine contractions Fundal pressure Abdominal palpation	Head compression resulting from the following: Uterine contractions Vaginal examination Fundal pressure Placement of internal mode of monitoring
Clinical significance	Acceleration with fetal movement signifies fetal well-being representing fetal alertness or arousal states	Reassuring pattern not associated with fetal hypoxemia, acidemia, or low Apgar scores
Nursing intervention	None required	None required

of the gravid uterus off the vena cava. Such lateral positioning allows better return of maternal blood flow to the heart, which in turn increases cardiac output and blood pressure.

Late decelerations caused by uteroplacental insufficiency can result from uterine hyperstimulation with oxytocin, pregnancy-induced hypertension, postdate or postterm pregnancy, amnionitis, small-for-gestational-age (SGA) fetus, maternal diabetes, placenta previa, abruptio placentae, conduction anesthetics (producing maternal hypotension), maternal cardiac disease, and maternal anemia. The clinical significance and nursing interventions are described in Table 20-5.

Variable Decelerations. *Variable deceleration* is defined as a visual abrupt decrease in FHR below the baseline. The decrease is 15 beats/min or more, lasts at least 15 seconds, and returns to baseline in less than 2 minutes from the time of onset (National Institute, 1997). Variable decelerations occur any time during the uterine contracting phase and are caused by compression of the umbilical cord. Table 20-5 contrasts late deceleration with variable deceleration.

The pattern of variable decelerations differs from those of early and late decelerations, which closely approximate the shape of the corresponding uterine contraction. Instead, variable decelerations often have a U or V shape, characterized by a rapid descent and ascent to and from the nadir (or depth) of the deceleration (Fig. 20-7, *C*). Some variable decelerations are preceded and followed by brief accelerations of the FHR, known as "shouldering," which is an appropriate compensatory response to compression of the umbilical cord.

Variable decelerations may be related to partial, brief compression of the cord. If encountered in the first stage of labor, they usually can be resolved by changing the mother's position, such as from one side to the other. Oxygen administration by face mask to the mother is sometimes helpful. Variable decelerations are most commonly found during the second stage of labor as a result of umbilical cord compression during fetal

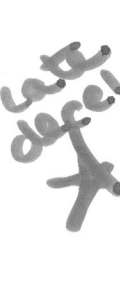

TABLE 20-5 **Late Decelerations and Variable Decelerations**

	LATE DECELERATION	VARIABLE DECELERATION
Description	Transitory gradual decrease in fetal heart rate (FHR) below baseline rate in contracting phase (see Fig. 20-7, *B*)	Abrupt decrease in FHR that is variable in duration, intensity, and timing related to onset of contractions (see Fig. 20-7, *C*)
Shape	Uniform; mirror images of uterine contraction; may be deep or shallow	Variable; characterized by sudden decrease in FHR in V, U, or W shape
Onset	Late in contraction phase; after peak of contraction; nadir of deceleration occurs after peak of contraction	Onset of deceleration to the beginning of nadir, <30 sec; decrease in FHR baseline is ≥15 beats/min, lasting ≥15 sec; variable times in contracting phase; often preceded by transitory acceleration
Recovery	Well after end of contraction	Return to baseline is rapid and <2 min from onset, sometimes with transitory acceleration or acceleration immediately before and after deceleration (shouldering or "overshoot"); slow return to baseline with severe variable decelerations
Deceleration	Usually proportional to amplitude of contraction; rarely decelerates to <100 beats/min; however, shallow late decelerations have the same significance	*Mild:* decelerates to any level, <30 sec with abrupt return to baseline *Moderate:* decelerates to ≥80 beats/min, any duration, with abrupt return to baseline *Severe:* decelerates to <60 beats/min for >60 sec, with slow return to baseline
Baseline	Often associated with loss of variability and increasing baseline rate	Mild variables usually associated with average baseline variability; moderate and severe variables often associated with decreasing variability and increasing baseline rate
Occurrence	Occurs with each contraction; may be observed at any time during labor	Variable; commonly observed late in labor with fetal descent and pushing
Cause	Uteroplacental insufficiency caused by the following: Uterine hyperactivity or hypertonicity Maternal supine hypotension Epidural or spinal anesthesia Placenta previa Abruptio placentae Hypertensive disorders Postmaturity Intrauterine growth restriction Diabetes mellitus Intraamniotic infection	Umbilical cord compression caused by the following: Maternal position with cord between fetus and maternal pelvis Cord around fetal neck, arm, leg, or other body part Short cord Knot in cord Prolapsed cord
Clinical significance	Nonreassuring pattern associated with fetal hypoxemia, acidemia, and low Apgar scores; considered ominous if persistent and uncorrected, especially when associated with fetal tachycardia and loss of variability	Variable decelerations occur in ~50% of all labors and usually are transient and correctable *Reassuring* variable decelerations last <45 sec; abruptly return to the FHR baseline; normal baseline rate continues; variability does not decrease *Nonreassuring* variable decelerations decrease to ≤70 beats/min for ≥60 sec; have a prolonged return to baseline; baseline rate increases, variability is absent Nonreassuring variable decelerations are associated with fetal acidemia, hypoxemia, and low Apgar scores; severe variable decelerations with average baseline variability just before birth are usually well tolerated

Continued

TABLE 20-5 Late Decelerations and Variable Decelerations—cont'd

	LATE DECELERATION	VARIABLE DECELERATION
Nursing intervention	Change maternal position (lateral) Correct maternal hypotension by elevating legs Increase rate of maintenance IV Discontinue oxytocin if infusing Administer oxygen at 8 to 10 L/min with tight face mask Fetal scalp or acoustic stimulation Assist with fetal oxygen saturation monitoring if ordered Assist with birth (cesarean or vaginal assisted) if pattern cannot be corrected	Change maternal position (side to side); if decelerations are severe, proceed with following measures: Discontinue oxytocin if infusing Administer oxygen at 8 to 10 L/min with tight face mask Assist with vaginal or speculum examination If cord is prolapsed, examiner will elevate fetal presenting part with cord between gloved fingers until cesarean birth is accomplished Assist with amnioinfusion if ordered Assist with fetal oxygen saturation monitoring if ordered Assist with birth (vaginal assisted or cesarean) if pattern cannot be corrected

descent. If repetitive variable decelerations occur during the second stage, it is important to discourage the woman from pushing with every contraction so that the fetus has time to recover. Variable decelerations are associated with neonatal depression only when cord compression is severe or prolonged (i.e., tight nuchal cord, short cord, knot in cord, prolapsed cord). Further descriptions of the types of variable decelerations, the clinical significance, and nursing interventions are given in Table 20-5.

Prolonged Decelerations. A **prolonged deceleration** is a visually apparent decrease in FHR below the baseline 15 beats/min or more and lasting more than 2 minutes but less than 10 minutes. A deceleration lasting more than 10 minutes is considered a baseline change (National Institute, 1997). Generally the benign causes are pelvic examination, application of a spiral electrode, rapid fetal descent, and sustained maternal Valsalva maneuver. Other, less benign, causes are progressive severe variable decelerations, sudden umbilical cord prolapse, hypotension produced by spinal or epidural analgesia or anesthesia, paracervical anesthesia, tetanic contraction, and maternal hypoxia, which may occur during a seizure. When the deceleration lasts longer than 1 to 2 minutes, a loss of variability with rebound tachycardia usually occurs. Occasionally a period of late decelerations follows. Prolonged decelerations usually are isolated events that end spontaneously. However, when a prolonged deceleration is seen late in the course of severe variable decelerations or during a prolonged series of late decelerations, the prolonged deceleration may occur just before fetal death.

NURSE ALERT

Nurses should notify the physician or nurse-midwife immediately and initiate appropriate treatment of nonreassuring patterns when they see a prolonged deceleration.

CARE MANAGEMENT

The care given to women being monitored by EFM or auscultation is the same as that given to the woman having a low risk labor. Care of the woman being monitored by internal methods may vary. FHR pattern recognition and intervention may require a nurse to have additional education and clinical experience.

Assessment and Nursing Diagnoses

The assessment of the woman includes the maternal temperature, pulse, respiratory rate, blood pressure, position, comfort, voiding pattern, status of membranes, uterine contraction pattern, cervical effacement and dilation, and emotional status. The fetal assessment includes the fetal presentation, fetal position, FHR, and identification of both reassuring and nonreassuring FHR patterns. A checklist may be used by the nurse to assess the FHR (Box 20-1). All of the assessment information must be documented in the woman's medical record.

Evaluation of the EFM equipment also must be done to ensure that the equipment is working properly and to allow an accurate assessment of the woman and fetus. A checklist for fetal monitoring equipment can be used to evaluate the equipment functions (Box 20-2).

Nursing diagnoses for the woman who is being monitored electronically for fetal status are based on assessment findings. Possible diagnoses include the following:

- *Decreased maternal cardiac output related to*
  –supine hypotension secondary to maternal position
- *Anxiety related to*
  –lack of knowledge concerning fetal monitoring during labor
  –restriction of mobility or movement during EFM
- *Impaired fetal gas exchange related to*
  –umbilical cord compression
  –placental insufficiency
- *Acute pain related to*
  –use of belts to position transducers
  –maternal position
  –vaginal examinations associated with application of maternal or fetal internal monitoring equipment or fetal blood sampling
- *Risk for fetal injury related to*
  –unrecognized hypoxemia, hypoxia, or anoxia
  –infection secondary to internal monitoring or scalp blood sampling

Expected Outcomes of Care

The primary goals of nursing care are to have a healthy fetal and maternal outcome. The interventions implemented to achieve these outcomes are determined by knowledge of fetal status and by standards for care. The planning process includes accommodating the wishes of the woman and family, answering questions, and explaining nursing interventions.

Expected outcomes for the pregnant woman and family and the fetus include the following:

- The pregnant woman and family will verbalize their understanding of the need for monitoring.
- The pregnant woman and the family will recognize and avoid situations that compromise maternal and fetal circulation.
- The fetus will not have any hypoxemic, hypoxic, or anoxic episodes.
- Should fetal compromise occur, it will be identified promptly, and appropriate nursing interventions such as intrauterine resuscitation will be initiated and the physician or nurse-midwife notified.

Plan of Care and Interventions

It is the responsibility of the nurse providing care to women in labor to assess FHR patterns, implement independent nursing interventions, document observations and actions according to the established standard of care, and report nonreassuring patterns to the primary care provider (e.g., physician, certified nurse-midwife). See Box 20-3 for a sample protocol for FHR monitoring, which contains guidelines for the care of the woman being monitored electronically for fetal status during labor.

Although the use of EFM can be reassuring to many parents, it can be a source of anxiety to some. Therefore the nurse must be particularly sensitive to and respond appropriately to the emotional, informational, and comfort

---

BOX 20-1 Checklist for Fetal Heart Rate Assessment

Client's name ______________________
Date/time ______________________

1. What is the baseline fetal heart rate (FHR)?
   _____ Beats/min
   Check one of the following as observed on the monitor strip:
   _____ Average baseline FHR (110 to 160 beats/min)
   _____ Tachycardia (>160 beats/min)
   _____ Bradycardia (<110 beats/min)
2. What is the baseline variability?
   _____ Moderate variability (6 to 25 beats/min)
   _____ Minimal variability (≤5 beats/min)
   _____ Absence of variability
   _____ Marked variability (>25 beats/min)
3. Are there any periodic or episodic changes in FHR?
   _____ Accelerations with fetal movement
   _____ Repetitive accelerations with each contraction
   _____ Early decelerations (head compression)
   _____ Late decelerations (uteroplacental insufficiency)
   _____ Variable decelerations (cord compression)
      _____ Mild
      _____ Moderate
      _____ Severe
   _____ Prolonged deceleration
4. What does the uterine activity panel show?
   _____ Frequency (beginning to beginning or peak to peak)
   _____ Duration (beginning to end)
   _____ Intensity (in mm Hg only with intrauterine catheter)
   _____ Resting tone (<15 mm Hg pressure)
   _____ Resting time ≥30 sec

COMMENTS: ______________________
____
PANEL NUMBER: ______________________
WHAT CAN BE OR SHOULD HAVE BEEN DONE:
____
____
____

Modified from Tucker, S. (2000). *Pocket guide to fetal monitoring and assessment* (4th ed.). St. Louis: Mosby.

BOX 20-2 Checklist for Fetal Monitoring Equipment

PREPARATION OF MONITOR

1. Is the paper inserted correctly?
2. Are transducer cables plugged into the appropriate outlet of the monitor?

ULTRASOUND TRANSDUCER

1. Has ultrasound transmission gel been applied to the transducer?
2. Was the FHR tested and noted on the monitor paper?
3. Does a signal light flash or an audible beep occur with each heartbeat?
4. Is the belt secure and snug but comfortable for the laboring woman?

TOCOTRANSDUCER

1. Is the tocotransducer firmly positioned at the site of the least maternal tissue?
2. Has it been applied without gel or paste?
3. Was the UA knob adjusted between the 10 and 20 mm Hg marks and noted on the monitor paper?
4. Was this setting done between contractions?
5. Is the belt secure and snug but comfortable for the laboring woman?

SPIRAL ELECTRODE

1. Is the connector attached firmly to the leg plate?
2. Is the spiral electrode attached to the presenting part of the fetus?
3. Is the inner surface of the leg plate covered with electrode gel (if necessary)?
4. Is the leg plate properly secured to the woman's thigh?

INTERNAL CATHETER/STRAIN GAUGE

1. Is the length line on the catheter visible at the introitus?
2. Is it noted on the monitor paper that a UA test was done?
3. Is the IUPC properly secured to the woman's thigh?

Modified from Tucker, S. (2000). *Pocket guide to fetal monitoring and assessment* (4th ed.). St. Louis: Mosby.

needs of the woman in labor and those of her family (Fig. 20-8 and Box 20-4).

Electronic Fetal Monitoring Pattern Recognition

Nurses must evaluate many factors to determine whether an FHR pattern is reassuring or nonreassuring. A complete description of FHR tracings includes both qualitative and quantitative descriptions of baseline rate and variability, presence of accelerations, periodic or episodic decelerations, and changes in the FHR pattern over time (National Institute, 1997). Nurses evaluate these factors based on other obstetric complications, progress in labor, and analgesia or anesthesia. They also must consider the estimated time interval until birth. Interventions are therefore based on clinical judgment of a complex, integrated process (Haggerty & Nuttall, 2000).

LEGAL TIP Fetal Monitoring Standards

Nurses who care for women during childbirth are legally responsible for correctly interpreting FHR patterns, initiating appropriate nursing interventions based on those patterns, and documenting the outcomes of those interventions. Perinatal nurses are responsible for the timely notification of the physician or nurse-midwife in the event of nonreassuring FHR patterns. Perinatal nurses also are responsible for initiating the institutional chain of command should differences in opinion arise among health care providers concerning the interpretation of the FHR pattern and the intervention required.

Nursing Management of Nonreassuring Patterns. The term **intrauterine resuscitation** is sometimes used to refer to those interventions initiated when a nonreassuring FHR pattern is noted; they are directed primarily toward improving uterine and intervillous space blood flow and secondarily toward increasing maternal oxygenation and cardiac output (Fanaroff & Martin, 2002). The following preventive interventions are described in this chapter: avoiding the supine position and encouraging maternal position changes; encouraging spontaneous short bursts of pushing in response to involuntary bearing-down urges; and encouraging pushing with mouth open and glottis open with vocalizing. Previously it was thought that the left lateral maternal position preferentially promoted maternal cardiac output, thereby enhancing blood flow to the fetus. However, it is now known that either the right or left lateral maternal position effectively enhances uteroplacental blood flow. The key issue is to avoid positioning the laboring woman on her back to reduce the risk of supine hypotension leading to decreased placental perfusion.

Compression of the umbilical cord vessels results in variable decelerations. Amnioinfusion is an intervention that can help relieve such pressure on a nonprolapsed umbilical cord. If maternal hypotension caused by acute hemorrhage (hypovolemia) occurs, the rapid infusion of blood volume expanders may be ordered. Until the infusion is established, the nurse can elevate the woman's legs. Blood pooled in the legs, especially that occurring as the result of sympathetic blockade (e.g., epidural anesthesia), will then drain quickly into the central venous circulation, and this will augment the effective intravascular volume (Fanaroff & Martin, 2002).

Oxytocin always should be infused as a piggyback connection near the indwelling needle. If FHR patterns change for any reason, oxytocin stimulation of the uterine muscle must be discontinued. This consists of turning off the IV line from the piggyback (containing oxytocin) and opening the primary infusion line.

BOX 20-3 Protocol for Fetal Heart Rate Monitoring

MATERNAL/FETAL ASSESSMENTS

Obtain a 20-min strip of EFM for all clients admitted to labor unit

Low Risk Client

Auscultate or assess tracing every 30 min in active phase of first stage of labor

Auscultate or assess tracing every 15 min in second stage

High Risk Client

Auscultate or assess tracing every 15 min in active phase and every 5 min in second stage

Auscultation: All Clients

Count baseline FHR in between contractions

Assess FHR during the contraction and for ≥30 sec after the contraction

Note increases or decreases of FHR

Assess FHR before ambulation

Interpret FHR data, nursing interventions, and client responses

Notify primary health care provider

EFM: All Clients

Assess and interpret baseline FHR, variability of FHR, and presence or absence of decelerations and accelerations

Assessments for All Clients

Assess uterine activity for frequency and duration, the intensity of contractions, and uterine resting tone

Assess FHR immediately after rupture of membranes, vaginal examinations, and any invasive procedure

MATERNAL CARE

Assist woman to a comfortable position other than supine

Change maternal position at least every 2 hr

EXTERNAL MONITORING

Ultrasound Transducer

Function

Monitors FHR with high-frequency sound waves.

Nursing Care

Tap transducer before use to ensure sound transmission.

Apply ultrasound transmission gel to transducer, clean abdomen and transducer, and reapply gel q2hr and prn.

Massage reddened skin areas gently and reposition belt or adhesive device q2hr and prn.

Auscultate FHR with stethoscope or fetoscope if in doubt as to validity of tracing.

Position and reposition transducer prn to ensure receipt of clear, interpretable FHR data.

Tocotransducer

Function

Monitors uterine activity via a pressure-sensing device placed on the maternal abdomen.

Nursing Care

Position and reposition q2hr and prn on the fundus, where there is the least maternal tissue.

Keep abdominal strap snug but comfortable for the laboring woman.

Adjust knob between contractions to print between 10 and 20 mm Hg on the monitor strip paper.

Palpate fundus every 30 to 60 min to assess strength of contraction; only frequency and duration of contractions can be assessed with tocotransducer.

Do not determine woman's need for analgesia based on uterine activity displayed on monitor strip.

Gently massage reddened areas under transducer and belt qhr and prn.

INTERNAL MONITORING

Spiral Electrode

Function

Obtains fetal ECG from presenting part and converts it into FHR.

Nursing Care

Ensure that the connector to the scalp electrode is appropriately attached to leg plate.

Reapply electrode paste to leg plate if needed.

Observe FHR tracing on monitor strip for variability.

Turn electrode counterclockwise to remove; never pull straight out from presenting part.

Administer perineal care after the woman voids during labor and prn.

Intrauterine Catheter

Function

Catheter (solid or fluid filled) that monitors intraamniotic pressure internally.

Nursing Care

Ensure that the length line on catheter is visible at introitus.

For closed-system catheters, set baseline rate between uterine contractions when uterus is relaxed.

Flush open-system catheter with sterile water before insertion and prn.

For open-system catheters, turn stopcock off to woman, then with pressure valve of strain gauge released, flush strain gauge, remove syringe, and set stylus to 0 line of chart paper; test further according to manufacturer's instructions q3-4hr and prn.

Continued

BOX 20-3 Protocol for Fetal Heart Rate Monitoring—cont'd

Check proper functioning by tapping catheter, asking woman to cough, or applying fundal pressure; observe appropriate inflection on strip chart.
Keep catheter or cable secured to woman's leg to prevent dislodgment.

REPORTABLE CONDITIONS

Presence of nonreassuring patterns:
- Severe variable decelerations
- Late decelerations
- Absence of variability
- Prolonged deceleration
- Severe bradycardia

Worsening of any pattern
Presence of identifiable fetal dysrhythmias
Difficulty in obtaining adequate FHR tracing or inadequate audible FHR

EMERGENCY MEASURES

Implement the following measures immediately in the event of the nonreassuring patterns:
Reposition client in lateral position to increase uteroplacental perfusion or relieve cord compression
Administer oxygen at 8 to 10 L/min or per hospital protocol by face mask
Discontinue oxytocin if infusing
Correct maternal hypovolemia by increasing IV rate per protocol or as ordered
Assess for bleeding or other cause of pattern change, such as maternal hypotension
Notify primary health care provider
Assist with other methods of assessment such as fetal oxygen saturation monitoring or interventions such as amnioinfusion
Anticipate emergency preparation for surgical intervention if nonreassuring pattern continues despite interventions

DOCUMENTATION*

Client Record: Auscultation

FHR baseline, rate and rhythm, increases or decreases

Client Record: EFM

Method of monitoring, change in method, and adjustments to equipment
FHR range, variability, presence of decelerations or accelerations
Uterine activity as determined by palpation or by external or internal monitoring
Interpretation of FHR data, nursing interventions, and client responses
Notification of primary health care provider

Monitor Strip

Client identification data
Assessments, procedures, and interventions (medications, etc.)
Notification of primary health care provider
Significant occurrences (sterile vaginal examination, rupture of membranes, etc.)
Adjustments of the monitor equipment

*If computer charting system is used, follow institutional policies and system guidelines/protocols.

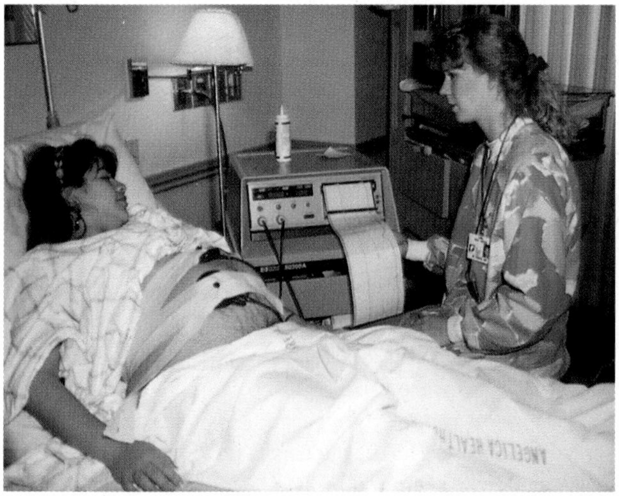

FIG. 20-8 Nurse explains electronic fetal monitoring as ultrasound transducer monitors the fetal heart rate. (Courtesy Marjorie Pyle, RNC, Lifecircle, Costa Mesa, CA.)

Nurses must assign priorities to interventions to maximize the efficacy of the intrauterine resuscitation. The *first priority* is to open the maternal and fetal vascular systems; the *second priority* is to increase blood volume; and the *third priority* is to optimize oxygenation of the circulating blood volume. For example, to relieve an acute FHR deceleration, the nurse can do the following:

- Assist the woman to the side-lying position if she is not already in a lateral position.
- Increase the maternal blood volume by increasing the rate of the primary IV infusion or by raising the woman's legs.
- Provide oxygen by face mask.

Some interventions are specific to the FHR pattern. Nursing interventions appropriate for the management of tachycardia and bradycardia are given in Table 20-2, and those appropriate for the management of increased or decreased variability are given in Table 20-3. No specific nursing interventions are required for the management of FHR

BOX 20-4 Client/Family Teaching When Electronic Fetal Monitor Is Used

The following guidelines relate to client teaching and the functioning of the monitor:

Explain the purpose of monitoring.
Explain each procedure.
Provide rationale for maternal position other than supine.
Explain that fetal status can be continuously assessed by electronic fetal monitoring (EFM), even during contractions.
Explain that the lower tracing on the monitor strip paper shows uterine activity; the upper tracing shows the fetal heart rate (FHR).
Reassure woman and partner that prepared childbirth techniques can be implemented without difficulty.
Explain that, during external monitoring, effleurage can be performed on sides of abdomen or upper portion of thighs.
Explain that breathing patterns based on the time and intensity of contractions can be enhanced by the observation of uterine activity on the monitor strip paper, which shows the onset of contractions.
Note peak of contraction; knowing that contraction will not get stronger and is half over is usually helpful.
Note diminishing intensity.
Coordinate with appropriate breathing and relaxation techniques.
Reassure woman and partner that the use of internal monitoring does not restrict movement, although she is confined to bed.*
Explain that use of external monitoring usually requires the woman's cooperation during positioning and movement.
Reassure woman and partner that use of monitoring does not imply fetal jeopardy.
Reassure her that the equipment is removed periodically to permit the applicator sites to be washed and other care to be given.

*Portable telemetry monitors allow the FHR and uterine contraction patterns to be observed on centrally located display stations. These portable units permit ambulation during electronic monitoring.

acceleration or early deceleration (see Table 20-4). However, late and some types of variable FHR decelerations require aggressive intervention (see Table 20-5). The primary health care provider decides whether medical intervention should be instituted, what intervention is indicated, or whether immediate vaginal or cesarean birth should be performed.

Other Methods of Assessment and Intervention

Other methods of assessment and intervention are designed to be used in conjunction with EFM in an effort to identify and intervene in the presence of a nonreassuring FHR. These methods include FHR response to stimulation, fetal oxygen saturation monitoring, fetal blood sampling, amnioinfusion, and tocolysis. Umbilical cord acid-base determination is an assessment technique that is a useful adjunct to the Apgar score in assessing the immediate condition of the newborn.

Fetal Heart Rate Response to Stimulation. Stimulation of the fetus is done to elicit an acceleration of the FHR of 15 beats/min for at least 15 seconds (Tucker, 2000). The two methods of fetal stimulation currently in practice are scalp stimulation (using digital pressure during a vaginal examination) and vibroacoustic stimulation (using an artificial larynx or fetal acoustic stimulation device over the fetal head for 1 to 2 seconds). An FHR acceleration usually indicates fetal well-being. If the fetus does not have an acceleration, however, it does not necessarily indicate fetal compromise, but further evaluation of fetal well-being is needed.

Fetal Oxygen Saturation Monitoring. Continuous monitoring of fetal oxygen saturation ($FSpO_2$) or **fetal pulse oximetry (FPO)** is a method of fetal assessment that was approved for clinical use by the Food and Drug Administration in May 2000 (Porter, 2000). FPO works in a way similar to the pulse oximetry used in children and adults. A specially designed sensor is inserted next to the fetal cheek or temple area to assess oxygen saturation. The sensor is then connected to a monitor, and the data are displayed on the uterine activity panel of the fetal monitor tracing. The normal range of oxygen saturation in the adult is 95% to 100%. The normal range for the healthy fetus is 30% to 70% (Simpson & Porter, 2001) with the cutoff value for the critical threshold of $FSpO_2$ at 30% (Garite et al., 2000).

FPO may be used if certain criteria are met, including a single fetus at least 36 weeks' gestation in a vertex presentation with a nonreassuring FHR pattern. The membranes should be ruptured, the cervix dilated at least 2 cm, and the fetal station at least a minus 2 or less (Garite et al., 2000). The value of $FSpO_2$ monitoring is that in the event of nonreassuring FHR patterns, it could support the decision about whether labor should continue or whether to intervene with an expeditious assisted vaginal or cesarean birth of the fetus. The American College of Obstetricians and Gynecologists has not endorsed the use of FPO in clinical practice and recommends further clinical research (ACOG, 2001).

When the use of FPO becomes more widely practiced, the labor nurse's role will expand to include this type of monitoring in practice (Porter, 2000). Simpson and Porter (2001) suggested that nurses will be involved in identifying potential candidates for monitoring, inserting the sensor (according to state nurse practice acts and institutional policies), interpreting data, documenting findings, and communicating with the primary health care provider.

Fetal Scalp Blood Sampling. Sampling of the fetal scalp blood was designed to assess the fetal pH, PO_2, and PCO_2. The procedure is performed by obtaining a sample of fetal scalp blood through the dilated cervix after the membranes have ruptured. The scalp is swabbed with a disinfecting solution before making the puncture, and the sample is then collected. However, the blood gas values vary so rapidly with transient circulatory changes that fetal blood sampling is seldom performed. When used, it is usually in tertiary centers with the capability for repetitive sampling and rapid report of results. The circulatory changes that cause the variability and thus undermine the utility of this procedure are maternal acidosis or alkalosis, caput succedaneum, the stage of labor, and the time relation of scalp sampling to UCs.

Amnioinfusion. **Amnioinfusion** is used during labor either to supplement the amount of amniotic fluid to reduce the severity of variable decelerations caused by cord compression or to dilute meconium-stained amniotic fluid with saline or lactated Ringer's solution (Hofmeyr, 2002; Schmidt, 1997). The procedure to supplement amniotic fluid is indicated for clients with oligohydramnios, secondary to uteroplacental insufficiency, premature rupture of membranes, or postmaturity, who are at risk for variable decelerations because of umbilical cord compression.

Oligohydramnios is an abnormally small amount of amniotic fluid or the absence of amniotic fluid. Without the buffer of amniotic fluid, the umbilical cord can easily become compressed during contractions or fetal movement, diminishing the flow of blood between the fetus and placenta, as evidenced by variable decelerations. Amnioinfusion replaces the "cushion" for the cord and relieves both the frequency and intensity of variable decelerations.

Amnioinfusion also is indicated in the presence of moderate to thick meconium to dilute and flush out the meconium with the intent of avoiding meconium-aspiration syndrome in the neonate (Hofmeyr, 2002).

Risks of amnioinfusion are overdistention of the uterine cavity and increased uterine tone. Techniques of amnioinfusion treatment vary, but usually fluid is administered through an IUPC. The woman's membranes must be ruptured for the IUPC placement. The fluid is administered by attaching plastic (IV) tubing to a liter of normal saline or lactated Ringer's solution through a port in the IUPC. Double-lumen IUPCs are preferred because the IUP can be monitored without stopping the procedure. The fluid is usually warmed with a blood warmer before administration for the preterm or SGA fetus (American College of Obstetricians and Gynecologists, 1995). The flow rate can be by bolus or continuous flow or by a combination of these two methods.

Intensity and frequency of UCs should be continually assessed during the procedure. The recorded uterine resting tone during amnioinfusion will appear higher than normal because of resistance to outflow and turbulence at the end of the catheter. The true resting tone can be checked by discontinuing the amnioinfusion when using a single-lumen IUPC (Tucker, 2000).

Tocolytic Therapy. **Tocolysis** (relaxation of the uterus) can be achieved through the administration of drugs that inhibit UCs. This therapy can be used as an adjunct to other interventions in the management of fetal stress when the fetus is exhibiting nonreassuring patterns associated with increased uterine activity. Tocolysis improves blood flow through the placenta by inhibiting UCs (Brown, 1998). Tocolysis may be considered by the primary health care provider and implemented when other interventions to reduce uterine activity, such as maternal position change and discontinuance of an oxytocin infusion, have no effect on diminishing the UCs. A tocolytic drug such as magnesium sulfate or terbutaline can be administered IV to decrease uterine activity. If the FHR pattern improves, the woman may be allowed to continue labor; if there is no improvement, immediate surgical delivery may be needed.

Umbilical Cord Acid-Base Determination. In assessing the immediate condition of the newborn after birth, a sample of cord blood is a useful adjunct to the Apgar score. The procedure is generally done by withdrawing blood from the umbilical artery and having the blood tested for pH, PCO_2, and PO_2. Metabolic acidosis can cause a low Apgar score.

Client and Family Teaching

Part of the nurse's role includes acting as a partner with the woman to achieve a high-quality birthing experience. In addition to teaching and supporting the woman and her family with understanding of the laboring and birth process, breathing techniques, use of equipment, and pain management techniques, the nurse can assist with two factors that have an effect on fetal status: pushing and positioning. The nurse should provide information and support to the woman in regard to these two factors.

Maternal Positioning. Maternal supine hypotensive syndrome is caused by the weight and pressure of the gravid uterus on the ascending vena cava when the woman is in a supine position. This decreases venous return to the woman's heart and cardiac output and subsequently reduces her blood pressure. The low maternal blood pressure decreases intervillous space blood flow during UCs and results in fetal hypoxemia. This is reflected on the fetal monitor as a nonreassuring FHR pattern, usually late decelerations. The nurse should solicit the woman's cooperation in avoiding the supine position. The woman should be encouraged to maintain a side-lying position or semi-Fowler's position with a lateral tilt to the uterus.

Discouraging the Valsalva Maneuver. The **Valsalva maneuver** can be described as the process of making a forceful bearing-down attempt while holding one's breath with a closed glottis and tightening the abdominal muscles. This process stimulates the parasympathetic division of the autonomic nervous system, producing a vagal response, and results in the decrease of the maternal heart rate and blood pressure. Prolonged pushing in this manner can decrease placental blood flow, alter maternal and fetal oxygenation, decrease the fetal pH and PO_2, increase the fetal P_{CO_2}, and increase the likelihood of fetal hypoxemia, as reflected in FHR pattern changes.

During the second stage of labor, when the woman needs to push, an alternative to breath holding with a closed glottis is to perform the open-mouth and open-glottis breathing-pushing technique. The nurse should instruct the woman to keep her mouth and glottis open and to let air escape from the lungs during the pushing process. This may result in an audible grunting sound and will prevent the Valsalva maneuver. Some providers of care prefer the laboring-down process or delayed pushing, which is to refrain from pushing in the early second stage of labor. The natural forces of labor contractions are used to move the fetus down the birth canal, and then focused pushing is used for a short period to expel the fetus from the birth canal.

Documentation

Clear and complete documentation on the woman's monitor strip is started before the initiation of monitoring and consists of identifying information plus other relevant data. This documentation is continued and updated according to institutional protocol as monitoring progresses. In some institutions, observations noted and interventions implemented are recorded on the monitor strip to produce a comprehensive document that chronicles the course of labor and the care rendered. In other institutions, this documentation is confined to the labor flow record or computer chart. Advocates of documenting on both the medical record and the EFM strip cite as advantages of this approach the ease of writing directly on the strip while at the bedside or inputting the data on a computer-based documentation system and the improved accuracy in documenting critical events and the interventions implemented. Others believe that charting on the EFM strip constitutes duplicate documentation of the same information noted in the medical record, and thus it is unnecessary additional paperwork for the nurse.

One way of documenting that frequent maternal-fetal assessments have been done at the bedside is either to initial the EFM strip or to depress the "mark" button during these assessments. Data-entry devices are now available with some EFM systems; assessments are keyed in and subsequently printed on the strip. A disadvantage of documenting on both the EFM strip and the medical record is that frequently the times noted for events and interventions on the EFM strip do not correlate with what is later documented in the medical record. These inaccuracies can lead those involved in the retrospective review process carried out during litigation to infer that documentation errors have occurred. Therefore if institutional policy mandates documentation on both the monitor strip and the medical record, it is critically important for the nurse to make sure the times and notations of events and interventions recorded in each place agree. No one method of documentation is right; rather the nurse must be aware of and follow individual institutional policies, as well as participate in formulating such policies (McCartney, 2002). Many of the aspects of care and events that can be documented on the client's medical record or the monitor strip are listed in Box 20-5.

Evaluation

Evaluation is a continuous process. The nurse can assume that care was effective when the outcomes for care have been achieved (see Plan of Care).

BOX *20-5* **Documentation**

OBSERVATIONS

Maternal

Vital signs: BP, TPR
Oxygen saturation if monitored
Uterine activity: frequency, duration, intensity, resting tone
Behavior: anxiety, irritability, fear of losing control
Breathing pattern
Position; activity (ambulating, BRP, use of birthing ball, etc.)
Rupture of membranes; time, color, amount, odor
Voidings; nausea, vomiting
Urge to push; bearing down; pushing

Fetal

FHR, variability, periodic/episodic changes
Fetal movement
Oxygen saturation if monitored
Presentation, position, station

ADJUSTMENTS

Relocation of transducers
Replacement of electrode
Replacement of IUPC
Adjustment or flushing of IUPC
Testing of monitor
Monitor paper changes; time lapse
Interruption/removal of monitoring equipment

INTERVENTIONS

Maternal position change
Administration of oxygen
Parenteral fluids; changes in flow rate
Amnioinfusion
Fetal scalp stimulation
Medication administration
Oxytocin
Analgesics
Anesthetics
Tocolytics
Primary health care provider notification, reason, and response
Birth data

Plan of Care: EFM During Labor

NURSING DIAGNOSIS Maternal anxiety related to lack of knowledge about use of electronic monitor

Expected Outcomes *The client will exhibit increased understanding about fetal monitoring and signs of reduced anxiety (i.e., absence of physical indicators, absence of perceived threat, and absence of feelings of dread).*

Nursing Interventions/*Rationales*

Explain and demonstrate to woman and labor support partner how the electronic monitor (internal or external) works in assessing FHR and in detecting and assessing quality of uterine contractions *to remove fear of unknown and ensure that woman can move with the monitor.*

When making adjustment to the monitor, explain to the couple what is being done and why, *because information increases understanding and allays anxiety.*

Explain that although a side-lying position or Fowler's position provides for optimal monitoring, position changes decrease discomfort; therefore encourage frequent changes in position (other than supine) and explain any monitoring adjustments that are being made as a result *to reduce discomfort and allay anxiety.*

NURSING DIAGNOSIS Risk for fetal injury related to inaccurate placement of transducers/electrodes, misinterpretation of results, or failure to use other assessment techniques to monitor fetal well-being

Expected Outcomes *Fetal well-being is adequately assessed, and any fetal compromise is identified immediately.*

Nursing Interventions/*Rationales*

Carefully follow guidelines and checklist for application and initiation of monitoring *to ensure proper placement of monitoring devices and production of accurate output from monitoring device.*

Check placement throughout monitoring process *to ensure that devices remain correctly placed.*

Regularly assess and record results of EFM (FHR and variability, decelerations, accelerations, uterine activity, contractions, uterine resting tone) *to provide consistent and timely evaluation of fetal well-being and progress of labor.*

Auscultate FHR and palpate contractions on a regular basis *to provide a cross-check on the EFM output and ensure fetal well-being.*

NURSING DIAGNOSIS Risk for maternal injury related to incorrect placement of external or internal monitors or misinterpretation of contraction pattern

Expected Outcome *Maternal well-being is assessed continuously and any alterations identified promptly.*

Nursing Interventions/*Rationales*

Palpate uterine contractions *to correlate data with electronic monitoring results.*

Periodically recheck placement *to verify that all monitoring devices are accurately placed.*

Assess uterine activity, contraction pattern, and baseline *to provide ongoing evaluation and basis for further interventions.*

Use correct aseptic technique for insertion of internal monitors *to prevent infection.*

Monitor maternal temperature, as well as color, odor, and amount of amniotic fluid, *to determine indicators of infection.*

NURSING DIAGNOSIS Risk for impaired physical mobility related to restriction of movement with monitoring devices

Expected Outcome *Woman will be able to change positions and ambulate at intervals.*

Nursing Interventions/*Rationales*

Discontinue continuous EFM at intervals *to change position and increase mobility.*

Encourage woman to change position and reposition monitor as needed *to decrease complications of immobility.*

Place external monitor manually at intervals *to collect data while woman is out of bed.*

KEY POINTS

- Fetal well-being during labor is gauged by the response of the FHR to UCs.
- FHR characteristics include the baseline FHR and periodic changes in the FHR.
- The monitoring of fetal well-being includes FHR assessment, watching for meconium-stained amniotic fluid, and assessment of maternal vital signs and uterine activity.
- It is the responsibility of the nurse to assess FHR patterns, implement independent nursing interventions, and report nonreassuring patterns to the physician or nurse-midwife.
- The Association of Women's Health, Obstetric, and Neonatal Nurses and the American College of Obstetricians and Gynecologists have established and published health care provider standards and guidelines for fetal heart monitoring.
- The emotional, informational, and comfort needs of the woman and her family must be addressed when the mother and her fetus are being monitored.
- Documentation is initiated and updated according to institutional protocol.

CRITICAL THINKING EXERCISES

1. While caring for a woman in early labor, you identify a pattern of repetitive FHR decelerations from the baseline FHR.
   a. Outline your approach in determining whether the pattern is reassuring or nonreassuring.
   b. List the nursing interventions that should be implemented for nonreassuring repetitive late decelerations.
   c. List the nursing interventions that should be implemented for nonreassuring variable decelerations.
2. Review two actual monitor strips of women who have given birth. If possible, request to see a monitor strip of a woman who had an uncomplicated vaginal birth and a strip of a woman who had a cesarean birth because of fetal distress.
   a. For each of these fetal monitor strips, determine the following:
      - The baseline rate and variability of the FHR
      - Periodic changes, if any
      - The contraction frequency, duration, intensity, and resting tone
   b. Identify the type of nonreassuring FHR pattern that prompted the cesarean birth.
   c. Corroborate your findings in a clinical conference.
3. You will be assigned to a woman who has very little information about the methods used to assess the fetus during labor. Develop a plan of education in an outline format that covers:
   a. The auscultatory method of fetal assessment
   b. The external mode of EFM
   c. The internal mode of EFM

RESOURCES

American College of Nurse-Midwives
818 Connecticut Ave., NW, Suite 900
Washington, DC 20006
202-728-9860
www.midwife.org

American College of Obstetricians and Gynecologists
409 12th St. SW
Washington, DC 20024
800-762-2264
www.acog.com

Association of Women's Health, Obstetric, and Neonatal Nurses (AWHONN)
2000 L St., NW, Suite 740
Washington, DC 20036
800-673-8499 (United States)
800-245-0231 (Canada)
www.awhonn.org

National Association of Parents and Professionals for Safe Alternatives in Childbirth (NAPSAC)
P.O. Box 267
Marble Hill, MO 63764
314-238-2010
www. napsac.org

National Institute of Child Health and Human Development (NICHD)
National Institutes of Health
9000 Rockville Pike
Bldg. 31, Room 2A32
Bethesda, MD 20892
301-496-4000
www.nih.gov

REFERENCES

Albers, L. (2001). Monitoring the fetus in labor: Evidence to support the methods. *Journal of Midwifery and Women's Health, 46*(6), 366-373.

American College of Obstetricians and Gynecologists. (1995). *Fetal heart rate patterns: Monitoring, interpretation, and management. ACOG Technical Bulletin No. 207.* Washington, DC: ACOG.

American College of Obstetricians and Gynecologists. (2001). *Fetal pulse oximetry. ACOG Committee Opinion No. 248.* Washington, DC: ACOG.

Association of Women's Health, Obstetric, and Neonatal Nurses. (1997). *Fetal heart monitoring principles and practice* (2nd ed.). Dubuque, IA: Kendall/Hunt.

Association of Women's Health, Obstetric, and Neonatal Nurses. (1998). *Clinical competencies and education guide: Fetal surveillance in antepartum and intrapartum nursing practice* (3rd ed.). Washington, DC: AWHONN.

Brown, C. (1998). Intrapartal tocolysis: An option for acute intrapartal fetal crisis. *Journal of Obstetric, Gynecologic, and Neonatal Nursing, 27*(3), 257-261.

Chez, B., Harvey, M., & Harvey, C. (2000). Intrapartum fetal monitoring: Past, present, and future. *Journal of Perinatal and Neonatal Nursing, 14*(3), 1-18.

Fanaroff, A., & Martin, R. (2002). *Neonatal-perinatal medicine: Diseases of the fetus and infant* (7th ed.). St. Louis: Mosby.

Feinstein, N. (2000). Fetal heart rate auscultation: Current and future practice. *Journal of Obstetric, Gynecologic, and Neonatal Nursing, 29*(3), 306-315.

Feinstein, N., Sprague, A., & Trepanier, M. (2000). *Fetal heart rate auscultation.* Washington, DC: AWHONN.

Garite, T. (2000). A multicenter controlled trial of fetal pulse oximetry in the intrapartum management of nonreassuring fetal heart rate patterns. *American Journal of Obstetrics and Gynecology, 183*(5), 1049-1058.

Goodwin, L. (2000). Intermittent auscultation of the fetal heart rate: A review of general principles. *Journal of Perinatal and Neonatal Nursing, 14*(3), 53-61.

Haggerty, L., & Nuttall, R. (2000). Experienced obstetric nurses' decision-making in fetal risk situations. *Journal of Obstetric, Gynecologic, and Neonatal Nursing, 29*(5), 480-490.

Harvey, C. (1997). Coming to terms: Electronic fetal monitoring update. *AWHONN Lifelines, 1*(3), 49-51.

Hofmeyr, G. (2002). Amnioinfusion for meconium-stained liquor in labour. (Cochrane Review). *The Cochrane Library*. Oxford: Update Software.

King, T., & Parer, J. (2000). The physiology of fetal heart rate patterns and perinatal asphyxia. *Journal of Perinatal and Neonatal Nursing, 14*(3), 19-39.

McCartney, P. (2002). Electronic fetal monitoring and the legal medical record. *MCN American Journal of Maternal and Child Nursing, 27*(4), 249.

National Institute of Child Health and Human Development Research Planning Workshop (1997). Electronic fetal heart rate monitoring: Research guidelines for interpretation. *American Journal of Obstetrics and Gynecology, 177*(6), 1385-1390.

Parer, J., & King, T. (2000). Fetal heart rate monitoring: Is it salvageable? *American Journal of Obstetrics and Gynecology, 182*(4), 982-987.

Porter, M. (2000). Fetal pulse oximetry: As adjunct to electronic fetal heart rate monitoring. *Journal of Obstetric, Gynecologic, and Neonatal Nursing, 29*(5), 537-548.

Schmidt, J. (1997). Fluid check: Making the case for intrapartum amnioinfusion. *AWHONN Lifelines, 1*(5), 46-51.

Simpson, K., & Knox, G. (2000). Risk management and electronic fetal monitoring: Decreasing risk of adverse outcomes and liability exposure. *Journal of Perinatal and Neonatal Nursing, 14*(3), 40-52.

Simpson, K., & Porter, M. (2001). Fetal oxygen saturation monitoring: Using this new technology for fetal assessment during labor. *AWHONN Lifelines, 5*(2), 26-33.

Thacker, S., Stroup, D., & Chang, M. (2001). Continuous electronic heart rate monitoring for fetal assessment during labor. (Cochrane Review). *The Cochrane Library 2.* Oxford: Update Software.

Tucker, S. (2000). *Pocket guide to fetal monitoring and assessment* (4th ed.). St. Louis: Mosby.

CHAPTER 21

Karen A. Piotrowski

Nursing Care During Labor

http://evolve.elsevier.com/Lowdermilk/MatWmnHlth/

LEARNING OBJECTIVES

- Review the factors included in the initial assessment of the woman in labor.
- Describe the ongoing assessment of maternal progress during each stage of labor.
- Recognize the physical and psychosocial findings indicative of maternal progress during labor.
- Describe fetal assessment during labor.
- Identify signs of developing complications during labor.
- Develop a comprehensive plan of care relevant to each stage of labor.
- Discuss the nurse's role in managing care for the woman and her significant others (support person[s], family) during each stage of labor.
- Analyze the influence of cultural and religious beliefs and practices on the process of labor and birth.
- Discuss research findings on the importance of support from family, partner, doula, and nurse in facilitating maternal progress during labor and birth.
- Describe the role and responsibilities of the nurse in an emergency childbirth situation.
- Evaluate the impact of perineal trauma on the woman's reproductive and sexual health.
- Analyze the nurse's role as advocate in reducing the incidence of routine episiotomy.

The labor process is an exciting and anxious time for the woman and her significant others (support persons, family). In a relatively short period, they experience one of the most profound changes in their lives.

For most women, labor begins with the first uterine contraction, continues with hours of hard work during cervical dilation and birth, and ends as the woman and her significant others begin the attachment process with the newborn. Nursing care management focuses on assessment and support of the woman and her significant others throughout labor and birth, with the goal of ensuring the best possible outcome for all involved.

FIRST STAGE OF LABOR

CARE MANAGEMENT

The **first stage of labor** begins with the onset of regular uterine contractions and ends with full cervical effacement and dilation. Care begins when the woman reports one or more of the following:

- Onset of progressive, regular uterine contractions that increase in frequency, strength, and duration
- Blood-tinged mucoid vaginal discharge **(bloody** or **pink show)** indicating that the mucus plug (operculum) has passed
- Fluid discharge from the vagina **(spontaneous rupture of membranes** [SROM; SRM])

The first stage of labor consists of the following three phases: the **latent phase** (up to 3 cm of dilation), the **active phase** (4 to 7 cm of dilation), and the **transition phase** (8 to 10 cm of dilation). Most nulliparous women seek admission to the hospital in the latent phase because they have not experienced labor before and are unsure of the "right" time to come in. Multiparous women usually do not come to the hospital until they are in the active phase. Even though no two labors are identical, women who have given birth before appear less anxious about the process, unless their previous experience has been negative.

The nurse uses the nursing process as a framework for managing the care of women and their significant others during all stages of labor. Nurses should involve the laboring woman as a partner in the formulation of an individualized plan of care. This helps preserve the woman's sense of control and participation in her own childbirth experience and helps enhance the woman's self-esteem and level of satisfaction (Proctor, 1998).

Women often have lingering impressions of their childbirth experiences. Caregivers who are respectful, supportive, available, protective, encouraging, kind, patient, professional, calm, and comforting help these women to remember their childbirth experiences in positive terms. Frustrations women feel regarding their childbirth experiences stem from pain, lack of control, lack of knowledge, or the negative behaviors of some caregivers (Fowles, 1998; Hanson, VandeVusse, & Harrod, 2001; Tumblin & Simkin, 2001).

Assessment and Nursing Diagnoses

Assessment begins at the first contact with the woman, whether by telephone or in person. Many women call the hospital or birthing center first to receive validation that it is all right for them to come in for evaluation or admission. The manner in which the nurse communicates with the woman during this first contact can set the tone for a positive birth experience. A caring attitude by the nurse encourages the woman to verbalize questions and concerns. If possible, the nurse should have the woman's prenatal record in hand when speaking to her or admitting her for evaluation of labor. Copies of records are often filed on the perinatal unit at some time during the woman's third trimester.

Certain factors are assessed initially to determine whether the woman is in true or false labor and whether she should come for further assessment or admission (Varney, 1997) (see Teaching for Self-Care box).

TEACHING FOR SELF-CARE

How to Distinguish True Labor from False Labor

TRUE LABOR

Contractions
- Occur regularly, becoming stronger, lasting longer, and occurring closer together.
- Become more intense with walking.
- Usually felt in lower back, radiating to lower portion of abdomen.
- Continue despite use of comfort measures.

Cervix (by vaginal examination)
- Shows progressive change (softening, effacement, and dilation signaled by the appearance of bloody show).
- Moves to an increasingly anterior position.

Fetus
- Presenting part usually becomes engaged in the pelvis. This results in increased ease of breathing; at the same time, the presenting part presses downward and compresses the bladder, resulting in urinary frequency.

FALSE LABOR

Contractions
- Occur irregularly or become regular only temporarily.
- Often stop with walking or position change.
- Can be felt in the back or abdomen above the navel.
- Often can be stopped through the use of comfort measures.

Cervix (by vaginal examination)
- May be soft but there is no significant change in effacement or dilation or evidence of bloody show.
- Is often in a posterior position.

Fetus
- Presenting part is usually not engaged in the pelvis.

BOX 21-1 Telephone Interview with Woman in Latent Phase of Labor

The perinatal nurse performs the following steps of the nursing process:

ASSESSMENT
- Gathers data regarding the woman's status, including signs and symptoms indicative of true or false labor.
- Discusses instructions given by the woman's primary health care provider regarding when to come for admission.

PLANNING AND IMPLEMENTATION
- Decides whether the woman will come for labor assessment and admission or be encouraged to stay at home until contractions increase in duration, frequency, and intensity.
- Assures the woman that she is welcome to call the perinatal unit at any time to discuss her labor status.
- Answers questions the woman and her family may have regarding labor or provides instruction as needed (e.g., which entrance of the hospital to enter).
- Suggests a variety of positions she can assume to maximally enhance uteroplacental and renal blood flow (e.g., side-lying position) and enhance the progress of labor (e.g., upright positions and ambulation).
- Suggests diversional activities, such as walking, reading, watching television, talking to friends.
- Suggests measures to maintain comfort, such as a warm shower, back or foot massage.
- Discusses the oral intake of foods and fluids appropriate for early labor (light foods or fluids or clear liquids depending on the preference of her primary health care provider).
- Instructs the woman to come in immediately if membranes rupture, bleeding occurs, or fetal movements change.

EVALUATION
- Evaluates whether instructions and information have been understood by the woman by asking her to verbalize her understanding.

The pregnant woman may call the primary health care provider or come to the hospital while in false labor or early in the latent phase of the first stage of labor. She may feel discouraged on learning that the contractions that feel so strong and regular to her are not true contractions because they are not causing cervical dilation or are still not strong or frequent enough for admission.

If the woman lives near the hospital, she may be asked to stay home or return home to allow labor to progress (i.e., until the uterine contractions are more frequent and intense). The ideal setting for the low risk woman at this time is the familiar environment of her home. The nurse can use a telephone interview (Box 21-1) to assess the woman's status and to give instructions regarding the optimal time for admission and to reinforce teaching regarding the signs that require immediate notification of the primary health care provider. Measures the woman and her significant others can use to enhance the progress of labor, reduce anxiety, and maintain comfort should be described.

A warm shower can be relaxing for the woman in early labor; however, warm baths should be avoided until the cervix is approximately 5 cm dilated, because water immersion in early labor could prolong the labor process and increase the use of oxytocin to stimulate uterine contractions and epidural analgesia for pain reduction (Eriksson, Mattsson, & Ladfors, 1997; Mackey, 2001; Odent, 1997). Soothing back, foot, and hand massage or a warm drink of preferred liquids such as tea or milk can help the woman to rest and even to sleep, especially if false or early labor is occurring at night.

Diversional activities such as walking outdoors or in the house, reading, watching television, doing needlework, or talking with friends can reduce the perception of early discomfort, help the time pass, and reduce anxiety (Austin & Calderon, 1999; Varney, 1997).

The woman who lives at a considerable distance from the hospital may be admitted in early labor. The same measures used by the woman at home should be offered to the hospitalized woman in early labor.

Admission to Labor Unit

When the woman arrives at the perinatal unit, assessment is the top priority (Fig. 21-1). The nurse first performs a screening assessment by using the techniques of interview and physical assessment and reviews the laboratory and diagnostic test findings to determine the health status of the woman and her fetus and the progress of her labor. The primary health care provider is notified, and if the woman is admitted, a detailed systems assessment is done.

When the woman is admitted, she usually is moved from an observation area to the labor room; the labor, delivery, and recovery (LDR) room; or the labor, delivery, recovery, and postpartum (LDRP) room. Because first impressions are important, the woman and her partner are welcomed by name and introduced to the staff members who will be involved in the woman's care. Women often express concern regarding the number of persons intruding on their labor experience, especially if the role of the person and purpose for his or her presence are not clearly identified (Hanson et al., 2001).

If the woman wishes, her partner is included in the assessment and admission process. Significant others not participating in this process may be directed to the appropriate waiting area, if that is the policy of the unit. Family-centered care is the trend in maternity today. This approach views labor as wellness and the woman and her support persons as active participants in the process of labor and birth. LDR or LDRP rooms are essential components of family-centered care, and the woman is encouraged to have anyone she wishes present for her support. After birth, the mother, baby, and support persons are permitted to stay together to celebrate the arrival of a new family member (Zwelling & Phillips, 2001).

The woman is asked to undress and put on her own gown or a hospital gown. Her personal belongings are put away safely or given to family members, according to agency policy. Often women who participate in expectant parents classes bring a Birth Bag or Lamaze bag with them. Tennis balls or rolling pins for counterpressure, a pillow for comfort and reminder of home, an object for a focal point (e.g., meaningful picture, stuffed animal), and rice bags for warm packs may be included in her bag.

The nurse orients the woman and her partner to the layout and operation of the unit and room. This includes the use of the call light and telephone system, the location of personal storage areas in the bedside and over-the-bed tables, and how to adjust lighting in the room.

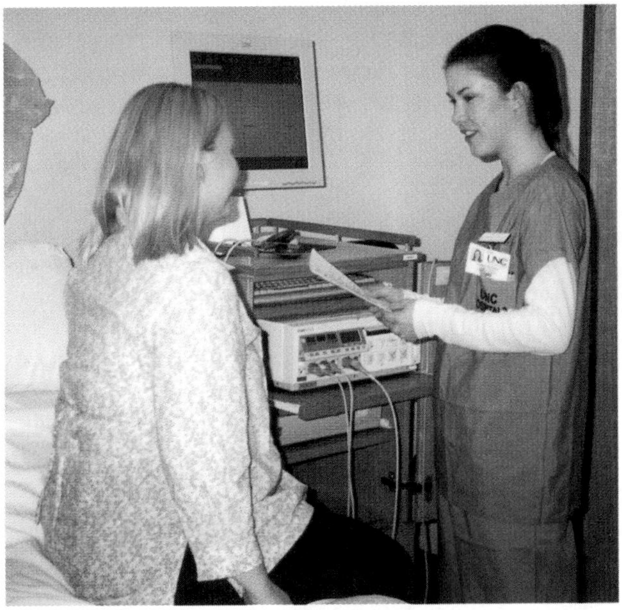

FIG. 21-1 Woman being assessed for admission to the labor and birth unit. (Courtesy Dee Lowdermilk, Chapel Hill, NC.)

The woman is told how to notify the nurse of her wish to use the bathroom or to ambulate. An admissions bracelet is placed on the woman's wrist, as well as an allergy bracelet (usually colored), when relevant. The nurse should reassure the woman that she is in competent, caring hands, that she and her partner can ask questions related to her care and the status of herself and her fetus at any time during labor, and that questions will be answered.

The nurse can minimize the woman's anxiety by explaining terms commonly used during labor. The woman's interest, response, and prior experience guide the depth and breadth of these explanations.

Admission Data

Admission forms such as the one in Figure 21-2 can provide guidelines for the acquisition of important assessment information when a woman in labor is being evaluated or admitted. Additional sources of data include (1) the prenatal record, (2) the initial interview, (3) physical examination to determine baseline physiologic parameters, (4) laboratory and diagnostic test results, (5) expressed psychosocial and cultural factors, and (6) the clinical evaluation of labor status.

Prenatal Data. The nurse reviews the prenatal record to identify the woman's individual needs and risks. Incomplete information regarding a woman's prenatal health status could adversely affect the quality and safety of the care provided to her and her fetus or newborn during labor and birth and in the postpartum period. Use of standardized worksheets and flow sheets developed by health care providers and computer access to antepartal health records are strategies to facilitate the gathering of information relevant to the safe and effective management of care during labor (Hill, Lowery, & Chez, 1998).

If the woman has not had any prenatal care or her prenatal record is unavailable, certain baseline information must be obtained. If the woman is having discomfort, the nurse should ask questions between contractions when the woman can concentrate more fully on her answers. At times the partner or support person(s) may need to be secondary sources of essential information.

It is important to know the woman's age so that the plan of care can be tailored to the needs of her age group. For example, a 14-year-old girl and a 40-year-old woman have different but specific needs, and their ages place them at risk for different problems. Height and weight relations are important to determine because a weight gain greater than that recommended may place the woman at a higher risk for cephalopelvic disproportion and cesarean birth. This is especially true for women who are petite and have gained 16 kg or more. Other factors to consider are her general health status, current medical conditions or allergies, respiratory status, and previous surgical procedures.

Her obstetric and pregnancy history are carefully noted. These include gravidity, parity, and problems such as history of vaginal bleeding, pregnancy-induced hypertension (PIH), anemia, gestational diabetes, infections (e.g., bacterial or sexually transmitted), and immunodeficiency.

If this is not the woman's first labor and birth experience, it is important to note the characteristics of her previous experiences. This information includes the duration of previous labors, the type of anesthesia used, the kind of birth (e.g., spontaneous vaginal, forceps-assisted, vacuum-assisted, or cesarean birth) and the condition of the newborn. The woman's perception of her previous labor and birth experiences should be explored because it may influence her attitude toward her current experience. Women can retain long-term memories of their childbirth experiences. The memory of labor and birth events including their behavior and that of health care providers (e.g., physician, midwife, nurses, doula, partner) can affect a woman's postpartum emotional adjustment, self-esteem, and ability to parent effectively (Hanson et al., 2001).

It is important to confirm the expected date of birth (EDB). Other data in the prenatal record include patterns of maternal weight gain, physiologic measurements such as maternal vital signs (blood pressure; temperature, pulse, respiration); fundal height, baseline fetal heart rate (FHR), and laboratory and diagnostic test results. Laboratory tests include the woman's blood type and Rh factor, a complete or partial blood cell count (CBC, hemoglobin, and hematocrit), the 50-g blood glucose test, determination of the rubella titer, serologic tests (Venereal Disease Research Laboratories [VDRL] or rapid plasma reagin [RPR] test) for syphilis, hepatitis B surface antigen (HBsAg), culture for group B streptococci, and urinalysis. Additional tests may include a tuberculosis screen with purified protein derivative (PPD), screening for the human immunodeficiency virus (HIV), and a screen for sickle cell trait or other genetic disorders (e.g., maternal serum α-fetoprotein). Diagnostic tests include amniocentesis, nonstress test (NST), contraction stress test (CST), biophysical profile (BPP), and ultrasound examination.

Interview. The woman's primary complaint or reason for coming to the hospital is determined in the interview. Her primary complaint may be that her bag of waters (BOW, amniotic membranes) ruptured, with or without contractions. The woman may have come in for an obstetric check, which is a period of observation reserved for women who are unsure about the onset of their labor. This allows time on the unit for the diagnosis of labor without official admission and minimizes or avoids cost to the client when used by the hospital and approved by the woman's health insurance plan.

Even the experienced mother may have difficulty determining the onset of labor. The woman is asked to recall the events of the previous days and to describe the following:

- Time and onset of contractions and progress in terms of frequency and duration
- Location and character of discomfort from contractions (e.g., back pain, suprapubic discomfort)

Obstetric Admitting Record **Page 1 of 2**

Basic Admission Data Date ___ / ___ / ___ Time ________
☐ Ambulatory ☐ Direct admit ☐ Stretcher
☐ Wheelchair ☐ Transfer from________

G	T	Pt	A	L	LMP / /	EDD / /	Age
						EDD By fetal assessment / /	

Race/Ethnicity________
Occupation________ Education________
Marital status S M Sep D W Religion________

MD/CNM Tel no	Support person/Relationship Tel no

Reasons for Admission
☐ **Onset of labor**
☐ Induction of labor
☐ Spontaneous abortion
☐ Cesarean section
☐ Primary ☐ Repeat
(reason for primary________)
☐ VBAC
☐ Tubal ligation
☐ Vaginal bleeding
☐ PROM
☐ Preterm labor
Detail reasons for admission________

Observation evaluation
☐ Fetal status
☐ Ultrasound
☐ Amniocentesis
☐ NST
☐ CST
☐ Medical complications ________
☐ Obstetric complications ________

Patient Triage Data
Contractions ☐ **None** ☐ Palpation ☐ Tocotransducer
Frequency________ Duration________ Intensity________
Began on___ / ___ / ___ Time________
Membranes ☐ **Intact** ☐ Bulging
☐ Ruptured (Date___ / ___ / ___ Time________)
Fluid ☐ Clear ☐ Bloody ☐ Foul smelling
☐ Meconium stained ☐ No foul odor
Vaginal bleeding ☐ **None** ☐ Normal show
☐ Bleeding (describe________)

Cervical Exam
Station________ Effacement________ Dilatation________ cms
Presentation
☐ Vertex ☐ Transverse lie
☐ Face/Brow ☐ Compound
☐ Breech (type________) ☐ Unknown
Medication allergy/Sensitivity ☐ **None**
☐ Identify________
Other allergy/Sensitivity ☐ **None**
☐ Identify________

Patient Care Data

Personal Effects	Disposition		
Item	With patient	With support person	Other (describe)

Illness (≤ 14 days prior to admission) ☐ **None**
☐ Type/Treatment________
Recent Exposure to Communicable Disease ☐ **None**
☐ Type/Date________ ___ / ___ / ___
Last Oral Intake
Fluids___ / ___ / ___ Time________
Solids___ / ___ / ___ Time________
Medications ☐ **None**

Type/Dose	Last taken	With patient No	With patient Yes	Disposition
________	________	☐	☐	________

Alcohol/Drug use ☐ No ☐ Yes
Substances Amt/Day Last used
________ ________ ___ / ___ / ___ Time________
________ ________ ___ / ___ / ___ Time________

Plans for Birth and Hospital Stay
Support person present in L&D ☐ No ☐ Yes________
Other family members in L&D ☐ No ☐ Yes________
Anesthesia ☐ **None**
☐ Local ☐ Epidural ☐ Spinal ☐ General
Delivery site
☐ DR ☐ Birthing room ☐ LDR ☐ LDRP ☐ OR
Personal requests________
Adoption ☐ No
☐ Yes Contact with infant ☐ No ☐ Yes
Adoption contact________
Feeding preference ☐ Breast ☐ Bottle
Room preference ☐ Private ☐ Semi-Private
☐ Rooming-In
☐ Tubal ligation Authorization signed ☐ Yes ☐ No
☐ Circumcision Authorization signed ☐ Yes ☐ No

Psychosocial Data
Communication Deficit ☐ **None**
☐ Identify________
Other children ☐ No ☐ Yes Age/Sex________
________, ________, ________, ________

Partner involved ☐ Yes ☐ No

Admitting signature________ Time________

Continued

FIG. 21-2 Obstetric admitting record. (Permission to use and/or reproduce this copyrighted material has been granted by the owner, Hollister, Inc., Libertyville, IL.)

Obstetric Admitting Record **Page 2 of 2**

Psychosocial Data (Cont'd.)

Basic needs met	Yes	No	If no, explain
Housing	☐	☐	
Clothing	☐	☐	
Food	☐	☐	
Transportation	☐	☐	

Free from apparent physical/emotional abuse ☐Yes ☐No

If no, explain__________

Life Stress	No	Yes	If no, explain
Living	☐	☐	
Working	☐	☐	
Serious illness	☐	☐	

Self Care Needs ☐None ☐Needs help with__________

Emotional status ☐Happy ☐Ambivalent ☐Anxious ☐Depressed ☐Angry

Discharge Planning Data

Discharge planning initiated ☐**Yes** ☐No

Discharge needs identified__________

Social service referral ☐No ☐Yes __/__/__

Planned length of stay______days

Significant Prenatal Data

Prenatal Records Available on Admission

☐**Yes** ☐No

Source of prenatal data__________

First prenatal visit__/__/__

Attended prenatal classes ☐**Yes** ☐No

Infant care provider:

Lab Findings ☐**None**

Blood type & Rh	
Rubella titer	
Serology	
HbSAg	

Fetal Assessment Tests ☐**None**

Date	Test	Result
/		
/		
/		
/		

Maternal Problems Identified ☐**None**

	Active	Resolved
1.	☐	☐
2.	☐	☐
3.	☐	☐

Fetal Problems Identified ☐**None**

	Active	Resolved
1.	☐	☐
2.	☐	☐
3.	☐	☐

Physical Assessment

Detail all abnormal findings

Height		Wt pregrav/grav	
Temp	Pulse	Resp	BP

System	Normal	Abnormal
HEENT	☐	☐
Neurologic	☐	☐
Skin	☐	☐
Breasts	☐	☐
Extremities	☐	☐
Cardiovascular	☐	☐
Respiratory	☐	☐
Abdomen	☐	☐
Gastrointestinal	☐	☐
Urinary	☐	☐
Genitalia	☐	☐

Specimens obtained (check all that apply)

Urine test	Time	Results	Blood test	Time	Results
☐Urinalysis			☐Hgb		
☐C + S			☐Hct		
☐Glucose			☐VDRL/RPR		
☐Albumin			☐Type/Screen		
☐Ketones			☐		
☐pH			☐		
☐Blood			☐		

Fetal Evaluation Data

Fundal height______cms FHR______

Estimated fetal weight______

☐Fetoscope ☐Doppler ☐Fetal monitor ☐Other

Weeks gestation (est)

By dates______wks

By ultrasound______wks

Date__/__/__

Multiple gestation ☐**No** ☐Yes

Infant	Presentation	Position
1.		
2.		
3.		

Initial Problems Identified ☐**None**

1.
2.
3.

Physician/CNM__________

Notified by__________

Date__/__/__Time______

Admitting signature

Examiner signature

Date__/__/__Time______

FIG. 21-2, cont'd For legend see page 545.

- Persistence of contractions despite changes in maternal position and activity (e.g., walking or lying down)
- Presence and character of vaginal discharge or show
- The status of amniotic membranes, such as a gush or seepage of fluid **(rupture of membranes [ROM]).** If there has been a discharge that may be amniotic fluid, she is asked the date and time the fluid was first noted and the fluid characteristics (e.g., amount, color, unusual odor). In many instances, a sterile speculum examination and a nitrazine (pH) or fern test can confirm that the membranes are ruptured (see Procedure box).

These descriptions help the nurse assess the degree of progress in the process of labor. Bloody or pink show is distinguished from bleeding by the fact that it is pink and feels sticky because of its mucoid nature. It is scant to begin with and increases with effacement and dilation of the cervix. A woman may report a scant brownish to bloody discharge that may be attributed to cervical trauma resulting from vaginal examination or coitus within the last 48 hours.

In case general anesthesia may be required in an emergency, it is important to assess the woman's respiratory status. The nurse determines this by asking the woman if she has a "cold" or related symptoms (e.g., "stuffy nose," sore throat, or cough). The status of allergies is rechecked, including allergies to medications routinely used in obstetrics, such as meperidine (Demerol) or lidocaine (Xylocaine). Some allergic responses cause swelling of the mucous membranes of the respiratory tract, which could interfere with breathing and the administration of inhalation anesthesia.

Because vomiting and subsequent aspiration into the respiratory tract can complicate an otherwise normal labor, the nurse records the time and type of the woman's last solid and liquid intake.

Any information not found in the prenatal record is obtained during the admission assessment. Pertinent data include the birth plan (Box 21-2), the choice of infant feeding method, the type of pain management, and the name of the pediatrician. A client profile is obtained that identifies the woman's preparation for childbirth, the support person or family members desired during childbirth and their availability, and ethnic or cultural expectations and needs. The woman's use of alcohol, drugs, and tobacco before or during pregnancy should be determined. Screening of the neonate for substances abused by the mother may be required. After birth, the nurse would assess the neonate for signs indicating maternal substance use during pregnancy (e.g., abstinence syndrome, size, and appearance).

The nurse reviews the birth plan; if no written plan has been prepared, the nurse helps the woman formulate a birth plan by describing options available and finds out the woman's wishes and preferences. The nurse prepares the woman for the possibility that changes may be needed in her plan as labor progresses and assures her that information will be provided so that she can make informed decisions. The nurse uses the information in the birth plan to individualize the care given the woman during labor.

The nurse should discuss with the woman and her partner their plans for preserving childbirth memories by using photography and videotaping. Health care agencies and

PROCEDURE
Tests for Rupture of Membranes

NITRAZINE TEST FOR pH

Explain procedure to woman/couple.

Procedure

Wash hands.

Use **nitrazine test** paper, a dye-impregnated test paper for determining pH. (Differentiates amniotic fluid, which is slightly alkaline, from urine and purulent material [pus], which are acidic.)

Wearing a sterile glove lubricated with water, place a piece of test paper at the cervical os.

OR

Use a sterile, cotton-tipped applicator to dip deep into vagina to pick up fluid; touch applicator to test paper. (Procedure may be done during speculum examination.)

Read results:

Membranes probably intact: identifies vaginal and most body fluids that are acidic:

Yellow	pH 5.0
Olive-yellow	pH 5.5
Olive-green	pH 6.0

Membranes probably ruptured: identifies amniotic fluid that is alkaline:

Blue-green	pH 6.5
Blue-gray	pH 7.0
Deep blue	pH 7.5

Realize that false test results are possible because of presence of bloody show, insufficient amniotic fluid, or semen.

Provide pericare as needed.

Remove gloves and wash hands.

Document Results

Positive or negative.

TEST FOR FERNING OR FERN PATTERN

Explain procedure to woman/couple.

Wash hands, apply sterile gloves, obtain specimen of fluid (usually during sterile speculum examination).

Spread a drop of fluid from vagina on a clean glass slide with a sterile, cotton-tipped applicator.

Allow fluid to dry.

Examine slide under microscope: observe for appearance of **ferning** (a frondlike crystalline pattern) (do not confuse with cervical mucus test, when high levels of estrogen cause the ferning).

Observe for absence of ferning. (Alerts staff to possibility that amount of specimen was inadequate or that specimen was urine, vaginal discharge, or blood.)

Provide pericare as needed.

Remove gloves and wash hands.

Document Results

Positive or negative.

BOX 21-2 **The Birth Plan**

The birth plan should include the woman's/couple's preferences related to the following:
- Presence of birth companions such as the partner, older children, parents, friends, a doula, and the role each will play
- Presence of other persons such as students, male attendants, interpreters
- Clothing to be worn
- Environmental modifications such as lighting, music, privacy, focal point, items from home such as pillows
- Labor activities such as preferred positions for labor and for birth, ambulation, birth balls, showers and whirlpool baths, oral food and fluid intake
- Repertoire of comfort and relaxation measures
- Labor and birth medical interventions such as pharmacologic pain relief measures, intravenous therapy, electronic monitoring, induction or augmentation measures, episiotomy
- Care and handling of the newborn immediately after birth such as cutting of the cord, eye care, breastfeeding
- Cultural and religious requirements related to the care of the mother, newborn, and placenta

The childbirth.org website (http://www.childbirth.org) provides couples with an interactive birth plan along with examples of birth plans.

insurance companies have voiced concern that this type of recording of childbirth events could be used in court should the couple sue the health care agency or health care providers. The nurse can promote the appropriate use of cameras during labor and birth, including who and what will be recorded, the method that will be used, and the person who will perform the task. Protection of privacy and safety and infection control are major concerns. Policies should be in place that address such issues as use of flash photography in the presence of combustible gases and where the person who is recording the labor and birth should stand. The woman's record should reflect that the childbirth was recorded. Consideration should be given to the woman's reaction to viewing the video after birth. She may need help in interpreting the events, behaviors, and reactions she sees depicted in the video, because her impression of her childbirth experience, including her behavior, can have a profound effect on her future labor and birth experiences. Women may have an idealized view of what their birth video will depict, based on childbirth videos viewed during an expectant childbirth class (Cesario, 1998; Hanson et al., 2001).

During this initial interview, the approximate time of the onset of true labor is confirmed, and information on the woman's current clinical condition is obtained.

Psychosocial Factors. The woman's general appearance and behavior (and that of her partner) provide valuable clues to the type of supportive care she will need. However, the nurse should keep in mind that general appearance and behavior may vary, depending on the stage and phase of labor (Table 21-1). Psychosocial factors to assess include the following:

Verbal interactions. Does the woman ask questions? Can she ask for what she needs? Does she talk to her support person(s)? Does she talk freely with the nurse or respond only to questions?

Body language. Is she relaxed or tense? What is her anxiety level? How does she react to being touched by the nurse or support person? Does she change positions or lie rigidly still? Does she avoid eye contact? Does she look tired? How much rest has she had during the past day?

Perceptual ability. Does she understand what the nurse says? Is there a language barrier? Are repeated explanations necessary because her anxiety level interferes with her ability to comprehend? Can she repeat what she has been told or demonstrate her understanding?

Discomfort level. To what degree does the woman describe what she is experiencing? How does she react to a contraction? Are any nonverbal pain messages seen? Does she complain to the nurse or her partner? Can she ask for comfort measures?

Women with a History of Sexual Abuse. Memories of sexual abuse can be triggered during labor by intrusive procedures such as vaginal examinations; loss of control; being confined to bed and "restrained" by monitors, intravenous (IV) lines, and epidurals; being watched by students; and having intense sensations in the uterus and genital area, especially at the time when she must push the baby out. Women who are abuse survivors may fight the labor process by reacting in panic or anger toward care providers, may take control of everyone and everything related to their childbirth, may surrender by being submissive and dependent, or may retreat by mentally dissociating themselves from the sensations of labor and birth (Rhodes & Hutchinson, 1994).

The nurse can help these women to associate the sensations they are experiencing with the process of childbirth and not with their past abuse. The woman's sense of control should be maintained by explaining all procedures and why they are needed, validating her needs and paying close attention to her requests, proceeding at the woman's pace by waiting for her to give permission to touch her, accepting her often extreme reactions to labor, and protecting her privacy by limiting the amount of exposure of her body and the number of persons involved in her care. It is recommended that all laboring women be cared for in this manner, because it is not unusual for a woman to choose not to reveal a history of sexual abuse. These care measures can help a woman to perceive her childbirth experience

TABLE 21-1 **Woman's Responses and Support Person's Actions During First Stage of Labor**

WOMAN'S RESPONSES	NURSE/SUPPORT PERSON'S ACTIONS*
DILATION OF CERVIX 0-3 CM (LATENT) (contractions 30-45 sec long, 5-30 min apart, mild to moderate)	
Mood: alert, happy, excited, mild anxiety	Provides encouragement, feedback for relaxation, companionship
Settles into labor room; selects focal point	Assists woman to cope with contractions
Rests or sleeps, if possible	Encourages use of focusing techniques
Uses breathing techniques	Helps to concentrate on breathing techniques
Uses effleurage, focusing, and relaxation techniques	Uses comfort measures
	Assists woman into comfortable position
	Informs woman of progress; explains procedures and routines
	Gives praise
	Offer fluids, food, ice chips as ordered
DILATION OF CERVIX 4-7 CM (ACTIVE) (contractions 40-70 sec long, 3-5 min apart, moderate to strong)	
Mood: seriously labor oriented, concentration and energy needed for contractions, alert, more demanding	Acts as buffer; limits assessment techniques to between contractions
	Assists woman to cope with contractions
	Encourages woman as needed to help her maintain breathing techniques
Continues relaxation, focusing techniques	Uses comfort measures
Uses breathing techniques	Assists with frequent position changes, emphasizing side-lying and upright positions
	Encourages voluntary relaxation of muscles of back, buttocks, thighs, and perineum; effleurage
	Applies counterpressure to sacrococcygeal area
	Encourages and praises
	Keeps woman aware of progress
	Offers analgesics as ordered
	Checks bladder; encourages her to void
	Gives oral care; offers fluids, food, ice chips as ordered
DILATION OF CERVIX 8-10 CM (TRANSITION) (contractions 45-90 sec long, 2-3 min apart, strong)	
Mood: irritable, intense concentration, symptoms of transition (e.g., nausea, vomiting)	Stays with woman; provides constant support
	Assists woman to cope with contractions
Continues relaxation, needs greater concentration to do this	Reminds, reassures, and encourages woman to reestablish breathing pattern and concentration as needed
Uses breathing techniques	Alerts woman to begin breathing pattern before contraction becomes too intense
Uses 4:1 breathing pattern if using psychoprophylactic techniques	Prompts panting respirations if woman begins to push prematurely
	Uses comfort measures
Uses panting to overcome response to urge to push if appropriate	Accepts woman's inability to comply with instructions
	Accepts irritable response to helping, such as counterpressure
	Supports woman who has nausea and vomiting; gives oral care as needed; gives reassurance regarding signs of end of first stage
	Uses relaxation techniques (effleurage and voluntary relaxation)
	Keeps woman aware of progress

*Provided by nurses and support persons in collaboration with the nurse.

in positive terms and to parent her new baby effectively (Heritage, 1998; Waymire, 1997).

Stress in Labor. The way in which women and their support person or family members approach labor is related to the manner in which they have been socialized to the childbearing process. Their reactions reflect their life experiences regarding childbirth–physical, social, cultural, and religious. Society communicates its expectations regarding acceptable and unacceptable maternal behaviors during labor and birth. These expectations may be used by some women as the basis for evaluating their own actions during childbirth. An idealized perception of labor and birth may be a source of guilt and a sense of failure if the woman finds the process less than joyous, especially when the pregnancy is unplanned or is the product of a shaky or terminated relationship. Often women have heard horror stories or have seen friends or relatives going through labors that appear anything but easy. Multiparous women will often base their expectations of the present labor on their previous childbirth experiences. Feelings a woman has about her pregnancy and fears regarding childbirth should be discussed. This is especially important if the woman is a primigravida who has not attended childbirth classes or is a multiparous woman who has had a previous negative childbirth experience. Major fears and concerns relate to the process and effects of childbirth, maternal and fetal well-being, and the attitude and actions of the health care staff. Unresolved fears increase a woman's stress and can inhibit the process of labor as a result of the inhibiting effects of catecholamines associated with the stress response on uterine contractions (Melender, 2002).

High expectations for childbirth often result in greater satisfaction and a greater sense of fulfillment with the childbirth experience. Conversely, women who have lower expectations often have less positive perceptions of their childbirth experience (Nichols, 1996).

Women in labor usually have a variety of concerns that they will voice if asked but rarely volunteer. To correct misinformation, it is important for the nurse to ask the woman what she expects or to suggest that the woman ask her primary health care provider about an issue. The following are common concerns of women in labor: Will my baby be all right? Will I be able to stand labor? Will my labor be long? How will I act? Will I need medication? Will it work for me? Will my partner or someone be there to support me? Do I have to have an IV?

The nurse's responsibility to the woman in labor with regard to these concerns is to answer her questions or find out the answers, to provide support for her and her support person or family, to take care of her in partnership with those persons the woman wants as her support team, and to serve as their advocate. According to McKay and Smith (1993), women equate emotional support with information giving. Nurses are perceived as supportive when they explain things in detail by using positive terms and provide accurate information and specific directions. Women feel empowered when they are given information they can understand and that shows support for their efforts. This feeling of empowerment gives women the sense that they have the freedom to participate fully in their labor and birth and fosters a positive perception of the experience. In contrast, a woman's level of anxiety and fear may increase when she does not understand what is being said. The woman who is unfamiliar with expressions such as "bloody show," "the membranes ruptured," "scalp electrode," and "baby's lying on the cord" could panic. Many such expressions sound violent and could conjure up thoughts of injury or pain.

The nurse communicates to the woman that she is not expected to act in any particular way and that the process will end in the birth of her baby, which is the only expectation she should have. Women need to be able to behave in a manner that is natural for them and be able to "let go" (Waldenström et al., 1996). The woman's views and expectations regarding the nurse's role as caregiver should be determined. The nurse-client relationship will become increasingly important as labor progresses. Women need to trust in their own innate ability to give birth, and nurses need to support and protect the woman's efforts to achieve this outcome (Bryanton, Fraser-Davey, & Sullivan, 1994; Lothian, 2001).

Women prepare themselves for labor in a variety of ways. Some go to childbirth education classes, some read books and talk to friends and relatives about childbirth, and some prepare elaborate birth plans spelling out their wishes for labor and birth. The longer the list of "wishes," however, the greater the likelihood that expectations will not be met. It is the nurse's responsibility to integrate the woman's desires into the plan of care as much as possible. The nurse can help make sure various aspects of the birth plan are observed by reviewing the plan with the physician or midwife and telling the woman to remind her primary health provider in advance about what she wants.

The father, coach, or significant other(s) also experiences stress during labor. The nurse can assist and support these individuals by identifying their needs and expectations and by helping make sure these are met. The nurse can ascertain what role the support person intends to fulfill and whether he or she is prepared for that role by making observations and asking such questions as, "Has the couple attended childbirth classes?" "What role does this person expect to play?" "Does he or she do all the talking?" "Is he or she nervous, anxious, aggressive, or hostile?" "Does he or she look hungry, tired, worried, or confused?" "Does he or she watch television, sleep, or stay out of the room instead of paying attention to the woman?" "Where does he or she sit?" "Does he or she touch the woman; what is the character of the touch?" The nurse should be sensitive to the needs of support persons and provide teaching and support as appropriate. Often the support this person is able to give the laboring woman is in direct proportion to the support he or she receives from the nurses and other health care providers (Nichols, 1993).

Cultural Factors. It is important to note the woman's ethnic or cultural and religious background to anticipate nursing interventions that should to be added or eliminated from the individualized plan of care (Fig. 21-3). The woman should be encouraged to request specific generic caregiving behaviors and practices that are important to her. If a special request contradicts usual practices in that setting, the woman or the nurse can ask the woman's primary health care provider to write an order to accommodate the special request. For example, in many cultures, it is unacceptable to have a male caregiver examine a pregnant woman. In some cultures, it is traditional to take the placenta home; in others, the woman is given only certain nourishments during labor. Some women believe that cutting her body, as with an episiotomy, allows her spirit to leave her body and that rupturing the membranes prolongs, not shortens, labor. It is important that the rationale for required care measures be carefully explained (Mattson, 2000) (see Cultural Consideration box).

Cultural beliefs and values can influence a woman's reliance on her primary health care provider during labor as well as her desire to participate in making decisions about the care she receives (Callister, Vehvilainen-Julkunen, & Lauri, 1996). Native American women, who view childbirth as a natural event, may find the high-technology environment of a hospital frightening and a disruption of the balance and harmony that are critical for a positive birth experience. They often prefer to be surrounded by a large number of family members, especially the grandparents, and become anxious in the presence of a large number of health care providers who come into the labor room and loudly discuss the progress of labor with each other (Molina, 2001).

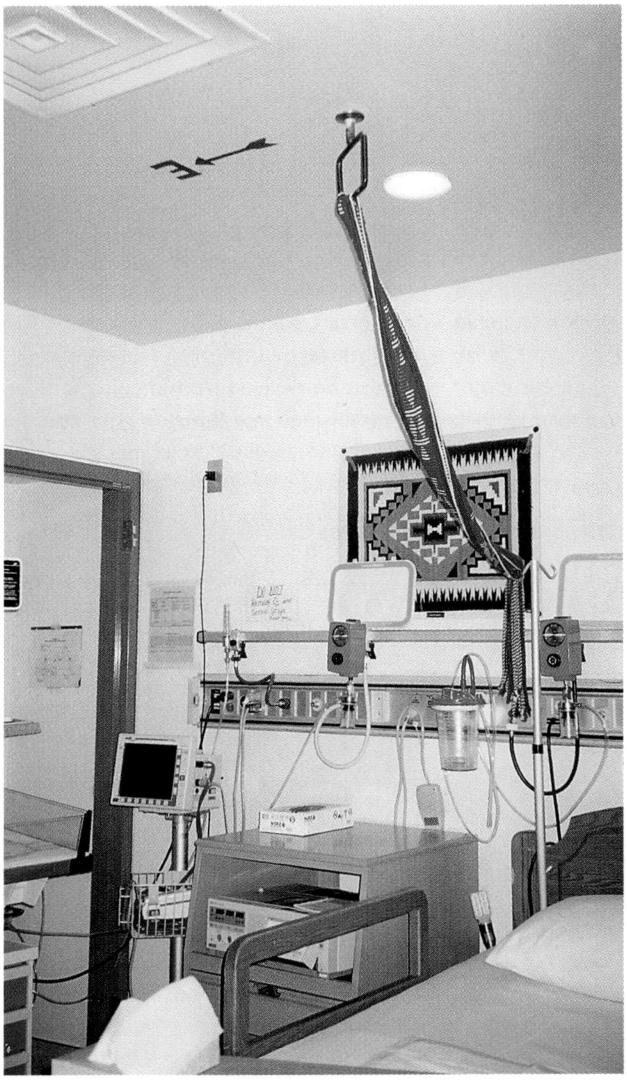

FIG. 21-3 Birthing room specific to a Native American population. Note the arrow pointing east, the rug on the wall, and the cord hanging from the ceiling. (Courtesy Patricia Hess, San Francisco, CA; Chinle Comprehensive Health Care Center, Chinle, AZ.)

In assessing a woman's cultural and religious preferences, Callister (1995) suggested that the nurse ask questions regarding the following:

- Value and meaning placed on the childbirth experience
- View of childbirth as a wellness or illness experience and as a private or social event
- Practices regarding diet, medications, activity, and emotional and physical support
- Appropriate maternal and paternal behaviors
- Birth companions–who they should be and what they should do
- Views regarding the newborn and the newborn's care immediately after birth

Within cultures, women may have the "right" way to behave in labor instilled in them and to react to the pain experienced in that way. These behaviors can range from total silence to moaning or screaming, but they are not in and of themselves a gauge of the degree of pain. A woman who moans with contractions may not be in as much physical pain as a woman who is silent but winces during

CULTURAL CONSIDERATIONS

Birth Practices in Different Cultures

SOUTH KOREA
Stoic response to labor pain; fathers usually not present.

JAPAN
Natural childbirth methods practiced; may labor silently; may eat during labor; father may be present.

CHINA
Stoic response to pain; fathers usually not present; side-lying position preferred for labor and birth, because this position is thought to reduce infant trauma.

INDIA
Natural childbirth methods preferred; father is usually not present; female relatives usually present.

IRAN
Father not present; prefers female support and female caregivers.

MEXICO
May be stoic about discomfort until second stage, then may request pain relief; fathers and female relatives may be present.

LAOS
May use squatting position for birth; fathers may or may not be present; prefer female attendants.

From D'Avanzo, C. & Geissler, E. (2003). *Pocket guide to cultural assessment.* (3rd ed.). St. Louis: Mosby.

contractions (Table 21-2). Some women feel it is shameful to scream or cry out in pain if a man is present. If the woman's support person is her mother, she may perceive the need to "behave" more strongly than if her support person is the father of the baby. She will perceive herself as failing or succeeding on the basis of her ability to adhere to these "standards" of behavior. Conversely, a woman's behavior in response to pain may influence the support received from significant others. In some cultures, women who lose control and cry out in pain may be scolded, whereas in other cultures, support persons will become more helpful (Choudhry, 1997; Weber, 1996).

Culture and Father Participation. A companion is an important source of support, encouragement, and comfort for women during childbirth. The nurse managing the care of pregnant women should help these women identify the person or persons they wish to be their supportive companions during childbirth. The choice of birth companion is influenced by the woman's cultural and religious background and by trends in the society in which she lives. For example, in Western societies, the father is viewed as the ideal birth companion. For European-American couples, attending childbirth classes together has become a traditional, expected activity. Laotian (Hmong) husbands traditionally are active participants in the labor process, often by supporting their wife's position, catching the baby as it emerges, cutting the cord, and burying the placenta (Lipson, Dibble, & Minarik, 1996). A Mormon woman expects her husband to be present during her labor and to lay his hands on her head in a blessing that imparts strength, comfort, and well-being for safe passage through childbirth (Callister, 1992,

TABLE 21-2 **Sociocultural Basis of Pain Experience**

WOMAN IN LABOR	NURSE
PERCEPTION OF MEANING	
Origin: Cultural concept of and personal experience with pain; for example: Pain in childbirth is inevitable, something to be endured. Pain in childbirth can be avoided completely. Pain in childbirth is punishment for sin. Pain in childbirth can be controlled.	Origin: Cultural concept of and personal experience with pain; in addition, nurse becomes accustomed to working with certain "expected" pain trajectories. For example, in obstetrics, pain is expected to increase as labor progresses, be intermittent, and have an end point; relief can be derived from medications once labor is well established and fetus or newborn can cope with amount and elimination of medications; relief can also come from woman's knowledge, attitude, and support from family or friends.
COPING MECHANISMS	
Woman may exhibit the following behaviors: Be traditionally vocal or nonvocal; crying out or groaning, or both, may be part of her ritual response to pain. Use counterstimulation to minimize pain (e.g., rubbing, applying heat, or applying counterpressure). Use relaxation, distraction, or autosuggestion as pain-countering techniques. Resist any use of "needles" as modes of administering pain relief agents.	Nurse may respond by Using self effectively (e.g., using tone of voice, closeness in space, and touch as media for conveying message of interest and caring). Using avoidance, belittling, or other distracting actions as protective device for self. Using pharmacologic resources at hand judiciously. Using comfort measures. Assuming accountability for control and management of pain.
EXPECTATIONS OF OTHERS	
Nurse may be seen as someone who will accept woman's statement of pain and act as her advocate. Medical personnel may be expected to relieve woman of all pain sensations. Nurse may be expected to be interested, gentle, kind, and accepting of behavior exhibited.	Only certain verbal or nonverbal responses to pain may be accepted as appropriate responses. Couple that is prepared for childbirth may be expected to refuse medication and to wish to "do everything on their own." Woman's definition of pain may not be accepted; that is, woman may wish to experience and participate in controlling pain or may not be able to accept any pain as reasonable.

1995). In some cultures, the father may be available, but his presence in the labor room with the mother may not be considered appropriate, or he may be present but resist active involvement in her care. Such behavior could be misconstrued by the nursing staff to represent a lack of concern, caring, or interest. Latina women expect their male partner to be present at their bedside during labor, to talk to them, keep them calm, and tell them everything is going to be okay and not to worry. The men are expected to show love and affection by telling the women they love them, by hugging them, and by holding their hands. However, Latino men do not become actively involved in giving their partners care during labor by performing such activities as backrubs and helping with pushing (Khazoyan & Anderson, 1994). Lantican and Corona (1992) identified the importance of the affectional bond Mexican-American and Filipina women have with their female relatives when it comes to home-related activities such as childbearing. This also is true for the women of many other cultural groups. The presence of another woman or women is highly desired at such occasions. Women who come from some of these cultures and who give birth in the hospital like to have at least one woman present for assistance. Vietnamese, Chinese, and Indian women prefer a female companion during childbirth and are very concerned about their modesty (Choudhry, 1997; D'Avanzo & Geissler, 2003). Islamic women also are very modest and would not accept the presence of a man during childbirth, not even the father (Woods, 1991). The religious beliefs of some Orthodox Jews forbid the father to touch his wife during labor or to be present at the birth. Instead, while he prays, the female members of the laboring woman's family act as supportive childbirth companions (Callister, 1995; De Sevo, 1997). In India, women are attended by other women, and in rural areas, by a local untrained midwife or dai. Men usually are not present and in some cases may not be allowed to see the face of their child until certain prayers are said or an astrologically appropriate time is reached (Choudhry, 1997).

The Non–English-Speaking Woman in Labor. A woman's level of anxiety in labor increases when she does not understand what is happening to her or what is being said. Some misunderstanding may occur with English-speaking women and cause some stress, but the effect of misunderstanding on non–English-speaking women is much more dramatic. These women often feel a complete loss of control over their situation if no health care provider is present who speaks their language. They can panic and withdraw or become physically abusive when someone tries to do something they perceive might harm them or their babies. Sometimes a support person is able to serve as an interpreter. However, this must be done with caution because the interpreter may not be able to convey exactly what the nurse or others are saying or what the woman is saying and thus increases the woman's stress level even more.

Ideally, a bilingual nurse will care for the woman. Alternatively, an employee or volunteer interpreter may be contacted for assistance (see Box 2-3). Ideally, the interpreter is from the woman's culture. For some women, a female interpreter may be more acceptable. If no one in the hospital is able to interpret, a service can be called so that interpretation can take place over the telephone. Another alternative is for the labor and birth unit staff to prepare a set of cards with graphic illustrations that depict common situations. These cards can be used to communicate with non–English-speaking women. Even when the nurse has limited ability to communicate verbally with the woman, in most instances, the nurse's efforts to communicate are meaningful and appreciated by the woman. Speaking slowly and avoiding complex words and medical terms can help a woman and her partner to understand (Mattson, 2000) (see Guidelines/Guías box).

GUIDELINES/GUÍAS

Labor Assessment

What time did the contractions begin?
¿A qué hora le empezaron las contracciones?

How far apart are the contractions?
¿Con qué frecuencia tiene las contracciones?

Have the membranes ruptured? When?
¿Se le rompió la fuente? ¿Cuándo?

What color was the fluid? Red? Pink?
¿Qué color tenía el líquido? ¿Rojo? ¿Rosado?

Have you had bleeding?
¿Ha sangrado?

How much? A cupful? A tablespoonful? A teaspoonful?
¿Cuánto? ¿Una taza? ¿Una cucharada? ¿Una cucharadita?

When was the last time you ate or drank anything?
¿Cuándo fue la última vez que comió o bebió algo?

Have you had any problems with this pregnancy?
¿Ha tenido algún problema con este embarazo?

Are you taking any medications?
¿Está tomando alguna medicación?

Are you allergic to penicillin or other medicines?
¿Es alérgica a la penicilina u otras medicinas?

Please sign this consent form.
Por favor, firme esta forma de consentimiento.

Physical Examination

During the admission process, the physical examination begins with a vaginal examination to rule out imminent birth. The nurse proceeds with the remainder of the initial physical examination to confirm the onset of true labor. The initial physical examination includes a general systems assessment; performance of Leopold's maneuvers to determine fetal presentation and position and the point of maximal intensity (PMI) for auscultating the FHR; assessment of fetal status; assessment of uterine contractions; and vaginal examination to assess the status of cervical effacement and dilation, fetal descent, and amniotic membranes and fluid. The most vital aspect of the assessment is the determination of fetal status. The findings of the admission physical examination serve as a baseline for assessing the woman's progress from that point.

It is important to obtain as many related pieces of information as possible before planning and implementing care. Women often focus on the nature of their contractions as the clearest indicator of how far advanced their labor is. However, the findings from the vaginal examination are more valid indicators of the phase of labor, especially for nulliparous women. ROM significantly affects the woman's plan of care because, once this occurs, the membranes can no longer protect the intrauterine cavity and fetus from infectious organisms that can travel up the birth canal. The risk of umbilical cord prolapse exists once the membranes have ruptured if the presenting part is not engaged.

The information yielded by a complete and accurate assessment during the initial examination serves as the basis for determining whether the woman should be admitted and what her ongoing care should be. Expected maternal progress and minimal assessment guidelines during the first stage of labor are presented in Table 21-3 and the Care Path for the low risk woman in the first stage of labor.

The assessment procedures described in the following paragraphs can be used as a basis for teaching women and their significant others. The equipment needed, the nursing actions involved, and the rationale for each procedure can be shared with the woman. The nurse should thoroughly wash her hands before performing any of these

TABLE 21-3 Expected Maternal Progress in First Stage of Labor

PHASES MARKED BY CERVICAL DILATION*			
CRITERION	**0-3 CM (LATENT)**	**4-7 CM (ACTIVE)**	**8-10 CM (TRANSITION)**
Duration†	About 6-8 hr	About 3-6 hr	About 20-40 min
Contractions			
Strength	Mild to moderate	Moderate to strong	Strong to very strong
Rhythm	Irregular	More regular	Regular
Frequency	5-30 min apart	3-5 min apart	2-3 min apart
Duration	30-45 sec	40-70 sec	45-90 sec
Descent			
Station of presenting part	Nulliparous: 0 Multiparous: 0 to −2 cm	Varies: +1 to +2 cm Varies: +1 to +2 cm	Varies: +2 to +3 cm Varies: +2 to +3 cm
Show			
Color	Brownish discharge, mucous plug, or pale pink mucus	Pink to bloody mucus	Bloody mucus
Amount	Scant	Scant to moderate	Copious
Behavior and appearance‡	Excited; thoughts center on self, labor, and baby; may be talkative or silent, calm or tense; some apprehension; pain controlled fairly well; alert, follows directions readily; open to instructions	Becomes more serious, doubtful of control of pain, more apprehensive; desires companionship and encouragement; attention more inner directed; fatigue evidenced; malar (cheeks) flush; has some difficulty following directions	Pain described as severe; backache common; frustration, fear of loss of control, and irritability surface; vague in communications; amnesia between contractions; writhing with contractions; nausea and vomiting, especially if hyperventilating; hyperesthesia; circumoral pallor, perspiration of forehead and upper lips; shaking tremor of thighs; feeling of need to defecate, pressure on anus

*In the nullipara, effacement is often complete before dilation begins; in the multipara, it occurs simultaneous with dilation.

†Duration of each phase is influenced by such factors as parity, maternal emotions, position, level of activity, fetal size, and presentation position. For example, the labor of a nullipara tends to last longer, on average, than the labor of a multipara. Women who ambulate and assume upright positions or change positions frequently during labor tend to experience a shorter first stage. Descent is often prolonged in breech presentations and occiput posterior positions.

‡Women who have epidural analgesia for pain relief may not demonstrate some of these behaviors.

procedures. Handwashing also is important after the examinations are completed. Standard Precautions should guide all assessment and care measures (Box 21-3). The assessment findings are explained to the woman whenever possible. Throughout labor, accurate documentation, following agency policy, is done as soon as possible after a procedure has been performed (Fig. 21-4).

General Systems Assessment. A brief systems assessment is performed. This includes an assessment of the heart, lungs, and skin; an examination to determine the

Care Path Low Risk Woman in First Stage of Labor

CARE MANAGEMENT	CERVICAL DILATION 0-3 CM (LATENT)	4-7 CM (ACTIVE)	8-10 CM (TRANSITION)
I. ASSESSMENT MEASURES*	**Frequency**	**Frequency**	**Frequency**
• Blood pressure, pulse, respirations	Every 30-60 min	Every 30 min	Every 15-30 min
• Temperature†	Every 4 hr	Every 4 hr	Every 4 hr
• Uterine activity	Every 30-60 min	Every 15-30 min	Every 10-15 min
• Fetal heart rate (FHR)	Every 30-60 min	Every 15-30 min	Every 15-30 min
• Vaginal show	Every 30-60 min	Every 30 min	Every 15 min
• Behavior, appearance, mood, energy level of woman; condition of partner	Every 30 min	Every 15 min	Every 5 min
• Vaginal examination‡	As needed to identify progress	As needed to identify progress	As needed to identify progress
II. PHYSICAL CARE MEASURES§	Stay at home for as long as possible Relaxation measures; rest and sleep if at night Activity—ambulation; emphasize upright positions Diversional activities Nourishment—light foods and full liquids Void every 2 hr Perform basic hygiene measures	Coach breathing techniques Encourage effleurage Assist in using relaxation techniques between contractions Encourage ambulation, upright positions Assist with position changes Use comfort measures desired by woman: massage, hot/cold packs, touch, etc. Initiate hydrotherapy (shower, bath, jacuzzi) Provide nourishment as desired Encourage voiding every 2 hr Assist with hygiene, perineal care Provide pharmacologic pain relief as indicated Provide relief for partner	Coach breathing techniques Reduce touch if increased sensitivity is noted Help to relax between contractions Assist with position changes Use comfort measures according to acceptance level Continue hydrotherapy if effective Provide clear liquids: sips, ice chips Encourage voiding every 2 hr Provide hygiene measures, emphasizing mouth and perineal care Provide pharmacologic pain relief as indicated Prepare for birth
III. EMOTIONAL SUPPORT	Review birth plan Review process of labor—what to expect, pain management techniques available Redemonstrate breathing techniques Keep informed: progress, procedures	Provide feedback about performance Reduce distractions during contractions Role model comfort measures Reassure, encourage, praise Take charge, talk through contraction until control regained Continue to keep informed	Provide continuous support Reduce distractions Role model care measures to assist partner Continue reassurance, praise, and encouragement Keep informed Take charge as needed

*Full assessment using interview, physical examination, and laboratory testing is performed on admission. Subsequently, frequency of assessment is determined by the risk status of the maternal-fetal unit. More frequent assessment is required in high risk situations. Frequency of assessment and method of documentation are also determined by agency policy, which is usually based on the recommended care standards of medical and nursing organizations.

†If membranes have ruptured, the temperature should be assessed every 1 to 2 hr; assess orally or tympanically between contractions.

‡Perform vaginal examination at admission and thereafter only when signs indicate that progress has occurred (e.g., significant increase in frequency, duration, and intensity of contractions; rupture of membranes; perineal pressure); strict aseptic technique should be used. In the presence of vaginal bleeding, the primary health care provider performs the examination under a double setup in a delivery room, or an ultrasonography is performed to determine placental location.

§Physical care measures are performed by the nurse working together with the woman's partner and significant others. The woman is capable of greater independence in the latent phase but needs more assistance during the active and transition phases.

BOX 21-3 Standard Precautions During Childbirth

Birth is a time when nurses and other health care providers are exposed to a great deal of maternal and newborn blood and body fluids. Observation of Standard Precautions is necessary to prevent the transmission of infection. Perinatal infections most often are transmitted through contact with body fluids. The Standard Precautions applicable to childbirth include the following:

- Wash hands before and after putting on gloves and performing procedures.
- Wear gloves (clean or sterile, as appropriate) when performing procedures that require contact with the woman's genitalia and body fluids, including bloody show (e.g., during vaginal examination, amniotomy, hygienic care of the perineum, insertion of an internal scalp electrode and intrauterine pressure monitor, and catheterization).
- Wear a mask that has a shield or protective eyewear, and cover gown when assisting with the birth. Cap and shoe covers are worn for cesarean birth but are optional for vaginal birth in a birthing room. Gowns worn by the primary health care provider who is attending the birth should have a waterproof front and sleeves and should be sterile.
- Drape the woman with sterile towels and sheets as appropriate. Explain to the woman what can and cannot be touched.
- Help the woman's partner put on appropriate coverings for the type of birth, such as cap, mask, gown, and shoe covers. Show the partner where to stand and what can and cannot be touched.
- Wear gloves and gown when handling the newborn immediately after birth.
- Use an appropriate method to suction the newborn's airway, such as a bulb syringe, mechanical wall suction, or De Lee oral suction device that prevents the newborn's mucus from getting into the user's mouth or airway.

presence and extent of edema of the legs, face, hands, or sacrum; and testing of deep tendon reflexes and for clonus.

Vital Signs. Vital signs (temperature, pulse, respirations, and blood pressure) are assessed on admission, and the initial values are used as the baseline for comparison with subsequent values. If the blood pressure is elevated, it should be reassessed 30 minutes later, between contractions, using a correct-size blood pressure cuff to obtain a reading after the woman has relaxed. To prevent supine hypotension and fetal distress, the woman should be encouraged to lie on her side and not supine (Fig. 21-5 on p. 561). Her temperature is monitored so that signs of infection or a fluid deficit (e.g., dehydration associated with inadequate intake of fluids) can be identified. The woman's intake and output should be measured at least every 8 hours. Urinary protein and ketone levels may be determined by using a dipstick each time the woman voids.

Leopold's Maneuvers (Abdominal Palpation). **Leopold's maneuvers** are performed with the woman briefly lying on her back (see Procedure box and Fig. 21-6 on p. 562). These maneuvers help identify the (1) number of fetuses; (2) presenting part, fetal lie, and fetal attitude; (3) degree of the presenting part's descent into the pelvis; and (4) expected location of the PMI of the fetal heart tones (FHTs) on the woman's abdomen.

Assessment of FHR and Pattern. It is important for the nurse to understand the relation between the location of the PMI of the FHTs and fetal presentation, lie, and position. A high risk for childbirth complications may be revealed by variations in these findings. The PMI of the FHTs is the location on the maternal abdomen where FHTs are heard the loudest. It is usually directly over the fetal back. The PMI also is an aid in determining the fetal presentation and position (Fig. 21-7 on p. 563). In a vertex presentation, FHTs are usually heard below the mother's umbilicus in either the right or left lower quadrant of the abdomen; in a breech presentation, FHTs are usually heard above the mother's umbilicus (Fig. 21-7, *A*, and Fig. 21-8, *C* on p. 563). As the fetus descends and rotates internally, the FHTs are heard lower and closer to the midline of the maternal abdomen. The PMI of the fetus in the right occipitoanterior (ROA) position moves to the midline just over the symphysis pubis (Fig. 21-8, *A* and *B*). Just before birth, the fetal position is occipitoanterior (OA), and the fetal back is directly above the symphysis pubis. Diagrams of the PMI for different presentations and positions are presented in Fig. 21-7. Assessments recommended for determining fetal status in the low risk woman during each stage of labor are summarized in the Care Paths. The FHR and pattern also must be assessed (1) immediately after ROM, because this is the most common time for the umbilical cord to prolapse; (2) after any change in the contraction pattern or maternal status; and (3) before and after medicating the woman or performing a procedure (Tucker, 2000).

Assessment of Uterine Contractions. A general characteristic of effective labor is regular uterine activity, but uterine activity is not directly related to labor progress. **Uterine contractions** are the primary powers that act involuntarily to expel the fetus and the placenta from the uterus. Several methods are used to evaluate uterine contractions, including the woman's subjective description, palpation and timing of contractions by a health care provider, and electronic monitoring.

Each contraction exhibits a wavelike pattern. It begins with a slow increment (the "building up" of a contraction from its onset), gradually reaches an acme (intrauterine

Text continued on p. 561.

Labor Progress Chart

Admit date	Admit time	Blood type and Rh	Age	G	T	P	A	L	EDB __/__/__ LMP __/__/__	Membranes ☐ **Intact** ☐ Ruptured SROM AROM ☐ Bulging Date __/__/__ Time ____
__/__/__										

Current date __/__/__	**Time →**																		
Vital signs	Temperature																		
	Pulse																		
	Respiration																		
	Blood pressure																		
Maternal	Deep tendon reflexes (L/R)	/	/	/	/	/	/	/	/	/	/	/	/	/	/	/	/	/	/
	Urine (Protein/sugar)	/	/	/	/	/	/	/	/	/	/	/	/	/	/	/	/	/	/
	Vaginal bleeding																		
Uterine activity	Monitor mode																		
	Frequency																		
	Duration																		
	Intensity																		
	Resting tone																		
	Peak IUP																		
	MVUs																		
Fetal Assessment	Monitor mode																		
	Baseline (FHR)																		
	STV																		
	LTV																		
	Accelerations																		
	Decelerations																		
	Strip number																		
	Membranes																		
	Fluid																		
Intake/Output (cc's/Hr)	IV																		
	PO																		
	Urine																		
	Emesis																		
Cont meds	Pitocin mU/min																		
	$MgSO_4$ gms/hr																		
	Ritodrine mg/min																		
	Terbutaline mg/hr																		
Intervention	Position change																		
	O_2 L/min																		
	IV bolus																		
Initials																			

Abbreviations/Key	Vaginal bleeding	Monitor mode uterine activity	MVUs montevideo units	Monitor mode fetal	STV short term variability
	NS = Normal show ABN = Frank vaginal Bleeding	P = Palpation E = External I = Internal	The sum of the peak of each uterine contraction minus resting tone, in a 10 minute period.	A = Auscultation (fetoscope) D = Doppler E = External I = Internal	STV + = Present (roughness of tracing line present) STV Ø = Absent (tracing line is smooth)

Continued

FIG. 21-4 Labor progress chart. (Permission to use and/or reproduce this copyrighted material has been granted by the owner, Hollister, Inc., Libertyville, IL.)

Labor Progress Chart

Medication Allergy/Sensitivity ☐ **None**

(Identify)__________

Chart______ of______

LVT (long term variability)
0-2 BPM = Absent
3-5 BPM = Minimal
6-25 BPM = Average
>25 BPM = Marked

Accelerations
+ = 15 BPM ↑ × 15 sec
0 = Absent

Decelerations
N = None
E = Early
V = Variable
L = Late
P = Prolonged

Membranes
I = Intact
B = Bulging
R = Ruptured

Fluid
C = Clear
M = Meconium stained
B = Bloody
F = Foul smelling
NF = Not foul smelling

FIG. 21-4, cont'd For legend see page 557.

Labor Progress Chart

Station	Mark X	Dilation •	
	Time →		
	Mark X •	10	
	-4	9	
	-3	8	
	-2	7	
	-1	6	
	0	5	
	+1	4	
	+2	3	
	+3	2	
Effacement % and/or position			
Examined by:			

IV Record

Start date	Time	Solution	Amount (cc's)	Medication/Dose added	Initials	Infused date	Time	Amount infused

Teaching

Topic	Date time	Comments
Oriented		
Labor review		
Support person		
Pre-Op		
Safety		

Interval Medications

Date time	Medication/Dose	Route	Site	Initials

Initials	Signature

Progress Notes

Date	Time	

Continued

FIG. 21-4, cont'd For legend see page 557.

Labor Progress Chart

Progress Notes (Cont'd.)

Date	Time	

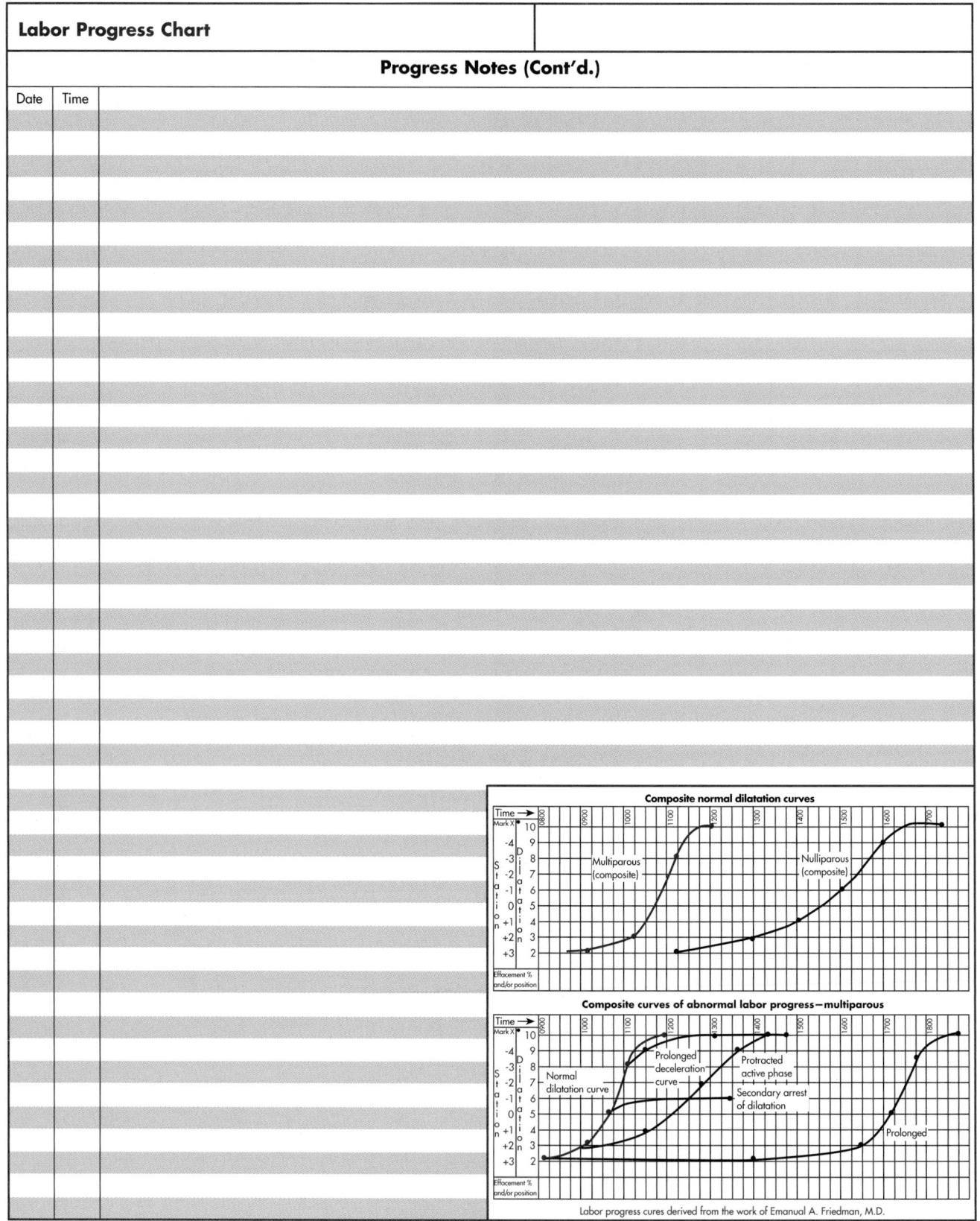

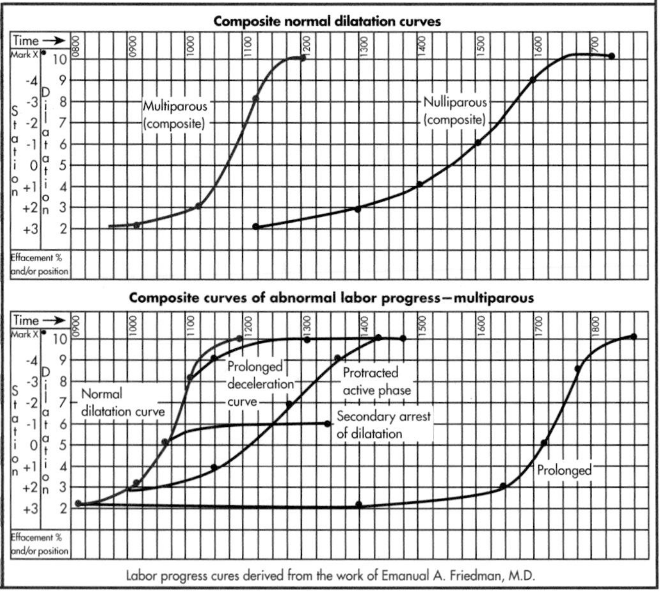
Composite normal dilatation curves
Time →
Mark X
Station
Dilatation
-4 -3 -2 -1 0 +1 +2 +3
10 9 8 7 6 5 4 3 2
0800 0900 1000 1100 1200 1300 1400 1500 1600 1700
Multiparous (composite)
Nulliparous (composite)
Effacement % and/or position
Composite curves of abnormal labor progress—multiparous
0900 1000 1100 1200 1300 1400 1500 1600 1700 1800
Normal dilatation curve
Prolonged deceleration curve
Protracted active phase
Secondary arrest of dilatation
Prolonged
Labor progress cures derived from the work of Emanual A. Friedman, M.D.

FIG. 21-4, cont'd For legend see page 557.

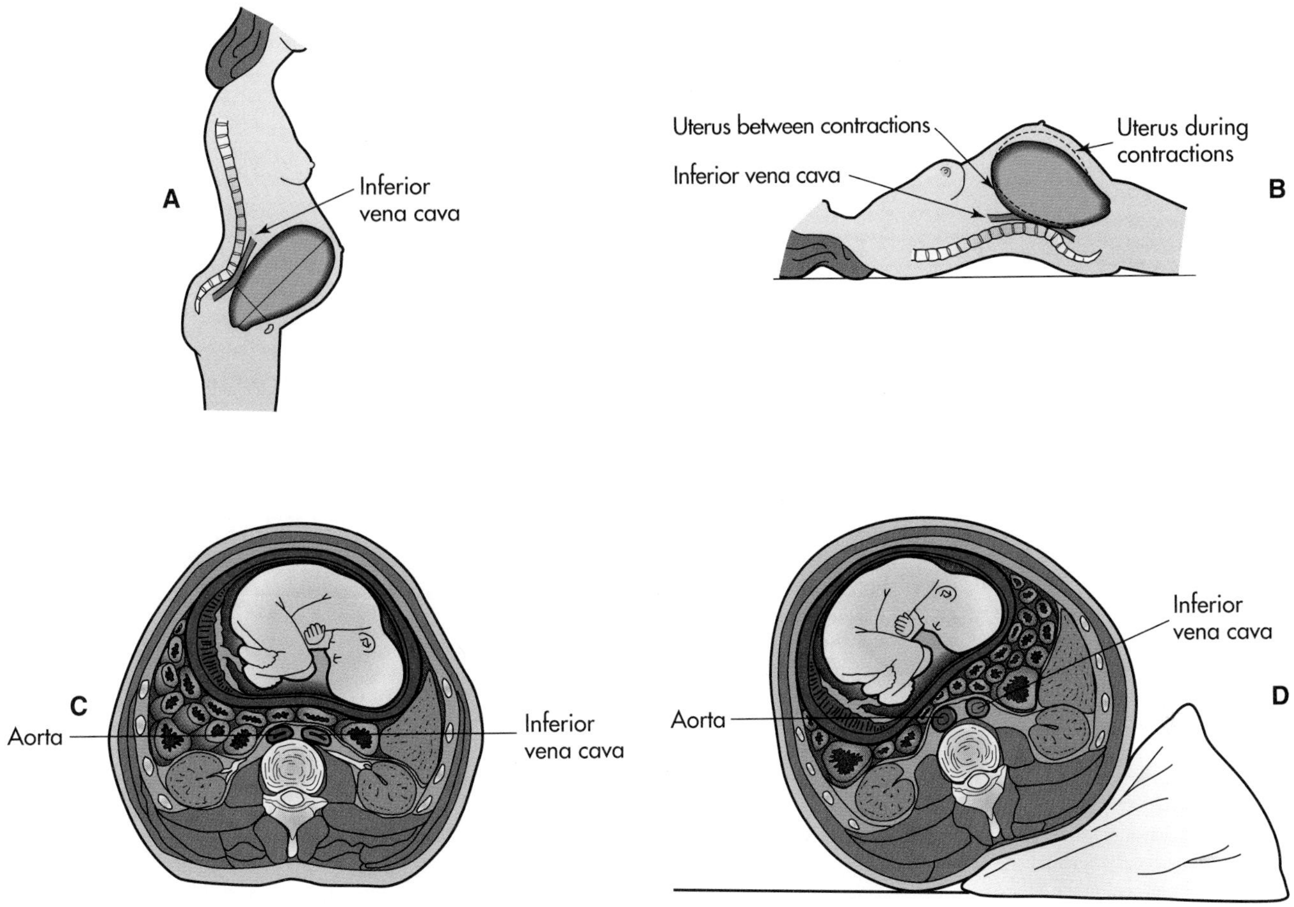
A
Inferior vena cava
Uterus between contractions
Uterus during contractions
Inferior vena cava
B
C
Aorta
Inferior vena cava
Aorta
Inferior vena cava
D

FIG. 21-5 Supine hypotension. Note relation of pregnant uterus to ascending vena cava in standing position **(A)**, and in the supine position **(B)**. **C,** Compression of aorta and inferior vena cava with woman in supine position. **D,** Compression of these vessels is relieved by placement of a wedge pillow under the woman's right side.

pressure less than 80 mm Hg), and then diminishes rapidly (decrement, the "letting down" of the contraction). An interval of rest (intrauterine pressure less than 20 mm Hg with a duration of at least 30 seconds) ends when the next contraction begins (Tucker, 2000). The outward appearance of the woman's abdomen during and between contractions and the pattern of a typical uterine contraction are shown in Figure 21-9.

A uterine contraction is described in terms of the following characteristics:

- **Frequency of uterine contractions:** How often uterine contractions occur; the time that elapses from the beginning of one contraction to the beginning of the next or from the peak of one contraction to the peak of the next (if using electronic monitoring)
- **Intensity of uterine contractions:** The strength of a contraction at its peak
- **Duration of uterine contractions:** The time that elapses between the onset and the end of a contraction
- **Resting tone of uterine contractions:** The tension in the uterine muscle between contractions

Uterine contractions are assessed by palpation or by an external or internal electronic monitor. Frequency and duration can be measured by all three methods of uterine activity monitoring. The accuracy of determining intensity varies by the method used. Palpation is more subjective and is a less precise way of determining the intensity of uterine contractions (Arrabal & Naegy, 1996). The following terms are used to describe what is felt on palpation:

- *Mild:* Slightly tense fundus that is easy to indent with fingertips (feels like touching finger to tip of nose)
- *Moderate:* Firm fundus that is difficult to indent with fingertips (feels like touching finger to chin)
- *Strong:* Rigid, boardlike fundus that is almost impossible to indent with fingertips (feels like touching finger to forehead)

Women in labor tend to describe the pain of contractions in terms of the sensations they are experiencing in

PROCEDURE

Leopold Maneuvers and Determination of the Points of Maximal Intensity for FHTs

LEOPOLD MANEUVERS

Wash hands.

Ask woman to empty bladder.

Position woman supine with one pillow under her head and with her knees slightly flexed.

Place small rolled towel under woman's right or left hip to displace uterus off major blood vessels (prevents supine hypotensive syndrome; see Fig. 21-5).

If right-handed, stand on woman's right, facing her:

1. Identify fetal part that occupies the fundus. The head feels round, firm, freely movable, and palpable by ballottement; the breech feels less regular and softer. This maneuver identifies fetal lie (longitudinal or transverse) and presentation (cephalic or breech) (Fig. 21-6, *A*).
2. Using palmar surface of one hand, locate and palpate the smooth convex contour of the fetal back and the irregularities that identify the small parts (feet, hands, elbows). This maneuver helps identify fetal presentation (Fig. 21-6, *B*).
3. With right hand, determine which fetal part is presenting over the inlet to the true pelvis. Gently grasp the lower pole of the uterus between the thumb and fingers, pressing in slightly (Fig. 21-6, *C*). If the head is presenting and not engaged, determine the attitude of the head (flexed or extended).
4. Turn to face the woman's feet. Using both hands, outline the fetal head (Fig. 21-6, *D*) with the palmar surface of the fingertips. When the presenting part has descended deeply, only a small portion of it may be outlined. Palpation of the cephalic prominence helps identify the attitude of the head. If the cephalic prominence is found on the same side as the small parts, this means that the head must be flexed and the vertex is presenting (Fig. 21-6, *D*). If the cephalic prominence is on the same side as the back, this indicates that the presenting head is extended and the face is presenting (Fig. 21-6, *D*).

Document fetal presentation, position, and lie and whether presenting part is flexed or extended, engaged, or free floating. Use hospital's protocol for documentation (e.g., "Vtx, LOA, floating").

DETERMINATION OF PMI OF FHT

Wash hands.

Perform Leopold maneuvers.

Auscultate fetal heart tones (FHTs) based on fetal presentation identified with Leopold maneuvers. The PMI is the location where the FHTs are heard the loudest, usually over the fetal back (see Figs. 21-7 and 21-8).

Chart PMI of FHTs using a two-line figure to indicate the four quadrants of the maternal abdomen, as follows: right upper quadrant (RUQ), left upper quadrant (LUQ), left lower quadrant (LLQ), and right lower quadrant (RLQ):

RUQ	LUQ
RLQ	LLQ

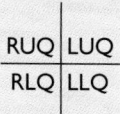

The umbilicus is the reference point for the quadrants (point where the lines cross). The PMI for the fetus in vertex presentation, in general flexion with the back on the mother's right side, commonly is found in the mother's right lower quadrant and is recorded with an "X" or with the FHT, as follows:

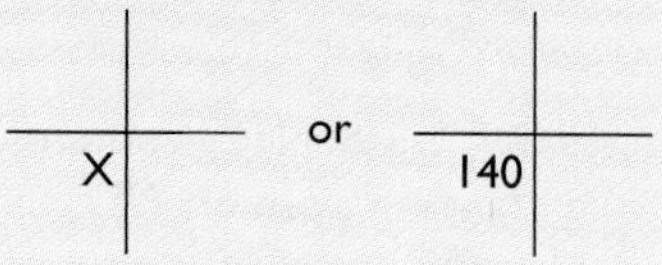
X
or
140

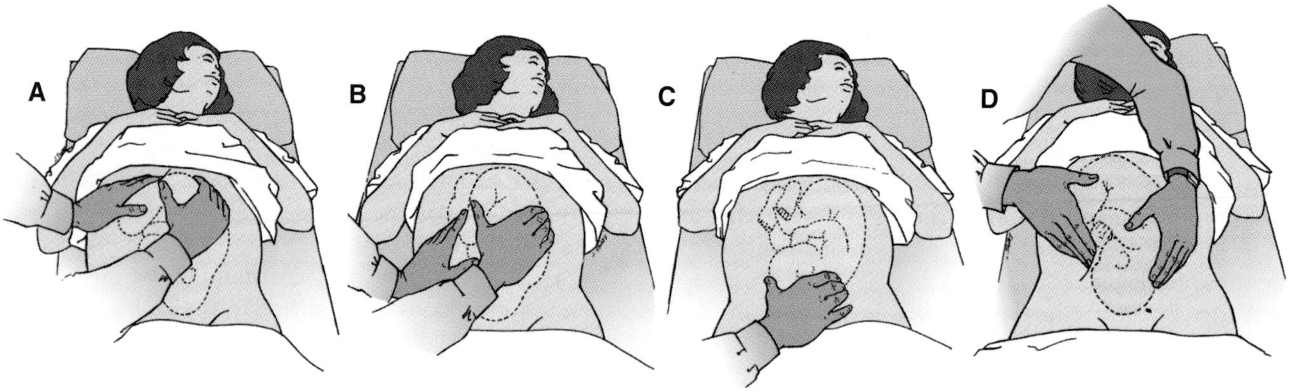
A
B
C
D

FIG. 21-6 Leopold maneuvers.

the lower abdomen or back, which may be unrelated to the firmness of the uterine fundus. Thus their assessment of the strength of their contractions can be less valid than that of the health care provider, although the amount of discomfort reported is valid.

External electronic monitoring provides information about the relative strength of the uterine contractions. Internal electronic monitoring with an intrauterine pressure catheter is the most reliable way of assessing the intensity of uterine contractions.

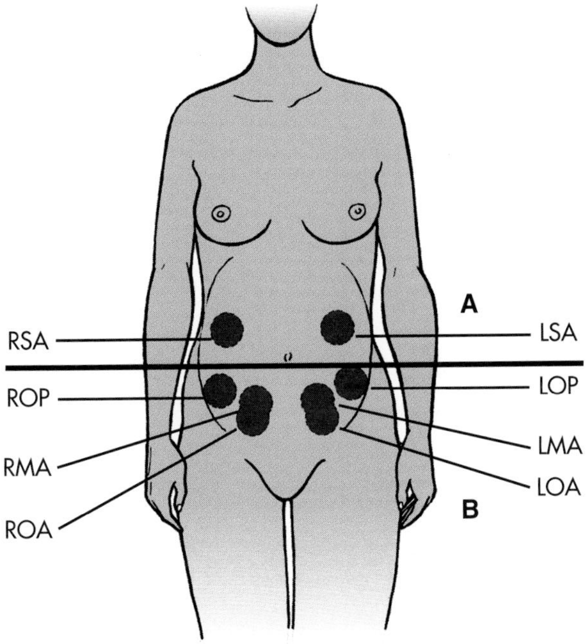
A
RSA
LSA
ROP
LOP
RMA
LMA
LOA
ROA
B

FIG. 21-7 Areas of maximal intensity of fetal heart tones (FHTs) for differing positions: *RSA*, right sacrum anterior; *ROP*, right occipitoposterior; *RMA*, right mentum anterior; *ROA*, right occipitoanterior; *LSA*, left sacrum anterior; *LOP*, left occipitoposterior; *LMA*, left mentum anterior; *LOA*, left occipitoanterior. **A,** Presentation is usually *breech* if FHTs are heard *above* umbilicus. **B,** Presentation is usually *vertex* if FHTs are heard *below* umbilicus.

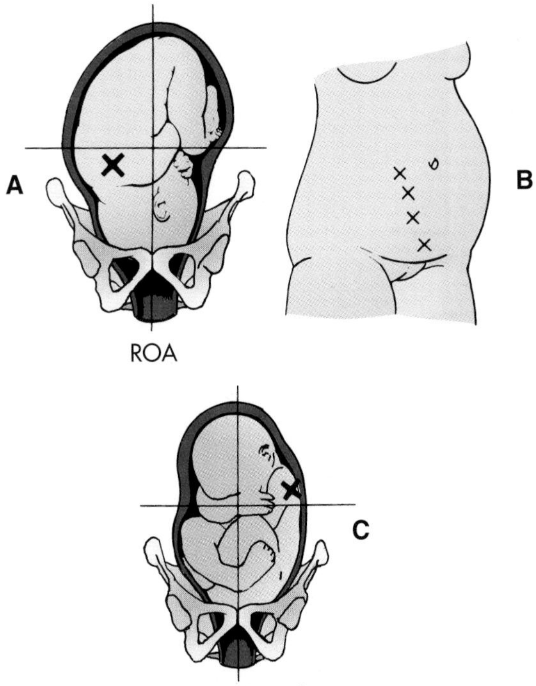
A
B
ROA
C
Complete breech
Lie: Vertical
Presentation: Breech (sacrum and feet presenting)
Reference point: Sacrum (with feet)
Attitude: General flexion

FIG. 21-8 Location of the fetal heart tones (FHTs). **A,** With fetus in right occipitoanterior (ROA) position. **B,** Changes in location of point of maximal intensity of FHTs as fetus undergoes internal rotation from ROA to OA and descent for birth. **C,** With fetus in left sacrum posterior position. (**A** and **C** courtesy Ross Laboratories, Columbus, OH.)

On admission, a 20- to 30-minute baseline monitoring of uterine contractions and the FHR and pattern usually is done (Scott et al., 1999). The minimal assessment times during the various phases of labor are given in the Care Paths on pp. 555 and 584, and the findings expected as labor progresses are summarized in Tables 21-3 and 21-7.

The nurse's responsibility in the monitoring of uterine contractions is to ascertain whether they are powerful and frequent enough to accomplish the work of expelling the fetus and the placenta.

NURSE ALERT

If the characteristics of contractions are found to be abnormal, either exceeding or falling below what is considered acceptable in terms of the standard characteristics, the nurse should report this to the primary health care provider.

Cervical Effacement, Dilation, Fetal Descent. Uterine activity must be considered in the context of its effect on cervical effacement and dilation and on the degree of descent of the presenting part (see Chapter 18). The effect on the fetus also must be considered. The progress of labor can be effectively verified through the use of graphic charts *(partograms)* on which cervical dilation and station (descent) are plotted. This type of graphic charting assists in early identification of deviations from expected labor patterns. Figure 21-10 provides examples of partograms. Hospitals and birthing centers may develop their own graphs for recording assessments. Such graphs may include not only data on dilation and descent but also data on maternal vital signs, FHR, and uterine activity.

NURSE ALERT

It is important for the nurse to recognize that active labor can actually last longer than the expected labor patterns. This finding should not be a cause for concern unless the maternal-fetal unit exhibits signs of distress (e.g., nonreassuring FHR patterns, maternal fever).

Vaginal Examination. The vaginal examination reveals whether the woman is in true labor and enables the examiner to determine whether the membranes have ruptured. Because this examination is often stressful and uncomfortable

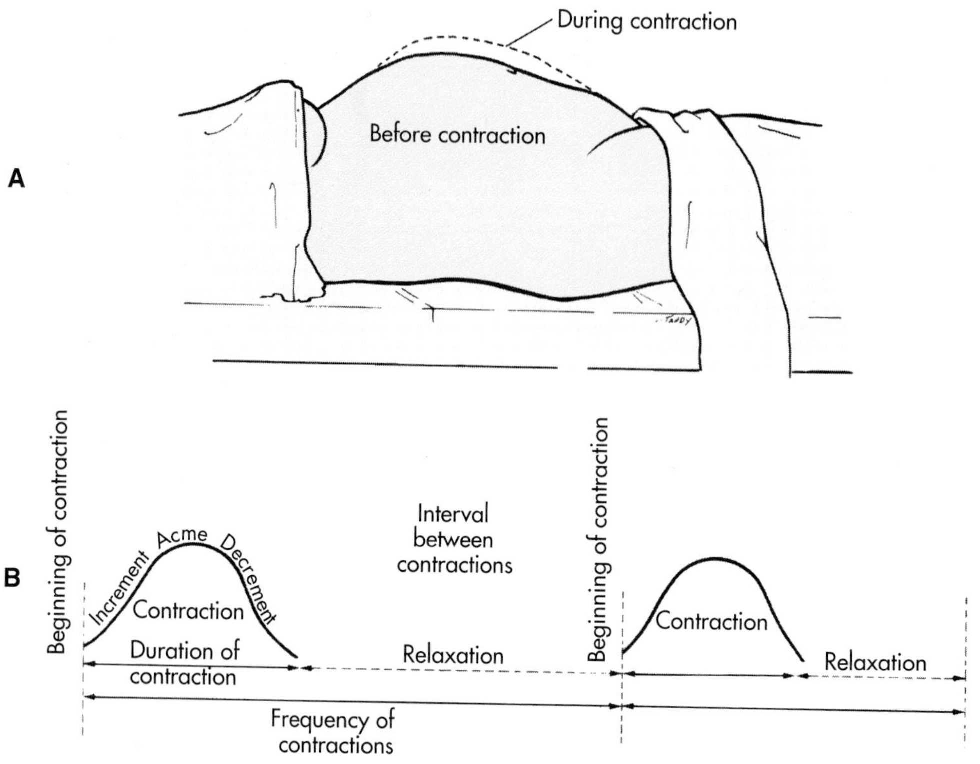
A
During contraction
Before contraction
B
Beginning of contraction
Increment
Acme
Decrement
Contraction
Duration of contraction
Interval between contractions
Relaxation
Beginning of contraction
Contraction
Relaxation
Frequency of contractions

FIG. 21-9 Assessment of uterine contractions. **A,** Abdominal contour before and during uterine contraction. **B,** Wavelike pattern of contractile activity.

for the woman, it should be performed only when indicated by the status of the woman and her fetus. For example, a vaginal examination should be performed on admission, when significant change has occurred in uterine activity, on maternal perception of perineal pressure or the urge to bear down, when membranes rupture, or when variable decelerations of the FHR are noted. A full explanation of the examination and support of the woman are important factors in reducing the stress and discomfort associated with the examination. Chapter 5 describes a typical vaginal examination. Steps in the vaginal examinations of the woman in labor include the following:

1. Use a sterile glove and antiseptic solution or soluble gel; use water for lubrication during the initial examination if ROMs is suspected and a Nitrazine test is required.
2. Position the woman to prevent supine hypotension (see Fig. 21-5). Cleanse the perineum and vulva if needed.
3. Ask the woman for permission to touch her before proceeding (Waymire, 1997) and explain that she will feel insertion of the nurse's index and middle fingers into the vagina. Perform the examination gently, with concern for the woman's comfort. Acknowledge the woman's expressions of pain or discomfort and anxiety.
4. Assess status of the following (Fig. 21-11):
   a. Dilation, effacement, and position (e.g., posterior, mid, anterior) of cervix
   b. Presenting part, position, station, and if vertex, any molding of the head
   c. Membranes–intact, bulging, or ruptured; amniotic fluid–color, clarity, and odor
5. Discuss the findings of the examination with the woman or couple.
6. Document the findings and report them to the primary health care provider.

Laboratory and Diagnostic Tests

Analysis of Urine Specimen. A clean-catch urine specimen may be obtained to gather further data about the pregnant woman's health. It is a convenient and simple procedure that can provide information about her hydration status (e.g., specific gravity, color, amount), nutritional status (e.g., ketones), infection status (e.g., leukocytes), or the status of possible complications such as PIH, shown by finding protein in the urine. The results can be obtained quickly and help the nurse determine appropriate interventions to implement.

Blood Tests. The blood tests performed vary with the hospital protocol and the woman's health status. An example of a minimal assessment is a hematocrit determination, in which the specimen is centrifuged in the perinatal unit. Blood can be obtained by a finger stick or from the hub of a catheter used to start an IV line. More comprehensive blood

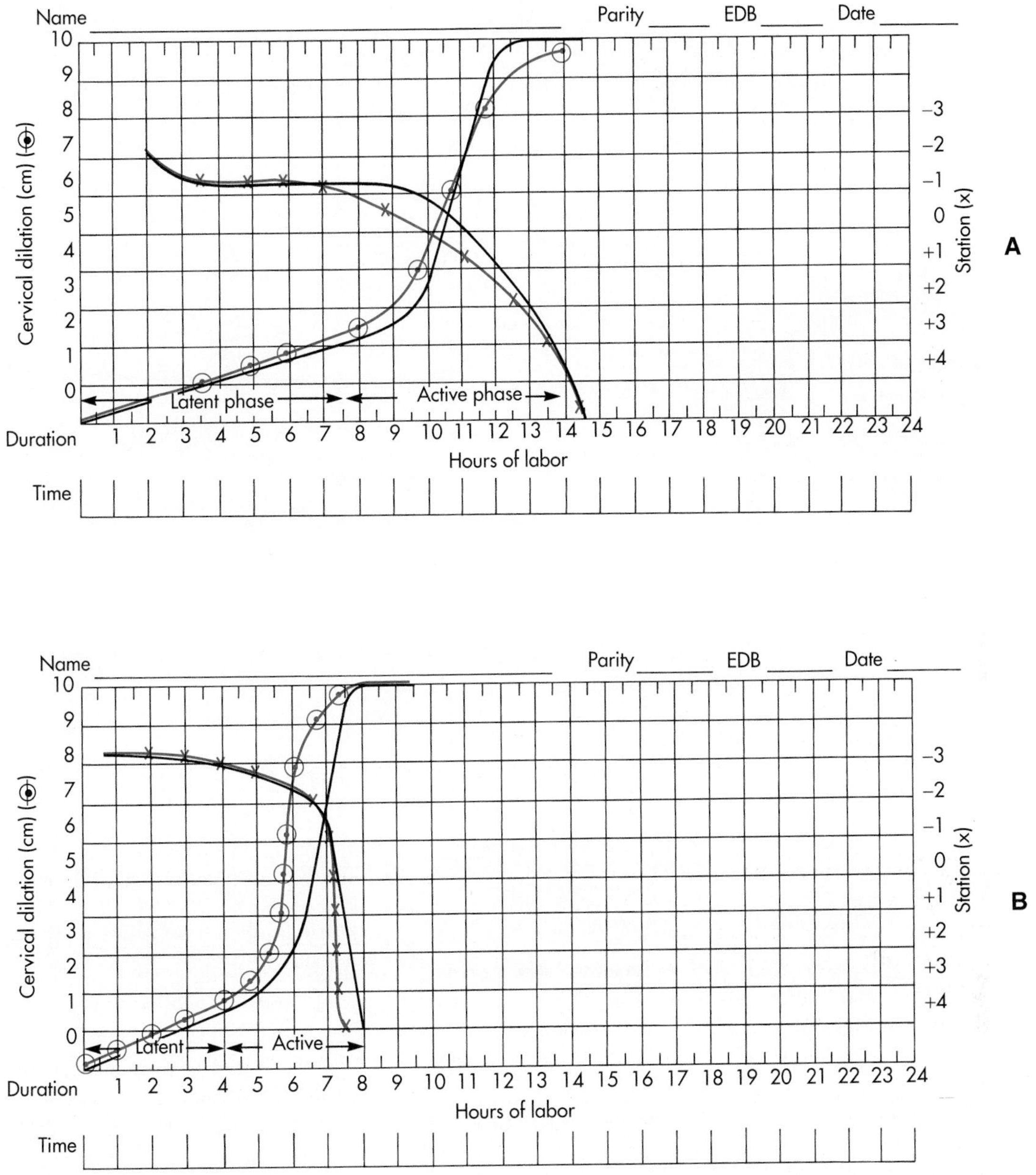
Name
Parity
EDB
Date
Cervical dilation (cm)
Station (x)
Latent phase
Active phase
Duration
Hours of labor
Time
A
Name
Parity
EDB
Date
Cervical dilation (cm)
Station (x)
Latent
Active
Duration
Hours of labor
Time
B

FIG. 21-10 Partogram for assessment of patterns of cervical dilation and descent. Individual woman's labor patterns *(colored)* superimposed on prepared labor graph *(black)* for comparison. **A,** Labor of a nulliparous woman. **B,** Labor of a multiparous woman. The rate of cervical dilation is plotted with the circled plot points. A line drawn through these symbols depicts the slope of the curve. Station is plotted with Xs. A line drawn through the Xs reveals the pattern of descent.

assessments such as white blood cell count, red blood cell count, the hemoglobin level, hematocrit, and platelet values are included in a CBC. A CBC may be ordered for women with a history of infection, anemia, PIH, and other disorders.

If the woman's blood type has not been verified, blood is drawn for the purpose of determining the type and Rh factor. If blood typing has already been done, the primary health care provider may choose not to repeat the test. If obvious signs of immunocompromise or substance abuse are present, other blood tests may be ordered.

Assessment of Amniotic Membranes and Fluid. Labor is initiated at term by SROM in approximately 25% of pregnant women. A lag period, rarely exceeding 24 hours, may precede the onset of labor. Membranes (the bag of waters) also can rupture spontaneously any time during labor, but most commonly in the transition phase of the first stage of labor.

NURSE ALERT

The umbilical cord may prolapse when the membranes rupture. The FHR and pattern should be monitored closely for several minutes immediately after ROM to ascertain fetal well-being, and the findings should be documented.

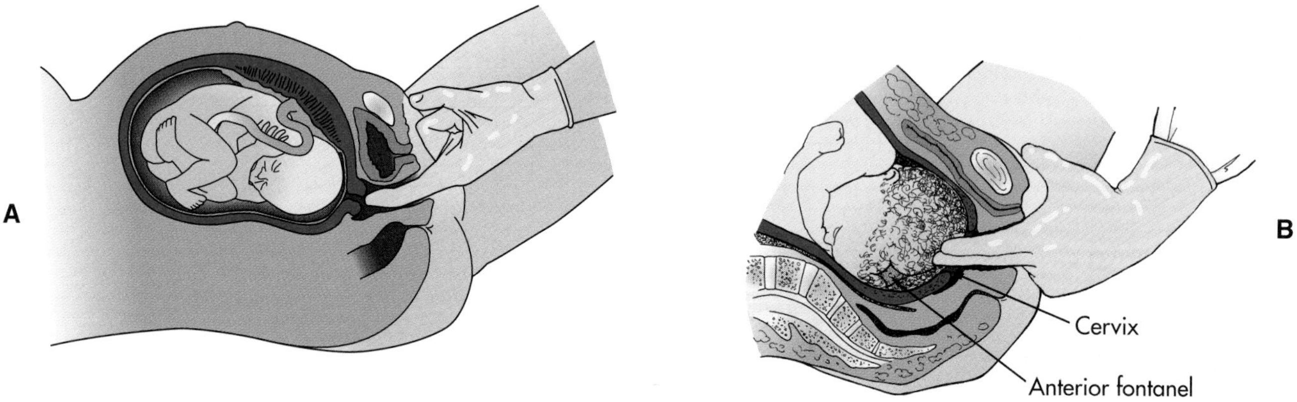
A
B
Cervix
Anterior fontanel

FIG. 21-11 Vaginal examination. **A,** Undilated, uneffaced cervix; membranes intact. **B,** Palpation of sagittal suture line. Cervix effaced and partially dilated.

TABLE 21-4 **Assessment of Amniotic Fluid Characteristics**

CHARACTERISTIC OF FLUID	NORMAL FINDING	DEVIATION FROM NORMAL FINDING	CAUSE OF DEVIATION FROM NORMAL
Color	Pale, straw colored; may contain white flecks of vernix caseosa, lanugo, scalp hair	Greenish brown color	Hypoxic episode in fetus results in meconium passage into fluid May be normal finding in breech presentations related to pressure exerted on fetal abdominal wall during descent
		Yellow-stained fluid	Fetal hypoxia ≥36 hr before ROM; fetal hemolytic disease; intrauterine infection
		Port wine colored	Bleeding associated with premature separation of the placenta (abruptio placentae)
Viscosity and odor	Watery; no strong odor	Thick, cloudy, foul-smelling	Intrauterine infection Large amount of meconium can make fluid thick
Amount (normally varies with gestational age)	400 ml (20 wk gestation)	>2000 ml (32 to 36 wk gestation)	Hydramnios; associated with congenital anomalies of the fetus when fetus cannot drink or fluid is trapped in the body (e.g., fetal gastrointestinal obstruction or atresias); increased risk with maternal pregestational or gestational diabetes mellitus
	1000 ml (36 to 38 wk gestation)	<500 ml (32 to 36 wk gestation)	Oligohydramnios; associated with incomplete or absent kidney; obstruction of urethra; fetus cannot secrete or excrete urine

ROM, Rupture of membranes.

The tests used to assess amniotic fluid are discussed in the Procedure box on p. 547, and the characteristics of the fluid are described in Table 21-4. **Artificial rupture of membranes** (AROM, ARM), or **amniotomy,** may be done to augment or induce labor or to facilitate placement of internal monitors when fetal status indicates the need for some form of direct assessment (e.g., insertion of a fetal scalp electrode or an intrauterine pressure catheter).

Infection. When membranes rupture, microorganisms from the vagina can then ascend into the amniotic sac, causing chorioamnionitis and placentitis to develop. For this reason, maternal temperature and vaginal discharge are assessed frequently (every 1 to 2 hours) so that an infection developing after ROM can be identified early. Even when membranes are intact, however, microorganisms may ascend and cause PROM. There is controversy regarding whether prophylactic antibiotic therapy can protect against infection (chorioamnionitis), which involves both the maternal and fetal sides of the membrane. Prophylactic antibiotics for prelabor ROM at term or preterm is a form of care of unknown effectiveness (Enkin et al., 2000).

The nurse's responsibility is to report findings promptly to the primary health care provider and to document findings in the labor record and on the monitor strip. If abnormal findings are noted, continuous electronic monitoring usually is implemented and maintained for the duration of labor. The presence of meconium-stained amniotic fluid alerts the nurse to the need to observe fetal status more closely. After birth, the newborn may be at risk for an alteration in respiratory status if meconium is aspirated into the lungs with the first breath.

Signs of Potential Problems. Assessment findings serve as a baseline for evaluating the woman's subsequent progress during labor. Although some problems of labor are anticipated, others may appear unexpectedly during the clinical course of labor (see Signs of Potential Complications box).

SIGNS OF POTENTIAL COMPLICATIONS

Labor

- Intrauterine pressure of ≥80 mm Hg (determined by intrauterine pressure catheter monitoring) or resting tone of ≥20 mm Hg
- Contractions consistently lasting ≥90 sec
- Contractions consistently occurring ≤2 min apart
- Contractin interval <30 sec
- Fetal bradycardia, tachycardia, persistently decreased variability, or late or severe variable deceleration
- Irregular FHR; suspected fetal dysrhythmias
- Appearance of meconium-stained or bloody fluid from the vagina
- Arrest in progress of cervical dilation or effacement, descent of the fetus, or both
- Maternal temperature of ≥38° C
- Foul-smelling vaginal discharge
- Persistent bright or dark-red vaginal bleeding

Nursing Diagnoses

Nursing diagnoses determine the types of nursing actions needed to implement a plan of care. When establishing nursing diagnoses, the nurse should analyze the significance of findings ascertained during the assessment.

- *Impaired verbal communication related to*
  - –language barrier
- *Risk for injury (maternal and fetal) related to*
  - –undiagnosed prenatal conditions associated with inadequate prenatal care
  - –inadequate powers of labor
- *Impaired physical mobility related to*
  - –advanced station of fetal presenting part
  - –fetal monitoring
  - –epidural analgesia
- *Impaired fetal gas exchange related to*
  - –maternal position
  - –maternal hypotension
  - –maternal hypertension
  - –intense uterine contractions
  - –compression of umbilical cord
- *Situational low self-esteem (maternal) related to*
  - –inability to meet self-expectations concerning performance during childbirth
  - –loss of control during labor
- *Fear related to*
  - –triggering of memories associated with history of sexual abuse
- *Situational low self-esteem (father or partner) related to*
  - –unrealistic expectations regarding role as labor coach
  - –perceived ineffectiveness in meeting the needs of the laboring woman

Expected Outcomes of Care

It is important for the nurse and woman to set and assign priorities to expected outcomes that focus on the woman, fetus, and her significant others. Appropriate nursing and client actions are then determined so that these expected outcomes can be met. Planning with the woman is essential to ensure the achievement of expected outcomes and to maintain her sense of control over her own childbirth experience. Expected outcomes for the woman in the first stage of labor are that the woman will accomplish the following:

- Express satisfaction with the assistance of her support person(s), family, and nursing staff.
- Actively participate in the labor process.
- Continue normal progression of labor while the FHR and pattern remains reassuring and without signs of distress.
- Maintain adequate hydration status through oral or IV intake.

- Void at least every 2 hours to prevent bladder distention.
- Verbalize discomfort and indicate the need for measures that help reduce discomfort and promote relaxation.
- Express satisfaction with her performance during labor.

Plan of Care and Interventions

Standards of Care

Standards of care guide the nurse in preparing for and implementing procedures with the expectant mother (Box 21-4). Protocols for care based on standards include the following tasks:

- Check the primary health care provider's orders.
- Review the primary health care provider's orders for completeness and correctness (e.g., the dose and route of the analgesic to be administered).
- Check labels on IV solutions, drugs, and other materials used for nursing care.
- Check the expiration date on any packs of supplies used for procedures.
- Ensure that information on the woman's identification band is accurate (e.g., the band is the appropriate color for allergies).
- Use an empathic approach when giving care (see Guidelines/Guias box):
  –use words the woman can understand when explaining procedures; repeat as necessary.

BOX 21-4 **Care Plan Using Protocols and Nursing Standards**

CARE PLAN FOR LABOR

MARY JAMES
UNIT NO. 4587024

Date Initiated: _______ Time: _______ RN: _______

OUTCOME STANDARDS:

1. Client will demonstrate normal labor progress while the fetus tolerates the labor process without demonstrating nonreassuring signs. Date met: ______
2. Client will participate in decisions about her care. Date met: ______
3. Client and her partner will verbalize knowledge of labor process and their expectations for the birth experience. Date met: ______

INITIATED Date/RN	PROBLEM	NURSING INTERVENTIONS	DISCONTINUED
	Impaired maternal/fetal gas exchange	Implement fetal monitoring per protocol or orders from health care provider	Date/RN
	Risk related to labor progress: • Impaired urinary elimination • Impaired tissue integrity related to birth	Provide nursing care per hospital procedure manual Implement labor care per protocol or care path Notify primary health care provider of problems (see Signs of Potential Complications box) Provide care for vaginal birth per hospital procedure manual Provide immediate care for newborn per hospital procedure manual Implement care for fourth stage of labor per protocol or care path	
	Anxiety related to maternal/fetal status	Encourage woman and her partner to express their concerns Keep couple informed of labor progress Involve woman in decision making regarding her care	
	Deficient knowledge about labor/procedures	Explain procedures in terms woman can understand	
	Acute pain related to process of labor	Promote use of relaxation techniques Provide comfort measures Offer pain medications as ordered Evaluate response to pain relief measures	
	Other problems:		

–respect the woman's individual needs and behaviors.
–establish rapport with the woman and her significant others.
–be kind, caring, and competent when performing necessary procedures.
–be aware that pain and discomfort are as the woman describes them.
–carry out appropriate comfort measures such as mouth care and back care
–include the support persons in the care as desired by the woman and the support persons
–recognize that a woman's current childbirth experience and the actions of nurses and other health care providers can have a positive or negative effect on the woman's future childbirth experiences.

- Use Standard Precautions, including precautions for invasive procedures (see Box 21-3).
- Document care according to hospital guidelines, and communicate information to the primary health care provider when indicated.

GUIDELINES/GUÍAS

Care During Labor

Lie down, please.
Acuéstese, por favor.

I am going to take your vital signs.
Le voy a tomar sus signos vitales.

I'm going to listen to the baby's heartbeat.
Voy a escuchar los latidos del corazón del bebé.

This is a fetal monitor.
Este es un monitor del feto.

I need to examine you.
Necesito examinarle.

Do you need to use the bathroom?
¿Necesita usar el baño?

Would you like some pain medication?
¿Desea medicina para calmar el dolor?

Roll over on your side, please.
Póngase al lado, por favor.

Relax.
Relájese.

Breathe deeply.
Respire profundamente.

Push.
Puje.

Don't push.
No puje.

Grab your knees and push.
Agarre las rodillas y puje.

You're doing fine.
Bien. Muy bien.

Congratulations!
¡Felicidades!

You have a beautiful boy.
Usted tiene un niño precioso.

You have a beautiful girl.
Usted tiene una niña preciosa.

Physical Nursing Care During Labor

The physical nursing care rendered to the woman in labor is an essential component of her care. The current emphasis on evidence-based practice supports the management of care by using this approach to enhance the safety, effectiveness, and acceptability of the physical care measures chosen to support the woman during labor and birth (Enkin et al., 2000). The various physical needs, the requisite nursing actions, and the rationale for care are presented in Table 21-5, the Plan of Care on p. 571, and the Care Path on p. 555.

General Hygiene. Women in labor should be offered the use of showers or jacuzzis, if they are available, to enhance the feeling of well-being and to minimize the discomfort of contractions. Women also should be encouraged to wash their hands after voiding and to perform self-hygiene measures. Linen should be changed if it becomes wet or stained with blood, and linen savers (Chux) should be used and changed as needed.

Nutrient and Fluid Intake

Oral Intake. Traditionally the laboring woman has been offered only clear liquids or ice chips or given nothing by mouth during the active phase of labor to minimize the risk of anesthesia complications and their sequelae should general anesthesia be required in an emergency. These sequelae include the aspiration of gastric contents and resultant compromise in oxygen perfusion, which may endanger the lives of the mother and fetus. This practice is being challenged today because regional anesthesia is used more often than general anesthesia, even for emergency cesarean births. Women are awake during regional anesthesia and are able to participate in their own care and protect their airway.

Although gastric emptying is slowed as a result of labor, stress, and the use of narcotics or sedatives, fasting does not cause gastric contents to be eliminated and may even cause them to become more acidic. In addition, fasting is identified by many laboring women as a stressor with which they must cope and a source of frustration during labor related to a loss of control with regard to meeting their own nourishment needs (Fowles, 1998).

An adequate intake of fluids and calories is required to meet the energy demands and fluid losses associated with childbirth. The progress of labor slows, and ketosis develops if these demands are not met and fat is metabolized. Reduced energy for bearing-down efforts (pushing) increases the risk for a forceps- or vacuum-assisted birth. This is most likely to occur in women who begin to labor early in the morning after a night without caloric intake. When women are permitted to consume fluids and food freely,

TABLE 21-5 **Physical Nursing Care During Labor**

NEED	NURSING ACTIONS	RATIONALE
GENERAL HYGIENE		
Showers/bed baths, jacuzzi bath	Assess for progress in labor	Determines appropriateness of the activity
	Supervise showers closely if woman is in true labor	Prevents injury from fall; labor may be accelerated
	Suggest allowing warm water to flow over back	Aids relaxation; increases comfort
Perineum	Cleanse frequently, especially after rupture of membranes and when show increases	Enhances comfort and reduces risk of infection
Oral hygiene	Offer toothbrush or mouthwash or wash the teeth with an ice-cold, wet washcloth as needed	Refreshes mouth; helps counteract dry, thirsty feeling
Hair	Brush, braid per woman's wishes	Improves morale; increases comfort
Handwashing	Offer washcloths before and after voiding and as needed	Maintains cleanliness; prevents infection
Face	Offer cool washcloth	Provides relief from diaphoresis; cools and refreshes
Gowns/linens	Change prn; fluff pillows	Improves comfort; enhances relaxation
NUTRIENT AND FLUID INTAKE		
Oral	Offer fluids and solid foods, following orders of primary health care provider and desires of laboring woman	Provides hydration and calories; enhances positive emotional experience and maternal control
IV	Establish and maintain IV as ordered	Maintains hydration; provides venous access for medications
ELIMINATION		
Voiding	Encourage voiding at least every 2 hr	A full bladder may impede descent of presenting part; overdistention may cause bladder atony and injury, as well as postpartum voiding difficulty
Ambulatory woman	Allow ambulation to bathroom according to orders of primary health care provider, if:	
	The presenting part is engaged	Reinforces normal process of urination
	The membranes are not ruptured	Precautionary measure to protect against prolapse of umbilical cord
	The woman is not medicated	Precautionary measure to protect against injury
Woman on bed rest	Offer bedpan	Prevents complications of bladder distention and ambulation
	Allow tap water to run; pour warm water over the vulva; give positive suggestion	Encourages voiding
	Provide privacy	Shows respect for woman
	Put up side rails on bed	Prevents injury from fall
	Place call bell within reach	
	Offer washcloth for hands	Maintains cleanliness; prevents infection
	Wash vulvar area	Maintains cleanliness; enhances comfort; prevents infection
Catheterization	Catheterize according to orders of primary health care provider or hospital protocol if measures to facilitate voiding are ineffective	Prevents complications of bladder distention
	Insert catheter between contractions	Minimizes discomfort
	Avoid force if obstacle to insertion is noted	"Obstacle" may be caused by compression of urethra by presenting part
Bowel elimination—sensation of rectal pressure	Help the woman ambulate to bathroom or offer bedpan, after careful assessment	Prevents misinterpretation of rectal pressure from the presenting part as the need to defecate
	Perform vaginal examination	Determine degree of descent of presenting part
	Cleanse perineum immediately after passage of stool	Reduces risk of infection and sense of embarrassment

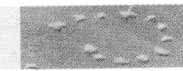

Plan of Care Labor and Birth

NURSING DIAGNOSIS Anxiety related to labor and the birthing process

Expected Outcome *Woman exhibits decreased signs of anxiety.*

Nursing Interventions/*Rationales*

Orient woman and significant others to labor and birth unit and explain admission protocol *to allay initial feelings of anxiety.*

Assess woman's knowledge, experience, and expectations of labor; note any signs or expressions of anxiety, nervousness, or fear *to establish a baseline for intervention.*

Discuss the expected progression of labor and describe what to expect during the process *to allay anxiety associated with the unknown.*

Actively involve woman in care decisions during labor, interpret sights and sounds of environment (monitor sights and sounds, unit activities), and share information on progression of labor (vital signs, FHR, dilation, effacement) *to increase her sense of control and allay fears.*

NURSING DIAGNOSIS Acute pain related to increasing frequency and intensity of contractions

Expected Outcome *Woman exhibits signs of ability to cope with discomfort.*

Nursing Interventions/*Rationales*

Assess woman's level of pain and strategies that she has used to cope with pain *to establish a baseline for intervention.*

Encourage significant other to remain as support person during labor process *to assist with support and comfort measures, because measures are often more effective when delivered by a familiar person.*

Instruct woman and support person in use of specific techniques such as conscious relaxation, focused breathing, effleurage, massage, and application of sacral pressure *to increase relaxation, decrease intensity of contractions, and promote use of controlled thought and direction of energy.*

Provide comfort measures such as frequent mouth care to prevent dry mouth, application of damp cloth to forehead, and changing of damp gown or bed covers *to relieve discomfort associated with diaphoresis; positioning to reduce stiffness.*

Explain what analgesics and anesthesia are available for use during labor and birth *to provide knowledge to help woman make decisions about pain control.*

NURSING DIAGNOSIS Risk for impaired urinary elimination related to sensory impairment secondary to labor

Expected Outcome *Bladder does not show signs of distention.*

Nursing Interventions/*Rationales*

Palpate the bladder superior to the symphysis on a frequent basis *to detect a full bladder that occurs from increased fluid intake and inability to feel urge to void.*

Encourage frequent voiding (at least every 2 hours) and catheterize if necessary *to avoid bladder distention because it impedes progress of fetus down birth canal and may result in trauma to the bladder.*

Assist to bathroom or commode to void if appropriate and provide privacy *to facilitate bladder emptying with an upright position (natural) and relaxation.*

NURSING DIAGNOSIS Risk for ineffective individual coping related to birthing process

Expected Outcome *Woman actively participates in the birth process with no evidence of injury to her or her fetus.*

Nursing Interventions/*Rationales*

Constantly monitor events of second-stage labor and birth, including physiologic responses of woman and fetus, emotional responses of woman and partner, *to ensure maternal, partner, and fetal well-being.*

Provide ongoing feedback to woman and partner *to allay anxiety and enhance participation.*

Continue to provide comfort measures and minimizing distractions *to decrease discomfort and aid in focus on the birth process.*

Encourage woman to experiment with various positions *to assist downward movement of fetus.*

Ensure that woman takes deep cleansing breaths before and after each contraction *to enhance gas exchange and oxygen transport to the fetus.*

Encourage woman to push spontaneously when urge to bear down is perceived during a contraction *to aid descent and rotation of fetus.*

Encourage woman to exhale, holding breath for short periods while bearing down *to avoid holding breath and triggering a Valsalva maneuver and increasing intrathoracic and cardiovascular pressure and decreasing perfusion of placental oxygen, placing the fetus at risk.*

Have woman take deep breaths and relax between contractions *to reduce fatigue and increase effectiveness of pushing efforts.*

Have mother pant as fetal head crowns *to control birth of head.*

Explain to woman and labor partner what is expected in the third stage of labor *to enlist cooperation.*

Have woman maintain her position *to facilitate delivery of the placenta.*

NURSING DIAGNOSIS Fatigue related to energy expenditure required during labor and birth

Expected Outcome *Woman's energy levels are restored.*

Nursing Interventions/*Rationales*

Educate woman and partner about need for rest and help them plan strategies (e.g., restricting visitors, increasing role of support systems performing functions associated with daily routines) that allow specific times for rest and sleep *to ensure that woman can restore depleted energy levels in preparation for caring for a new infant.*

Monitor woman's fatigue level and the amount of rest received *to ensure restoration of energy.*

NURSING DIAGNOSIS Risk for deficient fluid volume related to decreased fluid intake and increased fluid loss during labor and birth

Expected Outcomes *Fluid balance is maintained, and there are no signs of dehydration.*

Nursing Interventions/*Rationales*

Monitor fluid loss (i.e., blood, urine, perspiration) and vital signs; inspect skin turgor and mucous membranes for dryness *to evaluate hydration status.*

Administer oral/parenteral fluid per physician/nurse-midwife orders *to maintain hydration.*

Monitor the fundus for firmness after placental separation *to ensure adequate contraction and prevent further blood loss.*

they typically regulate their own oral intake, eating light foods (e.g., eggs, yogurt, ice cream, dry toast and jelly, fruit) and drinking fluids during early labor and tapering off to the intake of clear fluids and sips of water or ice chips as labor intensifies and the second stage approaches. Common practice is to allow clear liquids (e.g., water, tea, apple juice, clear sodas, gelatin, broth) during early labor, tapering off to ice chips and sips of water as labor progresses and becomes more active. Food and fluid consumed orally during labor can meet a laboring woman's hydration and energy demands more effectively and safely than fluid administered intravenously. In addition, the woman's sense of control and level of comfort are enhanced (Ludka & Roberts, 1993; Scheepers et al., 2001; Varney, 1997). The CNM Data Group (1999) found that a woman's culture may influence what she will eat and drink during labor. In addition, women who used nonpharmacologic pain relief measures and labored in nonhospital settings were more likely to eat and drink during labor.

Withholding food and fluids in labor is a form of care unlikely to be beneficial and that offering oral fluids is demonstrably useful and should be encouraged (Enkin et al., 2000). Nurses should follow the orders of the woman's primary health care provider when offering the woman food or fluids during labor. As advocates, however, nurses can facilitate change by informing others of the current research findings that support the safety and effectiveness of the oral intake of food and fluid during labor and by initiating such research themselves.

Intravenous Intake. Fluids are administered intravenously to the laboring woman to maintain hydration, especially when a labor is long and the woman is unable to ingest a sufficient amount of fluid orally or if she is receiving epidural or intrathecal anesthesia. However, routine use of IV fluids during labor is a form of care that is unlikely to be beneficial and may be harmful (Enkin et al., 2000). In most cases, an electrolyte solution without glucose is adequate and does not introduce excess glucose into the bloodstream. The latter is important because an excessive maternal glucose level results in fetal hyperglycemia and fetal hyperinsulinism. After birth, the neonate's high levels of insulin will then deplete his or her glucose stores, and hypoglycemia will result. Infusions containing glucose can also reduce sodium levels in both the woman and the fetus, leading to transient neonatal tachypnea (Ludka & Roberts, 1993). If maternal ketosis occurs, the primary health care provider may order an IV solution containing a small amount of dextrose to provide the glucose needed to assist in fatty acid metabolism.

NURSE ALERT

Nurses should carefully monitor the intake and output of laboring women receiving IV fluids because they also face an increased danger of hypervolemia as a result of the fluid retention that occurs during pregnancy.

Elimination

Voiding. Voiding every 2 hours should be encouraged. A distended bladder may impede descent of the presenting part, inhibit uterine contractions, and lead to decreased bladder tone or atony after birth. Women who receive epidural analgesia or anesthesia are especially at risk for the retention of urine, and the need to void should be assessed more frequently in them.

The woman should be assisted to the bathroom to void, unless the primary health care provider has ordered bed rest; the woman is receiving epidural analgesia or anesthesia; internal monitoring is being used; or, in the nurse's judgment, ambulation would compromise the status of the laboring woman, her fetus, or both. External monitoring can usually be interrupted for the woman to go to the bathroom.

Catheterization. If the woman is unable to void and her bladder is distended, she may need to be catheterized. Most hospitals have protocols that rely on the nurse's judgment concerning the need for catheterization. Before performing the catheterization, the nurse should clean the vulva and perineum because vaginal show and amniotic fluid may be present. If there appears to be an obstacle that prevents advancement of the catheter, this is most likely the presenting part. If the catheter cannot be advanced, the nurse should stop the procedure and notify the primary health care provider of the difficulty.

Bowel Elimination. Most women do not have bowel movements during labor because of decreased intestinal motility. Stool that has formed in the large intestine often is moved downward toward the anorectal area by the pressure exerted by the fetal presenting part as it descends. This stool is often expelled during second-stage pushing and birth. However, the passage of stool with bearing-down efforts increases the risk of infection and may embarrass the woman, thereby reducing the effectiveness of these efforts. To prevent these problems, the nurse should immediately cleanse the perineal area to remove any stool, while reassuring the woman that the passage of stool at this time is a normal and expected event, because the same muscles used to expel the baby also expel stool. Routine use of an enema to empty the rectum is considered to be harmful or ineffective and should be eliminated (Enkin et al., 2000).

When the presenting part is deep in the pelvis, even in the absence of stool in the anorectal area, the woman may feel rectal pressure and think she needs to defecate. If the woman expresses the urge to defecate, the nurse should perform a vaginal examination to assess cervical dilation and station. When a multiparous woman experiences the urge to defecate, this often means birth will follow quickly.

Ambulation and Positioning. Freedom of maternal movement and choice of position throughout labor are forms of care likely to be beneficial for the laboring woman and should be encouraged (Enkin et al., 2000).

The potential advantages of ambulation include enhanced uterine activity, distraction from labor's discomforts, enhanced maternal control, and an opportunity for

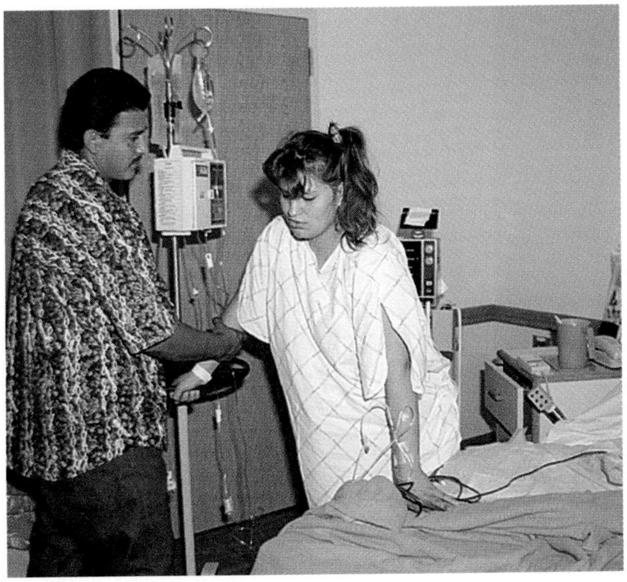

FIG. 21-12 Woman preparing to walk with partner. (Courtesy Marjorie Pyle, RNC, Lifecircle, Costa Mesa, CA.)

close interaction with the woman's partner and care provider as they help her to walk. Ambulation is associated with a reduced rate of operative birth (i.e., cesarean birth, use of forceps, and vacuum extraction) and less frequent use of opioid analgesics (Albers et al., 1997).

Bloom and colleagues (1998) found that although walking did not shorten the duration of labor, it did not impair the process or result in harm to the mother or fetus. They concluded that women should be allowed to choose to walk or not walk as they felt comfortable.

Walking, sitting, or standing during labor is more comfortable than lying down and facilitates the progress of labor (Simkin & Ancheta, 2000). Ambulation should be encouraged if membranes are intact, if the fetal presenting part is engaged after ROM, and if the woman has not received medication for pain (Fig. 21-12). Ambulation may be contraindicated, however, because of maternal or fetal status. The woman also may find it comfortable to stand and lean forward on her partner, doula, or nurse for support at times during labor (Fig. 21-13, *A*).

When the woman lies in bed, she will usually change her position spontaneously as labor progresses (Albers et al., 1997). If she does not change position every 30 to 60 minutes, she should be assisted to do so. The side-lying (lateral) position is preferred because it promotes optimal uteroplacental and renal blood flow and increases fetal oxygen saturation (Fig. 21-14, *B*). If the woman wants to lie supine, the nurse may place a pillow under one hip as a wedge to prevent the uterus from compressing the aorta and vena cava (see Fig. 21-5). Sitting is not contraindicated unless it adversely affects fetal status, which can be determined by checking the FHR and pattern. If the fetus is in the occiput posterior position, it may be helpful to encourage the woman to squat during contractions, because this position increases pelvic diameter, allowing the head to rotate to a more anterior position (Fig. 21-14, *A*). A hands-and-knees position during contractions also is recommended to facilitate the rotation of the fetal occiput from a posterior to an anterior position, as gravity pulls the fetal back forward (Fig. 21-13, *B*).

Much research continues to be directed toward acquiring a better understanding of the physiologic and psychologic effects of maternal position in labor. The variety of positions that are recommended for the laboring woman are described in Box 21-5.

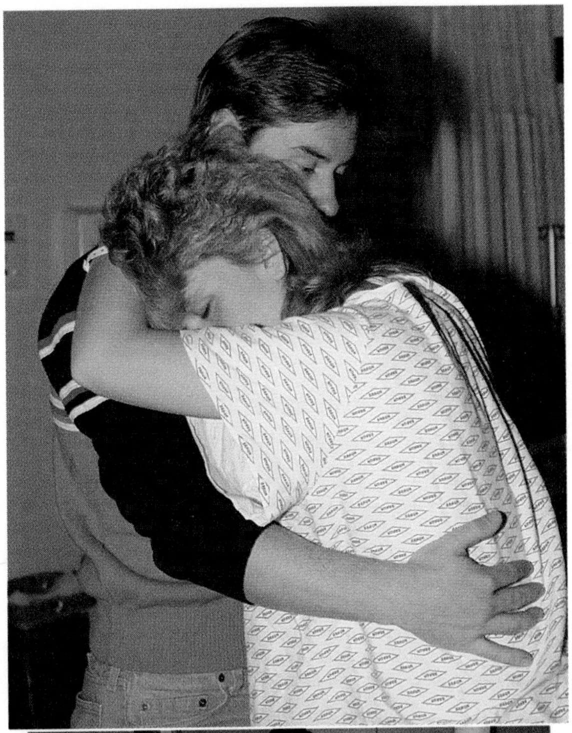

A

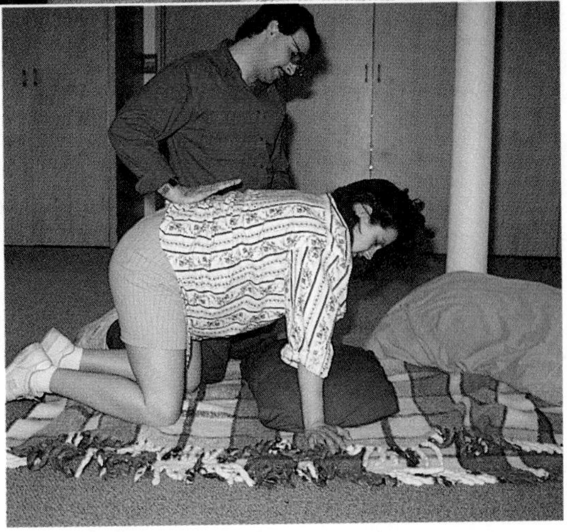

B

FIG. 21-13 **A,** Woman standing and leaning forward with support. **B,** Woman in hands-and-knees position. (Courtesy Marjorie Pyle, RNC, Lifecircle, Costa Mesa, CA.)

A

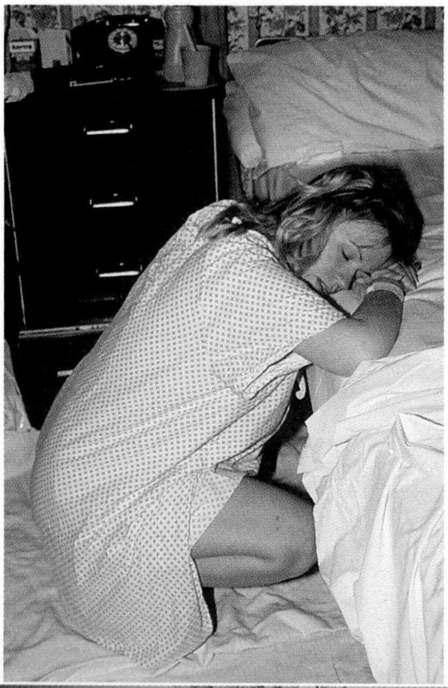

B

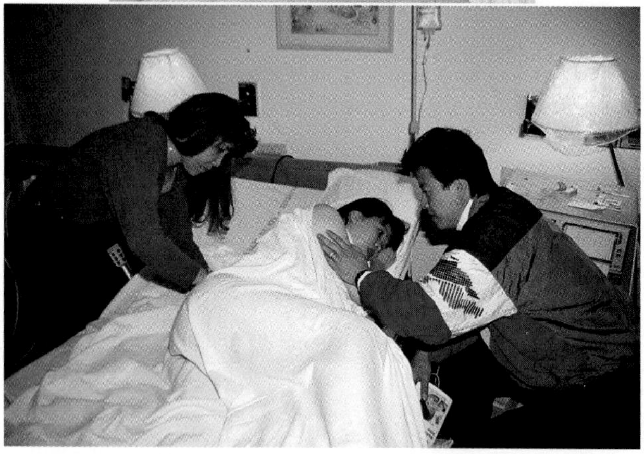

FIG. 21-14 Maternal positions for labor. **A,** Squatting. **B,** Lateral position. Support person is applying sacral pressure while partner provides encouragement. (Courtesy Marjorie Pyle, RNC, Lifecircle, Costa Mesa, CA.)

A birth ball (gymnastic ball, also used in physical therapy) can be used to support a woman's body as she assumes a variety of labor and birth positions (Fig. 21-15). The woman can sit on the ball while leaning over the bed, or she can lean over the ball to support her upper body and reduce stress on her arms and hands when she assumes a hands-and-knees position. The birth ball can encourage pelvic mobility and pelvic and perineal relaxation when the woman sits on the firm yet pliable ball and rocks in rhythmic movements. Warm compresses applied to the perineum and lower back can maximize this relaxation and comfort effect. The birth ball should be large enough so that when the woman sits, her knees are bent at a 90-degree angle and her feet are flat on the floor and approximately 2 feet apart (Perez, 1998).

Supportive Care During Labor and Birth

Support during labor and birth involves emotional support, physical care and comfort measures, and provision of advice and information (Davies & Hodnett, 2002; Miltner, 2000). Effective support provided to women during labor can result in shorter labors; reduced rates of complications and surgical or obstetric interventions (e.g., cesarean births, labor augmentations and inductions, episiotomies, forceps- and vacuum-assisted births); and enhanced self-esteem and satisfaction (Gagnon & Waghorn, 1999; Miltner, 2000). Physical, emotional, and psychologic support of the woman during labor and birth is a beneficial form of care demonstrated by clear research evidence (Enkin et al., 2000) (see Evidence-Based Practice box).

Labor rooms should be airy, clean, and homelike. The laboring woman should feel safe in this environment and free to be herself and to use the comfort and relaxation measures she prefers. To enhance relaxation, bright overhead lights should be turned off when not needed, and noise and intrusions should be kept to a minimum. The temperature is controlled to ensure the laboring woman's comfort. The room should be large enough to accommodate a comfortable chair for the woman's partner, the monitoring equipment, and hospital personnel. Couples may be encouraged to bring extra pillows to make the hospital surroundings more homelike and to facilitate position changes. Women often state that this type of an environment helps them view their childbirth experience as normal and not related to illness (Proctor, 1998). Environmental modifications should reflect the preferences of the woman, including the number of visitors and availability of a telephone, television, and music. Nurses should ensure that each woman labors in an optimal birth environment (Hanson et al., 2001).

Labor Support by the Nurse. The nurse can alleviate a woman's anxiety by explaining unfamiliar terms, providing information and explanations without her having to ask, and preparing her for sensations she will experience and procedures that will follow. By encouraging the woman or couple to ask questions and by providing honest, understandable answers, the nurse can play an important role in helping the woman achieve a satisfying birth experience (Miltner, 2002; Proctor, 1998; Tomlinson & Bryan, 1996).

Supportive nursing care for a woman in labor includes the following:

- Helping the woman maintain control and participate to the extent she wishes in the birth of her infant
- Meeting the woman's expected outcomes for her labor
- Acting as the woman's advocate, supporting her decisions and respecting her choices as appropriate, and relating her wishes as needed to other health care providers
- Helping the woman conserve her energy
- Helping control the woman's discomfort

BOX 21-5 **Some Maternal Positions* During Labor and Birth**

SEMIRECUMBENT POSITION

With woman sitting with her upper body elevated to at least a 30° angle, place wedge or small pillow under hip to prevent vena caval compression and reduce likelihood of supine hypotension (see Fig. 21-18, *B*)

- The greater the angle of elevation, the more gravity or pressure is exerted that promotes fetal descent, the progress of contractions, and the widening of pelvic dimensions.
- Convenient for rendering care measures and for external fetal monitoring.

LATERAL POSITION (SEE FIG. 21-14, *B* & 21-18, *A*)

Have woman alternate between left and right side-lying position, and provide abdominal and back support as needed for comfort.

- Removes pressure from the vena cava and back; enhances uteroplacental perfusion and relieves backache.
- Makes it easier to perform back massage or counterpressure.
- Associated with less frequent, but more intense, contractions.
- Obtaining good external fetal monitor tracings may be more difficult.
- May be used as a birthing position.
- Takes pressure off perineum, allowing it to stretch gradually.
- Reduces risk for perineal trauma.

UPRIGHT POSITION

The gravity effect enhances the contraction cycle and fetal descent: the weight of the fetus places increasing pressure on the cervix; the cervix is pulled upward, facilitating effacement and dilation; impulses from the cervix to the pituitary gland increase, causing more oxytocin to be secreted; and contractions are intensified, thereby applying more forceful downward pressure on the fetus, but they are less painful.

- Fetus is aligned with pelvis, and pelvic diameters are widened slightly.
- Effective upright positions include the following:
  - Ambulation (see Fig. 21-12).
  - Standing and leaning forward with support provided by coach (see Fig. 21-13, *A*), end of bed, back of chair, or birth ball (see Fig. 21-15); relieves backache and facilitates application of counterpressure or back massage
  - Sitting up in bed, chair, birthing chair, on toilet or bedside commode
  - Squatting (see Fig. 21-14, *A*)

HANDS-AND-KNEES POSITION—IDEAL POSITION FOR POSTERIOR POSITIONS OF THE PRESENTING PART (SEE FIG. 21-13, *B*)

Assume an "all fours" position in bed or on a covered floor; allows for pelvic rocking.

- Relieves backache characteristic of "back labor."
- Facilitates internal rotation of the fetus by increasing mobility of the coccyx, increasing the pelvic diameters, and using gravity to turn the fetal back and rotate the head.

*Assess the effect of each position on the laboring woman's comfort and anxiety level, progress of labor, and FHR pattern. Alternate positions every 30 to 60 min, allowing woman to take control of her position changes.

- Acknowledging the woman's efforts, as well as those of her partner, during labor and providing positive reinforcement
- Protecting the woman's privacy and modesty

The nurse serves as a coach to the woman in the absence of other support persons or as an assistant coach to the support persons present. To do this, the nurse must have a thorough knowledge of breathing and relaxation techniques.

Couples who have attended childbirth education programs that teach the psychoprophylactic approach will know something about the labor process, coaching techniques, and comfort measures. The nurse should play a supportive role and keep such a couple informed of the progress. A review and repeated demonstration of methods learned in class and practiced in the familiar environment of their home without the pain and discomfort of labor and without the anxiety of being in an unfamiliar environment may be needed. It is important that the

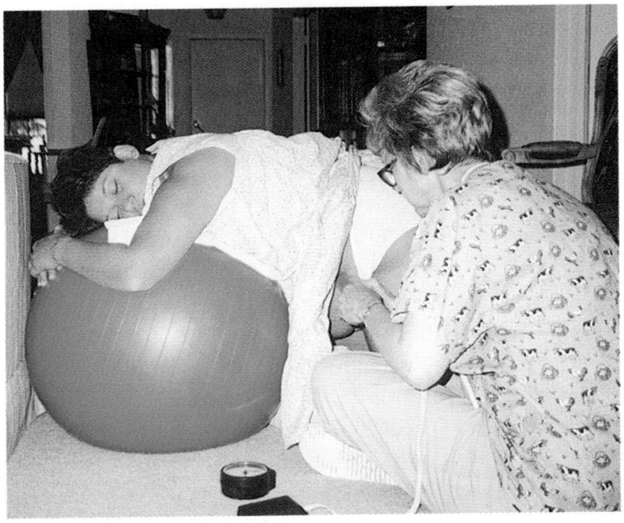

FIG. 21-15 Laboring woman using birth ball. (Courtesy Polly Perez, Cutting Edge Press, Johnson, VT.)

EVIDENCE-BASED PRACTICE

SUPPORT DURING LABOR

BACKGROUND

Support during labor and birth has been a practice throughout history as women have been cared for by family and friends who provided emotional support and comfort. However, the impact of such support was not a topic of research until the 1970s.

The effect of labor support on maternal and fetal outcomes has been the topic of over 30 published reports and reviews since 1980 and 4 meta-analyses since 1992. Fourteen of the studies were randomized clinical trials carried out in the United States, Canada, Mexico, Guatemala, and South Africa.

OBJECTIVES

Sauls (2002) reviewed 11 randomized controlled trials and 4 meta-analyses that compared continuous labor support with usual care during labor in relation to birth outcomes, maternal outcomes, and newborn outcomes.

In the individual studies, not all of the results were substantiated as statistically significant because of small sample sizes and lack of statistical power. Despite these limitations, all of the studies found evidence of beneficial effects of labor support, including reduced use of analgesia, shorter labor, and lower rates of cesarean births and operative vaginal births. Improved fetal/neonatal outcomes included higher Apgar scores, lower neonatal intensive care unit admissions, higher rates of exclusive breastfeeding, and higher rates of maternal-infant attachment. Emotional benefits to the mother included positive feelings about the labor, increased satisfaction with the birth process, increased bonding with the infant, more positive feelings about mothering, and higher self-esteem (Sauls, 2002).

Findings of the four meta-analyses were similar. Klaus et al. (1992) combined five randomized clinical trials investigating continuous labor support that included 1252 primiparous women at term in uncomplicated pregnancies. The researchers found that for women who had continuous labor support, cesarean birth rates were decreased by 50%, labor length was reduced by 25%, oxytocin use was decreased by 40%, pain medication use was reduced by 30%, forceps use was decreased by 40%, and requests for epidural analgesia were reduced by 60%. Decreased maternal anxiety and depression, increased breastfeeding, and increased satisfaction with partners were also reported.

Zhang et al. (1996) combined four studies of labor support in young, low-income, primiparous women and found that labor support had positive effects on birth outcomes. These outcomes included shorter labors, 50% more vaginal births, and decreased need for analgesia, forceps, and cesarean births. Increased mother-infant attachment, higher rates of breastfeeding, and more satisfaction with labor and birth were also reported but were not compared statistically.

Scott, Berkowitz, and Klaus (1999) combined data from 11 clinical trials that compared continuous support with intermittent support on five birth outcomes. Continuous support was associated with shorter labors, decreased use of anesthesia and oxytocin augmentation, and reduced use of forceps and cesarean births. Intermittent support was not found to be better than no support.

Hodnett (2001) reviewed 14 randomized trials that included 5000 patients and compared continuous support with usual care. Women with support used less pain medication, had fewer operative vaginal births and cesarean births, and gave birth to more infants with Apgar scores greater than 7. The women also had more positive perceptions of their labor and birth and were more likely to breastfeed exclusively.

CLINICAL IMPLICATIONS

In practice, labor nurses spend most of their time with clients doing technologic tasks and only about 10% of their time providing supportive care. Reasons frequently given by labor nurses for not giving more supportive care include inadequate staffing, the physical environment of the unit, negative staffing attitudes toward supportive care, and lack of management support.

If intrapartal nurses are to incorporate findings of these studies into practice, the nurse needs to value supportive care and work in an environment that also values professional supportive care. Supportive behaviors that are helpful for different types of mothers (e.g., adolescent, high risk, low risk) need to be identified. Classes or workshops that teach labor support strategies as well as the benefits of supportive care may increase the nurse's skill as well as the valuing of supportive care. Further research on professional labor support versus lay support and cost-effectiveness of professional labor support is needed.

Sources: Hodnett, E. (2001). Caregiver support for women during childbirth (Cochrane Review). In *The Cochrane Library,* Issue 3, Oxford, UK: Update Software; Klaus, M. et al. (1992). Maternal assistance and support in labor: Father, nurse, midwife, or doula? *Clinical Consultations in Obstetrics and Gynecology, 4*(4), 211-217; Sauls, D. (2002). Effects of labor support on mothers, babies, and birth outcomes. *Journal of Obstetric, Gynecologic, and Neonatal Nursing, 31*(6), 733-741; Scott, K., Berkowitz, G., & Klaus, M. (1999). A comparison of intermittent and continuous support during labor: A meta-analysis. *American Journal of Obstetrics and Gynecology, 180*, 1054-1059; Zhang, J. et al. (1996). Continuous labor support from labor attendants for primparous women: A meta-analysis. *Obstetrics and Gynecology, 88*(4, Part 2), 739-744.

nurse caution the woman not to begin patterned breathing techniques during the latent phase of labor because this practice has been associated with an increase in the level of fatigue the woman experiences as labor progresses (Pugh et al., 1998).

Even when expectant parents have not attended childbirth classes, the nurse can teach them various techniques during the early phase of labor. In this case, the nurse may provide more of the coaching and supportive care.

Breathing and relaxation techniques should be simple and performed with the woman until the support person feels ready to take on a more active coaching role. Comfort measures can be demonstrated by the nurse while encouraging the support person to assist and the laboring woman to express her needs and feelings. "Expert watching" or active role modeling can help the partner to learn effective comfort measures (Hodnett, 1996; Tomlinson & Bryan, 1996).

Comfort measures vary with the situation (Fig. 21-16). The nurse can draw on the couple's repertoire of comfort measures learned during the pregnancy. Such measures include maintaining a comfortable, supportive atmosphere

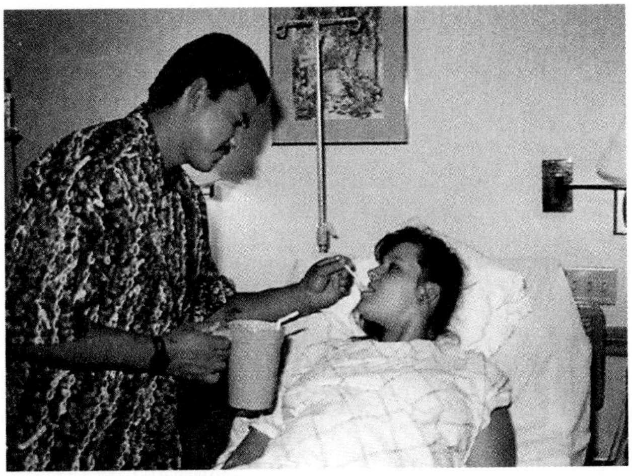

FIG. 21-16 Partner providing comfort measures. (Courtesy Marjorie Pyle, RNC, Lifecircle, Costa Mesa, CA.)

in the labor and birth area; using touch therapeutically (e.g., heat or cold applied to the lower back in the event of back labor, a cool cloth applied to the forehead); providing nonpharmacologic measures to relieve discomfort; administering analgesics when necessary; and most of all, just being there (see Table 21-1; see also the Care Paths on pp. 555 and 584). See Chapter 19 for a full discussion of both pharmacologic and nonpharmacologic comfort measures.

Most women in labor respond positively to touch. They appreciate gentle handling by staff members. Back rubs and counterpressure may be offered, especially if the woman is experiencing back labor. A support person may be taught to exert counterpressure against the woman's sacrum over the occiput of the head of a fetus in a posterior position (see Fig. 21-14, *B*). The back pain is caused by the occiput pressing on spinal nerves, and counterpressure lifts the occiput off these nerves, thereby providing some relief from pain. Once counterpressure is initiated, the woman usually asks her partner to continue doing this for each following contraction. The partner will need to be relieved after a while, however, because exerting counterpressure is hard work. Hand and foot massage also can be soothing and relaxing (Simkin & Ancheta, 2000).

The woman's perception of the soothing qualities of touch changes as labor progresses. Many women become more sensitive to touch (hyperesthesia) as labor progresses. This is a typical response during the transition phase (see Table 21-3). They may tell their coach to leave them alone or not to touch them. The partner who is unprepared for this normal response may feel rejected and may react by withdrawing active support. The nurse can reassure him or her that this response is a positive indication that the first stage is ending and the second stage is approaching. Women with increased sensitivity to touch may have a positive response when touched on surfaces of the body where hair does not grow, such as the forehead, the palms of the hands, and the soles of the feet.

The woman in labor may exhibit a variety of reactions and needs support from her partner and the nurse no matter what her reactions. Critical comments directed toward the woman are unwarranted and inappropriate (see Table 21-1).

Relaxation measures for use during labor are often learned in childbirth classes and through life experiences. They include guided imagery, music, and soothing massage

Music, taped or live, can cue rhythmic breathing and enhance relaxation, thereby reducing stress and anxiety and even relieving pain. Nurses can be advocates for the implementation of this complementary therapy by developing protocols for the use of music, assessing a woman's desire to use music and what type of music to use, and mobilizing the musical talents of the woman, her significant others, and even health care providers (Olson, 1998).

These techniques can provide comfort, prevent fatigue, and help the woman conserve energy for the expulsive work of the second stage of labor. Today, many health care providers advocate the use of warm water or hydrotherapy (e.g., whirlpool baths or jacuzzis, showers) for its soothing, relaxing effects and its ability to reduce discomfort and enhance the progress of labor, especially during the first 1 to 2 hours of immersion (Odent, 1997). Many birthing units have baths with air jets. The buoyancy of the warm water in a bath, with or without air jets, provides support for tense muscles and allows the woman to move freely and change her position. The relaxing and soothing effect that the warm water has on muscles yields immediate benefits during labor and also reduces the aftereffects of tense muscles during the immediate postpartum period. Other benefits associated with hydrotherapy during labor include enhanced progress of cervical dilation, diminished pain, decreased use of analgesia, reduced perineal trauma and operative birth, and increased maternal satisfaction. Maternal, fetal-newborn, and caregiver infection; hyperthermia; fetal hypoxia; newborn water aspiration; and tearing of the cord are theoretic risks that must be addressed (Mackey, 2001). Immersion in water to relieve pain in labor is a form of care of unknown effectiveness requiring further research (Enkin et al., 2000).

It is recommended that the use of a whirlpool bath or jacuzzi begins when the woman is in active labor with cervical dilation of at least 5 cm, because initiation of this method in the latent phase could slow contractions or stop them temporarily (Eriksson et al., 1997). The temperature of the water should be maintained at body temperature or lower (e.g., 37° C or lower) to prevent maternal and fetal hyperthermia. Women should be encouraged to drink oral fluids while in the bath to maintain fluid balance and the beneficial effects of the hydrotherapy on the progress of the labor. A support person should be with the woman at all times while she is in the bath. After approximately

2 hours, the effectiveness of hydrotherapy seems to diminish. Contractions become more intense or the contractions may decrease in efficiency. Getting out of the bath and ambulating may help to reestablish an effective contraction pattern, at which point the woman may reenter the bath (Eriksson et al., 1997; Mackey, 2001; Odent, 1997). Newborns who are born, either accidentally or intentionally, while women are immersed in the water do not begin to breathe until removed from the water. Most authorities recommend that the birth occur out of the water; if it occurs in the water, the newborn's head should be lifted immediately above the water. The rest of the body may be removed or allowed to remain in the water to maintain body temperature and to ease the transition to extrauterine life. It may take as long as 1 minute for breathing to begin. Resuscitation is unnecessary if the newborn's heart rate is normal and muscle tone is good (Mackey, 2001; Odent, 1997) (Fig. 21-17). Standard precautions should guide use of personal protective equipment and cleansing of the tub. Further research is needed regarding water immersion during labor and birth to establish a protocol for its use, to validate the beneficial effects, and to determine whether detrimental effects occur and if they can be prevented. Showers also can enhance relaxation and reduce pain when warm water is directed over the laboring woman's lower back and abdomen (Simkin & Ancheta, 2000).

Labor Support by the Father or Partner. Although another woman or a man other than the father may be the woman's partner, the father of the baby is usually the support person during labor. He often is able to provide the comfort measures and touch that the laboring woman needs. When the woman becomes focused on her pain, sometimes the partner can persuade her to try nonpharmacologic variations of comfort measures. In addition, he usually is able to interpret the woman's needs and desires to staff members.

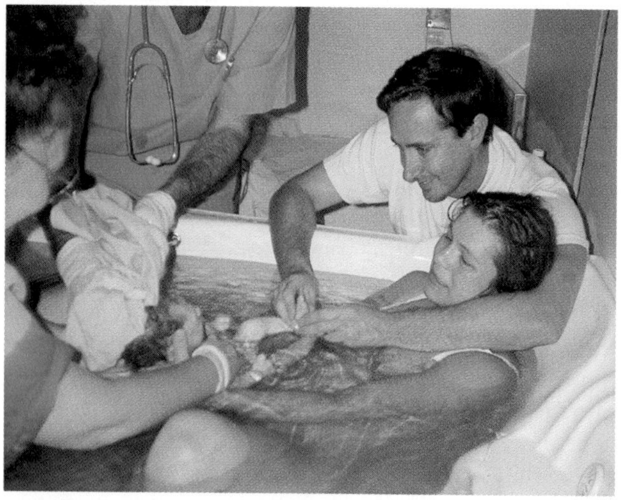

FIG. 21-17 Water birth. (Courtesy Global Maternal/Child Health Association, Inc., Wilsonville, OR.)

Throughout the past 30 years, childbirth preparation education has been widely available. The father's ideal role was thought to be that of labor coach, and he was expected actively to help the woman cope with labor. However, this expectation may be unrealistic, because some men have concerns about their labor-coaching abilities. Men can assume one of at least three different roles during labor and birth: coach, teammate, or witness (Chapman, 1992). As a *coach*, the father actively assists the woman during and after contractions. Men who are coaches express a strong need to be in control of themselves and of the labor experience. Women also express a great desire for the father to be physically involved in labor. The father who acts as the *teammate* assists the woman during labor and birth by responding to requests for physical or emotional support, or both. Teammates usually adopt the follower or helper role and look to the woman or nurse to tell them what to do. Women express a strong desire to have the father present and willing to help in any way. The father who acts as a *witness* acts as a companion, giving emotional and moral support. He watches the woman labor and give birth, but he often sleeps, watches television, or leaves the room for long periods. Witnesses believe that there is little they can do to help the woman physically and look to the nurses and health care providers to be in charge of the experience. Women do not expect more of this type of father than to just be present.

The degree of mutuality (level of interdependency and sharing) and understanding (the ability to know each other's needs) in a couple's relationship determines which role the father adopts. The coach and teammate roles are often assumed by men in couples with a high degree of mutuality. Men in couples in which mutuality is low tend to adopt the witness role. Because the father can participate in labor and birth in different ways, the nurse should encourage him to adopt the role most comfortable for him and for the woman, rather than to assume an unnatural role. Participation in the birth is ego building. The father can be of assistance; his presence is important.

The feelings of a first-time father change as labor progresses. Although he is often calm at the onset of labor, feelings of fear and helplessness begin to dominate as labor becomes more active and the father realizes that labor is more work than he anticipated. The first-time father may feel excluded as birth preparations begin during the transition phase. Once the second stage begins and birth nears, the father's focus changes from the woman to the baby who is about to be born (Box 21-6).

The father will be exposed to many sights and smells he may never before have experienced. It is therefore important to tell him what to expect and to make him comfortable about leaving the room to regain his composure should something occur that surprises him. Before he leaves the room, provision should be made for someone else to support the woman during his absence. Staff members should tell the father that his presence is helpful and encourage him to be involved in the care of the woman to the extent to which he is comfortable. Reassure him that he is not assuming the responsibility for observation and management of his partner's labor, but that his responsibility is to support her as the labor progresses. Suggest alternative comfort measures when those he is using are no longer helpful or are rejected by his partner (Hodnett, 1996; Tomlinson & Bryan, 1996).

Supporting both the father and the woman in labor elevates the nurse's role. It is another step forward for a nurse from merely providing custodial care to enacting a therapeutic role. Support of the father reflects the nurse's orientation and commitment to each person, the family, and the community. Therapeutic nursing actions convey several important concepts to the father: first, that the father is of value as a person; second, that he can learn to be a partner in the woman's care; and third, that childbearing is a partnership.

Ways in which the nurse can support the father-partner are detailed in Box 21-7. A well-informed father can make an important contribution to the health and well-being of the mother and child, their family interrelationship, and his self-esteem.

Labor Support by the Grandparents. When grandparents act as labor coaches, it is especially important to support and treat them with respect. They may have a way to deal with pain relief based on their experience. They should be encouraged to help as long as their actions do not compromise the status of the mother or the fetus. One example of an acceptable practice would be giving the woman herbal teas during labor. The nurse acts as a role model for parents by treating grandparents with dignity and respect, by acknowledging the value of the grandparents' contributions to parental support, and by recognizing the difficulty parents have in witnessing their child's discomfort or crisis, regardless of the age of the child. If they have never witnessed a birth, the nurse may need to provide explanations of what is happening. Many of the activities used to support fathers also are appropriate for grandparents.

When possible, the nurse offers the grandparents emotional support. A nurse can show such support by offering them liquid refreshment and by initiating discussion with open-ended questions or statements, such as, "It is sometimes hard to watch a daughter in labor." Nursing actions that provide support for the grandparents can have a therapeutic effect on all members of the family. In turn, a strong, supportive family unit is important for the optimal growth and development of its newest member.

Labor Support by Doulas. Continuity of care has been cited by women as a critical component of a satisfying childbirth experience. These women expressed concern regarding a change in their caregiver when a new shift began (Proctor, 1998). This need can be met by an especially trained, experienced female labor attendant called a **doula.**

BOX 21-6 A Father's Presence at Birth

I attended childbirth classes before I was married, so my husband didn't have that experience when I was pregnant. He functioned in the "witness" role during labor; although he provided no comfort measures, he was there during the labor, which was very important to me. I knew I wanted him in the delivery room, even though he had said that he didn't want to be there.

When it was time to transfer to the delivery room, the obstetrician said, "OK, Bill, let's go change clothes." My husband was too shy to say he didn't want to go, so shortly he and the doctor came into the delivery room. Bill sat at my head and observed. When the baby's head emerged, the doctor and nurse agreed that the baby looked like Bill. After the baby was born, Bill was the first to hold her. He later commented that if we ever had another baby, he would be in the delivery room because it wouldn't be fair to the baby if he weren't there.

BOX 21-7 Guidelines for Supporting the Father

- Orient to the labor room and the unit; explain location of the cafeteria, toilet, waiting room, and nursery; visiting hours; names and functions of personnel present.
- Inform him of sights and smells he can expect to encounter; encourage him to leave the room if necessary.
- Respect his or the couple's decision about the degree of his involvement. Offer them freedom to make decisions.
- Tell him when his presence has been helpful and continue to reinforce this throughout labor.
- Offer to teach him comfort measures.
- Inform him frequently of the progress of the labor and the woman's needs. Keep him informed about procedures to be performed.
- Prepare him for changes in the woman's behavior and physical appearance.
- Remind him to eat; offer him snacks and fluids if possible.
- Relieve him of the job of support person as necessary. Offer him blankets if he is to sleep in a chair by the bedside.
- Acknowledge the stress experienced by each partner during labor and birth and identify normal responses.
- Attempt to modify or eliminate unsettling stimuli, such as extra noise and extra light.

The doula provides a continuous, one-on-one caring presence throughout the labor and birth of the woman she is attending. This is a beneficial form of care (Enkin et al., 2000). The primary role of the doula is to focus on the laboring woman and provide physical and emotional support by using soft, reassuring words; touching, stroking, and hugging; administering comfort measures to reduce pain and enhance relaxation; and walking with the woman, helping her to change positions, and coaching her bearing-down efforts. Doulas provide information and explain procedures and events. They advocate for the woman's right to participate actively in the management of her labor (Kayne, Greulich, & Albers, 2001).

The doula also supports the woman's partner, who often feels unqualified to be the sole labor support. The doula can encourage and praise the partner's efforts, create a partnership as caregivers, and provide respite care. Doulas also facilitate communication between the laboring woman and her partner, as well as between the couple and the health care team (Perez & Herrick, 1998; Simkin & Way, 1998; Tumblin & Simkin, 2001; Zhang et al., 1996).

Continuous care provided by doulas significantly reduces the cesarean birth rate; duration of labor; use of oxytocin, analgesics, and forceps; and requests for epidural anesthesia. Laboring women also reported a higher level of satisfaction with their childbirth experience and greater success with breastfeeding (Klaus, Kennell, & Klaus, 1993). Long-term benefits of doula care are reflected in more positive maternal feelings regarding their parenting ability and closer interaction with their infants up to 1 year after birth (Landry et al., 1998; Trowell, 1993).

The role of the nurse and the doula are complementary. They should work together as a team with the doula providing supportive nonmedical care measures and with the nurse focusing on monitoring the status of the maternal-fetal unit; implementing clinical care protocols, including pharmacologic interventions; and documenting assessment findings, actions, and responses.

Siblings During Labor and Birth. The preparation of siblings for acceptance of the new child helps promote the attachment process. Such preparation and participation during pregnancy and labor may help the older children accept this change. The older child or children who know themselves to be important to the family become active participants. Rehearsal for the event before labor is essential.

The age and developmental level of children influence their responses; therefore preparation for the children to be present during labor is adjusted to meet each child's needs. The child younger than 2 years shows little interest in pregnancy and labor; for the older child, such preparation may reduce fears and misconceptions. Parents need to be prepared for labor and birth themselves and feel comfortable about the process and the presence of their children. Most parents have a "feel" for their children's maturational level and their physical and emotional ability to observe and cope with the events of the labor and birth process. Preparation can include a description of the anticipated sights, events (e.g., ROM, monitors, IV infusions), smells, and sounds; a labor and birth demonstration; a tour of the birthing unit; and an opportunity to be around a real newborn. Children must learn that their mother will be working hard during labor and birth. She will not be able to talk to them during contractions. She may groan, scream, grunt, and pant at times as well as say things she would not say otherwise (e.g., "I can't take this anymore;" "Take this baby out of me;" or "This pain is killing me"). They can be told that labor is uncomfortable, but that their mother's body is made for the job. Storybooks about the birth process can be read to or by children to prepare them for the event. Films are available for preparing preschool and school-age children to participate in the labor and birth experience. Most agencies require that a specific person be designated to watch over the children who are participating in their mother's childbirth experience, to provide them with support, explanations, diversions, and comfort as needed. Health care providers involved in attending women during birth must be comfortable with the presence of children and the unpredictability of their questions, comments, and behaviors.

Emergency Interventions

Emergency conditions that require immediate nursing intervention can arise with startling speed. Interventions for a nonreassuring FHR, inadequate uterine relaxation, vaginal bleeding, infection, and prolapse of the cord are detailed in the Emergency box.

Evaluation

Evaluation of progress and outcomes is a continuous activity during the first stage of labor. The nurse must carefully evaluate each interaction with the mother-to-be and her family and critically appraise how well the expected outcomes of care are being met.

SECOND STAGE OF LABOR

The **second stage of labor** is the stage in which the infant is born. This stage begins with full cervical dilation (10 cm) and complete effacement (100%) and ends with the baby's birth. The force exerted by uterine contractions, gravity, and maternal bearing-down efforts facilitates achievement of the expected outcome of a spontaneous, uncomplicated vaginal birth.

The second stage comprises three phases: the latent, descent, and transition phases. These phases are characterized by maternal verbal and nonverbal behaviors, uterine activity, the urge to bear down, and fetal descent.

The latent phase is a period of rest and relative calm (i.e., "laboring down"). During this early phase, the fetus continues to descend passively through the birth canal and rotate to an anterior position as a result of ongoing uterine contractions. The woman is quiet and often relaxes with her

EMERGENCY

Interventions for Emergencies

SIGNS	INTERVENTIONS*
Nonreassuring FHR Pattern • Fetal bradycardia (FHR <110 beats/min for >10 min)† • Fetal tachycardia (FHR >160 beats/min for >10 min in term pregnancy)§ • Irregular FHR, abnormal sinus rhythm shown by internal monitor • Persistent decrease in baseline FHR variability without an identified cause • Late, severe variable, and prolonged deceleration patterns • Absence of FHTs	Notify primary health care provider‡ Change maternal position Discontinue oxytocin (Pitocin) infusion, if being infused Increase IV fluid rate, if fluid being infused per protocol order Administer oxygen at 8 to 10 L/min by snug face mask Check maternal temperature for elevation Start an IV line if one is not in place Assist with amnioinfusion if ordered Stimulate fetal scalp or use sound stimulation
Inadequate Uterine Relaxation • Intrauterine pressure >75 mm Hg (shown by intrauterine pressure catheter monitoring) • Contractions consistently lasting >90 sec • Contraction interval <2 min	Notify primary health care provider‡ Discontinue oxytocin infusion, if being infused Change woman to side-lying position Increase IV fluid rate, if fluid is being infused Administer oxygen at 8 to 10 L/min by snug face mask Start an IV line if one is not in place Palpate and evaluate contractions Give tocolytics (terbutaline), as ordered
Vaginal Bleeding • Vaginal bleeding (bright red, dark red, or in an amount in excess of that expected during normal cervical dilation) • Continuous vaginal bleeding with FHR changes • Pain; may or may not be present	Notify primary health care provider‡ Anticipate emergency (stat) cesarean birth *Do NOT perform a vaginal examination*
Infection • Foul-smelling amniotic fluid • Maternal temperature >38° C in presence of adequate hydration (straw-colored urine) • Fetal tachycardia >160 beats/min for >10 min	Notify primary health care provider‡ Institute cooling measures for laboring woman Start an IV line if one is not in place Assist with or perform collection of catheterized urine specimen and amniotic fluid sample and send to the laboratory for urinalysis and cultures
Prolapse of Cord • Fetal bradycardia with variable deceleration during uterine contraction • Woman reports feeling the cord after membranes rupture • Cord lies alongside or below the presenting part of the fetus; can be seen or felt in or protruding from the vagina • Major predisposing factors: – Rupture of membranes with a gush – Loose fit of presenting part in lower uterine segment – Presenting part not yet engaged – Breech presentation	Call for assistance Have someone notify the primary health care provider immediately Glove the examining hand quickly and insert two fingers into the vagina to the cervix; with one finger on either side of the cord or both fingers to one side, exert upward pressure against the presenting part to relieve compression of the cord Place a rolled towel under the woman's hip Place woman in extreme Trendelenburg or modified Sims position or knee-chest position Wrap the cord loosely in a sterile towel saturated with warm sterile normal saline if the cord is protruding from the vagina Administer oxygen at 8 to 10 L/min by face mask until birth is accomplished Start IV fluids or increase existing drip rate Continue to monitor FHR by internal fetal scalp electrode, if possible Do not attempt to replace cord into cervix Prepare for immediate birth (vaginal or cesarean)

*Because emergency situations are often frightening events, it is important for the nurse to explain to the woman and her support person what is happening and how it is being managed.
†Practice is to intervene within 2 to 30 min of FHR , <110 beats/min.
‡In most emergency situations, nurses take immediate action, following a protocol and standards of nursing practice. Another person can notify the primary health care provider, or this can be done by the nurse as soon as possible.
§Nonreassuring sign when associated with late decelerations or absence of variability, especially of >180 beats/min.

eyes closed between contractions. The urge to bear down is not well established and may not be experienced at all or only during the acme of a contraction. Allowing a woman to rest during this phase, and waiting until the urge to push intensifies, has been found to reduce maternal fatigue, conserve energy for bearing-down efforts, and provide optimal maternal and fetal outcomes (Minato, 2000). Coaching a woman to push before her body signals readiness can result in a prolonged period of active pushing with limited to no progress. The woman may become dependent on her coach or nurses to tell her when and how to push (Roberts, 2002). However, women who have epidural analgesia may not feel the urge to bear down and will need coaching.

The descent phase or the phase of active pushing is characterized by strong urges to bear down as the **Ferguson reflex** is activated when the presenting part presses on the stretch receptors of the pelvic floor. At this point, the fetal station is usually 1+, and the position is anterior. This stimulation causes the release of oxytocin from the posterior pituitary gland, which provokes stronger expulsive uterine contractions. The woman becomes more focused on bearing-down efforts, which become rhythmic. She changes positions frequently to find a more comfortable pushing position. The woman often announces the onset of contractions and becomes more vocal as she bears down. The urge to bear down intensifies as descent progresses.

In the *transition phase,* the presenting part is on the perineum, and bearing-down efforts are most effective for promoting birth. The woman may be more verbal about the pain she is experiencing; she may scream or swear and may act out of control (Roberts, 2002).

The nurse encourages the woman to "listen" to her body as she progresses through the phases of the second stage of labor. When a woman listens to her body to tell her when to bear down, she is using an internal locus of control and often feels more satisfied with her efforts to give birth to her baby. Her sense of self-esteem and accomplishment is enhanced, and her efforts become more effective. The woman's trust in her own body and her ability to give birth to her baby should be fostered (Mayberry et al., 2000).

If a woman is confined to bed, especially in a recumbent position, the rhythmic urge to bear down is delayed because gravity is not being used to press the presenting part against the pelvic floor. Being moved to another room and placed on a delivery table in the lithotomy position, as has been the custom in North America, also has an inhibiting effect on the urge to bear down. Today, Western societies have adopted the birthing practice of most non-Western societies where labor and birth occur in the same room and women use various positions for bearing down, such as side-lying, kneeling, squatting, sitting, or standing.

Duration of Second Stage

The duration of the second stage of labor is influenced by several factors, such as the effectiveness of the primary and secondary powers of labor; the type and amount of analgesia or anesthesia used; the physical and emotional condition, position, activity level, parity, and pelvic adequacy of the laboring woman; the size, presentation, and position of the fetus; and the nature and source of support the woman receives.

For many multiparous women, birth occurs within minutes of complete dilation, perhaps only one push later. Nulliparous women usually push for 1 to 2 hours before giving birth. If the woman has been given epidural analgesia, pushing can last more than 2 hours. Epidural analgesia blocks or reduces the urge to bear down and limits the woman's ability to attain an upright position to push. By adjusting dosages to the lowest effective level, allowing the epidural to wear off at full dilation or after 1 hour of pushing, or using mixtures containing an opioid-agonist analgesic and a local anesthetic, the woman is able more fully to perceive the urge to bear down, to move more freely, and to attain an upright position with assistance as a result of increased strength and sensation in her legs. This approach can enhance the ability to bear down effectively and achieve an uncomplicated vaginal birth (Mayberry et al., 2000; Shermer & Raines, 1997). However, women also will have an increase in distress and the severity of pain. This results in an increase in sympathetic activity and the release of catecholamines. Catecholamines inhibit uterine contractions, potentially prolonging the second stage of labor. Allowing these women a "laboring down" period for fetal descent and rotation may result in a more positive outcome (Roberts, 2002).

Commonly, a second stage of more than 2 hours may be considered prolonged in women without regional analgesia and is reported to the primary health care provider. By using assessment findings such as the FHR and pattern, the descent of the presenting part, the quality of the uterine contractions, and the status of the woman, premature intervention with episiotomy or forceps- or vacuum-assisted birth can be avoided. If the status of the maternal-fetal unit is reassuring and progress is continuing, interventions to end the second stage of labor are unwarranted. Less emphasis should be placed on a definite time limit for the second stage. The duration of active pushing has been found to be more relevant to the newborn's condition at birth than the duration of the second stage of labor itself (d'Entremont, 1996; Minato, 2000; Peterson & Besuner, 1997; Roberts, 2002).

CARE MANAGEMENT

Assessment and Nursing Diagnoses

The only certain objective sign that the second stage of labor has begun is the inability to feel the cervix during vaginal examination, indicating that the cervix is fully dilated and effaced. The precise moment that this occurs is not easily determined because it depends on when a vaginal examination is performed to validate full dilation and effacement. This makes timing of the actual duration of the second stage difficult (Roberts, 2002).

Other signs that suggest the onset of the second stage include the following:

- Sudden appearance of sweat on upper lip
- An episode of vomiting
- Increased bloody show
- Shaking of extremities
- Increased restlessness; verbalization (e.g., "I can't go on")
- Involuntary bearing-down efforts

These signs commonly appear at the time the cervix reaches full dilation (Scott et al., 1999); however, women with an epidural block may not exhibit such signs. Other indicators for each phase of the second stage are given in Table 21-6.

Women can begin to experience an irresistible urge to bear down before full dilation. For some women, this occurs as early as 5-cm dilation. This is most often related to the station of the presenting part below the level of the ischial spines of the maternal pelvis. This occurrence creates a conflict between the woman, whose body is telling her to push, and her health care providers, who believe that pushing the fetal presenting part against an incompletely dilated cervix will result in cervical edema and lacerations, as well as a slowing down of labor progress. The premature urge to bear down must be evaluated as a phase of labor progress possibly indicating the onset of the second stage of labor. In addition, the consequences of pushing against a partially dilated cervix must be determined with research findings. When a woman pushes in relation to the degree of cervical dilation should be based on research evidence rather than on tradition or routine practice. It may be safe and effective for a woman to push with the urge to bear down at the acme of a contraction if her cervix is soft, retracting, and 8 cm or more

TABLE 21-6 **Expected Maternal Progress in Second Stage of Labor**

CRITERION	LATENT PHASE (AVERAGE DURATION, 10-30 MIN)	DESCENT PHASE (AVERAGE DURATION VARIES)*	TRANSITION PHASE (AVERAGE DURATION 5-15 MIN)
Contractions Magnitude (intensity)	Period of physiologic lull for all criteria; period of peace and rest "laboring down"	Significant increase	Overwhelmingly strong Expulsive
Frequency		2-2.5 min	1-2 min
Duration		90 sec	90 sec
Descent, station	0 to +2	Increases and Ferguson reflex† activated, +2 to +4	Rapid, +4 to birth Fetal head visible in introitus
Show: color and amount		Significant increase in dark red bloody show	Bloody show accompanies birth of head
Spontaneous bearing-down efforts	Slight to absent, except during acme of strongest contractions	Increased urge to bear down	Greatly increased
Vocalization	Quiet; concern over progress	Grunting sounds or expiratory vocalization; announces contractions	Grunting sounds and expiratory vocalizations continue; may scream or swear
Maternal behavior	Experiences sense of relief that transition to second stage is finished Feels fatigued and sleepy Feels a sense of accomplishment and optimism, because the "worst is over" Feels in control	Senses increased urge to push Alters respiratory pattern: has short 4- to 5-sec breath holds with regular breaths in between, 5 to 7 times per contraction Makes grunting sounds or expiratory vocalizations Frequent repositioning	Describes extreme pain Expresses feelings of powerlessness Shows decreased ability to listen or concentrate on anything but giving birth Describes **ring of fire** (burning sensation of acute pain as vagina stretches and fetal head crowns) Often shows excitement immediately after birth of head

Source: Roberts, J. (2002). The "push" for evidence: Management of the second stage. *Journal of Midwifery and Women's Health, 47*(1), 2-15; Simkin, P., & Ancheta, R. (2000). *The labor progress handbook.* Malden, MA: Blackwell Science.

*Duration of descent phase can vary depending on maternal parity, effectiveness of bearing-down effort, and presence of spinal anesthesia or epidural analgesia.

†Pressure of presenting part on stretch receptors of pelvic floor stimulates release of oxytocin from posterior pituitary, resulting in more intense uterine contractions.

Care Path Low Risk Woman in Second and Third Stages of Labor

CARE MANAGEMENT	SECOND STAGE OF LABOR	THIRD STAGE OF LABOR
I. ASSESSMENT MEASURES*	**FREQUENCY**	**FREQUENCY**
• Blood pressure, pulse, respirations	Every 5-30 min	Every 15 min
• Uterine activity	Assess every contraction	Assess for placental separation
• Bearing-down effort	Assess each effort	
• Fetal heart rate (FHR)	Every 5-15 min	Perform Apgar at 1 and 5 min
• Vaginal show	Every 15 min	Assess bleeding until placental expulsion
• Signs of fetal descent: urge to bear down, perineal bulging, crowning	Every 10-15 min	
• Behavior, appearance, mood, energy level of woman; condition of partner	Every 10-15 min	Assess response to completion of childbirth process, reaction to newborn
II. PHYSICAL CARE MEASURES†	**Latent phase:** Assist to rest in position of comfort Encourage relaxation to conserve energy Promote urge to push; if delayed: ambulation, shower, pelvic rock, position changes **Descent phase:** Assist to bear down effectively Help to use recommended positions that facilitate descent Encourage correct breathing during bearing-down efforts Help to relax between contractions Provide comfort measures as needed Cleanse perineum immediately if fecal material is expelled **Transition phase:** Assist to pant during contraction to avoid rapid birth of head Coach to gently bear down between contractions	Assist to bear down to facilitate delivery of separated placenta Administer oxytocic as ordered Provide pain relief as needed Provide hygiene and comfort measures as needed
III. EMOTIONAL SUPPORT	Keep informed of progress of fetal descent Provide feedback for bearing-down efforts Explain purpose if medications given Role model comfort measures Provide continuous nursing presence Create a quiet, calm environment Reassure, encourage, praise Take charge as needed, until mother regains confidence in ability to birth her baby Offer mirror to watch birth	Keep informed about progress of placental separation Explain purpose if medications given Describe status of perineal tissue and inform if repair is needed Introduce parents to their baby Assess and care for newborn within view of parents; delay eye prophylaxis to facilitate eye contact Provide private time for family to bond with their new baby and help them to create memories Encourage breastfeeding if desired

*Frequency of assessment is determined by the risk status of the maternal-fetal unit. More frequent assessment is required in high risk situations. Frequency of assessment and method of documentation are also determined by agency policy, which is usually based on the recommended care standards of medical and nursing organizations.

†Physical care measures are performed by the nurse working together with the woman's partner and significant others.

dilated and if the fetus is at 1+ station and rotating to an anterior position (Bergstrom et al., 1997; Roberts, 2002; Varney, 1997).

Assessment is continuous during the second stage of labor. Professional standards and agency policy determine the specific type and timing of assessments, as well as the way in which findings are documented. The Care Path for the second and third stages of labor indicates typical assessments and the recommended frequency for their performance. Signs and symptoms of impending birth (see Table 21-6) may appear unexpectedly, requiring immediate action by the nurse (Box 21-8).

BOX 21-8 Guidelines for Assistance at the Emergency Birth of a Fetus in the Vertex Presentation

1. The woman usually assumes the position most comfortable for her. A lateral position is often recommended.
2. Reassure the woman that birth is usually uncomplicated and easy in these situations. Use eye-to-eye contact and a calm, relaxed manner. If there is someone else available, such as the partner, that person could help support the woman in the position, assist with coaching, and compliment her on her efforts.
3. Wash your hands and put on gloves, if available.
4. Place under woman's buttocks whatever clean material is available.
5. Avoid touching the vaginal area to decrease the possibility of infection.
6. As the head begins to crown, you should do the following:
   a. Tear the amniotic membrane if it is still intact.
   b. Instruct the woman to pant or pant-blow, thus minimizing the urge to push.
   c. Place the flat side of your hand on the exposed fetal head and apply *gentle* pressure toward the vagina to prevent the head from "popping out." The mother may participate by placing her hand under yours on the emerging head. Note: Rapid delivery of the fetal head must be prevented because a rapid change of pressure within the molded fetal skull follows, which may result in dural or subdural tears and may cause vaginal or perineal lacerations.
7. After the birth of the head, check for the umbilical cord. If the cord is around the baby's neck, try to slip it over the baby's head or pull it *gently* to get some slack so that you can slip it over the shoulders.
8. Support the fetal head as restitution (external rotation) occurs. After restitution, with one hand on each side of the baby's head, exert *gentle* pressure downward so that the anterior shoulder emerges under the symphysis pubis and acts as a fulcrum; then, as *gentle* pressure is exerted in the opposite direction, the posterior shoulder, which has passed over the sacrum and coccyx, emerges.
9. Be alert! Hold the baby securely because the rest of the body may emerge quickly. The baby will be slippery!
10. Cradle the baby's head and back in one hand and the buttocks in the other. Keep the head down to drain away the mucus. Use a bulb syringe, if one is available, to remove mucus from the baby's mouth.
11. Dry the baby quickly to prevent rapid heat loss. Keep the baby at the same level as the mother's uterus until the end of the cord stops pulsating. Note: It is important to keep the baby at the same level as the mother's uterus to prevent the baby's blood from flowing to or from the placenta and the resultant hypovolemia or hypervolemia. Also, do not "milk" the cord.
12. Place the baby on the mother's abdomen, cover the baby (remember to keep the head warm, too) with the mother's clothing, and have her cuddle the baby. Compliment her (them) on a job well done, and on the baby, if appropriate.
13. Wait for the placenta to separate; *do not* tug on the cord. Note: Injudicious traction may tear the cord, separate the placenta, or invert the uterus. Signs of placental separation include a slight gush of dark blood from the introitus, lengthening of the cord, and change in the uterine contour from a discoid to globular shape.
14. Instruct the mother to push to deliver the separated placenta. Gently ease out the placental membranes using an up-and-down motion until the membranes are removed. If birth occurs outside a hospital setting, to minimize complications, do not cut the cord without proper clamps and a sterile cutting tool. Inspect the placenta for intactness. Place the baby on the placenta and wrap the two together for additional warmth.
15. Check the firmness of the uterus. Gently massage the fundus and demonstrate to the mother how she can massage her own fundus properly.
16. If supplies are available, clean the mother's perineal area and apply a peripad.
17. In addition to gentle massage of the fundus, the following measures can be taken to prevent or minimize hemorrhage:
    a. Put the baby to the mother's breast as soon as possible. Sucking or nuzzling and licking the nipple stimulates the release of oxytocin from the posterior pituitary. Note: If the baby does not or cannot nurse, manually stimulate the mother's nipples.
    b. Do not allow the mother's bladder to become distended. Assess the bladder for fullness and encourage her to void if fullness is found.
    c. Expel any clots from the mother's uterus.
18. Comfort or reassure the mother and her family or friends. Keep the mother and the baby warm. Give her fluids if available and tolerated.
19. If this is a multifetal birth, identify the infants in order of birth (using letters *A, B,* etc.).
20. Make notations regarding the following aspects of the birth:
    a. Fetal presentation and position
    b. Presence of cord around neck (nuchal cord) or other parts and number of times cord encircled part
    c. Color, character, and amount of amniotic fluid, if rupture of membranes occurs immediately before birth
    d. Time of birth
    e. Estimated time of determination of Apgar score (e.g., 1 and 5 min after birth), resuscitation efforts implemented, and ultimate condition of baby
    f. Sex of baby
    g. Time of placental expulsion, as well as the appearance and completeness of the placenta
    h. Maternal condition: affect, amount of bleeding, and status of uterine tonicity
    i. Any unusual occurrences during the birth (e.g., maternal or paternal response, verbalizations, or gestures in response to birth of baby)

Nursing diagnoses that represent potential areas for concern during the second stage of labor include the following:

- *Risk for injury to mother and fetus related to*
  - –persistent use of Valsalva maneuver during bearing-down efforts
- *Acute pain related to*
  - –bearing-down efforts and distension of the perineum
- *Anxiety related to*
  - –inability to control defecation during bearing-down efforts
  - –deficient knowledge regarding and inexperience with perineal sensations associated with the urge to bear down
- *Risk for infection related to*
  - –prolonged ROM
  - –perineal trauma
- *Situational low self-esteem (maternal) related to*
  - –deficient knowledge regarding normal, beneficial effects of vocalization during bearing-down efforts
  - –inability to carry out plan for birth without medication
- *Situational low self-esteem (partner or father) related to*
  - –inability to support woman during bearing-down efforts

Expected Outcomes of Care

Planning for the second and third stages of labor is done during the first stage of labor. Previously determined expected outcomes may be modified as these stages progress. Expected outcomes for the woman in the second stage of labor are that the woman will accomplish the following:

- Actively participate in the process of giving birth
- Sustain no injury to herself or her fetus during the labor and birth process
- Accept comfort and support measures from significant others and health care providers as needed

Plan of Care and Interventions

The nurse continues to monitor maternal-fetal status and events of the second stage and provide comfort measures for the mother, such as positioning; providing mouth care; maintaining clean, dry bedding; and keeping extraneous noise, conversation, and other distractions (e.g., laughing, talking of attending personnel in or outside the labor area) to a minimum. The woman is encouraged to indicate other support measures she would like (Table 21-7, Care Path for Low Risk Woman in Second and Third Stages of Labor on p. 584, and Plan of Care for Labor and Birth on p. 571).

In the hospital, birth may occur in an LDR, LDRP, or delivery room. If the mother is to be transferred to the delivery room for birth, the nurse accomplishes the transfer early enough to avoid rushing the woman. The birth area also is readied for the birth.

Preparing for Birth

Maternal Position. There is no single position for childbirth. Labor is a dynamic, interactive process involving the woman's uterus, pelvis, and voluntary muscles. In addition, angles between the baby and the woman's pelvis constantly change as the infant turns and flexes down the birth canal. The woman may want to assume various positions for childbirth, and she should be encouraged and assisted in attaining and maintaining her position(s) of choice. Hanson (1998a) found that sitting and side-lying are the two most common positions assumed by women for their bearing-down efforts and birth.

Birth attendants play a major role in influencing a woman's choice of positions for birth, with midwives tending to advocate the nonlithotomy positions for the second stage of labor (Hanson, 1998b). Upright positions facilitate birth and fetal descent and reduce the duration of the second stage of labor and the need for episiotomy, forceps, or vacuum extractor as a result of the following mechanisms (Gupta & Nikodem, 2000; Shermer & Raines, 1997):

- Straighten the longitudinal axis of the birth canal
- Use gravity to direct the fetal head toward the pelvic inlet, thereby facilitating descent
- Enlarge pelvic dimensions and restrict the encroachment of the sacrum and coccyx into the pelvic outlet
- Increase uteroplacental circulation, resulting in more intense, efficient uterine contractions
- Enhance the woman's ability to bear down effectively, thereby minimizing maternal exhaustion

The upright positions may, however, slightly increase the risk for second-degree lacerations and a blood loss greater than 500 ml. Further investigation is needed to determine the exact mechanism for these outcomes (Shorten, Donsante, & Shorten, 2002).

Squatting is highly effective in facilitating the descent and birth of the fetus. It is considered to be one of the best positions for the second stage of labor (Mayberry et al., 2000; Roberts, 2002). Women should assume a modified, supported squat until the fetal head is engaged, at which time a deep squat can be used. A firm surface is required for this position, and the woman will need side support (see Fig. 21-14, *A*). In a birthing bed, a squat bar is available that she can use to help support herself. A birth ball can help a woman maintain the squatting position. The fetus will be aligned with the birth canal, and pelvic and perineal relaxation will be facilitated as she sits on the ball or holds it in front of her for support as she squats (Perez, 1998).

When a woman uses the standing position for bearing down, her weight is borne on both femoral heads, allowing the pressure in the acetabulum to cause the transverse diameter of the pelvic outlet to increase by up to 1 cm. This can be helpful if descent of the head is delayed because the occiput has not rotated from the lateral (transverse diameter of pelvis) to the anterior position (Biancuzzo, 1993). Birthing chairs or rocking chairs

TABLE 21-7 **Woman's Responses and Support Person's Actions During Second Stage of Labor**

WOMAN'S RESPONSES*	NURSE/SUPPORT PERSON'S ACTIONS†
LATENT PHASE	
Experiences a short period of peace and rest	Encourages woman to "listen" to her body Continues support measures allowing woman to rest Suggests an upright position to encourage progression of descent if descent phase does not begin after 20 min
DESCENT PHASE	
Senses increased urgency to bear down as Ferguson reflex is activated Notes increase in intensity of uterine contractions—alters respiratory pattern: short 4- to 5-sec breath holds, 5 to 7 times per contraction Makes grunting sounds or expiratory vocalizations	Encourages respiratory pattern of short breath holds and open glottis pushing Stresses normality and benefits of grunting sounds and expiratory vocalizations Encourages bearing-down efforts with urge to push Encourages/suggests maternal movement and position changes (upright, if descent is not occurring) Encourages woman to "listen" to her body regarding movement and position change if descent is occurring Discourages long breath holds (no longer than 5 to 7 sec) If birth is to occur in a delivery room, transfers woman to delivery room early to avoid rushing or, if permitted, offers her option of walking to delivery room Places woman in lateral recumbent position to slow descent if descent is too fast
TRANSITIONAL PHASE	
Behaves in manner similar to behavior during transition in first stage (8-10 cm) Experiences a sense of severe pain and powerlessness Shows decreased ability to listen Concentrates on birth of baby until head is born Experiences contractions as overwhelming in intensity Reports feeling ring of fire as head crowns Maintains respiratory pattern of three to five 7-sec breath holds per contraction, followed by forced expiration Eases head out with short expirations Responds with excitement and relief after head is born	Encourages slow, gentle pushing Explains that "blowing away the contraction" facilitates a slower birth of the head Provides mirror to help woman see or touch the emerging fetal head (best to extend over two to three contractions) to help her understand the perineal sensations Coaches woman to relax mouth, throat, and neck to promote relaxation of pelvic floor Applies warm compress to perineum to promote relaxation

*Woman's responses will be altered if epidural analgesia is being administered.
†Provided by nurses and support persons in collaboration with the nurse.

may be used to provide women with a good physiologic position to enhance her bearing-down efforts during childbirth, although some women feel restricted by a chair. The upright position also provides a potential psychologic advantage in that it allows the mother to see the birth as it occurs and to maintain eye contact with the attendant. Most birthing chairs are designed so that if an emergency occurs, the chair can be adjusted to the horizontal or the Trendelenburg position.

Oversized beanbag chairs and large floor pillows may be used for both labor and birth. They can mold around and support the mother in whatever position she selects. These chairs are of particular value for mothers who wish to be actively involved in the birth process. Birthing stools can be used to support the woman in an upright position similar to squatting. Women may want to sit on the toilet or commode during pushing because they are concerned about stool incontinence during this stage. These women must be closely monitored, however, and removed from the toilet before birth becomes imminent. Because sitting on chairs, stools, toilets, or commodes can increase perineal edema and blood loss, it is important to assist the woman to change her position every 10 to 15 minutes (Shermer & Raines, 1997).

The side-lying position, with the upper part of the woman's leg held by the nurse or coach or placed on a pillow, is an effective position for the second stage of labor (Fig. 21-18, *A*). Women using the lateral position have

A

B

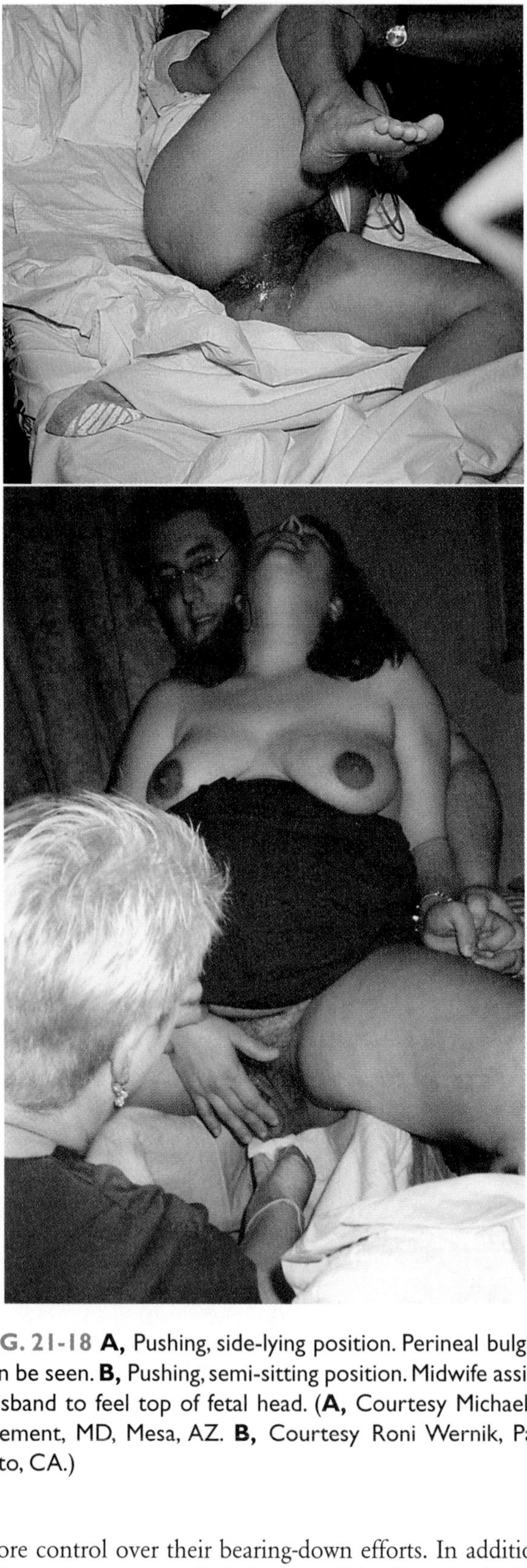

FIG. 21-18 A, Pushing, side-lying position. Perineal bulging can be seen. **B,** Pushing, semi-sitting position. Midwife assists husband to feel top of fetal head. (**A,** Courtesy Michael S. Clement, MD, Mesa, AZ. **B,** Courtesy Roni Wernik, Palo Alto, CA.)

more control over their bearing-down efforts. In addition, a slower, more controlled descent of the fetus results in a reduced risk of perineal trauma (Gupta & Nickodem, 2000). Some women prefer a semi-sitting (semi-recumbent) position. To maintain good uteroplacental circulation and to

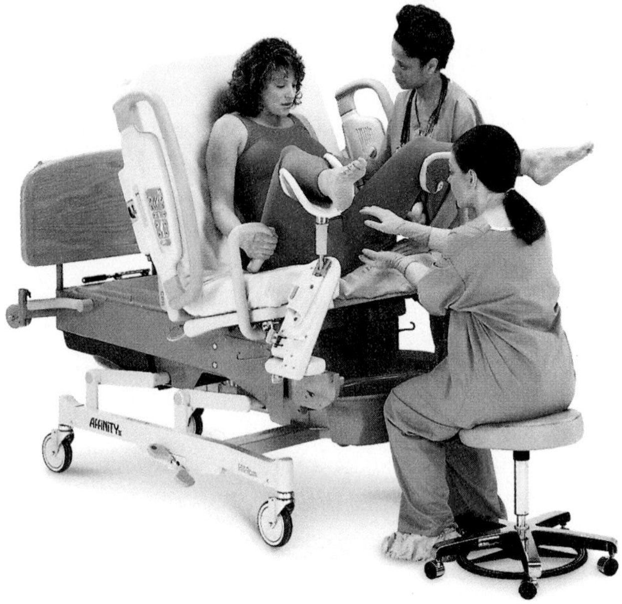
AFFINITY

FIG. 21-19 Birth bed. (Courtesy Hill-Rom, Batesville, IN.)

enhance the woman's bearing-down efforts in this position, the woman's back and shoulders should be elevated to at least a 30-degree angle, and a wedge should be placed under one hip (Fig. 21-18, *B*). The episiotomy rate for nulliparas has been found to be highest in this position (Shorten, Donsante, & Shorten, 2002).

The hands-and-knees position, along with pelvic rocking and abdominal stroking, is an effective position for birth because it enhances placental perfusion, helps rotate the fetus from a posterior to an anterior position, and may facilitate the birth of the shoulders, especially if the fetus is large. Perineal trauma also may be reduced (Gannon, 1992; Simkin & Ancheta, 2000) (see Fig. 21-13, *B*).

The birthing bed is commonly used today and can be set for different positions according to the woman's needs (Figs. 21-19 and 21-20). The woman can squat, kneel, sit, recline, or lie on her side, choosing the position most comfortable for her without having to climb into bed for the birth. At the same time, there is excellent exposure for examinations, electrode placement, and birth. The bed also can be positioned for the administration of anesthesia and is ideal to help women receiving an epidural to assume different positions to facilitate birth. The bed can be used to transport the woman to the operating room if a cesarean birth is necessary. Squat bars, over-the-bed tables, birth balls, and pillows can be used for support.

Bearing-Down Efforts. As the fetal head reaches the pelvic floor, most women experience the urge to bear down. Reflexively the woman will begin to exert downward pressure by contracting her abdominal muscles while relaxing her pelvic floor. This bearing down is an involuntary response to the Ferguson reflex.

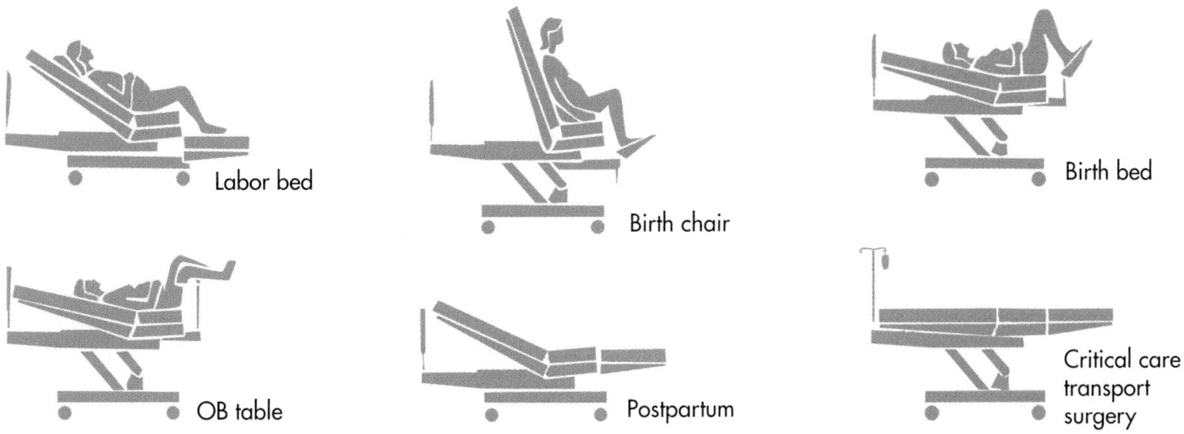
Labor bed
Birth chair
Birth bed
OB table
Postpartum
Critical care
transport
surgery

FIG. 21-20 The versatility of today's birthing bed makes it practical in a variety of settings. Note: OB table used for *lithotomy position.* (Courtesy Hill-Rom, Batesville, IN.)

When coaching women to push, the nurse should encourage them to push as they feel like pushing (instinctive, spontaneous pushing) rather than to give a prolonged push on command. Women will usually begin to push naturally as the contraction increases in intensity and the Ferguson reflex strengthens. The nurse should monitor the woman's breathing so that the woman does not hold her breath for more than 5 to 7 seconds at a time and should remind her to ventilate her lungs fully by taking deep cleansing breaths before and after each contraction. Bearing down while exhaling (open-glottis pushing) and taking breaths between bearing-down efforts help maintain adequate oxygen levels for the mother and fetus and results in approximately five pushes during a contraction, with each push lasting about 5 seconds (Mayberry et al., 2000). Women who use spontaneous pushing are less likely to have second- or third-degree lacerations or episiotomies (Hodnett, 1996; Roberts, 2002; Sampselle & Hines, 1999).

A strong expiratory grunt or groan (vocalization) often accompanies pushing when the woman exhales as she pushes. This natural vocalization by women during open-glottis bearing-down efforts is likely to be discouraged by nurses in part to "conserve the woman's energy" but also as a result of concern that it will seem to other nurses and clients that the woman has lost control or the nurse has lost control of the client (Peterson & Besuner, 1997).

Prolonged breath-holding, or sustained, directed bearing down, which is still a common practice, may trigger the **Valsalva maneuver,** which occurs when the woman closes the glottis (closed-glottis pushing), thereby increasing intrathoracic and cardiovascular pressure, reducing cardiac output, and inhibiting perfusion of the uterus and the placenta. In addition, breath-holding for more than 5 to 7 seconds causes the perfusion of oxygen across the placenta to be diminished, resulting in fetal hypoxia. This approach to bearing down is harmful or ineffective and should be discouraged (Enkin et al., 2000).

A woman may reach the second stage of labor and then experience a lack of readiness to complete the process and give birth to her child. McKay and Barrows (1991) identified several factors that may inhibit the woman's voluntary bearing-down efforts:

- Doubts about her readiness to be a mother
- Reluctance to care for another baby
- Desire to wait for support person or primary health care provider to arrive
- Fear or anxiety regarding the unfamiliar or painful sensations of the second stage of labor and pushing
- Embarrassment regarding behaviors during pushing, including sounds made and the passage of stool
- Giving up and not wanting to proceed any further toward a vaginal birth
- Fear that the baby will be in danger once it emerges from the protective intrauterine environment

By recognizing that a woman may experience a need to hold back the birth of her baby, the nurse can then address the woman's concerns and effectively coach the woman during this stage of labor.

To ensure the slow birth of the fetal head, the woman is encouraged to control the urge to bear down by coaching her to take panting breaths or to exhale slowly through pursed lips as the baby's head crowns. At this point, the woman needs simple, clear directions from one person.

Amnesia between contractions often is pronounced in the second stage, and the woman may have to be roused to get her to cooperate in the bearing-down process. Parents who have attended childbirth education classes may have devised a set of verbal cues for the laboring woman to follow. It is helpful for them to have these cues printed on a card that can be attached to the head of the bed so that the nurse can better substitute as coach if the partner has to leave.

Fetal Heart Rate and Pattern. As noted previously, the FHR must be checked. If the baseline rate begins to slow, if there is a loss of variability, or if deceleration patterns develop (e.g., late, variable), prompt treatment must be initiated. The woman can be turned on her side to reduce the pressure of the uterus against the ascending vena cava and descending aorta (see Fig. 21-5), and oxygen can be administered by mask at 8 to 10 L/min (Tucker, 2000). This is often all that is necessary to restore a reassuring pattern. If the FHR and pattern does not become reassuring immediately, the primary health care provider should be notified quickly because medical intervention to hasten the birth may be indicated.

Support of the Father or Partner. During the second stage, the woman needs continuous support and coaching (see Table 21-7). Because the coaching process can be physically and emotionally tiring for support persons, the nurse offers them nourishment and fluids and encourages them to take short breaks. If birth occurs in an LDR or LDRP room, the partner may be allowed to wear street clothes or be required to wear a clean scrub outfit, cap, and mask (for the birth). The support person who attends the birth in a delivery room is instructed to put on a cover gown or scrub clothes, mask, hat, and shoe covers, as required by agency policy. The nurse also specifies support measures that can be used for the laboring woman and points out areas of the room in which the partner can move freely.

Partners are encouraged to be present at the birth of their infants if this is in keeping with their cultural and personal expectations and beliefs. In this way the psychologic closeness of the family unit is maintained, and the partner can continue to provide the supportive care given during labor. The woman and her partner need to have an equal opportunity to initiate the attachment process with the baby.

LEGAL TIP Documentation

Documentation of all observations (e.g., maternal vital signs, FHR and pattern, progress of labor) and nursing interventions, including client response, should be done concurrent with care. The course of labor and the maternal-fetal response may change without warning. It is important that all documentation be accurate, complete, timely, and according to agency policy.

Supplies, Instruments, and Equipment. To prepare for birth in any setting, the birthing table is usually set up during the transition phase for nulliparous women and during the active phase for multiparous women.

The birthing table is prepared, and instruments are arranged on the instrument table (Fig. 21-21). Standard procedures are followed for gloving, identifying and opening sterile packages, adding sterile supplies to the instrument table, unwrapping sterile instruments, and handing them to the primary health care provider. The crib or radiant warmer and equipment are readied for the support and stabilization of the infant (Fig. 21-22).

The items used for birth may vary among different facilities; therefore each facility's procedure manual should be consulted to determine the protocols specific to that facility.

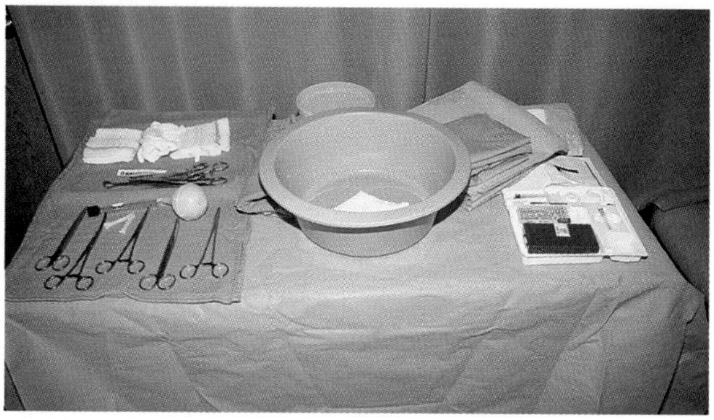

FIG. 21-21 Instrument table. (Courtesy Marjorie Pyle, RNC, Lifecircle, Costa Mesa, CA.)

The nurse estimates the time until the birth will occur and notifies the primary health care provider if he or she is not in the client's room. Even the most experienced nurse can miscalculate the time left before birth occurs; thus every nurse who attends a woman in labor must be prepared to assist with an emergency birth if the primary health care provider is not present (see Box 21-8).

Birth in a Delivery Room or Birthing Room

The woman will need assistance if she must move from the labor bed to the delivery table (Fig. 21-23). The various positions assumed for birth in a delivery room are the Sims or lateral position in which the attendant supports the upper part of the woman's leg, the dorsal position (supine position with one hip elevated), and the lithotomy position.

The **lithotomy position** has been the position most commonly used for birth in Western cultures, although this practice is slowly changing. The lithotomy position makes it more convenient for the primary health care provider to deal with complications that arise (see Fig. 21-20). To place the woman in this position, her buttocks are brought to the edge of the table and her legs are placed in stirrups. Care must be taken to pad the stirrups, to raise and place both legs simultaneously, and to adjust the shanks of the stirrups so that the calves of the legs are supported. There should be no pressure on the popliteal space. If the stirrups are not the same height, ligaments in the woman's back can be strained as she bears down, leading to considerable discomfort in the postpartum period. The lower portion of the table may be dropped down and rolled back under the table.

It should be noted that the routine use of a supine or lithotomy position for labor and birth has been identified as a clearly harmful or ineffective practice and should be discouraged (Enkin et al., 2000).

The maternal position for birth in a birthing room varies from a lithotomy position with the woman's legs in

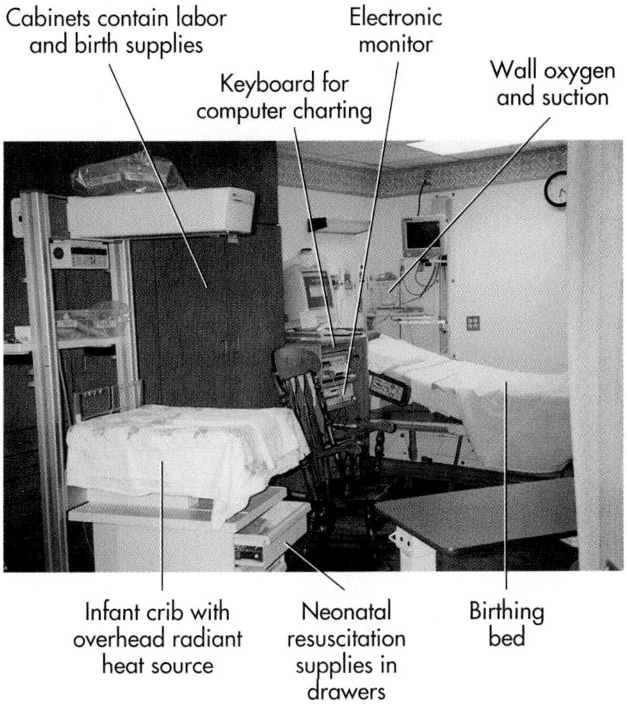
Cabinets contain labor and birth supplies
Electronic monitor
Keyboard for computer charting
Wall oxygen and suction
Infant crib with overhead radiant heat source
Neonatal resuscitation supplies in drawers
Birthing bed

FIG. 21-22 Birthing room. (Courtesy Dee Lowdermilk, Chapel Hill, NC.)

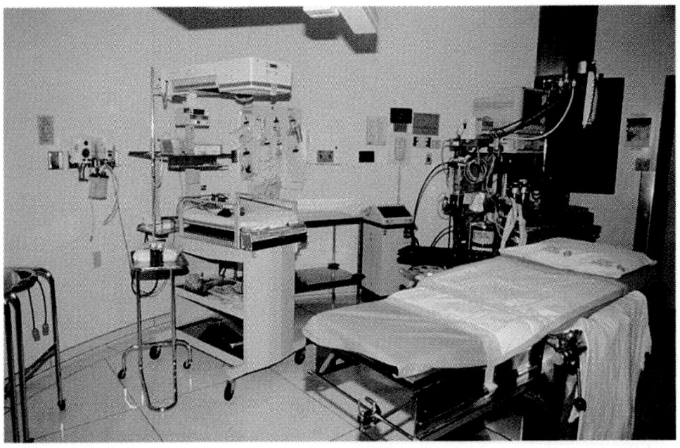

FIG. 21-23 Delivery room. (Courtesy Michael S. Clement, MD, Mesa, AZ.)

stirrups, to one in which her feet rest on footrests while she holds onto a squat bar, to a side-lying position with the woman's upper leg supported by the coach, nurse, or squat bar. The foot of the bed can be removed so that the primary health care provider attending the birth can gain better perineal access for performing an episiotomy, delivering a large baby, using forceps or vacuum extractor, or getting access to the emerging head to facilitate suctioning. Otherwise the foot of the bed is left in place and lowered slightly to form a ledge that allows access for birth and that also serves as a place to lay the newborn (see Fig. 21-19).

Once the woman is positioned for birth either in a delivery room or birthing room, the vulva and perineum may be cleansed. Hospital protocols and the preferences of primary health care providers for cleansing may vary.

The circulating nurse (usually the same nurse as the labor nurse) continues to coach and encourage the woman. The nurse auscultates the FHR or evaluates the monitor tracing every 5 to 15 minutes, depending on whether the woman is at low or high risk for problems or per protocol of the birthing facility, or continuously monitors the FHR with electronic monitoring. The primary health care provider is kept informed of the rate and pattern of the FHR (Tucker, 2000). An oxytocic medication such as oxytocin (Pitocin) may be prepared so that it is ready to be administered after expulsion of the placenta. Standard Precautions should always be followed as care is administered during the process of labor and birth (see Box 21-3).

In the delivery room, the primary health care provider puts on a cap, a mask that has a shield or protective eyewear, and shoe covers. Hands are scrubbed, a sterile gown (with waterproof front and sleeves) is donned, and gloves are put on. Nurses attending the birth also may need to wear caps, protective eyewear, masks, gowns, and gloves. The woman may then be draped with sterile drapes. In the birthing room, Standard Precautions are observed, but the amount and types of protective coverings worn by those in attendance may vary.

Nursing contact with the parents is maintained by touching, verbal comforting, explaining the reasons for care, and sharing in the parents' joy at the birth of their child.

Mechanism of Birth: Vertex Presentation

The three phases of the spontaneous birth of a fetus in a vertex presentation are (1) birth of the head, (2) birth of the shoulders, and (3) birth of the body and extremities (see Chapter 18).

With voluntary bearing-down efforts, the head appears at the introitus (Fig. 21-24). **Crowning** occurs when the widest part of the head (the biparietal diameter) distends the vulva just before birth. The birth attendant may apply mineral oil to the perineum and stretch it as the head is crowning. Immediately before birth, the perineal musculature becomes greatly distended. If an **episiotomy** (incision into the perineum to enlarge vaginal outlet) is necessary, it is done at this time to minimize soft tissue damage. Local anesthetic is administered prior to the episiotomy.

The physician or nurse midwife may use a hands-on approach to control the birth of the head, believing that guarding the perineum results in a gradual birth that will prevent fetal intracranial injury, protect maternal tissues, and reduce postpartum perineal pain. This approach involves (1) applying pressure against the rectum, drawing it downward to aid in flexing the head as the back of the

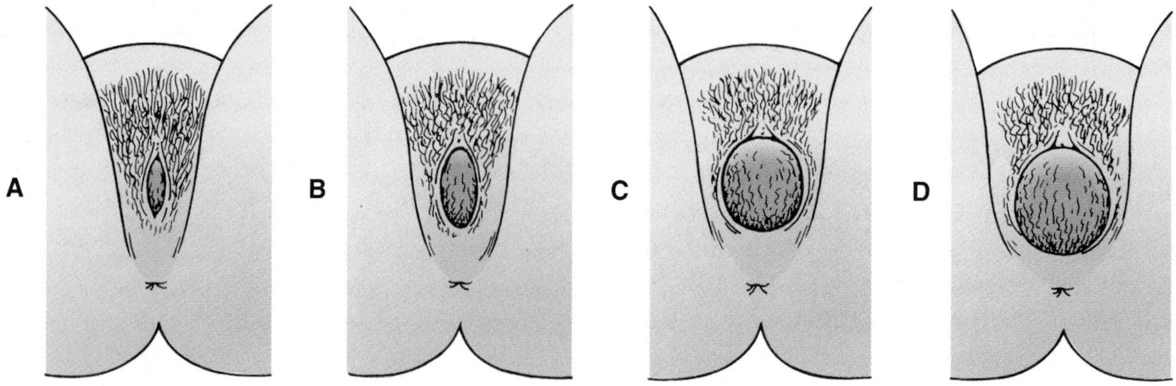
A
B
C
D

FIG. 21-24 Beginning birth with vertex presenting. **A,** Anteroposterior slit. **B,** Oval opening. **C,** Circular shape. **D,** Crowning.

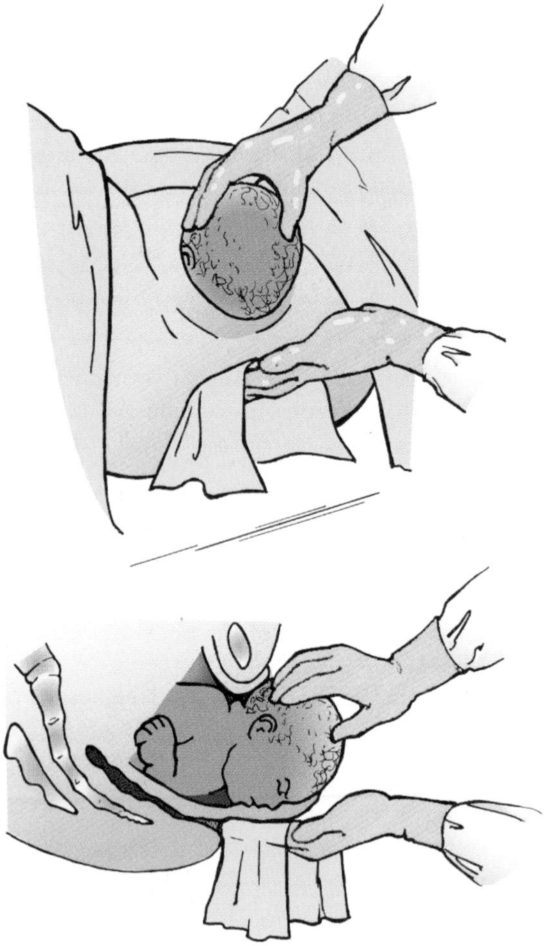

FIG. 21-25 Birth of head with modified Ritgen maneuver. Note control to prevent too rapid birth of head.

neck catches under the symphysis pubis; (2) then applying upward pressure from the coccygeal region (modified **Ritgen maneuver)** (Fig. 21-25) to extend the head during the actual birth, thereby protecting the musculature of the perineum; and (3) assisting the mother with voluntary control of the bearing-down efforts by coaching her to pant while letting uterine forces expel the fetus.

Some health care providers use a hands-poised (hands-off) approach when attending a birth. In this approach, hands are prepared to place light pressure on the fetal head to prevent rapid expulsion. Hands are not placed on the perineum or used to assist with birth of the shoulders and body.

The hands-on and hands-poised approaches have similar results in terms of perineal trauma and condition of the newborn. However, perineal pain is slightly less at 10 days postpartum when the hands-on approach is used (McCandlish, 2001). Guarding the perineum is a form of care likely to be beneficial (Enkin et al., 2000).

The umbilical cord often encircles the neck **(nuchal cord)** but rarely so tightly as to cause hypoxia. After the head is born, gentle palpation is used to feel for the cord. If present, the cord should be slipped gently over the head (Fig. 21-26). If the loop is tight or if there is a second loop, the cord is clamped twice, cut between the clamps, and unwound from around the neck before the birth is allowed to continue. Mucus, blood, or meconium in the nasal or oral passages may prevent the newborn from breathing. To eliminate this problem, moist gauze sponges are used to wipe the nose and mouth. A bulb syringe is first inserted into the mouth and oropharynx to aspirate contents, and then the nares are cleared in the same fashion while the head is supported.

If meconium has been present in the amniotic fluid during labor, preparations are made for wall suction, or in some cases, a De Lee suction apparatus is placed on the sterile field for use. Fluids are withdrawn from the infant's mouth and nose before the first breath is taken to prevent meconium aspiration. Use of the De Lee device with oral suction to withdraw fluid from the infant should be avoided unless the suction device is designed so that it can keep mucus from entering the user's airway.

The time of birth is the precise time when the entire body is out of the mother. This time must be recorded on the record.

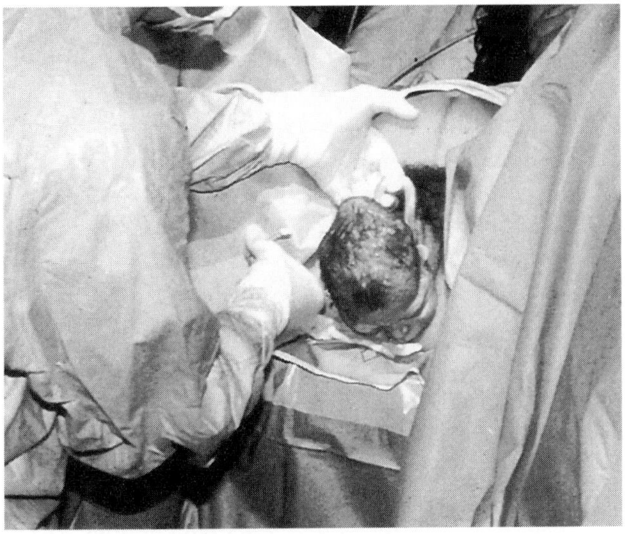

FIG. 21-26 Loosening nuchal cord (umbilical cord around neck). (Courtesy Marjorie Pyle, RNC, Lifecircle, Costa Mesa, CA.)

If the newborn's condition is not compromised, it may be placed on the mother's abdomen immediately after birth and covered with a warm, dry blanket. The cord may be clamped at this time, and the primary health care provider may ask if the woman's partner would like to cut the cord. If so, the partner is given a sterile pair of scissors and instructed to cut the cord 1 inch (2.5 cm) above the clamp.

Use of Fundal Pressure. Fundal pressure is the application of gentle, steady pressure against the fundus of the uterus to facilitate the vaginal birth. Historically it has been used when the administration of analgesia and anesthesia decreased the woman's ability to push during the birth, in cases of shoulder dystocia, and when second-stage fetal bradycardia or other nonreassuring FHR patterns were present. Use of fundal pressure by nurses is not advised because there is no standard technique available for this maneuver, and no current legal, professional, or regulatory standards exist for its use. In cases of shoulder dystocia, fundal pressure is not recommended: the all-fours position (Gaskin maneuver), suprapubic pressure, and maternal position changes are among the recommended interventions (Bruner et al., 1998; Cosner, 1996; Naef & Morrison, 1994; Piper & McDonald, 1994) (see Chapter 36).

Immediate Assessments and Care of the Newborn

The care given immediately after the birth focuses on assessing and stabilizing the newborn. The nurse's primary responsibility at this time is the infant, because the primary health care provider is involved with the delivery of the placenta and the care of the mother. The nurse must watch the infant for any signs of distress and initiate appropriate interventions should any appear.

A brief assessment of the newborn can be performed while the mother is holding the infant. This includes checking the infant's airway and Apgar score. Maintaining a patent airway, supporting respiratory effort, and preventing cold stress by drying the newborn and covering the newborn with a warmed blanket or placing him or her under a radiant warmer are the major priorities in terms of the newborn's immediate care. Further examination, identification procedures, and care can be postponed until later in the third stage of labor or early in the fourth stage.

Perineal Trauma Related to Childbirth

Lacerations

Most acute injuries and lacerations of the perineum, vagina, uterus, and their support tissues occur during childbirth. Some injuries to the supporting tissues, whether they were acute or nonacute and whether they were repaired or not, may lead to genitourinary and sexual problems later in life (e.g., pelvic relaxation, uterine prolapse, cystocele, rectocele, dyspareunia, urinary and bowel dysfunction).

Some damage occurs during every birth to the soft tissues of the birth canal and adjacent structures. The tendency to sustain lacerations varies with each woman; that is, the soft tissue in some women may be less distensible. Damage usually is more pronounced in nulliparous women because the tissues are firmer and more resistant than are those in multiparous women. Heredity also may be a factor. For example, the tissue of light-skinned women, especially those with reddish hair, is not so readily distensible as that of darker-skinned women, and healing may be less efficient. The perineal skin and vaginal mucosa may appear intact, but numerous small lacerations in underlying muscle and its fascia may be obscured. Damage to pelvic supports usually is readily apparent and is repaired after birth.

Immediate repair promotes healing, limits residual damage, and decreases the possibility of infection. Immediately after birth, the cervix, vagina, and perineum are inspected to look for damage. In addition, during the early postpartum period, the nurse and primary health care provider continue to inspect the perineum carefully and evaluate lochia and symptoms to identify any previously missed damage.

Perineal Lacerations. Perineal lacerations usually occur as the fetal head is being born. The extent of the laceration is defined in terms of its depth:

1. *First degree:* Laceration that extends through the skin and structures superficial to muscles
2. *Second degree:* Laceration that extends through muscles of the perineal body
3. *Third degree:* Laceration that continues through the anal sphincter muscle
4. *Fourth degree:* Laceration that also involves the anterior rectal wall

Perineal injury often is accompanied by small lacerations on the medial surfaces of the labia minora below the

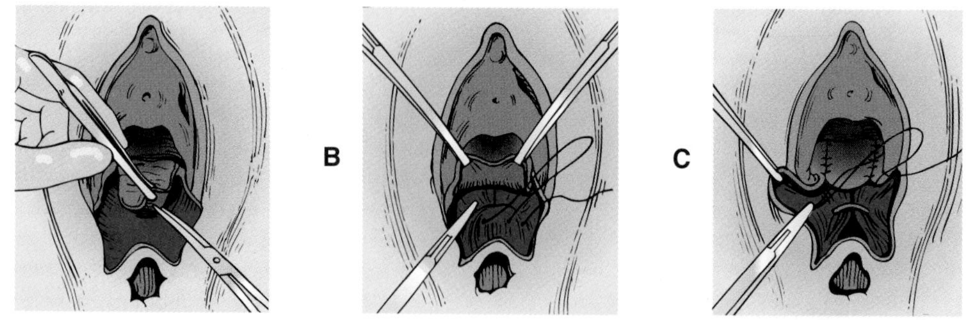
A
B
C

FIG. 21-27 Perineal lacerations. **A,** Bilateral sulcus tears, periurethral tear, and separation of anal sphincter. **B,** Exposure and approximation of levator ani structures. **C,** Approximation of torn bulbocavernous muscle.

pubic rami and to the sides of the urethra (periurethral) and clitoris. Lacerations in this highly vascular area often result in profuse bleeding. Such lacerations must be repaired with absorbable suture (Fig. 21-27).

Special attention must be paid to third- and fourth-degree lacerations so that the woman retains fecal continence. Measures are taken to promote soft stools (e.g., roughage, fluid, activity, and stool softeners) to increase the woman's comfort and foster healing. Antimicrobial therapy may be instituted in some cases. Enemas and suppositories are contraindicated for these women.

When the levator ani (including the iliococcygeal and pubococcygeal muscles, which form the sling-like support of the pelvic viscera) is not involved, simple perineal injuries usually heal without permanent disability, regardless of whether they were repaired. However, the vaginal introitus may gape if torn or severed (episiotomy) ends of superficial perineal muscles (e.g., the bulbocavernosus) are not well approximated during repair.

The ends of the torn or severed anal sphincter muscles must be repaired adequately to prevent fecal incontinence (Fig. 21-28). It is easier to repair a new perineal injury to prevent sequelae than it is to correct long-term damage.

Vaginal and Urethral Lacerations. Vaginal lacerations often occur in conjunction with perineal lacerations. Vaginal lacerations tend to extend up the lateral walls (sulci) and, if deep enough, involve the levator ani. Additional injury may occur high in the vaginal vault near the level of the ischial spines. Vaginal vault lacerations may be circular and may result from forceps rotation, especially in the presence of cephalopelvic disproportion, rapid fetal descent, or precipitate birth.

Cervical Injuries. Cervical injuries occur when the cervix retracts over the advancing fetal head. These cervical lacerations occur at the lateral angles of the external os; most are shallow, and bleeding is minimal. More extensive lacerations may extend to the vaginal vault or beyond it into the lower uterine segment; serious bleeding may occur. Extensive lacerations may follow hasty attempts to enlarge the cervical opening artificially or to deliver the fetus before full cervical dilation is achieved. Injuries to the cervix can have adverse effects on future pregnancies and childbirths.

Episiotomy

An episiotomy is an incision made in the perineum to enlarge the vaginal outlet. It is performed more commonly in the United States and Canada than in Europe. The side-lying position for birth, used routinely in Europe, causes less tension on the perineum, making possible a gradual stretching of the perineum with fewer indications for episiotomies.

Clear evidence exists that routine performance of an episiotomy for birth is a form of care that is likely to be harmful or ineffective (Enkin et al., 2000). The routine performance of episiotomies has been declining. From 1980 to 1998, the number of episiotomies performed in the United States declined from more than 2 million to 1.2 million, reflecting a 39% reduction. The greatest decline occurred in the 1990s, most likely related to the clear evidence regarding the harmful effects of episiotomy in terms of increased postpartum pain, blood loss, risk for infection, and occurrence of third- and fourth-degree lacerations (Weeks & Kozak, 2001). The practice in many settings now is to support the perineum manually during birth and allow the perineum to tear rather than perform an episiotomy. Tears are often smaller than an episiotomy, are repaired easily or not at all, and heal quickly. Conversely, episiotomy incisions extend into pelvic floor muscles, take longer to heal, and are more painful than lacerations (McGinnis, Norr, & Nacion, 1991; Paciornik, 1990; Woolly, 1995). The pain and discomfort resulting from episiotomies can interfere with mother-infant interaction, breastfeeding, reestablishment of sexual relationship with partner, and even emotional recovery after birth.

Proponents of the use of episiotomy believe it shortens the second stage of labor if the well-being of the woman or fetus is in jeopardy, facilitates vacuum- or forceps-assisted birth, prevents cerebral hemorrhage stemming from capil-

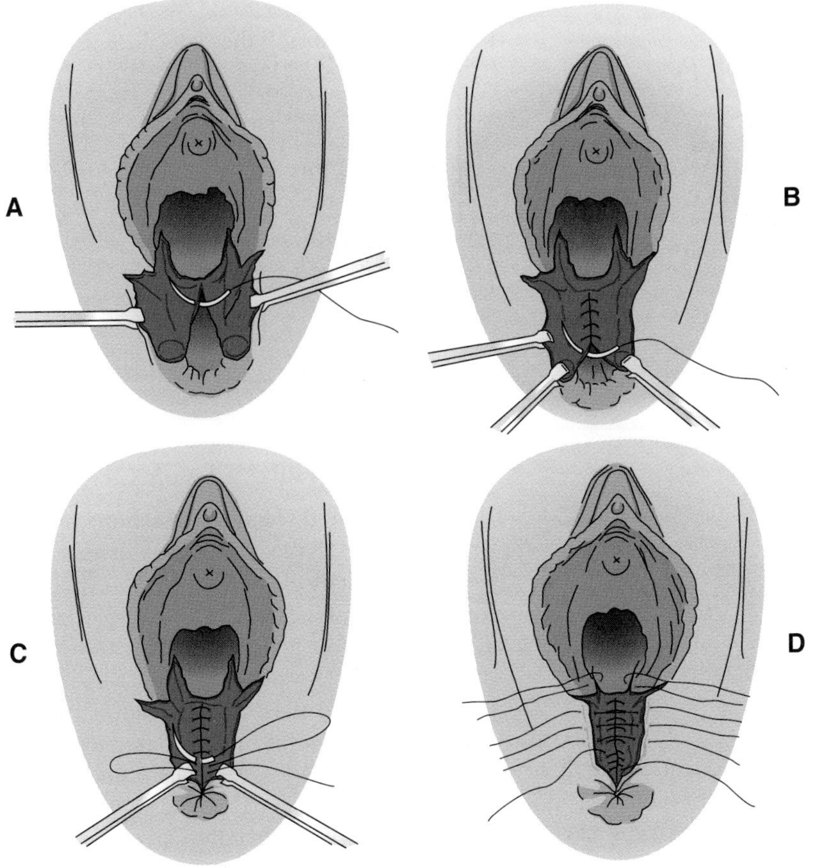
A
B
C
D

FIG. 21-28 Repair of fourth-degree laceration. **A,** Repair of rectal mucosa, with inverted sutures buried in muscles of rectal wall. **B,** Sutures of levator muscles to be buried; ends of sphincter drawn forward: first step in suturing sphincter. **C,** Second step of suturing sphincter: beginning figure-of-eight sutures. **D,** Sphincter suture completed and ready for tying. Remainder of perineal repair done in usual manner.

lary fragility during the birth of a preterm infant, facilitates the birth of a large infant (more than 4000 g), or facilitates most forceps-assisted breech births. However, research does not support the claims that episiotomies reduce risk for fetal cerebral hemorrhage or distress or shorten the second stage of labor. Further investigation is required to determine whether episiotomies are of actual benefit in the instances cited (Woolley, 1995).

The type of episiotomy is designated by the site and direction of the incision (Fig. 21-29). Midline (median) episiotomy is most commonly used in the United States. It is effective, easily repaired, and generally the least painful. However, midline episiotomies also are associated with a higher incidence of third- and fourth-degree lacerations (Labreque et al., 1997; Woolley, 1995). Sphincter tone is usually restored after primary healing and a good repair.

Mediolateral episiotomy is used in operative births when the need for posterior extension is likely. Although a fourth-degree laceration may be prevented, a third-degree laceration may occur. The blood loss also is greater and the repair more difficult and painful than with midline episiotomies. It is also more painful in the postpartum period, and the pain lasts longer.

Risk factors associated with perineal trauma (e.g., episiotomy, lacerations) include nulliparity, maternal position, pelvic inadequacy (e.g., narrow subpubic arch with a constricted outlet), fetal malpresentation and position (e.g., breech, occiput posterior position), large (macrosomic) infants, use of instruments to facilitate birth, prolonged second stage of labor, fetal distress, and rapid labor in which there is insufficient time for the perineum to stretch. Women of Caucasian and Asian races and those who have private insurance and care have higher rates of episiotomies. The rate of episiotomies also is higher when obstetricians rather than nurse midwives attend births. (Albers et al., 1996; Hueston, 1996; Lydon-Rochelle, Albers, & Teaf, 1995; Shorten et al., 2002).

Alternative measures for perineal management, such as warm compresses, manual support, and massage (e.g.,

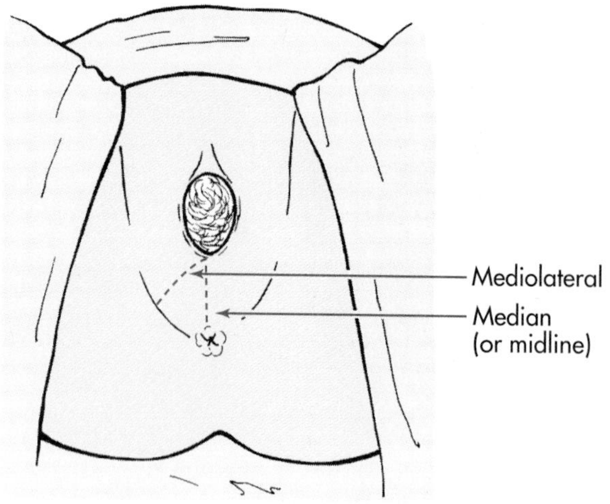
Mediolateral
Median
(or midline)

FIG. 21-29 Types of episiotomies.

prenatal and intrapartum), have been shown to reduce, to varying degrees, the incidence of episiotomies, but further research is recommended (Albers et al., 1996; Lydon-Rochelle et al., 1995; Renfrew et al., 1998). Use of Kegel exercises in the prenatal and postpartum periods improves and restores the tone and strength of the perineal muscles. Health practices, including good nutrition and appropriate hygienic measures, help maintain the integrity and suppleness of the perineal tissue. Nurses acting as advocates can encourage women to use alternative birthing positions that reduce pressure on the perineum (e.g., lateral position) and to use spontaneous bearing-down efforts. In addition, nurses can educate other health care providers about measures to preserve perineal integrity and to be more flexible in defining the maximal limit for the duration of the second stage of labor as long as the maternal-fetal unit is stable (Maier & Maloni, 1997).

Emergency Childbirth

Even under the best of circumstances, there probably will come a time when the perinatal nurse will be required to assist with the birth of an infant without medical assistance. Because it is neither possible nor desirable to prevent impending birth, the perinatal nurse must be able to function independently and be skilled in the safe birth of a vertex fetus (see Box 21-8).

A lateral Sims position may be the position of choice for birth when (1) the birth is progressing rapidly, and there is insufficient time for slow distention of the perineum; (2) the fetal head seems too large to pass through the introitus without laceration, and episiotomy is not possible; or (3) the apparent size of the fetus is consistent with possible shoulder dystocia. In the lateral Sims position, less stress is placed on the perineum, and better visualization of the perineum is possible as the upper leg is supported by the woman's partner or the nurse (see Fig. 21-18, *A*). In the event of shoulder dystocia, the lateral Sims position increases the space needed for birth.

Evaluation

During the second stage of labor, the nurse evaluates the degree to which expected outcomes are being met, for example, the extent to which the woman has actively participated in the labor process, whether she or her fetus has sustained any injury during the labor process, the degree to which her birth plan has been fulfilled, and the extent to which she has been able to obtain comfort and support from her support person.

THIRD STAGE OF LABOR

The **third stage of labor** lasts from the birth of the baby until the placenta is expelled. The goal in the management of the third stage of labor is the prompt separation and expulsion of the placenta, achieved in the easiest, safest manner.

The placenta is attached to the decidual layer of the basal plate's thin endometrium by numerous fibrous anchor villi–much in the same way as a postage stamp is attached to a sheet of postage stamps. After the birth of the fetus, strong uterine contractions cause the placental site to shrink markedly. This causes the anchor villi to break and the placenta to separate from its attachments. Normally the first few strong contractions that occur 5 to 7 minutes after the baby's birth cause the placenta to be sheared away from the basal plate. A placenta cannot detach itself from a flaccid (relaxed) uterus because the placental site is not reduced in size.

Placental Separation and Expulsion

Placental separation is indicated by the following signs (Fig. 21-30):

- A firmly contracting fundus
- A change in the uterus from a discoid to a globular ovoid shape as the placenta moves into the lower uterine segment
- A sudden gush of dark blood from the introitus
- Apparent lengthening of the umbilical cord as the placenta descends to the introitus
- The finding of vaginal fullness (the placenta) on vaginal or rectal examination or of fetal membranes at the introitus

Depending on the preferences of the primary health care provider, an expectant or active approach may be used to manage the third stage of labor. Expectant management (watchful waiting) involves the natural, spontaneous separation and expulsion of the placenta by efforts of the mother with clamping and cutting of the cord after pulsation ceases. It may involve the use of gravity or nipple stimulation to facilitate separation and

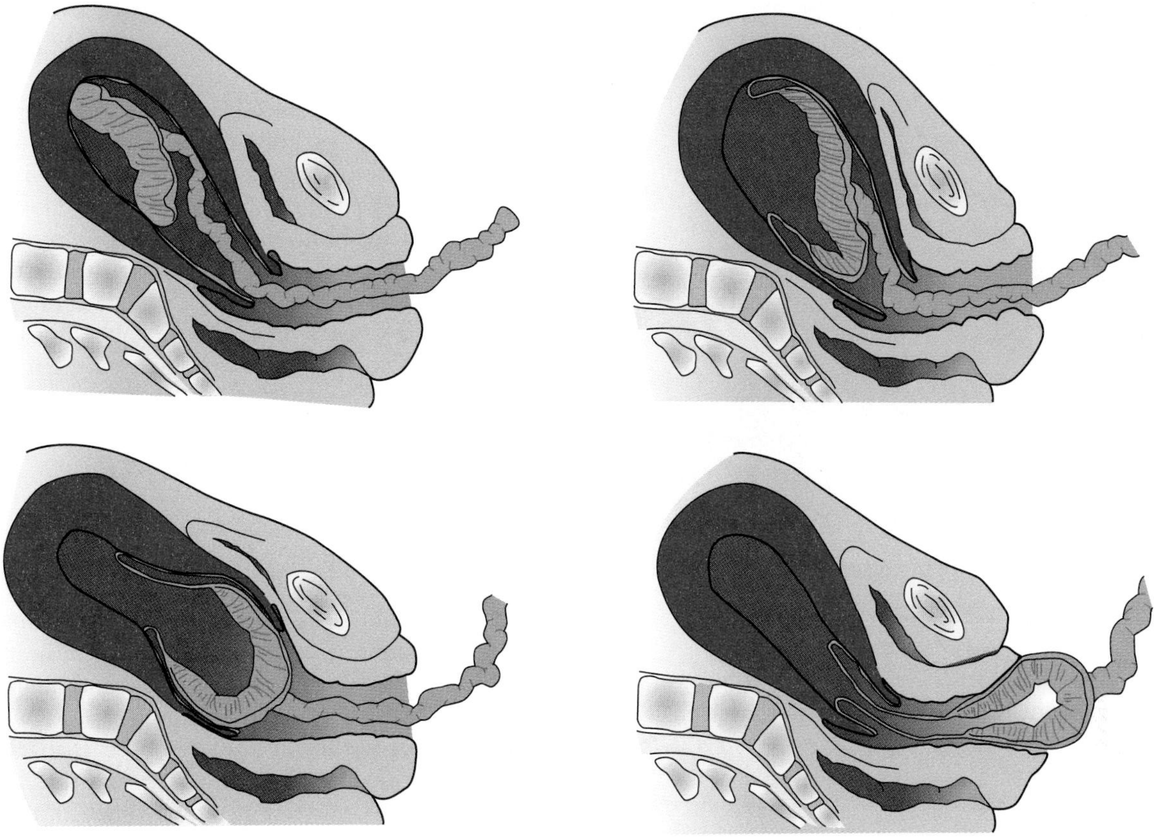
A
B
C
D

FIG. 21-30 Third stage of labor. **A,** Placenta begins to separate in central portion accompanied by retroplacental bleeding. Uterus changes from discoid to globular shape. **B,** Placenta completes separation and enters lower uterine segment. Uterus is globular shape. **C,** Placenta enters vagina, cord is seen to lengthen, and there may be an increase in bleeding. **D,** Expulsion (delivery) of placenta and completion of third stage.

expulsion, but no oxytocic (uterotonic) medications are given. A quiet, relaxed environment that supports close skin-to-skin contact between mother and newborn also promotes the release of endogenous oxytocin. Active management facilitates placenta separation and expulsion with administration of one or more oxytocic (uterotonic) medications after the birth of the anterior shoulder of the fetus, clamping and cutting of the umbilical cord immediately, and delivery of the placenta by application of controlled cord traction when signs of separation are noted. Research findings support the superiority of active management in terms of less blood loss and reduced risk of hemorrhage and other complications of the third stage of labor (Brucker, 2001; Prendiville, Elbourne, & McDonald, 2000; Rogers et al., 1998). Active management of the third stage of labor is a beneficial form of care (Enkin et al., 2000).

To assist in the delivery of the placenta, the woman is instructed to push when signs of separation have occurred. If possible, the placenta should be expelled by maternal effort during a uterine contraction. Alternate compression and elevation of the fundus, plus minimal, controlled traction on the umbilical cord, may be used to facilitate delivery of the placenta and amniotic membranes. Oxytocics may be administered after the placenta is removed because they stimulate the uterus to contract, thereby helping to prevent hemorrhage.

NURSE ALERT

If an oxytocic medication is ordered (e.g., 10 to 20 units of oxytocin [Pitocin] diluted in an IV solution, 10 units of Pitocin given as an intramuscular injection, or 0.2 mg of methylergonovine maleate [Methergine] injected intramuscularly), the nurse administers the medication in the dose, by the route, and at the time, indicated by the primary health care provider.

Whether the placenta first appears by its shiny fetal surface (Schultze mechanism) or turns to show its dark

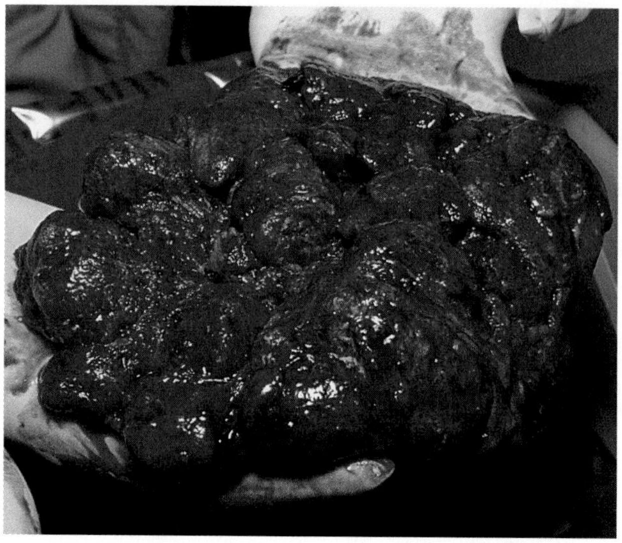

FIG. 21-31 Examination of the placenta. (Courtesy Michael S. Clement, MD, Mesa, AZ.)

roughened maternal surface first (Duncan mechanism) is of no clinical importance.

Collaborative Care

Placental Examination and Disposal

After the placenta and the amniotic membranes emerge, the primary health care provider examines them for intactness to ensure that no portion remains in the uterine cavity (i.e., no fragments of the placenta or membranes are retained) (Fig. 21-31).

Some women and their families may have culturally based beliefs regarding the care of the placenta and the manner of its disposal after birth, viewing the care and disposal of the placenta as a way of protecting the newborn from bad luck and illness. Requests by the woman to take the placenta home and dispose of it according to her customs may be at odds with health care agency policies, especially those related to infection control and the disposal of biologic wastes. Many cultures follow specific rules regarding the disposal of the placenta in terms of method (burning, drying, burying, eating), site for disposal (in or near the home), and timing of disposal (immediately after birth, time of day, astrologic signs). Disposal rituals may vary according to the gender of the child and the length of time before another child is desired. If eaten, the placenta can be a means of restoring a woman's well-being after birth or ensuring high-quality breast milk. Health care providers can provide culturally sensitive health care by encouraging women and their families to express their wishes regarding the care and disposal of the placenta and by establishing a policy to fulfill these requests (Choudhry, 1997; Howard & Berbiglia, 1997; Molina, 2001; Schneiderman, 1998).

Maternal Physical Status

Physiologic changes after birth are profound. The cardiac output increases rapidly as maternal circulation to the placenta ceases and the pooled blood from the lower extremities is mobilized. The pulse rate slows in response to the change in cardiac output and tends to remain slightly slower than the prepregnancy rate for approximately 1 week.

Soon after the birth, the woman's blood pressure usually returns to prepregnancy levels. Several factors contribute to an elevated blood pressure at this time: the excitement of the second stage, certain medications, and the time of day (blood pressure is highest during the late afternoon). Analgesics and anesthetics may cause hypotension to develop in the hour after birth.

Signs of Potential Problems

The major risk for women during the third stage of labor is postpartum hemorrhage. When the primary health care provider completes the delivery of the placenta, the nurse observes the mother for signs of excessive blood loss, including alteration in vital signs, pallor, light-headedness, restlessness, decreased urinary output, and alteration in level of consciousness and orientation.

Because of the rapid cardiovascular changes taking place (e.g., the increased intracranial pressure during pushing and the rapid increase in cardiac output), the risk of rupture of a preexisting cerebral aneurysm and the risk of formation of pulmonary emboli are greater than usual during this period. Another dangerous, unpredictable problem that may occur is the formation of an amniotic fluid embolism (see Chapter 36).

Women with a history of cardiac disorders are at increased risk for cardiac decompensation and pulmonary edema as a result of the circulatory changes associated with the birth of the fetus and expulsion of the placenta. The nurse should carefully assess the woman's respiratory pattern and effort, especially in the early postpartum period.

Nursing diagnoses that may be appropriate for the third stage of labor include the following:

- *Risk for infection related to*
  - –second-degree perineal laceration associated with birth
- *Anxiety related to*
  - –deficient knowledge regarding the separation and expulsion of the placenta
  - –the occurrence of perineal trauma and the need for repair
- *Compromised family coping related to*
  - –birth of infant whose gender was not preferred by the parents
  - –unexpected birth of an infant with serious congenital anomalies
- *Situational low self-esteem related to*
  - –perceived inability to meet personal expectations regarding performance during childbirth

Care After Placental Delivery

When the third stage is complete and any lacerations are repaired or an episiotomy is sutured, the vulvar area is gently cleansed with warm water or normal saline, and a perineal pad or an ice pack is applied to the perineum (some agencies or primary health care providers may require the use of sterile technique for perineal care immediately after birth). The birthing bed or table is repositioned, and the woman's legs are lowered simultaneously from the stirrups if she gave birth in a lithotomy position. Drapes are removed, and dry linen is placed under the woman's buttocks; she is provided with a clean gown and a blanket, which is warmed, if needed. She is assisted into her bed if she is to be transferred from the birthing area to the recovery area; assistance also is necessary to move the woman from the birthing table onto a bed if the woman has had anesthesia and does not have full use of her lower extremities. The side rails are raised during the transfer. She may be given the baby to hold during the transfer or the father or partner may carry the baby or transport it in a crib, either to the nursery or to the recovery area. If the woman labors, gives birth, and recovers in the same bed and room, she is refreshed following the protocol already described. Maternal and neonatal assessments for the fourth stage of labor are instituted. When fourth-stage recovery is complete, the woman may be transferred via wheelchair to a room on the postpartum unit. Box 21-9 summarizes normal vaginal childbirth.

Care of the Family During the Third Stage

Most parents enjoy being able to handle, hold, explore, and examine the baby immediately after birth. Both parents can assist with the thorough drying of the infant. The infant may be wrapped in a receiving blanket and placed on the woman's abdomen. If skin-to-skin contact is desired, the unwrapped infant may be placed on the woman's abdomen and then covered with a warm blanket.

Holding the newborn next to her skin helps the mother maintain the baby's body heat and provides skin-to-skin contact; care must be taken to keep the head warm. Stockinette caps are sometimes used to cover the newborn's head.

Many women wish to begin breastfeeding their newborns at this time to take advantage of the infant's alert state *(first period of reactivity)* and to stimulate the production of oxytocin that promotes contraction of the uterus. Others prefer to wait until the newborn, parents, and older siblings are together in the recovery area. In some cultures, breastfeeding is not considered acceptable until the milk comes in.

The woman usually feels some discomfort while the primary health care provider carries out the postbirth vaginal examination. The nurse can assist the woman to use breathing and relaxation or distraction techniques to assist her in dealing with the discomfort. During this time, the nurse assesses the newborn's physical condition; the baby can be weighed and measured, given eye prophylaxis and a vitamin K injection, given an identification bracelet, wrapped in warm blankets, and then given to the partner or back to the mother to hold when she is ready.

Family-Newborn Relationships

The woman's reaction to the sight of her newborn may range from excited outbursts of laughing, talking, and even crying to apparent apathy. A polite smile and nod may be her only acknowledgment of the comments of nurses and the primary health care provider. Occasionally the reaction is one of anger or indifference; the woman turns away from the baby, concentrates on her own pain, and sometimes makes hostile comments. These varied reactions can arise from pleasure, exhaustion, or deep disappointment. When evaluating parent-newborn interactions after birth, the nurse also should consider the cultural characteristics of the woman and her family and the expected behaviors of that culture. In some cultures, the birth of a male child is preferred, and women may grieve when a female child is born (Choudhry, 1997).

Whatever the reaction and its cause may be, the woman needs continuing acceptance and support from all staff. Notation regarding the parents' reaction to the newborn can be made in the recovery record. Nurses can assess this reaction by asking themselves such questions as, "How do the parents look?" "What do they say?" "What do they do?" Further assessment of the parent-newborn relationship can be conducted as care is given during the period of recovery. This is especially important if warning signs (e.g., passive or hostile reactions to the newborn, disappointment with sex or appearance of the newborn, absence of eye contact, or limited interaction of parents with each other) were noted immediately after birth. The nurse may find it helpful to discuss any warning signs that may have been noted with the woman's primary health care provider.

Siblings, who may have appeared only remotely interested in the final phases of the second stage, tend to experience renewed interest and excitement when the newborn appears. They can be encouraged to hold the baby (Fig. 21-32).

Parents usually respond to praise of their newborn. Many need to be reassured that the dusky appearance of their baby's extremities immediately after birth is normal until circulation is well established. If appropriate, the nurse should explain the reason for the molding of the newborn's head. Information about hospital routine can be communicated. It is important, however, for nurses to recognize that the cultural background of the parents may influence their expectations regarding the care and handling of their newborn immediately after birth. For example, some traditional Southeast Asians believe that the head should not be touched because it is the most

BOX 21-9 Normal Vaginal Childbirth

FIRST STAGE

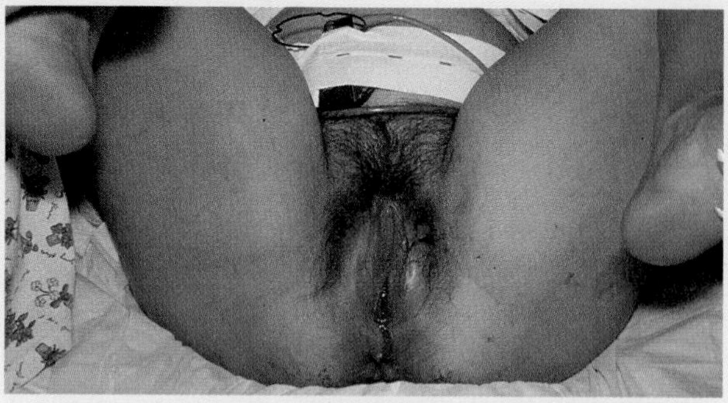

Anteroposterior slit. Vertex visible during contraction.

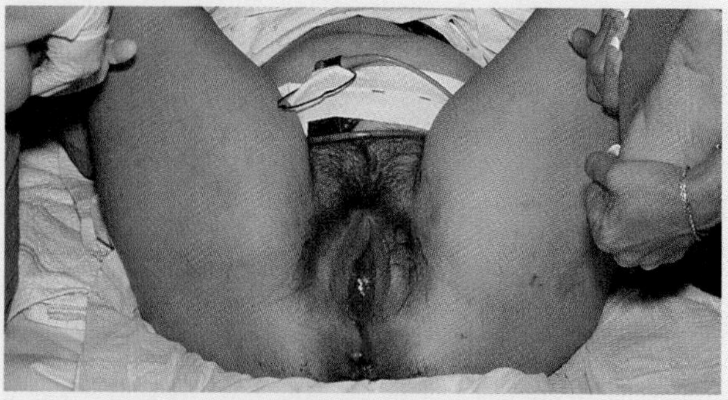

Oval opening. Vertex presenting. Note: nurse *(on left)* is wearing gloves but support person *(on right)* is not.

SECOND STAGE

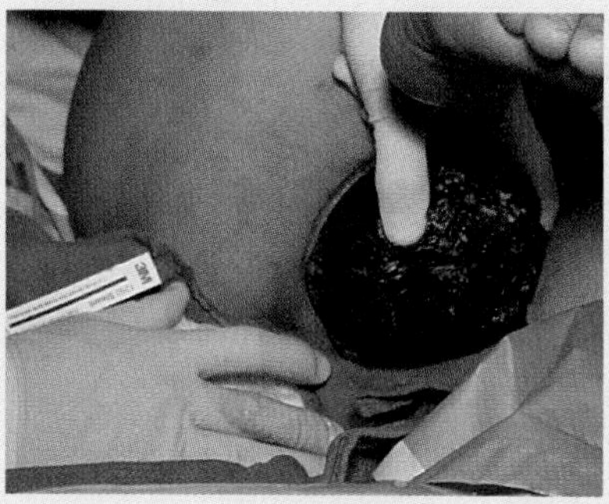

Crowning.

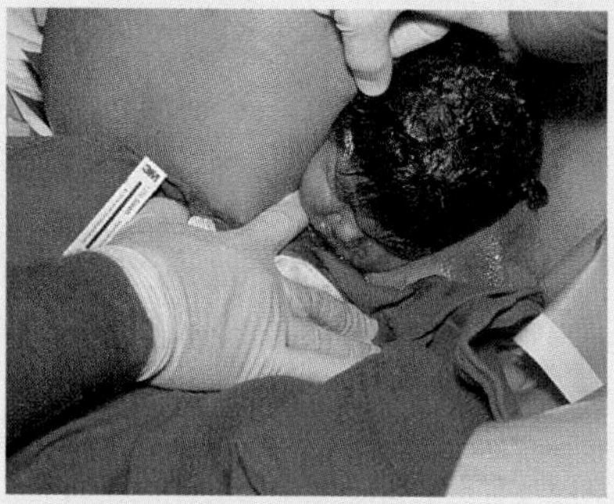

Nurse-midwife using Ritgen maneuver as head is born by extension.

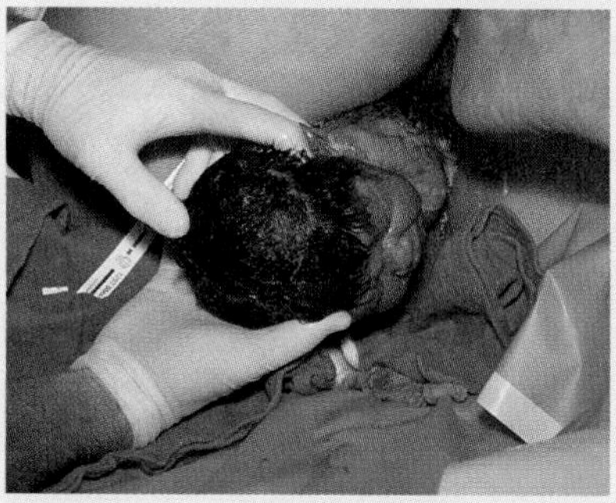

After nurse-midwife checks for nuchal cord, she supports head during external rotation and restitution.

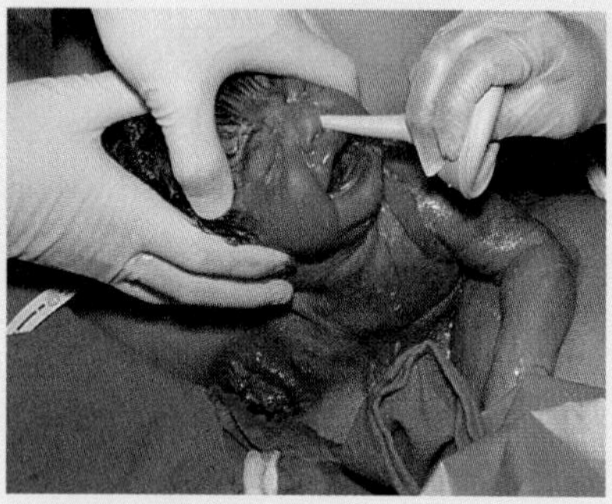

Use of bulb syringe to suction mucus.

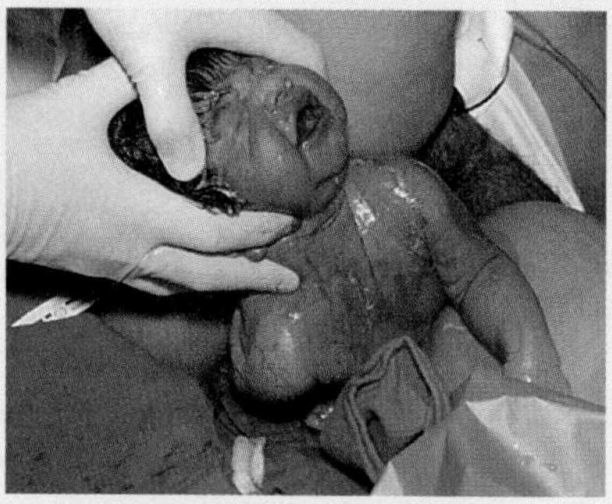

Birth of posterior shoulder.

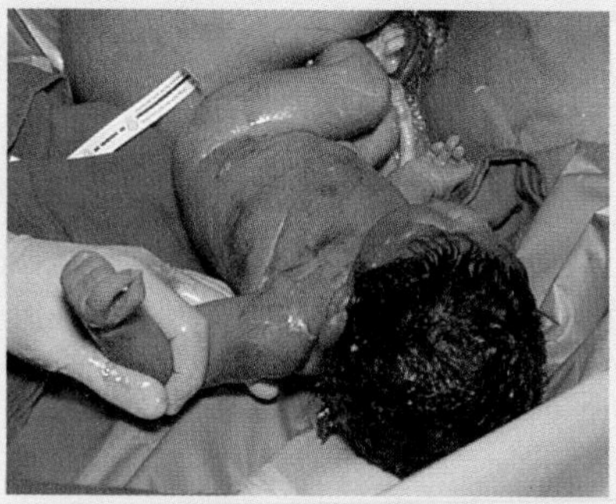

Birth of newborn by slow expulsion.

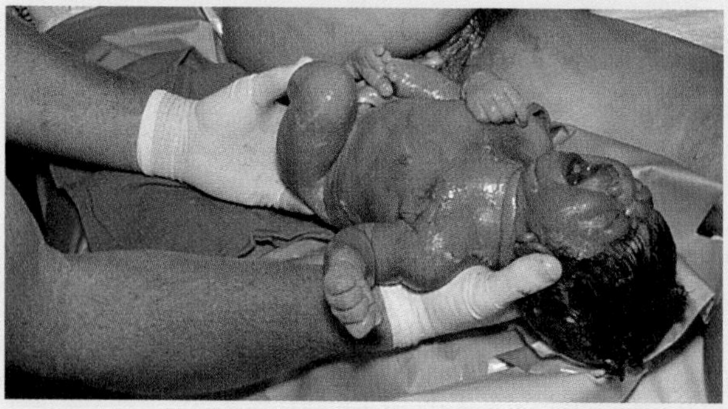

Second stage complete. Note that newborn is not completely pink yet.

Courtesy Michael S. Clement, MD, Mesa, AZ.

THIRD STAGE

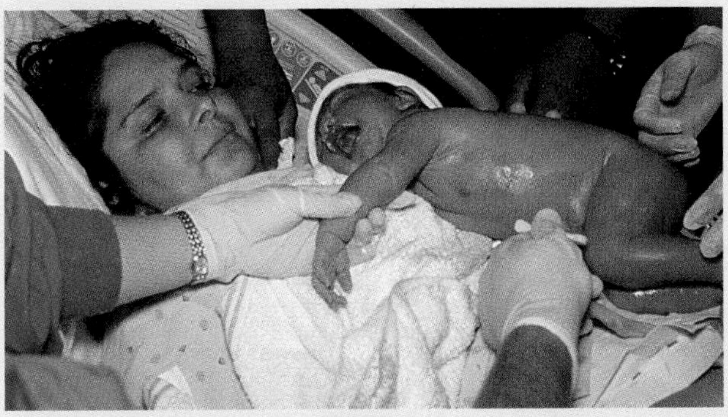

Newborn placed on mother's abdomen while cord is clamped and cut.

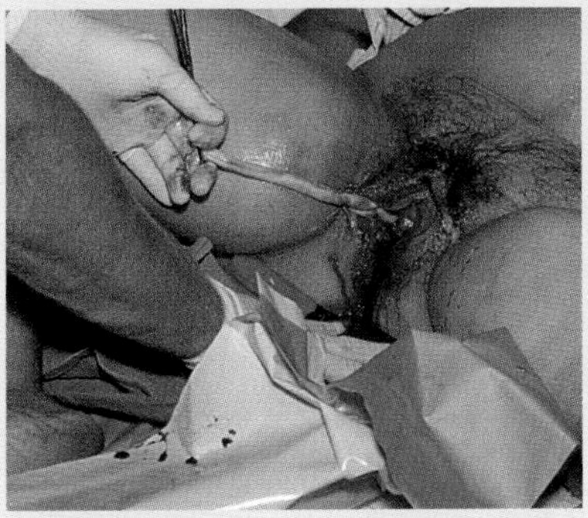

Note increased bleeding as placenta separates.

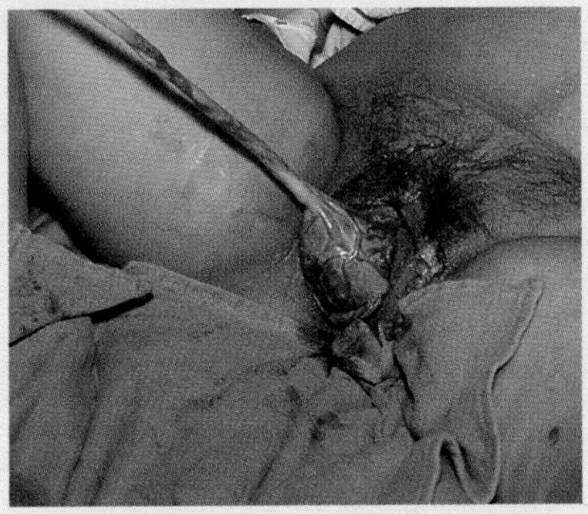

Expulsion of placenta.

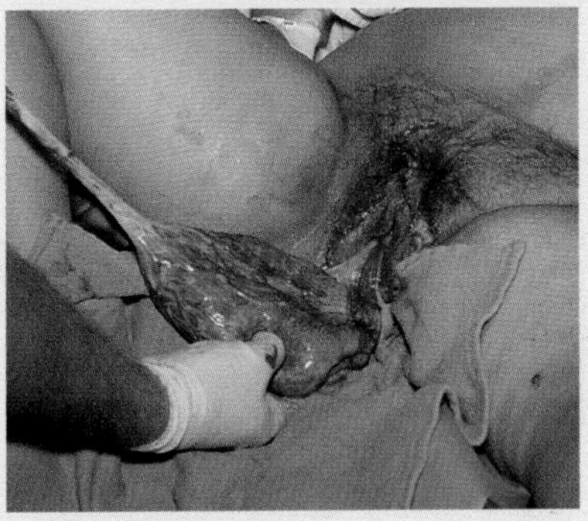

Expulsion is complete, marking the end of the third stage.

THE NEWBORN

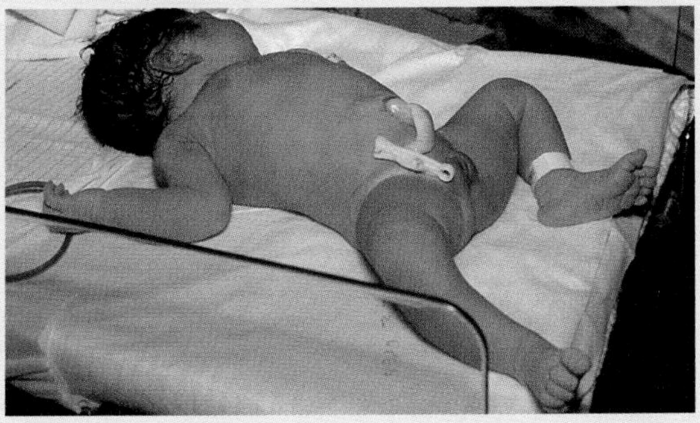

Newborn awaiting assessment. Note that color is almost completely pink.

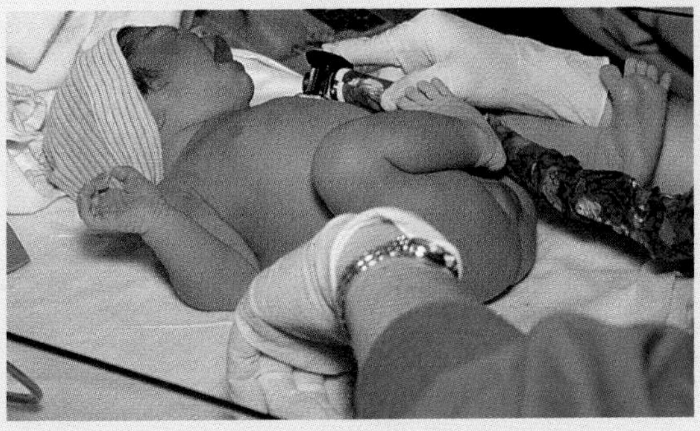

Newborn assessment under radiant warmer.

Parents admiring their newborn.

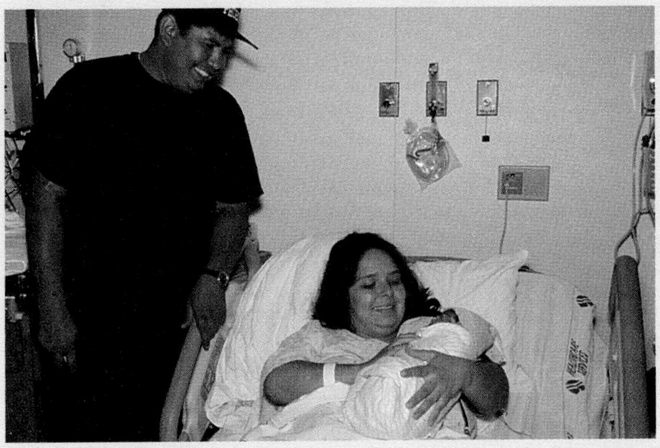

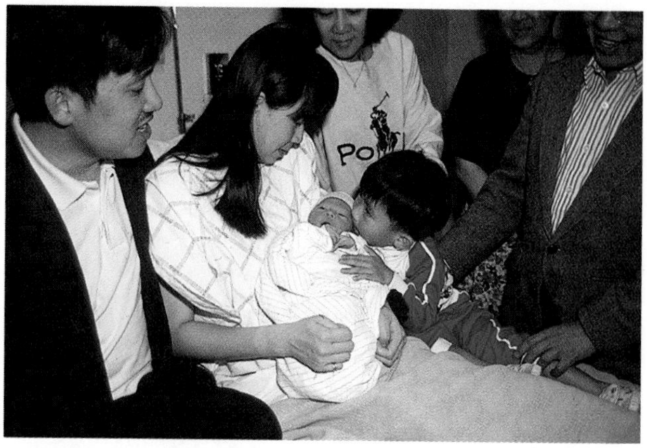

FIG. 21-32 Big brother becomes acquainted with new baby sister. (Courtesy Marjorie Pyle, RNC, Lifecircle, Costa Mesa, CA.)

sacred part of a person's body. They also believe that praise of the baby is dangerous because jealous spirits may then cause the baby harm or take it away (D'Avanzo & Geissler, 2003). Hospital staff members, by their interest and concern, can provide the environment for making this a satisfying experience for parents, family, and significant others.

Determining a woman's satisfaction with and impressions of her childbirth experience is a critical component in the provision of high-quality maternal-newborn health care that meets the individual needs of women and families using these services (Fowles, 1998; Young, 1998). In addition, reviewing the childbirth experience with someone who will listen, support, and explain has been found to reduce the degree of postpartum depression experienced by many women during the first week or so after birth (Wessely, 1998).

KEY POINTS

- The onset of labor may be difficult to determine for both nulliparous and multiparous women.
- The familiar environment of her home is most often the ideal place for a woman during the latent phase of the first stage of labor.
- The nurse assumes much of the responsibility for assessing the progress of labor and for keeping the primary health care provider informed about progress in labor and deviations from expected findings.
- The FHR and pattern reveal the fetal response to the stress of the labor process.
- Meconium-stained amniotic fluid is not always indicative of fetal distress associated with hypoxia.
- Assessment of the laboring woman's urinary output and bladder is critical to ensure her progress and to prevent injury to the bladder.
- Regardless of the actual labor and birth experience, the woman's or couple's perception of the birth experience is most likely to be positive when events and performances are consistent with expectations, especially in terms of maintaining control and adequacy of pain relief.
- The woman's level of anxiety may increase when she does not understand what is being said to her about her labor because of the medical terminology used or because of a language barrier.
- Coaching, emotional support, and comfort measures assist the woman to use her energy constructively in relaxing and working with the contractions.
- The progress of labor is enhanced when a woman changes her position frequently during the first stage of labor.
- Doulas provide a continuous supportive presence during labor that can have a positive effect on the process of childbirth and its outcome.
- The cultural beliefs and practices of a woman and her significant others, including her partner, can have a profound influence on their approach to labor and birth.
- The nurse who is aware of particular sociocultural aspects of helping and coping acts as an advocate or protective agent for the woman or couple during labor.
- The quality of the nurse-client relationship is a factor in the woman's ability to cope with the stressors of the labor process.
- Women with a history of sexual abuse often experience profound stress and anxiety during childbirth.
- Inability to palpate the cervix during vaginal examination indicates that complete effacement and full dilation have occurred and is the only certain, objective sign that the second stage has begun.
- Women may have an urge to bear down at various times during labor; for some it may be before the cervix is fully dilated, and for others, it may not occur until the active phase of the second stage of labor.
- When allowed to respond to the rhythmic nature of the second stage of labor, the woman normally changes body positions, bears down spontaneously, and vocalizes (open-glottis pushing) when she perceives the urge to push (Ferguson reflex).
- Women should bear down several times during a contraction using the open-glottis pushing method; sustained closed-glottis pushing should be avoided because oxygen transport to the fetus will be inhibited.
- Nurses can use the role of advocate to prevent routine use of episiotomy and to reduce the incidence of lacerations by empowering women to take an active role in their birth and educating health care providers about approaches to managing childbirth that reduce the incidence of perineal trauma.

KEY POINTS—cont'd

- Objective signs indicate that the placenta has separated and is ready to be expelled; excessive traction (pulling) on the umbilical cord, before the placenta has separated, can result in maternal injury.
- Siblings present for labor and birth need preparation and support for the event.
- Most parents/families enjoy being able to handle, hold, explore, and examine the baby immediately after the birth.
- Nurses should observe the progress in the development of parent-child relationships and be alert for warning signs that may appear during the immediate postpartum period.
- After an emergency childbirth out of the hospital, stimulation of the mother's nipple manually or by the infant's suckling stimulates the release of oxytocin from the maternal posterior pituitary gland; oxytocin stimulates the uterus to contract and thereby prevents hemorrhage.
- A woman benefits from reviewing her childbirth experience with the nurse who managed her care during the process of labor and birth.

CRITICAL THINKING EXERCISES

1. You have been asked to present a class to a group of pregnant adolescents. The topic of your class is, "Labor: how to know when it is starting and what to do when it does." Prepare a detailed outline of the content of your class and create teaching methods (e.g., role-playing scenarios, handouts, anatomic models, and illustrations) that reflect the developmental status of adolescents and ensure that these young women will arrive for assistance with their labor and birth at an appropriate time.
2. Imagine that you are the nurse manager of a Birthing Center that will open in 2 weeks. During the development of protocols for your center, you discover research studies that indicate that a woman's memories of her behavior and the events during childbirth linger for a long period and affect her future childbirth experiences. Devise a plan that would ensure that all women who give birth at your Birthing Center have the opportunity to form positive memories of their childbirth that will help rather than hinder future experiences.
3. You are a staff nurse on the labor and birth unit of a local hospital. After attending a nursing seminar related to evidence-based care during childbirth, you recognize that the care management of laboring women on your unit does not support a woman's need to take charge of her labor. Identify three changes that you would propose to give women the ability to maintain control of and to make decisions about their labor. Discuss the research evidence that supports each change that you propose. Outline the process that you would use as a catalyst for change on your unit.

RESOURCES

American College of Nurse Midwives
818 Connecticut Ave. NW, Suite 900
Washington, DC 20006
202-728-9860
www.midwife.org

Association of Labor Assistants and Childbirth Educators (ALACE)
P.O. Box 390436
Cambridge, MA 02139
617-441-2500
www.alace.org

Childbirth Graphics
P.O. Box 21207
Waco, TX 76702-1207
800-299-3366
www.childbirthgraphics.com

Childbirth Organization
www.childbirth.org

Coalition for Improving Maternity Services (CIMS)
c/o ASPO/Lamaze
1200 19th Street NW, S-300
Washington, DC 20036
www.clicked.com/babytime/index.html

Doulas of North America (DONA)
P.O. Box 626
Jasper, IN 47547
888-788-DONA
www.dona.com

Gentlebirth
www.gentlebirth.org

Global Maternal/Child Health Association and Waterbirth International
P.O. Box 1400
Wilsonville, OR 97070
503-673-0026
www.waterbirth.org

National Association of Parents and Professionals for Safe Alternatives in Childbirth (NAPSAC)
Route 4, Box 646
Marble Hill, MO 63764
573-238-2010
www.napsac.org

International Childbirth Education Association, Inc. (ICEA)
P.O. Box 20048
Minneapolis, MN 55420
952-854-8660
www.icea.org

Journal of Midwifery and Women's Health (formerly Journal of Nurse-Midwifery)
Elsevier Science, Inc.
655 Avenue of the Americas
New York, NY 10010
212-989-5800
www.elsevier.com

Journal of Perinatal and Neonatal Nursing
Aspen Publishers, Inc.
7201 McKinney Circle
Frederick, MD 21704
800-234-1660
www.aspenpublishers.com

Midwives Alliance of North America (MANA)
4805 Lawrenceville Hwy.
Suite 116-279
Lilburn, GA 30047
888-923-6262
www.mana.org

National Association of Childbearing Centers (NACC)
3123 Gottschall Road
Perkiomenville, PA 18074
215-234-8068
www.birthcenters.org

Online Birth Center (OBC)
www.moonlily.com/obc

REFERENCES

Albers, L. et al. (1996). Factors related to perineal trauma in childbirth. *Journal of Nurse Midwifery, 41*(4), 269-276.

Albers, L. et al. (1997). The relationship of ambulation in labor to operative delivery. *Journal of Nurse Midwifery, 42*(1), 4-8.

Arrabal, P., & Naegy, D. (1996). Is manual palpation of uterine contractions accurate? *American Journal of Obstetrics and Gynecology, 114*(1 pt 1), 217-219.

Austin, D., & Calderon, L. (1999). Triaging patients in the latent phase of labor. *Journal of Nurse Midwifery, 44*(6), 585-591.

Bergstrom, L. et al. (1997). "I gotta push. Please let me push." Social interactions during the change from first to second stage of labor. *Birth, 24*(3), 173-180.

Biancuzzo, M. (1993). Six myths of maternal posture during labor. *MCN American Journal of Maternal Child Nursing, 18*(5), 264-269.

Bloom, S. et al. (1998). Lack of effect of walking on labor and delivery. *New England Journal of Medicine, 339*(2), 76-79.

Brucker, M. (2001). Management of the third stage of labor: An evidence-based approach. *Journal of Midwifery and Women's Health, 46*(6), 381-392.

Bruner, J. et al. (1998). All-fours maneuver for reducing shoulder dystocia during labor. *Journal of Reproductive Medicine, 43*(5), 439-443.

Bryanton, J., Fraser-Davey, H., & Sullivan, P. (1994). Women's perception of nursing support during labor. *Journal of Obstetric, Gynecologic, and Neonatal Nursing, 23*(8), 638-644.

Callister, L. (1992). The meaning of the childbirth experience to the Mormon woman. *Journal of Perinatal Education, 1*(1), 50-57.

Callister, L. (1995). Cultural meanings of childbirth. *Journal of Obstetric, Gynecologic, and Neonatal Nursing, 24*(4), 327-331.

Callister, L., Vehvilainen-Julkunen, K., & Lauri, S. (1996). Cultural perceptions of childbirth. *Journal of Holistic Nursing, 14*(1), 66-78.

Carbonne, B. et al. (1996). Maternal position during labor: Effects on fetal oxygen saturation measured by pulse oximetry. *Obstetrics and Gynecology, 88*(5), 797-800.

Cesario, S. (1998). Should cameras be allowed in the delivery room? *MCN American Journal of Maternal Child Nursing, 23*(2), 87-91.

Chapman, L. (1992). Expectant father's roles during labor and birth. *Journal of Obstetric, Gynecologic, and Neonatal Nursing, 21*(2), 114-120.

Choudhry, U. (1997). Traditional practices of women from India: Pregnancy, childbirth, and newborn care. *Journal of Obstetric, Gynecologic, and Neonatal Nursing, 26*(5), 533-539.

CNM Data Group, 1996 (1999). Oral intake in labor: Trends in midwifery practice. *Journal of Nurse Midwifery, 44*(2), 135-138.

Cosner, K. (1996). Use of fundal pressure during second-stage labor: A pilot study. *Journal of Nurse Midwifery, 41*(4), 334-337.

Cosner, K., & deJong, E. (1993). Physiologic second-stage labor. *MCN American Journal of Maternal Child Nursing, 18*(1), 38-43.

D'Avanzo, C., & Geissler, E. (2003). *Pocket guide to cultural assessment* (3rd ed.). St. Louis: Mosby.

Davies, B., & Hodnett, E. (2002). Labor support: Nurses' self-efficacy and views about factors influencing implementation. *Journal of Obstetric, Gynecologic, and Neonatal Nursing, 31*(1), 48-56.

d'Entremont, M. (1996). Directed pushing in the second stage of labour. *Modern Midwife, 6*(6), 12-16.

De Sevo, M. (1997). Keeping the faith: Jewish traditions in pregnancy and childbirth. *AWHONN Lifelines, 1*(4), 46-49.

Enkin, M. et al. (2000). *A guide to effective care in pregnancy and childbirth* (3rd ed.). Oxford, New York: Oxford University Press.

Eriksson, M., Mattsson, L., & Ladfors, L. (1997). Early or late bath during the first stage of labour: A randomized study of 200 women. *Midwifery, 13*(3), 146-148.

Fowles, E. (1998). Labor concerns of women 2 months after delivery. *Birth, 25*(4), 235-240.

Gagnon, A., & Waghorn, K. (1999). One-to-one nurse labor support of nulliparous women stimulated with oxytocin. *Journal of Obstetric, Gynecologic, and Neonatal Nursing, 28*(4), 371-376.

Gannon, J. (1992). Delivery on the hands and knees: A case study approach. *Journal of Nurse Midwifery, 37*(1), 48-52.

Gupta, J., & Nikodem, V. (2000). Women's position during second stage of labor (Cochrane Review). *The Cochrane Library*, Issue 4, Oxford: Update Software.

Hanson, L. (1998a). Second stage positioning in nurse midwifery practices. Part 1: Position use and preferences. *Journal of Nurse Midwifery, 43*(5), 320-324.

Hanson, L. (1998b). Second stage positioning in nurse midwifery practices. Part 2: Factors affecting use. *Journal of Nurse Midwifery, 43*(5), 326-330.

Hanson, L., VandeVusse, L., & Harrod, K. (2001). The theater of birth: Scenes from women's scripts. *Journal of Perinatal and Neonatal Nursing, 15*(2), 18-35.

Heritage, C. (1998). Working with childhood sexual abuse survivors during pregnancy, labor, and birth. *Journal of Obstetric, Gynecologic, and Neonatal Nursing, 27*(6), 671-677.

Hill, V., Lowery, L., & Chez, R. (1998). Charting progress: Taking steps toward better documentation in the L&D. *AWHONN Lifelines, 2*(1), 43-46.

Hodnett, E. (1996). Nursing support of the laboring woman. *Journal of Obstetric, Gynecologic, and Neonatal Nursing, 25*(3), 257-264.

Hodnett, E. (2001). Caregiver support for women during childbirth (Cochrane Review). In *The Cochrane Library,* Issue 3, Oxford, UK: Update Software.

Howard, J., & Berbiglia, V. (1997). Caring for childbearing Korean women. *Journal of Obstetric, Gynecologic, and Neonatal Nursing, 26*(6), 665-671.

Hueston, W. (1996). Factors associated with the use of episiotomy during vaginal delivery. *Obstetrics and Gynecology, 87*(6), 1001-1005.

Kayne, M., Greulich, M., & Albers, L. (2001). Doulas: An alternative yet complementary addition to care during childbirth. *Clinical Obstetrics and Gynecology, 44*(4), 692-703.

Khazoyan, C., & Anderson, N. (1994). Latina's expectations for their partners during childbirth. *MCN American Journal of Maternal Child Nursing, 19*(4), 226-229.

Klaus, M. et al. (1992). Maternal assistance and support in labor: Father, nurse, midwife, or doula? *Clinical Consultations in Obstetrics and Gynecology, 4*(4), 211-217.

Klaus, M., Kennell, J., & Klaus, P. (1993). *Mothering the mother.* Redwood City, CA: Addison-Wesley.

Labrecque, M. et al. (1997). Association between median episiotomy and severe perineal lacerations in primiparous women. *Canadian Medical Association Journal, 156*(6), 797-802.

Landry, S. et al. (1998). The effects of doula support during labor on mother-infant interaction at 2 months. *Pediatric Research, 43,* 13A.

Lantican, L., & Corona, D. (1992). Comparison of the social support networks of Filipinos and Mexican American primigravidas. *Health Care for Women International, 13*(4), 329-338.

Lipson, J., Dibble, S., & Minarik, P. (1996). *Culture and nursing care: A pocket guide.* San Francisco: UCSF Nursing Press.

Lothian, J. (2001). Back to the future: Trusting birth. *Journal of Perinatal and Neonatal Nursing, 15*(3), 13-22.

Ludka, L., & Roberts, C. (1993). Eating and drinking in labor, a literature review. *Journal of Nurse Midwifery, 38*(4), 199-207.

Lydon-Rochelle, M., Albers, L., & Teaf, D. (1995). Perineal outcomes and nurse-midwifery management. *Journal of Nurse Midwifery, 40*(1), 13-18.

Mackey, M. (2001). Use of water in labor and birth. *Clinical Obstetrics and Gynecology, 44*(4), 733-749.

Maier, J., & Maloni, J. (1997). Nurse advocacy for selective versus routine episiotomy. *Journal of Obstetric, Gynecologic, and Neonatal Nursing, 26*(2), 155-161.

Mattson, S. (2000). Working toward cultural competence: Making first steps through cultural assessment. *AWHONN Lifelines, 4*(4), 41-43.

Mayberry, L. et al. (2000). *Second stage labor management: Promotion of evidence-based practice and a collaborative approach to patient care.* Washington, D.C.: Association of Women's Health, Obstetric, and Neonatal Nurses.

McCandlish, R. (2001). Perineal trauma: Prevention and treatment. *Journal of Midwifery and Women's Health, 46*(6), 396-401.

McGuinnes, M., Norr, K., & Nacion, K. (1991). Comparison between different perineal outcomes on tissue healing. *Journal of Nurse Midwifery, 36*(3), 192-198.

McKay, S., & Barrows, T. (1991). Holding back: Maternal readiness to give birth. *MCN American Journal of Maternal Child Nursing, 16*(5), 250-254.

McKay, S., & Smith, S. (1993). "What are they talking about? Is something wrong?" Information sharing during the second stage of labor. *Birth, 20*(3), 142-147.

Melender, H. (2002). Experiences of fears associated with pregnancy and childbirth: A study of 329 pregnant women. *Birth, 29*(2), 101-111.

Miltner, R. (2000). Identifying labor support actions of intrapartum nurses. *Journal of Obstetric, Gynecologic, and Neonatal Nursing, 29*(5), 491-499.

Miltner, R. (2002). More than support: Nursing interventions provided to women in labor. *Journal of Obstetric, Gynecologic, and Neonatal Nursing, 31*(6), 753-761.

Minato, J. (2000). Is it time to push? Examining rest in second-stage labor. *AWHONN Lifelines, 4*(6), 20-23.

Molina, J. (2001). Traditional Native American practices in obstetrics. *Clinical Obstetrics and Gynecology, 44*(4), 661-670.

Naef, R., & Morrison, J. (1994). Guidelines for the management of shoulder dystocia. *Journal of Perinatology, 14*(6), 435-441.

Nichols, F. (1996). The meaning of the childbirth experience: A review of the literature. *Journal of Perinatal Education, 5*(4), 71-77.

Nichols, M. (1993). Paternal perspectives of the childbirth experience. *Maternal Child Nursing Journal, 21*(3), 99-108.

Odent, M. (1997). Can water immersion stop labor? *Journal of Nurse Midwifery, 42*(5), 414-416.

Olson, S. (1998). Bedside musical care: Applications in pregnancy, childbirth, and neonatal care. *Journal of Obstetric, Gynecologic, and Neonatal Nursing, 27*(5), 569-575.

Paciornik, M. (1990). Commentary: Arguments against episiotomy and in favor of squatting for birth. *Birth, 17*(2), 104-105.

Perez, P. (1998). *Using the Gymnastik Ball in pregnancy, labor, birth, and postpartum.* Katy, TX: Cutting Edge Press.

Perez, P., & Herrick, L. (1998). Doulas: Exploring their roles with parents, hospitals, and nurses. *AWHONN Lifelines, 2*(2), 54-55.

Peterson, L., & Besuner, P. (1997). Pushing techniques during labor: Issues and controversies. *Journal of Obstetric, Gynecologic, and Neonatal Nursing, 26*(6), 719-726.

Piper, D., & McDonald, P. (1994). Management of anticipated and actual shoulder dystocia. *Journal of Nurse Midwifery, 39*(2 suppl), 91S-105S.

Prendiville, W., Elbourne, D., & McDonald, S. (2000). Active versus expectant management in the third stage of labour. *Cochrane Database System Review* (2), CD000007.

Proctor, S. (1998). What determines quality in maternity care? Comparing the perceptions of childbearing women and midwives. *Birth, 25*(2), 85-93.

Pugh, L. et al. (1998). First stage of labor management: An examination of patterned breathing and fatigue. *Birth, 25*(4), 241-245.

Renfrew, M. et al. (1998). Practices that minimize trauma to the genital tract in childbirth: A systematic review of the literature. *Birth, 25*(3), 143-160.

Rhodes, N., & Hutchinson, S. (1994). Labor experiences of childhood sexual abuse survivors. *Birth, 21*(4), 213-220.

Roberts, J. (2002). The "push" for evidence: Management of the second stage. *Journal of Midwifery and Women's Health, 47*(1), 2-15.

Rogers, J. et al. (1998). Active versus expectant management of third stage labour: The Hinchingbrooke randomized controlled trial. *Lancet, 351*(9104), 693-699.

Sampselle, C., & Hines, S. (1999). Research exchange: Spontaneous pushing during birth: Relationship to perineal outcomes. *Journal of Nurse Midwifery, 44*(1), 36-39.

Sauls, D. (2002). Effects of labor support on mothers, babies, and birth outcomes. *Journal of Obstetric, Gynecologic, and Neonatal Nursing, 31*(6), 733-741.

Scheepers, H. et al (2001). Eating and drinking in labor: The influence of caregiver advice on women's behavior. *Birth, 28*(2), 119-123.

Schneiderman, J. (1998). Rituals of placenta disposal. *MCN American Journal of Maternal Child Nursing, 23*(3), 142-143.

Scott, J. et al. (1999). *Danforth's obstetrics and gynecology* (8th ed.). Philadelphia: Lippincott Williams & Wilkins.

Scott, K., Berkowitz, G., & Klaus, M. (1999). A comparison of intermittent and continuous support during labor: A meta-analysis. *American Journal of Obstetrics and Gynecology, 180,* 1054-1059.

Shermer, R., & Raines, D. (1997). Positioning during the second stage of labor: Moving back to basics. *Journal of Obstetric, Gynecologic, and Neonatal Nursing, 26*(6), 727-734.

Shorten, A., Donsante, J., & Shorten, B. (2002). Birth position, accoucheur, and perineal outcomes: Informing women about choices for vaginal birth. *Birth, 29*(1), 18-27.

Simkin, P., & Ancheta, R. (2000). *The labor progress handbook.* Malden, MA: Blackwell Science.

Simkin, P., & Way, K. (1998). *Doulas of North America Position Paper: The doula's contribution to modern maternity care.* Seattle: DONA.

Thomson, A. (1993). Pushing techniques in the second stage of labour. *Journal of Advanced Nursing, 18*(2), 171-177.

Tomlinson, P., & Bryan, A. (1996). Family centered intrapartum care: Revisiting an old concept. *Journal of Obstetric, Gynecologic, and Neonatal Nursing, 25*(4), 331-337.

Trowell, J. (1993). Emergency cesarean section: A research study of the mother/child relationship of a group of women admitted expecting a normal vaginal delivery. *Child Abuse and Neglect, 7,* 387-394.

Tucker, S. (2000). *Pocket guide to fetal monitoring* (4th ed.). St. Louis: Mosby.

Tumblin, A., & Simkin, P. (2001). Pregnant women's perception of their nurse's role during labor and delivery. *Birth, 28*(1), 52-56.

Varney, H. (1997). *Varney's midwifery* (3rd ed.). Sudbury, MA: Jones & Bartlett.

Waldenström, U. et al. (1996). The childbirth experience: A study of 295 new mothers. *Birth, 23*(3), 144-153.

Waymire, V. (1997). A triggering time: Childbirth may recall sexual abuse memories. *AWHONN Lifelines, 1*(2), 47-50.

Weber, S. (1996). Cultural aspects of pain in childbearing women. *Journal of Obstetric, Gynecologic, and Neonatal Nursing, 25*(1), 67-72.

Weeks, J., & Kozak, L. (2001). Trends in the use of episiotomy in the United States: 1980-1998. *Birth, 28*(3), 152-160.

Wessely, S. (1998). Commentary: Reducing distress after normal childbirth. *Birth, 25*(4), 220-221.

Woods, A. (1991). Nurse midwifery in rural Pakistan. *Journal of Nurse Midwifery, 36*(4), 249-252.

Woolley, R. (1995). Benefits and risks of episiotomy: A review of the English-language literature since 1980: Part I and part II. *Obstetrical and Gynecological Survey, 50*(11), 806-835.

Young, D. (1998). First class delivery: The importance of asking women what they think about their maternity care. *Birth, 25*(2), 71-72.

Zhang, J. et al. (1996). Continuous labor support from labor attendant for primiparous women: A meta-analysis. *Obstetrics and Gynecology, 88*(4), 739-744.

Zwelling, E., & Phillips, C. (2001). Family-centered maternity care in the new millennium: Is it real or is it imagined? *Journal of Perinatal and Neonatal Nursing, 15*(3), 1-12.

CHAPTER 22

Kitty Cashion

Postpartum Physiology

http://evolve.elsevier.com/Lowdermilk/MatWmnHlth/

LEARNING OBJECTIVES

- Describe the anatomic and physiologic changes that occur during the postpartum period.
- Identify characteristics of uterine involution and lochial flow and describe ways to measure them.
- Compare expected values for vital signs and blood pressure, deviations from normal findings, and probable causes of the deviations.

The postpartum period is the interval between the birth of the newborn and the return of the reproductive organs to their normal nonpregnant state. This period is sometimes referred to as the puerperium, or fourth trimester of pregnancy. Although the puerperium has traditionally been considered to last 6 weeks, this time frame varies among women. The physiologic changes that occur as the processes of pregnancy are reversed, although distinctive, are considered normal. Many factors, including the mother's energy level and degree of comfort, the health of the newborn, and the care and encouragement given by health professionals, contribute to the mother's response to her infant during this time. To provide care during the recovery period that is beneficial to the mother, her infant, and her family, the nurse must synthesize knowledge of maternal anatomy and physiology, the newborn's physical and behavioral characteristics, infant care activities, and the family response to the birth of the child. This chapter focuses on anatomic and physiologic changes that occur in the woman during the postpartum period.

REPRODUCTIVE SYSTEM AND ASSOCIATED STRUCTURES

Uterus

Involution Process

The return of the uterus to a nonpregnant state after birth is known as **involution.** This process begins immediately after expulsion of the placenta with contraction of the uterine smooth muscle.

At the end of the third stage of labor, the uterus is in the midline, about 2 cm below the level of the umbilicus, with the fundus resting on the sacral promontory. At this time, the uterus weighs about 1000 g.

Within 12 hours, the fundus may be approximately 1 cm above the umbilicus (Fig. 22-1). By 24 hours postpartum, the uterus is about the same size it was at 20 weeks' gestation (Resnik, 1999). Involution progresses rapidly during the next few days. The fundus descends about 1 to 2 cm every 24 hours. By the sixth postpartum day, the fundus is normally located halfway between the symphysis pubis and the umbilicus. Within 2 weeks after childbirth, the uterus once again lies in the true pelvis.

The uterus, which at full term is approximately 11 times its prepregnancy weight, involutes to about 500 grams by 1 week after birth and 350 g by 2 weeks after birth. At 6 weeks it has returned to its nonpregnant size of 50 to 60 g (see Fig. 22-1).

Increased estrogen and progesterone levels are responsible for stimulating the massive growth of the uterus during pregnancy. Prenatal uterine growth is the result of both hyperplasia, an increase in the number of muscle cells, and hypertrophy, enlargement of the existing cells. Postpartally the decrease in the secretion of these hormones causes **autolysis,** which is the self-destruction of excess hypertrophied tissue. The additional cells laid down during pregnancy remain, however, and account for the fact that uterine size increases slightly after each pregnancy.

Subinvolution is the failure of the uterus to return to a nonpregnant state. The most common causes of subinvolution are retained placental fragments and infection.

A

B

C

D

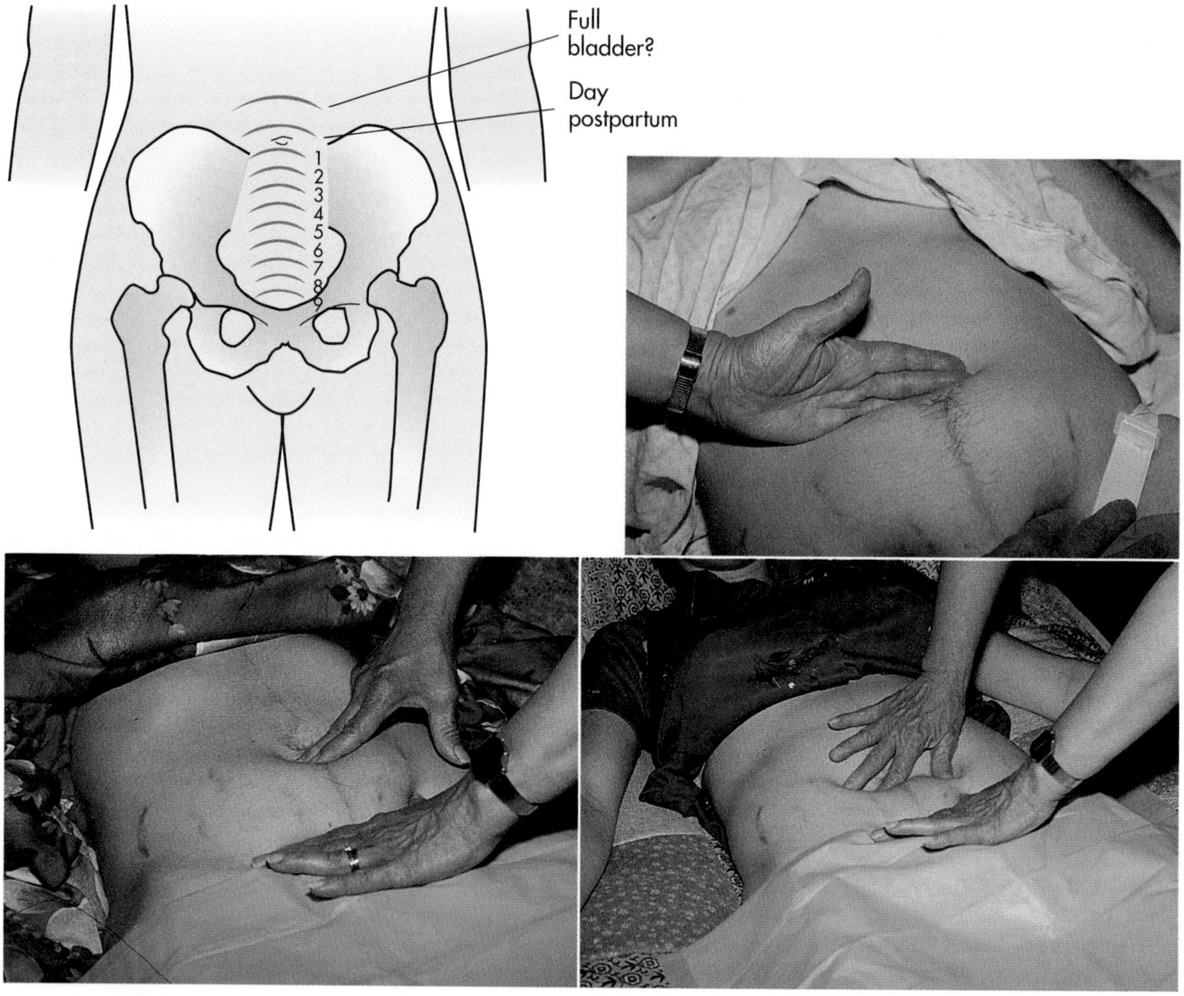
Full
bladder?
Day
postpartum
1
2
3
4
5
6
7
8
9

FIG. 22-1 Assessment of involution of uterus after childbirth. **A,** Normal progress, days 1 through 9. **B,** Size and position of uterus 2 hours after childbirth. **C,** Two days after childbirth. **D,** Four days after childbirth. (**B, C,** and **D** courtesy Marjorie Pyle, RNC, Lifecircle, Costa Mesa, CA.)

Contractions

Postpartum hemostasis is achieved primarily by compression of intramyometrial blood vessels as the uterine muscle contracts, rather than by platelet aggregation and clot formation. The hormone oxytocin, which is released from the pituitary gland, strengthens and coordinates these uterine contractions, which compress blood vessels and thereby promote hemostasis. During the first 1 to 2 postpartum hours, uterine contractions may decrease in intensity and become uncoordinated. Because it is vital that the uterus remain firm and well contracted, exogenous oxytocin (Pitocin) is usually administered intravenously or intramuscularly immediately after expulsion of the placenta. Mothers who plan to breastfeed may be encouraged to put the baby to breast immediately after birth as well, because suckling stimulates the release of oxytocin.

Afterpains

In first-time mothers, uterine tone is increased, so the fundus generally remains firm. Periodic relaxation and vigorous contraction are more common in subsequent pregnancies and may cause uncomfortable cramping called **afterpains** (afterbirth pains) that persist throughout the early puerperium. Afterpains are more noticeable after births in which the uterus was greatly distended (e.g., a large baby, multifetal gestation). Breastfeeding and exogenous oxytocic medication usually cause these afterpains to intensify, because both stimulate uterine contractions.

Placental Site

Immediately after the placenta and membranes are expelled, vascular constriction and thrombosis cause the placental site to be reduced to an irregular nodular and elevated area.

Upward growth of the endometrium causes the sloughing of necrotic tissue and prevents the scar formation characteristic of normal wound healing. This unique healing process enables the endometrium to resume its usual cycle of changes and to permit implantation and placentation in future pregnancies. Endometrial regeneration is completed by postpartum day 16, except at the placental site (Resnik, 1999). Regeneration at the placental site usually is not complete until 6 weeks after birth.

Lochia

Postchildbirth uterine discharge, commonly called **lochia,** is initially bright red, changing later to a pinkish red or reddish brown. It may contain small clots of blood.

For the first 2 hours after birth, the amount of uterine discharge should be about that of a heavy menstrual period. After that time, the lochial flow should steadily decrease.

Lochia rubra consists mainly of blood and decidual and trophoblastic debris. The flow pales, becoming pink or brown after 3 to 4 days (lochia serosa). **Lochia serosa** consists of old blood, serum, leukocytes, and tissue debris. The median duration of lochia serosa discharge is 22 to 27 days (Bowes & Katz, 2002). In most women, about 10 days after childbirth, the drainage becomes yellow to white (lochia alba). **Lochia alba** consists of leukocytes, decidua, epithelial cells, mucus, serum, and bacteria. Lochia alba may continue to drain from the vaginal opening for up to and beyond 6 weeks after childbirth (Visness, Kennedy, & Ramos, 1997).

It is difficult to judge the amount of lochial flow based only on observation of perineal pads (see Chapter 23). Any estimation of lochial flow is inaccurate and incomplete without considering the time factor. For example, the woman who saturates a peripad in 1 hour or less is bleeding much more than the woman who saturates a peripad in 8 hours.

If the woman receives an oxytocic medication, regardless of the route of administration, the flow of lochia is usually scant until the effects of the medication wear off. The amount of lochia is usually less after cesarean births. The flow of lochia usually increases with ambulation and breastfeeding. Lochia tends to pool in the vagina when the woman is lying in bed; the woman may then experience a gush of blood when she stands. This gush should not be confused with hemorrhage.

Persistence of lochia rubra early in the postpartum period suggests continued bleeding as a result of retained fragments of the placenta or membranes. Recurrence of bleeding 7 to 14 days after birth is from the healing placental site. About 10% to 15% of women will still be experiencing normal lochia serosa discharge at their 6-week postpartum examination (Bowes & Katz, 2002). In the majority of women, however, the continued flow of lochia serosa or lochia alba by 3 to 4 weeks after birth may indicate endometritis, particularly if this is accompanied by fever, pain, or abdominal tenderness. Lochia should smell like normal menstrual flow; an offensive odor usually indicates infection.

It is important to remember that not all postpartal vaginal bleeding is necessarily lochia. Another common source of vaginal bleeding after birth is unrepaired vaginal or cervical lacerations. Table 22-1 distinguishes between lochial and nonlochial bleeding.

TABLE 22-1 **Lochial and Nonlochial Bleeding**

LOCHIAL BLEEDING	NONLOCHIAL BLEEDING
Lochia usually trickles from the vaginal opening. The steady flow is greater as the uterus contracts.	If the bloody discharge spurts from the vagina, there may be cervical or vaginal tears in addition to the normal lochia.
A gush of lochia may result as the uterus is massaged. If it is dark, it has been pooled in the relaxed vagina; the amount soon lessens to a trickle of bright red lochia (in the early puerperium).	If the amount of bleeding continues to be excessive and bright red, a cervical or vaginal tear may be the source.

Cervix

The cervix is soft immediately after birth. Within 2 to 3 postpartum days, however, it has shortened, become firm, and regained its form (Resnik, 1999). The cervix up to the lower uterine segment remains edematous, thin, and fragile for several days after birth. The ectocervix (that portion of the cervix that protrudes into the vagina) appears bruised and has some small lacerations, constituting an optimal condition for the development of infection. The cervical os, which is dilated to 10 cm during labor, closes gradually. It may still be possible to introduce two fingers into the cervical os for the first 4 to 6 postpartum days; however, only the smallest curette may be introduced by the end of 2 weeks. The external cervical os never regains its prepregnancy appearance; it is no longer shaped like a circle but appears as a jagged slit often described as a "fish mouth." Lactation delays the production of cervical and other estrogen-influenced mucus and mucosal characteristics.

Vagina and Perineum

The estrogen deprivation that occurs after the birth is responsible for causing the thinness of the vaginal mucosa and the absence of rugae. The greatly distended, smooth-walled vagina gradually returns to its prepregnancy size by

6 to 10 weeks after childbirth (Resnik, 1999). Rugae reappear within 3 weeks, although they are never as prominent as they are in the nulliparous woman. Most rugae may be permanently flattened. The mucosa remains atrophic in the lactating woman, at least until menstruation begins again. Thickening of the vaginal mucosa occurs with the return of ovarian function. The reduced estrogen levels also are responsible for causing a decreased amount of vaginal lubrication. Localized dryness and coital discomfort (dyspareunia) may persist until ovarian function returns and menstruation resumes. Use of a water-soluble lubricant that can help reduce discomfort during intercourse is usually recommended.

Initially the introitus is erythematous and edematous, especially in the area of the episiotomy or laceration repair. It is usually barely distinguishable from that of a nulliparous woman, however, if lacerations and an episiotomy have been carefully repaired, hematomas are prevented or treated early, and the woman observes good hygiene during the first 2 weeks after birth.

Most episiotomies are visible only if the woman is lying on her side with her buttock raised or if she is placed in the lithotomy position. A good light source is essential for visualization of some episiotomies. An episiotomy heals the same way as any surgical incision. Signs of infection (pain, redness, warmth, swelling, or discharge) or the loss of approximation (separation of the incision edges) may occur. Healing should occur within 2 to 3 weeks.

Hemorrhoids (anal varicosities) are commonly seen. Women often experience associated symptoms such as itching, discomfort, and bright red bleeding with defecation. Hemorrhoids usually decrease in size within 6 weeks of childbirth.

Pelvic Muscular Support

The supporting structure of the uterus and vagina may be injured during childbirth and may contribute to gynecologic problems later. The supportive tissues of the pelvic floor that are torn or stretched during childbirth may require up to 6 months to regain tone. Women are often encouraged to do Kegel exercises (p. 125) after birth to help strengthen perineal muscles and promote healing. The term **pelvic relaxation** refers to the lengthening and weakening of the fascial supports of pelvic structures. These structures include the uterus, upper posterior vaginal wall, urethra, bladder, and rectum. Although pelvic relaxation can occur in any woman, it is usually a direct but delayed complication of childbirth (see Chapter 12).

ENDOCRINE SYSTEM

Placental Hormones

Significant hormonal changes occur during the postpartal period. Expulsion of the placenta results in dramatic decreases of the hormones produced by that organ. Decreases in human chorionic somatomammotropin (hCS; also called human placental lactogen [hPL]), estrogens, cortisol, and the placental enzyme insulinase cause the diabetogenic effects of pregnancy to be reversed, resulting in significantly lower blood sugar levels in the immediate puerperium. Mothers with type 1 diabetes will thus be likely to require much less insulin for several days after birth. Because these normal hormonal changes make the puerperium a transitional period for carbohydrate metabolism, it is more difficult to interpret the results of glucose tolerance tests at this time.

Estrogen and progesterone levels decrease markedly after expulsion of the placenta, reaching their lowest levels 1 week into the postpartum period. Decreased estrogen levels are associated with breast engorgement and with the diuresis of excess extracellular fluid that has accumulated during pregnancy. The estrogen levels in nonlactating women begin to increase by 2 weeks after birth and are higher by postpartum day 17 than in women who breastfeed (Bowes & Katz , 2002).

Pituitary Hormones and Ovarian Function

Lactating and nonlactating women differ considerably in the time of the first ovulation and the reestablishment of menstruation. The persistence of elevated serum prolactin levels in breastfeeding women appears to be responsible for suppressing ovulation. Because levels of follicle-stimulating hormone (FSH) have been shown to be identical in lactating and nonlactating women, it is thought that ovulation is suppressed in lactating women because the ovary does not respond to FSH stimulation when increased prolactin levels are present (Bowes & Katz, 2002).

Prolactin levels in blood increase progressively throughout pregnancy. In women who breastfeed, prolactin levels remain elevated into the sixth week after birth (Bowes & Katz, 2002). Serum prolactin levels are influenced by the frequency of breastfeeding, the duration of each feeding, and the degree to which supplementary feedings are used. The individual differences in the strength of the infant's sucking stimulus probably also affect prolactin levels. This emphasizes the fact that breastfeeding is not a reliable form of birth control. After birth, prolactin levels decline in nonlactating women, reaching the prepregnant range by the third postpartum week (Bowes & Katz, 2002).

Ovulation occurs as early as 27 days after birth in nonlactating women, with a mean time of about 70 to 75 days (Bowes & Katz, 2002). About 70% of nonbreastfeeding women resume menstruating by 3 months after birth (Resnik, 1999). The mean time to ovulation in women who breastfeed is about 6 months (Bowes & Katz, 2002), although women who breastfeed for less than 28 days will ovulate at about the same time as women who do not breastfeed at all (Resnik, 1999). In lactating women, both the resumption of ovulation and the return of menses are determined in large part by breastfeeding patterns (Resnik, 1999). The fact that many women ovulate before their first postpartum menstrual period occurs reemphasizes the need for discussion of contraceptive options early in the puerperium (Rebar, 1999).

The first menstrual flow after childbirth is usually heavier than normal. Within three to four cycles, the amount of menstrual flow has returned to the woman's prepregnant volume.

ABDOMEN

When the woman stands during the first days after birth, her abdominal muscles protrude and give her a still-pregnant appearance. During the first 2 weeks after birth, the abdominal wall is relaxed. It takes approximately 6 weeks for the abdominal wall to return almost to its prepregnancy state. The skin regains most of its previous elasticity, but some striae may persist. The return of muscle tone depends on previous tone, proper exercise, and the amount of adipose tissue. Occasionally, with or without overdistention because of a large fetus or multiple fetuses, the abdominal wall muscles separate, a condition termed **diastasis recti abdominis** (see Fig. 14-13). Persistence of this defect may be disturbing to the woman, but surgical correction is rarely necessary. With time, the defect becomes less apparent.

URINARY SYSTEM

The hormonal changes of pregnancy (i.e., high steroid levels) may be partly responsible for causing an increase in renal function, whereas the diminishing steroid levels after birth may partly explain the reduced renal function that occurs during the puerperium. Kidney function returns to normal within a month after birth. About 2 to 8 weeks is required for the pregnancy-induced hypotonia and dilation of the ureters and renal pelves to return to the prepregnant state (Cunningham et al., 2001). In a small percentage of women, dilation of the urinary tract may persist for 3 months, which increases the chance for the development of a urinary tract infection.

Urine Components

The renal glycosuria induced by pregnancy disappears, but lactosuria may occur in lactating women. The blood urea nitrogen (BUN) level increases during the puerperium as autolysis of the involuting uterus occurs. This breakdown of excess protein in the uterine muscle cells also results in a mild (+1) proteinuria for 1 to 2 days after childbirth in about 50% of women (Simpson & Creehan, 2001). Ketonuria may occur in women with an uncomplicated birth or after a prolonged labor with dehydration.

Postpartal Diuresis

Within 12 hours of birth, women begin to lose the excess tissue fluid that has accumulated during pregnancy. One mechanism responsible for reducing these retained fluids is the profuse diaphoresis that often occurs, especially at night, for the first 2 or 3 days after childbirth. Postpartal diuresis, caused by decreased estrogen levels, removal of increased venous pressure in the lower extremities, and loss of the remaining pregnancy-induced increase in blood volume, is another mechanism by which the body rids itself of excess fluid. The fluid loss through perspiration and the increased urinary output accounts for a weight loss of approximately 2.25 kg during the puerperium. This elimination of excess fluid accumulated during pregnancy is sometimes referred to as reversal of the water metabolism of pregnancy.

Urethra and Bladder

Trauma to the urethra and bladder may occur during the birth process as the infant passes through the pelvis, so the bladder wall may be hyperemic and edematous, often with small areas of hemorrhage. Clean-catch or catheterized urine specimens after birth often reveal hematuria from bladder trauma. The urethra and urinary meatus also may be edematous.

Birth-induced trauma, increased bladder capacity after childbirth, and the effects of conduction anesthesia combine to cause a decrease in the urge to void. In addition, pelvic soreness from the forces of labor, vaginal lacerations, or an episiotomy reduces or alters the voiding reflex. Decreased voiding, along with postpartal diuresis, may result in bladder distention. Immediately after birth, excessive bleeding can occur if the bladder becomes distended because this pushes the uterus up and to the side and prevents the uterus from firmly contracting. Later in the puerperium, overdistention can make the bladder more susceptible to infection and impede the resumption of normal voiding (Cunningham et al., 2001). With adequate emptying of the bladder, bladder tone is usually restored 5 to 7 days after childbirth.

GASTROINTESTINAL SYSTEM

Appetite

The mother is usually hungry shortly after giving birth and can tolerate a light diet. Most new mothers are ravenously hungry after full recovery from analgesia, anesthesia, and fatigue. Requests for extra portions of food and frequent snacks are not uncommon.

Bowel Evacuation

A spontaneous bowel evacuation may be delayed until 2 to 3 days after childbirth. This can be explained by decreased muscle tone in the intestines during labor and the immediate puerperium, prelabor diarrhea, lack of food, or dehydration. The mother often anticipates discomfort during the bowel movement because of perineal tenderness as a result of an episiotomy, lacerations, or hemorrhoids and therefore resists the urge to defecate.

Regular bowel habits should be reestablished when bowel tone returns.

Operative vaginal birth (forceps or vacuum use) and anal sphincter lacerations are associated with an increased risk of postpartum anal incontinence. If it occurs, anal incontinence is often temporary and may resolve within 6 months (Bowes & Katz, 2002). Women should be taught during pregnancy about episiotomy and its possible sequelae. Pelvic floor (Kegel) exercises should be encouraged.

BREASTS

Promptly after childbirth, there is a reduction in the concentrations of hormones that stimulated breast development during pregnancy (estrogen, progesterone, human chorionic gonadotropin, prolactin, cortisol, and insulin). The time it takes for these hormones to return to prepregnancy levels is determined in part by whether the mother breastfeeds her infant.

Breastfeeding Mothers

As lactation is established, a mass (lump) may be felt in the breast. Unlike the lumps associated with fibrocystic breast changes or cancer, which may be consistently palpated in the same location, a filled milk sac will shift position from day to day. Before lactation begins, the breasts feel soft, and a yellowish fluid, *colostrum,* can be expressed from the nipples. After lactation begins, the breasts feel warm and firm. Tenderness may persist for about 48 hours after the start of lactation. Bluish-white milk with a skim milk appearance (true milk) can be expressed from the nipples. The nipples are examined for erectility and signs of irritation, such as cracks, blisters, or reddening.

Nonbreastfeeding Mothers

Generally the breasts feel nodular (in nonpregnant women, they feel granular). The nodularity is bilateral and diffuse.

Prolactin levels decrease rapidly. Colostrum is excreted for the first few days after childbirth. Palpation of the breast on the second or third day, as milk production begins, may reveal tissue tenderness in some women. On the third or fourth postpartum day, *engorgement* may occur; the breasts become distended (swollen), firm, tender, and warm to the touch (caused by vasocongestion). Breast distention is primarily caused by the temporary congestion of veins and lymphatics rather than by an accumulation of milk. Milk is present but should not be expressed. Axillary breast tissue (the tail of Spence) and any accessory breast or nipple tissue along the milk line also may be involved. Engorgement resolves spontaneously, and discomfort usually decreases within 24 to 36 hours. A breast binder or tight bra, ice packs, or mild analgesics may be used to relieve discomfort. Nipple stimulation is avoided. If suckling is never begun (or is discontinued), lactation ceases within a few days to a week.

CARDIOVASCULAR SYSTEM

Blood Volume

The changes in blood volume after birth depend on several factors, such as blood loss during childbirth and the amount of extravascular water (physiologic edema) mobilized and subsequently excreted. Blood loss results in an immediate but limited decrease in total blood volume. Thereafter most of the blood volume increase during pregnancy (1000 to 1500 ml) is eliminated within the first 2 weeks after birth, with return to nonpregnant values by 6 months postpartum (Simpson & Creehan, 2001).

Pregnancy-induced hypervolemia (an increase in blood volume of at least 35% more than prepregnancy values near term (Bowes & Katz, 2002) allows most women to tolerate a considerable blood loss during childbirth. Many women lose approximately 500 ml of blood during vaginal birth of a single fetus and about twice this amount during cesarean birth (Resnik, 1999).

The readjustments in the maternal vasculature after childbirth are dramatic and rapid. The woman's response to blood loss during the early puerperium differs from that in a nonpregnant woman. Three postpartum physiologic changes help protect the woman from excessive blood loss: (1) elimination of uteroplacental circulation reduces the size of the maternal vascular bed by 10% to 15%; (2) loss of placental endocrine function removes the stimulus for vasodilation; and (3) mobilization of extravascular water stored during pregnancy increases blood volume. Thus hypovolemic shock usually does not occur in women who experience a normal blood loss during the early puerperium.

Cardiac Output

The pulse rate, stroke volume, and cardiac output increase throughout pregnancy. Immediately after the birth, they remain elevated or increase even higher for 30 to 60 minutes as the blood that was shunted through the uteroplacental circuit suddenly returns to the maternal systemic venous circulation (Bowes & Katz, 2002). Data are scant regarding the exact return of cardiac hemodynamic levels to nonpregnant levels, but in recent studies, researchers found that cardiac output remained significantly elevated in both nulliparous and multiparous normal women a year after the birth (Bowes & Katz, 2002).

Vital Signs

Few alterations in vital signs are seen under normal circumstances. There may be a small, transient increase in both systolic and diastolic blood pressure lasting about

TABLE 22-2 **Vital Signs After Childbirth**

NORMAL FINDINGS	DEVIATIONS FROM NORMAL FINDINGS AND PROBABLE CAUSES
Temperature	
During first 24 hours may increase to 38° C as a result of dehydrating effects of labor. After 24 hours, the woman should be afebrile.	A diagnosis of puerperal sepsis is suggested if an increase in maternal temperature to 38° C is noted after the first 24 hours after childbirth and recurs or persists for 2 days. Other possibilities are mastitis, endometritis, urinary tract infections, and other systemic infections.
Pulse	
Pulse, along with stroke volume and cardiac output, remains elevated for the first hour or so after childbirth. It then begins to decrease at an unknown rate. By 8 to 10 weeks after childbirth, the pulse has returned to a nonpregnant rate.	A rapid pulse rate or one that is increasing may indicate hypovolemia as a result of hemorrhage.
Respirations	
The respiratory rate should decrease to within the woman's normal prebirth range by 6 to 8 weeks after childbirth.	Hypoventilation may occur after an unusually high subarachnoid (spinal) block or epidural narcotic after a cesarean birth.
Blood Pressure	
Blood pressure is altered slightly if at all. Orthostatic hypotension, as indicated by feelings of faintness or dizziness immediately after standing up, can develop in the first 48 hours as a result of the splanchnic engorgement that may occur after birth.	A low or decreasing blood pressure may indicate the existence of hypovolemia secondary to hemorrhage; however, it is a late sign, and other symptoms of hemorrhage usually alert the staff. An increased reading may result from excessive use of vasopressor or oxytocic medications. Because preeclampsia can persist into or occur first in the postpartum period, routine evaluation of blood pressure is needed. If a woman complains of headache, hypertension must be ruled out as a cause before analgesics are administered.

4 days after the birth (Bowes & Katz, 2002) (Table 22-2). Respiratory function returns to the nonpregnant state by 6 to 8 weeks after birth. After the uterus is emptied, the diaphragm descends, the normal cardiac axis is restored, and the point of maximum impulse (PMI) and the electrocardiogram (ECG) are normalized.

Blood Components

Hematocrit and Hemoglobin

During the first 72 hours after childbirth, a greater loss in plasma volume than in the number of blood cells is found. This results in an increase in the hematocrit and hemoglobin levels by the seventh day after birth. No accelerated red blood cell (RBC) destruction occurs during the puerperium, but any excess will disappear gradually in accordance with the life span of the RBC. The exact time when the RBC volume returns to nonpregnant values is not known, but it is within normal limits when measured 8 weeks after childbirth (Bowes & Katz, 2002).

White Blood Cell Count

Normal leukocytosis of pregnancy averages about 12,000/mm^3. During the first 10 to 12 days after childbirth, however, values of between 20,000 and 25,000/mm^3 are common. Neutrophils are the most numerous white blood cells (WBCs). This leukocytosis, coupled with the normal increase in erythrocyte sedimentation rate, may obscure the diagnosis of acute infections at this time.

Coagulation Factors

Clotting factors and fibrinogen levels are normally increased during pregnancy and remain elevated in the immediate puerperium. This hypercoagulable state, combined with the vessel damage that occurs during childbirth and the immobility of the woman during recovery, increases the risk of thromboembolism (blood clots), especially after cesarean birth. Fibrinolytic activity also increases during the first few days after childbirth (Bowes & Katz, 2002). Levels of factors I, II, VIII, IX, and X decrease to nonpregnant levels within a few days.

Fibrin split products, probably released from the placental site, also can be found in maternal blood.

Varicosities

Varicosities (varices) of the legs and vulva and around the anus (hemorrhoids) that appear during pregnancy regress (empty) rapidly immediately after childbirth. Total or near-total regression of the varices is expected after childbirth.

NEUROLOGIC SYSTEM

Neurologic changes during the puerperium result from a reversal of maternal adaptations to pregnancy and from trauma during labor and childbirth.

Pregnancy-induced neurologic discomforts abate after birth. The elimination of physiologic edema through the diuresis that occurs after childbirth relieves carpal tunnel syndrome by easing the compression of the median nerve. The periodic numbness and tingling of fingers that afflict 5% of pregnant women usually disappear after childbirth unless lifting and carrying the baby aggravates the condition. Headache requires careful assessment. Postpartum headaches may be caused by various conditions, including postpartum-onset preeclampsia, stress, and the leakage of cerebrospinal fluid into the extradural space during placement of the needle for administration of epidural or spinal anesthesia. Headaches last from 1 to 3 days to several weeks, depending on the cause and effectiveness of the treatment.

MUSCULOSKELETAL SYSTEM

Adaptations of the mother's musculoskeletal system during pregnancy are reversed in the puerperium. These adaptations include the relaxation and subsequent hypermobility of the joints and the change in the mother's center of gravity in response to the enlarging uterus. The joints are completely stabilized by 6 to 8 weeks after birth. Although all other joints return to their normal prepregnancy state, however, those in the parous woman's feet do not. The new mother may notice a permanent increase in her shoe size.

INTEGUMENTARY SYSTEM

Chloasma of pregnancy usually disappears at the end of pregnancy. Hyperpigmentation of the areolae and linea nigra may not regress completely after childbirth but may be permanent in some women. Stretch marks on breasts, abdomen, hips, and thighs may fade but usually do not disappear.

Vascular abnormalities such as spider angiomas (nevi), palmar erythema, and epulis generally regress in response to the rapid decline in estrogens after the end of pregnancy. For some women, spider nevi persist indefinitely.

Hair growth slows during the postpartum period. Some women may actually experience hair loss, because the amount of hair lost is temporarily more than the amount regrown. The abundance of fine hair seen during pregnancy usually disappears after birth; however, any coarse or bristly hair that appears during pregnancy usually remains. Fingernails return to their nonpregnant consistency and strength.

The profuse diaphoresis that occurs in the immediate postpartum period is the most noticeable change in the integumentary system.

IMMUNE SYSTEM

No significant changes in the maternal immune system occur during the postpartum period. The mother's need for rubella vaccination or for prevention of Rh isoimmunization is determined.

KEY POINTS

- Postpartum physiologic changes allow the woman to tolerate considerable blood loss at birth.
- The uterus involutes rapidly after birth, returning to the true pelvis within 2 weeks.
- The rapid decrease in estrogen and progesterone levels after expulsion of the placenta is responsible for triggering many of the anatomic and physiologic changes in the puerperium.
- Assessment of lochia and fundal height is essential to monitor the progress of normal involution and to identify potential problems.
- The time it takes for the hormones that stimulated breast development during pregnancy to return to prepregnancy levels is determined in part by whether the woman breastfeeds her infant.
- Under normal circumstances, few alterations in vital signs are seen after childbirth.
- Activation of blood-clotting factors, immobility, and sepsis predispose the woman to thromboembolism.
- Marked diuresis, decreased bladder sensitivity, and overdistention of the bladder can lead to problems with urinary elimination.

CRITICAL THINKING EXERCISES

1. You receive a phone call from Marcy, who states, "I had my baby 10 days ago. I had just about quit bleeding, but today I've noticed a lot of bright red blood. What should I do?"
   - **a.** What possible causes might there be for Marcy's increased vaginal bleeding?
   - **b.** What questions would you want to ask her over the phone?
   - **c.** What advice would you give her concerning her situation?
2. Assess the accuracy of subjective estimates of blood loss.
   - **a.** Pour measured amounts of a red fluid (or expired blood from the blood bank, if available) on perineal pads or on plastic-backed underpads.
   - **b.** Ask nursing students, maternity nurses, medical students, obstetricians, nurse-midwives, and anesthesiologists to make independent assessments of the volume.
   - **c.** Calculate the percentage of correct responses among the total group and within each category of observer.
   - **d.** Compare the results. Do profession, area of specialization, or years of experience correlate with more reliable estimates? Were people more likely to overestimate or underestimate the amount? Were the estimates for perineal pads or for underpads different? Were the errors in judgment large enough to raise concern about the accuracy of estimates of blood loss?

RESOURCES

American College of Nurse-Midwives (ACNM)
818 Connecticut Ave. NW, Suite 900
Washington, DC 20006
202-728-9860
www.midwife.org

American College of Obstetricians and Gynecologists (ACOG)
409 12th St. SW
Washington, DC 20024
800-762-2264
www.acog.org

Association of Women's Health, Obstetric, and Neonatal Nurses (AWHONN)
200 L St. NW, Suite 740
Washington, DC 20036
800-673-8499 (U.S.)
800-245-0231 (Canada)
www.awhonn.org

Coping with the Overall Pregnancy Experience (COPE)
37 Clarendon St.
Boston, MA 02116
617-357-5588

Maternity Center Association, Inc
281 Park Ave. South, 5th Floor
New York, NY 10010
212-777-5000

REFERENCES

Bowes, W., & Katz, V. (2002). Postpartum care. In S. Gabbe, J. Niebyl, & J. Simpson (Eds.), *Obstetrics: Normal and problem pregnancies* (4th ed.). New York: Churchill Livingstone.

Cunningham, F. et al. (2001). *Williams obstetrics* (21st ed.). New York: McGraw-Hill.

Rebar, R. (1999). The breast and the physiology of lactation. In R. Creasy & R. Resnik (Eds.), *Maternal-fetal medicine* (4th ed.). Philadelphia: W.B. Saunders.

Resnik, R. (1999). The puerperium. In R. Creasy & R. Resnik (Eds.), *Maternal-fetal medicine* (4th ed.). Philadelphia: W.B. Saunders.

Simpson, K., & Creehan, P. (2001). *AWHONN's perinatal nursing* (2nd ed.). Philadelphia: J.B. Lippincott.

Visness, C., Kennedy, K., & Ramos, R. (1997). The duration and character of postpartum bleeding among breast-feeding women. *Obstetrics and Gynecology, 89*(2), 159-163.

CHAPTER 23

Kitty Cashion

Nursing Care of the Postpartum Woman

http://evolve.elsevier.com/Lowdermilk/MatWmnHlth/

LEARNING OBJECTIVES

- Identify the priorities of maternal care given during the fourth stage of labor.
- Identify common selection criteria for safe early postpartum discharge.
- Compare and contrast the pros and cons of early postpartum discharge.
- Give examples of physical and psychosocial nursing diagnoses pertaining to women in the postpartum period.
- Identify expected outcomes for postpartum physical and psychosocial care.
- Summarize nursing interventions to prevent infection and excessive bleeding.
- Summarize nursing interventions to promote normal bladder and bowel patterns and care for the breasts of women who are breastfeeding or bottle-feeding.
- Examine the influence of cultural expectations on postpartum adjustment.
- Determine the nurse's responsibilities related to discharge teaching and preparation for home care.
- Describe the nurse's role in these postpartum follow-up strategies: home visits, telephone follow-up, warm lines and help lines, support groups, and referrals to community resources.

The goal of nursing care in the immediate postpartum period is to assist women and their partners during their initial transition to parenting. The approach to the care of women after birth is wellness oriented. Consequently, in the United States, most women remain hospitalized no more than 1 or 2 days after giving birth, and some, for as few as 6 hours. Because there is so much important information to be shared with these women in a very short time, it is vital that their care be thoughtfully planned and provided. The nurse provides care that focuses on the woman's physiologic recovery, her psychologic well-being, and her ability to care for herself and her new baby. In addition, the nurse considers the needs of other family members and includes strategies in the plan of care to assist the family in adjusting to the new baby. This chapter focuses on using the nursing process to meet both the mother's and the family's needs during this crucial time.

FOURTH STAGE OF LABOR

The first 1 to 2 hours after birth, sometimes referred to as the **fourth stage of labor,** is a crucial time for the mother and newborn. Both not only are recovering from the physical process of birth but also are becoming acquainted with each other and with additional family members. During this time, maternal organs start to undergo readjustment to the nonpregnant state, and the functions of body systems begin to stabilize. Meanwhile, the newborn continues to make the transition from an intrauterine to extrauterine existence. The nurse's role during the fourth stage of labor is to monitor the recovery of the new mother and infant, to identify and manage promptly any deviations from the normal processes that may occur, and to promote and support parent-infant attachment.

The fourth stage of labor is an excellent time to begin breastfeeding because the infant is in an alert state and ready to nurse. Breastfeeding at this time also promotes the contraction of the uterus and the prevention of maternal hemorrhage. Getting breastfeeding off to a good start is encouraging for the mother; it also is physiologically vital for the infant. Colostrum loosens mucus and acts as a laxative, thus promoting the rapid elimination of meconium. It also decreases the likelihood of hypoglycemia, reduces the severity of physiologic hyperbilirubinemia, and provides important immunologic benefits.

In most centers, the mother remains in the labor and birth area during this recovery time. In an institution where labor, delivery, and recovery (LDR) rooms are used, the woman stays in the same room where she gave birth. In traditional settings, women are taken from the delivery room to a separate recovery area for observation.

Arrangements for the care of the newborn vary during the fourth stage of labor. In many settings, the baby remains at the mother's bedside, and the labor or birth nurse cares for both of them. In other institutions, the baby is taken to the nursery for several hours of observation after an initial bonding period with the parents (Fig. 23-1).

Assessment

If the recovery nurse has not previously cared for the new mother, her assessment begins with an oral report from the nurse who attended the woman during labor and birth and a review of the prenatal, labor, and birth records. Of primary importance are conditions that could predispose the mother to hemorrhage, such as precipitate labor, a large baby, grand multiparity, or induced labor. For healthy women, hemorrhage is probably the most dangerous potential complication.

To help the nurse provide comprehensive care, use of a worksheet or recovery record is suggested. Figure 23-2 illustrates an easy-to-use flow sheet that has the essential immediate postpartum and anesthesia recovery assessments. During the first hour in the recovery room, physical assessments of the mother are frequent. All factors except temperature are assessed every 15 minutes for 1 hour. Temperature is assessed at the beginning and end of the recovery period. After the fourth 15-minute assessment, if all parameters have stabilized within the normal range, the process is usually repeated every 30 minutes during the second hour. Box 23-1 and Fig. 23-3 describe the physical assessment of the mother during the fourth stage.

During the fourth stage of labor, many postpartum women experience intense tremors that resemble shivering from a chill. They are commonly seen after birth and are not related to infection. Several theories have been offered to explain these tremors or shivering, such as their being the result of a sudden release of pressure on pelvic nerves after birth, a response from a fetus-to-mother transfusion that occurred during placental separation, a reaction to maternal adrenaline production during labor and birth, or a reaction to epidural anesthesia. The nurse can help women who experience these chills by providing warm blankets and reassurance that the chills or tremors are common, self-limiting, and last only a short while.

The nutritional status of the woman is assessed. Restriction of food and fluid intake and the loss of fluids (blood, perspiration, or emesis) during labor cause many women to express a strong desire to eat or drink soon after birth. In the absence of complications, a woman who has given birth vaginally, has recovered from the effects of the anesthetic, and has stable vital signs, a firm uterus, and small to moderate lochial flow may have fluids and a regular diet as desired (American Academy of Pediatrics & American College of Obstetricians and Gynecologists, 1997).

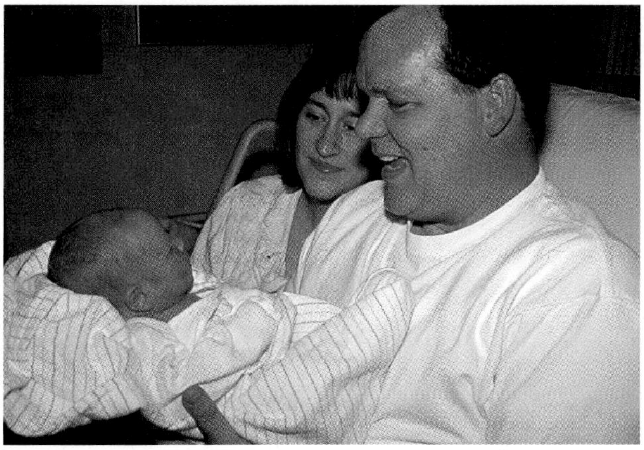

FIG. 23-1 Mother and father get acquainted with their newborn. (Courtesy Michael S. Clement, MD, Mesa, AZ.)

Postanesthesia Recovery

The woman who has given birth by cesarean or has received regional anesthesia for a vaginal birth requires special attention during the recovery period. Obstetric recovery areas are held to the same standard of care that would be expected of any other postanesthesia recovery room (AAP & ACOG, 1997). A recovery from anesthesia requires the nurse to have available cardiopulmonary support and emergency supplies. A postanesthesia recovery (PAR) score is determined for each client on her arrival and is updated as part of every 15-minute assessment. Components of the PAR score include activity, respirations, blood pressure, level of consciousness, and color.

NURSE ALERT
Regardless of her obstetric status, no woman should be discharged from the recovery area until she has completely recovered from the effects of anesthesia.

If the woman received general anesthesia, she should be awake and alert, oriented to time, place, and person. Her respiratory rate should be within normal limits, and her oxygen saturation levels at least 95%, as measured by a pulse oximeter. If the woman received epidural or spinal anesthesia, she should be able to raise her legs, extended at the knees, off the bed, or to flex her knees, place her feet flat on the bed, and raise her buttocks well off the bed. The numb or tingling, prickly sensation should be entirely gone from her legs. Women vary greatly in regard to length of time required to recover from regional anesthesia. Often it takes several hours for these anesthetic effects to disappear.

Transfer from the Recovery Area

After the initial recovery period has been completed, the woman may be transferred to a postpartum room in the same or another nursing unit. In facilities with labor,

DIAGNOSIS:________________

PHYSICIAN:________________

ANESTHESIA:________________

ANESTHETIST:________________

ARMBANDS:________ mother ________ infant

CLOTHING:________ c̄ family ________ c̄ patient

ALLERGIES:________________

PAR SCORE: ADM: DC:					
ACTIVITY					
RESPIRATION					
BLOOD PRESSURE					
CONSCIOUS LEVEL					
COLOR					
TOTAL					

Activity	
Able to move 4 extremities voluntarily or on command	2
Able to move 2 extremities voluntarily or on command	1
Able to move 0 extremities voluntarily or on command	0
Respiration	
Able to deep breathe and cough freely	2
Dyspnea or limited breathing	1
Apneic	0
Blood Pressure	
BP ± mm Hg of preanesthetic level	2
BP ± 25-50 mm HG of preanesthetic level	1
BP ± Greater than 50 mm HG of preanesthetic level	0
Conscious Level	
Fully aware	2
Arousable on calling	1
Not responding	0
Color	
Pink	2
Pale, dusky, blotchy, jaundiced, other	1
Cyanotic	0

Pain Scales
Wong Baker = WB
Numeric = N
Simple Descriptive = SD

Pain Characteristics
Location
Duration
Aggravating/Alleviating fx
Nature - dull, gnawing, hot, achy, sharp, burning, throbbing, shooting, stabbing

Observation Codes

A - Anxious	D - Depressed	H - Relaxed
B - Agitated, Restless	E - Crying	V - VS Charge
	R - Restless	W - Withdrawn
C - Confused	G - Grimace	O - Other

Results Code
0 - No pain present
1 - Improved but still in pain
2 - No improvement

Pain Management Intervention
P - Pharmacological
NP - Non pharmacological

VITAL SIGNS:													
	TIME												
	BP												
	PULSE												
	RESP / O_2 Sat												
	TEMP												
FUNDUS FB-FINGERBREADTH B-BOGGY FM-FIRM MD-MIDLINE	FUNDUS												
LOCHIA CL-CLOTS MOD-MODERATE SM-SMALL LG-LARGE	LOCHIA												
BLADDER D-DISTENDED F-FOLEY ND-NON-DISTENDED	BLADDER												
EPISIOTOMY/INCISION NL-NORMAL D-DRY ABNL-ABNORMAL I-INTACT	EPIS / INC												
CLEAR CL WHEEZING W DIMINISHED	BREATH SOUNDS												
q 1° / q Shift	DTR / PROTEIN												
O_2 liters/min													
JP drain cc/hr													
INTAKE													
OUTPUT													
Pain Scale													
Observation Code													
Pain Management Intervention													
Results Code													
INITIALS													

PCA

PCA Medication, Concentration and Volume

____

Loading Dose ________

Continuous Rate ______ 4 hour limit ________

Lockout Interval ________________

RN __________ RN __________

____ / ____ / ____ ____:____ am / pm

Meds / IV / Rate	Time / Initial
	/
	/
	/
	/

INTAKE TOTAL
Shift 7A 3P 11P

OUTPUT TOTAL
Shift 7A 3P 11P

IV _____ cc LTC
@ D/C

Homan's Sign Pos☐ Neg☐

BONDING
☐ appropriate
☐ inappropriate
☐ NA (explain)

Social Services Notified
___/___/___
___:___ am/pm

TEACHING
☐ fundal massage
☐ TC & DB
☐ breast feeding
☐ assistance on 1st ambulation
☐ Pain Scale
☐ PCA pump

Signatures/Initials

DISCHARGE NOTE

Report Called To: ________________

ANESTHESIA D/C:

EPIDURAL CATHETER: IN OUT NA

THE MED **Regional Medical Center at Memphis**

MATERNITY RECOVERY ROOM RECORD

FORM NO. 68622 (10/01) White (Chart) Yellow (Pharmacy)

FIG. 23-2 An example of a maternity recovery room record. (Courtesy The Regional Medical Center at Memphis [The Med], Memphis, TN.)

BOX 23-1 Assessment During Fourth Stage of Labor

Before beginning the assessment, wash hands thoroughly, assemble necessary equipment, and explain the procedure to the woman.

BLOOD PRESSURE

Measure blood pressure per assessment schedule. Be sure to use the proper-sized cuff.

PULSE

Assess rate and regularity.

TEMPERATURE

Determine temperature.

FUNDUS

Put on clean examination gloves.
Position woman with knees flexed and head flat.
Just below the umbilicus, cup hand and press firmly into abdomen. At the same time, stabilize the uterus at the symphysis with the opposite hand.
If fundus is firm (and bladder is empty), with uterus in midline, measure its position relative to woman's umbilicus. Lay fingers flat on abdomen under umbilicus; measure how many fingerbreadths (fb) or centimeters (cm) fit between the umbilicus and top of fundus. If the fundus is above the umbilicus, this is recorded as plus fb or cm; if below, as minus fb or cm.
If the fundus is not firm, massage it gently to help it contract and expel any clots before measuring the distance from the umbilicus.
Place hands appropriately; massage gently only until firm.
Expel clots while keeping hands placed as shown in Fig. 23-3. With upper hand, apply firm pressure downward toward vagina; observe perineum for amount and size of expelled clots.

BLADDER

Assess distention by noting location and firmness of uterine fundus and by observing and palpating bladder. A distended bladder is seen as a rounded suprapubic bulge that is dull to percussion and fluctuates like a water-filled balloon. When the bladder is distended, the uterus is usually boggy in consistency, well above the umbilicus, and to the woman's right side.
Assist woman to void spontaneously. Measure amount of urine voided.
Catheterize as necessary.
Reassess after voiding or catheterization to make sure the bladder is not palpable and the fundus is firm and in the midline.

LOCHIA

Observe lochia on perineal pads and on linen under the woman's buttocks. Determine amount and color; note size and number of clots and odor.
Observe perineum for source of bleeding (e.g., episiotomy, lacerations).

PERINEUM

Ask or assist woman to turn on her side and flex upper leg on hip.
Lift upper buttock.
Observe perineum in good lighting.
Assess episiotomy site or laceration repair for intactness, hematoma, edema, bruising, redness, and drainage.
Assess for presence of hemorrhoids.

delivery, recovery, postpartum (LDRP) rooms, the woman stays in the same room and the nurse who provides care during the recovery period usually continues the care for the woman. Women who have received general or regional anesthesia must be cleared for transfer from the recovery area by a member of the anesthesia care team.

In preparing the transfer report, the recovery nurse uses information from the records of admission, birth record, and recovery. Information usually communicated to the postpartum nurse includes identity of the primary health care provider; gravidity and parity; age; anesthetic used; any medications given; duration of labor and time of rupture of membranes; oxytocin induction or augmentation; type of birth and repair; blood type and Rh status; group B streptococcus (GBS) status; status of rubella immunity; human immunodeficiency virus (HIV), syphilis, and hepatitis B serology test results; intravenous (IV) infusion of any fluids; physiologic status since birth; description of the fundus, lochia, bladder, and perineum; sex and weight of the infant; time of birth; pediatrician; chosen method of feeding; any abnormalities noted; and assessment of initial parent-infant interaction.

Most of this information also is documented for the nursing staff in the newborn nursery. In addition, specific information should be provided regarding the infant's Apgar scores, weight, voiding and stooling, and whether fed since birth. Nursing interventions that have been completed (e.g., eye prophylaxis, vitamin K injection) also must be recorded.

Table 23-1 gives examples for documenting this information before the transfer of the woman from the recovery area.

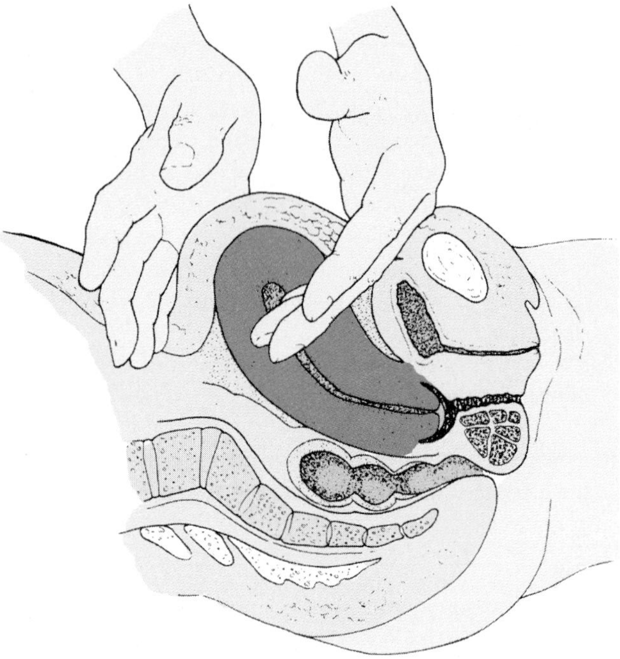

FIG. 23-3 Palpating fundus of uterus during the fourth stage of labor. Note that upper hand is cupped over the fundus; lower hand dips in above symphysis pubis and supports uterus while massaging it gently.

Women who give birth in birthing centers may go home within a few hours after the woman's and infant's conditions are stable.

DISCHARGE: BEFORE 24 HOURS AND AFTER 48 HOURS

Early postpartum discharge, shortened hospital stay, and 1-day maternity stay are all terms for the decreasing length of stay of mothers and their newborns after a low risk birth. The trend of shortened hospital stay (24 hours or less for a woman who had an uncomplicated vaginal birth and about 72 hours for a woman who had an uncomplicated cesarean birth) is based largely on efforts to reduce health care costs (economic factors) coupled with consumer demands to have less medical intervention and more family-centered experiences (Ferguson & Engelhard, 1997; Wilkerson, 1996), all of which has increasingly affected numbers of maternity clients and the nurses who provide their care.

Laws Relating to Discharge

Health care providers expressed concern that some medical problems do not show up in the first 24 hours after birth and that new mothers have not sufficiently learned how to care for their newborns and identify newborn health problems such as jaundice and dehydration related to breastfeeding difficulties (Havens & Hannan, 1996). The first day after birth is not a time conducive to learning for many women (Brown & Johnson, 1998). There also was concern that shortened hospital stays would increase maternal hospital readmission for infection, hypertension, and hemorrhage in women who gave birth vaginally.

The widespread concern for the potential increase in adverse maternal-child outcomes from hospital early discharge practices led the American College of Obstetricians and Gynecologists (ACOG), the American Academy of Pediatrics (AAP), and other professional health care organizations to promote the enactment of federal and various state maternity length-of-stay bills to ensure adequate care for both the mother and the newborn. The passage of the landmark Newborns' and Mothers' Health Protection Act of 1996 provided minimum federal standards for health plan coverage for mothers and their newborns (Ferguson & Engelhard, 1997). Under the Act, all health plans were required to allow the new mother and newborn to remain in the hospital for a minimum of 48 hours after a normal vaginal birth and for 96 hours after a cesarean birth unless the attending provider, in consultation with the mother, decided on early discharge.

Research studies to determine the appropriate length of hospital stay for newborns seem to support this legislation. One large study (Liu et al., 1997) found that newborns discharged early (less than 30 hours after birth) were more likely to be rehospitalized for jaundice, dehydration, and infection within 1 month of life than were newborns discharged later (30 to 72 hours after birth). Edmonson, Stoddard, and Owens (1997) were unable to find any significant reason for newborn readmission; however, they concluded that readmission was more likely among babies who were firstborn, breastfed, or born to unmarried and poorly educated women.

Conversely, several early postpartum hospital discharge programs that provided extensive prenatal preparation and postpartum follow-up found it generally safe for mothers who gave birth vaginally and their newborns to be discharged less than 48 hours after birth (Fishbein & Burggraf, 1998; Williams & Cooper, 1996).

Proponents of early postpartum discharge cite the following advantages of the practice:

- Reinforces the concept of childbirth as a normal physiologic event.
- Allows shorter separations between mothers and other children.
- Extends a couple's sense of control and participation beyond the birth itself.
- Capitalizes on the security of the home environment during the stressors of early parenting.
- Decreases unnecessary exposure to the pathogens in the hospital environment.
- Allows beds on the maternity service to be used more effectively (i.e., quick turnover in clients or greater availability for clients with a complication).

TABLE 23-1 **Recovery Nurse's Report**

ITEM	EXAMPLE OF DOCUMENTATION OF MOTHER	EXAMPLE OF DOCUMENTATION OF NEWBORN
Type of labor and birth: unusual observations, if any, of the placenta	Spontaneous or assisted (forceps) vaginal birth; vertex presentation	Spontaneous or assisted (forceps, vacuum extractor) vaginal birth in vertex presentation; time of ROM
Gravidity and parity, age	G1, P1, age 22 yr; 39 wk of gestation	G1, P1, age 22 yr; 39 wk of gestation
Anesthesia and analgesia used	None; epidural, low spinal, local	None; epidural, low spinal, or local
Condition of perineum	Episiotomy; repair of lacerations; intact	
Events since birth	Vital signs, BP, fundus, lochia, intake and output, medications (dosage, time of administration, and results), response to newborn, observation of family interactions, including siblings, if present	Nursed at breast for ____ min. Voided × 1; meconium stool × 1 Eye prophylaxis given Vitamin K injection given Held by siblings who are happy (or have other response to newborn)
Condition and sex of newborn; other information	Time of birth; Apgar at 1 and 5 min; weight; whether breastfeeding or bottle feeding; sex of the baby	Time of birth; Apgar scores at 1 and 5 min Sex; weight; name of pediatrician; breastfeeding or bottle feeding; mother's hepatitis B status and GBS status; whether mother received $MgSO_4$; time of last systemic analgesia
Relevant information from prenatal record	Need for rubella vaccination; presence of infections; hepatitis B status; HIV status; blood type; Rh status; GBS status and treatment if positive	Unremarkable pregnancy
Miscellaneous information: IV drip	If IV drip is infusing, rate of infusion, medications added (e.g., oxytocin [Pitocin]), whether to keep open or discontinue after completion of bag that is hung	
Social factors	If woman is releasing baby for adoption, whether she wants to see baby, breastfeed, allow visitors, or other preferences she may have	Baby up for adoption; to stay in NBN until discharge

BP, Blood pressure; *GBS,* group B streptococcus; *HIV,* human immunodeficiency virus; *NBN,* newborn nursery; *ROM,* rupture of membranes.

- Allows more time for mother/father/partner/infant and other family members to bond (Fig. 23-4).
- Creates less disruption in the daily life of the family.
- Promotes active involvement of family and support persons in assisting the mother and newborn (Fig. 23-5).

Opponents of early postpartum discharge cite the following disadvantages of the practice:

- Complications (maternal or newborn) may go unrecognized.
- Families may be or feel unprepared for the reality they face once the baby is at home.
- The mother is fatigued from the labor and childbirth process.
- The mother is experiencing postpartum pain or discomfort.
- The length of time for learning after the birth in the hospital setting is decreased.
- A vulnerability and crisis potential exists for both women and families.

The protest against early discharge becomes more powerful in the conventional health care arena in which care does not include a home care visit and there is a long interval between discharge and the first follow-up examination.

Criteria for Discharge

Early discharge and postpartum home care can be a safe and satisfying option for women and their families when it is comprehensive and based on individual needs (Wilkerson, 1996). However, early discharge is not appropriate for every mother and newborn (AAP & ACOG, 1997). Hospital stays must be long enough to identify problems and to ensure that the woman is sufficiently recovered and prepared to care for herself and

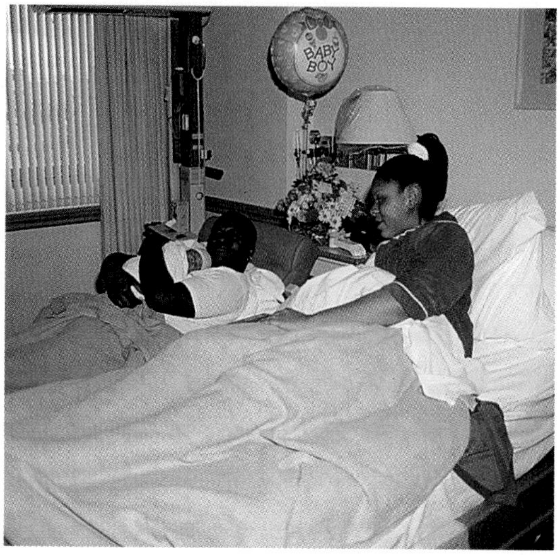
BABY BOY

FIG. 23-4 Bonding and attachment begun early after birth are fostered in the postpartum period. (Courtesy Marjorie Pyle, RNC, Lifecircle, Costa Mesa, CA.)

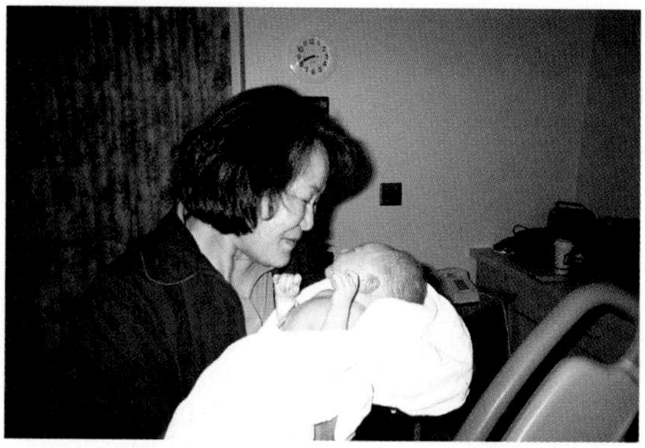

FIG. 23-5 Active involvement of grandmother provides support for the mother and newborn. (Courtesy Shannon Perry, San Jose, CA.)

the baby at home. By applying predetermined criteria for identifying low risk in mothers and newborns (Box 23-2), the length of hospitalization can be based on the medical need for care in an acute care setting or in consideration of the ongoing care needed in the home environment (AAP & ACOG, 1997; Weekly & Neumann, 1997).

In collaboration with other health care providers, the nurse is instrumental in determining whether the mother and newborn meet the criteria for early discharge. Because care paths provide the nurse with an organized approach toward meeting essential maternal-newborn care and teaching goals within a limited time frame, they can be useful in helping to prepare the woman and family for early discharge and home care. An example of a care path for the progression of postpartum physical, psychosocial, and self-care changes and for the teaching needs of women after uncomplicated, vaginal birth within a 24-hour time frame is found on pp. 624-625. A similar format can be used for a cesarean birth care path with time frame adjustments accounting for a longer hospital stay (e.g., 3 to 4 days) (Simpson & Creehan, 2001). Other methods such as postpartum order sets and maternal-newborn teaching checklists (Fig. 23-6) can also be used to accomplish designated client care and educational outcomes.

Hospital-based maternity nurses continue to play invaluable roles as caregivers, teachers, and client and family advocates in developing and implementing effective home care strategies. With coordination, clinical care and education can be planned and provided throughout pregnancy, during the hospital stay, and in the home after discharge to ensure the family's continued well-being.

CARE MANAGEMENT: PHYSICAL NEEDS

Assessment and Nursing Diagnoses

A *focused physical assessment*, including measurement of vital signs, is performed on admission to the postpartum unit. If the woman's vital signs are within normal limits, they will likely be assessed every 4 to 8 hours for the remainder of her hospitalization. Other components of the initial assessment include the mother's emotional status, energy level, degree of physical discomfort, hunger, and thirst. Intake and output assessments should always be done if an IV infusion or a urinary catheter is in place. If the woman gave birth by cesarean, the incisional dressing should be assessed as well. To some degree, her knowledge level concerning self-care and infant care also can be determined at this time.

Ongoing Physical Assessment

The postpartum woman should be evaluated thoroughly during each nursing shift throughout hospitalization (see Guidelines/Guías box on p. 627). Physical assessments include evaluation of the breasts, uterine fundus, lochia, perineum, bladder and bowel function, vital signs, and legs. If a woman has an IV line in place, her fluid and hematologic status should be evaluated before it is removed. Signs of potential problems that may be identified during the assessment process are listed in the Signs of Potential Complications box on p. 627.

Routine Laboratory Tests

Several laboratory tests may be performed in the immediate postpartum period. Hemoglobin and hematocrit values are often requested on the first postpartum day to assess effects of blood loss during childbirth, especially after cesarean birth. In some hospitals, a clean-catch or catheterized urine specimen may be obtained and sent for routine urinalysis or culture and sensitivity, especially

BOX 23-2 **Criteria for Early Discharge**

MOTHER

Uncomplicated pregnancy, labor, vaginal birth, and postpartum course
No evidence of premature rupture of membranes
Blood pressure and temperature stable and within normal limits
Ambulating unassisted
Voiding adequate amounts without difficulty
Hemoglobin >10 g
No significant vaginal bleeding; perineum intact or no more than second-degree episiotomy or laceration repair; uterus is firm
Received instructions on postpartum self-care

INFANT

Term infant (38 to 42 weeks) with weight appropriate for gestational age
Normal findings on physical assessment
Temperature, respirations, and heart rate within normal limits and stable for the 12 hours preceding discharge
At least two successful feedings completed (normal sucking and swallowing)
Urination and stooling have occurred at least once
No evidence of significant jaundice in the first 24 hours after the birth
No excessive bleeding at the circumcision site for at least 2 hours
Screening tests performed according to state regulations; tests to be repeated at follow-up visit if done before the infant is 24 hours old
Initial hepatitis B vaccine given or scheduled for first follow-up visit
Laboratory data reviewed: maternal syphilis and hepatitis B status; infant or cord blood type and Coombs' test results if indicated

GENERAL

No social, family, or environmental risk factors identified
Family or support person available to assist mother and infant at home
Follow-up scheduled within 1 week if discharged before 48 hours after the birth
Documentation of skill of mother in feeding (breast or bottle), cord care, skin care, perineal care, infant safety (use of car seat, sleeping positions), and recognizing signs of illness and common infant problems

Source: American Academy of Pediatrics. (1995). Hospital stay for healthy term infants. *Pediatrics, 96*(4), 788-790; Weekly, S., & Neumann, M. (1997). Speaking up for baby: The case for individualized neonatal discharge plans. *AWHONN Lifelines, 1*(1), 24-29.

if an indwelling urinary catheter was inserted during the intrapartum period. In addition, if the woman's rubella and Rh status are unknown, tests to determine her status and need for possible treatment should be performed at this time.

Nursing Diagnoses

Although all women experience similar physiologic changes during the postpartum period, certain factors make each woman's experience unique. From a physiologic standpoint, the length and difficulty of the labor, type of birth (vaginal or cesarean), presence of episiotomy or lacerations, and whether the mother plans to breastfeed or bottle feed are important factors to be investigated with each woman. After analyzing the data obtained during the assessment process, the nurse establishes nursing diagnoses that will guide the plan of care. Examples of nursing diagnoses commonly established for the postpartum woman include the following:

- *Risk for infection related to*
  –childbirth trauma to tissues
- *Risk for constipation related to*
  –postchildbirth discomfort
  –decreased intake of solid food and/or fluids
- *Disturbed sleep pattern related to*
  –discomforts of postpartum period
  –long labor process
  –infant care and hospital routine
- *Acute pain related to*
  –involution of uterus
  –hemorrhoids
  –engorged breasts
- *Risk for injury related to*
  –effects of anesthesia
- *Ineffective breastfeeding related to*
  –maternal discomfort
  –infant positioning

Expected Outcomes of Care

The nursing plan of care includes both the postpartum woman and her infant, even if the nursery nurse retains primary responsibility for the infant. In many hospitals, **couplet care** (also called *mother and baby care* or *single-room maternity care*) is practiced. Nurses in these settings have been educated in both mother and infant care and function as the primary nurse for both mother and infant, even if the infant is kept in the nursery. This approach is a variation of **rooming-in,** in which the mother and child room

Text continued on p. 627

Care Path 24-Hour Vaginal Birth Without Complications

Date of Birth: ______________

Hour of Birth: ______________

The uncomplicated vaginal birth client's admission/discharge is based on a 24-hr length of stay after birth based on individual needs.

Time: ______

	RECOVERY	ADM. TO PP UNIT—8 HOUR	9-16 HOURS	17-24 HOURS/DISCHARGE
PRIMARY PHYSIOLOGIC FOCUS	Woman will have normal vital signs as documented on flowsheet.	Woman will have normal VS and moderate lochia rubra.	Woman will have normal VS and minimal lochia rubra.	Woman will have normal VS and minimal lochia rubra.
	NA MET VARIANCE	NA MET VARIANCE	NA MET VARIANCE	NA MET VARIANCE
	Vital signs every 15 min × 1 hr, then every 4 hr. Assess perineum/episiotomy. Ice pack prn. Assess lochia.	Vital signs every 4 hr. Assess perineum/episiotomy. Ice pack prn. Assess lochia.	Vital signs every shift. Assess perineum/episiotomy. Ice pack prn. Assess lochia.	Vital signs every shift. Assess perineum/episiotomy. Ice pack prn. Assess lochia.
	RECOVERY	ADM. TO PP UNIT—8 HOURS	9-16 HOURS	17-24 HOURS/DISCHARGE
IVs/LABWORK/ MEDICATIONS	Woman will have appropriate lab work done and medication given by time of transfer to Mother/Baby Unit.	Woman will begin to verbalize understanding of hepatitis status and medication requirements.	Woman will have appropriate lab work done by 16 hr PP.	Woman will have appropriate lab work done and appropriate medications initiated.
	NA MET VARIANCE	NA MET VARIANCE	NA MET VARIANCE	NA MET VARIANCE
	CBC, if not done before birth. Urine drug screen if ordered. U/A—dipstick. (Send to lab, if abnormal.)	Review hepatitis B status. Medication regimen initiated.	CBC. Review rubella status. Review Hgb and Hct.	Fe Tab. Prenatal vitamin. Rubella vaccine, if appropriate. RhoGAM, if indicated. Laxative.
	RECOVERY	ADM. TO PP UNIT—8 HOURS	9-16 HOURS	17-24 HOURS/DISCHARGE
NUTRITION/ ELIMINATION	Woman will be up to bathroom before transfer.	Woman will resume normal nutritional status and bladder function.	Woman will resume normal nutritional status and bladder function.	Woman will have normal bowel and bladder function.
	NA MET VARIANCE	NA MET VARIANCE	NA MET VARIANCE	NA MET VARIANCE
	Assess bladder fullness. Assist to bathroom. Assess for tolerance of PO intake.	Encourage ambulation. Encourage PO fluids. Assist to bathroom as needed. Assess bladder function. Encourage PO intake.	Encourage ambulation. Encourage PO fluids. Assist to bathroom as needed. Assess bladder function. Encourage PO intake.	Encourage ambulation. Encourage PO fluids. Assist to bathroom as needed. Laxative prn.
	RECOVERY	ADM. TO PP UNIT—8 HOURS	9-16 HOURS	17-24 HOURS/DISCHARGE
PSYCHOSOCIAL	Woman/family will begin attachment behaviors with newborn.	Woman/family will demonstrate appropriate attachment behaviors.	Family will verbalize comfort with new infant.	Family will verbalize comfort with new infant.
	NA MET VARIANCE	NA MET VARIANCE	NA MET VARIANCE	NA MET VARIANCE
	Encourage mother/family members to hold and touch infant. Provide skin-to-skin contact of mother/infant. Provide mother the opportunity to breastfeed, if applicable.	Offer flexible rooming-in with infant. Allow verbalization of woman's feelings. Assess discharge needs and need for social service consult.	Reinforce interventions.	Reinforce interventions. Completion of birth certificate. Arrange for home visit.

Care Path 24-Hour Vaginal Birth Without Complications—cont'd

	RECOVERY	ADM. TO PP UNIT—8 HOURS	9-16 HOURS	17-24 HOUR/DISCHARGE
SELF-CARE ACTIVITY	Woman will begin self-care activities as tolerated.	Woman will be up to bathroom/shower with assistance.	Woman will be up to bathroom/shower independently.	Woman will be up to bathroom/shower independently.
	NA MET VARIANCE	NA MET VARIANCE	NA MET VARIANCE	NA MET VARIANCE
	Instruct woman in pericare and pad changes.	Reinforce proper pericare. Instruct on use of sitz bath. Encourage woman to shower.	Reinforce proper pericare. Reinforce use of sitz bath.	Reinforce proper pericare. Reinforce use of sitz bath.
	RECOVERY	ADM. TO PP UNIT—8 HOURS	9-16 HOURS	17-24 HOURS/DISCHARGE
TEACHING/ DISCHARGE PLANNING	Woman will begin to verbalize and/or demonstrate self-care and infant-care activities.	Woman will begin to verbalize and/or demonstrate infant and self-care activities.	Woman/family will demonstrate appropriate infant-care activities.	Woman/family will demonstrate appropriate infant-care activities.
	NA MET VARIANCE	NA MET VARIANCE	NA MET VARIANCE	NA MET VARIANCE
	Date:			
	Initials:			
	Teaching to include: Breastfeeding latch-on and positioning, if applicable. Appropriate handwashing techniques. Cough and deep breathing exercises. Instruct in pain-relief techniques/medication.	Teaching to include: Breastfeeding/formula initial feeding information. Breast care. Perineal care. Proper nutrition. Safety issues reviewed.	Teaching to include: Attendance at mother/baby-care class. Breast care or formula information. Newborn channel. Lactation consult prn. Appropriate handwashing techniques.	Teaching to include: Reinforcement of teaching from mother/baby class. Plans for self/infant follow-up. Review IHSP.* Review Baby Net program. Telephone number for follow-up questions. Home-going meds and purposes.
	1.	1.	1.	1.
	2.	2.	2.	2.
	3.	3.	3.	3.
	4.	4.	4.	4.

Variance Documentation: ______________________________

____

____

____

____

____

*IHSP denotes a test done to determine whether follow-up is needed in the Infant Hearing Screening Program (IHSP).

Abbott Northwestern Hospital
A HealthSpan™ Organization
SELF/FAMILY LEARNING CHECKLIST

Patient Name, Social Security #, Date of Birth

I learn best by: ☐ *Group classes* ☐ *Individual instruction* ☐ *Video instruction* ☐ *Reading it myself*

Please indicate your desired learning needs by placing a check in one of the columns next to each topic.

KEY *1 = Most important to learn before I go home*
2 = I already know

(Please DATE when learning need is met.)

CARING FOR YOURSELF	1	2	DATE
Episiotomy and perineal care			
Vaginal discharge			
Hemorrhoids/Constipation			
Breast care			
Nutrition			
Activity			
Post partal exercises			
Return of menstruation			
Family planning			
Blood clots			
Post partum emotions			
Post partum warning signs			
Cesarean Birth			
Incisional care			
AFTER DISCHARGE			
When to call health care provider			
OTHER			
Working mothers			
Day care			
Sibling adjustment			
Single parent support			
Time out for parents			
Infant safety and security			
Infant As A Person Class			
New Parent Connection			

CARING FOR BABY	1	2	DATE
Diapering			
Baby bath, skin and cord care			
Circumcised/uncircumcised care			
Burping			
Bowel movements/wet diapers			
Sleeping habits			
Newborn behavior			
Jaundice			
Signs of illness			
Car seat safety			
General infant safety/poison control			
Signs/symptoms of dehydration			
Bulb syringe			
BREAST FEEDING			
Sore nipples			
Positioning			
Frequency of feedings			
Expressing/storing milk			
Engorgement			
Feeding water			
Nursing while working			
Weaning			
BOTTLE FEEDING			
Types of formula			
Preparing formula			
Frequency of feedings			

MEDICATIONS AT HOME

MEDICATIONS	STRENGTH	DOSAGE	FREQUENCY	PURPOSE/SPECIAL INSTRUCTIONS
			times per day	
			times per day	
			times per day	

RESOURCES
REFERRALS
☐ *Physician Discharge Instructions* ______
☐ *Home Care Agency* ______
☐ *Other Referrals* ______

VALUABLES: ☐ *Returned* ☐ *None* **MEDICATIONS:** ☐ *Returned* ☐ *None* ☐ *Room checked for belongings*

Patient verbalized understanding of discharge information received.

PATIENT OR SUPPORT PERSON ______ NURSE'S SIGNATURE ______ DATE ______

SELF/FAMILY LEARNING CHECKLIST

SELF/FAMILY LEARNING CHECKLIST

FIG. 23-6 Self/family learning checklist. (Copyright Abbott Northwestern Hospital of Allina Health System, Minneapolis and St. Paul, MN.)

GUIDELINES/GUÍAS

Postpartum Physical Assessment

Are you planning to breastfeed or bottle feed?
¿Piensa darle pecho o biberón al bebé?

Lie down.
Acuéstese.

I am going to take your vital signs.
Le voy a tomar sus signos vitales.

I need to take your blood pressure.
Necesito tomarle la presión de sangre.

Do you need to use the bathroom?
¿Necesita usar el baño?

I need to examine you.
Necesito examinarle.

Spread your knees and legs apart.
Abra las rodillas y las piernas.

Roll over on your side.
Póngase al lado.

Would you like some pain medication?
¿Desea medicina para calmar el dolor?

Would you like to take a sitz bath?
¿Desea tomar un baño de asiento?

SIGNS OF POTENTIAL COMPLICATIONS

Physiologic Problems

TEMPERATURE
More than 38° C after the first 24 hr

PULSE
Tachycardia or marked bradycardia

BLOOD PRESSURE
Hypotension or hypertension

ENERGY LEVEL
Lethargy, extreme fatigue

UTERUS
Deviated from the midline, boggy consistency, remains above the umbilicus after 24 hr

LOCHIA
Heavy, foul odor, bright red bleeding that is not lochia

PERINEUM
Pronounced edema, not intact, signs of infection, marked discomfort

LEGS
Homan's sign positive; painful, reddened area; warmth on posterior aspect of calf

BREASTS
Redness, heat, pain, cracked and fissured nipples, inverted nipples, palpable mass

APPETITE
Lack of appetite

ELIMINATION
Urine: inability to void, urgency, frequency, dysuria; bowel: constipation, diarrhea

REST
Inability to rest or sleep

together, and mother and nurse share the care of the infant. The organization of the mother's care must take the newborn into consideration. The day actually revolves around the baby's feeding and care times.

Expected outcomes for the postpartum period are based on the nursing diagnoses identified for the individual woman. Examples of common expected outcomes for physiologic needs are that the woman will do the following:

- Remain free from infection.
- Demonstrate normal involution and lochial characteristics.
- Remain comfortable and injury free.
- Demonstrate normal bladder and bowel elimination patterns.
- Demonstrate knowledge of breast care for breastfeeding and bottle feeding, as appropriate.
- Protect the health of future pregnancies and children.
- Integrate the newborn into the family.

Plan of Care and Interventions

Once the nursing diagnoses are formulated, the nurse plans with the woman what nursing measures will be appropriate and which are to be given priority. During her hospital stay the mother is encouraged to assume increasing responsibility for her self-care and her infant's care. As the woman and her partner provide more care for herself and the baby, the nurse's role changes from one of providing direct care to one of teaching, encouragement, and support.

The nursing plan of care will include periodic assessments to detect deviations from normal physical changes, measures to relieve discomfort or pain, safety measures to prevent injury or infection, and teaching and counseling measures designed to promote the woman's feelings of competence in self-care and baby care. Family members are included in the teaching. The nurse evaluates continuously and is ready to change the plan if indicated. Almost all hospitals use standardized care plans as a base. The nurse's ability to adapt the standardized plan to specific medical and nursing diagnoses results in individualized client care. Caution is advised against total reliance on a standardized plan; by doing so, the uniqueness of the individual may be overlooked.

Nurses assume many roles while implementing the nursing plan of care. They provide direct physical care, teach mother and baby care, and provide anticipatory guidance and counseling. Perhaps most important, they nurture the woman by providing encouragement and support as she begins to assume the many tasks of motherhood. Nurses who take the time to "mother the mother" do much to increase feelings of self-confidence in new mothers.

The first step in providing individualized care is to confirm the woman's identity by checking her wristband. At the same time, the infant's identification number is matched with the corresponding band on the mother's and, in some instances, the father's wrist. The nurse demonstrates caring and respect by determining how the mother wishes to be addressed and then notes her preference in her record and in her nursing plan of care.

The woman and her family are oriented to their surroundings. Familiarity with the unit, routines, resources, and personnel reduces one potential source of anxiety: the unknown. The mother is reassured by knowing whom and how she can call for assistance and what she can expect in the way of supplies and services. If the woman's usual daily routine before admission differs from the facility's routine, the nurse works with the woman to develop a mutually acceptable routine.

Infant abduction from hospitals in the United States has increased in the past few years. The mother should be taught to check the identity of any person who comes to remove the baby from her room. Hospital personnel usually wear picture identification badges. On some units, all staff members wear matching scrubs or special badges. Other units use closed-circuit television, computer monitoring systems, or fingerprint identification pads. As a rule, the baby is never carried in a staff member's arms between the mother's room and the nursery but is always wheeled in a bassinet, which also contains baby care supplies. Clients and nurses must work together to ensure the safety of newborns in the hospital environment.

Implementation of the nursing plan of care involves putting into practice specific activities that should result in achieving the expected outcomes planned for each individual woman (see Plan of Care).

Prevention of Infection

One important means of preventing infection is maintenance of a clean environment. Bed linens should be changed as needed. Disposable pads should be changed frequently. Women should avoid walking about barefoot to avoid contaminating bed linens when they return to bed. Supervision of use of equipment to prevent cross-contamination also is necessary. For example, a common sitz bath or heat lamp must be scrubbed after each woman's use. Staff members are another important part of the hospital environment. Personnel must be conscientious about their handwashing techniques to prevent cross-infection. Standard Precautions must be practiced. Staff members with colds, coughs, or skin infections (e.g., a cold sore on the lip [herpes simplex virus, type 1]) must follow hospital protocol when in contact with postpartum women. In many hospitals, staff with open herpetic lesions, strep throat, conjunctivitis, upper respiratory infections, or diarrhea are encouraged to avoid contact with mothers and infants by staying home until the condition is no longer contagious.

Proper care of the episiotomy site and any perineal lacerations prevents infection in the genitourinary area and aids the healing process. Educating the woman to wipe from front to back (urethra to anus) after voiding or defecating is a simple first step. In many hospitals, a squeeze bottle filled with warm water or antiseptic solution is used after each voiding to cleanse the perineal area (Box 23-3). The woman should also be taught to change her perineal pad from front to back each time she voids or defecates and to wash her hands thoroughly before and after doing so (Fig. 23-7).

Prevention of Excessive Bleeding

The most frequent cause of excessive bleeding after childbirth is **uterine atony,** failure of the uterine muscle to contract firmly. The two most important interventions for preventing excessive bleeding, therefore, are maintaining good uterine tone and preventing bladder distention. If uterine atony occurs, the relaxed uterus distends with blood and clots, and blood vessels in the placental site are not clamped off; thus excessive bleeding results.

Excessive blood loss after childbirth also may be caused by vaginal or vulvar hematomas, unrepaired lacerations of the vagina or cervix, and retained placental fragments.

NURSE ALERT

A perineal pad saturated in 15 minutes or less and/or pooling of blood under the buttocks are indications of excessive blood loss, requiring immediate assessment, intervention, and notification of the primary health care provider.

Accurate visual estimation of blood loss is an important nursing responsibility. Blood loss is usually described subjectively as scant, light, moderate, or heavy (profuse). Figure 23-8 shows examples of perineal pad saturation corresponding to each of these descriptions.

Luegenbiehl (1997) studied the ability of nurses to assess blood loss visually with precision. She found that nurses in general are inaccurate and tend to overestimate, rather than underestimate, blood loss. Luegenbiehl also found that different brands of peripads vary in their saturation volume and soaking appearance. For example, blood placed on some brands tends to soak down into the pad, whereas blood tends to spread outward on other brands. She strongly recommends that nurses determine saturation volume and soaking appearance for the peripad brands used at their institution to improve accuracy of blood-loss estimation.

More objective estimates of blood loss include weighing blood clots and items saturated with blood (1 ml

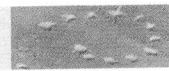

Plan of Care Postpartum Care—Vaginal Birth

NURSING DIAGNOSIS Risk for deficient fluid volume related to uterine atony/hemorrhage

Expected Outcomes *Fundus is firm, lochia is moderate, and there is no evidence of hemorrhage.*

Nursing Interventions/*Rationales*

Monitor lochia (color, amount, consistency) and count and weigh sanitary pads if lochia is heavy *to evaluate amount of bleeding.*

Monitor and palpate fundus for location and tone *to determine status of uterus and dictate further interventions because atonic uterus is most common cause of postpartum hemorrhage.*

Monitor intake and output, assess for bladder fullness, and encourage voiding *because a full bladder interferes with involution of the uterus.*

Monitor vital signs (increased pulse and respirations, decreased blood pressure) and skin temperature and color *to detect signs of hemorrhage/shock.*

Monitor postpartum hematology studies *to assess effects of blood loss.*

If fundus is boggy, apply gentle massage and assess tone response *to promote uterine contractions and increase uterine tone.* (Do not overstimulate because doing so can cause fundal relaxation.)

Express uterine clots *to promote uterine contraction.*

Explain to the woman the process of involution and teach her to assess and massage the fundus and to report any persistent bogginess *to involve her in self-care and increase sense of self-control.*

Administer oxytocic agents per physician/nurse-midwife order and evaluate effectiveness *to promote continuing uterine contraction.*

Administer fluids, blood, blood products, or plasma expanders as ordered *to replace lost fluid and lost blood volume.*

NURSING DIAGNOSIS Acute pain related to postpartum physiologic changes (hemorrhoids, episiotomy, breast engorgement, cracked/sore nipples)

Expected Outcome *Woman exhibits signs of decreased discomfort.*

Nursing Interventions/*Rationales*

Assess location, type, and quality of pain *to direct intervention.*

Explain to the woman the source and reasons for the pain, its expected duration, and treatments *to decrease anxiety and increase sense of control.*

Administer prescribed pain medications *to provide pain relief.*

If pain is perineal (episiotomy, hemorrhoids), apply ice packs in the first 24 hours *to reduce edema and vulvar irritation and reduce discomfort;* encourage sitz baths using cool water first 24 hours *to reduce edema* and warm water thereafter *to promote circulation;* apply witch hazel compresses *to reduce edema;* teach woman to use prescribed perineal creams, sprays, or ointments *to depress response of peripheral nerves;* teach woman to tighten buttocks before sitting and to sit on flat, hard surfaces *to compress buttocks and reduce pressure on the perineum.* (Avoid donuts and soft pillows as they separate the buttocks and decrease venous blood flow, increasing pain.)

If pain is from breasts and woman is breastfeeding, encourage use of a supportive bra *to increase comfort;* ascertain that infant has latched on correctly *to prevent sore nipples;* vary infant position during feeding *to prevent sore nipples.*

If breasts are engorged, have woman use warm compresses or take a warm shower before breastfeeding *to stimulate milk flow and relieve stasis.*

If nipples are sore, have woman air-dry nipples after feeding *to toughen nipples,* apply breast creams as prescribed *to soften nipples and relieve irritation* and wear breast shields in her bra *to relieve irritation.*

If pain is from breast and woman is not breastfeeding, encourage use of a tight supportive bra or breast binder and application of ice packs *to reduce lactation and decrease heaviness.*

NURSING DIAGNOSIS Disturbed sleep pattern related to excitement, discomfort, and environmental interruptions

Expected Outcome *Woman sleeps for uninterrupted periods of time and feels rested after waking.*

Nursing Interventions/*Rationales*

Establish woman's routine sleep patterns and compare with current sleep pattern, exploring things that interfere with sleep, *to determine scope of problem and direct interventions.*

Individualize nursing routines to fit woman's natural body rhythms (i.e., wake/sleep cycles), provide a sleep-promoting environment (i.e., darkness, quiet, adequate ventilation, appropriate room temperature), prepare for sleep using woman's usual routines (i.e., back rub, soothing music, warm milk), teach use of guided imagery and relaxation techniques *to promote optimum conditions for sleep.*

Avoid things or routines (i.e., caffeine, foods that induce heartburn, fluids, strenuous mental/physical activity) *that may interfere with sleep.*

Administer sedation or pain medication as prescribed *to enhance quality of sleep.*

Advise woman/partner to limit visitors and activities *to avoid further taxation and fatigue.*

Teach woman to use infant nap time as a time for her also *to nap and replenish energy and decrease fatigue.*

NURSING DIAGNOSIS Risk for impaired urinary elimination related to perineal trauma and effects of anesthesia

Expected Outcomes *Woman will void within 6 to 8 hr after birth and empty bladder completely.*

Nursing Interventions/*Rationales*

Assess position and character of uterine fundus and bladder *to ascertain if any further interventions are indicated because of displacement of the fundus or distention of the bladder.*

Measure intake and output *to assess any evidence of dehydration and subsequent decreased anticipated urine output.*

Encourage voiding by walking woman to bathroom, running water over perineum, running water in sink, providing privacy *to encourage voiding.*

Encourage oral intake *to replace any fluids lost at delivery and prevent dehydration.*

Catheterize as necessary with indwelling or straight method *to ensure bladder emptying and allow uterine involution.*

BOX 23-3 Interventions for Episiotomy, Lacerations, and Hemorrhoids

Explain both procedure and rationale before implementation.

CLEANSING

Wash hands before and after cleansing perineum and changing pads.
Wash perineum with mild soap and warm water at least once daily.
Cleanse from symphysis pubis to anal area.
Apply peripad from front to back, protecting inner surface of pad from contamination.
Wrap soiled pad and place in covered waste container.
Change pad with each void or defecation or ≥4 times per day.
Assess amount and character of lochia with each pad change.

ICE PACK

Apply a covered ice pack to perineum from front to back.

1. During first 2 hr to decrease edema formation and increase comfort
2. After the first 2 hr after the birth to provide anesthetic effect

SQUEEZE BOTTLE

Demonstrate for and assist woman; explain rationale.
Fill bottle with tap water warmed to ≈38° C (comfortably warm on the wrist).
Instruct woman to position nozzle between her legs so that squirts of water reach perineum as she sits on toilet seat. Explain that it will take whole bottle of water to cleanse perineum.
Remind her to blot dry with toilet paper or clean wipes.
Remind her to avoid contamination from anal area.
Apply clean pad.

SITZ BATH

Built-in Type

Prepare bath by thoroughly scrubbing with cleaning agent and rinsing.
Pad with towel before filling.
Fill one-half to one-third full with water of correct temperature: 38° C to 40.6° C. Some women prefer cool sitz baths. Ice is added to water to lower the temperature to the level comfortable for the woman.
Encourage woman to use at least twice a day for 20 min.
Place call bell within easy reach.
Teach woman to enter bath by tightening gluteal muscles and keeping them tightened and then relaxing them after she is in the bath.
Place dry towels within reach.
Ensure privacy.
Check woman in 15 min; assess pulse as needed.

Disposable Type

Clamp tubing and fill bag with warm water.
Raise toilet seat, place bath in bowl with overflow opening directed toward back of toilet.
Place container above toilet bowl.
Attach tube into groove at front of bath.
Loosen tube clamp to regulate rate of flow: fill bath to about one-half full; continue as above for built-in sitz bath.

SURGI-GATOR

Assemble Surgi-Gator (see Fig. 23-6).
Instruct woman regarding use and rationale.
Follow package directions.
Instruct woman to sit on toilet with legs apart and to put nozzle so tip is just past the perineum, adjusting placement as needed.
Remind her to return her applicator to her bedside stand.

TOPICAL APPLICATIONS

Apply anesthetic cream or spray: use sparingly 3 to 4 times per day.
Offer witch hazel pads (Tucks) after voiding or defecating; woman pats perineum dry from front to back, then applies witch hazel pads to hemorrhoids.

blood equals 1 g) by using devices that catch and measure blood flowing from the vagina, and establishing the milliliters of blood it takes to saturate perineal pads being used (Johnson & Johnson, 1996; Luegenbiehl, 1997); however, these methods are not common practice.

NURSE ALERT

The nurse always checks under the mother's buttocks as well as on the perineal pad. Blood may flow between the buttocks onto the linens under the mother although the amount on the perineal pad is slight; thus excessive bleeding goes undetected.

Blood pressure is not a reliable indicator of impending shock from early hemorrhage. More sensitive means of identifying shock are provided by respirations, pulse, skin condition, and urinary output (Benedetti, 2002). The frequent physical assessments performed during the fourth stage of labor are designed to provide prompt identification of excessive bleeding (see Emergency box).

Maintenance of Uterine Tone. A major intervention to restore good tone is stimulation by gently massaging the uterine fundus until it is firm (see Fig. 23-3). Fundal massage may cause a temporary increase in the amount of

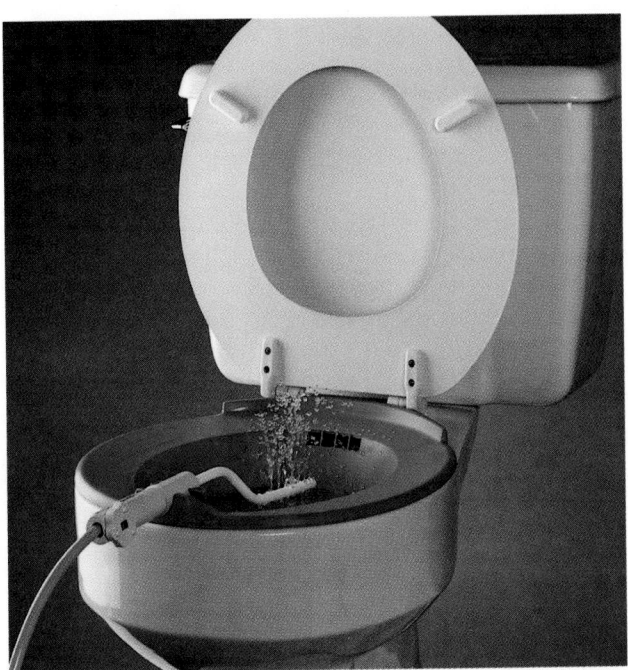

FIG. 23-7 Hygienic sitz bath (Surgi-Gator) for perineal care. (Courtesy Andermac, Inc., Yuba City, CA.)

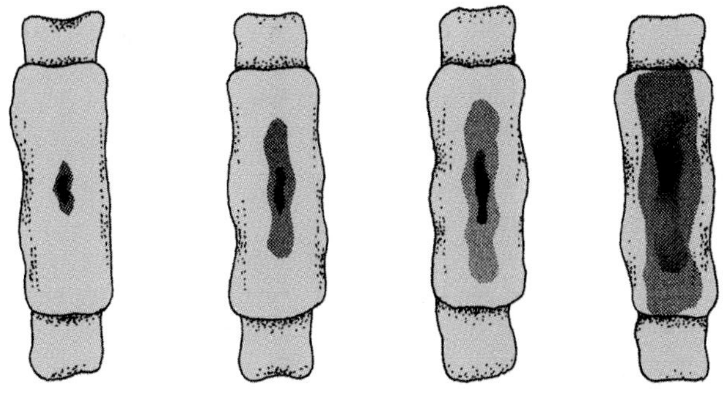

FIG. 23-8 Blood loss after birth is assessed by the extent of perineal pad saturation as (from left to right) scant (<2.5 cm); light (<10 cm); moderate (>10 cm); or heavy (one pad saturated within 2 hours).

vaginal bleeding seen as pooled blood leaves the uterus. Clots also may be expelled. Client education is extremely important in maintaining uterine tone. Fundal massage can be a very uncomfortable procedure. Understanding the causes and dangers of uterine atony and the purpose of fundal massage can help the woman to be more cooperative. Teaching the woman to do fundal self-massage enables her to maintain some control and decreases her anxiety. The uterus may remain boggy even after massage and expulsion of clots. If this occurs, it is a major warning sign of uterine atony. The nurse must remain with the client and summon help, including notifying the primary health care provider immediately. Additional interventions likely to be used are administration of IV fluids and oxytocic medications (drugs that stimulate contraction of the uterine smooth muscle). Table 37-1 contains information about common oxytocic medications.

LEGAL TIP Client Abandonment

In an emergency situation, the nurse must remain with the client and call for help. Leaving the client can lead to a charge of client abandonment.

Prevention of Bladder Distention. A full bladder causes the uterus to be displaced above the umbilicus and well to one side of the midline in the abdomen. It also prevents the uterus from contracting normally. Nursing interventions focus on helping the woman to empty her bladder spontaneously as soon as possible. The first priority is to assist the woman to the bathroom or onto a bedpan if she is unable to ambulate. Having the woman listen to running water, placing her hands in warm water, or pouring water from a squeeze bottle over her perineum may stimulate voiding. Other techniques include assisting the woman into the shower or sitz bath and encouraging her to void or placing spirits of peppermint in a bedpan under

EMERGENCY
Hypovolemic Shock

SIGNS AND SYMPTOMS

- Persistent significant bleeding—perineal pad soaked within 15 min; *may not be accompanied by a change in vital signs or maternal color or behavior.*
- Woman states she feels weak, light-headed, "funny," "sick to my stomach," or "sees stars."
- Woman begins to act anxious or exhibits air hunger.
- Woman's skin turns ashen or grayish.
- Skin feels cool and clammy.
- Pulse rate increases.
- Blood pressure declines.

INTERVENTIONS

- Notify primary health care provider.
- If uterus is atonic, massage gently and expel clots to cause uterus to contract; compress uterus manually, as needed, by using two hands. Add oxytocic agent to IV drip, as ordered.
- Give oxygen by face mask or nasal prongs at 8 to 10 L/min.
- Tilt the woman to her side or elevate the right hip; elevate her legs to a ≥30-degree angle.
- Provide additional or maintain existing IV infusion of lactated Ringer's solution or normal saline solution to restore circulatory volume.
- Administer blood or blood products, as ordered.
- Monitor vital signs.
- Insert an indwelling urinary catheter to monitor perfusion of kidneys.
- Administer emergency drugs, as ordered.
- Prepare for possible surgery or other emergency treatments or procedures.
- Chart incident, medical and nursing interventions instituted, and results of treatments.

the woman. The vapors may relax the urinary meatus and trigger spontaneous voiding. Administering analgesics, if ordered, may be indicated because some women may fear voiding because of the anticipated pain. If these measures are unsuccessful, a sterile catheter may be inserted to drain the urine.

Evaluation of the woman's responses to intervention is an ongoing part of the nursing process. All responses to interventions should be carefully recorded. If the expected outcomes are not met or new needs emerge, modify the plan of care accordingly. For example, if the uterus is firm and the bladder empty, something other than uterine atony is causing the excessive bleeding. Further assessment is necessary to determine the cause and correct the problem. See Chapter 37 for further discussion of postpartum hemorrhage.

Promotion of Comfort, Rest, Ambulation, and Exercise

Comfort. Most women have some degree of discomfort during the immediate postpartum period. Common causes of discomfort include afterbirth pains, episiotomy or perineal lacerations, hemorrhoids, and breast engorgement. The woman's description of the type and severity of her pain is the nurse's best guide in choosing an appropriate intervention. To confirm the location and extent of discomfort, the nurse inspects and palpates areas of pain as appropriate for redness, swelling, discharge, and heat and observes for body tension, guarded movements, and facial tension. Blood pressure, pulse, and respirations may be elevated in response to acute pain. Diaphoresis may accompany severe pain. A lack of objective symptoms does not necessarily mean there is no pain, because there also may be a cultural component to the expression of pain. Nursing interventions are intended to eliminate the pain sensation entirely or reduce it to a tolerable level that allows the woman to care for herself and her baby. Nurses may use both nonpharmacologic and pharmacologic interventions to promote comfort. Depending on reported severity, nonpharmacologic measures should be used either alone or in combination with pharmacologic interventions. Pain relief is enhanced by using more than one method or route.

Nonpharmacologic Interventions. **Afterbirth pains** are the menstrual-like cramps felt by many women as the uterus contracts after childbirth. Warmth, distraction, deep breathing, imagery, therapeutic touch, relaxation, and interaction with the infant may decrease the discomfort associated with these uterine contractions.

Simple interventions that can decrease the discomfort associated with an episiotomy or perineal lacerations include encouraging the woman to lie on her side whenever possible and to use a pillow when sitting. Other interventions include application of an ice pack; topical applications (if ordered); dry heat; cleansing with a squeeze bottle; and a cleansing shower, tub bath, or sitz bath. Many of these interventions also are effective for hemorrhoids, especially ice packs, sitz baths, and topical applications (such as witch hazel pads). Box 23-3 gives more specific information about these interventions.

The discomfort associated with engorged breasts may be lessened by the application of either ice or heat to the breasts, application of cold cabbage leaves to the breasts, and the wearing of a well-fitted support bra. Decisions about specific interventions for relieving engorgement are based on whether the woman chooses to breastfeed or bottle feed (see Chapter 27).

Pharmacologic Interventions. Most primary health care providers routinely order a variety of analgesics to be administered as needed, including both narcotic and nonnarcotic (nonsteroidal antiinflammatory medications) choices, with their dosage and time-frequency ranges. Topical application of antiseptic or anesthetic ointment or sprays is a common pharmacologic intervention.

Patient-controlled analgesia (PCA) pumps and continuous epidural analgesia infusions are technologies frequently used to provide postpartum pain relief after cesarean birth. The nurse should carefully monitor all women receiving opioids because respiratory depression and decreased intestinal motility are side effects. Many women want to participate in decisions about analgesia. Severe pain, however, may interfere with active participation in choosing pain relief measures. If an analgesic is to be given, the nurse must make a clinical judgment of the type, dosage, and frequency from the medications ordered. The woman is informed of the prescribed analgesic and its common side effects; this teaching is documented.

Breastfeeding mothers often have concerns about the effects on the infant of taking an analgesic. Although nearly all medications present in maternal circulation also are found in breast milk, many analgesics (e.g., ibuprofen, acetaminophen) commonly used during the postpartum period are considered relatively safe for breastfeeding mothers (American Academy of Pediatrics, 2001). Often the timing of medications can be adjusted to minimize infant exposure. A mother may be given pain medication at the time of or immediately after breastfeeding, for example, so that the interval between medication administration and the next nursing period is as long as possible. The decision to administer medications of any kind to a breastfeeding mother must always be made by carefully weighing the woman's need for the medication against actual or potential risks to the infant.

If acceptable pain relief has not been obtained in 1 hour and there has been no change in the initial assessment, the nurse may contact the primary care provider for additional pain relief orders or further directions. Unrelieved pain results in fatigue, anxiety, and a worsening perception of the pain. It might also indicate the presence of a previously unknown or untreated problem. Further assessment and treatment will likely be necessary to determine the cause of the pain and correct it.

Rest. The excitement and exhilaration felt after the birth of the infant may make rest difficult. The new mother, who often is anxious about her ability to care for her infant or is uncomfortable, may also have difficulty sleeping. In the days that follow, the demands of the infant, along with the influence of the hospital environment and routines, contribute to alterations in her sleep pattern.

Fatigue. Fatigue is common in the postpartum period (Pugh et al., 1999) and involves both physiologic components associated with long labors, cesarean birth, anemia, and breastfeeding and psychologic components related to depression and anxiety. Infant behavior also can be related to fatigue, particularly with mothers of more difficult infants.

Interventions must be planned to meet the woman's individual needs for sleep and rest. Backrubs, other comfort measures, and medication for sleep for the first few nights may be necessary. Support and encouragement in mothering behaviors help reduce anxiety. Hospital and nursing routines also may be adjusted to meet individual needs. In addition, the nurse can help the family limit visitors and provide a comfortable chair or bed for the partner.

Ambulation. Early ambulation is successful in reducing the incidence of thromboembolism and in promoting the woman's more rapid recovery of strength. Confinement to bed is not required for the woman who had general anesthesia, epidural or spinal anesthesia, or local anesthesia such as a pudendal block. Free movement is permitted once the anesthetic wears off, unless an analgesic has been administered. After the initial recovery period is over, the mother is encouraged to ambulate frequently.

NURSE ALERT

Having a hospital staff or family member present the first time the woman gets out of bed after childbirth is wise because she may feel weak, dizzy, faint, or light-headed.

The rapid decrease in intraabdominal pressure after birth results in a dilation of blood vessels supplying the intestines, which is known as splanchnic engorgement, and causes blood to pool in the viscera. This condition contributes to the development of orthostatic hypotension and may occur when the woman who has recently given birth sits or stands, first ambulates, or takes a warm shower or sitz bath. The nurse also must consider the baseline blood pressure; amount of blood loss; and type, amount, and timing of analgesic or anesthetic medications administered when assisting a woman to ambulate.

Prevention of thrombus (clot formation) is part of the nursing plan of care. Women who must remain in bed after giving birth are at an increased risk for the development of thrombus. If a woman remains in bed longer than 8 hours (e.g., postpartum $MgSO_4$ therapy for preeclampsia), exercise to promote circulation in the legs is indicated by using the following routine:

- Alternate flexion and extension of feet.
- Rotate ankle in circular motion.
- Alternate flexion and extension of legs.
- Press back of knee to bed surface; relax.

If the woman is susceptible to thromboembolism, she is encouraged to walk about actively and discouraged from sitting immobile in a chair. Women with varicosities are encouraged to wear support hose. If a thrombus is suspected–as evidenced by a positive **Homan's sign** (complaint of pain in calf muscles when the foot is dorsiflexed) or warmth, redness, or tenderness in the suspected leg–the primary health care provider should be notified immediately; meanwhile the woman should be confined to bed, with the affected limb elevated on pillows.

Exercise. Most women who have just given birth are extremely interested in regaining their nonpregnant figures. Postpartum exercise can begin soon after birth, although the woman should be encouraged to start with simple exercises and gradually progress to more strenuous ones. Figure 23-9 illustrates a number of exercises appropriate for the new mother. Abdominal exercises are postponed until about 4 weeks after cesarean birth.

Kegel pelvic exercises to strengthen muscle tone are extremely important, particularly after vaginal birth. To perform them, the woman consciously contracts and relaxes the muscles around the vagina. Kegel exercises help women to regain the muscle tone that is often lost as pelvic tissues are stretched and torn during pregnancy and birth. Women who maintain muscle strength may benefit years later by maintaining urinary continence.

Women must learn to perform the Kegel exercises correctly (see Teaching for Self-Care box in Chapter 5). Studies have shown that approximately one fourth of all women who learn Kegel exercises do them incorrectly and may increase their risk of incontinence (Sampselle et al., 2000). This may occur when women inadvertently bear down on the pelvic floor muscles (Valsalva effort), thrusting the perineum outward. The health care provider can teach and assess the woman's technique during the pelvic examination at the 6-week checkup, inserting two fingers intravaginally and checking whether the pelvic floor muscles correctly contract and relax.

Promotion of Nutrition

During the hospital stay, most women display a good appetite and eat well; nutritious snacks are usually welcomed. Women may request that family members bring to the hospital favorite or culturally appropriate foods (Fig. 23-10). Cultural dietary preferences must be respected. This interest in food presents an ideal opportunity for nutritional counseling on dietary needs after pregnancy, such as for breastfeeding, preventing constipation and anemia, weight loss, and promoting healing and well-being (see Chapter 15). Prenatal vitamins and iron supplements are often continued until 6 weeks postpartum or the ordered supply has been used.

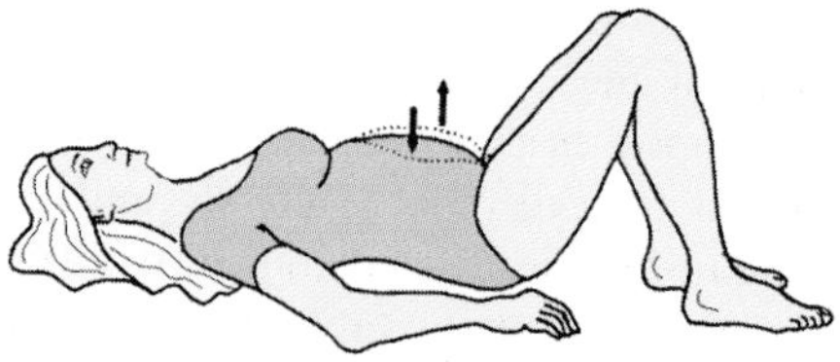

Abdominal Breathing. Lie on back with knees bent. Inhale deeply through nose. Keep ribs stationary and allow abdomen to expand upward. Exhale slowly but forcefully while contracting the abdominal muscles; hold for 3 to 5 seconds while exhaling. Relax.

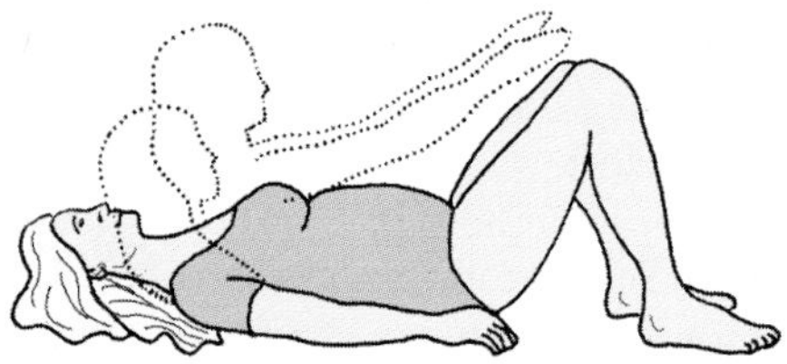

Reach for the Knees. Lie on back with knees bent. While inhaling, deeply lower chin onto chest. While exhaling, raise head and shoulders slowly and smoothly and reach for knees with arms outstretched. The body should only rise as far as the back will naturally bend while waist remains on floor or bed (about 6 to 8 inches). Slowly and smoothly lower head and shoulders back to starting position. Relax.

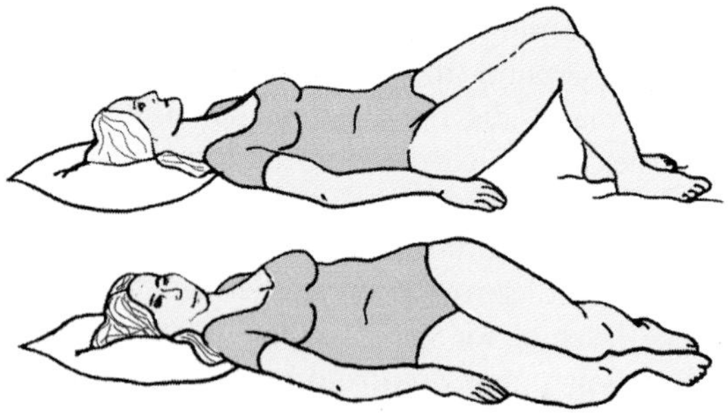

Double Knee Roll. Lie on back with knees bent. Keeping shoulders flat and feet stationary, slowly and smoothly roll knees over to the left to touch floor or bed. Maintaining a smooth motion, roll knees back over to the right until they touch floor or bed. Return to starting position and relax.

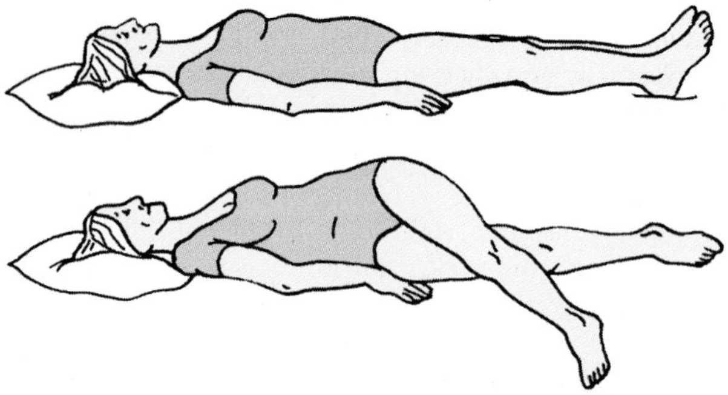

Leg Roll. Lie on back with legs straight. Keeping shoulders flat and legs straight, slowly and smoothly lift left leg and roll it over to touch the right side of floor or bed and return to starting position. Repeat, rolling right leg over to touch left side of floor or bed. Relax.

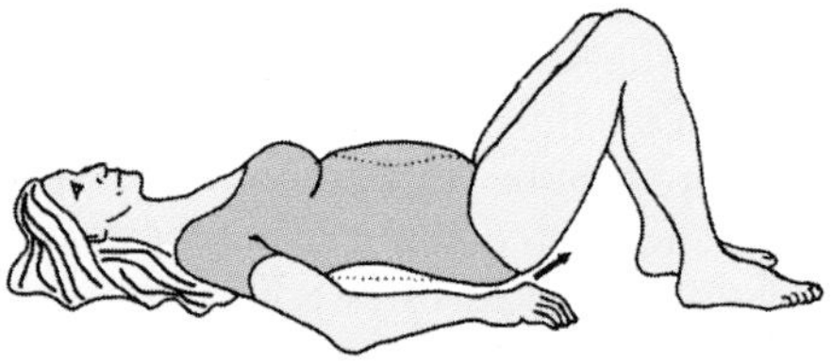

Combined Abdominal Breathing and Supine Pelvic Tilt (Pelvic Rock). Lie on back with knees bent. While inhaling deeply, roll pelvis back by flattening lower back on floor or bed. Exhale slowly but forcefully while contracting abdominal muscles and tightening buttocks. Hold for 3 to 5 seconds while exhaling. Relax.

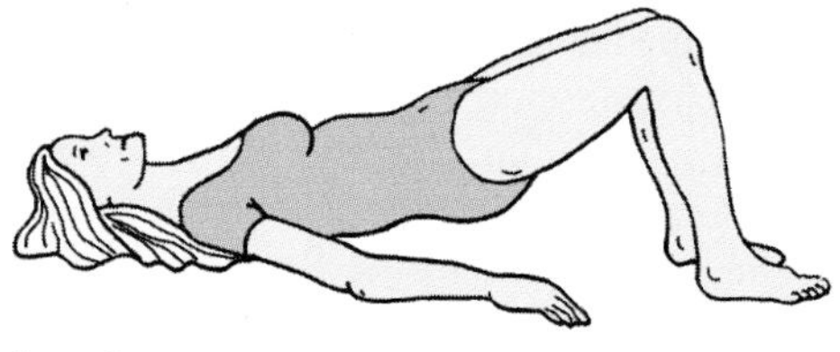

Buttocks Lift. Lie on back with arms at sides, knees bent, and feet flat. Slowly raise buttocks and arch back. Return slowly to starting position.

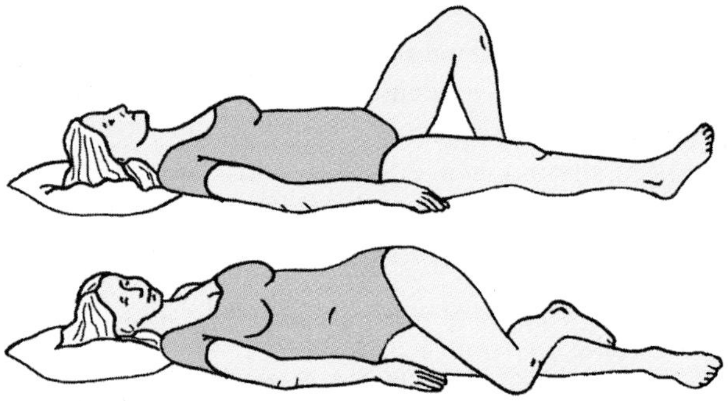

Single Knee Roll. Lie on back with right leg straight and left leg bent at the knee. Keeping shoulders flat, slowly and smoothly roll left knee over to the right to touch floor or bed and then back to starting position. Reverse position of legs. Roll right knee over to the left to touch floor or bed and return to starting position. Relax.

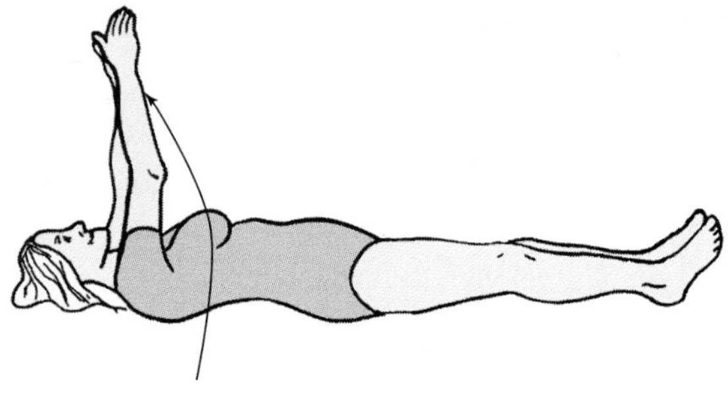

Arm Raises. Lie on back with arms extended at 90 degree-angle from body. Raise arms so they are perpendicular and hands touch. Lower slowly.

FIG. 23-9 Postpartum exercise should begin as soon as possible. The woman should start with simple exercises and gradually progress to more strenuous ones.

Promotion of Normal Bladder and Bowel Patterns

Bladder. After giving birth the mother should void spontaneously within 6 to 8 hours. The first several voidings should be measured to document adequate emptying of the bladder. A volume of at least 150 ml is expected for each voiding. Some women have difficulty in emptying the bladder, possibly as a result of diminished bladder tone, edema from trauma, or fear of discomfort. Nursing interventions for inability to void and bladder distention are discussed on pp. 631-632.

Bowel. Nursing interventions to promote normal bowel elimination include educating the woman about measures to avoid constipation. These interventions include ensuring adequate roughage and fluid intake and promoting exercise. Alerting the woman to side effects of medications such as narcotic analgesics (i.e., decreased gastrointestinal tract motility) may encourage her to implement measures to reduce the risk of constipation. Stool softeners or laxatives are often routinely ordered and may be necessary during the early postpartum period. With early discharge, a new mother is often at home before having a bowel movement.

Breastfeeding Promotion or Lactation Suppression

Breastfeeding Promotion. The first 2 hours after birth are an excellent time to encourage the mother to breastfeed. The infant is in an alert state and ready to nurse. Breastfeeding aids in the contraction of the uterus and prevention of maternal hemorrhage. This is a wonderful opportunity for the nurse to instruct the mother in breastfeeding and to assess the physical appearance of the breasts. (See Chapter 27 for further information on assisting the breastfeeding woman.)

Lactation Suppression. Suppression of lactation is necessary when the woman has decided not to breastfeed or in the event of neonatal death. One very important nonpharmacologic intervention is wearing a well-fitted support bra or breast binder continuously for at least the first 72 hours after giving birth. Women also should avoid any breast stimulation, including running warm water over the breasts, newborn suckling, or pumping of the breasts. A few nonbreastfeeding mothers experience severe breast *engorgement* (swelling of breast tissue caused by increased blood and lymph supply to the breasts before lactation). If breast engorgement occurs, it can usually be managed satisfactorily with nonpharmacologic interventions.

Ice packs to the breasts are helpful in decreasing the discomfort associated with engorgement. The woman should use a 15-minutes-on, 45-minutes-off schedule to prevent the rebound swelling that can occur if ice is used continuously, or she can place fresh cabbage leaves inside her bra. Cabbage leaves have been used to treat swelling in other cultures for years (Roberts, 1995). The exact mechanism of action is not known, but it is thought that naturally occurring plant estrogens or salicylates may be responsible for the effects. The leaves are replaced each time they wilt. A mild analgesic also may be necessary to help the mother through this uncomfortable time. Medications that were once prescribed for lactation suppression (estrogen, estrogen and testosterone, and bromocriptine) are no longer used.

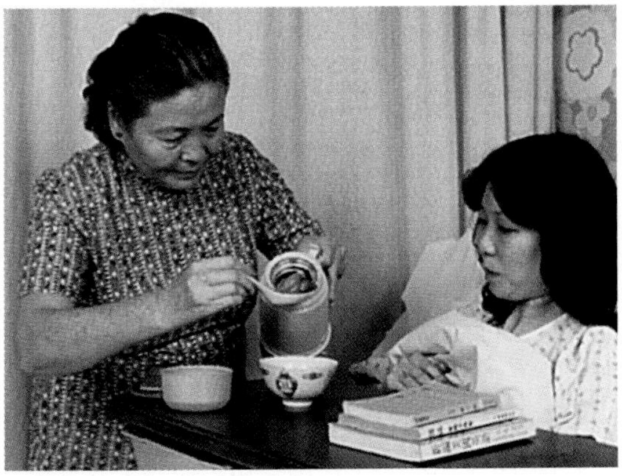

FIG. 23-10 Special foods are considered essential for recovery in the Asian culture. (Courtesy Concept Media, Irvine, CA).

Health Promotion of Future Pregnancies and Children

If the assessment data indicate the need, rubella vaccination and Rh immune globulin (RhoGAM) are administered during the puerperium. Failure to administer these products to women at risk of contracting rubella or developing Rh isoimmunization can seriously jeopardize the health of any future pregnancies and children.

Rubella Vaccination. For women who have not had rubella (10% to 20% of all women) or women who are serologically not immune (titer of 1:8 or enzyme immunoassay [EIA] level 0.8), a subcutaneous injection of rubella vaccine is recommended before discharge. Seroconversion occurs in approximately 90% of women vaccinated after birth. The live attenuated rubella virus is not communicable; therefore breastfeeding mothers can be vaccinated. However, because the virus is shed in urine and other body fluids, the vaccine should not be given if the mother or other household members are immunocompromised. Rubella vaccine is made from duck eggs, so a hypersensitivity reaction to the vaccine may develop in women who have allergies to these eggs, for which they will need adrenaline. A transient benign arthralgia or rash is common in vaccinated women. Because the vaccine may be teratogenic, the client must be informed about the vaccine (Legal Tip).

LEGAL TIP Rubella Vaccination

Informed consent for rubella vaccination in the postpartum period includes information about the possible side effects and the risk of teratogenic effects. Women must understand that they must practice contraception to avoid pregnancy for 2 to 3 months after being vaccinated.

Prevention of Rh Isoimmunization. Injection of Rh immune globulin (a solution of gamma-globulin that contains Rh antibodies) within 72 hours after birth prevents sensitization in the Rh-negative woman who has had a fetomaternal transfusion of Rh-positive red blood cells (RBCs) (see Medication Guide box). The Rh immune globulin promotes lysis of the fetal Rh-positive blood cells before the mother forms her own antibodies against them.

NURSE ALERT

Rh immune globulin is administered postpartally to all Rh-negative, antibody (Coombs') negative women who give birth to Rh-positive infants. Rh immune globulin is administered to the mother intramuscularly. It should never be given to an infant.

MEDICATION GUIDE

Rh Immune Globulin, RhoGAM, Gamulin Rh, HypRho-D

ACTION ■ Suppression of immune response in nonsensitized women with Rh-negative blood who receive Rh-positive blood cells because of fetomaternal hemorrhage, transfusion, or accident

INDICATIONS ■ Suppress antibody formation in women with Rh-negative blood after birth, miscarriage/pregnancy termination, abdominal trauma, ectopic pregnancy, amniocentesis, version, or chorionic villi sampling

DOSAGE/ROUTE ■ Standard dose, 1 vial (300 μg) IM in deltoid or gluteal muscle; microdose, 1 vial (50 μg) IM in deltoid muscle

ADVERSE EFFECTS ■ Myalgia, lethargy, localized tenderness and stiffness at injection site, possible allergic response

NURSING CONSIDERATIONS ■ Give standard dose to mother within 72 hr after birth if baby is Rh positive, at 28 wk of gestation as prophylaxis, or after an incident or exposure risk that occurs after 28 wk of gestation (e.g., amniocentesis, second trimester miscarriage or abortion, after version). ■ Give microdose for first trimester miscarriage or abortion, ectopic pregnancy, chorionic villi sampling. ■ Verify that the woman is Rh negative and has not been sensitized, that Coombs' test is negative, and that baby is Rh positive. Provide explanation to the woman about procedure, including the purpose, possible side effects, and effect on future pregnancies. Have the woman sign a consent form if required by agency. Verify correct dosage and confirm lot number and woman's identity before giving injection (verify with another RN or other procedure per agency policy); document administration per agency policy.

The administration of 300 μg (1 vial) of Rh immune globulin is usually sufficient to prevent maternal sensitization. If a large fetomaternal transfusion is suspected, however, the dosage needed should be determined by performing a **Kleihauer-Betke test,** which detects the amount of fetal blood in the maternal circulation. If more than 15 ml of fetal blood is present in maternal circulation, the dosage of Rh immune globulin must be increased.

A 1:1000 dilution of Rh immune globulin is crossmatched to the mother's RBCs to ensure compatibility. Because Rh immune globulin is usually considered to be a blood product, precautions similar to those used for transfusing blood are necessary when it is given. The identification number on the client's hospital wristband should correspond to the identification number found on the laboratory slip. The nurse also must check to see that the lot number on the laboratory slip corresponds to the lot number on the vial. Finally, the expiration date on the vial should be checked to ensure a usable product.

Rh immune globulin suppresses the immune response; therefore the woman who receives both Rh immune globulin and rubella vaccine must be tested at 3 months to see if she has developed rubella immunity. If not, the woman will need another dose of rubella vaccine.

Some disagree about whether Rh immune globulin should be considered a blood product. Health care providers should discuss the most recent information about this issue with women whose religious beliefs conflict with having blood products administered to them.

Evaluation

The nurse can be reasonably assured that care was effective if expected outcomes for care for physical needs have been met.

CARE MANAGEMENT: PSYCHOSOCIAL NEEDS

Meeting the psychosocial needs of new mothers involves planning care that considers the composition and functioning of the entire family. Nurses assess the parents' reactions to the birth experience, feelings about themselves, and interactions with the new baby and other family members. Specific interventions are then planned to increase the parents' knowledge and self-confidence as they assume the care and responsibility of the new baby and integrate a new member into their existing family structure in a way that meets their cultural expectations (see Chapters 24 and 28).

Assessment and Nursing Diagnoses

Impact of the Birth Experience

Many women indicate a need to examine the birth process itself and look at their own intrapartal behavior in retrospect. Their partners may express similar desires. During pregnancy the woman and her partner may have developed a specific birth plan that included a vaginal birth and very little medical intervention. If their birth experience was quite different (e.g., labor induction, epidural anesthesia, cesarean birth), both partners may need to mourn the loss of their expectations before they can adjust to the reality of their birth experience. Inviting them to review the events and describe how they feel helps the nurse assess how well they understand what happened and how well they have been able to put their childbirth experience into perspective.

Maternal Self-Image

An important assessment concerns the woman's self-concept, body image, and sexuality. How this new mother feels about herself and her body during the puerperium may affect her behavior and adaptation to parenting. The woman's self-concept and body image also may affect her sexuality.

Feelings related to sexual adjustment after childbirth are often a cause of concern for new parents. Women who have recently given birth may be reluctant to resume sexual intercourse for fear of pain or may worry that coitus could damage healing perineal tissue. Because many new parents are anxious for information but reluctant to bring up the subject, postpartum nurses should matter-of-factly include the topic of postpartum sexuality during their routine physical assessment. While examining the episiotomy site, for example, the nurse can say, "I know you're sore right now, but it probably won't be long until you (or you and your partner) are ready to make love again. Have you thought about what that might be like? Would you like to ask me questions?" This approach assures the woman and her partner that resuming sexual activity is a legitimate concern for new parents and indicates the nurse's willingness to answer questions and share information.

Maternal Adaptation

The psychosocial assessment also includes evaluating adaptation to parenthood, which represents a significant stress for many women. The majority (50% to 70%) of new mothers have a psychologic reaction after birth that is often referred to as "maternity or postpartum blues" or the *baby blues*. The cause of these baby blues is unknown, but may well be a transient response to the rapid role changes that occur as women adapt to motherhood. Symptoms vary widely from woman to woman, but can include behaviors such as weeping, insomnia, irritability, anxiety, forgetfulness, mood swings, and negative feelings toward the infant. These symptoms, which may be exacerbated by the sleep deprivation that often occurs during the puerperium, usually appear within the first week after birth and generally disappear by postpartum day 10. Extra rest, physical and emotional support, and sympathetic understanding from friends and family are usually sufficient to help women cope with this reaction (Bowes & Katz, 2002). It is important to remember that the baby blues are mild and short-lived. See Chapter 35 for a discussion of more severe postpartum depression.

Parent-Infant Interactions

Adaptation to parenthood also can be assessed by evaluating the mother's and father's reactions to and interactions with the new baby. Clues indicating successful adaptation begin to appear early in the postbirth period as parents react positively to the newborn infant and continue the process of establishing a relationship with him or her.

Parents are adapting well to their new role when they exhibit a realistic perception and acceptance of their newborn's needs and his or her limited abilities, immature social responses, and helplessness. Examples of positive parent-infant interactions include taking pleasure in their infant and in the tasks done for and with him or her, understanding their infant's emotional states and providing comfort, and reading their infant's cues for new experiences and sensing his or her fatigue level. See Chapter 24 for a more in-depth discussion of parenting.

Family Structure and Functioning

Another important component of the psychosocial assessment is examining the family composition and functioning. A woman's adjustment to her role as mother is affected greatly by her relationships with her partner, her mother and other relatives, and any other children. Nurses can help to ease the new mother's return home by identifying possible conflicts among family members and helping the woman plan strategies for dealing with these problems before discharge. Such a conflict could arise when couples have very different ideas about parenting. Dealing with the stresses of sibling rivalry and unsolicited grandparent advice also can affect the woman's transition to motherhood. Only by asking about the woman's relationship with other nuclear and extended family members can the nurse discover potential problems in such relationships and help to plan workable solutions for them.

Impact of Cultural Diversity

The final component of a complete psychosocial assessment is the client's cultural beliefs and values. Much of a woman's behavior during the postpartum period is strongly influenced by her cultural background. In today's world, where travel is commonplace, nurses are likely to come in contact with women from many different countries and cultures. The nurse must remember that all cultures have developed safe and satisfying methods of caring for new mothers and babies. Only by understanding and respecting the values and beliefs of each woman can the nurse design a plan of care to meet the individual needs.

The following is an example of one "clash of cultures." The nurse in this case was able to take this information and modify her plan of care to make it culturally relevant, and therefore more satisfying, for the woman.

A Vietnamese woman who had been in the United States for 4 years requested rooming-in facilities after childbirth. Instead of participating in the care of her infant, she refused to do so, remained in bed, wore a woolen cap, and appeared distressed and angry. The staff were puzzled and upset by her behavior. One nurse decided to put into effect her newly learned concepts concerning cross-cultural nursing. She began by praising the woman's ability to speak English and, after eliciting a smile, remarked, "Every country has developed good ways to look after mothers and babies. Would you tell me about the care in Vietnam?" There was an immediate response. The woman explained that in her country, women remained in bed for at least 10 days after birth, and the biggest danger to their health was getting a cold. The baby was kept in the room with his mother, but either a grandmother or nurse took complete charge of the care.

Sometimes the psychosocial assessment indicates serious actual or potential problems that must be addressed. The Signs of Potential Complications box lists several psychosocial needs that, at a minimum, warrant ongoing evaluation after hospital discharge. Clients exhibiting these needs should be referred to appropriate community resources for assessment and management.

After analyzing the data obtained during the assessment process, the nurse establishes nursing diagnoses to provide a guide for planning care. Nursing diagnoses related to psychosocial issues that are frequently established for the postpartum woman include the following:

- *Interrupted family processes related to*
  - –unexpected birth of twins
- *Impaired verbal communication related to*
  - –woman's hearing impairment
  - –woman's language not the same as nurse's
- *Impaired parenting related to*
  - –long, difficult labor
  - –unmet expectations of labor and the birth
- *Anxiety related to*
  - –newness of parenting role
- *Risk for situational low self-esteem related to*
  - –body image changes

Expected Outcomes of Care

The psychosocial plan of care for the postpartum woman includes all family members. The postnatal period is a crucial one for family adjustment. Developing a plan of care that recognizes family strengths and provides support for family weaknesses does much to help family members take on new tasks and responsibilities.

Expected psychosocial outcomes during the postpartum period are based on the nursing diagnoses identified for the individual woman and her family. Examples of common expected outcomes include that the woman (family) will do the following:

- Identify measures that promote a healthy personal adjustment in the postpartum period.
- Maintain healthy family functioning based on cultural norms and personal expectations.

Plan of Care and Interventions

The nurse functions in the roles of teacher, encourager, and supporter rather than doer while implementing the psychosocial plan of care for a postpartum woman. Implementation of the psychosocial plan of care involves carrying out specific activities to achieve the expected outcomes of care planned for each individual woman. Several topics that should be included in the psychosocial plan of care include promotion of parenting skills and family member adjustment to the newest member. Chapter 24 discusses these topics.

Cultural issues also must be considered when planning care. In contrast with allopathic medicine, many traditional health beliefs and practices occur among the different cultures within the North American population. Traditional health practices that are used to maintain health or to avoid illnesses deal with the whole person (body, mind, and spirit) and tend to be culturally based.

Women from various cultures may view health as a balance between opposing forces (e.g., yin versus yang), being in harmony with nature, or just "feeling good." Traditional practices may include the observance of certain dietary restrictions, clothing, or taboos for balancing the body; participation in certain activities such as sports and art for maintaining mental health; and use of silence, prayer, or meditation for developing spiritually. Practices (e.g., using religious objects, eating garlic) are used to protect oneself from illness and may involve avoiding people who are believed to create hexes or spells, or who have an evil eye.

SIGNS OF POTENTIAL COMPLICATIONS

Psychosocial Needs

Unable or unwilling to discuss labor and birth experience.
Refers to self as ugly and useless.
Excessively preoccupied with self (body image).
Markedly depressed.
Lacks a support system.
Partner and/or other family members react negatively to the baby.
Refuses to interact with or care for baby. For example, does not name baby, does not want to hold or feed baby, is upset by vomiting and wet or dirty diapers. (Cultural appropriateness of actions must be considered.)
Expresses disappointment over baby's sex.
Sees baby as messy or unattractive.
Baby reminds mother of family member or friend she doesn't like.

Restoration of health may involve a person taking folk medicines (e.g., herbs, animal substances) or using a traditional healer.

Childbirth occurs within this sociocultural context. Rest, seclusion, dietary restraints, and ceremonies honoring the mother are all common traditional practices that are followed for the promotion of the health and well-being of the mother and baby (Davis, 2001; Kridli, 2002; Lauderdale, 1999; Mattson, 2000).

Several common traditional health practices are used and beliefs held by women and their families during the postpartum period. In Southeast Asia, for example, the body is thought to be in a "cold" state after birth, because of the loss of blood, which is considered a "hot" substance (Davis, 2001). Therefore balance must be restored by increasing the return of yang forces present physically or symbolically in hot food, hot water, and warm air (Davis, 2001; Lauderdale, 1999.). Vietnamese, Cambodian, and Hmong women reported that if they did not follow the traditional diet or get sufficient rest after childbirth, they would likely become ill or develop serious health problems later in life (Davis, 2001).

Another common belief is that the mother and baby remain in a weak and vulnerable state for a period of several weeks after birth (Davis, 2001; Mattson, 2000). During this time, the mother may remain in a passive role, not take baths or showers, and stay in bed to prevent cold air from entering her body.

Women who have immigrated to the United States or other Western nations without their extended family may not have much help at home, thus making it extremely difficult for them to observe these activity restrictions (Davis, 2001). The Cultural Considerations box lists some common cultural beliefs about the postpartum period.

It is important that nurses consider all cultural aspects when planning care and not use their own cultural beliefs as the framework for that care. A nursing diagnosis of noncompliance is not appropriate for a client who has a language barrier or behaves culturally different from what is generally expected by nurses during postpartum care. Although the beliefs and behaviors of other cultures may seem different or strange, they should be encouraged as long as the mother wants to conform to them, and she and the baby have no ill effects. The nurse must determine whether a woman is using any folk medicine during the postpartum period because active ingredients in folk medicine may have adverse physiologic effects on the woman when ingested with prescribed medicines (Mattson, 2000). The nurse also should not assume that a mother desires to use traditional health practices that represent a particular cultural group merely because she is a member of that culture. Many young women who are first-generation or second-generation Americans follow their cultural traditions only when older family members are present or not at all.

Nursing must be culturally relevant. As in planning care to meet physiologic needs, standardized care plans must be adapted to meet the specific needs of the individual families. The nurse must be open and continue to learn about how best to meet the health needs of childbearing women with diverse cultural backgrounds.

Evaluation

The nurse can be reasonably assured that care was effective if expected outcomes for care for psychosocial needs have been met.

CULTURAL CONSIDERATIONS

Some Cultural Beliefs About the Postpartum Period

Chinese, Mexican, Korean, and Southeast Asian women may wish to eat only warm foods and drink hot drinks to replace blood loss and to restore the balance of hot and cold in their bodies. These women also may wish to stay warm and avoid bathing, exercises, and hair washing for 7 to 30 days after childbirth. Self-care may not be a priority; care by family members is preferred. The woman has respect for elders and authority. These women may wear abdominal binders. They may prefer not to give their babies colostrum.

Arabic women eat special meals designed to restore their energy. They are expected to stay at home for 40 days after delivery to avoid illness resulting from exposure to the outside air.

Haitian women may request to take the placenta home to bury or burn.

Muslim women follow strict religious laws on modesty and diet. A Muslim woman must keep her hair, body, arms to the wrist, and legs to the ankles covered at all times. She cannot be alone in the presence of a man other than her husband or a male relative. Observant Muslims will not eat pork or pork products and are obligated to eat meat slaughtered according to Islamic laws (halal meat). If halal meat is not available, kosher meat, seafood, or a vegetarian diet is usually accepted.

CONTRACEPTION

Birth control is government mandated in mainland China. Most Chinese women will have an intrauterine device inserted after the birth of their first child. Women do not want hormonal methods of contraception because they fear putting these medications in their bodies.

Saudi Arabian and Hispanic women will likely choose the rhythm method because most are Catholic.

(East) Indian men are encouraged to have voluntary sterilization by vasectomy.

Muslim couples may practice contraception by mutual consent as long as its use is not harmful to the woman. Acceptable contraceptive methods include foam and condoms, the diaphragm, and natural family planning.

Hmong women highly value and desire large families, which limits birth control practices.

Arabic women value large families, and sons are especially prized.

DISCHARGE TEACHING

Teaching for Self-Care; Signs of Complications

Bridging the gap between hospital and home care requires sensitive and knowledgeable nursing care. Discharge planning begins at the time of admission to the unit and should be reflected in the plan of care developed for each individual woman. For example, a great deal of the time during the hospital stay is usually spent in teaching about maternal and newborn care, because all women must be capable of providing basic care for themselves and their infants at the time of discharge. It also is crucial that every woman be taught to recognize physical signs and symptoms that might indicate problems and how to obtain advice and assistance quickly if these signs appear. The Signs of Potential Complications boxes on pp. 627 and 638 list several common indications of maternal physical and psychosocial problems in the postpartum period. (See Chapter 37 for more information on postpartum complications.) Before discharge, women also need basic instruction regarding the resumption of intercourse, prescribed medications, routine mother-baby checkups, and contraception (see Guidelines/Guías box).

New mothers may be too overwhelmed physically and emotionally to absorb and retain all this information in the brief time they are in the postpartum unit. Nurses must target their teaching on expressed needs of the woman. Giving the woman a list of topics and asking her to indicate her teaching needs will help the nurse maximize teaching efforts and may increase retention of information by the woman (Ruchala, 2000).

Just before the time of discharge, the nurse reviews the woman's chart to see that laboratory reports, medications, signatures, and so on are in order. Some hospitals have a checklist to follow before the woman's discharge. The nurse verifies that medications, if ordered, have arrived on the unit, that any valuables kept secure during

GUIDELINES/GUÍAS

Discharge Teaching

When you go to the bathroom, always wipe from front to back.
Cuando vaya al baño, séquese siempre de adelante hacia atrás.

Sit in a warm tub to relieve discomfort.
Siéntese en una bañera con agua tibia para aliviarse.

You will have moderate amounts of vaginal discharge.
Usted tendrá cantidades moderadas de sangrado vaginal.

It may last from 4 to 6 weeks.
Puede durar desde 4 a 6 semanas.

The color may vary from dark brown to red to pink.
El color puede variar entre café oscuro a rojo a rosado.

It may contain blood clots.
Es probable que contenga coágulos.

Use a sanitary pad instead of a tampon.
Use una toalla sanitaria en vez de un tampón.

Your menstrual period will not resume for 4 to 10 weeks.
Su periodo menstrual no regresará hasta 4 a 10 semanas más tarde.

If you are breastfeeding, it may take a little longer.
Si está amamantando, puede demorar un poco más.

It is possible to become pregnant while you are breastfeeding.
Es posible quedar embarazada mientras amamanta.

Avoid having sexual relations for 2 to 4 weeks after birth.
Evite las relaciones sexuales por 2 a 4 semanas después del parto.

Gradually increase activity to incorporate everyday routines.
Aumente las actividades gradualmente hasta llegar a su rutina normal.

Do your Kegel exercises.
Haga sus ejercicios Kegel.

Do not lift heavy objects (>10 pounds).
No levante objetos pesados (de más de diez libras).

Rest as often as possible.
Descanse mucho.

Rest when your baby sleeps.
Descanse cuando duerma su bebé.

Eat daily:
Diariamente comase:

4 servings of bread/cereals, fruits/vegetables (green), milk or foods made from milk, and 2 servings of meat. You need to drink 8 glasses of fluids a day to support breastfeeding.
4 porciones de pan/cereal, frutas/vegetales (verduras), leche o comidas del grupo de leche, y 2 porciones de carne. Tiene que beber 8 vasos de liquidos diariamente para soportar el dar de pecho.

Call your doctor (obstetrician) if you have:
Llame al médico de obstetricas si tenga cualquier de lo siguente:

- Fever >38° C
  Fiebre de 38° C o más
- Increased vaginal bleeding (more than a regular period)
  Aumento de desangre vaginal (más que una regla normal)
- Chills
  Escalofrío
- Painful, burning urination
  Orin que le duele o le quema
- Foul-smelling vaginal discharge
  Desangre vaginal de muy mal olor
- Increased pain or swelling
  Aumento de dolor o hinchazón
- Drainage or separation of incision (cesarean)
  Desangre o deshecho de la herida

the woman's stay have been returned to her and she has signed a receipt for them, and that the infant is ready to be discharged.

The nurse is careful not to administer any medication that would make the mother sleepy if she is the one who will be holding the baby on the way out of the hospital. In most instances, the woman is seated in a wheelchair and is usually given the baby to hold. Some families leave unescorted and ambulatory, depending on hospital protocol. The woman's possessions are gathered and taken out with her and her family. The woman's and the baby's identification bands are carefully checked. As the woman and the baby are assisted into the car, the nurse should make sure that there is a car seat in which to secure the baby.

Sexual Activity/Contraception

Many couples resume sexual activity before the traditional postpartum checkup 6 weeks after childbirth. Risk of hemorrhage and infection is minimal approximately 2 weeks postpartum. Couples may be anxious about the topic but feel uncomfortable and unwilling to bring it up. It is important that the nurse discuss the physical and psychologic effects that giving birth can have on lovemaking. The Teaching for Self-Care box contains helpful information about the resumption of sexual intercourse. Contraceptive options also should be discussed with women (and their partners, if present) before discharge so that they can make informed decisions about fertility management before resuming sexual activity. Waiting to discuss contraception at the 6-week checkup may be too late. It is possible, particularly in women who bottle feed, for ovulation to occur as soon as 1 month after birth. A woman who engages in unprotected sex risks becoming pregnant much sooner than she planned. Current contraceptive options are discussed in detail in Chapter 9. Women who are undecided about contraception at the time of discharge need information about using condoms with foam or creams until the 6-week checkup.

Prescribed Medications

Most women have at least one medication prescribed for their use after discharge. Many health care providers routinely have women continue to take their prenatal vitamins and iron during the 6-week postpartum period. It is especially important that women who are breastfeeding or who are discharged with a lower than normal hematocrit level take these medications as ordered. Women with extensive episiotomies (third or fourth degree) or vaginal lacerations are usually given stool softeners to take at home. Pain relief medications (analgesics or nonsteroidal antiinflammatory medications) may be prescribed, especially for women who had cesarean births. The nurse should make certain that the woman knows the route, dosage, and frequency of all ordered medications and the common side effects.

Routine Mother and Baby Checkups

Women who have had uncomplicated vaginal births are still commonly scheduled for the traditional 6-week postpartum examination. Women who have had cesarean births are often seen in the health care provider's office or clinic within 2 weeks after hospital discharge. The date and time for the follow-up appointment should be included in the discharge orders. If an appointment has not been made before the woman leaves the hospital, she should be encouraged to call the health care provider's office or clinic immediately and schedule an appointment herself.

Parents who have not already done so must make plans for newborn follow-up at the time of discharge. Most offices and clinics like to see newborns for an initial examination within the first week or by age 2 weeks. Again, if an appointment for a specific date and time was not made for the infant before leaving the hospital, the parents should be encouraged to call the office or clinic right away.

TEACHING FOR SELF-CARE

Resumption of Sexual Intercourse

- You can safely resume sexual intercourse by the second to fourth week after birth when bleeding has stopped and the episiotomy has healed. For the first 6 weeks to 6 months, the vagina does not lubricate well.
- Your physiologic reactions to sexual stimulation for the first 3 months after birth will be slower and less intense. The strength of the orgasm is reduced.
- A water-soluble gel, cocoa butter, or a contraceptive cream or jelly might be recommended for lubrication. If some vaginal tenderness is present, your partner can be instructed to insert one or more clean, lubricated fingers into the vagina and rotate them within the vagina to help relax it and to identify possible areas of discomfort. A position in which you have control of the depth of the insertion of the penis also is useful. The side-by-side or female-on-top position may be more comfortable.
- The presence of the baby influences postbirth lovemaking. Parents hear every sound made by the baby; conversely you may be concerned that the baby hears every sound you make. In either case, any phase of the sexual response cycle may be interrupted by hearing the baby cry or move, leaving both of you frustrated and unsatisfied. In addition, the amount of psychologic energy expended by you in child care activities may lead to fatigue. Newborns require a great deal of attention and time.
- Some women have reported feeling sexual stimulation and orgasms when nursing their babies. Nursing mothers often are interested in returning to sexual activity before nonnursing mothers.
- You should be instructed to correctly perform the Kegel exercises to strengthen your pubococcygeal muscle. This muscle is associated with bowel and bladder function and with vaginal feeling during intercourse.

Follow-Up After Discharge

Home Visits

The Association of Women's Health, Obstetric, and Neonatal Nurses (AWHONN) (1994) published guidelines for postpartum home care that describe comprehensive perinatal home care follow-up services. Although these services may be offered by hospitals, maternity centers, home care agencies, public health agencies, private physicians, or entrepreneurs, nurses are a constant presence in this care. The common goal of these services is to ensure that the mother, newborn, and family have an optimal opportunity to prepare for and enjoy safe, comprehensive, and high-quality perinatal care.

Home visits to new mothers and babies within a few days of discharge can help bridge the gap between hospital care and routine visits to health care providers. Nurses are able to assess the mother, infant, and home environment; answer questions and provide education; and make referrals to community resources if necessary. Home visits also may help decrease stress in new families and reduce the need for more expensive health care, such as nonroutine health care visits and rehospitalization (Brown & Johnson, 1998).

A referral form containing information about both mother and baby should be completed at hospital discharge and sent immediately to the home care agency. Figure 23-11 is an example of such a referral form.

The home visit is most commonly scheduled on the woman's second day home from the hospital, but it may be scheduled on the first, third, or fourth day home instead, depending on the individual family's situation and needs. Additional visits are planned throughout the first week, as needed. The home visits may be extended beyond that time if the family's needs warrant it and if a home visit is the most appropriate option for carrying out the follow-up care required to meet the specific needs identified.

A home visit progresses more effectively if it is preplanned and well organized. In advance, the nurse reviews the hospital's discharge summary, teaching plan, and any other records, including the physician's orders; this serves to structure the interview and physical assessment and hence provide continuity of care. Before the visit, the nurse also obtains directions to the family's home and gets a map, if necessary.

Telephone Follow-Up

As part of the routine follow-up of a woman and her infant after discharge from the hospital, many providers are implementing one or more postpartum telephone follow-up calls to their clients for assessment, health teaching, identification of complications to effect timely intervention, and referrals. Telephone follow-up may be part of the services offered by the hospital, private physician or clinic, or a private agency and may be either a separate service or combined with other strategies for extending postpartum care. If no home care follow-up is provided, then telephone follow-up may take its place. If the family has a home care visit, this follow-up is incorporated into that care. Telephonic nursing assessments are frequently used after a postpartum home care visit to reassess a woman's knowledge about the signs and symptoms of adequate hydration in breastfeeding or, after initiating home phototherapy, to assess the caregiver's knowledge regarding equipment complications.

Warm Lines

The warm line is another type of telephone link between the new family and concerned caregivers or experienced parent volunteers. A **warm line** is a help line or consultation service, not a crisis intervention line. The warm line is appropriately used for dealing with less extreme concerns that may seem urgent at the time the call is placed but are not actual emergencies. Calls to warm lines commonly relate to issues such as infant feeding, prolonged crying, or sibling rivalry. Often families will be given the telephone number for the nursery or the postpartum unit and encouraged to call if questions or concerns arise after hospital discharge.

Support Groups

A postpartum support group enables mothers and fathers to share with and support each other as they adjust to parenting. Many new parents find it reassuring to discover that they are not alone in their feelings of confusion and uncertainty. Often in a postpartum support group, an experienced parent can impart concrete information that can be valuable to other group members. Inexperienced parents may find themselves imitating the behavior of others in the group whom they perceive as particularly capable.

On occasion, postpartum women who have met earlier in prenatal clinics or on the hospital unit may begin to associate for mutual support. Members of Lamaze classes who attend a postpartum reunion may decide to extend their relationship during the fourth trimester. Realizing the value of group support, nurses may wish to make postpartum support groups available as a strategy for bridging the hospital and home experience.

Referral to Community Resources

At times the nurse will want to refer families needing extra attention for specific problems to appropriate agencies. Health departments and school systems can usually provide information about existing local resources, such as parent or professional support groups. National organizations also can be useful in providing published resource guides and lists of community service agencies specific to the group or condition they represent (see Resource list at the end of the chapter). Individual nurses will find it helpful to develop their own resource file of services that are frequently useful to postpartum families.

OB Homecare
Phone: 612-863-4478
Fax: 612-863-4568

POSTPARTUM HOME CARE REFERRAL

☐PHN Referral Made to ____________ County

Mother's Name: ______________________

Address/Phone where mother will be staying:

Address: ______________________

City: ______________________

Phone #:(______)______________

☐ **Address & Phone Verified**

Language Spoken: ☐ English ☐ Other: __________

Understands English: ☐ Well ☐ Poor

☐ Mother Needs Interpreter ☐ Hearing Impaired

Who interpreted in hospital: __________

Phone: (_____)__________

Mom's MD/Midwife: (Full Name) ______________

Phone #: (______)____________

Next Appt: ______________

MOTHER:

Gravida ____ T___ P___ A___ L___

Marital Status: S M W D Sep

Normal Maternal Exam: ☐Yes ☐No (explain below)

☐ Vaginal Birth ☐ C/Birth

Epis/Incision: ______________

Meds: ______________

Allergies: ______________

☐ Needs Large BP Cuff

OTHER ISSUES:

Diabetic: ______________

Hgb pp, if abnormal: ______________

Psycho/Social Issues:

☐ Parent/Child Interaction ☐ Limited Support System

☐ Mental Health Status ☐ Drug Use/Dependency

☐ Previous Losses ☐ Hx of Domestic Violence

☐ Other: ______________

Husband/Significant Other: ______________

Baby's Name: ______________ ☐M ☐F

Delivery Date/Time:_________@_________

Mother's Discharge Date/Time: _________@_________

Baby's MD (Full Name): ______________

Phone #: (______)____________

Next Appt: ______________

BABY:

Gestation: ________weeks ☐ Fetal Loss

Birth Weight: ________ Discharge wt: ________

Apgars: 1"______ 5"______

Feedings: ☐ Breast ☐ Bottle ☐ Both

Feeding Issues: ______________

____

Normal Infant Exam: ☐ Yes ☐ No (explain below)
Circumcised: ☐ Yes ☐ No

Additional Order:

☐ Home care to draw newborn screen
**Must send lab-slip home with family.

ADDITIONAL COMMENTS or
ABNORMAL FINDINGS FOR MOTHER OR BABY:

____

Mom aware of referral: ☐Yes ☐No **REFERRAL COMPLETED BY:** ______________

☐ ***Faxed to OB Homecare @-612-863-4568:*** ☐ ***Facesheet*** ☐ ***Referral***
☐ ***Faxed to PHN*** ____________ ***County:*** ☐ ***Facesheet*** ☐ ***Referral***
Currently being seen by PHN: ☐ Yes ☐ No

FIG. 23-11 Referral form. (Courtesy OB Homecare of Allina Hospitals and Clinics, Minneapolis, MN.)

KEY POINTS

- Postpartum care is modeled on the concept of health.
- Cultural beliefs and practices affect the client's response to the puerperium.
- The nursing plan of care includes assessments to detect deviations from normal, comfort measures to relieve discomfort or pain, and safety measures to prevent injury or infection.
- The nurse provides teaching and counseling measures designed to promote the woman's feelings of competence in self-care and baby care.
- The nurse must exhibit both clinical and decision-making skills to provide safe and effective physical care. Common nursing interventions include evaluating and treating the boggy uterus and the full urinary bladder, providing for pharmacologic and nonpharmacologic relief of pain and discomfort associated with the episiotomy or lacerations, and instituting measures to promote or suppress lactation.
- Nurses can help promote the health of the woman's future pregnancies and children by administering rubella vaccine and Rh immune globulin if indicated.
- Meeting the psychosocial needs of new mothers involves planning care that takes into consideration the composition and functioning of the entire family.
- Early postpartum discharge will continue to be the trend as a result of consumer demand, medical necessity, discharge criteria for low risk childbirth, and cost-containment measures.
- The short-stay option in perinatal care is safer when selection criteria are used to determine a woman's eligibility for early discharge and when home care follow-up is available.
- Home visits, telephone follow-up, warm lines, support groups, and referral to community resources—used either individually or in combination—are effective means of preventing crisis and facilitating physiologic and psychologic adjustments in the postpartum period.

CRITICAL THINKING EXERCISES

1. Maria is a 16-year-old primigravida who gave birth to an $8\frac{1}{2}$-pound boy 5 days ago by cesarean. You make a home visit on the day after she and the baby are discharged and find them home alone. The baby is screaming, and Maria looks exhausted. She tells you that she was "up all night with this brat," and that she is "bleeding and hurting a lot."
   - **a.** What other information would you want to obtain immediately from Maria?
   - **b.** After performing a physical assessment, what findings would cause you to recommend that Maria telephone her care provider or return to the hospital immediately?
   - **c.** Identify resources in your community that could provide assistance to Maria and her son.
   - **d.** What other factors must be considered before referring Maria and the baby to the agency(ies) identified in question c?
2. Kim is a 30-year-old Vietnamese woman who has just given birth to her fourth child, but first son. Kim speaks very limited English. When you do her discharge teaching, you find her alone, lying in bed, covered with several blankets. Her breakfast tray is untouched, and her water pitcher is full. Her son, who was circumcised several hours ago, is screaming in his bassinet, but Kim pays no attention to him.
   - **a.** What education related to self-care and infant care would you most want to communicate to Kim?
   - **b.** How could you provide adequate discharge teaching for Kim?
   - **c.** Based on your knowledge of Kim's culture, explain why you think she is behaving as she is.
   - **d.** What other information should you obtain in regard to Kim's home situation before discharging her and the baby?

RESOURCES

American Red Cross
430 17th St., NW
Washington, DC 20006
202-737-8300
www.redcross.org

Child Welfare League of America
440 First St., NW, Third Floor
Washington, DC 20001-2085
202-638-2952
202-638-4004 (fax)
www.cwla.org/default.htm

Depression After Delivery
P.O. Box 59973
Renton, WA 98508
206-283-9278
www.behavenet.com

HAND (Helping After Neonatal Death)
P.O. Box 341
Los Gatos, CA 95031
www.h-a-n-d.org

La Leche League
1400 N. Meacham Rd.
Schaumburg, IL 60168-4079
800-525-3243 (24-hour line)
www.lalecheleague.org

March of Dimes Birth Defects Foundation
National Foundation/March of Dimes
1275 Mamaroneck Ave.
White Plains, NY 10605
914-428-7100
888-663-4637 (MODIMES)
www.modimes.org

National Perinatal Association
101½ South Union St.
Alexandria, VA 22314-3323
703-549-5523

Nursing Mothers Council
Consult telephone directory for local chapters

Parent Soup
www.parentsoup.com

Planned Parenthood Federation of America, Inc.
810 Seventh Ave.
New York, NY 10019
800-230-PLAN
www.plannedparenthood.org

Positive Parenting
www.positiveparenting.com

Postpartum Education for Parents
P.O. Box 6154
Santa Barbara, CA 93160
www.sbpep.org/pepppd.htm

Special Supplemental Nutrition Program for Women, Infants, and Children (WIC)
Food and Consumer Service
3101 Park Center Dr., Room 819
Alexandria, VA 22302
703-305-2286
www.usda.gov/fns/wic.html

REFERENCES

American Academy of Pediatrics. (1995). Hospital stay for healthy term infants. *Pediatrics, 96*(4), 788-790.

American Academy of Pediatrics Committee on Drugs. (2001). The transfer of drugs and other chemicals into human milk. *Pediatrics, 108*(3), 776-789.

American Academy of Pediatrics & American College of Obstetricians and Gynecologists. (1997). *Guidelines for perinatal care* (4th ed.). Elk Grove Village, IL: American Academy of Pediatrics.

Association of Women's Health, Obstetric, and Neonatal Nurses (AWHONN). (1994). *Didactic content and clinical skills verification for professional nurse providers of perinatal home care.* Washington, DC: AWHONN.

Benedetti, T. (2002). Obstetric hemorrhage. In S. Gabbe, J. Niebyl, & J. Simpson (Eds.), *Obstetrics: Normal and problem pregnancies* (4th ed.). New York: Churchill Livingstone.

Bowes, W., & Katz, V. (2002). Postpartum care. In S. Gabbe, J. Niebyl, & J. Simpson (Eds.), *Obstetrics: Normal and problem pregnancies* (4th ed.). New York: Churchill Livingstone.

Brown, S., & Johnson, B. (1998). Enhancing early discharge with home follow-up: A pilot project. *Journal of Obstetric, Gynecologic, and Neonatal Nursing, 27*(1), 33-38.

Davis, R. (2001). The postpartum experience for Southeast Asian women in the United States. *MCN American Journal of Maternal Child Nursing, 26*(4), 208-213.

Edmonson, M., Stoddard, J., & Owens, L. (1997). Hospital readmission with feeding-related problems after early postpartum discharge of normal newborns. *Journal of the American Medical Association, 278*(4), 299-303.

Ferguson, S., & Engelhard, C. (1997). Short stay: The art of legislating quality and economy. *AWHONN Lifelines, 1*(1), 17-23.

Fishbein, E., & Burggraf, E. (1998). Early postpartum discharge: How are mothers managing? *Journal of Obstetric, Gynecologic, and Neonatal Nursing, 27*(2), 142-148.

Havens, D., & Hannan, C. (1996). Legislation to mandate maternal and newborn length of stay. *Journal of Pediatric Health Care, 10*(3), 141-144.

Johnson & Johnson. (1996). *Compendium of postpartum care.* Skillman, NJ: Johnson & Johnson Consumer Products, Inc.

Kridli, S. (2002). Health beliefs and practices among Arab women. *MCN American Journal of Maternal Child Nursing, 27*(3), 178-182.

Lauderdale, J. (1999). Childbearing and transcultural nursing care issues. In M. Andrews & J. Boyle (Eds.), *Transcultural concepts in nursing care* (3rd ed.). Philadelphia: Lippincott.

Liu, L. et al. (1997). The safety of newborn early discharge: the Washington State Experience. *Journal of the American Medical Association, 278*(4), 293-298.

Luegenbiehl, D. (1997). Improving visual estimation of blood volume on peripads. *MCN American Journal of Maternal Child Nursing, 22*(6), 294-298.

Mattson, S. (2000). Providing culturally competent care: Strategies and approaches for perinatal clients. *AWHONN Lifelines, 4*(5), 37-39.

Pugh, L. et al. (1999). Clinical approaches in the assessment of childbearing fatigue. *Journal of Obstetric, Gynecologic, and Neonatal Nursing, 28*(1), 74-80.

Roberts, K. (1995). A comparison of chilled cabbage leaves and chilled gel-paks in reducing breast engorgement. *Journal of Human Lactation, 11*(1), 17-20.

Ruchala, P. (2000). Teaching new mothers: Priorities of nurses and postpartum women. *Journal of Obstetric, Gynecologic, and Neonatal Nursing, 29*(3), 265-273.

Sampselle, C. et al. (2000). Continence for women: A test of AWHONN's evidence-based protocol in clinical practice. *Journal of Obstetric, Gynecologic, and Neonatal Nursing, 29*(1), 18-26.

Simpson, K., & Creehan, P. (2001). *AWHONN's perinatal nursing* (2nd ed.). Philadelphia: J.B. Lippincott.

Weekly, S., & Neumann, M. (1997). Speaking up for baby: The case for individualized neonatal discharge plans. *AWHONN Lifelines, 1*(1), 24-29.

Wilkerson, N. (1996). Appraisal of early discharge programs. *Journal of Perinatal Education, 5*(2), 1.

Williams, L., & Cooper, M. (1996). A new paradigm for postpartum care. *Journal of Obstetric, Gynecologic, and Neonatal Nursing, 25*(9), 745-749.

CHAPTER 24

Lienne D. Edwards

Transition to Parenthood

http://evolve.elsevier.com/Lowdermilk/MatWmnHlth/

LEARNING OBJECTIVES

- Discuss transition as a concept central to the discipline of nursing.
- Delineate parental and infant behaviors that affect parent-infant attachment.
- Discuss the critical attributes, antecedents, and consequences of parent-infant attachment.
- Describe sensual responses that strengthen attachment.
- Differentiate the three periods in parental role change after childbirth.
- Summarize six parental tasks and responsibilities during the transition to parenthood.
- Interpret infant behaviors that facilitate and inhibit parental attachment.
- Compare maternal adjustment and paternal adjustment.
- Delineate ways to facilitate parent-infant adjustment.
- Discuss the effects of the following on parental response: parental age (adolescence and older than 35 years), social support, culture, socioeconomic conditions, personal aspirations, and sensory impairment.
- Describe sibling adjustment.
- Describe grandparent adaptation.

Becoming a parent creates a period of change and instability for all men and women who decide to have children. This holds true whether parenthood is biologic or adoptive and whether the parents are married husband-wife couples, cohabiting couples, single mothers, single fathers, lesbian couples with one woman as biologic mother, or gay male couples who adopt a child. This period of developmental change is referred to as the **transition to parenthood.**

Transition is a concept central to the discipline of nursing. **Transition** is defined as a passage or process occurring over time involving development, flow, or movement from one state, condition, or place to another (Meleis, 1991; Schumacher & Meleis, 1994). Nurses often encounter clients during times of transition that occur because of developmental, situational, or health-illness events. The transition to parenthood is one such time.

Transition often entails profound change, such as changes in identities, roles, relationships, abilities, and patterns of behavior, and may have dramatic effects on the lives of the individuals and significant others involved (Schumacher & Meleis, 1994; Vehvilainen-Julkunen, 1995). Wide variation occurs in how individuals and families experience transition. Six conditions influence the transition experience (Schumacher & Meleis, 1994):

1. Meanings: Understanding the meaning of a transition from the perspective of those experiencing it is essential.
2. Expectations: People may or may not know what to expect of a transition, just as their expectations may or may not be realistic. Knowing what to expect realistically may help alleviate some of the stress associated with transitions.
3. Level of knowledge: Transitions often require new knowledge or skills. Individuals involved have degrees of uncertainty as they progress to increased levels of knowledge.
4. Environment: Facilitative resources external to the person are important for successful transition. Such resources include social support from spouse, partner, family, friends, and colleagues; effective communication; institutional support; and flexibility. Understanding the sociocultural context is important.
5. Level of planning: Success of a transition depends in part on the level of planning that occurs before and during the transition. Effective planning involves identification of needs, problems, and issues that may arise during the transition.
6. Emotional and physical well-being: A wide range of emotions accompanies transition, the more distressful ones attesting to the difficulties encountered during transition. As individuals and families work through the transition, they report feeling overwhelmed, anxious, insecure, frustrated, depressed, ambivalent, isolated, and lonely. Role conflict and low self-esteem also may

be experienced. Physical discomfort and bodily unpredictability can interfere with the assimilation of new information.

Indicators of healthy transition outcomes include the following:

- Subjective well-being: As successful transition occurs, emotional distress gives way to a sense of well-being. Individuals experience effective coping, managing one's emotions, personal integrity, increased self-esteem, growth, and role satisfaction.
- Role mastery: People achieve skilled role performance, empowerment, and comfort with the behaviors required in the new situation. When role mastery is reached, they feel competent and self-confident.
- Well-being of interpersonal relationships: Transitions involving one or more family members must be evaluated in terms of the whole family. Disagreements or family disruption may occur. As members move toward successful conclusion to the transition, family relationship well-being is restored or promoted. Outcomes include family adaptation, enhanced appreciation and closeness, meaningful interaction, and integration with the broader social networks and community.

A thorough understanding of the process parents go through during their transition to parenthood guides the nurse in helping family members adapt. This chapter reviews the transition to parenthood, including the parenting process and the adjustment of parents, siblings, and grandparents.

PARENTING PROCESS

Parenting is a process of role attainment and role transition that begins during pregnancy. The transition ends when the parent develops a sense of comfort and confidence in performing the parental role. The parenting process requires cognitive and affective skills and knowledge as well as motor skills. The infant's well-being and development depend on these components.

Skill and Knowledge Component

The first component in the process of parenting includes knowledge of and skill in childcare activities (see discussion in Chapter 28).

Affective Component

The emotional component in the parenting process probably stems from the parents' earliest experiences with a loving, accepting parent or parental figure, during which a sense of trust in and concern for others developed. In essence, parents "inherit" the ability to show concern and tenderness and then pass this ability to the next generation by providing for their children the kind of parent-child relationship they experienced. This includes an attitude of tenderness, awareness, and concern for the infant's needs and desires. This component of parenting profoundly affects the manner in which the practical aspects of child care are performed and the emotional response of the child to the care. A positive parent-child relationship is mutually rewarding. This relationship helps a person develop confidence in the expectations that others will be willing to help and that the person is worth helping.

PARENTAL ATTACHMENT, BONDING, AND ACQUAINTANCE

The process whereby parents come to love and accept a child and a child comes to love and accept a parent is referred to as **attachment** (see Plan of Care). By using the terms attachment and bonding, Klaus and Kennell originally proposed that, "There is a period shortly after birth that is uniquely important to mother-to-infant attachment in the human being" (Klaus & Kennell, 1997). They defined the phenomenon of **bonding** as a sensitive period in the first minutes and hours after birth when mothers and fathers must have close contact with their infants for "later development to be optimal" (Klaus & Kennell, 1976). Subsequently, Klaus and Kennell (1982) revised their theory of parent-infant bonding, modifying their claim of the critical nature of immediate contact with the infant after birth. They acknowledged the adaptability of human parents, stating that it took longer than minutes or hours for parents to form an emotional relationship with their infants. Nurse researchers of that time integrated both concepts of attachment and acquaintance into a conceptual framework of the bonding process.

The terms attachment and bonding continue to be used interchangeably, and confusion exists regarding the meaning and measurement of attachment. In an attempt to bring clarity to this issue, Goulet and colleagues (1998) presented an analysis of the concept of parent-infant attachment. These nurse scholars identified the critical attributes of attachment (i.e., those characteristics that must be present to recognize the concept in a naturalistic setting) (Walker & Avant, 1995). The critical attributes are proximity, reciprocity, and commitment. **Proximity** is the physical and emotional experience of the parents' being close to their infant. Parents seek proximity through touching, holding, and gazing. Parents also differentiate infant needs from their own needs and respond appropriately, in a sense detaching as well as attaching. **Reciprocity** is the process by which the infant's capabilities and behaviors elicit parents' response. The infant is an active partner in this interactional process. Parents who are sensitive and responsive to the infant's cues promote the infant's growth and development. **Commitment** is the enduring nature of the attachment relationship. Parents put the infant at the center of their lives and family and acknowledge their responsibility for the infant's welfare. Parents integrate the parental identity into

Plan of Care Multiparous Woman and Family

NURSING DIAGNOSIS Risk for impaired maternal-infant attachment related to stress of birth of second infant

Expected Outcome *Woman will demonstrate positive attachment toward the new infant.*

Nursing Interventions/*Rationales*

Identify any negative maternal and paternal behaviors *to provide baseline for interventions.*

Assist woman to identify positive coping methods *to provide ongoing support.*

Interpret newborn's behaviors to mother *to facilitate positive response to infant.*

Provide suggestions for introducing sibling(s) to newborn *to minimize sibling rivalry.*

Identify support systems and professional referrals *to promote expression of feelings and enhance maternal-infant attachment.*

NURSING DIAGNOSIS Ineffective family coping related to family disorganization

Expected Outcomes *Family will identify stressors and verbalize possible resources that will provide assistance during family role transition.*

Nursing Interventions/*Rationales*

Assess for prominent stressors in family environment *to determine plan of care.*

Assist family to identify positive coping strategies *to deal with family role transition.*

Encourage family to identify appropriate resources *to decrease family stress.*

NURSING DIAGNOSIS Fatigue related to multiple role demands

Expected Outcome *Woman will report increased energy level.*

Nursing Interventions/*Rationales*

Teach woman signs of fatigue *to recognize importance of immediate interventions.*

Promote consumption of balanced diet with adequate vitamins and iron *to prevent nutritional deficiencies that may cause fatigue.*

Assess availability of effective support systems *to provide meaningful assistance to the woman during this time of role transition.*

Suggest modification of infant's behavioral cycle to increase awake periods during the day and recommend sleeping when infant sleeps *to prevent excessive fatigue.*

NURSING DIAGNOSIS Caregiver role strain related to demands of mothering two children

Expected Outcome *The caregiver will develop a plan to decrease role strain.*

Nursing Interventions/*Rationales*

Discuss with woman and family a plan *to provide infant care at home to decrease role strain.*

Allow time to discuss role transition for second child *to prepare for realistic role changes in the household.*

Assist woman to develop time management plan for infant and self-care *to set realistic priorities.*

List ways in which other members of the household can assist with infant care and household duties *to decrease demands on the woman.*

Provide list of outside resources *to assist in decreasing caregiver role strain.*

the self and reorganize their lives to gain a sense of well-being (Goulet et al., 1998).

Goulet and colleagues (1998) delineated antecedents to and consequences of parent-infant attachment. Antecedents, or prerequisites for attachment to be established, include (1) awareness of previous attachments, (2) physical and psychologic availability, (3) acceptance of the pregnancy and the baby, and (4) making mutual acquaintance with the baby. A favorable environment is an enabler (i.e., a facilitator for the development of attachment). Consequences highlighting the importance of parent-infant attachment include (1) consolidation of parenting skills, (2) growth and development of the baby, and (3) establishment of a durable bond.

The process of attachment has been described as linear, beginning during pregnancy, intensifying during the early postpartum period, having developmental periods of progress and regression, and being constant and consistent once established. Components of the attachment process frequently observed in parents include favorable preconditions and identification and claiming of the infant by the parent (Mercer, 1983).

Favorable preconditions for attachment to begin and progress without unusual difficulty include the following:

- A parent's emotional health (including the ability to trust another person)
- A social support system encompassing mate, friends, and family
- A competent level of communication and care-giving skills
- Parental proximity to the infant
- Parent-infant fit (including infant state, temperament, and sex)

If any of these preconditions are not present or are distorted, nurses must intervene to facilitate the attachment process.

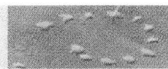

Attachment is developed and maintained by proximity and interaction with the infant, through which the parent becomes acquainted with the infant, identifies the infant as an individual, and claims the infant as a member of the family. Attachment is facilitated by positive feedback (i.e., social, verbal, and nonverbal responses, whether real or perceived, that indicate acceptance of one partner by the other). Attachment occurs through a mutually satisfying experience. A mother commented on her son's grasp reflex, "I put my finger in his hand, and he grabbed right on. It is just a reflex, I know, but it felt good anyway" (Fig. 24-1).

The concept of attachment has been extended to include **mutuality;** that is, the infant's behaviors and characteristics call forth a corresponding set of maternal behaviors and characteristics. The infant displays signaling behaviors such as crying, smiling, and cooing that initiate the contact and bring the caregiver to the child. These behaviors are followed by executive behaviors such as rooting, grasping, and postural adjustments that maintain the contact. The caregiver is attracted to an alert, responsive, cuddly infant and repelled by an irritable, apparently disinterested infant. Attachment occurs more readily with the infant whose temperament, social capabilities, appearance, and sex fit the parent's expectations. If the child does not meet these expectations, resolution of the parent's disappointment can delay the attachment process. A list of infant behaviors affecting parental attachment that continues to be a classic comprehensive reference is presented in Table 24-1. A corresponding list of parental behaviors that affect infant attachment is presented in Table 24-2.

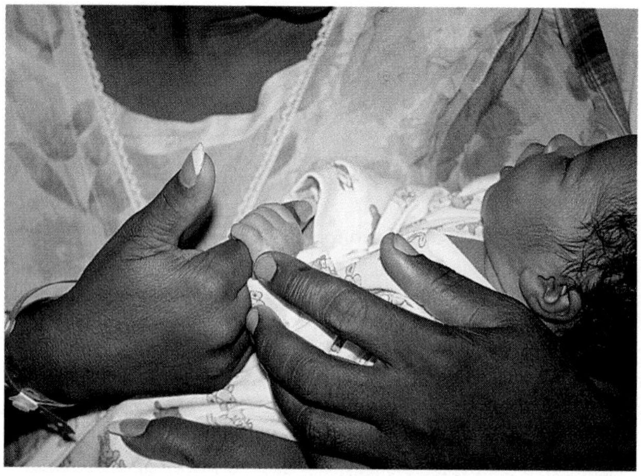

FIG. 24-1 Hands. (Courtesy Marjorie Pyle, RNC, Lifecircle, Costa Mesa, CA.)

An important part of attachment is **acquaintance** (Klaus & Kennell, 1983). Parents use eye contact (Fig. 24-2), touching, talking, and exploring to become acquainted with their infant during the immediate postpartum period. Adoptive parents undergo the same process when they first meet their new child. During this period, families engage in the **claiming process,** the identification of the new baby (Fig. 24-3). The child is first identified in terms of "likeness" to other family members, then in terms of "differences," and finally in terms of "uniqueness." The unique newcomer is thus incorporated into the family. Mothers and fathers scrutinize their infant carefully and point out characteristics that the child shares with other family members and that are indicative of a relationship between them. The claiming process is revealed by maternal comments such as the following: "Russ held him close and said, 'He's the image of his father,' but I found one part like me–his toes are shaped like mine."

TABLE *24-1* **Infant Behaviors Affecting Parental Attachment**

FACILITATING BEHAVIORS	INHIBITING BEHAVIORS
Visually alert; eye-to-eye contact; tracking or following of parent's face	Sleepy; eyes closed most of the time; gaze aversion
Appealing facial appearance; randomness of body movements reflecting helplessness	Resemblance to person parent dislikes; hyperirritability or jerky body movements when touched
Smiles	Bland facial expression; infrequent smiles
Vocalization; crying only when hungry or wet	Crying for hours on end; colicky
Grasp reflex	Exaggerated motor reflex
Anticipatory approach behaviors for feedings; sucks well; feeds easily	Feeds poorly; regurgitates; vomits often
Enjoys being cuddled, held	Resists holding and cuddling by crying, stiffening body
Easily consolable	Inconsolable; unresponsive to parenting, caretaking tasks
Activity and regularity somewhat predictable	Unpredictable feeding and sleeping schedule
Attention span sufficient to focus on parents	Inability to attend to parent's face or offered stimulation
Differential crying, smiling, and vocalizing; recognizes and prefers parents	Shows no preference for parents over others
Approaches through locomotion	Unresponsive to parent's approaches
Clings to parent; puts arms around parent's neck	Seeks attention from any adult in room
Lifts arms to parents in greeting	Ignores parents

From Gerson, E. (1973). *Infant behavior in the first year of life.* New York: Raven Press.

Conversely, some mothers react negatively. They "claim" the infant in terms of the discomfort or pain the baby causes. The mother interprets the infant's normal responses as being negative toward her and reacts to her child with dislike or indifference. She does not hold the child close or touch the child to be comforting; for example, "The nurse put the baby into Marie's arms. She promptly laid him across her knees and glanced up at the television. 'Stay still until I finish watching–you've been enough trouble already.'"

Over the years, attachment research has shown that neither the type of birth (vaginal, planned cesarean, unplanned cesarean) nor the type of infant feeding is related to parental attachment. Parents' perception of their own competence is an important predictor of parental attachment for mothers and fathers. Nurses can use

TABLE 24-2 **Parental Behaviors Affecting Infant Attachment**

FACILITATING BEHAVIORS	INHIBITING BEHAVIORS
Looks; gazes; takes in physical characteristics of infant; assumes *en face* position; eye contact	Turns away from infant; ignores infant's presence
Hovers; maintains proximity; directs attention to, points to infant	Avoids infant; does not seek proximity; refuses to hold infant when given opportunity
Identifies infant as unique individual	Identifies infant with someone parent dislikes; fails to discern any of infant's unique features
Claims infant as family member; names infant	Fails to place infant in family context or identify infant with family member; has difficulty naming
Touches; progresses from fingertip to fingers to palms to encompassing contact	Fails to move from fingertip touch to palmar contact and holding
Smiles at infant	Maintains bland countenance or frowns at infant
Talks to, coos, or sings to infant	Wakes infant when infant is sleeping; handles roughly; hurries feeding by moving nipple continuously
Expresses pride in infant	Expresses disappointment, displeasure in infant
Relates infant's behavior to familiar events	Does not incorporate infant into life
Assigns meaning to infant's actions and sensitively interprets infant's needs	Makes no effort to interpret infant's actions or needs
Views infant's behaviors and appearance in positive light	Views infant's behavior as exploiting, deliberately uncooperative; views appearance as distasteful, ugly

From Mercer, R. (1983). Parent-infant attachment. In L. Sonstegard, K. Kowalski, & B. Jennings (Eds.), *Women's health*, Vol. 2, *Childbearing*. New York: Grune & Stratton.

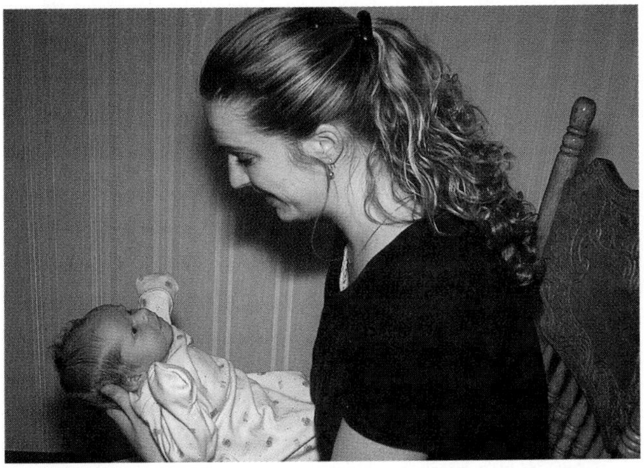

FIG. 24-2 Mother and baby make eye contact in *en face* position. (Courtesy Michael S. Clement, MD, Mesa, AZ.)

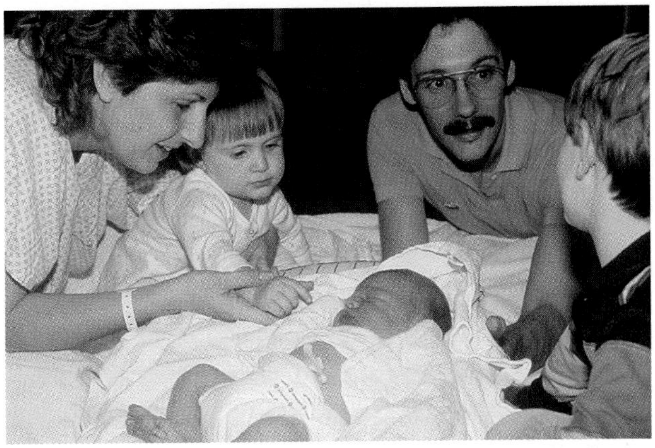

FIG. 24-3 Family members examine the new baby. They discuss how she resembles them and other family members. (Courtesy Marjorie Pyle, RNC, Lifecircle, Costa Mesa, CA.)

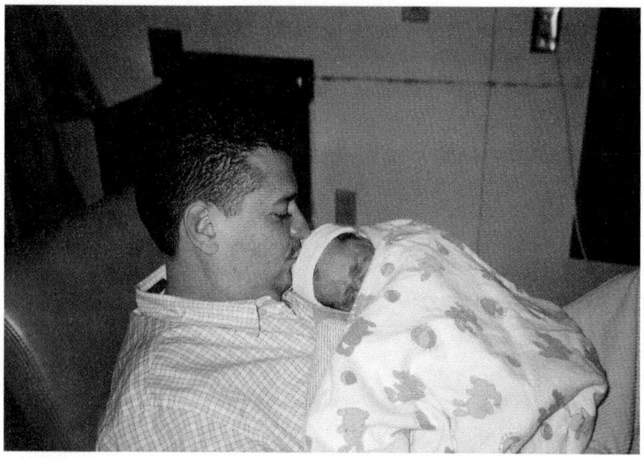

FIG. 24-4 Father kisses his newborn son. (Courtesy Shannon Perry, San Jose, CA.)

these findings to reassure mothers who have had unplanned cesarean births that they can bond as successfully with their infants as if they had had vaginal births. Through teaching and positive reinforcement, nurses can strengthen parents' sense of competence.

Nurses play an important role in facilitating parental attachment. They can enhance positive parent-infant contacts by heightening parental awareness of an infant's responses and ability to communicate. As parents attempt to become competent and loving in their role, nurses can bolster the parents' self-confidence and egos. Nurses are in prime positions to identify actual and potential problems and collaborate with other health care professionals who will care for the parents after discharge.

Nursing interventions related to the promotion of parent-infant attachment are numerous and varied. Table 24-3 lists examples of activities for parent-infant attachment interventions.

Assessment of Attachment Behaviors

One of the most important areas of assessment is careful observation of those behaviors thought to indicate the formation of emotional bonds between the newborn and family, especially the mother. Although the words *bonding* and *attachment* are sometimes referred to as separate phenomena, with bonding representing the development of emotional ties from parent to infant, and attachment representing the emotional ties from infant to parent, in this discussion, the words are used interchangeably to denote both processes.

Unlike physical assessment of the neonate, which has concrete guidelines to follow, assessment of parent-infant attachment requires much more skill in observation and interviewing. Rooming-in of mother and infant and liberal visiting privileges for father, siblings, and grandparents facilitate recognition of behaviors that demonstrate positive or negative attachment. Guidelines for assessment of attachment behaviors are presented in Box 24-1.

Talking to the parents uncovers many variables that can affect the development of attachment and parenting. What expectations do they have for this child? In other words, how similar are their predictions of the fantasy child and their realizations about the real child? Encourage them to talk about their relationship with their own parents, because the type of parenting that parents received as a child influences their child-rearing practices. Was this a planned pregnancy? How do they see the addition of a dependent family member affecting their lifestyle? What arrangements have they made in terms of such changes in lifestyle? What support system or significant others are available for assistance? What are their views regarding child rearing?

The labor process also significantly affects the immediate attachment of mothers to their newborn children. Factors such as a long labor, feeling tired or "drugged" after birth, and problems with breastfeeding can delay the development of initial positive feelings toward the newborn.

During pregnancy, and often even before conception occurs, parents develop an image of the "ideal" or "fantasy" infant. At birth the fantasy infant becomes the real infant. How closely the dream child resembles the real child influences the bonding process. Assessing such expectations during pregnancy and at the time of the infant's birth allows identification of discrepancies in the parents' view of the fantasy child versus the real child.

Because attachment involves a reciprocal interchange, observing the interaction between parent and infant is very important (Fig. 24-4). An excellent opportunity exists during feeding. A useful instrument for systematically describing the parent's and infant's behaviors is the Nursing Child Assessment Feeding Scale (NCAFS) (Barnard, 1994). It consists of 76 behavioral items; 50 items describe the parent's behavior regarding sensitivity to cues, response to child's distress, social-emotional growth fostering, and cognitive growth fostering. Twenty-six items focus on the child's behavior in terms of clarity of cues and responsiveness to parent. The results also can be shared with the parent to encourage discussion of feelings about the infant and to highlight behaviors of the dyad that foster successful interaction. The NCAFS is appropriate for use with infants during the first year.

PARENT-INFANT CONTACT

Since the early 1970s, consumers have strived for childbirth practices that promote the family as the focus of care. The alternatives of home birth, birthing centers, and family-centered maternity care units reflect parents' desires to share in the birth process and have more contact with their infants.

TABLE 24-3 **Examples of Parent-Infant Attachment Interventions**

INTERVENTION LABEL/DEFINITION	ACTIVITIES
Attachment Promotion Facilitation of development of parent-infant relationship	Provide opportunity for parent(s) to see, hold, and examine newborn immediately after birth Encourage parent(s) to hold infant close to body Assist parent(s) to participate in infant care Provide rooming-in in hospitals
Environmental Management: Attachment Process Manipulation of client's surroundings to facilitate development of parent-infant relationship	Create environment that fosters privacy Individualize daily routine to meet parent's needs Permit father/significant other to sleep in room with mother Develop policies that permit presence of significant others as much as desired
Family Integrity Promotion: Childbearing Family Facilitation of growth of individuals or families who are adding infant to family unit	Prepare parent(s) for expected role changes involved in becoming a parent Prepare parent(s) for responsibilities of parenthood Monitor effects of newborn on family structure Reinforce positive parenting behaviors
Lactation Counseling Use of interactive helping process to assist in maintenance of successful breastfeeding	Correct misconceptions, misinformation, and inaccuracies about breastfeeding Evaluate parent's understanding of infant's feeding cues (e.g., rooting, sucking, alertness) Determine frequency of feedings in relation to infant's needs Demonstrate breast massage and discuss its advantages to increasing milk supply
Parent Education: Infant Instruction on nurturing and physical care needed during first year of life	Determine parent(s) knowledge, readiness, and ability to learn about infant care Provide anticipatory guidance about developmental changes during first year of life Teach parent(s) skills to care for newborn Demonstrate ways in which parent(s) can stimulate infant's development Discuss infant's capabilities for interaction Demonstrate quieting techniques
Risk Identification: Childbearing Family Identification of individual or family likely to experience difficulties in parenting and assigning priorities to strategies to prevent parenting problems	Determine developmental stage of parent(s) Review prenatal history for factors that predispose client to complications Ascertain understanding of English or other language used in community Monitor behavior that may indicate problem with attachment Plan for risk-reduction activities in collaboration with individual or family

Modified from McCloskey, J., & Bulechek, G. (2000). *Nursing interventions classification* (3rd ed.). St. Louis: Mosby.

BOX 24-1 Assessing Attachment Behavior

- When the infant is brought to the parents, do they reach out for the infant and call the infant by name? (Recognize that in some cultures, parents may not name the infant in the early newborn period.)
- Do the parents speak about the infant in terms of identification—whom the infant looks like; what appears special about their infant over other infants?
- When parents are holding the infant, what kind of body contact is there—do parents feel at ease in changing the infant's position; are fingertips or whole hands used; are there parts of the body they avoid touching or parts of the body they investigate and scrutinize?
- When the infant is awake, what kinds of stimulation do the parents provide—do they talk to the infant, to each other, or to no one; how do they look at the infant—direct visual contact, avoidance of eye contact, or looking at other people or objects?
- How comfortable do the parents appear in terms of caring for the infant? Do they express any concern regarding their ability or disgust for certain activities, such as changing diapers?
- What type of affection do they demonstrate to the newborn, such as smiling, stroking, kissing, or rocking?
- If the infant is fussy, what kinds of comforting techniques do the parents use, such as rocking, swaddling, talking, or stroking?

Early Contact

Early close contact may facilitate the attachment process between parent and child. This does not mean that a delay will inhibit this process (humans are too resilient for that), but additional psychologic energy may be needed to achieve the same effect. No scientific evidence has demonstrated that immediate contact after birth is essential for the human parent-child relationship. Research evidence continues to be conflicting.

Prodromidis and colleagues (1995) studied early and extended contact for young, unmarried, predominantly African-American, low-socioeconomic level mothers. They found that mothers who had early and extended contact (rooming-in) with their infants during the first 18 hours after birth looked at, talked to, and touched their newborns more than did mothers who had minimal contact (infant feedings only). Two studies by Troy (1993, 1995) produced conflicting results regarding time of first holding of the infant and the development of maternal attachment feelings. In one study, Troy (1993) demonstrated that feelings of attachment began when the infant was first held, regardless of how long after birth the holding occurred. In the second study, Troy (1995) found that the earlier after birth the mother holds her infant, the sooner she develops feelings of maternal attachment.

In a study of the timing of parents' first holding (also being skin-to-skin) of small preterm infants, Gloppestad (1998) found that fathers held their infants later than did the mothers, even though fathers saw their infants before the mothers did. Both mothers and fathers rated their experience of love significantly higher when holding their preterm infants skin-to-skin than when holding them wrapped in blankets.

Women who have had a long, difficult labor are often too exhausted to respond other than in a superficial way to the newborn. They may welcome the attention of others and be grateful that the infant is healthy, but their primary need centers on recovery from the physical and emotional aspects of pregnancy and childbirth. Infants born at risk as a result of either fetal or maternal disabilities are usually transferred to the intensive care nursery as quickly as possible. Concerns for their need for intensive medical and nursing interventions take priority over the need for close contact with the parents. Opportunities for parents to be with the infant in the intensive care nursery, to touch or hold the baby if at all possible, and to receive reports of the infant's progress must be part of the nursing plan of care.

Parents who desire but are unable to have early contact with their newborn can be reassured that such contact is not essential for optimal parent-infant interactions. Otherwise, adopted infants would not form the usual affectional ties with their parents. Nor does the mode of infant-mother contact after birth (skin-to-skin versus wrapped) appear to have any important effect. Nurses must counsel parents to assure them that the emotional bond to the infant is not necessarily weaker because they missed early contact or the contact was not skin to skin. Nurses must stress that the parent-infant relationship is a process that occurs over time.

Extended Contact

The provision of rooming-in facilities for the mother and her baby continues to be a prevalent aspect of family-centered care. The infant is transferred to the area from the transitional nursery (if the facility uses one) after showing satisfactory extrauterine adjustment. The father is encouraged to participate in the care of the infant, and siblings and grandparents also are encouraged to visit and become acquainted with the infant. Many hospitals have established family birth units such as labor-delivery-recovery (LDR) rooms, labor-delivery-recovery-postpartum (LDRP) rooms, and single-room maternity care (SRMC). The mother is accompanied by her partner during the birth of the infant, and all three may remain together until discharged around 48 hours after birth. Whether rooming-in or a family birth unit is the method of family-centered care, mothers and their partners are considered equal and integral parts of the developing family. Partners are encouraged to take as active a role as they wish. Some hospitals and birth centers arrange for the discharge of the mother and infant any time from 2 to 24 hours after the birth if the parents desire it and the condition of the mother and that of the child warrant it. Follow-up care with nursing personnel from a home health care agency is usually part of this plan.

Mother-baby care, also called couplet care, is another form of family-centered care. Care and teaching for the mother and baby are provided by a primary nurse, fostering family unity. Parents involved in this approach are likely to be more self-confident in care, and maternal attachment and role attainment are promoted.

Extended contact with the infant should be available for all parents but especially for those at risk for parenting inadequacies, such as adolescents and low-income women. Any activity that optimizes family-centered care is worthy of serious consideration by postpartum nurses.

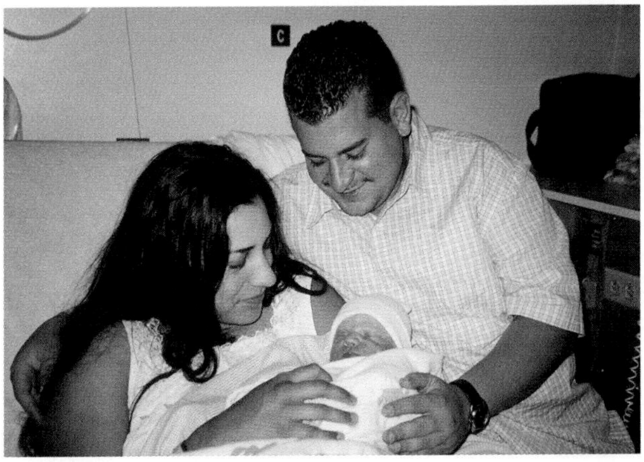

FIG. 24-5 Father, mother, and newborn getting to know each other. (Courtesy Shannon Perry, San Jose, CA.)

COMMUNICATION BETWEEN PARENT AND INFANT

Both partners in the interaction strengthen the parent-infant relationship through the use of sensual responses and abilities. The nurse should keep in mind that cultural variations may occur in these interactive behaviors used in communications between parent and infant (described later).

Touch

Parents and other caregivers use touch, or the tactile sense, extensively as a means of becoming acquainted with the newborn. Many mothers reach out for their infants as soon as they are born and the cord is cut. They lift them to their breasts, enfold them in their arms, and cradle them. Once the infant is close to them, they begin the exploration process with their fingertips, one of the most touch-sensitive areas of the body. For some mothers and other caregivers (fathers, nursing and medical students), studies have depicted a predictable pattern of touch behavior (Klaus & Kennell, 1982; Rubin, 1963; Tulman, 1985). The caregiver begins with a fingertip exploration of the infant's head and extremities. Within a short time, the caregiver uses the palm to caress the baby's trunk and eventually enfolds the infant. Gentle stroking motions are used to soothe and quiet the infant; patting or gently rubbing the infant's back is a comfort after feedings. Infants also pat the mother's breast as they nurse. Both seem to enjoy sharing each other's body warmth. There is a desire in parents to touch, pick up, and hold the infant (Fig. 24-5). They comment on the softness of the baby's skin and are aware of milia and rashes. As parents become increasingly sensitive to the infant's like or dislike of different types of touch, they draw closer to their baby.

Variations in touching behaviors have been noted in mothers from different cultural groups (Galanti, 1997; Inman, 1996; Jambunathan & Stewart, 1995; Jiménez, 1995). For example, minimal touching and cuddling is a traditional Southeast Asian practice thought to protect the infant from evil spirits. Because of tradition and spiritual beliefs, women in India and Bali have practiced infant massage since ancient times.

Eye-to-Eye Contact

Interest in having eye contact with the baby has been demonstrated repeatedly by parents. Some mothers remark that once their babies have looked at them, they feel much closer to them. Parents spend much time getting their babies to open their eyes and look at them. In American culture, eye contact appears to have a cementing effect on the development of a trusting relationship and is an important factor in human relationships at all ages. In other cultures, eye-to-eye contact may be perceived differently. For example, in Mexican culture, sustained direct eye contact is considered to be rude, immodest, and dangerous for some. This danger may arise from the *mal ojo* (evil eye), resulting from excessive admiration. Women and children are thought to be more susceptible to the *mal ojo* (D'Avanzo & Geissler, 2003).

As newborns become functionally able to sustain eye contact with their parents, time is spent in mutual gazing, often in the *en face* position (see Fig. 24-2). **En face,** "face-to-face," is a position in which the parent's face and the infant's face are approximately 8 inches apart and on the same plane. Nursing and medical practices that encourage this interaction should be implemented. Immediately after birth, for example, the infant can be positioned on the mother's abdomen or breasts with the mother's and the infant's faces on the same plane so that they can easily make eye contact. This would not be accomplished well with the infant lying in the mother's arms at her side. Lights can be dimmed so that the infant's eyes will open. Instillation of prophylactic antibiotic ointment in the infant's eyes can be delayed until the infant and parents have had some time together in the first hour after birth.

Voice

The shared response of parents and infants to each other's voices also is remarkable. Parents wait tensely for the first cry. Once that cry has reassured them of the baby's health, they begin comforting behaviors. As the parents talk in high-pitched voices, the infant is alerted and turns toward them.

Infants respond to higher-pitched voices and can distinguish their mother's voice from others soon after birth. Infants use their cries to signal hunger, pain, boredom, and tiredness. With experience, parents learn to distinguish such cries.

Odor

Another behavior shared by parents and infants is a response to each other's odor. Mothers comment on the smell of their babies when first born and have noted that each infant has a unique odor. Infants learn rapidly to distinguish the odor of their mother's breast milk.

Entrainment

Newborns move in time with the structure of adult speech. They wave their arms, lift their heads, and kick their legs, seemingly "dancing in tune" to a parent's voice. This means that culturally determined rhythms of speech have been ingrained in the infant long before spoken language is used to communicate. Carryover, or **entrainment,** occurs once the child begins to talk. This shared rhythm also gives the parent positive feedback and establishes a positive setting for effective communication.

Biorhythmicity

The fetus is in tune with the mother's natural rhythms, such as heartbeats. After birth, a crying infant may be soothed by being held in a position where the mother's heartbeat can be heard or by hearing a recording of a heartbeat. One of the newborn's tasks is to establish a personal rhythm, or **biorhythmicity.** Parents can help in this process by giving consistent loving care and by using their infant's alert state to develop responsive behavior and thereby increase social interactions and opportunities for learning. The more quickly parents become competent in child care activities, the more quickly their psychologic energy can be directed toward observing the communication cues the infant gives them.

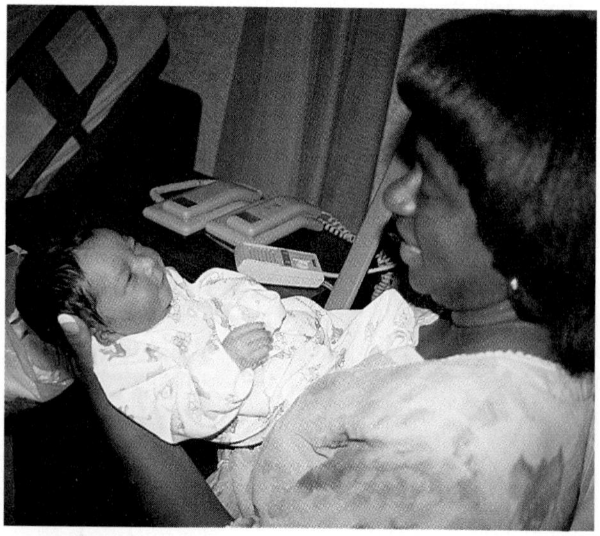

FIG. 24-6 Sharing a smile: example of synchrony. (Courtesy Marjorie Pyle, RNC, Lifecircle, Costa Mesa, CA.)

Reciprocity and Synchrony

Reciprocity is a type of body movement or behavior that provides the observer with cues. The observer or receiver interprets those cues and responds to them. Reciprocity often takes several weeks to develop with a new baby. For example, when the newborn fusses and cries, the mother responds by picking up and cradling the infant; the baby becomes quiet and alert and establishes eye contact; the mother verbalizes, sings, and coos while the baby maintains eye contact. The baby then averts the eyes and yawns; the mother decreases her active response. If the parent continues to stimulate the infant, the baby may become fussy.

Synchrony refers to the "fit" between the infant's cues and the parent's response. When parent and infant have a synchronous interaction, it is mutually rewarding (Fig. 24-6). Parents need time to interpret the infant's cues correctly. For example, after a certain time, the infant develops a specific cry in response to different situations such as boredom, loneliness, hunger, and discomfort. The parent may need assistance in deciphering these cries, along with trial-and-error interventions, before synchrony develops.

PARENTAL ROLE AFTER CHILDBIRTH

For the biologic parent, the parental role is enlarged and intensified at birth. The care and nurturing of the child were initiated well before birth. The mother who carried out the dictates of health (e.g., diet, rest, and exercise) for the "good of her baby," the partner who supported and sheltered her, and the parents who became aware of and attached to their unborn child were already functioning in the parental role before the birth. Even preconception decisions about whether and when to have a child influence mothers' and fathers' adjustment to the parental role.

The 6 weeks after birth form the **fourth trimester.** During the postpartum period, new tasks and responsibilities arise, and old behaviors must be modified or new ones added. The responses of mothers and their partners to the parental role change over time and tend to follow a predictable course. During the first 3 to 4 weeks of the fourth trimester, parents have to reorganize their relationship with the newborn. What was accomplished through the biologic process of pregnancy now requires an array of caregiving activities. The infant's needs for shelter, nourishment, protection, and socializing must be met. These early weeks are characterized by intense learning and need for nurturing.

The next few weeks are a time of drawing together and uniting the family unit. This period of consolidation involves negotiations as to roles (wife-husband, mother-father, mother-partner, parent-child, sibling-sibling). Family integrity and adaptation occur when transactions between spouses regarding roles and role relationships are successful.

Adaptation involves a stabilizing of tasks, a coming to terms with commitments. Parents demonstrate growing competence in childcare activities and are more attuned to their infant's behavior. Typically, the period from the decision to conceive through the first months of having a child is termed the transition to parenthood.

Transition to Parenthood

The transition to parenthood is frequently described as a time of disorder and disequilibrium, as well as satisfaction, for mothers and their partners (Rogan et al., 1997; Tomlinson, 1996). Usual methods of coping often seem ineffective. For example, some parents can be so distressed that they are unable to be supportive of each other. Men typically identify their spouses as their primary or only source of support. The transition can be harder for the fathers, who feel deprived because the mothers, who also are experiencing stress, cannot provide the usual level of support. Strong emotions such as helplessness, inadequacy, and anger that arise when dealing with a crying infant catch many parents unprepared. Conversely, parenthood allows adults to develop and display a selfless, warm, and caring side of themselves, which may not be expressed in other adult roles. To view the world through the eyes of a child and to be childlike (not childish) are two rich rewards of parenthood.

Historically the transition to parenthood was viewed as a crisis. The current perspective is that parenthood is a developmental transition (Tomlinson, 1996) rather than a major life crisis for the majority of families. The transition to parenthood is not a single static event but a dynamic, unfolding process (Levy-Shiff et al., 1998). A concept derived from the developmental crisis perspective but having relevance for the developmental transition theory is that at the point of crisis, a moment occurs when a person is mentally and physically prepared for, the culture is pushing for, and the person is reaching out to achieve some developmental change. The person is motivated for change. For the majority of mothers and their partners, the transition to parenthood is such a period and is viewed as an opportunity rather than a time of danger. Parents are stimulated to try new coping strategies as they work to master their new roles and reach new developmental levels. As they work through the transition, personal strength and resourcefulness are revealed (Rogan et al., 1997). Parents' appraisal of parenting as stressful, challenging, and within their control, as well as parents' coping strategies, all exhibit developmental change across the transition to parenthood. Parents display normative responses to the obvious situational demands of parenthood (Levy-Shiff et al., 1998). Five domains of family life combine to affect each parent's adaptation: feelings about self, relationship with family of origin, social support network, parent-infant relationship, and relationship with intimate partner (Cowan & Cowan, 1995).

Parental Tasks and Responsibilities

Parents must reconcile the actual child with the fantasy and dream child. This means coming to terms with the infant's physical appearance, sex, innate temperament, and physical status. If the real child differs greatly from the fantasy child, parents may delay acceptance of the child. In some instances, they may never accept the child.

Some parents are startled by the normal appearance of the neonate–size, color, molding of the head, or bowed appearance of the legs. Many fathers have commented that they thought the odd shape of the infant's head (molding) meant the infant would be mentally retarded.

Although many parents know the sex of the infant before birth because of the use of ultrasound assessments, for those who do not have this information, disappointment over the sex of the infant can take time to resolve. The parents may provide adequate physical care but find it difficult to be sincerely involved with the infant until this internal conflict has been resolved. As one mother remarked,

> I really wanted a boy. I know it is silly and irrational, but when they said, "She's a lovely little girl," I was so disappointed and angry–yes, angry–I could hardly look at her. Oh, I looked after her okay, her feedings and baths and things, but I couldn't feel excited. To tell the truth, I felt like a monster not liking my child. Then one day she was lying there, and she turned her head and looked right at me. I felt a flooding of love for her come over me, and we looked at each other a long time. It's okay now. I wouldn't change her for all the boys in the world.

Nursing care plans should include discussion about reconciliation of the real versus the fantasy child. Nurses should provide opportunities for parents to discuss their lack of parental feelings without fear of censure or ridicule. Often the expression of doubts and concerns provides relief and makes it easier for parents to deal with and resolve such feelings.

Parents need to establish the newborn as a person separate from himself or herself, that is, as someone having many dependency needs and requiring much nurturing. Nurses can discuss with parents that this acceptance of the infant as a separate being with many needs evolves over time. Parents who see the baby by ultrasound assessments during pregnancy may begin to appreciate earlier that the baby is a real–and separate–human being.

Parents need to become adept in the care of the infant, including caregiving activities, noting the communication cues given by the infant to indicate needs and responding appropriately to the infant's needs.

Parents need to establish reasonable evaluative criteria for assessing the success or failure of the care given the infant. Parents are surprisingly sensitive to infant responses. One father spoke about his first attempt to give his infant a kiss. At that moment, the infant turned her head. The father felt hurt, although he understood that the baby was totally unaware of her own movements. The infant's response to the parental care and attention may be interpreted by the parent as a comment on the quality of that care. Examples of infant behaviors that are interpreted by parents as positive responses to their care include being consoled easily, enjoying being cuddled, and making eye contact. Spitting frequently after feedings, crying, and being unpredictable may be perceived as negative responses to parental care. Continuation of these infant responses that are viewed as negative by the parent can result in alienation of parent and infant to the detriment of the infant.

Parents' self-efficacy (i.e., their belief that they have the ability to succeed at a challenging task) can affect a successful transition to parenthood. As maternal self-efficacy increases, so does a mother's satisfaction with her life situation and with her infant and infant care, her evaluation of the relationship with her husband, and her confidence in and satisfaction with parenting at 4 months after birth (Reece & Harkless, 1998). Mothers with higher self-efficacy report less postpartum stress. Mothers' self-efficacy tends to be higher than fathers' self-efficacy (Hudson, Elek, & Fleck, 2001; Reece & Harkless, 1998), as does their confidence, satisfaction, and support (Reece & Harkless, 1998). For fathers, higher self-efficacy is related to higher confidence in parenting, satisfaction with life situation (Reece & Harkless, 1998), and satisfaction with parenting (Hudson et al., 2001). Paternal self-efficacy, however, does not appear to be related to a father's postpartum stress at 4 months (Reece & Harkless, 1998).

Assistance, including advice by husbands, partners, wives, mothers, mothers-in-law, and professional workers, can be seen either as supportive or as an indication of how inept these people have judged the new parents to be. Criticism, real or imagined, of the new parents' ability to provide adequate physical care, nutrition, or social stimulation for the infant can prove devastating. By providing encouragement and praise for parenting efforts, nurses can bolster the new parents' confidence. Parents should feel safe discussing concerns about other peoples' criticisms with the nurses, who can help them practice assertiveness techniques to use with unwanted "critics." The nurses, as client advocates, also can use positive, nonjudgmental approaches to help critics direct their advice constructively.

Parents must establish a place for the newborn within the family group. Whether the infant is the firstborn or the last born, all family members must adjust their roles to accommodate the newcomer. The firstborn child needs support to accept a rival for parental affections. An older child needs help dealing with losing a favored position in the family hierarchy. The parents are expected to negotiate these changes.

Parents need to establish the primacy of their adult relationships to maintain the family as a group. Because this includes reorganizing many roles–for example, sexual, childcare, career, and community roles–time and energy must be provided for this vital task.

Maternal Adjustment

Three phases are evident as the mother adjusts to her parental role. These phases of **maternal adjustment** are characterized by dependent behavior, dependent-independent behavior, and interdependent behavior (Table 24-4).

TABLE 24-4 **Phases of Maternal Postpartum Adjustment**

PHASE	CHARACTERISTICS
Dependent: Taking-in*	• First 24 hr (range, 1 to 2 days) • Focus: self and meeting of basic needs • Reliance on others to meet needs for comfort, rest, closeness, and nourishment • Excited and talkative • Desire to review birth experience
Dependent-independent: Taking-hold*	• Starts second or third day; lasts 10 days to several weeks • Focus: care of baby and competent mothering • Desire to take charge • Still need for nurturing and acceptance by others • Eagerness to learn and practice—optimal period for teaching by nurses • Handling of physical discomforts and emotional changes • Possible experience with "blues"
Interdependent: Letting go*	• Focus: forward movement of family as unit with interacting members • Reassertion of relationship with partner • Resumption of sexual intimacy • Resolution of individual roles

*From Rubin, R. (1961). Basic maternal behavior. *Nursing Outlook 9*, 683-686.

Phases

Dependent Phase. During the first 24 to 48 hours after childbirth, the mother's dependency needs predominate. To the extent that others meet these needs, the mother is able to divert her psychologic energy to her infant rather than to focus it on herself. She needs "mothering" herself to "mother." Rubin (1961) aptly described these few days as the **taking-in phase:** a time when nurturing and protective care are required by the new mother. In Rubin's classic description, the taking-in phase lasted 2 to 3 days. Later studies by Ament (1990) and Wrasper (1996) supported Rubin's work, except that women were now found to move more rapidly through the taking-in phase. A strong taking-in phase was noted only in the first 24 hours after birth. Evans and colleagues (1998), in a study of women giving birth vaginally, found that both taking-in and taking-hold were present on the evening of birth. There were small decreases in taking-in and small increases in taking-hold between the evening of birth and the first morning.

For 24 hours after the birth, mature and apparently healthy women appear to suspend their involvement in everyday responsibilities. They rely on others to satisfy their needs for comfort, rest, nourishment, and closeness to their families and newborn.

This dependent phase is a time of great excitement during which parents need to verbalize their experience of pregnancy and birth. Focusing on, analyzing, and accepting these experiences help the parents move on to the next phase. Some parents use staff members or other mothers as an "audience," whereas others are more comfortable talking with family and friends about the pregnancy and birth experience.

Because anxiety and preoccupation with her new role often narrow a mother's perceptions, information may have to be repeated. The new mother may require reminders to rest or, conversely, to ambulate enough to promote recovery. Hospital or birth center routines may not necessarily be an important priority to the new mother; she may take showers when examinations are scheduled and be involved in a telephone conversation rather than "being ready" for the baby. Regulations seem cumbersome, and sometimes mothers and their families have difficulty accepting rules that interfere with their need to share reactions about their infant.

Physical discomfort from an episiotomy, sore nipples, hemorrhoids, afterpains, and occasionally a sprained coccygeal joint can interfere with the mother's need for rest and relaxation. The selective use of comfort measures and medication depends on the nurse. Many women hesitate to ask for medication, believing that any pain they experience is normal and to be expected; breastfeeding mothers may fear the effects of medication on the infant. Few have knowledge of the use of heat or cold to relieve local pain.

Dependent-Independent Phase

If the mother has received adequate nurturing in the first few hours or days, by the second or third day, her desire for independent action reasserts itself. In the dependent-independent phase, the mother alternates between a need for extensive nurturing and acceptance by others and the desire to "take charge" once again. She responds enthusiastically to opportunities to learn and practice baby care or, if she is an accomplished mother, to carry out or direct this care. Rubin (1961) described this phase as the **taking-hold phase,** noting that it lasts approximately 10 days. Several studies (Evans et al., 1998; Martell, 1996; Wrasper, 1996) found that contemporary women exhibit taking-hold behaviors sooner than did the women in Rubin's study; however, the peak and duration of the taking-hold phase were not determined. In Martell's study (1996), women exhibited some taking-in and taking-hold behaviors but not in the sequence of postpartum phases described originally by Rubin. Evans and colleagues (1998) found that taking-hold behaviors began increasing between the evening of birth and the first morning, despite high levels of sleep disturbance.

Childbirth preparation classes, early contact with the newborn, rooming-in, and early discharge are some of the current obstetric practices that seem to enhance taking-hold behaviors (Martell, 1996; Wrasper, 1996). Given these changes in health care and in women's lives, more research is needed to evaluate the effect of such changes on patterns of women's behaviors during the postpartum period.

Most mothers are discharged home during this dependent-independent phase. Contemporary mothers have short hospital stays, ranging from 6 to 48 hours for low risk, uncomplicated births and from 48 to 96 hours for a cesarean birth. Once home, mothers must continue to cope with physical adaptations and psychologic adjustments that most mothers describe as stressful (Horowitz & Damato, 1999).

In studies of the experience of low risk mothers (25 multiparas and 25 primiparas) during the first 2 postpartum weeks, the majority of mothers identified fatigue as their major physical concern (Ruchala & Halstead, 1994; Smith-Hanrahan & Deblois, 1995). This fatigue affected various aspects of their lives, such as their relationships with their husbands and other family members and household responsibilities. Lee and Zaffke (1999) reported that rates of fatigue increase from 20% before conception to 64% immediately after birth. Bozoky and Corwin (2002) found that women reporting greatest fatigue in the hospital continue to report high fatigue at home for the first 4 postpartum weeks.

Some studies indicate that primiparas experience more sleep disturbance and fatigue than do multiparas (Waters & Lee, 1996) and that this higher level of fatigue, especially in the morning, continues for several weeks (Troy & Dalgas-Pelish, 1997).

Because of the relation of fatigue to postpartum depression (PPD), nurses must screen women for psychologic and physical signs and symptoms of fatigue. The Modified Fatigue Screening Checklist (MFSC) (Pugh et al., 1999) is a screening tool with 30 statements to which the mother responds yes or no. Examples of the statements are "My brain feels hot and muddled" and "I can't straighten my posture." Maternity nurses working in hospital postpartum units, birth centers, obstetrics offices, and home care, as well as pediatric nurses who come in contact with mothers during newborn well checks, are in prime positions to screen new mothers for fatigue.

Because fatigue continues to be a major concern of women during the early weeks of parenthood, nurses must provide anticipatory guidance regarding sleep disturbance and fatigue, as well as suggestions for dealing with the fatigue. Another strategy for helping new mothers cope with fatigue is a self-care guide for postpartum fatigue such as the "Tiredness Management Guide" developed by Troy and Dalgas-Pelish (1995). This guide provides a list of eight sources of postpartum fatigue: infection; no chance to rest; inability to get everything done; interrupted sleep; feeling stressed, anxious, or other psychologic changes from demands placed on the mother; low hemoglobin; and social activities. For each source of fatigue, techniques are listed for the mother to use. Two of the techniques, suggested for no chance to rest, are (1) sit or lie in a comfortable position when you feed your baby, and (2) organize your day for rest between tiring activities. The self-care guide is grounded on the principle that adult learners are self-directed, oriented to tasks specific to their social roles, and motivated to learn when immediate application is needed, all of which fit the postpartum woman.

Other physical concerns of mothers are loss of weight or figure, pain from the episiotomy or cesarean incision, sexual relations, and hemorrhoids.

Although women express enjoyment during the early postpartum period, most describe the period as hectic and a time of adjustment. Primiparas report feeling uncertain, trapped, and overwhelmed by fatigue and lack of experience in infant care. Many multiparas describe their experience as being better than with previous births, primarily because of their comfort with caring for an infant.

Emotional concerns are a recurring theme, with mothers reporting feeling "down," being tense and irritable, feeling "blue," being depressed, and crying easily. Many who report feeling depressed say that it is transient, lasting less than a week. Mothers usually realize that the emotional changes are normal and ascribe them to fatigue, physical discomfort, the condition of their bodies, the infants' temperaments, and the impact of the infant on their freedom.

Mothers who report feeling confident in caring for their infants identify someone, usually their own mothers, who had influenced them or been a role model for infant care. Research indicates that, by 3 to 4 months after birth, most mothers feel competent with specific infant care and feeding skills and with overall parenting, and report strong positive perceptions of themselves as mothers (Fowles, 1998). By 4 months after the birth, fathers with higher infant care self-efficacy have higher satisfaction with parenting (Hudson et al., 2001).

Maternal concerns and stress during the postpartum period may be attenuated through breastfeeding. Groer, Davis, and Hemphill (2002), in their article exploring postpartum stress and the possible protective role of breastfeeding, discussed the evidence that breastfeeding may produce a diminished biologic stress response as well as a diminished psychologic perception of stress for the mother.

These findings have implications for nursing care. Nurses can discuss, before and after birth, the usual postpartum concerns that mothers experience and provide anticipatory guidance on coping strategies, such as resting when the infant sleeps and planning with an extended family member or friend to do the housework for the first week or two after the baby is born. Once a mother is home, periodic phone calls from a nurse who cared for her in the birth setting can provide the mother with an opportunity to vent her concerns and get support and advice from "her nurse." Nurses should plan additional supportive counseling for first-time mothers inexperienced in child care; women whose careers had provided outside stimulation; women who lack friends or family members with whom to share delights and concerns; and adolescent mothers. When possible, postpartum home visits are included in the plan of care. Nurses also can discuss the possible stress-diminishing benefit of breastfeeding.

Postpartum "Blues"

The "pink" period surrounding the first day or two after birth, characterized by heightened joy and feelings of well-being, is often followed by a "blue" period. Approximately 50% to 80% of women of all ethnic and racial groups experience the **postpartum blues** or "baby blues" (Sutter et al., 1997; Wood et al., 1997). During the blues, women are emotionally labile, often crying easily and for no apparent reason. This lability seems to peak around the fifth day, subsiding by the tenth day. Other symptoms of postpartum blues include depression, a let-down feeling, restlessness, fatigue, insomnia, headache, anxiety, sadness, and anger. A reduced level of circulating glucocorticoids or a subclinical hypothyroidism may exist during the puerperium. Biochemical, psychologic, social, and cultural factors have been explored as possible causes of the postpartum depressive state; however, the etiology remains unknown.

Whatever the cause, the early postpartum period appears to be one of emotional and physical vulnerability for new mothers, who may be psychologically overwhelmed by the reality of parental responsibilities. The mother may feel deprived of the supportive care she received from family members and friends during pregnancy. Some mothers regret the loss of the mother–unborn child relationship and mourn its passing. Still others have a let-down feeling when labor and birth are complete. Fatigue after childbirth is experienced by as many as 64% of women in the immediate postpartum period (Lee & Zaffke, 1999), is compounded by the around-the-clock demands of the new baby, and can accentuate the feelings of depression (Wood et al., 1997). Fatigue as early as 7 days after birth is predictive of depression at 28 days after birth (Bozoky & Corwin, 2002). Exhaustion is rated by women as one of the top four contributing factors to PPD (Small et al., 1994). Postpartum depressive symptoms can have a negative effect on maternal role attainment (Fowles, 1998). To help mothers cope with postpartum blues, nurses can suggest various strategies (see Teaching for Self-Care box).

"Am I Blue?" (Johnson & Johnson, 1996), a self-administered questionnaire, can help mothers to assess their level of "blues" and to decide when to seek advice from their nurse, nurse-midwife, or physician (Fig. 24-7). Nurse home visits and telephone follow-up calls are important to assess the mother's pattern of "blue" feelings and behavior over time. Educating women about normal newborn/infant growth and development can help new mothers develop realistic expectations about infant behavior (Wood et al., 1997), thus decreasing one source of postpartum stress.

Although the postpartum blues are usually mild and short lived, approximately 10% to 15% of women experience PPD (Wood et al., 1997). The symptoms can range from mild to severe, with women having "good days" and "bad days." All symptoms can be equally distressing and make the woman feel as if she is "going mad." PPD leaves the woman with feelings of failure, overwhelming guilt, loneliness, and low self-esteem. Nurses should teach women how to differentiate symptoms of the "blues" and PPD and urge women to report depressive symptoms promptly if they occur (see Chapter 35 for a discussion of PPD). PPD can go undetected because new mothers generally do not voluntarily admit to this kind of emotional distress out of embarrassment, guilt, or fear. Nurses must be active listeners and compassionate intermediaries in interactions with new mothers so that symptoms of depression can be recognized early, assessed, and treated. Through careful attention to holistic health histories, nurses can identify women who are at high risk for PPD (see Box 35-5).

Interdependent Phase

In this phase, interdependent behavior reasserts itself, and the mother and her family move forward as a unit with interacting members. The relationship of the partners, although altered by the introduction of a baby, resumes many of its former characteristics. A primary need is to establish a lifestyle that includes but in some respects also excludes the baby. The couple must share interests and activities that are adult in scope.

An important aspect of the adult couple relationship is sexual intimacy. Sexual interest and postpartum resumption of sexual behavior are influenced by biologic, psychologic, and social changes that accompany giving birth. Changes in a woman's sexuality after childbirth are related to hormonal shifts, increased breast size, uneasiness with a body that has yet to return to a prepregnant size, chronic fatigue related to sleep deprivation, and physical exhaustion (Bitzer & Alder, 2000). The early demands of breastfeeding a newborn frequently can cause the mother not to want to be touched in one more way, especially on her breasts. However, breastfeeding also is a sensual experience for some mothers, promoting relaxation and a sense of being at peace. This may preclude somewhat the woman's need for further sensual experiences.

Sexual desire that typically wanes for a woman in the latter part of pregnancy persists in the first postpartum weeks. Three months after birth, about 40% of women report little or no desire for sexual activity. Although the majority of couples do not engage in sexual intercourse for the first 4 to 6 postpartum weeks, 94% have resumed coitus by the second month (Bitzer & Alder, 2000). Some couples begin sexual activity early, as soon as it can be accomplished without discomfort, depending on factors such as the presence of an episiotomy, perineal tears, or caesarean incision and amount of vaginal dryness. Regardless of when a couple resumes sexual intercourse, they should consider the prevention of another pregnancy, at least until the woman's body has had time to complete the

TEACHING FOR SELF-CARE

Coping with Postpartum Blues

- Remember that the "blues" are normal.
- Get plenty of rest; nap when the baby does if possible. Go to bed early, and let friends know when to visit.
- Use relaxation techniques learned in childbirth classes (or ask the nurse to teach you and your partner some techniques).
- Do something for yourself. Take advantage of the time your partner or family members care for the baby—soak in the tub or go for a walk.
- Plan a day out of the house—go to the mall with the baby, being sure to take a stroller or carriage, or go out to eat with friends without the baby. Many communities have churches or other agencies that provide child-care programs such as Mothers' Morning Out.
- Talk to your partner about the way you feel—for example, about feeling tied down, how the birth met your expectations, and things that will help you.
- If you are breastfeeding, give yourself and your baby time to learn.
- Seek out and use community resources such as La Leche League or community mental health centers. One nationally recognized resource is:
  Postpartum Support International
  927 North Kellogg Avenue
  Santa Barbara, CA 93111
  805-967-7636
  www.chss.iup.edu/postpartum

Am I Blue?

Many new mothers feel anxious, sad, or angry about the changes in their lives after the birth of their new baby. It is perfectly normal to feel this way, but sometimes the feelings grow so strong that they make life difficult. This quiz lists many feelings and experiences of "blue" or depressed mothers. Mark how strong each of these feelings or experiences is for you, compared with what is normal for you. For example: Do you feel no anger [0]; mild (very little) anger [1]; moderate (some) anger [2]; or severe (very strong) anger [3] compared with the way you usually feel? Add up your total score when you are finished, and discuss the results with your health care provider.

0 = Not there at all 1 = Mild 2 = Moderate 3 = Severe	0	1	2	3
Anger				
Anxiety attacks: periods of very strong fear, shortness of breath, rapid heartbeat				
Increased or decreased appetite and/or weight gain or loss that doesn't seem normal				
Strong feeling that you need to get away, need more time for your own interests				
Problems in a relationship with a family member, lover, close friend, etc.				
Crying spells				
Less interest in your personal appearance				
Less motivation—less energy or interest in accomplishing goals				
Depression				
Fatigue—feeling tired or exhausted				
Fear of harming yourself or your baby				
Loss of your sense of humor				
Nervousness, feeling tense or edgy				
Feelings of guilt				
Feelings of panic				
Feeling alone or lonely; without the support of others				
Feeling no love, or not enough love, for your baby				
Feeling forgetful, distracted, absent-minded—having trouble concentrating				
Frustration				
Hopelessness				
Insomnia				
Feeling irritable, bad-tempered				
Loss of sexual desire and/or pleasure in sex				
Loss of self-respect or confidence—feeling like you don't count or can't do anything right				
Feeling confused, uncertain				
Mood swings—your moods and emotions change all the time				
Obsessive thoughts—ideas or feelings you can't stop from repeating in your mind				
Odd or frightening thoughts—thoughts or images that scare you or that you can't control				
Thoughts of suicide, feeling like you want to die				
Feeling sad, unhappy				
TOTAL				

SCORE:

0 – 31 = MILD BLUES

This will probably pass, but pay attention to your feelings and needs.

32 – 64 = MODERATE BLUES

You may want to ask for help from a close friend or family member, or ask the advice of your health care provider.

65 – 98 = SEVERE BLUES

You could be depressed; see your health care provider for a check-up and advice as soon as possible.

If you are afraid you might harm yourself or your baby—ask a health care provider you trust for help—you don't have to be alone!

FIG. 24-7 Am I Blue? (Courtesy Johnson & Johnson Consumer Products, Skillman, NJ.)

involution process and until she is emotionally and physically ready for another pregnancy. Before and after birth, nurses should review with new parents their plans for other pregnancies and their preferences for contraception. See Chapters 9 and 23 for discharge teaching on sexual activity and contraception.

Sexual intimacy enhances the adult aspect of the family, and the adult pair shares a closeness denied to other family members. Many new fathers speak of the alienation felt when they observe the intimate mother-infant relationship, and some are frank in expressing feelings of jealousy toward the infant. The resumption of sexual intimacy seems to bring the parents' relationship back into focus.

The interdependent phase, termed the **letting-go phase,** is often stressful for the parental pair (Cox et al., 1999). Interests and needs often diverge during this time. Women and their partners must resolve the effects on their relationship of their individual roles related to child rearing, homemaking, and careers. Mothers as well as their partners may take a more traditional role in an effort to adapt to parenthood. A special continuing effort must be undertaken to strengthen the adult-adult relationship as a basis for the family unit.

Little is known about postpartum maternal adjustment in the lesbian couple. Relationship satisfaction in lesbian parent couples appears related to egalitarianism, commitment, sexual compatibility, and communication skills, as well as the birth mother's decision for insemination by an anonymous sperm donor (Osterwell, 1991; Reimann, 1997b; Reimann, 1999). Similar to heterosexual parent couples, most lesbian parent couples voice concern about less time and energy for their relationship after the arrival of the baby (Gartrell et al., 1996), and stress occurs when one partner perceives the other as not doing her fair share of the domestic work (Reimann, 1997a). Both partners consider themselves to be equal parents of the baby who share actively in childrearing (Brewaeys et al., 1995) and use various models of division of labor to provide one full-time mother for as long is economically possible (Reimann, 1997a). A primary concern of co-mothers is the legal vulnerability of lesbian families confounded by their social invisibility (Reimann, 1999).

Lesbian couples face strong social sanctions regarding pregnancy and parenting. Their families may not have resolved the initial dismay and guilt over learning of their daughters' homosexuality, or they may disagree with the lesbian couple's decision to conceive and be parents. Lesbian parents deal with public ignorance, social and legal invisibility, and the lack of biologic connection to the child by using a variety of techniques. These techniques include carefully planning and accomplishing their transition to parenthood, displaying public acts of equal mothering, sharing parenting at home, establishing a distinct parenting role within the family, and supporting each partner's sense of identity as a mother (Reimann, 1997a; 1997b). In situations in which family support is limited or absent, the nurse can help lesbian couples locate more supportive social groups, lesbian or heterosexual.

Paternal Adjustment

Fathers go through a predictable three-stage process during the first 3 weeks of their transition to parenthood (Henderson & Brouse, 991) (Table 24-5). During this period, fathers feel intense emotions. Stage 1 (expectations) involves approaching the experience with preconceptions about what it will be like when the baby is home. In stage 2 (reality), some fathers realize that their expectations are not based on fact. Many fathers acknowledge that their expectations were of limited value once they were immersed in the reality of parenthood. Feelings that often accompany this reality are sadness, ambivalence, jealousy, frustration at not being able to participate in breastfeeding, and an overwhelming desire to be more involved, most of which are different from the feelings mothers report. Conversely, some fathers are pleasantly surprised at the ease and fun of parenting. Stage 3 (transition to mastery) involves a conscious decision to take control and become more actively involved in the infant's life.

First-time fathers perceive the first 4 to 10 weeks of parenthood in much the same way that mothers do, that is, as a period characterized by uncertainty, increased responsibility, disruption of sleep, and inability to control time needed to care for the infant and reestablish the marital dyad (see Research box). Fathers across cultures

TABLE 24-5 **Transition to Fatherhood: A Three-Stage Process**

STAGES	CHARACTERISTICS
Stage 1: Expectations	Father has preconceptions about what life will be like after baby comes home
Stage 2: Reality	Father realizes that expectations are not always based on fact Common feelings experienced are as follows: Sadness Ambivalence Jealousy Frustration Overwhelming desire to be more involved Some fathers are pleasantly surprised at ease and fun of parenting
Stage 3: Transition to mastery	Father makes conscious decision to take control and become more actively involved with infant

believe that fatherhood affects marriage deeply. Generally they feel that the marital quality is enhanced, especially the cohesiveness of the family unit, yet fathers express concerns about (1) decreased attention from their partners relative to their personal relationship, (2) the mother's lack of recognition of the father's desire to participate in decision making for the infant, and (3) limited time available to establish a relationship with their infants (Steinberg, Kruckman, & Steinberg, 2000). These concerns can precipitate feelings of jealousy of the infant. Discussing their needs with the partner and becoming more involved with their infants and partner can help alleviate such feelings of jealousy. A consistent finding in the literature is that fathers who feel affection and support in the relationships with their partners or mates are more involved with infant care, and their involvement is more responsive, affectionate, and developmentally stimulating (Anderson, 1996a; 1996b).

Father-Infant Relationship

In American culture, neonates have a powerful impact on their fathers, who become intensely involved with their babies (Fig. 24-8). The term used for the father's absorption, preoccupation, and interest in the infant is **engrossment.** Characteristics of engrossment include some of the sensual responses relating to touch and eye-to-eye contact discussed earlier and the father's keen awareness of features both unique and similar to himself that validate his claim to the infant. An outstanding response is one of strong attraction to the newborn. Fathers spend considerable time "communicating" with the infant and taking delight in the infant's response to them. A sense of increased self-esteem and a sense of being proud, bigger, more mature, and older are all experienced by fathers after seeing their baby for the first time.

The development of the father-infant relationship involves three process components: making a commitment, becoming connected, and making room for baby (Anderson, 1996a; 1996b) (Table 24-6). "Commitment" is the father's willingness to invest in and take responsibility for nurturing the relationship with his infant despite difficulties in parenting and other life demands. Fathers feel the reality of commitment when the pregnancy is confirmed, during the pregnancy or birth, when they assume responsibility for infant care, and when the infant responds to them. The helpless nature of the infant af-

RESEARCH

New Fathers at 6 Weeks

Much is written of the transition to the mothering role, but little has been investigated about what new fathers experience. They must integrate their new or expanding role into their old roles, be the main support person for the mother, commit and connect with the newborn, and be a man about it. Some men experience ambivalence, anxiety, powerlessness, and confusion and feel alone in their struggle. There may be a disconnection between the couples' expectations of roles and responsibilities that may strain their relationships.

One practical way to understand the status of new fathers is to measure how they are functioning. A team of Australian nurse midwives asked 204 new fathers about whether they had assumed or resumed their normal activities using the Inventory of Functional Status—Fathers. This questionnaire was designed to assess social aspects of functional status, including household, social and community, infant and child care, personal care, and work and educational activities.

At 6 weeks postpartum, 72% of the new fathers reported full resumption of the care of older children, followed by 66% for helping with household activities, 59% for resuming work-related activities, 36% for social/community involvement, 27% for educational obligations, and 14% for personal care (grooming, exercise). About 37% had assumed the desired involvement in infant care activities. Older fathers assumed more household activities but were less involved in social events and in personal care than younger fathers. The more children in the home, the less the father was involved in infant care, and the less satisfaction he expressed about fatherhood. Few fathers took on more household responsibilities than they had prior to the birth. The authors speculated that the Australian extended maternity leave policy may reduce the father's involvement in day-to-day responsibilities.

IMPLICATIONS FOR PRACTICE

All health care providers can support men in their transition to fatherhood by involving them as full partners, not just as helpers. Nurses can encourage couples to discuss expectations of parenting and support before birth, including negotiation of the division of household and infant care responsibilities. Nurses can advocate for parental leaves and encourage fathers to investigate opportunities for leaves and for finding a support group for fathers.

Reference: McVeigh, C., Baafi, M., & Williamson, M. (2002). Functional status after fatherhood: An Australian study. *Journal of Obstetric, Gynecologic, and Neonatal Nursing, 31*(2), 165-171.

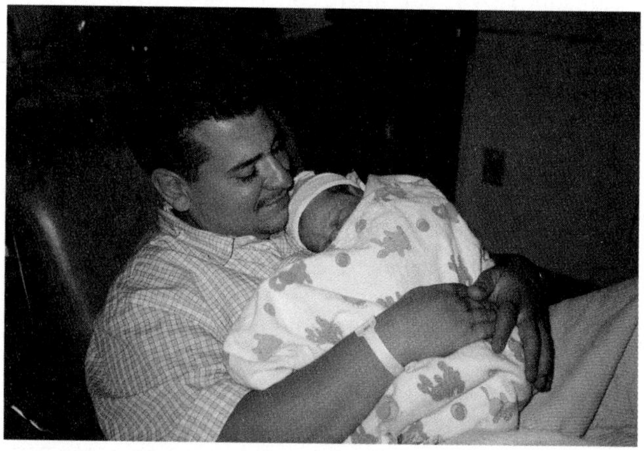

FIG. 24-8 Engrossment: Father absorbed in looking at his son. (Courtesy Shannon Perry, San Jose, CA.)

fects a sense of duty to nurture and protect the infant. Fathers want to get to know and be psychologically involved with their infants. Fathers identify rewards of developing a father-infant relationship, such as the infant's smile, increased self-esteem, gaining a new dimension in life, and finding the child within themselves.

"Becoming connected" appears to be the basic psychologic process in the development of the father-infant relationship. When meeting their infant for the first time, fathers experience feelings of joy, elation, awe, and wonderment. Some fathers feel an immediate bond, whereas others feel it once they touch and hold their infants. For others, the feelings of love and engrossment do not occur quickly, but gradually increase during the first 2 months of the infant's life. A turning point in the relationship development is when fathers perceive their infants as more responsive, predictable, and familiar.

In "making room for baby," fathers make changes in their work and social/personal time, in relationships with their wives, and within themselves so that they can be physically and emotionally available to their infants. Fathers identify the following as qualities a dad should have: to love, protect, and be emotionally present for the infant; to be supportive of their partners in the mothering role; and to use good communication skills.

Many studies on fathers of infants have focused on the amount of time fathers spend with their infants and what they do when they are with their infants. Two consistent findings are that (1) fathers spend less time than mothers with infants, and (2) fathers' interactions with infants tend to be characterized by stimulating social play rather than care taking. In the United States, fathers tend to take the lead in initiating play and to play in a rougher manner, whereas mothers tend to take the lead in caregiving activities. In India, fathers are not characterized as vigorous, playful partners. They appear to use more affectional display than very rough play with infants. The subtle and more open differences in stimulation from two sources, mother and father, provide a wider social experience for the infant.

Fathers can be sensitive and competent in caring for infants just as mothers can. Fathers' parental competence is associated with family functioning, partner relationship, emotional and informational support from partner, a sense of mastery, relationship with own father, knowledge of infant development, and having an "easy" infant. Fathers continue to report that parenting information directed specifically to fathers is not readily available and not offered typically by health care providers as it is for mothers (Steinberg et al., 2000).

Nurses can help fathers feel more competent in the parental role by teaching and providing information. Men entering parenthood with knowledge and realistic expectations may cope more successfully with the demands of a young infant and develop nurturing relationships with their infants. For nurses, dissemination of information can be a cost-effective intervention. Use of videos on infant cognitive and social capabilities and on early infant care and stimulation, as well as direct parent teaching methods such as exposure to newborn assessments and classes on parenting skills and infant behavioral cues, has been successful.

Impact of Fatherhood

For Caucasian, middle-class American husbands, first-time fatherhood is seen as a maturing event during which increased responsibility is assumed. Fathers report taking their work more seriously while trying to balance work and

TABLE 24-6 **Development of a Father-Infant Relationship: Process Components**

COMPONENT	CHARACTERISTICS
Making a commitment	Willingness to invest in and take responsibility for nurturing the relationship despite difficulties in parenting and other life demands Feel reality of commitment: at confirmation of pregnancy; during pregnancy and birth; when to provide infant care; when infant responds to them Helpless nature of infant affects a felt duty to nurture and protect Desire to get to know and be psychologically involved Rewarded by infant smile, increased self-esteem, gaining a new dimension in life, finding the child within self
Becoming connected	The basic psychologic process in the development of father-infant relationship First meeting with infant: feelings of joy, elation, awe, and wonderment Sense of a bond with the infant: may feel this at first meeting or when first touch/hold the infant or may develop gradually during the first 2 months Turning point: when perceives the infant as more responsive, predictable, and familiar
Making room for baby	Father makes changes in work and social/personal time, in relationship with wife/partner, and within self so more physically and emotionally available to infant

family demands. These men experience an identity change, developing images of themselves as fathers. Over time, they develop strong bonds with their infants and feel a sense of fulfillment and purpose in life (Anderson, 1996a; 1996b).

Canadian and Japanese men describe a similar perception of the impact of fatherhood (Steinberg et al., 2000). These men see parenthood as having a major effect on their personal relationship with their wives/partners and on the family's economic status, yet are confused on how to cope. They express concern about providing a sufficient income. Those who considered paternity leave resisted taking it because of financial considerations and, for some, because of workplace discrimination. Many of these Canadian and Japanese fathers perceive society as offering no special status to fatherhood, just added responsibility. As one French Canadian father said:

> Being a father demands a lot. A man works and then he goes back home to help the mother take care of the baby. Take care of whatever the mother cannot do because she is taking care of the baby. I don't think society in general see that. Especially in the workplace where men are career oriented, they expect the father to be career oriented. It is less now, but I think that there is still the expectation that the mother will take care of the baby and the father the finances. But it is not like that anymore. More and more fathers want to share the responsibility of childcare (Steinberg et al., 2000, p. 1269).

These fathers report a lack of health care information and parenting instruction directed to fathers. They state that they learn to be fathers by trial and error, by living the experience day by day, and that they turn to their wives/partners for confirmation that they are "fathering" correctly.

Studies investigating the impact of fatherhood on African-American men are sparse. One study on parental role attainment by African-American parents (Sank, 1991) provides nurses with some understanding of the father's experience. Self-concept was found to be the best predictor of these fathers' parental role attainment during the postpartum period. Fathers felt less competent with the skill and knowledge component of parenting than did the mothers, but they were at ease with the valuing and comfort component. Although these fathers did not see themselves as being as skillful as their partners in caring for infants, they valued parenthood and felt comfortable in the father role.

Despite their active involvement in the perinatal period, fathers tend to gravitate toward a more traditional division of family responsibilities. One reason for this return to more traditional roles may be the new father's concerns about his ability to support his new family financially.

Fathers can benefit from nursing interventions during the postpartum period just as mothers can. Nurses can arrange to teach infant care when the father is present and provide anticipatory guidance for fathers about the transition to parenthood. Separate prenatal and parenting classes and parenting support groups for fathers can provide them with an opportunity to discuss their concerns and have some of their needs met. Postpartum phone calls and home visits by the nurse must include time for assessment of the father's adjustment and needs.

Infant-Parent Adjustment

It has long been recognized that newborns participate actively in shaping their parents' reaction to them. Research has demonstrated that the behavioral characteristics of the infant influence parenting behaviors (Anderson, 1996a; Vehvilainen-Julkunen, 1995). The infant and the parent each have unique rhythms, behaviors, and response styles that are brought to every interaction. **Infant-parent interactions** can be facilitated in any of three ways: (1) modulation of rhythm, (2) modification of behavioral repertoires, and (3) mutual responsivity. Nurses can teach parents about these three aspects of infant-parent interaction through discussions, written materials, and videotapes on infant capabilities (e.g., *The Amazing Newborn*). A creative approach is to videotape the parent-infant pair during an interaction and then use the individualized tape to discuss the pair's rhythm, behavioral repertoire, and responsivity.

Rhythm

To modulate **rhythm,** both parent and infant must be able to interact. Therefore the infant must be in the alert state, one of the most difficult of the sleep-wake states to maintain. The alert state (Fig. 24-9) occurs most often during a feeding or in face-to-face play. The parent must work hard to help the infant maintain the alert state long enough and often enough for interactions to take place. The *en face* position (the parent's face is positioned in the same plane as that of the newborn) is usually assumed (Fig. 24-10, *D*). Multiparous mothers in particular are very sensitive and responsive to the infant's feeding rhythms. Mothers learn

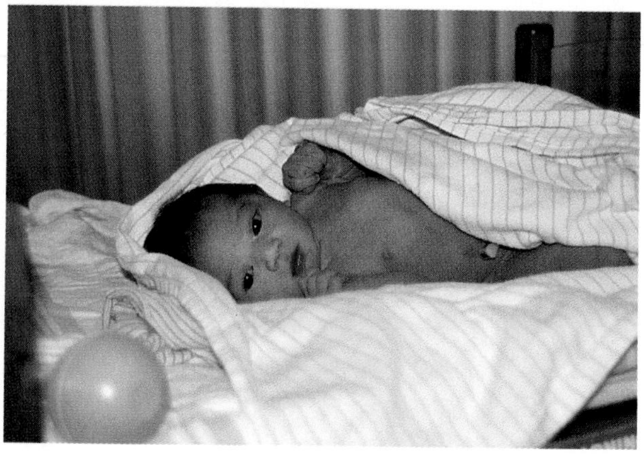

FIG. 24-9 Infant in alert state. (Courtesy Marjorie Pyle, RNC, Lifecircle, Costa Mesa, CA.)

to reserve stimulation for pauses in sucking activity and not to talk or smile excessively while the infant is sucking because the infant will stop feeding to interact with her. With maturity the infant can sustain longer interactions by modulating activity rhythms, that is, limb movement, sucking, gaze alternation, and habituation. Meanwhile, the parent becomes more attuned to the infant's rhythms and learns to modulate the rhythms, facilitating a rhythmic turn-taking interaction.

Behavioral Repertoires

Both the infant and the parent have a **repertoire of behaviors** they can use to facilitate interactions. Fathers and mothers engage in these behaviors depending on the extent of contact and caregiving of the infant.

The infant's behavioral repertoire includes gazing, vocalizing, and facial expressions. The infant is able to focus and follow the human face from birth and also is able to alternate the gaze voluntarily, looking away from the parent's face when understimulated or overstimulated (Fig. 24-10, *F*). One of the key responses for the parents to learn is to be sensitive to the infant's capacity for attention and inattention. Developing this sensitivity is especially important when interacting with preterm infants.

Body gestures form a part of the infant's "early language." Babies greet parents with waving hands (Fig. 24-10, *E*) or a reaching out of hands. They can raise an eyebrow or soften their expression to elicit loving attention. Game playing can stimulate them to smile or laugh. Pouting or crying, arching of the back, and general squirming usually signal the end of an interaction.

The parents' repertoire includes various types of interactive behaviors such as constantly looking at the infant and noting the infant's response. New parents often remark that they are exhausted from looking at the baby and smiling. Adults also "infantilize" their speech to help the infant "listen." They do this by slowing the tempo, speaking loudly and rhythmically, and emphasizing key words. Phrases are repeated frequently. Infantilizing does not mean using "baby talk," which involves distortion of sounds.

To communicate emotions to the infant, parents often use facial expressions such as slow and exaggerated looks of surprise, happiness, and confusion. Games such as "peek-a-boo" and imitation of the infant's behaviors are other means of interaction. For example, if the baby smiles, so does the parent; if the baby frowns, the parent responds in kind.

Responsivity

Contingent responses **(responsivity)** are those that occur within a specific time and are similar in form to a stimulus behavior. The adult has the feeling of having an influence on the interaction. Infant behaviors such as smiling, cooing, and sustained eye contact, usually in *en face* position, are viewed as contingent responses. The infant's responses act as rewards to the initiator and encourage the adult to continue with the game when the infant responds

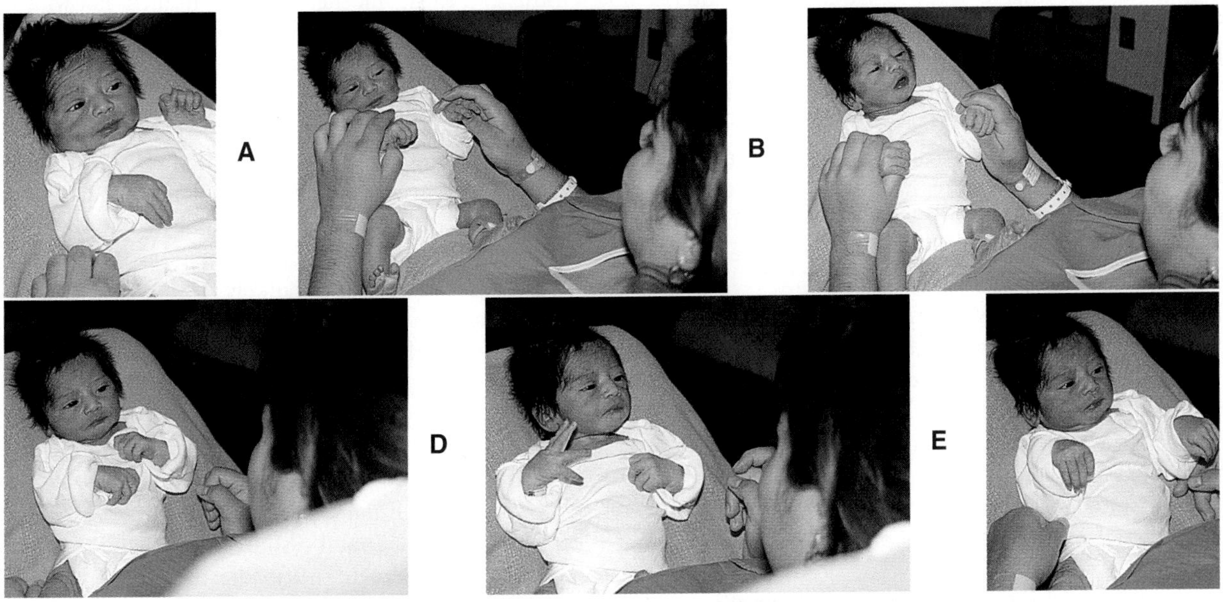
A
B
C
D
E
F

FIG. 24-10 Holding newborn in *en face* position, mother works to alert her daughter, 6 hours old. **A,** Infant is quiet and alert. **B,** Mother begins talking to daughter. **C,** Infant responds, opens mouth like her mother. **D,** Infant gazes at her mother. **E,** Infant waves hand. **F,** Infant glances away, resting. Hands relax. (Courtesy Marjorie Pyle, RNC, Lifecircle, Costa Mesa, CA.)

positively. When the adult imitates the infant, the infant appears to enjoy it. A progression occurs in the types of behaviors that parents present for the baby to imitate; for example, in early interactions, the parent will grimace rather than laugh, which is in keeping with the infant's developmental level. Such "turnabout" behaviors sustain interactions and promote harmony in the relationship.

FACTORS INFLUENCING PARENTAL RESPONSES

How parents respond to the birth of their child is influenced by various factors, including age, social networks, socioeconomic conditions, and personal aspirations for the future.

Age

Maternal age has a definite effect on the outcome of pregnancy. The mother and fetus are both at highest risk when the mother is an adolescent or is older than 35 years.

The Adolescent Mother

Although it is biologically possible for the adolescent female to become a parent, her egocentricity and concrete thinking interfere with her ability to parent effectively. The very young adolescent mother is inexperienced and unprepared to recognize the early signs of illness, potential danger, or household hazards. She may inadvertently neglect her child. The higher mortality rates among the infants of adolescent mothers are attributed to the inexperience, lack of knowledge, and immaturity of the mothers, causing them to be unable to recognize a problem and obtain the necessary resources to rectify the situation. Nevertheless, in most instances, with adequate support and developmentally appropriate teaching, adolescents can learn effective parenting skills.

The developmental tasks of parenthood include (1) reconciling the imagined infant with the actual infant, (2) becoming adept at caregiving activities, (3) being aware of the infant's needs, and (4) establishing oneself and one's infant as a family.

The transition to parenthood may be difficult for adolescent parents. Coping with the developmental tasks of parenthood is often complicated by the unmet developmental needs and tasks of adolescence. Some young parents may have difficulty accepting a changing self-image and adjusting to new roles related to the responsibilities of infant care. Other adolescent parents, however, may have higher self-concepts than their nonparenting peers (Alpers, 1998; Dalla & Gamble, 2000). Self-concept of pregnant and parenting teens appears to vary in relation to age, years of schooling, types of schools attended, income sources, and receipt of public assistance (Alpers, 1998). Nurses developing or implementing teen parenting programs should have occasional checkpoints in place throughout their programs to reassess the self-concept of adolescent parents and the types of socioeconomic supports these teens use.

As adolescent parents move through the transition to parenthood, they may feel "different" from their peers, excluded from "fun" activities, and prematurely forced to enter an adult social role. The conflict between their own desires and the infant's demands, in addition to the low tolerance for frustration that is typical of adolescence, further contribute to the normal psychosocial stress of childbirth. Less maternal education is associated with less favorable maternal responses to distress and infant behavior (Dalla & Gamble, 2000; Diehl, 1997).

Maintaining a relationship with the baby's father is beneficial for the teen mother and her infant. A close and satisfying relationship is positively correlated with maternal-fetal and maternal-infant attachment (Bloom, 1998). The involvement of the baby's father is related to appropriate maternal behaviors and positive mother-infant relationship (Diehl, 1997).

Some differences between adolescent and adult mothers have been observed. Adolescent mothers provide warm and attentive physical care; however, they use less verbal interaction than do older parents, tend to be less responsive, and interact less positively with their infants than do older mothers. Interventions emphasizing verbal and nonverbal communication skills between mother and infant are important. Such intervention strategies must be concrete and specific because of the cognitive level of adolescents. Although some observers suggest that some adolescents may use more aggressive behaviors, a higher incidence of child abuse has not been documented. In comparison with adult mothers, teenage mothers have a limited knowledge of child development. They tend to expect too much of their children too soon and often characterize their infants as being fussy. This limited knowledge may cause teenagers to respond to their infants inappropriately.

Many young mothers pattern their maternal role on what they themselves experienced. Therefore nurses need to determine the kind of support that people close to the young mother are able and prepared to give, as well as the kinds of community aid available to supplement this support. Many teen mothers can identify a source of social support, with the predominant source being their own mothers. Navajo adolescent mothers who had social support (emotional and instrumental) from their own mothers felt able to focus on both the adolescent and the maternal roles without neglecting either role (Dalla & Gamble, 2000). Rural adolescent mothers who reported firm encouragement and resources to pursue their life aspirations had more resilient adjustments to parenthood than did adolescent mothers who did not have this type of support (Camarena et al., 1998).

The need for continued assessment of the new mother's parenting abilities during this postbirth period is essential. In addition, continued support should be provided by involving the grandparents and other family members, as well as home visits and group sessions for discussion of infant care and parenting problems. Outreach programs concerned with self-care, parent-child interactions, child injuries, and failure to thrive, in addition to programs that provide prompt and effective community intervention, prevent more serious problems from occurring. As the adolescent performs her mothering role within the framework of her family, she may need to address dependence versus independence issues. The adolescent's family members also may need help adapting to their new roles.

The Adolescent Father

As with the adolescent mother, the nurse must be aware of the male adolescent's cognitive-developmental levels, values, and culture. The more successful outreach programs also address cultural diversity in teenage fathers.

The adolescent father and mother face immediate developmental crises, which include completing the developmental tasks of adolescence, making a transition to parenthood, and sometimes adapting to marriage. These transitions can be stressful. The nurse may initiate interaction with the adolescent father by asking him to be present when postpartum home visits are made and to accompany the mother and the baby to well baby checks at the clinic or pediatrician's office. With the adolescent mother's agreement, the nurse may contact the father directly. The decision to include the young father in all aspects of the care is based on assessment in the following four areas: (1) the couple's relationship; (2) levels of stress, concern, and coping; (3) educational and vocational goals; and (4) the level of health education knowledge. Adolescent fathers need support to discuss their emotional responses to the pregnancy. The nurse's nonjudgmental attitude is essential for open communication. The father's feelings of guilt, powerlessness, or bravado should be recognized because of their negative consequences for both the parents and the child. Counseling of adolescent fathers must be reality oriented. Topics such as finances, child care, parenting skills, and the father's role in the birth experience must be discussed. Teenage fathers also need to know about reproductive physiology and birth control options.

The adolescent father may continue to be involved in an ongoing relationship with the young mother and his baby. In many instances, he also plays an important role in the decisions about childcare and raising the child. The nurse supports the young father by helping him develop realistic perceptions of his role as "father to a child." The nurse encourages him to use coping mechanisms that are not detrimental to his own, his partner's, or his child's well-being. The nurse enlists support systems, parents, and professional agencies on his behalf. The father is encouraged to be involved in decisions regarding future contraception and safer sex practices.

Maternal Age Older Than 35 Years

Women older than 35 years have always continued their childbearing either by choice or because of a lack or failure of contraception during the perimenopausal years. Added to this group are women who have postponed pregnancy because of careers or other reasons, as well as women of infertile couples who finally become pregnant with the aid of technologic advances.

Researchers have examined the adjustment of midlife mothers to parenthood (Garrison et al., 1997; Poelker & Baldwin, 1999; Welles-Nystrom, 1997). Many mothers 35 years of age and older reported having a hard time coping, especially with irregular sleep patterns and the fussy periods babies have in the late afternoon and early evening. Mothers admitted to unrealistic preconceptions about parenting and high expectations of their ability to cope with the demands of motherhood, as the following report indicates:

> I was surviving, not living, for the first 3 months. I couldn't get over how dramatically my life changed. I had thought the baby would adjust to our lifestyle. I didn't understand that everyone had to adapt.

Other 35+ mothers, however, found that their preparedness, by delaying motherhood, enhanced their adaptation to parenthood. They felt that midlife mothers had qualities that younger mothers might lack, such as greater life experience, patience and understanding, readiness to settle down, and more mature outlook on life.

A factor that helps older mothers adjust and see themselves as competent parents is support from their partners. Support from other family members and friends also is important for positive self-evaluation of parenting, a sense of well-being and satisfaction, and help in dealing with stress. Positive self-evaluation of parenting early in the transition to parenthood is associated with greater confidence and support in mothering at 1 year (Reece & Harkless, 1996).

Older mothers report having to adjust to changes in the relationships with their partners. Some women regarded the changes as negative (e.g., having less time together), whereas others see the changes as positive (e.g., feeling closer to their partners). Because many of these couples have been together for many years before the baby is born, the loss of the "just-the-two-of-us" aspect of the relationship may be stressful.

Changes in the sexual aspect of a relationship can be a stressor for new midlife parents. Mothers report that finding time and energy for a romantic rendezvous is more difficult. They attribute much of this to the reality of caring for an infant but also to the decreasing libido that normally accompanies getting older.

Work and career issues are sources of conflict for older mothers (Reece & Harkless, 1996). Conflicts emerge over being disinterested, worrying about giving enough attention to work with the distractions of a new baby, and anticipating what it will be like to return to work. A major factor causing stress about work is childcare.

Another major issue for older mothers with careers is the perception of loss of control (Poelker & Baldwin, 1999; Reece & Harkless, 1996). Mothers older than 35, compared with younger mothers, are at a different stage in their careers, having attained higher levels of education, career, and income. The loss of control experienced when going from the consistency of a work role to the inconsistency of the parent role is a surprise to many. Perhaps this is because of the women's previous achievements and high expectations of themselves (Reece & Harkless, 1996). Nurses should be aware of the older mother's sense of loss of control and of the preoccupation with juggling career and family. Nurses can provide anticipatory guidance during pregnancy and early parenthood, with special attention to the issues of career women. Helping the older mother have realistic expectations of herself and of parenthood is essential.

New mothers who also are perimenopausal may find it hard to distinguish fatigue, loss of sleep, decreased libido, or other physiologic symptoms as the cause of the changes in their sex lives. Although many women view menopause as a natural stage of life, for midlife mothers, this cessation of menstruation coincides with the state of parenthood. The changes of midlife and menopause can add more emotional and physical stress to older mothers' lives because of the time- and energy-consuming aspects of raising a young child. Resources that older parents may find helpful are listed in Resources at the end of the chapter.

Paternal Age Older Than 35 Years

Literature on the experiences of first-time fathers older than 35 years is sparse. However, in the available literature (Poelker & Baldwin, 1999; Cain, 1994), older fathers describe their experience of midlife parenting as wonderful but not without drawbacks. Midlife fathers, established in their careers, are ready to concentrate on family and parenting. To them, positive aspects of older parenthood include increased love and commitment between the spouses, a reinforcement of why one married in the first place, a feeling of being complete, experiencing of "the child" again in oneself, more financial stability than in younger years, and more freedom to focus on parenting rather than on career. A common theme is sharing: sharing joy, sharing in raising the child, sharing as a family. The main drawback of midlife parenting that these men report is the change that parenthood makes in the relationships with their partners. They miss the deeper and more selfish couple relationship and look forward to the time when they can have that again. Some fathers mention age as a disadvantage: "Sometimes I think I'm the oldest father in [the group]. I can't do quite as many physical things as I used to when I was younger." All fathers seem to qualify statements about the less desirable side of parenting with positive statements such as ". . . but, I would not change it for the world!" or "I can't imagine life not being a parent now."

Social Support

Social support is strongly related to positive adaptation by new parents, including adolescent parents, during the transition to parenthood (Merriwether-deVries, 2000). Social support is multidimensional and includes the number of members in a person's social network, types of support, perceived general support, actual support received, and satisfaction with support available and received. The type and satisfaction of support seem to be more important than the total number of support network members.

Postpartum women who have received social support from a doula, compared with women who did not have a doula, demonstrate a stronger self-esteem, less depression, more positive feelings for their infant, and increased ability to care for their infant during the transition to parenthood (Klaus & Kennell, 1997).

Across cultural groups, families and friends of new parents form an important dimension of the parent's social network. For example, the extended family unit is the single strongest unit in the lives of most Asians. Extended family members also are relied on heavily after childbirth by Jordanians (D'Avanzo & Geissler, 2003). Through seeking help within the social network, new mothers learn practices that are culturally valued and develop role competency (Pridham, 1997). However, one study of 94 Chinese women at 1 month after birth found that social support was not significantly related to maternal concerns, the primary concerns being about the maternal role (Cheng & Chen, 2001).

Social networks provide a support system on which parents can rely for assistance, but they also can be a source of conflict. Sometimes a large network can cause problems because it results in conflicting advice from numerous people. Grandparents or in-laws are most appreciated when they assist with household responsibilities and do not intrude into the parents' privacy or judge them critically.

Women who have given birth before may have different support needs from those of first-time mothers. First-time mothers may need more follow-up for parenting skills, including referral to community resources. Women with other children may be more realistic in anticipating physical limitations and the changes in roles and relationships. However, these experienced mothers express concerns over separation from their firstborn, loss of the exclusive relationship with the older child or children, and the challenge of caring for two or more children.

Because of the extent of restructuring and reorganization that occurs in a family with the birth of another child, the mothers' moods and fatigue in the postpartum period can be helped more by situation-specific support from family and friends than by general support. General support addresses feeling loved, respected, and valued. Situation-specific support relates to practical concerns such as physical needs and childcare. For example, the practical support of a grandparent bathing the infant can help lessen a second-time mother's feelings of loss by providing her time to be with her firstborn child. Second-time mothers report that practical support is the most useful and desirable type of support during the postpartum period.

Nurses must be aware that not all types of support are equally beneficial to mothers after birth, and therefore, should assess the presence and types of practical help available to new mothers. The assumption that second-time (experienced) mothers are "old pros" and therefore do not need help should be avoided. Because second-time mothers may expect this of themselves, nurses can help these mothers explore the differences associated with adding another child to the family and identify the types of support that they need the most. As Gottlieb and Mendelson (1995) suggested, there must be a "fit" between the availability of support and a parent's needs for the support to be effective, and support may change with changing situations.

Culture

Cultural beliefs and practices are important determinants of parenting behaviors. Culture defines what is socially acceptable in terms of eye contact, touch, and space (Lipson, Dibble, & Minarik, 1996). Culture influences the interactions with the baby as well as the parent's or family's caregiving style. For example, the provision for a period of rest and recuperation for the mother after birth is prominent in several cultures. Asian mothers must remain at home with the baby at least 30 days after birth and are not supposed to engage in household chores, including care of the baby. Many times the grandmother takes over the baby's care immediately, even before discharge from the hospital (D'Avanzo & Geissler, 2003). An example is the traditional Taiwanese ritual, *Tso-Yueh-Tzu* (translated "doing, within the first month postpartum"). Contemporary Taiwanese women still participate in *Tso-Yueh-Tzu*; however, they express concern over how to use this ritual better in their adaptation to their new role and in transitioning back to contemporary society (Liu-Chiang, 1995). While they work through their concern, these contemporary Taiwanese mothers focus on the "integration of the self." Jordanian mothers have a 40-day lying-in after birth during which their mothers or sisters care for the baby (D'Avanzo & Geissler, 2003). The Japanese tradition called *Satogairi-Bunben* requires a woman to return to her family of origin for rest during the last month of pregnancy and for the first 2 months after childbirth for recuperation. However, the modern Japanese woman now tends to stay with her husband during the early postpartum period or go to her family for a much shorter time. This change may be in part due to the family of origin living a distance away and, in keeping the tradition, the woman would have to choose between her husband and her family (Steinberg et al., 2000). Hispanics practice an intergenerational family ritual, *la cuarentena*. For 40 days after birth, the mother is expected to recuperate and get acquainted with her infant. Traditionally this involves many restrictions concerning food (spicy or cold foods, fish, pork, and citrus are avoided; tortillas and chicken soup are encouraged), exercise, and activities, including sexual intercourse. Abdominal binding is a traditional practice, and many women avoid tub bathing and washing their hair. Traditional Hispanic husbands do not expect to see their wives or infants until both have been cleaned and dressed after birth. *La cuarentena* incorporates individuals into the family, instills parental responsibility, and integrates the family during a critical life event (D'Avanzo & Geissler, 2003; Niska, Snyder, & Lia-Hoagberg, 1998).

Desire for and valuing of children is salient in all cultures. In Asian families, children are valued as a source of family strength and stability, are perceived as wealth, and are objects of parental love and affection. Infants almost always are given an affectionate "cradle" name that is used during the first years of life; for example, a Filipino girl might be called "Ling-Ling" and a boy "Bong-Bong." In the Yup'ik culture of the Alaskan Eskimos, where sharing has been necessary for survival throughout their history, children are looked on as security. There is no concept of illegitimacy; whether parents are married does not matter. Every child is welcomed and loved. Adoption is common and is usually within the extended family, for example, by grandparents (MacDonald-Clark & Boffman, 1995).

Differing cultural values can influence parents' interactions with health care professionals. For example, Asians are taught to be humble and obedient; to be outspoken is frowned on. They are brought up not to question authority figures (such as a nurse), to avoid confrontation, and to respect the yin/yang balance in nature. Because of these learned values, an Asian mother might not confront the nurse about the length of time it has taken to receive the medication requested for her episiotomy pain. A mother may nod and say, "Yes," in response to the nurse's directions for using an iced sitz bath but then will not use the sitz bath. The "yes," in this case, is a gesture of courtesy, meaning, "I'm listening"; it is not an indication of agreement to comply. The mother does not use the iced sitz bath because of her traditional avoidance of bathing and cold in the puerperium. Because all members of a cultural group do not necessarily adhere to traditional practices, validating which cultural practices are important to individual parents is important. Also refer to Table 2-2 for examples of some traditional cultural beliefs that may be important to parents from African-American, Asian, and Hispanic cultures.

Knowledge of cultural beliefs can help the nurse make more accurate assessments and diagnoses of observed parenting behaviors. For example, nurses may become concerned when they observe cultural practices that appear to reflect poor maternal-infant bonding. Algerian mothers may not unwrap and explore their infants as part of the acquaintance process because in Algeria, babies are wrapped tightly in swaddling clothes to protect them physically and psychologically (D'Avanzo & Geissler, 2003). The nurse may observe a Vietnamese woman who gives minimal care to her infant but refuses to cuddle or further interact with her baby. This apparent lack of interest in the newborn is this cultural group's attempt to ward off "evil spirits" and actually reflects an intense love and concern for the infant (Galanti, 1997). An Asian mother might be criticized for almost immediately relinquishing the care of the infant to the grandmother and not even attempting to hold her baby when it is brought to her room. However, in Asian extended families, members show their support for a new mother's rest and recuperation by assisting with the care of the baby. Contrary to the guidance given to mothers in the United States about "nipple confusion," a mix of breastfeeding and bottle feeding is standard practice for Japanese mothers. This is out of concern for the mother's rest during the first 2 to 3 months and does not lead to any problems with lactation; breastfeeding is widespread and successful among Japanese women (Sharts-Hopko, 1995).

An example of a culture in which the norm of maternal behaviors with infants parallels what is expected in the United States is the Yup'ik culture of the Alaskan Eskimos. New Yup'ik mothers typically are observed to be quiet, loving, and gentle with their newborns, almost always holding their infants in a position where eye contact can be made. They are keenly aware of and responsive to their infants' cues. In one study, Yup'ik mothers scored higher on measures of responsiveness to infant cues, especially distress cues, than did the normative group (Caucasian, African-American, and Hispanic mothers) (MacDonald-Clark & Boffman, 1995).

Cultural beliefs and values give perspective to the meaning of childbirth for a new mother. Nurses can provide an opportunity for a new mother to talk about her perception of the meaning of childbearing. This may foster self-actualization, promote maternal role attainment, improve her relationship with her partner, and enrich the family perspective. In helping new families adjust to parenthood, nurses must provide culturally sensitive care by following principles that facilitate nursing practice within transcultural situations.

Socioeconomic Conditions

Socioeconomic conditions often determine access to available resources. Parents whose economic condition is made worse with the birth of each child and who are unable to use an effective method of fertility management may find childbirth complicated by concern for their own health and a sense of helplessness. Mothers who are single, separated, or divorced from their husbands or without a partner, family, and friends for whatever reason may view the birth of a child with dread. Serious financial problems may override any desire for mothering the infant. Nurses must be sensitive to the stressors that economically disadvantaged mothers have to contend with and consider these in efforts to foster mother-infant bonding (Sharts-Hopko, 1995). Nursing measures designed to help mothers in trying socioeconomic circumstances involve referral to social and economic community service agencies, as well as to health care agencies. A satisfactory outcome for such problems often requires long-term commitments from both the woman or couple and the community. Adequate situational supports must be instituted in the prenatal period.

Personal Aspirations

For some women, parenthood interferes with or blocks their plans for personal freedom or advancement in their careers. Resentment concerning this loss may not have been resolved during the prenatal period, and if it remains unresolved, it will spill over into caregiving activities. This may result in indifference and neglect of the infant, or in excessive concern and the setting of impossibly high standards by the mother for her own behavior or the child's performance.

In a study of first-time mothers with career commitments, Leonard (1993) found that the meaning and content of work and of motherhood, and the timing of return to work had a powerful influence in shaping the career woman's experience with the transition to parenthood. Women expected that having a baby would add a role to their repertoire of roles; however, the women experienced motherhood as "world-transforming," not simply additive. Returning to work was especially stressful to these career women, particularly if the work setting did not recognize the needs and responsibilities the women now had as mothers. If the women viewed their work as meaningful and if their income was economically important for their family, the stress they experienced was mitigated.

Role models that assist women in integrating work role and motherhood role may be helpful for new mothers; however, these role models are scarce (Hartrick, 1997; Miller, 1996). Mothers returning to work who do not identify with such role models appear to improvise and negotiate relationships to manage their careers and the care of their infants (Miller, 1996). Over time, new mothers progress to nurturing themselves and making new connections, to a time of reclaiming and discovery (Hartrick, 1997). Not all new mothers experience role conflict. Some have less role conflict because their careers provide a sense of self-fulfillment and self-worth, especially when they feel supported by their family and confident in child care arrangements.

Nursing intervention includes providing opportunities for mothers to express their feelings freely to an objective listener; to discuss measures to permit personal growth; and to learn about the care of their infant.

Nurses also can be proactive in influencing changes in work policies related to maternity and paternity leaves, varying models of work sharing, and "family friendly" work environments. Some corporations already structure their work sites to support new mothers (e.g., by providing on-site day-care facilities and breastfeeding rooms).

PARENTAL SENSORY IMPAIRMENT

In the early dialogue between the parent and child, each uses all senses–sight, hearing, touch, taste, and smell–to initiate and sustain the attachment process. A parent who has an impairment of one of the senses must maximize use of the remaining senses. Although these parents may need the assistance and support of a sighted or hearing person as well as other accommodations to their disability, they certainly can become skilled parents. It is important for nurses and other health care professionals to remember that these parents are people living with a disability, not "disabled parents."

Visually Impaired Parent

Visual impairment alone does not seem to have a negative impact on mothers' early parenting experiences. These mothers, just as sighted mothers, express the wonders of parenthood and encourage other visually impaired persons to become parents (Conley-Jung & Olkin, 2001). Mothers with disabilities tend to value the importance of performing parenting tasks in the perceived culturally usual way. Their maternal engagement also is facilitated by self-acceptance of their own unique differences in performing parenting tasks (Farber, 2000).

Although visually impaired mothers initially feel a pressure to conform to traditional, sighted ways of parenting, they soon adapt these ways and develop methods better suited to themselves (Conley-Jung & Olkin, 2001). Examples of activities that visually impaired mothers do differently include preparation of the infant's nursery, clothes, and supplies. Mothers may put an entire clothing outfit together and hang it in the closet rather than keeping the items separately in drawers. They might develop a labeling system for the infant's clothing and put diapering, bathing, and other care supplies where these will be easy to locate with minimal searching (Conley-Jung & Olkin, 2001). A strength that visually impaired parents have is a heightened sensitivity to other sensory outputs. A blind mother can tell when her infant is facing her because she can feel the baby's breath on her face.

Concerns expressed by visually impaired mothers include (1) their infant's safety; (2) the extra planning, time, and effort needed to accommodate their visual limitations beyond those parenting usually requires; (3) transportation; (4) handling other people's reactions; (5) providing proper guidance and discipline as the infant grows; and (5) missing out visually (Conley-Jung & Olkin, 2001). Visually impaired mothers use various strategies to cope with the reactions of others. They suggest being upfront and conveying a sense of openness; making people aware of the nature of the visual impairment early in the relationship; informing and educating people about visual impairment; focusing on the positive and ignoring negative messages; expressing anger; and laughing and joking (Conley-Jung & Olin, 2001).

One of the major difficulties of visually impaired parents is the skepticism, open or hidden, of health care professionals. Blind people sense reluctance on the part of others to acknowledge that they have a right to be parents. All too often, nurses and doctors lack the experience to deal with the childbearing and child-rearing needs of visually impaired mothers, as well as mothers with other disabilities (such as hearing impaired, physically impaired, and mentally challenged). Shyness, fear, or reluctance on the part of nurses can result in visually impaired parents being left alone or being involved in awkward conversations. The best approach by the nurse is to assess the mother's capabilities. From that basis, the nurse can make plans to assist the woman, often in much the same way as for a mother with sight. Visually impaired mothers have made suggestions for providing care for women such as themselves during childbearing (Box 24-2). Such approaches by the nurse can help avoid a sense of increased vulnerability on the mother's part.

Eye-to-eye contact is considered important in American culture. With a parent who is visually impaired, this critical factor in the parent-child attachment process is obviously missing. However, the blind parent, who may never have experienced this method of strengthening relationships, does not miss it. The infant will need other sensory input from that parent. An infant looking into the eyes of a mother who is blind may not be aware that the eyes are unseeing. Other people in the newborn's environment can participate in active eye-to-eye contact to supply this need. A problem may arise, however, if the visually impaired parent has an impassive facial expression. Her infant, making repeated unsuccessful attempts to engage in face play

BOX 24-2 Nursing Approaches for Working with Visually Impaired Parents

1. Parents who are blind need oral teaching by health care providers because maternity information is not accessible to blind people.
2. A visually impaired parent needs an orientation to the hospital room that allows the parent to move about the room independently. For example, "Go to the left of the bed and trail the wall until you feel the first door. That is the bathroom."
3. Parents who are blind need explanations of routines.
4. Parents who are blind need to feel devices (e.g., monitors, pelvic models) and to hear descriptions of the devices.
5. Visually impaired parents need "a chance to ask questions."
6. Visually impaired parents need the opportunity to hold and touch the baby after birth.
7. Nurses need to demonstrate baby care by touch and to follow with, "Now let me see you do it."
8. Nurses need to give instructions such as, "I'm going to give you the baby. The head is to your left side."

with the mother, will abandon the behavior with her and intensify it with the father or other people in the household. Nurses can provide anticipatory guidance regarding this situation and help the mother learn to nod and smile while talking and cooing to the infant.

Hearing-Impaired Parent

The parent who has a hearing impairment faces another set of problems, particularly if the deafness dates from birth or early childhood. The mother and her partner are likely to have established an independent household. A number of devices that transform sound into light flashes are now marketed and can be fitted into the infant's room to permit immediate detection of crying. Even if the parent is not speech trained, vocalizing can serve as both a stimulus and a response to the infant's early vocalizing. Deaf parents can provide additional vocal training by use of recordings and television so that from birth, the child is aware of the full range of the human voice. Young children acquire sign language readily, and the first sign used is as varied as the first word.

Section 504 of the Rehabilitation Act of 1973 requires that hospitals and other institutions receiving funds from the U.S. Department of Health and Human Services use various communication techniques and resources with the deaf, including having staff members or certified interpreters who are proficient in sign language. For example, provision of written materials with demonstrations and having nurses stand where the parent can read their lips (if the parent practices lip reading) can be used. A creative approach is for the nursing unit to develop videotapes in which information on postpartum care, infant care, and parenting issues is signed by an interpreter and spoken by a nurse. A videotape in which a nurse signs while speaking would be ideal.

SIBLING ADAPTATION

Because the family is an interactive, open unit, the addition of a new family member affects everyone in the family. Siblings are no exception. Older children have to assume new positions within the family hierarchy. The older child's goal is to maintain the lead position. Parents are faced with the task of caring for a new child while not neglecting the others. Parents need to distribute their attention in an equitable manner.

Reactions of siblings may result from temporary separation from the mother, changes in the mother's or father's behavior, or the siblings' response to the infant's coming home. Sibling reactions are manifested in behavioral changes. Positive behavioral changes include interest in and concern for the baby and increased independence. Regression in toileting and sleep habits, aggression toward the baby, and increased seeking of attention and whining are examples of negative behaviors.

The introduction of a baby into a family with one or more children challenges parents to promote acceptance of the baby by siblings (Fig. 24-11). Parents' attitudes toward the arrival of the baby can set the stage for the other children's reactions. In some families, parental support promotes sibling adjustment; in others, the needs of the sibling shape the parental support.

Because the baby absorbs the time and attention of the important people in the other children's lives, jealousy is to be expected once the initial excitement of having a new baby in the home is over. However, **sibling rivalry,** or negative behaviors in siblings, may have been overemphasized in the past. Developmentally appropriate behaviors in siblings are similar before and after the baby arrives. Firstborn children seem to continue their usual routines and are more pleased with the newborns and more understanding of the baby's need for care than the parents predict.

Parents, especially mothers, spend much time and energy promoting sibling acceptance of a new baby. Participating in sibling preparation classes makes a difference in the ability of mothers to cope with sibling behavior. Older children are actively involved in preparing for the infant, and this involvement intensifies after the birth of the child. Parents face a number of tasks related to sibling rivalry and adjustment. For example, parents have to manage the feeling of guilt because the older children are being deprived of parental time and attention. They also have to monitor the behavior of older children toward the more vulnerable infant and to divert aggressive behavior. Strategies that parents have used to facilitate acceptance of a new baby by siblings are presented in Box 24-3.

Siblings demonstrate acquaintance behaviors with the newborn. The acquaintance process depends on the in-

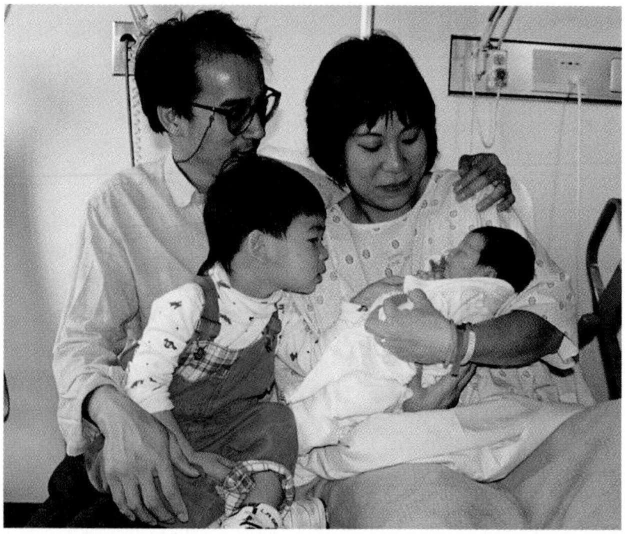

FIG. 24-11 Parent introduces "big" brother to infant daughter. (Courtesy Kim Molloy, Knoxville, IA.)

formation given to the child before the baby is born and on the child's cognitive development level. The initial behaviors of siblings with the newborn include looking at the infant and touching the head (Fig. 24-12). The initial adjustment of older children to a newborn takes time, and children should be allowed to interact at their own pace rather than being forced to do so. To expect a young child to accept and love a rival for the parents' affection assumes an unrealistic level of maturity. Sibling love grows as does other love (i.e., by being with another person and sharing experiences) (Fig. 24-13). The relationship that develops between siblings has been conceptualized as sibling attachment. This bond between siblings involves a secure base in which one child provides support for the other, is missed when absent, and is looked to for comfort and security.

Direct sibling contact does not place healthy newborns at risk for exposure to pathogenic organisms; therefore separation of newborns and older siblings does not appear to be justified.

BOX 24-3 **Strategies for Facilitating Sibling Acceptance of a New Baby**

1. Take your firstborn child on a tour of your hospital room and point out similarities to his or her birth. "This is like the room I was in with you, and the baby is in the same kind of bassinet that you were in."
2. Have a small gift from the baby to give to your older child each day.
3. Give the older child a T-shirt that says "I'm a big brother" (or "sister").
4. Arrange for your children to be in the first group (grandparents, sister) to see the newborn. Let them hold the baby in the hospital. One mother and father arranged for their firstborn son to be present at the births of his three brothers and to be the first one to hold them.
5. Plan time for both children. "When I get home, I'll arrange my day so that I can have the baby's care done in the morning while Sam (first child) is at school. Maybe the baby will sleep part of the afternoon and I can spend some time with Sam."
6. Fathers can spend time with the older sibling while mothers are taking care of the baby and vice versa. Siblings like to have time and attention from both parents.
7. Give preschool and early school-age siblings a newborn doll as "their baby" to care for. Give sibling a photograph of the new baby to take to school to show off "his" or "her" baby. Older siblings may enjoy the responsibility of helping care for the newborn, such as learning how to give the baby a bottle or to change a diaper. One mother let her preschooler help burp the new baby by patting on the baby's back. She figured her son could pat the baby fairly firmly without harming him and at the same time get out some pent-up aggressive feelings.

GRANDPARENT ADAPTATION

Grandparents are unique. They contribute to a sense of family continuity and provide maintenance of cultural traditions. They can educate their grandchildren about their roots and relate anecdotes about their parents. In turn, the presence of grandchildren often helps relieve the grandparents' loneliness and boredom. Grandparents who are free to love the grandchild can have a significant positive influence on the child's life (Fig. 24-14).

Just as the new parents go through a transition to parenthood, grandparents experience a transition to grandparenthood. Intergenerational relationships shift, and grandparents must deal with changes in practices and attitudes toward childbirth, child rearing, and men's and women's roles at home and in the workplace. The degree to which grandparents understand and accept current practices can influence how supportive they are perceived to be by their adult children.

While they are adjusting to grandparenthood, the majority of grandparents have normative middle- and old-age life transition issues, such as retirement and a move to smaller housing, and need support from their adult children. Some may feel regret about their limited involvement because of poor health or geographic distance. Maternal grandmothers, more than the other three grandparents, may have high expectations of themselves that cause them to be very self-critical.

The extent of involvement of grandparents in the care of the newborn depends on many factors (e.g., the willingness of the grandparents to become involved, the proximity of the grandparents, and ethnic and cultural expectations of the grandparents' role). If the new parents live in the United States, Asian grandparents, for example, typically are asked to come to the United States to care for the baby and the mother after birth and to care for the children once the parents return to work. In the United States, paternal grandparents, in contrast to those in other cultures, frequently consider themselves secondary to the maternal grandparents. Less seems expected of them, and they are initially less involved. Nevertheless, these grandparents are eager to help and express great pleasure in their son's fatherhood and his involvement with the baby. Support that they provide for their son can help the new father in being supportive of the new mother, thus influencing a smoother parental adjustment for the new parents.

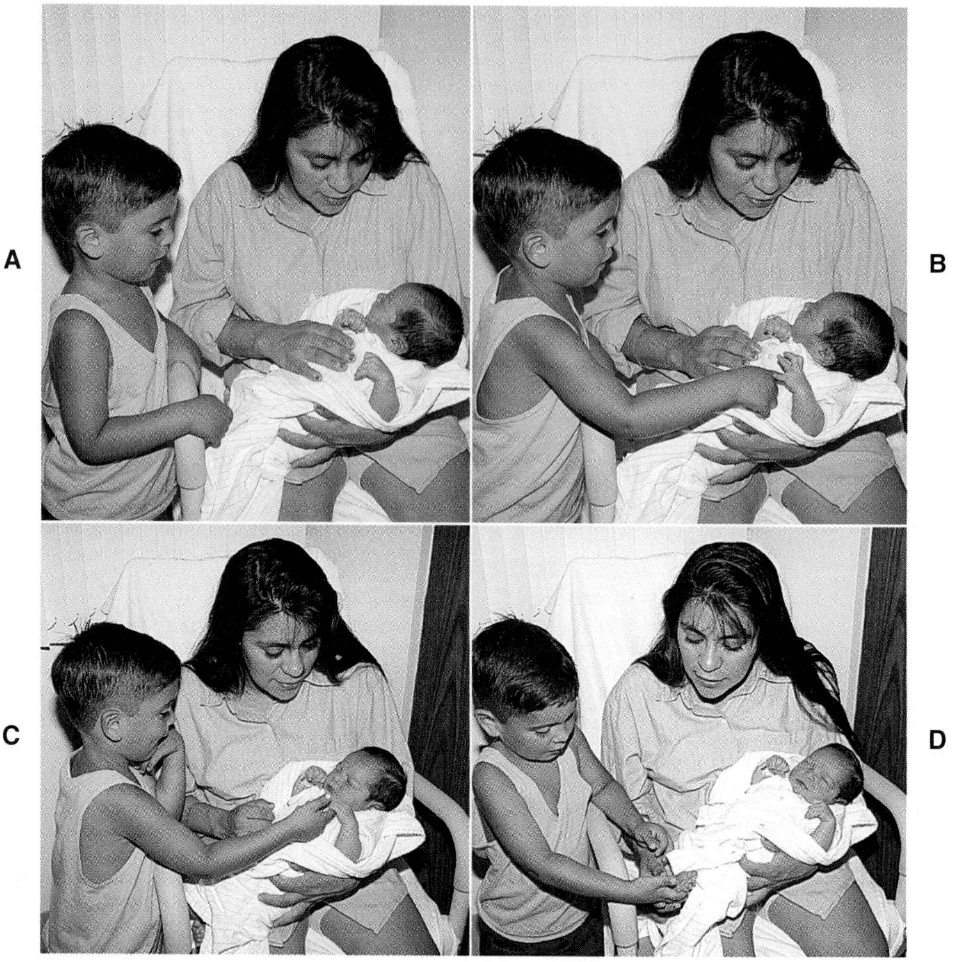

FIG. 24-12 First meeting. **A,** Boy with mother during first meeting with new sibling. **B,** First tentative touch. **C,** Testing with fingertip. **D,** Relationship more secure: it is now okay to hold with whole hand. (Courtesy Marjorie Pyle, RNC, Lifecircle, Costa Mesa, CA.)

For first-time parents, pregnancy and parenthood can reawaken old issues related to dependence versus independence. Some expectant parents may not plan on their parents' help immediately after the baby arrives. They may want time "to be a family," implying a couple-baby unit, not the intergenerational family network. Intergenerational help may be perceived as interference. Many new parents, contrary to their expectations, do call on their parents for help, especially the maternal grandmother (Steinberg et al., 2000). Many grandparents realize their adult children's wishes for autonomy, respect these wishes, and remain available to help when asked.

As parents are assisted in working through differing opinions and unresolved conflicts (e.g., feelings of dependence and control) between themselves and their parents, they can move toward mastery of the developmental tasks of adulthood. The support of grandparents can be a stabilizing influence for families undergoing developmental transitions such as childbearing and new parenthood. Grandparents can foster the learning of parental skills and preserve tradition. The maternal grandmother is an important model for child-rearing practices, a source of knowledge, and a support person. With teenage mothers, the regular assistance of grandparents with childcare has allowed these young mothers to continue their educations (Dalla & Gamble, 2000).

Nurses should be aware that the transition to parenthood and grandparenthood offers and demands new intergenerational adaptations. Rather than taking for granted intergenerational support between adult children and their parents, nurses must acknowledge the wide range of dynamic issues that enhance or mitigate experiences of intergenerational support. Early in pregnancy, a family assessment that includes an intergenerational perspective can identify whether grandparents are included in the couple's social support network and whether their support is wanted and helpful.

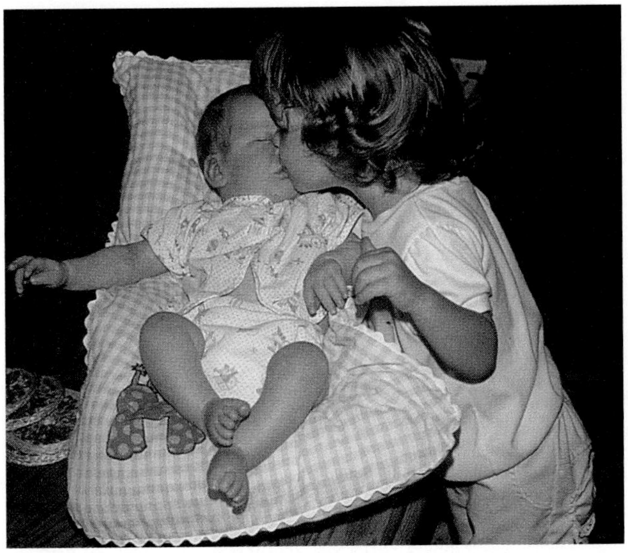

FIG. 24-13 Sister kisses her new brother. Family contacts are important for newborn and siblings. (Courtesy Marjorie Pyle, RNC, Lifecircle, Costa Mesa, CA.)

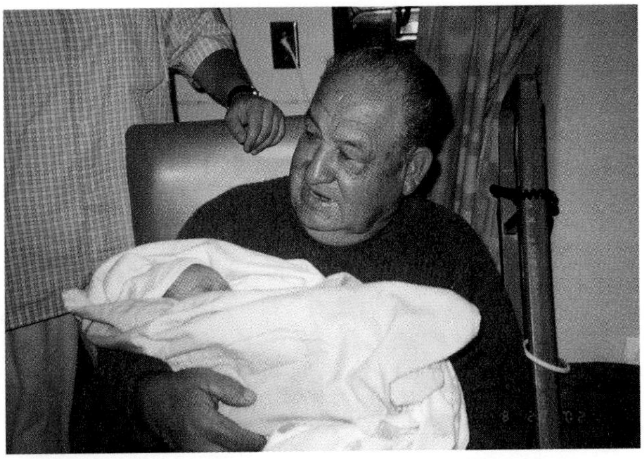

FIG. 24-14 Grandfather and new grandson get acquainted. (Courtesy Shannon Perry, San Jose, CA.)

One simple technique to help people span the generation gap is through a printed "letter to new parents" (written from the grandparents' perspective), which can be included in prenatal kits distributed in childbirth preparation classes and made available to all family members on the postpartum unit. Classes may help grandparents bridge the generation gap and understand their adult children's parenting concepts. Included in these classes would be information about up-to-date childbearing practices (especially family-centered care); infant care, feeding, and safety (car seats); and exploration of roles that grandparents play in the family unit. Both techniques can foster open discussion between the generations about the feelings and needs of parents and grandparents.

KEY POINTS

- The birth of a child necessitates changes in the existing interactional structure of a family.
- Either parent may exhibit "motherliness."
- Attachment is the process by which the parent and infant come to love and accept each other.
- Both partners in the parent-infant interaction strengthen attachment through the use of sensual responses or interactions.
- Early contact with the newborn is not essential for attachment to occur.
- For the biologic parent, the parental role does not begin at birth but rather enlarges and intensifies from the preconception decision to have a child.
- The father is considered an equal and integral part of the developing family.
- In adjusting to the parental role, the mother moves from a dependent state (taking in) to an interdependent state (letting go).
- Mothers may exhibit signs of postpartum blues (baby blues).
- Fathers experience emotions and adjustments during the transition to parenthood that are similar to, and distinctly different from, those of mothers.
- Modulation of rhythm, modification of behavioral repertoires, and mutual responsivity facilitate infant-parent adjustment.
- A primary need of parents is to establish a lifestyle that includes, but in some respects excludes, the baby.
- Many factors influence adaptation to parenthood (e.g., age, culture, socioeconomic level, and expectations of what the child will be like).
- Parents face a number of tasks related to sibling adjustment that require creative parental interventions.
- Grandparents can be a source of knowledge and support and can have a positive influence on the postpartum family.

CRITICAL THINKING EXERCISES

1. You are assigned to care for Karen (26 years old) and Doug (27 years old), who are first-time parents. Karen gave birth to a daughter 6 hours ago. Both Karen and Doug are visually impaired. Doug has been blind since birth, and Karen lost part of her sight as the result of a car accident when she was 16 years old; what she sees resembles shadows. Karen and Doug have college degrees. Doug teaches history in a community college; Karen worked as a phone counselor in a family crisis center until the last 2 weeks of her pregnancy. They plan to go home from the birth center tomorrow.
   - **a.** Should the nurse's approach with these parents be different from an approach used with sighted parents? Why or why not? If yes, in what ways?
   - **b.** How might Karen's and Doug's adjustments to the parental role be similar? Different?
   - **c.** Karen and Doug have read a lot about bonding and voice concern that their visual impairment will interfere with their daughter bonding with them. Respond to their concern.
   - **d.** Identify strategies that visually impaired parents can use to have a smoother transition to parenthood.
2. You are the nurse in a neighborhood health clinic that serves two communities whose residents are of a low socioeconomic level, living in subsidized housing, and are primarily Asian and Hispanic immigrants. At a regular meeting with the neighborhood advisory group, a priority identified is the need for a support group and parenting classes for new mothers and fathers. Several families have babies aged 2 weeks to 12 months, plus a few who are expecting babies during the next 8 months.
   - **a.** What are the common concerns/needs of these parents of newborns and infants? How does their cultural heritage influence transition to parenthood?
   - **b.** How will you determine what content to include in the classes? Outline the content for the parenting classes: state a rationale to justify each area of content. How will you design the support group? What should be the goal/purpose of the support group?
   - **c.** Identify community resources you will use for the support group and the parenting classes. How will the demographic and cultural characteristics of the residents of these communities influence the design and content of the support group and parenting classes?

RESOURCES

At-Home Dad (newsletter for fathers who stay at home)
61 Brightwood Ave.
North Andover, MA 01845-1702
E-mail: athomedad@aol.com

Baby-Friendly USA
8 Jan Sebastian Way, No. 13
Sandwich, MA 02563
508-888-8044
E-mail: hea@capecod.net

The Fatherhood Project at the Families and Work Institute
330 Seventh Ave.
New York, NY 10001
212-465-2044

FEMALE (Formerly Employed Mother at the Leading Edge)
P.O. Box 31
Elmhurst, IL 60126
630-941-3553

Institute for Responsible Fatherhood and Family Revitalization
1146 19th Street NW
Suite 800
Washington, DC 20036
800-7FATHER or 800-732-8437

International Association of Infant Massage (IAIM)
800-248-5432

La Leche League International
1400 North Meacham Road
Schaumburg, IL 60168-4079
847-519-7730
www.lalecheleague.org
(Local La Leche League groups are usually listed in city and town phone books)

Motherhood Maternity Health and Fitness Program
SBI Corporation
1106 Stratford Dr.
Carlisle, PA 17103
717-258-4641

Mothers at Home
8310A Old Courthouse Road
Vienna, VA 22182
703-827-5903

National Council for Adoption
202-328-5903

National Organization of Mothers of Twins Clubs, Inc.
P.O. Box 23188
Albuquerque, NM 87192
505-275-0955

Pink Inc.! Publishing
P.O. Box 866
Atlantic Beach, FL 32233-0866

Postpartum Support International
927 North Kellogg Avenue
Santa Barbara, CA 93111
805-967-7636
www.chss.iup.edu/postpartum

Protecting Your Newborn, Video and Instructor's Guide
Ford Motor Company and U. S. Department of Transportation National Highway Traffic Safety Administration (NHTSA)

Single Parent Resource Center
141 West 28th Street
Suite 302
New York, NY 10001
212-947-0221

REFERENCES

Alpers, R. (1998). The changing self-concept of pregnant and parenting teens. *Journal of Professional Nursing, 14*(2), 111-118.

Ament, L. (1990). Maternal tasks of the puerperium re-identified. *Journal of Obstetric, Gynecologic, and Neonatal Nursing, 19*(4), 330-335.

Anderson, A. (1996a). The father-infant relationship: Becoming connected. *Journal of Social and Pediatric Nursing, 1*(2), 83-92.

Anderson, A. (1996b). Factors influencing the father-infant relationship. *Journal of Family Nursing, 2*(3), 306-324.

Barnard, K. (1994). *NCAST feeding manual.* Seattle: University of Washington.

Bitzer, J., & Alder, J. (2000). Sexuality during pregnancy and the postpartum period. *Journal of Sex Education and Therapy, 25*(1), 49-58.

Bloom, K. (1998). Perceived relationship with the father of the baby and maternal attachment in adolescents. *Journal of Obstetric, Gynecologic, and Neonatal Nursing, 27*(4), 420-430.

Bozoky, I., & Corwin, E. (2002). Fatigue as a predictor of postpartum depression. *Journal of Obstetric, Gynecologic, and Neonatal Nursing, 31*(4), 436-443.

Brewaeys, A. et al. (1995). Lesbian mothers who conceived after donor insemination: A follow-up study. *Human Reproduction, 10*(10), 2731-2735.

Cain, M. (1994). *First time mothers, last chance babies: Parenting at 35.* Far Hills, NJ: New Horizon Press.

Camarena, P. et al. (1998). The nature and support of adolescent mothers' life aspirations. *Family Relations, 47*(2), 129-137.

Cheng, H., & Chen, C. (2001). Maternal concerns and social support during postpartum period. *Journal of Nursing Research (China), 9*(3), 322-332.

Conley-Jung, C., & Olkin, R. (2001). Mothers with visual impairments who are raising young children. *Journal of the Visually Impaired and Blind, 95*(1), 14-30.

Cowan, C., & Cowan, P. (1995). Interventions to ease the transition to parenthood: Why they are needed and what they can do. *Family Relations, 44*, 412-423.

Cox, M. et al. (1999). Marital perceptions and interactions across the transition to parenthood. *Journal of Marriage and the Family, 61*, 611-625.

Dalla, R., & Gamble, E. (2000). Mother, daughter, teenager–who am I? Perceptions of adolescent maternity in a Navajo reservation community. *Journal of Family Issues, 21*(2), 225-245.

D'Avanzo, C., & Geissler, E. (2003). *Pocket guide to cultural assessment* (3rd ed.). St. Louis: Mosby.

Denehy, J. (1992). Interventions related to parent-infant attachment. *Nursing Clinics of North America, 27*(2), 425-433.

Diehl, K. (1997). Adolescent mothers: What produces positive mother-infant interaction? *MCN: American Journal of Maternal Child Nursing, 22*, 89-95.

Evans, M. et al. (1998). Postpartum sleep in the hospital: Relationship to taking-in and taking-hold. *Clinical Nursing Research, 7*(4), 379-389.

Farber, R. (2000). Mothers with disabilities: In their own voice. *American Journal of Occupational Therapy, 54*(3), 260-268.

Fowles, E. (1998). The relationship between maternal role attainment and postpartum depression. *Health Care for Women International, 19*(1), 83-94.

Galanti, G. (1997). *Caring for patients from different cultures.* Philadelphia: University of Pennsylvania Press.

Garrison, M. et al. (1997). Delayed parenthood: An exploratory study of family functioning. *Family Relations, 46*, 281-290.

Gartrell, N. et al. (1996). The National Lesbian Family Study: Interview with prospective mothers. *American Journal of Orthopsychiatry, 66*(2), 272-281.

Gerson, E. (1973). *Infant behavior in the first year of life.* New York: Raven Press.

Gloppestad, K. (1998). Experiences of maternal love and paternal love when preterm infants were held skin-to-skin and wrapped in blankets. *Nursing Science Research Nordic Countries, 18*(1), 23-30.

Gottlieb, L., & Mendelson, M. (1995). Mothers' moods and social support when a second child is born. *Maternal-Child Nursing Journal, 23*(1), 3-14.

Goulet, C. et al. (1998). A concept analysis of parent-infant attachment. *Journal of Advanced Nursing, 28*(5), 1071-1081.

Groer, M., Davis, M., & Hemphill, J. (2002). Postpartum stress: Current concepts and the possible protective role of breastfeeding. *Journal of Obstetric, Gynecologic, and Neonatal Nursing, 31*(4), 411- 417.

Hartrick, G. (1997). Women who are mothers: The experience of defining self. *Health Care for Women International, 18*, 263-277.

Henderson, A., & Brouse, A. (1991). The experiences of new fathers during the first three weeks of life. *Journal of Advanced Nursing, 16*(3), 293-298.

Horowitz, J., & Damato, E. (1999). Mothers' perception of postpartum stress and satisfaction. *Journal of Obstetric, Gynecologic, and Neonatal Nursing, 28*(6), 595-605.

Hudson, D., Elek, S., & Fleck, M. (2001). First-time mothers' and fathers' transition to parenthood: Infant care self-efficacy, parenting satisfaction, and infant sex. *Issues in Comprehensive Pediatric Nursing, 24*, 31-43.

Inman, M. (1996). The power of touch: Infant massage therapy. *Childbirth Instructor Magazine, 8*(2), 28-32.

Jambunathan, J., & Stewart, S. (1995). Hmong women in Wisconsin: What are their concerns in pregnancy and childbirth? *Birth, 22*(4), 204-210.

Jiménez, S. (1995). The Hispanic culture, folklore, and perinatal health. *Journal of Perinatal Education, 4*(1), 9-16.

Johnson and Johnson. (1996). *Compendium of postpartum care.* Skillman, NJ: Johnson and Johnson Consumer Products.

Klaus, M. et al. (1972). Maternal attachment: Importance of first postpartum days. *New England Journal of Medicine, 286*, 460-463.

Klaus, M., & Kennell, J. (1976). *Maternal-infant bonding.* St. Louis: Mosby.

Klaus, M., & Kennell, J. (1982). *Parent-infant bonding* (2nd ed.). St. Louis: Mosby.

Klaus, M., & Kennell, J. (1983). *Bonding: The beginnings of parent-infant attachment.* St. Louis: Mosby.

Klaus, M., & Kennell, J. (1997). The doula: An essential ingredient of childbirth rediscovered. *Acta Pediatrica, 86*, 1034-1036.

Lee, K., & Zaffke, M. (1999). Longitudinal changes in fatigue and energy during pregnancy and the postpartum period. *Journal of Obstetric, Gynecologic, and Neonatal Nursing, 28*(2), 183-191.

Leonard, V. (1993). *Stress and coping in the transition to parenthood of first-time mothers with career commitments: An interpretive study.* Doctoral dissertation. University of California, San Francisco.

Levy-Shiff, R. et al. (1998). Cognitive appraisals, coping strategies, and support resources as correlates of parenting and infant development. *Developmental Psychology, 34*(6), 1417-1427.

Lipson, J., Dibble, S., & Minarik, P. (1996). *Culture and nursing care: A pocket guide.* San Francisco: UCSF Nursing Press.

Liu-Chiang, C. (1995). Postpartum worries: An exploration of Taiwanese primiparas who participate in the Chinese ritual of Tso-Yuen-Tzu. *Maternal Child Nursing Journal, 23*(4), 110-122.

MacDonald-Clark, N., & Boffman, J. (1995). Mother-child interaction among the Alaskan Eskimos. *Journal of Obstetric, Gynecologic, and Neonatal Nursing, 24*(5), 450-457.

Martell, L. (1996). Is Rubin's "taking-in" and "taking-hold" a useful paradigm? *Health Care for Women International, 17*(1), 1-13.

Meleis, A. (1991). *Theoretical nursing: Development and progress* (2nd ed.). Philadelphia: J.B. Lippincott.

Mercer, R. (1983). Parent-infant attachment. In L. Sonstegard, K. Kowalski, & B. Jennings (Eds.), *Women's health, Vol. 2, Childbearing.* New York: Grune & Stratton.

Merriwether-deVries, C. (2000). Adjustment to the role of motherhood among adolescent African American mothers. *Dissertation Abstracts International, A.: The Humanities and Social Sciences, 61*(3), 1183-A.

Miller, S. (1996). Questioning, resisting, acquiescing, balancing: New mothers' career reentry strategies. *Health Care for Women International, 17*, 109-131.

Niska, K., Snyder, M., & Lia-Hoagberg, B. (1998). Family ritual facilitates adaptation to parenthood. *Public Health Nursing, 15*(5), 329-337.

Osterwell, D. (1991). *Correlates of relationship satisfaction in lesbian couples who are parenting their first child together.* Doctoral dissertation, Berkeley, California School of Professional Psychology.

Poelker, D., & Baldwin, C. (1999). Postponed motherhood and the out-of-sync life cycle. *Journal of Mental Health Counseling, 21*(2), 136-148.

Pridham, K. (1997). Mothers' help seeking as care initiated in a social context. *Image: The Journal of Nursing Scholarship, 29*(1), 65-70.

Prodromidis, M. et al. (1995). Mothers touching newborns: A comparison of rooming-in versus minimal contact. *Birth, 22*(4), 196.

Pugh, L. et al. (1999). Clinical approaches to the assessment of maternal fatigue. *Journal of Obstetric, Gynecologic, and Neonatal Nursing, 28*, 74-80.

Reece, S., & Harkless, G. (1996). Divergent themes in maternal experience in women older than 35 years of age. *Applied Nursing Research, 9*(3), 148-153.

Reece, S., & Harkless, G. (1998). Self-efficacy, stress and parental adaptation: Applications to the care of childbearing families. *Journal of Family Nursing, 4*(2), 198-215.

Reimann, R. (1997a). Does biology matter? Lesbian couples' transition to parenthood and their division of labor. *Qualitative Sociology, 20*(2), 153-185.

Reimann, R. (1997b). *Will the "real" mother please stand up? Lesbian couples' transition to shared motherhood.* 1997 ASA Conference proceedings: Washington, D.C.: American Sociological Association.

Reimann, R. (1999). *Becoming lesbian mothers: Lesbian couples' transition to parenthood.* 1999 ASA Conference proceedings. Washington, D.C.: American Sociological Association.

Rogan, F. et al. (1997). "Becoming a mother": Developing a new theory of early motherhood. *Journal of Advanced Nursing, 25*, 877-885.

Rubin, R. (1961). Basic maternal behavior. *Nursing Outlook, 9*, 683-686.

Rubin, R. (1963). Maternal touch at first contact with the newborn infant. *Nursing Outlook, 11*, 828-831.

Ruchala, P., & Halstead, L. (1994). The postpartum experience of low-risk women: A time of adjustment and change. *Maternal-Child Nursing Journal, 22*(3), 83-89.

Sank, J. (1991). *Factors in the prenatal period that affect parental role attainment during the postpartum period in Black American mothers and fathers.* Doctoral dissertation, Austin: University of Texas.

Schumacher, K., & Meleis, A. (1994). Transitions: A central concept in nursing. *Image: Journal of Nursing Scholarship, 26*(2), 119-127.

Sharts-Hopko, N. (1995). Birth in the Japanese context. *Journal of Obstetric, Gynecologic, and Neonatal Nursing, 24*(14), 343-351.

Small, R. et al. (1994). Missing voices: What women say and do about depression after childbirth. *Journal of Reproductive Infant Psychology, 12*(2), 89-103.

Smith-Hanrahan, C., & Deblois, D. (1995). Postpartum early discharge. *Clinical Nursing Research, 4*(1), 50-66.

Steinberg, S., Kruckman, L., & Steinberg, S. (2000). Reinventing fatherhood in Japan and Canada. *Social Science Medicine, 50*, 1257-1272.

Sutter, A.L. et al. (1997). Postpartum blues and mild depressive symptomatology at days three and five after delivery: A French cross-sectional study. *Journal of Affective Disorders, 44*(1), 1-4.

Tomlinson, P. (1996). Marital relationship change in the transition to parenthood: A reexamination as interpreted through transition theory. *Journal of Family Nursing, 2*(3), 286-305.

Troy, N. (1993). Early contact and maternal attachment among women using public health care facilities. *Applied Nursing Research, 6*(4), 161-166.

Troy, N. (1995). The time of first holding of the infant and maternal self-esteem related to feelings of maternal attachment. *Women's Health, 22*(3), 59-72.

Troy, N., & Dalgas-Pelish, P. (1995). Development of a self-care guide for postpartum fatigue. *Applied Nursing Research, 8*(2), 92-101.

Troy, N., & Dalgas-Pelish, P. (1997). The natural evolution of postpartum fatigue among a group of primiparous women. *Clinical Nursing Research, 6*(2), 126-141.

Tulman, L. (1985). Mothers and unrelated persons' initial handling of newborn infants. *Nursing Research, 34*(4), 205-210.

Vehvilainen-Julkunen, K. (1995). Family training: Supporting mothers and fathers in the transition to parenthood. *Journal of Advanced Nursing, 22*, 731-737.

Walker, L., & Avant, K. (1995). *Strategies for theory construction in nursing* (3rd ed.). Norwalk, CT: Appleton & Lange.

Waters, M., & Lee, K. (1996). Differences between primigravidae and multigravidae mothers in sleep disturbances, fatigue, and functional status. *Journal of Nurse Midwifery, 41*(5), 364-367.

Welles-Nystrom, B. (1997). The meaning of postponed motherhood for women in the United States and Sweden: Aspects of feminism and radical timing strategies. *Health Care for Women International, 18*, 279-299.

Wood, A. et al. (1997). The downward spiral of postpartum depression. *MCN American Journal of Maternal Child Nursing, 22*(6), 308-317.

Wrasper, C. (1996). Discharge timing and Rubin's concept of puerperal change. *Journal of Perinatal Education, 5*(2), 13-23.

CHAPTER 25

Kathryn Rhodes Alden

Physiologic and Behavioral Adaptations of the Newborn

http://evolve.elsevier.com/Lowdermilk/MatWmnHlth/

LEARNING OBJECTIVES

- Describe the changes in the biologic system of the neonate during the transition to extrauterine life.
- Compare and contrast the four types of heat loss in a neonate and describe how to prevent heat loss.
- Elicit newborn reflexes and differentiate characteristic responses from abnormal responses.
- Describe the behavioral adaptations of the newborn, including sleep-wake states and periods of reactivity.
- Describe the sensory and perceptual functioning of the neonate.

The neonatal period includes the time from birth through day 28 of life. During this time the neonate must make many adjustments to extrauterine life. Many of these developmental tasks occur shortly after birth. Biologic tasks are those that involve (1) establishing and maintaining respirations; (2) adjusting to circulatory changes; (3) regulating temperature; (4) ingesting, retaining, and digesting nutrients; (5) eliminating waste; and (6) regulating weight. Behavioral tasks include (1) establishing a regulated behavioral tempo independent of the mother, which involves self-regulation of arousal, self-monitoring of changes in state, and patterning of sleep; (2) processing, storing, and organizing multiple stimuli; and (3) establishing a relationship with caregivers and the environment. The infant at term (between 38 and 42 weeks of gestation) normally makes these adjustments with little or no difficulty.

TRANSITION TO EXTRAUTERINE LIFE

Infants undergo phases of instability during the first 6 to 8 hours after birth. These phases are collectively called the **transition period** between intrauterine and extrauterine existence. To detect disorders in adaptation soon after birth, nurses must be aware of normal features of the transition period. Labor and immediate neonatal events stimulate a sympathetic response reflected by changes in heart rate, color, respiration, motor activity, gastrointestinal function, and temperature of the infant. Behavioral characteristics also change during this transition period.

The first phase of the transition period lasts up to 30 minutes after birth and is called the *first period of reactivity*. The newborn's heart rate increases rapidly to 160 to 180 beats/min but gradually decreases after 30 minutes or so to a baseline rate of between 100 and 120 beats/min. Respirations are irregular, with a rate between 60 and 80 breaths/min. Crackles may be present on auscultation; audible grunting, nasal flaring, and retractions of the chest also may be noted. In addition, brief periods of apnea (periodic breathing) may occur. Coincident with these changes in heart rate and respiratory rate, the infant is alert. The infant's behavior is marked by spontaneous startle reactions, tremors, crying, and movement of the head from side to side. This characteristic exploratory behavior is accompanied by a decrease in body temperature and generalized increase in motor activity, with an increase in muscle tone. Gastrointestinal manifestations of this first period of reactivity include the onset of bowel sounds, passage of meconium, and production of saliva.

After the first period of reactivity, the newborn either sleeps or has a marked decrease in motor activity. This period of decreased responsiveness, frequently accompanied by sleep, lasts for 60 to 100 minutes and is followed by a second period of reactivity.

The *second period of reactivity* occurs roughly between the fourth and eighth hours after birth. This period of reactivity lasts from 10 minutes to several hours. Periods of tachycardia and tachypnea occur, associated with increased muscle tone, skin color, and mucus production. Meconium is commonly passed at this time.

All newborns experience this transition, regardless of gestational age or type of birth. The length of time the periods last will vary depending on the amount and kind of stress experienced by the neonate before or after birth.

PHYSIOLOGIC ADAPTATIONS

Respiratory System

With the cutting of the umbilical cord, the infant must undergo rapid and complex changes. The most critical adjustment of a newborn at birth is the establishment of respirations. At term the lungs hold approximately 20 milliliters of fluid/kg. Air must be substituted for the fluid that filled the respiratory tract. During normal vaginal birth, some lung fluid is squeezed or drained from the newborn's trachea and lungs. With the first breath of air, the newborn begins a sequence of cardiopulmonary changes.

Initiation of Breathing

Initial breathing is probably the result of a reflex triggered by pressure changes, chilling, noise, light, and other sensations related to the birth process. In addition, the chemoreceptors in the aorta and carotid bodies initiate neurologic reflexes when arterial oxygen pressure (PO_2) decreases from 80 to 15 mm Hg, arterial carbon dioxide pressure (PCO_2) increases from 40 to 70 mm Hg, and arterial pH declines. In most cases, an exaggerated respiratory reaction follows within 1 minute of birth, and the infant takes a first gasping breath and cries.

Certain respiratory patterns are characteristic of the normal term newborn. After respirations are established, breaths are shallow and irregular, ranging from 30 to 60 breaths/min, with short periods of apnea (less than 15 seconds). These short periods of apnea occur most often during the active (rapid eye movement [REM]) sleep cycle and decrease in frequency and duration with age. Apneic periods longer than 15 seconds should be evaluated.

NURSE ALERT

Newborn infants are preferential nose breathers. The reflex response to nasal obstruction is to open the mouth to maintain an airway. This response is not present in most infants until 3 weeks after birth; therefore cyanosis or asphyxia may occur with nasal blockage.

Signs of Respiratory Distress

Most term infants breathe spontaneously and continue to have normal respirations; however, infants can manifest other problems through respiratory distress. Signs of respiratory distress may include nasal flaring, retractions (indrawing of tissue between the ribs, below the rib cage, or above the sternum and clavicles), or grunting with expirations. Any increased use of the intercostal muscles may be a sign of distress. Seesaw respirations, instead of normal abdominal respirations, are not normal and should be reported (Fig. 25-1, *B*). A respiratory rate that is less than 30 or greater than 60 breaths/min with the infant at rest must be reported to the pediatrician. The respiratory rate of the infant may be slowed or depressed by the analgesics or anesthetics administered to the mother during labor and birth. Apneic episodes also can be related to rapid warming or cooling of the infant; tachypnea may result from aspiration or a diaphragmatic hernia.

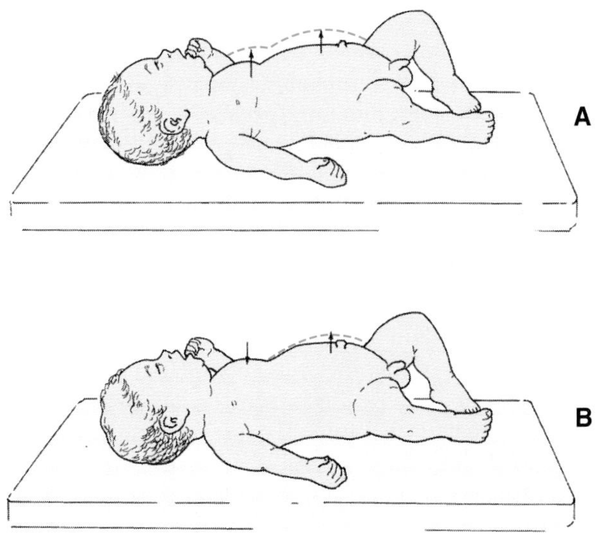
A
B

FIG. 25-1 Comparison of normal and seesaw respirations. **A,** Normal respiration. Chest and abdomen rise with inspiration. **B,** Seesaw respiration. Chest wall retracts and abdomen rises with inspiration. (Courtesy Mead Johnson & Co., Evansville, IN.)

Maintaining Adequate Oxygen Supply

During the first hour of life, the pulmonary lymphatics continue to remove large amounts of fluid. Removal of fluid also is a result of the pressure gradient from alveoli to interstitial tissue to blood capillary. Reduced vascular resistance accommodates this flow of lung fluid.

Abnormal respiration and failure to expand the lungs completely retard the movement of fetal lung fluid from alveoli and interstices into the pulmonary circulation. Retention of fluid interferes with the infant's ability to maintain adequate oxygenation.

Auscultation of the chest reveals loud, clear breath sounds that seem very near, because little chest tissue intervenes. The ribs of the infant articulate with the spine at a horizontal rather than a downward slope; consequently, the rib cage cannot expand with inspiration as readily as that of an adult. Neonatal respiratory function is largely a matter of diaphragmatic contraction. The negative intrathoracic pressure is created by the descent of the diaphragm, much as negative pressure is created in the barrel of a syringe when medication is drawn up by retracting the plunger. The newborn infant's chest and abdomen rise simultaneously with inspiration (Fig. 25-1, *A*). Characteristics of the respiratory system of the neonate and the effects of these characteristics on respiratory function are listed in Table 25-1.

The alveoli of the term infant's lungs are lined with **surfactant,** a phospholipid. Lung expansion augments surfactant secretion. Surfactant reduces surface tension, therefore requiring less pressure to keep the alveolus open, and maintains alveolar stability by changing surface tension as the size of the alveolus changes. The surfactant system develops as the infant develops in utero.

Fetal pulmonary maturity can be determined by examining amniotic fluid for lecithin/sphingomyelin ratio (L/S) and other phospholipid levels. Phosphatidylglycerol appears at 35 to 36 weeks; its presence is a more predictable indicator of lung maturity. The L/S ratio increases with gestational age. Mature fetal lungs have an L/S ratio greater than 2:1. Infants born before the L/S ratio is 2:1 will have varying degrees of respiratory distress.

Cardiovascular System

The cardiovascular system changes markedly after birth. The infant's first breath inflates the lungs and reduces pulmonary vascular resistance to the pulmonary blood flow. The pulmonary artery pressure decreases. This sequence is the major mechanism by which pressure in the right atrium declines. The increased pulmonary blood flow returned to the left side of the heart increases the pressure in the left atrium. This change in pressures causes a functional closure of the foramen ovale. During the first few days of life, crying may reverse the flow through the foramen ovale temporarily and lead to mild cyanosis.

The ductus arteriosus begins to constrict as pulmonary circulation increases and arterial oxygen tension increases. In term infants, the ductus arteriosus functionally closes within 24 hours; permanent closure may take several weeks. With the clamping and severing of the cord, the umbilical arteries, umbilical vein, and ductus venosus are functionally closed and are converted into ligaments within 2 to 3 months (Kliegman, 2002). Table 25-2 summarizes the cardiovascular changes at birth.

TABLE 25-1 Characteristics of the Respiratory System of the Neonate

CHARACTERISTIC	EFFECT ON FUNCTION
Lung elastic tissue and recoil is decreased	Lung compliance is decreased; more work and higher pressure are required to expand; risk of atelectasis
Limited movement of diaphragm	Respiratory movement less effective; risk of atelectasis
Preferential nose breather; larynx and epiglottis high	Can breathe and swallow at the same time; risk of airway obstruction; difficulty intubating
Airway passages small and compliant; high airway resistance; weak cough reflex	Risk of obstruction of airway and apnea
Surfactant system altered in immature infants	Atelectatic areas; work of breathing increased; risk of respiratory distress syndrome (RDS)
Respiratory control immature	Respirations irregular; unable to increase rate and depth of respirations rapidly

From Blackburn, S. (1992). Alterations of the respiratory system in the neonate: Implications for clinical practice. *Journal of Perinatal and Neonatal Nursing,* 6(2), 46-58.

Heart Rate and Sounds

The term newborn has a resting heart rate between 100 and 160 beats/min, with brief fluctuations above and below these values, usually noted during sleeping and waking states. Shortly after the first cry, the infant's heart rate may accelerate as high as 180 beats/min. The range of the heart rate in the term infant is about 85 to 100 beats/min during deep sleep and 120 to 160 beats/min while awake. A heart rate of 180 beats/min is not unusual when the infant cries. A heart rate that is either high (more than 160 beats/min) or low (fewer than 100 beats/min) should be reevaluated within 30 minutes to 1 hour or when the activity of the infant changes. Immediately after birth, the heart rate can be palpated by grasping the base of the umbilical cord.

By term the infant's heart lies midway between the crown of the head and the buttocks, and the axis is more transverse than that in an adult (Fig. 25-2). The apical impulse (point of maximal impulse [PMI]) in the newborn is at the fourth intercostal space and to the left of the midclavicular line. The PMI is often visible.

Apical pulse rates should be obtained on all infants. Auscultation should be for a full minute, preferably when the infant is asleep. Sinus arrhythmia (irregular heart rate) may be considered a physiologic phenomenon in infancy and an indication of good heart function.

Heart sounds during the neonatal period are of higher pitch, shorter duration, and greater intensity than those during adult life. The first sound is typically louder and duller than the second sound, which is sharp. Most heart murmurs heard during the first few days of life have no pathologic significance; they usually result from a patent ductus arteriosus, tricuspid regurgitation, or the acute angle of the pulmonary artery bifurcation (Lissauer, 2002).

Blood Pressure

The newborn infant's average systolic blood pressure is 60 to 80 mm Hg, and the average diastolic pressure is 40 to 50 mm Hg. A decrease in systolic blood pressure

(BP) of approximately 15 mm Hg during the first hour of life is common. Crying and movement result in changes in BP, especially in the systolic pressure. BP also is sensitive to the changes in blood volume that occur with the adaptations in circulation. The measurement of BP is best accomplished with a Doppler device and while the infant is at rest. The correct-size BP cuff must be used for accurate measurement of an infant's BP. When arm BP measurement is followed by leg BP measurement, different-sized cuffs may be needed because arms and legs are rarely the same size.

Blood Volume

The blood volume of the newborn depends on the amount of blood transferred placentally. The blood volume of the term infant is about 86 ml/kg of body weight. Immediately after birth, the total blood volume averages 300 ml, but this volume can increase by as much as 100 ml, depending on the length of time the infant is attached to the placenta. The preterm infant has a proportionately greater blood volume than that of the term newborn. This occurs because the preterm infant has a greater plasma volume, not a greater red blood

TABLE 25-2 **Cardiovascular Changes at Birth**

PRENATAL STATUS	POSTBIRTH STATUS	ASSOCIATED FACTORS
Primary Changes		
Pulmonary circulation: high pulmonary vascular resistance, increased pressure in right ventricle and pulmonary arteries	Low pulmonary vascular resistance; decreased pressure in right atrium, ventricle, and pulmonary arteries	Expansion of collapsed fetal lung with air
Systemic circulation: low pressures in left atrium, ventricle, and aorta	High systemic vascular resistance; increased pressure in left atrium, ventricle, and aorta	Loss of placental blood flow
Secondary Changes		
Umbilical arteries: patent, carrying of blood from hypogastric arteries to placenta	Functionally closed at birth; obliteration by fibrous proliferation possibly taking 2-3 mo, distal portions becoming lateral vesicoumbilical ligaments, proximal portions remaining open as superior vesicle arteries	Closure preceding that of umbilical vein, probably accomplished by smooth muscle contraction in response to thermal and mechanical stimuli and alteration in oxygen tension, mechanically severed with cord at birth
Umbilical vein: patent, carrying of blood from placenta to ductus venosus and liver	Closed, becoming ligamentum teres hepatis after obliteration	Closure shortly after umbilical arteries, hence blood from placenta possibly entering neonate for short period after birth, mechanically severed with cord at birth
Ductus venosus: patent, connection of umbilical vein to inferior vena cava	Closed, becoming ligamentum venosum after obliteration	Loss of blood flow from umbilical vein
Ductus arteriosus: patent, shunting of blood from pulmonary artery to descending aorta	Functionally closed almost immediately after birth, anatomic obliteration of lumen by fibrous proliferation requiring 1-3 mo, becoming ligamentum arteriosum	High systemic resistance increasing aortic pressure; low pulmonary resistance reducing pulmonary arterial pressure Increased oxygen content of blood in ductus arteriosus creating vasospasm of its muscular wall
Foramen ovale: formation of a valve opening that allows blood to flow directly to left atrium (shunting of blood from right to left atrium)	Functionally closed at birth, constant apposition gradually leading to fusion and permanent closure within a few months or years in majority of persons	Increased pressure in left atrium and decreased pressure in right atrium causing closure of valve over foramen

Modified from Wong, D. (1995). *Whaley and Wong's nursing care of infants and children* (5th ed.). St. Louis: Mosby.

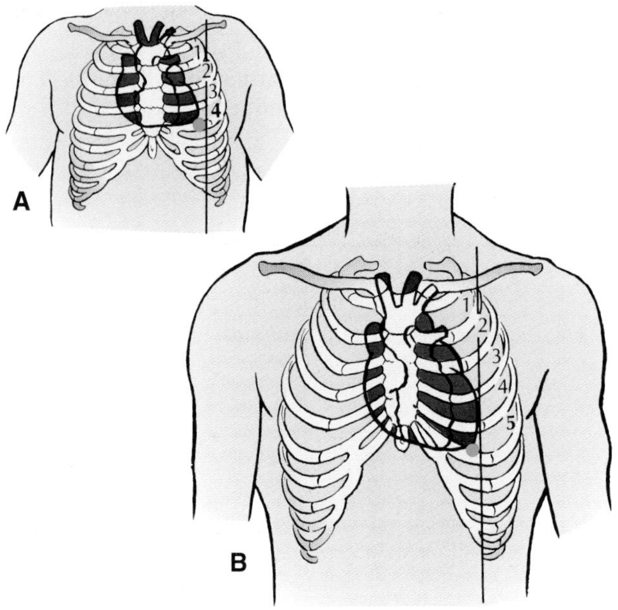
1
2
3
4
A
1
2
3
4
5
B

FIG. 25-2 Differences in locations of apical pulse in newborn from that of adult. **A,** Neonate. **B,** Adult.

cell (RBC) mass (Luchtman-Jones, Schwartz, & Wilson, 2002; Hockenberry et al., 2003).

Early or late clamping of the umbilical cord changes circulatory dynamics of the newborn. Early clamping of the cord reduces the mean blood volume, whereas late clamping expands the blood volume from the so-called placental transfusion. This, in turn, causes an increase in heart size, higher systolic blood pressure, and increased respiratory rate.

Hematopoietic System

The hematopoietic system of the newborn exhibits certain variations from that of the adult. Levels of RBCs and leukocytes differ, but platelet levels are relatively the same.

Red Blood Cells and Hemoglobin

Because fetal circulation is less efficient at oxygen exchange than the lungs, the fetus needs additional RBCs for transport of oxygen in utero. Therefore at birth, the average levels of RBCs and hemoglobin are higher than those in the adult. Cord blood of the term newborn may have a hemoglobin concentration of 14 to 24 g/dl (mean, 17 g/dl). The hematocrit ranges from 44% to 64% (mean, 55%). The RBC count is correspondingly elevated, ranging from 4.8 to 7.1 mm^3 (mean, 5.14). By 2 weeks of age, slight decreases in hemoglobin (mean, 16.5 g/dl), hematocrit (mean, 50%), and RBC count (mean, 4.2 mm^3) are found. At 3 months, hemoglobin ranges from 9.5 g/dl to 14.5 g/dl (mean, 12), and hematocrit ranges from 31% to 41% (mean, 36%) (Luchtman-Jones et al., 2002; Scott, 2002).

The initial blood values may be affected by delayed clamping of the cord, which results in an increase in hemoglobin level, RBC count, and hematocrit value. The source of the sample is another important factor because capillary blood yields higher values than venous blood. The time after birth when the blood sample was obtained also is significant; the slight increase in RBC numbers after birth is followed by a substantial decrease. At birth, 80% of the infant's blood contains fetal hemoglobin, but because of the shorter life span of the cells containing fetal hemoglobin, the percentage decreases to 55% by 5 weeks and to 5% by 20 weeks. Iron stores are generally sufficient to sustain normal RBC production for 5 months, and thus mild, brief anemia is not serious.

Leukocytes

Leukocytosis, with a white blood cell (WBC) count of approximately 18,000/mm^3 (range, 9000 to 30,000/mm^3), is normal at birth. The number of WBCs, predominantly polymorphonuclear leukocytes, increases to 23,000 to 24,000/mm^3 during the first day after birth. This early high WBC count of the newborn decreases rapidly, and a resting level of 12,000/mm^3 is normally maintained during the neonatal period (Scott, 2002). Serious infection is not well tolerated by the newborn, and a marked increase in the WBC count is unlikely, even in critical sepsis (infection). In most instances, sepsis is accompanied by a decline in WBCs, particularly in neutrophils. The activity of the bone marrow is accurately reflected by the number of circulating cells, both RBCs and WBCs.

Platelets

The platelet count ranges between 150,000 and 300,000/mm^3 and is essentially the same in newborns as in adults. The levels of factors II, VII, IX, and X, found in the liver, are decreased during the first few days of life because the newborn cannot synthesize vitamin K. However, bleeding tendencies in the newborn are rare, and unless the vitamin K deficiency is great, clotting is sufficient to prevent hemorrhage (Kliegman, 2002).

Blood Groups

The infant's blood group is genetically determined and established early in fetal life. However, during the neonatal period, a gradual increase occurs in the strength of the agglutinogens present in the RBC membrane. Cord blood samples may be used to identify the infant's blood type and Rh status.

Signs of Risk for Cardiovascular Problems

Close monitoring of the infant's vital signs is important for early detection of impending problems. Persistent tachycardia (more than 160 beats/min) may indicate respiratory distress syndrome (RDS), whereas persistent bradycardia (less than 120 beats/min) may be a sign of a congenital heart block. Any prolonged cyanosis other than in the hands or feet may indicate respiratory and/or cardiac problems. A difference between upper and lower extremity BP may be an early sign of coarctation of the aorta. The presence of jaundice may indicate ABO or Rh factor problems (see Chapter 39).

Thermogenic System

Next to establishing respirations, heat regulation is most critical to the newborn's survival. **Thermoregulation** is the maintenance of balance between heat loss and heat production. Newborns attempt to stabilize their internal body temperatures within a narrow range. Hypothermia from excessive heat loss is a common and dangerous problem in neonates. The newborn infant's ability to produce heat **(thermogenesis)** often approaches that of the adult; however, the tendency toward rapid heat loss in a cold environment is increased in the newborn and poses a hazard.

Thermogenesis

The shivering mechanism of heat production is rarely operable in the newborn. Nonshivering thermogenesis is accomplished primarily by metabolism of **brown fat,** which is unique to the newborn, and by increased metabolic activity in the brain, heart, and liver. Brown fat is located in superficial deposits in the interscapular region and axillae, as well as in deep deposits at the thoracic inlet, along the vertebral column, and around the kidneys. Brown fat has a richer vascular and nerve supply than does ordinary fat. Heat produced by intense lipid metabolic activity in brown fat can warm the newborn by increasing heat production as much as 100%. Reserves of brown fat, usually present for several weeks after birth, are rapidly depleted with cold stress. The less mature the infant, the less reserve of this essential fat is available at birth.

Heat Loss

Heat loss in the newborn occurs by four modes:

- *Convection* is the flow of heat from the body surface to cooler ambient air. Because of heat loss by convection, the ambient temperatures in the nursery are kept at approximately 24° C, and newborns are wrapped to protect them from the cold.
- *Radiation* is the loss of heat from the body surface to a cooler solid surface not in direct contact but in relative proximity. Nursery cribs and examining tables are placed away from outside windows to prevent this type of heat loss.
- *Evaporation* is the loss of heat that occurs when a liquid is converted to a vapor. In the newborn, heat loss by evaporation occurs as a result of vaporization of moisture from the skin. The process is invisible and is known as insensible water loss (IWL). This heat loss can be intensified by failure to dry the newborn directly after birth or by too-slow drying of the infant after a bath.
- *Conduction* is the loss of heat from the body surface to cooler surfaces in direct contact. When admitted to the nursery, the newborn is placed in a warmed crib to minimize heat loss.

Loss of heat must be controlled to protect the infant. Control of such modes of heat loss is the basis of caregiving policies and techniques.

Temperature Regulation

Anatomic and physiologic differences among the newborn, child, and adult are notable. The newborn's thermal insulation is less than that of an adult. The blood vessels are closer to the surface of the skin. Changes in environmental temperature alter the temperature of the blood, thereby influencing temperature regulation centers in the hypothalamus. Newborns have larger body surface–to–body weight (mass) ratios than do children and adults. The flexed position of the newborn helps guard against heat loss because it diminishes the amount of body surface exposed to the environment. Infants also can reduce the loss of internal heat through the body surface by constricting peripheral blood vessels.

Changes in environmental temperature can disturb body temperature. This may lead to serious consequences in the newborn. Brown fat metabolism is activated in response to changes in environmental temperature perceived by the thermal sensors in the newborn's skin, even when the temperature of the newborn is unchanged. When exposed to cold, the newborn may cry, become restless, and increase muscular activity to generate heat. However, crying increases workload and energy expenditure. Newborns also may increase their respiratory rates in an attempt to stimulate muscular activity.

Cold stress imposes metabolic and physiologic demands in all infants, regardless of gestational age and condition. The respiratory rate increases in response to the increased need for oxygen. In the cold-stressed infant, oxygen consumption and energy are diverted from maintaining normal brain and cardiac function and growth to thermogenesis for survival. If the infant cannot maintain an adequate oxygen tension, vasoconstriction jeopardizes pulmonary perfusion. As a consequence, the partial pressure of arterial oxygen (PaO_2) is decreased, and the blood pH declines. These changes aggravate existing RDS. Moreover, decreased pulmonary perfusion and oxygen tension may maintain or reopen the right-to-left shunt across the patent ductus arteriosus.

The basal metabolic rate increases with cold stress (Fig. 25-3). If cold stress is protracted, anaerobic glycolysis occurs, resulting in increased production of acids. Metabolic acidosis develops, and if a defect in respiratory function is present, respiratory acidosis also develops. Excessive fatty acids displace the bilirubin from the albumin-binding sites. The resulting increased level of circulating unbound bilirubin heightens the risk of kernicterus even at serum bilirubin levels of 10 mg/dl or less.

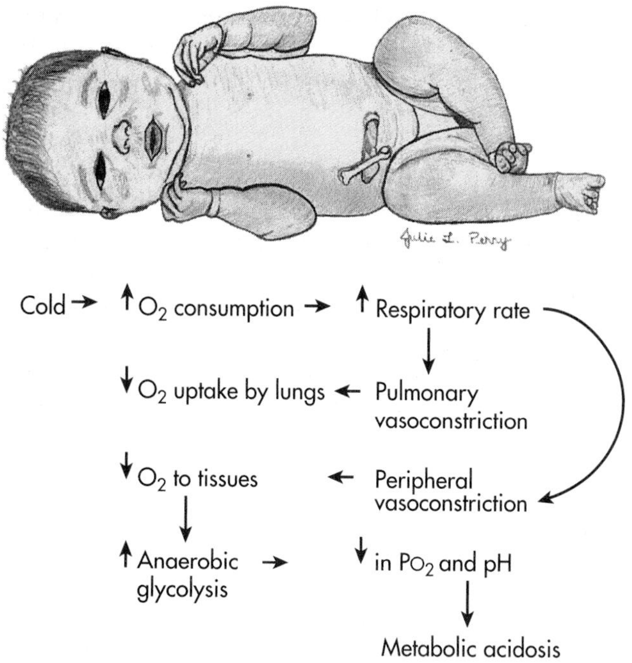

Cold → ↑ O_2 consumption → ↑ Respiratory rate
↓ O_2 uptake by lungs ← Pulmonary vasoconstriction
↓ O_2 to tissues ← Peripheral vasoconstriction
↑ Anaerobic glycolysis → ↓ in PO_2 and pH
Metabolic acidosis

FIG. 25-3 Effects of cold stress. When an infant is stressed by cold, oxygen consumption increases and pulmonary and peripheral vasoconstriction occur, thereby decreasing oxygen uptake by the lungs and oxygen to the tissues; anaerobic glycolysis increases; and there is a decrease in PO_2 and pH, leading to metabolic acidosis.

Hyperthermia develops more rapidly in the newborn than in the adult because of the larger surface area of an infant. Although newborns have 6 times as many sweat glands per unit area as adults, these glands do not function. Serious overheating of the newborn can cause cerebral damage from dehydration or heat stroke and death.

Renal System

At term gestation, the kidneys occupy a large portion of the posterior abdominal wall. The bladder lies close to the anterior abdominal wall and is an abdominal as well as a pelvic organ. In the newborn, almost all palpable masses in the abdomen are renal in origin.

A small quantity (approximately 40 ml) of urine is usually present at birth in the bladder of a term infant. Newborns should void within the first 24 hours of life.

NURSE ALERT

Noting and recording first voidings is important. An infant who has not voided by 24 hours should be assessed for adequacy of fluid intake, bladder distention, restlessness, and symptoms of pain. The pediatrician also should be notified.

The frequency of voiding varies according to the amount of fluid intake. It is expected that infants will void at least once during the first 24 hours, twice during the second 24 hours, and three times during the third 24 hours. Formula-fed infants may void more frequently; however, in breastfed infants, the urine output increases after the third or fourth day when the mother's milk has "come in." After the fourth day of life, all newborns should have at least six to eight voidings of straw-colored urine every 24 hours.

Term infants are unable to concentrate urine; therefore the specific gravity of the urine may range from 1.001 to 1.020 (Pagana & Pagana, 2002). The ability to concentrate urine fully is attained by about age 3 months. After the first voiding, the infant's urine may appear cloudy (because of mucus content) and have a much higher specific gravity, which decreases as fluid intake increases. Normal urine during early infancy is usually straw colored and almost odorless. Sometimes pink-tinged stains (brick dust) appear on the diaper. These stains are caused by uric acid crystals and are normal during the first few days, but if seen later can be a sign of dehydration. Blood may be found on a diaper of a female infant. This *pseudomenstruation* is caused by the withdrawal of maternal hormones. Male infants may have some bloody spotting from a circumcision. If there is no apparent cause of bleeding, the physician should be notified.

Loss of fluid through urine, feces, lungs, increased metabolic rate, and limited fluid intake results in a 5% to 10% loss of the birth weight (weight loss greater than 7% should be evaluated by the health care provider). This usually occurs during the first 3 to 5 days of life. If the mother is breastfeeding and her milk supply has not come in yet (which happens on the third or fourth day after birth), the neonate is usually protected from dehydration by its increased extracellular fluid volume. The neonate should regain the birth weight within 14 days after birth.

Because renal thresholds are low in the infant, bicarbonate concentration and buffering capacity are decreased, which may lead to acidosis and electrolyte imbalance.

Fluid and Electrolyte Balance

Approximately 40% of the body weight of the newborn is extracellular fluid. Each day the newborn takes in and excretes roughly 600 to 700 ml of water, which is 20% of the total body fluid or 50% of the extracellular fluid. The glomerular filtration rate of a newborn is approximately 30% to 50% that of the adult. This results in a decreased ability to remove nitrogenous and other waste products from the blood.

Sodium reabsorption is decreased as a result of a reduced sodium- or potassium-activated adenosine triphosphatase (ATPase) activity. The decreased ability to excrete excessive sodium results in hypotonic urine compared with plasma, with a higher concentration of sodium, phosphates, chloride, and organic acids and a lower concentration of bicarbonate ions. The infant has a higher renal threshold for glucose.

Signs of Risk for Renal System Problems

The renal system has a wide range of functions, and dysfunction can result from physiologic abnormalities ranging from the lack of a steady stream of urine to gross anomalies. Gross anomalies such as hypospadias and exstrophy of the bladder can be identified easily at birth. Enlarged or cystic kidneys may be identified as masses during abdominal palpation. Some kidney anomalies also can be detected by ultrasound examination during pregnancy.

Gastrointestinal System

The term newborn is capable of swallowing, digesting, metabolizing, and absorbing proteins and simple carbohydrates, and emulsifying fats. With the exception of pancreatic amylase, the characteristic enzymes and digestive juices are present even in low-birth-weight neonates.

In the adequately hydrated infant, the mucous membrane of the mouth is moist and pink. The hard and soft palates are intact. Retention cysts, small whitish areas (Epstein's pearls), may be found on the gum margins and at the juncture of the hard and soft palate. The cheeks are full because of well-developed sucking pads. These, like the labial tubercles (sucking calluses) on the upper lip, disappear when the sucking period is over, around the age of 12 months.

Even though sucking motions in utero have been recorded by ultrasonography, these motions are not coordinated in any infant who is less than 1500 g at birth or born before 32 weeks of gestation. Sucking behavior is influenced by neuromuscular maturity, maternal medications and anesthetics received during labor and birth, and the type of initial feeding.

A special mechanism present in normal newborns coordinates the breathing, sucking, and swallowing reflexes necessary for oral feeding. Sucking in the newborn takes place in small bursts of three to eight sucks at a time. In the term newborn, longer and more efficient sucking attempts occur a few hours after birth. The infant is unable to move food from the lips to the pharynx; therefore placing the nipple (breast or bottle) well inside the baby's mouth is necessary. Peristaltic activity in the esophagus is uncoordinated in the first few days of life. It quickly becomes a coordinated pattern in normal infants, and they swallow easily.

Teeth begin developing in utero, with enamel formation continuing until about age 10 years. Tooth development is influenced by neonatal or infant illnesses, medications, and illnesses of or medications taken by the mother during pregnancy. The fluoride level in the water supply also influences tooth development. Occasionally an infant may be born with one or more teeth. Native American infants are commonly born with teeth.

Bacteria are not present in the infant's gastrointestinal tract at birth. Soon after birth, oral and anal orifices permit entry of bacteria and air. Generally the highest bacterial concentration is found in the lower portion of the intestine, particularly in the large intestine. Normal colonic bacteria are established within the first week after birth, and normal intestinal flora help synthesize vitamin K, folate, and biotin. Bowel sounds can usually be heard shortly after birth.

The capacity of the stomach varies from 30 to 90 ml, depending on the size of the infant. The emptying time for the stomach is highly variable. Several factors, such as time and volume of feedings or type and temperature of food, may affect the emptying time. The cardiac sphincter is immature, and nervous control of the stomach is not well established, so some regurgitation may occur. Regurgitation during the first day or two of life can be decreased by avoiding overfeeding, by burping the infant, and by positioning the infant with the head slightly elevated.

Digestion

The infant's ability to digest carbohydrates, fats, and proteins is regulated by the presence of certain enzymes. Most of these enzymes are functional at birth. One exception is amylase, produced by the salivary glands after about 3 months and by the pancreas at about 6 months of age. This enzyme is necessary to convert starch into maltose. The other exception is lipase, also secreted by the pancreas; it is necessary for the digestion of fat. Thus the normal newborn is capable of digesting simple carbohydrates and proteins but has a limited ability to digest fats.

Further digestion and absorption of nutrients occur in the small intestine in the presence of pancreatic secretions, secretions from the liver through the common bile duct, and secretions from the duodenal portion of the small intestine.

Stools

At birth the lower intestine is filled with meconium. **Meconium** is formed during fetal life from the amniotic fluid and its constituents, intestinal secretions (including bilirubin), and cells (shed from the mucosa). Meconium is greenish black and viscous and contains occult blood. The first meconium passed is sterile, but within hours, all meconium passed contains bacteria. The majority of normal term infants pass meconium within the first 12 hours of life, and almost all do so by 24 hours. The number of stools varies during the first week, being most numerous between the third and sixth days. Newborns fed early pass stools sooner. Progressive changes in the appearance of stools and in the stooling pattern indicate a properly functioning gastrointestinal system (Box 25-1). Stooling also is an indicator of the adequacy of nutritional intake. For example, breastfed infants should have at least three stools per 24 hours after day 3 or 4 of life when the mother's milk is in.

Feeding Behaviors

Variations occur among infants regarding interest in food, symptoms of hunger, and amount ingested at one time. The amount of food that the infant takes in at any feeding

BOX 25-1 Change in Stooling Patterns of Newborns

MECONIUM

Infant's first stool: composed of amniotic fluid and its constituents, intestinal secretions, shed mucosal cells, and possibly blood (ingested maternal blood or minor bleeding of alimentary tract vessels).

Passage of meconium should occur within the first 24 to 48 hr, although it may be delayed up to 7 days in very low-birth-weight infants.

TRANSITIONAL STOOLS

Usually appear by third day after initiation of feeding; greenish brown to yellowish brown, thin, and less sticky than meconium; may contain some milk curds.

MILK STOOL

Usually appears by fourth day

In *breastfed infants*, stools are yellow to golden, are pasty in consistency, and have an odor similar to that of sour milk.

In *formula-fed infants*, stools are pale yellow to light brown, are firmer in consistency, and have a more offensive odor.

depends on the size, hunger level, and alertness of the infant. When an infant is put to breast, some feed immediately, whereas others require a learning period of up to 48 hours before breastfeeding is completely effective. Random hand-to-mouth movement and sucking of fingers are well developed at birth and intensified when the infant is hungry. Caregivers should be alert to these hunger cues.

Signs of Risk for Gastrointestinal Problems

The time, color, and character of the infant's first stool should be noted. A lack of passage of stool could indicate an inborn error of metabolism (e.g., cystic fibrosis) or a congenital disorder (e.g., Hirschsprung disease or an imperforate anus). An active rectal "wink" reflex (contraction of the anal sphincter muscle in response to touch) usually is a good sign of sphincter tone.

Some infants do not digest specific formulas well. If an infant is allergic to or unable to digest a formula, the stools may become very soft with a high water content that is seen as a distinct water ring around the stool on the diaper. Forceful ejection of stool and a water ring around the stool are signs of diarrhea. Care must be taken to avoid misinterpreting transitional stools for diarrhea. The loss of fluid in diarrhea can rapidly lead to fluid and electrolyte imbalance. Passage of meconium from the vagina or urinary meatus is a sign of a possible fistulous tract from the rectum.

Abdominal distention at birth usually indicates a serious disorder such as a ruptured viscus (from abdominal wall defects) or tumors. Distention that occurs later may be the result of overfeeding or may signal gastrointestinal disorders. A scaphoid (sunken) abdomen with bowel sounds heard in the chest and signs of respiratory distress indicate a diaphragmatic hernia.

The amount and frequency of regurgitation ("spitting up") after feedings must be recorded. Color change, gagging, and projectile (very forceful) vomiting occur in association with esophageal and tracheoesophageal anomalies.

Hepatic System

In the newborn the liver can be palpated about 1 cm below the right costal margin because it is enlarged and occupies about 40% of the abdominal cavity. The infant's liver plays an important role in iron storage, carbohydrate metabolism, conjugation of bilirubin, and coagulation.

Iron Storage

The infant's iron store in the liver is proportional to the body weight and, for the term infant, should be sufficient for the first 4 to 6 months. Preterm and small-for-date infants have lower iron stores, which are sufficient for only 2 to 3 months.

Carbohydrate Metabolism

At birth the newborn is cut off from its maternal glucose supply and, as a result, has an initial decrease in serum glucose levels. The newborn's increased energy needs, decreased hepatic release of glucose from glycogen stores, increased RBC volume, and increased brain size may initially contribute to the rapid depletion of stored glycogen within the first 24 hours after birth. In most healthy term newborns, blood glucose levels stabilize at 40 to 60 mg/dl during the first several hours after birth; by the third day of life, the blood glucose levels should be approximately 60 to 70 mg/dl. The initiation of feedings assists in the stabilization of the newborn's blood glucose levels. If the infant appears to be jittery or has tremors, the blood glucose level should be determined to rule out hypoglycemia.

Conjugation of Bilirubin

Bilirubin is a yellow pigment derived from the hemoglobin released with the breakdown of RBCs and the myoglobin in muscle cells. The hemoglobin is phagocytized by the reticuloendothelial cells, converted to bilirubin, and released in an unconjugated form. **Unconjugated bilirubin,** termed *indirect bilirubin*, is relatively insoluble and almost entirely bound to circulating albumin, a plasma protein. The unbound bilirubin can leave the vascular system and permeate other extravascular tissues (e.g., the skin, sclera, and oral mucous membranes). The resultant yellow coloring is termed jaundice.

In the liver, the unbound bilirubin is conjugated with glucuronide in the presence of the enzyme glucuronyl transferase. The conjugated form of bilirubin is excreted from liver cells as a constituent of bile. This form is termed *direct bilirubin* and is water soluble. Along with other components of bile, direct bilirubin is excreted into the biliary tract system that carries the bile into the duodenum. Bilirubin is converted to urobilinogen and stercobilinogen within the duodenum by the action of the bacterial flora. Urobilinogen is excreted in urine and feces; stercobilinogen is excreted in the feces (Fig. 25-4). The total serum bilirubin level is the sum of the levels of both conjugated (direct) and unconjugated (indirect) bilirubin.

Adequate serum albumin–binding sites are available unless the infant has asphyxia neonatorum (respiratory failure in the newborn), cold stress, or hypoglycemia. A mother's prebirth ingestion of medications such as sulfa drugs and aspirin can reduce the amount of serum albumin–binding sites in the newborn. Although the neonate has the functional capacity to convert bilirubin, physiologic hyperbilirubinemia commonly occurs in infants.

Physiologic Jaundice

Physiologic or **neonatal jaundice** or **hyperbilirubinemia** occurs in almost all newborn infants but is more severe in preterm infants (Frank, Cooper, & Merenstein, 2002). The incidence and severity of physiologic jaundice is increased in Asian and Native American infants (Hockenberry et al., 2003). Although neonatal jaundice is considered benign, bilirubin may accumulate to hazardous levels and lead to a pathologic condition. Physiologic jaundice results from characteristics of normal newborn physiology, such as increased bilirubin production due to increased RBC mass, shortened life span of the fetal RBCs, and liver immaturity. Newborns also tend to reabsorb bilirubin from the small intestine.

The infant who is diagnosed with physiologic jaundice appears to be otherwise well and exhibits signs of jaundice after age 24 hours. Clinically, the indirect-reacting bilirubin (unconjugated) is no more than 12 mg/dl by 3 days of age. In preterm infants, the peak is higher (15 mg/dl) and tends to occur later. The peak indirect bilirubin level may be higher in breastfed infants (15 to 17 mg/dl). Jaundice is considered to be pathologic if it appears before 24 hours of age, increases more than 0.5 mg/dl/hr, peaks at greater than 13 mg/dl in a term infant, or is associated with anemia and hepatosplenomegaly. Jaundice that appears before 24 hours of age always warrants immediate attention. Pathologic jaundice is usually caused by blood group incompatibility or infection, but may rarely be the result of RBC enzyme defects (glucose-6-phosphate dehydrogenase [G6PD, pyruvate kinase), RBC membrane disorders (spherocytosis, ovalocytosis), or hemoglobinopathy (thalassemia) (Frank et al., 2002).

NURSE ALERT

At any serum bilirubin level, the appearance of jaundice during the first 24 hours of life or persistence beyond day 7 usually indicates a pathologic process.

Jaundice appears in a cephalocaudal manner. It is generally first noticed in the head, especially the sclera and mucous membranes, and then progresses gradually to the thorax, abdomen, and extremities. It dissipates in the reverse order.

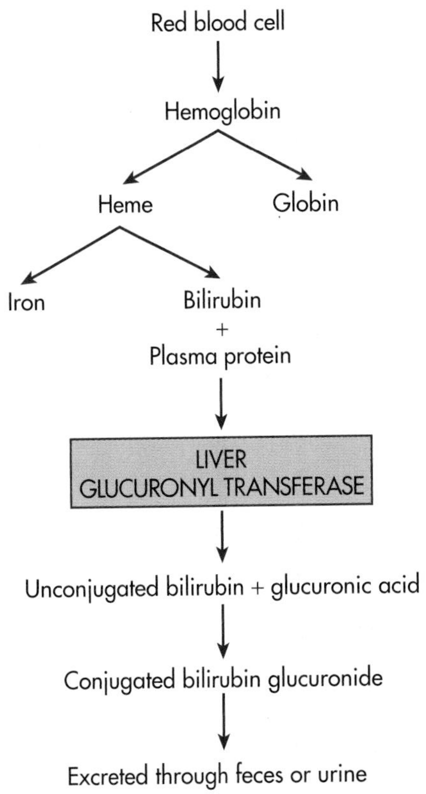

Red blood cell
Hemoglobin
Heme
Globin
Iron
Bilirubin
+
Plasma protein
LIVER
GLUCURONYL TRANSFERASE
Unconjugated bilirubin + glucuronic acid
Conjugated bilirubin glucuronide
Excreted through feces or urine

FIG. 25-4 Formation and excretion of bilirubin. (From Hockenberry, M. et al. [2003]. *Wong's nursing care of infants and children* [7th ed.]. St. Louis: Mosby.)

Feeding practices may influence the appearance and degree of physiologic hyperbilirubinemia. Early (within the first hour) and frequent feeding tends to keep the serum bilirubin level low by stimulating intestinal activity (the gastrocolic reflex) and passage of meconium.

Cold stress of the newborn may result in acidosis and increase the level of free fatty acids. In the presence of acidosis, albumin binding of bilirubin is weakened, and bilirubin is freed.

Kernicterus, or bilirubin encephalopathy, is the most serious complication of neonatal hyperbilirubinemia. It occurs when bilirubin is deposited in the basal ganglia and brainstem, disrupting neuronal function and metabolism. Kernicterus usually occurs when bilirubin levels are higher than 25 mg/dl, but may be noted with levels that are lower than 20 mg/dl in the presence of sepsis, meningitis, hypothermia, hypoglycemia, prematurity, and bilirubin-displacing drugs. In the acute stage of kernicterus, the infant is lethargic, hypotonic, and has a poor suck. If untreated, the infant becomes hypertonic (with backward arching of the neck and trunk), has a high-pitched cry, and may develop fever. If an infant survives kernicterus, there may be residual cerebral palsy, epilepsy, and mental retardation. Although neonatal jaundice is common and kernicterus is rare, in recent years, there has been a resurgence in the number of infants with kernicterus. This may be related to the shortened hospital stays after birth, an increase in the incidence of neonatal jaundice, and a lack of concern and attention to infants exhibiting signs of jaundice (Maisels, 2001) (see Chapter 39).

NURSE ALERT

In cases in which the infant is discharged from the hospital before 48 hours after birth or the infant is born at home, a professional attendant may not be available to assess pathologic increases in circulating unbound bilirubin. Therefore all parents need instruction in how to assess jaundice and when to call the health care provider.

Breastfeeding and Jaundice

Breastfeeding jaundice (early-onset jaundice) occurs in the first few days after birth and is associated with a lack of fluid and caloric intake related to ineffective breastfeeding patterns. Breast milk jaundice (late-onset jaundice) has been defined as a progressive indirect hyperbilirubinemia beyond the first week of life; it typically occurs after 3 to 5 days of age and peaks by about 2 weeks (Reiser, 2001). (See Chapter 27 for a discussion of this topic.)

Coagulation

The liver plays an important role in blood coagulation. Coagulation factors, which are synthesized in the liver, are activated by vitamin K. The lack of intestinal bacteria needed to synthesize vitamin K results in a transient blood coagulation deficiency between days 2 and 5 of life. The levels of coagulation factors slowly increase to reach adult levels by age 9 months. An injection of vitamin K soon after birth helps prevent clotting problems. Any bleeding problems noted in an infant should be reported immediately, and tests for clotting ordered.

Signs of Risk for Hepatic System Problems

Some problems such as kernicterus and hypoglycemia have already been discussed. The infant's hemoglobin levels must be assessed for anemia. Because infants may develop a coagulation deficiency, a male child who has been circumcised must be observed closely for signs of hemorrhage. Hemorrhage also could be caused by a clotting defect, indicating a serious problem such as hemophilia.

Immune System

The cells that provide the infant with immunity are developed early in fetal life; however, they are not activated for several months. For the first 3 months of life, the infant is protected by passive immunity received from the mother. Natural barriers such as the acidity of the stomach and the production of pepsin and trypsin, which maintain sterility of the small intestine, are not fully developed until age 3 to 4 weeks. The membrane-protective immunoglobulin A (IgA) is missing from the respiratory and urinary tracts, and unless the newborn is breastfed, it also is absent from the gastrointestinal tract. The infant begins to synthesize IgG, and about 40% of adult levels are reached by age 1 year. Significant concentrations of IgM are produced at birth, and adult levels are reached by age 9 months. The production of IgA, IgD, and IgE is much more gradual, and maximal levels are not attained until early childhood. The infant who is breastfed receives passive immunity through the colostrum and breast milk. The protection provided varies with the age and maturity of the infant and the mother's level of immunity (Lawrence, 1999).

Signs of Risk for Immune System Problems

All newborns and preterm newborns especially are at high risk for infection during the first several months of life. During this period, infection is one of the leading causes of morbidity and mortality. The newborn cannot limit the invading pathogen to the portal of entry because of the generalized hypofunctioning of the inflammatory and immune mechanisms. Any unusual discharges from the infant's eyes, nose, mouth, or other orifice must be investigated. If a rash appears, it must be evaluated closely; many normal rashes in the newborn are not associated with any infection. When an infant is septic, the usual response is respiratory distress. Infants must be protected from infections by the use of good handwashing techniques.

Integumentary System

All skin structures are present at birth. The epidermis and dermis are loosely bound and extremely thin. **Vernix caseosa** (a cheeselike, whitish substance) is fused with the epidermis and serves as a protective covering. The infant's skin is very sensitive and can be easily damaged. The term infant has an erythematous (red) skin for a few hours after birth, after which it fades to its normal color. The skin often appears blotchy or mottled, especially over the extremities. The hands and feet appear slightly cyanotic **(acrocyanosis);** this is caused by vasomotor instability, capillary stasis, and a high hemoglobin level. Acrocyanosis is normal and appears intermittently over the first 7 to 10 days, especially with exposure to cold.

The healthy term newborn is plump. Subcutaneous fat accumulated during the last trimester acts as insulation. The newborn's skin may be slightly tight, suggesting fluid retention. Fine lanugo hair may be noted over the face, shoulders, and back. Actual edema of the face and ecchymosis (bruising) or petechiae may be present as a result of face presentation or forceps-assisted birth.

Creases can be found on the palms of the hands. The simian line, a single palmar crease, is often found in Asian infants or in infants with Down syndrome. The soles of the feet should be inspected for the number of creases. Premature newborns have few if any creases. Increasing numbers of creases correlate with a greater maturity rating.

Caput Succedaneum

Caput succedaneum is a generalized, easily identifiable edematous area of the scalp, most commonly found on the occiput (Fig. 25-5, *A*). With vertex presentation, the sustained pressure of the occiput against the cervix results in compression of local vessels, thereby slowing venous return. The slower venous return causes an increase in tissue fluids within the skin of the scalp, and an edematous swelling develops. This boggy edematous swelling, present at birth, extends across suture lines of the fetal skull and disappears spontaneously within 3 to 4 days. Infants who are delivered with the assistance of vacuum extraction usually have a caput (and bruising) in the area where the cup was applied.

Cephalhematoma

Cephalhematoma is a collection of blood between a skull bone and its periosteum; therefore a cephalhematoma does not cross a cranial suture line (Fig. 25-5, *B*). Caput succedaneum and cephalhematoma often occur simultaneously.

Bleeding resulting in cephalhematoma may occur with spontaneous birth from pressure against the maternal bony pelvis. Low forceps birth and difficult forceps rotation and extraction also may cause bleeding. This soft, fluctuating, irreducible fullness of cephalhematoma does not pulsate or bulge when the infant cries. It appears several hours or the day after birth and may not become apparent until a caput succedaneum is absorbed. A cephalhematoma is usually largest on the second or third day, by which time the bleeding stops. The fullness of a cephalhematoma spontaneously resolves in 3 to 6 weeks. It is not aspirated because infection may develop if the skin is punctured. As the hematoma resolves, hemolysis of RBCs occurs, and jaundice may result. Hyperbilirubinemia may occur after the newborn is home.

Desquamation

Desquamation (peeling) of the skin of the term infant does not occur until a few days after birth. Its presence at birth is an indication of postmaturity.

Sweat and Oil Glands

Sweat glands are present at birth but do not respond to increases in ambient or body temperature. Some fetal sebaceous (oil) gland hyperplasia and secretion of sebum result from the hormonal influences of pregnancy. Vernix caseosa is a product of the sebaceous glands. Removal of the vernix is followed by desquamation of the epidermis in most infants. Distended, small, white sebaceous glands **(milia)** may be noticeable on the newborn face.

Mongolian Spots

Mongolian spots, bluish-black areas of pigmentation, may appear over any part of the exterior surface of the body, including the extremities. They are more commonly noted on the back and buttocks (Fig. 25-6). These pigmented areas are most frequently noted in babies whose ethnic origins are in the Mediterranean area, Latin America, Asia, or Africa. They are more common in dark-skinned individuals, regardless of race. They fade gradually over months or years. Mongolian spots have no clinical significance but can be mistaken for bruises.

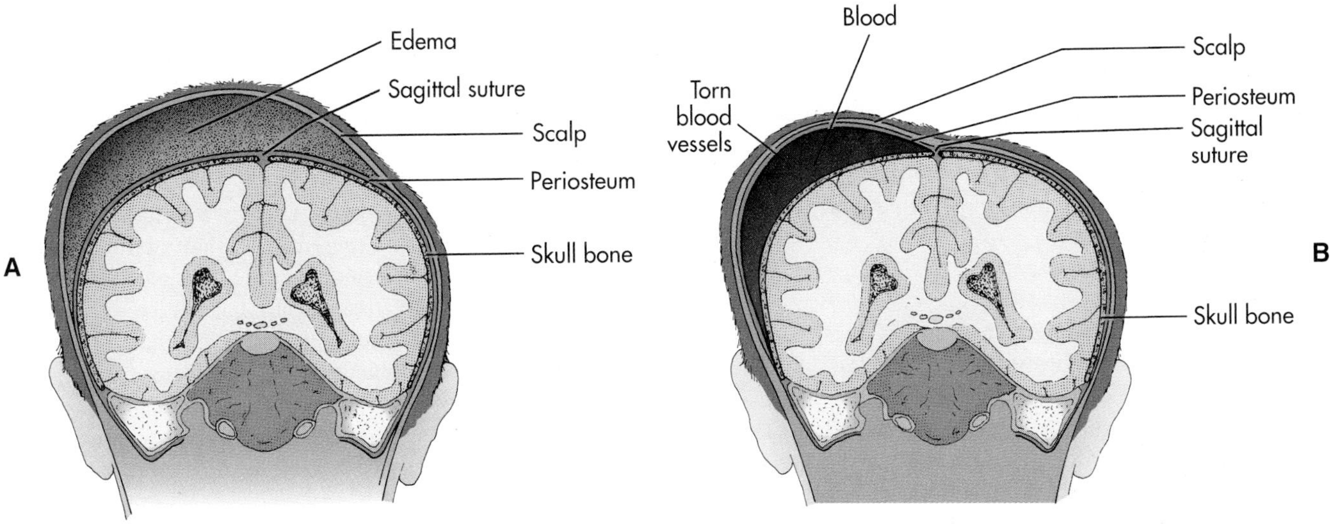
Edema
Sagittal suture
Scalp
Periosteum
Skull bone
A
Blood
Torn blood vessels
Scalp
Periosteum
Sagittal suture
Skull bone
B

FIG. 25-5 Differences between caput succedaneum and cephalhematoma. **A,** Caput succedaneum: edema of scalp noted at birth; crosses suture lines. **B,** Cephalhematoma: bleeding between periosteum and skull bone appearing within first 2 days; does not cross suture lines.

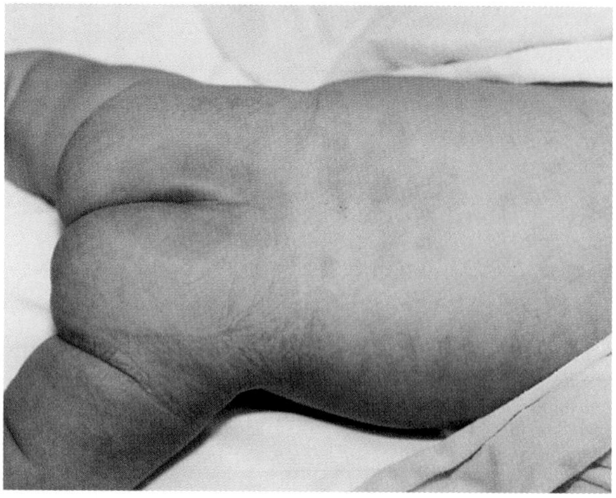

FIG. 25-6 Mongolian spot.

Nevi

Known as "stork bites" or "angel kisses," telangiectatic nevi are pink and easily blanched (Fig. 25-7, *A*). They may appear on the upper eyelids, nose, upper lip, lower occipital area, and nape of the neck. They have no clinical significance and fade by the second year of life.

The strawberry mark, or nevus vasculosus, is a common type of capillary hemangioma. It consists of dilated, newly formed capillaries occupying the entire dermal and subdermal layers with associated connective tissue hypertrophy. The typical lesion is a raised, sharply demarcated, bright or dark red, rough-surfaced swelling that resembles a strawberry. Lesions usually are single but may be multiple, with 75% occurring on the head. These lesions can remain until the child is of school age or sometimes even longer.

A port-wine stain, or nevus flammeus, is usually observed at birth and is composed of a plexus of newly formed capillaries in the papillary layer of the corium. It is red to purple; varies in size, shape, and location; and is not elevated. True port-wine stains do not blanch on pressure or disappear. They are most frequently found on the face.

Erythema Toxicum

A transient rash, **erythema toxicum,** is also called erythema neonatorum, "newborn rash," or "flea bite" dermatitis. It has lesions in different stages: erythematous macules, papules, and small vesicles (Fig. 25-7, *B*). The lesions may appear suddenly anywhere on the body. The rash is thought to be an inflammatory response. Eosinophils, which help decrease inflammation, are found in the vesicles. The rash is found in term neonates (gestational age of 36 weeks or more) during the first 3 weeks after birth. Although the appearance is alarming, the rash has no clinical significance and requires no treatment.

A

B

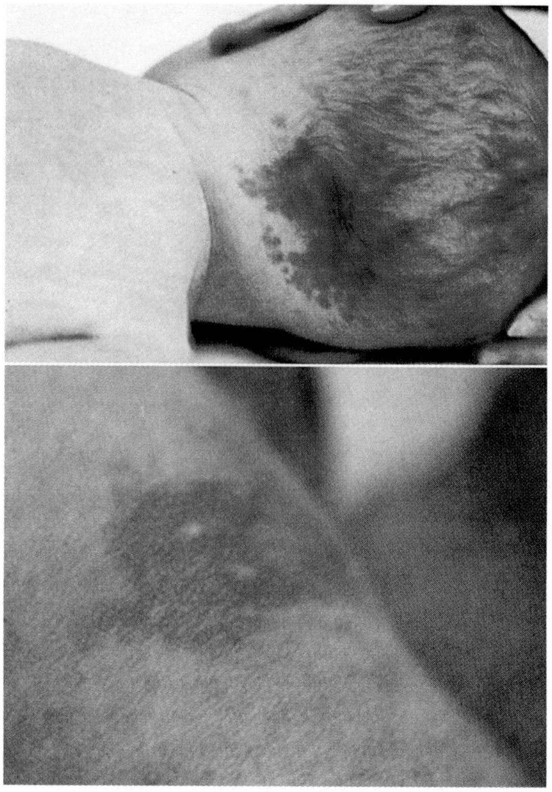

FIG. 25-7 A, Telangiectatic nevi (stork bite). **B,** Erythema toxicum (flea bite). (Courtesy Mead Johnson & Co., Evansville, IN.)

Signs of Risk for Integumentary Problems

Close observation of the newborn's skin color can lead to early detection of potential problems. Any pallor, plethora (deep purplish color from increased circulating RBCs), petechiae, central cyanosis, or jaundice should be noted and described. The skin should be examined for signs of birth injuries, such as forceps marks and lesions related to fetal monitoring. Bruises or petechiae may be present on the head, neck, and face of an infant born with a nuchal cord (cord around the neck) or in an infant who was a face presentation at birth. When bruises are present, the infant's bilirubin levels may be elevated. Petechiae may be present if increased pressure was applied to an area. Petechiae scattered over the infant's body should be reported to the pediatrician because their presence may indicate underlying problems such as low platelet count or infection. Unilateral or bilateral periauricular papillomas (skin tags) occur fairly frequently. Their occurrence is usually a family trait and of no consequence.

Reproductive System

Female

At birth the ovaries contain thousands of primitive germ cells. These represent the full complement of potential ova; no oogonia form after birth in term infants. The ovarian cortex, which is made up primarily of primordial follicles, occupies a larger portion of the ovary in the female newborn than in the female adult. From birth to sexual maturity, the number of ova decreases by approximately 90%.

An increase of estrogen during pregnancy followed by a decrease after birth results in a mucoid vaginal discharge and even some slight bloody spotting (pseudomenstruation). External genitals are usually edematous with increased pigmentation. In term newborn infants, the labia majora and minora cover the vestibule (Fig. 25-8, *A*). In preterm infants, the clitoris is prominent, and the labia majora are small and widely separated. Vaginal or hymenal tags are common findings and have no clinical significance. Vernix caseosa may be present between the labia.

If the female was born in the breech position, the labia may be edematous and bruised. The edema and bruising resolve in a few days; no treatment is necessary.

Male

The testes descend into the scrotum by birth in 90% of newborn boys. Although this percentage decreases with premature birth, by 1 year of age, the incidence of undescended testes in all boys is less than 1%.

A tight prepuce (foreskin) is common in newborns. The urethral opening may be completely covered by the prepuce, which may not be retractable for 3 to 4 years. Smegma, a white, cheesy substance, is commonly found under the foreskin. Small, white, firm lesions called epithelial pearls may be seen at the tip of the prepuce. By 28 to 36 weeks of gestation, the testes can be palpated in the inguinal canal, and a few rugae appear on the scrotum. At 36 to 40 weeks of gestation, the testes are palpable in the upper scrotum, and rugae appear on the anterior portion. After 40 weeks, the testes can be palpated in the scrotum, and rugae cover the scrotal sac. The postterm neonate has deep rugae and a pendulous scrotum. The scrotum is usually more deeply pigmented than the rest of the skin (Fig. 25-8, *B*), particularly in darker-skinned infants. Hydroceles, caused by an accumulation of fluid around the testes, may be present. They can be easily transilluminated with a light and usually decrease in size without treatment.

If the male infant was born in a breech presentation, the scrotum may appear very edematous and bruised. The swelling and discoloration resolve within a few days.

Swelling of Breast Tissue

Swelling of the breast tissue in infants of both sexes is caused by the hyperestrogenism of pregnancy. In a few infants, a thin discharge (witch's milk) can be seen. This condition has no clinical significance, requires no treatment, and subsides as the maternal hormones are eliminated from the infant's body within a few days.

The nipples should be symmetric on the chest. Breast tissue and areola size increase with gestation. The areola appears slightly elevated at 34 weeks of gestation. By 36 weeks, a breast bud of 1 to 2 mm is palpable and increases to 12 mm by 42 weeks.

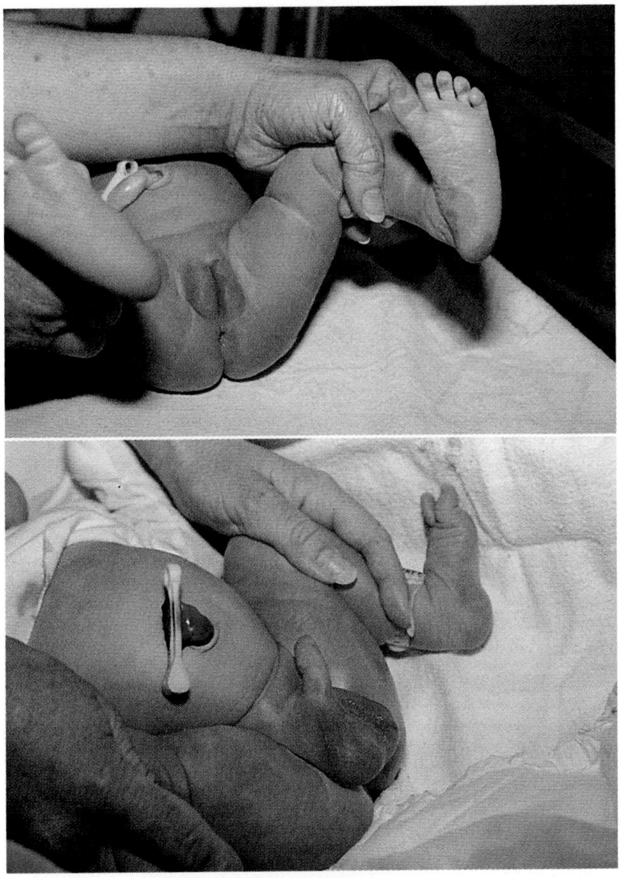

A

B

FIG. 25-8 External genitalia. **A,** Genitals in female term infant. Note mucoid vaginal discharge. **B,** Genitals in male infant. Uncircumcised penis. Rugae cover scrotum, indicating term gestation. Cord has been swabbed with ethylene blue to prevent infection. (Courtesy Marjorie Pyle, RNC, Lifecircle, Costa Mesa, CA.)

Signs of Risk for Reproductive System Problems

The infant must be closely inspected for ambiguous genitalia and other abnormalities. Normally in a female infant, the urethral opening is located behind the clitoris. Any deviation from this may mistakenly suggest that the clitoris is a small penis, which can occur in conditions such as adrenal hyperplasia. Nearly all female infants are born with hymenal tags; absence of such could indicate vaginal agenesis. Fecal discharge from the vagina indicates a rectovaginal fistula. Any of these findings must be reported to the physician for further evaluation.

The male infant's scrotum should always be palpated for the presence of testes. Inguinal hernias may be present and become more obvious when the infant cries. If the urinary meatus is not at the tip of the glans penis, hypospadias (urethral meatus opening on the underside of the penis) or epispadias (urethral meatus opening on the top of the penis) may be present. These problems are usually associated with other anomalies.

Skeletal System

The infant's skeletal system undergoes rapid development during the first year of life. At birth, more cartilage is present than ossified bone. Because of cephalocaudal (head-to-rump) development, the newborn looks somewhat out of proportion.

At term the head is one fourth the total body length. The arms are slightly longer than the legs. In the newborn, the legs are one third the total body length, but only 15% of the total body weight. As growth proceeds, the midpoint in head-to-toe measurements gradually descends from the level of the umbilicus at birth to the level of the symphysis pubis at maturity.

The face appears small in relation to the skull, which appears large and heavy. Cranial size and shape can be distorted by **molding** (the shaping of the fetal head by the overlapping of cranial bones to facilitate movement through the birth canal during labor) (Fig. 25-9).

A

B

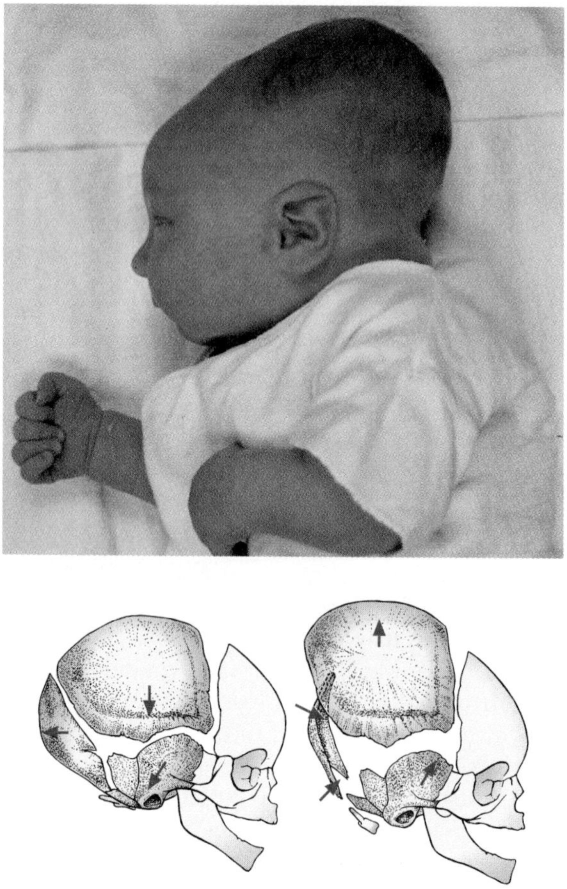

FIG. 25-9 Molding. **A,** Significant molding, soon after birth. **B,** Schematic of bones of skull when molding is present. (**A,** Courtesy Kim Molloy, Knoxville, IA.)

The bones in the vertebral column of the newborn form two primary curvatures, one in the thoracic region and one in the sacral region (Fig. 25-10, *A*). Both are forward, concave curvatures. As the infant gains head control at approximately age 3 months, a secondary curvature appears in the cervical region (Fig. 25-10, *B*).

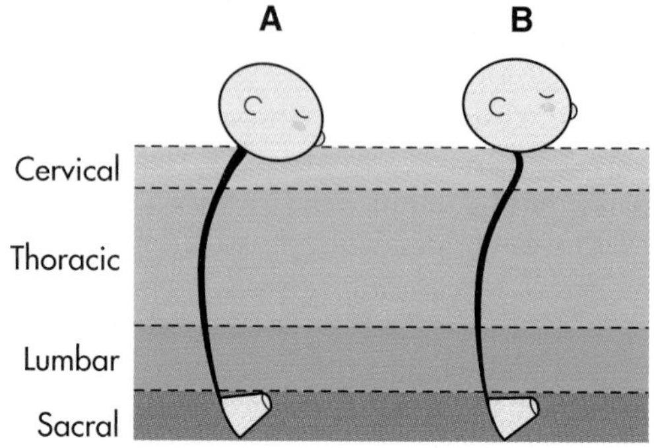
A
B
Cervical
Thoracic
Lumbar
Sacral

FIG. 25-10 Development of spinal curvatures. **A,** Newborn. **B,** Cervical secondary curvature. (From Wong, D. [1999]. *Whaley and Wong's nursing care of infants and children* [6th ed.]. St. Louis: Mosby.)

A

B

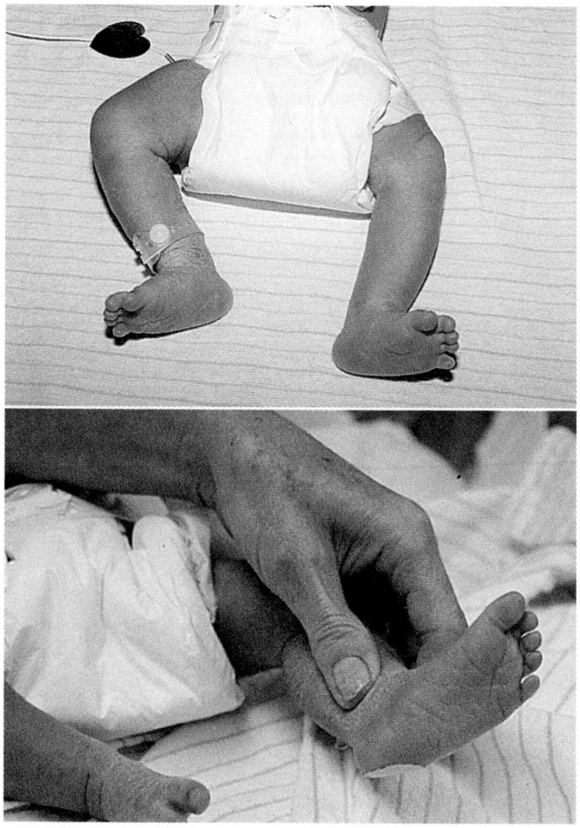

FIG. 25-11 Extremities. **A,** Bowed appearance of legs. **B,** Normal absence of arch in newborn's foot. (Courtesy Marjorie Pyle, RNC, Lifecircle, Costa Mesa, CA.)

In some newborns, a significant separation of the knees occurs when the ankles are held together, resulting in an appearance of bowlegs (Fig. 25-11, *A*). If an infant was in the frank breech position in utero, the legs may be extended and remain in this position for several weeks. The newborn is also very flat footed because no clearly apparent arch to the foot is present (Fig. 25-11, *B*).

The infant's extremities should be symmetric and of equal length. Fingers and toes should be equal in number and should have nails present. Extra digits (polydactyly) are sometimes found on hands or feet. Fingers or toes may be fused (syndactyly).

The infant's hips should be inspected for symmetry. Skin folds should be equal and symmetric. Hip integrity is assessed by using the Ortolani maneuver (Fig. 25-12). The examiner places the index and middle fingers of each hand over the greater trochanters of the hips at the same time. Downward pressure is exerted on the hips while the neonate's knees are flexed. The hips are flexed at least 70 degrees and then abducted. The motion should be smooth without any unusual clicks. The presence of a click, unequal movement, or uneven gluteal skin folds is considered a positive response, indicating that the hip is dislocated, and the physician should be notified.

The newborn's spine appears straight and can be easily flexed. The newborn can lift the head and turn it from side to side when prone. The vertebrae should appear straight and flat. The base of the spine should not have a dimple. If a dimple is noted, further inspection is required to determine whether a sinus is present. A pilonidal dimple, especially with a sinus and nevus pilosis (hairy nevus), is significant because it can be associated with spina bifida.

Signs of Risk for Skeletal Problems

Skeletal deformities may be congenital or drug induced. Clubfoot (talipes equinovarus), a deformity in which the foot turns inward and is fixed in a plantar-flexion position, and any absence of a limb or digit should be recorded and reported. Signs of congenital hip dislocation, additional digits or webbing of digits, and any other abnormality should be recorded and reported to the health care provider.

Neuromuscular System

Unlike the skeletal system, the neuromuscular system is almost completely developed at birth. The term newborn is a responsive and reactive being with remarkable sensory development and an amazing ability for self-organization and social interaction.

Growth of the brain after birth follows a predictable pattern of rapid growth during infancy and early childhood, more gradual growth during the remainder of the first decade, and minimal growth during adolescence. The cerebellum ends its growth spurt, which began at about 30 gestational weeks, by the end of the first year. This may be the reason the brain is vulnerable to nutritional deficiencies and trauma in early infancy.

The brain requires glucose as a source of energy and a relatively large supply of oxygen for adequate metabolism. Such requirements signal a need for careful assessment of the infant's respiratory status. The necessity for

A

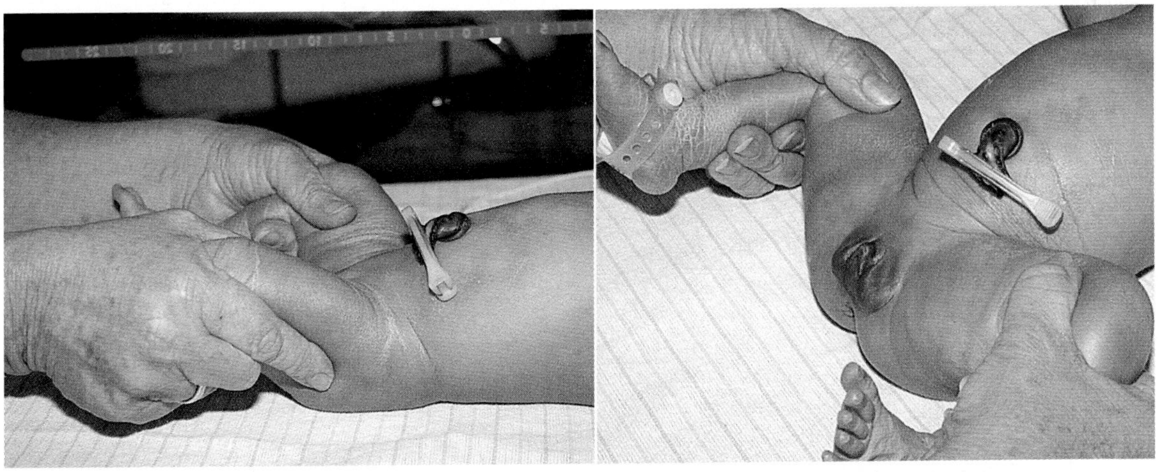

B

FIG. 25-12 Method of assessing for hip dysplasia or dislocation using the Ortolani maneuver. **A,** Examiner's middle fingers are placed over greater trochanter, and thumbs are placed over inner thigh opposite lesser trochanter. **B,** Gentle pressure is exerted to flex thigh on hip further, and thighs are rotated outward. If hip dysplasia is present, head of femur can be felt to slip forward in acetabulum and flip back when pressure is released and legs are returned to their original position. A click is sometimes heard (Ortolani sign). (Courtesy Marjorie Pyle, RNC, Lifecircle, Costa Mesa, CA.)

glucose requires attentiveness to those neonates who may have hypoglycemic episodes.

Spontaneous motor activity may be seen as transient tremors of the mouth and chin, especially during crying episodes, and of the extremities, notably the arms and hands. Transient tremors are normal and can be observed in nearly every newborn. These tremors should not be present when the infant is quiet and should not persist beyond 1 month of age. Persistent tremors or tremors involving the total body may indicate pathologic conditions. Marked tonicity, clonicity, and twitching of facial muscles are signs of seizure activity. Normal tremors, tremors of hypoglycemia, and central nervous system (CNS) disorders must be differentiated so that diagnostic workups and corrective care can be instituted as necessary.

Although it is limited, some neuromuscular control is present in the newborn. If newborns are placed face down on a firm surface, they will turn their heads to the side to maintain an airway. They attempt to hold their heads in line with their bodies if they are raised by their arms.

Newborn Reflexes

The newborn has many primitive reflexes. The times at which these reflexes appear and disappear reflect the maturity and intactness of the developing nervous system. The most common reflexes found in the normal newborn are described in Table 25-3.

Signs of Risk for Neuromuscular Problems

Any absence of a newborn reflex could indicate major neurologic problems. Birth trauma may cause nerve damage that results in facial asymmetry and paralysis. CNS depression, due to maternal medications received during labor and birth, also will influence neuromuscular functioning. Observation of the neonate for any abnormalities must be documented. A thorough physical examination of the newborn assists in detecting any potential complications (see Table 26-2).

Neurologic Assessment

The physical assessment includes a neurologic assessment of the newborn's reflexes (see Table 25-3). This provides useful information about the infant's nervous system and state of neurologic maturation. Many reflex behaviors are important for survival, for example, sucking and rooting. Other reflexes act as safety mechanisms, for instance, gagging, coughing, and sneezing. The assessment must be carried out as early as possible because abnormal signs present in the early neonatal period may disappear. They may reappear months or years later as abnormal functions.

BEHAVIORAL CHARACTERISTICS

The healthy infant must achieve behavioral and biologic tasks to develop normally. Behavioral characteristics form the basis of the social capabilities of the infant. Normal newborns differ in their activity levels, feeding patterns, sleeping patterns, and responsiveness. Parents' reactions to their newborns often are determined by these differences. Showing parents the unique characteristics of their infant assists parents to develop a more positive perception of the infant with increased interaction between infant and parent.

Behavioral responses, as well as physical characteristics, change during the period of transition. The Brazelton Neonatal Behavioral Assessment Scale (BNBAS) can be used to assess the infant's behavior systematically (Brazelton, 1999; Brazelton & Nugent, 1996). The BNBAS is an interactive examination that assesses the infant's response to 28 areas organized according to the clusters in Box 25-2. It is generally used as a research or diagnostic tool and requires special training.

In addition to use as initial and ongoing tools to assess neurologic and behavioral responses, the scales can be used to assess initial parent-infant relationships and as a guide for parents to help them focus on their infant's individuality and to develop a deeper attachment to their child. See Chapter 24 for further discussion of attachment.

Sleep-Wake States

Variations in the state of consciousness of infants are called *sleep-wake states* (Brazelton, 1999). The six states form a continuum from deep sleep to extreme irritability (Fig. 25-13 on p. 704): two sleep states (deep sleep and light sleep) and four wake states (drowsy, quiet alert, active alert, and crying). Each state has specific characteristics and state-related behaviors. The optimal state of arousal is the quiet alert state. During this state infants smile, vocalize, move in synchrony with speech, watch their parents' faces, and respond to people talking to them. The infants' reaction to internal and external stimuli and

BOX 25-2 Clusters of Neonatal Behaviors in BNBAS

Habituation: Ability to respond to and then inhibit responding to discrete stimulus (light, rattle, bell, pinprick) while asleep.
Orientation: Quality of alert states and ability to attend to visual and auditory stimuli while alert
Motor performance: Quality of movement and tone
Range of state: Measure of general arousal level or arousability of infant
Regulation of state: How infant responds when aroused
Autonomic stability: Signs of stress (tremors, startles, skin color) related to homeostatic (self-regulator) adjustment of the nervous system
Reflexes: Assessment of several neonatal reflexes

TABLE 25-3 **Assessment of Newborn's Reflexes**

REFLEX	ELICITING THE REFLEX	CHARACTERISTIC RESPONSE	COMMENTS
Sucking and rooting	Touch infant's lip, cheek, or corner of mouth with nipple	Infant turns head toward stimulus, opens mouth, takes hold, and sucks	Response is difficult if not impossible to elicit after infant has been fed; if response weak or absent, consider prematurity or neurologic defect Parental guidance: Avoid trying to turn head toward breast or nipple, allow infant to root; response disappears after 3 to 4* mo but may persist up to 1 yr
Swallowing	Feed infant; swallowing usually follows sucking and obtaining fluids	Swallowing is usually coordinated with sucking and usually occurs without gagging, coughing, or vomiting	If response is weak or absent, this may indicate prematurity or neurologic defect Sucking and swallowing are often uncoordinated in preterm infant
Grasp			
Palmar	Place finger in palm of hand	Infant's fingers curl around examiner's fingers, toes curl downward	Palmar response lessens by 3 to 4 mo; parents enjoy this contact with infant; plantar response lessens by 8 mo
Plantar	Place finger at base of toes		
Extrusion	Touch or depress tip of tongue	Newborn forces tongue outward	Response disappears about fourth month of life
Glabellar (Myerson's)	Tap over forehead, bridge of nose, or maxilla of newborn whose eyes are open	Newborn blinks for first four or five taps	Continued blinking with repeated taps is consistent with extrapyramidal disorder
Tonic neck or "fencing"	With infant falling asleep or sleeping, turn head quickly to one side	With infant facing left side, arm and leg on that side extend; opposite arm and leg flex (turn head to right, and extremities assume opposite postures)	Responses in leg are more consistent Complete response disappears by 3 to 4 mo, incomplete response may be seen until third or fourth year After 6 wk, persistent response is sign of possible cerebral palsy

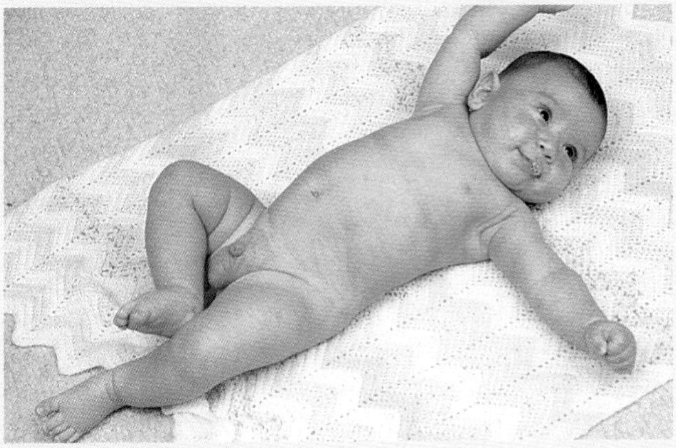

Classic pose in spontaneous tonic neck reflex. (Courtesy Marjorie Pyle, RNC, Lifecircle, Costa Mesa, CA.)

*All durations for persistence of reflexes are based on time elapsed after 40 wk of gestation, that is, if this newborn was born at 36 wk of gestation, add 1 mo to all time limits given.

Continued

REFLEX	ELICITING THE REFLEX	CHARACTERISTIC RESPONSE	COMMENTS
Moro	Hold infant in semisitting position, allow head and trunk to fall backward to an angle of at least 30 degrees Place infant on flat surface, strike surface to startle infant	Symmetric abduction and extension of arms are seen; fingers fan out and form a C with thumb and forefinger; slight tremor may be noted; arms are adducted in embracing motion and return to relaxed flexion and movement Legs may follow similar pattern of response Preterm infant does not complete "embrace"; instead, arms fall backward because of weakness	Response is present at birth; complete response may be seen until 8 wk; body jerk is seen only between 8 and 18 wk; response is absent by 6 mo if neurologic maturation is not delayed; response may be incomplete if infant is deeply asleep; give parental guidance about normal response Asymmetric response may connote injury to brachial plexus, clavicle, or humerus Persistent response after 6 mo indicates possible brain damage
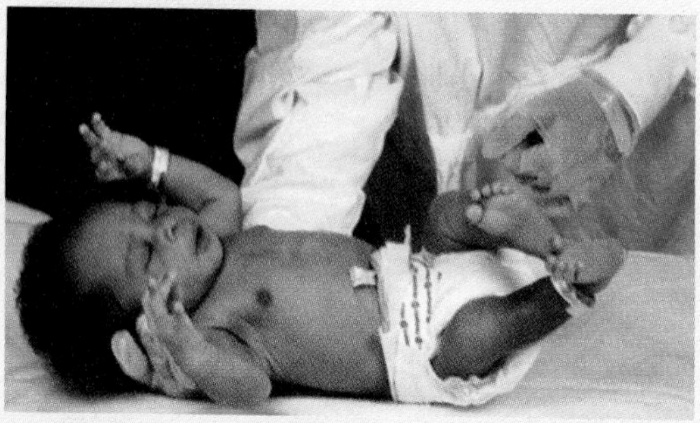		Moro reflex.	
Stepping or "walking"	Hold infant vertically, allowing one foot to touch table surface	Infant will simulate walking, alternating flexion and extension of feet; term infants walk on soles of their feet, and preterm infants walk on their toes	Response is normally present for 3 to 4 wk
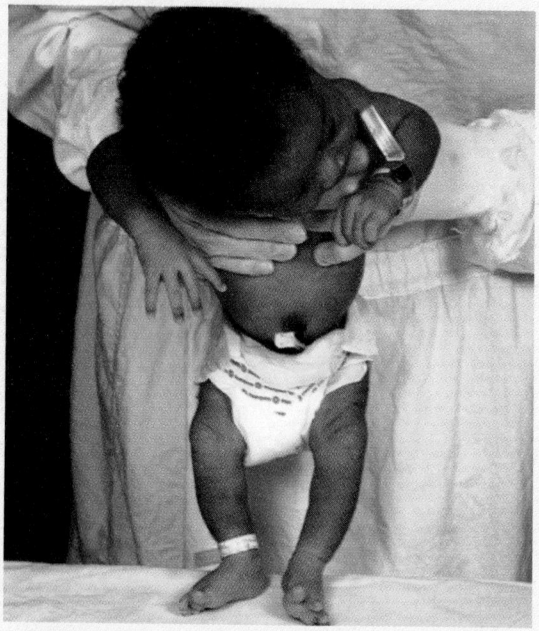		Stepping reflex. (From Dickason, E., Silverman, B., & Kaplan, J. [1998]. *Maternal-infant nursing care* [3rd ed.]. St. Louis: Mosby.)	

REFLEX	ELICITING THE REFLEX	CHARACTERISTIC RESPONSE	COMMENTS
Crawling	Place newborn on abdomen	Newborn makes crawling movements with arms and legs	Response should disappear about 6 wk of age
Deep tendon	Use finger instead of percussion hammer to elicit patellar, or knee jerk, reflex; newborn must be relaxed	Reflex jerk is present; even with newborn relaxed, nonselective overall reaction may occur	
Crossed extension	Infant should be supine; extend one leg, press knee downward, stimulate bottom of foot; observe opposite leg	Opposite leg flexes, adducts, and then extends	

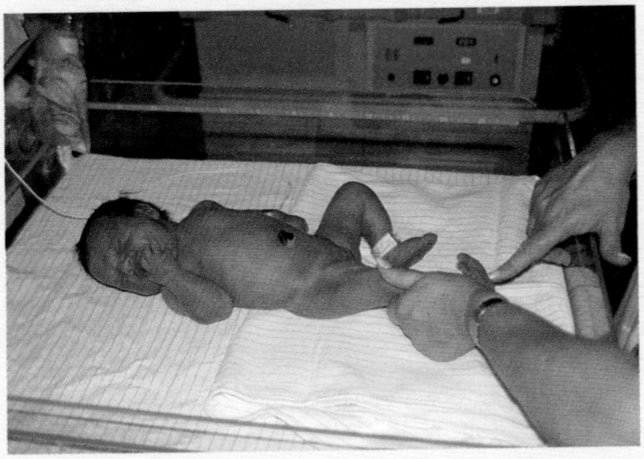

Crossed extension reflex. With the infant in supine position, examiner extends one leg of the infant and presses the knee down. Stimulation of sole of foot of fixated limb should cause free leg to flex, adduct, and extend as if attempting to push away stimulating agent. This reflex should be present during newborn period. (Courtesy Marjorie Pyle, RNC, Lifecircle, Costa Mesa, CA.)

REFLEX	ELICITING THE REFLEX	CHARACTERISTIC RESPONSE	COMMENTS
Startle	Perform sharp hand clap; best elicited if newborn is 24 to 36 hr old or older	Arms abduct with flexion of elbows, hands stay clenched	Response should disappear by 4 mo of age Response is elicited more readily in preterm newborn (inform parents of this characteristic)
Babinski sign (plantar)	On sole of foot, beginning at heel, stroke upward along lateral aspect of sole, then move finger across ball of foot	All toes hyperextend, with dorsiflexion of big toe—recorded as a positive sign	Absence requires neurologic evaluation, should disappear after 1 yr of age

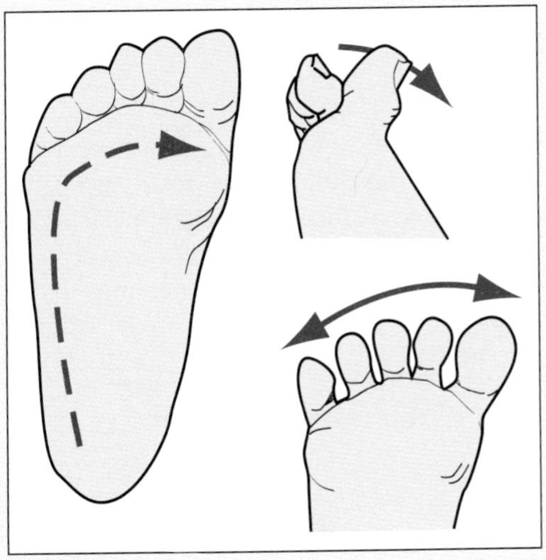

Babinski reflex. (From Hockenberry, M. et al. [2003]. *Wong's nursing care of infants and children* [7th ed.]. St. Louis: Mosby.)

Continued

TABLE 25-3 **Assessment of Newborn's Reflexes—cont'd**

REFLEX	ELICITING THE REFLEX	CHARACTERISTIC RESPONSE	COMMENTS
Pull-to-sit (traction)	Pull infant up by wrists from supine position with head in midline	Head will lag until infant is in upright position, then head will be held in same plane with chest and shoulder momentarily before falling forward; infant will attempt to right head	Response depends on general muscle tone and maturity and condition of infant
Trunk incurvation (Galant)	Place infant prone on flat surface, run finger down back about 4 to 5 cm lateral to spine, first on one side and then down other	Trunk is flexed, and pelvis is swung toward stimulated side	Response disappears by fourth week Absence suggests general depression of nervous system

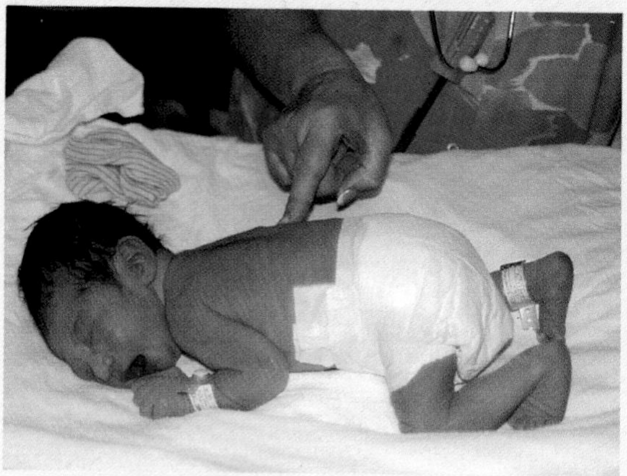

Trunk incurvation reflex. In prone position, infant responds to linear skin stimulus (blunt end of pin or finger) along paravertebral area by flexing the trunk and swinging the pelvis toward stimulus. With transverse lesions of cord, no response below the level of the lesion is present. Response may vary but should be obtainable in all infants, including preterm ones. If not seen in the first few days, it is usually apparent by 5 or 6 days. (Courtesy Marjorie Pyle, RNC, Lifecircle, Costa Mesa, CA.)

ability to control their responses while in these sleep-wake states reflect their ability to organize behavior.

Infants use purposeful behavior to maintain the optimal arousal state: (1) actively withdrawing by increasing physical distance, (2) rejecting by pushing away with hands and feet, (3) decreasing sensitivity by falling asleep or breaking eye contact by turning head, or (4) using signaling behaviors, such as fussing and crying. These behaviors permit infants to quiet themselves and reinstate readiness to interact.

The first 6 weeks of life involve a steady decrease in the proportion of active REM sleep to total sleep. A steady increase in the proportion of quiet sleep to total sleep also occurs. Periods of wakefulness increase. For the first few weeks the wakeful periods seem dictated by hunger, but soon a need for socializing appears as well. The newborn sleeps approximately 17 hours a day, with periods of wakefulness gradually increasing. By the fourth week of life, some infants stay awake from one feeding to the next.

Other Factors Influencing Behavior of Newborns

Gestational Age

The gestational age of the infant and level of CNS maturity affect the observed behavior. In an infant with an im-

TABLE 25-3 **Assessment of Newborn's Reflexes—cont'd**

REFLEX	ELICITING THE REFLEX	CHARACTERISTIC RESPONSE	COMMENTS
Magnet	Place infant in supine position, partially flex both lower extremities and apply pressure to soles of feet	Both lower limbs should extend against examiner's pressure	Absence suggests damage to spinal cord or malformation Reflex may be weak or exaggerated after breech birth
Additional newborn responses: Yawn, stretch, burp, hiccup, sneeze	These are spontaneous behaviors	May be slightly depressed temporarily because of maternal analgesia or anesthesia, fetal hypoxia, or infection	Parental guidance: Most of these behaviors are pleasurable to parents Parents need to be assured that behaviors are normal Sneeze is usually response to lint, etc., in nose and not an indicator of a cold No treatment is needed for hiccups; sucking may help

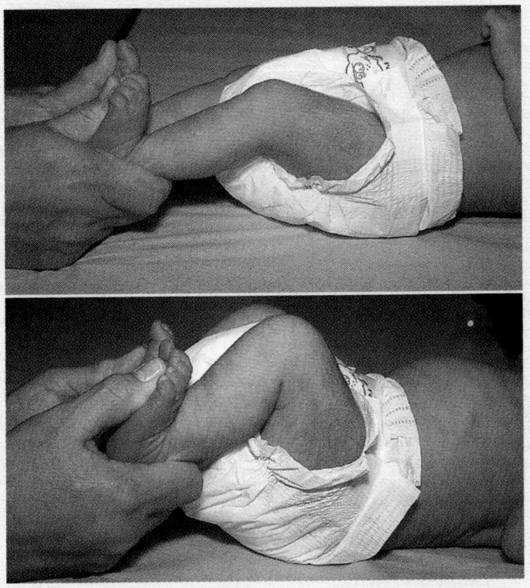

A

Magnet reflex. **A,** With child in supine position and lower limbs semiflexed, light pressure is applied with fingers to both feet. **B,** Normally, while the examiner's fingers maintain contact with the soles of the feet, the lower limbs extend. Weak reflex may be seen after breech presentation *without* extended legs or may indicate sciatic nerve stretch syndrome. Breech presentation *with* extended legs may evoke exaggerated response. (Courtesy Michael S. Clement, MD, Mesa, AZ.)

B

mature CNS, the entire body responds to a pinprick of the foot. The mature infant withdraws only the foot. CNS immaturity is reflected in reflex development and sleep-wake cycles. Preterm infants have brief periods of alertness but have difficulty maintaining this state. Premature or sick infants show fatigue or stress sooner than do term healthy infants.

Time

The time elapsed since birth affects the behavior of infants as they attempt to become organized initially. Time elapsed since the previous feeding and time of day also may influence infants' responses.

Stimuli

Environmental events and stimuli affect the behavioral responses of infants. The newborn responds differently to animate and inanimate stimuli. Nurses in intensive care nurseries observe that infants respond to loud noises, bright lights, monitor alarms, and tension in the unit. If a mother is tense and has a fast heart beat while feeding an infant, the infant will have an increase in heart rate that is similar to the mother's.

Medication

Analgesic and anesthetic medications administered to the mother during labor may affect the newborn's neurologic status and behavior. Narcotics are likely to cause CNS depression and hypotonia and may even cause apnea (Kliegman, 2002). These medications also can affect the infant's sucking ability, at the breast or from a bottle (Lawrence, 1999; Riordan et al., 2000).

Sensory Behaviors

From birth, infants possess sensory capabilities that indicate a state of readiness for social interaction. Infants effectively use behavioral responses in establishing their first dialogues. These responses, coupled with the newborns' "baby appearance" (e.g., facial proportions of forehead and eyes larger than the lower portion of the face) and their small size and helplessness, rouse feelings of wanting to hold, protect, and interact with them.

Vision. Compared with other sensory systems, the visual system is the least mature at term gestation. Development of the visual system continues for the first 6 months. The pupils react to light, the blink reflex is easily stimulated, and the corneal reflex is activated by light touch. Infants are sensitive to light, preferring low illumination. If the room is darkened, they will open their eyes wide and look about. Newborns respond to a flash of bright light by frowning, blinking, and withdrawing the head by arching the entire body.

Newborns have the ability to fixate and will track a high-contrast object horizontally and vertically. Infants seem attentive to the human face and will track their parents' eyes. Parents often comment on how exciting this behavior is.

Visual acuity is difficult to determine, although it appears that the clearest visual distance for the newborn is approximately 19 cm, which is about the distance the infant's face is from the mother's face as she breastfeeds or cuddles. Newborns prefer to look at patterns rather than plain surfaces, even if the latter are brightly colored, and they prefer more complex patterns to simple ones (Brazelton, 1999; Gupta, Hamming, & Miller, 2002).

Hearing. As soon as the amniotic fluid drains from the ear, the infant's hearing is similar to that of an adult. This may occur as early as 1 minute after birth. Loud sounds of about 90 decibels cause the infant to respond with a startle reflex. The newborn responds to low-frequency sounds such as a heartbeat or lullaby by decreasing motor activity or stopping crying. High-frequency sound elicits an alerting reaction.

The infant responds readily to the mother's voice. Studies indicate a selective listening to maternal voice sounds and rhythms during intrauterine life that prepares newborns for

A B C

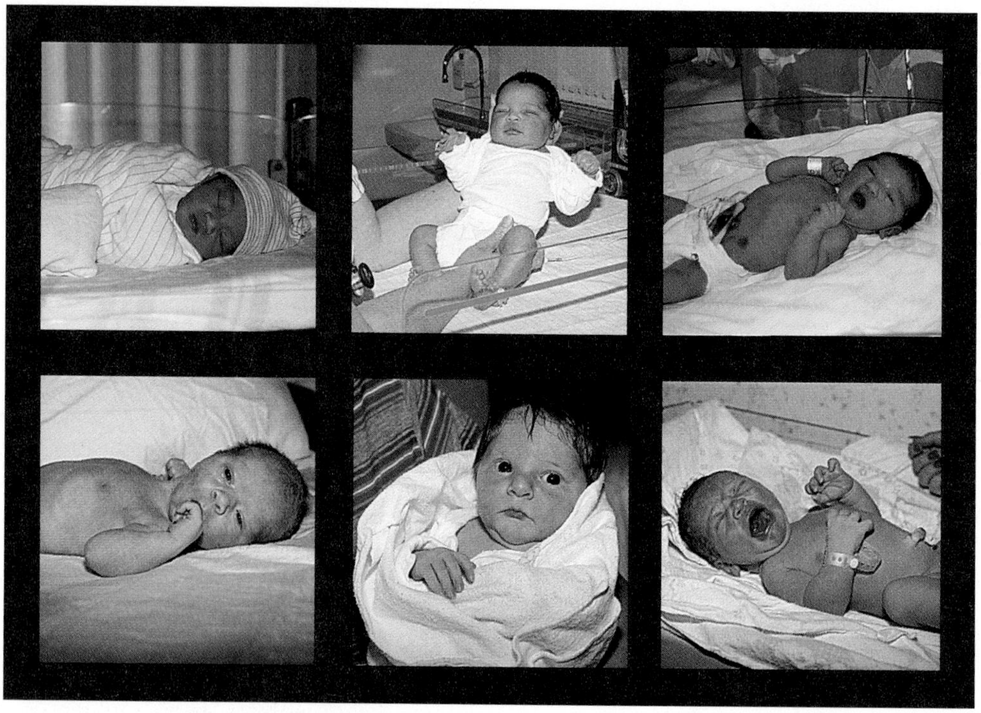

D E F

FIG. 25-13 Summary of newborn sleep-wake states. States of consciousness: **A,** Deep sleep, **B,** Light sleep. **C,** Drowsy. **D,** Quiet alert. **E,** Active alert. **F,** Crying. (Courtesy Marjorie Pyle, RNC, Lifecircle, Costa Mesa, CA.)

recognition and interaction with their primary caregivers—their mothers. Newborns are accustomed in the uterus to hearing the regular rhythm of the mother's heartbeat. As a result, they respond by relaxing and ceasing to fuss and cry if a regular heartbeat simulator is placed in their cribs.

The internal and middle portions of the ear are larger at birth, but the external canal is small. The mastoid process and bony parts of the external canal have not developed; therefore the tympanic membrane and facial nerve are very close to the surface and can be easily damaged. Hearing loss is common at birth; 1 to 3 of every 1000 well newborn infants have bilateral hearing loss (American Academy of Pediatrics Task Force on Newborn and Infant Hearing, 1999). To identify affected infants, the hearing of all infants is screened before discharge (Knott, 2001) (see Fig. 26-6).

Smell. Newborns have a highly developed sense of smell and are responsive to odors that facilitate adaptation to the extrauterine environment. Newborns react to strong odors such as alcohol or vinegar by turning their heads away but are attracted to sweet smells. By the fifth day of life, newborn infants can recognize their mother's smell (Brazelton, 1999). Breastfed infants are able to smell breast milk and can differentiate their mother from other lactating women (Lawrence, 1999).

Taste. The newborn can distinguish between tastes, and various types of solutions elicit differing facial expressions. A tasteless solution produces no response; a sweet solution elicits eager sucking. A sour solution causes a puckering of the lips, and a bitter liquid produces a grimace. Newborns prefer glucose water to plain water (Lawrence, 1999).

Young infants are particularly oriented toward the use of their mouths, both for meeting their nutritional needs for rapid growth and for releasing tension through sucking. The early development of circumoral sensation, muscle activity, and taste would seem to be preparation for survival in the extrauterine environment.

Touch. The infant is responsive to touch on all parts of the body. The face (especially the mouth), the hands, and the soles of the feet appear to be the most sensitive. Reflexes can be elicited by stroking the infant. The newborn's responses to touch suggest that this sensory system is well prepared to receive and process tactile messages. Touch and motion are essential to normal growth and development; however, each infant is unique, and variations can be seen in newborns' responses to touch. Birth trauma or stress and depressant drugs taken by the mother decrease the infant's sensitivity to touch or painful stimuli.

Response to Environmental Stimuli

Temperament. Classic studies identified individual variations in the primary reaction pattern of newborns and described them as temperament. Their style of behavioral response to stimuli is guided by the temperament affecting the newborn's sensory threshold, ability to habituate, and response to maternal behaviors. The newborn possesses individual characteristics that affect selective responses to various stimuli present in the internal and external environment.

Habituation. Habituation is a protective mechanism that allows the infant to become accustomed to environmental stimuli. Habituation is a psychologic and physiologic phenomenon whereby the response to a constant or repetitive stimulus is decreased. In the term newborn, this can be demonstrated in several ways. Shining a bright light into a newborn's eyes will cause a startle or squinting the first 2 to 3 times. The third or fourth flash will elicit a diminished response, and by the fifth or sixth flash, the infant ceases to respond (Brazelton, 1999). The same response pattern holds true for the sounds of a rattle or a pinprick to the heel. A newborn presented with new stimuli becomes wide eyed and alters its gaze for a time but will eventually show a diminished interest.

The ability to habituate also allows the newborn to select stimuli that promote continued learning about the social world, thus avoiding overload. The intrauterine experience seems to have programmed the newborn to be especially responsive to human voices, soft lights, soft sounds, and sweet tastes.

The newborn quickly learns the sounds in a newborn nursery and the home and is able to sleep in their midst. The selective responses of the newborn indicate cerebral organization capable of remembering and making choices. The ability to habituate depends on state of consciousness, hunger, fatigue, and temperament. These factors also affect consolability, cuddliness, irritability, and crying.

Consolability. Newborns vary in their ability to console themselves or to be consoled. In the crying state, most newborns initiate one of several ways to reduce their distress. Hand-to-mouth movements are common, with or without sucking, as well as alerting to voices, noises, or visual stimuli.

Cuddliness. Cuddliness is especially important to parents because they often gauge their ability to care for the child by the child's responses to their actions. The degree varies to which newborns will mold into the contours of the persons holding them. Babies are soothed and become alert with the vestibular stimulation of being picked up and moved.

Irritability. Some newborns cry longer and harder than others. For some the sensory threshold seems low. They are readily upset by unusual noises, hunger, wetness, or new experiences, and thus respond intensely. Others with a high sensory threshold require a great deal more stimulation and variation to reach the active, alert state.

Crying. Crying in an infant may signal hunger, pain, desire for attention, or fussiness. Most mothers learn to distinguish among the cries. The duration of crying is highly variable in each infant; newborns may cry for as little as 5 minutes or as much as 2 hours or more per day. The amount of crying peaks in the second month and then decreases. The diurnal rhythm of crying typically includes more crying in the evening hours. Crying does not seem to differ with different caregivers.

KEY POINTS

- By term, the infant's various anatomic and physiologic systems have reached a level of development and functioning that permits a physical existence apart from the mother. The infant has sensory capabilities that indicate a state of readiness for social interaction.
- Several significant differences exist between the respiratory, renal, and thermogenic systems in the newborn and those of an adult.
- At any serum bilirubin level, the appearance of jaundice during the first day of life or persistence of jaundice for more than 7 days usually indicates a pathologic process in term infants.
- Loss of heat in a newborn, even a healthy newborn, may result in acidosis and increase the level of free fatty acids, leading to cold stress.
- Many reflex behaviors are important for the newborn's survival.
- Individual personalities and behavioral characteristics of infants play major roles in their ultimate relationships with their parents.
- Sleep-wake states and other factors influence the newborn's behavior.
- Each newborn has a predisposed capacity to handle the multitude of stimuli in the external world.

CRITICAL THINKING EXERCISES

1. In your clinical rotation in the newborn nursery, observe at least five infants (of various ethnicity if possible in your setting). Notice the presence of normal variations such as vernix caseosa, milia, caput succedaneum, and Mongolian spots. What proportion of the infants had some of these normal variations? Speak to the parents of one of the infants. Had the parents noticed the normal variations? Had anyone explained the cause or significance of the variation? What questions did the parent have? What did this tell you about the needs of parents for education?
2. Observe three newborn infants over a several-hour period (such as during a day in the nursery during a clinical rotation). How often, at what time of the day, and for how long do the infants cry? What stimulates them to cry? Do baby boys cry more than baby girls? What measures do the parents (or nurses) use to soothe the infant? Are they able to distinguish among the baby's cries? Prepare teaching materials on "helpful hints" about how to soothe an infant. Discuss these hints with the parents. What did you learn from this teaching encounter?
3. Prepare a discharge teaching guide for parents on normal physical findings of a newborn and how to recognize deviations from normal that require intervention. Identify deviations that parents should report to their pediatric care provider. Be sure to discuss jaundice and how to determine when to call the care provider. Include information on interventions that parents can implement.

RESOURCES

Academy of Neonatal Nursing
2777 Yulupa Ave., No. 166
Santa Rosa, CA 94505-8584
707-568-2168
www.academyonline.org

Advances in Neonatal Care
Saunders
The Curtis Center
Independence Square West
Philadelphia, PA 19106-3399
800-654-2452
www.advancesinneonatalcare.org

American Academy of Pediatrics
141 Northwest Point Blvd.
Elk Grove, IL 60007-1098
www.aap.org

Journal of Perinatal and Neonatal Nursing
Aspen Publishers, Inc.
7201 McKinney Circle
Frederick, MD 21701
800-234-1660

National Association of Neonatal Nurses (NANN)
4700 W. Lake Avenue
Glenview, IL 60025-1485
800-451-3795
888-477-6266 (fax)
www.nann.org
E-mail: info@nann.org

Neonatal Network
1410 Neotomas Ave., Suite 107
Santa Rosa, CA 95405-7533
www.neonatalnetwork.com

REFERENCES

American Academy of Pediatrics Task Force on Newborn and Infant Hearing. (1999). Newborn and infant hearing loss: Detection and intervention. *Pediatrics, 103*(2), 527-530.

Blackburn, S. (1992). Alterations of the respiratory system in the neonate: Implications for clinical practice. *Journal of Perinatal and Neonatal Nursing,* 6(2), 46-58.

Brazelton, T. (1999). Behavioral competence. In G. Avery, M. Fletcher, & M. MacDonald (Eds.), *Neonatology: Pathophysiology and management of the newborn* (5th ed.). Philadelphia: Lippincott Williams & Wilkins.

Brazelton, T., & Nugent, K. (1996). *Neonatal behavioural assessment scale* (3rd ed.). London: MacKeith.

Dickason, E., Silverman, B., & Kaplan, J. (1998). *Maternal-infant nursing care* (3rd ed.). St. Louis: Mosby.

Frank, C., Cooper, S., & Merenstein, G. (2002). Jaundice. In G. Merenstein & S. Gardner (Eds.), *Handbook of neonatal intensive care* (5th ed.). St. Louis: Mosby.

Gupta, B., Hamming, N., & Miller, M. (2002). The eye: Diagnosis and evaluation. In A. Fanaroff & R. Martin (Eds.), *Neonatal-perinatal medicine* (7th ed.). St. Louis: Mosby.

Hockenberry, M. et al. (2003). *Wong's nursing care of infants and children* (7th ed.), St. Louis: Mosby.

Kliegman, R. (2002). Fetal and neonatal medicine. In R. Behrman & R. Kliegman (Eds.), *Nelson essentials of pediatrics* (4th ed.). Philadelphia: W.B. Saunders.

Knott, C. (2001). Universal newborn hearing screening coming soon: "Hear's why." *Neonatal Network, 20*(8), 25-33.

Lawrence, R. (1999). *Breastfeeding: A guide for the medical profession* (5th ed.). St. Louis: Mosby.

Lissauer, T. (2002). Physical examination and care of the newborn. In A. Fanaroff & R. Martin (Eds.), *Neonatal-perinatal medicine* (7th ed.). St. Louis: Mosby.

Luchtman-Jones, L., Schwartz, A., & Wilson, D. (2002). The blood and hematopoietic system. In A. Fanaroff & R. Martin (Eds.), *Neonatal-perinatal medicine* (7th ed.). St. Louis: Mosby.

Maisels, M. (2001). Neonatal jaundice and kernicterus. *Pediatrics, 108*, 763-765.

Pagana, K., & Pagana, T. (2002). *Mosby's manual of diagnostic and laboratory tests* (2nd ed.). St. Louis: Mosby.

Reiser, D. (2001). Hyperbilirubinemia. *AWHONN Lifelines, 5*(3), 55-61.

Riordan, J. et al. (2000). The effect of labor pain relief medication on neonatal suckling and breastfeeding duration. *Journal of Human Lactation, 16*(1), 7-12.

Scott, J. (2002). Hematology. In R. Behrman & R. Kliegman (Eds.), *Nelson essentials of pediatrics* (4th ed.). Philadelphia: W.B. Saunders.

Wong, D. (1995). *Whaley and Wong's nursing care of infants and children* (5th ed.). St. Louis: Mosby.

Wong, D. (1999). *Whaley and Wong's nursing care of infants and children* (6th ed.). St. Louis: Mosby.

CHAPTER 26

Kathryn Rhodes Alden

Nursing Care of the Newborn

http://evolve.elsevier.com/Lowdermilk/MatWmnHlth/

LEARNING OBJECTIVES

- Identify the purpose and components of the Apgar score.
- Identify the sequence to follow in assessment of the newborn.
- Recognize deviations from normal physiologic findings during examination of the newborn.
- Discuss nursing care management of the newborn in transition to extrauterine life.
- Explain what is meant by a safe environment.
- Discuss phototherapy and the guidelines for teaching parents about this treatment.
- Explain purposes for and methods of circumcision, the postoperative care of the circumcised infant, and parent teaching regarding circumcision.
- Review procedures for doing a heel stick, collecting urine specimens, assisting with venipuncture, and restraining the newborn.
- Evaluate pain in the newborn based on physiologic changes and behavioral observations.

The numerous biologic changes the neonate makes during the transition to extrauterine life are discussed in the preceding chapter. The first 24 hours are critical because respiratory distress and circulatory failure can occur rapidly and with little warning. Although most infants make the necessary biopsychosocial adjustment to extrauterine existence without undue difficulty, their well-being depends on the care they receive from others. This chapter describes assessment and care of the infant immediately after birth until discharge. A discussion of pain in the neonate and its management is included.

CARE MANAGEMENT: FROM BIRTH THROUGH THE FIRST 2 HOURS

Care begins immediately after birth and focuses on assessing and stabilizing the newborn's condition. The nurse has primary responsibility for the infant during this period, because the physician or midwife is involved with delivery of the placenta and caring for the mother. The nurse must be alert for any signs of distress and initiate appropriate interventions.

Assessment and Nursing Diagnoses

The initial assessment of the neonate is done at birth by using the Apgar score (Table 26-1) and a brief physical examination (Box 26-1). A gestational age assessment is done within 2 hours of birth (Fig. 26-1). A more comprehensive physical assessment is completed within 24 hours of birth (Table 26-2).

Apgar Score

The **Apgar score** permits a rapid assessment of the need for resuscitation based on five signs that indicate the physiologic state of the neonate: (1) *heart rate,* based on auscultation with a stethoscope; (2) *respiratory rate,* based on observed movement of the chest wall; (3) *muscle tone,* based on degree of flexion and movement of the extremities; (4) *reflex irritability,* based on response to gentle slaps on the soles of the feet; and (5) *color,* described as pallid, cyanotic, or pink. Each item is scored as a 0, 1, or 2. Evaluations are made 1 and 5 minutes after birth. Scores of 0 to 3 indicate severe distress; scores of 4 to 6 indicate moderate difficulty; and scores of 7 to 10 indicate that the infant should have no difficulty adjusting to extrauterine life. Apgar scores do not predict future neurologic outcome, but the 5-minute score does correlate with the degree of risk for neonatal morbidity and mortality (Casey, McIntire, & Leveno, 2001; Juretschke, 2000).

Initial Physical Assessment

The nurse must anticipate likely variations in the infant at birth based on antenatal conditions and intrapartal events. For example, the nurse must be cognizant of the gesta-

TABLE 26-1 **Apgar Score**

SIGN	SCORE 0	1	2
Heart rate	Absent	Slow (<100)	>100
Respiratory rate	Absent	Slow, weak cry	Good cry
Muscle tone	Flaccid	Some flexion of extremities	Well flexed
Reflex irritability	No response	Grimace	Cry
Color	Blue, pale	Body pink, extremities blue	Completely pink

tional age of the infant, whether the mother is a substance abuser or has diabetes, if the amniotic fluid was meconium stained, or whether forceps were used. Each of these factors may affect the condition of the infant.

The *initial physical assessment* includes a brief review of systems (see Box 26-1):

1. *External:* Note skin color, staining, peeling, or wasting (dysmaturity); note any birthmarks; note length of nails and creases on soles of feet; check for presence of breast tissue; assess nasal patency by covering one nostril at a time while observing respirations and color; note meconium staining of cord, skin, fingernails, or amniotic fluid (staining may indicate fetal hypoxia; offensive odor may indicate intrauterine infection)
2. *Chest:* Palpate for point of maximal impulse (PMI) and auscultate for rate and quality of heart tones and murmurs; note character of respirations and presence of crackles or rhonchi; note equality of breath sounds on each side of chest by holding stethoscope in each axilla
3. *Abdomen:* Verify presence of a rounded abdomen and absence of anomalies; note number of vessels in cord
4. *Neurologic:* Check muscle tone and reflex reaction; assess Moro reflex; palpate anterior fontanel for fullness or bulge; note by palpation the presence and size of the fontanels and sutures
5. *Other observations:* Note gross structural malformations obvious at birth

The initial examination of the newborn can occur while the nurse is drying and wrapping the infant, or observations can be made while the infant is lying on the mother's abdomen or in her arms immediately after birth. Efforts should be directed to minimizing interference in the initial parent-infant acquaintance process. If the infant is breathing easily, has good color, and is normal in appearance, then further examination can be delayed until after the parents have had an opportunity to interact with the infant.

Routine procedures and the admission process can be carried out in the mother's room or in a separate nursery. Box 26-2 on p. 727 shows an example of newborn routine orders.

BOX 26-1 **Initial Physical Assessment by Body System**

CNS [ ] moves extremities, muscle tone good
[ ] symmetric features, movement
[ ] suck, rooting, Moro response, grasp reflexes good
[ ] anterior fontanel soft and flat

CV [ ] heart rate strong and regular
[ ] no murmurs heard
[ ] pulses strong/equal bilaterally

RESP [ ] lungs clear to auscultation bilaterally
[ ] no retractions or nasal flaring
[ ] respiratory rate, 30-60 breaths/min
[ ] chest expansion symmetric
[ ] no upper airway congestion

GU [ ] male: urethral opening at tip of penis; testes descended bilaterally
[ ] female: vaginal opening apparent

GI [ ] abdomen soft, no distention
[ ] cord attached and clamped
[ ] anus appears patent

ENT [ ] eyes clear
[ ] palates intact
[ ] nares patent

SKIN Color [ ] pink [ ] acrocyanotic
[ ] no lesions or abrasions
[ ] no peeling
[ ] birthmarks ____________
[ ] caput/molding
[ ] vacuum "cap"
[ ] forceps marks
[ ] other

Comments:
____
____
____
____
____

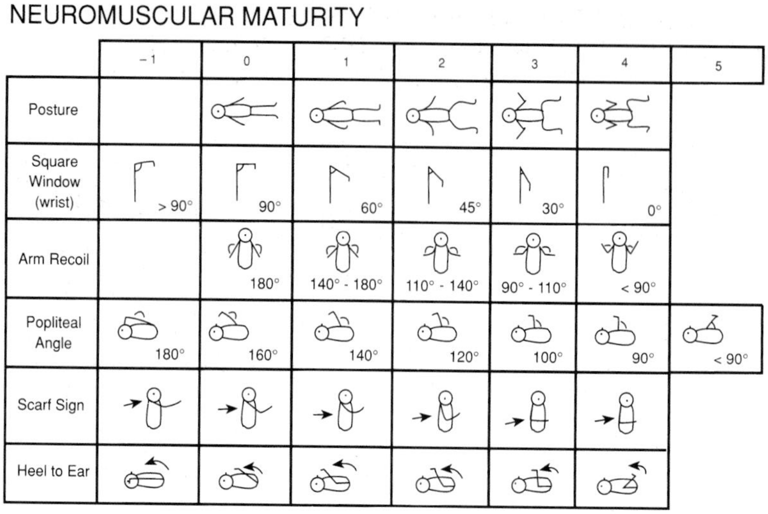

NEUROMUSCULAR MATURITY
-1
0
1
2
3
4
5
Posture
Square Window (wrist)
> 90°
90°
60°
45°
30°
0°
Arm Recoil
180°
140° - 180°
110° - 140°
90° - 110°
< 90°
Popliteal Angle
180°
160°
140°
120°
100°
90°
< 90°
Scarf Sign
Heel to Ear

A PHYSICAL MATURITY

Skin	sticky friable transparent	gelatinous red, translucent	smooth pink, visible veins	superficial peeling or rash, few veins	cracking pale areas rare veins	parchment deep cracking no vessels	leathery cracked wrinkled
Lanugo	none	sparse	abundant	thinning	bald areas	mostly bald	
Plantar Surface	heel-toe 40-50 mm: -1 <40 mm: -2	>50 mm no crease	faint red marks	anterior transverse crease only	creases ant. 2/3	creases over entire sole	
Breast	imperceptible	barely perceptible	flat areola no bud	stippled areola 1-2 mm bud	raised areola 3-4 mm bud	full areola 5-10 mm bud	
Eye/Ear	lids fused loosely: -1 tightly: -2	lids open pinna flat stays folded	sl. curved pinna; soft; slow recoil	well-curved pinna; soft but ready recoil	formed & firm instant recoil	thick cartilage ear stiff	
Genitals (male)	scrotum flat, smooth	scrotum empty faint rugae	testes in upper canal rare rugae	testes descending few rugae	testes down good rugae	testes pendulous deep rugae	
Genitals (female)	clitoris prominent labia flat	prominent clitoris small labia minora	prominent clitoris enlarging minora	majora & minora equally prominent	majora large minora small	majora cover clitoris & minora	

MATURITY RATING

score	weeks
-10	20
-5	22
0	24
5	26
10	28
15	30
20	32
25	34
30	36
35	38
40	40
45	42
50	44

FIG. 26-1 Estimation of gestational age. **A,** New Ballard Scale for newborn maturity rating. Expanded scale includes extremely premature infants and has been refined to improve accuracy in more mature infants. (From Ballard, J. et al. [1991]. New Ballard Score, expanded to include extremely premature infants. *Journal of Pediatrics 119*[3], 417-423.).

Nursing diagnoses are established after analysis of the findings of the physical assessment and may include the following:

- *Ineffective airway clearance related to*
  –airway obstruction with mucus
- *Impaired gas exchange related to*
  –hypothermia
- *Ineffective thermoregulation related to*
  –heat loss to the environment
- *Risk for infection related to*
  –umbilical cord stump
  –fetal scalp electrode sites

Expected Outcomes of Care

Expected outcomes can apply to both the infant and the caregiver. The expected outcomes for the newborn during the immediate recovery period include that the infant will achieve the following:

- Maintain effective breathing patterns.
- Maintain effective thermoregulation.
- Remain free from infection.
- Receive necessary nutrition for growth.

Expected outcomes for the parents include that they will do the following:

- Begin to attain knowledge, skill, and confidence relevant to infant care activities.
- Begin to integrate the infant into the family.

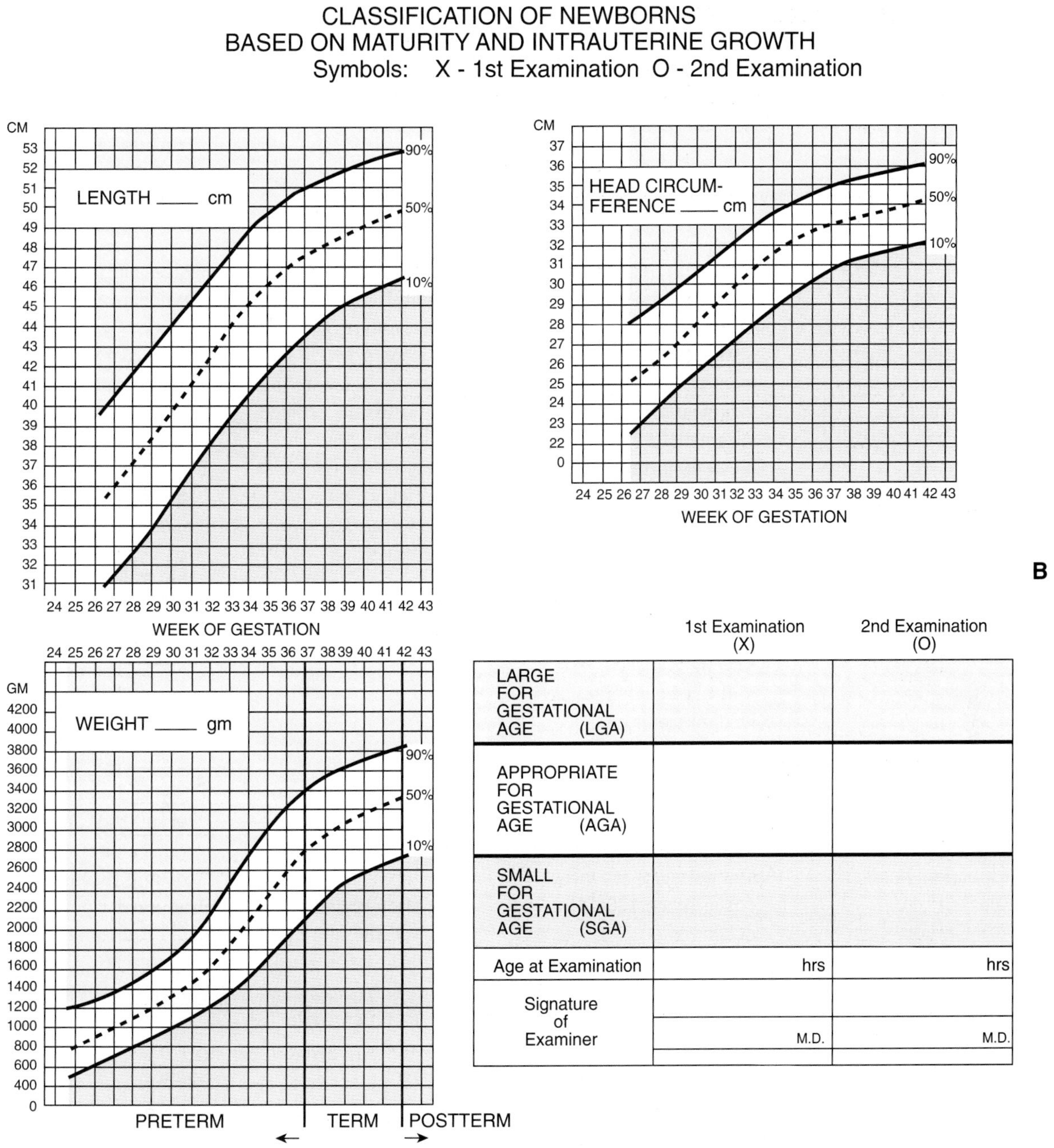
CLASSIFICATION OF NEWBORNS
BASED ON MATURITY AND INTRAUTERINE GROWTH
Symbols: X - 1st Examination O - 2nd Examination
CM
LENGTH ____ cm
90%
50%
10%
WEEK OF GESTATION
HEAD CIRCUM-
FERENCE ____ cm
B
GM
WEIGHT ____ gm
PRETERM
TERM
POSTTERM
1st Examination (X)
2nd Examination (O)
LARGE FOR GESTATIONAL AGE (LGA)
APPROPRIATE FOR GESTATIONAL AGE (AGA)
SMALL FOR GESTATIONAL AGE (SGA)
Age at Examination
hrs
hrs
Signature of Examiner
M.D.
M.D.

FIG. 26-1, cont'd Estimation of gestational age. **B,** Newborn classification based on maturity and intrauterine growth. (Modified from Lubchenco, L., Hansman, C., & Boyd, E. [1966]. Intrauterine growth in length and head circumference as estimated from live births at gestational ages from 26 to 42 weeks. *Journal of Pediatrics, 37*[3], 403-408; and Battaglia, F., & Lubchenco, L. [1967]. A practical classification of newborn infants by weight and gestational age. *Journal of Pediatrics, 71*[2], 159-167.)

Plan of Care and Interventions

Changes can occur rapidly in newborns immediately after birth. Assessment must be followed quickly by the implementation of appropriate care.

Stabilization and Resuscitation

Generally, the normal term infant born vaginally has little difficulty clearing the air passages. Most secretions are moved by gravity and brought to the oropharynx by the cough reflex, to be drained or swallowed. If the infant has excess mucus in the respiratory tract, the mouth and nasal passages may be suctioned with a bulb syringe (see Procedure box and Fig. 26-2 on p. 727); routine suctioning is not necessary (Waltman, 2000). The nurse may perform gentle percussion over the chest wall by using a soft circular mask or a percussion cup to aid in loosening secretions before suctioning (Fig. 26-3 on p. 727). The infant who is coughing and choking on the secretions

Text continued on p. 726

TABLE 26-2 **Physical Assessment of Newborn**

AREA ASSESSED AND APPRAISAL PROCEDURE	NORMAL FINDINGS		DEVIATIONS FROM NORMAL RANGE: POSSIBLE PROBLEMS (ETIOLOGY)
	AVERAGE FINDINGS	NORMAL VARIATONS	
Posture			
Inspect newborn before disturbing for assessment Refer to maternal chart for fetal presentation, position, and type of birth (vaginal, surgical), because newborn readily assumes prenatal position	Vertex: arms, legs in moderate flexion; fists clenched Resistance to having extremities extended for examination or measurement, crying possible when attempted Cessation of crying when allowed to resume curled-up fetal position Normal spontaneous movement bilaterally asynchronous (legs moving in bicycle fashion) but equal extension in all extremities	Frank breech: legs straighter and stiff, newborn assuming intrauterine position in repose for a few days Prenatal pressure on limb or shoulder possibly causing temporary facial asymmetry or resistance to extension of extremities	Hypotonia, relaxed posture while awake (prematurity or hypoxia in utero, maternal medications) Hypertonia (drug dependence, central nervous system [CNS] disorder) Opisthotonos (CNS disturbance) Limitation of motion in any of extremities (see pp. 724-725)
Vital Signs			
Check heart rate and pulses: Thorax (chest) Inspection Palpation Auscultation Apex: mitral valve Second interspace, left of sternum: pulmonic valve Second interspace, right of sternum: aortic valve Junction of xiphoid process and sternum: tricuspid valve	Visible pulsations in left midclavicular line, fifth intercostal space Apical pulse, fourth intercostal space 120-160 beats/min Quality: *first sound* (closure of mitral and tricuspid valves) and *second sound* (closure of aortic and pulmonic valves) sharp and clear	100 beats/min (sleeping) to 180 beats/min (crying); possibly irregular for brief periods, especially after crying Murmurs, especially over base or at left sternal border in interspace 3 or 4 (foramen ovale anatomically closing at ~1 yr)	Tachycardia: persistent, ≥160 beats/min (respiratory distress syndrome [RDS]) Bradycardia: persistent, ≤120 beats/min (congenital heart block) Murmurs (possibly functional) Arrhythmias: irregular rate Sounds Distant (pneumomediastinum) Poor quality Extra Heart on right side of chest: Dextrocardia, often accompanied by reversal of intestines
For femoral pulse palpation, place fingers along inguinal ligament about midway between symphysis pubis and iliac crest; feel bilaterally simultaneously	Femoral pulses equal and strong		Weak or absent femoral pulses (hip dysplasia, coarctation of aorta, thrombophlebitis)

TABLE 26-2 **Physical Assessment of Newborn—cont'd**

AREA ASSESSED AND APPRAISAL PROCEDURE	NORMAL FINDINGS		DEVIATIONS FROM NORMAL RANGE: POSSIBLE PROBLEMS (ETIOLOGY)
	AVERAGE FINDINGS	NORMAL VARIATONS	
Vital Signs—cont'd			
Obtain temperature: Axillary: method of choice until age 6 yr Electronic: thermistor probe (avoid taping over bony area)	Axillary: 37° C Temperature stabilized by 8-10 hr of age Undeveloped shivering mechanism	36.5° C to 37.2° C Heat loss: 200 kcal/kg/min from evaporation, conduction, convection, radiation	Subnormal (prematurity, infection, low environmental temperature, inadequate clothing, dehydration) Increased (infection, high environmental temperature, excessive clothing, proximity to heating unit or in direct sunshine, drug addiction, diarrhea and dehydration) Temperature not stabilized by 10 hr after birth (if mother received magnesium sulfate, newborn less able to conserve heat by vasoconstriction; maternal analgesics possibly reducing thermal stability in newborn)
Check respiratory rate and effort:			
Observe respirations when infant is at rest Count respirations for full minute Check apnea monitor Listen for sounds audible without stethoscope Observe respiratory effort	40 breaths/min Tendency to be shallow and irregular in rate, rhythm, and depth when infant is awake No sounds audible on inspiration or expiration Breath sounds: bronchial; loud, clear, near	30-60 breaths/min Possibly appearing to be Cheyne-Stokes with short periods of apnea and no evidence of respiratory distress First period (reactivity): 50-60/min Second period: 50-70/min Stabilization (1-2 days): 30-40/min	Apneic episodes: >15 sec (preterm infant: "periodic breathing," rapid warming or cooling of infant) Bradypnea: <25/min (maternal narcosis from analgesics or anesthetics, birth trauma) Tachypnea: >60/min (RDS, aspiration syndrome, diaphragmatic hernia) Sounds Crackles, rhonchi, wheezes (fluid in lungs) Expiratory grunt (narrowing of bronchi) Distress evidenced by nasal flaring, retractions, chin tug, labored breathing (RDS, fluid in lungs)

Continued

TABLE 26-2 **Physical Assessment of Newborn—cont'd**

AREA ASSESSED AND APPRAISAL PROCEDURE	NORMAL FINDINGS: AVERAGE FINDINGS	NORMAL FINDINGS: NORMAL VARIATONS	DEVIATIONS FROM NORMAL RANGE: POSSIBLE PROBLEMS (ETIOLOGY)
Vital Signs—cont'd			
Attain blood pressure (BP) (usually assessed only if a problem is suspected) Check electronic monitor BP cuff: BP cuff width affects readings, use cuff 2.5 cm wide and palpate radial pulse	78/42 (approximately) At birth Systolic: 60-80 mm Hg Diastolic: 40-50 mm Hg At 10 days Systolic: 95-100 mm Hg Diastolic: slight increase	Variation with change in activity level: awake, crying, sleeping	Difference between upper and lower extremity pressures (coarctation of aorta) Hypotension (sepsis, hypovolemia) Hypertension (coarctation of aorta)
Weight*			
Put protective liner cloth or paper in place and adjust scale to 0 Weigh at same time each day Protect newborn from heat loss	Female, 3400 g Male, 3500 g Regain birth weight within first 2 weeks	2500-4000 g Acceptable weight loss: ≤10% Second baby weighs more than first	Weight ≤2500 g (prematurity, small for gestational age, rubella syndrome) Weight ≥4000 g (large for gestational age, maternal diabetes, heredity—normal for these parents) Weight loss >10% (dehydration)
Length			
Measure length from top of head to heel; measuring is difficult in term infant because of presence of molding, incomplete extension of knees	50 cm	45-55 cm	<45 cm or >55 cm (chromosomal aberration, heredity—normal for these parents)

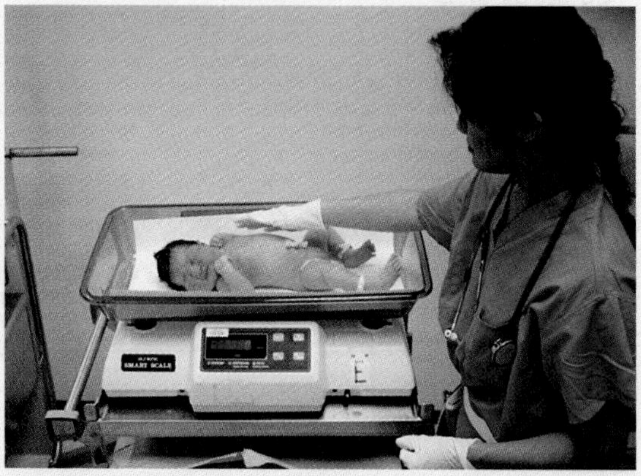

Weighing the infant. Note that a hand is held over infant as a safety measure. The scale is covered to protect against cross infection. (Courtesy Kim Molloy, Knoxville, IA.)

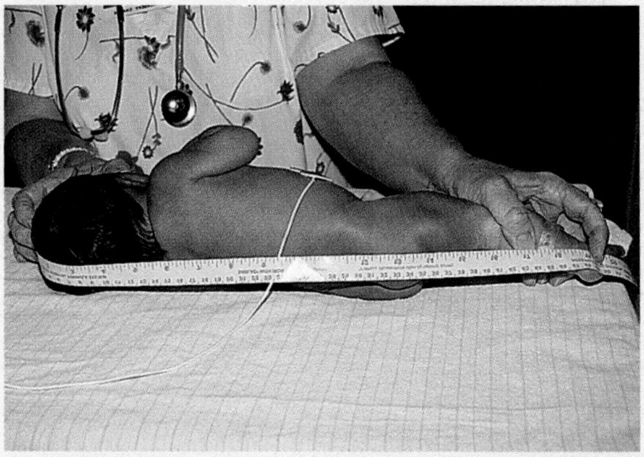

Length, crown to rump. To determine total length, include length of legs. If measurements are taken before the infant's initial bath, wear gloves. (Courtesy Marjorie Pyle, RNC, Lifecircle, Costa Mesa, CA.)

*Note: Weight, length, and head circumference all should be close to the same percentile for any newborn.

TABLE 26-2 **Physical Assessment of Newborn—cont'd**

AREA ASSESSED AND APPRAISAL PROCEDURE	NORMAL FINDINGS: AVERAGE FINDINGS	NORMAL FINDINGS: NORMAL VARIATONS	DEVIATIONS FROM NORMAL RANGE: POSSIBLE PROBLEMS (ETIOLOGY)
Head Circumference			
Measure head at greatest diameter: occipitofrontal circumference May need to remeasure on second or third day after resolution of molding and caput succedaneum	33-35 cm Circumference of head and chest approximately the same for first 1 or 2 days after birth	32-36.8 cm	Small head ≤32 cm: microcephaly (rubella, toxoplasmosis, cytomegalic inclusion disease) Hydrocephaly: sutures widely separated, circumference ≥4 cm more than chest circumference Increased intracranial pressure (hemorrhage, space-occupying lesion)
Chest Circumference			
Measure at nipple line	2-3 cm less than head circumference, averages between 30 and 33 cm		≤30 cm (prematurity)

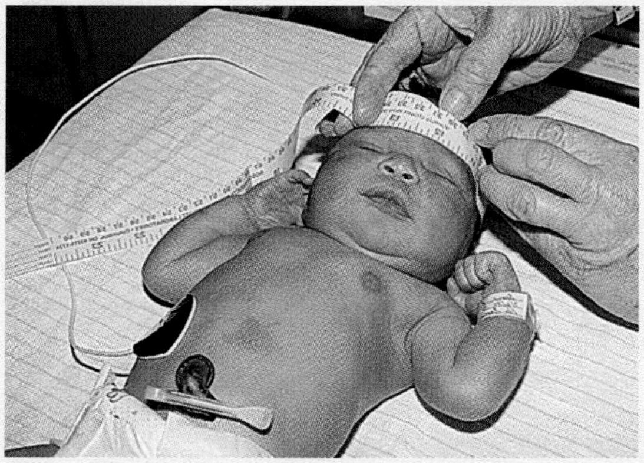

Circumference of head. (Courtesy Marjorie Pyle, RNC, Lifecircle, Costa Mesa, CA.)

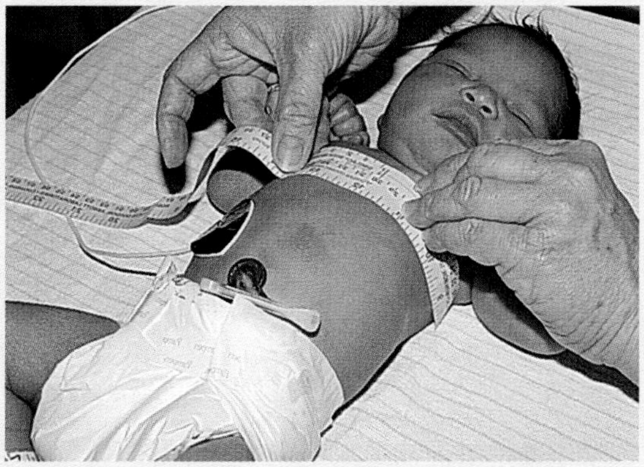

Circumference of chest. (Courtesy Marjorie Pyle, RNC, Lifecircle, Costa Mesa, CA.)

AREA ASSESSED AND APPRAISAL PROCEDURE	NORMAL FINDINGS: AVERAGE FINDINGS	NORMAL FINDINGS: NORMAL VARIATONS	DEVIATIONS FROM NORMAL RANGE: POSSIBLE PROBLEMS (ETIOLOGY)
Abdominal Circumference			
Not usually measured unless specific indication	Abdomen enlargement after feeding because of lax abdominal muscles Same size as chest		Enlarging abdomen between feedings (abdominal mass or blockage in intestinal tract)

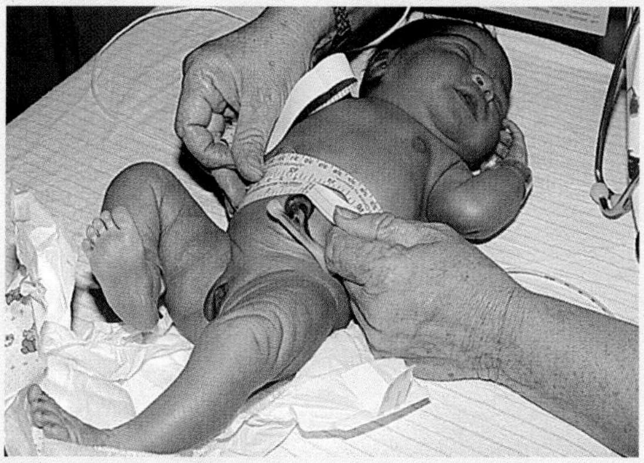

Abdominal circumference. (Courtesy Marjorie Pyle, RNC, Lifecircle, Costa Mesa, CA.)

Continued

TABLE 26-2 **Physical Assessment of Newborn—cont'd**

AREA ASSESSED AND APPRAISAL PROCEDURE	NORMAL FINDINGS		DEVIATIONS FROM NORMAL RANGE: POSSIBLE PROBLEMS (ETIOLOGY)
	AVERAGE FINDINGS	NORMAL VARIATONS	
Skin			
Check color: Inspect and palpate Inspect naked newborn in well-lit, warm area without drafts; natural daylight provides best lighting Inspect newborn when quiet and when active	Generally pink Varying with ethnic origin, skin pigmentation beginning to deepen right after birth in basal layer of epidermis Acrocyanosis, especially if chilled	Mottling Harlequin sign Plethora Telangiectases ("stork bites" or capillary hemangiomas) (see Fig. 25-7, *A*) Erythema toxicum/ neonatorum ("newborn rash") (see Fig. 25-7, *B*) Milia	Dark red (prematurity, polycythemia) Pallor (cardiovascular problem, CNS damage, blood dyscrasia, blood loss, twin-to-twin transfusion, nosocomial infection) Cyanosis (hypothermia, infection, hypoglycemia, cardiopulmonary diseases, cardiac, neurologic, or respiratory malformations)
		Petechiae over presenting part	Petechiae over any other area (clotting factor deficiency, infection)
		Ecchymoses from forceps in vertex births or over buttocks, genitalia, and legs in breech births	Ecchymoses in any other area (hemorrhagic disease, traumatic birth)
Check for jaundice	None at birth	Physiologic jaundice in 50% of term infants after first 24 hr	Gray (hypotension, poor perfusion) Jaundice within first 24 hr (Rh isoimmunization)
Check birthmarks: Inspect and palpate for location, size, distribution, characteristics, color	Transient hyperpigmentation Areolae Genitals Linea nigra	Mongolian spotting (see Fig. 25-6) Infants of African-American, Asian, and Native American origin: 70% Infants of Caucasian origin: 9%	Hemangiomas Nevus flammeus: port-wine stain Nevus vasculosus: strawberry mark Cavernous hemangiomas
Check condition: Inspect and palpate for intactness, smoothness, texture, edema	No skin edema Opacity: few large blood vessels visible indistinctly over abdomen	Slightly thick; superficial cracking, peeling, especially of hands, feet No visible blood vessels, a few large vessels clearly visible over abdomen Some fingernail scratches	Edema on hands, feet; pitting over tibia Texture thin, smooth, or of medium thickness; rash or superficial peeling visible Numerous vessels very visible over abdomen (prematurity) Texture thick, parchment-like; cracking, peeling (postmaturity) Skin tags, webbing Papules, pustules, vesicles, ulcers, maceration (impetigo, candidiasis, herpes, diaper rash)

TABLE 26-2 **Physical Assessment of Newborn—cont'd**

AREA ASSESSED AND APPRAISAL PROCEDURE	NORMAL FINDINGS: AVERAGE FINDINGS	NORMAL FINDINGS: NORMAL VARIATONS	DEVIATIONS FROM NORMAL RANGE: POSSIBLE PROBLEMS (ETIOLOGY)
Skin—cont'd			
Assess hydration and consistency			
Weigh infant routinely Inspect and palpate Gently pinch skin between thumb and forefinger over abdomen and inner thigh to check for turgor Check subcutaneous fat deposits (adipose pads) over cheeks, buttocks	Dehydration: loss of weight best indicator After pinch released, skin returns to original state immediately	Normal weight loss after birth: $\leq$10% of birth weight Possibly puffy Variation in amount of subcutaneous fat	Loose, wrinkled skin (prematurity, postmaturity, dehydration: fold of skin persisting after release of pinch) Tense, tight, shiny skin (edema, extreme cold, shock, infection) Lack of subcutaneous fat, prominence of clavicle or ribs (prematurity, malnutrition)
Check voiding	Voiding within 24 hr of birth Voiding 6-10 times per day after 4 days of life		
Check vernix caseosa:			
Observe amount		Variation in amount; usually more found in creases, folds	Absent or minimal (postmaturity) Excessive (prematurity)
Observe its color and odor before bath or wiping	Whitish, cheesy, odorless		Yellow color (possible fetal anoxia > 36 hr before birth, Rh or ABO incompatibility) Green color (possible in utero release of meconium or presence of bilirubin) Odor (possible intrauterine infection)
Assess lanugo:			
Inspect for this fine, downy hair, including its amount, distribution	Over shoulders, pinnas of ears, forehead	Variation in amount	Absent (postmaturity) Excessive (prematurity, especially if lanugo abundant and long and thick over back)
Head			
Palpate skin	See Skin	Caput succedaneum, possibly showing some ecchymosis (see Fig. 25-5, *A*)	Cephalhematoma (see Fig. 25-5, *B*)
Inspect shape, size	Making up one fourth of body length Molding (see Fig. 25-9)	Slight asymmetry from intrauterine position Lack of molding (prematurity, breech presentation, cesarean birth)	Molding Severe molding (birth trauma) Indentation (fracture from trauma) (see Fig. 38-3)

Continued

TABLE 26-2 **Physical Assessment of Newborn—cont'd**

AREA ASSESSED AND APPRAISAL PROCEDURE	NORMAL FINDINGS: AVERAGE FINDINGS	NORMAL FINDINGS: NORMAL VARIATONS	DEVIATIONS FROM NORMAL RANGE: POSSIBLE PROBLEMS (ETIOLOGY)
Head—cont'd			
Palpate, inspect, measure fontanels	Anterior fontanel 5 cm diamond, increasing as molding resolves Posterior fontanel triangle, smaller than anterior	Variation in fontanel size with degree of molding Difficulty in feeling fontanels possible because of molding	Fontanels Full, bulging (tumor, hemorrhage, infection) Large, flat, soft (malnutrition, hydrocephaly, retarded bone age, hypothyroidism) Depressed (dehydration)
Palpate sutures	Palpable and unjoined sutures	Possible overlap of sutures with molding	Sutures Widely spaced (hydrocephaly) Premature closure
Inspect pattern, distribution, amount of hair; feel texture	Silky, single strands lying flat; growth pattern toward face and neck	Variation in amount	Fine, woolly (prematurity) Unusual swirls, patterns, hairline or coarse, brittle (endocrine or genetic disorders)
Eyes			
Check placement on face	Eyes and space between eyes each one third the distance from outer-to-outer canthus	Epicanthal folds: normal racial characteristic	Epicanthal folds when present with other signs (chromosomal disorders such as Down, *cri-du-chat* syndromes)
Check for symmetry in size, shape	Symmetric in size, shape		
Check eyelids for size, movements, blink	Blink reflex	Edema if silver nitrate instilled; also may occur with instillation of erythromycin and tetracycline	
Assess for discharge	None	Some discharge if silver nitrate used	Discharge: purulent (infection)
Evaluate eyeballs for size, shape	No tears Both present and of equal size, both round, firm	Occasional presence of some tears Subconjunctival hemorrhage	Agenesis or absence of one or both eyeballs Small eyeball (rubella syndrome)

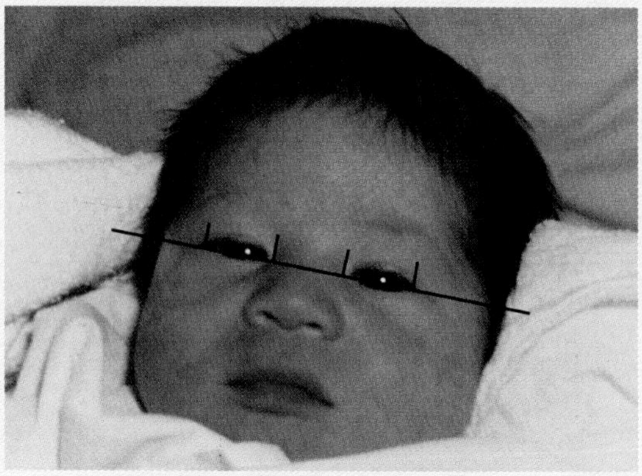

Eyes. In pseudostrabismus, inner epicanthal folds cause the eyes to appear misaligned; however, corneal light reflexes are perfectly symmetric. Eyes are symmetric in size and shape and are well placed.

TABLE 26-2 **Physical Assessment of Newborn—cont'd**

AREA ASSESSED AND APPRAISAL PROCEDURE	NORMAL FINDINGS: AVERAGE FINDINGS	NORMAL FINDINGS: NORMAL VARIATONS	DEVIATIONS FROM NORMAL RANGE: POSSIBLE PROBLEMS (ETIOLOGY)
Eyes—cont'd			Lens opacity or absence of red reflex (congenital cataracts, possibly from rubella) Lesions: coloboma, absence of part of iris (congenital) Pink color of iris (albinism) Jaundiced sclera (hyperbilirubinemia)
Check pupils	Present, equal in size, reactive to light		Pupils: unequal, constricted, dilated, fixed (intracranial pressure, medications, tumors)
Evaluate eyeball movement	Random, jerky, uneven, focus possible briefly, following to midline	Transient strabismus or nystagmus until third or fourth month	Persistent strabismus Doll's eyes (increased intracranial pressure) Sunset (increased intracranial pressure)
Assess eyebrows: amount of hair, pattern	Distinct (not connected in midline)		Connection in midline (Cornelia de Lange syndrome)
Nose			
Observe shape, placement, patency, configuration of bridge of nose	Midline Apparent lack of bridge, flat, broad Some mucus but no drainage Preferential nose breather Sneezing to clear nose	Slight deformity from passage through birth canal	Copious drainage, with or without regular periods of cyanosis at rest and return of pink color with crying (choanal atresia, congenital syphilis) Malformed (congenital syphilis, chromosomal disorder) Flaring of nares (respiratory distress)
Ears			
Observe size, placement on head, amount of cartilage, open auditory canal	Correct placement: line drawn through inner and outer canthi of eyes reaching to top notch of ears (at junction with scalp) Well-formed, firm cartilage	Size: small, large, floppy Darwin's tubercle (nodule on posterior helix)	Agenesis Lack of cartilage (prematurity) Low placement (chromosomal disorder, mental retardation, kidney disorder) Preauricular tags Size: possibly overly prominent or protruding ears
Assess hearing	Responses to voice and other sounds	State (e.g., alert, asleep) influencing response	Deaf: no response to sound

Continued

TABLE 26-2 **Physical Assessment of Newborn—cont'd**

Ears—cont'd

A B C

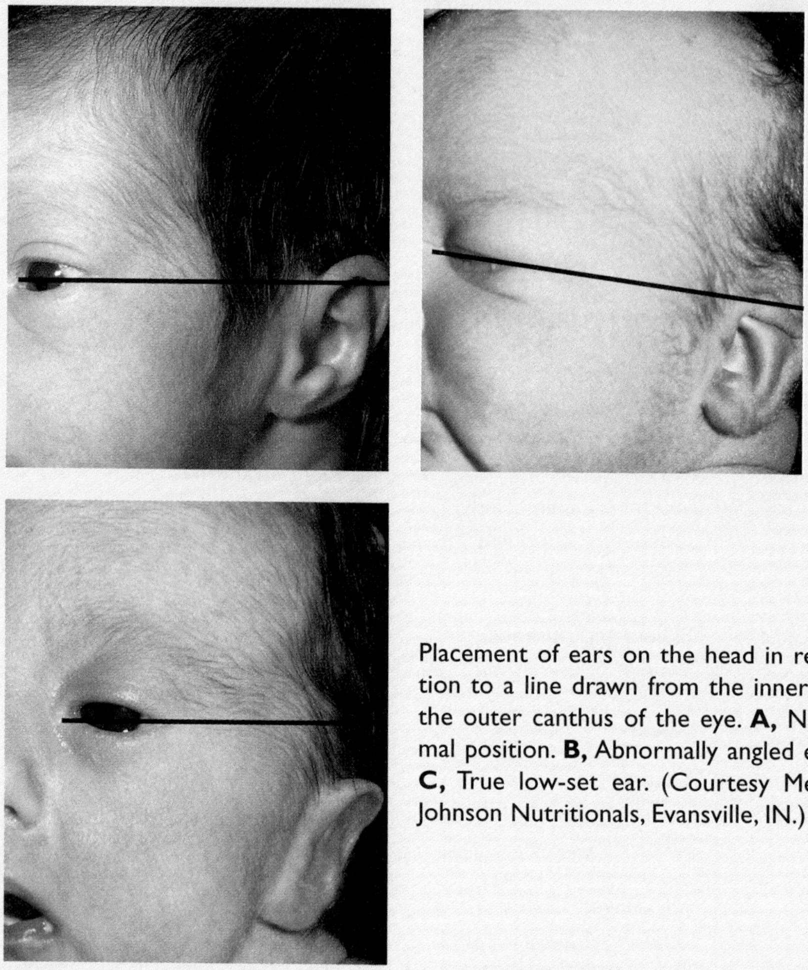

Placement of ears on the head in relation to a line drawn from the inner to the outer canthus of the eye. **A,** Normal position. **B,** Abnormally angled ear. **C,** True low-set ear. (Courtesy Mead Johnson Nutritionals, Evansville, IN.)

AREA ASSESSED AND APPRAISAL PROCEDURE	NORMAL FINDINGS: AVERAGE FINDINGS	NORMAL FINDINGS: NORMAL VARIATONS	DEVIATIONS FROM NORMAL RANGE: POSSIBLE PROBLEMS (ETIOLOGY)
Facies			
Observe overall appearance of face	"Normal" appearance, well-placed, proportionate, symmetric features	Positional deformities	Infant appearance "odd" or "funny" Usually accompanied by other features such as low-set ears, other structural disorders (hereditary, chromosomal aberration)
Mouth			
Inspect and palpate Check placement on face Assess lips for color, configuration, movement	Symmetry of lip movement	Transient circumoral cyanosis	Gross anomalies in placement, size, shape (cleft lip and/or palate, gums) Cyanosis, circumoral pallor (respiratory distress, hypothermia) Asymmetry in movement of lips (cranial nerve VII paralysis)

TABLE 26-2 **Physical Assessment of Newborn—cont'd**

AREA ASSESSED AND APPRAISAL PROCEDURE	NORMAL FINDINGS: AVERAGE FINDINGS	NORMAL FINDINGS: NORMAL VARIATONS	DEVIATIONS FROM NORMAL RANGE: POSSIBLE PROBLEMS (ETIOLOGY)
Mouth—cont'd			
Check gums	Pink gums	Inclusion cysts (Epstein pearls—Bohn nodules, whitish, hard nodules on gums or roof of mouth)	Teeth: predeciduous or deciduous (hereditary)
Assess tongue for attachment, mobility, movement, size	Tongue not protruding, freely movable, symmetric in shape, movement	Short frenulum	Macroglossia (prematurity, chromosomal disorder)
Evaluate cheeks	Sucking pads inside cheeks		Thrush: white plaques on cheeks or tongue that bleed if touched (*Candida albicans*)
Assess palate (soft, hard): Arch Uvula	Soft and hard palates intact Uvula in midline	Anatomic groove in palate to accommodate nipple, disappearance by 3 to 4 yr of age Epstein pearls	Cleft hard or soft palate
Assess chin	Distinct chin		Micrognathia (Pierre Robin or other syndrome)
Evaluate saliva for amount, character	Mouth moist		Excessive saliva (esophageal atresia, tracheoesophageal fistula)
Check reflexes: Rooting Sucking Extrusion	Reflexes present	Reflex response dependent on state of wakefulness and hunger	Absent (prematurity)
Neck			
Inspect and palpate length	Short, thick, surrounded by skin folds; no webbing		Webbing (Turner syndrome)
Check sternocleidomastoid muscles, movement and position of head	Head held in midline (sternocleidomastoid muscles equal), no masses Freedom of movement from side to side and flexion and extension, no movement of chin past shoulder	Transient positional deformity apparent when newborn is at rest: passive movement of head possible	Restricted movement, holding of head at angle (torticollis [wryneck], opisthotonos) Absence of head control (prematurity, Down syndrome)
Assess trachea for position and thyroid gland	Thyroid not palpable		Masses (enlarged thyroid) Distended veins (cardiopulmonary disorder)
Chest			
Inspect and palpate Shape	Almost circular, barrel shaped	Tip of sternum possibly prominent	Bulging of chest, unequal movement (pneumothorax, pneumomediastinum) Malformation (funnel chest—pectus excavatum)
Check respiratory movements	Symmetric chest movements, chest and abdominal movements synchronized during respirations	Occasional retractions, especially when crying	Retractions with or without respiratory distress (prematurity, RDS)

Continued

AREA ASSESSED AND APPRAISAL PROCEDURE	NORMAL FINDINGS		DEVIATIONS FROM NORMAL RANGE: POSSIBLE PROBLEMS (ETIOLOGY)
	AVERAGE FINDINGS	NORMAL VARIATONS	
Chest—cont'd			
Evaluate clavicles	Clavicles intact		Fracture of clavicle (trauma); crepitus (see Fig. 38-4)
Assess ribs	Rib cage symmetric, intact; moves with respirations		Poor development of rib cage and musculature (prematurity)
Assess nipples for size, placement, number	Nipples prominent, well formed; symmetrically placed		Nipples Supernumerary, along nipple line Malpositioned or widely spaced
Check breast tissue	Breast nodule: approximately 6 mm in term infant	Breast nodule: 3-10 mm Secretion of witch's milk	Lack of breast tissue (prematurity)
Auscultate: Heart sounds and rate and breath sounds (see Vital signs)			Sounds: bowel sounds (see Abdomen, below)
Abdomen			
Inspect, palpate, and smell umbilical cord	Two arteries, one vein Whitish gray Definite demarcation between cord and skin, no intestinal structures within cord Dry around base, drying Odorless		One artery (renal anomalies) Meconium stained (intrauterine distress) Bleeding or oozing around cord (hemorrhagic disease) Redness or drainage around cord (infection, possible persistence of urachus)
	Cord clamp in place for 24 hr	Reducible umbilical herniation	Hernia: herniation of abdominal contents into area of cord (e.g., omphalocele); defect covered with thin, friable membrane, possibly extensive
Inspect size of abdomen and palpate contour	Rounded, prominent, dome-shaped because abdominal musculature not fully developed Liver possibly palpable 1-2 cm below right costal margin No other masses palpable No distention	Some diastasis of abdominal musculature	Gastroschisis: fissure of abdominal cavity Distention at birth (ruptured viscus, genitourinary masses or malformations: hydronephrosis, teratomas, abdominal tumors) Mild (overfeeding, high gastrointestinal tract obstruction) Marked (lower gastrointestinal tract obstruction, imperforate anus) Intermittent or transient (overfeeding) Partial intestinal obstruction (stenosis of bowel)

AREA ASSESSED AND APPRAISAL PROCEDURE	NORMAL FINDINGS: AVERAGE FINDINGS	NORMAL FINDINGS: NORMAL VARIATONS	DEVIATIONS FROM NORMAL RANGE: POSSIBLE PROBLEMS (ETIOLOGY)
Abdomen—cont'd			Visible peristalsis (obstruction) Malrotation of bowel or adhesions Sepsis (infection)
Auscultate bowel sounds and note number, amount, and character of stools; note behavior—crying, fussiness—before or during elimination	Sounds present within 1-2 hr after birth Meconium stool passing within 24-48 hr after birth		Scaphoid, with bowel sounds in chest and respiratory distress (diaphragmatic hernia)
Assess color		Linea nigra possibly apparent and caused by hormone influence during pregnancy	
Check movement with respiration	Respirations primarily diaphragmatic, abdominal and chest movement synchronous		Decreased abdominal breathing (intrathoracic disease, diaphragmatic hernia) "Seesaw" (respiratory distress)
Genitalia			
Female (see Fig. 25-8)			
Inspect and palpate General appearance Clitoris Labia majora	Female genitals Usually edematous Usually edematous, covering labia minora in term newborns	Increased pigmentation caused by pregnancy hormones Edema and ecchymosis after breech birth	Ambiguous genitals—enlarged clitoris with urinary meatus on tip, fused labia (chromosomal disorder, maternal drug ingestion) Stenosed meatus
Labia minora	Possible protrusion over labia majora	Blood-tinged discharge from pseudomenstruation caused by pregnancy hormones	
Discharge Vagina	Smegma Open orifice Mucoid discharge Hymenal/vaginal tag	Some vernix caseosa between labia possible	Labia majora widely separated and labia minora prominent (prematurity) Absence of vaginal orifice or imperforate hymen Fecal discharge (fistula)
Urinary meatus	Beneath clitoris, difficult to see—to watch for voiding	Rust-stained urine (uric acid crystals)*	
Male (see Fig. 25-8)			
Inspect and palpate General appearance Penis Urinary meatus as slit	Male genitals Meatus at tip of penis	Increased size and pigmentation caused by pregnancy hormones	Ambiguous genitals Urinary meatus not on tip of glans penis (hypospadias, epispadias) Round meatal opening

*To determine whether rust color is caused by uric acid or blood, rinse diaper under running warm tap water; uric acid washes out, blood does not.

Continued

TABLE 26-2 **Physical Assessment of Newborn—cont'd**

AREA ASSESSED AND APPRAISAL PROCEDURE	NORMAL FINDINGS		DEVIATIONS FROM NORMAL RANGE: POSSIBLE PROBLEMS (ETIOLOGY)
	AVERAGE FINDINGS	NORMAL VARIATONS	
Genitalia—cont'd			
Male—cont'd			
Prepuce	Prepuce (foreskin) covering glans penis and not retractable	Prepuce removed if circumcised Wide variation in size of genitals	
Scrotum Rugae (wrinkles)	Large, edematous, pendulous in term infant; covered with rugae	Scrotal edema and ecchymosis if breech birth Hydrocele, small, noncommunicating	Scrotum smooth and testes undescended (prematurity, cryptorchidism) Hydrocele Inguinal hernia
Testes	Palpable on each side	Bulge palpable in inguinal canal	Undescended (prematurity)
Check urination	Voiding within 24 hr, stream adequate, amount adequate	Rust-stained urine (uric acid crystals)*	
Check reflexes:			
Erection	Erection possibly occurring spontaneously and when genitals touched		
Cremasteric	Testes retracted, especially when newborn is chilled		
Extremities			
Make a general check: Inspect and palpate Degree of flexion Range of motion Symmetry of motion Muscle tone	Assuming of position maintained in utero Attitude of general flexion Full range of motion, spontaneous movements	Transient (positional) deformities	Limited motion (malformations) Poor muscle tone (prematurity, maternal medications, CNS anomalies) Positive scarf sign
Check arms and hands: Inspect and palpate Color Intactness Appropriate placement	Longer than legs in newborn period Contours and movement symmetric	Slight tremors sometimes apparent Some acrocyanosis, especially when chilled	Asymmetry of movement (fracture/crepitus, brachial nerve trauma, malformations) Asymmetry of contour (malformations, fracture) Amelia or phocomelia (teratogens) Palmar creases Simian line with short, incurved little fingers (Down syndrome)
Check number of fingers	Five on each hand Fist often clenched with thumb under fingers		Webbing of fingers: syndactyly Absence or excess of fingers Strong, rigid flexion; persistent fists; positioning of fists in front of mouth constantly (CNS disorder)

*To determine whether rust color is caused by uric acid or blood, rinse diaper under running warm tap water; uric acid washes out, blood does not.

TABLE 26-2 **Physical Assessment of Newborn—cont'd**

AREA ASSESSED AND APPRAISAL PROCEDURE	NORMAL FINDINGS: AVERAGE FINDINGS	NORMAL FINDINGS: NORMAL VARIATONS	DEVIATIONS FROM NORMAL RANGE: POSSIBLE PROBLEMS (ETIOLOGY)
Extremities—cont'd			
Palpate humerus	Intact		Fractured humerus
Evaluate joints Shoulder Elbow Wrist Fingers	Full range of motion, symmetric contour		Increased tonicity, clonicity, prolonged tremors (CNS disorder)
Check reflex: grasp			
Check legs and feet:			
Inspect and palpate Color Intactness Length in relation to arms and body and to each other	Appearance of bowing because lateral muscles more developed than medial muscles	Feet appearing to turn in but can be easily rotated externally, positional defects tending to correct while infant is crying	Amelia (or absence of limbs), phocomelia (or shortened limbs) (chromosomal defect, teratogenic effect)
Number of toes	Five on each foot	Acrocyanosis	Webbing, syndactyly (chromosomal defect) Absence or excess of digits (chromosomal defect, familial trait)
Femur	Intact femur		Femoral fracture (difficult breech birth)
Head of femur as legs are flexed and abducted, placement in acetabulum (see Fig. 25-12)	No click heard, femoral head not overriding acetabulum		Congenital hip dysplasia/dislocation
Major gluteal folds	Major gluteal folds even		
Soles of feet	Soles well lined (or wrinkled) over two thirds of foot in term infants		Soles of feet Few lines (prematurity) Covered with lines (postmaturity)
	Plantar fat pad giving flat-footed effect		Congenital clubfoot Hypermobility of joints (Down syndrome)
Evaluate joints Hip Knee Ankle Toes	Full range of motion, symmetric contour		Yellowed nail beds (meconium staining) Temperature of one leg differing from that of the other (circulatory deficiency, CNS disorder)
Check reflexes (see Table 25-3)			Asymmetric movement (trauma, CNS disorder)
Back			
Assess anatomy:			
Inspect and palpate Spine Shoulders Scapulae Iliac crests Base of spine—pilonidal area	Spine straight and easily flexed Infant able to raise and support head momentarily when prone Shoulders, scapulae, and iliac crests lining up in same plane	Temporary minor positional deformities, correction with passive manipulation	Limitation of movement (fusion or deformity of vertebra) Pigmented nevus with tuft of hair, location anywhere along the spine, often associated with spina bifida occulta

Continued

TABLE 26-2 **Physical Assessment of Newborn—cont'd**

AREA ASSESSED AND APPRAISAL PROCEDURE	NORMAL FINDINGS: AVERAGE FINDINGS	NORMAL FINDINGS: NORMAL VARIATONS	DEVIATIONS FROM NORMAL RANGE: POSSIBLE PROBLEMS (ETIOLOGY)
Back—cont'd			
			Spina bifida cystica (meningocele, myelomeningocele)
Check reflexes (spinal related) Test trunk incurvation reflex	Trunk flexed and pelvis swings to stimulated side	May not be apparent in first few days but is usually present in 5-6 days	If transverse lesion is present, no response below lesion; absence of response: nervous system abnormality or general depression
Test magnet reflex	Lower limbs extend as pressure applied to feet with legs in semiflexed position	Weak or exaggerated response with breech presentation	Absence: suggestive of spinal cord damage or malformation
Anus			
Inspect and palpate Placement Number Patency Test for sphincter response (active "wink" reflex) Observe for following: Abdominal distention Passage of meconium Passage of fecal drainage from surrounding orifices	One anus with good sphincter tone Passage of meconium within 24 hr after birth Good "wink" reflex of anal sphincter	Passage of meconium within 48 hr of birth	Low obstruction: anal membrane High obstruction: anal or rectal atresia Drainage of fecal material from vagina in female or urinary meatus in male (rectal fistula)
Stools			
Observe frequency, color, consistency	Meconium followed by transitional and soft yellow stools		No stool (obstruction) Frequent watery stools (infection, phototherapy)

should be supported with the head to the side. Deeper suctioning may be necessary to remove excessive or tenacious mucus from the infant's nasopharynx (see Procedure box).

Relieving Airway Obstruction. A choking infant needs immediate attention. Often, simply repositioning the infant and suctioning the mouth and nose with the bulb syringe eliminates the problem. The infant should be positioned with the head slightly lower than the body to facilitate gravity drainage. The nurse also should listen to the infant's respiration and lung sounds with a stethoscope to determine whether there are crackles and wheezes. If the lungs are clear, the bulb syringe is used to clear the mouth and nose. If the bulb syringe does not provide relief, mechanical suction can be used.

If these measures do not relieve the obstruction, the nurse gives the infant back blows and chest thrusts (see Emergency: Relieving Airway Obstruction, p. 806). All personnel working with infants must have current infant cardiopulmonary resuscitation (CPR) certification. Many institutions offer infant CPR courses to new parents before discharge. Because cardiac and respiratory arrest can occur in infants, careful monitoring is necessary so that rapid treatment can be initiated.

Maintaining an Adequate Oxygen Supply. Four conditions are essential for maintaining an adequate oxygen supply:

- A clear airway
- Respiratory efforts
- A functioning cardiopulmonary system

BOX 26-2 Routine Newborn Admission Orders

Vital signs: on admission and q30min ×2, q1hr ×2, then q8hr
Weight, length, and head and chest circumference on admission; then weigh daily
Tetracycline or erythromycin ophthalmic ointment, 5 mg/g, 1- to 2-cm line in lower conjunctiva of each eye (ou)
Vitamin K, 1.0 mg IM
Hematocrit by warm heel stick within 3 to 8 hours of age; call health care provider if <44 or >72
Dextrostix prn; notify health care provider if <40 mg/dl; offer early D5W PO or breastfeeding
Feedings: sterile water ×1 by nurse within first 4 hr of life; if tolerated, begin formula q3-4hr on demand
(Breastfeeding on demand may be initiated immediately after birth without initial sterile water feeding.)
Rooming-in as desired and infant's condition permits
Newborn screen for phenylketonuria (PKU), thyroxine (T_4), and galactosemia or other screening tests as ordered ≥24 hr after first feeding

PROCEDURE

Suctioning with a Bulb Syringe

The mouth is suctioned first to prevent the infant from inhaling pharyngeal secretions by gasping as the nares are touched.
The bulb is compressed (see Fig. 26-2) and inserted into one side of the mouth. The center of the infant's mouth is avoided because this could stimulate the gag reflex.
The nasal passages are suctioned one nostril at a time.
When the infant's cry does not sound as though it is through mucus or a bubble, suctioning can be stopped. The bulb syringe should always be kept in the infant's crib.
The parents should be given demonstrations on how to use the bulb syringe and asked to perform a return demonstration.

- Heat support (exposure to cold stress increases oxygen needs)

Signs of potential complications related to abnormal breathing are shown in the Signs of Potential Complications box.

Maintenance of Body Temperature

Effective neonatal care is based on the maintenance of an optimal thermal environment. Cold stress is detrimental to the newborn; it increases the need for oxygen and may upset the acid-base balance. The infant may react by increasing the respiratory rate and may become cyanotic. Ways to stabilize the newborn's body temperature include

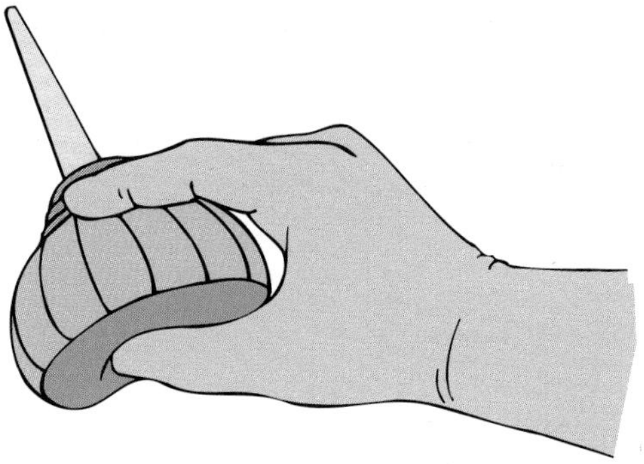

FIG. 26-2 Bulb syringe. Bulb must be compressed before insertion.

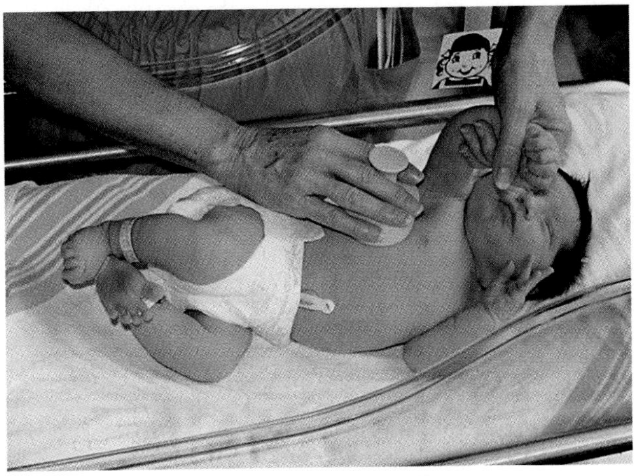

FIG. 26-3 Chest percussion. Nurse performs gentle percussion over the chest wall by using a percussion cup to aid in loosening secretions before suctioning. (Courtesy Shannon Perry, San Jose, CA.)

PROCEDURE

Suctioning with a Nasopharyngeal Catheter with Mechanical Suction Apparatus

To remove excessive or tenacious mucus from the infant's nasopharynx:
If wall suction is used, adjust the pressure to <80 mm Hg. Proper tube insertion and suctioning for ≤5 sec per tube insertion help prevent laryngospasms and oxygen depletion.
Lubricate the catheter in sterile water and then insert either orally along the base of the tongue or up and back into the nares.
After the catheter is properly placed, create suction by placing your thumb over the control as the catheter is carefully rotated and gently withdrawn.
Repeat the procedure until the infant's cry sounds clear and air entry into the lungs is heard by stethoscope.

SIGNS OF POTENTIAL COMPLICATIONS

Abnormal Newborn Breathing

- Bradypnea: respirations (≤25/min)
- Tachypnea: respirations (≥60/min)
- Abnormal breath sounds: crackles, rhonchi, wheezes, expiratory grunt
- Respiratory distress: nasal flaring, retractions, chin tug, labored breathing

placing the infant directly on the mother's abdomen and covering with a warm blanket; drying and wrapping the newborn in warmed blankets immediately after birth, keeping the head well covered, and keeping the ambient temperature of the nursery at 24° C.

If the infant does not remain with the parents during the first 1 to 2 hours after birth, the thoroughly dried, unclothed infant can be placed under a radiant heat panel or warmer until the body temperature stabilizes. The infant's skin temperature is used as the point of control in a warmer with a servocontrolled mechanism. The control panel usually is maintained between 36° C and 37° C. This setting should maintain the infant's skin temperature at approximately 36.5° C. A thermistor probe (automatic sensor) is taped to the right upper quadrant of the abdomen immediately below the right intercostal margin (never over a bone). This will ensure detection of minor changes resulting from peripheral vasoconstriction, vasodilation, or increased metabolism long before a change in core body temperature develops. The other end of the probe cord is attached to the control panel. The sensor must be checked periodically to make sure it is securely attached to the infant's skin. An axillary temperature should be taken every hour until the newborn's temperature stabilizes. By the twelfth hour, the newborn's temperature should stabilize within the normal range.

During all procedures, heat loss must be avoided or minimized for the newborn; therefore examinations and activities are performed with the newborn under a heat panel. The initial bath is postponed until the newborn's skin temperature reaches 36.5° C.

Even a normal term infant in good health can become hypothermic. Birth in a car on the way to the hospital, a cold birthing room, or inadequate drying and wrapping immediately after birth may cause **hypothermia.** Warming the hypothermic infant is accomplished with care. Rapid warming or cooling may cause apneic spells and acidosis in an infant; therefore the warming process is monitored to progress slowly over a period of 2 to 4 hours.

Immediate Interventions

It is the nurse's responsibility to perform certain interventions immediately after birth to provide for the safety of the newborn.

Identification. Information on the matching identification bracelets applied immediately after birth to the newborn and mother (and in some institutions, the father or significant other) should include name, sex, date and time of birth, and identification number, according to hospital protocol. Infants also are footprinted by using a form that includes the mother's fingerprints, name, and date and time of birth. These identification procedures must be performed before the mother and infant are separated.

Therapeutic Interventions

Eye Prophylaxis. The instillation of a prophylactic agent in the eyes of all neonates is mandatory in the United States as a precaution against **ophthalmia neonatorum** (Fig. 26-4). This is an inflammation of the eyes resulting from gonorrheal or chlamydial infection contracted as the newborn passes through the mother's infected birth canal. The agent used for prophylaxis varies according to hospital protocols, but the usual agents are forms of erythromycin and tetracycline. Canadian hospitals have not recommended the use of silver nitrate since 1986. Its use in the United States is minimal because silver nitrate does not protect against chlamydial infection and can cause chemical conjunctivitis. In some institutions, eye prophylaxis is delayed until an hour or so after birth so that eye contact and parent-infant attachment and bonding are facilitated. The Centers for Disease Control and Prevention specifies that it should be given as soon as possible after birth; if instillation is delayed, there should be a monitoring process in place to ensure that all newborns are treated (Workowski & Levine, 2002) (see Medication Guide box). In some Canadian institutions, the parents may sign a form refusing such eye prophylaxis. In the United States, if the family objects to this treatment, the primary care provider asks the parents to sign an informed consent form, and their refusal is noted in the neonate's record.

Vitamin K Administration. Administering vitamin K intramuscularly is routine in the newborn period. A single parenteral dose of 0.5 to 1 mg of vitamin K is given soon after birth to prevent hemorrhagic disorders (Kliegman, 2002). Vitamin K is not produced in the gastrointestinal (GI) tract until after microorganisms are introduced. By day 8, normal newborns are able to produce their own vitamin K (see Medication Guide box).

Umbilical Cord Care. The care of the umbilical cord is the same as that for any surgical wound. The goal of care is prevention and early identification of hemorrhage or infection. The umbilical cord stump is an excellent medium for bacterial growth and can easily become infected.

NURSE ALERT

If bleeding from the blood vessels of the cord is noted, the nurse checks the clamp (or tie) and applies a second clamp next to the first one. If bleeding is not stopped immediately, the nurse calls for assistance.

Hospital protocol directs the time and technique for routine cord care. The stump and base of the cord should

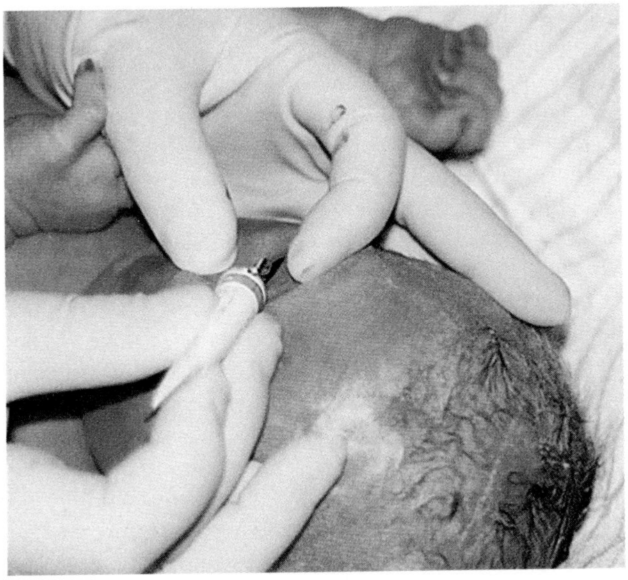

FIG. 26-4 Instillation of medication into eye of newborn. Thumb and forefinger are used to open the eye; medication is placed in the lower conjunctiva from the inner to the outer canthus. (Courtesy Marjorie Pyle, RNC, Lifecircle, Costa Mesa, CA.)

be assessed for edema, redness, and purulent drainage with each diaper change. The cord clamp is removed after 24 hours when the cord is dry (Fig. 26-5).

Promote Parent-Infant Interaction

Today's childbirth practices strive to promote the family as the focus of care. Parents generally desire to share in the birth process and have early contact with their infants. Early contact between mother and newborn can be important in developing future relationships. It also has a positive effect on the duration of breastfeeding. The physiologic benefits of early mother-infant contact include increased oxytocin and prolactin levels in the mother and activation of sucking reflexes in the infant. The infant can be put to breast soon after birth. The process of developing active immunity begins as the infant ingests flora from the mother's skin.

Evaluation

Evaluation of the effectiveness of immediate care of the newborn is based on the previously stated outcomes.

CARE MANAGEMENT: FROM 2 HOURS AFTER BIRTH UNTIL DISCHARGE

The infant's admission to the nursery may be delayed, or it may never actually occur. Depending on the routine of the hospital, the infant frequently remains in the labor area and is then transferred to either the nursery or the

MEDICATION GUIDE

Eye Prophylaxis: Erythromycin Ophthalmic Ointment, 0.5%, and Tetracycline Ophthalmic Ointment, 1%

ACTION ▪ These antibiotic ointments are both bacteriostatic and bactericidal. They provide prophylaxis against *Neisseria gonorrhoeae* and *Chlamydia trachomatis*.

INDICATION ▪ These medications are applied to prevent ophthalmia neonatorum in newborns of mothers who are infected with gonorrhea and conjunctivitis in newborns of mothers infected with chlamydia.

NEONATAL DOSAGE ▪ Apply a 1- to 2-cm ribbon of ointment to the lower conjunctival sac of each eye; also may be used in drop form.

ADVERSE REACTIONS ▪ May cause chemical conjunctivitis that lasts 24 to 48 hours; vision may be blurred temporarily.

NURSING CONSIDERATIONS ▪ Administer within 1 to 2 hr of birth. Wear gloves. Cleanse eyes if necessary before administration. Open eyes by putting a thumb and finger at the corner of each lid and gently pressing on the periorbital ridges. Squeeze the tube and spread the ointment from the inner canthus of the eye to the outer canthus. Do not touch the tube to the eye. After 1 min, excess ointment may be wiped off. Observe eyes for irritation. Explain treatment to parents.

Eye prophylaxis for ophthalmia neonatorum is required by law in all states of the United States.

MEDICATION GUIDE

Vitamin K: Phytonadione (AquaMEPHYTON, Konakion)

ACTION ▪ This intervention provides vitamin K because the newborn does not have the intestinal flora to produce this vitamin in the first week after birth. It also promotes formation of clotting factors (II, VII, IX, X) in the liver.

INDICATION ▪ Vitamin K is used for prevention and treatment of hemorrhagic disease in the newborn.

NEONATAL DOSAGE ▪ Administer a 0.5- to 1-mg (0.25 to 0.5 ml) dose intramuscularly within 2 hr of birth; may be repeated if newborn shows bleeding tendencies.

ADVERSE REACTIONS ▪ Edema, erythema, and pain at injection site may occur rarely; hemolysis, jaundice, and hyperbilirubinemia have been reported, particularly in preterm infants.

NURSING CONSIDERATIONS ▪ Wear gloves. Administer in the middle third of the vastus lateralis muscle by using a 25-gauge, 5/8-inch needle. Inject into skin that has been cleaned, or allow alcohol to dry on puncture site for 1 min to remove organisms and prevent infection. Stabilize leg firmly, and grasp muscle between the thumb and fingers. Insert the needle at a 90-degree angle; aspirate, and inject medication slowly if there is no blood return. Massage the site with a dry gauze square after removing needle to increase absorption. Observe for signs of bleeding from the site.

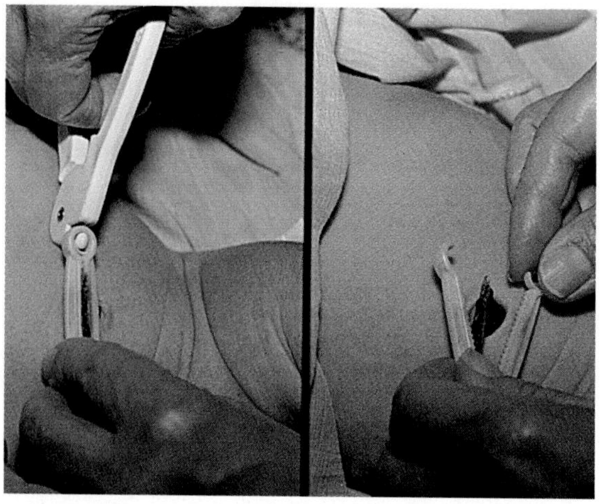

FIG. 26-5 With special scissors, remove clamp after cord dries (about 24 hours). (Courtesy Marjorie Pyle, RNC, Lifecircle, Costa Mesa, CA.)

postpartum unit with the mother. Many hospitals have adopted variations of single-room maternity care (SRMC) in which one nurse provides care for the mother and newborn. SRMC allows the infant to remain with the parents after the birth. Many of the procedures, such as assessment of weight and measurement (i.e., circumference of head and chest, length), instillation of eye medications, intramuscular administration of vitamin K, and physical assessment, may be accomplished in the labor and birth unit. This requires that nurses who work in an SRMC unit; labor, delivery, and recovery (LDR) room; or labor, delivery, recovery, and postpartum (LDRP) room must be knowledgeable and competent in delivery of intrapartal, neonatal, and postpartum nursing care. If an infant is transferred to the nursery, the infant's identification is verified by the nurse receiving the infant, who places the baby in a warm environment and begins the admission process.

Regardless of the physical organization for care, many hospitals have a small holding nursery, which is available for procedures or on the request of the mother who wishes her infant to be placed there. This setup promotes parent-infant bonding while still allowing the new parents some time to be alone.

Baseline Measurements of Physical Growth

The examiner records baseline measurements to help assess the progress of the neonate and to determine the neonate's growth patterns. These may be recorded on growth charts. The following measurements are made.

Weight. The newborn is usually weighed shortly after birth. The totally unclothed neonate is placed in the center of the scale, which is usually covered with a disposable pad or diaper to prevent heat loss from conduction. The nurse should place one hand over (but not touching) the neonate to prevent the infant from falling off the scales (see Table 26-2). The infant is commonly weighed at the same time every day during the hospital stay.

The birth weight of a term infant ranges from 2500 to 4000 g. Neonates normally lose about 5% to 10% of their birth weight during the first 3 to 5 days after birth because of the excretion of fluids through the lungs, urinary bladder, and bowels, and the low level of intake during the first few days of life. Weight loss in excess of 7% should be evaluated by the health care provider. Birth weight should be regained by age 10 to 14 days.

Circumferences and Length. The head is measured at the widest part, which is the occipitofrontal diameter (see Table 26-2). The tape measure is placed around the head at the infant's eyebrows.

The chest circumference usually measures about 2 cm less than the head circumference. Frequently the chest is the same size as the head but should not exceed it. The tape is placed around the infant's chest at the nipple line (see Table 26-2).

Abdominal circumference is measured by placing the tape around the abdomen (see Table 26-2). Measurements vary with the size of the infant. The abdomen should be cylindrical and protrude slightly. Abdominal measurements are not always taken but should be made when abdominal distention is suspected.

The length may be difficult to measure because of the flexed posture of the newborn (see Table 26-2). The examiner places the newborn on a flat surface and extends the leg until the knee is flat against the surface. Placing the head against a perpendicular surface and extending the leg may assist with this measurement.

Assessment

Gestational Age Assessment

The assessment of physical and neurologic findings to determine gestational age should optimally be done between 2 and 12 hours after birth. If the tests are done earlier while the infant is recovering from the stress of birth, muscle movements may reflect fatigue; for example, the arm recoil is slower. After 48 hours, some significant changes are found. For instance, the plantar creases on the soles of the feet appear to become more numerous and visible as the skin loses fluid and dries.

Assessment of gestational age is important because perinatal morbidity and mortality are related to gestational age and birth weight. The simplified Assessment of Gestational Age (Ballard, Novak, & Driver, 1979) is commonly used to assess gestational age of infants between 35 and 42 weeks. It assesses six external physical and six neuromuscular signs. Each sign has a number score, and the cumulative score correlates with a maturity rating of 26 to 44 weeks of gestation. The score is accurate to plus or minus 2 weeks and is accurate for infants of all races.

The *New Ballard Score,* a revision of the original scale, can be used with newborns as young as 20 weeks of gestation. The tool has the same physical and neuromuscular sections but includes -1 to -2 scores that reflect signs of extremely premature infants, such as fused eyelids; imperceptible breast tissue; sticky, friable, transparent skin; no lanugo; and square-window (flexion of wrist) angle greater than 90 degrees (see Fig. 26-1, *A*). The scale overestimates gestational age by 2 to 4 days in infants younger than 37 weeks of gestation, especially at gestational ages of 32 to 37 weeks (Ballard et al., 1991).

Classification of Newborns by Gestational Age and Birth Weight. A normal range of birth weights exists for each gestational week (see Fig. 26-1, *B*), but the birth weights of preterm, term, postterm, or postmature newborns also may be outside these normal ranges. Birth weights are classified in the following ways:

- **Large for gestational age (LGA).** Weight is above the 90th percentile (or two or more standard deviations above the norm) at any week.
- **Appropriate for gestational age (AGA).** Weight falls between the 10th and 90th percentile for infant's age.
- **Small for gestational age (SGA).** Weight is below the 10th percentile (or two or more standard deviations below the norm) at any week.
- **Low birth weight (LBW).** Weight of 2500 g or less at birth. These newborns have had either less than the expected rate of intrauterine growth or a shortened gestation period. Preterm birth and LBW commonly occur together (e.g., less than 32 weeks of gestation and birth weight of less than 1200 g).
- **Very low birth weight (VLBW).** Weight of 1500 g or less at birth.
- **Intrauterine growth restriction (IUGR)** is the term applied to the fetus whose rate of growth does not meet expected norms.

Newborns are classified according to their gestational ages in the following ways:

- **Preterm or premature.** Born before completion of 37 weeks of gestation, regardless of birth weight.
- **Term.** Born between the beginning of week 38 and the end of week 42 of gestation.
- **Postterm (postdate).** Born after completion of week 42 of gestation.
- **Postmature.** Born after completion of week 42 of gestation and showing the effects of progressive placental insufficiency.

Maternal Effects on Gestational Age Assessment and Birth Weight. Some maternal conditions can affect the results of the gestational assessment. For instance, any infant who has had oxygen deprivation during labor will show poor muscle tone. Infants in respiratory distress tend to be flaccid and assume a "frog-leg" posture. Even though an infant may look large, such as the infant of a diabetic mother, it may respond more like a premature infant. The infant of a mother who has been receiving magnesium sulfate will tend to be somewhat lethargic.

Physical Assessment

A complete physical examination is done within 24 hours. The parents' presence during this examination encourages discussion of parental concerns and actively involves the parents in the health care of their infant from birth. It also affords the nurse an opportunity to observe parental interactions with the infant.

The area used for the examination should be well-lighted, warm, and free from drafts. The infant is undressed as needed and placed on a firm, warmed, flat surface or under a radiant warmer. The physical assessment should begin with a review of the maternal history and prenatal and intrapartal records. This provides a background for the recognition of any potential problems.

The assessment includes general appearance, behavior, vital signs measurement, and parent-infant interactions. The assessment should progress systematically from head to toe, with assessment and evaluation of each system (i.e., cardiovascular, respiratory, and so on). Descriptions of any variations from normal findings and all abnormal findings are included. The findings provide a database for implementing the nursing process with newborns and providing anticipatory guidance for the parents. (Table 26-2 summarizes the newborn assessment.) Ongoing assessments of the newborn are made throughout the hospital stay, and an evaluation is performed before discharge.

Nursing Considerations in Assessment. The neonate's maturity level can be gauged by assessment of general appearance. Features to assess in the general survey include skin color, posture, state of alertness, cry, head size, lanugo, vernix caseosa, breast tissue, and sole creases. The normal resting position of the neonate is one of general flexion. The neck is short, and the abdomen is prominent.

The temperature, heart rate, and respiratory rate are always obtained. Blood pressure (BP) is not routinely assessed unless cardiac problems are suspected. An irregular, very slow, or very fast heart rate may indicate a need for BP measurements.

The axillary temperature is a safe, accurate substitute for the rectal temperature. Electronic thermometers have expedited this task and provide a reading within 1 minute. Taking an infant's temperature may cause the infant to cry and struggle against the placement of the thermometer in the axilla. Tympanic thermometers may be used after the newborn's ear canals are free of vernix and fluid. Before taking the temperature, the examiner may want to determine the apical heart rate and respiratory rate while the infant is quiet and at rest. The normal axillary temperature averages 37° C with a range from 36.5° C to 37.2° C.

The respiratory rate varies with the state of alertness after birth. Respirations are abdominal and can easily be counted by observing or lightly feeling the rise and fall of the abdomen. Neonatal respirations are shallow and irregular. It is important to count the respirations for a full minute to obtain an accurate count because of normal short periods of apnea. The examiner also should observe for symmetry of chest movements (see Table 26-2 for normal respiratory rates).

Apical pulse rates should be obtained on all infants. Auscultation should be for a full minute, preferably when the infant is asleep. The infant may need to be held and comforted during assessment. Auscultation of the heart sounds is difficult because of the rapid rate and effective transmission of respiratory sounds. However, the first (S_1) and second (S_2) sounds should be clear and well defined; the second sound is somewhat higher in pitch and sharper than the first. Murmurs are often heard in the newborn, especially over the base of the heart or at the left sternal border in the third or fourth interspace. These are usually functional murmurs due to incomplete closure of fetal shunts. Any murmur or other unusual sounds should be recorded and reported. See Table 26-2 for normal heart rates.

If blood pressure is measured, a Doppler (electronic) monitor facilitates this procedure. It is important to use the correct size BP cuff. Neonatal BP usually is highest immediately after birth and decreases to a minimum by 3 hours after birth. It then begins to increase steadily and reaches a plateau between 4 and 6 days after birth. This measurement is usually equal to that of the immediate postbirth BP. BP may be measured in both arms and legs to detect any discrepancy between the two sides or between the upper and lower body. A discrepancy of 10 mm Hg or more between the arms and legs may signal a cardiac defect such as coarctation of the aorta.

Skin color varies with racial background, pigmentation, and physiologic changes. Texture and opacity of the skin vary with gestation. Observations should include color and color changes during activity, familial and racial features, rashes, milia, anomalies or deformities, birthmarks, jaundice, petechiae, forceps or vacuum-cup marks, internal scalp electrode site, tone, and hydration status. Location, size, color, characteristics, and distribution of variations in the appearance of the skin should be noted and recorded.

Acrocyanosis is characterized by bluish discoloration of the hands and feet. This normal condition is caused by vasomotor instability and poor peripheral circulation. To distinguish between true cyanosis and acrocyanosis, the examiner vigorously rubs the sole of the infant's foot. If the sole turns pink, the discoloration is caused by acrocyanosis. It will not turn pink with true cyanosis. In addition, acrocyanosis should disappear when the infant cries. True cyanosis, or central cyanosis, appears as bluish discoloration and pallor of the lips and around the mouth.

The fontanels are inspected, palpated, and measured. The anterior fontanel is located at the junction of the sagittal and coronal sutures and is diamond shaped. The fontanel usually feels soft and may pulsate. It should be not bulging or depressed but flush with the level of the skull. The posterior fontanel is a triangular depression located at the junction of the lambdoidal and sagittal sutures. The posterior fontanel is often not palpable. Molding may give the neonate's head an asymmetric appearance (see Fig. 25-9). Parents should be reassured that this will go away and that nothing need be done to the head.

Facial asymmetry may occur from fetal positioning in utero; asymmetry usually disappears spontaneously over time. The mouth should appear at the midline, and its size should be appropriate for the face. When the neonate cries, there should be symmetric mouth and facial movement. The chin normally is slightly receding. The hard and soft palates are assessed with the gloved little finger of the examiner. At the same time, the suck reflex can be assessed.

The eyes are most easily examined when the infant is in a quiet, alert state. The sclerae should be clear and white or may appear slightly yellow in dark-skinned infants. The conjunctivae should be clear and may be somewhat bluish. The iris color should be distributed evenly. Occasionally, subconjunctival hemorrhage, a result of the pressure the infant experiences while traversing the birth canal during labor and birth, may be seen. Tears are not usually produced until 2 months of age.

The pupils are examined with a penlight or flashlight and with room lights dim. The pupils should be round, centered in the iris, and constrict equally bilaterally when exposed to light in a darkened room. A newborn's eyes do not accommodate. To assess for the red reflex, the examiner places the penlight or ophthalmoscope directly in front of the pupil and turns on the light. If the red reflex is visible, there is no congenital cataract present.

Transient strabismus (pseudostrabismus) and nystagmus (constant, involuntary cyclic movement of the eyeball) may be seen until the third or fourth month; it persists until the eye muscles develop sufficiently to act in coordination (see Table 26-2). When the neonate's head is rotated from side to side, the eyes do not follow in response to head movements. This doll's-eye phenomenon persists for about 10 days.

The ears are inspected for symmetric shape and size. The top of the ear should align with the inner and outer canthi of the eyes (see Table 26-2). Skin tags, pinpoint holes, and sinus tracts along the helix or preauricular surface may be minor abnormalities. The neonate's hearing should be checked. A loud noise should elicit the startle reflex or crying. Formal hearing screening of all infants is conducted in the newborn nursery (see Fig. 26-6). At 36 weeks of gestation, the upper two thirds of the pinna is incurved, and the pinna recoils instantly. In the term neonate, the pinna has well-defined incurving. Old blood and vernix may be in the ear canal for several days, and therefore the tympanic membrane may not be visible.

Because the neonate cannot coordinate tongue movements well, the tongue often falls backward, occluding the oral airway. Consequently, the neonate is a preferential nose breather who depends on patent nares (nostrils). To assess the nares for patency, the examiner occludes them one at a time and holds the mouth closed. The neonate should be able to breathe through the open naris. The neonate's nose also is examined for size, shape, mucous membrane integrity, and discharge. The nose should be midline on the face. The mucous membranes will appear pink and moist with no copious drainage.

The oral cavity should be inspected, but it is best to avoid doing this soon after a feeding because the gag reflex could be stimulated, causing vomiting and subsequent aspiration. The mouth should be inspected to determine if the oral mucous membranes are pink and moist. Natal teeth, Epstein's pearls, and cysts on the gums are noted. The rooting reflex can be elicited by stroking the corner of the neonate's mouth or the cheek. The tongue should be freely movable and symmetric in shape and movement. To check for tongue extrusion, touch the tongue lightly. Occasionally a neonate may have difficulty fully extruding the tongue; this is usually due to a shortened frenulum (ankyloglossia or "tongue tie"). To assess intactness of the hard and soft palates, insert a gloved finger into the infant's mouth. This also stimulates the suck reflex, and the intensity of the reflex can be evaluated.

The posterior pharynx is easiest to see when the neonate is crying. Saliva is usually scant because the salivary glands are immature. The presence of excessive saliva in a neonate should alert the nurse to the possibility of tracheoesophageal fistula or esophageal atresia.

The neck should appear symmetric and without webbing; it also should be flexible enough to allow the head to move freely and equally to each side.

The chest should appear smaller than the abdomen. As the infant breathes, chest movement should be symmetric. Respirations should be nonlabored, without retractions. The ribs should be flexible and symmetric, with no palpable masses. The xiphoid process may be palpable at the bottom of the sternum and may be visible in a thin neonate.

The chest is auscultated for heart and lung sounds. A murmur should be reported to the health care provider. Breath sounds should be clear and equal bilaterally, although fine crackles may be audible immediately after birth, especially in infants born by cesarean birth.

When palpating the clavicles, the examiner moves the fingers slowly over the anterior clavicular surface. If a mass or lump is detected, the examiner tries to move the neonate's arm gently while palpating with the other hand. A grating sensation and uneven movement of two juxtaposed bone fragments indicate a fracture. If a fractured clavicle is present, the infant will usually have limited movement of the arm on the affected side.

Assess breast tissue through observation and palpation. To measure breast tissue, palpate the nipple gently with one finger or place the second and third fingers on either side of the nipple. The amount of breast tissue is measured between the two fingers. Breast tissue and areola size increase with gestational age. The nipples are inspected for spacing and number. Supernumerary nipples may appear as darkened spots just below or beside natural nipples. Any discharge from the nipples is noted.

The abdomen should appear larger than the chest and should have a symmetric, slightly rounded contour. Peristaltic waves normally are not visible; however, the abdomen should move visibly during breathing. Auscultation of the abdomen is performed before palpation and percussion. Bowel sounds are noted in all four quadrants. To promote relaxation and comfort during palpation, the examiner flexes the neonate's legs in the fetal position. If the neonate has an asymmetric abdomen, which suggests an internal mass, great caution must be used during the assessment. The liver edge may be palpated just below the costal margin.

The abdomen should be percussed just after the neonate voids to prevent misleading findings. Percussion should reveal tympany (a clear, hollow note like that of a drum) below the left costal margin, reflecting a gastric bubble. Most other abdominal areas also should be tympanic. However, dullness should be percussed over the liver, spleen, and bladder. Percussion delineates the borders of these organs to detect enlargement, indicated by increased areas of dullness. Decreased areas of dullness suggest fluid or air where solid tissue is expected.

The posterior position of the kidneys makes them less accessible to palpation. If they cannot be palpated with one hand, bimanual palpation is used. In this technique, the examiner places one hand behind the neonate's back while palpating the abdomen with the fingertips of the other hand. The kidney should be felt between the hands.

Unless the bladder is distended, it should not be visible. The bladder may be percussed just above the symphysis pubis. The presence of urine will produce a tympanic sound. Pressing on the bladder may induce voiding or expression of urine. The time of the first voiding should be noted.

The umbilical cord remnant should appear bluish white and contain two arteries and one vein. The umbilical cord is clamped or tied at birth, and the clamp or tie is usually removed when the cord is dry in approximately 24 hours. The umbilical cord begins to dry, shrivels, and blackens by the second or third day of life. The umbilicus should be inspected frequently for signs of infection (foul odor, redness, and purulent drainage), granuloma (small, red, raw-appearing polyp where the umbilical cord separates), bleeding, and discharge. The cord normally falls off by 2 weeks after birth. By the time the neonate is 1 month old, the umbilicus should be healed.

To assess the back, the examiner positions the neonate prone and inspects for spinal alignment, enlargement, and masses. The back should be straight. The sacrum is examined for dimpling, a tuft of hair, or bulges. The vertebral column is palpated for enlargement and signs of pain.

The perineum should be smooth and without dimpling or extra orifices. The anus should be midline and patent. The anal sphincter is assessed by lightly stroking the anus with a cotton-tipped applicator and observing anal constriction–a reaction called the anal wink. Passage of meconium indicates patency of the rectum, which should be noted.

In the male neonate, the genitalia should be assessed for testicular descent, scrotal size, and number of rugae (skin folds). Hydroceles are a common finding and usually decrease without intervention. If the male neonate is circumcised, he must be observed for signs of bleeding and ability to void.

The female genitalia should be assessed for signs of gestational maturity. The degree to which the labia majora and minora have come together and reduced the visual prominence of the labia minora and clitoris reflects the stage of the infant's maturity. The labia majora may appear edematous. A vaginal tag is often noted at the vaginal orifice. Mucoid discharge from the vagina is normal.

The extremities are inspected for length, symmetry relative to each other and to the body as a whole, equality, muscle tone, and range of motion. Normally the term neonate has a full range of motion, which can be tested either actively or passively. The number of digits, palmar and plantar creases, and abnormalities such as webbing of the hands and feet are noted.

To assess leg length, the examiner extends the legs simultaneously. The legs should be equal length, with symmetric skin folds. The examiner inspects the legs in both the prone and supine positions.

A neurologic assessment of the newborn's reflexes (see Table 25-1) provides useful information about the infant's nervous system and state of neurologic maturation. The assessment must be carried out as early as possible because abnormal signs present in the early neonatal period may disappear. They may reappear months or years later as abnormal functions.

Common Problems in the Newborn

Mechanical Birth Trauma. Birth trauma constitutes any physical injury sustained by a newborn during labor and birth. Many injuries are minor and readily resolve in the neonatal period without treatment. Other types of trauma require some form of intervention. A few are serious enough to be fatal. Several factors predispose an infant to birth trauma (Pressler & Hepworth, 2000). *Maternal factors* include uterine dysfunction that leads to prolonged or precipitate labor, preterm or postterm labor, and cephalopelvic disproportion. Injury may result from dystocia caused by fetal macrosomia, multifetal gestation, abnormal or difficult presentation, and congenital anomalies. *Intrapartum events* that can result in scalp injury include the use of intrapartum monitoring of the fetal heart rate (FHR) and fetal scalp sampling. Obstetric birth techniques also can cause injury. These include forceps-assisted birth, vacuum extraction, version and extraction, and cesarean birth.

Soft-Tissue Injuries. Caput succedaneum and cephalhematoma are described in Chapter 25 (see Fig. 25-4).

Subconjunctival and retinal hemorrhages result from rupture of capillaries caused by increased pressure during birth (see also Chapter 25). These hemorrhages clear within 5 days after birth and usually present no further problems; however, parents need explanation and reassurance that these injuries will resolve without sequelae.

Erythema, ecchymoses, petechiae, abrasions, lacerations, or edema of buttocks and extremities may be present. Localized discoloration may appear over presenting parts and may result from the application of forceps or the vacuum extractor. Ecchymoses and edema may appear anywhere on the body.

Bruises over the face may be the result of face presentation (see Fig. 38-1). In a breech presentation, bruising and swelling may be seen over the buttocks or genitalia (see Fig. 38-2). The skin over the entire head may be ecchymotic and covered with petechiae caused by a tight nuchal cord. Petechiae (pinpoint hemorrhagic areas) acquired during birth may extend over the upper trunk and face. These lesions are benign if they disappear within 2 or 3 days of birth and no new lesions appear. Ecchymoses and petechiae may be signs of a more serious disorder, such as thrombocytopenic purpura.

NURSE ALERT

To differentiate hemorrhagic areas from skin rashes and discolorations, try to blanch the skin with two fingers. Petechiae and ecchymoses do not blanch because extravasated blood remains within the tissues, whereas skin rashes and discolorations do.

Trauma resulting from dystocia occurs to the presenting part. Forceps injury and bruising from the vacuum cup occur at the site where the instruments were applied. In a forceps injury, commonly a linear mark appears across both sides of the face in the shape of the forceps blades. The affected areas are kept clean to minimize the risk of infection. With the increased use of the vacuum extractor and the use of padded forceps blades, the incidence of these lesions may be significantly reduced (Mangurten, 2002).

Accidental lacerations may be inflicted with a scalpel during a cesarean birth. These cuts may occur on any part of the body but are most often found on the scalp, buttocks, and thighs. Usually they are superficial and only must be kept clean. Butterfly adhesive strips can hold together the edges of more serious lacerations. Rarely are sutures needed.

Skeletal Injuries. Fracture of the clavicle (collarbone) is the most common fracture during birth; the break usually occurs in the middle third of the bone (see Fig. 38-4 and discussion in Chapter 38).

Fractures of the humerus and femur may occur during a difficult birth, but such fractures in newborns generally heal rapidly. Immobilization is accomplished with slings, splints, swaddling, and other devices.

The infant's immature, flexible skull can withstand a great deal of molding before fracture results. Fractures may occur during difficult births and result from the head pressing on the bony pelvis or from the injudicious application of forceps. The location of a skull fracture determines whether it is insignificant or fatal (see Fig. 38-3 and discussion in Chapter 38).

Dislocations due to birth trauma are rare. True dislocations, such as of the hip or knee, are most likely congenital malformations or the result of intrauterine positioning (Mangurten, 2002). See Chapter 39 for a discussion of congenital hip dysplasia.

Parents need emotional support when it comes to handling a newborn with skeletal injuries because they are often fearful of hurting their newborn. Parents are encouraged to practice handling, changing, and feeding the injured newborn under the guidance of the nursing staff. This increases the parents' knowledge and confidence, in addition to facilitating attachment. A plan for follow-up therapy is developed with the parents so that the times and arrangements for therapy are convenient for them.

Physiologic Problems

Physiologic Jaundice. Virtually all term newborns have physiologic jaundice (become yellowish) during the first 3 days of life (see Chapter 25). Serum bilirubin levels of less than 5 mg/dl usually are not reflected in visible skin jaundice.

Every newborn is assessed for jaundice. The blanch test helps differentiate cutaneous jaundice from skin color. To do the test, apply pressure with a finger over a bony area (e.g., the nose, forehead, sternum) for several seconds to empty all the capillaries in that spot. If jaundice is present, the blanched area will look yellow before the capillaries refill. The conjunctival sacs and buccal mucosa also are assessed, especially in darker-skinned infants. It is better to assess for jaundice in daylight, because artificial lighting and reflection from nursery walls can distort the actual skin color.

Jaundice is noticeable first in the head and then progresses gradually toward the abdomen and extremities because of the newborn infant's circulatory pattern (cephalocaudal developmental progression). If jaundice is suspected, evaluation of serum bilirubin level is needed.

Hypoglycemia. *Hypoglycemia* during the early newborn period of a term infant is defined as a blood glucose concentration of less than 35 mg/dl or as a plasma concentration of less than 40 mg/dl. It occurs because at birth, when the cord is cut, the newborn abruptly loses its glucose supply. The glucose level normally declines during the first hours after birth. Because hypoglycemia may be asymptomatic, a blood glucose test is often done soon after birth and repeated at age 4 hours. More frequent testing is required if the newborn is in an at-risk group (i.e., infant of diabetic mother, LGA, SGA, or LBW) or has been exposed to stressors such as birth trauma, cold, perinatal asphyxia, or tocolysis to inhibit preterm labor. These infants should be checked for hypoglycemia frequently during the first 4 hours after birth and every 4 hours thereafter until the risk period has passed (Ogata, 1999).

Signs of hypoglycemia include jitteriness; an irregular respiratory effort; cyanosis; apnea; a weak, high-pitched cry; feeding difficulty; hunger; lethargy; twitching; eye rolling; and seizures. The signs may be transient and recurrent.

Hypoglycemia in the low risk term infant is usually eliminated by feeding the infant. Occasionally the intravenous administration of glucose is required.

Hypocalcemia. *Hypocalcemia* (blood calcium levels of less than 7 mg/dl) may occur in newborns of diabetic mothers or in those who had perinatal asphyxia or trauma, and in LBW and preterm infants. Early-onset hypocalcemia occurs within the first 72 hours after birth. Signs of hypocalcemia include jitteriness, edema, apnea, intermittent cyanosis, and abdominal distention.

In most instances, early-onset hypocalcemia is self-limiting and resolves within 1 to 3 days. Treatment includes early feeding and, occasionally, the administration of calcium supplements.

Jitteriness is a symptom of both hypoglycemia and hypocalcemia; therefore hypocalcemia must be considered if the therapy for hypoglycemia proves ineffective. In many newborns, jitteriness remains despite therapy and cannot be explained by hypoglycemia or hypocalcemia (DeMarini & Tsang, 2002).

Laboratory and Diagnostic Tests

Routine Testing. Blood glucose levels are measured, and urinalysis is performed commonly in newborns. Other tests may be performed as needed, including the measurement of bilirubin levels, complete blood count (CBC), newborn screening tests, and drug tests. Standard laboratory values for a term newborn are given in Box 26-3.

Newborn Genetic Screening. Before hospital discharge, a heel-stick blood sample is obtained to detect a variety of congenital conditions. Mandated by U.S. law, newborn genetic screening is an important public health program that is aimed at early detection of genetic diseases that result in severe health problems if not treated early. All states screen for phenylketonuria (PKU) and hypothyroidism, but each state determines whether other tests are performed. Other genetic defects that are included in some screening programs include galactosemia, cystic fibrosis, maple syrup urine disease, and sickle cell disease (see Chapter 3). It is recommended that the screening test be repeated at age 1 to 2 weeks if the initial specimen was obtained when the infant was younger than 24 hours (Glass, 1999; Zinn, 2002).

BOX 26-3 **Standard Laboratory Values in the Neonatal Period**

	NEONATAL
1. HEMATOLOGIC VALUES	
Clotting factors	
Activated clotting time (ACT)	2 min
Bleeding time (Ivy)	2 to 7 min
Clot retraction	Complete 1 to 4 hr
Fibrinogen	125 to 300 mg/dl*

	TERM	PRETERM
Hemoglobin (g/dl)	14 to 24	15 to 17
Hematocrit (%)	44 to 64	45 to 55
Reticulocytes (%)	0.4 to 6	Up to 10
Fetal hemoglobin (% of total)	40 to 70	80 to 90
Red blood cells (RBCs)/μl†	4.8×10^6 to 7.1×10^6	
Platelet count/μl	150,000 to 300,000	120,000 to 180,000
White blood cells (WBCs)/μl	9000 to 30,000	10,000 to 20,000
Neutrophils (%)	54 to 62	47
Eosinophils and basophils (%)	1 to 3	
Lymphocytes (%)	25 to 33	33
Monocytes (%)	3 to 7	4
Immature WBC (%)	10	16

**dl* refers to deciliter (1 dl = 100 ml); this conforms to the SI system (standardized international measurements).
†*μl* refers to microliter.

			NEONATAL
2. BIOCHEMICAL VALUES			
Bilirubin, direct			0 to 1 mg/dl
Bilirubin, total	Cord:		<2 mg/dl
	Peripheral blood:	0 to 1 day	6 mg/dl
		1 to 2 days	8 mg/dl
		2 to 5 days	12 mg/dl
Blood gases		Arterial:	pH 7.31 to 7.49
			P_{CO_2} 26 to 41 mm Hg
			P_{O_2} 60 to 70 mm Hg
		Venous:	pH 7.31 to 7.41
			P_{CO_2} 40 to 50 mm Hg
			P_{O_2} 40 to 50 mm Hg
Serum glucose			40 to 60 mg/dl

	NEONATAL
3. URINALYSIS	
Color	Clear, straw
Specific gravity	1.001 to 1.020
pH	5 to 7
Protein	Negative
Glucose	Negative
Ketones	Negative
RBCs	0 to 2
WBCs	0 to 4
Casts	None

Volume: 24 to 72 ml/kg excreted daily in the first few days; by week 1, 24-hr urine volume close to 200 ml.
Protein: may be present in first 2 to 4 days.
Osmolarity (mOsm/L): 100 to 600.

Some data from Hockenberry, M. et al. (2003). *Wong's nursing care of infants and children* (7th ed.). St. Louis: Mosby; Pagana, K., & Pagana, T. (2002). *Mosby's manual of diagnostic and laboratory tests* (2nd ed.). St. Louis: Mosby.

Newborn Hearing Screening. Universal newborn hearing screening is required by law in more than 30 states and is performed routinely in other states. Infants in the neonatal intensive care unit (NICU) and those with other risk factors are screened in many settings where universal screening is not routinely done. Newborn hearing screening is completed before hospital discharge, and infants who do not pass are referred for repeated testing within the next 2 to 8 weeks. The practice of universal hearing screening reduces the age at which infants with hearing loss are identified and treated (Joint Committee on Infant Hearing, 2000) (Fig. 26-6).

Collection of Specimens

Ongoing evaluation of a newborn often requires obtaining blood by the heel-stick or venipuncture method or the collection of a urine specimen.

Heel Stick. Most blood specimens are drawn by laboratory technicians. Nurses, however, may be required to perform heel sticks to obtain blood for glucose monitoring and to measure hematocrit levels. The same technique is needed to obtain a blood sample for newborn genetic screening tests.

It may be helpful to warm the heel before the sample is taken, because the application of heat for 5 to 10 minutes helps dilate the vessels in the area. A cloth soaked with warm water and wrapped loosely around the foot can effectively warm the foot (Fig. 26-7, *A*). Disposable heel warmers also are available from a variety of companies but should be used with care to prevent burns. Nurses should wear gloves when collecting any specimen. The nurse first cleanses the area with alcohol, restrains the infant's foot with his or her free hand, and then punctures the site. A spring-loaded automatic puncture device causes less pain and requires fewer punctures than a manual lance blade.

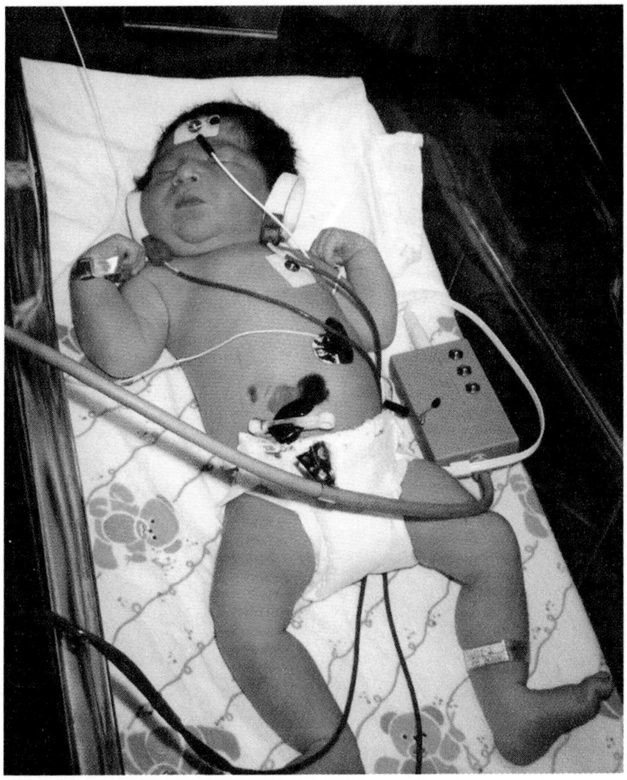

FIG. 26-6 Hearing screening in the newborn nursery. (Courtesy Dee Lowdermilk, Chapel Hill, NC.)

The most serious complication of an infant heel stick is necrotizing osteochondritis resulting from lancet penetration of the bone (Meehan, 1998). To prevent this, the stick should be made at the outer aspect of the heel and should penetrate no deeper than 2.4 mm (Hockenberry et al., 2003). To identify the appropriate puncture site, the nurse should draw an imaginary line from between the fourth and fifth toes that runs parallel to the lateral aspect of the heel, where the stick should be made; a line can also be drawn from the great toe that runs parallel to the medial aspect of the heel, another site for a stick (Fig. 26-7, *B*). Repeated trauma to the walking surface of the heel can cause fibrosis and scarring that may lead to problems with walking later in life.

After the specimen has been collected, pressure should be applied with a dry gauze square, but no further alcohol should be applied because this will cause the site to continue to bleed. The site is then covered with an adhesive bandage. The nurse ensures proper disposal of equipment used, reviews the laboratory slip for correct identification, and checks the specimen for accurate labeling and routing.

A heel stick is traumatic for the infant and causes pain. After several heel sticks, infants often withdraw their feet when they are touched. To reassure the infant and promote feelings of safety, the neonate should be cuddled and comforted when the procedure is complete.

Venipuncture. A venipuncture is less painful than a heel stick for blood sampling (Shah & Ohlsson, 2001). Venous blood samples can be drawn from antecubital, saphenous, superficial wrist, and rarely, scalp veins. If an intravenous site is used to obtain a blood specimen, it is important to consider the type of infusion fluid, because mixing of the blood sample with the fluid can alter the results.

When venipuncture is required, positioning of the needle is extremely important. Although regular venipuncture needles may be used, some prefer butterfly needles. It is necessary to be very patient during the procedure, because the blood return in small veins is slow, and consequently the small needle must remain in place longer. The mummy restraint commonly is used to help secure the infant (Fig. 26-8).

For *external jugular venipuncture,* "mummy" the infant as necessary, and then lower the infant's head over a rolled towel, the edge of a table, or your knee, and stabilize. For *femoral venipuncture,* place your hands over the infant's knees, but avoid pressing your fingers over the inner aspect of the thigh. Both of these positions ensure the safety of

A

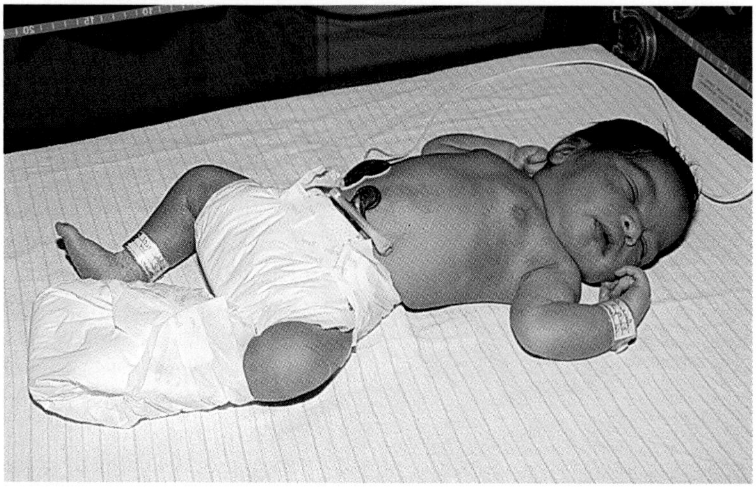

B

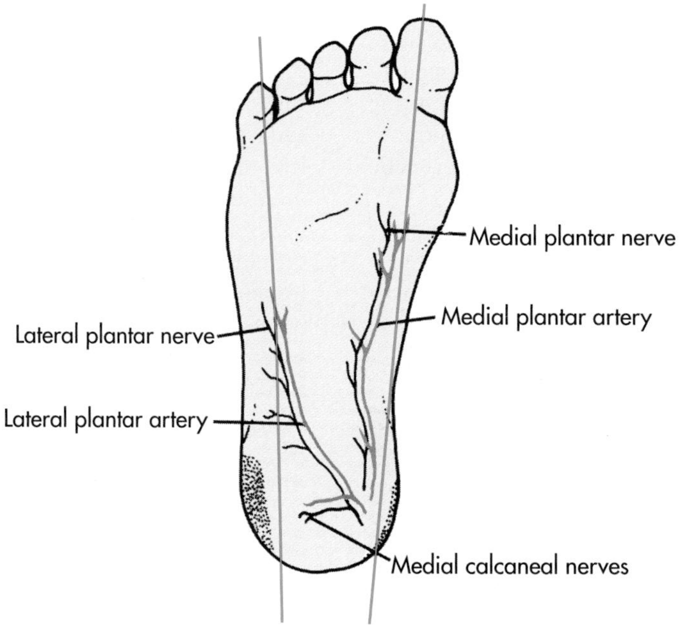
Medial plantar nerve
Medial plantar artery
Lateral plantar nerve
Lateral plantar artery
Medial calcaneal nerves

FIG. 26-7 Heel stick. **A,** Newborn with foot wrapped for warmth to increase blood flow to extremity before heel stick. **B,** Heel-stick sites (*shaded areas*) on infant's foot for obtaining samples of capillary blood. (**A** courtesy Marjorie Pyle, RNC, Lifecircle, Costa Mesa, CA.)

the infant and exposure of the puncture sites (Fig. 26-9, *A*). If the radial vein is used, the infant's arm is exposed and held securely in place. The nurse also may restrain the infant (see Restraining the Infant on p. 741).

If venipuncture or arterial puncture is being performed for blood gas studies, crying, fear, and agitation will affect the values; therefore every effort must be made to keep the infant quiet during the procedure. For blood gas studies, the blood sample tubes are packed in ice (to reduce blood cell metabolism) and are taken immediately to the laboratory for analysis.

Pressure must be maintained over an arterial or femoral vein puncture with a dry gauze square for at least 3 to 5 minutes to prevent bleeding from the site. For an hour after any venipuncture, the nurse should then observe the infant frequently for evidence of bleeding or hematoma formation at the puncture site. The infant's tolerance of the procedure also should be recorded. The infant should be cuddled and comforted when the procedure is completed.

Obtaining a Urine Specimen. Examination of urine is a valuable laboratory tool for infant assessment; the way in which the urine specimen is collected may influence the results. The urine sample should be fresh and analyzed within 1 hour of collection.

A variety of urine collection bags are available, including the Hollister U-Bag (Fig. 26-10). These are clear plastic,

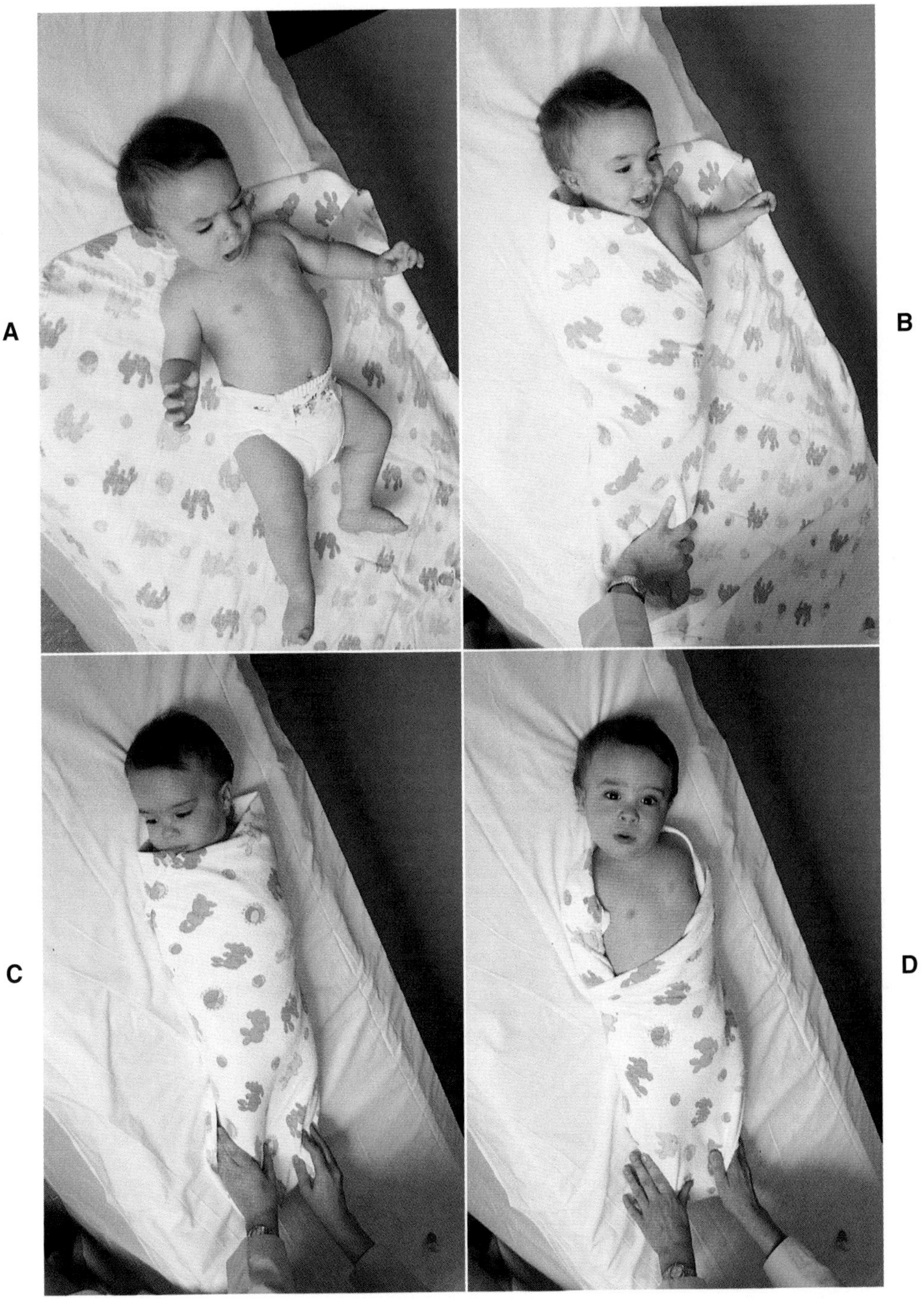
A
B
C
D

FIG. 26-8 Application of mummy restraint. **A,** Infant is placed on folded corner of blanket. **B,** One corner of blanket is brought across body and secured beneath the body. **C,** Second corner is brought across body and secured, and lower corner is folded and tucked or pinned in place. **D,** Modified mummy restraint with chest uncovered. (From Hockenberry, M. et al. (2003). *Wong's nursing care of infants and children* [7th ed.]. St. Louis: Mosby.)

single-use bags with an adhesive material around the opening at the point of attachment.

To prepare the infant, the nurse removes the diaper and places the infant in a supine position. The genitalia, perineum, and surrounding skin are washed and thoroughly dried because the adhesive on the bag will not stick to moist, powdered, or oily skin surfaces. The protective paper is removed to expose the adhesive (Fig. 26-10, *A*). In female infants, the perineum is first stretched to flatten skin folds, and then the adhesive area on the

A

B

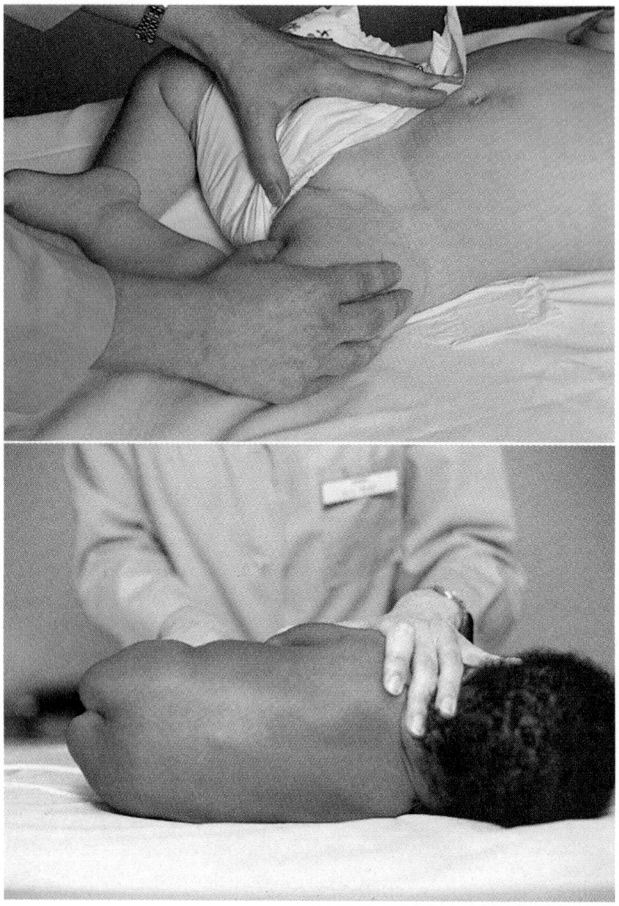

FIG. 26-9 **A,** Restraining infant for femoral vein puncture. **B,** Modified side-lying position for lumbar puncture. (From Hockenberry, M. et al. (2003). *Wong's nursing care of infants and children* [7th ed.]. St. Louis: Mosby.)

bag is pressed firmly onto the skin all around the urinary meatus and vagina. (NOTE: Start with the narrow portion of the butterfly-shaped adhesive patch.) Starting the application at the bridge of skin separating the rectum from the vagina and working upward is most effective (Fig. 26-10, *B*). In male infants, the penis and scrotum are tucked through the opening into the collection bag before removing the protective paper from the adhesive and pressing it firmly onto the perineum, making sure the entire adhesive is firmly attached to skin and the edges of the opening do not pucker (Fig. 26-10, *C*). This helps ensure a leak-proof seal and decreases the chance of contamination from stool. Cutting a slit in the diaper and pulling the bag through the slit also may help prevent leaking.

The diaper is carefully replaced, and the bag is checked frequently. When a sufficient amount of urine (this amount varies according to the test done) appears, the bag is removed. The infant's skin is observed for signs of irritation while the bag is in place. The specimen can be aspirated with a syringe or drained directly from the bag. For draining, the bag is held in the one hand and tilted to keep urine away from the tab. The tab is then removed and the urine drained into a clean receptacle (Fig. 26-10, *D*).

Collection of a 24-hour specimen can be a challenge; the infant may need to be restrained. The 24-hour urine bag is applied in the manner just described, and the urine is drained into a receptacle. The collection tube can be shortened or capped (Fig. 26-10, *E*). During the collection, the infant's skin is observed closely for signs of irritation and for lack of a proper seal.

For some types of urine tests, urine can be aspirated directly from the diaper by means of a syringe without a

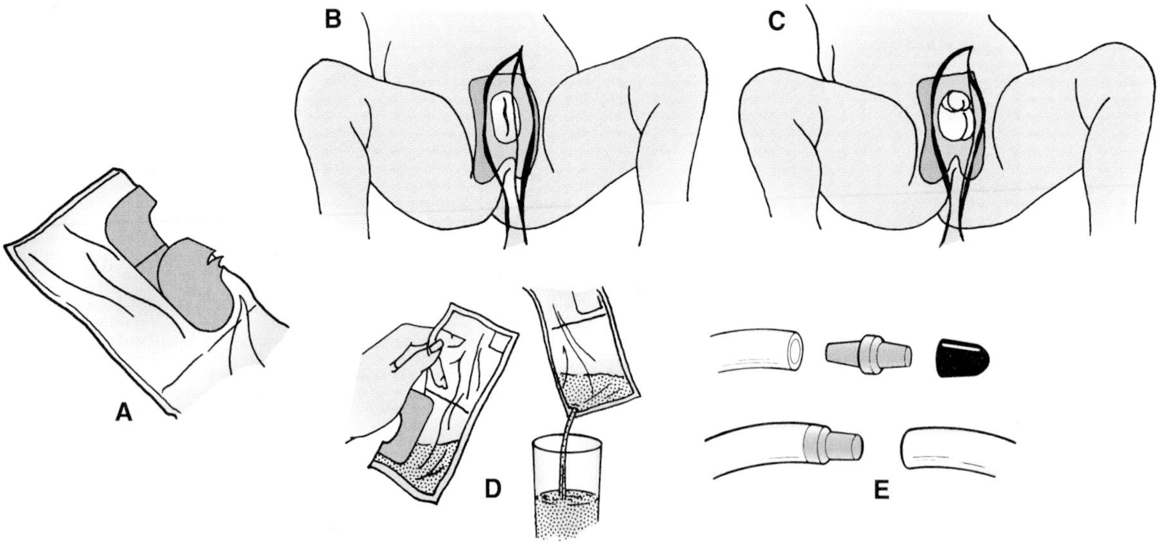
B
C
A
D
E

FIG. 26-10 Collection of urine specimen. **A,** Protective paper is removed from the adhesive surface. **B,** Applied to girls. **C,** Applied to boys. **D,** Cut to drain urine. **E,** Collection tube. (Permission to use and/or reproduce this copyrighted material has been granted by the owner, Hollister, Inc., Libertyville, IL.)

needle. If the diaper has absorbent gelling material that traps urine, a small gauze dressing or some cotton balls can be placed inside the diaper and the urine aspirated from them (Hockenberry et al., 2003).

Restraining the Infant. Infants may need to be restrained to (1) protect the infant from injury, (2) facilitate examinations, and (3) limit discomfort during tests, procedures, and specimen collections (see Figs. 26-8 and 26-9). These special considerations must be kept in mind when restraining an infant:

- Apply restraints and check them to make sure they are not irritating the skin or impairing circulation.
- Maintain proper body alignment.
- Apply restraints without using knots or pins if possible. If knots are necessary, make the kind that can be released quickly. Use pins with care so that there is no danger of their puncturing or pressing against the infant's skin.
- Check the infant hourly, or more frequently if indicated.

Restraint Without Appliance. The nurse may restrain the infant by using the hands and body. Figure 26-9, *B*, illustrates ways to restrain an infant in this manner.

Nursing Diagnoses

Possible nursing diagnoses for the newborn from 2 hours after birth until discharge include the following:

- *Ineffective breathing pattern related to*
  - obstructed airway
- *Impaired gas exchange related to*
  - hypothermia
- *Ineffective thermoregulation related to*
  - heat loss to the environment
- *Acute pain related to*
  - circumcision
  - heel sticks, venipuncture

Possible nursing diagnoses for the parents are as follows:

- *Readiness for enhanced family coping related to*
  - knowledge of newborn's social capabilities
  - knowledge of newborn's dependency needs
  - knowledge of biologic characteristics of the newborn
- *Situational low self-esteem related to*
  - misinterpretation of newborn's behavioral cues

Examples of nursing diagnoses derived from specific assessment findings are listed in the Plan of Care.

Expected Outcomes of Care

The expected outcomes for newborn care relate to the infant and parents. The outcomes for the infant expect that the infant will do the following:

- Maintain an effective breathing pattern.
- Maintain effective thermoregulation.
- Remain free from infection.
- Establish adequate elimination patterns
- Experience minimal pain.

For the parents, expected outcomes will include the following:

- Continue to attain knowledge, skill, and confidence relevant to infant care activities.
- State understanding of biologic and behavioral characteristics of their newborn.
- Have opportunities to intensify their relationship with the infant.
- Continue to integrate the infant into the family.

Plan of Care and Interventions

In the inpatient setting, priorities of care must be established and a systematic teaching plan devised for infant care. One way to accomplish this is to use critical path case management. A care path may be developed to cover the changes expected in the infant during the first several days of life (see Care Path). When variations from the care path occur, further assessment and intervention may be necessary.

Protective Environment

The provision of a protective environment is basic to the care of the newborn. The construction, maintenance, and operation of nurseries in accredited hospitals are monitored by national professional organizations such as the American Academy of Pediatrics and local or state governing bodies. In addition, hospital personnel develop their own policies and procedures for protecting the newborns under their care. Prescribed standards cover areas such as the following:

- *Environmental factors:* Provision of adequate lighting, elimination of potential fire hazards, safety of electrical appliances, adequate ventilation, and controlled temperature (i.e., warm and free of drafts) and humidity (lower than 50%).
- *Measures to control infection:* Adequate floor space to permit the positioning of bassinets at least 60 cm apart, handwashing facilities, and areas for cleaning and storing equipment and supplies.

Only those personnel directly involved in the care of mothers and infants are allowed in this area, thereby reducing the opportunities for the transmission of pathogenic organisms.

NURSE ALERT

Personnel are instructed to use good handwashing techniques; handwashing between each infant handling is the single most important measure in the prevention of neonatal infection.

Health care personnel must wear gloves when handling the infant until blood and amniotic fluid have been removed from its skin, when drawing blood (e.g., heel stick), when caring for a fresh wound (e.g., circumcision), and during diaper changes.

Plan of Care Normal Newborn

NURSING DIAGNOSIS Risk for ineffective airway clearance related to excess mucus production/improper positioning

Expected Outcomes *Neonate's airway remains patent; breath sounds are clear, and no respiratory distress is evident.*

Nursing Interventions/*Rationales*

Teach parents that gagging, coughing, and sneezing are normal neonatal responses *that assist the neonate in clearing airways.*

Teach parents feeding techniques that prevent overfeeding and distention of the abdomen and to burp neonate frequently *to prevent regurgitation and aspiration.*

Position neonate on back when sleeping *to prevent suffocation.*

Suction mouth and nasopharynx with bulb syringe as needed; clean nares of crusted secretions *to clear airway and prevent aspiration and airway obstruction.*

NURSING DIAGNOSIS Risk for imbalanced body temperature related to larger body surfaces in relationship to mass

Expected Outcome *Neonate temperature remains in range of 36.5° C to 37.2° C.*

Nursing Interventions/*Rationales*

Maintain neutral thermal environment *to identify any changes in neonate's temperature that may be related to other causes.*

Monitor neonate's temperature frequently *to identify any changes promptly and ensure early interventions.*

Bathe neonate efficiently when temperature is stable, using warm water, drying carefully, and avoiding exposing neonate to drafts *to avoid heat losses from evaporation and convection.*

Report any alterations in temperature findings promptly *to assess and treat for possible infection.*

NURSING DIAGNOSIS Risk for infection related to immature immunologic defenses/environmental exposure

Expected Outcome *The neonate will be free from signs of infection.*

Nursing Interventions/*Rationales*

Review maternal record for evidence of any risk factors *to ascertain whether the neonate may be predisposed to infection.*

Monitor vital signs *to identify early possible evidence of infection, especially temperature instability.*

Have all care providers, including parents, practice good handwashing techniques before handling newborn *to prevent spread of infection.*

Provide prescribed eye prophylaxis *to prevent infection.*

Keep genital area clean and dry using proper cleansing techniques *to prevent skin irritation, cross-contamination, and infection.*

Keep umbilical stump clean and dry and keep exposed to air *to allow to dry and minimize chance of infection.*

If circumcised, keep site clean and apply diaper loosely *to prevent trauma and infection.*

Teach parents to keep neonate away from crowds and environmental irritants *to reduce potential sources of infection.*

NURSING DIAGNOSIS Risk for injury related to sole dependence on caregiver

Expected Outcome *Neonate remains free of injury.*

Nursing Interventions/*Rationales*

Monitor environment for hazards such as sharp objects, long fingernails of caretaker and neonate, and jewelry of caretaker that may be sharp *to prevent injury.*

Handle neonate gently and support head, ensure use of car seat by parents, teach parents never to place neonate on high surface unsupervised, and to supervise pet and sibling interactions *to prevent injury.*

Assess neonate frequently for any evidence of jaundice *to identify rising bilirubin levels, treat promptly, and prevent kernicterus.*

NURSING DIAGNOSIS Readiness for enhanced family coping related to anticipatory guidance regarding responses to neonate's crying

Expected Outcomes *Parents will verbalize understanding of methods of coping with neonate's crying and describe increased success in interpreting neonate's cries.*

Nursing Interventions/*Rationales*

Alert parents to crying as neonate's form of communication and that cries can be differentiated to indicate hunger, wetness, pain, and loneliness *to provide reassurance that crying is not indicative of neonate's rejection of parents and that parents will soon be able to interpret the different cries of their child.*

Differentiate self-consoling behaviors from fussing/crying *to give parents concrete examples of interventions.*

Discuss methods of consoling a neonate who has been crying, such as checking and changing diapers; talking softly to neonate; holding neonate's arms close to body; swaddling; picking neonate up; rocking; using a pacifier, feeding, or burping; *to provide anticipatory guidance.*

Visitors and health care providers such as nurses, physicians, parents, brothers and sisters, department supervisors, electricians, and housekeepers are expected to wash their hands before having contact with infants or equipment. Cover gowns are not necessary.

Individuals with infectious conditions are excluded from contact with newborns or must take special precautions when working with infants. This includes persons with upper respiratory tract infections, GI tract infections, and infectious skin conditions. Most agencies have now coupled this day-to-day self-screening of personnel with yearly health examinations.

- *Safety factors:* Many agencies have implemented security measures in response to infant abductions from nurseries. Examples of the measures include placing identification bracelets on infants and their parents and footprinting or taking identification pictures immediately after birth, before the infant leaves the mother's side. Personnel wear picture identification badges or other badges that identify them as newborn personnel. Mother-baby units may have infant tracking systems that will set off an alarm if a baby is left alone or is with unauthorized personnel. Mothers are instructed to be

Care Path Neonatal Adaptation to Extrauterine Life

	DAY 1	DAY 2	DAY 3	DAY 4	DAY 7	DAY 14
Weight		Loss of 5%-7% of birth weight	Gain of 150-300 g per day			Birth weight regained
Temperature	Stabilized at 37° C					
Feedings						
Volume						
Formula	15-60 ml	60-90 ml	60-90 ml	60-90 ml	60-90 ml	60-90 ml
Breast			Softening of at least one breast at each feeding			
Frequency						
Formula	6-10 times/24 hr		6-10 times/24 hr		6-10 times/24 hr	
Breast	8-12 times/24 hr		8-12 times/24 hr		8-12 times/24 hr	
Voiding	At least 1 time in first 24 hr	2-6 times/24 hr		6-8 times/24 hr		6-8 times/24 hr
Stools		Meconium; ≥1 time in first 48 hr	Transitional stool: 1-5/day	Yellow stool: 1-5/day		Yellow stool: 1-2/day
Sleep	16-20 hr/24 hr					16-20 hr/24 hr
Umbilical cord	Moist; clamped	Dry; clamp removed				Cord off
Circumcision	Red; sore	Yellow exudate covers glans	Healing	Healing		Healed
Color	Pink; acrocyanotic	Pink; slight jaundice	Peak of jaundice		Pink	
Bilirubin level	0-6 mg/dl	≤8 mg/dl	≤12 mg/dl		≤2 mg/dl	
Laboratory tests	Glucose when required; Hct	PKU, T_4, galactose				Repeat PKU, if needed
Medications	Eye prophylaxis and vitamin K within 2 hr of birth; HBIG within 12 hr of birth	HBV may be given any time after birth before discharge				

HBV, Hepatitis B vaccine; *Hct*, hematocrit, *PKU*, phenylketonuria.

certain they know the identity of anyone who cares for the infant and never to release the infant to anyone who is not wearing the appropriate identification.

Supporting Parents in the Care of Their Infant

The sensitivity of the caregiver to the social responses of the infant is basic to the development of a mutually satisfying parent-child relationship (Leitch, 1999). Sensitivity increases over time as parents become more aware of their infant's social capabilities (see Cultural Considerations box).

Social Interaction. The activities of daily care during the neonatal period are the best times for infant-family interactions. While caring for their baby, the mother and father can talk to the infant, play baby games, and caress and cuddle the child. In Figure 26-11, a mother, father,

CULTURAL CONSIDERATIONS

Cultural Beliefs and Practices

Nurses working with childbearing families from other cultures and ethnic groups must be aware of cultural beliefs and practices that are important to individual families. People with a strong sense of heritage may hold on to traditional health beliefs long after adopting other American lifestyle practices. These health beliefs may involve practices regarding the newborn. For example, some Asians, Hispanics, eastern Europeans, and Native Americans delay breastfeeding because they believe that colostrum is "bad." Some Hispanics and African-Americans place a belly band over the infant's navel. The birth of a male child is generally preferred by Asians and Indians, and some Asians and Haitians delay naming their infant (D'Avanzo & Geissler, 2003).

and infant are shown engaging in arousal, imitation of facial expression, and smiling. Too much stimulation should be avoided after feeding and before a sleep period. Older children's contact with a newborn must be supervised in terms of strength of hugs, the exploring of eyes and nose, and attempts to feed the baby (Fig. 26-12).

Infant Feeding. The infant may be put to breast shortly after birth or at least within 4 hours of birth. If the infant is to be bottle fed, a nurse may first offer it a few sips of sterile water to make certain its sucking and swallowing reflexes are intact and that there are no anomalies such as a tracheoesophageal fistula. Most infants are on demand feeding schedules and are allowed to feed when they awaken. Ordinarily mothers are encouraged to feed their infants every 3 to 4 hours during the day and only when the infant awakens during the night in the first few days after birth. Formula-fed infants usually eat approximately every 3 to 4 hours. Breastfed babies nurse more often than bottle-fed babies because breast milk is digested faster than formulas made from cow's milk, and the stomach empties sooner as a result. Water supplements are not recommended. For a thorough discussion of infant feeding, see Chapter 27.

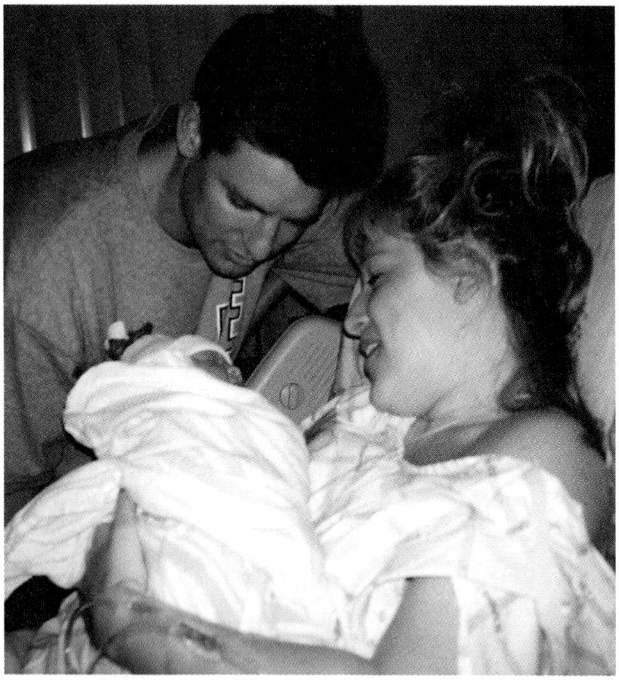

FIG. 26-11 Mother-father-baby interaction. (Courtesy Ellen Lewis, Irvine, CA.)

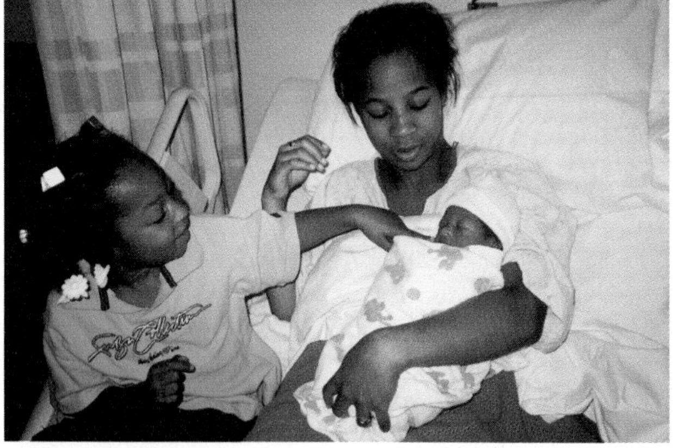

FIG. 26-12 Big sister meets baby brother for the first time. Note the fingertip touch. (Courtesy Shannon Perry, San Jose, CA.)

Therapeutic and Surgical Procedures

Intramuscular Injection. As discussed previously, it is routine to administer a single dose of 0.5 to 1 mg of vitamin K intramuscularly to an infant soon after birth (see Medication Guide box on p. 729).

Hepatitis B (Hep B) vaccination is recommended for all infants. Infants at highest risk of contracting hepatitis B are those born to women who come from Asia, Africa, South America, the South Pacific, or southern or eastern Europe (see Medication Guide). If the infant is born to an infected mother or to a mother who is a chronic carrier, hepatitis

MEDICATION GUIDE

Hepatitis B Vaccine (Recombivax HB, Engerix-B)

ACTION ■ Hepatitis B vaccine induces protective anti–hepatitis B antibodies in 95% to 99% of healthy infants who receive the recommended three doses. The duration of protection of the vaccine is unknown.

INDICATION ■ HBV is for immunization against infection caused by all known subtypes of hepatitis B virus.

NEONATAL DOSAGE ■ The usual dosage is Recombivax HB, 5 μg/0.5 ml, or Engerix-B, 10 μg/0.5 ml, at 0, 1, and 6 months. An alternate dosing schedule is 0, 1, 2, and 12 months and is usually for newborns whose mothers were hepatitis B surface antigen (HbsAg) positive.

ADVERSE REACTIONS ■ Common adverse reactions are rash, fever, erythema, swelling, and pain at injection site.

NURSING CONSIDERATIONS ■ Parental consent must be obtained before administration. Wear gloves. Administer in the middle third of the vastus lateralis muscle by using a 25-gauge, 5/8-inch needle. Inject into skin that has been cleaned, or allow alcohol to dry on puncture site for 1 min to remove organisms and prevent infection. Stabilize leg firmly and grasp muscle between the thumb and fingers. Insert the needle at a 90-degree angle; aspirate, and inject medication slowly if there is no blood return. Massage the site with a dry gauze square after removing needle to increase absorption. If the infant was born to HBsAg-positive mother, hepatitis B immune globulin (HBIG) should be given within 12 hr of birth in addition to the HB vaccine. Separate sites must be used.

vaccine and hepatitis B immune globulin (HBIG) should be administered within 12 hours of birth (see Medication Guide). The hepatitis vaccine is given in one site and the HBIG in another. For infants born to healthy women, the first dose of the vaccine may be given at birth or at age 1 or 2 months. Parental consent should be obtained before administering these vaccines.

In most cases, a 25-gauge, 5/8-inch needle should be used for the vitamin K and hepatitis vaccine injections. A 22-gauge needle may be necessary if thicker medications such as some penicillins are to be given.

Selection of the site for injection is important. Injections must be given in muscles large enough to accommodate the medication, and major nerves and blood vessels must be avoided. The muscles of newborns may not tolerate more than a 0.5 ml per intramuscular injection. The injection site for newborns is the vastus lateralis (Fig. 26-13). The dorsogluteal muscle is very small, poorly developed, and dangerously close to the sciatic nerve, which occupies a larger area in infants compared with older children. Therefore it is not recommended that it be used as an injection site until the child has been walking for at least 1 year.

Newborn infants offer little, if any, resistance to injections. Although they squirm and may be difficult to hold in position if they are awake, they can usually be restrained without the need for assistance from a second person if the nurse is experienced.

The neonate's leg should be stabilized. Gloves should be worn by the person giving the injection. The nurse cleanses the injection site with alcohol and then pinches up the infant's muscle between the thumb and forefinger. The needle is inserted into the vastus lateralis at a 90-degree angle. The muscle is released and the plunger of the syringe gently withdrawn. If no blood is aspirated, the medication is injected. If blood is aspirated, the needle is withdrawn and the injection is given in another site. After the injection has been given, the needle is withdrawn quickly and the site massaged with a gauze square to hasten absorption, unless contraindicated. It is not uncommon for blood to ooze from the injection site, but it is not necessary to cover the site with an adhesive bandage. Pressure should be applied until oozing stops.

MEDICATION GUIDE

Hepatitis B Immune Globulin (HBIG)

ACTION ▪ HBIG provides a high titer of antibody to hepatitis B surface antigen (HBsAg).

INDICATION ▪ The HBIG vaccine provides prophylaxis against infection in infants born of HBsAg-positive mothers.

NEONATAL DOSAGE ▪ Administer one 0.5-ml dose intramuscularly within 12 hr of birth.

ADVERSE REACTIONS ▪ Hypersensitivity may occur.

NURSING CONSIDERATIONS ▪ Must be given within 12 hr of birth. Wear gloves. Administer in the middle third of the vastus lateralis muscle by using a 25-gauge, 5/8-inch needle. Inject into skin that has been cleaned, or allow alcohol to dry on puncture site for 1 min to remove organisms and prevent infection. Stabilize leg firmly, and grasp muscle between the thumb and fingers. Insert the needle at a 90-degree angle; aspirate, and inject medication slowly if there is no blood return. Massage the site with a dry gauze square after removing needle to increase absorption. May be given at same time as hepatitis B vaccine but at a different site.

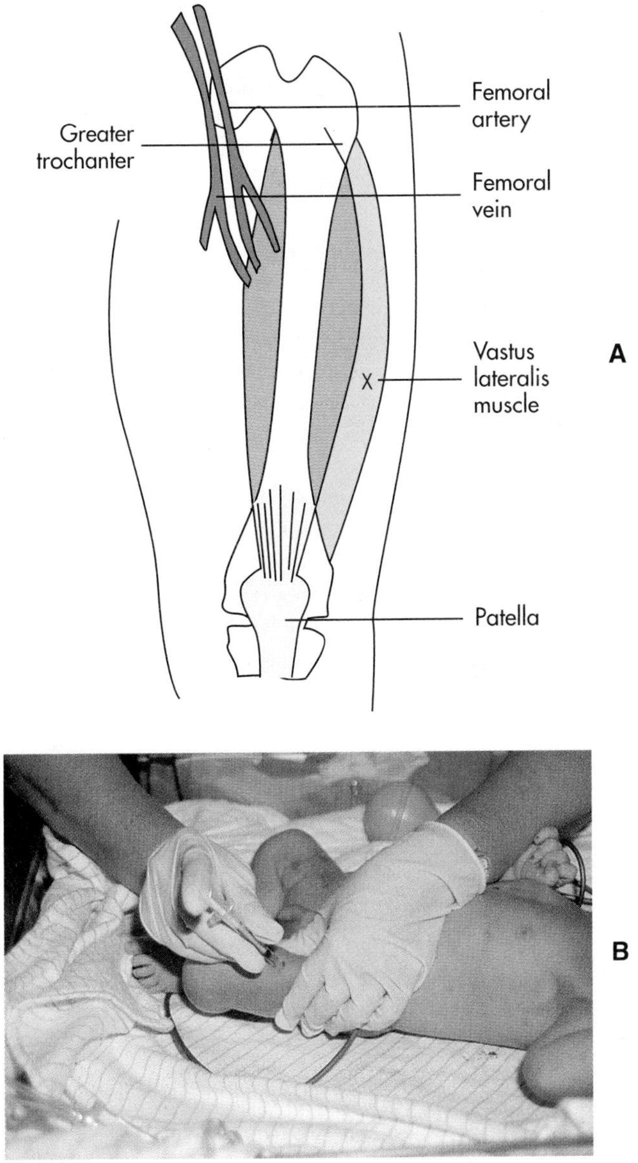
Greater trochanter
Femoral artery
Femoral vein
Vastus lateralis muscle
X
Patella
A
B

FIG. 26-13 Intramuscular injection. **A,** Acceptable intramuscular injection site for newborn infant. X, Injection site. **B,** Infant's leg stabilized for intramuscular injection. Nurse is wearing gloves to give injection. (**B** courtesy Marjorie Pyle, RNC, Lifecircle, Costa Mesa, CA.)

The nurse should always remember to comfort the infant after an injection and to discard equipment properly. It is important to record the name of the medication, the date and time of administration, the amount, the route, the site of injection, and the infant's tolerance of injection.

Therapy for Hyperbilirubinemia. The best therapy for hyperbilirubinemia is prevention. Because bilirubin is excreted in meconium, prevention can be facilitated by early feeding, which stimulates the passage of meconium. However, despite early passage of meconium, the term infant may have trouble conjugating the increased amount of bilirubin derived from disintegrating fetal red blood cells. As a result, the serum levels of unconjugated bilirubin may increase beyond normal limits, causing hyperbilirubinemia (see Chapter 25). The goal of treatment of hyperbilirubinemia is to help reduce the newborn's serum levels of unconjugated bilirubin. The two principal ways of doing this are phototherapy and exchange blood transfusion. Exchange transfusion treats those infants whose increased levels of bilirubin cannot be controlled by phototherapy.

Phototherapy. During **phototherapy** the unclothed infant is placed beneath a bank of lights. The distance may vary based on unit protocol and the type of light used. The infant is turned every 2 hours to expose all body surfaces to the light. This is done for several hours or days until the infant's serum bilirubin level decreases to within an acceptable range. The decision to discontinue therapy is based on the observation of a definite downward trend in the bilirubin values. After therapy has been terminated, the infant may have a rebound in bilirubin levels, which is usually harmless (Kliegman, 2002).

Several precautions must be taken while the infant is undergoing phototherapy. The lamp energy output should be monitored routinely during treatment with a photometer. The infant's eyes must be protected by an opaque mask to prevent overexposure to the light; the eye shield should cover the eyes completely but not occlude the nares. Before the mask is applied, the infant's eyes should be closed gently to prevent excoriation of the corneas. The mask should be removed during infant feedings so that the eyes can be checked and the parents can have visual contact with the infant (Maisels, 1999) (see Fig. 28-6).

To promote optimal skin exposure during phototherapy, the diaper may be left off, or a "string bikini" made from a disposable face mask may be used to cover the infant's genital area.

NURSE ALERT

Before its application, the metal strip must be removed from the face mask to prevent burning the infant. Lotions and ointments should not be applied to the infant because they absorb heat, and this can cause burns.

Phototherapy may cause the infant to sleep for longer than the usual 3- to 4-hour periods, but the infant must be kept on a regular feeding schedule to maintain hydration. When possible, it is best to hold the infant for feeding and to encourage parent-infant interaction during this time.

The number and consistency of stools are monitored. Because bilirubin breakdown increases gastric motility, which results in the formation of loose stools that can cause skin excoriation and breakdown, the infant's buttocks are cleaned after each stool to help maintain skin integrity.

During phototherapy, the infant's temperature may become elevated; this requires monitoring at least every 4 hours. The lights increase insensible water loss, placing the infant at risk for fluid loss and dehydration; therefore it is important that the infant be adequately hydrated. All aspects of the phototherapy rendered should be accurately recorded in the infant's chart.

An alternative device for phototherapy that is safe and effective is a fiberoptic panel attached to an illuminator. This fiberoptic blanket, which wraps light around the newborn's torso, delivers continuous phototherapy. While wearing it, the newborn can remain in the mother's room in an open crib or in her arms; follow unit protocol for the use of eye patches. The blanket also may be used for home care. Fiberoptic blankets may be used in combination with phototherapy lights to deliver "double phototherapy" (Maisels, 1999).

Exchange Transfusion. Exchange transfusion is usually reserved for infants at risk for kernicterus due to high bilirubin levels. Small amounts of cross-matched whole blood are transfused into the infant as equivalent amounts of the infant's blood are withdrawn and discarded. This is most often accomplished through an umbilical venous catheter. Potential complications of exchange transfusion include transfusion reaction, infection, metabolic instability, and complications related to placement of the umbilical catheter (Kliegman, 2002) (see Chapter 39).

Parent Education. Serum levels of bilirubin in the newborn continue to increase until the fifth day of life. Many parents leave the hospital within 24 hours, and some, as early as 6 hours after birth. Therefore parents must be able to assess the newborn's degree of jaundice. They should have written instructions for assessing the infant's condition and the name of the contact person to whom to report their findings. Some health care agencies have a nurse make a home visit to evaluate the infant's condition. If it proves necessary to measure the infant's bilirubin levels after discharge from the hospital, either the home care nurse may draw the blood specimen or the parents may take the baby to a laboratory for the determination (Box 26-4).

Circumcision. Circumcision of male infants is commonly performed in the United States, although there is controversy over its value. The American Academy of Pediatrics (AAP) Task Force on Circumcision (1999) noted that, although there is scientific evidence of potential medical benefits of circumcision, the data are not sufficient to recommend routine circumcision. The Task Force further recommended that if circumcision is performed, analgesia should be used.

BOX 26-4 **Hyperbilirubinemia**

DEFINITIONS

- *Hyperbilirubinemia:* higher levels of bilirubin than normal
- *Bilirubin:* end product of RBCs when they mature and break down
- *RBCs:* red blood cells
- *Jaundice:* yellow skin, sclerae, and mucous membranes caused by circulating bilirubin
- *Phototherapy:* the use of fluorescent light to break down the bilirubin in the skin into substances that can be excreted in the feces (stool) and urine
- *Bililites:* fluorescent lights used for phototherapy

HOW JAUNDICE HAPPENS

- When RBCs break down, they release bilirubin, which then circulates in the blood. The bilirubin combines with another substance in the liver. This combined substance moves through the blood to the kidneys and the intestines, where it is eliminated in the urine and the stool. The bilirubin gives the yellow color to urine and the brown color to the stool.
- Before birth, babies have more RBCs in each ounce of blood than adults have. The RBCs of the unborn infant also have a shorter life span (70 to 90 days) than do RBCs formed after birth (120 days). When the RBCs of a fetus break down, the bilirubin produced by this is carried by the fetus's blood, through the placenta, and to the mother's liver to be excreted.
- After birth, the infant's liver must get rid of the bilirubin. Even though a baby's liver functions well, it may not be able to get rid of all the bilirubin produced by breakdown of RBCs. Bilirubin then seeps out of the blood and into the tissues and the skin, coloring them yellow (jaundice). The blood level of bilirubin increases quickly up to the fifth day, and then it declines; the jaundice usually clears up by the end of the week.

THE DANGER OF EXCESS BILIRUBIN

- Some newborns seem to have extra bilirubin to excrete. High levels of bilirubin may cause damage to the brain.
- According to the American Academy of Pediatrics guidelines (1994), phototherapy is considered in a healthy term infant who is 1 to 2 days old if the total bilirubin level is $\geq$ 12 mg/dl, or it is instituted if the bilirubin level is $\geq$ 15 mg/dl. The infant is placed under phototherapy lights or on a fiberoptic bili blanket. This helps the infant eliminate the extra bilirubin and prevents damage to the brain.

CARING FOR THE INFANT

- The newborn is placed under a radiant warmer or in an isolette under phototherapy lights so that it can be kept warm and the nurse can observe it.
- The infant wears an eye mask to keep the light out of the eyes.
- The infant is undressed so that as much light as possible can reach the skin. The newborn may wear a "string bikini" as a small diaper, which is made out of a paper diaper or a face mask.
- The infant's temperature is taken often so that any changes in temperature can be noted, and the infant is not allowed to become too hot or too cold.
- The newborn is taken out from under the lights for feedings and cuddling. If a bili blanket is being used, the infant can be held and fed with the blanket in place.
- Blood is taken from the heel periodically to check the amount of bilirubin still in the newborn's blood, and the nurse or physician updates the parents about the results.

AFTER THE NEWBORN GOES HOME

The parents should be encouraged to ask any questions they have. The nurse gives them a telephone number to call at any hour with their questions. If therapy is continued at home, referral is made to home care, and appropriate teaching is done (see Chapter 28).

Circumcision is a matter of personal parental choice. Parents usually decide to have their newborn circumcised for one or more of the following reasons: hygiene, religious conviction, tradition, culture, or social norms. Regardless of the reason for the decision, parents should be given unbiased information and the opportunity to discuss the benefits and risks of the procedure (Van Ryzin, 2000). Risks include cold stress, hypoglycemia, aspiration, bleeding, infection, and, rarely, cutting off too much of the foreskin or the penis.

Expectant parents should begin learning about circumcision during the prenatal period, but circumcision often is not discussed with the parents before labor. In many instances, it is only when the mother is being admitted to the hospital or birth unit that parents are first confronted with the decision regarding circumcision. Because the stress of the intrapartal period makes this a difficult time for parental decision making, this is not an ideal time to broach the topic of circumcision and expect a well-thought-out decision.

Procedure. **Circumcision** involves removing the prepuce (foreskin) of the glans. The procedure is usually not done immediately after birth because of the danger of cold stress but is performed in the hospital before the infant's discharge. The circumcision of a Jewish male is performed on the eighth day after birth and is done at home, in a ceremony called a *bris*, unless the infant is not well. This timing is logical from a physiologic standpoint because clotting factors decrease somewhat immediately after birth and do not return to prebirth levels until the end of the first week.

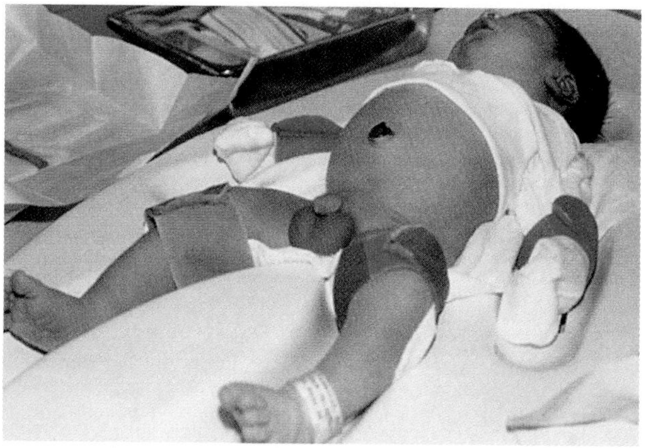

FIG. 26-14 "Circ board" restrains infant during circumcision. (Courtesy Marjorie Pyle, RNC, Lifecircle, Costa Mesa, CA.)

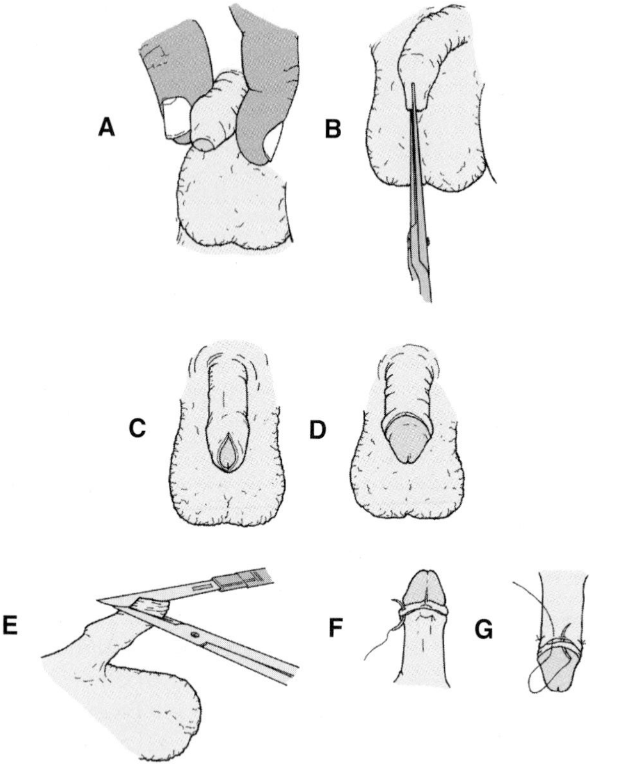
A
B
C
D
E
F
G

FIG. 26-15 Technique of circumcision. **A** to **D,** Prepuce is stripped and slit to facilitate its retraction behind glans penis. **E,** Prepuce is now clamped and excessive prepuce cut off. **F** and **G,** A very small needle and plain 2-0 or 3-0 catgut are used for suture material; some physicians prefer silk.

Formula feedings are usually withheld up to 4 hours before the circumcision to prevent vomiting and aspiration; breastfed infants may be allowed to nurse up until the procedure is done; this varies with unit protocol. To prepare the infant for the circumcision, he is positioned on a plastic restraint form (Fig. 26-14), and his penis is cleansed with soap and water or a preparatory solution such as povidone-iodine. The infant is draped to provide warmth and a sterile field, and the sterile equipment is readied for use.

Although some circumcision procedures require no special equipment or appliances (Fig. 26-15), numerous instruments have been designed for this purpose. Use of the Gomco, Yellen, or Mogen clamp (Fig. 26-16) may make this an almost bloodless operation. The procedure itself takes only a few minutes. After it is completed, a small petrolatum gauze dressing or a generous amount of petrolatum may be applied for the first day or two to prevent the diaper from adhering to the site. A PlastiBell also may be used for the circumcision. The advantages to its use are that it applies constant direct pressure to prevent hemorrhage during the procedure and afterward protects against infection, keeps the site from sticking to the diaper, and prevents pain with urination. To use the bell for circumcision, first fit it over the glans, tie the suture around the rim of the bell, and then cut away

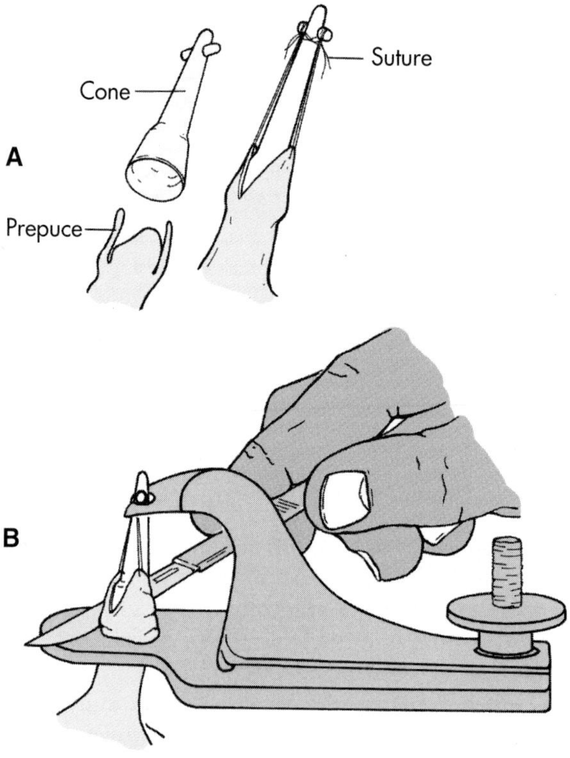
A
Cone
Suture
Prepuce
B

FIG. 26-16 Circumcision with Yellen clamp. **A,** Prepuce drawn over cone. **B,** Yellen clamp is applied, hemostasis occurs, and then prepuce (over cone) is cut away.

excess prepuce. The plastic rim remains in place for about a week until it falls off, after healing has taken place (Fig. 26-17). Petrolatum need not be applied when the PlastiBell is used.

Discomfort. Circumcision is painful, and the pain is manifested by both physiologic and behavioral changes in the infant. Three types of anesthesia/analgesia are used in newborns who undergo circumcisions. These include (from most effective to less effective) ring block, dorsal penile nerve block (DPNB), and topical anesthetic (AAP Task Force on Circumcision, 1999) (see Evidence-Based Practice box).

A ring block is the injection of buffered lidocaine administered subcutaneously on each side of the penile shaft. A DPNB includes subcutaneous injections of buffered lidocaine at the 2 o'clock and 10 o'clock positions at the base of the penis. The circumcision should not be done for at least 5 minutes after these injections.

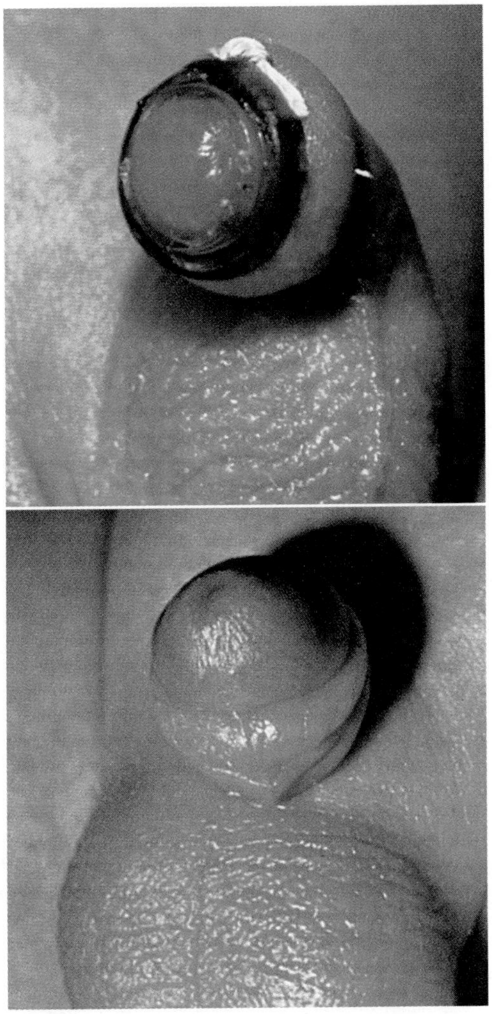
A
B

FIG. 26-17 Circumcision by using Hollister Plastibell. **A,** Suture around rim of Plastibell controls bleeding. **B,** Plastic rim and suture drop off in 7 to 10 days. (Permission to use and/or reproduce this copyrighted material has been granted by the owner, Hollister, Incorporated, Libertyville, IL.)

A topical cream containing prilocaine-lidocaine such as EMLA can be applied to the base of the penis at least 1 hour before the circumcision. The area where the prepuce attaches to the glans is well coated with the cream and then covered with a transparent occlusive dressing or finger cot. After the procedure, the cream is removed. Blanching or redness of the skin may occur (Taddio, Ohlsson, & Ohlsson, 2001)

Oral acetaminophen and comfort measures such as the infant sucking on a pacifier and talking to the infant in a soothing voice have not proven to be effective in pain reduction. However, pacifiers dipped in a concentrated glucose solution have been used during procedure with varying levels of effectiveness. None of these interventions is sufficient for the control of operative pain associated with circumcision; they are not recommended as the sole method of analgesia (AAP Task Force on Circumcision, 1999).

After the circumcision, the infant is comforted until he is quieted. If the parents were not present during the procedure, the infant is returned to them. The infant may be fussy for several hours, or he may be sleepy and difficult to awaken for feedings.

Care of the Newly Circumcised Infant. Bleeding is the most common complication of circumcision (AAP Task Force on Circumcision, 1999). The nurse checks the penis hourly for the next 12 hours to make sure no bleeding is occurring and voiding is normal. If bleeding is noted from the circumcision, the nurse applies gentle pressure to the site of bleeding with a folded sterile gauze square; absorbable gelatin sponge (Gelfoam) powder or sponge may be applied to stop bleeding. If bleeding is not easily controlled, a blood vessel may require ligation. In this event, one nurse notifies the physician and prepares the necessary equipment (circumcision tray and suture material), while another nurse maintains intermittent pressure until the physician arrives. If the parents take the baby home before the end of the 12-hour observation period, they must be instructed about postcircumcision care and when to notify the physician (see Teaching for Self-Care box on p. 793). Before the infant is discharged, the nurse checks to see that the parents have the physician's telephone number.

Nursing actions are planned and implemented to prevent infection. With each diaper change, the nurse gently washes the penis with warm water to remove urine and feces. If the clamp technique was used, fresh petrolatum is applied around the glans after each diaper change. The glans penis, which is normally dark red during healing, becomes covered with a yellow exudate in 24 hours. This is part of normal healing, not an infective process. No attempt is made to remove the exudate, which persists for 2 to 3 days. Parents should be

EVIDENCE-BASED PRACTICE

NEONATAL CIRCUMCISION PAIN MANAGEMENT

BACKGROUND

Circumcision is a painful procedure, causing physiologic and behavioral effects in newborns who are circumcised. Physiologic stress responses that have been identified during the procedure include elevated serum cortisol, elevated heart and respiratory rates, and decreased transcutaneous oxygen saturation levels. After the procedure, heart and respiratory rates remain elevated for a short time. Behavioral changes identified during the procedure include increased crying and facial patterning; for a short time after the circumcision, the infants have been found to be less alert, irritable, and not easily consoled; exhibit jerky body movement; and be difficult to feed (Macke, 2001).

Pain during circumcision can be reduced using anesthetics, and the infant is less irritable and more alert after the procedure. The American Academy of Pediatrics recommends the use of nonpharmacologic and pharmacologic interventions to prevent, reduce, or eliminate stress and pain during circumcision (Lannon et al., 1999).

OBJECTIVE

Evidence of pain management during neonatal circumcision was examined to establish a standard of practice for pain control. Interventions evaluated included the administration of acetaminophen, use of dorsal penile nerve block with buffered lidocaine, application of eutectic mixture of local anesthetic one hour before the procedure, offer of a pacifier dipped in a sugar solution, swaddling, and environmental modifications such as dim lights and soft music (Geyer et al., 2002).

SEARCH STRATEGY

Members of a multidisciplinary health care team at the Children's Hospital of Iowa reviewed the literature using various search strategies. Each member of the team was responsible for reviewing one specific intervention.

REVIEW OF THE EVIDENCE (GEYER ET AL., 2002)

Acetaminophen

Two randomized placebo-controlled trials of acetaminophen administration for newborn circumcision reported that pain during the procedures was not relieved by the acetaminophen; however, the drug did provide some degree of pain relief afterwards, particularly if it was given every 4 to 6 hours for 24 hours (Howard, Howard, & Weitzman, 1994; Macke, 2001).

Penile Nerve Block

Many studies of dorsal penile nerve block (DPNB) support the efficacy and safety of the procedure. It is effective in reducing fluctuations in vital signs and oxygen saturation levels during the circumcision. There have been no significant short-term complications found in 7000 infants studied over an 8-year period. The ring block is another type of nerve block that is performed at the mid-shaft of the penis and is also effective for newborn circumcision. No data were found that compared the efficacy of this method with DPNB.

Through many studies of pain in children, use of buffered lidocaine has been shown to decrease pain of injections without interfering with the efficacy of the anesthetic. Whether it decreases the pain response with DPNB is not known. The efficacy of using a slow injection speed, a small-gauge needle, and a warmed solution for nerve blocks is also unknown.

Eutectic Mixture of Local Anesthetic (EMLA)

EMLA cream applied to the penis 45 to 60 minutes before circumcision has been shown to improve heart rate, crying, and facial activity scores even though these measurements were still higher than the baseline measurements. EMLA was not found to provide postoperative analgesia equal to DPNB.

Sucrose Pacifier

A meta-analysis of 13 studies showed that giving oral sucrose decreased crying time of newborns during venipuncture and heel stick. Use of a pacifier dipped in sucrose before and during circumcision decreased behavioral pain responses, but the intervention was not found to be as effective as DPNB.

Swaddling

Swaddling the upper body of the infant during circumcision significantly decreased pain responses. Padding the restraint board also decreased signs of distress.

Modifying the Environment

Studies that shielded the eyes of newborns from bright light during painful procedures found that infants had fewer body movements and lower heart and respiratory rates. No specific studies of using soft music specifically for circumcision were found, but its use in studies of preterm infants having invasive procedures was associated with infants being less agitated and having higher oxygen saturation levels.

LIMITATIONS

Only a small number of clinical trials for any of the interventions to reduce circumcision pain were reported in the review. More evidence exists for the use of acetaminophen and DPNB than for any of the other methods.

CONCLUSIONS

Acetaminophen does not appear to control pain during circumcision, but postcircumcision administration of the drug does provide pain relief. It is likely to be a beneficial form of care. Whether it should be given before the procedure and continued every 4 to 6 hours for 24 hours or administered only after the procedure needs further study.

DPNB is effective for pain relief during neonatal circumcision and is a beneficial form of care. Studies comparing DPNB with ring nerve block are needed. There is substantial evidence that buffered lidocaine reduces injection pain, but its use has been studied minimally in relation to circumcision.

Using EMLA alone does not provide as much pain relief as nerve blocks. Whether its use enhances pain relief when combined with other methods needs to be studied.

Swaddling, offering a sucrose pacifier, and modifying the environment can reduce behavioral stress in newborns undergoing painful procedures such as heel stick and venipuncture and are likely to be beneficial adjuncts to other methods of analgesia used for circumcision. More studies are needed.

Reference: Geyer, J. et al. (2002). Evidence-based multidisciplinary protocol for neonatal circumcision pain management. *Journal of Obstetric, Gynecologic, and Neonatal Nursing, 31*(4), 403-410; Howard, C., Howard, F., & Weitzman, M. (1994). Acetaminophen analgesia in neonatal circumcision: The effect on pain. *Pediatrics, 93,* 641-646; Lannon, C. et al. (1999). *Circumcision policy statement* (No. RE9850). Elk Grove, IL: American Academy of Pediatrics; Macke, J. (2001). Analgesia for circumcision: Effects on newborn behavior and maternal-infant interactions. *Journal of Obstetric, Gynecologic, and Neonatal Nursing, 30*(5), 507-514.

taught to fan-fold the diaper so that it does not press on the circumcised area. They also should be encouraged to change the diaper at least every 4 hours to prevent it from sticking to the penis. It is also important to note that the infant is voiding sufficiently after the circumcision.

If the PlastiBell technique was used, the parents are instructed to observe the position of the plastic ring on the glans; it should remain on the glans (not on the shaft of the penis) and should fall off within 5 to 7 days.

Evaluation

The nurse can be reasonably assured that care was effective to the extent that the expected outcomes for care have been achieved.

PAIN IN NEONATES

Pain has physiologic and psychologic components. The psychologic component of pain and the diffuse total body response to pain exhibited by the neonate led many health care providers to believe that infants, especially preterm infants, do not experience pain. The central nervous system is well developed, however, as early as 24 weeks of gestations. The peripheral and spinal structures that transmit pain information are present and functional between the first and second trimester. The pituitary-adrenal axis also is well developed at this time, and a fight-or-flight reaction is observed in response to the catecholamines released in response to stress (American Academy of Pediatrics & Canadian Paediatric Society, 2000; Walden & Franck, 2003).

The physiologic response to pain in neonates can be life threatening. Pain response can decrease tidal volume, increase demands on the cardiovascular system, increase metabolism, and cause neuroendocrine imbalance. The hormonal-metabolic response to pain in a term infant has greater magnitude and shorter duration than that in adults. The newborn's sympathetic response to pain is less mature and thus less predictable than an adult's.

Assessment

The response to pain can be assessed in behavioral, physiologic/autonomic, and metabolic categories (Walden & Franck, 2003).

Behavioral Responses

The most common behavioral sign of pain is a vocalization or cry. The pain cry is distinctive: high pitched, and shrill. A cry face also is characteristic of an infant experiencing pain. Other facial features exhibited during pain include eye squeeze, brow contraction, deepened nasolabial furrows, a taut and quivering tongue, and open mouth. The infant will flex and adduct the upper body and lower limbs in an attempt to withdraw from the painful stimulus (Anand, Grunau, & Oberlander, 1997; Hadjistavropoulos et al., 1997). The preterm infant has a lower threshold for initiation of this flex response. An infant who receives a muscle-paralyzing agent such as vecuronium will be unable to mount a behavioral or visible pain response.

Physiologic/Autonomic Responses

Significant changes in heart rate, BP (increased or decreased), intracranial pressure, vagal tone, respiratory rate, and oxygen saturation occur during noxious stimuli (Walden & Franck, 2003).

Metabolic Responses

Infants release epinephrine, norepinephrine, glucagon, corticosterone, cortisol, 11-deoxycorticosterone, lactate, pyruvate, and glucose in response to pain (Walden & Franck, 2003).

Assessment and Management of Neonatal Pain

Pain should be assessed regularly (Walden, 2001). Several pain assessment tools have been developed to assess pain in the neonate. One pain assessment tool used by nurses in the NICU is the CRIES (see Table 40-3). This tool was developed for use by nurses who work with preterm and term infants. CRIES is an acronym for the physiologic and behavioral indicators of pain used in the tool: crying, requiring increased oxygen, increased vital signs, expression, and sleeplessness. Each indicator is scored from 0 to 2. The total possible pain score, which represents the worst pain, is 10. A pain score greater than 4 should be considered significant. This tool can be used on infants between ages 32 weeks of gestation and 20 weeks after birth (Pasero, 2002).

The goals of the management of neonatal pain are to (1) minimize the intensity, duration, and physiologic cost of the pain; and (2) maximize the neonate's ability to cope with and recover from the pain (Walden & Franck, 2003). Nonpharmacologic and pharmacologic strategies are used.

Nonpharmacologic Management

Containment, also known as swaddling, is effective in reducing excessive immature motor responses. This may provide comfort through other senses, such as thermal, tactile, and proprioceptive senses (Walden & Franck, 2003). Nonnutritive sucking is the most common comfort measure used; however, the effectiveness of nonnutritive sucking in reducing the pain response has been found to be limited and confined to the pain caused by certain procedures (Mohan et al., 1998). Sucrose may be effective in reducing response to procedural pain (Stevens & Ohlsson, 2001). Distraction with visual, oral, auditory, or tactile stimulation may be helpful in term or older infants (Walden & Franck, 2003). Skin-to-skin contact with the mother during painful procedures, such as heel-stick, reduces the pain reaction (Gibbons, 2000).

Pharmacologic Management

Pharmacologic agents are routinely used for adults during painful procedures. These same agents are now being used routinely for neonates to alleviate pain with procedures. Local anesthesia has become routine during procedures such as chest tube insertion and circumcision. Topical anesthesia has been used for circumcision, lumbar puncture, venipuncture, and heel sticks (Walden & Franck, 2003; Mohan et al., 1998). Nonopioid analgesia (acetaminophen) is effective for mild to moderate pain from inflammatory conditions. Opioids have been used as preprocedural analgesia. If the infant is not ventilated, the use of opioids is of concern because of the potential for these agents to cause respiratory depression (Walden & Franck, 2003).

KEY POINTS

- The immediate nursing assessment of the newborn includes Apgar scoring and a general evaluation of physical status.
- Nursing care of the newborn immediately after birth includes maintaining a patent airway, preventing heat loss, stabilizing the infant, and promoting parent-infant interaction.
- Nursing care of the newborn may include diagnostic and therapeutic procedures.
- Assessment of the newborn requires data from the prenatal, intrapartal, and postnatal periods.
- The newborn assessment should proceed systematically so that each system is thoroughly evaluated.
- Providing a protective environment is a key responsibility of the nurse and includes such measures as careful identification procedures, support of physiologic functions, measures to prevent infection, and restraining techniques.
- Circumcision is an elective surgical procedure.
- Pain in neonates must be assessed and managed.

CRITICAL THINKING EXERCISES

1. Investigate the law in your state regarding use of car seats; that is, until what weight or age must children use a car seat? (Check with the state highway patrol department to see if they have a car seat safety program.) What information is being given to new parents about car seat safety before hospital discharge? Does your community hold car seat safety clinics? Prepare a display on car seat safety for parents who bring their infants to a well-baby clinic. Go to area retail stores that sell baby equipment and examine the types of available car seats, including the various features and costs. Find out if there is a program in your community for lending car seats to low-income families. Brainstorm about ways to increase the proper use of car seats.
2. Explore the medical and nursing literature with regard to potential benefits and risks of circumcision. Check Internet sites about circumcision, and compare the information accessed with the medical literature to see if appropriate and correct information is being presented. Examine your own beliefs and preferences in relation to circumcision. Discuss the "pros and cons" with your classmates. Prepare a teaching module for first-time parents who are trying to decide whether to have their newborn son circumcised. Develop an information sheet to give parents regarding care of the newly circumcised infant.

RESOURCES

American Academy of Pediatrics
141 Northwest Point Blvd.
Elk Grove, IL 60007
847-228-5005
www.aap.org

National Healthy Mothers, Healthy Babies Coalition
121 North Washington St., Suite 300
Alexandria, VA 22314
703-836-6110
www.hmhb.org

National Institute of Child Health and Human Development (NICHD)
National Institutes of Health
9000 Rockville Pike
Bldg. 31, Room 2A32
Bethesda, MD 20892
301-496-4000
www.nih.gov

Neonatal Network
1410 Neotomas Ave., Suite 107
Santa Rosa, CA 95405
www.neonatalnetwork.com

REFERENCES

American Academy of Pediatrics and Canadian Paediatric Society. (2000). Prevention and management of pain and stress in the neonate. *Pediatrics, 105*(2), 454-461.

American Academy of Pediatrics Task Force on Circumcision. (1999). Circumcision policy statement. *Pediatrics, 103*(3), 686-693.

Anand, K., Grunau, R., & Oberlander, T. (1997). Developmental character and long-term consequences of pain in infants and children. *Child and Adolescent Psychiatric Clinics of North America, 6*(4), 703-724.

Ballard, J., Novak, K., & Driver, M. (1979). A simplified score for assessment of fetal maturity of newly born infants. *Journal of Pediatrics, 95*(5 Pt. 1), 769-774.

Ballard, J. et al. (1991). New Ballard score, expanded to include extremely premature infants. *Journal of Pediatrics, 119*(3), 417-423.

Battaglia, F., & Lubchenco, L. (1967). A practical classification of newborn infants by weight and gestational age. *Journal of Pediatrics, 71*(2), 159-163.

Casey, B., McIntire, D., & Leveno, K. (2001). The continuing value of the Apgar score for the assessment of newborn infants. *New England Journal of Medicine, 344*(7), 467-471.

D'Avanzo, C., & Geissler, E. (2003). *Pocket guide to cultural assessment* (3rd ed.). St. Louis: Mosby.

DeMarini, S., & Tsang, R. (2002). Disorders of calcium, phosphorus, and magnesium metabolism. In A. Faranoff & R. Martin (Eds.), *Neonatal-perinatal medicine* (7th ed.). St. Louis: Mosby.

Geyer, J. et al. (2002). Evidence-based multidisciplinary protocol for neonatal circumcision pain management. *Journal of Obstetric, Gynecologic, and Neonatal Nursing, 31*(4), 403-410.

Gibbons, S. (2000). Skin to skin contact with their mothers reduced pain reactions in healthy newborn infants during a heel lance. Commentary on Gray L., Watt, L., & Blass, E. Skin-to-skin contact is analgesic in healthy newborns. *Pediatrics, 105*, e14. *Evidence Based Nursing, 3*(3), 73.

Glass, S. (1999). Genetic screening. In P. Thureen, J. Deacon, P. O'Neill, & J. Hernandez (Eds.), *Assessment and care of the well newborn*. Philadelphia: W.B. Saunders.

Hadjistavropoulos, H. et al. (1997). Judging pain in infants: Behavioural, contextual, and developmental determinants. *Pain, 73*(3), 319-324.

Hockenberry, M. et al. (2003). *Wong's nursing care of infants and children* (7th ed.). St. Louis: Mosby.

Howard, C., Howard, F., & Weitzman, M. (1994). Acetaminophen analgesia in neonatal circumcision: The effect on pain. *Pediatrics, 93*, 641-646.

Joint Committee on Infant Hearing. (2000). Year 2000 position statement: Principles and guidelines for early hearing detection and intervention programs. *Pediatrics, 106*, 725-735.

Juretschke, L. (2000). Apgar scoring: Its use and meaning for today's newborn. *Neonatal Network, 19*(1), 17-19.

Kliegman, R. (2002). Fetal and neonatal medicine. In R. Behrman & R. Kliegman (Eds.), *Nelson essentials of pediatrics* (4th ed.). Philadelphia: W.B. Saunders.

Lannon, C. et al. (1999). *Circumcision policy statement* (No. RE9850). Elk Grove, IL: American Academy of Pediatrics.

Leitch, D. (1999). Mother-infant interaction: Achieving synchrony. *Nursing Research, 48*(1), 55-58.

Lubchenco, L., Hansman, C., & Boyd, E. (1966). Intrauterine growth in length and head circumference as estimated from live births at gestational ages from 26-42 weeks. *Journal of Pediatrics, 37*(3), 403-408.

Macke, J. (2001). Analgesia for circumcision: Effects on newborn behavior and maternal-infant interactions. *Journal of Obstetric, Gynecologic, and Neonatal Nursing, 30*(5), 507-514.

Maisels, M. (1999). Jaundice. In G. Avery, M. Fletcher, & M. MacDonald (Eds.), *Neonatology: Pathophysiology and management of the newborn* (5th ed.). Philadelphia: Lippincott Williams & Williams.

Mangurten, H. (2002). Birth injuries. In A. Faranoff & R. Martin (Eds.), *Neonatal-perinatal medicine* (7th ed.). St. Louis: Mosby.

Meehan, R. (1998). Heelsticks in neonates for capillary blood sampling. *Neonatal Network, 17*(1), 17-24.

Mohan, C. et al. (1998). Comparison of analgesics in ameliorating the pain of circumcision. *Journal of Perinatology, 18*(1), 13-14.

Ogata, E. (1999). Carbohydrate homeostasis. In G. Avery, M. Fletcher, & M. MacDonald (Eds.), *Neonatology: Pathophysiology and management of the newborn* (5th ed.). Philadelphia: Lippincott Williams & Williams.

Pagana, K., & Pagana, T. (2002). *Mosby's manual of diagnostic and laboratory tests* (2nd ed.). St. Louis: Mosby.

Pasero, C. (2002). Pain assessment in infants and young children: Neonates. *American Journal of Nursing, 102*(8), 61, 63, 65.

Pressler, J., & Hepworth, J. (2000). The conceptualization, measurement, and validation of transient mechanical birth trauma. *Clinical Nursing Research, 9*(3), 317-338.

Shah, V., & Ohlsson, A. (2001). Venipuncture versus heel lance for blood sampling in term neonates. *The Cochrane Library*, Issue 1, Oxford: Update Software.

Stevens, B., & Ohlsson, A. (2001). Sucrose for analgesia in newborn infants undergoing painful procedures. *The Cochrane Library*, Issue 1, Oxford: Update Software.

Taddio, A., Ohlsson, I., & Ohlsson, A. (2001). Lidocaine-prilocaine cream for analgesia during circumcision of newborn boys. *The Cochrane Library*, Issue 1, Oxford: Update Software.

Van Ryzin, L. (2000). The circumcision debate. *American Journal of Nursing, 100*(7), 24A-24B.

Walden, M. (2001). *Pain assessment and management: Guidelines for practice.* Glenview, IL: National Association of Neonatal Nurses.

Walden, M., & Franck, L. (2003). Identification, management, and prevention of newborn/infant pain. In C. Kenner & J. Latt (Eds.), *Comprehensive neonatal nursing: A physiologic perspective* (3rd ed.). Philadelphia: Saunders.

Waltman, P. (2000). Oronasopharyngeal bulb suction at birth: Effects on extrauterine adaptation of healthy, term newborns. Poster presentation, NANN 16th National Meeting, September 28-October 2, San Antonio, TX.

Workowski, K., & Levine, W. (2002). Sexually transmitted disease treatment guidelines, 2002. *Morbidity and Mortality Weekly Report, 51*(RR-6), 1-78.

Zinn, A. (2002). Inborn errors of metabolism. In A. Faranoff & R. Martin (Eds.), *Neonatal-perinatal medicine* (7th ed.). St. Louis: Mosby.

CHAPTER 27

Kathryn Rhodes Alden

Newborn Nutrition and Feeding

http://evolve.elsevier.com/Lowdermilk/MatWmnHlth/

LEARNING OBJECTIVES

- Describe current recommendations for feeding infants.
- Explain the nurse's role in helping families to choose an infant feeding method.
- Describe nutritional needs of infants.
- List newborn feeding-readiness cues and indicators of effective breastfeeding.
- Discuss benefits of breastfeeding for infants, mothers, families, and society.
- Describe the anatomy and physiology of breastfeeding.
- Identify nursing interventions to facilitate and promote successful breastfeeding.
- Identify common problems associated with breastfeeding and nursing interventions to help resolve them.
- Develop a teaching plan for the formula-feeding family.

Good nutrition in infancy fosters optimal growth and development. Infant feeding is more than the provision of nutrition; it is an opportunity for social, psychologic, and even educational interaction between parent and infant. It also can establish a basis for developing good eating habits that last a lifetime. Health supervision of infants requires knowledge of their nutritional needs.

Through preconception and prenatal education and counseling, nurses play an instrumental role in assisting parents with the selection of an infant feeding method, which ideally will be breastfeeding. Whether the parents choose to breastfeed or formula feed, nurses provide support and ongoing education. Education of parents is necessarily based on current research findings and standards of practice.

This chapter focuses on meeting nutritional needs for normal growth and development from birth to age 6 months, with emphasis on the neonatal period when feeding practices and patterns are being established. Both breastfeeding and formula feeding are addressed.

RECOMMENDED INFANT NUTRITION

The American Academy of Pediatrics (AAP) recommends that infants be breastfed exclusively for the first 6 months of life and that breastfeeding continue for at least 12 months (American Academy of Pediatrics Work Group on Breastfeeding, 1997). If infants are weaned before 12 months, they should receive iron-fortified infant formula.

NUTRIENT NEEDS

Choosing an Infant Feeding Method

Women who elect to breastfeed their infants most often do so because they are aware of the benefits to the infant. Many are seeking the unique bonding experience between mother and infant that is characteristic of breastfeeding. The support of the partner and family is a major factor in the mother's decision to breastfeed and in her ability to do so successfully (see Research box). Prenatal preparation ideally includes the father of the baby, giving him information about benefits of breastfeeding and how he can participate in infant care and nurturing. Parents who elect to formula feed often make this decision without complete information and understanding of the benefits of breastfeeding and the potential hazards of formula feeding. This may be owing to a lack of breastfeeding education and a failure of health care providers to promote and support breastfeeding. Cultural beliefs, as well as myths and misconceptions about breastfeeding, influence women's decision making. Other women select bottle feeding even though they are aware of the benefits of breastfeeding (Earle, 2000). Many women see bottle feeding as more convenient or less embarrassing than breastfeeding. Formula feeding is often viewed as a way to ensure that the father, other family members, and day-care providers can feed the baby. Some women lack confidence in their ability to produce an adequate quantity or quality of breast milk. Women who have had previous unsuccessful breastfeeding experiences may chose to formula feed subsequent infants. Breastfeeding is seen by some women as incompatible with an active social life, or they think that it will prevent them from going back to work. Modesty issues and significant societal barriers exist against breastfeeding in public. A major barrier for many women is the influence of family and friends; this is especially true for lower-income mothers, for whom bottle feeding is the norm. Occasionally, there is no other option except formula feeding, such as when a mother has had a bilateral mastectomy or extensive breast scarring. The mother may be taking medications that preclude breastfeeding, or the baby may be adopted (some adoptive mothers attempt breastfeeding and can often produce some amount of breast milk). Formula feeding is recommended for mothers who are infected with the human immunodeficiency virus (HIV).

To make an informed decision about an infant feeding method, parents must be presented with factual information about the nutritional and immunologic needs of the infant that *are* met by human milk, the potential benefits to the infant and the mother, and the inherent risks associated with infant formulas. The nurse must provide this information to parents in a nonjudgmental manner and respect their decision. Some health care professionals may attempt to avoid this responsibility with the rationalization that they do not want parents to feel guilty if they choose not to breastfeed. However, the nurse is required to give complete information about infant feeding to parents and to document having done so.

The key to encouraging mothers to breastfeed is education, beginning as early as possible during pregnancy and even before pregnancy. Prenatal breastfeeding classes are an excellent vehicle to relay important information to expectant parents. Each encounter with an expectant mother is an opportunity to dispel myths, clarify misinformation, and address personal concerns. Connecting expectant mothers with women who are breastfeeding or have successfully breastfed and are from similar backgrounds may be helpful. Peer counseling programs, such as those instituted by Women, Infants, and Children (WIC) programs, are beneficial, particularly in lower socioeconomic groups, where bottle feeding is common (Arlotti et al., 1998).

The postnatal period is not too late to educate parents about the benefits of breastfeeding. For those women with limited access to health care, the postpartum period may provide the first opportunity for education about breastfeeding. Even women who have indicated the desire to bottle feed may benefit from information about the differences in formula and breast milk for their infants. Offering these women the chance to try breastfeeding with the assistance of a nurse may influence a change in infant feeding practices.

It is the responsibility of the nurse and other health care professionals to promote feelings of competence and confidence in the breastfeeding mother and to reinforce the unequaled contribution she is making toward the health and well-being of her infant. Evidence-based guidelines for supporting breastfeeding are available for use by health care professionals (AWHONN, 1998; International Lactation Consultant Association, 1999) (Box 27-1).

RESEARCH

Men: Women's Strongest Ally for Breastfeeding

One of the goals of *Healthy People 2010* is to increase breastfeeding among all Americans. The most vulnerable families, the low-income and minority populations with high infant mortality rates, are still the least likely to breastfeed. Their infants lose the nutritional, immunologic, social, economic, psychologic, and developmental benefits of breast milk. Most decisions about breastfeeding are made prior to birth and are strongly influenced by the partner or the mother of the expectant mother.

To describe cultural differences in attitudes and knowledge about breastfeeding, nurse researchers questioned 100 men who were accompanying their pregnant partner at an inner city hospital obstetric unit or its prenatal clinic. The respondents were predominantly African American, with a high school education, employed and living with the partner and children.

Results of the study found that the attitudes of the men about breastfeeding were positive: 81% wanted their baby to be breastfed. They agreed that breastfeeding promotes bonding (90%), they would support their partner who wanted to breastfeed (96%), they have respect for women who breastfeed (97%), and breastfeeding would not interfere with their sexual relationship (98%). Most of the men knew that breast milk is healthier for infants (74%), but they were not always sure what specific benefits breast milk offers. Some (26%) believed that their partner could not breastfeed because she would not be able to follow a special diet. Some men (34%) were embarrassed by the idea of breastfeeding in public. Men were more supportive of their partners choosing to breastfeed if they were breastfed as infants.

IMPLICATION FOR PRACTICE

Nurses need to distribute information on specific benefits of breastfeeding and share this good news about men's attitudes to churches, schools, and community groups. It may be possible, as one respondent said, that African American couples "just don't bring the topic up during pregnancy." If so, then programs that encourage discussion and decision-making between women and their male partners may give women the support they did not know they had for breastfeeding.

Reference: Pollock, C., Bustamante-Forest, R., & Giarrantano, G. (2002). Men of diverse cultures: Knowledge and attitudes about breastfeeding. *Journal of Obstetric, Gynecologic, and Neonatal Nursing, 31*(6), 673-679.

Cultural Influences on Infant Feeding

Cultural beliefs and practices are significant influences on infant feeding methods. Although recognized cultural norms exist, one cannot assume that generalized observations about any cultural group hold true for all members of that group. Within the United States, many regional and ethnic cultures are found. Dealing effectively with these groups requires that the nurse be knowledgeable about and sensitive to the cultural factors influencing infant feeding practices.

Persons who have immigrated to the United States from poorer countries often choose to formula feed their infants because they believe it is a better, more "modern" method. Others adopt formula feeding because they want to adapt to American culture and perceive that it is the custom to bottle feed.

Among some cultural groups within the United States, breastfeeding rates have declined. As increasing numbers of families leave Native American reservations to reside in urban areas, the traditional practice of breastfeeding often shifts to formula feeding. The separation from female relatives who lend childbirth and lactation support may be a factor in the change in feeding practices (Houghton, 2001).

As many as 50 of 120 cultures studied by Morse, Jehle, and Gamble (1990) typically do not give colostrum to newborns and begin breastfeeding after the milk has "come in." This is true for some Filipinos, Hispanics, Vietnamese, Hmong, Koreans, and Nigerians. When breastfeeding is delayed until the milk is in, babies are given prelacteal food (Lefeber & Voorhoeve, 1999) (Table 27-1). Other cultures begin breastfeeding immediately and offer the breast each time the infant cries. Cultural attitudes regarding modesty and breastfeeding are important considerations.

BOX *27-1* **AWHONN's Guidelines for Breastfeeding Support**

- During pregnancy a breast assessment is performed that includes a breastfeeding history, a breast examination, and a medication-use history.
- A prenatal plan of care is developed to prepare the woman for lactation.
- Immediately after birth, the newborn is kept with the mother when possible so that breastfeeding can be initiated when the newborn is most receptive.
- After birth:
    - Assistance with latch-on and positioning are given as needed.
    - Encouragement of frequent feedings is reinforced.
    - Discharge instructions for knowing criteria for successful breastfeeding are given.
    - Information about community resources for breastfeeding is given.
- Especially for premature and low-birth-weight infants, breastfeeding is encouraged.

Adapted from AWHONN. (1998). *Standards and guidelines for professional nursing practice in the care of women and newborns* (5th ed.). Washington, DC: The Association.

Some cultures have specific beliefs and practices related to the mother's intake of foods that foster milk production. Korean mothers often eat seaweed soup and rice to enhance milk production. Hmong women believe that boiled chicken, rice, and hot water are the only appropriate nourishments during the first postpartum month. The balance between energy forces, hot and cold, or yin and yang, is integral to the diet of the lactating mother. Hispanics, Vietnamese, Chinese, East Indians, and Arabs often use this belief in choosing foods. "Hot" foods are considered best for new mothers; this does not necessarily relate to the temperature or spiciness of foods. For example, chicken and broccoli are considered "hot," whereas many fresh fruits and vegetables are considered "cold." Families often bring desired foods into the health care setting.

BREASTFEEDING RATES

Healthy People 2010 goals state that 75% of women will breastfeed at birth, 50% will continue for 6 months, and 25% will breastfeed for 1 year (Department of Health and Human Services, 2000). Although the United States has seen a gradual resurgence in breastfeeding initiation and continuance rates, the goals of *Healthy People 2010* have yet to be attained. After a low of 26.5% in 1970, breastfeeding initiation rates climbed to 58% in 1985, only to decline gradually to 51.5% in 1990. Since then, breastfeeding rates have steadily increased to 68.4% in 2000. Likewise, the number of infants still breastfeeding at 6 months has increased from 14.1% in 1970 to 31.4% in 2000. By age 1 year, only 17.6% of infants are still breastfed (Abbott Laboratories, 2001; Ryan, 1997).

Breastfeeding rates have increased across all demographic groups, although the most significant increases are seen among women who have historically been less likely to breastfeed. These individuals are typically young (younger than 25 years), lower income, African-American, primiparas, with grade school education or less, employed full time outside the home, residing in the South Atlantic region of the United States, mothers of low-birth-weight infants, and enrolled in the WIC program (Ryan, 1997).

The characteristics of women most likely to breastfeed have remained consistent over the years. These women are white, older than 30 years, college educated, with higher incomes, not employed outside the home or working only part-time, residents of western states, and not participating in the WIC program (Forste, Weiss, & Lippincott, 2001; Ryan, 1997).

BENEFITS OF BREASTFEEDING

Human milk is designed specifically for human infants and is nutritionally superior to any alternative. Breast milk is considered a living tissue because it contains almost

TABLE 27-1 **The Advised First Food for Newborn Babies in Countries of Africa, Asia, and Latin America**

	COUNTRY	PEOPLE	FIRST FOOD	RATIONALE
Africa	Ghana	Asante	Gin, rum, lime-juice palm	To clear the infant's throat
	Nigeria	Yoruba	Palm wine	
	South Africa	Pedi, Zulu, Sotho	Watery porridge, cow's milk, water dextrose/water mixture	To clear the infant's throat
	Zambia	Lozi, Mbunda	Light beer (mahel)	To clear the infant's bowel of meconium
Asia	Bangladesh		Mustard oil	To clean intestine of meconium
			Honey, sugar (gur or talmisri)	For ritual and/or medicinal purpose
			Sugar-water	
	India		Honey, water	To clean and purify the body
			Castor oil, herbs	To remove the fluids of the womb ingested by the newborn during birth
	Thailand	Karen	Rice	To learn the taste
	Indonesia	Minangkabau	Honey, coconut water	
			Rice water	To learn the taste
	Iran Jaya			
	Lowland		Sago, sago-porridge	To learn the taste
	Highland		Taro (yam), pork fat	To learn the taste
Latin America	Jamaica		Mint tea, castor oil	To cough up mucus
	Haiti		Castor oil	To clear the infant's bowel of meconium
	Guatemala	Maya, Ladinos	Tea, boiled with anise, sugar, onion stalk, garlic, salt, tea of chicoria	
	Bolivia		Wine, cow's milk, water with herbs or salt, coffee	

From Lefeber, Y., & Voorhoeve, H. (1999). Indigenous first feeding practices in newborn babies. *Midwifery, 15,* 97-100.

as many live cells as blood. It is bacteriologically safe and always fresh. The nutrients in breast milk are more easily absorbed than are those in formula.

Numerous research studies have identified the beneficial effects of human milk for infants during the first year of life. Long-term epidemiologic studies have shown that these benefits do not cease when the infant is weaned, but instead extend into childhood and beyond. Breastfeeding has many advantages for mothers, for families, and for society in general. In discussing the benefits of breastfeeding with parents, it is critical that nurses and other health care professionals have a thorough understanding of these benefits from both a physiologic and a psychosocial perspective. Benefits for the infant include the following:

- Breast milk enhances maturation of the gastrointestinal (GI) tract and contains immune factors that contribute to a lower incidence and severity of diarrheal illness, necrotizing enterocolitis, Crohn disease, and celiac disease (Barnard, 1997; Gianino et al., 2002; Lopez-Alarcon, Villalpando, & Fajardo, 1997; Scariati, Grummer-Strawn, & Fein, 1997).
- Breastfed infants receive specific antibodies and cell-mediated immunologic factors that help decrease the incidence and severity of otitis media, respiratory illnesses such as respiratory syncytial virus (RSV) and pneumonia, urinary tract infections, bacteremia, and bacterial meningitis (Bulkow et al., 2002; Cushing et al., 1998; Lopez-Alarcon et al., 1997).
- By reducing exposure to potential allergens, breastfeeding may reduce the risk of cow's milk allergy and eczema. Breastfeeding reduces the incidence of atopic dermatitis in infants with a family history (Gdalevich et al., 2001). Asthma, which is often of an allergic nature, is less frequent among children who were breastfed (Char-Yeung et al., 2000; Dell & To, 2001; Oddy et al., 1999)
- Breastfed infants are less likely to die of sudden infant death syndrome (McVea, Turner, & Peppler, 2000).
- Breast milk may have a protective effect against childhood lymphoma, leukemia, and insulin-dependent diabetes (Davis, 1998; Hypponen et al., 1999; Shu et al., 1999).
- Breast milk/breastfeeding may enhance cognitive development (Anderson, Johnstone, & Remley, 1999; Horwood & Fergusson, 1998; Vestergaard et al., 1999).

- Breastfeeding enhances jaw development, decreasing problems with malocclusions and malalignment of teeth (Page, 2001; Palmer, 1998).
- Breastfeeding may decrease the risk of childhood obesity (Fisher et al., 2000; VonKries et al., 1999).

Maternal benefits include the following:

- Women who breastfeed may have a decreased risk of breast cancer (Enger et al., 1998).
- Breastfeeding promotes uterine involution and is associated with a decreased risk of postpartum hemorrhage (Lawrence, 1999).
- Mothers who breastfeed experience lactational amenorrhea. Return of menses is usually delayed with increased frequency and exclusivity of breastfeeding. Breastfeeding also delays the return of fertility but is not considered to be an effective method of birth control (Lawrence, 1999).
- Mothers who are breastfeeding tend to return to their prepregnancy weight more quickly (King, 2000).
- Breastfeeding may provide some protection against the development of osteoporosis (Eisman, 1998).
- Breastfeeding provides a unique bonding experience and increases maternal role attainment (Lawrence, 1999).

Benefits to families and society include the following:

- Breastfeeding is convenient; breast milk does not need to be warmed and does not require a clean water supply or a clean serving container. No bottles or other necessary equipment must be purchased or cleaned. Breastfed babies are portable; when traveling, fewer supplies must be taken along.
- Breastfeeding saves money. The cost of formula far exceeds the cost of extra food for the lactating mother. Because breastfed infants have a lower incidence of illness and infection, health care costs are lower for families and federal, state, and local governments. Breastfeeding represents cost savings to employers: less time is lost from work by parents who must stay home with sick infants. Breastfeeding families who are eligible for WIC represent a cost savings to the government (Montgomery & Splett, 1998; Weimer, 2001).
- Intangible benefits for families and society include increased quality of life through psychologic benefits for mothers and infants, increased mothering behaviors, and more free time for interaction with family and friends.
- Breastfeeding benefits the environment. It is a natural resource that is renewable with each pregnancy. It requires no fossil fuels, and no advertising, shipping, or disposal is needed.

FEEDING READINESS

Term neonates are born with reflexes that facilitate feeding: **rooting,** sucking, and swallowing. Healthy newborns have experience with sucking on fingers and swallowing amniotic fluid for several weeks in utero but have made no connection between sucking and satiation. Neither have they needed to suck, swallow, and breathe before they emerged from the uterus. Although the majority of newborns do not feel hunger or thirst in the first hours after birth, they will suckle when given the opportunity.

Physical assessment of the newborn reveals signs that the baby is physiologically ready to begin feeding:

- Vital signs within normal limits
- Unlabored respirations; nares patent; no cyanosis
- Active bowel sounds
- No abdominal distention

When newborns feel hunger, they usually cry vigorously until their needs are met. Some infants, however, will withdraw into sleep because of discomfort associated with hunger. Babies exhibit **feeding-readiness cues** that can be recognized by a knowledgeable caregiver. Instead of waiting to feed until the infant is crying in a distraught manner or withdrawing into sleep, it is better to begin a feeding when the baby exhibits some of these cues (even during light sleep):

- Hand-to-mouth or hand-to-hand movements
- Sucking motions
- Rooting
- Mouthing

Babies normally consume small amounts of milk during the first 3 days of life. The breastfed infant receives colostrum, which is very concentrated and high in protein. Similarly, bottle-fed infants initially require small feedings. However, as the baby adjusts to extrauterine life and the digestive tract is cleared of meconium, milk intake increases from 15 to 30 ml per feeding in the first 24 hours to 60 to 90 ml by the end of the first week.

At birth and for several months thereafter, all of the secretions of the infant's digestive tract contain enzymes especially suited to the digestion of human milk. The ability to digest foods other than milk depends on the physiologic development of the infant. The capacities for salivary, gastric, pancreatic, and intestinal digestion increase with age, indicating that the natural time for introduction of solid foods may be around 6 months of age.

Babies are born with a tongue extrusion reflex that causes them to push out of the mouth anything placed on the tongue. This reflex disappears by 6 months–another indication of physiologic readiness for solids.

Early introduction of solids may make the infant more prone to food allergies. Regular feeding of solids can lead to decreased intake of breast milk or formula and may be associated with early cessation of breastfeeding.

NUTRIENT NEEDS

Fluids

The fluid requirement for normal infants is 100 to 140 ml of water per kilogram of body weight per 24 hours; however, during the first 24 hours after birth, most infants need only 60 to 80 ml/kg/24 hours (Kliegman, 2002). In general, neither breastfed nor formula-fed infants need to be fed water, not even those living in very hot climates. Breast milk contains 87% water, which easily meets fluid requirements. Feeding water to infants may only decrease caloric consumption at a time when infants are growing rapidly.

Infants have room for little fluctuation in fluid balance and should be monitored closely for fluid intake and water loss. Infants lose water through excretion of urine and insensibly through respiration. Under normal circumstances, infants are born with some fluid reserve, and some of the weight loss during the first few days is related to fluid loss. In some cases, however, infants do not have this fluid reserve, possibly because of inadequate maternal hydration during labor or birth.

Energy

Infants require adequate caloric intake to provide energy for growth, digestion, physical activity, and maintenance of organ metabolic function. For the first 3 months, the infant needs 110 kcal/kg/day. From 3 months to 6 months, the requirement is 100 kcal/kg/day. This decreases slightly to 95 kcal/kg/day from 6 to 9 months and increases to 100 kcal/kg/day from 9 months to 1 year (AAP, 1998).

Human milk provides 67 kcal/100 ml or 20 kcal/oz; the greatest amount of energy is provided by the fat content of breast milk. Infant formulas are made to simulate the caloric content of human milk; standard formulas contain 20 kcal/oz, with differences in composition varying among brands.

Carbohydrate

Because newborns have only small hepatic glycogen stores, carbohydrates should provide at least 40% to 45% of the total calories in the diet. Moreover, newborns may have a limited ability to carry out gluconeogenesis (the formation of glucose from amino acids and other substrates) and ketogenesis (the formation of ketone bodies from fat), the mechanisms that provide alternative sources of energy.

As the primary carbohydrate in human milk and cow's-milk formula, lactose is the most abundant carbohydrate in the diet of infants up to age 6 months. It provides calories in an easily available form. Its slow breakdown and absorption probably also increase calcium absorption. Corn syrup solids or glucose polymers have been added to infant formulas to supplement the lactose in the cow's milk and thereby provide sufficient carbohydrates.

Fat

For infants to acquire adequate calories from the limited amount of human milk or formula they are able to consume, at least 15% of the calories provided must come from fat (triglycerides). This fat must therefore be easily digestible. The fat in human milk is easier to digest and absorb than that in cow's milk because of the arrangement of the fatty acids on the glycerol molecule. Fat absorption also is related to the natural lipase activity present in human milk.

Cow's milk is used in most infant formulas, but the milk fat is removed, and another fat source such as corn oil, which can be digested and absorbed by the infant, is added in its place. If whole milk or evaporated milk without added carbohydrate is fed to infants, the resulting fecal loss of fat (and therefore loss of energy) may be excessive because the milk moves through the infant's intestines too quickly for adequate absorption to take place. This can lead to poor weight gain.

In addition to its energy contributions, fat also furnishes essential fatty acids (EFAs), which are required for growth and tissue maintenance. EFAs are components of cell membranes and precursors of some hormones. An inadequate intake of EFAs results in eczema and growth failure. The lack of EFAs in skim and low-fat milk is another reason infants should not be fed these products.

Protein

The protein requirement per unit of body weight is greater in the newborn than at any other time of life. The recommended daily allowance (RDA) for protein during the first 6 months is 2.2 g/kg.

The protein content of human milk, which is lower than that of unmodified cow's milk, is ideal for the newborn. Human milk contains far more lactalbumin in relation to casein than does cow's milk, and lactalbumin is more easily digested than casein. In addition, the amino acid composition of human milk is suited to the newborn's metabolic capabilities. For example, the phenylalanine and methionine levels are low, and cystine and taurine levels are high. The protein in some commercial formulas is modified so that the amount of lactalbumin, or whey, protein is increased and the relative proportion of casein is decreased to more closely approximate the protein composition of human milk.

Vitamins

Human milk contains all of the vitamins required for infant nutrition, with individual variations based on maternal diet and genetic differences. Vitamins are added to cow's-milk formulas to resemble levels found in breast milk. Although cow's milk contains adequate amounts of vitamin A and vitamin B complex, vitamin C (ascorbic acid) and vitamin E must be added.

Vitamin D also is added to commercial infant formulas. Human milk may be somewhat deficient in vitamin D, but supplementation may not be necessary, provided that the infant is exposed to sunlight for 30 minutes per week wearing only a diaper, or for 2 hours per week fully clothed but without a hat. To prevent rickets, supplementation is recommended for breastfed infants who are dark skinned with limited exposure to the sun, as well as for infants whose mothers eat vegetarian diets that exclude meat, fish, and dairy products. Infants of mothers who are strict vegans also should receive vitamin B_{12} supplements (Tershakovic & Stallings, 2002).

Vitamin K, required for blood coagulation, is produced by intestinal bacteria. However, the gut is sterile at birth, and a few days are needed for intestinal flora to become established and produce vitamin K. To prevent hemorrhagic problems in the newborn, an injection of vitamin K is given at birth to all newborns, regardless of feeding method.

Minerals

The mineral content of commercial infant formula is designed to reflect that of breast milk. Unmodified cow's milk is much higher in mineral content than is human milk, which also makes it unsuitable for infants during the first year of life. Minerals are typically highest in human milk during the first few days after birth and decrease slightly throughout lactation.

The ratio of calcium to phosphorus in human milk is 2:1, a proportion optimal for bone mineralization. Although cow's milk is high in calcium, the calcium-to-phosphorus ratio is low, resulting in decreased calcium absorption. Consequently, young infants fed unmodified cow's milk are at risk for hypocalcemia, seizures, and tetany. The calcium-to-phosphorus ratio in commercial infant formula is between that of human milk and cow's milk.

Iron levels are low in all types of milk; however, iron from human milk is better absorbed (50%) than that from cow's milk, iron-fortified formula, or infant cereals. Breastfed infants draw on iron reserves deposited in utero and benefit from the high lactose and vitamin C levels in human milk that facilitate iron absorption. The infant who is entirely breastfed normally maintains adequate hemoglobin levels for the first 6 months. After that time, iron-fortified cereals and other iron-rich foods are added to the diet. Infants who are weaned from the breast before 6 months of age and all formula-fed infants should receive an iron-fortified commercial infant formula until 12 months of age.

Fluoride levels in human milk and commercial formulas are low. This mineral, which is important in the prevention of dental caries, may cause spotting of the permanent teeth (fluorosis) in excess amounts. It is recommended that a fluoride supplement be given only to those infants not receiving fluoridated water after age 6 months (AAP, 1997).

OVERVIEW OF LACTATION

Breast Development

Each female breast is composed of approximately 15 to 20 segments (lobes) embedded in fat and connective tissues and well supplied with blood vessels, lymphatic vessels, and nerves (Fig. 27-1). Within each lobe are alveoli, the milk-producing cells, surrounded by myoepithelial cells, which contract to send the milk forward into the ductules. Each ductule enlarges into **lactiferous ducts** and **sinuses** where milk collects just behind the nipple. Each nipple has 15 to 20 pores through which milk is transferred to the suckling infant.

The size of the breast is not an accurate indicator of its ability to produce milk. Although nearly every woman can lactate, a small number have insufficient mammary gland development to breastfeed their infants exclusively. Typically, these women experience few breast changes during puberty or early pregnancy. In some cases, women may still be able to breastfeed and offer supplemental nutrition to support optimal infant growth. Devices are available to allow mothers to offer supplements while the baby is nursing at the breast (Fig. 27-2).

Because of the effects of estrogen and progesterone during pregnancy, the lobular components of the breast enlarge while the ductal system proliferates and differentiates. The nipples become more erect, and pigmentation of the areola increases. Nipples and areola may enlarge. The breasts increase in size and sensitivity and exhibit more prominent veins. Around week 16 of gestation, the alveoli begin producing colostrum (early milk) in response to human placental lactogen.

After the mother gives birth, a precipitate decrease in estrogen and progesterone levels triggers the release of **prolactin** from the anterior pituitary gland. During pregnancy, prolactin prepares the breasts to secrete milk and, during lactation, to synthesize and secrete milk. Prolactin levels are highest during the first 10 days after birth, gradually declining over time, but remaining above baseline levels for

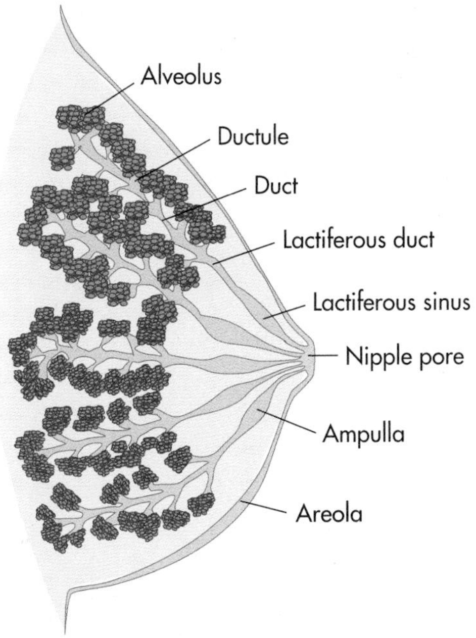
Alveolus
Ductule
Duct
Lactiferous duct
Lactiferous sinus
Nipple pore
Ampulla
Areola

FIG. 27-1 Detailed structural features of human mammary gland.

the duration of lactation. Prolactin is produced in response to infant suckling and emptying of the breasts (lactating breasts are never completely empty; milk is constantly being produced by the alveoli as the infant feeds) (Fig. 27-3, *A*). Milk production is a **supply-meets-demand system;** that is, as milk is removed from the breast, more is produced. Incomplete emptying of the breasts with feedings can lead to a decreased milk supply.

Oxytocin is the other hormone essential to lactation. As the nipple is stimulated by the suckling infant, the posterior pituitary is prompted by the hypothalamus to produce oxytocin. This hormone is responsible for the **milk-ejection reflex (MER),** or **let-down reflex** (Fig. 27-3, *B*). The myoepithelial cells surrounding the alveoli respond to oxytocin by contracting and sending the milk forward through the ducts to the nipple. Many "let-downs" can occur with each feeding session. The MER can be triggered by thoughts, sights, sounds, or odors that the mother associates with her baby (or other babies), such as hearing the baby cry. Many women report a tingling "pins and needles" sensation in the breasts as let-down occurs, although some mothers can detect milk ejection only by observing the sucking and swallowing of the infant. Let-down also may occur during sexual activity, because oxytocin is released during orgasm.

Oxytocin is the same hormone that stimulates uterine contractions during labor. Consequently, the laboring woman can experience let-downs that may be evidenced by leakage of colostrum. This readies the breast for immediate feeding by the infant after birth. Oxytocin has the important function of contracting the mother's uterus after birth to control postpartum bleeding and promote

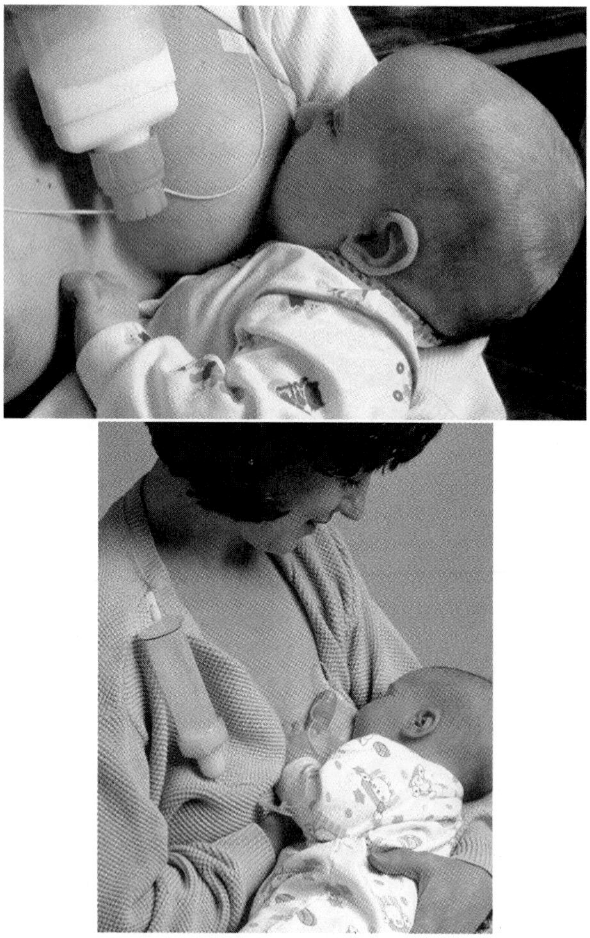

FIG. 27-2 Supplemental nursing system. (Courtesy Medela, Inc., McHenry, IL.)

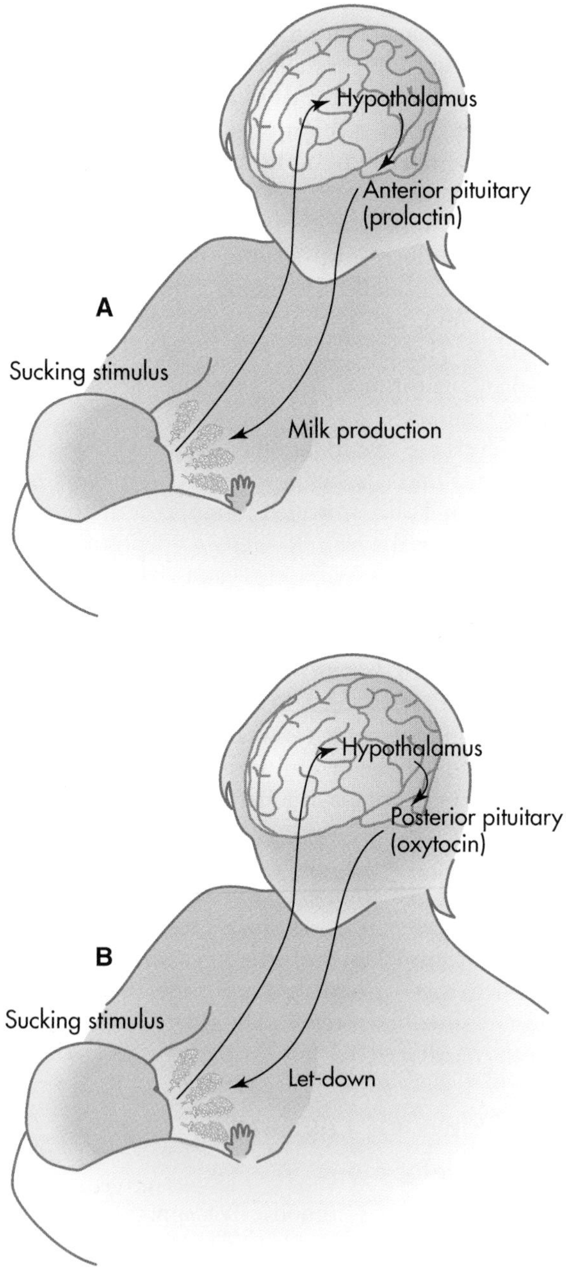
A
Hypothalamus
Anterior pituitary
(prolactin)
Sucking stimulus
Milk production
B
Hypothalamus
Posterior pituitary
(oxytocin)
Sucking stimulus
Let-down

FIG. 27-3 Maternal breastfeeding reflexes. **A,** Milk production. **B,** Let-down.

uterine involution. Thus mothers who breastfeed are at decreased risk for postpartum hemorrhage. These uterine contractions or "afterpains" that occur with breastfeeding can be painful during and after feeding for the first 3 to 5 days, particularly in multiparas.

Prolactin and oxytocin have been referred to as the "mothering hormones," because they are known to affect the postpartum woman's emotions, as well as her physical state. Many women report feeling thirsty or very relaxed during breastfeeding, probably as a result of these hormones.

The **nipple-erection reflex** is an integral part of lactation. When the infant cries, suckles, or rubs against the breast, the nipple becomes erect. This assists in the propulsion of milk through the lactiferous sinuses to the nipple pores. Nipple sizes, shapes, and ability to become erect vary with individuals. Some women have flat or **inverted nipples** that do not become erect with stimulation. Babies are usually able to learn to breastfeed successfully with any nipple. It is important that these infants not be offered bottles or pacifiers until breastfeeding is well established.

Uniqueness of Human Milk

Human milk is a highly complex, species-specific fluid uniquely designed to meet the needs of the human infant. It is a dynamic substance whose composition changes to meet the changing nutritional and immunologic needs of the infant as growth and development ensues. Breast milk is specific to the needs of each newborn; for example, the milk of preterm mothers differs in composition from that of mothers who give birth at term.

Human milk contains antimicrobial factors (antibodies) that provide some protection against a broad spectrum of bacterial, viral, and protozoan infections. Secretory immunoglobulin A (IgA) is the major antibody in human milk. Other factors in human milk that help protect against infection include lactoferrin, the bifidus factor, oligosaccharides, milk lipids, and milk leukocytes. Antiinflammatory agents, growth factors, hormones, and enzymes are found in human milk, many of which contribute to the maturation of the infant's intestine. Immunomodulating agents found in human milk are instrumental in preventing disease after infancy (Table 27-2).

TABLE 27-2 **Summary of Immune Properties of Breast Milk**

COMPONENT	ACTION
White Blood Cells	
B lymphocytes	Give rise to antibodies targeted against specific microbes
Macrophages	Kill microbes outright in baby's gut, produce lysozyme, and activate other components of the immune system
Neutrophils	May act as phagocytes, ingesting bacteria in baby's digestive system
T lymphocytes	Kill infected cells directly or send out chemical messages to mobilize other defenses
	Proliferate in the presence of organisms that cause serious illness in infants
	Manufacture compounds that can strengthen an infant's own immune response
Molecules	
Antibodies of secretory immunoglobulin A (IgA) class	Bind to microbes in infant's digestive tract and thereby prevent them from passing through walls of the gut into body tissues
B_{12}-binding protein	Reduces amount of vitamin B_{12}, which bacteria need to grow
Bifidus factor	Promotes growth of *Lactobacillus bifidus,* a harmless bacterium, in infant's gut. Growth of such nonpathogenic bacteria helps crowd out dangerous varieties
Fatty acids	Disrupts membranes surrounding certain viruses and destroys them
Fibronectin	Increases antimicrobial activity of macrophages; helps repair tissues that have been damaged by immune reactions in infant's gut
Gamma-interferon	Enhances antimicrobial activity of immune cells
Hormones and growth factors	Stimulates infant's digestive tract to mature more quickly. Once the initially "leaky" membranes lining the gut mature, infants become less vulnerable to microorganisms
Lactoferrin	Binds to iron; a mineral many bacteria need to survive. By reducing the available amount of iron, lactoferrin thwarts growth of pathogenic bacteria
Lysozyme	Kills bacteria by disrupting their cell walls
Mucins	Adheres to bacteria and viruses, thus keeping such microorganisms from attaching to mucosal surfaces
Oligosaccharides	Binds to microorganisms and bars them from attaching to mucosal surfaces

From Newman, J. (1995). How breast milk protects newborns. *Scientific American, 273*(6), 76-79.

Human milk composition and volumes vary according to the stage of lactation. In **lactogenesis** stage I, beginning in pregnancy, the breasts prepare for milk production. Colostrum is present in the breasts at this time. **Colostrum,** a clear yellowish fluid, is more concentrated than mature milk and is extremely rich in immunoglobulins. It has higher concentrations of protein and minerals but less fat than mature milk. The high protein level of colostrum facilitates binding of bilirubin, and the laxative action of colostrum promotes early passage of meconium. Colostrum gradually changes to mature milk; this is referred to as "the milk coming in" or as lactogenesis stage II. By day 3 to 5 after birth, most women have had this onset of copious milk secretion. Breast milk continues to change in composition for approximately 10 days, when the mature milk is established in stage III of lactogenesis (Lawrence, 1999).

Composition of mature milk changes during each feeding. As the infant nurses, the fat content of breast milk increases. Initially, a bluish-white foremilk is released that is part skim milk (about 60% of the volume) and part whole milk (about 35% of the volume). It provides primarily lactose, protein, and water-soluble vitamins. The hindmilk, or cream (about 5%), is usually let down 10 to 20 minutes into the feeding, although it may occur sooner. It contains the denser calories from fat necessary for ensuring optimal growth and contentment between feedings. Because of this changing composition of human milk during each feeding, it is important to breastfeed the infant long enough to supply a balanced feeding.

Milk production gradually increases as the baby grows. Babies have fairly predictable **growth spurts** (at about 10 days, 3 weeks, 6 weeks, 3 months, and 4 to 6 months), when more frequent feedings stimulate increased milk production. These growth spurts usually last 24 to 48 hours, and then the infants resume their usual feeding pattern.

CARE MANAGEMENT: THE BREASTFEEDING MOTHER AND INFANT

Effective management of the breastfeeding mother and infant requires that the caregivers be knowledgeable about the benefits of breastfeeding, as well as about basic anatomy and the physiology of breastfeeding, how to assist the mother with feeding, and interventions for common problems. Ongoing support of the mother enhances her self-confidence and promotes a satisfying and successful breastfeeding experience. Planning care for the breastfeeding couplet is based on thorough assessment of both the mother and infant.

Assessment and Nursing Diagnoses

Infant

Before the initiation of breastfeeding, the nurse must consider the following in preparing to assist the breastfeeding infant effectively:

- Maturity level: gestational age, term or preterm, birth weight (small for gestational age [SGA], large for gestational age [LGA])
- Labor and birth: length of labor, maternal medications (narcotics, magnesium sulfate [$MgSO_4$]); type of birth: vaginal (with or without use of vacuum extraction or forceps) or cesarean; type of anesthesia
- Birth trauma: fractured clavicle, bruising of face or head
- Maternal risk factors: diabetes, preeclampsia, infection, HIV, herpes, hepatitis B
- Congenital defects: cleft lip or palate, cardiac anomalies, Down syndrome or other genetic anomalies
- Physical stability: vital signs within normal limits, unlabored respirations, bowel sounds present
- State of alertness: awake, sleepy, crying

Assessment during feeding: the infant is assessed for the following by direct observation while breastfeeding:

- Latch-on (attachment of the infant to the breast for feeding)
- Position, alignment
- Sucking/swallowing

Assessment of the infant:

- Behavior after/between feedings: contented, sleepy
- Elimination patterns: within 24 hours after birth, at least one wet diaper and one stool; by day 3, three to four wet diapers and one or two stools that are beginning to change from meconium to yellowish; after day 4 (and mother's milk has "come in"), six to eight wet diapers and at least three stools per 24 hours (AAP, 1998).
- General assessment: presence of jaundice; weight loss of less than 10%; regain birth weight by age 10 to 14 days.

Mother

Before breastfeeding is begun, it is important that the nurse carefully assess the mother's knowledge of breastfeeding, as well as her physical and psychologic readiness to breastfeed. This assessment can be accomplished through interviews, discussion, and direct observation. Factors to consider include the following:

- Previous experience with breastfeeding: first baby; successful or unsuccessful breastfeeding with previous infants
- Knowledge about breastfeeding: prenatal classes, support groups, books/pamphlets, videos, friends/relatives who breastfed; knowledge about positioning, latch-on, frequency/duration of feedings, etc.
- Cultural factors: belief that colostrum is bad, modesty issues, language barrier
- Feelings about breastfeeding: anxious, fear of failure; confident, expecting success
- Physical features: development of breast tissue, protractility of nipples (flat or inverted), previous breast surgery, chronic illness, carpal tunnel syndrome, visual or hearing impairment, physical limitations
- Physical/psychologic readiness: risk factors, time since giving birth, type of birth, complications, perineal discomfort, level of pain, medications, mood (eager, cheerful), energy level (tired, exhausted)
- Support: father of baby or family members/friends and their knowledge about breastfeeding

As breastfeeding is becoming established, the nurse performs ongoing assessment of the mother and infant to determine appropriate interventions. During the time in the hospital, the nurse can help the mother to view each breastfeeding session as a "feeding lesson" or "practice session" that will foster maternal confidence and a satisfying breastfeeding experience for mother and baby. Items that should be assessed are the following:

- Condition of nipples: during feeding; mother feels a "tugging" sensation, but no pain after the initial latch-on; presence of soreness, redness, cracking, bleeding
- Transition to mature milk: milk is "in" by day 3 to 5
- Breasts feel softer or lighter after feeding
- Mother states she feels relaxed or sleepy during feeding
- Mother reports uterine cramping and/or increased lochia flow during/after feeding
- Mother appears comfortable with breastfeeding techniques, including positioning and latch-on

Nursing diagnoses for the breastfeeding woman include the following:

- *Effective breastfeeding related to*
  - –mother's knowledge of breastfeeding techniques
  - –mother's appropriate response to infant's feeding-readiness cues
  - –mother's ability to facilitate efficient breastfeeding
  - –mother's adequate fluid and caloric intake for breastfeeding
- *Risk for ineffective breastfeeding related to:*
  - –insufficient knowledge regarding newborn's reflexes and breastfeeding techniques
  - –lack of support by father of baby, family, friends
  - –lack of maternal self-confidence; anxiety, fear of failure
  - –poor infant sucking reflex
  - –difficulty waking sleepy baby

Expected Outcomes of Care

In planning care, the nurse discusses the desired outcomes with the parents. The expected outcomes include that the infant will do the following:

- Latch on and feed effectively at least 8 times per day.
- Gain weight appropriately.
- Remain well hydrated (have six to eight wet diapers and at least three bowel movements every 24 hours after day 4).
- Sleep or seem contented between feedings.

Examples of expected outcomes for the mother include that she will do the following:

- Verbalize/demonstrate understanding of breastfeeding techniques, including positioning and latch-on, signs of adequate feeding, self-care.
- Report no nipple discomfort with breastfeeding.
- Express satisfaction with the breastfeeding experience.
- Consume a nutritionally balanced diet with appropriate caloric and fluid intake to support breastfeeding.

Plan of Care and Interventions

Interventions are based on the expected outcomes and are influenced by the resources and time available to achieve the desired goals. In the early days after birth, interventions focus on helping the mother and the newborn initiate breastfeeding and achieve some degree of success/satisfaction before discharge from the hospital or birthing center. Interventions to promote successful breastfeeding include basics such as latch-on and positioning, signs of adequate feeding, and self-care measures such as prevention of engorgement. An important intervention is to provide the parents with a list of resources that they may contact after discharge from the hospital. Guidelines for Spanish-speaking clients are in the accompanying Guidelines/Guías box.

The ideal time to begin breastfeeding is within 1 hour after birth (AAP, 1997) when the infant is in the quiet, alert state. If this is not possible because of the effects of labor medications or anesthesia, it is advantageous to place the infant in skin-to-skin contact on the mother's chest for the first hour after birth. Each mother should receive instruction, assistance, and support in positioning and latching on until she is able to do so independently (see Guidelines/Guías box).

GUIDELINES/GUÍAS

Breastfeeding: Latching On

Do you want to breastfeed your baby?
¿Desea amamantar a su bebé?

I will help you.
Yo le ayudo.

Hold your baby's head close to your breast.
Sostenga la cabeza del bebé cerca del pecho.

Lightly touch your nipple to the baby's lower lip until he opens his mouth.
Con el pezón, toque ligeramente el labio inferior del bebé hasta que abra la boca.

Lift your breast to the baby's mouth.
Levante el seno hasta la boca del bebé.

Center your nipple and areola as far in the baby's mouth as possible.
Centre el pezón y la areola lo más que se pueda dentro de la boca del bebé.

Make sure the baby's tongue is under the nipple and the gums close around the areola.
Asegurese que la lengua del bebé está debajo del pezón y sus encías se cierren sobre la areola.

To change breasts, push one of your fingers into the corner of the baby's mouth.
Para cambiar al otro seno, introduzca un dedo en el ángulo de la boca del bebé.

This will break the suction and prevent the baby from biting the nipple.
Esto rompe la succión y impide que el bebé muerda el pezón.

Positioning

The four basic positions for breastfeeding are the football hold, cradle, modified cradle or across-the-lap, and side-lying positions (Fig. 27-4). Initially it is advantageous to use the position that most easily facilitates latch-on while allowing maximal comfort for the mother. The football hold is often recommended for early feedings because the mother can easily see the baby's mouth as she guides the infant onto the nipple. The football hold is usually preferred by mothers who gave birth by cesarean. The modified cradle or across-the-lap hold also works well for early feedings, especially with smaller babies. The side-lying position allows the mother to rest while breastfeeding and is often preferred by women with perineal pain and swelling. Cradling is the most common breastfeeding position for infants who have learned to latch on easily and feed effectively. Before discharge from the hospital, the mother may desire to try all of the positions so that she will feel confident in her ability to vary positions at home.

A

B

C

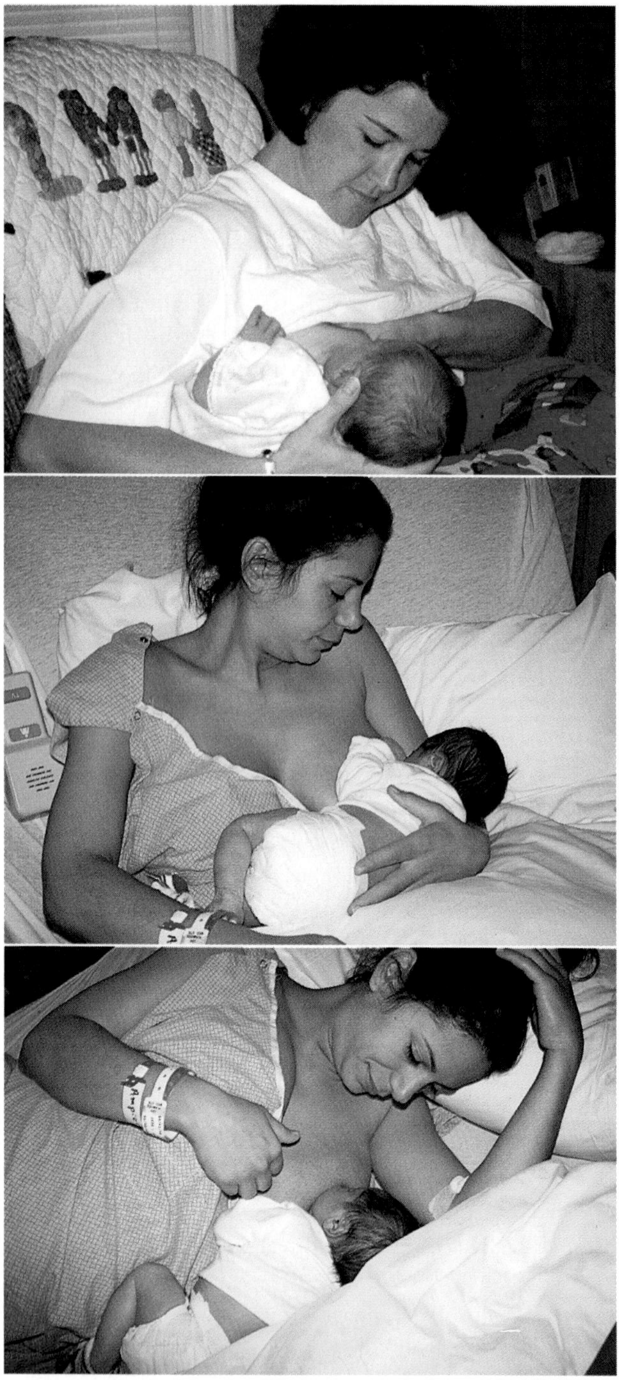

FIG. 27-4 Breastfeeding positions. **A,** Football hold. **B,** Cradling. **C,** Lying down. (**B** and **C** courtesy Marjorie Pyle, RNC, Lifecircle, Costa Mesa, CA.)

Whichever position is used, the mother should be comfortable. The infant is placed at the level of the breast, supported by pillows or folded blankets, turned completely on his or her side, and facing the mother so that the infant is "belly to belly," with the arms "hugging" the breast. The baby's mouth is directly in front of the nipple. It is important that the mother support the baby's neck and shoulders with her hand and not push on the occiput. Pushing on the back of the head may cause the newborn to bite, hyperextend the neck, or develop an aversion to being brought near the breast. The baby's body is held in correct alignment (ears, shoulders, and hips are in a straight line) during latch-on and feeding (Fig. 27-5).

Latch-On

In preparation for latch-on, it may be helpful for the mother to express a few drops of colostrum or milk manually and spread it over the nipple. This lubricates the nipple and may entice the baby to open the mouth as the milk is tasted.

To facilitate latch-on, the mother supports her breast in one hand with the thumb on top and four fingers underneath at the back edge of the areola. The breast is compressed slightly, as one might compress a large sandwich in preparing to take a bite, so that an adequate amount of breast tissue is taken into the mouth with latch-on (Weissinger, 1998). Most mothers need to support the breast during feeding for at least the first days until the infant is adept at feeding.

With the baby held close to the breast with the mouth directly in front of the nipple, the mother tickles the baby's lower lip with the tip of her nipple, stimulating the mouth to open. When the mouth is open wide and the tongue is down, the mother quickly pulls the baby onto the nipple. She brings the baby to the breast, not the breast to the baby. If the breast is pushed into the baby's mouth, the typical response is for the baby to close the mouth too soon, which precludes correct latch-on (see Fig. 27-5).

The amount of areola in the baby's mouth with correct latch-on depends on the size of the baby's mouth and the size of the areola and the nipple. In general, the baby's mouth should cover the nipple and an areolar radius of approximately 2 to 3 cm all around the nipple. (It is incorrect to tell all mothers that the baby should take the entire areola into the mouth with latch-on because areolae vary in size from very small to the size of a saucer.)

When the baby is latched on correctly, the nose, cheeks, and chin should all be touching the breast (Fig. 27-6). It is important for the mother not to pull the nipple out of the mouth when trying to create a breathing space for the baby's nose. Depressing the breast tissue around the baby's nose is not necessary. If she is worried about the baby's breathing, the mother can raise the baby's hips slightly to change the angle of the baby's head at the breast. The nurse should reassure the mother that if the baby cannot breathe, innate reflexes will prompt the baby to move the head and pull back to breathe.

When the baby is latched on correctly and sucking appropriately, (1) the mother reports a firm tugging sensation on her nipples, but no pinching or pain; (2) the baby sucks with cheeks rounded, not dimpled; (3) the baby's jaw glides smoothly with sucking; and (4) swallowing is audible. Sucking creates a vacuum in the intraoral cavity as the breast is compressed between the tongue and the palate. If the mother feels pinching or pain after the initial sucks or does not feel a strong tugging sensation on the nipple, the latch-on and positioning should be evaluated. If each suck is painful, the baby may be having difficulty keeping the tongue out over the lower gum ridge. Clicking or smacking may be audible when this occurs. The nurse can place a finger on the side of the baby's lower jaw, pulling down gently but firmly as the baby sucks, to help stabilize the jaw so that the tongue stays in place.

Any time the signs of adequate latch-on and sucking are not present, the baby should be taken off the breast and latch-on attempted again. To prevent nipple trauma as the baby is taken off the breast, the mother is instructed to break the suction by inserting a finger in the side of the baby's mouth between the gums and leaving it there until the nipple is completely out of the baby's mouth (Fig. 27-7).

Milk Ejection or Let-Down

As the baby begins sucking on the nipple, the let-down, or milk ejection, reflex is stimulated (see Fig. 27-3, *B*). The following signs indicate that let-down has occurred:

- The mother may feel a tingling sensation in the nipples, although many women never feel their milk let down.
- The baby's suck changes from quick, shallow sucks to a slower, more drawing, sucking pattern.
- Swallowing is heard as the baby sucks.
- The mother feels uterine cramping and may have increased lochia during and after feedings.
- The mother feels relaxed, even sleepy, during feedings.
- The opposite breast may leak.

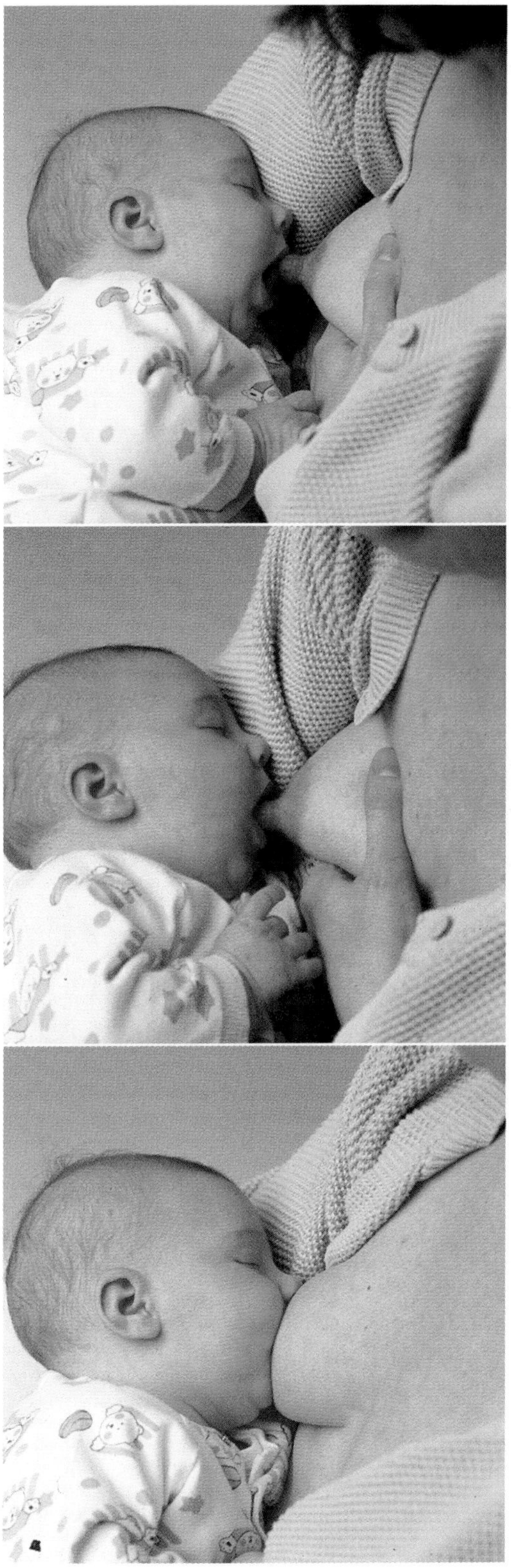

A

B

C

FIG. 27-5 Latching on. **A,** Tickle baby's lower lip with your nipple until he or she opens wide. **B,** Once baby's mouth is opened wide, quickly pull baby onto breast. **C,** Baby should have as much areola (dark area around nipple) in his or her mouth as possible, not just the nipple. (Courtesy Medela, Inc., McHenry, IL.)

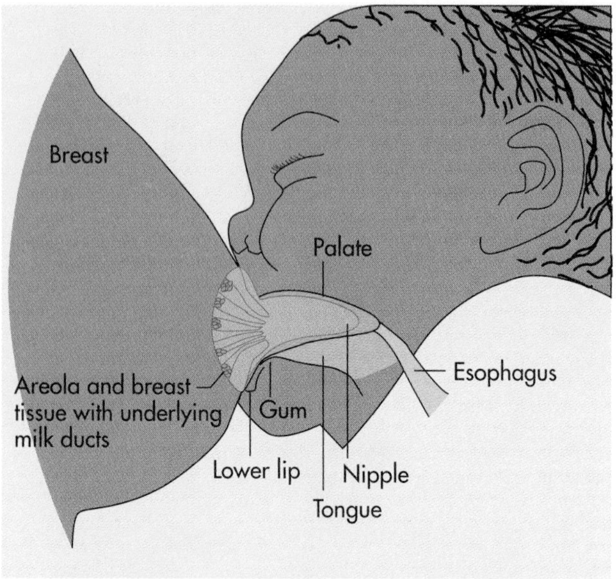
Breast
Palate
Esophagus
Areola and breast tissue with underlying milk ducts
Gum
Lower lip
Nipple
Tongue

FIG. 27-6 Correct attachment (latch-on) of infant at breast.

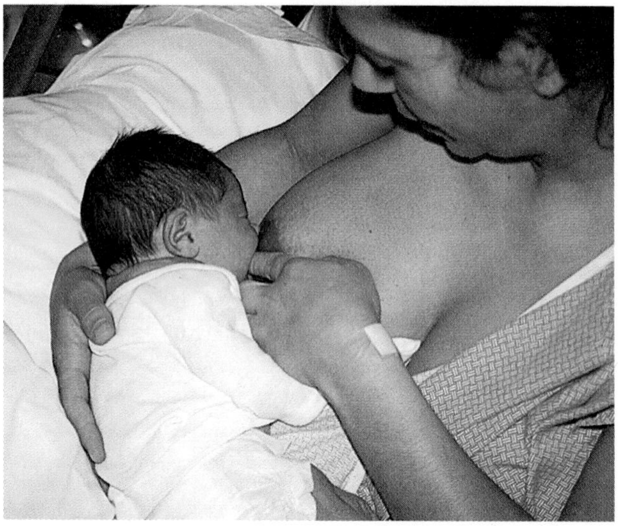

FIG. 27-7 Removing infant from the breast. (Courtesy Marjorie Pyle, RNC, Lifecircle, Costa Mesa, CA.)

Frequency of Feedings

Newborns need to breastfeed 8 to 12 times in a 24-hour period. Feeding patterns are variable because every baby is unique. Some infants will breastfeed every 2 to 3 hours throughout a 24-hour period. Others may *cluster-feed*, breastfeeding every hour or so for three to five feedings and then sleeping for 3 to 4 hours between clusters. During the first 24 to 48 hours after birth, most babies do not awaken this often to feed. It is important that parents understand that they should awaken the baby to feed at least every 3 hours during the day and at least every 4 hours at night. (Feeding frequency is determined by counting from the beginning of one feeding to the beginning of the next.) Once the infant is feeding well and gaining weight adequately, it is more appropriate to go to **demand feeding** when the infant determines the frequency of feedings. (With demand feeding, the infant should still receive at least eight feedings in 24 hours.)

Parents should be cautioned about attempting to place newborn infants on strict feeding schedules that are recommended by some contemporary child-rearing proponents. Incidents of dehydration, poor weight gain, and failure to thrive have been seen in infants whose parents adhered to a strict feeding schedule.

Infants should be fed whenever they exhibit feeding cues such as hand-to-mouth movements and mouth and tongue movements. Crying is a late sign of hunger, and babies may become frantic when they have to wait too long to feed. Some infants will shut down or go into a deep sleep when their needs are not met. Keeping the baby close is the best way to observe and respond to infant feeding cues. Newborns should remain with mothers during the recovery period after birth and room-in during the hospital stay. At home, babies should be kept nearby so that parents can observe signs that the baby is ready to feed.

Duration of Feedings

The duration of breastfeeding sessions is highly variable because the timing of milk transfer differs for each mother-baby pair. The average time for feeding is 30 to 40 minutes, or approximately 15 to 20 minutes per breast. Some mothers do one-sided nursing, in which the baby nurses only one breast at each feeding. In reality, instructing mothers to feed for a set number of minutes is inappropriate. It is better to teach mothers how to determine when a baby has finished a feeding: the baby's suck/swallow pattern has slowed, the breast is softened, and the baby appears content and may fall asleep or release the nipple.

If a baby seems to be feeding effectively and the urine output is adequate but the weight gain is not satisfactory, the mother may be switching to the second breast too soon. The high-lactose, low-fat foremilk may cause the baby to have explosive stools, gas pains, and inconsolable crying. Feeding on the first breast until it softens ensures that the baby will receive the hindmilk, which usually results in increased weight gain.

Indicators of Effective Breastfeeding

In the newborn period when breastfeeding is becoming established, it is important to teach parents the signs that breastfeeding is going well (Box 27-2). When they understand these signs, they will be more likely to recognize when problems arise and know when to seek assistance.

BOX 27-2 Indicators of Effective Breastfeeding During the First Week

INFANT

Physical Assessment

The baby is alert when awake and appears well hydrated, with normal skin turgor and moist mucous membranes. The fontanels are soft and flat, and the baby demonstrates a strong and coordinated suck. Periods of wakefulness and hunger alternate with periods of contentment/sleeping. Weight loss is less than 7% before discharge, and the infant gains 15 to 30 g/day after milk is "in." Birth weight should be regained by 10 to 14 days.

Feeding Frequency

The infant should breastfeed 8 to 12 times in 24 hours.

Feeding Behavior

Baby latches on easily and sucks with gliding jaw movements in bursts of 10 to 12 sucks/swallows at beginning of feeding, slowing to bursts of 2 to 3 sucks/swallows at end of feeding. Swallowing is audible. Baby appears relaxed during feeding and contented when finished.

Output

In the first 3 days of life, a newborn should have one wet diaper and one stool for each day of life. After day 4, when milk has come in, the baby should have six to eight wet diapers every 24 hours. The baby may stool with every feeding, but should minimally have three bowel movements every 24 hours. Stools transition from meconium to milk stools, becoming lighter in color by day 3, and by day 5, appearing mustard-yellow in color.

MOTHER

Physical Assessment

Nipples are intact (no redness, cracking, scabs, or bleeding), and nipple tenderness is minimal. Breasts are full, soft, and without engorgement, with no redness and minimal tenderness to palpation. The mother should have no fever.

Nursing Behavior

Milk is "in" by the third or fourth day. Breasts are full at beginning of feeding and soften as baby breastfeeds. Baby softens at least one breast per feeding. There should be no pinching or nipple pain with sucking, and the mother should feel a strong tugging sensation as the baby sucks.

Mother easily positions and latches baby on and experiences let-down with feeding. She may have a tingling sensation in the nipples as the milk lets down. During the first 4 or 5 days after birth, she may feel uterine cramping and have increased lochia. As she breastfeeds, the mother may be thirsty and experience leaking from the opposite breast. She should feel relaxed during feeding.

Supplements, Bottles, and Pacifiers

The American Academy of Pediatrics Work Group on Breastfeeding (1997) recommends that, unless a medical indication exists, no supplements should be given to breastfeeding infants. With sound breastfeeding knowledge and practice, supplements rarely are needed.

Situations that may necessitate supplementary feeding include such things as low birth weight, hypoglycemia, dehydration, or inborn errors of metabolism. Mothers may be unable to breastfeed because of severe illness or complications of birth, or they may be taking medications incompatible with breastfeeding.

Offering formula to a baby after breastfeeding just to "make sure the baby is getting enough" is normally unnecessary and should be avoided. This can contribute to low milk supply because the baby becomes overly full and does not breastfeed often enough. Supplementation interferes with the supply-meets-demand system of milk production. The parents may interpret the baby's willingness to take a bottle to mean that the mother's milk supply is inadequate. They need to know that a baby will automatically suck from a bottle, as the easy flow of milk from the nipple triggers the suck/swallow reflex.

Babies who receive supplementary feedings may develop **nipple confusion** (i.e., difficulty knowing how to latch on to the breast). This is because breastfeeding and bottle feeding require different skills. The way babies use their tongues, cheeks, and lips, as well as the sucking and swallowing patterns, are very different. Some babies can transition easily between breast and bottle, but some have considerable difficulty. It is impossible to predict which babies will adapt well and which ones will not; therefore it is best to avoid bottles until breastfeeding is well established, usually after 3 to 4 weeks. If supplementation is needed, devices such as supplemental nursing systems may be used, in which the baby can be supplemented while breastfeeding (see Fig. 27-2). Syringe feeding, finger feeding, and cup feeding are other methods for offering supplements to breastfed infants. If parents choose to use bottles, a slow-flow nipple is recommended. Although some parents combine breastfeeding and bottle feeding, many babies never take a bottle and go directly from the breast to a cup as they grow.

Pacifiers are not recommended until breastfeeding is well established. Their use has been associated with shorter duration of breastfeeding, sore nipples, and insufficient milk supply (Aarts et al., 1999; Howard et al., 1999; Kloeben-Tanwer, 2001). Newborns need to learn the association between sucking and satiation. Although some infants have nonnutritive sucking needs between feedings, it is best to wait to introduce a pacifier until the infant is proficient at breastfeeding.

Special Considerations

Sleepy Baby. During the first few days of life, some babies need to be awakened for feedings. Parents are instructed to be alert for behavioral signs or feeding cues such as rapid eye movements under the eyelids, sucking movements, or hand-to-mouth motions. When these signs are present, it is a good time to attempt breastfeeding. If the infant is awakened from a sound sleep, attempts at feeding are more likely to be unsuccessful. Unwrapping the baby, changing the diaper, sitting the baby upright, talking to the baby with variable pitch, gently massaging the baby's chest or back, and stroking the palms or soles may bring the baby to an alert state (Box 27-3).

Fussy Baby. Babies sometimes awaken from sleep crying frantically. Although they may be hungry, they cannot focus on feeding until they are calmed. The nurse can encourage parents to swaddle the baby, hold the baby close, talk soothingly, and allow the baby to suck on a clean finger until calm enough to latch on to the breast (Box 27-4).

BOX 27-3 Waking the Sleepy Newborn

- Lay the baby down and unwrap.
- Change the diaper.
- Hold the baby upright, turn from side to side.
- Talk to the baby.
- Gently, but firmly, massage the chest and back.
- Rub the baby's hands and feet.
- Do baby "sit-ups." Gently rock the baby from a lying to sitting position and back again until the eyes open.
- Adjust lighting up for stimulation or down to encourage the baby to open the eyes.
- Apply cool cloth to face.

BOX 27-4 Calming the Fussy Baby

- Swaddle the baby.
- Hold closely.
- Move or rock gently.
- Talk soothingly.
- Reduce environmental stimuli.
- Allow baby to suck on adult finger.
- Place baby skin-to-skin with mother.

Babies sometimes cry as soon as they are positioned for feeding. This may be the result of a bruised head or previously undetected fractured clavicle. Changing the feeding position may be needed.

If an infant required extensive suctioning at birth, an aversion to oral stimulation may occur, and the baby may scream and stiffen if anything approaches the mouth. Parents may need to spend time holding and cuddling the baby before attempting to breastfeed.

An infant may become fussy and appear discontented when sucking if the nipple does not extend far enough into the mouth. The feeding may begin with well-organized sucks and swallows, but the infant soon begins to pull off the breast and cry. It may be helpful for the mother to support her breast throughout the feeding so that the nipple stays in the same position as the feeding proceeds and the breast softens.

Fussiness may be related to GI distress (i.e., cramping and gas pains). This may occur in response to an occasional feeding of infant formula, or it may be related to something the mother has ingested. Although most mothers can consume their normal diet without affecting the baby, foods such as broccoli, cabbage, or onions may irritate some babies. Others may react to cow's-milk protein ingested by the mother. No standard foods should be avoided by all mothers when breastfeeding; each mother-baby couple responds individually. If gas is a problem, it may be helpful to give the baby liquid simethicone drops before feeding.

Parents should be taught that persistent crying or refusing to breastfeed can indicate illness, and the health care provider should be notified. Ear infections, sore throat, or oral thrush may cause the infant to be fussy and not breastfeed well.

Slow Weight Gain. Newborn infants typically lose about 5% of body weight before they begin to show weight gain. Weight loss of 7% in a breastfeeding infant during the first 3 days of life should be investigated (Lawrence, 1999). Thereafter they should begin to show a weight gain of 110 to 200 g per week or 20 to 28 g per day for the first 3 months. (Breastfed infants usually do not gain weight as quickly as formula-fed infants.) The infant who continues to lose weight after 5 days, who does not regain birth weight by 14 days, or whose weight is below the 10th percentile by 1 month should be evaluated and closely monitored by a health care provider.

Most often, slow weight gain is related to inadequate breastfeeding. Feedings may be short or infrequent, or the infant may be latching on incorrectly or sucking ineffectively or inefficiently. Other possibilities are illness/infection, malabsorption, or circumstances that increase the baby's energy needs such as congenital heart disease, cystic fibrosis, or simply being SGA.

Maternal factors may be the cause of slow weight gain. There may be a problem with inadequate emptying of the breasts, pain with feeding, or inappropriate timing of feedings. Inadequate glandular breast tissue or previous breast surgery may affect milk supply. Severe intrapartum or postpartum hemorrhage, illness, or medications may decrease milk supply. Stress and fatigue also may negatively affect milk production.

Usually the solution to slow weight gain is to improve the feeding technique. Positioning and latch-on are evaluated, and adjustments made. It may help to add a feeding or two in a 24-hour period. If the problem is a sleepy baby, parents are taught waking techniques.

Using *alternate breast massage* during feedings may help increase the amount of milk going to the infant. With this technique, the mother massages her breast from the chest wall to the nipple whenever the baby has sucking pauses. Some think this technique also may increase the fat content of the milk, which aids in weight gain.

When babies are calorie-deprived and need supplementation, expressed breast milk or formula can be given with a nursing supplementer (see Fig. 27-2), cup, syringe, or bottle. In most cases, supplementation is needed only for a short time until the baby gains weight and is feeding adequately.

If the baby's slow weight gain is related to the mother's milk supply, it must be determined if this is an actual or perceived problem and whether it is related to milk production or milk transfer to the infant. Maternal health habits should be assessed because such things as medications, smoking, stress, fatigue, or infection can decrease milk supply.

Jaundice. Jaundice (hyperbilirubinemia) in the newborn is discussed in detail in Chapter 25. Physiologic jaundice usually occurs after age 24 hours and peaks by the third day. This has been referred to as *early-onset jaundice* or *breastfeeding jaundice*, which in the breastfed infant may be associated with insufficient feeding and infrequent stooling. Colostrum has a natural laxative effect and promotes early passage of meconium. Bilirubin is excreted from the body primarily through the intestines. Infrequent stooling allows bilirubin in the stool to be reabsorbed into the infant's system, thus promoting hyperbilirubinemia. Infants who receive water or glucose water supplements are more likely to have hyperbilirubinemia, because only small amounts of bilirubin are excreted through the kidneys. Decreased caloric intake (less milk) is associated with decreased stooling and increased jaundice.

To prevent early-onset breastfeeding jaundice from occurring, babies should be breastfed frequently during the first several days of life. More frequent feedings are associated with lower bilirubin levels.

To treat early-onset jaundice, breastfeeding is evaluated in terms of frequency and length of feedings, positioning and latch-on, and the infant's ability to empty the breast. Factors such as a sleepy or lethargic baby or breast engorgement may interfere with effective breastfeeding and should be corrected. If the infant's intake of milk needs to be increased, a supplemental feeding device may be used to deliver additional breast milk or formula while the infant is nursing. Hyperbilirubinemia may reach levels that require treatment with phototherapy administered with a light or a fiberoptic blanket (see Chapter 26).

Late-onset jaundice or *breast milk jaundice* affects a few breastfed infants and develops in the second week of life, peaking at about age 10 days. These infants are typically thriving, gaining weight, and stooling normally; all pathologic causes of jaundice have been ruled out. It was once postulated that an enzyme in the milk of some mothers caused the bilirubin level to increase. It now appears that a factor in human milk increases the intestinal absorption of bilirubin. In most cases, no intervention is necessary, although some experts recommend temporary interruption of breastfeeding for 12 to 24 hours to allow bilirubin levels to decrease. During this time, the mother pumps her breasts, and the baby is offered alternative nutrition, usually formula (Lawrence, 1999).

Preterm Infants. Human milk is the ideal food for preterm infants, with benefits that are unique and in addition to those received by term, healthy infants. Breast milk enhances retinal maturation in the preterm infant and improves neurocognitive outcome. It also decreases the risk of necrotizing enterocolitis. Greater physiologic stability occurs with breastfeeding as compared with bottle feeding (Lawrence, 1999).

Mothers of preterm infants who are not able to breastfeed their infants should begin pumping their breasts as soon as possible after birth with a hospital-grade electric pump (Fig. 27-8). To establish an optimal milk supply, the mother should use a dual collection kit and pump 8 to 10 times daily for 10 to 15 minutes and/or until the milk flow has ceased for a few minutes. These women are taught proper handling and storage of breast milk to minimize bacterial contamination and growth (Meier, 1997).

The mothers of preterm infants receive specific emotional benefits in breastfeeding or providing breast milk for their babies. They report rewards in knowing they can provide the healthiest nutrition for the infant and believe that breastfeeding enhances feelings of closeness to the infant (Kavanaugh et al., 1997).

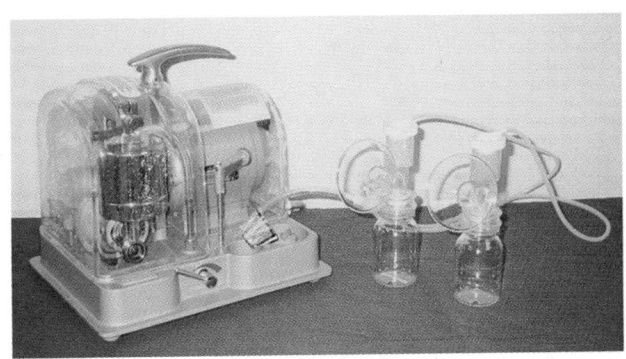

FIG. 27-8 Hospital-grade electric breast pump.

Breastfeeding Twins. Caring for twins takes some planning, but breastfeeding twins means that feedings are always ready instantly, and no one has to wash bottles and fix formula. Some mothers are able to feed both babies at once. The mother who is breastfeeding twins needs extra nourishment (200 to 500 kcal per day for each baby).

Each baby feeds from one breast per feeding, usually for about 20 to 30 minutes. Some mothers assign each baby a breast; others switch babies from one breast to the other, either on a schedule or randomly. The mother may find it easiest to use a modified demand feeding schedule. This involves feeding the first baby who wakes and then waking the second baby for feeding.

During the early weeks, parents may find it helpful to keep a record of feeding times and which breast was used first by which baby. If one twin nurses more vigorously than the other, the more vigorous baby should be alternated between breasts to equalize breast stimulation.

If the mother wants to feed the babies simultaneously, she may wish to experiment with positions. The easiest position to feed both babies is football hold (Fig. 27-9). Alternatively, one baby could be held in the football hold and the other in the cradle hold, or the babies could each be held in a cradling position.

Expressing and Storing Breast Milk

In some situations, expression of breast milk is necessary or desirable, such as when engorgement occurs, the mother and baby are separated (e.g., preterm or sick infant), the mother is employed outside the home and needs to maintain her milk supply, the nipples are severely sore or damaged, or the mother is leaving the infant with a caregiver and will not be present for feeding.

Because pumping and hand expression are rarely as efficient as a baby in removing milk from the breast, the milk supply should never be judged based on the volume expressed.

Hand Expression. After her hands are thoroughly washed, the mother places one hand on her breast at the edge of the areola. With her thumb above and fingers below, she presses in toward her chest wall and gently compresses the breast while rolling her thumb and fingers forward toward the nipple. These motions are repeated rhythmically until the milk begins to flow. The mother simply maintains steady, light pressure while the milk is flowing easily. The thumb and fingers should not pinch the breast or slip down to the nipple, and the mother should rotate her hand to reach all sections of the breast. After expressing milk from the second breast, she should return and express milk from the first breast, and then repeat the second breast until all readily available milk is expressed.

Pumping. For most women, it is advisable to initiate pumping only after the milk supply is well established and the infant is latching on and breastfeeding well. However, when breastfeeding is delayed after birth, pumping is started as soon as possible and continued regularly until the infant is able to breastfeed effectively.

Numerous ways exist to approach pumping. Some women pump on awakening in the morning, or when the baby has fed but did not completely empty the breast. Others choose to pump after feedings or may pump one breast while the baby is feeding from the other. Double pumping (pumping both breasts at the same time) saves time and may stimulate the milk supply more effectively than single pumping (Fig. 27-10).

The amount of milk obtained when pumping depends on the type of pump being used, the time of day, how long it has been since the baby breastfed, the mother's milk supply, how practiced she is at pumping, and her comfort level (pumping is uncomfortable for some women). Breast milk may vary in color and consistency, depending on the time of day, the age of the baby, and foods the mother has

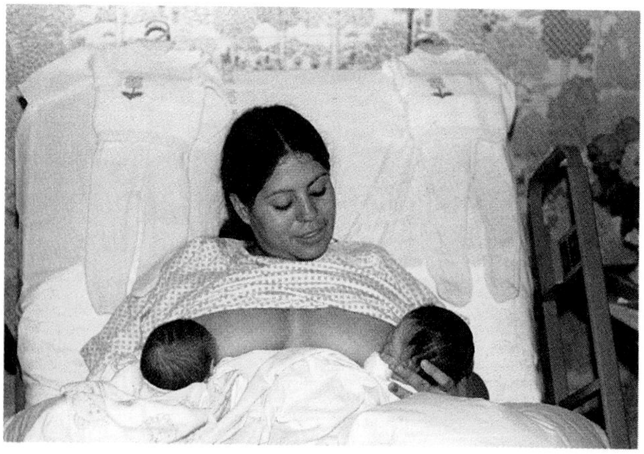

FIG. 27-9 Breastfeeding twins. (Courtesy Marjorie Pyle, RNC, Lifecircle, Costa Mesa, CA.)

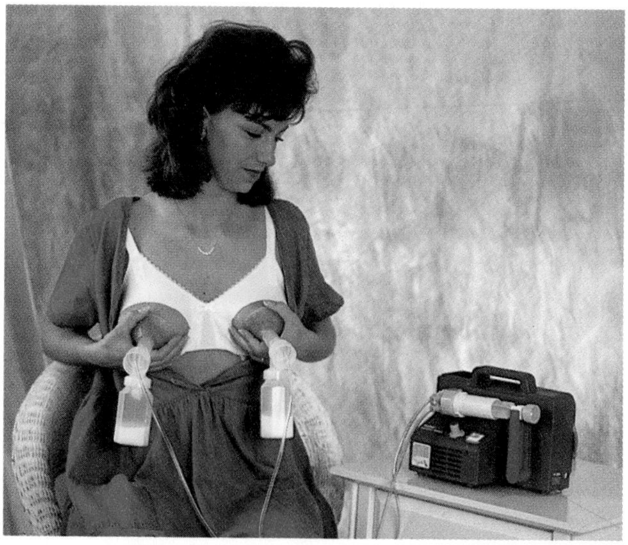

FIG. 27-10 Bilateral breast pumping. (Courtesy Medela, Inc., McHenry, IL.)

eaten (e.g., the milk may appear green after the mother eats a spinach salad).

Types of Pumps. Many types of breast pumps are available. Some are more effective than others, and they vary in price. Before purchasing or renting a breast pump, the mother would benefit from counseling by a nurse or lactation consultant to determine which pump best suits her needs (Biancuzzo, 1999).

Manual or hand pumps are least expensive and may be the most appropriate where portability and quietness of operation are important. These are most often used by mothers who are pumping for an occasional bottle (Fig. 27-11).

Full-service electric pumps, or hospital-grade pumps (see Fig. 27-8), are most similar to the sucking action and pressure of the breastfeeding infant. When breastfeeding is delayed after birth (e.g., the newborn is preterm or ill), or when mother and baby are separated for lengthy periods, these pumps are most appropriate. Because hospital-grade breast pumps are very heavy and expensive, portable versions of these pumps can be rented for home use.

Electric, self-cycling double pumps are efficient and easy to use. These pumps were designed for working mothers. Some of these pumps come with carry bags containing coolers to store pumped milk.

Smaller electric or battery-operated pumps also are available. Some have automatic suck/release cycling, and others require use of a finger to regulate strength and speed of suction. These are typically used when pumping is done occasionally, but some models are satisfactory for working mothers or others who pump on a regular basis.

Storage of Breast Milk. Breast milk can be safely stored in any clean glass or plastic container. Plastic bags especially designed for freezing breast milk can be purchased. Disposable bottle liners are easy and inexpensive to use when storing milk. When using bottle liners, double bagging is recommended to protect the milk most effectively.

For full-term, healthy infants, freshly expressed breast milk can be stored at room temperature for up to 8 hours. It can be refrigerated safely for 3 to 5 days. Milk can be frozen for 3 months in the freezer section of a refrigerator with a separate door, and for 6 to 12 months in a deep freeze (0° C). When storing breast milk, the container should be dated, and the oldest milk should be used first.

Frozen milk is thawed by placing the container in the refrigerator for gradual thawing or in warm water for faster thawing. It cannot be refrozen and should be used within 24 hours. After thawing, the container should be shaken to mix the layers that have separated (see Teaching for Self Care box).

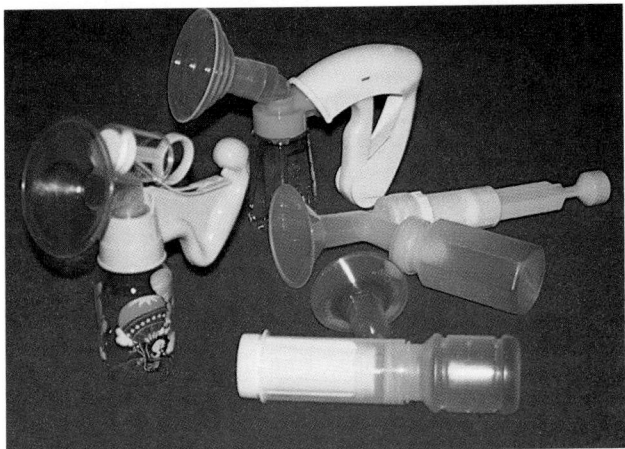

FIG. 27-11 Manual breast pumps. (Courtesy Marjorie Pyle, RNC, Lifecircle, Costa Mesa, CA.)

TEACHING FOR SELF-CARE

Breast Milk Storage Guidelines for Home Use

- Before expressing breast milk, wash your hands.
- Containers for storing milk should be washed in hot, soapy water and rinsed thoroughly; they can also be washed in a dishwasher. Plastic bags designed specifically for breast milk storage can be used; if using plastic disposable bottle liners, be sure to double-bag the milk.
- Write the date of expression on the container before storing the milk.
- It is acceptable to store breast milk in the refrigerator/freezer with other food items.
- When storing milk in a refrigerator/freezer, place the containers in the middle or back of the freezer, not in the door.
- Freeze milk in serving sizes of 2 to 4 ounces to avoid wasting.
- When filling a storage container that will be frozen, allow space at the top of the container for expansion.
- To thaw frozen breast milk, place the container in the refrigerator for gradual thawing or place the container under warm, running water for quicker thawing. Never boil or microwave.
- Milk thawed in the refrigerator can be stored for 24 hours. Milk thawed in warm water can be refrigerated for use within 4 hours.
- Thawed breast milk should never be refrozen.
- Shake the milk container before feeding baby, and test the temperature of the milk on the inner aspect of your wrist.
- Any unused milk left in the bottle after feeding must be discarded.
- Freshly expressed breast milk can be stored at room temperature (less than 78° F [25.6° C]) for up to 8 hours.
- Breast milk can be stored in the refrigerator for 3 to 5 days.
- Frozen breast milk can be stored for 2 weeks in a freezer compartment within a refrigerator.
- Frozen breast milk can be stored for up to 3 months in the freezer section with a separate door.
- Frozen breast milk can be stored for 6 to 12 months in a deep freeze (32° F [0° C] or lower)

From Lawrence, R. (1999). *Breastfeeding: A guide for the medical profession* (5th ed.). St. Louis: Mosby, and www.breastfeeding.com/workingmom/pumping/storage_guidelines.html.

Frozen milk is never thawed or heated in a microwave oven. Microwaving does not heat evenly and can cause encapsulated boiling bubbles to form in the center of the liquid. This may not be detected when drops of milk are checked for temperature. Babies have sustained severe burns to the mouth, throat, and upper GI tract as a result of microwaved milk (Lawrence, 1999).

Being Away From the Baby

Many women are able to combine breastfeeding successfully with employment, attending school, or other commitments. If feedings are missed, the milk supply may be affected. Some women's bodies adjust the milk supply to the times she is with the baby for feedings, whereas others find they must pump or the supply diminishes quickly. Businesses are increasingly making available rooms where mothers can nurse their infants or use breast pumps (Fig. 27-12).

Breastfeeding mothers who work outside the home often feel a special connection to their babies even when they are separated. It is easy to continue breastfeeding while working. Planning ahead makes the transition back to work after birth much smoother and easier for both mother and baby. Breastfed babies are healthier, and mothers are less likely to miss work; this is an added benefit for the family and the employer.

Weaning

Typically weaning is initiated at a time chosen by the mother or the infant. Weaning can be accomplished with little effort and no discomfort when it is done gradually. Abrupt weaning is likely to be distressing for both mother and baby, as well as physically uncomfortable for the mother.

Infant-led weaning means that the infant moves at his or her own pace in omitting feedings. Drinking from a cup and increasing the amount of solid foods substitute for breastfeeding and allow a gradual decrease in the mother's milk supply.

Mother-led weaning means that the mother decides which feedings to drop. This is most easily done by omitting the feeding of least interest to the baby or the one the infant is most likely to sleep through. It also can be the feeding most convenient for the mother to omit. After a week or more, another feeding is dropped, and so on, until the infant is weaned from the breast. Allowing time for the milk supply to adjust before omitting another feeding prevents discomfort for the mother as her supply gradually decreases.

Infants can be weaned directly from the breast to a cup. Bottles are usually offered to infants younger than 6 months. If the infant is weaned before age 1 year, formula should be fed to the infant instead of cow's milk.

If abrupt weaning is necessary, breast engorgement often occurs. The mother is instructed to take mild analgesics, wear a supportive bra, apply ice packs or cabbage leaves to the breasts, and pump if needed to increase comfort. Pumping should be avoided because the breasts should remain full enough to promote a decrease in the milk supply. If the mother is feeling severe discomfort from breast engorgement, she can be told to pump just enough to make her feel more comfortable but not enough to empty the breasts.

Many women feel that weaning is the end to a special, satisfying relationship with the infant and benefit from time to adapt to the changes. Sudden weaning may evoke feelings of guilt and disappointment; some women go through a grieving period after weaning. The nurse can assist the mother by discussing other ways to continue this nurturing relationship with the infant, such as skin-to-skin contact while bottle feeding, or holding and cuddling the baby. Support from the father of the baby and other family members is essential at this time.

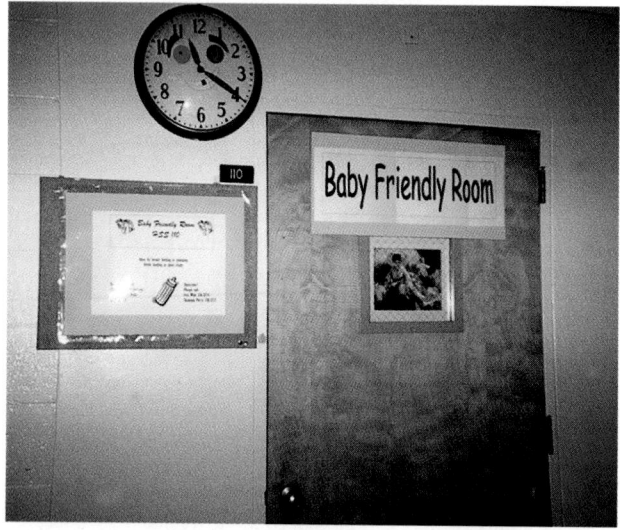
110
Baby Friendly Room

FIG. 27-12 Room on a university campus dedicated to parents and infants. The room contains comfortable furniture, a breast pump, a refrigerator, a baby changing table, and a television and VCR for instructional purposes. The room is available to students, faculty, and staff. (Courtesy Shannon Perry, San Jose, CA.)

Milk Banking

For those infants who cannot be breastfed but who also cannot survive except on human milk, banked donor milk is critically important. Because of the antiinfective and growth-promoting properties of human milk, as well as its superior nutrition, donor milk is used in many neonatal intensive care units for preterm or sick infants when the mother's own milk is not available. Donor milk also is used therapeutically for some medical purposes, such as in transplant recipients who are immunocompromised.

The Human Milk Banking Association of North America (HMBANA) has established annually reviewed guidelines for the operation of donor human milk banks. Donor milk banks collect, screen, process, and distribute the milk donated by breastfeeding mothers who are feeding their own infants and pumping a few ounces extra each day for the milk bank. All donors are screened both by interview and serologically for communicable diseases. Donor milk is stored frozen until it is heat processed to kill potential pathogens; then it is refrozen for storage until it is dispensed for use. The heat processing adds a level of protection for the recipient that is not possible with any other donor tissue or organ. Banked milk is dispensed only by prescription. A per-ounce fee is charged by the bank to pay for the processing costs, but the HMBANA guidelines prohibit payment to donors (see the Resource list at the end of this chapter).

Care of the Mother

Diet. The composition of human milk varies slightly among women, regardless of their diets. The mother's milk automatically contains everything the baby needs, except in rare cases of maternal nutrient deficiencies. For most women, only 200 to 500 extra calories per day must be added to the diet to provide adequate nutrients for the infant while also protecting the mother's body stores.

No specific foods or drinks must be either consumed or avoided. Lactating mothers should ideally consume a balanced diet of nutrient-dense foods. Adequate amounts of calcium, minerals, and fat-soluble vitamins are important. Breastfeeding mothers are encouraged to continue taking their prenatal vitamins until the baby is weaned.

If the breastfeeding mother is drinking enough fluids to quench her thirst, she is likely drinking enough to support lactation. Typically, women find that they are drinking as much as 2 to 3 quarts of fluid each day, with the choice of fluid depending on the mother's preference. Because of her increased need for fluids, the breastfeeding mother may wish to keep a drink within reach during feedings. An indicator of adequate fluid intake is the color of the mother's urine. If she is drinking enough fluids, her urine should be clear to light yellow throughout the day.

Weight Loss. Because it takes energy to produce milk, many mothers have a gradual weight loss while breastfeeding, as fat stores deposited during pregnancy are used. For overweight women, this can be an added incentive for breastfeeding. However, the mother who wants to diet while lactating should avoid losing large amounts of weight quickly because fat-soluble environmental contaminants to which she has been exposed are stored in her body's fat reserves, and these may be released into her milk. In addition, some mothers find that their milk supply decreases when their caloric intake is severely restricted. Most mothers find that they can lose about 1 kg per week without affecting their milk supply (King, 2000).

Exercise. There is no reason for a breastfeeding woman to restrict her physical activity. Women can continue to engage in activities such as hiking, jogging, swimming, and aerobics with no detrimental effect on the milk supply or composition. For comfort, mothers may find it beneficial to engage in exercise soon after breastfeeding, when their breasts are as empty as possible. Wearing a well-designed, supportive bra also may be helpful.

Rest. It is important for the breastfeeding mother to rest as much as possible, especially in the first 1 or 2 weeks after birth. Fatigue, stress, and worry can negatively affect milk production and let-down. The nurse can encourage the mother to sleep when the baby sleeps. Breastfeeding in a side-lying position promotes rest for the mother. Assistance with household chores and caring for other children can be done by the father, grandparents or other relatives, and friends.

Breast Care. The breastfeeding mother's normal routine bathing is all that is necessary to keep her breasts clean. Soap can have a drying effect on nipples, so she should be instructed to avoid washing the nipples with soap. (The small amount of soap that runs down her breasts while washing her face and neck or shampooing her hair is of no concern.)

Breast creams should not be used routinely because they may block the natural oil secreted by the Montgomery glands on the areola. Some breast creams contain alcohol, which may dry the nipples. Vitamin E oil or cream is not recommended for use on nipples because it is a fat-soluble vitamin, and a breastfeeding infant might consume enough vitamin E from the nipple to reach toxic levels. In addition, some people are allergic to vitamin E oil.

Modified lanolin with reduced allergens can be used safely on dry or sore nipples. Research has shown that lanolin is beneficial in moist wound healing of sore nipples (Brent et al., 1998). Because lanolin is made from sheep's wool, the nurse should ask the mother if she is allergic to wool before applying the lanolin. Lanolin is not recommended if it is suspected that nipple soreness may be due to a monilial infection. Antifungal creams are used to treat yeast infections on nipples.

The mother with flat or inverted nipples will likely benefit from wearing breast shells in her bra. These hard plastic devices exert mild pressure around the base of the nipple to encourage nipple eversion. It is advisable for women with flat or inverted nipples to begin wearing breast shells during the last month of pregnancy. Breast shells also are useful for sore nipples to keep the mother's bra or clothing from touching the nipples (Fig. 27-13).

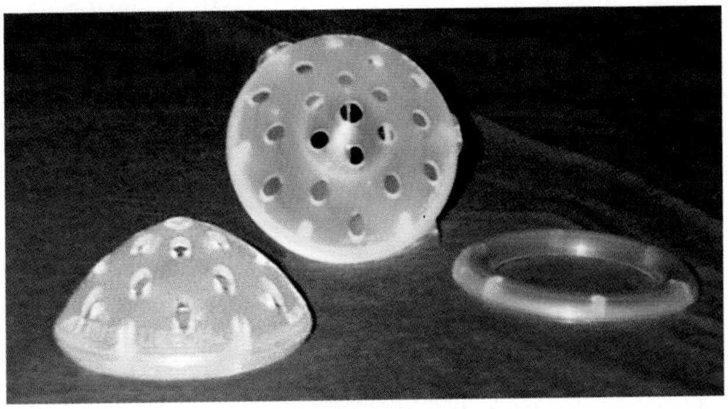

FIG. 27-13 Breast shells.

If a mother needs breast support, she will be uncomfortable unless she wears a bra, because the ligament that supports the breast (Cooper's ligament) will otherwise stretch and be painful. If she is comfortable without a bra, there is no reason for her to wear one. If a woman prefers to wear a bra, it should fit well, offer nonbinding support, and feel comfortable. Underwire bras or improperly fitting bras may contribute to clogged milk ducts. Mothers should be encouraged to breastfeed at least once daily without a bra on so that all milk ducts can empty well.

Leakage of milk between feedings is a problem for some women. Using breast pads (disposable or washable) inside a bra and wearing layered or printed tops can help camouflage the leakage. Plastic-lined breast pads are not recommended because they trap moisture and may contribute to sore nipples. To stop leakage, the mother can be alert to any sensation, such as tingling, that her milk is letting down. If this happens, she can usually stop the letdown by pressing straight back on her nipples. In public, she can fold her arms across her chest to apply pressure unobtrusively.

Although few cases of breast cancer are diagnosed during pregnancy or lactation, the breastfeeding woman should perform monthly breast self-examination (BSE). The woman who is not menstruating should choose a convenient date on which to do her BSE each month. She needs to become familiar with the normal nodularity of her lactating breasts so that she can detect anything unusual on examination. Nodules that match in location in both breasts are likely breast tissue. Nodules that increase and decrease in size are probably milk glands or ducts. Because lactating breasts are very dense, mammography is of limited diagnostic value. Should a suggestive nodule be discovered, a biopsy can usually be done without interrupting breastfeeding.

Effect of Menstruation. The return of menstrual periods varies among lactating women. The majority will resume menstruation by 6 months postpartum. Menstruation has no effect on breastfeeding. There are no hormonal effects on the infant, although some babies may seem fussy for the first day. The quality of the milk is not affected (Lawrence, 1999).

Sexual Sensations. Some women experience rhythmic uterine contractions during breastfeeding. Such sensations are not unusual because uterine contractions and milk ejection are both triggered by oxytocin. These uterine contractions may provoke sensations resembling an orgasmic response, which is disturbing to some mothers.

Breastfeeding and Contraception. Although breastfeeding confers a period of infertility, it is not considered an effective method of contraception. Breastfeeding delays the return of ovulation and menstruation; however, ovulation may occur even before the first menstrual period after birth. The breastfeeding woman who is relying on the lactational amenorrhea (LAM) method of birth control needs to be knowledgeable about ways to determine when ovulation occurs (i.e., basal body temperature, consistency of cervical mucus, and cervical position). Hormonal contraceptives, including pills, injectables, and implants, may cause a decrease in the milk supply and are best avoided during the first 6 weeks after birth. Oral contraceptives containing estrogen are not recommended for breastfeeding mothers. Progestin-only birth control pills are less likely to interfere with the milk supply. Some women find that the progestin-only injection (Depo-Provera) interferes with milk production, although others notice no alteration in the milk supply. Nonhormonal contraceptive methods (e.g., foam, condoms, nonhormonal intrauterine device [IUD], natural family planning, sterilization) are less likely to have a detrimental effect on breastfeeding.

Breastfeeding During Pregnancy. It is possible for a breastfeeding woman to conceive and continue breastfeeding throughout the pregnancy if there are no medical contraindications (e.g., risk of preterm labor). When the baby is born, colostrum is produced. The practice of breastfeeding a newborn and an older child is called *tandem nursing.* The nurse should remind the mother always to feed the infant first to ensure that the newborn is receiving adequate nutrition. The supply-meets-demand principle works in this situation, just as with breastfeeding multiples.

The Mother with Diabetes. The mother with diabetes is encouraged to breastfeed. In addition to benefits for the infant, and maternal satisfaction, breastfeeding has an antidiabetogenic effect. Blood glucose levels and insulin requirements are lower because of the carbohydrate used in milk production. During lactation, the woman may be able to eat more food and still take less insulin. However, insulin dosage must be adjusted as the baby is weaned. Some women with diabetes are at increased risk for sore nipples caused by monilial infections and may have an increased risk for mastitis.

Medications and Breastfeeding. Although there is much concern about the compatibility of drugs and breastfeeding, few drugs are absolutely contraindicated during lactation. In evaluating the safety of a specific medication during breastfeeding, the health care provider considers the pharmacokinetics of the drug in the maternal system, as well as the absorption, metabolism, distribution, storage, and excretion in the infant. The gestational and chronologic age of the infant, body weight, and breastfeeding pattern also are considered. Most medications do not cause problems for the infant, but breastfeeding mothers should be cautioned about taking any medications except those that are deemed essential. Breastfeeding women should check with their physician before taking any medication. If a breastfeeding mother is taking a medication that has questionable effect on the infant, she can be advised to take the medication just after nursing the baby or just before the infant is expected to sleep for a long time. The American Academy of Pediatrics published a report about the transfer of drugs and other chemicals in human milk; this report specifies possible effects of these substances on the infant and on lactation (AAP Committee on Drugs, 2001). Reference books are available, and websites describe the safety of specific medications during pregnancy.

Smoking may impair milk production; it also exposes infants to the effects of second-hand smoke. Mothers who continue to smoke tobacco when lactating should be advised not to smoke within 2 hours before breastfeeding and never to smoke in the same room with the infant (AAP Committee on Drugs, 2001).

Consumption of alcohol during lactation is approached with caution. Excessive amounts can have serious effects on the infant and can adversely affect the mother's MER. The level of alcohol in breast milk decreases over time, unlike the levels of many drugs that remain in milk until it is removed from the breasts. If a mother chooses to consume alcohol, she should be advised to minimize its effects by having only one drink, and to consume the drink immediately after breastfeeding. The mother who is pumping for a sick or preterm infant should avoid alcohol entirely until her infant is healthy (Lawrence, 1999).

Although only 1% of the caffeine ingested by the mother is passed into her breast milk, the infant's immature system limits the ability to excrete the caffeine. Caffeine accumulates in the infant's system and can cause irritability and poor sleeping patterns. For most women, two servings of caffeine a day does not cause untoward effects; however, some infants are sensitive to even small amounts of caffeine. Mothers of such infants should limit caffeine intake. Caffeine is found in coffee, tea, chocolate, and many soft drinks (Lawrence, 1999).

Herbs and herbal teas are becoming more widely used during lactation. Although some are considered safe, others contain pharmacologically active compounds that may have detrimental effects. A thorough maternal history should include the use of any herbal remedies. Each remedy should then be evaluated for its compatibility with breastfeeding. The regional poison control center may provide information on the active properties of herbs.

Environmental Contaminants. Except under unusual circumstances, breastfeeding is not contraindicated because of exposure to environmental contaminants such as DDT (an insecticide) and tetrachloroethylene (used in dry cleaning plants) (Lawrence, 1999).

Special Considerations

The breastfeeding mother may have some common problems. In the majority of cases, these complications are preventable if the mother receives appropriate education about breastfeeding. Early recognition and resolution of these problems is important to prevent interruption of breastfeeding and to promote the mother's comfort and sense of well-being. The nurse or lactation consultant is likely to be the first contact the mother makes when these problems arise. By using astute interview and assessment skills, the nurse can gather essential data related to these problems, make necessary referrals to the physician or nurse practitioner, and assist the mother in initiating the appropriate treatment plan. Emotional support provided by the nurse or lactation consultant is essential to help allay the mother's frustration and anxiety and to prevent early cessation of breastfeeding.

Engorgement. Engorgement usually occurs 3 to 5 days after birth when the milk "comes in" and lasts about 24 hours. It is a common response of the breasts to the sudden change in hormones and the presence of an increased volume of milk. Blood supply to the breasts increases and causes swelling of tissues surrounding the milk ducts. The ducts may be pinched shut, so that the milk does not flow. The breasts are firm, tender, hot, and may appear shiny and taut. The tenderness and swelling extends into the axilla. The areolae are firm, and the nipples may flatten. The unyielding areolae make it difficult for the infant to latch on. Because back pressure on full milk glands inhibits milk production, if milk is not removed from the breasts, the milk supply may diminish.

Preparing the mother for what to expect when the milk comes in may help prevent engorgement or minimize its severity. Breastfeeding the baby frequently, at least every 2 to 3 hours, as the milk is coming in may help prevent engorgement. The baby should be encouraged to feed at least 15 to 20 minutes on each breast or until one breast softens per feeding.

When engorgement occurs, the nurse should reassure the mother that this a temporary condition usually resolved within 24 hours. The mother is instructed to feed every 2 hours, massaging the breasts as the baby is feeding. The baby should feed on the first breast until it softens before switching to the other side. If the infant does not soften the second breast, the mother may use a breast pump to empty the breast. Pumping during engorgement will not cause a problematic increase in milk supply. A warm shower just before feeding or pumping can aid in relaxation and let-down.

Because of the swelling of breast tissue surrounding the milk glands and milk ducts, ice packs are recommended in a 15-to-20-minutes-on, 45-minutes-off rotation, between feedings. The ice packs should cover both breasts. Large bags of frozen peas or corn make easy packs and can be refrozen between uses.

Raw cabbage leaves placed over the breasts in between feedings may help reduce the swelling. The mother washes the cabbage leaves and places them in her refrigerator until they are cool. She then crushes the leaves and places them over the breasts for 15 to 20 minutes. This can be repeated for two or three sessions; frequent application of cabbage leaves can decrease milk supply. (They are often very effective for formula-feeding mothers who want their milk to "dry up.") Cabbage leaves should not be used if the mother is allergic to cabbage, sulfa drugs, or develops a skin rash (Lactation Education Resources, 2001).

Antiinflammatory medications, such as ibuprofen, may help reduce the pain and swelling associated with engorgement. Mothers often have a low-grade fever with engorgement and experience aching in their breasts, which ibuprofen can help remedy.

Sore Nipples. Mild nipple discomfort at the beginning of feedings or mild nipple tenderness during the first few days of breastfeeding is not abnormal. Severe soreness and abraded, cracked, or bleeding nipples are not normal and most often result from poor positioning, incorrect latch-on, improper suck, or a monilial infection. Many women expect breastfeeding to be painful, based on stories they have heard from family and friends. The nurse or lactation consultant must emphasize that breastfeeding should not be a painful experience; infant suckling should feel like a strong tugging sensation, but without pain or pinching. Limiting the time at the breast will not prevent sore nipples; the key to preventing sore nipples is correct breastfeeding technique.

For the first few days after birth, the mother may have some tenderness with the infant's initial sucks at the beginning of a feeding. This should quickly dissipate as the colostrum or milk begins to flow. To make the initial sucks less painful, the mother can express a few drops of colostrum or milk to moisten the nipple and areola before latch-on.

If the mother continues to experience nipple pain or discomfort after the first few sucks, it is necessary to help the mother evaluate the latch-on and baby's position at the breast to determine if the baby is well supported, is in straight body alignment, and has no pressure on the back of his or her head. The baby's nose, cheeks, and chin should touch the breast, and the mother should support the breast with her hand during the early feedings. The nurse helps the mother to reposition as necessary to try to resolve the nipple discomfort.

If the mother reports a pinching sensation on the nipple as the baby sucks, it may be helpful to pull down on the side of the baby's jaw gently during sucking to increase the amount of breast tissue in the baby's mouth. If the nipple pain continues, the mother needs to remove the baby from the breast, breaking suction with her finger in the baby's mouth. She then proceeds to attempt latch-on again, making sure the baby's mouth is open wide before the baby is pulled quickly to the breast (see Fig. 27-5). Often sore nipples are the result of the mother latching the baby onto the breast before the mouth is open wide.

The infant's suck can be assessed by the nurse or lactation consultant simply by inserting a clean gloved finger in the baby's mouth and stimulating the baby to suck. If the baby is not extruding the tongue over the lower gum, and the mother reports pain or pinching with sucking, the baby may have a short frenulum (commonly referred to as being "tongue-tied"). Sometimes this is corrected surgically to free the tongue for less painful, more effective breastfeeding (Messner, 2000).

The treatment for sore nipples is first to correct the cause. Once the problem is identified and corrected, sore nipples should heal within a few days, even though the baby continues to breastfeed regularly.

When sore nipples occur, it is more comfortable to start the feeding on the least sore nipple. Applying ice to the nipple for 2 to 3 minutes provides a numbing effect that increases comfort with latch-on. After feeding, the nipples are wiped with water to remove the baby's saliva. A few drops of milk can be expressed, rubbed into the nipple, and allowed to air dry.

Rapid healing of sore nipples is critical to relieve the mother's discomfort, maintain breastfeeding, and prevent mastitis. Moist wound-healing techniques seem to accelerate healing by allowing sore nipples to "breathe" while moisturizing the skin and protecting against insensible water loss. Purified lanolin helps sore nipples by retaining the skin's natural moisture and protecting the nipple from further abrasion. It is applied to nipples after feeding and need not be removed for the next feeding. (Mothers with history of wool allergy should not use lanolin until a skin test is done). An antibiotic ointment may be recommended if nipples are cracked, abraded, or bleeding; this must be washed off before the feeding. A recent technique for sore nipples is hydrogel dressings. These create a soothing, moist healing environment by using a glycerin-based gel or saline-based hydrophilic polymer to provide a healing environment and bacterial barrier. Hydrogel pads are applied to the sore nipples after feeding, pumping, or bathing; they will not wipe off onto clothing or stick to sore nipples. They can be rinsed and reused for several days. Hydrogel also is available in a cream (Lactation Education Resources, 2001).

If nipples are extremely sore or damaged, and the mother cannot tolerate breastfeeding, she may be advised to use an electric breast pump for 24 to 48 hours to allow the nipples to begin healing before resuming breastfeeding. It is important that the mother use a pump that will effectively empty the breasts; a rental pump is likely the best choice (see Fig. 27-10).

Sore nipples should be open to air as much as possible. Breast shells worn inside the bra allow air to circulate, while keeping clothing off sore nipples (see Fig. 27-13).

Flexible nipple shields have been marketed as a treatment for sore nipples; however, they do not protect the nipple and can actually chafe the nipple as the baby sucks. The danger of the baby not receiving adequate milk flow through the shield exists because it is difficult for most infants to get far enough back on the breast to compress the lactiferous sinuses adequately and get the milk to flow. In special situations, nipple shields are useful; however, they should be used only by trained lactation consultants who closely monitor the infant's intake of milk and growth.

Monilial Infections. Nipple soreness that is not resolved by the previously mentioned methods may be due to a **monilial** (yeast) **infection.** Sore nipples that occur after the newborn period are often due to a yeast infection.

The mother usually reports sudden onset of severe nipple pain and tenderness, burning or stinging, and may have sharp, shooting, burning pains into the breasts during and after feedings. The nipples appear somewhat pink and shiny or may be scaly or flaky; there may be a visible rash, small blisters, or thrush. Most often, the pain is out of proportion to the appearance of the nipple. Yeast infections of the nipples and breast can be excruciatingly painful and can lead to early cessation of breastfeeding if not recognized and treated promptly.

Babies may or may not exhibit symptoms of monilial infection. Oral thrush and a red, raised diaper rash are common indications of a yeast infection. An affected infant is often very fussy and gassy. When feeding, the baby is likely to pull off the breast soon after starting to feed, crying with apparent pain. The infant may be biting or gumming at the breast.

The most common predisposing factors for yeast infection of the breast include previous antibiotic use, vaginal yeast infections, and nipple damage.

Mothers and babies must be treated simultaneously, even if the infant has no visible signs of infection. Treatment for mother is typically an antifungal cream applied to the nipples after feedings. Most pediatricians prescribe an oral antifungal medication, such as Nystatin, for infants. Treatment of mother and baby should continue for at least 7 days after symptoms begin to improve. Careful handwashing is essential to prevent the spread of yeast. Family members may have symptoms of yeast infections and should receive appropriate treatment. Jock itch and finger or toenail fungus are types of yeast infections. Other children in the family may have diaper rash due to yeast (Hoover, 2001).

Plugged Milk Ducts. A milk duct may become plugged or clogged, causing a red, tender area or small lump in the breast, which may or may not be tender. This area typically does not empty or soften with feeding or pumping. A small white blister or "pearl" may be seen on the tip of the nipple; this is the curd of milk blocking the flow. The mother is afebrile and has no generalized symptoms.

Plugged ducts are most often the result of inadequate emptying of the breast. This may be due to poor breastfeeding, delayed or missed feedings, always using the same position for feeding, clothing that is too tight, or poorly fitting or underwire bra.

Application of warm compresses to the affected area and to the nipple before feeding helps promote emptying of the breast and release of the plug. (A disposable diaper filled with warm water makes an easy compress.) Soaking in a warm bath before feeding may be helpful. If there is a small white "pearl" or blister on the tip of the nipple, it can be opened with a sterile needle, and the thick white substance can be expressed.

Frequent feeding is recommended, with the baby beginning the feeding on the affected side to foster more complete emptying. The mother is advised to massage the affected area while the baby nurses or while she is pumping. Varying feeding positions and feeding without wearing a bra may be useful in resolving a plugged duct. Positioning the baby with the chin pointing toward the affected area of the breast may be helpful.

If the mother develops fever or flulike symptoms, she may have mastitis and should notify her health care provider. Plugged milk ducts do not necessarily cause mastitis, but milk stasis may increase the susceptibility to a breast infection. For women with recurrent plugged milk ducts, taking oral lecithin capsules may be helpful (Newman, 1998).

Mastitis. A breast infection, or **mastitis,** is characterized by the sudden onset of flulike symptoms such as fever, chills, body aches, and headache. (Flulike symptoms in a breastfeeding mother should be considered indicative of mastitis, until proven otherwise.) Localized breast pain and tenderness usually is accompanied by a warm, reddened area on the breast, often resembling the shape of a pie wedge. Mastitis most commonly occurs in the upper outer quadrant of the breast; it may affect one or both breasts.

Certain factors may predispose a woman to mastitis. Inadequate emptying of the breasts is common, related to engorgement, plugged ducts, a sudden decrease in the number of feedings, abrupt weaning, or wearing underwire bras. Sore, cracked nipples may lead to mastitis by providing a portal of entry for causative organisms (*Staphylococcus, Streptococcus,* and *Escherichia coli* are most common) (Osterman & Rahm, 2000). Stress and fatigue, ill family members, breast trauma, and poor maternal nutrition also are predisposing factors for mastitis (Fetherston, 1998).

Breastfeeding mothers should be taught the signs of mastitis before they are discharged from the hospital after birth, and they need to know to call the health care provider promptly if the symptoms occur. Treatment includes antibiotics such as cephalexin or dicloxacillin, and analgesics/antipyretic medications such as ibuprofen. The mother is advised to rest as much as possible, and she should feed the baby or pump frequently, striving to empty the affected side adequately. Warm compresses to the breast before feeding or pumping may be useful. Adequate fluid intake and a balanced diet are important for the mother with mastitis.

Complications of mastitis include breast abscess, chronic mastitis, or fungal infections of the breast. Most complications can be prevented by early recognition and treatment.

Role of the Nurse in Promoting Successful Lactation

Providing a birth environment in which breastfeeding is initiated and supported is an important nursing responsibility. "Baby Friendly" status for a hospital is one means to promote a family-centered approach that facilitates breastfeeding. The Baby Friendly Hospital Initiative, sponsored by the World Health Organization and UNICEF, was founded to encourage institutions to offer optimal levels of care for lactating mothers. When a hospital achieves the "Ten Steps to Successful Breastfeeding for Hospitals," it is recognized as a Baby Friendly Hospital. The steps included the following: having a written breastfeeding policy, training staff, informing pregnant women about the benefits of breastfeeding, initiating breastfeeding within an hour of birth, helping mothers maintain lactation even when separated from their infants, giving newborns only breast milk to drink, rooming-in 24 hours a day, breastfeeding on demand, avoiding pacifiers, and promoting the establishment of breastfeeding support groups and referring mothers to them. Within such an environment, the *Healthy People 2010* and AAP goals for breastfeeding are more likely to be met (Hill, 2000).

Nurses working in a variety of perinatal settings can play a major role in breastfeeding education and support for new parents. In prenatal settings, nurses are often the first to inquire about the mother's plans regarding infant feeding. Nurses can educate the mother and her partner about the advantages of breastfeeding and explore reasons that they may prefer formula feeding. Current reading materials and information about prenatal classes are made available to expectant parents. At each encounter, the nurse offers to answer questions and provide additional information as needed. Assessment of the mother's breasts and nipples during pregnancy is important. The nurse should inquire about breast changes during pregnancy, such as enlargement of the breasts. Flat or inverted nipples are identified, and the mother is offered breast shells (see Fig. 27-13) to wear during the last month of pregnancy to encourage eversion of the nipples.

Prenatal education of the mother who plans to breastfeed includes information about nipple preparation. No special nipple preparation is necessary. The mother is advised to avoid using soap directly on her nipples. In previous years, women were told to pull on nipples and to rub them with a towel to "toughen" nipples for breastfeeding; women should be cautioned against these practices. The stimulation associated with pulling on nipples can prompt the release of oxytocin and result in preterm labor. Rubbing nipples with a towel can damage the outer layer of protective skin cells, which may increase the risk of sore nipples.

Through interviewing the pregnant woman and assessing the breasts, the nurse should determine if there have been any previous breast surgeries. Breast reduction or augmentation may interfere with the ability to produce milk and transfer it successfully to the baby. Interruption of milk ducts and the blood and nerve supply associated with various surgical techniques can affect the woman's ability to breastfeed. It is important to discuss concerns about previous breast surgery with the woman and to stress the need to monitor the breastfeeding baby carefully for signs of adequate intake.

In the immediate postpartum period, the nurse is instrumental in helping the mother initiate breastfeeding as soon as possible after birth. Encouraging parents to keep the baby in the mother's room (rooming in) allows the mother to learn to recognize feeding cues and to feed the baby when these cues are present. The nurse provides help with positioning and latch-on until the mother can do so independently. Explanations are given early on regarding frequency and duration of feedings, how to wake a sleepy baby, and how to determine if the baby is getting enough milk. Before discharge, the nurse verifies that the parents are knowledgeable about breastfeeding and are prepared for what to expect in the days ahead. For example, information about the transition to mature milk (milk coming in) and how to prevent engorgement is needed. The mother also is informed about prevention and treatment of sore nipples and about signs of mastitis.

Parents often expect that because breastfeeding is "natural," it comes naturally for both mother and baby. This misconception should be clarified early so that parents may view breastfeeding as a learning process. Then they are able to give themselves and their baby permission to learn, without unrealistic expectations. Nurses, physicians, and other health care providers who are knowledgeable about breastfeeding can offer needed support and encouragement to parents, helping to instill a sense of confidence.

Nurses often work in collaboration with lactation consultants in hospitals, physician offices, or community settings. Although the vast majority are registered nurses, lactation consultants come from a variety of backgrounds such as nutrition, physical or occupational therapy, home economics, psychology, social work, education, or the basic sciences. **Lactation consultants** have had specialized education, training, and clinical experience related to breastfeeding. Most lactation consultants are certified by the International Board of Lactation Consultant Examiners, having met specific criteria for academic and clinical experience and having passed the certifying examination. The professional organization for lactation consultants is the International Lactation Consultant Association (ILCA) and is open to anyone interested in breastfeeding. The organization publishes the *Journal of Human Lactation,* which includes research and clinical articles related to breastfeeding.

Follow-Up After Hospital Discharge. Problems with sore nipples, engorgement, and jaundice are likely to occur after discharge. It is the role of the nurse to educate and prepare the mother for problems she may encounter once she is home. Objective data should be used to assess breastfeeding; tools are available for this purpose (Johnson, Brennan, & Flynn-Tymkow, 1999). It is critical that the mother be given a list of resources for help with breastfeeding concerns and that she realize when to call for assistance. Community resources for breastfeeding mothers include lactation consultants in hospitals, physician offices, or in private practice; nurses in pediatric or obstetric offices; support groups such as La Leche League; and peer counseling programs (e.g., those offered through WIC) (see Resources at end of chapter.)

Telephone follow-up by hospital, birth center, or office nurses within the first day or two after discharge can provide a means to identify any problems and offer needed advice and support. The AAP recommends that infants discharged before age 48 hours be seen by a health care provider within 48 hours and have an office visit within 7 days after discharge. In some settings and circumstances, home care follow-up is available for mothers after hospital discharge. The readmission rate of infants who are breastfeeding is lower for those who receive a home visit than for those who do not (Johnson et al., 1999).

Evaluation

Evaluation is based on the expected outcomes, and the plan of care is revised as needed based on the evaluation (see Plan of Care).

FORMULA FEEDING

Infant formula is the means of nutrition that some parents choose for their babies. Formula also may be used to supplement breastfeeding if the mother's milk supply may be inadequate, or it may be fed to the baby when the mother will be away and wishes to leave a bottle of formula instead of expressed breast milk. Infant who are bottle fed gain more weight than breastfed babies in the first 3 to 6 months of life, but the differences do not last into the second year of life (Butte, Wong, Hopkinson, Smith, & Ellis, 2000).

Parent Education

Inexperienced mothers and fathers who are formula feeding their infants usually need teaching, counseling, and support. They may need assistance with the feeding process and with any problems they may have. Some parents who are formula feeding express concern that the baby will suffer as a result of their decision. Emphasis on the beneficial use of feeding times for close contact and socializing with the infant can help relieve some of this concern.

Plan of Care: Breastfeeding and Infant Nutrition

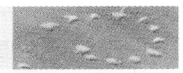

NURSING DIAGNOSIS Ineffective breastfeeding related to knowledge deficit of mother as evidenced by ongoing incorrect latch-on technique

Expected Outcomes *Mother will demonstrate correct latch-on technique. Infant will latch on and suck with gliding jaw movements and audible swallowing. Mother will report no nipple pain with infant suckling. Mother will express increased satisfaction with breastfeeding, and neonate will exhibit satisfaction of hunger and sucking needs.*

Nursing Interventions/*Rationales*

Assess mother's knowledge and motivation for breastfeeding *to acknowledge client's desire for effective outcome and provide starting point for teaching.*

Observe a breastfeeding session *to provide database for positive reinforcement and problem identification.*

Describe and demonstrate ways to stimulate the sucking reflex, various positions for breastfeeding, and the use of pillows during a session *to promote client and neonatal comfort and effective latch-on.*

Monitor neonatal position of mouth on areola and position of head and body *to give positive reinforcement for correct latch-on position or to correct poor latch-on position.*

Teach client ways to stimulate neonate to maintain an awake state by diapering, unwrapping, massaging, or burping *to complete a breastfeeding thoroughly and satisfactorily.*

Give client information regarding lactation diet, expression of milk by hand or pump, and storage of expressed breast milk *to provide basic information.*

Make sure client has written information on all aspects of breastfeeding *to reinforce verbal instructions and demonstrations.*

Refer to support groups and lactation consultant if needed *to provide further information and group support.*

NURSING DIAGNOSIS Ineffective infant feeding pattern related to inability to coordinate sucking and swallowing

Expected Outcome *Neonate will coordinate sucking and swallowing in order to accomplish an effective feeding pattern.*

Nursing Interventions/*Rationales*

Assess for factors that may contribute to ineffective sucking and swallowing *to provide a basis for plan of care.*

Teach mother to observe feeding readiness cues *to enhance effective feeding.*

Modify feeding methods as needed *to maintain hydration status and nutritional requirements.*

Promote a calm, relaxed atmosphere *to provide a pleasant breastfeeding experience for woman and neonate.*

Refer to lactation consultant *to provide specialized support.*

NURSING DIAGNOSIS Anxiety related to ineffective infant feeding pattern

Expected Outcome *Woman will report a decrease in anxiety level.*

Nursing Interventions/*Rationales*

Monitor anxiety level during feeding sessions *to provide a basis for care planning.*

Provide positive reinforcement for feeding pattern improvement *to decrease anxiety.*

Monitor weight, intake, and output *to provide information regarding effective feeding.*

Enlist assistance of support persons *to provide positive feedback for increasing skill.*

Provide information for lactation support *to decrease anxiety after discharge.*

Readiness for Feeding

The first feeding of formula is ideally given after the initial transition to extrauterine life is made. Feeding-readiness cues include such things as stability of vital signs, presence of bowel sounds, an active sucking reflex, and those described earlier for breastfed infants. The type of formula is usually determined by the pediatrician. Parents are advised to avoid switching formulas unless instructed to do so by the physician.

Before the first formula feeding, some institutions have the policy of offering sips of water to the newborn to assess patency of the GI tract and absence of tracheoesophageal fistula. If the infant sucks and swallows the water without difficulty, formula is then offered.

Feeding Patterns

Typically, a newborn will drink 15 to 30 ml of formula per feeding during the first 24 hours, with the intake gradually increasing during the first week of life. The newborn infant should be fed at least every 3 to 4 hours, even if that requires waking the baby for the feedings. The infant showing an adequate weight gain can be allowed to sleep at night and fed only on awakening. Most newborns need six to eight feedings in 24 hours, and the number of feedings decreases as the infant matures. Usually by 3 to 4 weeks after birth, a fairly predictable feeding pattern has developed. Scheduling feedings arbitrarily at predetermined intervals may not meet a baby's needs, but initiating feedings at convenient times often moves the baby's feedings to times that work for the family.

Mothers will usually notice increases in the infant's appetite at 7 to 10 days, 3 weeks, 6 weeks, 3 months, and 6 months. These appetite spurts correspond to growth spurts. The amount of formula per feeding should be increased by about 30 ml to meet the baby's needs at these times.

Feeding Technique

Parents who choose formula feeding often need education regarding feeding techniques. During feedings they should be encouraged to sit comfortably, holding the infant closely in a semiupright position. Feedings provide opportunities to bond with the baby through touching, talking, singing, or reading to the infant. Parents should consider feedings as a time of peaceful relaxation with the baby (Fig. 27-14).

A bottle should never be propped with a pillow or other inanimate object and left with the infant. This practice may result in choking, and it deprives the infant of important interaction during feeding. Moreover, propping the bottle has been implicated in causing nursing bottle caries, or decay of the first teeth resulting from continuous bathing of the teeth with carbohydrate-containing fluid as the infant sporadically sucks the nipple.

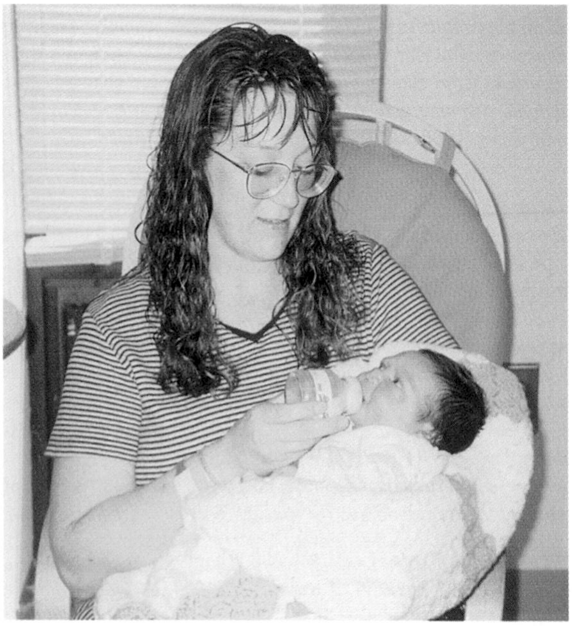

FIG. 27-14 Mother bottle feeding her 1-day-old infant.

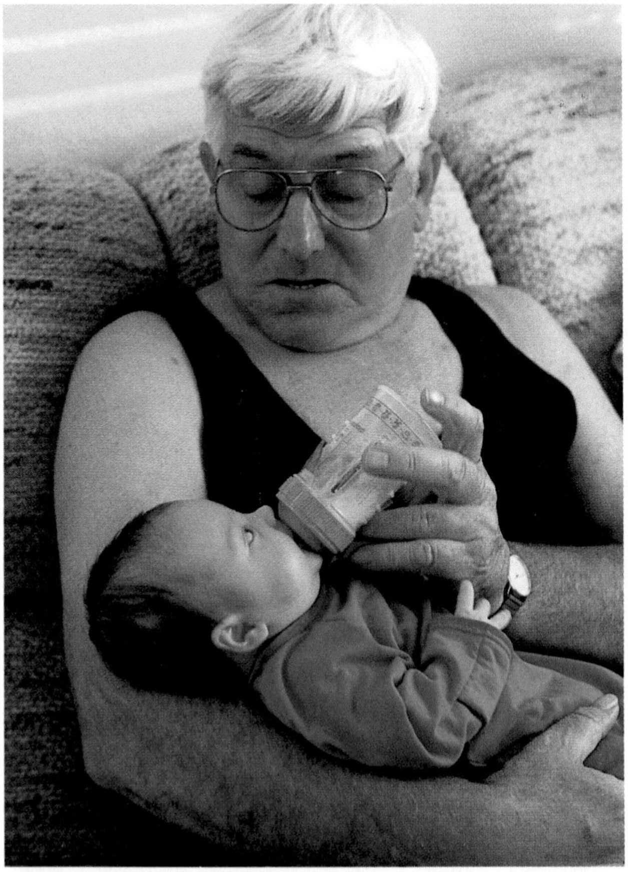

FIG. 27-15 Grandfather feeding infant granddaughter. Note angle of bottle that ensures that milk covers nipple area. (Courtesy Kim Molloy, Knoxville, IA.)

The bottle should be held so that fluid fills the nipple and none of the air in the bottle is allowed to enter the nipple (Fig. 27-15). When the infant falls asleep, turns aside the head, or ceases to suck, it is usually an indication that enough formula has been taken to satisfy the baby. Parents should be taught to look for these cues and avoid overfeeding, which can contribute to obesity.

Most infants swallow air when fed from a bottle and should be given a chance to burp several times during a feeding (Fig. 27-16) (see Guidelines/Guías box).

Bottles and Nipples

Various brands and styles of bottles and nipples are available to parents. Most babies will feed well with any bottle and nipple. It is important that the bottles and nipples be washed in warm soapy water, using a bottle and nipple brush to facilitate thorough cleansing. Careful rinsing is necessary. Boiling of bottles and nipples is not needed unless there is some question about the safety of the water supply.

GUIDELINES/GUÍAS

Burping

Position #1 (Fig. 27-16, *B*)
Posición #1

Hold your baby up, head on your shoulder.
Ponga su bebé con la cabeza muy alta sobre su hombro.

Put one arm under the baby's bottom.
Ponga un brazo debajo de las nalgas del bebé.

With the other hand, pat or rub the baby's back.
Con la otra mano, dé leves palmaditas o sobe la espalda del bebé.

Position #2 (Fig. 27-16, *A*)
Posición #2

Sit your baby up in your lap.
Siente al bebé sobre su regazo.

Hold the head and back with one hand.
Con una mano, sostenga la cabeza y la espalda del bebé.

Hold the chin and front with the other.
Con la otra mano, sostenga la barbilla y la parte delantera del bebé.

Rock the baby's upper body back and forth.
Mueva la parte superior del bebé hacia adelante y hacia atrás.

Or pat the baby's back.
O dé suaves palmaditas a la espalda del bebé.

Position #3 (Fig. 27-16, *C*)
Posición #3

Lay your baby face down on your lap.
Coloque al bebé boca abajo sobre su regazo.

Hold the baby's head with one hand.
Con una mano, sostenga la cabeza del bebé.

Rub or pat the baby's back.
Sobe o dé suaves palmaditas a la espalda del bebé.

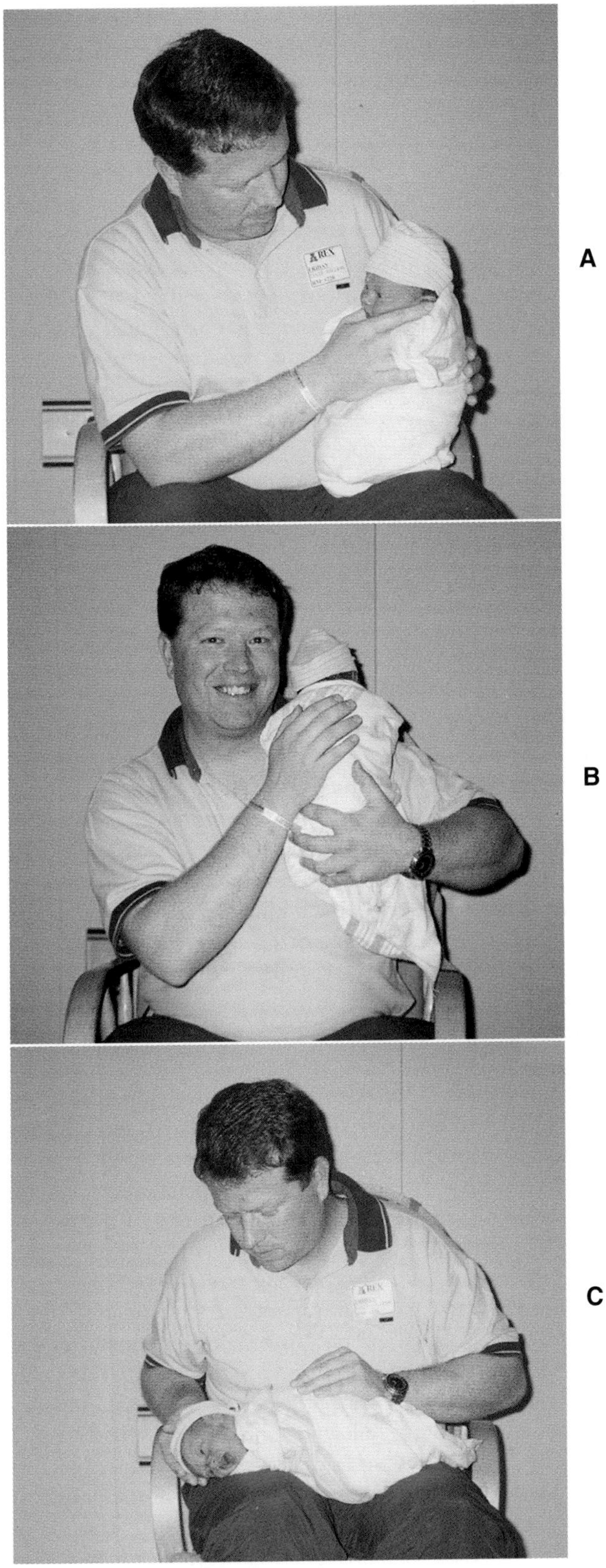
A
B
C

FIG. 27-16 Positions for burping an infant. **A,** Sitting. **B,** On the shoulder. **C,** Across the lap.

Infant Formulas

Commercial Formulas. Because human milk is species specific to meet the needs of the human infant, it is used as the standard for all infant formulas. Commercial infant formulas are designed to resemble human milk as closely as possible, although none has ever duplicated it.

Infants who are not breastfed should be given commercial formulas. If this is too expensive, the family would likely be eligible for services through the WIC program, which provides iron-fortified commercial infant formula. Cow's milk is the basis for most infant formulas, although soy-based and other specialized formulas are available for the infant who cannot tolerate cow's milk.

Commercial formulas are available in three forms: powder, concentrate, and ready-to-feed. All are equivalent in terms of nutritional content, but they vary considerably in cost:

- Powdered formula is the least expensive type. It is easily mixed by using one scoop for every 60 ml of water.
- Concentrated formula is more expensive than powder. It is diluted with equal parts of water and can be stored in the refrigerator for 48 hours after opening.
- Ready-to-feed formula is the most expensive but easiest to use. The desired amount is poured into the bottle. The opened can is safely refrigerated for 48 hours. This type of formula can be purchased in individual disposable bottles for the most convenient feeding.

Special Formulas. Some infants have an allergic reaction to cow's-milk formula. They may have diarrhea, rash, colic, or vomiting, and, in extreme cases, failure to thrive. Some of these infants may better tolerate a soy-milk formula; however, some may be allergic to soy protein. If hypersensitivity to cow's-milk protein is suspected, a hydrolyzed casein formula may be recommended; however, special formulas are very expensive. Some women may be able to begin breastfeeding or, in life-threatening cases, obtain human milk through a milk bank, at least temporarily.

Evaporated Milk. Although evaporated milk is concentrated and less expensive than commercial formula, the mixing of evaporated milk and water to feed a baby is no longer recommended because evaporated milk does not provide adequate nutrition for an infant.

Unmodified Cow's Milk. Unmodified cow's milk is not suited to the nutritional needs of the human infant in the first year of life. Specific concerns include the excessive amounts of calcium, phosphorus, and other minerals it contains; an imbalance of calcium and phosphorus; its excessive protein content; the poor absorption of the fat it contains; and its low iron concentration. In addition, its use in infants is apt to cause microscopic hemorrhages that lead to GI blood loss. This blood loss, as well as the low levels of iron in the milk, increases the likelihood of iron-deficiency anemia.

Formula Preparation

The commercial infant formula must include directions for preparation and use with pictures and symbols for the benefit of persons who cannot read. Some manufacturers are translating the directions into various languages, such as Spanish, French, Vietnamese, Chinese, and Arabic to prevent misunderstanding and errors in formula preparation.

NURSE ALERT

It is important to impress on families that the proportions must not be altered—neither diluted to expand the amount of formula nor concentrated to provide more calories.

Although manufacturers of commercial formula include directions for preparing their products, the nurse should review formula preparation with the parents. It is especially important that formula be mixed properly. The newborn's kidneys are immature, and giving the infant overly concentrated formula may provide protein and minerals in amounts that exceed the kidney's excretory ability. In contrast, if the formula is diluted too much (sometimes done in an effort to save money), the infant does not consume enough calories and does not grow well.

Sterilization of formula rarely is recommended for those families with access to a safe public water supply. Instead, the formula is prepared with attention to cleanliness. When water from a private well is used, parents should be advised to contact the health department to have a chemical and bacteriologic analysis of the water done before using the water in formula preparation. The presence of nitrates, excess fluoride, or bacteria may be harmful to the infant.

If the sanitary conditions in the home appear unsafe, it would be better to recommend the use of ready-to-feed formula or to teach the mother to sterilize the formula. The two traditional methods for sterilization are terminal heating and the aseptic method. In the terminal-heating method, the prepared formula is placed in the bottles, which are topped with the nipples placed upside down and covered with the caps, and then sealed loosely with the rings. The bottles are then boiled together in a water bath for 25 minutes. In the aseptic method, the bottles, rings, caps, nipples, and any other necessary equipment, such as a funnel, are boiled separately, after which the formula is poured into the bottles. Any formula left in the bottle after the feeding should be discarded because the baby's saliva has mixed with it. (Instructions for formula preparation and feeding are provided in the Teaching for Self-Care box.)

Vitamin and Mineral Supplementation

Commercial iron-fortified formula has all of the nutrients the infant needs for the first 6 months of life. After 6 months, the only mineral supplementation required is 0.25 mg of fluoride daily if the local water supply is not fluoridated (AAP, 1997).

Weaning

The bottle-fed infant will gradually learn to use a cup, and the parents will find that they are preparing fewer bottles. Often the bottle feeding before bedtime is the last one to

TEACHING FOR SELF-CARE

Formula Preparation and Feeding

FORMULA PREPARATION

- Wash your hands and clean the bottle, nipple, and can opener carefully before preparing formula.
- If new nipples seem too hard, they can be softened by boiling them in water for 5 minutes before use.
- Read the label on the container of formula and mix it exactly according to the directions.
- Use tap water to mix concentrated or powdered formula unless directed otherwise by your baby's physician or nurse.
- Test the size of the nipple hole by holding a prepared bottle upside down. The formula should drip from the nipple. If it runs in a stream, the hole is too big and should not be used. If it has to be shaken for the formula to come out, the hole is too small. You can either buy a new nipple or enlarge the hole by boiling the nipple for 5 minutes with a sewing needle inserted in the hole.
- If a nipple collapses when your baby sucks, loosen the nipple ring a little to let in air.
- Opened cans of ready-to-feed or concentrated formula should be covered and refrigerated. Any unused portions must be discarded after 48 hours.
- Bottles or cans of unopened formula can be stored at room temperature.
- If the formula is refrigerated, warm it by placing the bottle in a pan of hot water. Never use a microwave to warm any food to be given to a baby. Test the temperature of the formula by letting a few drops fall on the inside of your wrist. If the formula feels comfortably warm to you, it is the correct temperature.

FEEDING TECHNIQUES AND TIPS

- Newborns should be fed at least every 3 to 4 hours and should never go longer than 4 hours without feeding until a satisfactory pattern of weight gain is established. This may take 2 weeks. If a baby cries or fusses between feedings, check to see if the diaper should be changed, and if the baby needs to be picked up and cuddled. If the baby continues to cry and acts hungry, go ahead and feed. Babies do not get hungry on a regular schedule.
- Babies gradually increase the amount of milk they drink with each feeding. The first day or so, most newborns consume 15 to 30 ml (one-half to 1 ounce) with each feeding. This amount increases as the infant grows. If any formula remains in the bottle as the feeding ends, that milk must be thrown away, because saliva from the baby's mouth can cause the formula to spoil.
- It is a good idea to keep a feeding diary, writing down the amount of formula the baby drinks with each feeding for the first week or so. Also record the wet diapers and bowel movements the baby is having. Take this "diary" with you when you take the baby for the first pediatrician visit.
- For feeding, hold the baby close in a semireclining position. Talk to the baby during the feeding. This is a great time for social interaction and cuddling.
- Place the nipple in the baby's mouth on the tongue. It should touch the roof of the mouth to stimulate the baby's sucking reflex. Hold the bottle like a pencil. Keep the bottle tipped so that the nipple stays filled with milk and the baby does not suck in air.
- It is normal for babies to take a few sucks and then pause briefly before continuing to suck again. Some newborns take longer to feed than others. Be patient. It may be necessary to keep the baby awake and to encourage sucking. Moving the nipple gently in the baby's mouth may stimulate sucking.
- Newborns are apt to swallow air when sucking. Give the baby opportunities to burp several times during a feeding. As the baby gets older, you will know better when it is necessary to stop for burping.
- After the first 2 or 3 days, the stools of a formula-fed infant are yellow and soft, but formed. The baby may have a stool with each feeding in the first 2 weeks, although this may decrease to one or two stools each day.

SAFETY TIPS

- Babies should be held and never left alone while feeding. Never prop the bottle. The baby might inhale formula or choke on any that was spit up. Babies who fall asleep with a propped bottle of milk or juice may be prone to cavities when the first teeth come in.
- Know how to use the bulb syringe and how to help a baby who is choking.

remain. Babies have a strong need to suck, and the baby who has the bottle taken away too early or abruptly will compensate with nonnutritive sucking on his or her fingers, thumb, a pacifier, or even his or her own tongue. Weaning from a bottle should therefore be done gradually because the baby has learned to rely on the comfort that sucking provides.

Introducing Solid Foods

The infant receives the right balance of nutrients from breast milk or formula during the first 4 to 6 months. It is not true that the feeding of solids will help the infant sleep through the night. Introduction of solid foods before the infant is 4 to 6 months of age may result in overfeeding and decreased intake of breast milk or formula. The infant cannot communicate feeling full as can an older child, who is able to turn the head away. The proper balance of carbohydrate, protein, and fat for an infant to grow properly is in the breast milk or formula.

The infant's individual growth pattern should help determine the right time to start solids. The primary health care provider will advise when to introduce solid foods. The schedule for introducing solid foods and the types of foods to serve will be discussed during well-baby supervision visits with the pediatrician or pediatric nurse practitioner.

KEY POINTS

- Human breast milk is species specific and is the recommended form of nutrition for infants. It provides immunologic protection against many infections and diseases.
- Breast milk changes in composition with each stage of lactation, during each feeding, and as the infant grows.
- During the prenatal period, parents should be informed of the benefits of breastfeeding for infants, mothers, families, and society.
- Infants should be breastfed as soon as possible after birth and at least 8 to 12 times per day thereafter.
- Specific, measurable indicators show that the infant is breastfeeding effectively.
- Breast milk production is based on a supply-meets-demand principle: the more the infant nurses, the greater the milk supply.
- Commercial infant formulas provide satisfactory nutrition for most infants.
- All infants should be held for feedings.
- Parents should be instructed about the types of commercial infant formulas, proper preparation for feeding, and correct feeding technique.
- Unmodified cow's milk is inappropriate for infants during the first year of life.
- Solid foods should be started after age 6 months.
- Nurses must be knowledgeable about feeding methods and provide education and support for families.

CRITICAL THINKING EXERCISES

1. Mary was discharged from the birthing center at 48 hours postpartum with her newborn son, Matthew. He is now 4 days old, and she has brought him to the clinic for a follow-up visit. She states that her milk came in yesterday, and her breasts have been hard and painful. It has been difficult to latch the baby on. She reports that breastfeeding is very painful and that her nipples are so sore she "can hardly stand to feed the baby." Matthew has had only one wet diaper and one bowel movement in the last 24 hours. Describe what assessments the nurse should make, and devise a teaching plan for Mary and Matthew.
2. Tynaya is a 22-year-old African-American mother who delivered a 9 pound baby girl 2 hours ago. She has decided to breastfeed her newborn baby girl and attempted the first feeding right after the baby was born. The baby latched on and sucked vigorously for 15 minutes. Tynaya did not attend any prenatal breastfeeding classes, but has read a little about breastfeeding. Her mother is telling her she needs to give the baby a bottle after she nurses so they can be sure she is getting enough to eat. Discuss the plan of care for Tynaya and her daughter. (Be sure to include Tynaya's mother.) What type of education is needed? How can Tynaya determine if her baby is getting enough to eat?
3. Su Lin is an Asian-American who gave birth to a 7-pound baby boy yesterday. She says she wants to breastfeed, but you notice on the baby's chart that he has had bottles all during the night. When you ask Su about this, she says she has "no milk." Discuss appropriate assessment, intervention, and education for Su.

RESOURCES

American Academy of Pediatrics
141 Northwest Point Blvd.
Elk Grove, IL 60007-1098
800-422-4784
www.aap.org

Breastfeeding resources
www.parentsplace.com/expert/lactation/

Bright Future Lactation Resource Centre
www.bflrc.com

Dr. Thomas Hale (medications and breastfeeding)
neonatal.ttuhsc.edu/lact/

International Lactation Consultant Association
4101 Lake Boone Trail, Suite 201
Raleigh, NC 27607
919-787-5181
919-787-4916 (fax)
users.erols.com/ilca

Journal of Human Lactation
Sage Publications
2455 Teller Road
Thousand Oaks, CA 91320
805-499-9774
805-375-1700
www.sagepub.com

Lact-Aid *(provides information and services to promote breastfeeding)*
P.O. Box 1066
Athens, TN 37303
614-744-9090

RESOURCES—cont'd

Lactation Education Resources
www.leron-line.com

La Leche League
1400 N. Meacham Rd.
Schaumburg, IL 60168-4079
800-525-3243 (24-hour line)
www.lalecheleague.org

MOTHERS' MILK BANKS

Lactation Support Service
Children's and Women's Milk Bank
British Columbia Children's Hospital
Vancouver, British Columbia, Canada V6H 3V4
604-875-2345, ext. 7607

Mothers' Milk Bank
Presbyterian/St. Luke's Medical Center
Denver, CO 80218
303-869-1888

Mothers' Milk Bank
Valley Medical Center
San Jose, CA 95128
408-998-4550

Mothers' Milk Bank
WakeMed
3000 New Bern Avenue
Raleigh, NC 27610
919-350-8599
919-350-8923 (fax)

Nursing Mothers Advisory Council
www.nursingmoms.net
E-mail: nmac@phillyburbs.com

The Breastfeeding and Human Lactation Study Center
University of Rochester School of Medicine and Dentistry
Department of Pediatrics, Box 777
601 Elmwood Avenue
Rochester, NY 14642
716-275-0088
716-461-3614 (fax)

Special Care Nursery Mothers' Milk Bank
Christiana Care Health Services
4755 Ogletown Stanton Rd.
P.O. Box 6001
Newark, DE 19718
302-733-2340

Special Supplemental Nutrition Program for Women, Infants, and Children (WIC)
Food and Consumer Service
3103 Park Center Dr., Room 819
703-305-2286

REFERENCES

Aarts, C. et al. (1999). Breastfeeding patterns in relation to thumb sucking and pacifier use. *Pediatrics, 104*(4), e50.

Abbott Laboratories. (2001). *Mother's survey.* Ross Products Division.

American Academy of Pediatrics (AAP). (1998). *Pediatric nutrition handbook* (4th ed.). Elk Grove Village, IL: American Academy of Pediatrics.

American Academy of Pediatrics Committee on Drugs. (2001). The transfer of drugs and other chemicals into human milk. *Pediatrics, 108*(3), 776-789.

American Academy of Pediatrics Work Group on Breastfeeding. (1997). Breastfeeding and the use of human milk. *Pediatrics, 100*(6), 1035-1039.

Anderson, J., Johnstone, B., & Remley, D. (1999). Breastfeeding and cognitive development: A meta-analysis. *American Journal of Clinical Nutrition, 70*, 525-535.

Arlotti, J. et al. (1998). Breastfeeding among low-income women with and without peer support. *Journal of Community Health Nursing, 15*(3), 163-178.

Association of Women's Health, Obstetric, and Neonatal Nurses (AWHONN). (1998). *Standards and guidelines for professional nursing practice in the care of women and newborns* (5th ed.). Washington, DC: The Association.

Barnard, J. (1997). Gastrointestinal disorders due to cow's milk consumption. *Pediatric Annals, 26*(4), 244-250.

Biancuzzo, M. (1999). Selecting pumps for breastfeeding mothers. *Journal of Obstetric, Gynecologic, and Neonatal Nursing, 28*(4), 417-426.

Brent, N. et al. (1998). Sore nipples in breastfeeding women: A clinical trial of wound dressings vs. conventional care. *Archives of Pediatric and Adolescent Medicine, 152*(11), 1077-1082.

Bulkow, L. et al. (2002). Risk factors for severe respiratory syncytial virus infection among Alaska native children. *Pediatrics, 109*(2), 210-216.

Butte, N. et al. (2000). Infant feeding mode affects early growth and body composition. *Pediatrics, 106*(6), 1355-1366.

Char-Yeung, M. et al. (2000). A randomized control study of the effectiveness of a multifaceted intervention program in the primary prevention of asthma in high risk infants. *Archives of Pediatric and Adolescent Medicine, 154*(7), 657-663.

Cushing, A. et al. (1998). Breastfeeding reduces risk of respiratory illness in infants. *American Journal of Epidemiology, 147*(9), 863-870.

Davis, M. (1998). Review of the evidence for an association between infant feeding and childhood cancer. *International Journal of Cancer Supplement 11*, 29-33.

Dell, S., & To, T. (2001). Breastfeeding and asthma in young children: Findings from a population-based study. *Archives of Pediatric and Adolescent Medicine, 155*(11), 1261-1265.

Department of Health and Human Services. (2000). *Healthy People 2010: Conference edition: Vol. 2 Objectives for improving health.* Washington, DC: Department of Health and Human Services. Available at www.health.gov/healthypeople/document/default.htm.

Earle, S. (2000). Why some women do not breast feed: Bottle feeding and fathers' role. *Midwifery, 16*(4), 323-330.

Eisman, J. (1998). Relevance of pregnancy and lactation to osteoporosis. *Clinical Perinatology, 25*(2), 303-326.

Enger, S. et al. (1998). Breastfeeding experience and breast cancer risk among postmenopausal women. *Cancer Epidemiology, Biomarkers, and Prevention, 7*(5), 365-369.

Fetherston, C. (1998). Risk factors for lactational mastitis. *Journal of Human Lactation, 14*(2), 101-109.

Fisher, J. et al. (2000). Breastfeeding through the first year predicts maternal control in feeding and subsequent toddler energy intake. *Journal of the American Dietetic Association, 100*, 641-646.

Forste, R., Weiss, J., & Lippincott, A. (2001). The decision to breastfeed in the United States: Does race matter? *Pediatrics, 108*, 291-296.

Gdalevich, M. et al. (2001). Breastfeeding and the onset of atopic dermatitis in childhood: A systematic review and meta-analysis of prospective studies. *Journal of the American Academy of Dermatology, 45*(4), 520-527.

Gianino, P. et al. (2002). Incidence of nosocomial rotavirus infections, symptomatic and asymptomatic, in breastfed and nonbreastfed infants. *Journal of Hospital Infection, 50*(1), 13-17.

Hill, P. (2000). Update on breastfeeding: *Healthy People* objectives. *MCN American Journal of Maternal Child Nursing, 25*, 248-251.

Hoover, K. (2001). Yeast infections of the nipples and breasts. *Medela Messenger, 18*(3), 11-12.

Horwood, L., & Fergusson, D. (1998). Breastfeeding and later cognitive and academic outcomes. *Pediatrics, 10*(1), e9.

Houghton, M. (2001). Breastfeeding practices of Native-American mothers participating in WIC. *Journal of the American Dietetic Association, 101*(2), 245-247.

Howard, C. et al. (1999). The effects of early pacifier use on breastfeeding duration. *Pediatrics, 103*(3), e33.

Hypponen, E. et al. (1999). Infant feeding, early weight gain, and risk of type I diabetes. *Diabetes Care, 22*(12), 1961-1965.

International Lactation Consultant Association. (1999). *Evidence-based guidelines for breastfeeding management during the first fourteen days.* Raleigh, NC: The Association.

Johnson, T., Brennan, R., & Flynn-Tymkow, C. (1999). A home visit program for breastfeeding education and support. *Journal of Obstetric, Gynecologic, and Neonatal Nursing, 28*(5), 480-485.

Kavanaugh, K. et al. (1997). The rewards outweigh the efforts: Breastfeeding outcomes for mothers of preterm infants. *Journal of Human Lactation, 13*(1), 15-21.

King, D. (2000). Statistics: Weight loss and lactation. *International Journal of Childbirth Education, 15*(3), 44.

Kliegman, R. (2002). Fetal and neonatal medicine. In R. Behrman & R. Kliegman (Eds.), *Nelson essentials of pediatrics.* Philadelphia: W.B. Saunders.

Kloeben-Tanwer, A. (2001). Pacifier use is associated with shorter breastfeeding duration among low-income women. *Pediatrics, 108*, 526.

Lactation Education Resources. (2001). Available at www.leron-line.com.

Lawrence, R. (1999). *Breastfeeding: A guide for the medical profession* (5th ed.). St. Louis: Mosby.

Lefeber, Y., & Voorhoeve, H. (1999). Indigenous first feeding practices in newborn babies. *Midwifery, 15*, 97-100.

Lopez-Alarcon, M., Villalpando, S., & Fajardo, A. (1997). Breastfeeding lowers the frequency and duration of acute respiratory infections and diarrhea in infants under six months of age. *Journal of Nutrition, 127*(3), 436-443.

McVea, K., Turner, P., & Peppler, D. (2000). The role of breastfeeding in sudden infant death syndrome. *Journal of Human Lactation, 16*(1), 13-20.

Meier, P. (1997). *Professional guide to breastfeeding premature infants.* Columbus, OH: Ross Products Division, Abbott Laboratories.

Messner, A. et al. (2000). Ankyloglossia: Incidence and associated feeding difficulties. *Archives of Otolaryngology: Head and Neck Surgery, 126*(1), 36-39.

Montgomery, D., & Splett, P. (1998). *The economic benefits of breastfeeding infants enrolled in the WIC program: Twelve month follow-up study.* Final report submitted to the USDA Food and Consumer Service.

Morse, J., Jehle, C., & Gamble, D. (1990). Initiating breastfeeding: A world survey of the timing of postpartum breastfeeding. *International Journal of Nursing Studies, 27*(3), 303-313.

Newman, J. (1995). How breast milk protects newborns. *Scientific American, 273*(6), 76-79.

Newman, J. (1998). *Blocked ducts and mastitis.* www.bflrc.com (accessed 5/27/2002).

Oddy, W. et al. (1999). Association between breastfeeding and asthma in 6-year-old children: Findings of a prospective birth cohort study. *British Medical Journal, 319*, 815-819.

Osterman, K., & Rahm, V. (2000). Lactation mastitis: Bacterial cultivation of breast milk, symptoms, treatment, and outcome. *Journal of Human Lactation, 16*(4), 297-302.

Page, D. (2001). Breastfeeding is early functional jaw orthopedics. *Functional Orthodontics, 18*(3), 24-27.

Palmer, B. (1998). The influence of breastfeeding on the development of the oral cavity. *Journal of Human Lactation, 14*(2), 93-98.

Ryan, A. (1997). The resurgence of breastfeeding in the United States. *Pediatrics, 99*(4), e12.

Scariati, P., Grummer-Strawn, L., & Fein, S. (1997). A longitudinal analysis of infant morbidity and the extent of breastfeeding in the United States. *Pediatrics, 99*(6), e5.

Shu, X. et al. (1999). Breastfeeding and the risk of childhood acute leukemia. *Journal of the National Cancer Institute, 91*, 1765-1772.

Terschakovic, A., & Stallings, V. (2002). Pediatric nutrition and nutritional disorders. In R. Behrman & R. Kliegman (Eds.), *Nelson essentials of pediatrics.* Philadelphia: W.B. Saunders.

Vestergaard, M. et al. (1999). Duration of breastfeeding and development milestones during the latter half of infancy. *Acta Paediatrica, 88*, 1327-1332.

VonKries, R. et al. (1999). Breastfeeding and obesity: Cross sectional study. *British Medical Journal, 319*, 147-150.

Weimer, J. (March 2001). *The economic benefits of breastfeeding: A review and analysis. Food Assistance and Nutrition Research Report No. 18.* Washington, DC: Food and Rural Economics Division, Economic Research Service, U.S. Department of Agriculture.

Weissinger, D. (1998). A breastfeeding teaching tool using a sandwich analogy for latch-on. *Journal of Human Lactation, 14*(1), 51-56.

CHAPTER 28

Shannon E. Perry

Care of the Newborn at Home

http://evolve.elsevier.com/Lowdermilk/MatWmnHlth/

LEARNING OBJECTIVES

- Review the anticipatory guidance nurses provide parents before discharge.
- Discuss nursing care management for assisting parents in the care of the infant during the first weeks at home.
- Explain continuing care of the infant who was circumcised.
- Describe infant cardiopulmonary resuscitation (CPR).
- Discuss home phototherapy and the guidelines for teaching parents about this treatment.

Mothers and infants are ordinarily discharged from the place of birth (hospital, birthing center) between 6 and 48 hours after birth. The time of discharge depends on the condition of the mother and infant, whether breastfeeding is established, preferences of the parents, and insurance coverage. This chapter addresses the care of the infant in the first 6 weeks after birth.

Before discharge, the nurse provides anticipatory guidance related to feeding, elimination, care of the circumcised infant, crying, behavior, sleeping, signs of illness, and community resources, including support groups. Many hospitals have 24-hour in-house television channels where infant care topics can be viewed. When the opportunity presents, a bath demonstration may be provided. A sample Infant Teaching/Discharge Record is in Figure 28-1. Note that the parents can check the information that is most important to them, enabling the nurse to focus her teaching.

The infant must be secured in a car seat for the trip home. Infants younger than 37 weeks of gestation should be observed in a car seat for a period before discharge. The infant is monitored for apnea, bradycardia, and a decrease in SaO_2. It may be necessary to place blanket rolls on either side of the infant for support of the head and trunk. To prevent slumping, the back-to-crotch strap distance should be 14 cm. If necessary, a rolled blanket can be placed between the infant and the crotch strap.

Although the nurse is not responsible for securing the infant in the car seat, she should query the parents about whether the car seat is present and properly installed. Hospitals often have car seat classes for parents and/or provide information about the laws in the state. Highway safety departments provide instruction in proper installation of car seats for infants. If parents do not have a car seat, the nurse should be able to provide information about resources in the hospital or community where patients may borrow or be given a car seat.

It is usually best if siblings remain at home during the trip home so that the parents can concentrate on the mother and the care and safety of the newborn. When the mother arrives home, the father can carry the baby into the house while the mother greets the siblings. Siblings need some undivided attention on this first day as well as every day. This often provides the father an opportunity to spend time with the children that he otherwise might not have.

PROTECTIVE ENVIRONMENT

The provision of a **protective environment** is basic to the care of the infant. Environmental factors include adequate lighting, elimination of potential fire hazards, safety of electrical appliances, adequate ventilation, and controlled temperature (warm and free of drafts) and humidity (lower than 50%). The bassinet or crib should be placed on an inner wall to prevent cold stress by radiation. For the first few weeks at home, the bassinet is commonly placed in the parents' bedroom so that they can easily hear the infant. As the parents become more secure, the bassinet may be moved to the infant's own room or to one shared with a sibling.

INFANT TEACHING/DISCHARGE RECORD

Our nursing staff wish to give you the information you want and need most during your stay with us. Please look over the following list of educational topics and complete the form by putting a check in the column that most applies to you, using the following scale:

IMPRINT AREA

1 = Most important to learn before I go home 2 = I would like to review 3 = I already know or am comfortable with

SELF-ASSESSMENT CHECKLIST		1	2	3	PATIENT EDUCATION Date/Time	PATIENT EDUCATION Nurse Int.
BABY CARE						
Crying as Communication	Hunger, pain from not burping or gas, need for diaper change, too warm, too cold.					
Hiccoughs and Sneezing	Normal.					
Bath Sponge/Tub	Bath as needed.					
Soaps	Mild (Dove, Neutrogena, baby care products.)					
Nail Care	Emery board.					
Cord Care	Keep dry. Fold diaper below cord. Cord falls off 1–2 weeks.					
Skin Care/Diaper Rash	Air dry, zinc oxide. Call advice if no improvement in 2 days.					
Diaper Change	Wash girls front to back.					
Genitals	Vaginal care—white or pink discharge, cheesy material, normal.					
Circumcision Care	Remove Vaseline gauze after 4° if present. Vaseline applied to diaper as needed for 24°.					
Uncircumcised Baby Care	No need to retract foreskin.					
Elimination	Meconium first, then seedy soft yellow. Urinates 6–8 times/day.					
Axillary Temperature	Normal axillary temp. 97.6° F. Call advice if over 100° F.					
Clothing	Flame retardant. Dress comfortably. Do not overdress.					
Positioning	Side or back, **NOT STOMACH**.					
Bulb Syringe/Choking	Keep within reach/use to clear nose and mouth.					
Handwashing	Viruses and bacteria easily transmitted through hands. Wash frequently.					
Environment	Smoke free, smoke detector.					
Car Seat	Calif. Vehicle Code #27365.5. Follow manufacturer's directions for installation.					
BREASTFEEDING	See Breastfeeding Information Guide.					
Latching on	Breastfeeding. Demand feed, usually every 1 1/2–3 hours around the clock. Be flexible.					
Positioning Mom/Baby	• Frequency: 8–12 times in 24 hours.					
Frequency & Lengths of	• Duration: 10–15 minutes of swallowing at each breast each feeding.					
Care of Breasts/Nipples	• Sore nipples: check latch, vary positions; air dry; shorter, more frequent nursing. • Breast engorgement: hot soaks or hot showers, hand express, frequent nursing.					
Breast Pump/Pumping Storage	• Supplements: not necessary.					
BOTTLE FEEDING	Bottle feeding. Demand feed, usually every 3–4 hours. Be sure tongue is under nipple.					
Latching on & Positioning	• Clean bottles and nipples with hot, soapy water or dishwasher. • No need to sterilize.					
Positioning	• May use tap or bottled water to mix formula.					
Frequency & Lengths of	• Refrigerate extra feeding in quantities taken per feeding. • Do not microwave formula.					
Formula Preparation	• Do not prop bottle.					

SEEK MEDICAL ADVICE FOR THE FOLLOWING:

- Redness, discharge or foul odor from circumcision or umbilical cord.
- Less than 4 wet diapers/day by 4 days old.
- Less than 6–8 wet diapers/day by 6 days old.
- Frequent, explosive, watery stools that soak through the diaper.
- Axillary temperature of less than 97.4° F or greater than 100° F.
- Poor feeding, weak suck, no interest in eating.
- Yellow coloring of skin (jaundice) or whites of eyes.
- Vomiting forcefully several times (not just spitting up).
- Very irritable or excessive sleepiness.

Special instructions or comments: ____________

☐ Home Health referral: ____________

☐ Mother verbalizes understanding of discharge instructions.

MOTHER'S SIGNATURE | DATE

RN INITIALS	RN SIGNATURE	RN INITIALS	RN SIGNATURE

ID BAND # | M.R. # | ***Staple 1 Infant ID Band Here.***

I acknowledge receipt of my baby and have received educational instructions and materials. MOTHER'S SIGNATURE

DISCHARGE	DISCHARGE	CARRIED OUT BY		NURSE'S SIGNATURE
Date________ Time________	To________ With________	☐	☐ Mother ☐ Nurse	

01737-2 (REV. 12-96) DISTRIBUTION: WHITE = MOTHER'S CHART • CANARY = BABY'S CHART • PINK = MOTHER

FIG. 28-1 Infant Teaching/Discharge Record. (Courtesy Kaiser Permanente, Redwood City, CA.)

All visitors should wash their hands before touching the infant. Persons with infectious conditions including upper respiratory infections, gastrointestinal (GI) tract infections, and infectious skin conditions should be excluded from contact with the newborn. Some health care providers recommend that infants not be taken out in crowds, particularly when there is an increased risk for being exposed to communicable diseases such as the flu or colds.

Knowledge of and Skill in Child Care Activities

Parents must learn skills such as feeding, holding, clothing, and bathing the infant and protecting the baby from harm (see Research box). The ability to perform these task-oriented activities competently and confidently does not appear automatically with the birth of a child. Many parents must learn to do these tasks, and this learning process can be difficult. However, almost all parents become adept in caregiving activities when they have the desire to learn and the support of others.

Nurses can help inexperienced parents feel confident and competent in their new roles. They can provide opportunities for parents to practice child care tasks in the hospital, birth setting, or in the home, where assistance and feedback are available. Nursing approaches and strategies can enhance parents' self-concept by helping them feel more comfortable and confident in their parenting skills.

CARE MANAGEMENT: PRACTICAL SUGGESTIONS FOR THE FIRST WEEKS AT HOME

Numerous changes occur during the first weeks of parenthood. Care management should be directed toward helping parents cope with infant care, role changes, altered lifestyle, and changes in family structure resulting from the addition of a new baby. Parents may have inadequate or incorrect understanding of what to expect in the early postpartum weeks. Developing skill and confidence in caring for an infant can be especially anxiety provoking.

Nurses, especially those making postpartum visits to parents' homes, are in a prime position to help new families. The nurse's role becomes primarily one of teacher-supporter, focusing on enabling new parents to become capable of self-care and infant care and of meeting the needs of the family unit.

Assessment and Nursing Diagnoses

Assessment should include a psychosocial assessment focusing on parent-infant attachment, adjustment to the parental role, sibling adjustment, social support, and education needs, as well as mother's and baby's physical adaptation (see Chapter 24). Early home visits are an excellent opportunity for the nurse to assess beginnings of successful or harmful parenting behaviors. Parents demonstrating loving and nurturing behaviors with their infant need to be given positive reinforcement. Parents who interact in inappropriate or abusive ways with their

RESEARCH

Back to Sleep Campaign Effects on Infant Sleep Placement

The most common cause of infant death after the neonatal period is sudden infant death syndrome (SIDS). After research showed a strong association between prone sleep position and SIDS, the American Academy of Pediatrics recommended the nonprone positioning of infants. Since 1992, the Back to Sleep campaign has been credited with significantly decreasing SIDS mortality rates. Through educational programs, posters, and public health messages, new parents have been encouraged to place their infant supine to sleep, with a few medical exceptions.

Researchers are still tracking this behavior modification. From one ongoing population-based study, the Pregnancy Risk Assessment Monitoring System (PRAMS), researchers analyzed data obtained between 1996 and 1998, representing 55,263 infants. During this period, SIDS rates declined steadily. The PRAMS data showed that the prevalence of prone sleeping declined from 27% to 19%, and the recommended supine position increased from 31% to 49%. The data show dramatic compliance with the guidelines by Hispanics, with a corresponding decrease in SIDS in this population. African-American infants began with the highest rate of prone sleeping and the lowest rate of supine sleeping and remained virtually unchanged throughout the study period. The relative rate for SIDS declined in all other groups but actually increased slightly for African-Americans during this period, to more than twice the rate of non-Hispanic whites. Other risk factors for infants sleeping supine included infants in large families (>3 children), lower maternal age and education, and infant birth weight less than 1500 grams.

IMPLICATION FOR PRACTICE

Nurses can reinforce the public health message that the supine position is recommended to decrease the risk of SIDS, especially in vulnerable populations. African-Americans and other risk groups must be targeted for education and counseling. Family assessments can be done in the postpartum period to reveal factors that may impact how the decision is made regarding infant sleep position and interventions carried out to encourage adherence to the supine position for infant sleep.

Reference: Pollack, H., & Frohna, J. (2002). Infant sleep after the Back to Sleep campaign. *Pediatrics, 109*(4), 608-614.

infant should be monitored more closely, and an appropriate mental health practitioner or professional social worker should be notified.

Home visits often offer an opportunity to involve all family members. The mother, father, siblings, and even grandparents may ask questions and express concerns. The nurse can share her assessments and observations and develop a plan of care collaboratively with the family. Nursing diagnoses pertinent to the period of transition to parenthood include the following:

- *Readiness for enhanced family coping related to*
  - –Positive attitude and realistic expectations for the newborn and adapting to parenthood
  - –Verbalizing positive factors in lifestyle change
- *Risk for impaired parenting related to*
  - –Lack of knowledge of infant care
  - –Feelings of incompetence or lack of confidence
  - –Unrealistic expectations of infant
  - –Fatigue from interrupted sleep
- *Parental role conflict related to*
  - –Role transition and role attainment
  - –Unwanted pregnancy
  - –Lack of resources to support parenting (e.g., no paid leave)
- *Risk for impaired parent-infant attachment related to*
  - –Postpartum complications
  - –Neonatal complications/anomalies

Expected Outcomes of Care

A plan of care is formulated in collaboration with the family, incorporating their priorities and preferences, to meet their specific needs. Expected outcomes for effective transition to parenthood include that the parents will do the following:

- Interact with the infant in a loving and nurturing way.
- Demonstrate behaviors that reflect appreciation of sensory and behavioral capacities of the infant.
- Respond appropriately to infant cues.
- Verbalize increasing confidence and competence in feeding, diapering, dressing, and sensory stimulation of the infant.
- Identify deviations from normal in the infant that should be brought to the immediate attention of the primary health care provider.
- Describe or demonstrate emergency procedures and verbalize ways of getting emergency help.

Plan of Care and Interventions

Instructions for the First Days at Home

Parents, especially first-time parents, must be helped to anticipate what the transition from hospital to home will be like. Anticipatory guidance can help prevent a shock of reality that might negate the parents' joy or cause them undue stress. Even the simplest strategies can provide enormous support. Classes in the prenatal period or during the postpartum stay are helpful. Written information reinforcing education topics is helpful to provide to parents, as is a list of available community resources, both local and national (see Resources list at the end of this chapter). An excellent resource for the nurse is the Compendium of Postpartum Care, developed by Johnson & Johnson Products, Inc., in association with the Association of Women's Health, Obstetric, and Neonatal Nurses (1996). Postpartum nurses will find the "Patient Handouts" section especially useful. It includes handouts on topics such as rest and exercise, emotional well-being during adaptation to parenthood, understanding the blues, and what to expect and do regarding the infant's health. Instructions for the first days at home should minimally include activities of daily living, dealing with visitors, and activity and rest.

Activities of Daily Living. Given the demands of a newborn, the mother's discomfort or fatigue associated with giving birth, and a busy homecoming day, even small details of daily life can become stressful. Such things as using disposable diapers or having a diaper service for the first week or so, preparing frozen and/or microwavable dinners, or getting takeout meals can decrease stress by eliminating at least one or two parental responsibilities during the first few days at home.

Planning for discharge soon after an infant feeding ensures that the couple will have adequate time to get home and relatively settled before the next feeding. Offering a sample carton of premixed bottles for the formula-fed infant prevents the rushed preparation of formula.

Visitors. New parents are often inadequately prepared for the reality of bringing a new infant home because they romanticize the homecoming. One mother stated,

> By the time we drove an hour through traffic, my stitches were hurting, and all I wanted was a warm sitz bath and some private time with Bill and the baby, in that order. Instead, a carload of visitors pulled into the driveway as we were unbuckling the baby from his car seat. I thought I would surely cry.

The nurse can help parents explore ways, in advance, to assert their need to limit visitors. When family and friends ask what they can do to help, new parents can suggest they prepare and bring them a meal or pick up items at the store. Parents can work out a signal for alerting the partner that the mother is becoming tired or uncomfortable and needs the partner to invite the visitors to another room or to leave. Some mothers find that wearing a robe and not appearing ready for company leads visitors to stay a shorter time. A sign on the front door saying, "Mother and baby resting. . . .Please do not disturb" may be useful.

Activity and Rest. Because mothers have reported fatigue as a major problem during the first few weeks after giving birth, mothers should be encouraged to limit their activities and be realistic about their level of fatigue. Activities should not be sustained for long periods. Family, friends, and neighbors can be solicited for support and help with meals, housecleaning, picking up other children, etc. Rest periods throughout the day are important. Mothers can nap when the baby sleeps. Adequate nutrition also is important for postpartum recovery and for dealing with fatigue. Because many women are anemic or have a low normal hemoglobin and hematocrit, providing a list of foods high in iron may be useful. Increasing fiber and fluid intake helps reestablish bowel function.

Physical Care and Safety

Providing practical suggestions for infant care can help parents adjust to parenthood. Mothers and fathers want to feel capable and confident in the physical care of their infant. The nurse should assess each parent's need for instruction on care, such as care of the circumcised infant, bathing, clothing, and safety (see Guidelines/Guías box).

Cord Care. The cord should be kept clean and dry by folding the diaper below the cord to allow drying (AWHONN, 2001; Dore et al., 1998). The cord can be cleansed with water as necessary. Routine use of alcohol until the cord drops off is not recommended, because this practice may delay separation (Zuspan & Garner, 2000).

Care of the Circumcised Infant Male. The infant is often circumcised the day of discharge. The infant is observed to assure that excessive bleeding does not occur and that the infant voids at least once before discharge (see Teaching for Self-Care box). Petroleum jelly is applied to the penis with each diaper change for at least the first 24 hours after circumcision to prevent the diaper from adhering to the penis. The penis is kept clean with gentle cleansing with warm water. The diaper is applied loosely. A yellow exudates covers the glans within 24 hours. This is normal and will persist for 2 to 3 days. No attempt should be made to remove it. Circumcision is painful; the infant may be fussy and should be comforted. A prescription for oral acetaminophen may be written and the medication given as needed if the infant is not consoled.

Infant Bathing. The infant bath time provides a wonderful opportunity for parent-infant social interaction. Some fathers consider this their own special time with

GUIDELINES/GUÍAS

Daily Care

BATHING

Bathing 2 or 3 times a week is enough, using a mild soap like Johnson's, Dove, Tone, or Purpose. Sponge bathe the baby until the umbilical cord falls off and the belly button looks healed. Never leave the baby alone in the tub or sink!

Necesita bañar a su bebé dos o tres veces a la semana. Use un jabón suave como Johnson's, Dove, Tone, o Purpose. Lávelo con un paño o con una esponja de cuerpo suave hasta que se caiga el cordón umbilical y parece ser curado y seco el ombligo. ¡Nunca deje al bebé solo el la bañera o en el lavabo!

CLOTHING

The best clothing is soft and made of cotton. Dress your baby lightly when indoors and on hot days. Too many layers of clothing or blankets can make the baby too hot. On cold days, cover the baby's head when you go outdoors.

La mejor ropa para su bebé debe ser suave y hecha de algodón. No le ponga mucha ropa al bebé cuando esté dentro de la casa o en los días calientes. Demasiada ropa o mantas puede darle calor al bebé. En los días de frío, póngale una capa en la cabeza.

CAR SEATS

Use a real car seat (not a baby carrier for the house). It should face the rear of the car until the baby is 1 year old. Always place the car seat in the back seat of the car. Make sure the shoulder straps are snug enough that they don't fall off the baby's shoulders. Car seats are required until 4 years of age.

Use un asiento de coche que está hecho para un coche. El asiento debe mirar hacia la parte atrás del coche hasta que el bebé tenga un año. Siempre ponga el bebé en el asiento atrás del coche. Los cinturones deben estar apretados pero no deben limitar los movimientos del bebé. Se requiere por ley usar los asientos de coche hasta que el bebé tenga cuatro años.

TEACHING FOR SELF-CARE

Circumcision

- Wash hands before touching the newly circumcised penis.

CHECK FOR BLEEDING

- Check circumcision for bleeding every hour for the first 12 hr after the procedure.
- If bleeding occurs, apply gentle pressure with a folded sterile gauze square. If bleeding does not stop with pressure, notify primary health care provider.

OBSERVE FOR URINATION

- Check to see that the infant urinates after being circumcised.
- Infant should have a wet diaper 6 to 10 times per 24 hr.

KEEP AREA CLEAN

- Change diaper and inspect circumcision at least every 4 hr.
- Wash penis gently with warm water to remove urine and feces. Apply petrolatum to the glans with each diaper change (omit petrolatum if Plastibell was used).
- Use soap only after circumcision is healed.
- Fanfold diaper to prevent pressure on the circumcised area.

CHECK FOR INFECTION

- Glans penis is dark red after circumcision, then becomes covered with yellow exudate in 24 hr. This is normal and will persist for 2 to 3 days. Do not attempt to remove it.
- Redness, swelling, or discharge indicate infection. Notify primary health care provider if you think the circumcision area is infected.

PROVIDE COMFORT

- Circumcision is painful. Handle the area gently.
- Provide extra holding, feeding, and opportunities for nonnutritive sucking for a day or two.

A

B

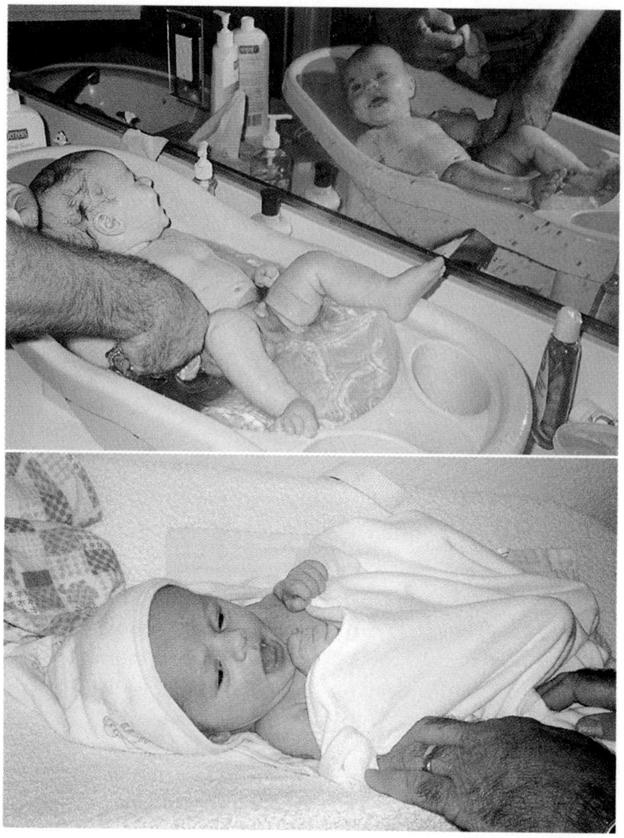

FIG. 28-2 **A,** Baths can be special times for babies and parents. **B,** After the bath, the baby is gently dried to minimize heat loss. (Courtesy Leslie Canerday, Phoenix, AZ.)

their babies. While bathing their baby, parents can talk to and caress and cuddle the infant, and engage in arousal and imitation of facial expressions and smiling (Fig. 28-2).

Sponge baths are usually used until the infant's umbilical cord falls off and the umbilicus is healed (see Teaching for Self-Care box). Bathing the newborn by immersion has been found to allow less heat loss and provoke less crying; however, most health care providers suggest that tub bathing be delayed until the umbilical cord falls off, which occurs at about 10 to 14 days after birth (Box 28-1). Newborns do not need a bath every day (Franck, Quinn, & Zahr, 2000). The face, creases under the arms and neck, and diaper area need more attention. Parents can pick a time for the bath that is easy for them and when the baby is awake, usually before a feeding.

Some parents question whether the use of soap, lotion, oil, and powder is necessary or advised. An important consideration in skin cleansing is preservation of the skin's acid mantle. The acid mantle is formed from the uppermost horny layer of the epidermis, sweat, superficial fat, metabolic products, and external substances such as amniotic fluid, microorganisms, and cosmetics. By 4 days of age, the newborn skin surface becomes more acidic, falling to within the bacteriostatic range (pH 5). Thus in the early newborn period, only plain, warm water should be used. Alkaline soaps (such as Ivory), oils, powders, and many lotions alter the acid mantle and provide a medium for bacterial growth. Use of commercial diaper wipes should be avoided because they can alter the acid mantle (AWHONN, 2001). Powders are not recommended, because the infant can inhale powder and experience respiratory distress (Darmstadt & Dinulos, 2000). If parents use powder, it should be shaken onto the parent's hand and smoothed onto the skin of the infant. Emollients such as Aquaphor (petrolatum based) ointment can be used for dry flaky skin (AWHONN, 2001).

Diaper Rash. To avoid diaper rash, the diaper area should be kept clean and dry by frequent diaper changes and gentle and thorough cleansing of the genitalia with warm water (AWHONN, 2001). If diaper rash occurs, zinc oxide may be used; powders and A&D ointment should be avoided. Antifungal ointments are used only when prescribed (AWHONN, 2001). Plastic pants should be left off until the diaper area heals.

Infant Clothing. Parents commonly ask how warmly they should dress their infant. A simple rule of thumb is to dress the child as the parents would dress themselves, adding or subtracting clothes and wraps for the infant as necessary. A shirt and diaper may be sufficient clothing for the young infant. A bonnet is needed to protect the scalp and to minimize heat loss if it is cool or to protect against sunburn and to shade the infant's eyes if it is sunny and hot. Sunglasses for infants are available. Wrapping the infant snugly in a blanket maintains body temperature and promotes a feeling of security. Overdressing in warm temperatures can cause discomfort and prickly heat rash. Underdressing in cold weather also can cause discomfort; cheeks, fingers, and toes can easily become frostbitten.

Infants have sensitive skin; therefore new clothes should be washed before putting them on the infant. Baby clothes should be washed separately with a mild detergent and hot water. A double rinse usually removes traces of the potentially irritating cleansing agent or acid residue from urine or stool. If possible, the clothing and bed linens are dried in the sun to neutralize residue. Parents who have to use coin-operated machines in laundromats to wash and dry clothes may find it expensive or impossible to wash and rinse the baby's clothes well.

Bedding requires frequent changing. The top of a plastic-coated mattress should be washed frequently, and the crib or bassinet should be dusted with a damp cloth. The infant's toilet articles may be kept convenient for use in a box, basket, or plastic carrier. Keeping moistened cotton balls in a container near the bassinet or bed to clean the infant's diaper area saves time and steps for the parents.

Infant Safety. Providing for the safety of an infant is not a matter of just using common sense. New parents may not be aware of many potential dangers to their

TEACHING FOR SELF-CARE

Sponge Bathing

FITTING BATHS INTO FAMILY'S SCHEDULE

Give a bath at any time convenient to you but not immediately after a feeding period because the increased handling may cause regurgitation.

PREVENTING HEAT LOSS

The temperature of the room should be 24° C (75° F), and the bathing area should be free of drafts.

Control heat loss during the bath to conserve the infant's energy. Bathing the infant quickly, exposing only a portion of the body at a time, and thorough drying are all parts of the bathing technique.

GATHERING SUPPLIES AND CLOTHING BEFORE STARTING

Clothing suitable for wearing indoors: diaper, shirt; stretch suit or nightgown optional

Unscented, mild soap

Pins, if needed for diaper, closed and placed well out of baby's reach

Cotton balls

Towels for drying infant and a clean washcloth

Receiving blanket

Tub for water

BATHING THE BABY

Bring infant to bathing area when all supplies are ready.

Never leave the infant alone on bath table or in bath water, not even for a second! If you have to leave, take the infant with you or put back into crib.

Test temperature of the water. It should feel pleasantly warm to the inner wrist 36.6° to 37.2° C (98° to 99° F).

Do not hold infant under running water—water temperature may change, and infant may be scalded or chilled rapidly.

Wash infant's head before unwrapping and undressing to prevent heat loss.

Cleanse the eyes from the inner canthus outward, using separate parts of a clean washcloth for each eye. For the first 2 to 3 days, a discharge may result from the reaction of the conjunctiva to the substance (erythromycin) used as a prophylactic measure against infection. Any discharge should be considered abnormal and reported to the health care provider.

Wash the scalp with water and mild soap; rinse well and dry thoroughly (Fig. 27-30). Scalp desquamation, called *cradle cap*, often can be prevented by removing any scales with a fine-toothed comb or brush after washing. If condition persists, the health care provider may prescribe an ointment to massage into the scalp.

Creases under the chin and arms and in the groin may need daily cleansing. The crease under the chin may be exposed by elevating the infant's shoulders 5 cm and letting the head drop back.

Cleanse ears and nose with twists of moistened cotton or a corner of the washcloth. Do not use cotton-tipped swabs because they may cause injury.

Undress baby and wash body and arms and legs. Pat dry gently. Baby may be tub bathed after the cord drops off and umbilicus and circumcised penis are completely healed.

PREVENTING SKIN TRAUMA

The fragile skin can be injured by too vigorous cleansing.

If stool or other debris has dried and caked on the skin, soak the area to remove it. Do not attempt to rub it off, because abrasion may result. Gentleness, patting dry rather than rubbing, and use of a mild soap without perfumes or coloring are recommended. Chemicals in the coloring and perfume can cause rashes on sensitive skin.

CARE OF THE CORD

Cleanse around base of the cord where it joins the skin with soap and water. Notify the health care provider of any odor, discharge, or skin inflammation around the cord. The clamp is removed when the cord is dry (approximately 24 hr). The diaper should not cover the cord because a wet or soiled diaper will slow or prevent drying of the cord and foster infection. When the cord drops off after a week to 10 days, small drops of blood may be seen when the baby cries. This will heal by itself. It is not dangerous.

CARE OF HANDS AND FEET

Wash and dry between the fingers and toes.

Do not cut fingernails and toenails immediately after birth. The nails have to grow out far enough from the skin so that the skin is not cut by mistake. If the baby scratches himself or herself, apply loosely fitted mitts over each of the baby's hands. Do so as a last resort, however, because it interferes with the baby's ability for self-consolation sucking on thumb or finger. When the nails have grown, the fingernails and toenails can be cut more easily with manicure scissors (preferably scissors with rounded tips) when the infant is asleep. Nails should be kept short.

CLEANSING GENITALS

Cleanse the genitals of infants daily and after voiding or defecating. For girls, the genitals may be cleansed by separating the labia and gently washing from the pubic area to the anus. For uncircumcised boys, gently pull back (retract) the foreskin. Stop when resistance is felt. Wash and rinse the tip (glans) with soap and warm water, and replace the foreskin. The foreskin must be returned to its original position to prevent constriction and swelling. In most newborns, the inner layer of the foreskin adheres to the glans and the foreskin cannot be retracted. By age 3 years in 90% of boys, the foreskin can be retracted easily without causing pain or trauma. For others, the foreskin is not retractable until adolescence. As soon as the foreskin is partly retractable and the child is old enough, he can be taught self-care. Once healed, the circumcised penis does not require any special care other than cleansing with diaper changes.

BOX 28-1 Tub Bathing

- See guidelines for sponge bathing.
- Place liner on bottom of tub to prevent infant from slipping.
- Add up to 5 inches of comfortably warm water (36.6° C to 37.2° C—pleasantly warm to your inner wrist) or water deep enough to cover the shoulders to prevent heat loss from evaporation.
- Undress baby. Lower infant slowly into water.
- Wash face and shampoo hair as for sponge bath. • Hold baby safely with fingers under the baby's armpit, with your thumb around the shoulder. Use the other hand to support the baby's bottom and legs.
- Wash the front of the baby.
- Go from front to back between the legs. Rinse with a wet washcloth.
- Wash the baby's back with your free hand lathered with soap.
- Rinse well with the wet washcloth.
- Remove infant from the water, and gently pat dry. Wrap in a warm blanket and leave wrapped for up to 10 minutes before dressing. Dressing immediately if the baby is still damp will get clothes wet and cause heat loss. After dressing, wrap in a warm blanket (Varda & Behnke, 2000).

BOX 28-2 Tips for Keeping Your Baby Safe

- Never leave your baby alone on a bed, couch, or table. Even newborns can move enough to reach the edge eventually and fall off.
- Never put your baby on a cushion, pillow, beanbag, or waterbed to sleep. Your baby may suffocate. Do not keep pillows, large floppy toys, or loose plastic sheeting in the crib.
- Do not place your infant on his or her stomach to sleep during the first few months of life. The American Academy of Pediatrics advises against this prone position because it has been associated with an increased incidence of sudden infant death syndrome (SIDS). The back-lying position is recommended. The infant may be rolled slightly to the side with a rolled blanket to the back.
- When using an infant carrier, stay within arm's reach when the carrier is on a high place, such as a table, sofa, or store counter. If at all possible, place the carrier on the floor near you.
- Infant carriers do not keep your baby safe in a car. Always place your baby in an approved car safety seat when traveling in a motor vehicle (car, truck, bus, or van). Car safety seats are recommended for travel on trains and airplanes as well. Use the car seat for every ride. Your baby should be in a rear-facing infant car seat from birth to 20 pounds, and the car seat should be in the back seat of the car (see Fig. 28-3). This is especially important in vehicles with front passenger air bags, because when air bags inflate, they can be fatal for infants and toddlers (see Fig. 28-4).
- When bathing your baby, never leave him or her alone. Newborns and infants can drown in 1 to 2 inches of water.
- Be sure that your hot water heater is set at 49° C or less. Always check bathwater temperature with your elbow before putting your baby in the bath.
- Do not tie anything around your baby's neck. Pacifiers tied around the neck with a ribbon or string may strangle your baby.
- Check your baby's crib for safety. Slats should be no more than 2.5 inches apart. The space between the mattress and sides should be less than 2 finger widths. There should be no decorative knobs on the bedposts.
- Keep crib or playpen away from window blind and drapery cords; your baby could strangle on them.
- Keep crib and playpen well away from radiators, heat vents, and portable heaters. Linens in crib or playpen could catch fire if in contact with these heat sources.
- Install smoke detectors on every floor of your home. Check them once a month to be sure they work. Change batteries at least once a year.
- Avoid exposing your baby to cigarette or cigar smoke in your home or other places. Passive exposure to tobacco smoke greatly increases the likelihood that your infant will have respiratory symptoms and illnesses.
- Be gentle with your baby. Do not pick your baby up or swing your baby by the arms or throw him or her up in the air.

infant (e.g., window blind cords near the crib or a parent throwing an infant in the air during play). Nurses should provide parents with concrete instructions on infant safety (Box 28-2; see Resources list).

Use of Car Seat. Infants should travel only in federally approved rear-facing safety seats secured in the rear seat (Fig. 28-3). The safest area of the car is in the back seat. A car seat that faces the rear gives the best protection for the disproportionately weak neck and heavy head of an infant. In this position, the force of a frontal crash is spread over the head, neck, and back; the back of the car seat supports the spine.

NURSE ALERT
Infants should use a rear-facing car seat from birth to 20 pounds and to age 1 year.

The car seat is secured by using the vehicle seat belts; the infant is secured by using the harness system in the car seat. If the infant must ride in the front seat, the air bag must be turned off to prevent injury from the air bag.

NURSE ALERT
In cars equipped with air bags, rear-facing infant seats must not be placed in the front seat. Because these types of infant seats fit close to the dashboard, serious injury can occur if the air bag inflates (Fig. 28-4).

Nonnutritive Sucking

Sucking is the infant's chief pleasure; however, sucking may not be satisfied by breastfeeding or formula feeding alone. Sucking is such a strong need that infants who are deprived of sucking, such as those with a cleft lip, will suck on their tongues. Some newborns are born with sucking pads on their fingers that developed during in utero sucking. Several benefits of nonnutritive sucking have been documented, such as an increased weight gain in premature infants, decreased crying, and decreased length of hospital stay (Pinelli & Symington, 2001).

Problems arise when parents are concerned about the sucking of fingers, thumb, or pacifier and try to restrain this natural tendency. Before giving advice, nurses should investigate the parents' feelings and base the guidance they give on the information elicited. For example, some parents may see no problem with the use of a finger but may find the use of a pacifier objectionable. In general, there is no need to restrain either practice, unless thumb sucking persists past 4 years of age or past the time when the permanent teeth erupt. Parents are advised to consult with their pediatrician and pediatric nurse practitioner about their concerns.

To decrease an infant's dependence on nonnutritive sucking, the feeding time can be prolonged. One way of doing this in bottle-fed infants is to use a small-holed, firm nipple because this necessitates stronger sucking and slows the feeding. A parent's excessive use of the pacifier to calm the child should be explored. It is not unusual for parents to place a pacifier in their infant's mouth as soon as it begins to cry, thus only reinforcing a pattern of distress-relief.

If parents choose to let their infant use a pacifier, they must be aware of certain safety considerations before purchasing one. A homemade or poorly designed pacifier can be dangerous because the entire object may be aspirated if it is small, or a portion may become lodged in the pharynx. Improvised pacifiers, such as those commonly made in

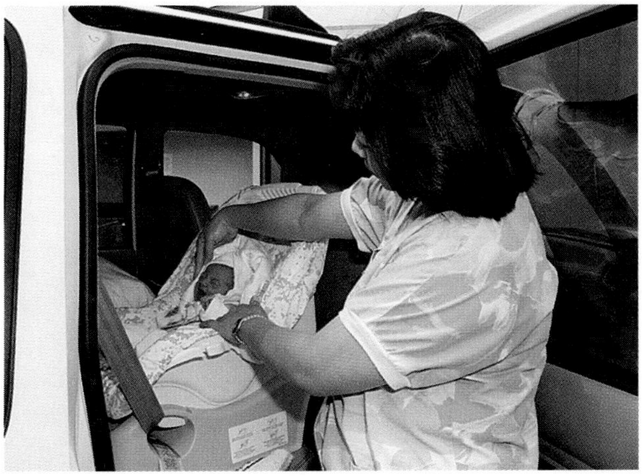

FIG. 28-3 Rear-facing infant seat in rear seat of car. (Courtesy Marjorie Pyle, RNC, Lifecircle, Costa Mesa, CA.)

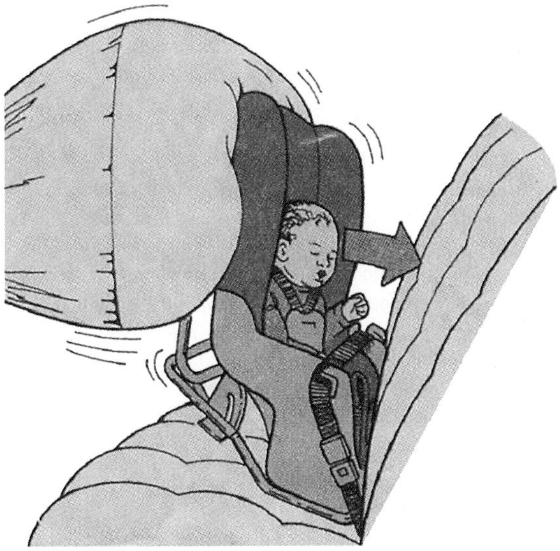

FIG. 28-4 An airbag could strike a child safety seat, causing serious injury to the child. (Redrawn from Health Alert [1994]. *AAP News,* 10[4], 22.)

hospitals from a padded nipple, also pose dangers because the nipple may separate from the plastic collar and be aspirated. Safe pacifiers are made of one piece that includes a shield or flange that is large enough to prevent entry into the mouth and a handle that can be grasped (Fig. 28-5).

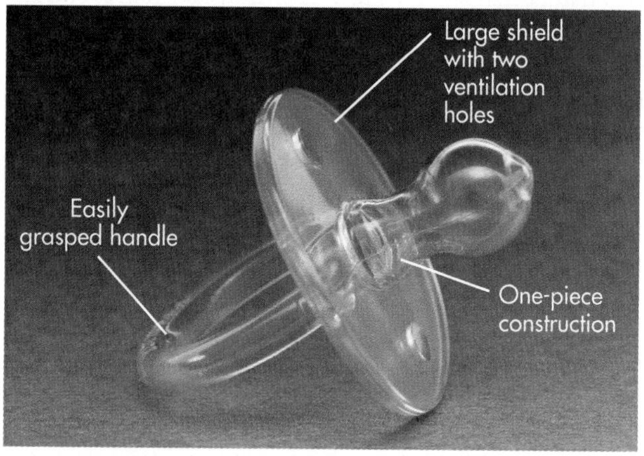
Large shield with two ventilation holes
Easily grasped handle
One-piece construction

FIG. 28-5 Design of safe pacifier. (In Wong, D. [1999]. *Whaley & Wong's nursing care of infants and children* [6th ed.]. St. Louis: Mosby.)

Anticipatory Guidance Regarding the Newborn

Anticipatory guidance helps prepare new parents for what to expect as their newborn grows and develops. Parents with realistic expectations of infant needs and behavior are prepared better to adjust to the demands of a new baby and to parenthood itself (see Guidelines/Guías box).

New parents can be overwhelmed by a large volume of information and may become anxious. Anticipatory guidance should include the following: newborn sleep-wake cycles, interpretation of crying and quieting techniques, infant developmental milestones, sensory enrichment/infant stimulation, recognizing signs of illness, and well-baby follow-up and immunizations. Printed materials and audiotapes or videotapes for parents to take home are helpful. These resources (1) reinforce content discussed in the hospital, (2) allow parents another chance to review the material in private and at their own pace, and (3) provide new information not covered in the hospital.

Development of Day-Night Routines. Nurses can help prepare new parents for the fact that most newborns cannot tell the difference between night and day and must learn the rhythm of day-night routines. Nurses should provide basic suggestions for settling a newborn and for help-

GUIDELINES/GUÍAS

General Advice

CRYING

Babies cry when they are hungry; need to burp; have a wet diaper; feel cold, hot, tired, bored, or overstimulated; and (rarely) when they are sick or in pain. After a while, you will learn the meaning of your baby's different cries. Be careful not to feed him or her every time he or she cries, because overfeeding causes tummy aches. Check to see if he or she needs burping or a new diaper. It is not harmful to let a baby cry for short periods (5 to 10 minutes). This may be what he or she needs to fall asleep.

Todos los bebés lloran cuando tienen hambre; cuando necesitan eructar; cuando necesitan que le cambia el pañal; cuando tienen calor o frío; cuando están cansados, aburridos, o sobreestimulados; y cuando están enfermos o tienen un dolor. Después de un tiempo, usted aprenderá los modos varios que tiene su bebé de llorar y podrá distinguir entre cada uno de ellos para saber lo que necesita. No le dé de comer cada vez que llore porque si come demasiado le puede dar dolor de estómago. Mire a ver si está mojado el pañal o si necesita eructar. No le hará ningún daño al bebé si llora por cinco o diez minutos. Puede ser que esto sea justo lo que necesita para quedarse dormido.

SLEEPING

Most babies can sleep through most of the night without a feeding by 4 to 5 months of age. You can help your baby sleep by keeping things quiet and dark at night. Both you and the baby will usually sleep better and wake up less often if he or she is sleeping in a separate bed. If your baby stirs at night but doesn't fully wake up, give him or her a chance to fall back asleep by himself or herself. Only get him or her up if he or she stays wide awake and seems hungry. The baby should sleep on the back for safety. Babies sleeping on their tummies seem to be more prone to crib death.

La mayoría de los bebés pueden dormir la noche entera sin comer cuando tienen algunos meses de edad. Un domicilio quieto y calmo ayuda a su bebé dormir tranquilo. Se duermen mejor (y se despiertan menos) si usted y el bebé están en camas separadas. Si se despierta el bebé durante la noche, dele la oportunidad de dormirse de nuevo. Pero si se queda despierto y tiene hambre, atiéndalo. La posición de dormir más segura para los infantes es en la espalda con la boca para arriba. Los bebés que duermen en los estómagos con la boca para abajo tienen un riesgo más grande de morir en la camita de niño.

SPITTING UP

Most babies spit up a little after feedings. If your baby is gaining weight, this is normal. It helps to keep your baby upright and quiet for a few minutes after feedings. If your baby seems to be spitting up a lot, bring him or her to your doctor for a weight check.

La mayoría de los bebés echan a fuera un poco de la leche después de comer o cuando eructan. Esto es normal si su bebé está aumentando de peso. Es bueno mantenerlo recto y quieto por unos minutos después de darle de comer. Si parece que está echando mucha leche o si lo hace con mucha frecuencia, llévelo al doctor para que lo pese.

ing him or her develop a predictable routine. Examples of such suggestions include

- In the late afternoon, bring the baby out to the center of family activity. Keep the baby there for the rest of the evening. If the baby falls asleep, let the baby do so in the infant seat or in someone's arms. Save the crib or bassinet for nighttime sleep.
- Give the baby a bath right before bedtime. This soothes the baby and helps him or her expend energy.
- Feed the baby for the last evening time around 11 PM and put him or her to bed in the crib or bassinet.
- For nighttime feedings and diaper changes, keep a small night-light on to avoid turning on bright lights. Talk in soft whispers (if at all) and handle the baby gently and only as absolutely necessary to feed and diaper. Nighttime feedings should be all business and no play. Babies usually go back to sleep if the room is quiet and dark.

A predictable, stable routine gradually develops for most babies; however, some babies never develop one. New parents will find it easier if they are willing to be flexible and to give up some control during those early weeks.

Interpretation of Crying and Quieting Techniques. Crying is an infant's first social communication. Some babies cry more than others, but all babies cry. They cry to communicate that they are hungry, uncomfortable, wet, ill, or bored, and sometimes for no apparent reason at all. Crying increases to about 2½ hours per day, peaks in the second month of life, and decreases after that time. Infants with high intensity and low distractibility cry more than other infants (Blum et al., 2002) (Box 28-3). However, caretaking behaviors of mothers of children who cry more are not different from behaviors of mothers whose infants cry less (St. James-Roberts, Conroy, & Wilsher, 1996).

The longer parents are around their infants, the easier it becomes to interpret what a cry means. Many infants, especially between ages 3 and 12 weeks, have a fussy period during the day, often in the late afternoon or early evening when everyone is naturally tired. Environmental tension adds to the length and intensity of crying spells. Babies also have periods of vigorous crying which no comforting helps. These periods of crying may last for long stretches until the infants seem to cry themselves to sleep. Possibly the infants are trying to discharge enough energy so that they can settle themselves down. The nurse should reinforce for new parents that time and infant maturation will take care of these types of cries.

Crying because of colic is a common concern of new parents. Babies with colic cry inconsolably for several hours, pull their legs up to their stomach, and pass large amounts of gas. No one really knows what colic is or why babies have it. Parents can be encouraged to contact their nurse practitioner or pediatrician if they are concerned that their baby has colic.

Certain types of sensory stimulation can calm and quiet infants and help them get to sleep. Important characteristics of this sensory stimulation—whether tactile, vestibular, auditory, or visual—appear to be that the stimulation is mild, slow, rhythmic, and consistently and regularly presented. Tactile stimulation can include warmth, patting, back rubbing, and covering the skin with textured cloth. Swaddling to keep arms and legs close to the body (as in utero) provides widespread and constant tactile stimulation and a sense of security. Vestibular stimulation is especially effective and can be accomplished by mild rhythmic movement such as rocking or by holding the infant upright, as on the parent's shoulder.

The nurse can teach parents a number of strategies that help quiet a fussy baby, prevent crying, and induce quiet attention or sleep (Boxes 28-4 and 28-5).

BOX 28-3 Early Infancy Temperament Questionnaire

The Early Infancy Temperament Questionnaire (EITQ) is designed for assessment of temperament of infants from ages 1 to 4 months. The EITQ is a 76-item parent questionnaire. It assesses the nine temperament categories originally identified in the New York Longitudinal Study. For this questionnaire, the Revised Infant Temperament Questionnaire was adapted to be developmentally appropriate for the young infant. The nine temperament categories showed no differences between female and male infants. With this tool, clinicians can more reliably assess infant temperament to assist in better understanding the contribution of temperament to problems in the infant.

Reference: Medoff-Cooper, B., Carey, W., & McDevitt, S. (1993). The early infancy temperament questionnaire. *Journal of Developmental and Behavioral Pediatrics, 14*, 230-235.

BOX 28-4 How to Swaddle an Infant

1. Fold down the top corner of the blanket. Position the infant on the blanket, with the infant's neck near the fold.
2. Bring the blanket around the infant's right side and across the infant, tucking the corner under the left side.
3. Bring the bottom of the blanket up to the infant's chest.
4. Bring the remaining corner of the blanket across the infant, tucking the corner under the infant's right side. The infant should be wrapped securely but not tightly; some room should be left for the infant to move.

BOX 28-5 Infant Quieting Techniques

- Many newborns feel insecure in the center of a large crib. They prefer a small, warm, soft space that reminds them of intrauterine life. Try a smaller bed, such as a bassinet, portable crib, buggy, or cradle, or use a rolled-up blanket to turn a corner of the big crib into a smaller place.
- Carry your baby in a frontpack or backpack.
- Swaddle your newborn snugly in a receiving blanket. Swaddling keeps your newborn's arms and legs close to his or her body, similar to the intrauterine position. It makes the newborn feel more secure.
- Prewarm the crib sheets with a hot water bottle or heating pad that you remove before putting your baby to bed. Some babies startle when placed on a cold sheet.
- Some newborns need extra sucking to soothe themselves to sleep. Breastfeeding mothers may prefer to let their infant suckle at the breast as a soothing technique. Other mothers choose to use a pacifier. Stroke the pacifier against the roof of the baby's mouth to encourage him or her to suck it during the first 2 weeks. Around age 3 months, infants become able to find and suck their thumbs consistently as a way of self-consoling.
- A rhythmic, monotonous noise simulating the intrauterine sounds of your heartbeat and blood flow may help your infant settle down. Some parents have found that putting the baby in a portable crib beside the dishwasher or washing machine helps settle a fussy baby.
- Movement often helps quiet a baby. Take your baby for a ride in the car, or take your baby for an outing in a stroller or carriage. Rock your baby in a rocking chair or cradle.
- Place your baby on his or her stomach across your lap; pat and rub his or her back while gently bouncing your legs or swaying them from left to right.
- Babies enjoy close skin-to-skin contact. A combination of this and warm water often helps soothe a fussy baby. Fill your tub with warm water. Get in and let the baby lie on your chest so that the baby is immersed in the water up to his or her neck. Cuddle the baby close.
- Let your baby see your face. Talk to your baby in a soothing voice.
- Your baby may simply be bored. Bring him or her into the room where you and the rest of the family are. Change your baby's position; many babies like to be upright, such as being held up on your shoulder.

Developmental Milestones. Knowledge of infant growth and development helps parents have realistic expectations of what an infant can do. When parents understand and appreciate the limitations and developing abilities of their infant, adjustment to parenthood can go more smoothly. Emphasizing the individuality of the infant enhances the capacity of the family to offer their infant an optimally nurturing environment (Brazelton, 1995).

Brazelton (1995) suggested the concept of "touch-points" for intervention, that is, points at which a change in the system (baby, parent, and family) is brought about by the baby's spurts in development (cognitive, motor, or emotional). Immediately before each spurt in development, there is a predictable short period of disorganization in the baby. Parents are likely to feel disorganized and stressed as well. Because these periods of disorganization are predictable, nurses can offer parents anticipatory guidance to help them understand what happens with infant development and to prepare them for the subsequent spurts in development.

Two touch-points occur during the early postpartum-newborn period: one soon after birth and another at 2 to 3 weeks (Brazelton, 1995). In the hospital or at a home visit during the first week, the nurse can use Brazelton's Neonatal Behavioral Assessment Scale (Brazelton & Nugent, 1996) to demonstrate to parents their baby's amazing repertoire of abilities. In this way, parents begin to appreciate their baby's individuality and become more sensitive to their baby's behavioral cues.

It also is helpful for nurses to provide parents with information on month-by-month infant growth and development. Written information that parents can refer to later is especially helpful. See Table 28-1 for a summary of infant growth and development during the first 2 to 3 months.

Infant Stimulation. Interacting with their parents is an important way in which infants learn about themselves and their environment. Nurses can teach parents a variety of ways to stimulate their infant's development and to enrich the infant's learning environment. Home health nurses are in a prime position to evaluate the home environment and to make suggestions to parents for promotion of their baby's physical, cognitive, and emotional development. Suggestions for teaching infants during the first few months are presented in Boxes 28-6 and 28-7. Table 28-2 presents suggestions for visual, auditory, tactile, and kinetic stimulation.

TABLE 28-1 **Growth and Development During Infancy**

1 MO	2 MO	3 MO
Physical		
Weight gain of 150 to 210 g weekly for first 6 mo Length gain of 2.5 cm monthly for first 6 mo Head circumference increases by 1.5 cm monthly for first 6 mo Primitive reflexes present and strong Doll's eye reflex and dance reflex fading Preferential nose breathing (most infants)	Posterior fontanel closed Crawling reflex disappears	Primitive reflexes fading
Gross Motor		
Assumes flexed position with pelvis high but knees not under abdomen when prone (at birth, knees flexed under abdomen)* Can turn head from side to side when prone; lifts head momentarily from bed* Has marked head lag, especially when pulled from lying to sitting position Holds head momentarily parallel and in midline when suspended in prone position Assumes asymmetric tonic neck reflex position when supine When held in standing position, body limp at knees and hips In sitting position, back is uniformly rounded; absence of head control	Assumes less flexed position when prone—hips flat, legs extended, arms flexed, head to side* Less head lag when pulled to sitting position Can maintain head in same plane as rest of body when held in ventral suspension When prone, can lift head almost 45 degrees off table When held in sitting position, head is held up but bobs forward Assumes asymmetric tonic neck reflex position intermittently	Able to hold head more erect when sitting, but still bobs forward Has only slight head lag when pulled to sitting position Assumes symmetric body positioning Able to raise head and shoulders from prone position to a 45- to 90-degree angle from table; bears weight on forearms When held in standing position, able to bear slight fraction of weight on legs Regards own hand
Fine Motor		
Hands predominantly closed Grasp reflex strong Hand clenches on contact with rattle	Hands often open Grasp reflex fading	Actively holds rattle but will not reach for it* Grasp reflex absent Hands kept loosely open Clutches own hand; pulls at blanket and clothes
Sensory		
Able to fixate on moving object in range of 45 degrees when held at a distance of 20 to 25 cm Visual acuity approaches 20/100† Follows light to midline Quiets when hears a voice	Binocular fixation and convergence to near objects beginning When supine, follows dangling toy from side to point beyond midline Visually searches to locate sounds Turns head to side when sound is made at level of ear	Follows object to periphery (180 degrees)* Locates sound by turning head to side and looking in same direction* Begins to have ability to coordinate stimuli from various sense organs
Vocalization		
Cries to express displeasure Makes small throaty sounds Makes comfort sounds during feeding	Vocalizes, distinct from crying* Crying becomes differentiated Coos Vocalizes to familiar voice	Squeals aloud to show pleasure* Coos, babbles, chuckles Vocalizes when smiling "Talks" a great deal when spoken to Less crying during periods of wakefulness

From Hockenberry, M. et al. (2003). *Wong's nursing care of infants and children* (7th ed.). St. Louis: Mosby.

Continued

*Milestones that represent essential integrative aspects of development that lay the foundation for the achievement of more advanced skills.

†Degree of visual acuity varies according to vision measurement procedure used.

TABLE 28-1 **Growth and Development During Infancy—cont'd**

1 MO	2 MO	3 MO
Socialization/Cognition		
Is in sensorimotor phase—stage I, use of reflexes (birth to 1 mo), and stage II, primary circular reactions (1 to 4 mo) Watches parent's face intently as she or he talks to infant	Demonstrates social smile in response to various stimuli*	Displays considerable interest in surroundings Ceases crying when parent enters room Can recognize familiar faces and objects, such as feeding bottle Shows awareness of strange situations

BOX 28-6 **Teaching Your Newborn**

- Newborns learn things every day. You can teach your newborn by playing with him or her and giving your newborn toys that help him or her to learn.
- Talk to your baby a lot. Tell your baby what is going on in the room ("Listen to the dog barking."). Label objects that you see or use ("Here's the washcloth.") and describe things you are doing ("Let's put the shirt over Kerry's head!").
- Look at your baby's face and make eye contact. Play face-making games: smile, stick out your tongue, open your eyes wide. As your baby gets older, he or she will try to imitate these facial expressions.
- Babies like music and rhythmic movement. Rock or swing your baby as you sing to him or her in a gentle voice.
- Acknowledge your baby's attempts to "answer" your talking and singing. He or she will respond to you by looking in your direction, making eye contact, moving his or her arms and legs, and/or making sounds.
- Babies like bright colors and vivid contrasts. Show your baby pictures and objects that are black and white, bright primary colors (red, blue, yellow, green), and/or large patterns. Keep colorful mobiles and toys where your baby can see them.
- Babies like to be held upright. Holding your newborn on your shoulder lets your baby look around his or her world and provides vestibular stimulation. Let your baby lift his or her head for a few seconds. Keep your hand ready to support your baby's head.

BOX 28-7 **Teaching Your 1- to 2-Month-Old Infant**

At age 1 to 2 months, your infant is gaining more control of his or her movements: more head control, even holding an object briefly in his or her hand. Your baby also is becoming more social. He or she demonstrates behaviors to engage you in interaction: smiling, cooing, making longer eye contact, and following you with his or her eyes.

During these months you can help your baby learn if you

- Put your baby on his or her stomach on a blanket on the floor. Lie on your stomach facing your baby. Talk to your baby to get him or her to raise his or her head to see you.
- Roll your baby onto his or her back and play with your baby's legs. Move the legs in a bicycle-riding motion. Try to get your baby to kick his or her legs.
- Play hand games, such as pat-a-cake, with your baby; kiss your baby's fingers; place your baby's hands on your face. Bring your baby's hands in front of his or her eyes as you play; get your baby to look at his or her hands.
- Encourage your baby to watch and follow things with his or her eyes. Use a noise-making toy, such as a rattle or a chime, or a brightly colored object about 12 inches from his or her eyes; move it slowly to one side and then the other. Objects hanging from a play frame are good for your baby to watch while he or she is on his or her back or sitting in an infant seat.
- Continue to talk and sing a lot to your baby. Continue to tell your baby what you are doing with him or her and what is going on in the immediate environment.
- Keep your baby near you during times when the family usually is together, such as at mealtimes. Infant seats, especially ones that bounce or rock, and infant swings are good to use at these times.

TABLE 28-2 **Play During Infancy: From Birth Through 3 Months**

AGE (MO)	VISUAL STIMULATION	AUDITORY STIMULATION	TACTILE STIMULATION	KINETIC STIMULATION
Suggested Activities				
Birth to 1	Look at infant at close range Hang bright, shiny object within 20 to 25 cm of infant's face and in midline Hang mobiles with black-and-white contrast designs	Talk to infant, sing in soft voice Play music box, radio, television Have ticking clock or metronome nearby	Hold, caress, cuddle Keep infant warm See if infant likes to be swaddled	Rock infant, place in cradle Use carriage for walks
2 to 3	Provide bright objects Make room bright with pictures or mirrors on walls Take infant to various rooms while doing chores Place infant in infant seat for vertical view of environment	Talk to infant Include in family gatherings Expose to various environmental noises other than those of home Use rattles, wind chimes	Caress infant while bathing, at diaper change Comb hair with a soft brush	Use infant swing Take in car for rides Exercise body by moving extremities in swimming motion Use cradle gym

From Hockenberry, M. et al. (2003). *Wong's nursing care of infants and children* (7th ed.). St. Louis: Mosby.

BOX 28-8 **Benefits of Infant Massage**

PSYCHOSOCIAL DOMAIN

Benefits to the Infant of Receiving Massage
- Promotes bonding and attachment
- Promotes body/mind/spirit connection
- Increases self-esteem
- Increases sense of love, acceptance, respect, and trust
- Enhances communication

Benefits to the Parent of Giving Massage
- Improves ability to read infant cues
- Improves synchrony between caregiver and infant
- Promotes bonding
- Increases confidence in parenting
- Increases communication—verbal and nonverbal
- Improves relaxation
- Provides time to share and quality time
- Promotes parenting skills

PHYSIOLOGIC/PHYSICAL GROWTH DOMAIN

Benefits to the Infant of Receiving Massage
- Improves relaxation and release of accumulated stress
- Stimulates circulation
- Strengthens digestive, circulatory, and GI systems, which can lead to weight gain
- Reduces discomfort from teething, congestion, gas, colic, and emotional stress
- Improves muscle tone/coordination
- Increases elimination, circulation, and respiration
- Improves sleep patterns
- Increases hormonal function

Benefits to the Parent of Giving Massage
- Improves sense of well-being
- Reduces blood pressure
- Reduces stress
- Improves overall health

From Schneider, E. (1997). Touch communication: The power of infant massage. *Massage Magazine, 68*, 40.

Another method of sensory enrichment that parents can learn to use is infant massage. This type of nurturing touch can help create a loving bond between the infant and parent and has been shown to contribute to the physical and emotional well-being of the massage giver and receiver (Schneider, 1996, 1997) (Box 28-8). Infant massage is not manipulative, but a gentle, warm communication done with the infant, not to the infant. The focus is on reciprocal interaction between infant and parent; the parent talks to the infant, asks permission to start the massage, questions the infant, and facilitates dialogue.

One of the most important skills for the parents is the improved ability to read their infant's cues (Schneider, 1997). Positive cues include eye contact, smiling, looking at the parent's face, babbling or cooing, and smooth movements of arms and legs. Negative cues from the infant include pulling away, frowning, grimacing, turning the head away, arching the back, crying, squirming, and flailing the arms and legs. Increased ability to read their infant's cues can increase parental confidence and self-esteem, thereby assisting adaptation to parenthood.

Well-Baby Follow-Up and Immunizations. Parents should be advised to plan for their infant's health follow-up care at the following ages: 2 to 4 weeks, and then every 2 months until 6 to 7 months; then every 3 months until 18 months, at 2 years, at 3 years, at preschool, and every 2 years thereafter. These well-baby follow-up visits with a nurse practitioner or pediatrician are important for the parents, as well as for the infant. They provide a time for parents to have questions answered, to receive reassurance about their adaptation to parenthood, and to receive anticipatory guidance for the ensuing weeks before the next well-baby visit.

The schedule for immunizations should be reviewed with parents (Table 28-3). An infant's ability to protect himself or herself against antigens by the formation of antibodies develops sequentially; therefore the infant must be developmentally capable of responding to these antibodies. This is the reason for planning sequential immunizations for infants.

TABLE 28-3 **Recommended Childhood Immunization Schedule**

VACCINES	AGE (THROUGH 18 MO)
DtaP (diphteria, tetanus, pertussis)	2, 4, 6 mo
Hep B (Hepatitis B)	Birth, 1-4 mo, 6-18 mo
HBIG (Hepatitis immune globulin)	Within 12 hours of birth if mother is HbsAG positive
Haemophilus influenzae type b	2, 4, 6, 12-15 mo
IPV (inactivated polio)	2, 4, 6-18 mo
MMR (measles, mumps, rubella)	12-15 mo
Varicella	12-18 mo
PCV (Pneumococcal)	2, 4, 6 mo

Data from Hockenberry, M. et al. (2003). *Wong's Nursing care of infants and children* (7th ed.). St. Louis: Mosby.

For additional information, see the National Immunization Program Website at www.cdc.gov/nip or call the National Immunization Hotline at 800-232-2522 (English) or 800-232-0233 (Spanish).

A form of passive immunity is already present in colostrum and breast milk. These antibodies are specific for microbes present in the mother's GI tract and protect against overgrowth as fresh colonization occurs in the term newborn.

The active ingredients in immunizations for diphtheria-pertussis-tetanus (DPT), hepatitis B, rubella, measles, and mumps, as well as the inactivated poliovirus vaccine (IPV), do not appear to be altered by breast milk and should be given according to the regular recommended schedule (Lawrence, 1999).

Recognizing Signs of Illness. As well as explaining the need for well-baby follow-up visits, the nurse should discuss with parents the signs of illness in newborns (Box 28-9). Parents should be advised to call their nurse practitioner or pediatrician immediately if they notice

BOX 28-9 **Signs of Illness to Report Immediately**

- Fever: temperature above 38° C axillary (under arm for 3 to 4 min); also, a continual increase in temperature
- Hypothermia: temperature below 36.6° C axillary
- Poor feeding or little interest in food: refusal to eat for two feedings in a row
- Vomiting: more than one episode of forceful vomiting or frequent vomiting (over a 6-hr period)
- Diarrhea: two consecutive green, watery stools (Note: Stools of breastfed infants are normally looser than stools of formula-fed infants. Diarrhea will leave a water ring around the stool, whereas breastfed stools will not.)
- Decreased bowel movement: less than two soiled diapers per day after 48 hr or fewer than three soiled diapers per day by day 5 of life
- Decreased urination: no wet diapers for 18 to 24 hr or fewer than six to eight wet diapers per day
- Breathing difficulties: labored breathing with flared nostrils or absence of breathing for more than 15 sec (Note: A newborn's breathing is normally irregular and between 30 to 40 breaths/min. Count the breaths for a full minute.)
- Cyanosis whether accompanying a feeding or not
- Lethargy: sleepiness, difficulty waking, or periods of sleep longer than 6 hr (Most newborns sleep for short periods, usually from 1 to 4 hr, and wake to be fed.)
- Inconsolable crying (attempts to quiet not effective) or continuous high-pitched cry
- Bleeding or purulent drainage from umbilical cord or circumcision
- Drainage developing in the eyes

such signs and to ask about over-the-counter medications, such as acetaminophen for infants, to keep at home (see Plan of Care).

Cardiopulmonary Resuscitation. Parents should receive instruction in relieving airway obstruction (see Emergency box) and CPR (see Emergency box). Often classes are offered in hospitals and clinics during the prenatal period or to parents of newborns. Such instruction is especially important for parents whose infants were preterm or had cardiac or respiratory problems. Babysitters also should learn CPR.

Evaluation

Evaluation is based on the expected outcomes of care. The plan is revised as needed, based on the evaluation findings.

HOME PHOTOTHERAPY

Healthy term infants may at times be discharged home and need phototherapy for hyperbilirubinemia (Fig. 28-6). Candidates for home phototherapy include those infants who are healthy and active with no signs and symptoms of other complications; the parents or other caregivers must be

Plan of Care: Home Care Follow-up: Transition to Parenthood

NURSING DIAGNOSIS Deficient knowledge of infant care related to lack of experience/lack of support

Expected Outcomes *Infant care routines are adequate, and infant appears healthy.*

Nursing Interventions/*Rationales*

Observe infant care routines (bathing, diapering, feeding, play) *to evaluate parental ease with care and adequacy of techniques.*

Observe infant appearance (height-weight ratio, head circumference, fontanels, skin tone and turgor); assess infant's vital signs, overall tone, reflexes, and age-appropriate developmental skills *to evaluate for signs indicative of inadequate care.*

Explore available support systems for infant care *to determine adequacy of existing system.*

Demonstrate troublesome care routines and have involved family members return demonstration *to facilitate improvements in care.*

Provide ongoing follow-up as needed *to remediate identified potential and actual care deficits.*

NURSING DIAGNOSIS Disturbed sleep pattern related to infant demands and environmental interruptions

Expected Outcomes *Woman sleeps for uninterrupted periods and feels rested on waking.*

Nursing Interventions/*Rationales*

Discuss woman's routine and specify things that interfere with sleep *to determine scope of problem and direct interventions.*

Explore ways woman and significant others can make environment more conducive to sleep (e.g., privacy, darkness, quiet, back rubs, soothing music, warm milk); teach use of guided imagery and relaxation techniques *to promote optimal conditions for sleep.*

Eliminate things or routines (e.g., caffeine, foods that induce heartburn, strenuous mental/physical activity) *that may interfere with sleep.*

Advise family to limit visitors and activities *to avoid further taxation and fatigue.*

Have family plan specific times to care for the newborn to allow mother time to sleep; have mother learn to use infant nap time as a time for her to nap as well *to replenish energy and decrease fatigue.*

NURSING DIAGNOSIS Risk for impaired home maintenance related to addition of new family member/inadequate resources/inadequate support systems

Expected Outcome *Home exhibits signs of safe and functional environment.*

Nursing Interventions/*Rationales*

Observe the home environment (e.g., available living space and sleeping arrangements; adequacy of facilities for food preparation and storage, hygiene and toileting; overall state of repair; cleanliness; presence of safety hazards) *to determine adequacy and effective use of resources.*

Observe arrangements for the newborn, such as sleeping space, care equipment and supplies (bathing, changing, feeding, transportation) *to determine adequacy of resources.*

Explore who is responsible for cooking, cleaning, child care, and newborn care and determine whether the mother seems adequately rested *to determine adequacy of support systems.*

Identify and arrange referrals to needed social agencies (e.g., Aid to Families with Dependent Children [AFDC], Women, Infants, and Children [WIC] program, food pantries) *to address resource deficits (finances, supplies, equipment).*

NURSING DIAGNOSIS Risk for interrupted family processes related to inclusion of new family member

Expected Outcome *Infant is successfully assimilated into family structure.*

Nursing Interventions/*Rationales*

Explore with family the ways that the birth and neonate have changed family structure and function *to evaluate functional and role adjustment.*

Observe family interaction with the newborn and note degree of bonding, evidence of sibling rivalry, and involvement in newborn care *to evaluate acceptance of newest family member.*

Clarify identified misinformation and misperceptions *to promote clear communication.*

Assist family to explore options for solutions to identified problems *to promote effective problem resolution.*

Support family efforts as they move toward adjusting and incorporating the new member *to reinforce new functions and roles.*

If needed, make referrals to appropriate social services or community agencies *to ensure ongoing support and care.*

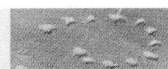

EMERGENCY

Relieving Airway Obstruction

Back blow and chest thrusts are used to clear an airway obstructed by a foreign body.

BACK BLOWS

Position the infant prone over forearm with the head down and the infant's jaw firmly supported.

Rest the supporting arm on the thigh.

Deliver four back blows forcefully between the infant's shoulder blades with the heel of the free hand.

TURN INFANT

Place the free hand on the infant's back to sandwich the baby between both hands; one hand supports the neck, jaw, and chest, while the other supports the back.

Turn the infant over, and place the head lower than the chest, supporting the head and neck.

Alternative position: Place the infant face down on your lap with the head lower than the trunk; firmly support the head. Apply back blows, and then turn the infant as a unit.

CHEST THRUSTS

Provide four downward chest thrusts on the lower third of the sternum.

Remove foreign body, if it is visible.

OPEN AIRWAY

Open airway with the head tilt–chin lift maneuver, and attempt to ventilate.

Repeat the sequence of back blows, turning, and chest thrusts.

Continue these emergency procedures until signs of recovery occur:

Palpable peripheral pulses return.

The pupils become normal in size and are responsive to light.

Mottling and cyanosis disappear.

Record the time and duration of the procedure and the effects of this intervention.

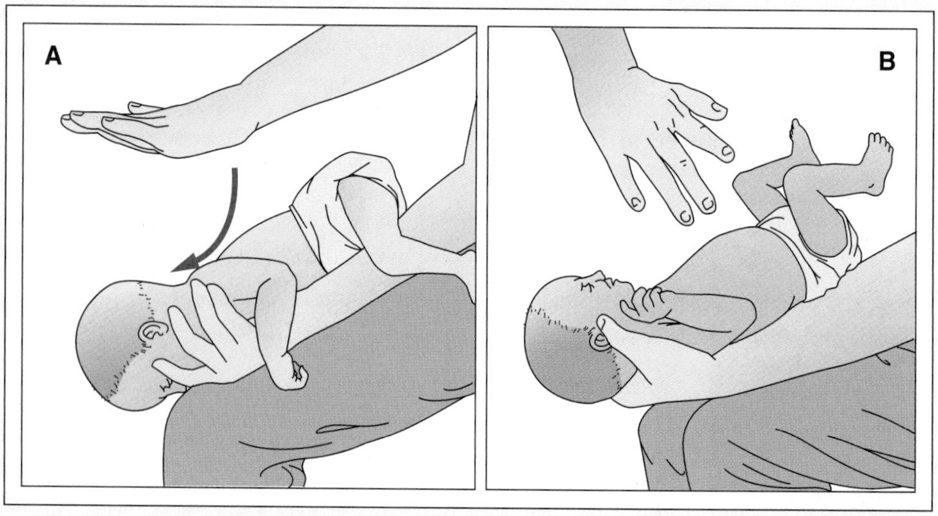
A
B

Back blows and chest thrust in infant to clear airway obstruction. **A,** Back blow. **B,** Chest thrust.

willing and able to assume responsibility for therapy maintenance and monitoring, and the home environment should be adequate with a telephone, heat, and electricity (University of California San Francisco Home Health Care [UCSF], 2001). Client considerations for administering home phototherapy are included in Box 28-10. Home health care nurses are usually responsible for assessing the parents' or other caregivers' willingness to use the equipment and monitor the infant (Box 28-11) and making home visits to assess the infant's response to therapy, including obtaining blood specimens for measuring bilirubin levels. The company that provides the home therapy equipment is responsible for setting up the phototherapy unit and teaching the parents/caregivers how to use the equipment. The home care nurse schedules home visits to assess the infant's response to therapy including weight, feeding, output, and temperature stability. Additional education of parents may be necessary; their understanding of the therapy and their responsibilities is assessed. Blood may be drawn for laboratory work, and results reported to the primary health care provider (UCSF Home Health Care, 2001). When therapy is discontinued, follow-up visits for monitoring may be ordered. The equipment company is called to arrange for pick-up of the phototherapy unit (UCSF Home Health Care, 2001).

EMERGENCY

Cardiopulmonary Resuscitation (CPR)

Wash hands before and after touching infant and equipment. Wear gloves, if possible.

ASSESS RESPONSIVENESS

Observe color; tap or gently shake shoulders.

Yell for help; if alone, perform CPR for 1 min before calling for help again.

POSITION INFANT

Turn the infant onto back, supporting the head and neck.

Place the infant on firm, flat surface.

AIRWAY

Open the airway with the head tilt–chin lift method.

Place one hand on the infant's forehead, and tilt the head back.

Place the fingers of other hand under the bone of the lower jaw at the chin.

BREATHING

Assess for evidence of breathing:

Observe for chest movement.

Listen for exhaled air.

Feel for exhaled air flow.

To breathe for infant:

Take a breath.

Place mouth over the infant's nose and mouth to create a seal.

NOTE: When available, a mask with a one-way valve should be used.

Give two slow breaths (1 to 1.5 sec/breath), pausing to inhale between breaths.

NOTE: Gently puff the volume of air in your cheeks into infant. Do not force air.

The infant's chest should rise slightly with each puff; keep fingers on the chest wall to sense air entry.

CIRCULATION

Assess circulation:

Check pulse of the brachial artery while maintaining the head tilt.

If the pulse is present, initiate rescue breathing. Continue doing once every 3 sec or 20 times/min until spontaneous breathing resumes.

If the pulse is absent, initiate chest compressions and coordinate them with breathing.

Chest compression

There are two systems of chest compression. Nurses should know both methods.

Maintain the head tilt and

1. Place thumbs side-by-side in the middle third of the sternum with fingers around the chest and supporting the back.
   - Compress the sternum 1.25 to 2 cm.
2. Place index finger of hand just under an imaginary line drawn between the nipples. Place the middle and ring fingers on the sternum adjacent to the index finger.
   - Using the middle and ring fingers, compress the sternum approximately 1.25 to 2.5 cm.

Avoid compressing the xiphoid process.

Release the pressure without moving the thumbs/fingers from the chest.

Repeat at least 100 times/min, doing five compressions in 3 sec or less.

Perform 10 cycles of five compressions and one ventilation.

After the cycles, check the brachial artery to determine whether there is a pulse.

Discontinue compressions when the infant's spontaneous heart rate reaches or exceeds 80 beats/min.

Record the time and duration of the procedure and the effects of intervention.

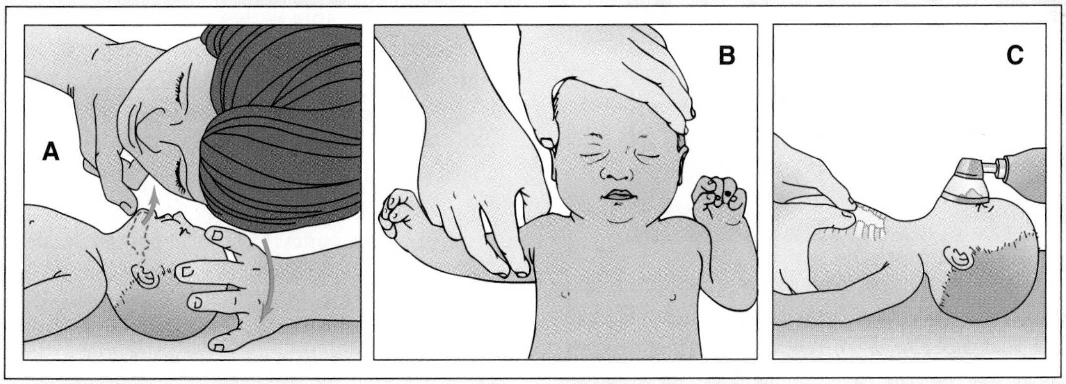
A
B
C

A, Opening airway with head tilt–chin lift method. **B,** Checking pulse of brachial artery. **C,** Side-by-side thumb placement for chest compressions in newborn.

Source: Stapleton, E. et al. (2001). *Fundamentals of BLS for healthcare providers.* Dallas, TX: American Heart Association.

A

B

C

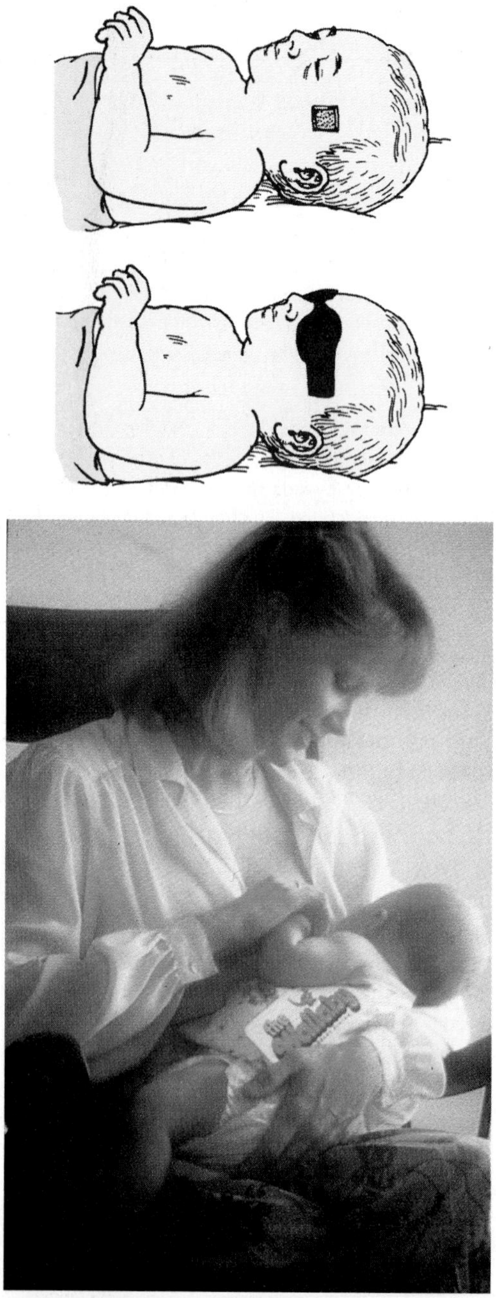

FIG. 28-6 Eyepatches for newborns receiving phototherapy. **A,** Small Velcro patch stuck to both sides of head. **B,** Eye cover sticks to Velcro patch, which reduces movement of eye cover and facilitates removal for feedings. **C,** A mother can breastfeed her baby without interrupting phototherapy. Eye patches are worn when infant is under bililights but not when a biliblanket is used. (**C,** Courtesy Respironics, Inc., Pittsburgh, PA.)

BOX 28-10 Considerations for Administering Infant Home Phototherapy

Infant >36 weeks' gestation
Infant age >24 hr
Birthweight >2300 g
Breast or bottle feeding well
Weight loss <10% of birth weight
Stooling and voiding by 24 hr of age; continued adequate amount
Not at risk for sepsis
Blood work results
- Coombs <1+
- ABO compatible or evidence of resolving initial hyperbilirubinemia
- Central hematocrit <65%
- Direct bilirubin <1.5 mg/100 ml
- If bilirubin history is known
  - <10 mg/100 ml at 24 hr
  - <15 mg/100 ml at 48 hr
  - <20 mg/100 ml at 72 hr

From University of California San Francisco Home Health Care.

BOX 28-11 Parent Information for Home Phototherapy Using a Biliblanket

Notify your child's health care provider if
- A notable change is seen in activity level
- The infant's temperature is not maintained at >97° F or <100° F
- The infant is feeding poorly
- The infant is not voiding ≥6 times per day or does not void within a 6-hr period
- Infant vomits two or more feedings

Notify your Home Care Agency if
- Phototherapy is discontinued
- An equipment malfunction occurs

Information for parents:
- As much of the infant's skin as possible should be in direct contact with the lighted section of the pad. The infant's back or chest should be placed directly on the pad, with the tip of the pad at the shoulder and the cable at the feet
- Follow the equipment supplier's instructions regarding safety and use of the phototherapy unit
- Phototherapy can be discontinued for brief periods without harming your baby
- Temperature instability may occur when starting and stopping phototherapy and when collecting laboratory specimens
- Effects of phototherapy may include changes in frequency and color of the infant's stools and rash due to an increase in the number of loose stools

From University of California San Francisco Home Health Care.

KEY POINTS

- Anticipatory guidance helps prepare new parents for what to expect.
- Topics to include in parent teaching include feeding, elimination, care of the circumcised infant, crying, behavior, sleeping, signs of illness, and community resources including support groups.
- Parents may need assistance in providing a protective environment for the infant.
- Instruction in infant CPR is often provided to new parents.
- Nurses are responsible for teaching parents about home phototherapy when it is ordered and for monitoring the infant's response to therapy.

CRITICAL THINKING EXERCISES

1. Joy is a 21-year-old primiparous single mother of a 2-week-old baby; Joy called the nurse advice line. She was distraught and crying, stating, "My baby is crying all the time, and I don't know what to do. I fed him and changed him and he just keeps crying. What is the matter with him? I can't stand his crying anymore." What should the nurse's initial response be? What are some causes of infant crying? What questions should the nurse ask? To what resources can Joy be referred? Make a handout listing ways to soothe infants that could be distributed to parents.
2. The home care nurse made a home visit when Mariah was 1 week old. The infant was in a crib near an outside window. Mariah's mother said she placed a pillow under Mariah's head to keep it from being flat. When you observed the infant, she was sleeping on her abdomen, and several blankets were scattered in the crib. When you weighed her, you noted that she had regained her birth weight. From your observations, what positive comments can you make to the mother about Mariah? What advice could be given to Mariah's mother to provide a protective environment for Mariah? What changes in her environment should be suggested?

RESOURCES

At-Home Dad (newsletter for fathers who stay at home)
61 Brightwood Avenue
North Andover, MA 01845-1702
E-mail: athomedad@aol.com

The Fatherhood Project at the Families and Work Institute
330 Seventh Avenue
New York, NY 10001
212-465-2044

The Institute for Responsible Fatherhood and Family Revitalization
1146 19th Street NW
Suite 800
Washington, DC 20036
800-732-8437 or 800-7-FATHER

Infant Massage: A Handbook for Loving Parents
Vimala McClure
International Association of Infant Massage (IAIM)
800-248-5432

La Leche League International
1400 North Meacham Road
Schaumburg, IL 60168-4079
847-519-7730
(Local La Leche League groups are usually listed in city and town phone books)

Motherhood Maternity Health and Fitness Program
SBI Corporation
1106 Stratford Drive
Carlisle, PA 17013
717-258-4641

Neonatology on the Web
www.neonatology.org

Pink Inc.! Publishing
P.O. Box 866
Atlantic Beach, FL 32233-0866
904-731-7120

Postpartum Support International
927 North Kellogg Avenue
Santa Barbara, CA 93111
805-967-7636

Protecting Your Newborn, Video and Instructor's Guide (1997)
Ford Motor Company and the U.S. Department of Transportation National Highway Traffic Safety Administration (NHTSA)
Auto Safety Hotline 800-424-9393
www.nhtsa.dot.gov

Single Parent Resource Center
141 West 28th Street
Suite 302
New York, NY 10001
212-947-0221

REFERENCES

Association of Women's Health, Obstetrics, and Neonatal Nurses (AWHONN). (2001). *Neonatal skin care evidence-based clinical practice guidelines.* Washington, DC: AWHONN.

Blum, N. et al. (2002). Maternal ratings of infant intensity and distractibility: Relationship with crying duration in the second month of life. *Archives of Pediatric and Adolescent Medicine, 156*(3), 286-290.

Brazelton, T. (1995). Working with families: Opportunities for early intervention. *Pediatric Clinics of North America, 42*(1), 1-9.

Brazelton, T., & Nugent, J. (1996). *Neonatal behavioural assessment scale* (3rd ed.). London: MacKeith.

Darmstadt, G., & Dinulos, J. (2000). Neonatal skin care. *Pediatric Clinics of North America, 47*, 757-782.

Dore, S. et al. (1998). Alcohol versus natural drying for newborn cord care. *Journal of Obstetric, Gynecologic, and Neonatal Nursing, 27*, 621-627.

Franck, L., Quinn, D., & Zahr, L. (2000). Effects of less frequent bathing of preterm infants on skin flora and pathogen colonization. *Journal of Obstetric, Gynecologic, and Neonatal Nursing, 29*, 584-589.

Hockenberry, M. et al. (2003). *Wong's nursing care of infants and children* (7th ed.). St. Louis: Mosby.

Johnson & Johnson. (1996). *Compendium of postpartum care.* Skillman, NJ: Johnson & Johnson Consumer Products.

Lawrence, R. (1999). *Breastfeeding: A guide for the medical profession* (5th ed.). St. Louis: Mosby.

Medoff-Cooper, B., Carey, W., & McDevitt, S. (1993). The early infancy temperament questionnaire. *Journal of Development and Behavioral Pediatrics, 14*, 230-235.

Pinelli, J., & Symington, A. (2001). Non-nutritive sucking for the promotion of physiologic stability and nutrition in preterm infants. *The Cochrane Library,* Issue 1, Oxford: Update Software.

Schneider, E. (1996). The power of touch: Massage for infants. *Infants and Young Children, 8*(3), 40-55.

Schneider, E. (1997). Touch communication: The power of infant massage. *Massage Magazine, 68*, 40.

St. James-Roberts, I., Conroy, S., & Wilsher, K. (1996). Bases for maternal perceptions of infant crying and colic behaviour. *Archives of Disease in Childhood, 75*(5), 375-384

Stapleton, E. et al. (2001). *Fundamentals of BLS for healthcare providers.* Dallas, TX: American Heart Association.

University of California San Francisco Home Health Care. (2001). *Guidelines for home therapy.* San Francisco: University of California.

Varda, K., & Behnke, R. (2000). The effect of timing of initial bath on newborn's temperature. *Journal of Obstetric, Gynecologic, and Neonatal Nursing, 29*, 27-32.

Wong, D. (1999). *Whaley and Wong's nursing care of infants and children* (6th ed.). St. Louis: Mosby.

Zuspan, J., & Garner, P. (2000). Topical umbilical cord care at birth. (Cochrane Review). *The Cochrane Library*, Issue 3. Oxford: Update Software.

CHAPTER 29

Cynthia Garrett

Assessment for Risk Factors

http://evolve.elsevier.com/Lowdermilk/MatWmnHlth/

LEARNING OBJECTIVES

- Explore the scope of high risk pregnancy.
- Discuss regionalization of health care services.
- Examine risk factors identified through client history, physical examination, and diagnostic techniques.
- Describe diagnostic techniques and the implications of findings.
- Explain diagnostic techniques and test results to clients and their families.

Approximately 500,000 of the 4 million births that occur in the United States each year will be categorized as high risk because of maternal or fetal complications. Identification of the risks, together with appropriate and timely intervention during the perinatal period, can prevent morbidity and mortality among mothers and infants.

With the changing demographics in the United States, more women and families can be identified as at risk because of factors other than biophysical criteria. The increasing numbers of homeless, single, or uninsured pregnant women who have no access to prenatal care during any stage of pregnancy and the behaviors and lifestyles that pose a risk to the health of the mother and fetus contribute to the problem (U.S. Department of Health and Human Services, 2000).

Care of these high risk clients requires the unified efforts of medical and nursing personnel. The high risk client and the factors associated with a diagnosis of high risk are identified in this chapter; diagnostic techniques used to monitor the maternal-fetal unit are emphasized.

DEFINITION AND SCOPE OF THE PROBLEM

A **high risk pregnancy** is one in which the life or health of the mother or fetus is jeopardized by a disorder coincidental with or unique to pregnancy. For the mother, the high risk status arbitrarily extends through the puerperium (30 days after childbirth). Postbirth maternal complications are usually resolved within 1 month of birth, but perinatal morbidity may continue for months or years.

Advances in the management of disorders that affect pregnant women have resulted in a significant decrease in maternal mortality and morbidity rates. In the United States, maternal mortality rates remained the same between 1980 and 1998 at 7 to 8 per 100,000; in 2000 the rate was 9.8, but this increase was attributed to a change in reporting rather than to an actual increase (Minino et al., 2002).

However, the decline in perinatal mortality and morbidity is not so significant and must be examined when the scope of high risk pregnancy is being considered. Infant mortality rates have shown improvement, dropping from 10 per 1000 live births in 1970 to 6.9 per 1000 live births in 2000, the lowest ever recorded in the United States. Compared with other developed countries the United States still ranks poorly in infant mortality (Hoyert et al., 2001).

High risk pregnancy is a critical problem for modern medical and nursing care. The new social emphasis on the quality of life and the wanted child has resulted in a reduction of family size and the number of unwanted pregnancies. At the same time, technologic advances have facilitated pregnancies in previously infertile couples. As a consequence, emphasis is on the safe birth of normal infants who can develop to their potential. Scientific and technologic advances have allowed perinatal health care to reach a level far beyond that previously available.

The diagnosis of high risk imposes a situational crisis on the family (e.g., loss of pregnancy before the anticipated date, development of gestational diabetes mellitus with its potential complications, or birth of a neonate who does not meet cultural, societal, or familial norms and expectations).

Maternal Health Problems

The leading causes of maternal death attributable to pregnancy differ over the world. In general, three major causes have persisted for the last 50 years: hypertensive disorders, infection, and hemorrhage. The three leading causes of maternal mortality today are pregnancy-induced hypertension, pulmonary embolism, and hemorrhage. Factors that are strongly related to maternal death include age (younger than 20 years and 35 years or older), lack of prenatal care, low educational attainment, unmarried status, and nonwhite race. African-American maternal mortality rates are more than 3 times higher than those for Caucasian women (Minino et al., 2002). Even though the United States maternal death rate remained between 7 and 8 per 100,000 live births in the 1990s, the goal set by Healthy People 2010 was no more than 3.3 maternal deaths per 100,000 live births (U.S. Department of Health and Human Services, 2000). Reaching this goal will be a significant challenge.

Although the overall number of maternal deaths is small, maternal mortality remains a significant problem because a high proportion of deaths are preventable, primarily through improving the access to and use of prenatal care services. Nurses can be instrumental in educating the public about the importance of obtaining early and regular care during pregnancy.

Fetal and Neonatal Health Problems

Fetal and neonatal health problems are described under certain categories: fetal death, neonatal death, perinatal death, perinatal death rate, and infant mortality. (Definitions for these terms are found in Chapter 1.) The incidence of each disorder that results in infant mortality is expressed as the number of deaths per 1000 live births. The infant mortality rate includes neonatal deaths.

The leading cause of death in the neonatal period is congenital anomalies (Hoyert et al., 2001). Other causes of neonatal death include disorders related to short gestation and low birth weight, sudden infant death, respiratory distress syndrome, and the effects of maternal complications. Racial differences in the infant mortality rates continue to challenge public health experts. Increased rates of survival during the neonatal period have resulted largely from high quality prenatal care and the improvement in perinatal services, including technologic advances in neonatal intensive care and obstetrics. These factors may account for at least a 50% reduction in mortality in neonates weighing less than 1500 g (Richardson et al., 1998). However, antepartum fetal deaths account for approximately 50% of all perinatal mortality.

What can be done to prevent antepartum fetal deaths? Some factors are presumed avoidable such as failure to respond appropriately to abnormalities of pregnancy and labor. Such abnormalities may include results of fetal growth or fetal well-being assessments, significant maternal weight loss, or decreased fetal movements (Druzin, Gabbe, & Reed, 2002). Additionally, commitment at national, state, and local levels is required to reduce the infant mortality rate. More research is needed to identify the extent to which financial, educational, sociocultural, and behavioral factors individually and collectively affect perinatal morbidity and mortality. Barriers to care must be removed and perinatal services modified to meet contemporary health care needs (Dooley, Freels, & Turnock, 1997).

Regionalization of Health Care Services

Early and ongoing risk assessment is a crucial component of perinatal care. Conditions associated with perinatal morbidity and mortality can be prevented, treated, or referred to more skilled health care providers. Factors to consider when determining a client's risk status include resources available locally to treat the condition, availability of appropriate facilities for transport if needed, and determination of the best match for the client's needs.

Not all facilities develop and maintain the full spectrum of services required for high risk perinatal clients. As a consequence, the concept of regionalization of health

GUIDELINES/GUÍAS

High Risk Factors

HIGH RISK ASSESSMENT	POTENTIAL PROBLEM
Have you had any problems with this pregnancy? *¿Ha tenido algún problema con este embarazo?*	General assessment
Have you had blurred vision? *¿Ha tenido la vista borrosa?*	PIH
Have you had severe headaches? *¿Ha tenido dolores fuertes de cabeza?*	PIH
Have you had difficulty breathing? *¿Ha tenido dificultad para respirar?*	Cardiac disease
Have you had heart palpitations? *¿Ha tenido palpitaciones del corazón?*	Cardiac disease
Have you been vomiting? *¿Ha estado vomitando?*	Hyperemesis gravidarum
Have you had any infections? *¿Ha tenido alguna infección?*	STIs/vaginal infections
Have you had swelling? *¿Ha tenido hinchazón?*	PIH
Were all your pregnancies term? *¿Llegaron a las cuarenta semanas todos sus embarazos?*	Preterm labor
Have you ever had diabetes? *¿Ha tenido diabetes?*	Diabetes
Have you ever had high blood pressure? *¿Ha tenido presión alta?*	PIH
Have you ever had anemia? *¿Ha tenido anemia?*	Anemia
Do you take drugs? Prescription medicine? *¿Toma drogas? ¿Medicina recetada?*	Substance abuse
Do you drink alcohol? Smoke? *¿Toma alcohol? ¿Fuma?*	Substance abuse

care services–facilities within a geographic region organized to provide different levels of care–emerged.

However, regionalization alone has not consistently improved perinatal outcomes (Dooley et al., 1997). Furthermore, managed care markets and other financial pressures have forced some providers to be more competitive. To meet this challenge, facilities began to extend the kind of perinatal services offered. Perinatal services in some areas were duplicated, creating an imbalance in the provision of services within a geographic area.

Clearer guidelines were established regarding the level of care that could be expected at any given facility. In ambulatory settings, providers must distinguish themselves by the level of care they provide. *Basic care* is provided by obstetricians, family physicians, certified nurse midwives, and other advanced practice clinicians approved by local governance. Routine risk-oriented prenatal care, education, and support is provided. Providers offering *specialty care* are obstetricians who must provide fetal diagnostic testing and management of obstetric and medical complications in addition to basic care. *Subspecialty care* is provided by maternal-fetal medicine specialists and includes the aforementioned in addition to genetic testing, advanced fetal therapies, and management of severe maternal and fetal complications (American Academy of Pediatrics/American College of Obstetricians and Gynecologists [AAP/ACOG], 1997).

In hospital settings, perinatal services also are designated as basic, specialty, or subspecialty. Criteria for basic perinatal services include care of all clients admitted to the service, with an established triage system for high risk clients who should be transferred to a higher level of care; ability to perform a cesarean birth within 30 minutes of a decision to do so; availability of blood and blood products; availability of radiology, anesthesia, and laboratory services on a 24-hour basis; presence of nursery and postpartum care; resuscitation and stabilization of all neonates born in hospital; availability of transport for all sick neonates; family visitation; and data collection and retrieval (AAP/ACOG, 1997).

Specialty hospital care includes these requirements in addition to care of high risk mothers and fetuses, stabilization of ill neonates before transfer, and care of preterm infants with a birth weight of 1500 g or more. Women in preterm labor or those with impending births of 32 weeks of gestation or less should be transferred for subspecialty care. Other criteria for subspecialty care include comprehensive prenatal services, research and educational support, and use of high risk technologies. Collaboration among providers to meet the client's needs is the key in reducing perinatal morbidity and mortality (AAP/ACOG, 1997).

Assessment of Risk Factors

Pregnancies can be designated as high risk for any of several undesirable outcomes. Those considered to be at risk for uteroplacental insufficiency carry a serious threat for fetal growth restriction, intrauterine fetal death, intrapartum death, intrapartum fetal distress, and various types of neonatal morbidity.

In the past, risk factors were evaluated only from a medical viewpoint; thus only adverse medical, obstetric, or physiologic conditions were considered to place the woman at risk. Today, a more comprehensive approach to high risk pregnancy is used, and the factors associated with high risk childbearing are grouped into broad categories based on threats to health and pregnancy outcome (see Guidelines/Guías box). Categories of risk are biophysical, psychosocial, sociodemographic, and environmental (Gilbert & Harmon, 2003) (Box 29-1).

BOX 29-1 Categories of High Risk Factors

BIOPHYSICAL FACTORS

1. *Genetic considerations*. Genetic factors may interfere with normal fetal or neonatal development, result in congenital anomalies, or create difficulties for the mother. These factors include defective genes, transmissible inherited disorders and chromosome anomalies, multiple pregnancy, large fetal size, and ABO incompatibility.
2. *Nutritional status*. Adequate nutrition, without which fetal growth and development cannot proceed normally, is one of the most important determinants of pregnancy outcome. Conditions that influence nutritional status include the following: young age; three pregnancies in the previous 2 years; tobacco, alcohol, or drug use; inadequate dietary intake because of chronic illness or food fads; inadequate or excessive weight gain; and hematocrit value <33%.
3. *Medical and obstetric disorders*. Complications of current and past pregnancies, obstetric-related illnesses, and pregnancy losses put the client at risk (see Box 29-3).

PSYCHOSOCIAL FACTORS

1. *Smoking*. A strong, consistent, causal relation has been established between maternal smoking and reduced birth weight. Risks include low-birth-weight infants, higher neonatal mortality rates, increased miscarriages, and increased incidence of premature rupture of membranes. These risks are aggravated by low socioeconomic status, poor nutritional status, and concurrent use of alcohol.
2. *Caffeine*. Birth defects in humans have not been related to caffeine consumption. High intake (three or more cups of coffee per day) has been related to a slight decrease in birth weight.

Continued

3. *Alcohol.* Although its exact effects in pregnancy have not been quantified and its mode of action is largely unexplained, alcohol exerts adverse effects on the fetus, resulting in fetal alcohol syndrome, fetal alcohol effects, learning disabilities, and hyperactivity.
4. *Drugs.* The developing fetus may be adversely affected by drugs through several mechanisms. They can be teratogenic, cause metabolic disturbances, produce chemical effects, or cause depression or alteration of CNS function. This category includes medications prescribed by a health care provider or bought over the counter, as well as commonly abused drugs such as heroin, cocaine, and marijuana. (See Chapter 35 for more information about drug and alcohol abuse.)
5. *Psychologic status.* Childbearing triggers profound and complex physiologic, psychologic, and social changes, with evidence to suggest a relation between emotional distress and birth complications. This risk factor includes conditions such as specific intrapsychic disturbances and addictive lifestyles; a history of child or spouse abuse; inadequate support systems; family disruption or dissolution; maternal role changes or conflicts; noncompliance with cultural norms; unsafe cultural, ethnic, or religious practices; and situational crises.

SOCIODEMOGRAPHIC FACTORS

1. *Low income.* Poverty underlies many other risk factors and leads to inadequate financial resources for food and prenatal care, poor general health, increased risk of medical complications of pregnancy, and greater prevalence of adverse environmental influences.
2. *Lack of prenatal care.* Failure to diagnose and treat complications early is a major risk factor arising from financial barriers or lack of access to care; depersonalization of the system resulting in long waits, routine visits, variability in health care personnel, and unpleasant physical surroundings; lack of understanding of the need for early and continued care or cultural beliefs that do not support the need; and fear of the health care system and its providers.
3. *Age.* Women at both ends of the childbearing age spectrum have a higher incidence of poor outcomes; however, age may not be a risk factor in all cases. Both physiologic and psychologic risks should be evaluated.
   a. *Adolescents.* More complications are seen in young mothers (younger than 15 years), who have a 60% higher mortality rate than those older than 20 years, and in pregnancies occurring <6 years after menarche. Complications include anemia, pregnancy-induced hypertension (PIH), prolonged labor, and contracted pelvis and cephalopelvic disproportion. Long-term social implications of early motherhood are lower educational status, lower income, increased dependence on government support programs, higher divorce rates, and higher parity.
   b. *Mature mothers.* The risks to older mothers are not from age alone but from other considerations such as number and spacing of previous pregnancies; genetic disposition of the parents; and medical history, lifestyle, nutrition, and prenatal care. The increased likelihood of chronic diseases and complications that arises from more invasive medical management of a pregnancy and labor combined with demographic characteristics put an older woman at risk. Medical conditions more likely to be experienced by mature women include hypertension and PIH, diabetes, extended labor, cesarean birth, placenta previa, abruptio placentae, and mortality. Her fetus is at greater risk for low birth weight and macrosomia, chromosomal abnormalities, congenital malformations, and neonatal mortality.
4. *Parity.* The number of previous pregnancies is a risk factor associated with age and includes all first pregnancies, especially a first pregnancy at either end of the childbearing age continuum. The incidence of PIH and dystocia is higher with a first birth.
5. *Marital status.* The increased mortality and morbidity rates for unmarried women, including a greater risk for PIH, are often related to inadequate prenatal care and a younger childbearing age.
6. *Residence.* The availability and quality of prenatal care varies widely with geographic residence. Women in metropolitan areas have more prenatal visits than do those in rural areas, who have fewer opportunities for specialized care and consequently a higher incidence of maternal mortality. Health care in the inner city, where residents are usually poorer and begin childbearing earlier and continue for longer, may be of lower quality than in a more affluent neighborhood.
7. *Ethnicity.* Although ethnicity by itself is not a major risk, race is an indicator of other sociodemographic risk factors. Nonwhite women are more than 3 times as likely as Caucasian women to die of pregnancy-related causes. African-American babies have the highest rates of prematurity and low birth weight, with the infant mortality rate among African-Americans being more than double that for Caucasians.

ENVIRONMENTAL FACTORS

Various environmental substances can affect fertility and fetal development, the chance of a live birth, and the child's subsequent mental and physical development. Environmental influences include infections, radiation, chemicals such as pesticides, therapeutic drugs, illicit drugs, industrial pollutants, cigarette smoke, stress, and diet. Paternal exposure to mutagenic agents in the workplace has been associated with an increased risk of miscarriage.

BOX 29-2 Antepartum Cultural Assessment

All cultures recognize pregnancy as a special transitional period, and particular customs and beliefs dictate behavior during this time. In the antepartum period, the nurse should assess the following:

- Beliefs of whether pregnancy is a state of illness or health
- Behavioral expectations of the mother and of the health care provider
- Dietary prescriptions or restrictions (e.g., hot/cold balance theory, pica)
- Activity restrictions or prescriptions (e.g., use of massage)
- Availability of advice (e.g., from whom and at what time advice will be sought and when prenatal care will begin [if at all])
- Considerations of modesty

Biophysical risks include factors that originate within the mother or fetus and affect the development or functioning of either one or both. Examples include genetic disorders, nutritional and general health status, and medical or obstetric-related illnesses.

Psychosocial risks comprise maternal behaviors and adverse lifestyles that have a negative effect on the health of the mother or fetus. These risks may include emotional distress and disturbed interpersonal relationships, as well as inadequate social support and unsafe cultural practices (Box 29-2).

Sociodemographic risks arise from the mother and her family. These risks may place the mother and fetus at risk. Examples include lack of prenatal care, low income, marital status, and ethnicity (see Box 29-1).

Environmental factors include hazards in the workplace and the woman's general environment and may include noxious chemicals, radiation, infections, and pollutants.

Risk factors are interrelated and cumulative in their effects. Box 29-3 lists specific pregnancy problems and risk

BOX 29-3 Specific Pregnancy Problems and Related Risk Factors

PRETERM LABOR
Age younger than 16 or older than 35 years
Low socioeconomic status
Maternal weight <50 kg
Poor nutrition
Previous preterm birth
Incompetent cervix
Uterine anomalies
Smoking
Drug addiction and alcohol abuse
Pyelonephritis, pneumonia
Multiple gestation
Anemia
Abnormal fetal presentation
Preterm rupture of membranes
Placental abnormalities
Infection
Abdominal surgery in current pregnancy
History of cervical surgery

POLYHYDRAMNIOS
Diabetes mellitus
Multiple gestation
Fetal congenital anomalies
Isoimmunization (Rh or ABO)
Nonimmune hydrops
Abnormal fetal presentation

INTRAUTERINE GROWTH RESTRICTION (IUGR)
Multiple gestation
Poor nutrition
Maternal cyanotic heart disease
Prior pregnancy with IUGR
Maternal collagen diseases
Chronic hypertension
Pregnancy-induced hypertension
Recurrent antepartum hemorrhage
Smoking
Maternal diabetes with vascular problems
Fetal infections
Fetal cardiovascular anomalies
Drug addiction and alcohol abuse
Fetal congenital anomalies
Hemoglobinopathies

OLIGOHYDRAMNIOS
Renal agenesis (Potter's syndrome)
Prolonged rupture of membranes
IUGR
Intrauterine fetal death

POSTTERM PREGNANCY
Anencephaly
Placental sulfatase deficiency
Perinatal hypoxia, acidosis
Placental insufficiency

CHROMOSOMAL ABNORMALITIES
Maternal age 35 years or older
Balanced translocation (maternal and paternal)

From DeCherney, A., & Pernoll, M. (Eds.). (1994). *Current obstetric and gynecologic diagnosis and treatment* (8th ed.). Norwalk, CT: Appleton & Lange.

factors. Risk factors for the postpartum woman and newborn are shown in Box 29-4.

The development of a comprehensive database for pregnancy risk assessment will help generate appropriate nursing diagnoses. For example, use of functional health patterns can be the basis for an assessment tool (Box 29-5).

BIOPHYSICAL ASSESSMENT

The major expected outcome of all antepartum testing is the detection of potential fetal compromise. Ideally the technique used identifies fetal compromise before intrauterine asphyxia of the fetus so that the health care provider can take measures to prevent or minimize adverse perinatal outcomes. No single test can provide this

BOX 29-4 Factors That Place the Postpartum Woman and Neonate at High Risk

MOTHER

- Hemorrhage
- Infection
- Abnormal vital signs
- Traumatic labor or birth
- Psychosocial factors

INFANT (FOR ADMISSION TO NICU)

High Risk

- Infants who continue with or develop signs of RDS or other respiratory distress
- Asphyxiated infants (Apgar score <6 at 5 min), resuscitation required at birth
- Preterm infants, dysmature infants
- Infants with cyanosis or suspected cardiovascular disease, persistent cyanosis
- Infants with major congenital malformations requiring surgery, chromosomal anomalies
- Infants with convulsions, sepsis, hemorrhagic diathesis, or shock
- Meconium aspiration syndrome
- CNS depression for >24 hr
- Hypoglycemia
- Hypocalcemia
- Hyperbilirubinemia

Moderate Risk

- Dysmaturity
- Prematurity (weight between 2000 and 2500 g)
- Apgar score <5 at 1 min
- Feeding problems
- Multifetal birth
- Transient tachypnea
- Hypomagnesemia or hypermagnesemia
- Hypoparathyroidism
- Failure to gain weight
- Jitteriness or hyperactivity
- Cardiac anomalies not requiring immediate catheterization
- Heart murmur
- Anemia
- CNS depression for <24 hr

CNS, Central nervous system; *NICU,* neonatal intensive care unit; *RDS,* respiratory distress syndrome.

BOX 29-5 Assessment for High Risk Pregnancy with Functional Health Patterns

For each of the following functional health patterns, the nurse includes questions that will provide data about the individual woman, her family, her community, and her cultural practices and beliefs:

- *Health perception/health management pattern.* Current health, medical history, family medical history, environmental/chemical exposure, family decision making about health, community resources, beliefs about health care during pregnancy
- *Nutritional-metabolic pattern.* Nutritional status, knowledge of pregnancy needs, pregnancy discomforts, community resources (WIC), cultural eating practices
- *Elimination pattern.* Urinary and bowel patterns, family or cultural practices (laxatives), community waste/sanitation services
- *Activity-exercise pattern.* Usual exercise, recreation, community resources, cultural practices or taboos for activities during pregnancy
- *Sleep-rest pattern.* Usual sleep patterns, use of remedies, family sleep arrangements, cultural beliefs about sleep and rest in pregnancy
- *Cognitive-perceptual pattern.* Communication problems, knowledge deficits about pregnancy and birth (individual and family), community resources for support for high risk pregnant clients, cultural beliefs about pain and its management
- *Self-perception/self-concept pattern.* Body image, responses of family to high risk pregnancy, housing conditions, cultural practices about parenting
- *Role-relationship pattern.* Feelings of security, occupation, hobbies, family living arrangements, community resources
- *Sexuality-reproductive pattern.* Sexual activities, problems, restrictions, obstetric history, current obstetric status, cultural beliefs about sexual practices during pregnancy
- *Coping-stress pattern.* Life stressors, losses experienced, coping mechanisms, support systems, community resources, spiritual or religious practices or beliefs that are important

Data from Gilbert, E., & Harmon, J. (2003). *Manual of high risk pregnancy and delivery* (3rd ed.). St. Louis: Mosby; Gordon, M. (2002). *Manual of nursing diagnosis* (10th ed.). St. Louis: Mosby.

information. Assessment tests should be selected based on their effectiveness, and the results must be interpreted in light of the complete clinical picture. The most reliable evidence for effectiveness is provided by randomized controlled trials (ACOG, 1999). Nurses can be informed about the most recent research on fetal assessment by using an up-to-date systematic review such as the Cochrane Database of Systematic Reviews (Enkin et al., 2001). Table 29-1 lists the evidence for recommending care for fetal assessment screening based on this database.

Daily Fetal Movement Count

Assessment of fetal activity by the mother is a simple yet valuable method for monitoring the condition of the fetus. The **daily fetal movement count (DFMC)** (also called "kick counts") can be done at home, is noninvasive, is simple to understand, and usually does not interfere with a daily routine. The DMFC is frequently used to monitor the fetus in pregnancies complicated by conditions that may affect fetal oxygenation. These conditions include but are not limited to pregnancy-induced hypertension or chronic hypertension and diabetes. The presence of movements is generally a reassuring sign of fetal health.

During the last trimester, the fetus spends 10% of its time making gross fetal body movements. Approximately 30 of these movements occur each hour over a 40-minute period of fetal activity. Movements peak between 9:00 PM and 1:00 AM when maternal glucose levels are lowest. Maternal monitoring of fetal movements may give information about pending fetal asphyxia. Decreases in fetal oxygenation are linked to decreases in gross fetal body movements (Druzin et al., 2002).

Several protocols are used for counting. Generally it is recommended that mothers count fetal activity 2 or 3 times daily for 60 minutes each time. Except for establishing a very low number of daily fetal movements or a trend toward decreased motion, the clinical value of the absolute number of fetal movements has not been established, except in the situation in which fetal movements cease entirely for 12 hours (the *fetal alarm signal*). A count of fewer than three fetal movements within 1 hour warrants further evaluation by nonstress or contraction stress testing, biophysical profile, or a combination of these. Women should be taught the significance of the presence and/or absence of fetal movements, the procedure for counting that is to be used, how to record findings on a DFM record, and when to notify their health care provider.

TABLE *29-1* **Fetal Assessment Screening: Recommendations for Care**

FETAL ASSESSMENT TEST	RECOMMENDATION/CONCLUSION
• Doppler ultrasound use in pregnancy at high risk for fetal compromise • Ultrasound use to estimate gestational age in first and early second trimesters • Ultrasound use to confirm suspected multiple pregnancy • Ultrasound use for placental location in suspected placenta previa • Ultrasound use to assess amniotic fluid volume • Early second trimester amniocentesis for identification of chromosomal abnormalities • Transabdominal instead of transvaginal chorionic villus sampling (CVS)	Beneficial effects Effects likely to be beneficial
• Formal systems of risk scoring • Routine use of early ultrasound • CVS versus amniocentesis for diagnosing chromosomal abnormalities • Serum alpha-fetoprotein screening for neural tube defects • Triple screen test for Down syndrome and neural tube defects	Trade-off between beneficial and adverse effects
• Placental grading by ultrasound to improve perinatal outcome • Biophysical profile for fetal surveillance • Routine fetal movement counts to improve perinatal outcome	Unknown effectiveness
• Routine use of ultrasound for fetal anthropometry (body measurements) in late pregnancy • Use of Doppler ultrasound screening in all pregnancies • Measurement of placental hormones (estriol and human placental lactogen)	Unlikely to be beneficial
• Nipple stimulation test to improve perinatal outcome • Nonselective nonstress test to improve perinatal outcome • Contraction stress test to improve perinatal outcome	Likely to be ineffective or harmful

Source: Enkin, M. et al. (2001). Effective care in pregnancy and childbirth: A synopsis. *Birth, 28*(1), 41-51.

NURSE ALERT

In assessing fetal movements, it is important to remember that they are usually not present during the fetal sleep cycle; they may be temporarily reduced if the woman is taking depressant medications, drinking alcohol, or smoking a cigarette; and they do not decrease as the woman nears term. Obesity decreases the ability of the mother to assess fetal movement.

Ultrasonography

Sound is a form of wave energy that causes small particles in a medium to oscillate. The frequency of sound, which refers to the number of peaks or waves that move over a given point per unit of time, is expressed in hertz (Hz). Sound with a frequency of 1 cycle, or one peak per second, has a frequency of 1 Hz. When directional beams of sound strike an object, an echo is returned. The time delay between the emission of the sound and the return of the echo and the direction of the echo are noted. From these data, the distance and location of an object can be calculated (Manning, 1999).

Diagnostic ultrasonography is an important, safe technique in antepartum fetal surveillance. Diagnostic ultrasonography provides critical information to health care providers regarding fetal activity and gestational age, normal versus abnormal fetal growth curves, visual assistance with which invasive tests may be performed more safely, fetal and placental anatomy, and fetal well-being (Chervenak & Gabbe, 2002). **Ultrasound** is sound frequency higher than that detectable by humans (greater than 20,000 Hz). Diagnostic ultrasound instruments operate within a frequency range of 2 to 10 million Hz (or 2 to 10 MHz), which is below the range used by sonar and radar equipment. Ultrasound images are a reflection of the strength of the sending beam, the strength of the returning echo, and the density of the medium (e.g., muscle [uterus], bone, tissue [placenta], fluid, or blood through which the beam is sent and returned) (Chervenak & Gabbe, 2002).

Ultrasound examination can be done abdominally or transvaginally during pregnancy. Both produce a three-dimensional view from which a pictorial image is obtained. Abdominal ultrasonography is more useful after the first trimester when the pregnant uterus becomes an abdominal organ. For the procedure, the woman usually should have a full bladder to get a better image of the fetus. Transmission gel or paste is applied to the abdomen before a transducer is moved over the skin to enhance transmission and reception of the sound waves.

Transvaginal ultrasonography, in which the probe is inserted into the vagina, allows pelvic anatomy to be evaluated in greater detail and intrauterine pregnancy to be diagnosed earlier (Cunningham et al., 2001). A transvaginal ultrasound examination is well tolerated by most clients because it alleviates the need for a full bladder. It is especially useful in obese women whose thick abdominal layers cannot be penetrated adequately by an abdominal approach. Transvaginal ultrasonography is optimally used in the first trimester to detect ectopic pregnancies, monitor the developing embryo, help identify abnormalities, and help establish gestational age. In some instances, it may be used as an adjunct to abdominal scanning to evaluate preterm labor in second- and third-trimester pregnancies (Cook & Ellwood, 2000).

Levels of Ultrasonography

Perinatal care providers and ultrasonographers have come to a tentative agreement on terminology describing two different levels of ultrasonography. The basic screening or limited examination is used most frequently and can be performed by ultrasonographers or other health care professionals, including nurses, who have had special training. Indications for limited ultrasonography are described in detail in the next section; its primary use is to detect fetal viability, determine the presentation of the fetus, assess gestational age, locate the placenta, examine the fetal anatomy for malformations, and determine amniotic fluid volume. Targeted or comprehensive examinations are performed if a woman is suspected of carrying an anatomically or a physiologically abnormal fetus. Indications for a comprehensive examination include abnormal findings on clinical examination, especially with polyhydramnios or oligohydramnios, elevated alpha-fetoprotein (AFP) levels, and a history of offspring with anomalies that can be detected by ultrasound examination. Comprehensive ultrasonography is performed by highly trained and experienced personnel.

Indications for Use

Major indications for obstetric sonography appear by trimester in Table 29-2. During the first trimester, ultrasound examination is performed to obtain information on (1) number, size, and location of gestational sacs; (2) presence or absence of fetal cardiac and body movements; (3) presence or absence of uterine abnormalities (e.g., bicornuate uterus or fibroids) or adnexal masses (e.g., ovarian cysts or an ectopic pregnancy); (4) date of pregnancy (by measuring the crown-rump length); and (5) presence and location of an intrauterine contraceptive device.

During the second and third trimesters, information on the following conditions is sought: (1) fetal viability, number, position, gestational age, growth pattern, and anomalies; (2) amniotic fluid volume; (3) placental location and maturity; (4) uterine fibroids and anomalies; (5) adnexal masses; and (6) cervical length (Fig. 29-1, *A*).

Ultrasonography provides earlier diagnoses, allowing therapy to be instituted early in the pregnancy, thereby decreasing the severity and duration of morbidity, both physical and emotional, for the family. For instance, early diagnosis of a fetal anomaly gives the family choices such as (1) intrauterine surgery or other therapy for the fetus, (2) termination of the pregnancy, or (3) preparation for the care of an infant with a disorder.

TABLE 29-2 **Major Uses of Ultrasonography During Pregnancy**

FIRST TRIMESTER	SECOND TRIMESTER	THIRD TRIMESTER
Confirm pregnancy	Establish or confirm dates	Confirm gestational age
Confirm viability	Confirm viability	Confirm viability
Determine gestational age	Detect polyhydramnios, oligohydramnios	Detect macrosomia
Rule out ectopic pregnancy	Detect congenital anomalies	Detect congenital anomalies
Detect multiple gestation	Detect intrauterine growth restriction (IUGR)	Detect IUGR
Visualization during chorionic villus sampling	Confirm placenta placement	Determine fetal position
Detect maternal abnormalities such as bicornuate uterus, ovarian cysts, fibroids	Visualization during amniocentesis	Detect placenta previa or abruptio placentae
		Visualization during amniocentesis, external version
		Biophysical profile
		Amniotic fluid volume assessment
		Doppler flow studies
		Detect placental maturity

Fetal Heart Activity. Fetal heart activity can be demonstrated as early as 6 to 7 weeks by real-time echo scanners and at 10 to 12 weeks by Doppler mode. By 9 to 10 weeks, gestational trophoblastic disease can be diagnosed. Fetal death can be confirmed by lack of heart motion, the presence of fetal scalp edema, and maceration and overlap of the cranial bones.

Gestational Age. Gestational dating by ultrasonography is indicated for conditions such as (1) uncertain dates for the last normal menstrual period, (2) recent discontinuation of oral contraceptives, (3) bleeding episode during the first trimester, (4) uterine size that does not agree with dates, and (5) other high risk conditions.

During the first 20 weeks of gestation, ultrasonography provides an accurate assessment of gestational age because most normal fetuses grow at the same rate. Accuracy is increased as the fetus ages because more than one variable is measured. The four methods of fetal age estimation used include (1) determination of gestational sac dimensions (at about 8 weeks), (2) measurement of crown-rump length (between 7 and 12 weeks), (3) measurement of the **biparietal diameter (BPD)** (after 12 weeks), and (4) measurement of femur length (after 12 weeks). Fetal BPD at 36 weeks should be approximately 8.7 cm. Term pregnancy and fetal maturity can be diagnosed with some confidence if the biparietal measurement by ultrasound examination is greater than 9.8 cm (Fig. 29-2 and Table 29-3), especially when this is combined with appropriate femur length measurement.

In later gestational periods, serial measurements can provide a more accurate determination of fetal age. Two and preferably three composite measurements are recommended, at least 2 weeks apart, and these are plotted against standard fetal growth curves. This method, when applied between 24 and 32 weeks of gestation, yields an estimation error of 10 days more or less than the actual age (Manning, 1999).

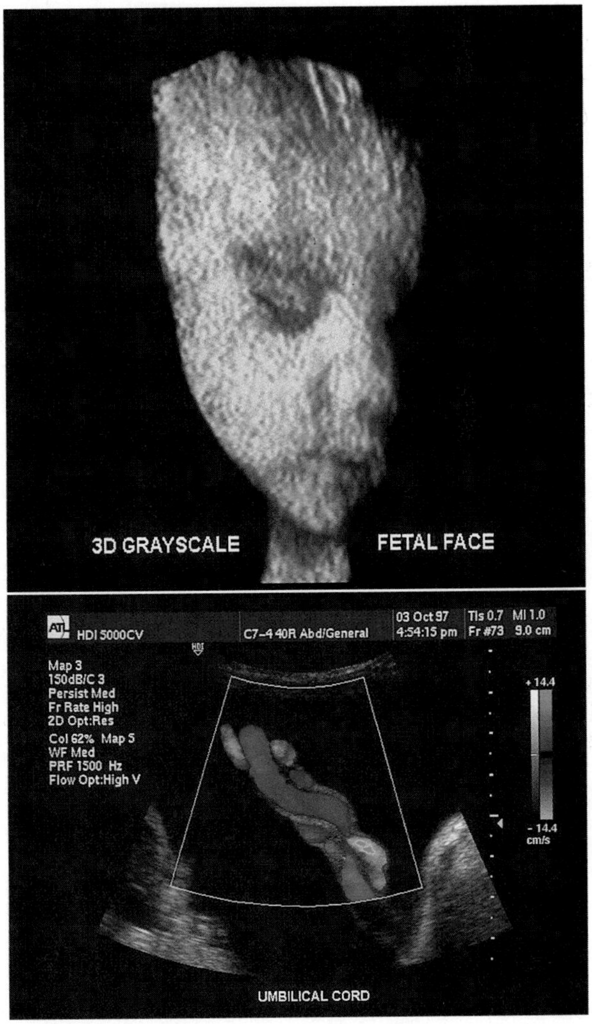
3D GRAYSCALE
FETAL FACE
HDI 5000CV
C7-4 40R Abd/General
03 Oct 97
4:54:15 pm
UMBILICAL CORD

A

B

FIG. 29-1 Two views of the fetus during ultrasonography. **A,** Fetal face (20 wk). **B,** Umbilical cord (26 wk). (Courtesy Advanced Technology Laboratories, Bothell, WA.)

Fetal Growth. Fetal growth is determined by both intrinsic growth potential and environmental factors. Conditions that require ultrasound assessment of fetal growth include (1) poor maternal weight gain or pattern of weight gain, (2) previous intrauterine growth restriction (IUGR), (3) chronic infections, (4) ingestion of drugs (tobacco, alcohol, over-the-counter, and street drugs), (5) maternal diabetes mellitus, (6) hypertension, (7) multifetal pregnancy, and (8) other medical or surgical complications.

Serial evaluations of BPD, limb length, and abdominal circumference (AC) can differentiate between size discrepancy resulting from inaccurate dates, true IUGR, and macrosomia. IUGR may be symmetric (the fetus being small in all parameters) or asymmetric (head and body growth varying). Symmetric IUGR reflects a chronic or long-standing insult and may be caused by low genetic growth potential, intrauterine infection, undernutrition, heavy smoking, or chromosomal aberration. Asymmetric growth suggests an acute or late-occurring deprivation, such as placental insufficiency resulting from hypertension, renal disease, or cardiovascular disease. Reduced fetal growth is still one of the most frequent conditions associated with stillbirth (Fig. 29-3).

Macrosomic infants (those weighing 4000 g or more) are at increased risk for dystocia, traumatic injury, and asphyxia during birth. In addition, fetal macrosomia associated with maternal glucose intolerance or diabetes carries an increased risk of intrauterine fetal death. Macrosomia in the infant of a diabetic mother is asymmetric and characterized by increases in fat and muscle in the abdomen and shoulders, while head circumference remains normal. Macrosomia in an infant whose mother is obese without glucose intolerance results in symmetric changes—excessive growth of abdominal and head circumferences (Chervenak & Gabbe, 2002).

long painful birth

Fetal Anatomy. Anatomic structures that can be identified by ultrasonography (depending on the gestational age) include the following: head (including ventricles and

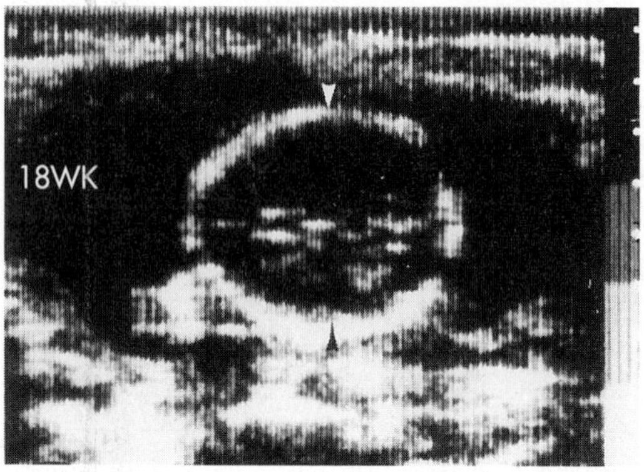
18WK

FIG. 29-2 Real-time image of fetal biparietal diameters at 18 wk. (From Athey, P., & Hadlock, F. [1985]. *Ultrasound in obstetrics and gynecology* [2nd ed.]. St. Louis: Mosby.)

TABLE 29-3 **Correlation of Fetal Weight and BPD**

BPD (CM)	ESTIMATED FETAL WEIGHT (G)
8.2	2290
8.5	2500
8.8	2730
9.4	3180
10.0	3630
10.6	4070

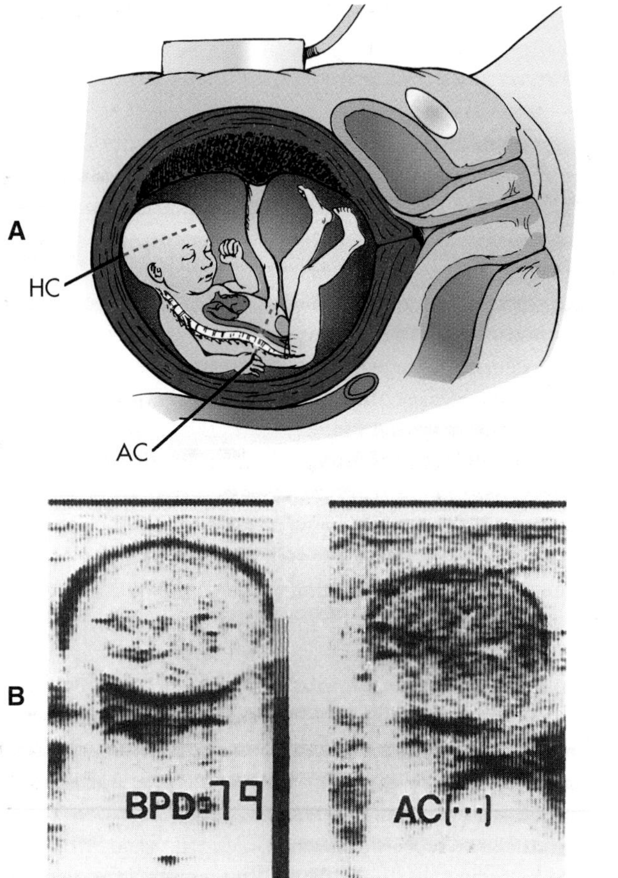
A
HC
AC
B
BPD
AC

FIG. 29-3 **A,** Appropriate planes of sections (*dotted lines*) for head circumference (*HC*), and abdominal circumference (*AC*). **B,** Real-time ultrasound image demonstrates typical head and body images that correspond to planes in **A.** By use of these two images, biparietal diameter (BPD) (7.9 cm), head circumference (30 cm), abdominal circumference (28 cm), and estimated fetal weight (1840 g) in this normal 32-week fetus can be determined. (From Athey, P., & Hadlock, F. [1985]. *Ultrasound in obstetrics and gynecology* [2nd ed.]. St. Louis: Mosby.)

blood vessels), neck, spine, heart, stomach, small bowel, liver, kidneys, bladder, and limbs. Ultrasonography permits the confirmation of normal anatomy, as well as the detection of major fetal malformations. The presence of an anomaly may influence the location of birth (e.g., a delivery room versus a labor-delivery-recovery room or a subspecialty center versus a basic care center) and the method of birth to optimize neonatal outcomes.

The number of fetuses and their presentations also may be assessed by ultrasonography, allowing plans for therapy and mode of birth to be made in advance.

Fetal Genetic Disorders and Physical Anomalies. A prenatal screening technique called fetal nuchal translucency (FNT) screening uses ultrasound measurement of fluid in the nape of the fetal neck between 10 and 14 weeks' gestation to identify possible fetal abnormalities. A finding of abnormal fluid collection that is greater than 2.5 mm is considered abnormal, whereas a measurement of 3 mm or greater is highly indicative of genetic disorders and/or physical anomalies. If the FNT is abnormal, diagnostic genetic testing is recommended (Beamer, 2001).

Placental Position and Function. The pattern of uterine and placental growth and the fullness of the maternal bladder influence the apparent location of the placenta by ultrasonography. During the first trimester, differentiation between the endometrium and small placenta is difficult. By 14 to 16 weeks, the placenta is clearly defined, but if it is seen to be low lying, its relation to the internal cervical os can sometimes be dramatically altered by varying the fullness of the maternal bladder. In approximately 15% to 20% of all pregnancies in which ultrasound scanning is performed during the second trimester, the placenta seems to be overlying the os, but the incidence of placenta previa at term is only 0.5%. Thus the diagnosis of placenta previa can seldom be confirmed before 27 weeks, primarily because of the elongation of the lower uterine segment as pregnancy advances.

Another use for ultrasonography is grading of placental maturation (Box 29-6). Calcium deposits are of significance in postterm pregnancies because as they increase, the available surface area that can be adequately bathed by maternal blood decreases. The point at which this results in fetal wastage and hypoxia cannot be determined precisely; however, the effects are usually observable by 42 weeks and are progressive (Gilbert & Harmon, 2003).

Adjunct to Other Invasive Tests. The safety of amniocentesis is increased when the positions of the fetus, placenta, and pockets of amniotic fluid can be identified accurately. Ultrasound scanning has reduced risks previously associated with amniocentesis, such as fetomaternal hemorrhage from a pierced placenta. Percutaneous umbilical blood sampling and chorionic villus sampling also are guided by ultrasonography to identify the cord and chorion frondosum accurately (see Fig. 29-1, *B*).

Fetal Well-Being

Physiologic parameters of the fetus that can be assessed with ultrasound scanning include amniotic fluid volume, vascular waveforms from the fetal circulation, heart motion, fetal breathing movements, fetal urine production, and fetal limb and head movements. Assessment of these parameters, singly or in combination, yields a fairly reliable picture of fetal well-being. The significance of these findings is discussed in the following sections.

Doppler Blood Flow Analysis. One of the major advances in perinatal medicine is the ability to study blood flow noninvasively in the fetus and placenta. **Doppler ultrasound** is a helpful adjunct in the management of pregnancies at risk because of hypertension, IUGR, diabetes mellitus, multiple fetuses, or preterm labor (Miller, 1998).

When a sound wave is reflected from a moving target, there is a change in frequency of the reflected wave relative to the transmitted wave. This is called the *Doppler effect*. An ultrasound beam scattered by a group of red blood cells (RBCs) is an example of this effect. The velocity of the RBCs can be determined by measuring the change in the frequency of the sound wave reflected off the cells.

The shifted frequencies can be displayed as a plot of velocity versus time, and the shape of these waveforms can be analyzed to give information about blood flow and resistance in a given circulation. Velocity waveforms from umbilical and uterine arteries, reported as systolic/diastolic (S/D) ratios, can be first detected at 15 weeks of pregnancy. Because of the progressive decline in

BOX 29-6 Placental Grading

Third-trimester grading of placental maturation can be accomplished by ultrasound scanning. The placenta undergoes detectable maturational changes throughout gestation; a relation has been noted between advancing placental grade and fetal pulmonary maturity. Placentas are graded 0, I, II, and III (with grade III placentas being the most mature) on the basis of the identification and distribution of calcium deposits within the fetal portion (Manning, 1999). Ultrasound examination can identify changes in the chorionic plate, placental substance, and basal layer of the placenta that correspond to the various grades: (1) grade 0 placentas are seen in the first and second trimesters, (2) grade I placentas appear between 30 and 32 weeks and may even persist until term, (3) grade II placentas are observed at around 36 weeks and persist until term in 45% of pregnancies, and (4) grade III placentas are seen at 38 weeks and reflect the greatest maturation. However, only a small number of placentas are grade III.

resistance in both the umbilical and uterine arteries, this ratio decreases as pregnancy advances. Most fetuses will achieve an S/D ratio of 3 or less by 30 weeks. Persistent elevation of S/D ratios after 30 weeks is associated with IUGR, usually resulting from uteroplacental insufficiency (UPI) (Druzin et al., 2002). In postterm pregnancies evaluated by Doppler umbilical flow studies, an elevated S/D ratio indicates a poorly perfused placenta. Abnormal results also are seen with certain chromosome abnormalities (trisomy 13 and 18) in the fetus and with lupus erythematosus in the mother. Exposure to nicotine from maternal smoking also has been reported to increase the S/D ratio (Fig. 29-4).

Fetal

Biophysical Profile. Real-time ultrasound permits detailed assessment of the physical and physiologic characteristics of the developing fetus and cataloging of normal and abnormal biophysical responses to stimuli. The **biophysical profile (BPP)** is a noninvasive dynamic assessment of a fetus that is based on acute and chronic markers of fetal disease. The BPP includes fetal breathing movements (FBMs), fetal movements, fetal tone, fetal heart rate (FHR) patterns by means of a nonstress test, and **amniotic fluid volume (AFV).** Abnormalities in AFV are frequently associated with fetal disorders. Subjective determinants of oligohydramnios (decreased fluid) include the absence of fluid pockets in the uterine cavity and the impression of crowding of small fetal parts. An objective criterion of decreased AFV is met if the largest pocket of fluid measured in two perpendicular planes is less than 1 cm. In polyhydramnios (increased fluid), subjective criteria include multiple large pockets of fluid, the impression of a floating fetus, and free movement of fetal limbs. The diagnosis may be made when the largest pocket of fluid exceeds 8 cm in two perpendicular planes (Chervenak & Gabbe, 2002).

The total AFV can be evaluated by a method in which the depths (in centimeters) of the amniotic fluid in all four quadrants surrounding the maternal umbilicus are totaled, providing an **amniotic fluid index (AFI).** An AFI less than 5 cm indicates oligohydramnios; 5 to 19 cm is considered a normal measurement; and a measurement greater than 20 cm reflects polyhydramnios (Chervenak & Gabbe, 2002). Oligohydramnios is associated with congenital anomalies (such as renal agenesis), growth restriction, and fetal distress during labor. Polyhydramnios is associated with neural tube defects, obstruction of the fetal gastrointestinal tract, multiple fetuses, and fetal hydrops.

The BPP may therefore be considered a physical examination of the fetus, including determination of vital signs. The fetal response to central hypoxia is alteration in movement, muscle tone, breathing, and heart rate patterns. The presence of normal fetal biophysical activities indicates that the central nervous system (CNS) is functional, and the fetus therefore is not hypoxemic (Manning, 1999). BPP variables and scoring are detailed in Table 29-4.

The BPP is an accurate indicator of impending fetal death. Fetal acidosis can be diagnosed early with a nonreactive NST and absent FBMs. An abnormal BPP score and oligohydramnios are indications that labor should be in-

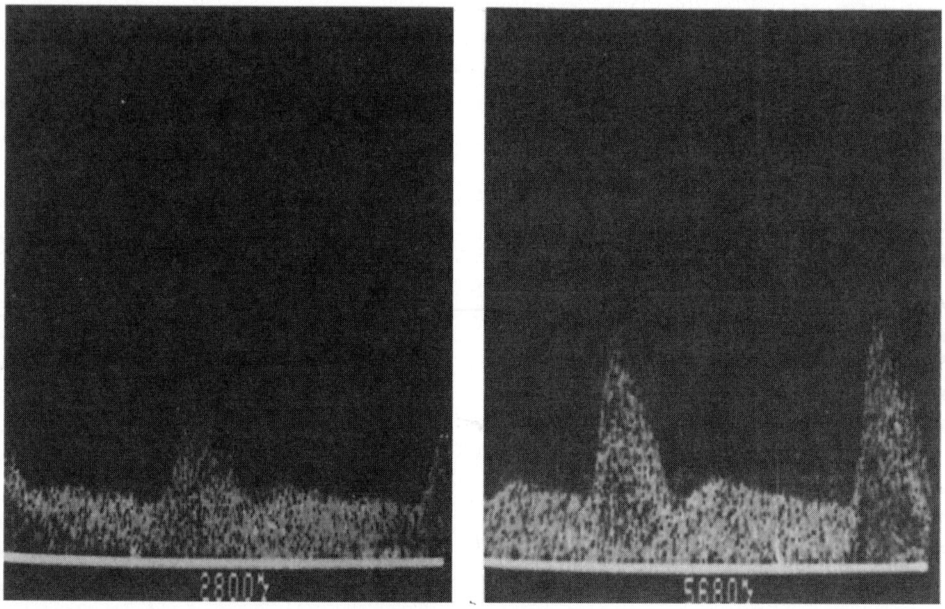

A

B

FIG. 29-4 Normal and abnormal uteroplacental vessels at 34 weeks. **A,** Normal S/D ratio of 2.1. **B,** S/D ratio of 3.4. (From Schulman, H. [1990]. Doppler ultrasound. In R. Eden & F. Boehm [Eds.], *Assessment and care of the fetus: Physiological, clinical, and medicolegal principles.* Norwalk, CT: Appleton & Lange.)

duced (Manning, 1999). Fetal infection in women whose membranes rupture prematurely (at less than 37 weeks of gestation) can be diagnosed early by changes in biophysical activity that precede the clinical signs of infection and indicate the necessity for immediate birth. When the BPP score is normal and the risk of fetal death low, intervention is indicated only for obstetric or maternal factors.

Nursing Role

Although a growing number of nurses perform ultrasound scans and BPPs in certain centers, the main role of nurses is in counseling and educating women about the procedure (see Research box). Providing accurate information regarding the procedure is imperative to allay the mother's anxiety. Although ultrasound scanning has become a widely used diagnostic tool, recommendations for the procedure are based on expectations of a fetal problem and therefore may cause concern. Women should be provided ample opportunity to ask questions and be reassured that the procedure is safe. In the 30 years that diagnostic ultrasonography has been used, no conclusive evidence of any harmful effects on humans has emerged. Although the possibility of unidentified biologic effects exists, the benefits to the client of prudent use of diagnostic ultrasonography appear to outweigh any possible risk (Chervenak & Gabbe, 2002).

LEGAL TIP Performance of Limited Ultrasound Examinations

Nurses who have the training and competence may perform limited ultrasound examinations if it is within the scope of practice in their state or area and consistent with regulations of the agencies in which they practice (Treanor, 1998). Limited ultrasound examinations include identification of fetal number, fetal presentation, fetal cardiac activity, location of the placenta, and BPP, including AFV assessment. Women should be informed about the limited information provided by these examinations. They are not meant to evaluate or identify fetal anomalies, assess fetal age, or estimate fetal weight. The obstetric health care provider is responsible for obtaining a more comprehensive ultrasound examination when complete client assessment is necessary (AWHONN, 1998).

For an abdominal ultrasound, the woman is usually directed to come for the examination with a full bladder because it supports the uterus in position for the imaging. She is then positioned with small pillows under her head and knees. The display panel is positioned so that the woman and/or her partner can observe the images on the screen if they desire.

A transvaginal ultrasound may be performed with the woman in a lithotomy position or with her pelvis elevated by towels, cushions, or a folded pillow. This pelvis tilt is

TABLE 29-4 **Biophysical Profile**

VARIABLES	NORMAL (SCORE = 2)	ABNORMAL (SCORE = 0)
Fetal breathing movements	One or more episodes in 30 min, each lasting ≥30 sec	Episodes absent or no episode ≥30 sec in 30 min
Gross body movements	Three or more discrete body or limb movements in 30 min (episodes of active continuous movement being considered as a single movement)	Less than three episodes of body or limb movements in 30 min
Fetal tone	One or more episodes of active extension with return to flexion of fetal limb(s) or trunk, opening and closing of hand being considered normal tone	Slow extension with return to flexion, movement of limb in full extension, or fetal movement absent
Reactive fetal heart rate	Two or more episodes of acceleration (≥15 beats/min) in 20 min, each lasting ≥15 sec and associated with fetal movement	Less than two episodes of acceleration or acceleration of <15 beats/min in 20 min
Qualitative amniotic fluid volume	One or more pockets of fluid measuring ≥1 cm in two perpendicular planes	Pockets absent or pocket <1 cm in two perpendicular planes
Score		
Normal	8-10 (if Amniotic Fluid Index is adequate)	
Equivocal	6	
Abnormal	<4	

Data from Manning, F. (1995). Dynamic ultrasound-based fetal assessment: The fetal biophysical profile score. *Clinical Obstetrics and Gynecology, 38*(1), 26-44; Mattson, S., & Smith, J. (2000). *Core curriculum for maternal-newborn nursing* (2nd ed.). Philadelphia: W.B. Saunders.

RESEARCH

Preparing Parents for Ultrasound

One of the most common and high-profile antenatal screening tests is the ultrasound scan. It provides a real-time image of the developing fetus and immediate feedback as to its well-being. Ultrasound has become a much-anticipated part of prenatal care. To evaluate the literature about research of women's views concerning ultrasound, a British team reviewed 74 studies from 18 countries. They found that women and their families were attracted to an ultrasound scan as a powerful confirmation of their pregnant status and were reassured by the images. They were not worried about maternal or fetal safety of having an ultrasound scan.

However, women often did not have enough information about the purpose of the scan and were either shocked by an adverse or equivocal finding or were unrealistically reassured that everything was fine. Some women would have declined the scan had they known it could detect a problem. Women were sometimes unsettled by the bedside manner of the technicians and became especially anxious if the scans indicated further study. Having an image of the fetus made some women more worried because of the increased feeling of attachment. In the event of bad news about the fetus, some women had more difficulty coping with the loss after having seen the fetus on ultrasound. In the event of fetal death, some regretted having viewed it, while others were comforted by having an image to mourn.

IMPLICATIONS FOR PRACTICE

Expectant parents who are well-informed about ultrasound uses and limitations can make an informed choice having a scan. The nurse can help them have realistic expectations and prepare them for adverse findings. Well-informed clinicians can provide nonjudgmental counseling and referrals should there be a need.

Reference: Garcia, J. et al. (2002). Women's views of pregnancy ultrasound: A systematic review. *Birth, 29*(4), 225-247.

optimal to image the pelvic structures. A protective cover such as a condom, the finger of a clean rubber surgical glove, or a special probe cover provided by the manufacturer is used to cover the transducer probe. The probe is lubricated with a water-soluble gel and placed in the vagina either by the examiner or by the woman herself. During the examination, the position of the probe or the tilt of the examining table may be changed so that the complete pelvis is in view. The procedure is not physically painful, although the woman will feel pressure as the probe is moved.

Magnetic Resonance Imaging

Magnetic resonance imaging (MRI) is a noninvasive radiologic technique used for obstetric and gynecologic diagnosis. Like computerized tomography (CT), MRI provides excellent pictures of soft tissue. Unlike CT, ionizing radiation is not used; thus vascular structures within the body can be visualized and evaluated without injection of an iodinated contrast medium, thus eliminating any known biologic risk. Like sonography, MRI is noninvasive and can provide images in multiple planes, but there is no interference from skeletal, fatty, or gas-filled structures, and imaging of deep pelvic structures does not require a full bladder.

With MRI, the examiner can evaluate (1) fetal structure (CNS, thorax, abdomen, genitourinary tract, musculoskeletal system) and overall growth, (2) placenta (position, density, and presence of gestational trophoblastic disease), (3) quantity of amniotic fluid, (4) maternal structures (uterus, cervix, adnexa, and pelvis), (5) biochemical status (pH, adenosine triphosphate content) of tissues and organs, and (6) soft tissue, metabolic, or functional anomalies.

The woman is placed on a table in the supine position and slid into the bore of the main magnet, which is similar in appearance to a CT scanner. Depending on the reason for the study, the procedure may take from 20 to 60 minutes, during which time the woman must be perfectly still except for short respites. Because of the long time needed to produce MRIs, the fetus will probably move, which will obscure anatomic details. The only way to ensure that this does not occur is to administer a sedative to the mother, but this approach should be reserved for selected cases in which visualization of fetal detail is critical.

MRI has little effect on the fetus; concerns that the FHR or fetal movement would decrease have not been supported (Poutamo et al., 1998).

BIOCHEMICAL ASSESSMENT

Biochemical assessment involves biologic examination (e.g., as chromosomes in exfoliated cells) and chemical determinations (e.g., lecithin/sphingomyelin [L/S] ratio and bilirubin level) (Table 29-5). Procedures used to obtain the needed specimens include amniocentesis, percutaneous umbilical blood sampling, chorionic villus sampling, and maternal sampling (see Ethical Considerations box).

Amniocentesis

Amniocentesis is performed to obtain amniotic fluid, which contains fetal cells. Under direct ultrasonographic visualization, a needle is inserted transabdominally into the uterus, amniotic fluid is withdrawn into a syringe, and the various assessments are performed. Amniocentesis is possible after week 14 of pregnancy, when the uterus becomes an abdominal organ, and sufficient amniotic fluid is available for testing (Fig. 29-5). Indications for the procedure include prenatal diagnosis of genetic disorders or congenital anomalies (neural tube defects in particular), assessment of pulmonary maturity, and diagnosis of fetal hemolytic disease.

TABLE 29-5 **Summary of Biochemical Monitoring Techniques**

TEST	POSSIBLE FINDINGS	CLINICAL SIGNIFICANCE
Maternal Blood		
Coombs' test	Titer of 1:8 and increasing	Significant Rh incompatibility
AFP	See below	See below
Amniotic Fluid Analysis		
Color	Meconium	Possible hypoxia or asphyxia
Lung profile		Fetal lung maturity
L/S ratio	>2:1	
Phosphatidylglycerol	Present	
Creatinine	>2 mg/dl	Gestational age >36 weeks
Bilirubin (ΔOD, 450/nm)	<0.015	Gestational age >36 weeks, normal pregnancy
	High levels	Fetal hemolytic disease in Rh isoimmunized pregnancies
Lipid cells	>10%	Gestational age >35 weeks
AFP	High levels after 15-week gestation	Open neural tube or other defect
Osmolality	Decline after 20-week gestation	Advancing nonspecific gestational age
Genetic disorders	Dependent on cultured cells for karyotype and enzymatic activity	Counseling possibly required
Sex-linked		
Chromosomal		
Metabolic		

Complications in the mother and fetus occur in fewer than 1% of the cases and include the following:

- Maternal: Hemorrhage, fetomaternal hemorrhage with possible maternal Rh isoimmunization, infection, labor, abruptio placentae, inadvertent damage to the intestines or bladder, and amniotic fluid embolism. Because of the possibility of fetomaternal hemorrhage, it is standard practice after an amniocentesis to administer Rh$_o$D immune globulin (RhoGAM) to the woman who is Rh negative.
- Fetal: Death, hemorrhage, infection (amnionitis), direct injury from the needle, miscarriage or preterm labor, and leakage of amniotic fluid.

Many of the complications have been minimized or eliminated by using ultrasonography to direct the procedure.

Indications for Use

Genetic Concerns. Prenatal assessment of genetic disorders is indicated in women older than 35 years, with a previous child with a chromosomal abnormality, or with a family history of chromosomal anomalies. Inherited errors of metabolism (such as Tay-Sachs disease, hemophilia, and thalassemia) and other disorders for which marker genes are known also may be detected. Fetal cells are cultured for karyotyping of chromosomes (see Chapter 3). Karyotyping also permits determination of fetal sex, which is important if an X-linked disorder (occurring almost always in a male fetus) is suspected.

ETHICAL CONSIDERATIONS

Fetal Rights

Amniocentesis, PUBS, and CVS are prenatal tests used for diagnosing fetal defects in pregnancy. They are invasive and carry risks to the mother and fetus. A consideration of abortion is linked to the performance of these tests because there is no treatment for genetically affected fetuses; thus the issue of fetal rights is a key ethical concern in prenatal testing for fetal defects.

Biochemical analysis of enzymes in amniotic fluid can detect inborn errors of metabolism. For example, **AFP** levels in amniotic fluid are assessed as a follow-up for elevated levels in maternal serum. High AFP levels in amniotic fluid help confirm the diagnosis of a neural tube defect such as spina bifida or anencephaly or an abdominal wall defect such as omphalocele. The elevation results from the increased leakage of cerebrospinal fluid into the amniotic fluid through the closure defect. AFP levels may also be elevated in a normal multifetal pregnancy and with intestinal atresia, presumably caused by lack of fetal swallowing.

A concurrent test that finds the presence of acetylcholinesterase almost always indicates a fetal defect (Scioscia, 1999). In such instances, follow-up ultrasound examination is recommended.

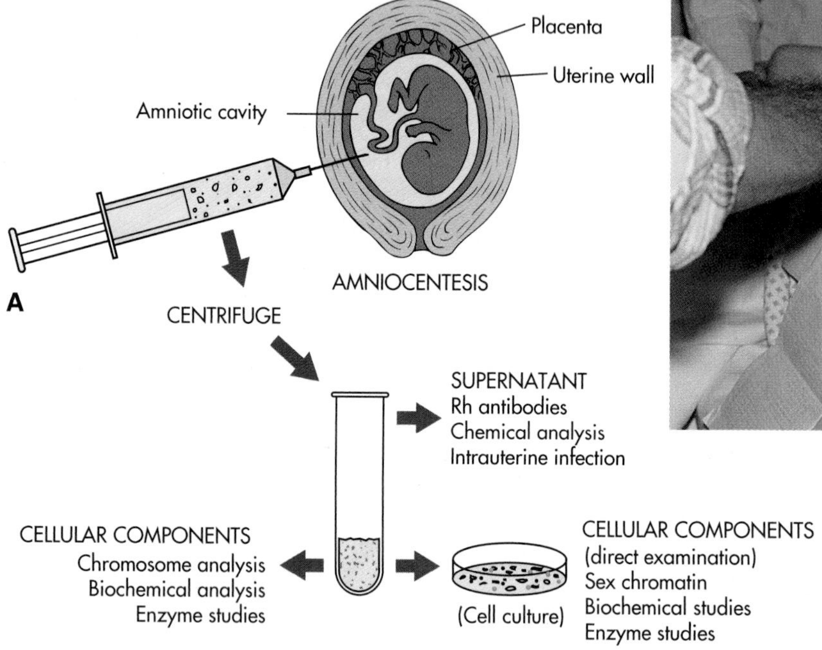
Placenta
Uterine wall
Amniotic cavity
AMNIOCENTESIS
A
CENTRIFUGE
SUPERNATANT
Rh antibodies
Chemical analysis
Intrauterine infection
CELLULAR COMPONENTS
Chromosome analysis
Biochemical analysis
Enzyme studies
CELLULAR COMPONENTS
(direct examination)
Sex chromatin
Biochemical studies
Enzyme studies
(Cell culture)

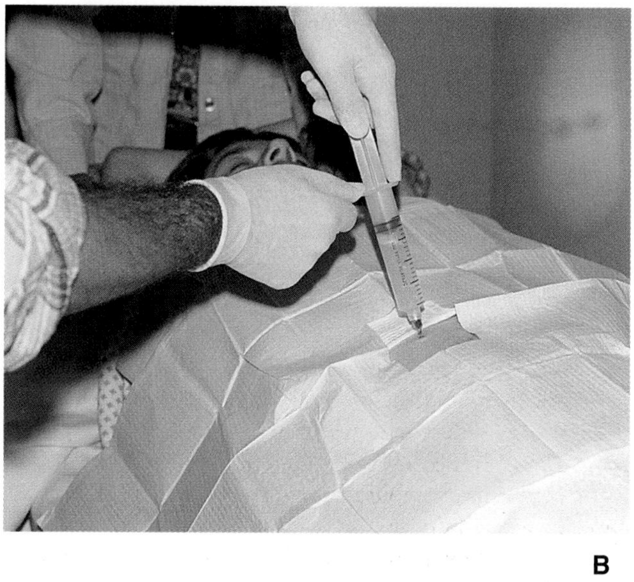
B

FIG. 29-5 A, Amniocentesis and laboratory use of amniotic fluid aspirant. **B,** Transabdominal amniocentesis. (**B,** Courtesy Marjorie Pyle, RNC, Lifecircle, Costa Mesa, CA.)

Fetal Maturity. Accurate assessment of fetal maturity is possible through examination of amniotic fluid or its exfoliated cellular contents. The laboratory tests described are determinants of term pregnancy and fetal maturity (see Table 29-4).

Fetal Hemolytic Disease. Another indication for amniocentesis is the identification and follow-up of fetal hemolytic disease in cases of isoimmunization. The procedure is usually not done until the mother's antibody titer reaches 1:8 and is increasing. However, percutaneous umbilical blood sampling is now the procedure of choice to evaluate and treat fetal hemolytic disease.

Meconium. The presence of meconium in the amniotic fluid is usually determined by visual inspection of the sample. The significance of meconium in the fluid varies depending on when it is found.

Antepartal Period. Meconium in the amniotic fluid before the beginning of labor is not usually associated with an adverse fetal outcome. The finding may be the result of acute and subsequently corrected fetal stress, chronic continuing stress, or simply the physiologic passage of meconium. Because there has been some association between meconium in amniotic fluid in the third trimester and hypertensive disorders and postmaturity, the fetus should undergo further antepartum evaluation if the birth is not imminent (Glantz & Woods, 1999).

Intrapartal Period. Intrapartal meconium-stained amniotic fluid is an indication for more careful evaluation by electronic fetal monitoring (EFM) and perhaps fetal scalp blood sampling. The presence of meconium, however, should not be the sole indicator for intervention.

Three possible reasons for the passage of meconium during the intrapartal period are as follows: (1) it is a normal physiologic function that occurs with maturity (meconium passage being infrequent before weeks 23 or 24, with an increased incidence after 38 weeks), (2) it is the result of hypoxia-induced peristalsis and sphincter relaxation, and (3) it may be a sequel to umbilical cord compression–induced vagal stimulation in mature fetuses.

The following criteria have been proposed for evaluating meconium-stained amniotic fluid during the intrapartal period (Scott et al., 1999):

1. *Consistency.* A thick, fresh consistency is more likely to be the result of fetal stress.
2. *Timing.* Thick, fresh meconium passed for the first time in late labor and in association with nonremediable severe variable or late FHR decelerations is an ominous sign. The presence of meconium alone, however, is not necessarily a sign of fetal distress.
3. *Presence of other indicators.* Meconium passage and nonremediable severe variable or late FHR decelerations (especially with poor baseline variability), with or with-

out acidosis confirmed by scalp blood sampling, are ominous signs of fetal distress.

NURSE ALERT

The birth team should be ready to suction the nasopharynx of the neonate carefully at the time of birth, ideally before the first breath is taken. Suctioning at this time effectively reduces the incidence and severity of meconium aspiration in the neonate.

Percutaneous Umbilical Blood Sampling

Direct access to the fetal circulation during the second and third trimesters is possible through **percutaneous umbilical blood sampling (PUBS),** or cordocentesis, which is the most widely used method for fetal blood sampling and transfusion. PUBS involves the insertion of a needle directly into a fetal umbilical vessel under ultrasound guidance. Ideally, the umbilical cord is punctured 1 to 2 cm from its insertion into the placenta (Fig. 29-6) (Simpson, 2002). At this point the cord is well anchored and will not move, and the risk of maternal blood contamination (from the placenta) is slight. Generally, 1 to 4 ml of blood is removed and tested immediately by the Kleihauer-Betke procedure to ensure that it is fetal in origin. Indications for use of PUBS include prenatal diagnosis of inherited blood disorders, karyotyping of malformed fetuses, detection of fetal infection, determination of the acid-base status of fetuses with IUGR, and assessment and treatment of isoimmunization and thrombocytopenia in the fetus (Harmon, 1999). Complications that can occur include leaking of blood from the puncture site, cord laceration, thromboembolism, preterm labor, premature rupture of membranes, and infection (Simpson, 2002).

In fetuses at risk for isoimmune hemolytic anemia, PUBS permits precise identification of fetal blood type and RBC count and may prevent the need for further intervention. If the fetus is positive for the presence of maternal antibodies, a direct blood test can confirm the degree of anemia resulting from hemolysis. Intrauterine transfusion of severely anemic fetuses can be done 4 to 5 weeks earlier than through the intraperitoneal route.

Follow-up includes continuous FHR monitoring for several minutes to 1 hour and a repeated ultrasound examination 1 hour later to ensure that no further bleeding or hematoma formation has occurred.

Chorionic Villus Sampling

The combined advantages of earlier diagnosis and rapid results have made **chorionic villus sampling (CVS)** a popular technique for genetic studies, although some risks to the fetus exist. Although indications for CVS are similar to those for amniocentesis, second trimester amniocentesis appears to be safer than CVS (Alfirevic, Gosden, & Neilson, 2000). The benefits of earlier diagnosis must be weighed against the increased risk of pregnancy loss and risk of anomalies.

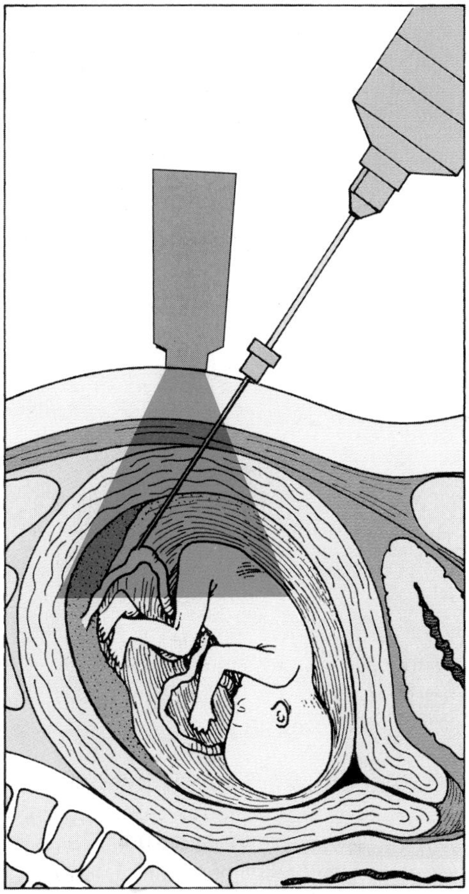

FIG. 29-6 Technique for percutaneous umbilical blood sampling guided by ultrasound.

The procedure is performed between 10 and 12 weeks of gestation and involves the removal of a small tissue specimen from the fetal portion of the placenta (Fig. 29-7). Because chorionic villi originate in the zygote, this tissue reflects the genetic makeup of the fetus.

CVS procedures can be accomplished either transcervically or transabdominally. In transcervical sampling, a sterile catheter is introduced into the cervix under continuous ultrasonographic guidance, and a small portion of the chorionic villi is aspirated with a syringe. The aspiration cannula and obturator must be placed at a suitable site, and rupture of the amniotic sac must be avoided.

If the abdominal approach is used, an 18-gauge spinal needle with stylet is inserted under sterile conditions through the abdominal wall into the chorion frondosum under ultrasound guidance. The stylet is then withdrawn, and the chorionic tissue is aspirated into a syringe (see Fig. 29-7).

Complications of the procedure include vaginal spotting or bleeding immediately afterward, miscarriage (in 0.3% of cases), rupture of membranes (in 0.1% of cases),

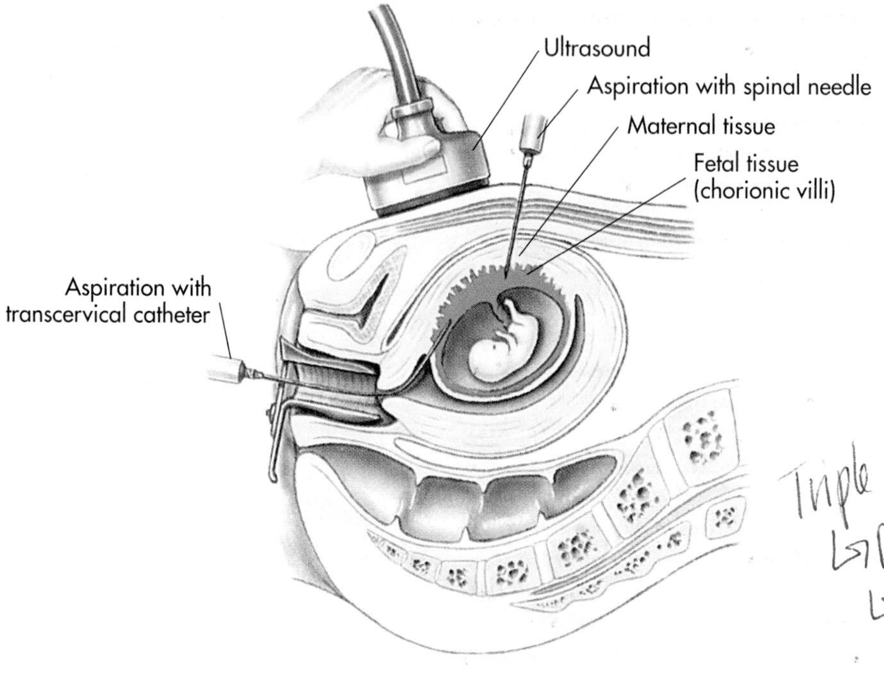
Ultrasound
Aspiration with spinal needle
Maternal tissue
Fetal tissue
(chorionic villi)
Aspiration with
transcervical catheter

FIG. 29-7 Chorionic villus sampling. (Courtesy Medical and Scientific Illustration, Crozet, VA.)

and chorioamnionitis (in 0.5% of cases). Because of the possibility of fetomaternal hemorrhage, women who are Rh negative should receive immune globulin (RhoGAM) to avoid isoimmunization (Gilbert & Harmon, 2003). An increased risk of limb anomalies (transverse digital anomalies) has been noted when CVS is done before 10 weeks of gestation (Wilson, 2000).

Maternal Assays

Alpha-fetoprotein

Maternal serum AFP (MSAFP) levels have been used as a screening tool for neural tube defects (NTDs) in pregnancy. Through this technique, approximately 80% to 85% of all open NTDs and open abdominal wall defects can be detected early in pregnancy. Screening is recommended for all pregnant women (ACOG, 1999).

The cause of NTDs is not well understood, but 95% of all affected infants are born to women with no family history of similar anomalies. The defect occurs in 1 to 2 per 1000 births in most parts of the United States. The birth of one affected child increases the risk of NTD recurrence in future pregnancies to 1% to 5% (Cunningham et al., 2001; Scioscia, 1999).

AFP is produced by the fetal liver, and increasing levels are detectable in the serum of pregnant women from 14 to 34 weeks. Although amniotic fluid AFP is diagnostic for NTD, MSAFP is a screening tool only and identifies candidates for the more definitive procedures of amniocentesis and ultrasound examination. MSAFP screening can be done with reasonable reliability any time between 15 and 22 weeks of gestation (16 to 18 weeks being ideal) (ACOG, 1999).

Once the maternal level of AFP is determined, it is compared with normal values for each week of gestation. Values also should be correlated with maternal age, weight, race, and whether the woman has insulin-dependent diabetes. If findings are abnormal, follow-up procedures include genetic counseling for families with a history of NTD, repeated AFP, ultrasound examination, and possibly, amniocentesis (Ross & Elias, 1997).

Down syndrome and probably other autosomal trisomies are associated with lower-than-normal levels of MSAFP and amniotic fluid AFP. The **triple-marker test** also is performed at 16 to 18 weeks of gestation and uses the levels of three maternal serum markers, MSAFP, unconjugated estriol, and human chorionic gonadotropin (hCG), in combination with maternal age to calculate a new risk. In the presence of a fetus with Down syndrome, the MSAFP and unconjugated estriol levels are low, whereas the hCG level is elevated. With these two additional screening tests, approximately 60% of cases of Down syndrome can be identified. Other maternal markers are being investigated as predictors of fetal abnormalities as well. Serum pregnancy-associated placental protein A (PAPP-A) is low in Down syndrome, whereas another substance, inhibin-A, is elevated in Down syndrome and other trisomies (Simpson, 2002).

As with MSAFP, these tests are screening procedures only and are not diagnostic. A definitive examination of amniotic fluid for AFP and chromosomal analysis combined with ultrasound visualization of the fetus is necessary for diagnosis; however, using these tests can reduce the number of amniocenteses needed (Egan et al., 2000).

Coombs' Test

Coombs' test for Rh incompatibility is discussed in Chapter 39. If the maternal titer for Rh antibodies is greater than 1:8, amniocentesis for determination of bilirubin in amniotic fluid is indicated to establish the severity of fetal hemolytic anemia. Coombs' test also can detect other antibodies that may place the fetus at risk for incompatibility with maternal antigens.

ELECTRONIC FETAL MONITORING

Indications

First- and second-trimester antepartal assessment is directed primarily at the diagnosis of fetal anomalies. The goal of third-trimester testing is to determine whether the intrauterine environment continues to be supportive to the fetus. The testing is often used to determine the timing of childbirth for women at risk for **uteroplacental insufficiency (UPI;** the gradual decline in delivery of needed substances by the placenta to the fetus). Gradual loss of placental function results first in inadequate nutrient delivery to the fetus, leading to IUGR. Subsequently, respiratory function also is compromised, resulting in fetal hypoxia. Common indication for both the **nonstress test (NST)** and the **contraction stress test (CST)** are listed in Box 29-7.

No clinical contraindications exist for the NST, but results may not be conclusive if gestation is 26 weeks or less. Absolute contraindications for the CST are the following: rupture of membranes, previous classic incision for cesarean birth, preterm labor, placenta previa, and abruptio placentae. Other conditions in which CST may be contraindicated are multifetal pregnancy, previous preterm labor, hydramnios, more than 36 weeks of gestation, and incompetent cervix. As a rule, reactive patterns with the NST or negative results with the CST are associated with favorable outcomes.

Fetal Responses to Hypoxia and Asphyxia

Observable fetal responses to hypoxia or asphyxia are the clinical basis for testing with electronic fetal monitoring. Hypoxia or asphyxia elicits a number of responses in the fetus. Blood flow is redistributed to certain vital organs. This series of responses (redistribution of blood flow favoring vital organs, decrease in total oxygen consumption, and switch to anaerobic glycolysis) is a temporary mechanism that enables the fetus to survive up to 30 minutes of limited oxygen supply without decompensation of vital organs. However, during more severe asphyxia or sustained hypoxemia, these compensatory responses are no longer maintained, and a decrease in the cardiac output, arterial blood pressure, and blood flow to the brain and heart occurs (Parer, 1999), with characteristic FHR patterns reflecting these changes.

BOX 29-7 Indications for Electronic Fetal Monitoring Assessment Using NST and CST

- Maternal diabetes mellitus
- Chronic hypertension
- Hypertensive disorders in pregnancy
- IUGR
- Sickle cell disease
- Maternal cyanotic heart disease
- Postmaturity
- History of previous stillbirth
- Decreased fetal movement
- Isoimmunization
- Meconium-stained amniotic fluid at third-trimester amniocentesis
- Hyperthyroidism
- Collagen disease
- Older pregnant woman
- Chronic renal disease

Variability

Considerable evidence supports the clinical belief that FHR variability indicates an intact nervous pathway through the cerebral cortex, midbrain, vagus nerve, and cardiac conduction system. With 98% accuracy in predicting fetal well-being, the presence of normal FHR variability is a reassuring indicator. Inputs from various areas of the brain decrease after cerebral asphyxia, leading to a decrease in variability after failure of the fetal hemodynamic compensatory mechanisms to maintain cerebral oxygenation (Parer, 1999).

Nonstress Test

The NST is the most widely applied technique for antepartum evaluation of the fetus. It is an ideal screening test and is the primary method of antepartum fetal assessment at most sites. The basis for the NST is that the normal fetus will produce characteristic heart rate (HR) patterns in response to fetal movement. In the healthy fetus with an intact CNS, 90% of gross fetal body movements are associated with accelerations of the FHR. The acceleration with movement response may be blunted by hypoxia, acidosis, drugs (analgesics, barbiturates, and beta-blockers), fetal sleep, and some congenital anomalies (Tucker, 2000). The NST can be performed easily and quickly in an outpatient setting because it is noninvasive, relatively inexpensive, and has no known contraindications. Disadvantages center around the high rate of false-positive results for nonreactivity as a result of fetal sleep cycles, chronic tobacco smoking, medications, and fetal immaturity. The test also is slightly less sensitive in detecting fetal compromise than are the CST or BPP.

Procedure

The woman is seated in a reclining chair (or in semi-Fowler position) with a slight left tilt to optimize uterine perfusion and avoid supine hypotension. The FHR is recorded with a Doppler transducer, and a tocodynamometer is applied to detect uterine contractions or fetal movements. The tracing is observed for signs of fetal activity and a concurrent acceleration of FHR. If evidence of fetal movement is not apparent on the tracing, the woman may be asked to depress a button on a hand-held event marker connected to the monitor when she feels fetal movement. The movement is then noted on the tracing. Because almost all accelerations are accompanied by fetal movement, the movements need not be recorded for the test to be considered reactive. The test is usually completed within 20 to 30 minutes, but it may take longer if the fetus must be awakened from a sleep state.

It has been suggested that the woman drink orange juice or be given glucose to increase her blood sugar level and thereby stimulate fetal movements. This practice is common; however, research has not proven this practice to be effective (McCarthy & Narrigan, 1995). Some sources suggest that fetal movements increase when maternal glucose levels are low. Other methods that have been used to stimulate fetal activity, such as manipulating the woman's abdomen or using a transvaginal light, have not been very effective either. Only vibroacoustic stimulation has had some impact (Marden et al., 1997).

Interpretation

Generally accepted criteria for a reactive tracing are as follows:

- Two or more accelerations of 15 beats/min lasting for 15 seconds over a 20-minute period
- Normal baseline rate
- Long-term variability amplitude of 10 or more beats per minute

If the test does not meet the criteria after 40 minutes, it is considered nonreactive (Fig. 29-8 and Table 29-6), in which case further assessments are needed with a CST or BPP. The current recommendation is that the NST be performed twice weekly (after 28 weeks of gestation) with women who have diabetes or are at risk for having a fetal death (Druzin et al., 2002).

Vibroacoustic Stimulation

Vibroacoustic stimulation (also called fetal acoustic stimulation test) is another method of testing antepartum FHR response and is sometimes used in conjunction with the NST. The test takes approximately 15 minutes to complete, with the fetus monitored for 5 to 10 minutes before stimulation to obtain a baseline FHR. If the fetal baseline pattern is nonreactive, the sound source (usually a laryngeal stimulator) is then activated for 3 seconds on the maternal abdomen over the fetal head. Monitoring continues for another 5 minutes, after which the monitor tracing is assessed. A test is considered reactive if there is an immediate and sustained increase in long-term variability and HR accelerations. The accelerations produced may have a significant increase in duration. The test may be repeated at 1-minute intervals up to 3 times when there is no response. Further evaluation is needed with BPP or CST if the pattern is still nonreactive (Druzin et al., 2002).

Contraction Stress Test

The CST is one of the first electronic methods to be developed for assessment of fetal health. It was devised as a graded stress test of the fetus, and its purpose was to identify the jeopardized fetus that was stable at rest but showed evidence of compromise after stress. Uterine contractions decrease uterine blood flow and placental

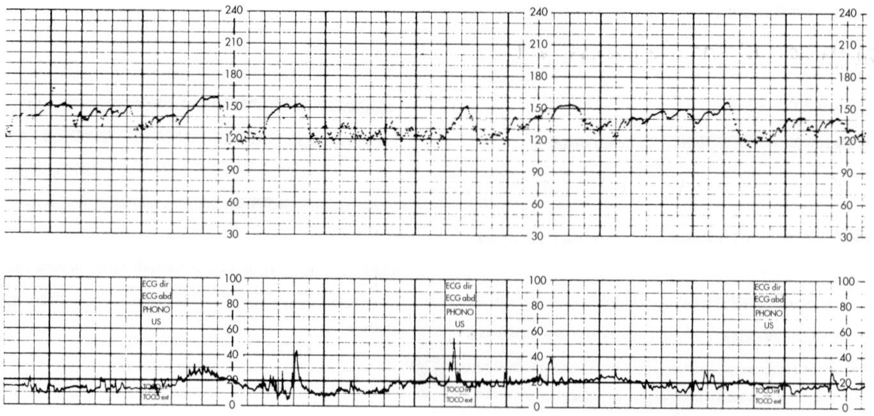
240
210
180
150
120
90
60
30
100
80
60
40
20
0
ECG dir
ECG abd
PHONO
US
TOCO ext

FIG. 29-8 Reactive NST (fetal heart rate acceleration with movement). (From Tucker, S. [2000]. *Pocket guide to fetal monitoring and assessment* [4th ed.]. St. Louis: Mosby.)

perfusion. If this decrease is sufficient to produce hypoxia in the fetus, a deceleration in FHR will result, beginning at the peak of the contraction and persisting after its conclusion (late deceleration).

NURSE ALERT

In a healthy fetoplacental unit, uterine contractions usually do not produce late decelerations, whereas if there is underlying uteroplacental insufficiency, contractions will produce late decelerations.

The CST provides an earlier warning of fetal compromise than the NST and with fewer false-positive results. In addition to the contraindications described earlier, the CST is more time consuming and expensive than the NST. It also is an invasive procedure if oxytocin stimulation is required. It is frequently used.

Procedure

The woman is placed in semi-Fowler position or sits in a reclining chair with a slight left tilt to optimize uterine perfusion and avoid supine hypotension. She is monitored electronically with the fetal ultrasound transducer and uterine tocodynamometer. The tracing is observed for 10 to 20 minutes for baseline rate, long-term variability, and the possible occurrence of spontaneous contractions. The two methods of CST are the nipple-stimulated contraction test and the oxytocin-stimulated contraction test.

Nipple-Stimulated Contraction Test. Several methods of nipple stimulation have been described. In one approach, the woman applies warm, moist washcloths to both breasts for several minutes. The woman is then asked to massage one nipple for 10 minutes. Massaging the nipples causes a release of oxytocin from the posterior pituitary. An alternative approach is for her to massage the nipple for 2 minutes, rest for 5 minutes, and repeat the cycles of massage and rest as necessary to achieve adequate uterine activity. When adequate contractions or hyperstimulation (defined as uterine contractions lasting more than 90 seconds or five or more contractions in 10 minutes) occurs, stimulation should be stopped (Druzin et al., 2002).

Oxytocin-Stimulated Contraction Test. Exogenous oxytocin also can be used to stimulate uterine contractions. An intravenous (IV) infusion is begun with a scalp needle. The oxytocin is diluted in an IV solution (e.g., 10 U in 1000 ml fluid), infused into the tubing of the main IV device through a piggyback port, and delivered by an infusion pump to ensure accurate dosage. One method of oxytocin infusion is to begin at 0.5 mU/min and increase the dose by 0.5 mU/min at 15-minute to 30-minute intervals until three uterine contractions of good quality are observed within a 10-minute period. A rate of 10 mU/min is usually adequate to elicit uterine contractions (Druzin et al., 2002).

Interpretation

If no late decelerations are observed with the contractions, the findings are considered negative (Fig. 29-9, *A*). Repetitive late decelerations render the test results positive (Fig. 29-9, *B*, and Table 29-7).

After interpretation of the FHR pattern, the oxytocin infusion is halted, and the maintenance IV solution infused until uterine activity has returned to the prestimulation level. If the CST is negative, the IV device is removed, and the fetal monitor disconnected. If the CST is positive, continued monitoring and further evaluation of fetal well-being are indicated.

NURSING ROLE IN ANTEPARTAL ASSESSMENT FOR RISK

The nurse's role is that of educator and support person when the woman is undergoing such examinations as ultrasonography, MRI, CVS, PUBS, and amniocentesis. In some instances, the nurse may assist the physician with the

TABLE 29-6 **Interpretation of the Nonstress Test**

RESULT	INTERPRETATION	CLINICAL SIGNIFICANCE
Reactive	Two or more accelerations of FHR of 15 beats/min lasting ≥15 sec, associated with each fetal movement in 20-min period	As long as twice-weekly NSTs remain reactive, most high risk pregnancies are allowed to continue
Nonreactive	Any tracing with either no FHR accelerations or accelerations <15 beats/min or lasting <15 sec throughout any fetal movement during testing period	Further indirect monitoring may be attempted with abdominal fetal electrocardiography in effort to clarify FHR pattern and quantitate variability; external monitoring should continue, and CST or BPP should be done
Unsatisfactory	Quality of FHR recording not adequate for interpretation	Test is repeated in 24 hr or CST is done, depending on clinical situation

BPP, Biophysical profile; *CST,* contraction stress test; *FHR,* fetal heart rate; *NST,* nonstress test.

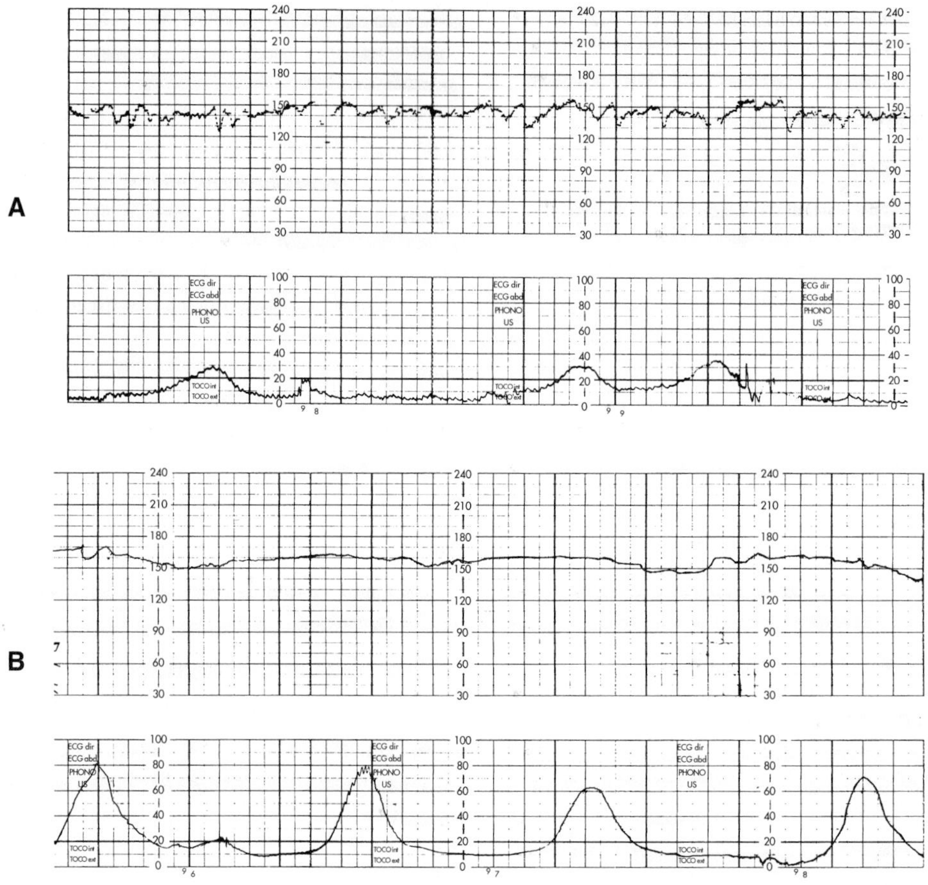

FIG. 29-9 Contraction stress test. **A,** Negative CST. **B,** Positive CST. (From Tucker, S. [2000]. *Pocket guide to fetal monitoring and assessment* [4th ed.]. St. Louis: Mosby.)

procedure. In many settings, nurses perform NSTs, CSTs, and BPPs; conduct an initial assessment; and begin necessary interventions for nonreassuring patterns. These nursing procedures are accomplished after additional education and training, under guidance of established protocols, and in collaboration with obstetrics providers (Treanor, 1998). Client teaching, which is an integral component of this role, involves preparing the woman for the procedure, interpreting the findings, and providing psychosocial support when needed (Lowe et al., 1998).

Psychologic Considerations

All women who undergo antepartal assessments are at risk for real and potential problems and may be in an anxious frame of mind. In most instances, the tests are ordered because of suspected fetal compromise, deterioration of a maternal condition, or both. In the third trimester, pregnant women are most concerned about protecting themselves and their fetuses and consider themselves most vulnerable to outside influences. The label of high risk will increase this sense of vulnerability.

PSYCHOLOGIC IMPLICATIONS OF HIGH RISK PREGNANCY

When a woman is diagnosed with a high risk pregnancy, she and her family will likely experience stress related to the diagnosis. The woman may exhibit various psychologic responses including anxiety, low self-esteem, guilt, frustration, and inability to function. The development of a high risk pregnancy also can affect parental attachment, accomplishment of the tasks of pregnancy, and family adaptation to the pregnancy (Ramer & Frank, 2001).

Women with complicated pregnancies perceive their risks as higher than do women with uncomplicated pregnancies (Gupton, Heaman, & Cheung, 2001). If the mother has to be placed on bed rest for pregnancy complications, separation from family, finances, and worry about children and home creates further stress (Maloni, Brezinski-Tomasi, & Johnson, 2001). Concerns about the fetus, uncertainty, and lack of control add to the stress of the experience (Gupton, Heamon, & Ashcroft, 1997). If hospitalization becomes necessary, further stress is generated. Mothers often feel more depressed

TABLE 29-7 **Guide for Interpretation of the CST**

INTERPRETATION	CLINICAL SIGNIFICANCE
Negative No late decelerations, with minimum of three uterine contractions lasting 40 to 60 sec within 10-min period (see Fig. 29-9, *A*)	Reassurance that the fetus is likely to survive labor should it occur within 1 wk; more frequent testing may be indicated by clinical situation
Positive Persistent and consistent late decelerations occurring with more than half of contractions (see Fig. 29-9, *B*)	Management lies between use of other tools of fetal assessment such as BPP and termination of pregnancy; a positive test result indicates that fetus is at increased risk for perinatal morbidity and mortality; physician may perform expeditious vaginal birth after successful induction or may proceed directly to cesarean birth; decision to intervene is determined by fetal monitoring and presence of FHR reactivity
Suspicious Late decelerations occurring in less than half of uterine contractions once adequate contraction pattern established	NST and CST should be repeated within 24 hr; if interpretable data cannot be achieved, other methods of fetal assessment must be used*
Hyperstimulation Late decelerations occurring with excessive uterine activity (contractions more often than every 2 min or lasting >90 sec) or persistent increase in uterine tone	
Unsatisfactory Inadequate uterine contraction pattern or tracing too poor to interpret	

*Applies to results noted as suspicious, hyperstimulation, or unsatisfactory.

and lonely, more concerned about children and their care, and greater stress over being confined (Gupton & Heamon, 1998).

If the woman is fearful for her own well-being, she may continue to feel ambivalence about the pregnancy or not accept the reality of the pregnancy. She may not be able to complete preparations for the baby or go to childbirth classes if she is on bed rest or hospitalized. The family may become frustrated because they cannot engage in these activities that prepare them for parenthood.

Antepartal hospitalization is an added stressor for the high risk pregnant woman and her family. The woman may be lonely because she is separated from her home and family. She may feel powerless and unable to make decisions for herself because her care is out of her control. Likewise, preparation for the birth process may be out of control of the woman and her family. Unexpected procedures and care for the woman or fetus may take priority over the usual birth plan and may not allow choices that would have been selected if the pregnancy had been normal.

Attachment to the newborn can be affected if the mother or newborn is ill after the birth. Early contact may not be possible. Time, support, and intervention by the health care team may be necessary to help the family begin the attachment process.

The nurse can help the woman and her family regain control and balance in their lives by providing support and encouragement, providing information about the pregnancy problem and its management (see Resources list at the end of this chapter), and providing opportunities to make as many choices as possible about the woman's care.

The impact of the effects of a specific pregnancy complication and its management is discussed in the following chapters in this unit.

KEY POINTS

- A high risk pregnancy is one in which the life or well-being of the mother or infant is jeopardized by a biophysical or psychosocial disorder coincidental with or unique to pregnancy.
- Biophysical, sociodemographic, psychosocial, and environmental factors place the pregnancy and fetus or neonate at risk.
- Psychosocial perinatal warning indicators include characteristics of the parents, the child, their support systems, and family circumstances.
- Maternal and perinatal mortality rates for Caucasians are considerably lower than for other ethnic groups in the United States.
- Mortality rate decreases when risk is identified early and intensive care is applied.
- Biophysical assessment techniques include fetal movement counts, ultrasonography, and MRI.
- Biochemical monitoring techniques include amniocentesis, PUBS, CVS, and MSAFP.
- Reactive NSTs and negative CSTs suggest fetal well-being.
- Most assessment tests have some degree of risk for the mother and fetus and usually cause some anxiety for the woman and her family.

CRITICAL THINKING EXERCISES

1. You are asked to review several pregnant clients' charts before the start of a weekly high risk clinic. On one chart, you note that the woman is anemic, smokes one and one-half packs of cigarettes a day, is in an abusive relationship, and works with noxious chemicals in her job. Describe your teaching plan to discuss her pregnancy risks.
2. Formulate a teaching plan for a woman who has been advised to monitor fetal activity at home. Include the times when monitoring is to take place, and instruct her on the way to count movements, the best time of day to complete the counts, and when to notify her health care provider.
3. Mary has been sent from her obstetric provider's office to your center for a BPP to be performed. She is worried about this test and its implications for the rest of her pregnancy and the health of her fetus. Explain the procedure and the rationale for doing the BPP.
4. Prepare a nursing care plan for families who are experiencing a high risk pregnancy. Include restriction of activities (e.g., bed rest, stopping work and or driving, the potential impact of family separation due to hospitalization). Identify strategies to lessen the impact of a high risk pregnancy on the family.

RESOURCES

Healthy Mothers, Healthy Babies Coalition
409 12th St. SW
Washington, DC 20024
202-863-2458

March of Dimes Birth Defects Foundation
National Foundation/March of Dimes
1275 Mamaroneck Ave.
White Plains, NY 10605
914-428-7100
888-663-4637 (MODIMES)
www.modimes.org

National Clearinghouse for Human Genetic Disease
*(Provides information about inherited diseases)*National Center for Education in Maternal and Child Health
38th and R Sts. NW
Washington, DC 20057

National Institute of Child Health and Human Development (NICHD)
National Institutes of Health
9000 Rockville Pike
Bldg. 31, Room 2A32
Bethesda, MD 20892
301-496-4000
www.nih.gov

Parenthood after Thirty
451 Vermont
Berkeley, CA 94707
415-524-6635

Spina Bifida Association of America
4590 McArthur Blvd. NW, Suite 250
Washington, DC 20007-4226
800-621-3141

REFERENCES

Alfirevic, Z., Gosden, C., & Neilson, J. (2000). Chorionic villus sampling versus amniocentesis for prenatal diagnosis. (Cochrane Review). In *The Cochrane Library*, Issue 1, 2001. Oxford: Update Software Ltd.

American Academy of Pediatrics/American College of Obstetricians and Gynecologists (AAP/ACOG). (1997). *Guidelines for perinatal care* (4th ed.). Elk Grove Village, IL: AAP/ACOG.

American College of Obstetricians and Gynecologists (ACOG) (1999). *Antepartum fetal surveillance. Technical Bulletin Number 9.* Washington, DC: ACOG.

Association of Women's Health, Obstetric and Neonatal Nurses (AWHONN). (1998). *Nursing practice competencies and educational guidelines for limited ultrasound examination in obstetric and gynecology/infertility settings* (2nd ed.). Washington, DC: AWHONN.

Athey, P., & Hadlock, F. (1985). *Ultrasound in obstetrics and gynecology* (2nd ed.). St. Louis: Mosby.

Beamer, L. (2001). Fetal nuchal translucency: A prenatal screening tool. *Journal of Obstetric, Gynecologic, and Neonatal Nursing, 30*(4), 376-385.

Chervenak, F., & Gabbe, S. (2002). Obstetric ultrasound: Assessment of fetal growth and anatomy. In S. Gabbe, J. Niebyl, & J. Simpson (Eds.), *Obstetrics: Normal and problem pregnancies* (4th ed.). New York: Churchill Livingstone.

Cook, C., & Ellwood, D. (2000). The cervix as a predictor of preterm delivery in "at-risk" women. *Ultrasound in Obstetrics and Gynecology, 15*(2), 109-113.

Cunningham, F. et al. (2001). *Williams obstetrics* (21st ed.). New York: McGraw-Hill.

DeCherney, A., & Pernoll, M. (Eds.). (1994). *Current obstetric and gynecologic diagnosis and treatment* (8th ed.). Norwalk, CT: Appleton & Lange.

Dooley, S., Freels, S., & Turnock, B. (1997). Quality assessment of perinatal regionalization by multivariate analysis: Illinois, 1991-1993. *Obstetrics and Gynecology, 89*, 193-198.

Druzin, M., Gabbe, S., & Reed, K. (2002). Antepartum fetal evaluation. In S. Gabbe, J. Niebyl, & J. Simpson (Eds.), *Obstetrics: Normal and problem pregnancies* (4th ed.). New York: Churchill Livingstone.

Egan. J. et al. (2000). Efficacy of screening for fetal Down syndrome in the United States: 1974 to 1997. *Obstetrics and Gynecology, 96*(6), 979-985.

Enkin, M. et al. (2001). Effective care in pregnancy and childbirth: A synopsis *Birth, 28*(1), 41-51.

Gilbert, E., & Harmon, J. (2003). *Manual of high risk pregnancy and delivery* (3rd ed.). St. Louis: Mosby.

Glantz, J., & Woods, J. (1999). Significance of amniotic fluid meconium. In R. Creasy & R. Resnik (Eds.), *Maternal-fetal medicine* (4th ed.). Philadelphia: W.B. Saunders.

Gordon, M. (2002). *Manual of nursing diagnosis* (10th ed.). St. Louis: Mosby.

Gupton, A., Heaman, M., & Cheung, L. (2001). Complicated and uncomplicated pregnancies: Women's perception of risk. *Journal of Obstetric, Gynecologic, and Neonatal Nursing, 30*(2), 192-201.

Gupton, A., & Heaman, M. (1998). Perceptions of bed rest by women with high-risk pregnancies: A comparison between home and hospital. *Birth, 25*(4), 252-258.

Gupton, A., Heaman, M., & Ashcroft, T. (1997). Bed rest from the perspective of the high-risk pregnant woman. *Journal of Obstetric, Gynecologic, and Neonatal Nursing, 26*(4), 423-430.

Harmon, C. (1999). Percutaneous fetal blood sampling. In R. Creasy & R. Resnik (Eds.), *Maternal-fetal medicine* (4th ed.). Philadelphia: W.B. Saunders.

Harmon, C., Menticoglous, S., & Manning, F. (2000). Assessing fetal health. In D. James et al. (Eds.), *High risk pregnancy management options* (2nd ed.). Philadelphia: W.B. Saunders.

Hoyert, D. et al. (2001). Annual summary of vital statistics, 2000. *Pediatrics, 108*(6), 1241-1255.

Lowe, S. et al. (1998). Routine use of ultrasound during pregnancy. *Nurse Practioner, 23*(10), 60, 63-66, 71.

Maloni, J., Brezinski-Tomasi, J., & Johnson, L. (2001). Antepartum bed rest: Effect upon the family. *Journal of Obstetric, Gynecologic, and Neonatal Nursing, 30*(2), 67-77.

Manning, F. (1995). Dynamic ultrasound-based fetal assessment: The fetal biophysical profile score. *Clinical Obstetrics and Gynecology, 38*(1), 26-44.

Manning, F. (1999). General principles and applications of ultrasound. In R. Creasy & R. Resnik (Eds.), *Maternal-fetal medicine* (4th ed.). Philadelphia: W.B. Saunders.

Marden, D. et al. (1997). A randomized controlled trial of a new fetal acoustic stimulation test for fetal well-being. *American Journal of Obstetrics and Gynecology, 176*(6), 1386-1388.

Mattson, S., & Smith, J. (2000). *Core curriculum for maternal-newborn nursing* (2nd ed.). Philadelphia: W.B. Saunders.

McCarthy, K., & Narrigan, D. (1995). Is there scientific support for the use of juice to facilitate the nonstress test? *Journal of Obstetric, Gynecologic, and Neonatal Nursing, 24*(4), 303-306.

Miller, D. (1998). Antepartum testing. *Clinical Obstetrics and Gynecology, 41*(3), 647-653.

Minino, A. et al. (2002). Deaths: Final data for 2000. *National Vital Statistics Report, 50*(15), 1-119.

Parer, J. (1999). Fetal heart rate. In R. Creasy & R. Resnik (Eds.), *Maternal-fetal medicine* (4th ed.). Philadelphia: W.B. Saunders.

Poutamo, J. et al. (1998). MRI does not change fetal cardiotocographic parameters. *Prenatal Diagnosis, 18*, 1149-1154.

Ramer, L., & Frank, B. (2001). *Pregnancy: Psychosocial perspectives* (3rd ed). White Plains, NY: March of Dimes.

Richardson, D. et al. (1998). Declining severity adjusted mortality: Evidence of improving neonatal intensive care. *Pediatrics, 102*, 893-899.

Ross, H., & Elias, S. (1997). Maternal serum screening for fetal genetic disorders. *Obstetrics and Gynecology Clinics of North America, 24*(1), 33-47.

Schulman, H. (1990). Doppler ultrasound. In R. Eden & F. Boehm (Eds.), *Assessment and care of the fetus: Physiological, clinical, and medicolegal principles.* Norwalk, CT: Appleton & Lange.

Scioscia, A. (1999). Prenatal genetic diagnosis. In R. Creasy & R. Resnik (Eds.), *Maternal-fetal medicine* (4th ed.). Philadelphia: W.B. Saunders.

Scott, J. et al. (Eds.). (1999). *Danforth's obstetrics and gynecology* (8th ed.). Philadelphia: Lippincott Williams & Wilkins.

Simpson, J. (2002). Genetic counseling and prenatal diagnosis. In S. Gabbe, J. Niebyl, & J. Simpson (Eds.), *Obstetrics: Normal and problem pregnancies* (4th ed.). New York: Churchill Livingstone.

Treanor, C. (1998). Exploring nurses' roles in limited ultrasound. *AWHONN Lifelines, 2*, 13-14.

Tucker, S. (2000). *Pocket guide to fetal monitoring and assessment* (4th ed.). St. Louis: Mosby.

United States Department of Health and Human Services. (2000). *Healthy People 2010.* (Conference Edition) (Vol. 1-2). Washington, DC: U.S. Government Printing Office.

Wilson, R. (2000). Amniocentesis and chorionic villus sampling. *Current Opinion in Obstetrics and Gynecology, 12*(2), 81-86.

CHAPTER 30

Judith H. Poole

Hypertensive Disorders in Pregnancy

http://evolve.elsevier.com/Lowdermilk/MatWmnHlth/

LEARNING OBJECTIVES

- Differentiate among gestational hypertension, preeclampsia/eclampsia, and chronic hypertension.
- Review etiologic theories of preeclampsia.
- Describe the pathophysiology of preeclampsia.
- Evaluate maternal, fetal, and newborn morbidity and mortality attributable to the hypertensive disorders of pregnancy.
- Identify assessment techniques for preeclampsia.
- Differentiate between the management of the woman with mild preeclampsia and the woman with severe preeclampsia.
- Describe HELLP syndrome, including appropriate nursing actions.
- Identify the priorities for management of eclamptic seizures.
- Evaluate the use of anticonvulsant and antihypertensive therapies.

Providing safe and effective care for the client at high risk requires a joint effort from all members of the health care team, with each member contributing unique skills and talents to provide optimal outcomes for mother and infant. This chapter focuses on the classification and theories of hypertensive disorders of pregnancy and their associated sequelae. Gestational hypertensive disorders, including preeclampsia and eclampsia, and chronic hypertension complicate pregnancy. Preeclampsia and eclampsia are the primary focus of the chapter. Pathophysiology is discussed as it affects maternal organ systems and the pregnancy. This background provides a working basis for early identification of the onset or worsening of the hypertensive condition and helps guide nurses in selecting timely and appropriate nursing interventions for preventing injury to the woman and fetus.

SIGNIFICANCE AND INCIDENCE

Hypertensive disorders of pregnancy are the most common medical complication reported during pregnancy (Martin et al., 2002). A significant contributor to maternal and perinatal morbidity and mortality, preeclampsia complicates approximately 12% to 20% of all pregnancies not terminating in first trimester miscarriages, depending on the populations and definitions used (ACOG, 2002; Egerman & Sibai, 1999; Walker, 2000). The rate of pregnancy-related hypertension has risen steadily, by about 30% to 40%, since 1990 for all ages, races, and ethnic groups to the current rate of 38.8 per 1000 live births (Martin et al., 2002). Rates for chronic hypertension have increased moderately (7.6 per 1000), whereas the rate for eclampsia has declined (3.1 per 1000 live births) (Martin et al., 2002). Age distribution remains U-shaped with women younger than 20 years and older than 40 years having the highest rates of occurrence for hypertension. Maternal race also influences the rate of pregnancy-associated hypertension, with the highest rates seen between Native American (48.2 per 1000) and African-American (41.7 per 1000) women. Asian or Pacific Islander women have the lowest rate for hypertension complicating pregnancy (20.5 per 1000) (Martin et al., 2002).

MORBIDITY AND MORTALITY

In the United States, pregnancy-associated hypertension is a leading cause of maternal death. The reported maternal death rate in 2000 was 9.8 per 100,000 (Minino et al., 2002). The overall rate of reported maternal death from preeclampsia/eclampsia is 1.8 per 100,000, which is the leading cause-specific cause of death identified (Minino et al., 2002). However, there is a large disparity between rates of maternal death by race, in that African-American women are more likely to die of preeclampsia than are women of all other races (Minino et al., 2002). Preeclampsia predisposes the woman to potentially lethal complications, including eclampsia, abruptio placentae, disseminated intravascular coagulation (DIC), acute renal failure, hepatic failure, adult respiratory distress syndrome (ARDS), and cerebral hemorrhage (ACOG, 2002; National High Blood Pressure Education Program Working Group on High Blood Pressure in Pregnancy [Working Group], 2000; Report of the National High Blood Pressure Education Program [Summary Report], 2000).

Hypertension (chronic and pregnancy induced) complicating pregnancy increases the woman's risk for a cesarean birth, which further increases the risk of morbidity and mortality. The final report of birth certificate data for 2000 indicated that of the total rates of cesarean birth for selected conditions, 42.9% were for women with chronic hypertension, 38.1% for women with pregnancy-associated hypertension, and 48.8% for women with eclampsia (Martin et al., 2002). When primary indications were reported, the rates of cesarean births are as follows: 32.6% for women with chronic hypertension, 32.7% for women with pregnancy-associated hypertension, and 43.9% for women with eclampsia (Martin et al., 2002).

Preeclampsia occurs primarily after the second trimester of pregnancy, representing a great danger to the fetus and neonate. Preeclampsia contributes significantly to intrauterine fetal death (IUFD) and perinatal mortality (ACOG, 2002; Summary Report, 2000; Working Group, 2000). Causes of perinatal death related to preeclampsia are uteroplacental insufficiency (UPI) and abruptio placentae, which lead to intrauterine death, preterm birth, and low birth weight (Roberts, 1999).

Eclampsia (characterized by seizures) from profound cerebral effects of preeclampsia is the major maternal hazard. As a rule, maternal and perinatal morbidity and mortality are highest among cases in which eclampsia is seen early in gestation (before 28 weeks); maternal age is older than 25 years; the woman is a multigravida; and chronic hypertension or renal disease is present. The fetus of the eclamptic woman is at increased risk from abruptio placentae, preterm birth, intrauterine growth restriction (IUGR), and acute hypoxia.

CLASSIFICATION

Current terminology used to describe the hypertensive disorders of pregnancy is associated with imprecise usage, causing confusion for health care providers caring for women with hypertensive complications during pregnancy and childbirth. The classification system most commonly used in the United States today is based on reports from the American College of Obstetricians and Gynecologists (2002) and the National High Blood Pressure Education Program Working Group on High Blood Pressure in Pregnancy (2000). This classification system is summarized in Table 30-1.

Gestational Hypertension

Gestational hypertension is the onset of hypertension without proteinuria after week 20 of pregnancy (ACOG, 2002; Summary Report, 2000; Working Group, 2000). Gestational hypertension is a nonspecific term that replaces the term *pregnancy-induced hypertension* or PIH. Chronic hypertension and gestational hypertension may occur independently or simultaneously. Gestational hypertension is further classified according to the maternal organ systems affected.

The final diagnosis and differentiation between gestational hypertension and preeclampsia is made in the postpartum period. If the woman has not developed preeclampsia and her blood pressure (BP) returns to normal values by 12 weeks after delivery, the woman is said to have *transient hypertension*. If BP values remain elevated, then the diagnosis of chronic hypertension is made (ACOG, 2002;

TABLE 30-1 **Classification of Hypertensive States of Pregnancy**

TYPE	DESCRIPTION
Gestational hypertension	Blood pressure elevation detected first time after mid-pregnancy without proteinuria. (Previously known as pregnancy-induced hypertension or PIH)
Transient hypertension	Gestational hypertension with no signs of preeclampsia present at the time of birth and hypertension resolves by 12 weeks postpartum. This is a retrospective diagnosis
Preeclampsia	Pregnancy-specific syndrome that usually occurs after 20 weeks' gestation and is determined by gestational hypertension plus proteinuria
Eclampsia	The occurrence of seizures in a woman with preeclampsia that cannot be attributed to other causes
Chronic hypertension	Hypertension that is present and observable before pregnancy or that is diagnosed before week 20 of gestation
Preeclampsia superimposed on chronic hypertension	Chronic hypertension with new proteinuria or an exacerbation of hypertension (previously well controlled) or proteinuria, thrombocytopenia, or increases in hepatocellular enzymes

Adapted from American College of Obstetricians and Gynecologists. (2002). *Diagnosis and management of preeclampsia and eclampsia: ACOG Practice Bulletin Number 33.* Washington, DC: ACOG; Blackburn, S. (2003). *Maternal, fetal, & neonatal physiology: A clinical perspective* (2nd ed.). St. Louis: W.B. Saunders; National High Blood Pressure Education Program Working Group on High Blood Pressure in Pregnancy (Working Group). (2000). *NIH Publication No. 00-3029.* Bethesda, MD: National Institutes of Health, National Heart, Lung, and Blood Institute.

Summary Report, 2000; Working Group, 2000). The presence of transient hypertension may be predictive of the eventual development of essential hypertension.

Preeclampsia

Preeclampsia, a pregnancy-specific syndrome in which hypertension develops after 20 weeks of gestation in a previously normotensive woman, is a multisystem, vasospastic disease process of reduced organ perfusion characterized by the presence of hypertension and proteinuria (ACOG, 2002; Summary Report, 2000; Working Group, 2000). Preeclampsia is usually categorized as mild or severe in terms of management (Table 30-2).

An elevated BP is often the first sign of preeclampsia to develop. ***Hypertension***, whether gestational or chronic, is defined as a systolic BP greater than 140 mm Hg, or a diastolic BP greater than 90 mm Hg, or a mean arterial pressure (MAP) greater than 105 mm Hg (ACOG, 2002; Summary Report, 2000; Working Group, 2000). The diagnosis of a new onset of hypertension during pregnancy is based on at least two measurements that meet the criteria for gestational BP elevation.

Elevations over prepregnancy values are no longer considered diagnostic for preeclampsia. However, women who demonstrate an increase of 30 mm Hg systolic or 15 mm Hg diastolic warrant closer observation if the BP elevation occurs with proteinuria and hyperuricemia (uric acid of 6 mg/dl or more) (ACOG, 2002; Summary Report, 2000; Working Group, 2000).

One of the difficulties in diagnosing hypertension has been a lack of standardization in BP measurement. Accurate and consistent BP assessment is important for establishing a baseline and monitoring subtle changes throughout the pregnancy. BP readings are affected by maternal position

TABLE 30-2 **Differentiation Between Mild and Severe Preeclampsia**

	MILD PREECLAMPSIA	SEVERE PREECLAMPSIA
MATERNAL EFFECTS		
Blood pressure	BP reading of 140/90 mm Hg ×2, ≥4-6 hr apart, no more than 1 wk apart	Rise to ≥160/110 mm Hg on two separate occasions
Mean arterial pressure (MAP)	>105 mm Hg	>105 mm Hg
Proteinuria		
Quantitative 24-hr analysis	Proteinuria of ≥0.3 g in a 24-hr specimen	Proteinuria of >2 g in 24 hr
Qualitative dipstick	≥30 mg/dl (≥/+) on dipstick	2+ to 3+ protein on dipstick
Reflexes	May be normal	Hyperreflexia ≥3+, possible ankle clonus
Urine output	Output matching intake, ≥30 ml/hr or <650 ml/24 hr	20 ml/hr or <400 ml to 500 ml/24 hr
Headache	Absent/transient	Severe
Visual problems	Absent	Blurred, photophobia, blind spots on funduscopy
Irritability/changes in affect	Transient	Severe
Epigastric pain	Absent	Present
Serum creatinine	Normal	Elevated
Thrombocytopenia	Absent	Present
AST elevation	Normal or minimal	Marked
FETAL EFFECTS		
Placental perfusion	Reduced	Decreased perfusion expressing as IUGR in fetus; FHR: late decelerations
Premature placental aging	Not apparent	At birth, placenta appearing smaller than normal for duration of pregnancy, premature aging apparent with numerous areas of broken syncytia, ischemic necroses (white infarcts) numerous, intervillous fibrin deposition (red infarcts)

AST, Aspartate aminotransferase; *FHR,* fetal heart rate; *IUGR,* intrauterine growth restriction.
American College of Obstetricians and Gynecologists. (2002). *Diagnosis and management of preeclampsia and eclampsia. ACOG Practice Bulletin Number 33.* Washington, DC: ACOG.
Report of the National High Blood Pressure Education Program Working Group on High Blood Pressure in Pregnancy. (2002). *American Journal of Obstetrics and Gynecology, 183*(1), S1-S22.

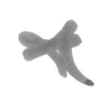

and measurement techniques. Consistency must be ensured in that proper equipment and cuff size are used, the woman is correctly positioned with a rest period before recording the pressure, and that Korotkoff phase V (disappearance of sound) is recorded (ACOG, 2002; Summary Report, 2000; Working Group, 2000). Korotkoff phase IV (muffling sound) is typically 5 to 10 mm Hg higher than phase V. Ideally, BP measurements should be recorded with the woman in a semi-Fowler position with the arm at heart level. If the initial measurement indicates an elevation, the woman should be allowed to relax and have a repeated measurement, again in a semi-Fowler position (ACOG, 2002; Summary Report, 2000; Working Group, 2000). The main point to remember is that BP measurements should be taken in a consistent manner. Assessment focuses on trends, not on a single reading. Box 30-1 presents recommendations for standardizing this procedure.

BOX *30-1* **Protocol for Blood Pressure Measurement**

- Measure blood pressure in the same arm with the woman in the same position each time (e.g., seated or in a 30-degree tilt on her left side).
- After positioning, allow the woman ≥5 min of quiet rest before blood pressure measurement, to encourage relaxation.
- If the woman is seated, her arm should be resting on a surface at the level of her heart.
- If woman is in a lateral position, the lower arm should be positioned so the woman is not lying on the arm, and the blood pressure is then taken in the dependent arm. This more closely approximates the arterial pressure, whereas using the arm of the opposite side will falsely reduce the measurement.
- Use the proper-sized cuff (cuff should cover ~80% of the upper arm).
- In women who have an upper arm too large for a standard-size cuff (cuff is too short), the more accurate measure is obtained by taking the blood pressure with the cuff placed on the forearm, and Korotkoff phase V is recorded at the radial artery.
- Maintain a slow, steady deflation rate.
- Take the average of two readings ≥6 hours apart to minimize recorded blood pressure variations across time.
- Use Korotkoff phase V (disappearance of sound) for recording the diastolic value (some sources recommend recording both phase IV [the muffled sound] and phase V).
- Use accurate equipment.
- If interchanging manual and electronic devices, use caution in interpreting different blood pressure values.

Proteinuria is defined as a concentration of ≥30 mg/dl (≥1+ on dipstick measurement) or more in at least two random urine specimens collected at least 6 hours apart, with no evidence of urinary tract infection (ACOG, 2002; Summary Report, 2000; Working Group, 2000). In a 24-hour specimen, *proteinuria* is defined as a concentration of ≥0.3 g per 24 hours. Because of the discrepancy between random protein determinations, current recommendations are that the diagnosis of proteinuria be based on a 24-hour urine collection if possible or a timed collection corrected for creatinine excretion if a 24-hour specimen is not feasible (ACOG, 2002; Summary Report, 2000; Working Group, 2000).

Pathologic edema is clinically evident, generalized accumulation of fluid of the face, hands, or abdomen that is not responsive to 12 hours of bed rest. It also may be manifested as a rapid weight gain of more than 2 kg in 1 week. However, edema occurs in too many normal pregnancies to be used as a marker for preeclampsia; therefore the presence of edema is no longer considered diagnostic of preeclampsia (ACOG, 2002; Sibai & Rodriguez, 1999; Summary Report, 2000; Working Group, 2000).

Severe Preeclampsia

Severe preeclampsia is the presence of any one of the following in the woman diagnosed with preeclampsia: (1) systolic BP of at least 160 mm Hg or a diastolic BP of at least 110 mm Hg; (2) proteinuria >2 g protein excreted in a 24-hour specimen, or greater than 2+ to 3+ on dipstick measurement; proteinuria ≥5 g/24-hr specimen or ≥3+ on dipstick are criteria used by ACOG (2002); (3) oliguria, less than 400 ml to 500 ml of urine output over a 24-hour period; (4) cerebral or visual disturbances, such as altered level of consciousness, headache, scotomata, or blurred vision; (5) hepatic involvement, including epigastric pain or elevated liver enzymes; (6) thrombocytopenia with a platelet count less than 100,000/mm^3; (7) pulmonary or cardiac involvement; (8) development of eclampsia; (9) development of the HELLP syndrome; (10) increased serum creatinine (≥1.2 mg/dl unless known to be elevated; or (11) certain cases of severe fetal growth restriction (ACOG, 2002; Sibai, 2002b; Summary Report, 2000; Working Group, 2000).

Eclampsia

Eclampsia is the onset of seizure activity or coma in the woman diagnosed with preeclampsia, with no history of preexisting pathology that can result in seizure activity (ACOG, 2002; Roberts, 1999; Summary Report, 2000; Working Group, 2000). A seizure can be the initial sign for a pregnancy complicated by preeclampsia.

Chronic Hypertension

Chronic hypertension is defined as hypertension present before the pregnancy or diagnosed before week 20 of gestation. Hypertension that persists longer than 12 weeks postpartum also is classified as chronic hypertension.

severe HTN = diastolic > 110

There is no widely accepted definition of mild hypertension. Severe hypertension is usually defined as a diastolic BP of 110 mm Hg or higher (ACOG, 2002; Summary Report, 2000; Working Group, 2000). Preconception counseling is recommended for women with respect to the increased risk of superimposed preeclampsia and lifestyle adjustments that may be necessary.

Chronic Hypertension with Superimposed Preeclampsia

Women with chronic hypertension may acquire preeclampsia or eclampsia. **Chronic hypertension with superimposed preeclampsia** is defined with the following findings:

- In women with hypertension and no proteinuria early in pregnancy (before 20 weeks), new-onset proteinuria, defined as the urinary excretion of 0.3 g or greater in a 24-hour specimen
- In women with hypertension and proteinuria before 20 weeks' gestation
- Sudden increase in proteinuria
- A sudden increase in BP in a woman whose hypertension has previously been well controlled
- Thrombocytopenia
- An increase in hepatocellular markers for hepatic dysfunction (ACOG, 2002; Roberts, 1999; Summary Report, 2000; Working Group, 2000).

PREECLAMPSIA

Etiology

Proposed causes of hypertension in pregnancy are multiple and have been the subject of extensive research and much speculation. The ultimate cause remains unknown.

Preeclampsia is a condition unique to human pregnancy; signs and symptoms develop only during pregnancy and disappear quickly after birth of the fetus and placenta. No single client profile identifies the woman who will have preeclampsia. However, certain high risk factors are associated with development of the disease: primigravidity, multifetal pregnancy, and morbid obesity (Box 30-2).

Several major concepts contribute to current theories regarding the etiology of preeclampsia: vasoconstrictor tone, abnormal prostaglandin action, endothelial cell dysfunction, coagulation abnormalities, abnormal trophoblast invasion, and dietary deficiencies or excesses (Dekker & Sibai, 1998; Sibai, 2002b). Immunologic factors and genetic disposition may play an important role (Dekker & Sibai, 1999).

In part, vasospasms are the underlying mechanism for the signs and symptoms of preeclampsia. Vasospasms result from an increased sensitivity to circulating pressors, such as angiotensin II, and possibly an imbalance between the prostaglandins prostacyclin and thromboxane A_2 (ACOG, 2002; Summary Report, 2000; Working Group, 2000).

Endothelial cell dysfunction, believed to result from decreased placental perfusion, may account for many preeclampsia changes, as depicted in Fig. 30-1. In addition to endothelial damage, arteriolar vasospasm may contribute to an increased capillary permeability. This increases edema and further decreases intravascular volume, predisposing the woman with preeclampsia to pulmonary edema (Roberts, 1999).

The relation of the immune system to preeclampsia suggests that immunologic factors play an important role in the development of preeclampsia (Sibai, 2002b). The presence of foreign protein, the placenta, or the fetus may trigger an adverse immunologic response. This theory is supported by the increased incidence of preeclampsia or

BOX 30-2 Risk Factors Associated with the Development of Preeclampsia

- Chronic renal disease
- Chronic hypertension
- Family history of preeclampsia
- Multifetal gestation
- Primigravidity or new partner
- Maternal age younger than 19 years or 40 years or older
- Diabetes
- Rh incompatibility
- Obesity

Data from American College of Obstetricians and Gynecologists. (2002). *Diagnosis and management of preeclampsia and eclampsia. ACOG Practice Bulletin Number 33.* Washington, DC: ACOG; National High Blood Pressure Education Program Working Group on High Blood Pressure in Pregnancy [Working Group]. (2000). NIH Publication No. 00-3029. Bethesda, MD: National Institutes of Health, National Heart, Lung, and Blood Institute; Roberts, J. (1999). Pregnancy-related hypertension. In R. Creasy & R. Resnik (Eds.), *Maternal-fetal medicine* (4th ed.). Philadelphia: W.B. Saunders.

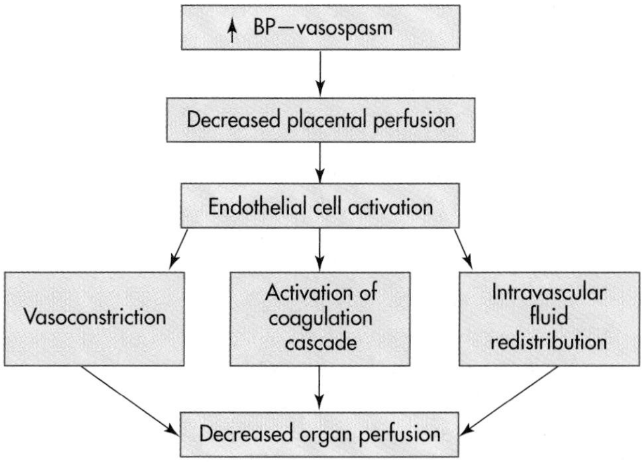
↑ BP—vasospasm
Decreased placental perfusion
Endothelial cell activation
Vasoconstriction
Activation of coagulation cascade
Intravascular fluid redistribution
Decreased organ perfusion

FIG. 30-1 Etiology of preeclampsia: Endothelial cell dysfunction.

eclampsia in first-time mothers (first exposure to fetal tissue) and multiparous women pregnant by a new partner (different genetic material) (Li & Wi, 2000). The protective role of the immunologic response is poorly understood. Preeclampsia may be an immune complex disease in which the maternal antibody system is overwhelmed from excessive fetal antigens in the maternal circulation. This theory seems compatible with the high incidence of preeclampsia among women exposed to a large mass of trophoblastic tissue as seen in twins and hydatidiform moles.

Genetic predisposition may be another immunologic factor. Dekker (2001) reported a greater frequency of preeclampsia and eclampsia among daughters and granddaughters of women with a history of eclampsia, which suggests an autosomal recessive gene controlling the maternal immune response. Paternal factors also are being examined (Robillard, 2002).

Diets inadequate in nutrients, especially protein, calcium, sodium, magnesium, and vitamins E and C, may be an etiologic factor in preeclampsia. Proponents of this theory prescribe high-protein diets without caloric or sodium restriction in prevention and treatment of this disorder (Stone, 1998). However, data are inconclusive for an association between diet and the development of preeclampsia.

Pathophysiology

Preeclampsia progresses along a continuum from mild disease to severe preeclampsia, HELLP syndrome, or eclampsia. The pathophysiology of preeclampsia reflects alterations in the normal adaptations of pregnancy. Normal physiologic adaptations to pregnancy include increased

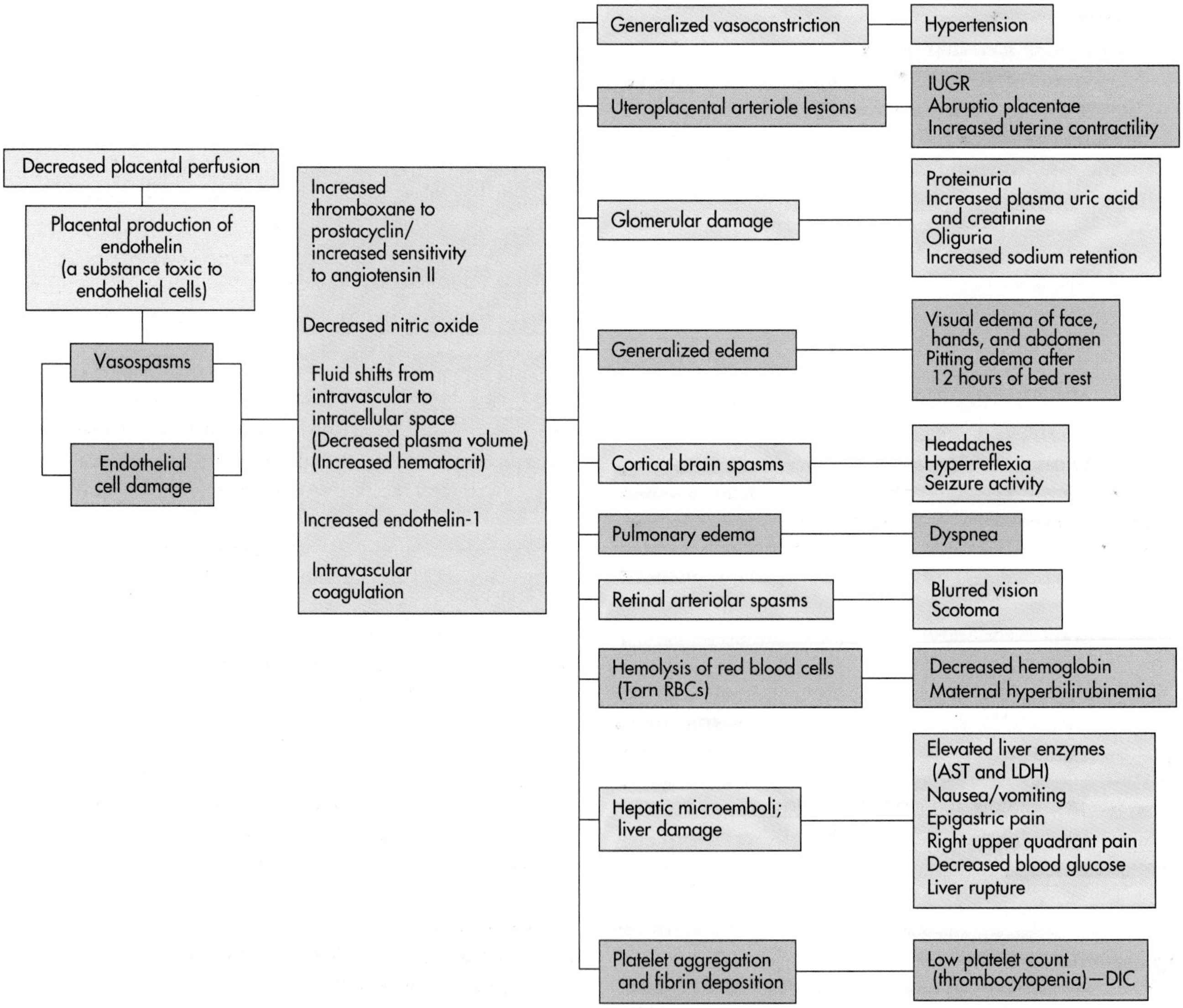
Decreased placental perfusion
Placental production of endothelin (a substance toxic to endothelial cells)
Vasospasms
Endothelial cell damage
Increased thromboxane to prostacyclin/ increased sensitivity to angiotensin II
Decreased nitric oxide
Fluid shifts from intravascular to intracellular space (Decreased plasma volume) (Increased hematocrit)
Increased endothelin-1
Intravascular coagulation
Generalized vasoconstriction
Hypertension
Uteroplacental arteriole lesions
IUGR
Abruptio placentae
Increased uterine contractility
Glomerular damage
Proteinuria
Increased plasma uric acid and creatinine
Oliguria
Increased sodium retention
Generalized edema
Visual edema of face, hands, and abdomen
Pitting edema after 12 hours of bed rest
Cortical brain spasms
Headaches
Hyperreflexia
Seizure activity
Pulmonary edema
Dyspnea
Retinal arteriolar spasms
Blurred vision
Scotoma
Hemolysis of red blood cells (Torn RBCs)
Decreased hemoglobin
Maternal hyperbilirubinemia
Hepatic microemboli; liver damage
Elevated liver enzymes (AST and LDH)
Nausea/vomiting
Epigastric pain
Right upper quadrant pain
Decreased blood glucose
Liver rupture
Platelet aggregation and fibrin deposition
Low platelet count (thrombocytopenia)—DIC

FIG. 30-2 Pathophysiology of preeclampsia. (Modified from Gilbert, E., & Harmon, J. [2003]. *Manual of high risk pregnancy and delivery* [3rd ed.]. St. Louis: Mosby.)

blood plasma volume, vasodilation, decreased systemic vascular resistance, elevated cardiac output, and decreased colloid osmotic pressure (Box 30-3).

Preeclampsia is quite different from chronic hypertension. Pathologic changes in the endothelial cells of the glomeruli (glomeruloendotheliosis) are uniquely characteristic of preeclampsia, particularly in nulliparous women (85%). The main pathogenic factor is not an increase in BP but poor perfusion as a result of vasospasm. **Arteriolar vasospasm** diminishes the diameter of blood vessels, which impedes blood flow to all organs and increases BP (Summary Report, 2000; Working Group, 2000). Function in organs such as the placenta, kidneys, liver, and brain is depressed by as much as 40% to 60%. The pathophysiologic sequelae are shown in Figure 30-2.

Impaired placental perfusion leads to early degenerative aging of the placenta and possible IUGR of the fetus. Reduced kidney perfusion decreases the glomerular filtration rate and leads to degenerative glomerular changes and oliguria. Protein, primarily albumin, is lost in the urine. Uric acid clearance is decreased; however, blood urea nitrogen (BUN), serum creatinine, and serum uric acid levels increase. Sodium and water are retained. Plasma colloid osmotic pressure decreases as serum albumin levels decrease. Intravascular volume is reduced as fluid moves out of the intravascular compartment, resulting in hemoconcentration, increased blood viscosity, and tissue edema. The hematocrit value increases as fluid leaves the intravascular space. In severe preeclampsia, blood volume may decrease to or below nonpregnancy levels; severe edema develops, and rapid weight gain is seen.

Decreased liver perfusion causes impaired function. Hepatic edema and subcapsular hemorrhage, felt by the pregnant woman as epigastric or right upper quadrant pain, is one sign of impending eclampsia (convulsion). Liver enzyme levels (e.g., aspartate aminotransferase [AST]) increase in the wake of liver damage.

Arteriolar vasospasms and decreased blood flow to the retina lead to visual symptoms such as scotomata (blind spots) and blurring. The same pathologic condition leads to cerebral edema and hemorrhages, as well as to increased central nervous system (CNS) irritability, which manifests as headache, hyperreflexia, positive ankle clonus, and occasionally the development of eclampsia. Changes in affect (changes in emotion, mood, and consciousness) are typical symptoms of cerebral edema and increasing intracranial pressure (Scott et al., 1999).

If the hypertension is difficult to bring under control, cardiac and pulmonary complications can occur. Heart failure, a common cause of maternal death attributed to preeclampsia, is rare among young, otherwise healthy women (Scott et al., 1999). Sudden circulatory collapse and shock may occur in women with a history of repeated hypertensive pregnancies.

Typically, pulmonary edema caused by preeclampsia is associated with severe generalized edema. Intravenous (IV) fluid infusion is an iatrogenic cause of fluid overload. A weak, rapid pulse; increased respiratory rate; reduced BP; and pulmonary crackles suggest circulatory failure. Pulmonary edema and congestive heart failure are the only accepted indications for diuretic therapy during pregnancy (Scott et al., 1999). Diuretic therapy further reduces intervillous blood flow (placental perfusion), which may lead to serious fetal jeopardy. Impaired intervillous perfusion is the main cause of perinatal morbidity and mortality associated with hypertension (Scott et al., 1999).

BOX 30-3 Normal Physiologic Adaptations to Pregnancy

CARDIOVASCULAR

↑ Blood volume; plasma volume expansion greater than red cell mass expansion, leading to physiologic anemia of pregnancy

↓ Total peripheral resistance, decreases in blood pressure readings and MAP

↑ Cardiac output resulting from increased blood volume, slight increase in heart rate to compensate for peripheral relaxation

↑ Oxygen consumption

Physiologic edema related to ↓ plasma colloid osmotic pressure and ↑ venous capillary hydrostatic pressure

HEMATOLOGIC

↑ Clotting factors, predisposing to DIC and clotting

↓ Serum albumin resulting in decreases in colloid osmotic pressure, predisposing to pulmonary edema

RENAL

↑ Renal plasma flow and glomerular filtration rate

ENDOCRINE

↑ Estrogen production resulting in ↑ renin–angiotensin II–aldosterone secretion

↑ Progesterone production blocking aldosterone effect (slight ↓ Na)

↑ Vasodilator prostaglandins resulting in resistance to angiotensin II (slight ↓ blood pressure)

MAP, Mean arterial pressure; *DIC,* disseminated intravascular coagulation.

HELLP Syndrome

HELLP syndrome is a laboratory diagnosis for a variant of severe preeclampsia that involves hepatic dysfunction, characterized by *hemolysis* (H), *elevated liver enzymes* (EL), and *low platelets* (LP) (ACOG, 2002). A diagnosis of HELLP syndrome is associated with an increased risk for adverse perinatal outcomes, including placental abruption, acute renal failure, subcapsular hepatic hematoma, hepatic rupture, recurrent preeclampsia, preterm birth, and fetal and maternal death (ACOG, 2002).

HELLP syndrome appears in only 2% to 12% of severely preeclamptic women, or about 1 in 1000 pregnancies

TABLE 30-3 **Common Laboratory Changes in Preeclampsia**

	NORMAL	PIH	HELLP
Hemoglobin/hematocrit	12-16 g/dl 37% to 47%	May increase	Decreased
Platelets	150,000-400,000/mm^3	Unchanged	<100,000/mm^3
PT/PTT	12-14 sec/60-70 sec	Unchanged	Unchanged
Fibrinogen	150-400 mg/dl	300-600 mg/dl	Decreased
Fibrin split products (FSP)	Absent	Absent	Present
Blood urea nitrogen	10-20 mg/dl	<10 mg/dl	Increased
Creatinine	0.5-1.1 mg/dl	<1 mg/dl	Increased
Lactate dehydrogenase (LDH)	45-90 U/L	Unchanged	Increased
Aspartate aminotransferase (AST)	4-20 U/L	Unchanged	Increased
Alanine aminotransferase (ALT)	3-21 U/L	Unchanged	Increased
Creatinine clearance	80-125 ml/min	130-180 ml/min	Decreased
Burr cells/schistocytes	Absent	Absent	Present
Uric acid	2-6.6 mg/dl	4.5-6 mg/dl	>10 mg/dl
Bilirubin (total)	0.1-1 mg/dl	Unchanged or increased	Increased

PT, Prothrombin time; *PTT,* partial thromboplastin time; *PIH,* pregnancy-induced hypertension.

(Stone, 1998). Although the exact mechanism is unknown, HELLP syndrome is thought to arise as a result of changes occurring with preeclampsia (see Fig. 30-2). Arteriolar vasospasm, endothelial damage, and platelet aggregation with resultant tissue hypoxia are the underlying mechanisms for the pathophysiology of HELLP syndrome. A circulating immunologic component may be the underlying cause. Maternal mortality rates have been reported as high as 24%. Perinatal mortality rates range from 79 to 367 per 1000 live births (Portis et al., 1997).

Most commonly, HELLP syndrome is seen in older, Caucasian, multiparous women. About 90% of women report a history of malaise for several days. Many women (65%) have epigastric or right upper quadrant abdominal pain (possibly related to hepatic ischemia), and nausea and vomiting develop in approximately half. It is extremely important to understand that many women with HELLP syndrome may not have signs or symptoms of severe preeclampsia. For example, many of these women are normotensive or have only slight elevations in BP. Proteinuria also may be absent. As a result, women with HELLP syndrome are often misdiagnosed with a variety of other medical or surgical disorders (Sibai, 2002b).

HELLP syndrome is a laboratory, not a clinical, diagnosis. To have a diagnosis of HELLP syndrome, a woman's platelet count must be less than 100,000/mm^3, her liver enzyme levels (AST and alanine aminotransferase [ALT]) must be elevated, and there must be some evidence of intravascular hemolysis (burr cells on peripheral smear or elevated bilirubin level) (Stone, 1998). A unique form of coagulopathy (not DIC) occurs with HELLP syndrome. The platelet count is low, but coagulation factor assays, prothrombin time (PT), partial thromboplastin time (PTT), and bleeding time remain normal (Stone, 1998).

Recognition of the clinical and laboratory findings associated with HELLP syndrome is important if early, aggressive therapy is to be initiated to prevent maternal and neonatal mortality. Complications reported with HELLP syndrome include renal failure, pulmonary edema, ruptured liver hematoma, DIC, and placental abruption (Sibai, 2002b). Common laboratory findings in preeclampsia are listed in Table 30-3.

CARE MANAGEMENT

Assessment and Nursing Diagnoses

Hypertensive disorders of pregnancy can occur without warning or with the gradual development of symptoms. Because the cause is unknown and proven methods to prevent the illness are nonexistent, a key goal is early detection of the disease to prevent the catastrophic maternal and fetal sequelae. One strategy to meet this goal is the identification of individuals at high risk at the initial prenatal visit (see Box 30-1). During each subsequent visit, the woman is assessed for signs or symptoms that suggest the onset or presence of preeclampsia.

Obstetric conditions associated with increased placental mass, such as multifetal gestation and hydatidiform moles, and chronic medical disorders, such as hypertension, collagen vascular disease, and diabetes mellitus, lead to a greater risk of preeclampsia (Roberts, 1999).

Interview

The nurse reviews the woman's admission form and prenatal record. The nurse conducts the interview to clarify, expand, or complete the form. Medical history is re-

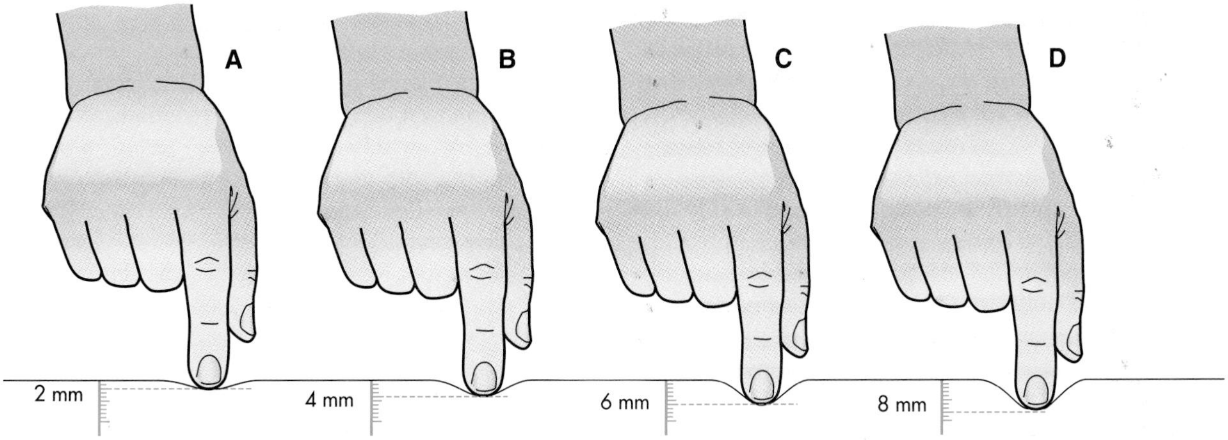
A
B
C
D
2 mm
4 mm
6 mm
8 mm

FIG. 30-3 Assessment of pitting edema of lower extremities. **A,** 1+. **B,** 2+. **C,** 3+. **D,** 4+.

viewed, especially the presence of diabetes mellitus, renal disease, and hypertension. Family history is explored for occurrence of preeclamptic or hypertensive conditions, diabetes mellitus, and other chronic conditions. The social and experiential history provides information about the woman's marital status, nutritional status, cultural beliefs, activity level, and health habits such as smoking and alcohol consumption. Limited data suggest that smoking may demonstrate a protective effect against the development of preeclampsia. However, smoking during pregnancy is detrimental to perinatal outcomes, and women should be counseled to stop.

A review of systems adds to the database for detecting BP changes from baseline and the presence of proteinuria. Noting whether the woman is having unusual, frequent, or severe headaches; visual disturbances; or epigastric pain also is important. Abnormal weight gain and pattern of weight gain and increased signs of edema may be noted even though they may not be specifically diagnostic signs of preeclampsia.

Physical Examination

Personnel caring for pregnant women must be consistent in taking and recording BP measurements in the standardized manner (see Box 30-1). If electronic BP devices are used, a manual reading should be taken to validate the electronic device reading. Electronic BP devices show a widening of the pulse pressure as compared with manual readings; the MAP, however, remains unchanged (Marx et al., 1993). Electronic BP devices are less accurate in high-flow states such as pregnancy or in hypertensive/hypotensive states.

Observation of edema in addition to hypertension warrants additional investigation. Edema is assessed for distribution, degree, and pitting. If periorbital or facial edema is not obvious, the pregnant woman is asked whether it was present when she awoke. Edema may be described as dependent or pitting.

Dependent edema is edema of the lowest or most dependent parts of the body, where hydrostatic pressure is greatest. If a pregnant woman is ambulatory, this edema may first be evident in the feet and ankles. If the pregnant woman is confined to bed, the edema is more likely to occur in the sacral region.

Pitting edema is edema that leaves a small depression or pit after finger pressure is applied to the swollen area. The pit, which is caused by movement of fluid to adjacent tissue away from the point of pressure, normally disappears within 10 to 30 seconds. Although the amount of edema is difficult to quantify, the method described in Figure 30-3 may be used to record relative degrees of edema formation.

Symptoms reflecting CNS and visual system involvement usually accompany facial edema. Although it is not a routine assessment during the prenatal period, evaluation of the fundus of the eye yields valuable data. An initial baseline finding of normal eye grounds assists in differentiating preexisting disease from a new disease process (Fig. 30-4). The woman may not have other symptoms such as epigastric pain or oliguria. Respirations are assessed for crackles, which may indicate pulmonary edema, a sign associated with severe preeclampsia.

Deep tendon reflexes (DTRs) are evaluated if preeclampsia is suspected. The biceps and patellar reflexes and ankle clonus are assessed and the findings recorded (Fig. 30-5; Table 30-4). The evaluation of DTRs is especially important if the woman is being treated with magnesium sulfate; absence of DTRs is an early indication of impending magnesium toxicity. To elicit the biceps reflex, the examiner strikes a downward blow over the thumb, which is situated over the biceps tendon. Normal response is flexion of the arm at the elbow, described as a 2+ response (see Table 30-4). The patellar reflex is elicited with the woman's legs hanging freely over the end of the examining table or with the woman lying on her left side with the knee slightly flexed. A blow with a percussion hammer is dealt directly to the patellar tendon, inferior to the patella. Normal response is the extension or kicking out of the leg. To assess for hyperactive reflexes **(clonus)** at the ankle joint, the examiner supports the leg with the knee flexed. With one hand, the examiner sharply dorsiflexes the foot, maintains the position for a moment, and then releases the foot. Normal *(negative clonus)* response is elicited when no rhythmic oscillations (jerks) are felt while the foot is held in dorsiflexion. When the foot is released, no oscillations are seen as the foot drops to the plantar-flexed position. Abnormal *(positive clonus)* response is recognized by rhythmic oscillations of one or more "beats" felt when the foot is in dorsiflexion and seen as the foot drops to the plantar-flexed position.

An important assessment is determination of fetal status. Uteroplacental perfusion is decreased in women with preeclampsia, placing the fetus in jeopardy. The fetal heart rate (FHR) is assessed for baseline rate, variability, and accelerations, which indicate an intact, oxygenated fetal CNS. Abnormal baseline rate, decreased or absent variability, and late or variable decelerations are indications of fetal intolerance to the intrauterine environment. Biophysical monitoring, such as nonstress testing, contraction stress testing, biophysical profile, and serial ultrasonography, is used to assess fetal status.

Doppler flow velocimetry studies are being used to evaluate maternal and fetal well-being (see Chapter 29). Measuring the velocity of blood flow through the uterine artery, umbilical artery, or both assesses uteroplacental perfusion. Abnormal uterine artery Doppler flow is associated with risk of IUGR in women with HELLP syndrome (Bush, O'Brien, & Barton, 2001). However, the usefulness in predicting preeclampsia is described as limited by Chien and others

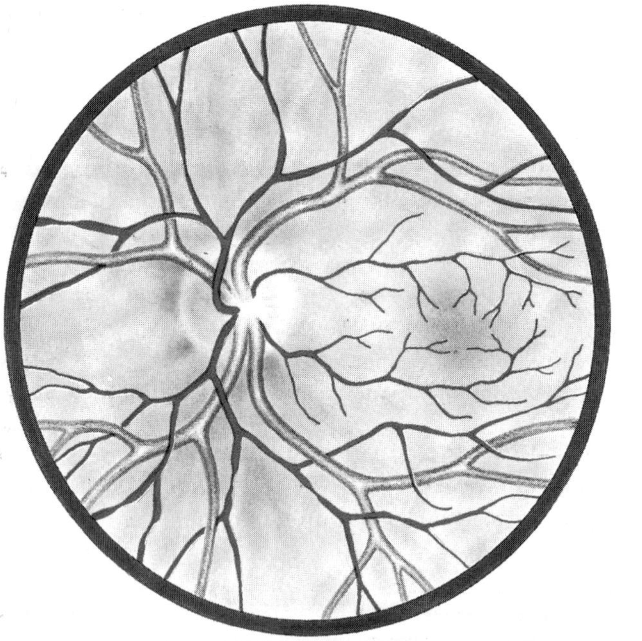

FIG. 30-4 Funduscopic evidence of severe preeclampsia: arteriospasm, edema, hemorrhages, arteriovenous nicking, and exudates.

TABLE 30-4 **Assessing Deep Tendon Reflexes**

GRADE	DEEP TENDON REFLEX RESPONSE
0	No response
1+	Sluggish or diminished
2+	Active or expected response
3+	More brisk than expected, slightly hyperactive
4+	Brisk, hyperactive, with intermittent or transient clonus

From Seidel, H. et al. (2003). *Mosby's guide to physical examination* (5th ed.). St. Louis: Mosby.

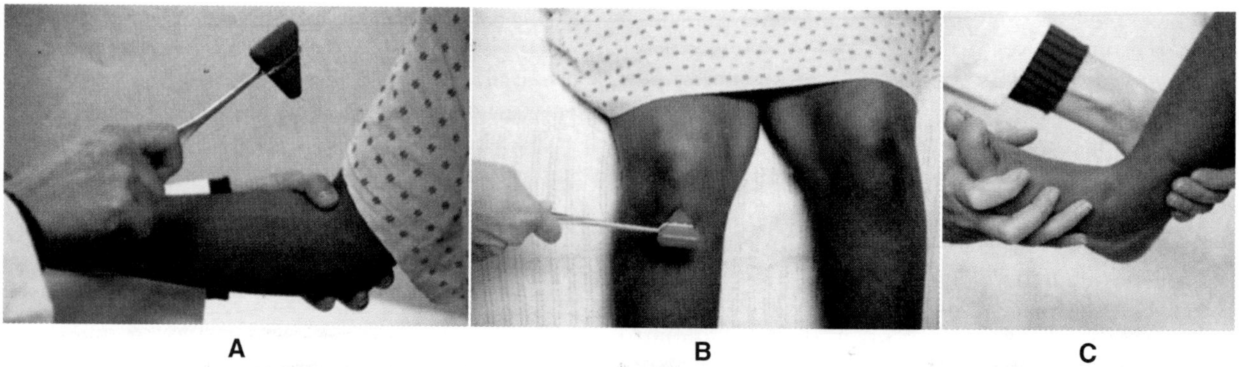
A
B
C

FIG. 30-5 **A,** Biceps reflex. **B,** Patellar reflex with client's legs hanging freely over end of examining table. **C,** Test for ankle clonus. (From Seidel, H. et al. [2003]. *Mosby's guide to physical examination* [5th ed.]. St. Louis: Mosby.)

(2000). Currently this diagnostic test is not recommended as a general screening test for preeclampsia (Sibai, 2002b).

Uterine tonicity is evaluated for signs of labor and abruptio placentae. If labor is suspected, a vaginal examination for cervical changes is indicated. Women with hypertension are at increased risk for an abruption.

NURSE ALERT

Uterine tenderness in the presence of increasing tone may be the earliest finding of an abruption. Idiopathic preterm contractions also may be an early sign.

During the physical examination, the pregnant woman is examined for signs of progression of mild preeclampsia to severe preeclampsia or eclampsia. Signs of worsening liver involvement, renal failure, worsening hypertension, cerebral involvement, and developing coagulopathies must be assessed and documented. Respirations are assessed for crackles or diminished breath sounds, which may indicate pulmonary edema. Warning signs of preeclampsia and the differentiation of mild from severe preeclampsia are summarized in Table 30-2. Noninvasive assessment parameters include level of consciousness, BP, hemoglobin oxygen saturation (pulse oximetry), electrocardiographic findings, and urine output. Invasive hemodynamic monitoring may be indicated in selected clients (ACOG, 2002). Eclampsia is usually preceded by various premonitory symptoms and signs, including headache, severe epigastric pain, hyperreflexia, and hemoconcentration. However, convulsions can appear suddenly and without warning in a woman in seemingly stable condition who has only minimal BP elevation.

The convulsions that occur in eclampsia are frightening to observe. Increased hypertension and tonic contraction of all body muscles (seen as arms flexed, hands clenched, legs inverted) precede the tonic-clonic convulsions (Fig. 30-6). During this stage, muscles alternately relax and contract. Respirations are halted and then begin again with a long, deep, stertorous inhalation. Hypotension follows, and coma ensues. Nystagmus and muscular twitching persist for a time. Disorientation and amnesia cloud the immediate recovery. Oliguria and anuria are notable. Seizures may recur within minutes of the first convulsion, or the woman may never have another. During the convulsion the mother and fetus are not receiving oxygen, so eclamptic seizures produce a marked metabolic insult to both mother and fetus.

Laboratory Tests

The nurse assists in obtaining a number of blood and urine specimens to aid in the diagnosis and treatment of preeclampsia, HELLP syndrome, and chronic hypertension. Baseline laboratory test information is useful in cases of early diagnosis of preeclampsia, because it can be compared with later results to evaluate progression and severity of disease (see Table 30-3). An initial blood specimen is obtained for the following tests to assess the disease process and its effect on renal and hepatic functioning:

- Complete blood cell count (including a platelet count)
- Clotting studies (including bleeding time, PT, PTT, and fibrinogen)
- Liver enzymes (lactate dehydrogenase [LDH], AST, ALT)
- Chemistry panel (BUN, creatinine, glucose, uric acid)
- Type and screen, possible crossmatch

The hematocrit, hemoglobin, and platelet levels are monitored closely for changes indicating a worsening of client status. Because hepatic involvement is a possible complication, serum glucose levels are monitored if liver function tests indicate elevated liver enzymes. Once the platelet count decreases below 100,000/mm^3, coagulation profiles are needed to identify developing DIC (Sibai, 2002b).

Proteinuria is determined from dipstick testing of a clean-catch or catheterized urine specimen. A reading of 2+ or 3+ on two or more occasions at least 6 hours apart should be followed by a 24-hour urine collection. A 24-hour collection for protein and creatinine clearance is more reflective of true renal status. Proteinuria is usually a late sign in the course of preeclampsia (Working Group, 2000).

Renal laboratory assessments include monitoring trends in serum creatine and BUN levels. As renal function becomes compromised, renal excretion of creatinine and other waste products, including magnesium sulfate, decreases. As renal excretion decreases, serum levels for creatinine, BUN, uric acid, and magnesium increase.

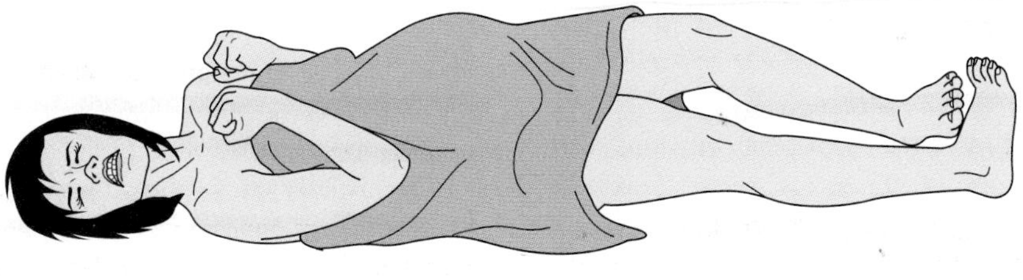

FIG. 30-6 Eclampsia (convulsions or seizures).

Nursing Diagnoses

Nursing diagnoses for the woman with hypertensive disorders in pregnancy may include the following:

- *Anxiety related to*
  - –preeclampsia and its effect on woman and infant
- *Deficient knowledge related to*
  - –management (diet, medications, activity restrictions)
- *Ineffective individual/family coping related to*
  - –woman's restricted activity and concern over a complicated pregnancy
  - –woman's inability to work outside the home
  - –transfer of the woman to a tertiary center for more intensive management
- *Powerlessness related to*
  - –inability to prevent or control condition and outcomes
- *Ineffective tissue perfusion related to*
  - –hypertension
  - –cyclic vasospasms
  - –cerebral edema
  - –hemorrhage
- *Risk for impaired gas exchange related to*
  - –magnesium sulfate therapy
  - –pulmonary edema
- *Risk for decreased alteration in cardiac output related to*
  - –excessive hypertensive therapy
  - –cardiac involvement of the disease process
- *Risk for injury to fetus related to*
  - –uteroplacental insufficiency
  - –preterm birth
  - –abruptio placentae
- *Risk for injury to mother related to*
  - –CNS irritability secondary to cerebral edema, vasospasm, decreased renal perfusion
  - –magnesium sulfate and antihypertensive therapies

Expected Outcomes of Care

Planning of care follows medical diagnosis, choice of home or hospital management, and the woman's and family's resources. A plan is developed mutually with the woman if possible and should be individually tailored and related specifically to the needs of the client and her family. Expected outcomes for care of clients with hypertensive disorders of pregnancy include that the woman will do the following:

- Recognize and immediately report signs and symptoms indicative of worsening condition.
- Adhere to the medical regimen to minimize risk to herself and her fetus.
- Identify and use available support systems.
- Verbalize her fears and concerns to cope with the condition and situation.
- Develop no signs of eclampsia and its complications.
- Give birth to a healthy infant.
- Develop no sequelae to her condition or its management.

Plan of Care and Interventions

Nursing actions are derived from medical management, health care provider directives, and nursing diagnoses. The most effective therapy is prevention. Early prenatal care, identification of pregnant women at risk for preeclampsia, and recognition and reporting of physical warning signs are essential components in the optimization of maternal and perinatal outcomes. The role of the nurse's skills in assessing the client for factors and symptoms of preeclampsia cannot be overestimated.

Nurses can do much in the advocacy role. Measurements should be taken to improve public education and access to antepartal care. Counseling, referral to community resources, mobilization of support systems, nutrition counseling, and information about normal adaptation to pregnancy are essential preventive components of care. The nurse's role as educator is important in informing the woman about her condition and responsibilities in preeclampsia management, whether in the home or hospital.

The goals of therapy are to (1) ensure maternal safety and (2) have the woman give birth to a healthy newborn, as close to term as possible, who will not require prolonged intensive care. At or near term, the plan of care for a woman with preeclampsia is most likely to be induction of labor, preceded, if necessary, by cervical ripening.

When preeclampsia is diagnosed in a woman who is at less than 37 weeks of gestation, however, immediate delivery may not be in the best interest of the fetus. In this situation, the initial intervention is usually a thorough evaluation of both the maternal and fetal condition. Women may be hospitalized during this initial evaluation, or the evaluation may be done in a high risk clinic or the physician's office. A multidisciplinary plan of care is then developed, based on the assessment findings. Whenever possible, the plan should take into account the wishes of the woman and her family.

Emotional and psychologic support are essential in assisting the woman and her family to cope. Their perception of the disease process, the reasons for it, and the care received will affect their compliance with and participation in therapy. The family will need to use coping mechanisms and support systems to help them through this crisis. A plan of care specifically designed for the woman with preeclampsia is superimposed on the nursing care all women need during labor and the birth process.

Mild Preeclampsia and Home Care

If the woman has mild preeclampsia (BP is stable, urine protein is less than 300 mg in a 24-hour collection, and no subjective complaints), she may be managed expectantly, usually at home. The maternal-fetal condition should be assessed 2 to 3 times per week. Many agencies are available to provide this assessment in the home. Arrangements for this service may be made, depending on the woman's insurance coverage. If home nursing care is not possible, the woman may be asked to perform self-assessment daily, including weight, urine dipstick protein determinations, BP measurement, and fetal movement counting (Lowdermilk & Grohar, 1998). In addition, she will be asked to report immediately the development of any subjective symptoms (see Teaching for Self-Care box). In this case, she will probably return to the physician's office or high risk clinic at least twice each week for continued fetal assessment.

The fetal condition also is closely monitored because the only reason for expectant management of preeclampsia is to allow additional time for fetal growth and maturation. An ultrasound for evaluation of fetal growth should be obtained at diagnosis and repeated every 3 weeks. Fetal movement is counted daily. Other fetal assessment tests include a nonstress test once or twice a week, and a biophysical profile as needed. Fetal jeopardy as evidenced by inappropriate growth or abnormal testing necessitates immediate delivery (ACOG, 2002; Summary Report, 2000; Working Group, 2000).

Activity Restriction. Bed rest in the lateral recumbent position is a traditional therapy for preeclampsia that may improve uteroplacental blood flow during pregnancy. However, recommendations for bed rest for all pregnant women at high risk are becoming more controversial. Maloni (1994) documented adverse physiologic outcomes related to complete bed rest, including cardiovascular deconditioning; diuresis with accompanying fluid, electrolyte, and weight loss; muscle atrophy; and psychologic stress. These changes begin on the first day of bed rest and continue for the duration of therapy. Sibai (2002b) recommends rest at home, rather than strict bed rest, and allows women hospitalized with mild preeclampsia to be out of bed.

Bed rest has been shown to be beneficial in decreasing BP and promoting diuresis. Women with mild preeclampsia feel reasonably well; boredom from the restriction is therefore common. Diversionary activities, visits from friends, telephone conversations, and creation of a comfortable and convenient environment are just a few ways of coping with this boredom (see Teaching for Self-Care box). Gentle exercise (e.g., range of motion, stretching, Kegel, pelvic tilts) is important in maintaining muscle tone, blood flow, regularity of bowel function, and a sense of well-being (Cunningham, 2001; Maloni, 1998). Relaxation techniques can help reduce the stress associated with the high risk condition and prepare the woman for labor and birth.

Diet. Diet and fluid recommendations are much the same as for healthy pregnant women. The efficacy of a high-protein diet, avoidance of foods high in sodium, and foregoing additional salt at the table have not been proven (Sibai, 2002b). Because pregnant women with hypertension have a lower plasma volume than do normotensive women, sodium restriction is not necessary. Women need salt for maintenance of blood volume and placental perfusion. The exception may be the woman with chronic hypertension that was successfully controlled with a low-salt diet before the pregnancy. Adequate fluid intake helps

TQ

TEACHING FOR SELF-CARE

Assessing and Reporting Clinical Signs of Preeclampsia

Report immediately any increase in your blood pressure, protein in urine, weight gain, decreased fetal movement.*

Take your blood pressure on the same arm in a sitting position each time for consistent and accurate readings. Support arm on a table in a horizontal position at heart level.

Use the same scale, wearing the same clothes, at the same time each day, after voiding, before breakfast, for reliable daily weights.

Dipstick test your clean-catch urine sample to assess proteinuria; report frequency or burning on urination.

Assess your baby's activity daily. Decreased activity (three or fewer movements per hour) may indicate fetal compromise.

It is important to keep your scheduled prenatal appointments so that any changes in your or your baby's condition can be detected immediately.

Keep a daily log or diary of your assessments for your home health care nurse, or bring it with you to your next prenatal visit.

*Thresholds for blood pressure, weight gain, fetal movement counts, and proteinuria are set by the physician or institutional protocol.

TEACHING FOR SELF-CARE

Coping with Bed Rest

In bed, lie on your side. This allows more blood to get to your uterus (womb) and baby. The bed or sofa should be near a window and a bathroom.

Increase your fluid intake to 8 glasses/day and add roughage (bran, fruits, leafy vegetables) to your diet to decrease constipation. Keep a bowl of fruit and a large container full of water close by.

Include diversionary activities, such as puzzles, reading, and crafts, to reduce boredom. Place a box or table within reach to store magazines, books, telephone, etc.

Do gentle exercises, such as circling your hands and feet or gently tensing and relaxing arm and leg muscles. This improves muscle tone, circulation, and sense of well-being.

Encourage family participation in your care.

Have significant others assist you with care of the house, children, etc.

Use relaxation to help cope with stress. Relax your body one muscle at a time, or imagine some pleasant scene, word, or image. Soothing music can also help you relax.

maintain optimal fluid volume and aids in renal perfusion and filtration. The nurse uses assessment data regarding the woman's diet to counsel her as needed in areas of deficiency (see Teaching for Self-Care box).

Successful home care requires the woman to be well educated about preeclampsia and motivated to follow the plan of care. She also must be reliable about keeping appointments. For home care to be effective, the home environment must be assessed and the woman's ability to assume responsibility determined. In addition, the effects of illness, language, age, culture, beliefs, and support systems must be considered. The woman's support systems must be mobilized and involved in planning and implementing her care. During the period of instruction for the woman and her family, time must be allowed for assimilation of information, questions, and concerns. A client's understanding is usually directly associated with compliance with the prescribed treatment program. Methods for enhancing learning include visual aids, videotapes, handouts, and demonstrations with return demonstrations (see Plan of Care).

TEACHING FOR SELF-CARE

Nutrition

- Eat a nutritious, balanced diet (60 to 70 g protein; 1200 mg calcium; and adequate zinc, magnesium, and vitamins). Consult with registered dietitian on the diet best suited for you as an individual.
- There is no sodium restriction; however, consider limiting excessively salty foods (luncheon meats, pretzels, potato chips, pickles, sauerkraut).
- Eat foods with roughage (whole grains, raw fruits, and vegetables).
- Drink six to eight 8-oz glasses of water per day.
- Avoid alcohol, and limit caffeine intake.

Severe Preeclampsia and HELLP Syndrome

If the woman's condition worsens or she already has severe preeclampsia or HELLP syndrome and is critically ill, she should receive appropriate management (usually in a tertiary care center), ranging from immediate birth to conservative management of the pregnancy (ACOG, 2002; Leicht & Harvey, 1999; Summary Report, 2000; Working Group, 2000). Recognition of the clinical and laboratory

Plan of Care — Mild Preeclampsia: Home Care

NURSING DIAGNOSIS Risk for injury related to signs of preeclampsia

Expected Outcomes *Client will demonstrate ability to assess self and fetus for signs of worsening preeclampsia; no adverse sequelae will occur as result of preeclamptic condition.*

Nursing Interventions/*Rationales*

- Review warning signs/symptoms of preeclampsia *to ensure adequate knowledge base exists for decision making.*
- Assess home environment, including woman's ability to assume self-care responsibilities, support systems, language, age, culture, beliefs, and effects of illness, *to determine if home care is viable option.*
- Teach woman how to do a self-assessment for clinical signs of preeclampsia (take and record blood pressure, measure urine protein, maintain daily weight log, assess edema formation, assess fetal activity) *to provide immediate evidence of a worsening condition.*
- Teach woman to report any increases in blood pressure, ≥+2 proteinuria, weight gain, and decreased fetal activity to her health care provider immediately *to prevent worsening of preeclamptic condition.*
- Teach woman about use of rest and relaxation as palliative treatment options *to decrease blood pressure and promote diuresis.*

NURSING DIAGNOSIS Fear/anxiety related to preeclampsia and its effect on the fetus

Expected Outcome *Client's feelings and symptoms of fear/anxiety will decrease/ease.*

Nursing Interventions/*Rationales*

- Provide a calm, soothing atmosphere and teach family to provide emotional support *to facilitate coping.*
- Encourage verbalization of fears *to decrease intensity of emotional response.*
- Involve woman and family in the management of her preeclamptic condition *to promote a greater sense of control.*
- Help woman identify and use appropriate coping strategies and support systems *to reduce fear/anxiety.*
- Explore use of desensitization strategies such as progressive muscle relaxation, visual imagery, or thought stopping *to reduce fear-related emotions and related physical symptoms.*

NURSING DIAGNOSIS Deficient diversional activity related to imposed bed rest

Expected Outcome *Client will verbalize diminished feelings of boredom.*

Nursing Interventions/*Rationales*

- Assist woman to creatively explore personally meaningful activities that can be pursued from the bed *to ensure activities that have meaning, purpose, and value to the individual.*
- Maintain emphasis on personal choices of woman *to promote control and minimize imposition of routines by others.*
- Evaluate what support and system resources are available in the environment *to assist in providing diversional activities.*
- Explore ways for woman to remain an active participant in home management and decision making *to promote control.*
- Engage support of family and friends in carrying out chosen activities and making necessary environmental alterations *to ensure success.*
- Teach woman about stress-management and relaxation techniques *to help manage tension of confinement.*

findings of severe preeclampsia or HELLP syndrome is important if early, aggressive therapy is to be initiated to prevent maternal and perinatal mortality. An unfavorable (uneffaced and undilated) cervix, resulting from the gestational age and the aggressive nature of this disorder, supports cesarean birth. Prolonged induction of labor could increase maternal morbidity.

Important components of management include the administration of magnesium sulfate as prophylaxis against seizures and an antihypertensive agent if diastolic BP is higher than 100 to 110 mm Hg.

Hospital Care. The woman with severe preeclampsia or HELLP syndrome has multiple problems and provides a complex challenge for the health care team. Nursing care must focus on both mother and fetus.

Antepartum care focuses on stabilization and preparation for birth. The woman may be admitted to an antepartum or a labor and birth unit, depending on the hospital. If the woman's condition is severe, she may be placed in an intensive care unit for any necessary hemodynamic monitoring. Maternal and fetal surveillance, client education regarding the disease process, and supportive measures directed toward the woman and her family are initiated. Assessments include review of the cardiovascular system, pulmonary system, renal system, hematologic system, and CNS. Fetal assessments for well-being (e.g., nonstress test, biophysical profile, fetal movement counts) are important because of the potential for hypoxia related to uteroplacental insufficiency. Baseline laboratory assessments include metabolic studies for liver enzyme (AST, ALT, LDH) determination, complete blood count with platelets, coagulation profile to assess for DIC, and electrolyte studies to establish renal functioning.

Weight is usually measured on admission and every day thereafter. An indwelling urinary catheter facilitates monitoring of renal function and effectiveness of therapy. If appropriate, vaginal examination may be done to check for cervical changes. Abdominal palpation establishes uterine tonicity and fetal size, activity, and position. Electronic monitoring to determine fetal status is initiated at least once a day. The nurse's skill in implementing the techniques described here can be reassuring to the woman and her family. The woman's room must be close to staff and emergency drugs, supplies, and equipment. Noise and external stimuli must be minimized. Seizure precautions are taken (Box 30-4).

Bed rest or restricted activity is commonly ordered even though there is lack of scientific evidence to support the efficacy of such restriction (Enkin et al., 2001; Working Group, 2000). The nurse's ingenuity may be called on to help the woman cope physically and psychologically with the side effects of immobility and an environment limited in stimuli and support. Thromboembolic events, a risk factor during normal pregnancy, pose an even greater risk with preeclampsia (see Plan of Care).

Intrapartum nursing care of the woman with severe preeclampsia or HELLP syndrome involves continuous monitoring of maternal and fetal status as labor progresses. The assessment and prevention of tissue hypoxemia and hemorrhage, both of which can lead to permanent compromise of vital organs, continue throughout the intrapartum and postpartum periods (Leicht & Harvey, 1999).

Magnesium Sulfate. One of the important goals of care for the woman with severe preeclampsia is prevention or control of convulsions. Magnesium sulfate ($MgSO_4$) is the drug of choice in the prevention and treatment of convulsions caused by preeclampsia or eclampsia (ACOG, 2002; Magpie Trial Collaborative Group, 2002). Results from the Magpie Trial Collaborative Group (2002) indicate that the use of magnesium sulfate in the management of preeclampsia halves the risk of eclampsia and probably reduces the risk of maternal death. The routine use of magnesium sulfate is indicated for severe preeclampsia, HELLP syndrome, or eclampsia; however, no data support routine use of magnesium sulfate for women diagnosed with mild preeclampsia or gestational hypertension (Summary Report, 2000; Working Group, 2000).

Magnesium sulfate is administered as a secondary infusion to the main IV line by volumetric infusion pump. An initial loading dose of 4 to 6 g magnesium sulfate diluted in 100 ml IV fluid per protocol or physician's order is infused over a 15- to 30-minute period. This dose is followed by a maintenance dose of magnesium sulfate diluted in an IV solution per physician's order (e.g., 40 g magnesium sulfate in 1000 ml lactated Ringer's solution) and administered by infusion pump at 1 to 3 g/hr (Gilbert & Harmon, 2003; Mandeville & Troiano, 1999). This dose should maintain a therapeutic serum magnesium level of 4 to 8 mg/dl. Serum magnesium levels are obtained if signs of toxicity are present or there is renal dysfunction. No data exist to support the routine of drawing

BOX 30-4 Hospital Precautionary Measures

Environment
- Quiet
- Nonstimulating
- Lighting subdued

Seizure precautions
- Suction equipment tested and ready to use
- Oxygen administration equipment tested and ready to use

Call button within easy reach

Emergency medication tray immediately accessible
- Hydralazine or other antihypertensive medication and magnesium sulfate in or adjacent to woman's room
- Calcium gluconate immediately available

Emergency birth pack accessible

Plan of Care Severe Preeclampsia: Hospital Care

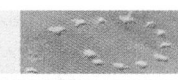

NURSING DIAGNOSIS Risk for injury to mother and fetus related to CNS irritability

Expected Outcomes *Client will show diminished signs of CNS irritability (e.g., DTRs 2+, absence of clonus) and have no convulsions.*

Nursing Interventions/*Rationales*

Establish baseline data (e.g., DTRs, clonus) *to use as basis for evaluating effectiveness of treatment.*

Administer IV $MgSO_4$ per physician's orders *to decrease hyperreflexia and minimize risk of convulsions.*

Monitor maternal vital signs, FHR, urine output, DTRs, IV flow rate, and serum levels of $MgSO_4$ *to assess for and prevent* $MgSO_4$ *toxicity (e.g., depressed respirations, oliguria, sudden drop in blood pressure, hyporeflexia, fetal distress).*

Have calcium gluconate at bedside if needed *as antidote for* $MgSO_4$ *toxicity.*

Maintain a quiet, darkened environment *to avoid stimuli that may precipitate seizure activity.*

NURSING DIAGNOSIS Ineffective tissue perfusion related to preeclampsia secondary to arteriolar vasospasm

Expected Outcomes *Client will exhibit signs of increased vasodilation (diuresis, decreased edema, weight loss).*

Nursing Interventions/*Rationales*

Establish baseline data (weight, degree of edema) *to use as basis for evaluating effectiveness of treatment.*

Administer IV $MgSO_4$ per physician order, *which serves to relax vasospasms and increase renal perfusion.*

Place woman on bed rest in a side-lying position *to maximize uteroplacental blood flow, reduce blood pressure, and promote diuresis.*

Monitor intake and output, edema, and weight *to assess for evidence of vasodilation and increased tissue perfusion.*

NURSING DIAGNOSIS Risk for
- Excess fluid volume related to increased sodium retention secondary to administration of $MgSO_4$
- Impaired gas exchange related to pulmonary edema secondary to increased vascular resistance
- Decreased cardiac output related to use of antihypertensive drugs
- Injury to fetus related to uteroplacental insufficiency secondary to use of antihypertensive medications

Expected Outcomes *Client will exhibit signs of normal fluid volume (balanced intake and output, normal serum creatinine levels, normal breath sounds); adequate oxygenation (normal respirations; fully oriented to person, time, and place); normal range of cardiac output (normal pulse rate and rhythm); and fetal well-being (adequate fetal movement, normal FHR).*

Nursing Interventions/*Rationales*

Monitor woman for signs of fluid volume excess (increased edema, decreased urine output, elevated serum creatinine level, weight gain, dyspnea, crackles) *to prevent complications.*

Monitor woman for signs of impaired gas exchange (increased respirations, dyspnea, altered blood gases, hypoxemia) *to prevent complications.*

Monitor woman for signs of decreased cardiac output (altered pulse rate and rhythm) *to prevent complications.*

Monitor fetus for signs of difficulty (decreased fetal activity, decreased FHR) *to prevent complications.*

Record findings and report signs of increasing problems to physician *to enable timely interventions.*

CNS, Central nervous system; *FHR,* fetal heart rate; *DTR,* deep tendon reflex.

serial serum magnesium levels, although levels are often checked daily (Gilbert & Harmon, 2003) (Box 30-5).

After the loading dose, a transient reduction of the arterial BP may occur as a result of relaxation of smooth muscle.

NURSE ALERT

The woman's BP, pulse, and respiratory status should be monitored closely while the loading dose is being administered IV and every 15 to 30 minutes at other times, depending on the stability of the woman's condition. Administration of magnesium sulfate is continued for at least the first 12 to 24 postpartum hours to prevent the occurrence of seizures.

Intramuscular (IM) magnesium sulfate is rarely used because the absorption rate cannot be controlled, injections are painful, and tissue necrosis may occur. The IM route may be used with some women who are being transported to a tertiary care center. The IM dose is 4 to 5 g given in each buttock, a total of 10 g (with 1% procaine possibly being added to the solution to reduce injection pain), and can be repeated at 4-hour intervals. Z-track technique should be used for the deep IM injection, followed by gentle massage at the site.

Magnesium sulfate interferes with the release of acetylcholine at the synapses, decreasing neuromuscular irritability, depressing cardiac conduction, and decreasing CNS irritability. Because magnesium circulates free and unbound to protein and is excreted in the urine, accurate recordings of maternal urine output must be obtained.

Diuresis within 24 to 48 hours is an excellent prognostic sign. It is considered evidence that perfusion of the kidney has improved as a result of relaxation of arteriolar spasm. With improved perfusion, fluid moves from interstitial spaces to the intravascular bed, and edema is reduced. Diuresis results in weight loss. Although diuresis generally indicates improvement, diuresis in the presence of worsening clinical status may indicate impending renal failure. As renal function declines and serum creatinine levels increase, renal filtration is compromised. The woman can excrete large volumes of urine (more than 200 ml/hr) but will not excrete magnesium sulfate.

IM 4-5g/buttock q4h z track

BOX 30-5 Protocol for Care of Client with Preeclampsia Receiving Magnesium Sulfate

MAGNESIUM SULFATE ADMINISTRATION

Client and Family Teaching

Explain technique, rationale, and reactions to expect
- Route and rate
- Purpose of "piggyback"

Reasons for use
- Tailor information to client's readiness to learn
- Explain that it is to prevent disease progression
- Explain that it is to prevent seizures

Reactions to expect from medication
- Initially client will feel flushed, hot, sedated, especially during the bolus
- Sedation will continue

Monitoring to anticipate
- Maternal: blood pressure, pulse, DTRs, level of consciousness, urine output (indwelling catheter likely), presence of headache, visual disturbances, epigastric pain
- Fetal: FHR and activity

Administration
- Verify physician order
- Position woman in side-lying position
- Prepare solution and administer with an infusion control device (pump)
- Piggyback a solution of 40 g magnesium sulfate in 1000 ml of lactated Ringer's solution with an infusion control device at the ordered rates: loading dose: initial bolus of 4-6 g over 15 to 30 min; maintenance dose: 1-3 g/hr

Maternal and Fetal Assessments
- Monitor blood pressure, pulse, respiratory rate, FHR, and contractions every 15-30 min, depending on client condition
- Monitor intake and output, proteinuria, DTRs, presence of headache, visual disturbances, and epigastric pain at least hourly
- Restrict hourly fluid intake to a total of 100 to 125 ml/hr; urinary output should be ≥30 ml/hr

Reportable Conditions
- Blood pressure: systolic, 160 mm Hg; diastolic, 110 mm Hg, or both
- Respiratory rate: 12 breaths/min
- Urinary output <30 ml/hr
- Presence of headache, visual disturbances, or epigastric pain
- Increasing severity or loss of DTRs, increasing edema, proteinuria
- Any abnormal laboratory values (magnesium levels, platelet count, creatinine clearance, levels of uric acid, AST, ALT, prothrombin time, partial thromboplastin time, fibrinogen, fibrin split products)
- Any other significant change in maternal or fetal status

Emergency Measures
- Keep emergency drug tray at bedside with calcium gluconate and intubation equipment
- Keep side rails up
- Keep lights dimmed, and maintain a quiet environment

Documentation
- All of the above

DTR, Deep tendon reflex; *FHR,* fetal heart rate; *AST,* aspartate aminotransferase; *ALT,* alanine aminotransferase.

Because magnesium sulfate is a CNS depressant, the nurse assesses for signs and symptoms of magnesium toxicity (see Box 30-5). Serum magnesium levels are obtained on the basis of the woman's response and if any signs of toxicity are present. Early symptoms of toxicity include nausea, a feeling of warmth, flushing, muscle weakness, decreased reflexes, and slurred speech.

NURSE ALERT

Loss of patellar reflexes, respiratory depression, oliguria, and decreased level of consciousness are signs of magnesium toxicity. Actions are needed to prevent respiratory or cardiac arrest. If magnesium toxicity is suspected, the infusion should be discontinued immediately. Calcium gluconate, the antidote for magnesium sulfate, also may be ordered (10 ml of a 10% solution, or 1 g) and given by slow IV push (usually by the physician) over at least a 3-minute period to avoid undesirable reactions such as dysrhythmias, bradycardia, and ventricular fibrillation.

relax uterus

Because magnesium sulfate also is a tocolytic agent, its use may increase the duration of labor.

NURSE ALERT

A preeclamptic woman receiving magnesium sulfate may need augmentation with oxytocin during labor. The amount of oxytocin needed to stimulate labor may be more than that needed for a woman who is not receiving magnesium sulfate.

Magnesium sulfate is not thought to affect FHR variability in a healthy term fetus and is rarely toxic in the healthy term neonate whose weight is within normal range for gestational age. Toxic levels in the fetus can, however, cause marked slowing of respirations and hyporeflexia after birth. Neonatal hypermagnesemia can be treated with calcium and exchange transfusion with citrated blood, or the neonate may require assisted mechanical ventilation until serum levels have normalized.

Fetal effects of MgSO4

Ca Gluconate is the Antidote for MgSO4!! 1g IV push over 3min

EMERGENCY

Eclampsia

TONIC-CLONIC CONVULSION SIGNS

Stage of invasion: 2-3 sec, eyes are fixed, twitching of facial muscles occurs

Stage of contraction: 15-20 sec, eyes protrude and are bloodshot, all body muscles are in tonic contraction

Stage of convulsion: Muscles relax and contract alternately (clonic), respirations are halted and then begin again with long, deep, stertorous inhalation, coma ensues

INTERVENTION

Keep airway patent: Turn head to one side, place pillow under one shoulder or back if possible

Call for assistance

Protect with side rails up

Observe and record convulsion activity

AFTER CONVULSION OR SEIZURE

Do not leave unattended until fully alert

Observe for postconvulsion coma, incontinence

Use suction as needed

Administer oxygen via face mask at 10 L/min

Start IV fluids and monitor for potential fluid overload

Give magnesium sulfate or anticonvulsant drug as ordered

Insert indwelling urinary catheter

Monitor blood pressure

Monitor fetal and uterine status

Expedite laboratory work as ordered to monitor kidney function, liver function, coagulation system, and drug levels

Provide hygiene and a quiet environment

Support and keep woman and family informed

Be prepared to assist with delivery when woman is in stable condition

If eclampsia develops after the initiation of magnesium sulfate therapy, the treatment of choice is to administer an additional 2 g of magnesium sulfate by IV push over a period of 3 to 5 minutes (Leicht & Harvey, 1999) (see Emergency box). Occasionally it is necessary to repeat the dose because the woman will experience additional seizures. Rarely the woman will continue to have seizures despite adequate blood magnesium levels. In that case, other anticonvulsants may be used. Diazepam is sometimes used to stop or shorten eclamptic seizures; however, this drug can cause phlebitis and venous thrombosis. If administered too rapidly, it also can lead to apnea or cardiac arrest.

Both sodium amobarbital and diazepam have fetal and neonatal effects as well. The FHR pattern demonstrates a loss of variability, a reflection of decreased fetal oxygenation. High levels of these drugs in the neonate depress sucking ability, cause hypotonia, and may result in temperature instability. The neonate's respiratory rate may be decreased. Careful surveillance of both maternal and fetal or neonatal status is warranted.

Control of Blood Pressure. For the severely hypertensive preeclamptic woman, antihypertensive medications are usually ordered to reduce the BP (systolic BP, 160 to 180 mm Hg; diastolic BP, 100 to 110 mm Hg). Initiation of antihypertensive therapy reduces maternal morbidity and mortality associated with left ventricular failure and cerebral hemorrhage. Because a degree of maternal hypertension is necessary to maintain uteroplacental perfusion, antihypertensive therapy must not decrease the arterial pressure too much or too rapidly. The target range for the diastolic pressure is therefore 90 to 100 mm Hg (Leicht & Harvey, 1999).

Intravenous hydralazine remains the antihypertensive agent of choice for the treatment of hypertension in severe preeclampsia. Intravenous labetalol hydrochloride also may be used (ACOG, 2002; Summary Report, 2000; Working Group, 2000). The choice of agent used depends on client response and physician preference. Table 30-5 compares antihypertensive agents used to treat hypertension in pregnancy. Nifedipine may be used as an antihypertensive agent in nonacute settings; however, the use for the control of severe hypertension or during a hypertensive crisis is contraindicated.

NURSE ALERT

When administering antihypertensive therapy, the nurse must remember that the drug effects are dependent on intravascular volume. Because preeclampsia is associated with contracted intravascular volume, initial doses should be given with caution, and maternal response monitored closely.

Eclampsia

Immediate Care. The immediate care during a convulsion is to ensure a patent airway (see Emergency box). When convulsions occur, the woman is turned onto her side to prevent aspiration of vomitus and supine hypotension syndrome. After the convulsion ceases, food and fluid are suctioned from the glottis or trachea, and oxygen is administered by face mask. Magnesium sulfate or other anticonvulsant is given as ordered. If an IV infusion is not in place, one is begun with a large-bore needle. Time, duration, and description of convulsions are recorded, and any urinary or fecal incontinence is noted. The fetus is monitored for adverse effects. Transient fetal bradycardia and decreased FHR variability are common.

Aspiration is a leading cause of maternal morbidity and mortality after eclamptic seizure. After initial stabilization and airway management, the nurse should anticipate orders for a chest radiograph and possibly arterial blood gases to rule out the possibility of aspiration.

A rapid assessment of uterine activity, cervical status, and fetal status is performed after a convulsion. During the convulsion, membranes may have ruptured; the cervix may have dilated, because the uterus becomes hypercontractile and hypertonic; and birth may be imminent. If not, once a woman's seizure activity and BP are controlled, a decision should be made regarding whether birth should take place. The more serious the condition of the woman, the greater the need to proceed to birth. The route of birth–that is, in-

TABLE 30-5 **Pharmacologic Control of Hypertension in Pregnancy**

ACTION	TARGET TISSUE	EFFECTS: MATERNAL	EFFECTS: FETAL	NURSING ACTIONS
HYDRALAZINE (APRESOLINE, NEOPRESOL)				
Arteriolar vasodilator	Peripheral arterioles: to decrease muscle tone, decrease peripheral resistance; hypothalamus and medullary vasomotor center for minor decrease in sympathetic tone	Headache, flushing, palpitation, tachycardia, some decrease in uteroplacental blood flow, increase in heart rate and cardiac output, increase in oxygen consumption, nausea and vomiting	Tachycardia; late decelerations and bradycardia if maternal diastolic pressure <90 mm Hg	Assess for effects of medications, alert mother (family) to expected effects of medications, assess blood pressure frequently because precipitate decrease can lead to shock and perhaps abruptio placentae; assess urinary output; maintain bed rest in a lateral position with side rails up; use with caution in presence of maternal tachycardia
LABETALOL HYDROCHLORIDE (NORMODYNE)				
Beta-Blocking agent causing vasodilation without significant change in cardiac output	Peripheral arterioles (see hydralazine)	Minimal: flushing, tremulousness; minimal change in pulse rate	Minimal, if any	See hydralazine; less likely to cause excessive hypotension and tachycardia; less rebound hypertension than hydralazine
METHYLDOPA (ALDOMET)				
Maintenance therapy if needed: 250-500 mg orally every 8 hr (alpha$_2$-receptor agonist)	Postganglionic nerve endings: interferes with chemical neurotransmission to reduce peripheral vascular resistance, causes CNS sedation	Sleepiness, postural hypotension, constipation; rare: drug-induced fever in 1% of women and positive Coombs' test result in 20%	After 4 mo maternal therapy, positive Coombs' test result in infant	See hydralazine
NIFEDIPINE (PROCARDIA)				
Calcium-channel blocker	Arterioles: to reduce systemic vascular resistance by relaxation of arterial smooth muscle	Headache, flushing; possible potentiation of effects on CNS if administered concurrent with magnesium sulfate, may interfere with labor	Minimal	See hydralazine; use caution if client also getting magnesium sulfate

CNS, Central nervous system.

duction of labor versus cesarean birth—depends on maternal and fetal condition. If fetal lungs are not mature and the birth can be delayed for 48 hours, steroids such as betamethasone may be given.

The woman may have been incontinent of urine and stool during the convulsion; she will need assistance with hygiene and a change of gown. Oral care with a soft toothbrush may be of comfort.

NURSE ALERT

Immediately after a seizure, the woman may be very confused and can be combative, necessitating the temporary use of restraints. It may take several hours for the woman to regain her usual level of mental functioning. The health care provider explains procedures briefly and quietly. The woman is never left alone. The family also is kept informed of management, rationale for treatment, and the woman's progress.

Determination of central venous pressure or pulmonary arterial wedge pressure (Swan-Ganz catheter) may occasionally be required for accurate fluid monitoring in the presence of pulmonary edema or acute renal failure (ACOG, 2002) (see Chapter 34). No oral intake is permitted if the woman is convulsing or has symptoms of severe preeclampsia. An indwelling catheter is required for accurate measurement of urinary output. For correction of hypovolemia, crystalloids (0.9% saline solution or lactated Ringer's solution) are infused IV at a rate that maintains a urine output of at least 25 to 30 ml/hr, and the maternal response is recorded.

Medications (e.g., magnesium sulfate) are given as directed. The woman's response is monitored and recorded, and all drugs, dosages, and times are noted. Laboratory tests are ordered to assess for HELLP syndrome and to have blood typed and crossmatched for administration of packed red blood cells as needed. Blood is kept available for emergency transfusion; abruptio placentae, with accompanying hemorrhage and shock, often occurs in women with eclampsia. Other tests include determination of electrolyte levels, liver function battery, and complete hemogram and clotting profile, including platelet count and fibrin split product levels (to assess for DIC).

Postpartum Nursing Care

After birth the symptoms of preeclampsia or eclampsia resolve quickly, usually within 48 hours; however, symptoms have been reported up to several weeks after birth. The hematopoietic and hepatic complications of HELLP syndrome may persist longer. These clients often show an abrupt decrease in platelet count, with a concomitant increase in LDH and AST levels, after a trend toward normalization of values has begun. Generally the laboratory abnormalities seen with HELLP syndrome resolve in 72 to 96 hours.

The nursing care of the woman with hypertensive disease differs from that required in the usual postpartum period in a number of respects. The following variations in the nursing process are described.

Careful assessment of the woman with a hypertensive disorder continues throughout the postpartum period. Blood pressure is measured at least every 4 hours for 48 hours or more frequently as the woman's condition warrants. Even if no convulsions occurred before the birth, they may occur within this period. Magnesium sulfate infusion is usually continued 12 to 24 hours after the birth. The same assessments continue until the medication is discontinued.

NURSE ALERT

The woman is at risk for a boggy uterus and a large lochia flow as a result of the magnesium sulfate therapy. Uterine tone and lochia flow must be monitored closely.

The preeclamptic woman is hemoconcentrated and unable to tolerate excessive postpartum blood loss. Oxytocin or prostaglandin products are used to control bleeding. Ergot products (e.g., Ergotrate and Methergine) are contraindicated because they increase BP. The woman is asked to report symptoms such as headaches and blurred vision. The nurse assesses affect, level of consciousness, BP, pulse, and respiratory status before an analgesic is given for headache. Magnesium sulfate potentiates the action of narcotics, CNS depressants, and calcium-channel blockers; these drugs must be administered with caution. The woman may need to continue an antihypertensive medication regimen if her diastolic BP exceeds 100 mm Hg at discharge.

The woman's and family's responses to labor, birth, and the neonate are monitored. Interactions and involvement in the care of the neonate are encouraged to the extent that the woman and her family desire. In addition, the woman and her family need opportunities to discuss their emotional response to complications. The nurse provides information concerning the prognosis. Preeclampsia and eclampsia do not necessarily recur in subsequent pregnancies (recurrence rate is approximately 30%), but prenatal care is essential for assessment and early intervention.

Prevention

Numerous clinical trials described various methods to prevent preeclampsia. The etiology continues to be unknown. Some of the strategies to prevent preeclampsia that have been or are being studied are described in the following paragraph. However, until a cause is discovered, prevention remains elusive.

Efforts to prevent or reduce the incidence of preeclampsia have used dietary supplementation and pharmacologic interventions. Large randomized clinical trials have not proven the use of low-dose aspirin to be a beneficial form of care (Caritis et al., 1998). Mattar and Sibai (1999) reviewed more than 70 studies of interventions for the prevention of preeclampsia. These studies included the use of calcium, magnesium, zinc, and fish oil dietary supplementation. None of these interventions demonstrated a benefit in reducing the incidence or severity of preeclampsia in healthy pregnant women. Antihypertensive agents, diuretics, and low-salt diets also have been studied in numerous clinical trials with no beneficial results related to prevention (Sibai, 1998). Vitamin C, 1000 mg, and vitamin E, 400 mg, and exercise may be of some benefit, although continued research with large randomized trials is needed (ACOG, 2002; Atallah, Hofmeyr, & Duley, 2002; Yeo & Davidge, 2000; Zhang et al., 2002). Continued research in prevention is needed because no strategies have been proven to have beneficial effects. Most are of unknown effectiveness or are not likely to be beneficial. Nurses should be aware of the strategies being studied and use the most reliable evidence about the results so that they can counsel pregnant women about interventions that are likely to be beneficial. One resource is the Cochrane Pregnancy and Childbirth Database.

Evaluation

Evaluation of the effectiveness of care of the woman with preeclampsia is based on the expected outcomes.

CHRONIC HYPERTENSION

Chronic hypertension occurs in up to 5% of pregnant women, with the incidence higher in African-American women and all women older than 40 years (Livingston & Sibai, 2001). Chronic hypertension in pregnancy is associated with increased incidence of abruptio placentae and superimposed preeclampsia, and adverse pregnancy outcomes are increased in women in whom these complications develop (Sibai, 2002a). Postpartum complications include pulmonary edema, renal failure, and hypertensive encephalopathy (Sibai, 2002a). The risk of perinatal deaths is increased, as are the rates of preterm birth and small-for-gestational-age (SGA) infants in women with chronic hypertension (Livingston & Sibai, 2001).

Women with chronic hypertension ideally should be screened before conception or at the first prenatal visit. Medications that could have adverse effects on the fetus should be discussed and may be discontinued or changed to another medication. Based on the history and physical findings, women with chronic hypertension are identified as either at high or low risk for pregnancy complications (Sibai, 2002a). Women who are high risk are usually managed with antihypertensive therapy and frequent assessments of maternal and fetal well-being. Methyldopa (Aldomet) is usually the drug of choice, although beta-blockers and calcium channel blockers also are used (Working Group, 2000). Antihypertensive therapy may or may not be beneficial for women who are at low risk for complications (Sibai, 2002a).

Lifestyle changes may be necessary; for example, limiting sodium in the diet, limiting exercise during pregnancy, not smoking or using alcohol, limiting caffeine, and losing weight in the preconception period if overweight (Gilbert & Harmon, 2003). The woman should be taught how to monitor her BP.

The time of birth is individualized, but a woman at low risk can usually wait until her cervix is favorable for induction at 40 to 41 weeks of gestation. The woman at high risk should not continue her pregnancy past 40 weeks (Livingson & Sibai, 2001). In the postpartum period, women with chronic hypertension, especially if at high risk, should be monitored for signs of complications such as renal failure, pulmonary edema, heart failure, and encephalopathy. All antihypertensive drugs are found in breast milk. If the woman wishes to breastfeed and needs medication to control her BP, methyldopa is the usual choice.

KEY POINTS

- Hypertensive disorders during pregnancy are a leading cause of worldwide infant and maternal morbidity and mortality.
- The cause of PIH is unknown, and there are no known reliable tests for predicting which women are at risk for preeclampsia.
- Preeclampsia is a multisystem disease rather than only an increase in BP.
- Failure of trophoblastic invasion of spiral arterioles is proposed as the triggering mechanism that eventually leads to vasospasm and organ ischemia; the cure is delivery of the fetus and placenta.
- The pathologic changes of preeclampsia, involving every organ system in the body, are present long before clinical manifestations are evident.
- Historic risk factors (e.g., first pregnancy or pregnancy of new genetic makeup, history of vascular disease, and multiple gestation) are associated with a higher incidence of preeclampsia.
- Progression of hypertensive disorders during pregnancy is unpredictable; mild hypertension must therefore be taken seriously and managed as for preeclampsia.
- Once preeclampsia becomes clinically evident, therapeutic intervention is palliative (bed rest, diet); this may slow the progression of the disease and allow the pregnancy to continue.
- Home care management is an option only for women whose condition is stable and who are able to comply with the medical regimen, reliably perform self-monitoring, and immediately recognize and report abnormal signs and symptoms.

KEY POINTS—cont'd

- HELLP syndrome can occur in women with severe preeclampsia and is considered life threatening.
- Magnesium sulfate, the anticonvulsive agent of choice for preventing eclampsia, requires careful monitoring of reflexes, respirations, and urinary output; its antidote, calcium gluconate, should be available at the bedside.
- The intent of emergency interventions for eclampsia is to prevent self-injury, ensure adequate oxygenation, reduce aspiration risk, establish seizure control with magnesium sulfate, and correct maternal acidemia.
- Chronic hypertension in pregnancy is associated with abruptio placentae and superimposed preeclampsia.

CRITICAL THINKING EXERCISES

1. Betty, a 42-year-old woman, comes into clinic for a routine prenatal visit at 34 weeks of gestation. She is pregnant with twins. You find that her blood pressure is 150/96, she has 2+ proteinuria on a urine dipstick, and she has gained 5 pounds since her last clinic visit 10 days ago.
   a. During your initial assessment, what risk factors and other signs and symptoms of preeclampsia might you find?
   b. Develop a plan for Betty's care at home.
   c. What would you teach her about diet, rest, self-assessment, and fetal assessment?
   d. What danger signs should Betty be told to report immediately?
2. Review three charts of postpartum clients who were diagnosed during pregnancy or labor with preeclampsia. Did the women have mild or severe preeclampsia, and what evidence was present for you to make that determination? Evaluate the management of each woman based on the information in this chapter.
3. Examine the research on aspirin therapy, calcium supplementation, and vitamin C and E supplementation as preventive measures against preeclampsia. How beneficial are these therapies? What advice can nurses give pregnant women about prevention of preeclampsia?

RESOURCES

American College of Obstetricians and Gynecologists
409 12th St. SW
Washington, DC 20024
800-762-2264
www.acog.com

The Cochrane Collaboration
www.cochrane.org

COPE (Coping with the Overall Pregnancy/Parenting Experience)
37 Clarendon St.
Boston, MA 02116
617-357-5588

International Society for the Study of Hypertension in Pregnancy (ISSHP)
www.ncl.ac.uk/isshp/

National Bed Rest Support Group
Sidelines
P.O. Box 1808
Laguna Beach, CA 92652
714-497-2265
www.sidelines.org

National Heart, Lung, and Blood Institute
www.nhlbi.nih.gov

REFERENCES

American College of Obstetricians and Gynecologists. (2002). *Diagnosis and management of preeclampsia and eclampsia. ACOG Practice Bulletin Number 33.* Washington, DC: ACOG.

Atallah, A., Hofmeyr, G., & Duley, L. (2002). Calcium supplementation during pregnancy for preventing hypertensive disorders and related problems (Cochrane Review). *The Cochrane Library,* Issue 4. Oxford: Update Software.

Blackburn, S. (2003). *Maternal, fetal, & neonatal physiology: A clinical perspective* (2nd ed). St. Louis: W.B. Saunders.

Bush, K., O'Brien, J., & Barton, J. (2001). The utility of umbilical artery Doppler investigation in women with HELLP (hemolysis, elevated liver enzymes, and low platelets) syndrome. *American Journal of Obstetrics and Gynecology, 184*(6), 1087-1089.

Caritis, S. et al. (1998). Low-dose aspirin to prevent preeclampsia in women at high risk. *New England Journal of Medicine, 338*(11), 7011-7015.

Chein, P. et al. (2000). How useful is uterine artery Doppler flow velocimetry in the prediction of pre-eclampsia, intrauterine growth retardation and perinatal death? An overview. *British Journal of Obstetrics and Gynecology, 107*(2), 196-208.

Cunningham, E. (2001). Coping with bed rest. *AWHONN Lifelines, 5*(5), 50-55.

Dekker, G. (2001). Prevention of preeclampsia. In B. Sibai (Ed.), *Hypertensive disorders in women.* Philadelphia: W.B. Saunders.

Dekker, G., & Sibai, B. (1998). Etiology and pathogenesis of preeclampsia: Current concepts. *American Journal of Obstetrics and Gynecology, 179*(5), 1359-1375.

Dekker, G., & Sibai, B. (1999). The immunology of preeclampsia. *Seminars in Perinatology, 23*(1), 24-33.

Egerman, R., & Sibai, B. (1999). HELLP syndrome. *Clinical Obstetrics and Gynecology, 42*(2), 381-389.

Enkin, M. et al. (2001). Effective care in pregnancy and childbirth: A synopsis. *Birth, 28*(1), 41-51.

Gilbert, E., & Harmon, J. (2003). *Manual of high risk pregnancy and delivery* (3rd ed.). St. Louis: Mosby.

Leicht, T., & Harvey, C. (1999). Hypertensive disorders in pregnancy. In L. Mandeville & C. Harvey (Eds.), *AWHONN's high risk and critical care intrapartum nursing* (2nd ed.). Philadelphia: J.B. Lippincott.

Li, D., & Wi, S. (2000). Changing paternity and the risk of preeclampsia/eclampsia in subsequent pregnancy. *American Journal of Epidemiology, 151*(1), 57-62.

Livingston, J., & Sibai, B. (2001). Chronic hypertension in pregnancy. *Obstetrics and Gynecology Clinics, 28*(3), 1-15.

Lowdermilk, D., & Grohar, J. (1998). *High risk antepartal home care.* White Plains, NY: March of Dimes.

Magpie Trial Collaborative Group. (2002). Do women with preeclampsia, and their babies, benefit from magnesium sulfate? The Magpie Trial: A randomized placebo-controlled trial. *Lancet, 359,* 1877-1890.

Maloni, J. (1994). Home care of the high risk pregnant woman requiring bed rest. *Journal of Obstetric, Gynecologic, and Neonatal Nursing, 23*(8), 696-706.

Maloni, J. (1998). *Antepartum bed rest: Case studies, research and nursing care.* Washington, DC: AWHONN.

Mandeville, L., & Troiano, N. (1999). *AWHONN's high risk and critical care intrapartum nursing* (2nd ed.). Philadelphia: J.B. Lippincott.

Martin J. et al. (2002). Births: Final data for 2000. *National Vital Statistics Report, 50*(5), 1-104.

Marx, G. et al. (1993). Automated blood pressure measurements in laboring women: Are they reliable? *American Journal of Obstetrics and Gynecology, 168,* 796-798.

Mattar, F., & Sibai, B. (1999). Prevention of preeclampsia. *Seminars in Perinatology, 23*(1), 58-64.

Minino, A. et al. (2002). Deaths: Final data for 1998. *National Vital Statistics Report, 50*(15), 1-120.

National High Blood Pressure Education Program Working Group on High Blood Pressure in Pregnancy [Working Group]. (2000). *NIH Publication No. 00-3029.* Bethesda, MD: National Institutes of Health, National Heart, Lung, and Blood Institute.

Portis, R. et al. (1997). HELLP syndrome (hemolysis, elevated liver enzymes, and low platelets) pathophysiology and anesthetic considerations. *American Association of Nurse Anesthetists Journal, 65*(1), 37-47.

Report of the National High Blood Pressure Education Program Working Group on High Blood Pressure in Pregnancy [Summary Report]. (2000). *American Journal of Obstetrics and Gynecology, 183*(1), S1-S22.

Roberts, J. (1999). Pregnancy-related hypertension. In R. Creasy & R. Resnik (Eds.), *Maternal-fetal medicine* (4th ed.). Philadelphia: W.B. Saunders.

Robillard, P. (2002). Interest in preeclampsia for researchers in reproduction. *Journal of Reproduction Immunology, 53*(1-2), 279-287.

Scott, J. et al. (1999). *Danforth's obstetrics and gynecology* (8th ed.). Philadelphia: Lippincott Williams & Wilkins.

Seidel, H. et al. (2003). *Mosby's guide to physical examination* (5th ed.). St. Louis: Mosby.

Sibai, B. (2002a). Chronic hypertension in pregnancy. *Obstetrics and Gynecology, 100*(2), 369-377.

Sibai, B. (2002b). Hypertension in pregnancy. In S. Gabbe, J. Niebyl, & J. Simpson (Eds.), *Obstetrics: Normal and problem pregnancies* (4th ed.). New York: Churchill Livingstone.

Sibai, B. (1998). Prevention of preeclampsia: A big disappointment. *American Journal of Obstetrics and Gynecology, 179*(5), 1275-1278.

Sibai, B., & Rodriguez, J. (1999). Preeclampsia: Diagnosis and management. In E. Reece et al. (Eds.), *Medicine of the fetus and mother.* Philadelphia: J.B. Lippincott.

Stone, J. (1998). HELLP syndrome: Hemolysis, elevated liver enzymes, and low platelets. *Journal of the American Medical Association, 280*(6), 559-562.

Walker, J. (2000). Preeclampsia. *Lancet, 356,* 1260-1265.

Yeo, S., & Davidge, S. (2001). Possible beneficial effect of exercise, by reducing oxidative stress, on the incidence of preeclampsia. *Journal of Womens' Health and Gender Based Medicine, 10*(10), 983-989.

Zhang, C. et al. (2002). Vitamin C and the risk of preeclampsia: Results from dietary questionnaire and plasma assay. *Epidemiology, 13*(4), 409-416.

CHAPTER 31

S. Kim Genovese

Antepartal Hemorrhagic Disorders

http://evolve.elsevier.com/Lowdermilk/MatWmnHlth/

LEARNING OBJECTIVES

- Differentiate among causes, signs and symptoms, possible complications, and management of miscarriage, ectopic pregnancy, incompetent cervix, and hydatidiform mole.
- Compare and contrast abruptio placentae and placenta previa in relation to signs and symptoms, complications, and management.
- Discuss clotting disorders in pregnancy, with emphasis on disseminated intravascular coagulation.
- Revise plans of care for the woman with an unruptured ectopic pregnancy versus a ruptured ectopic pregnancy.
- Review the physiology of a hydatidiform mole and the risk factors for the woman's immediate health future.
- Examine the role of the nurse in the health care team approach to the treatment of bleeding disorders.

Maternal adaptations in the hematologic and cardiovascular systems during pregnancy result in a hypervolemic state, with concomitant decreases in systemic and pulmonary vascular resistance. Increases in plasma volume and red blood cell mass occur as early as 4 to 8 weeks of gestation and serve to (1) meet the metabolic demands of the mother and fetus, (2) protect against the potentially deleterious impairment in venous return caused by the pressure of an enlarging uterus, and (3) safeguard the mother against the effects of blood loss at birth. Any bleeding in pregnancy may therefore jeopardize both maternal and fetal well-being. Maternal blood loss decreases oxygen-carrying capacity, which predisposes the woman to increased risk for hypovolemia, anemia, infection, and preterm labor and adversely affects oxygen delivery to the fetus. Fetal risks from maternal hemorrhage include blood loss or anemia, hypoxemia, hypoxia, anoxia, and preterm birth. If the bleeding involves fetal blood loss, the effects are exponential because of the smaller fetal blood volume.

Hemorrhagic disorders in pregnancy are medical emergencies; the incidence and type of bleeding vary by trimester. In the first trimester, most bleeding is a result of miscarriage and ectopic pregnancy. Approximately 50% of bleeding in the third trimester is caused by placenta previa and abruptio placentae (Cunningham et al., 2001). Antepartal hemorrhage is a leading cause of maternal death, with ectopic pregnancy rupture and abruptio placentae being responsible for most maternal deaths (Chichakli et al., 1999). Prompt assessment and intervention by the health care team is essential to save the life of the woman and fetus.

EARLY PREGNANCY BLEEDING

Bleeding during early pregnancy is alarming to the woman and of concern to health care providers. The common bleeding disorders of early pregnancy include spontaneous abortion (miscarriage), incompetent cervix, ectopic pregnancy, and hydatidiform mole (molar pregnancy).

Miscarriage (Spontaneous Abortion)

A pregnancy that ends before 20 weeks of gestation is defined as a **spontaneous abortion.** This 20-week marker is considered to be the point of viability, when a fetus may survive in an extrauterine environment. A fetal weight less than 500 g also may be used to define an abortion (Cunningham et al., 2001).

A spontaneous abortion, commonly called a miscarriage, results from natural causes. **Miscarriage** is suggested as a more appropriate term to use with clients because abortion may be an insensitive term to use with families who are grieving a pregnancy loss (Freda, 1999). The term miscarriage is used throughout this discussion. The term *abortion* is used when discussing therapeutic or elective induced abortion (see Chapter 9).

Incidence and Etiology

Approximately 10% to 15% of all clinically recognized pregnancies end in miscarriage (Simpson, 2002). An early miscarriage is one that occurs before 12 weeks of gestation. At least 50% of all clinically recognized pregnancy losses result from chromosomal abnormalities (Simpson, 2002). The majority (more than 90%) of miscarriages occur early, before 8 weeks of gestation (Simpson, 2002). Possible causes include endocrine imbalance (as in women who have luteal phase defects or insulin-dependent diabetes mellitus with high blood glucose levels in the first trimester), immunologic factors (e.g., antiphospholipid antibodies), infections (e.g., bacteriuria and *Chlamydia trachomatis*), systemic disorders (e.g., lupus erythematosus), and genetic factors (Cunningham et al., 2001; Gilbert & Harmon, 2003).

A late miscarriage occurs between 12 and 20 weeks of gestation. It usually results from maternal causes, such as advancing maternal age and parity, chronic infections, premature dilation of the cervix and other anomalies of the reproductive tract, chronic debilitating diseases, inadequate nutrition, and recreational drug use (Cunningham et al., 2001). Little can be done to avoid genetically caused pregnancy loss, but correction of maternal disorders, immunization against infectious diseases, adequate early prenatal care, and treatment of pregnancy complications can do much to prevent miscarriage.

Types

The types of miscarriage include threatened, inevitable, incomplete, complete, and missed. Miscarriage (both early and late) can recur; all but the threatened miscarriage can lead to infection (Fig. 31-1).

Clinical Manifestations

Signs and symptoms of miscarriage depend on the duration of pregnancy. The presence of uterine bleeding, uterine contractions, or uterine pain is an ominous sign during early pregnancy and must be considered a threatened miscarriage until proven otherwise.

If miscarriage occurs before the sixth week of pregnancy, the woman may report a heavy menstrual flow. Miscarriage that occurs between weeks 6 and 12 of pregnancy causes moderate discomfort and blood loss. After week 12, miscarriage is typified by more severe pain, similar to that of labor, because the fetus must be expelled. Diagnosis of the type of miscarriage is based on the signs and symptoms present (Table 31-1).

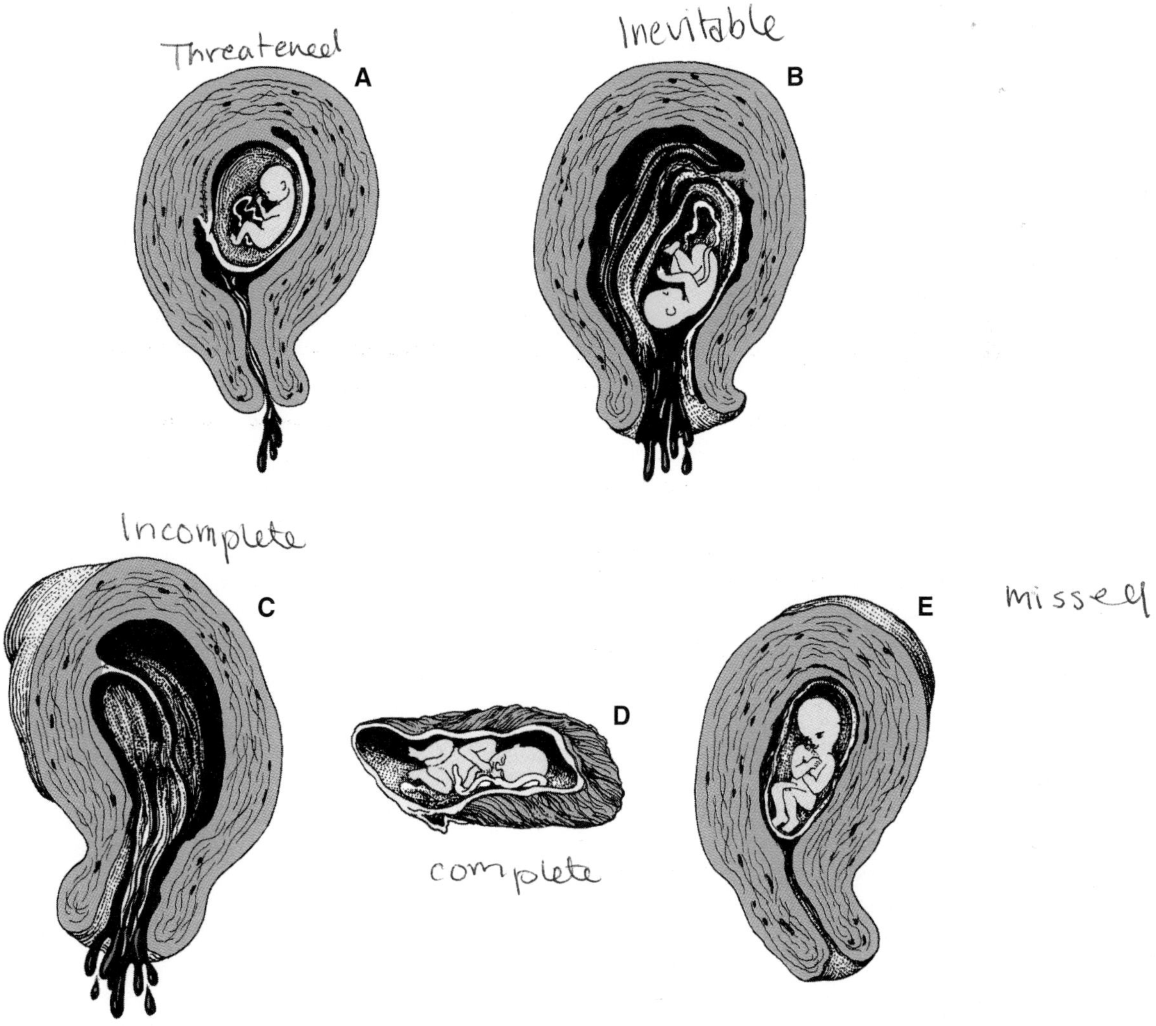
A
B
C
D
E

FIG. 31-1 Miscarriage. **A,** Threatened. **B,** Inevitable. **C,** Incomplete. **D,** Complete. **E,** Missed.

Symptoms of a *threatened* miscarriage (see Fig. 31-1, *A*) include spotting of blood but with the cervical os closed. Mild uterine cramping may be present.

Inevitable (see Fig. 31-1, *B*) and *incomplete* (see Fig. 31-1, *C*) miscarriages involve a moderate to heavy amount of bleeding with an open cervical os. Tissue may be present with the bleeding. Mild to severe uterine cramping may be present. An inevitable miscarriage is often accompanied by rupture of membranes (ROM) and cervical dilation; passage of the products of conception will occur. An incomplete miscarriage involves the expulsion of the fetus with retention of the placenta (Cunningham et al., 2001).

In a *complete* miscarriage (see Fig. 31-1, *D*), all fetal tissue is passed, the cervix is closed, and there may be slight bleeding. Mild uterine cramping may be present.

The term *missed* miscarriage (see Fig. 31-1, *E*) refers to a pregnancy in which the fetus has died, but the products of conception are retained in utero for up to several weeks.

TABLE 31-1 **Assessing Miscarriage and the Usual Management**

TYPE OF MISCARRIAGE	AMOUNT OF BLEEDING	UTERINE CRAMPING	PASSAGE OF TISSUE	CERVICAL DILATION	MANAGEMENT
Threatened	Slight, spotting	Mild	No	No	Bed rest, sedation, and avoidance of stress and orgasm usually recommended. Further treatment depends on woman's response to treatment
Inevitable	Moderate	Mild to severe	No	Yes	Prompt termination of pregnancy is accomplished, usually by dilation and curettage
Incomplete	Heavy, profuse	Severe	Yes	Yes, with tissue in cervix	
Complete	Slight	Mild	Yes	No	No further intervention may be needed if uterine contractions are adequate to prevent hemorrhage and there is no infection
Missed	None, spotting	None	No	No	If spontaneous evacuation of the uterus does not occur within 1 mo, pregnancy is terminated by method appropriate to duration of pregnancy. Blood clotting factors are monitored until uterus is empty. DIC and incoagulability of blood with uncontrolled hemorrhage may develop in cases of fetal death after the twelfth week, if products of conception are retained for >5 wk.
Septic	Varies, usually malodorous	Varies	Varies	Yes, usually	Immediate termination of pregnancy by method appropriate to duration of pregnancy. Cervical culture and sensitivity studies are done, and broad-spectrum antibiotic therapy (e.g., ampicillin) is started. Treatment for septic shock is initiated if necessary.
Recurrent	Varies	Varies	Yes	Yes, usually	Varies, depends on type. Prophylactic cerclage may be done if premature cervical dilation is the cause

Adapted from Gilbert, E., & Harmon, J. (2003). *Manual of high risk pregnancy and delivery* (3rd ed.). St. Louis: Mosby.
DIC, Disseminated intravascular coagulation.

It may be diagnosed by ultrasonic examination after the uterus stops increasing in size or even decreases in size. No bleeding or cramping may be present, and the cervical os remains closed.

Recurrent early (habitual) miscarriage is the loss of three or more previable pregnancies. Women having three or more miscarriages are at increased risk for preterm birth, placenta previa, and fetal anomalies in subsequent pregnancies (Cunningham et al., 2001).

Miscarriage can become septic, although this is not a common occurrence. Symptoms of a septic miscarriage include fever and abdominal tenderness. Vaginal bleeding, which may be slight to heavy, is usually malodorous.

CARE MANAGEMENT

Whenever a woman has vaginal bleeding early in pregnancy, a thorough assessment should be performed (Box 31-1). The data to be collected include pain, bleeding, and date of last menstrual period (LMP) to determine the approximate length of gestation. The initial database includes vital signs (a temperature higher than 38° C may indicate infection), previous pregnancies, previous pregnancy losses, type and location of pain, quantity and nature of bleeding, allergies, and emotional status (see Box 31-1). The woman may be anxious and fearful regarding what may happen to her and to her pregnancy.

BOX 31-1 Assessment of Bleeding in Pregnancy

INITIAL DATABASE
Chief complaint
Vital signs
Gravidity, parity
Last menstrual period/estimated date of birth
Pregnancy history (previous and current)
Allergies
Nausea and vomiting
Pain (onset, quality, precipitating event, location)
Bleeding or coagulation problems
Level of consciousness
Emotional status

EARLY PREGNANCY
Confirmation of pregnancy
Bleeding (bright or dark, intermittent or continuous)
Pain (type, intensity, persistence)
Vaginal discharge

LATE PREGNANCY
Estimated date of birth
Bleeding (quantity, associated pain)
Vaginal discharge
Amniotic membrane status
Uterine activity
Abdominal pain
Fetal status/viability

Various laboratory findings are characteristic of miscarriage. Evaluation of human chorionic gonadotropin (hCG), a placental hormone, is used in the diagnosis of pregnancy and pregnancy loss. Human chorionic gonadotropin is produced by the syncytiotrophoblast, and the beta subunit of hCG (beta-hCG) can be detected in maternal plasma and urine 8 to 9 days after ovulation if the woman is pregnant. In early pregnancy, the concentration of beta-hCG should double every 1.4 to 2.0 days until about 60 or 70 days of gestation (Cunningham et al., 2001). Before 8 weeks of gestation, if miscarriage is suspected, measurement of two serum quantitative beta-hCG levels is performed 48 hours apart. If a normal pregnancy is present, the beta-hCG level doubles in this time. Ultrasonography can then be used to determine the presence of a viable gestational sac. With considerable or persistent blood loss, anemia is likely (hemoglobin level less than 11 g/dl). If infection is present, the white blood cell count (WBC) is greater than 12,000/mm^3. Sedimentation rate is not helpful for differential diagnostic purposes because an increased sedimentation rate occurs with pregnancy, anemia, or infection.

The following nursing diagnoses are appropriate for the woman experiencing a miscarriage:

- *Anxiety/fear related to*
  - –unknown outcome and unfamiliarity with medical procedures
- *Deficient fluid volume related to*
  - –excessive bleeding secondary to miscarriage
- *Acute pain related to*
  - –uterine contractions
- *Anticipatory grieving related to*
  - –unexpected pregnancy outcome
- *Situational low self-esteem related to*
  - –inability to carry a pregnancy successfully to term gestation
- *Risk for infection related to*
  - –surgical treatment
  - –dilated cervix

Expected Outcomes of Care

Expected outcomes of care for the woman experiencing miscarriage may include that the woman will do the following:

- Discuss the impact of the loss on her and her family.
- Identify and use available support systems.
- Display no signs or symptoms of complications (e.g., hemorrhage or infection).
- Identify health promotion measures that decrease her risk of miscarriage and state understanding of reasons for diagnostic and genetic follow-up if needed.
- Report relief from pain.

Plan of Care and Interventions

Medical/Surgical Management

Medical management (see Table 31-1) depends on the classification of the miscarriage and on signs and symptoms. Traditionally, threatened miscarriages have been managed with bed rest and supportive care. Follow-up treatment depends on whether the threatened miscarriage progresses to actual miscarriage, or symptoms subside and the pregnancy remains intact. **Dilation and curettage (D&C)** is a surgical procedure in which the cervix is dilated and a curette is inserted to scrape the uterine walls and remove uterine contents. A D&C is commonly performed to treat inevitable and incomplete miscarriage. The nurse reinforces explanations, answers any questions or concerns, and prepares the woman for surgery.

Dilation and evacuation, performed after 16 weeks of gestation, consists of wide cervical dilation followed by instrumental removal of the uterine contents.

Before either surgical procedure is performed, a full history should be obtained, and general and pelvic examinations should be performed. General preoperative and postoperative care is appropriate for the woman requiring surgical intervention. Analgesics and anesthesia appropriate to the procedure are used.

For late incomplete, inevitable, or missed miscarriages (16 to 20 weeks), prostaglandins may be administered into the amniotic sac or by vaginal suppository to induce or augment labor and cause the products of conception to be expelled. Intravenous (IV) oxytocin also may be used.

Nursing Care

Immediate nursing care focuses on physiologic stabilization. Typical orders to be followed are initiation of an IV line, request for blood testing of hemoglobin and hematocrit, blood type and Rh, and indirect Coombs screen. An ultrasound examination is performed for diagnostic confirmation.

Nursing care is similar to care for any woman whose labor is being induced (see Chapter 36). Special care may be needed for management of side effects of prostaglandin such as nausea and vomiting and diarrhea. If the products of conception are not passed in entirety, the woman may be prepared for manual or surgical evacuation of the uterus.

After evacuation of the uterus, 10 to 20 U of oxytocin in 1000 ml of fluids may be given to prevent hemorrhage. For excessive bleeding, ergot products such as ergonovine or a prostaglandin derivative such as carboprost tromethamine may be given to contract the uterus. Three or four doses of ergonovine, 0.2 mg orally or intramuscularly every 4 hours, may be given if the woman is not hypotensive. A 25-mg dose of carboprost may be given intramuscularly every 15 to 90 minutes for as many as eight doses (Cunningham et al., 2001). Antibiotics are given as necessary. Analgesics, such as antiprostaglandin agents, may decrease discomfort from cramping. Transfusion therapy may be required for shock or anemia. The woman who is Rh negative and does not have isoimmunization is given an intramuscular injection of $Rh_0(D)$ immune globulin within 72 hours of the miscarriage.

Psychosocial aspects of care focus on what the pregnancy loss means to the woman and her family. Hutti, dePacheco, and Smith (1998) found that responses of women after miscarriage ranged from no grief to intense long-lasting grief. Explanations are provided regarding the nature of the miscarriage, expected procedures, and possible future implications for childbearing.

As with other fetal or neonatal losses, the woman should be offered the option of seeing the products of conception. She also may want to know what the hospital does with the products of conception or whether she needs to make a decision about final disposition of fetal remains.

NURSE ALERT

Procedures for disposition of the fetal remains vary from hospital to hospital and state to state. The nurse should know what the usual procedures are in his or her setting.

Home Care

The woman will likely be discharged home within a few hours after a D&C or as soon as vital signs are stable, vaginal bleeding remains minimal, and she has recovered from anesthesia. Discharge teaching emphasizes the need for rest. If significant blood loss has occurred, iron supplementation may be ordered. Teaching includes information about normal physical findings, such as cramping, type and amount of bleeding, resumption of sexual activity, and family planning (see Teaching for Self-Care box).

TEACHING FOR SELF-CARE

Discharge Teaching for the Woman After Early Miscarriage

- Advise the woman to report any heavy, profuse, or bright red bleeding to health care provider.
- Reassure the woman that a scant, dark discharge may persist for 1 to 2 weeks.
- To reduce the risk of infection, remind the woman not to put anything into the vagina for 2 weeks or until bleeding has stopped (e.g., no tampons, no vaginal intercourse). She should take antibiotics as prescribed.
- Advise the woman to eat foods high in iron and protein.
- Acknowledge that the woman has experienced a loss and that time is required for recovery. She may have mood swings and depression.
- Refer the woman to support groups, clergy, or professional counseling as needed.
- Advise the woman that attempts at pregnancy should be postponed for at least 2 months to allow her body to recover.

From Gilbert, E., & Harmon, J. (2003). *Manual of high risk pregnancy and delivery* (3rd ed.). St. Louis: Mosby.

Follow-up care should assess the woman's physical and emotional recovery. Referrals to local support groups should be provided as needed (see the Resource list at the end of this chapter).

Follow-up phone calls after a loss are important. The woman may appreciate a phone call on what would have been her due date. These calls provide opportunities for the woman to ask questions, seek advice, and receive information to help process her grief.

Incompetent Cervix (Recurrent Premature Dilation of the Cervix)

Another cause of late miscarriage is **incompetent cervix (recurrent premature dilation of the cervix),** which has traditionally been defined as passive and painless dilation of the cervix during the second trimester. This definition assumes an "all or nothing" role for the cervix; it is either "competent" or "incompetent." Current research contends that cervical competence is variable and exists as a continuum that is determined in part by cervical length. Other related factors include composition of the cervical tissue and the individual circumstances associated with the pregnancy in terms of maternal stress and lifestyle. Iams (2002) referred to this condition as abnormal or reduced cervical competence. Freda (1999) suggested the term *recurrent premature dilation of the cervix.*

Etiology

Etiologic factors include a history of previous cervical lacerations during childbirth, excessive cervical dilation for curettage or biopsy, or the woman's mother's ingestion of diethylstilbestrol during pregnancy with the woman. Other instances may result from a congenitally short cervix or cervical or uterine anomalies. Reduced cervical competence is a clinical diagnosis, based on history. Short labors and recurring loss of the pregnancy at progressively earlier gestational ages are characteristics of reduced cervical competence. Ultrasound examination is used to diagnose this condition objectively. A short cervix (less than 20 mm in length) is indicative of reduced cervical competence. Often, but not always, the short cervix is accompanied by **cervical funneling,** or effacement of the internal cervical os (Iams, 2002).

Collaborative Care

Medical/Surgical Management. Conservative management consists of bed rest, hydration, and tocolysis (inhibition of uterine contractions). A cervical **cerclage** may be performed. During gestation, a McDonald cerclage, band of homologous fascia, or nonabsorbable ribbon (Mersilene) may be placed around the cervix beneath the mucosa to constrict the internal os of the cervix (Fig. 31-2).

Prophylactic cerclage is placed at 10 to 14 weeks of gestation, after which the woman is told to refrain from intercourse, prolonged (more than 90-minute) standing, and heavy lifting. She is monitored during the course of her pregnancy with ultrasound scans to assess for cervical shortening and funneling. The cerclage is electively removed (usually an office or a clinic procedure) when the woman reaches 37 weeks of gestation, or it may be left in place, and a cesarean birth performed. Approximately 80% to 90% of pregnancies treated with cerclage result in live, viable births (Iams, 2002). If removed, the cerclage must be replaced with each successive pregnancy.

A woman whose reduced cervical competence is diagnosed during the current pregnancy may undergo emergency cerclage placement. Risks of the procedure include premature rupture of membranes (ROM), preterm labor, and chorioamnionitis. Because of these risks, and because bed rest and tocolytic therapy can be used to prolong the pregnancy, cerclage is rarely performed after 25 weeks of gestation (Iams, 2002).

Nursing Care. The nurse assesses the woman's feelings about her pregnancy and her understanding of reduced cervical competence. It also is important to evaluate the woman's support systems. Because the diagnosis of reduced cervical competence is usually not made until the woman has lost one or two pregnancies, she may feel guilty or to blame for this impending loss. It is therefore important to assess for previous reactions to stresses and appropriateness of coping responses. The woman needs the support of her health care providers, as well as that of her family.

If a cervical cerclage is performed, the nurse monitors the woman postoperatively for contractions, ROM, and

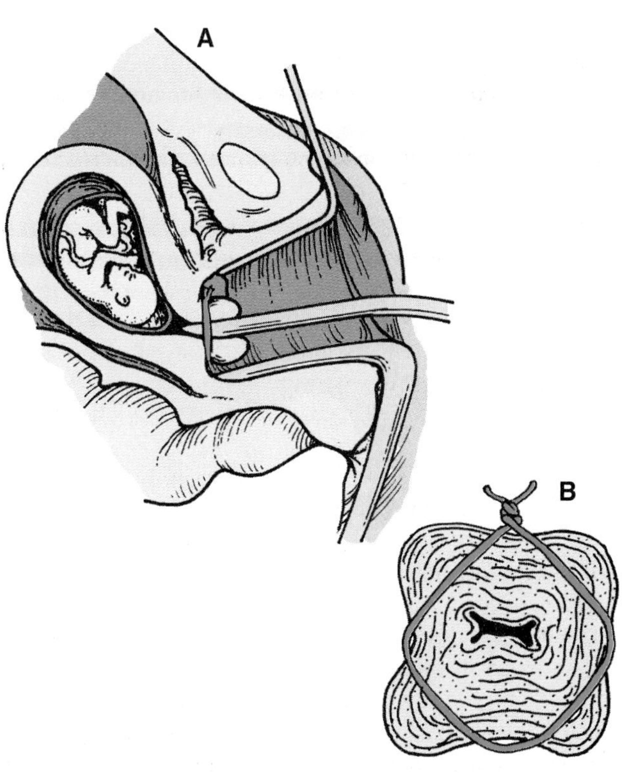
A
B

FIG. 31-2 **A,** Cerclage correction of premature dilation of the cervical os. **B,** Cross-sectional view of closed internal os.

signs of infection. Discharge teaching focuses on continued monitoring of these aspects at home. Home uterine monitoring may be indicated with follow-up from a home health agency.

Home Care. The woman must understand the importance of activity restriction at home and the need for close observation and supervision. Instruction includes the rationale for bed rest or activity restriction and warning signs of preterm labor, ROM, and infection to report (Lowdermilk & Grohar, 1998). The woman must be instructed on the importance of taking oral tocolytic medication if prescribed, the expected response, and possible side effects. Tocolytics may be given prophylactically to prevent uterine contractions and further dilation of the cervix. If home uterine monitoring is implemented, the woman is taught how to apply a uterine contraction monitor and transmit the monitor tracing by telephone to the monitoring center. Nurses at the monitoring center assess the tracing for contractions, answer questions, provide emotional support and education, and report information to the woman's physician or nurse-midwife. The woman should know the signs that would warrant immediate transfer to the hospital, including strong contractions less than 5 minutes apart, ROM, severe perineal pressure, and an urge to push (Health Care Resources, 1997). If management is unsuccessful and the fetus is born before viability, appropriate grief support should be provided. If the fetus is born prematurely, appropriate anticipatory guidance and support will be necessary.

Ectopic Pregnancy

Incidence and Etiology

Ectopic pregnancy is one in which the fertilized ovum is implanted outside the uterine cavity (Fig. 31-3). It accounts for 2% of all pregnancies in the United States (Flystra, 1998).

Approximately 95% of ectopic pregnancies occur in the uterine (fallopian) tube, with most located on the ampullar or largest portion of the tube. Other sites include the abdominal cavity (3% to 4%), ovary (1%), and cervix (1%).

Ectopic pregnancy is responsible for 10% of all maternal mortality, and it is the leading pregnancy-related cause of first trimester maternal mortality (Simpson, 2002). Moreover, ectopic pregnancy is a leading cause of infertility. Only about 60% of women who have been treated for ectopic pregnancy are able to conceive afterward, and approximately 40% of those pregnancies are ectopic (Powell & Spellman, 1996).

The reported incidence of ectopic pregnancy is increasing as a result of improved diagnostic techniques, such as more sensitive beta-hCG assays and the availability of transvaginal ultrasound. An increased incidence of sexually transmitted infections, better treatment of pelvic inflammatory disease (which formerly would have caused sterility), increased numbers of tubal sterilizations, and surgical reversal of tubal sterilizations also have resulted in more ectopic pregnancies (Simpson, 2002).

Ectopic pregnancy is classified according to site of implantation (e.g., tubal or ovarian). The uterus is the only organ capable of containing and sustaining a term pregnancy. However, abdominal pregnancy with birth by laparotomy may result in a living infant in 5% to 25% of such pregnancies (Fig. 31-4); the risk of deformity is as high as 40% (Gilbert & Harmon, 2003).

Clinical Manifestations

A missed period, adnexal fullness, and tenderness may suggest an unruptured tubal pregnancy. The tenderness can progress from a dull pain to a colicky pain when the tube stretches. Pain may be unilateral, bilateral, or diffuse over the abdomen. Dark red or brown abnormal vaginal bleed-

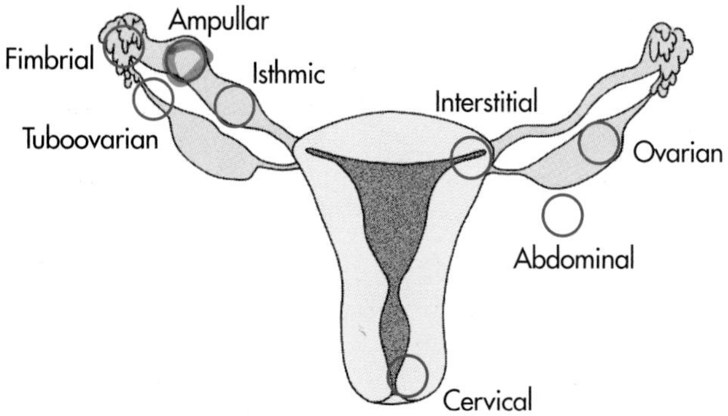

Ampullar
Fimbrial
Isthmic
Tuboovarian
Interstitial
Ovarian
Abdominal
Cervical

FIG. 31-3 Sites of implantation of ectopic pregnancies. Order of frequency of occurrence is ampulla, isthmus, interstitium, fimbria, tuboovarian ligament, ovary, abdominal cavity, and cervix (external os).

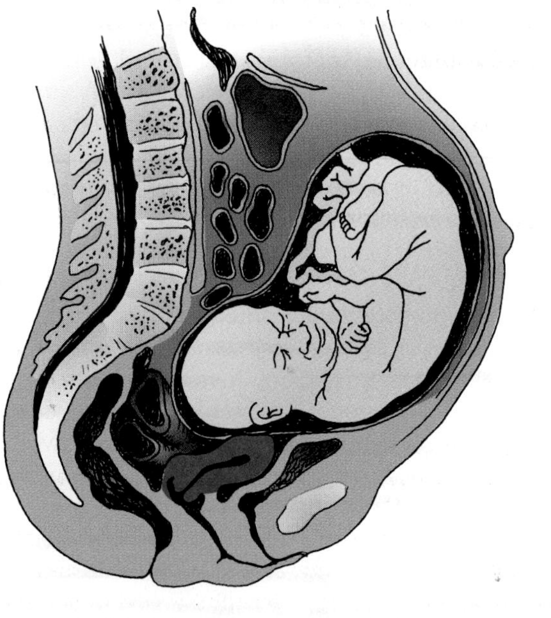

FIG. 31-4 Ectopic pregnancy, abdominal.

ing occurs in 50% to 80% of women. If the ectopic pregnancy ruptures, pain increases. This pain may be generalized, unilateral, or acute deep lower quadrant pain caused by blood irritating the peritoneum. Referred shoulder pain can occur as a result of diaphragmatic irritation caused by blood in the peritoneal cavity. The woman may exhibit signs of shock related to the amount of bleeding in the abdominal cavity and not necessarily related to obvious vaginal bleeding. An ecchymotic blueness around the umbilicus **(Cullen's sign)**, indicating hematoperitoneum, may develop in an undiagnosed ruptured intraabdominal ectopic pregnancy.

Collaborative Care

The differential diagnosis of ectopic pregnancy involves consideration of numerous disorders that share many signs and symptoms. The physician, nurse-midwife, or nurse practitioner must consider miscarriage, ruptured corpus luteum cyst, appendicitis, salpingitis, ovarian cysts, torsion of the ovary, and urinary tract infection (Table 31-2). The key to early detection of ectopic pregnancy is having a high index of suspicion for this condition. Any woman with complaints of abdominal pain, vaginal spotting or bleeding, and a positive pregnancy test should undergo screening for ectopic pregnancy. Laboratory screening includes determination of serum progesterone and beta-hCG levels. If either of these values is lower than would be expected for a normal pregnancy, the woman is asked to return within 48 hours for serial measurements. At this time, the woman also will undergo transvaginal ultrasound to confirm intrauterine or tubal pregnancy (Gracia & Barnhart, 2001).

The woman also should be assessed for the presence of active bleeding, which is associated with tubal rupture. If internal bleeding is present, assessment may reveal vertigo, shoulder pain, hypotension, and tachycardia. A vaginal examination should be performed only once, and then with great caution. Approximately half of clients with a tubal pregnancy have a palpable mass on examination. It is possible to rupture the mass during a bimanual examination, so gentleness is critical (Simpson, 2002).

Removal of the ectopic pregnancy by salpingostomy is possible before rupture. Residual tissue is dissolved with a dose of methotrexate postoperatively. Methotrexate is a folic acid analogue that destroys the rapidly dividing cells (DeLoia, Stewart-Akers, & Creinin, 1998). It also may be used in a single-dose intramuscular injection to treat unruptured pregnancies (Lipscomb et al., 1998). It has been shown to produce results similar to those of surgical therapy, in terms of high success rate, low complication rate, and good reproductive potential (Simpson, 2002).

Advanced ectopic abdominal pregnancy requires laparotomy as soon as the woman has been stabilized for operation. If the placenta of a second- or third-trimester abdominal pregnancy is attached to a vital organ, such as the liver, separation is usually not attempted because of the risk of hemorrhage. The cord is cut flush with the placenta, and the abdomen is closed, with the placenta left in place. Degeneration and absorption of the placenta usually occur without complication, although infection and intestinal obstruction may occur. Methotrexate may be given to dissolve the residual tissue (Cunningham et al., 2001).

Hospital Care. If surgery is planned, general preoperative and postoperative care is appropriate for the woman with an ectopic pregnancy. Vital signs (pulse, respirations, and blood pressure) are assessed preoperatively every 15 minutes or as needed, according to severity of the bleeding and the woman's condition. Preoperative laboratory tests include determination of blood type and Rh factor, complete blood cell count, and serum quantitative beta-hCG assay. Ultrasonography is used to confirm an extrauterine pregnancy. Blood replacement may be necessary. The nurse verifies the woman's Rh and antibody status and administers $Rh_0(D)$ immune globulin if appropriate. The woman should be encouraged to verbalize her feelings related to the loss. Referral to community resources may be appropriate.

Home Care. Hemodynamically stable women with ectopic pregnancies are eligible for methotrexate therapy if the mass is unruptured and measures less than 4 cm in diameter by ultrasonography (Simpson, 2002). Methotrexate therapy avoids surgery and is a safe, effective, and cost-conscious way of managing many cases of tubal pregnancy. Management is almost always accomplished on an outpatient basis.

The woman is informed how the medication works, what adverse effects are possible, whom to call if she has concerns or if problems develop, and the importance of follow-up care. After receiving the single methotrexate injection, the woman must return at least weekly for follow-up laboratory studies for an average of 2 to 8 weeks until beta-hCG titers decrease. During that time, she is instructed to put nothing in the vagina (no tampons, douches, or intercourse) and to avoid sun exposure because the drug will make her more photosensitive.

NURSE ALERT

The woman receiving methotrexate therapy who drinks alcohol and takes vitamins containing folic acid (e.g., prenatal vitamins) increases her risk of having side effects of the drug or exacerbating the ectopic rupture.

Future fertility should be discussed. Any woman who has been diagnosed with an ectopic pregnancy should be told to contact her health care provider as soon as she suspects that she might be pregnant, because of the increased risk for recurrent ectopic pregnancy. These women may need referral to grief or infertility support groups. In addition to the loss of the current pregnancy, they are faced with the possibility of future pregnancy losses and infertility.

TABLE 31-2 **Differential Diagnosis of Ectopic Pregnancy**

	ECTOPIC PREGNANCY	APPENDICITIS	SALPINGITIS	RUPTURED OVARIAN CYST	MISCARRIAGE
Pain	Unilateral cramps and tenderness before rupture May be colicky after rupture Sudden sharp abdominal pelvic pain Abdominal tenderness	Epigastric, periumbilical, then right lower quadrant pain, tenderness localizing at McBurney's point, rebound tenderness	Usually in both lower quadrants with or without rebound Mild to severe pelvic pressure	Unilateral, becoming general with progressive bleeding, dull cramping	Mild uterine cramps to severe uterine pain
Nausea and vomiting	Occasionally before, frequently after rupture	Usual, precedes shift of pain to right lower quadrant	Infrequent	Rare	Almost never
Menstruation	Some aberration, missed period, spotting	Unrelated to menses	Hypermenorrhea, metrorrhagia, or both	Period delayed, then bleeding, often with pain	Amenorrhea, then spotting, then brisk bleeding
Temperature, pulse, and blood pressure	37.2°-37.8° C, pulse variable, normal before and rapid after rupture, ↓BP after rupture	37.2°-37.8° C, pulse rapid	37.2°-40° C, pulse elevated in proportion to fever	Not >37.2° C, pulse normal unless blood loss marked, then rapid	To 37.2° C Signs of shock related to obvious bleeding
Pelvic examination	Unilateral tenderness, especially on movement of cervix, crepitant mass on one side or in cul-de-sac; dark red or brown vaginal discharge	No masses, rectal tenderness high on right side No vaginal discharge	Bilateral tenderness on movement of cervix Purulent discharge	Tenderness over affected ovary, no masses	Cervix open or closed, uterus slightly enlarged, irregularly softened, tender with infection, vaginal bleeding
Laboratory findings	White blood cell count (WBC) to 15,000/mm³ Pregnancy test positive Ultrasound to rule out pregnancy after 6 wk	WBC 10,000-18,000/mm³ (rarely normal) Pregnancy test negative	WBC 15,000-30,000/mm³ Pregnancy test negative	WBC normal to 10,000/mm³ Pregnancy test negative unless also pregnant Ultrasound will show ovarian cyst	WBC normal Pregnancy test positive

Modified from Gilbert, E., & Harmon, J. (2003). *Manual of high risk pregnancy and delivery* (3rd ed.). St. Louis: Mosby.

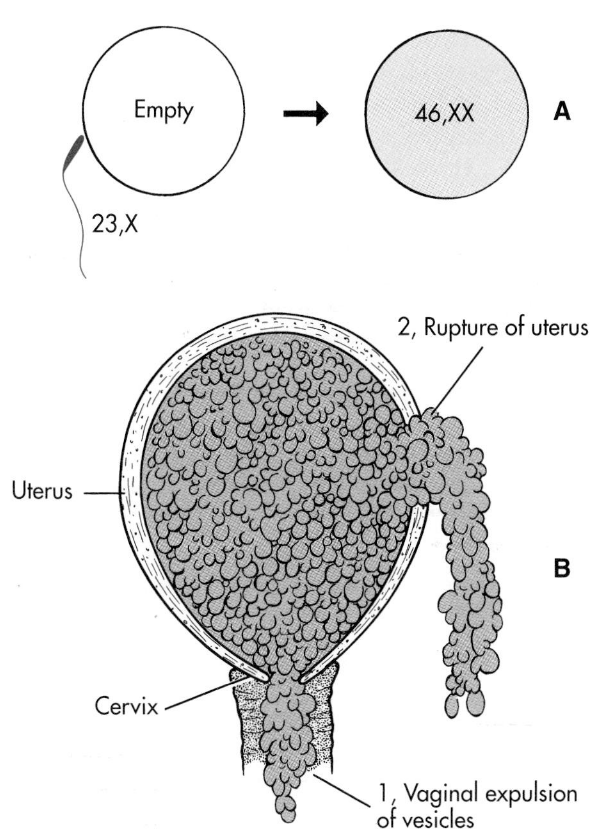
Empty
46,XX
A
23,X
2, Rupture of uterus
Uterus
B
Cervix
1, Vaginal expulsion of vesicles

FIG. 31-5 **A,** Chromosomal origin of complete mole. Single sperm (*color*) fertilizes an "empty" ovum. Reduplication of sperm's 23,X set gives completely homozygous diploid 46,XX. Similar process follows fertilization of empty ovum by two sperm with two independently drawn sets of 23,X or 23,Y; both karyotypes of 46,XX and 46,XY can therefore result. **B,** Uterine rupture with hydatidiform mole. *1,* Evacuation of mole through cervix. *2,* Rupture of uterus and spillage of mole into peritoneal cavity (rare).

Hydatidiform Mole (Molar Pregnancy)

Hydatidiform mole (molar pregnancy) is a gestational trophoblastic disease. The two distinct types of hydatidiform moles are complete (or classic) mole and partial mole.

Incidence and Etiology

Hydatidiform mole occurs in 1 in 1200 pregnancies in the United States, but a higher incidence has been reported in Asian countries (Berman, DiSaia, & Brewster, 1999). The etiology is unknown, although there may be an ovular defect or nutritional deficiency. Women at higher risk for hydatidiform mole formation are those who have undergone ovulation stimulation with clomiphene (Clomid) and those who are in their early teens or older than 40 years. The risk of a second mole is 1% to 2%.

Types

The complete mole results from fertilization of an egg with a lost or inactivated nucleus (Fig. 31-5, *A*). The nucleus of a sperm (23,X) duplicates itself (resulting in the diploid number, 46,XX) because the ovum has no genetic material or the material is inactive. The mole resembles a bunch of white grapes (Fig. 31-5, *B*). The hydropic (fluid-filled) vesicles grow rapidly, causing the uterus to be larger than expected for the duration of the pregnancy. Usually the complete mole contains no fetus, placenta, amniotic membranes, or fluid. Maternal blood has no placenta to receive it; hemorrhage into the uterine cavity and vaginal bleeding therefore occur. In about 20% of cases of complete mole, progression toward choriocarcinoma occurs.

For a partial mole, chromosomal studies often show a karyotype of 69,XXY; 69,XXX; or 69,XYY. This occurs as a result of two sperm fertilizing an apparently normal ovum (Fig. 31-6). Partial moles often have embryonic or fetal parts and an amniotic sac. Congenital anomalies are

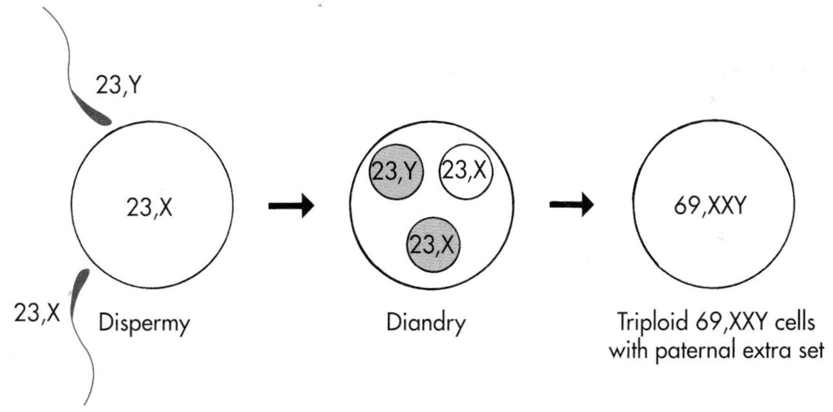
23,Y
23,X
23,X
Dispermy
23,Y
23,X
23,X
Diandry
69,XXY
Triploid 69,XXY cells with paternal extra set

FIG. 31-6 Chromosomal origin of triploid partial mole. Normal ovum with 23,X haploid set is fertilized by two sperms to give total of 69 chromosomes. Sex configuration of XXY, XXX, or XYY is possible.

usually present. The potential for malignant transformation is less than 6% (Copeland & Landon, 2002).

Clinical Manifestations

The clinical manifestations of a complete hydatidiform mole in the early stages cannot be distinguished from those of normal pregnancy. Vaginal bleeding occurs later in almost 95% of cases. The vaginal discharge may be dark brown (resembling prune juice) or bright red, either scant or profuse, continuing for only a few days or intermittently for weeks. Early in pregnancy, the uterus in about half of affected women is significantly larger than expected from menstrual dates. The percentage of women with an excessively enlarged uterus increases as length of time since LMP increases. Approximately 25% of affected women have a uterus smaller than would be expected from menstrual dates.

Anemia from blood loss, excessive nausea and vomiting (hyperemesis gravidarum), and abdominal cramps caused by uterine distention are relatively common findings. Preeclampsia occurs in about 15% of cases, usually between 9 and 12 weeks of gestation, but any symptoms of gestational hypertension before 24 weeks of gestation may suggest hydatidiform mole. Hyperthyroidism and pulmonary embolization of trophoblastic elements occur less commonly but are serious complications of hydatidiform mole. Partial moles cause few of these symptoms and may be mistaken for an incomplete or missed miscarriage.

Collaborative Care

Medical-Surgical Management. Although most moles abort spontaneously, suction curettage offers a safe, rapid, and effective method of evacuation of hydatidiform mole if necessary (Gilbert & Harmon, 2003). Induction of labor with oxytocic agents or prostaglandins is not recommended because of the increased risk of embolization of trophoblastic tissue (Copeland & Landon, 2002). Administration of $Rh_0(D)$ immune globulin to women who are Rh negative is necessary to prevent isoimmunization.

Nursing Care. Nursing assessments during prenatal visits should include observation for signs of molar pregnancy during the first 24 weeks. If hydatidiform mole is suspected, ultrasonography and serial beta-hCG immunoassays will be used to confirm the diagnosis. The sonographic pattern of a molar pregnancy is characterized by a diffuse "snowstorm" pattern. A beta-hCG titer will remain high or increase above normal peak after the time at which it normally decreases (70 to 100 days) (Cunningham et al., 2001).

The nurse provides the woman and her family with information about the disease process, the necessity for a long course of follow-up, and the possible consequences of the disease. The nurse helps the woman understand and cope with pregnancy loss and recognize that the pregnancy was abnormal. The woman and her family are encouraged to express their feelings, and information is provided about support groups or counseling resources if needed. Explanations about the importance of the need to postpone a subsequent pregnancy and contraceptive counseling are provided to emphasize the importance of consistent and reliable use of the method chosen.

NURSE ALERT

To avoid confusion with signs of pregnancy, pregnancy should be avoided for 1 year. Any contraceptive method except an intrauterine device is acceptable. Oral contraceptives are highly effective.

Home Care. Follow-up management includes frequent physical and pelvic examinations along with biweekly measurements of beta-hCG level until the level decreases to normal and remains normal for 3 weeks. Monthly measurements are taken for 6 months and then every 2 months for a total of 1 year. A rising titer and an enlarging uterus may indicate choriocarcinoma (see Chapter 12). Referral to community support resources may be needed (see Resources at the end of this chapter).

LATE PREGNANCY BLEEDING

Late pregnancy bleeding disorders include placenta previa, premature separation of placenta (abruptio placentae), and variations in the cord insertion and the placenta. Expedient assessment for and diagnosis of the cause of bleeding are essential to reduce maternal and perinatal morbidity and mortality (Fig. 31-7).

Placenta Previa

Placenta previa is the condition in which the placenta is implanted in the lower uterine segment near or over the internal cervical os. The degree to which the internal cervical os is covered by the placenta has traditionally been used to classify three types of placenta previa (Fig. 31-8). Placenta previa often is described as total if the internal os is entirely covered by the placenta when the cervix is fully dilated. Partial placenta previa implies incomplete coverage of the internal os. Marginal placenta previa indicates that only an edge of the placenta extends to the internal os but may extend onto the os during dilation of the cervix during labor. The term *low-lying placenta* is used when the placenta is implanted in the lower uterine segment but does not reach the os.

Vasa previa is the result of a velamentous insertion (see Cord Insertion and Placental Variations on p. 877, later in this chapter) of the umbilical cord. With vasa previa, the umbilical vein and arteries are not surrounded by Wharton's jelly and have no supportive tissue. The umbilical blood vessels are thus at risk for laceration at any time, but laceration occurs most frequently during ROM (Clark, 1999). The sudden appearance of bright red blood at the time of ROM (spontaneous or artificial) and a sudden change in the fetal heart rate without other known risk factors should immediately alert the nurse to the possibility of vasa previa.

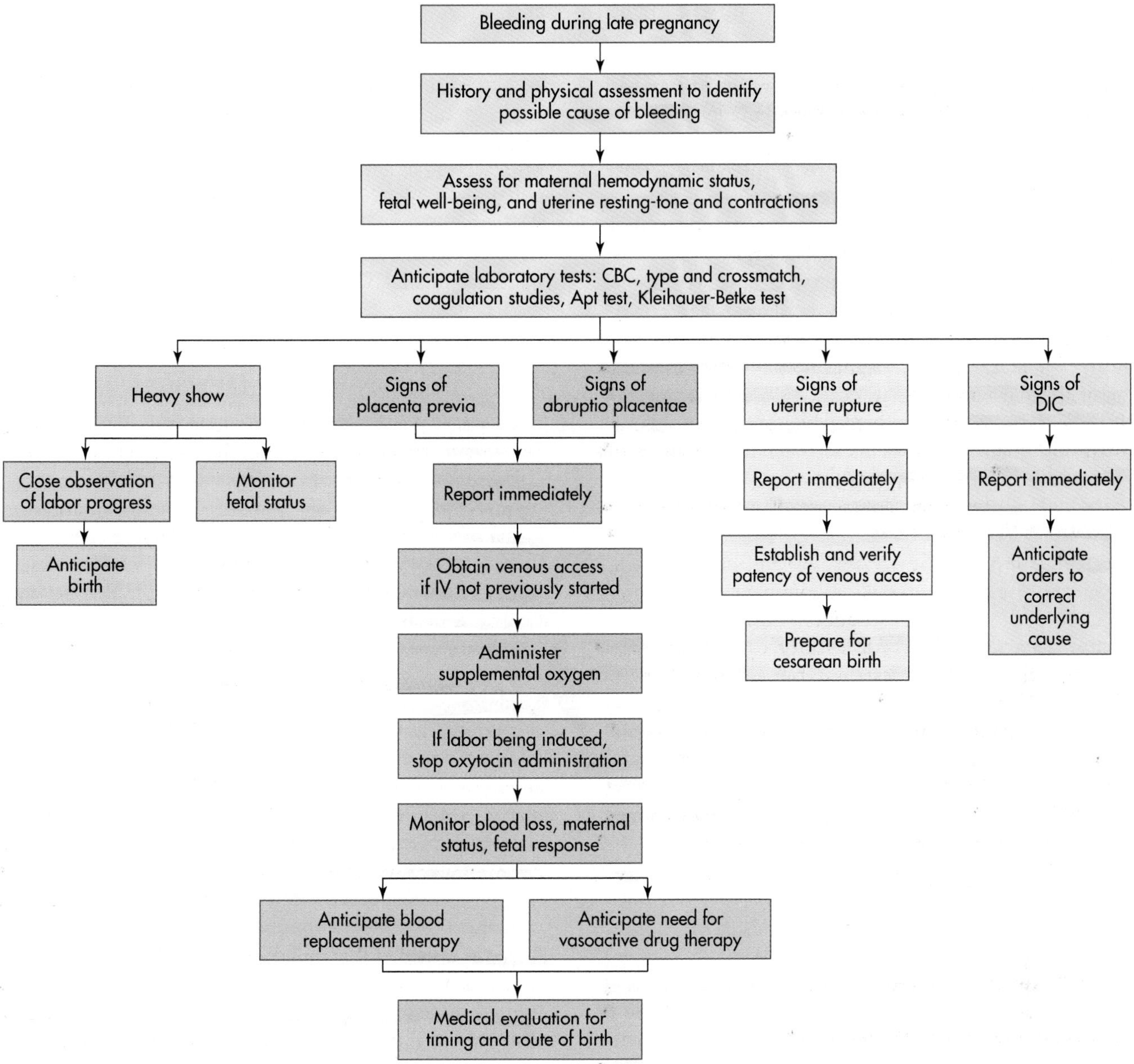

Bleeding during late pregnancy
History and physical assessment to identify possible cause of bleeding
Assess for maternal hemodynamic status, fetal well-being, and uterine resting-tone and contractions
Anticipate laboratory tests: CBC, type and crossmatch, coagulation studies, Apt test, Kleihauer-Betke test
Heavy show
Signs of placenta previa
Signs of abruptio placentae
Signs of uterine rupture
Signs of DIC
Close observation of labor progress
Monitor fetal status
Anticipate birth
Report immediately
Obtain venous access if IV not previously started
Administer supplemental oxygen
If labor being induced, stop oxytocin administration
Monitor blood loss, maternal status, fetal response
Anticipate blood replacement therapy
Anticipate need for vasoactive drug therapy
Medical evaluation for timing and route of birth
Report immediately
Establish and verify patency of venous access
Prepare for cesarean birth
Report immediately
Anticipate orders to correct underlying cause

FIG. 31-7 Bleeding during late pregnancy. *CBC,* Complete blood count; *DIC,* disseminated intravascular coagulation; *IV,* intravenous.

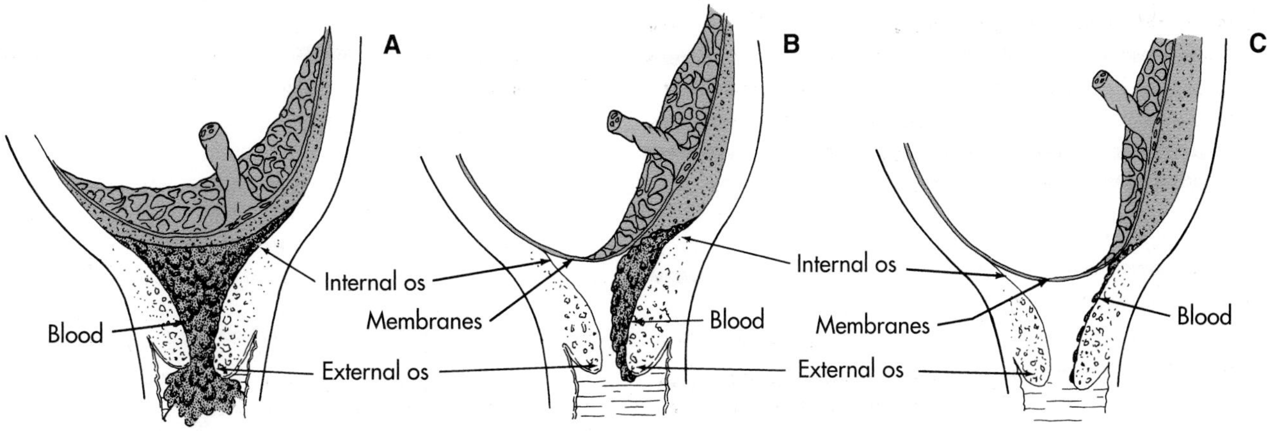

A
B
C
Internal os
Internal os
Blood
Membranes
Blood
Membranes
Blood
External os
External os

FIG. 31-8 Types of placenta previa after onset of labor. **A,** Complete, or total. **B,** Incomplete, or partial. **C,** Marginal, or low lying.

Although it occurs rarely, vasa previa is associated with high incidence of fetal morbidity and mortality because of the potential for fetal exsanguination (Benedetti, 2002). Diagnosis before birth is unusual, although examiners have reported palpating a pulsing vessel. Vasa previa also may be noted on ultrasonographic examination or by direct visualization (Cunningham et al., 2001).

Incidence and Etiology

The incidence of placenta previa is approximately 0.5% of births (Clark, 1999). The most important risk factors are previous placenta previa, previous cesarean birth, and induced abortion, possibly related to endometrial scarring (Ananth, Smulian, & Vintzileos, 1997). The risk also increases with multiple gestation (because of the larger placental area), closely spaced pregnancies, maternal age older than 35 years, African or Asian ethnicity, smoking, and cocaine use (Clark, 1999).

Clinical Manifestations

Approximately 70% of women with placenta previa have painless vaginal bleeding; 20% have vaginal bleeding associated with uterine activity. Previa should be suspected whenever vaginal bleeding occurs after 24 weeks of gestation. This bleeding is associated with the stretching and thinning of the lower uterine segment that occurs during the third trimester. Placental attachment is gradually disrupted, and bleeding occurs when the uterus is not able to contract adequately and stop blood flow from open vessels (Benedetti, 2002). The initial bleeding is usually a small amount and stops as clots form; however, it can recur at any time (Table 31-3). It is bright red.

Vital signs may be normal, even with heavy blood loss, because a pregnant woman can lose up to 40% of blood volume without showing signs of shock. Clinical presentation and decreasing urinary output may be better indicators of acute blood loss than are vital signs alone. The fetal heart rate will be reassuring unless there is a major detachment of the placenta (Gilbert & Harmon, 2003).

Abdominal examination usually reveals a soft, relaxed, nontender uterus with normal tone. If the fetus is lying longitudinally, the fundal height is usually greater than expected for gestational age because the low placenta hinders descent of the presenting fetal part. Leopold maneuvers may reveal a fetus in an oblique or breech position or lying transverse because of the abnormal site of placental implantation.

Maternal and Fetal Outcome

Maternal morbidity is about 5%, and mortality is less than 1% with placenta previa (Clark, 1999). Complications associated with placenta previa include preterm ROM, preterm labor and birth, surgery-related trauma to structures adjacent to the uterus, anesthesia complications, blood transfusion reactions, overinfusion of fluids, abnormal placental attachments, postpartum hemorrhage, anemia, thrombophlebitis, and infection (Crane et al., 2000).

The greatest risk of fetal mortality is caused by preterm birth. Other fetal risks include malpresentation and congenital anomalies (Gilbert & Harmon, 2003). Infants who are small for gestational age or have intrauterine growth restriction also have been associated with placenta previa; this association may be related to poor placental exchange or hypovolemia resulting from maternal blood loss and maternal anemia (Clark, 1999).

CARE MANAGEMENT

Assessment and Nursing Diagnoses

A woman with third-trimester vaginal bleeding requires immediate evaluation. Necessary history data include gravidity, parity, estimated date of birth, general status, bleeding (quantity, precipitating event, associated pain), vital signs, and fetal status (see Box 31-1). Abdominal assessment reveals a soft, relaxed, nontender uterus with normal tone. Laboratory studies include a complete blood cell count, determination of blood type and Rh factor, coagulation profile, and possible type and crossmatch.

The standard for diagnosis of placenta previa is a transabdominal ultrasonographic examination. This study is accurate 93% to 97% of the time, with false-negative and false-positive results occurring as a result of factors such as an engaged cephalic presentation, a posteriorly implanted placenta, maternal obesity, and compression of the lower uterine segment by an overdistended bladder. Transvaginal ultrasound also is used for placental location, particularly when the exact relation of the lower placental margin to the internal os is not clearly seen with transabdominal examination (Clark, 1999). If ultrasonographic scanning reveals a normally implanted placenta, a speculum examination is performed to rule out local causes of bleeding (e.g., cervicitis, polyps, or carcinoma of the cervix), and a coagulation profile is obtained to rule out other causes of bleeding. If expectant management is to be implemented, a vaginal speculum examination by the health care provider is postponed until fetal viability has been reached (preferably after 34 weeks of gestation). If a pelvic examination is needed before that time, anticipate the possibility that an immediate cesarean birth may be required. The woman is taken to a delivery or operating room set up for cesarean birth because profound hemorrhage can occur during the examination. This type of vaginal examination, known as the *double-setup procedure*, is not done often.

Potential nursing diagnoses for the woman with a placenta previa include the following:

- *Decreased cardiac output related to*
  –excessive blood loss secondary to placenta previa
- *Deficient fluid volume related to*
  –excessive blood loss secondary to placenta previa
- *Risk for excess fluid volume related to*
  –fluid resuscitation

TABLE 31-3 **Summary of Findings: Abruptio Placentae and Placenta Previa**

	ABRUPTIO PLACENTAE			
	GRADE 1 MILD SEPARATION (10% TO 20%)	GRADE 2 MODERATE SEPARATION (20% TO 50%)	GRADE 3 SEVERE SEPARATION (>50%)	PLACENTA PREVIA
Bleeding, external, vaginal	Minimal	Absent or moderate	Absent to moderate	Minimal to severe and life-threatening
Total amount of blood loss	<500 ml	1000-1500 ml	>1500 ml	Varies
Color of blood	Dark red	Dark red	Dark red	Bright red
Shock	Rare; none	Mild shock	Common, often sudden, profound	Uncommon
Coagulopathy	Rare; none	Occasional DIC	Frequent DIC	None
Uterine tonicity	Normal	Increased, may be localized to one region or diffuse over uterus, uterus fails to relax between contractions	Tetanic, persistent uterine contraction, boardlike uterus	Normal
Tenderness (pain)	Usually absent	Present	Agonizing, unremitting uterine pain	Absent
Ultrasonographic findings				
Location of placenta	Normal, upper uterine segment	Normal, upper uterine segment	Normal, upper uterine segment	Abnormal, lower uterine segment
Station of presenting part	Variable to engaged	Variable to engaged	Variable to engaged	High, not engaged
Fetal position	Usual distribution*	Usual distribution*	Usual distribution*	Commonly transverse, breech, or oblique
Gestational or chronic hypertension	Usual distribution*	Commonly present	Commonly present	Usual distribution*
Fetal effects	Normal fetal heart rate pattern	Nonreassuring fetal heart rate pattern	Nonreassuring fetal heart rate pattern; death can occur	Normal fetal heart rate pattern

**Usual distribution* refers to the usual variations of incidence seen when there is no concurrent problem.
DIC, Disseminated intravascular coagulation.

- *Ineffective peripheral tissue perfusion related to*
  –hypovolemia and shunting of blood to central circulation
- *Risk for injury (fetal) related to*
  –decreased placental perfusion secondary to placenta previa
- *Anxiety/fear related to*
  –maternal condition and pregnancy outcome
- *Deficient knowledge related to*
  –hospitalization and treatment regimens
- *Interrupted family processes related to*
  –mother's condition and hospitalization
- *Anticipatory grieving related to*
  –actual/perceived threat to self, pregnancy, or infant
- *Risk for infection related to*
  –anemia, hemorrhage, placenta previa, and transfusions
- *Risk for injury (mother) related to*
  –invasive monitoring procedures and treatment

Expected Outcomes of Care

Expected outcomes for the woman with placenta previa may include the following. The woman will:

- Verbalize understanding of her condition and its management.
- Identify and use available support systems.
- Demonstrate compliance with prescribed activity limitations.

- Develop no complications related to bleeding.
- Give birth to a healthy infant at or near term.

Plan of Care and Interventions

Hospital Care

Active Management. Once placenta previa has been diagnosed, a management plan is developed based on gestational age, amount of bleeding, and fetal condition. If the woman is at term (longer than or equal to 37 weeks of gestation) and in labor or bleeding persistently, immediate delivery by cesarean is almost always indicated. In women with partial or marginal previas who have minimal bleeding, vaginal birth may be attempted. Vaginal birth also may be indicated for previable gestations or births involving intrauterine fetal demise (Benedetti, 2002).

If cesarean birth is undertaken, the nurse continuously assesses maternal and fetal status while preparing the woman for surgery. Maternal vital signs are assessed frequently for decreasing blood pressure, increasing pulse rate, changes in level of consciousness (LOC), and oliguria. Fetal assessment is maintained by continuous electronic fetal monitoring to assess for signs of hypoxia.

Blood loss may not cease with the birth of the infant. The large vascular channels in the lower uterine segment may continue to bleed because of that segment's diminished muscle content. The natural mechanism to control bleeding so characteristic of the upper part of the uterus—the interlacing muscle bundles, the "living ligature" contracting around open vessels—is absent in the lower part of the uterus. Postpartum hemorrhage may therefore occur even if the fundus is contracted firmly.

Emotional support for the woman and her family is extremely important. The actively bleeding woman is concerned not only for her own well-being but for the well-being of her fetus. All procedures should be explained, and a support person should be present. The woman should be encouraged to express her concerns and feelings. If the woman and her support person or family desire pastoral support, the nurse can notify the hospital chaplain service or provide information about other supportive resources.

Expectant Management. If the woman is at less than 36 weeks of gestation, not in labor, and the bleeding is mild or has stopped, expectant management is generally the treatment of choice to give the fetus time to mature in utero. Expectant management consists of rest and close observation. The woman is usually placed on bed rest, although she may be allowed bathroom privileges and limited activity (up in a wheelchair for an hour or so daily). Bleeding is assessed by checking the amount of bleeding on perineal pads, bed pads, and linens. Weighing pads, although not often used, is one way to assess blood loss more accurately: 1 g represents 1 ml blood.

Ultrasonographic examinations may be done every 2 to 3 weeks. Fetal surveillance may include nonstress testing (NST) or biophysical profiles once or twice weekly. Serial laboratory values are evaluated for decreasing hemoglobin and hematocrit levels and changes in coagulation values. Venous access with an IV infusion or heparin lock may be placed in case blood or blood component therapy is needed. Antepartum steroids (betamethasone) may be ordered to promote fetal lung maturity if the woman is at less than 34 weeks of gestation. No vaginal or rectal examinations are performed, and the woman is placed on pelvic rest (nothing in the vagina). Once she reaches 37 weeks of gestation, and fetal lung maturity is documented, cesarean birth can be scheduled.

During her hospitalization, the woman with placenta previa should always be considered a potential emergency, because massive blood loss with resulting hypovolemic shock can occur quickly if bleeding resumes. The possibility always exists that she may require an emergency cesarean for birth. Placenta previa in a preterm gestation may be an indication for transfer to a tertiary perinatal center, because many community hospitals are not equipped to perform emergency cesarean births 24 hours per day, 7 days per week.

Home Care. Criteria for home care management vary among primary perinatal providers and home care agencies and are usually determined on a case-by-case basis. To be considered for home care referral, the woman must be in stable condition with no evidence of active bleeding and must have resources to be able to return to the hospital immediately if active bleeding resumes (Lowdermilk & Grohar, 1998).

She must have close supervision by family or friends in the home. The woman should be taught how to assess fetal and uterine activity and bleeding and told to avoid intercourse, douching, and enemas. She should limit her activities according to the advice of her physician and be advised to keep all appointments for fetal testing, laboratory assessments, and prenatal care. Visits by a perinatal home care nurse may be arranged (Lowdermilk & Grohar, 1998).

If hospitalization or home care with activity restriction is prolonged, the woman may have concerns about her work- or family-related responsibilities or may become bored with inactivity. She should be encouraged to participate in her own care and decisions about care as much as possible. Provision of diversionary activities or encouragement to participate in activities she enjoys and can do during bed rest is needed (see Teaching for Self-Care activities in Chapter 30, p. 849). Participation in a support group made up of other women on bed rest while hospitalized may be a helpful coping mechanism (Maloni & Kutil, 2000).

Evaluation

The expected outcomes of care are used to evaluate the care for the woman with placenta previa (see Plan of Care).

Premature Separation of Placenta

Premature separation of the placenta, also termed **abruptio placentae,** is the detachment of part or all of the placenta from its implantation site (Fig. 31-9). Separation occurs in the area of the decidua basalis after 20 weeks of pregnancy and before the birth of the baby.

Plan of Care: Placenta Previa

NURSING DIAGNOSIS Decreased cardiac output related to bleeding secondary to placenta previa

Expected Outcome *Client will exhibit signs of increased blood volume and restoration of cardiac output (i.e., normal pulse and blood pressure; normal heart and breath sounds; normal skin color, tone, and turgor; normal capillary refill).*

Nursing Interventions/*Rationales*

Palpate uterus for tenderness and tone; assess bleeding rate, amount, color, degree of bleeding, CBC values, and coagulation profile *to determine severity of situation.* Do not perform vaginal examination *because it may stimulate further bleeding.*

Establish baseline data for cardiac output (vital signs; heart and breath sounds; skin color, tone, turgor; capillary refill; level of consciousness; urinary output; pulse oximetry) *to use as basis for evaluating effectiveness of treatment.*

Initiate intravenous therapy or blood transfusions and medications per physician order *to restore blood volume and prevent organ compromise to mother and fetus.*

Place woman on bed rest *to decrease oxygen demands.*

Monitor vital signs, intake and output, hemodynamic status, and laboratory values *to evaluate treatment response.*

Provide emotional support to woman and her family (e.g., explain procedures and their rationale; explain what is happening and what to expect; keep support person present) *to allay fears and provide the family with some sense of control.*

After stabilization, teach woman home management, including bed rest, watching for spotting/bleeding, close follow-up with her health care provider, and preparation for immediate return to hospital if needed *to prevent or stem further complications.*

NURSING DIAGNOSIS Risk for injury to the fetus related to decreased uterine/placental perfusion secondary to bleeding

Expected Outcome *Client will exhibit ongoing signs of fetal well-being (i.e., adequate fetal movement, normal fetal heart rate, reactive NST, normal biophysical profile [BPP]).*

Nursing Interventions/*Rationales*

Monitor fetus daily for signs of tachycardia, decreased movement, loss of reactivity on NST *to identify and treat changes in fetal status early.*

Obtain BPP per physician order *to assess for signs of chronic asphyxia.*

Maintain maternal side-lying position *to prevent compression of aorta and vena cava.*

NURSING DIAGNOSIS Risk for infection related to anemia and bleeding secondary to placenta previa

Expected Outcome *Client will show no signs of intrauterine infection.*

Nursing Interventions/*Rationales*

Monitor vital signs for elevated temperature, pulse, and blood pressure; monitor laboratory results for elevated white blood cell count, differential shift; check for uterine tenderness and malodorous vaginal discharge *to detect early signs of infection resulting from exposure of placental tissue.*

Provide/teach perineal hygiene *to decrease the risk of ascending infection.*

CBC, Complete blood count; *NST,* nonstress test.

Incidence and Etiology

Premature separation of the placenta is a serious event that accounts for significant maternal and fetal morbidity and mortality. Maternal hypertension is probably the most consistently identified risk factor for abruption (Benedetti, 2002). Cocaine also is a risk factor, which is likely in part because cocaine use is associated with the development of hypertension (Andres & Day, 2000). Blunt external abdominal trauma, most often the result of motor vehicle accidents or maternal battering, is an increasingly significant cause of placental abruption (Benedetti, 2002). Maternal smoking and poor nutrition may be associated with an increased risk (Kramer et al., 1997). In the past, maternal age older than 35 years and parity, short umbilical cord, and folic acid deficiency were all thought to increase risk; however, more recent research has failed to confirm this (Benedetti, 2002). Abruption is more likely to occur in twin gestation (Ananth et al., 2001). There is a significant (5% to 17%) recurrence risk for placental abruption. A woman who has had two previous premature separations has a recurrence risk of 25% in the next pregnancy (Benedetti, 2002).

Classification Systems

The most common classification of placental abruption is according to type and severity. This classification system grades an abruption as follows (Clark, 1999):

Grade 1. The woman has vaginal bleeding perhaps with uterine tenderness and mild tetany, but neither mother nor baby is in distress. Approximately 10% to 20% of the total placental surface area is detached.

Grade 2. The woman has uterine tenderness and tetany, with or without external evidence of bleeding. The mother is not in shock, but there is fetal distress. Approximately 20% to 50% of the total surface area is detached.

Grade 3. Uterine tetany is severe; the woman is in shock (although the bleeding may not be obvious); and the fetus is dead. Often the woman has coagulopathy. Greater than 50% of the placental surface area detaches (Gilbert & Harmon, 2003).

These grades are often classified as mild (grade 1), moderate (grade 2), and severe (grade 3). This classification system is summarized in Table 31-3.

Clinical Manifestations

The separation may be partial or complete, or only the margin of the placenta may be involved. Bleeding from the placental site may dissect (separate) the membranes from the decidua basalis and flow out through the vagina; it may remain concealed (retroplacental hemorrhage); or it may do both (see Fig. 31-9). Clinical symptoms vary with degree of separation (see Table 31-3).

Classic symptoms of abruptio placentae include vaginal bleeding, abdominal pain, and uterine tenderness and contractions. Vaginal bleeding is present in as many as 70% to 80% of women with abruption (Clark, 1999). Although abdominal pain and uterine tenderness are characteristic for this complication, either finding may be absent in the presence of a silent abruption (Cunningham et al., 2001). Bleeding may result in maternal hypovolemia (shock, oliguria, anuria) and coagulopathy. Mild to severe uterine hypertonicity is present. Pain is mild to severe and localized over one region of the uterus or diffuse over the uterus with a boardlike abdomen.

Extensive myometrial bleeding damages the uterine muscle. If blood accumulates between the separated placenta and the uterine wall, it may produce a **Couvelaire uterus.** The uterus appears purplish and copper colored, it is ecchymotic, and contractility is lost. Shock may occur and is out of proportion to blood loss. Laboratory findings include a positive *Apt test* result (blood in amniotic fluid); a decrease in hemoglobin and hematocrit levels (which may appear later); and a decrease in coagulation factor levels. Clotting defects (e.g., disseminated intravascular coagulation [DIC]) develop in 10% to 30% of clients (most within 8 hours of hospital admission). A *Kleihauer-Betke stain* may be ordered to determine the presence of fetal-to-maternal bleeding (transplacental hemorrhage).

Maternal, Fetal, and Neonatal Outcomes

The maternal mortality rate approaches 1% for abruptio placentae; this condition remains a leading cause of maternal death. The mother's prognosis depends on the extent of placental detachment, overall blood loss, degree of DIC, and time between placental detachment and birth.

Maternal complications are associated with the abruption or its treatment. Hemorrhage, hypovolemic shock, hypofibrinogenemia, and thrombocytopenia are associated with severe abruption. Couvelaire uterus, DIC, and infection may occur. Renal failure and pituitary necrosis (Sheehan's syndrome) may result from ischemia. In rare cases, women who are Rh negative can become sensitized if fetal-to-maternal hemorrhage occurs and the fetal blood type is Rh positive.

Perinatal mortality rates range from 15% to 30%. Mortality occurs as a result of fetal hypoxia, preterm birth, and status as small for gestational age. Risks of neurologic defects are increased (Cunningham et al., 2001).

Collaborative Care

Abruptio placentae should be strongly suspected in the woman who has a sudden onset of intense, usually localized, uterine pain, with or without vaginal bleeding. Initial assessment is much the same as that for placenta previa. Physical examination usually reveals abdominal pain, uterine tenderness, and contractions. The fundal height may be measured over time, because increasing fundal height indicates concealed bleeding. Vaginal bleeding is present in about 80% of cases (Benedetti, 2002). Approximately 60% of live fetuses exhibit nonreassuring signs on the electronic fetal heart monitor, such as loss of variability and late decelerations; uterine hyperstimulation and increased resting tone may also be noted on the monitor tracing (Benedetti, 2002). Many women demonstrate coagulopathy, as evidenced by abnor-

Abruptio placentae (premature separation)

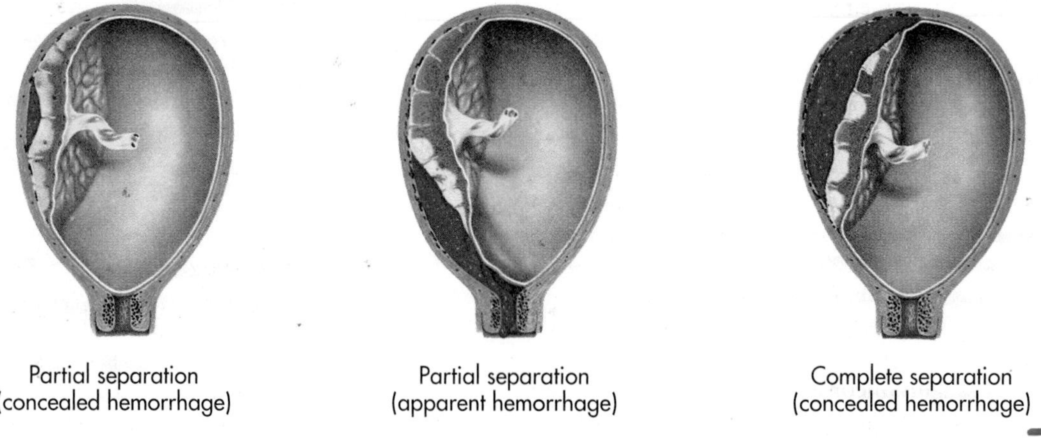

Partial separation (concealed hemorrhage) | Partial separation (apparent hemorrhage) | Complete separation (concealed hemorrhage)

FIG. 31-9 Abruptio placentae. Premature separation of normally implanted placenta.

mal clotting studies (fibrinogen, platelet count, prothrombin time [PT], partial thromboplastin time [PTT], fibrin split products). Sonographic examination is used to rule out placenta previa; however, it is not always diagnostic for abruption. A retroplacental mass may be detected with ultrasonographic examination, but negative findings do not rule out a life-threatening abruption (Clark, 1999; Cunningham et al., 2001). Better imaging technology has made it possible to demonstrate ultrasonographic evidence of hemorrhage in more than 50% of cases of confirmed placental abruption (Benedetti, 2002).

Nursing diagnoses and expected outcomes of care are similar to those described for placenta previa.

Hospital Care. Treatment depends on the severity of blood loss and fetal maturity and status. If the abruption is mild and the fetus is less than 36 weeks of gestation and not in distress, expectant management may be implemented. The woman is hospitalized and observed closely for signs of bleeding and labor. The fetal status also is monitored with intermittent fetal heart rate monitoring and NST or biophysical profiles until fetal maturity is determined or until the woman's condition deteriorates and immediate birth is indicated. Use of corticosteroids to accelerate fetal lung maturity is appropriately included in the plan of care for expectant management (ACOG, 1998; NIH, 2000). Women who are Rh-negative may be given $Rh_0(D)$ immune globulin if fetal-to-maternal hemorrhage occurs and the fetal blood is Rh positive.

Delivery is the treatment of choice if the fetus is at term gestation or if the bleeding is moderate to severe and mother or fetus is in jeopardy. At least one large-bore (16-gauge) IV line should be started. Maternal vital signs are monitored frequently to observe for signs of declining hemodynamic status, such as increasing pulse rate and decreasing blood pressure. Serial laboratory studies include hematocrit or hemoglobin determinations and clotting studies. Continuous electronic fetal monitoring is mandatory. An indwelling Foley catheter is inserted for continuous assessment of urine output, an excellent indirect measure of maternal organ perfusion (Benedetti, 2002).

Blood and fluid volume replacement will most likely be ordered, with a goal of maintaining the urine output at 30 ml/hr or more, and the hematocrit, at 30% or more. If this goal is not reached despite vigorous attempts at replacement, hemodynamic monitoring may be necessary (Benedetti, 2002). Fresh frozen plasma or cryoprecipitate may be given to maintain the fibrinogen level at a minimum of 100 to 150 mg/dl.

Vaginal birth is usually feasible and is especially desirable in cases of fetal death. Cesarean birth should be reserved for cases of fetal distress or other obstetric indications. Cesarean birth should not be attempted when the woman has severe and uncorrected coagulopathy because it may result in surgically uncontrollable bleeding (Benedetti, 2002).

Nursing care of clients experiencing moderate-to-severe abruption is demanding because it requires meticulous assessment of maternal and fetal condition, as described previously. Information about abruptio placentae, including cause, treatment, and expected outcome, is given to the woman and her family. Emotional support also is extremely important because the woman and her family may be experiencing fetal loss in addition to the woman's critical illness.

Home Care. Women with abruptio placentae are usually not managed out of the hospital because the placenta can separate further at any time, and immediate intervention or delivery may be necessary.

Cord Insertion and Placental Variations

Velamentous insertion of the cord is a rare placental anomaly associated with placenta previa and multiple gestation. The cord vessels begin to branch at the membranes and then course onto the placenta (Fig. 31-10, *A*). ROM or traction on the cord may tear one or more of the fetal vessels. As a result, the fetus may rapidly bleed to death. **Battledore** (marginal) **insertion of the cord** (Fig. 31-10, *B*) increases the risk of fetal hemorrhage, especially after marginal separation of the placenta.

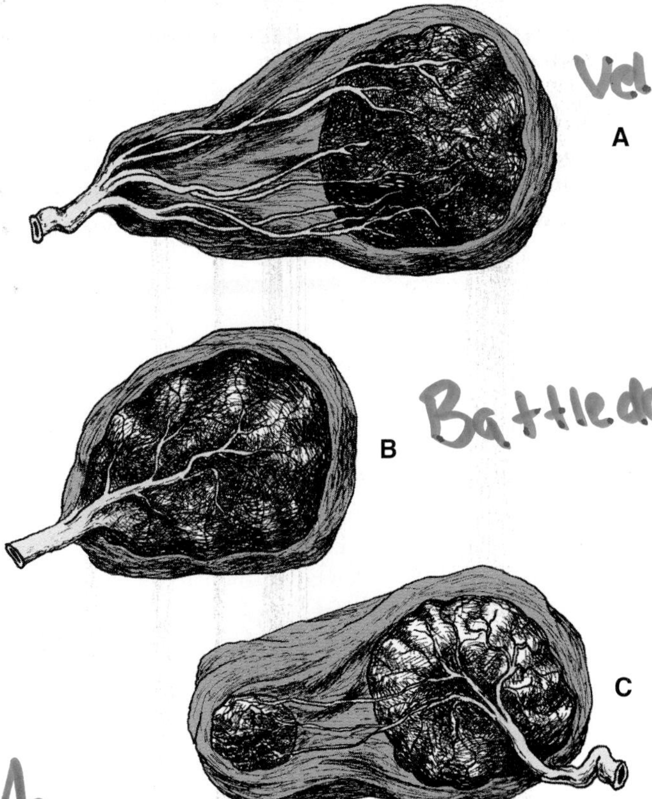
A
B
C

FIG. 31-10 Cord insertion and placental variations. **A,** Velamentous insertion of cord. **B,** Battledore placenta. **C,** Placenta succenturiate.

Rarely the placenta may be divided into two or more separate lobes, resulting in **succenturiate placenta** (Fig. 31-10, *C*). Each lobe has a distinct circulation; the vessels collect at the periphery, and the main trunks eventually unite to form the vessels of the cord. Blood vessels joining the lobes may be supported only by the fetal membranes and are therefore in danger of tearing during labor, birth, or expulsion of the placenta. During recovery of the placenta, one or more of the separate lobes may remain attached to the decidua basalis, preventing uterine contraction and increasing the risk of postpartum hemorrhage.

CLOTTING DISORDERS IN PREGNANCY

Normal Clotting

Normally a delicate balance (homeostasis) exists between the opposing hemostatic and fibrinolytic systems. The hemostatic system is involved in the life-saving process. This system stops the flow of blood from injured vessels, in part through the formation of insoluble fibrin, which acts as a hemostatic platelet plug. The phases of the coagulation process involve an interaction of the coagulation factors in which each factor sequentially activates the factor next in line, the "cascade effect" sequence. The fibrinolytic system is the process through which the fibrin is split into fibrinolytic degradation products and circulation is restored.

Clotting Problems

A history of abnormal bleeding, inheritance of unusual bleeding tendencies, and a report of significant aberrations of laboratory findings indicate a bleeding or clotting problem. For the pregnant woman, bleeding disorders are suspected if the woman has gestational hypertension, HELLP syndrome, retained dead fetus syndrome, amniotic fluid embolism, sepsis, or hemorrhage. Determination of hemostasis is made by testing the usual mechanisms for the control of bleeding, the function of platelets, and the necessary clotting factors. Most clotting disorders are more a concern in the immediate postpartum period. Recognition in the antepartal period may decrease hemorrhagic problems (see Chapter 37).

Disseminated Intravascular Coagulation. DIC is a pathologic form of diffuse clotting that consumes large amounts of clotting factors, causing widespread external bleeding, internal bleeding, or both. It is important to understand that DIC is always a secondary diagnosis. In the obstetric population, HELLP syndrome and gram-negative sepsis are examples of conditions that can trigger DIC because of widespread damage to vascular integrity. Medical management is discussed in Chapter 37.

The nurse caring for the pregnant woman at risk for DIC must be aware of risk factors. Careful and thorough assessment is required, with particular attention to signs of bleeding (petechiae, oozing from injection sites, and hematuria). Because renal failure is one consequence of DIC, urinary output is carefully monitored by using an indwelling Foley catheter. Vital signs are assessed frequently.

The pregnant woman will be maintained in a side-lying tilt to maximize blood flow to the uterus. Oxygen may be administered through a tight-fitting, rebreathing mask at 10 to 12 L/min, or per hospital protocol or physician order. Blood and blood products must be administered safely.

The educational and emotional needs of the woman and her family must be recognized and supported. They need information about her condition and explanations of procedures and will most likely be very anxious about the health of mother and baby.

KEY POINTS

- Blood loss during pregnancy should always be regarded as a warning sign until the cause is determined.
- Some miscarriages occur for unknown reasons, but fetal or placental maldevelopment and maternal factors account for many others.
- The type of miscarriage directs care management.
- Ectopic pregnancy is a significant cause of maternal morbidity and mortality, even in developed countries.
- The two distinctive types of hydatidiform mole are complete and partial.
- Premature separation of the placenta and placenta previa are differentiated by type of bleeding, uterine tonicity, and presence or absence of pain.
- Clotting disorders are associated with many obstetric complications.
- Management of late pregnancy bleeding requires immediate evaluation; care is based on gestational age, amount of bleeding, and fetal condition.

CRITICAL THINKING EXERCISES

1. Carrie, a 23-year-old pregnant client, is admitted to the emergency room complaining of abdominal pain, vaginal bleeding and dizziness after being involved in an automobile accident.
   a. Describe the position this client should be in as you begin your assessment.
   b. What critical pieces of information are needed in progressing with a history and physical examination?
   c. What is a collaborative diagnosis for this client?
2. The nurse is preparing discharge instructions for Mari, who has just had surgery for the evacuation of a hydatiform mole. What critical information does this client need to comprehend before discharge?
3. Joi is at 32 weeks' gestation. She awoke from sleep at home and is having bright red vaginal bleeding. She denies uterine contractions, but is crying and distraught. After her transport to the L&D unit per ambulance, you are to admit her to the unit.
   a. How will you proceed, and what will you include in her assessment?
   b. What type of examination should the nurse omit on this client?
   c. Define an anticipated plan of care for this client.

RESOURCES

American College of Obstetricians and Gynecologists
409 12th St. SW
Washington, DC 20024
800-762-2264
www.acog.com

COPE (Coping with the Overall Pregnancy/Parenting Experience)
37 Clarendon St.
Boston, MA 02116
617-357-5588

Pregnancy and Infant Loss
1421 East Wayzata Blvd., Suite 40
Wayzata, MN 55391
614-473-9372

REFERENCES

American College of Obstetricians and Gynecologists. (1998). *Antenatal corticosteroid therapy for fetal maturation. ACOG Committee Opinion No. 210.* Washington, DC: ACOG.

Ananth, C., Smulian, J., & Vintzileos, A. (1997). The association of placenta previa with history of cesarean delivery and abortion: A meta-analysis. *Obstetrics and Gynecology, 177*(5), 1071-1078.

Ananth, C. et al. (2001). Placental abruption among singleton and twin births in the United States: Risk factor profiles. *American Journal of Epidemiology, 153*(8), 771-778.

Andres, R., & Day, M. (2000). Perinatal complications associated with maternal tobacco use. *Seminars in Neonatology, 5*(3), 231-234.

Benedetti, T. (2002). Obstetric hemorrhage. In S. Gabbe, J. Niebyl, & J. Simpson (Eds.), *Obstetrics: Normal and problem pregnancies* (4th ed.). New York: Churchill Livingstone.

Berman, M., DiSaia, P., & Brewster, W. (1999). Pelvic malignancy, gestational trophoblastic neoplasm, and nonpelvic malignancies. In R. Creasy & R. Resnik (Eds.), *Maternal-fetal medicine* (4th ed.). Philadelphia: W.B. Saunders.

Chichakli, L. et al. (1999). Pregnancy-related mortality in the United States due to hemorrhage: 1979-1992. *Obstetrics and Gynecology, 94*, 721.

Clark, S. (1999). Placenta previa and abruptio placentae. In R. Creasy & R. Resnik (Eds.), *Maternal-fetal medicine* (4th ed.). Philadelphia: W.B. Saunders.

Copeland, L., & Landon, M. (2002). Malignant diseases and pregnancy. In S. Gabbe, J. Niebyl, & J. Simpson (Eds.), *Obstetrics: Normal and problem pregnancies* (4th ed.). New York: Churchill Livingstone.

Crane, J. et al. (2000). Maternal complications with placenta previa. *American Journal of Perinatology, 17*(2), 101-105.

Cunningham, F. et al. (2001). *Williams obstetrics* (21st ed.). New York: McGraw-Hill.

DeLoia, J., Stewart-Akers, A., & Creinin, M. (1998). Effects of methotrexate on trophoblast proliferation and local immune responses. *Human Reproduction, 13*(4), 1063-1069.

Flystra, D. (1998). Tubal pregnancy: A review of current diagnosis and treatment. *Obstetrical and Gynecological Survey, 53*(5), 320-328.

Freda, M. (1999). The power of words. *MCN, the American Journal of Maternal Child Nursing, 24*(2), 63.

Gilbert, E., & Harmon, J. (2003). *Manual of high risk pregnancy and delivery* (3rd ed.). St. Louis: Mosby.

Gracia, C., & Barnhart, K. (2001). Diagnosing ectopic pregnancy: Decision analysis comparing six strategies. *Obstetrics and Gynecology, 97*(3), 464-470.

Health Care Resources. (1997). *Handbook of high risk perinatal home care.* St. Louis: Mosby.

Hutti, M., dePacheco, M., & Smith, M. (1998). A study of miscarriage: Development and validation of the Perinatal Grief Intensity Scale. *Journal of Obstetric, Gynecologic, and Neonatal Nursing, 27*(5), 547-555.

Iams, J. (2002). Preterm birth. In S. Gabbe, J. Niebyl, & J. Simpson (Eds.), *Obstetrics: Normal and problem pregnancies* (4th ed.). New York: Churchill Livingstone.

Kramer, M. et al. (1997). Etiologic determinants of abruptio placentae. *Obstetrics and Gynecology, 89*(2), 221-226.

Lipscomb, G. et al. (1998). Analysis of three hundred fifteen ectopic pregnancies treated with single-dose methotrexate. *American Journal of Obstetrics and Gynecology, 178*(6), 1354-1358.

Lowdermilk, D., & Grohar, J. (1998). *High risk antepartal home care.* White Plains, NY: March of Dimes.

Maloni, J., & Kutil, R. (2000). Antepartum support groups for women hospitalized in bed rest. *MCN, the American Journal of Maternal Child Nursing, 25*(4), 204-210.

National Institutes of Health Consensus Development Conference. (2000). *Statement on repeated courses of corticosteroids, August 17-18, 2000,* Bethesda, MD. Available at consensus.nih.gov.

Powell, W., & Spellman, J. (1996). Medical management of the patient with an ectopic pregnancy. *Journal of Perinatal and Neonatal Nursing, 9*(4), 31-43.

Simpson, J. (2002). Fetal wastage. In S. Gabbe, J. Niebyl, & J. Simpson (Eds.), *Obstetrics: Normal and problem pregnancies* (4th ed.). New York: Churchill Livingstone.

CHAPTER 32

Kitty Cashion

Endocrine and Metabolic Disorders

http://evolve.elsevier.com/Lowdermilk/MatWmnHlth/

LEARNING OBJECTIVES

- Differentiate the types of diabetes mellitus and their respective risk factors in pregnancy.
- Compare insulin requirements during pregnancy, the postpartum period, and lactation.
- Identify maternal and fetal risks or complications associated with diabetes in pregnancy.
- Develop a plan of care for the pregnant woman with pregestational or gestational diabetes.
- Explain the effects of hyperemesis gravidarum on maternal and fetal well-being.
- Discuss care management for the woman with hyperemesis gravidarum.
- Compare the management of a pregnant woman with hyperthyroidism with one who has hypothyroidism.
- Examine the effects of maternal phenylketonuria on pregnancy outcome.
- Explain care management for the woman with phenylketonuria.

Endocrine and metabolic disorders, which often complicate pregnancy, require careful management to promote maternal and fetal well-being and a positive pregnancy outcome. Diabetes mellitus is the most common endocrine disorder associated with pregnancy. Hyperemesis gravidarum and disorders of the thyroid, although encountered less often, also require careful planning for care. Phenylketonuria, an inborn error of metabolism, is a relatively new disorder of women of reproductive age, and it has significant implications for pregnancy outcome.

Providing sound, effective nursing care that meets the unique maternal and fetal needs prompted by these endocrine and metabolic conditions can be challenging. The primary objective of nursing care must be to guide and support the woman and her family in achieving the optimal outcome for both the pregnant woman and the fetus. The nurse serves as teacher, counselor, and support person to assist the woman and her family in achieving the best possible outcome and in dealing with the problems and disappointments that may arise.

DIABETES MELLITUS

Before the discovery of insulin in 1922, it was uncommon for a woman with diabetes to give birth to a healthy baby. Many women of childbearing age were infertile or sterile, and the miscarriage rate was as high as 30% (Langer, 2000). Both maternal and infant mortality rates also were high, nearly 50%. Stillbirth was the primary cause of perinatal mortality (Inzucchi, 1999).

Advances in medicine have greatly improved perinatal outcome. Today the perinatal mortality rate for well-managed diabetic pregnancies, excluding major congenital malformations, is about the same as that for any other pregnancy (Landon, Catalano, & Gabbe, 2002). The incidence of major congenital malformations in infants born to women with diabetes has not changed significantly over time. Experts have concluded that the key to an optimal pregnancy outcome is strict maternal glucose control before conception, as well as throughout the gestational period. Consequently, much emphasis is placed on preconception counseling for women with diabetes.

Despite the advances in care, pregnancy complicated by diabetes is still considered at high risk. It is most successfully managed by a multidisciplinary approach involving the obstetrician, internist or diabetologist, neonatologist, nurse, nutritionist, and social worker. A favorable outcome of diabetic pregnancy requires commitment and active participation by the woman and her family. The woman must comply with a schedule of frequent prenatal visits, strict adherence to the dietary regimen, regular self-monitoring of her blood glucose level, frequent laboratory evaluation, intensive fetal surveillance, and possible hospitalization.

Care of the pregnant woman with diabetes requires that the nurse fully understand the normal physiologic responses to pregnancy and the altered metabolism of diabetes. Furthermore, the nurse must understand the relation between pregnancy and diabetes, including psychosocial implications, to assess the woman accurately, plan for her care, and intervene appropriately.

Pathogenesis

Diabetes mellitus is a group of metabolic diseases characterized by hyperglycemia resulting from defects in insulin secretion, insulin action, or both (Expert Committee on the Diagnosis and Classification of Diabetes Mellitus, 2003). Insulin, produced by the beta cells in the islets of Langerhans in the pancreas, regulates blood glucose levels by enabling glucose to enter adipose and muscle cells, where it is used for energy. Insulin also stimulates protein synthesis and storage of free fatty acids. When insulin is insufficient or ineffective in promoting glucose uptake by the muscle and adipose cells, glucose accumulates in the bloodstream, and hyperglycemia results. Hyperglycemia causes hyperosmolarity of the blood, which attracts intracellular fluid into the vascular system, resulting in cellular dehydration and expanded blood volume. Consequently the kidneys function to excrete large volumes of urine (polyuria) in an attempt to regulate excess vascular volume and to excrete the unusable glucose (glycosuria). Polyuria, along with cellular dehydration, causes excessive thirst (polydipsia).

The body compensates for its inability to convert carbohydrate (glucose) into energy by burning proteins (muscle) and fats. However, the end products of this metabolism are ketones and fatty acids, which, in excess quantities, produce ketoacidosis and acetonuria. Weight loss occurs as a result of the breakdown of fat and muscle tissue. This tissue breakdown causes a state of starvation that compels the individual to eat excessive amounts of food (polyphagia).

Over time, diabetes causes significant changes in both the microvascular and macrovascular circulations. These structural changes affect a variety of organ systems, particularly the heart, eyes, kidneys, and nerves. Complications resulting from diabetes include premature atherosclerosis, retinopathy, nephropathy, and neuropathy.

Diabetes may be caused by either impaired insulin secretion, when the beta cells of the pancreas are destroyed by an autoimmune process, or by inadequate insulin action in target tissues at one or more points along the metabolic pathway. Both of these conditions are frequently present in the same person, and it is unclear which, if either, abnormality is the primary cause of the disease (Expert Committee on the Diagnosis and Classification of Diabetes Mellitus, 2003).

Classification

The criteria for the diagnosis and classification of diabetes were extensively revised in 1997 by an international Expert Committee working under the sponsorship of the American Diabetes Association (ADA). The current classification system includes four groups: type 1 diabetes, type 2 diabetes, other specific types (e.g., diabetes caused by infection or drug-induced diabetes), and gestational diabetes mellitus. A major change proposed by the Expert Committee was a move away from a system that classified the disease by its pharmacologic management to one based on disease etiology (Expert Committee on the Diagnosis and Classification of Diabetes Mellitus, 2003).

Type 1 diabetes includes those cases that are primarily due to pancreatic islet beta cell destruction and that are prone to ketoacidosis. People with type 1 diabetes usually have an absolute insulin deficiency. Type 1 diabetes includes cases currently thought to be caused by an autoimmune process, as well as those for which the cause is unknown (Expert Committee on the Diagnosis and Classification of Diabetes Mellitus, 2003).

Type 2 diabetes is the most prevalent form of the disease and includes individuals who have insulin resistance and usually relative (rather than absolute) insulin deficiency. Specific etiologies for type 2 diabetes are unknown at this time. Type 2 diabetes often goes undiagnosed for years because hyperglycemia develops gradually and often is not severe enough for the person to recognize the classic signs of polyuria, polydipsia, and polyphagia. Many people in whom type 2 diabetes develops are obese or have an increased amount of body fat distributed primarily in the abdominal area. Other risk factors for the development of type 2 diabetes include aging, a sedentary lifestyle, hypertension, and prior gestational diabetes. Type 2 diabetes often has a strong genetic predisposition (Expert Committee on the Diagnosis and Classification of Diabetes Mellitus, 2003).

Pregestational diabetes mellitus is the label sometimes given to type 1 or type 2 diabetes that existed before pregnancy.

Gestational diabetes mellitus (GDM) is any degree of glucose intolerance with the onset or first recognition occurring during pregnancy. This definition is appropriate whether or not insulin is used for treatment or the diabetes persists after pregnancy. It does not exclude the possibility that the glucose intolerance preceded the pregnancy. Women with gestational diabetes should be reclassified 6 weeks or more after the pregnancy ends (Expert Committee on the Diagnosis and Classification of Diabetes Mellitus, 2003).

Metabolic Changes Associated with Pregnancy

Normal pregnancy is characterized by complex alterations in maternal glucose metabolism, insulin production, and metabolic homeostasis. During normal pregnancy, adjustments in maternal metabolism allow adequate nutrition for both the mother and the developing fetus. Glucose, the primary fuel used by the fetus, is transported across the placenta through the process of carrier-mediated facilitated diffusion. This means that the glucose levels in the fetus are directly proportional to maternal levels. Although glucose crosses the placenta, insulin does not. By the tenth week of gestation, the embryo or fetus secretes its own insulin at levels adequate to use the glucose obtained from the mother; thus as maternal glucose levels increase, fetal glucose levels are increased, resulting in increased fetal insulin secretion.

During the first trimester of pregnancy, the pregnant woman's metabolic status is significantly influenced by the increasing levels of estrogen and progesterone. These hormones stimulate the beta cells in the pancreas to increase insulin production, which promotes increased peripheral use of glucose and decreased blood glucose, with fasting levels being reduced by approximately 10% (Fig. 32-1, *A*). A concomitant increase occurs in tissue glycogen stores and a decrease in hepatic glucose production, which further encourage lower fasting glucose levels. As a result of these normal metabolic changes of pregnancy, women who are diabetic and are insulin dependent are prone to hypoglycemia during the first trimester.

During the second and third trimesters, pregnancy exerts a "diabetogenic" effect on the maternal metabolic status (Fig. 32-1, *B, C*). The major hormonal changes result in a decreased tolerance to glucose, an increased insulin resistance, decreased hepatic glycogen stores, and an increased hepatic production of glucose. Increasing levels of human placental lactogen, estrogen, progesterone, prolactin, cortisol, and insulinase increase insulin resistance through their actions as insulin antagonists. Insulin resistance is a glucose-sparing mechanism that ensures an abundant supply of glucose for the fetus. Maternal insulin requirements gradually increase from about 18 to 24 weeks' gestation to about 36 weeks' gestation. At this time insulin requirements usually level off until labor begins.

At birth, expulsion of the placenta prompts an abrupt decrease in levels of circulating placental hormones, cortisol, and insulinase (Fig. 32-1, *D*). Maternal tissues quickly regain their prepregnancy sensitivity to insulin. For the nonbreastfeeding mother, the prepregnancy insulin-carbohydrate balance usually returns in about 7 to 10 days (Fig. 32-1, *E*). Lactation uses maternal glucose; thus the breastfeeding mother's insulin requirements will remain low as long as she is nursing (Fig. 32-1, *F*).

Pregestational Diabetes Mellitus

Women with pregestational diabetes may have either type 1 or type 2 diabetes, with type 1 now the more common diagnosis. In the future, as the incidence of type 2 diabetes increases in the general population, it may become the more prevalent form of the disease in childbearing-aged women. About 2 in 1000 pregnancies are currently

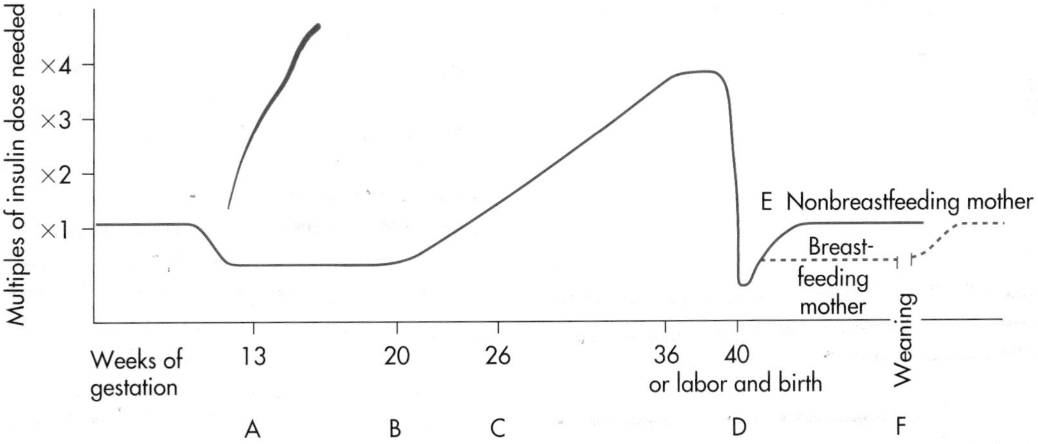
Multiples of insulin dose needed
×4
×3
×2
×1
E Nonbreastfeeding mother
Breast-
feeding
mother
Weaning
Weeks of
gestation
13
20
26
36
40
or labor and birth
A
B
C
D
F

FIG. 32-1 Changing insulin needs during pregnancy. **A,** First trimester: Insulin need is reduced because of increased insulin production by pancreas and increased peripheral sensitivity to insulin; nausea, vomiting, and decreased food intake by mother and glucose transfer to embryo or fetus contribute to hypoglycemia. **B,** Second trimester: Insulin needs begin to increase as placental hormones, cortisol, and insulinase act as insulin antagonists, decreasing insulin's effectiveness. **C,** Third trimester: Insulin needs may double or even quadruple but usually level off after 36 weeks of gestation. **D,** Day of birth: Maternal insulin requirements decrease drastically to approach prepregnancy levels. **E,** Breastfeeding mother maintains lower insulin requirements, as much as 25% less than prepregnancy; insulin needs of nonbreastfeeding mother return to prepregnancy levels in 7 to 10 days. **F,** Weaning of breastfeeding infant causes mother's insulin needs to return to prepregnancy levels.

estimated to be complicated by pregestational diabetes (Inzucchi, 1999). Fetal risks for women with type 1 and type 2 diabetes are about the same. Maternal risks, however, tend to be greater in type 1 diabetics. Their blood sugar control is usually more erratic because of their absolute lack of insulin production. They also are more likely to have the vascular, retinal, or renal complications that often accompany the disease, because their duration of illness is usually longer than that of women with type 2 diabetes (Inzucchi, 1999).

Preconception Counseling

Preconception counseling, which is recommended for all women of reproductive age with diabetes, is associated with an improved pregnancy outcome (Landon et al., 2002; Moore, 1999). Under ideal circumstances, the pregestational diabetic woman is counseled before the time of conception to plan the optimal time for pregnancy, establish glycemic control before conception, and diagnose any vascular complications of diabetes (see Evidence-Based Practice box). Unfortunately, it has been estimated that in the United States, fewer than 20% of women with diabetes participate in preconception counseling (Landon et al., 2002).

The woman's partner should be included in the counseling to assess the couple's level of understanding related to the effects of pregnancy on the diabetic condition and of the potential complications of pregnancy as a result of diabetes. The couple also should be informed of the anticipated alterations in management of diabetes during pregnancy and the need for a multidisciplinary team approach to health care. Financial implications of diabetic pregnancy and other demands related to frequent maternal and fetal surveillance should be discussed. Contraception is another important aspect of preconception counseling to assist the couple in planning effectively for pregnancy.

Preconception counseling is particularly important because strict metabolic control before conception and in the early weeks of gestation is instrumental in decreasing the risk of congenital anomalies (Landon et al., 2002; Langer, 2000; Moore, 1999).

Some types of oral hypoglycemic agents (sulfonylureas such as tolbutamide) may have teratogenic effects on the fetus; they should be discontinued in the preconception period in women with type 2 diabetes (Hagay & Reece, 1999). These women are started on insulin before pregnancy when the pregnancy is planned, or as soon as the pregnancy is diagnosed when it is unplanned.

Maternal Risks and Complications

Although maternal morbidity and mortality rates have improved significantly, the pregnant woman with diabetes remains at risk for the development of significant complications during pregnancy. Risk assessment is best done by evaluating the woman's blood glucose and blood vessels. Women with excellent glucose control and no blood vessel disease should have good pregnancy outcomes (Landon et al., 2002).

Poor glycemic control around the time of conception and in the early weeks of pregnancy may be associated with an increased incidence of early pregnancy loss in women with diabetes (Inzucchi, 1999). Those women with good glycemic control before conception and in the first trimester are no more likely than are women who do not have diabetes to have a miscarriage (Moore, 1999).

Poor glycemic control later in pregnancy, particularly in women without vascular disease, increases the rate of fetal macrosomia. Macrosomia occurs in 40% to 50% of diabetic pregnancies (Landon et al., 2002). These large infants tend to have a disproportionate increase in shoulder and trunk size. Because of this, the risk of shoulder dystocia is greater in these babies than in other macrosomic infants. Thus women with diabetes face an increased likelihood of cesarean birth because of failure to progress or descend, or operative vaginal birth (birth using episiotomy, forceps, or vacuum extractor) (Moore, 1999).

Hypertensive disorders, such as preeclampsia or eclampsia, occur much more frequently in women with pregestational diabetes, particularly in those who already have renal dysfunction (Inzucchi, 1999). Preterm labor/birth also is more likely to occur, especially with more severe diabetes, elevated glucose levels, and genital or urinary tract infections. The risk for indicated preterm delivery also is greater in women with pregestational diabetes (Cunningham et al., 2001; Inzucchi, 1999).

Hydramnios (polyhydramnios) occurs about 10 times more often in diabetic than in nondiabetic pregnancies. **Hydramnios**–amniotic fluid more than 2000 ml–increases the possibility of compression of maternal abdominal blood vessels (vena cava and aorta), causing supine hypotension. Maternal dyspnea may result from upward pressure on the diaphragm by the distended uterus. Premature rupture of membranes (PROM) and the onset of preterm labor are associated with hydramnios. Overdistention of the uterus caused by hydramnios may increase the incidence of postpartum hemorrhage.

Infections are more common and more serious in pregnant women with diabetes. Disorders of carbohydrate metabolism alter the body's normal resistance to infection. The inflammatory response, leukocyte function, and vaginal pH all are affected. Vaginal infections, particularly monilial vaginitis, are more common. Urinary tract infections (UTIs) also are more prevalent. Infection is serious because it causes increased insulin resistance and may result in ketoacidosis. Postpartum infection is more common among women who are insulin dependent.

Ketoacidosis occurs most often during the second and third trimesters, when the diabetogenic effect of pregnancy is the greatest. When the maternal metabolism is stressed by illness or infection, the woman is at increased risk for

EVIDENCE-BASED PRACTICE

PRECONCEPTION CARE

BACKGROUND

In the United States over 60% of pregnancies are unintended and almost a fifth of pregnant women do not seek prenatal care before the end of the first trimester. Few women seek preconception care, although about 70% of women between the ages of 18 and 39 receive preventive health services each year.

A healthy pregnancy outcome is related to the woman's health status and lifestyle and history before conception. Waiting to seek care until after conception may be too late for effective preventive care since the period of greatest sensitivity to environmental exposures and maternal health conditions is between 3 and 8 weeks of gestation.

A comprehensive review of evidence on preconception care published before 1990 led to recommendations for content and delivery of preconception care (ACOG, 1995; Cefalo & Moos, 1995). However many of the recommendations were based on expert opinions and not clinical evidence.

OBJECTIVE

Korenbrot and others (2002) systematically reviewed data from published research trials of preconception services to determine if there has been any evidence since 1990 demonstrating an impact on pregnancy or its outcomes by implementation of clinical or behavioral interventions provided before pregnancy.

SEARCH STRATEGY

Studies published between 1990 and 1999 and posted on Medline were reviewed. Over 40 preconception risk conditions were searched. More than 470 articles were found; 89 were selected for data extraction, but only 19 research trials met the review criteria and only 4 problems were identified. These included pregnancies with any preconception risk conditions, anatomical congenital anomalies, diabetes mellitus, and hyperphenylalaninemia.

EVIDENCE

Pregnancy with Any Preconception Risk Conditions

Only two clinical trials were found. Preconception services that were studied were provision of risk assessment, patient education about identified risk, counseling about contraception use during risk reduction, and referrals for patients with identified risks. There was some evidence that women who received preconception care had fewer unintended pregnancies, but there was limited evidence that women with risk conditions had interventions to reduce these risks before pregnancy.

Anatomical Congenital Anomalies

Five studies provided evidence that the risk for neural tube defects (NTDs) was reduced by periconceptional intake of folic acid. Diet supplementation was recommended to obtain the amount of folate needed.

Diabetes Mellitus

Seven studies provided evidence about the effects of preconception screening of women with diabetes mellitus to detect baseline blood glucose levels, counsel and educate the women about pregnancy and blood sugar control, and monitor and follow blood sugar control. Women who had better control before pregnancy had better control during pregnancy, they had fewer hospital admissions during pregnancy, and their babies had fewer anomalies and fewer NICU admissions.

Hyperphenylalaninemia (HPA)

Four studies reviewed preconception services for women with HPA. These included screening to detect phenylalanine levels in women who have HPA and education and counseling regarding preconception and prenatal dietary control of phenylalanine levels. Dietary restriction before pregnancy and in early pregnancy was found to be associated with improved neonatal outcomes and fewer anomalies.

LIMITATIONS

There were only a small number of clinical trials identified for preconception preventive interventions. This limited amount of data since 1990 does not support a revision of the current preventive services recommendations. Many interventions identified before 1990 have yet to be studied in clinical trials.

CONCLUSIONS

Support for screening sexually active women of reproductive age for risk conditions is supported by this review. There is still a need for research on interventions to improve access to preconception care.

The recommendation for supplementation with 0.4 mg of folic acid a day before pregnancy is beneficial. If a woman has previously given birth to a baby with an NTD, 4 mg a day is recommended.

For women with metabolic conditions, preconception services that helped them avoid unintended pregnancies and offered nutritional assessments and counseling and screening to detect blood glucose or phenylalanine levels decreased risks during pregnancy for the woman and her fetus.

While this review strengthens the evidence for preconception care in these four specific areas, more research is needed to determine what interventions will improve pregnancy outcomes in other areas.

Reference: American College of Obstetricians and Gynecologists. (1995). Preconceptional care. *ACOG Technical Bulletin Number 205,* Washington, DC: ACOG; Cefalo, R., & Moos, M. (1995). *Preconceptional health care: A practical guide.* St. Louis: Mosby; Korenbrot, C. et al. (2002). Preconception care: A systematic review. *Maternal and Child Health Journal, 6*(2), 75-88.

diabetic ketoacidosis (DKA). The use of beta-sympathomimetic drugs (e.g., terbutaline [Brethine]) or corticosteroids also may contribute to the risk for hyperglycemia and subsequent DKA (Cunningham et al., 2001; Hagay & Reece, 1999). DKA also may occur because of the woman's failure to take insulin appropriately (Inzucchi, 1999). The onset of previously undiagnosed diabetes during pregnancy is another cause of DKA. DKA may occur with blood glucose levels barely exceeding 200 mg/dl, compared with 300 to 350 mg/dl in the nonpregnant state. In response to stress factors such as infection or illness, **hyperglycemia** occurs as a result of increased hepatic glucose production and decreased peripheral glucose use. Stress hormones, which act to impair insulin action and further contribute to insulin deficiency, are released. Fatty acids are mobilized from fat stores to enter into the circulation, and as they are oxidized, ketone bodies are released into the peripheral circulation. The woman's buffering system is unable to compensate, and metabolic acidosis develops. The excessive blood glucose and ketone bodies result in osmotic diuresis with subsequent loss of fluid and electrolytes, volume depletion, and cellular dehydration. Prompt treatment of DKA is necessary to prevent maternal coma and death. Ketoacidosis at any time during pregnancy can lead to intrauterine fetal death; it is also a cause of preterm labor. The perinatal mortality rate is about 20% with maternal ketoacidosis (Cunningham et al., 2001) (Table 32-1).

The risk of **hypoglycemia** also is increased. Early in pregnancy, when hepatic production of glucose is diminished and peripheral use of glucose is enhanced, hypoglycemia occurs frequently, often during sleep. Later in pregnancy, as insulin doses are adjusted to maintain normoglycemia, hypoglycemia also may result. Women with

TABLE *32-1* **Differentiation of Hypoglycemia (Insulin Shock) and Hyperglycemia (Diabetic Ketoacidosis)**

CAUSES	ONSET	SYMPTOMS	INTERVENTIONS
HYPOGLYCEMIA (INSULIN SHOCK)			
Excess insulin Insufficient food (delayed or missed meals) Excessive exercise or work Indigestion, diarrhea, vomiting	Rapid (regular insulin) Gradual (modified insulin or oral hypoglycemic agents)	Irritability Hunger Sweating Nervousness Personality change Weakness Fatigue Blurred or double vision Dizziness Headache Pallor; clammy skin Shallow respirations Rapid pulse Laboratory values Urine: negative for sugar and acetone Blood glucose: ≤60 mg/dl	Check blood glucose level when symptoms first appear Eat or drink 10-15 g simple carbohydrate immediately Recheck blood glucose level in 15 min, and eat or drink another 10-15 g simple carbohydrate if glucose remains low Recheck blood glucose level in 15 min Notify primary health care provider if no change in glucose level If woman is unconscious, administer 50% dextrose IV push, 5%-10% dextrose-in-water IV drip, or glucagon Obtain blood and urine specimens for laboratory testing
HYPERGLYCEMIA (DIABETIC KETOACIDOSIS [DKA])			
Insufficient insulin Excess or wrong kind of food Infection, injuries, illness Emotional stress Insufficient exercise	Slow (hours to days)	Thirst Nausea or vomiting Abdominal pain Constipation Drowsiness Dim vision Increased urination Headache Flushed, dry skin Rapid breathing Weak, rapid pulse Acetone (fruity) breath odor Laboratory values Urine: positive for sugar and acetone Blood glucose: ≥200 mg/dl	Notify primary health care provider Administer insulin in accordance with blood glucose levels Give IV fluids such as normal saline solution or one-half normal saline solution; potassium when urinary output is adequate; bicarbonate for pH <7 Monitor lab testing of blood and urine

a prepregnancy history of severe hypoglycemia are at increased risk for severe hypoglycemia during gestation. Mild to moderate hypoglycemic episodes do not appear to have significant deleterious effects on fetal well-being. The long-term fetal effects of severe maternal hypoglycemia are as yet uncertain (Hagay & Reece, 1999).

Fetal and Neonatal Risks

Despite the improvements in care of the pregnant woman with diabetes, sudden and unexplained stillbirth is still a significant risk for her fetus (Cunningham et al., 2001; Inzucchi, 1999). The other major cause of perinatal deaths in pregnancies complicated by pregestational diabetes is congenital anomalies. The incidence of congenital anomalies in infants is 6% to 10%, a twofold to sixfold increase over that of the general population (Landon et al., 2002). Cardiac defects are the most common anomalies, followed by central nervous system and skeletal defects (Hagay & Reece, 1999).

Other problems that cause significant neonatal morbidity include macrosomia, hypoglycemia, respiratory distress syndrome, polycythemia, and hyperbilirubinemia (Inzucchi, 1999; Landon et al., 2002). See Chapter 38 for further discussion of neonatal risks associated with maternal diabetes.

CARE MANAGEMENT

Assessment and Nursing Diagnoses

Interview

When a pregnant woman with diabetes initiates prenatal care, a thorough evaluation of her health status is completed. In addition to the routine prenatal assessment, a detailed history regarding the onset and course of the diabetes and its management and the degree of glycemic control before pregnancy is obtained. Effective management of the diabetic pregnancy depends on the woman's adherence to a plan of care. For the woman to care for her diabetes on a daily basis, she must have an adequate understanding of her disease and the prescribed regimen. Thus with the initial prenatal visit, the woman's knowledge regarding diabetes and pregnancy, potential maternal and fetal complications, and the plan of care are thoroughly assessed. With subsequent visits, follow-up assessments are completed. Data from these assessments are used to identify the woman's specific learning needs. The support person's knowledge of diabetes also is assessed, and teaching needs are identified.

The woman's emotional status is assessed to determine how she is coping with pregnancy superimposed on preexisting diabetes. Although normal pregnancy typically evokes some degree of stress and anxiety, pregnancy designated "high risk" serves to compound anxiety and stress levels. Fear of maternal and fetal complications is a major concern. Strict adherence to the plan of care necessitates alterations in patterns of daily living and may be an additional source of stress.

The woman's support system is assessed to identify those people significant to the pregnant woman and their role in her life. It is important to assess reactions of the family members and partner to the pregnancy and to the strict management plan and their involvement in the treatment regimen. Socioeconomic factors also are reviewed. Any area of emotional stress is identified because such stress can precipitate complications.

Physical Examination

At the initial visit, a thorough physical examination assesses the woman's current health status. In addition to the routine prenatal examination, specific efforts are made to assess the effects of the diabetes. A baseline electrocardiogram (ECG) may be done to assess cardiovascular status. Evaluation for retinopathy is done, with follow-up by an ophthalmologist each trimester and more frequently if retinopathy is diagnosed. Blood pressure is monitored carefully throughout pregnancy because of the increased risk for preeclampsia. The woman's weight gain also is monitored at each visit. Fundal height is measured, noting any abnormal increase in size for dates, which may indicate hydramnios or fetal macrosomia.

Laboratory Tests

Routine prenatal laboratory examinations include assessment of baseline renal function with a 24-hour urine collection for total protein excretion and creatinine clearance. Urinalysis and culture are performed on the initial prenatal visit and throughout the pregnancy to assess for the presence of UTI, which is common in diabetic pregnancy. At each visit, urine also is tested for the presence of glucose and ketones. Because of the risk of coexisting thyroid disease, thyroid function tests also may be performed (see later discussion of thyroid disorders).

For the woman with pregestational type 1 or type 2 diabetes, laboratory tests may assess past glycemic control. At the initial prenatal visit, **glycosylated hemoglobin A$_{1C}$** level may be measured. With prolonged hyperglycemia, some of the hemoglobin remains saturated with glucose for the life of the red blood cell (RBC); therefore a test for glycosylated hemoglobin provides a measurement of glycemic control over time, specifically over the previous 4 to 6 weeks. Regular measurements of glycosylated hemoglobin provide data for altering the treatment plan and lead to improvement of glycemic control. Values for the measurement of hemoglobin A$_{1C}$, the most commonly used index of glycosylated hemoglobin, are as follows (Pagana & Pagana, 2002):

- Adult/elderly: 2.2% to 4.8%
- Good diabetic control: 2.5% to 5.9%

- Fair diabetic control: 6% to 8%
- Poor diabetic control: Greater than 8%

Fasting blood glucose and/or random (1 to 2 hours after eating) glucose levels may be assessed during antepartum visits (Fig. 32-2). Blood glucose self-monitoring records also may be reviewed.

Nursing diagnoses for the woman with pregestational diabetes include the following:

- *Deficient knowledge related to*
  - –diabetic pregnancy, management, and potential effects on pregnant woman and fetus
- *Risk for ineffective coping related to*
  - –woman's responsibility in managing her diabetes during pregnancy
- *Anxiety, fear, dysfunctional grieving, powerlessness, disturbed body image, situational low self-esteem, spiritual distress, ineffective role performance, interrupted family processes related to*
  - –stigma of being labeled "diabetic"
  - –effects of diabetes and its potential sequelae on the pregnant woman and the fetus
- *Risk for noncompliance related to*
  - –lack of understanding of diabetes and pregnancy
  - –lack of financial resources to purchase blood glucose–monitoring equipment/supplies or insulin and necessary supplies
  - –insufficient funds or lack of transportation to grocery store to follow dietary regimen
- *Risk for injury to fetus related to*
  - –uteroplacental insufficiency
  - –birth trauma
- *Risk for injury to mother related to*
  - –improper insulin administration
  - –hypoglycemia and hyperglycemia
  - –cesarean or operative vaginal birth
  - –postpartum infection
- *Imbalanced nutrition: less or more than body requirements related to*
  - –noncompliance with dietary regimen
  - –knowledge deficit regarding increased nutritional needs during pregnancy

Expected Outcomes of Care

Expected outcomes of care for the pregnant woman with pregestational diabetes include that she will do the following:

- Demonstrate/verbalize understanding of diabetic pregnancy, the plan of care, and the importance of glycemic control.
- Follow the plan of care.
- Achieve and maintain glycemic control.
- Demonstrate effective coping.
- Experience no complications (maternal morbidity or mortality).
- Give birth to a healthy infant at term.

Plan of Care and Interventions

Antepartum

Because of her high risk status, the woman with diabetes is monitored much more frequently and thoroughly than are other pregnant women. During the first and second trimesters of pregnancy, her routine prenatal care visits may be scheduled every 1 to 2 weeks. Throughout the last trimester, she will probably be seen 1 to 2 times each week. In the past, routine hospitalization for management of the diabetes, such as insulin dose changes, was common. With the availability of better home glucose monitoring and the growing reluctance of third-party payers to reimburse for hospitalization, however, pregnant women with diabetes are now generally managed as outpatients. Some client and family education and maternal and fetal assessment may be done in the home, depending on the woman's insurance coverage and care provider preference.

Achieving and maintaining constant **euglycemia** (normal blood glucose level, also called normogylcemia), with blood glucose levels in the range of 60 to 120 mg/dl (Table 32-2), is the primary goal of medical therapy for the

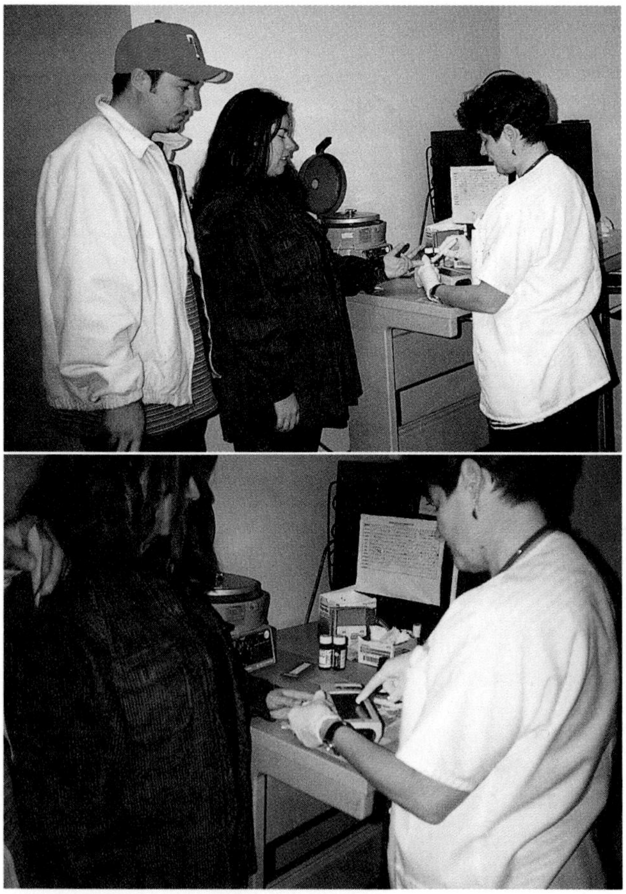

A

B

FIG. 32-2 **A,** Clinic nurse collects blood to determine glucose level. **B,** Nurse interprets glucose value displayed by monitor. (Courtesy Dee Lowdermilk, UNC Ambulatory Care Clinics, Chapel Hill, NC)

pregnant woman with diabetes. Euglycemia is achieved through a combination of diet, insulin, exercise, and blood glucose determinations. Providing the woman with the knowledge, skill, and motivation she needs to achieve and maintain excellent blood glucose control is the primary nursing goal.

Achieving euglycemia requires commitment on the part of the woman and her family to make the necessary lifestyle changes, which can sometimes seem overwhelming. Maintaining tight blood glucose control necessitates that the woman follow a consistent daily schedule. She must get up and go to bed, eat, exercise, and take insulin at the same time each day. Blood glucose measurements are done frequently to determine how well the major components of therapy–diet, insulin, and exercise–are working together to control blood glucose levels.

In addition to the routine prenatal care provided to all pregnant women, the woman with diabetes will receive additional counseling. She should wear a medical identification bracelet at all times and should carry insulin, syringes, and "glucose boosters" with her whenever she is away from home. She also should be given written instructions for reporting the development of problems such as nausea, vomiting, and infections, including directions for reaching her health care provider by phone at night and on weekends and holidays (see Teaching for Self-Care: Treatment for Hypoglycemia).

Because the woman with diabetes is at risk for infections, eye problems, and neurologic changes, foot care and general skin care are important. A daily bath that includes good perineal care and foot care is important. For dry skin, lotions, creams, or oils can be applied. Tight clothing should be avoided. Shoes or slippers should be worn at all times, should fit properly, and are best worn with socks or stockings. Feet should be inspected regularly; toenails should be cut straight across, and professional help should be sought for any foot problems. Extremes of temperature should be avoided.

TABLE 32-2 **Target Blood Glucose Levels During Pregnancy**

TIME OF MEASUREMENT	TARGET GLUCOSE LEVEL (MG/DL)*
Fasting	60 to 90
Premeal (lunch, dinner)	60 to 105
Bedtime	90 to 120
Postmeal	
1 hr	100 to 120
2 hr	90 to 120
2 AM to 4 AM	60 to 120

*Add 15% if plasma values are used.

Source: American Diabetes Association. (2000). *Medical management of pregnancy complicated by diabetes* (3rd ed.). Alexandria, VA: The Association.

Diet. The woman with pregestational diabetes has probably previously had nutritional counseling regarding management of the diabetes. Because pregnancy precipitates special nutritional concerns and needs, the woman must be educated to incorporate these changes into dietary planning. Nutritional counseling is usually provided by a registered dietitian.

Dietary management during diabetic pregnancy must be based on blood (not urine) glucose levels. The diet is individualized to allow increased fetal and metabolic requirements, with consideration of such factors as prepregnancy weight and dietary habits, overall health, ethnic background, lifestyle, stage of pregnancy, knowledge of nutrition, and insulin therapy. The dietary goal is to provide weight gain consistent with a normal pregnancy, to prevent ketoacidosis, and to minimize widely fluctuating blood glucose levels.

Energy needs are usually calculated on the basis of 30 to 35 calories per kilogram of ideal body weight, with the average diet including 2200 (first trimester) to 2500 calories (second and third trimesters). Total calories may be distributed among three meals and one evening snack, or more commonly, three meals and at least two snacks. Meals should be eaten on time and never skipped. Snacks must be carefully planned in accordance with insulin therapy to avoid fluctuations in blood glucose levels. A large bedtime snack of at least 25 g of carbohydrate with some protein is recommended to help prevent hypoglycemia and starvation ketosis during the night.

TEACHING FOR SELF-CARE

Treatment for Hypoglycemia

- Be familiar with signs and symptoms of hypoglycemia (nervousness, headache, shaking, irritability, personality change, hunger, blurred vision, sweaty skin, tingling of mouth or extremities).
- Check blood glucose level immediately when hypoglycemic symptoms occur.
- If blood glucose is <60 mg/dl, immediately eat or drink something that contains 10 to 15 g of simple carbohydrate. Examples:
  - ½ cup (4 ounces) unsweetened fruit juice
  - ½ cup (4 ounces) regular (not diet) soda
  - 5 to 6 Life Savers candies
  - 1 tablespoon honey or corn (Karo) syrup
  - 1 cup (8 ounces) milk
  - 2 to 3 glucose tablets
- Rest for 15 min, then recheck blood glucose.
- If glucose level is still <60 mg/dl, eat or drink another serving of one of the "glucose boosters" listed above.
- Wait 15 min, then recheck blood glucose. If it is still <60 mg/dl, notify health care provider immediately.

Source: American Diabetes Association. (2000). *Medical management of pregnancy complicated by diabetes* (3rd ed.). Alexandria, VA: The Association; Becton Dickinson & Co. (1997). *Controlling low blood sugar reactions*. Franklin Lakes, NJ: Becton Dickinson.

The ratio of carbohydrate, protein, and fat is important to meet the metabolic needs of the woman and the fetus. Approximately 50% to 60% of the total calories should be carbohydrate, with a minimum of 250 g/day. Simple carbohydrates are limited; complex carbohydrates that are high in fiber content are recommended because the starch and protein in such foods help regulate the blood glucose level as a result of more sustained glucose release. Protein intake should constitute 12% to 20% of the total kilocalories, and 20% to 30% of the daily caloric intake should come from fat, with no more than 10% saturated fats (see Teaching for Self-Care: Dietary Management of Diabetic Pregnancy). Weight gain for most women should be about 12 kg during the pregnancy (Gilbert & Harmon, 2003).

Exercise. Although it has been shown that exercise enhances the use of glucose and decreases insulin need in nonpregnant women with diabetes, limited data exist regarding exercise in pregnancy. Any prescription of exercise during diabetic pregnancy should be done by the primary health care provider and should be closely monitored to prevent complications. For those women with vasculopathy, only mild exercise is recommended because exercise causes a redistribution of blood flow, which increases the potential for ischemic injury to the placenta and already compromised organs. Women with vasculopathy also typically depend completely on exogenous insulin and are at greater risk for wide fluctuations in blood glucose levels and ketoacidosis, which can be worsened by exercise.

When exercise is prescribed by the health care provider as part of the treatment plan, careful instructions are given to the woman. She should be told that exercise need not be vigorous to be beneficial: 15 to 30 minutes of walking 4 to 6 times a week is satisfactory for most pregnant women. Other exercises that may be recommended are non–weight-bearing activities such as arm ergometry or use of a recumbent bicycle. The best time for exercise is after meals, when the blood glucose level is increasing. If the woman exercises when the insulin is peaking or engages in prolonged exercise without carbohydrate intake, hypoglycemia may result. Hyperglycemia may occur when exercise is done when insulin action is waning. To monitor the effect of insulin on blood glucose levels, the woman can measure blood glucose before, during, and after exercise.

The woman should be aware of the possibility of uterine contractions during exercise and stop immediately if they are detected.

Insulin Therapy. Adequate insulinization of the pregnant woman is the primary factor in the maintenance of normoglycemia during pregnancy, thus ensuring proper glucose metabolism of the mother and fetus. Insulin requirements during pregnancy change dramatically as the pregnancy progresses, necessitating frequent adjustments in insulin dosage. In the first trimester, little or no change occurs in prepregnancy insulin requirements; however, insulin dosage may need to be decreased because of hypoglycemia. During the second and third trimesters, because

TEACHING FOR SELF-CARE

Dietary Management of Diabetic Pregnancy

- Follow the prescribed diet plan.
- Eat a well-balanced diet, including daily food requirements for a normal pregnancy.
- Divide daily food intake between three meals and two to four snacks, depending on individual needs.
- Eat a substantial bedtime snack to prevent a severe drop in blood glucose level during the night.
- Limit the intake of fats if weight gain occurs too rapidly.
- Take daily vitamins and iron as prescribed by the health care provider.
- Avoid foods high in refined sugar.
- Eat consistently each day; never skip meals or snacks.
- Reduce the intake of saturated fat and cholesterol.
- Eat foods high in dietary fiber.
- Avoid alcohol and caffeine.

TEACHING FOR SELF-CARE

Administration of Insulin

PROCEDURE FOR MIXING NPH (INTERMEDIATE-ACTING) AND REGULAR (SHORT-ACTING) INSULIN

- Wash hands thoroughly and gather supplies. Be sure the insulin syringe corresponds to the concentration of insulin you are using.
- Check insulin bottle to be certain it is the appropriate type and check the expiration date.
- Gently rotate (do not shake) the insulin vial to mix the insulin.
- Wipe off rubber stopper of each vial with alcohol.
- Draw into syringe the amount of air equal to total dose.
- Inject air equal to NPH (intermediate-acting) dose into NPH vial. Remove syringe from vial.
- Inject air equal to regular insulin dose into regular insulin vial.
- Invert regular insulin bottle and withdraw regular insulin dose.
- Without adding more air to NPH vial, carefully withdraw NPH dose.

PROCEDURE FOR SELF-INJECTION OF INSULIN

- Select proper injection site (remember to rotate sites).
- Injection site should be clean. Use of alcohol is not necessary. If alcohol is used, let it dry before injecting.
- Pinch the skin up to form a subcutaneous pocket and, holding the syringe like a pencil, puncture the skin at a 45- to 90-degree angle. If there is a great deal of fatty tissue at the site, spread the skin taut and inject the syringe at a 90-degree angle.
- Slowly inject the insulin.
- As you withdraw the needle, cover the injection site with sterile gauze and apply gentle pressure to prevent bleeding.
- Record insulin dosage and time of injection.

of insulin resistance, dosage must be increased to maintain target glucose levels.

For the woman with type 1 pregestational diabetes who has typically been accustomed to one injection per day of intermediate-acting insulin, multiple daily injections of mixed insulin are a new experience. The woman with type 2 diabetes previously treated with oral hypoglycemics is faced with the task of learning to self-administer injections of insulin. The nurse is instrumental in education and support with regard to insulin administration and adjustment of insulin dosage to maintain normoglycemia (see Teaching for Self-Care: Administration of Insulin).

More types of insulin are available today than ever before. Beef and pork insulin have largely been replaced by biosynthetic human insulin preparations (Humulin or Novolin), which are less likely to cause antibody formation. Clients with new onset of diabetes are almost always started on this type of insulin. Lispro (Humalog) is a rapid-acting insulin preparation that has an onset of action within 15 minutes of injection and peaks in 2 to 3 hours. Advantages of lispro include convenience, because it is injected immediately before mealtime; less hyperglycemia after meals; and fewer hypoglycemic episodes. Lispro insulin has a total duration of action of 3 to 4 hours (Inzucchi, 1999; Landon et al., 2002) (Table 32-3).

Insulin-dependent diabetes is managed in most women with two to three injections per day. Usually two thirds of the daily insulin dose, with longer-acting (NPH) and short-acting (regular) insulin combined in a 2:1 ratio, is given before breakfast. Sometimes the remaining one third, again a combination of longer-acting and short-acting insulin, is administered in the evening before dinner. To reduce the risk of hypoglycemia during the night, separate injections often are administered, with short-acting insulin given before dinner, followed by longer-acting insulin at bedtime. Another alternative insulin regimen that works well for some women is to administer short-acting insulin before each meal and longer-acting insulin at bedtime (Hagay & Reece, 1999; Landon et al., 2002).

Although subcutaneous insulin injections are still more commonly used, increasing numbers of pregnant women are now using continuous insulin infusion systems. The insulin "pump" is designed to mimic more closely the function of the pancreas in secreting insulin (Fig. 32-3). This portable, battery-powered device is worn, like a pager, during most daily activities. The pump infuses regular insulin at a set basal rate and has the capacity to deliver up to four different basal rates in 24 hours. It also delivers bolus doses of insulin before meals to control postprandial blood glucose levels. A fine-gauge plastic catheter is inserted into subcutaneous tissue, usually in the abdomen, and attached to the pump syringe by connecting tubing. The subcutaneous catheter and connecting tubing are changed every 2 to 3 days. Although the insulin pump is convenient and generally provides good glycemic control, complications such as DKA, infection, or hypoglycemic coma can still develop. Use of the insulin pump requires a knowledgeable, motivated client, skilled health care providers, and 24-hour availability of emergency assistance (Hagay & Reece, 1999; Landon et al., 2002; Moore, 1999).

Monitoring Blood Glucose Levels. Blood glucose testing at home is the commonly accepted method for monitoring blood glucose levels and the most important tool available to the woman to assess her degree of glycemic control. In addition, this monitoring provides motivation to continue the prescribed treatment plan, and the data obtained facilitate interaction with the health care team in maintaining glycemic control and minimizing fetal risk.

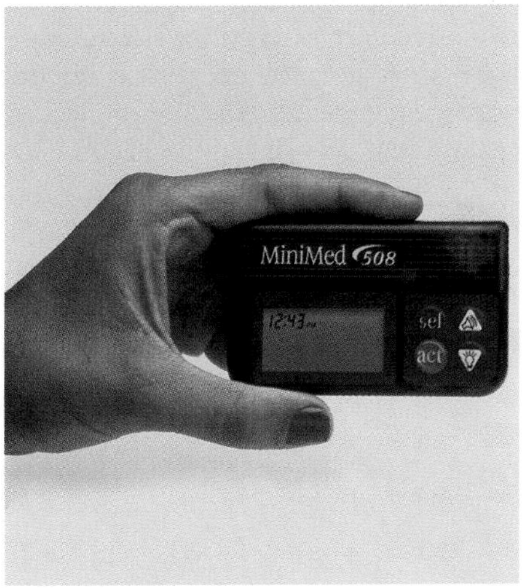
MiniMed 508
sel
act

FIG. 32-3 Insulin pump shows basal rate for pregnant women with diabetes. (Courtesy MiniMed, Inc., Sylmar, CA)

TABLE 32-3 **Insulin Administration During Pregnancy: Expected Time of Action**

TYPE OF INSULIN	ONSET	PEAK	DURATION
Lispro (rapid acting)	Within 15 min	2-3 hr	3-4 hr
Regular (short acting)	30 min	3-4 hr	6-8 hr
Intermediate acting	2-4 hr	4-12 hr	12-24 hr
Long acting	3-4 hr	14-24 hr	24-36 hr

Women with pregestational diabetes are often familiar with self-monitoring of blood glucose levels because it is typically included in the management plan for type 1 and some cases of type 2 diabetes. However, a thorough assessment of the woman's knowledge and skill related to blood glucose testing is essential to ensure accurate monitoring of glucose levels during pregnancy. The nurse observes the woman performing blood glucose monitoring to determine her accuracy and comfort with the system. The family also is included in the assessment and in subsequent instruction.

Pregnancy demands more frequent and judicious monitoring than many women have practiced previously. Willingness to comply with the monitoring schedule is essential to the management plan. Home glucose monitoring should be done by using a glucose reflectance meter, which is battery powered and determines the blood glucose level by the amount of light reflected from a reacted test strip. Most insurance companies will cover the cost of a meter and necessary supplies. To perform blood glucose monitoring, a drop of blood is obtained by a finger stick and placed on a test strip. After a specified amount of time, the glucose level can be read by the meter (see Teaching for Self-Care: Testing Blood Glucose Level).

Meters incorporate memory to store a large number of readings; however, the woman is still encouraged to keep written records of glucose levels. She should bring her written records, her meter containing stored test results, or both with her to each appointment. It is important that the monitoring equipment be checked for accuracy at intervals by comparing the woman's results on her machine with the results of a laboratory test done at the same time on a capillary whole blood sample.

TEACHING FOR SELF-CARE

Testing Blood Glucose Level

- Gather supplies, check expiration date, and read instructions on testing materials. Prepare glucose reflectance meter for use according to manufacturer's directions.
- Wash hands in warm water (warmth increases circulation).
- Select site on side of any finger (all fingers should be used in rotation).
- Pierce site with lancet (may use automatic, spring-loaded, puncturing device). Cleaning the site with alcohol is not necessary.
- Drop hand down to side; with other hand gently squeeze finger from hand to fingertip.
- Allow blood to drop onto testing strip. Be sure to cover entire reagent area.
- Determine blood glucose value using the glucose reflectance meter, following manufacturer's instructions.
- Record results.
- Repeat daily as instructed by health care provider and as needed for signs of hypoglycemia or hyperglycemia.

Source: American Diabetes Association. (2000). *Medical management of pregnancy complicated by diabetes* (3rd ed.). Alexandria, VA: The Association.

Blood glucose levels are routinely measured at various times throughout the day, such as before breakfast, lunch, and dinner; 2 hours after each meal; at bedtime; and in the middle of the night. The health care provider will determine for each woman the number and timing of routine blood glucose determinations. Because hyperglycemia is to be avoided, postprandial measurements are often performed.

NURSE ALERT

Hyperglycemia will most likely be identified in 2-hour postprandial values, because blood glucose levels peak about 2 hours after a meal.

Special circumstances may necessitate more frequent testing. Women are instructed to check glucose levels at any sign of hypoglycemia or hyperglycemia. When there is any readjustment in insulin dosage or diet, more frequent measurement of blood glucose is warranted. If nausea, vomiting, or diarrhea occurs, or if any infection is present, the woman will probably be asked to monitor her blood glucose levels more closely.

Target levels of blood glucose during pregnancy are lower than nonpregnant values. Acceptable fasting levels are generally between 60 and 90 mg/dl, and 2-hour postprandial levels should be between 90 and 120 mg/dl (see Table 32-2) (ADA, 2000). The woman should be told to report episodes of hypoglycemia (less than 60 mg/dl) and hyperglycemia (greater than 200 mg/dl) to her health care provider immediately so that adjustments in diet or insulin therapy can be made (ADA, 1998).

Pregnant women with diabetes are much more likely to have hypoglycemia than hyperglycemia, because the goal of therapy is to maintain the blood glucose in a narrow, low-normal range of 60 to 120 mg/dl. Although a blood glucose level greater than 120 mg/dl is considered too high for a pregnant woman, it will not produce the classic signs and symptoms of hyperglycemia. Conversely, many women will have signs and symptoms of hypoglycemia with blood glucose levels below 60 mg/dl (see Table 32-1).

Most episodes of mild or moderate hypoglycemia can be treated with oral intake of 10 to 15 g of simple carbohydrate (see Teaching for Self-Care: Treatment for Hypoglycemia). If severe hypoglycemia occurs, in which the woman has a decrease or loss of consciousness or an inability to swallow, she will require a parenteral injection of glucagon or intravenous (IV) glucose (ADA, 1998; Becton Dickinson & Co., 1997). Because hypoglycemia can develop rapidly and because impaired judgment can be associated with even moderate episodes, it is vital that family members, friends, and work colleagues be able to recognize signs and symptoms quickly and initiate proper treatment if necessary (Becton Dickinson & Co., 1997).

Although hyperglycemia is less likely to occur in compliant clients, it is still a dangerous complication. Hyperglycemia can rapidly progress to DKA. Women and family members should be particularly alert for signs and symptoms of hyperglycemia, especially when infections or other illnesses occur (see Table 32-1 and Teaching for Self-Care: What to Do When Illness Occurs).

Fetal Surveillance. Diagnostic techniques for fetal surveillance are often performed to assess fetal growth and well-being. The goals of fetal surveillance are to detect fetal compromise as early as possible and to prevent intrauterine fetal death or unnecessary preterm birth. The majority of fetal surveillance measures are concentrated in the third trimester, when the risk of fetal compromise is greatest.

Early in pregnancy, efforts are made to determine the estimated date of birth. A baseline sonogram is done during the first trimester to assess gestational age. Follow-up ultrasound examinations are usually performed during the pregnancy, as often as every 4 to 6 weeks, to monitor fetal growth; estimate fetal weight; and detect hydramnios, macrosomia, and congenital anomalies.

Because diabetic pregnancies are at greater risk for neural tube defects (e.g., spina bifida, anencephaly, microcephaly), measurement of maternal serum alpha-fetoprotein is performed between 16 and 18 weeks of gestation. This is often done in conjunction with a detailed ultrasound study to examine the fetus for neural tube defects.

Fetal echocardiography may be performed between 18 and 22 weeks of gestation to detect cardiac anomalies. Some practitioners repeat this fetal surveillance test at 34 weeks. Doppler studies of the umbilical artery may be performed in women with vascular disease to detect placental compromise.

Maternal evaluation of fetal movements (kick counts) is used primarily as a screening technique in fetal surveillance. Few research studies have investigated the use of this method in diabetic pregnancies.

TEACHING FOR SELF-CARE

What to Do When Illness Occurs

- Be sure to take insulin even though appetite and food intake may be less than normal. (Insulin needs are increased with illness or infection.)
- Call the health care provider and relay the following information:
  - Symptoms of illness (e.g., nausea, vomiting, diarrhea)
  - Fever
  - Most recent blood glucose level
  - Urine ketones
  - Time and amount of last insulin dose
- Increase oral intake of fluids to prevent dehydration.
- Rest as much as possible.
- If unable to reach health care provider and blood glucose exceeds 200 mg/dl with urine ketones present, seek emergency treatment at the nearest health care facility. Do not attempt to self-treat for this.

A commonly used measure of fetal well-being is the nonstress test, typically beginning around 28 to 32 weeks of gestation (see Chapter 29). After 32 weeks, testing may be done twice weekly. For the woman with vascular disease, testing may begin earlier and continue more frequently. In the presence of a nonreactive nonstress test, a contraction stress test or fetal biophysical profile may be used to evaluate fetal well-being (Hagay & Reece, 1999; Landon et al., 2002; Moore, 1999).

Complications Requiring Hospitalization. Occasionally it becomes necessary to hospitalize a woman with diabetes during pregnancy. A few days in the hospital early in pregnancy may be required to complete baseline cardiovascular, renal, and ophthalmologic evaluations and balance diet and insulin to achieve satisfactory glucose control. Infection, which can lead to hyperglycemia and DKA, is an indication for hospitalization, regardless of gestational age. At any time during the pregnancy, women who fail to maintain acceptable blood glucose levels may be hospitalized. A few days in a controlled environment often greatly increases compliance with diet and insulin therapy, resulting in marked improvement in blood glucose levels. Hospitalization during the third trimester for closer maternal and fetal observation may be indicated for women whose diabetes is poorly controlled or who also have hypertension (Cunningham et al., 2001).

Determination of Birth Date and Mode of Birth. Today the majority of diabetic pregnancies are allowed to progress to term (38 to 40 weeks of gestation), as long as good metabolic control is maintained and all parameters of antepartum fetal surveillance remain within normal limits. Reasons to proceed with delivery before term include poor metabolic control, worsening hypertensive disorders, fetal macrosomia, or fetal growth restriction (Hagay & Reece, 1999; Landon et al., 2002; Moore, 1999).

Many practitioners plan elective labor induction between 38 and 40 weeks, provided that maternal glucose levels are well controlled. To confirm fetal lung maturity before birth, an amniocentesis may be performed in pregnancies earlier than 39 weeks. For the pregnancy complicated by diabetes, fetal lung maturation is better predicted by the amniotic fluid phosphatidylglycerol than by the lecithin/sphingomyelin ratio. If the fetal lungs are still immature, birth should be postponed as long as the results of fetal assessment remain reassuring. Birth despite poor fetal lung maturity may be essential when testing suggests fetal compromise or if the maternal complications of preeclampsia, deteriorating vision due to proliferative retinopathy, or worsening renal function should develop (Landon et al., 2002).

The mode of birth for women with pregestational diabetes is a subject of controversy among practitioners. The cesarean rate for these women is exceedingly high, around 45%. Cesarean birth is often performed when antepartum testing suggests fetal distress or the estimated fetal weight is 4000 to 4500 g. When induction of labor is desired and the cervix fails to respond, cesarean birth often is necessary (Hagay & Reece, 1999; Landon et al., 2002; Moore, 1999).

Intrapartum

During the intrapartum period, the woman with pregestational diabetes must be monitored closely to prevent complications related to dehydration, hypoglycemia, and hyperglycemia. Most women use large amounts of energy (calories) to accomplish the work and manage the stress of labor and birth; however, this calorie expenditure varies with the individual. Blood glucose levels and hydration must be carefully controlled during labor. An IV line is inserted for infusion of a maintenance fluid, such as lactated Ringer's or 5% dextrose in lactated Ringer's solution. Insulin may be administered by continuous infusion or intermittent subcutaneous injection. Determinations of blood glucose levels are made every hour, and fluids and insulin are adjusted to maintain plasma blood glucose levels at 70 to 90 mg/dl or capillary whole blood glucose levels at 60 to 80 mg/dl. It is essential that these target glucose levels be maintained because hyperglycemia during labor can precipitate metabolic problems, particularly hypoglycemia, in the neonate (ADA, 2000).

During labor, continuous fetal heart monitoring is necessary. The woman should assume a side-lying position during bed rest in labor to prevent supine hypotension because of a large fetus or polyhydramnios. Labor is allowed to progress without intervention, provided normal rates of cervical dilation, fetal descent, and fetal well-being are maintained. Failure to progress may indicate a macrosomic infant and cephalopelvic disproportion, necessitating a cesarean birth. The woman is observed and treated during labor for diabetic complications such as hyperglycemia, ketosis, ketoacidosis, and glycosuria. During second stage labor, the nurse should be alert for the possibility of shoulder dystocia if delivery of a macrosomic infant is attempted and be prepared to assist with maneuvers to free the fetal shoulder that is lodged behind the symphysis pubis (see Chapter 36). A neonatologist, pediatrician, or neonatal nurse practitioner may be present at the birth to initiate assessment and neonatal care.

If a cesarean birth is planned, it should be scheduled in the early morning to facilitate glycemic control. The morning dose of insulin should be withheld and the woman given nothing by mouth. Epidural anesthesia is recommended because hypoglycemia can be detected earlier if the woman is awake (Hagay & Reece, 1999; Landon et al., 2002).

Postpartum

In the immediate postpartum period, insulin requirements decrease substantially because the major source of insulin resistance, the placenta, has been removed. Women with type 1 diabetes may require only half the prenatal insulin dose on the first postpartum day, provided that they are eating a full diet. It takes several days after birth to reestablish carbohydrate homeostasis. Blood glucose levels are monitored in the postpartum period, and insulin dosage is adjusted accordingly. Blood glucose levels do not require as tight control after birth. Usually insulin is not given until the blood glucose level is greater than 200 mg/dl (Hagay & Reece, 1999). The woman who is insulin dependent must realize the importance of eating on time, even if the baby needs feeding or other pressing demands exist. Women with type 2 diabetes often require no insulin in the postpartum period and are able to maintain normoglycemia through diet alone or with oral hypoglycemics.

Possible postpartum complications include preeclampsia-eclampsia, hemorrhage, and infection. Hemorrhage is a possibility if the mother's uterus was overdistended (hydramnios, macrosomic fetus) or overstimulated (oxytocin induction). Postpartum infections such as endometritis are more likely to occur in a woman with diabetes.

Mothers are encouraged to breastfeed. In addition to the advantages of maternal satisfaction and pleasure, breastfeeding has an antidiabetogenic effect. Many mothers with diabetes find that their glucose levels are easier to control. Insulin requirements may be half the prepregnancy levels because of the carbohydrate used in human milk production. Because glucose levels are lower, breastfeeding women are at increased risk for hypoglycemia, especially in the early postpartum period and after breastfeeding sessions (Hagay & Reece, 1999; Landon et al., 2002; Moore, 1999).

The mother may have early breastfeeding difficulties. Poor metabolic control may delay lactogenesis and contribute to decreased milk production (Moore, 1999). Because many women give birth by cesarean, the effects of anesthesia and postoperative discomfort may delay maternal attachment and make breastfeeding more difficult. In addition, initial contact and opportunity to breastfeed the infant are often delayed because many institutions place infants of mothers with diabetes in neonatal intensive care units or special care nurseries for observation during the first few hours after birth. Support and assistance from nursing staff and lactation specialists can facilitate the mother's early experience with breastfeeding and encourage her to continue.

Research studies suggest that infants who are exclusively breastfed are less likely to develop diabetes and that exposure to cow's milk products before age 8 days is an important risk factor for the disease. Because children born to women who have diabetes are at increased risk for diabetes to develop, this information further supports the importance of encouraging all women with diabetes to breastfeed (Moore, 1999).

The new mother needs information about contraception. Although family planning is important for all women, it is essential for the woman with diabetes to safeguard her own health and to promote optimal outcomes in future pregnancies. Because excellent glucose control at conception is crucial for all diabetics, the importance of conscientiously using a reliable contraceptive method until another pregnancy is desired should be stressed. No one best form of contraception succeeds for diabetic women. Instead, emphasis should be placed on consistent use of a reliable and effective birth control method (Inzucchi, 1999).

The barrier methods are often recommended as safe, inexpensive options that have no inherent risks for women with diabetes (Landon et al., 2002). However, barrier methods are not so effective as some other forms of contraception.

Use of oral contraceptives is controversial because of the risk of thromboembolic and vascular complications and the effect on carbohydrate metabolism. In women without vascular disease or other risk factors, combination low-dose oral contraceptives may be prescribed. Close monitoring of blood pressure and lipid levels is necessary to detect complications (Cunningham et al., 2001; Inzucchi, 1999; Landon et al., 2002). Progestin-only oral contraceptives also may be used, because they minimally affect carbohydrate metabolism (Cunningham et al., 2001; Landon et al., 2002).

Some health care providers are reluctant to use intrauterine contraceptive devices (IUDs) in women with diabetes because of concerns about infection. However, this method has been used successfully by these woman (Cunningham et al., 2001; Landon et al., 2002).

Opinion is divided about the use of long-acting parenteral or implantable progestins, such as Depo-Provera and Norplant. Some authorities recommend their use, especially in women who may not be compliant with daily dosing for oral contraceptives or appropriate follow-up care (Inzucchi, 1999). Others believe that these methods may adversely affect diabetic control (Landon et al., 2002).

The woman and her partner should be informed that the risks associated with pregnancy increase with the duration and severity of the diabetic condition and that pregnancy may contribute to vascular changes associated with diabetes. Therefore sterilization should be discussed with the woman who has completed her family or who has significant vasculopathy (Cunningham et al., 2001; Inzucchi, 1999).

Evaluation

Evaluation of the care of the pregnant woman with pregestational diabetes is based on the previously stated expected outcomes of care, which are closely associated with the degree of maternal metabolic control during pregnancy (see Plan of Care).

Gestational Diabetes Mellitus

Gestational diabetes mellitus (GDM) complicates 2% to 5% of all pregnancies in the United States and accounts for 90% of all cases of diabetic pregnancy. Although the incidence of GDM seems to be increasing in general, its prevalence varies by racial and ethnic groups. GDM is more likely to occur among Hispanic, Native American, Asian, and African-American populations than in Caucasians (Inzucchi, 1999; Landon et al., 2002). Women with GDM are at significant risk of developing glucose intolerance later in life; about 50% will be diagnosed as diabetic within 5 years (Inzucchi, 1999; Landon et al., 2002). This is especially true of women whose GDM is diagnosed early in pregnancy and who also are obese (Landon et al., 2002). Classic risk factors for GDM include maternal age older than 30 years; obesity; family history of type 2 diabetes; and an obstetric history of an infant weighing more than 9 pounds, hydramnios, unexplained stillbirth, miscarriage, or an infant with congenital anomalies. Other factors include hypertensive disorders, recurrent monilial vaginitis, and glucosuria on two consecutive visits to the clinic or office (ADA, 2003).

Maternal-Fetal Risks

Women with GDM have twice the risk of developing hypertensive disorders compared with normal pregnant women (Metzger & Coustan, 1998). They also have increased risk for fetal macrosomia, which can lead to increased rates of perineal lacerations, episiotomy, and cesarean birth (Jones & Stone, 1998). Infants born to women with GDM are at risk for macrosomia with associated shoulder dystocia and birth trauma. GDM also places the neonate at increased risk for hypoglycemia, hypocalcemia, hyperbilirubinemia, thrombocytopenia, polycythemia, and respiratory distress syndrome (Jones & Stone, 1998; Metzger & Coustan, 1998).

The overall incidence of congenital anomalies among infants of women with gestational diabetes approaches that of the general population because gestational diabetes usually develops after week 20 of pregnancy—after the critical period of organogenesis (first trimester) has passed.

Collaborative Care

Nurses involved in prenatal care delivery can be instrumental in the identification of women with GDM. Although protocols regarding which women will undergo screening and exactly how the screening will be done vary among care providers, nurses are often responsible for ensuring that the screen is performed on the identified group of women at the proper gestational age. Careful adherence to screening protocols is crucial to identify women with GDM correctly.

Screening for Gestational Diabetes Mellitus. The American College of Obstetricians and Gynecologists (ACOG) recommends that all pregnant women be screened for GDM, either by history, clinical risk factors, or laboratory screening of blood glucose levels (ACOG, 2001). Based on history and clinical risk factors, some women are at such low risk for the development of GDM that glucose testing is not cost-effective. This group at low risk includes normal-weight women younger than 25 years who have no family history of diabetes, are not members of an ethnic or a racial group known to have a high prevalence of the disease, and have no previous history of abnormal glucose tolerance or adverse obstetric outcomes usually associated with GDM (ACOG, 2001; Expert Committee, 2003). The Expert Committee on the Diagnosis and Classification of Diabetes Mellitus (2003) states that screening is unnecessary in these groups. Women at high risk for

Plan of Care Pregnancy Complicated by Pregestational Diabetes

NURSING DIAGNOSIS Deficient knowledge related to lack of recall of information as evidenced by client questions and concerns

Expected Outcome *Client will be able to verbalize important information regarding diabetes, its management, and potential effects on the pregnant woman and fetus.*

Nursing Interventions/*Rationales*

Assess client's current knowledge base regarding disease process, management, effects on pregnancy and fetus, and potential complications *to provide database for further teaching.*

Review the pathophysiology of diabetes, effects on pregnancy and fetus, and potential complications *to promote client recall of information and compliance with treatment plan.*

Review procedure for insulin administration, demonstrate procedure for blood glucose monitoring and insulin measurement and administration, and obtain return demonstration *to establish client comfort and competence with procedures.*

Discuss diet and exercise as prescribed by diabetologist *to promote self-care.*

Review signs and symptoms of complications of hypoglycemia and hyperglycemia and appropriate interventions *to promote prompt recognition of complications and self-care.*

Provide contact numbers for health care team for prompt interventions and answers to questions on an ongoing basis *to promote client and health team collaboration.*

NURSING DIAGNOSIS Risk for fetal injury related to elevated maternal glucose levels

Expected Outcomes *Fetus will remain free of injury and be born at term in a healthy state.*

Nursing Interventions/*Rationales*

Assess client's current diabetic control *to identify risk for fetal mortality and congenital anomalies.*

Monitor fundal height during each prenatal visit *to identify appropriate fetal growth.*

Monitor for signs and symptoms of pregnancy-induced hypertension *to identify early manifestations because pregnant women with diabetes are more at risk.*

Assess fetal movement and heart rate during each prenatal visit, and perform weekly nonstress tests during the last 4 weeks of pregnancy *to assess fetal well-being.*

Review procedure for blood glucose testing and insulin administration *to promote self-care.*

NURSING DIAGNOSIS Anxiety related to threat to maternal and fetal well-being as evidenced by client verbal expressions of concern

Expected Outcomes *Client will identify sources of anxiety and report feeling less anxious.*

Nursing Interventions/*Rationales*

Through therapeutic communication, promote an open relationship with client *to promote client trust.*

Listen to client's feelings and concerns *to assess for any misconception or misinformation that may be contributing to anxiety.*

Review potential dangers by providing factual information *to correct any misconceptions or misinformation.*

Encourage client to share concerns with her health care team *to promote client and team collaboration in her care.*

NURSING DIAGNOSIS Risk for imbalanced nutrition: less than body requirements related to inability to ingest nutrients that are needed for pregnancy complicated by diabetes

Expected Outcomes *Client will verbalize understanding of dietary needs during pregnancy, gain weight that is consistent with a normal pregnancy, and maintain blood sugar levels between 65 and 130 mg/dl.*

Nursing Interventions/*Rationales*

Assess caloric intake and dietary pattern using 24 hour recall *to evaluate client understanding and/or adherence to dietary regimen.*

Review importance of regularity of meals and snacks *to promote compliance with treatment plan.*

Review blood glucose monitoring *to determine if client is competent with procedure.*

Weigh client at each prenatal visit *to assess appropriate weight gain.*

Refer to dietitian for individualized counseling if needed *to plan diet that assists the woman to maintain normoglycemia and to gain the appropriate amount of weight.*

developing GDM should be screened at the first prenatal visit and again at 24 to 28 weeks' gestation (ADA, 2003).

The screening test (Glucola screening) most often used in North America consists of a 50-g oral glucose load, followed by a plasma glucose determination 1 hour later. Screening should be performed at 24 to 28 weeks of gestation. It is not necessary that the woman be fasting. A glucose value of 140 mg/dl or greater is usually considered a positive screen.

A positive Glucola screen requires follow-up with a 3-hour oral glucose tolerance test (OGTT). The 3-hour OGTT is administered after an overnight fast and at least 3 days of unrestricted diet (at least 150 g of carbohydrate) and physical activity. The woman is instructed to avoid caffeine because it tends to increase glucose levels and to abstain from smoking for 12 hours before and during the test. A fasting blood glucose level is determined before giving a 100-g glucose load. Blood glucose levels are then determined 1, 2, and 3 hours later. The woman is diagnosed with gestational diabetes if two or more values are met or exceeded (Fig. 32-4). The 100-g glucose load is preferred over the 2-hour, 75-g glucose load.

Nursing diagnoses and expected outcomes of care for the woman with GDM are basically the same as those for women with pregestational diabetes, except that the time frame for planning may be shortened with GDM because the diagnosis is usually made later in pregnancy.

Antepartum Care. When the diagnosis of gestational diabetes is made, treatment begins immediately, allowing little or no time for the woman and her family to adjust to the diagnosis before they are expected to participate in the

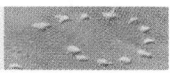

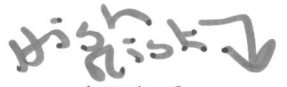

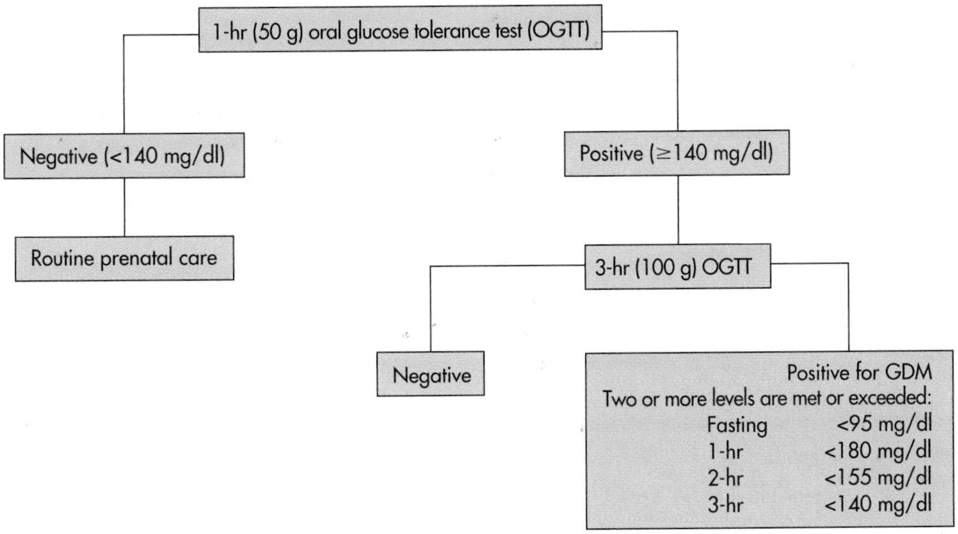
1-hr (50 g) oral glucose tolerance test (OGTT)
Negative (<140 mg/dl)
Positive (≥140 mg/dl)
Routine prenatal care
3-hr (100 g) OGTT
Negative
Positive for GDM
Two or more levels are met or exceeded:
Fasting <95 mg/dl
1-hr <180 mg/dl
2-hr <155 mg/dl
3-hr <140 mg/dl

FIG. 32-4 Screening and diagnosis for gestational diabetes. (Source: American Diabetes Association. [2003]. Position statement: Gestational diabetes mellitus. *Diabetes Care* *26*[suppl 1], S103-S105.)

treatment plan. This is in contrast to the woman with pregestational diabetes, who may have had years to learn about the disease and to adapt to dietary modifications, self-monitoring of glucose, and insulin administration. With each step of the treatment plan, the nurse and other health care providers should educate the woman and her family, providing detailed and comprehensive explanations to ensure understanding, participation, and adherence to the necessary interventions. Potential complications should be discussed, and the need for maintenance of normoglycemia throughout the remainder of the pregnancy is reinforced. It may be reassuring for the woman and her family to know that gestational diabetes typically disappears when the pregnancy is over.

As with pregestational diabetes, the aim of therapy in women with GDM is meticulous blood glucose control. Fasting blood glucose levels should be between 60 and 90 mg/dl, and 2-hour postprandial blood levels should be between 90 and 120 mg/dl (ADA, 2000).

Diet. Dietary modification is the mainstay of treatment for GDM. The woman with GDM is given a standard diabetic diet immediately on diagnosis (see previous discussion). Some authorities recommend fewer calories for overweight or morbidly obese women, believing that such a diet will cause less hyperglycemia and reduce the need for insulin (Landon et al., 2002; Metzger & Coustan, 1998).

Exercise. Exercise in women with GDM appears to be safe. It helps reduce blood glucose levels and may be instrumental in eliminating the need for insulin (see previous discussion).

Monitoring Blood Glucose Levels. Regular blood glucose monitoring is necessary to determine whether euglycemia can be maintained by diet and exercise. However, the optimal frequency and timing of blood glucose monitoring has not been established (ACOG, 2001). Some women with GDM are provided with reflectance meters and encouraged to perform frequent self-monitoring at home, or monitoring may be done only at the clinic or office visit.

Insulin Therapy. It is important to understand that up to 20% of women with GDM will require insulin during the pregnancy to maintain adequate blood glucose levels, despite compliance with the prescribed diet (Inzucchi, 1999). Therefore the nurse should never assume that increased blood glucose levels in the woman with GDM have been caused by dietary indiscretion alone without first taking a thorough history.

Women who repetitively exceed glucose thresholds for fasting and 2-hour postprandial values are usually started on insulin therapy. Again, there is no consensus regarding the exact glucose values that warrant insulin use (ACOG, 2001; Landon et al., 2002). The woman and her family should be taught the necessary skills to manage insulin administration (see previous discussion). Langer et al., (2000) compared the use of glyburide, a second-generation oral hypoglycemic agent, and insulin in women with GDM. They found similar improvement in maternal glucose levels in both groups. Furthermore, the incidence of fetal macrosomia and neonatal hypoglycemia in the two study groups also was similar. More studies must be done, however, before oral hypoglycemic agents become widely used in GDM.

Fetal Surveillance. There is no standard recommendation for fetal surveillance in pregnancies complicated by GDM. Women whose blood glucose levels are well controlled by diet are at low risk for fetal death. Many practitioners do not routinely perform antepartum fetal testing on them so long as their fasting and 2-hour postprandial blood glucose levels remain within normal limits, and they have no other risk factors. Usually these women are allowed to progress to term and spontaneous labor without intervention. Once the woman reaches 40 weeks of gestation, fetal surveillance once or twice weekly is usually instituted (ACOG, 2001; Landon et al., 2002; Metzger & Coustan, 1998).

Women with GDM whose blood glucose levels are not well controlled or who require insulin therapy, have hypertension, or have a history of previous stillbirth generally receive more intensive fetal biophysical monitoring. There is no standard recommendation regarding initiation of testing. Nonstress tests and biophysical profiles are often performed weekly, beginning anywhere from 32 to 36 weeks of gestation (ACOG, 2001; Landon et al., 2002; Metzger & Coustan, 1998).

Intrapartum Care. During the labor and birth process, blood glucose levels are monitored at least every 2 hours to maintain levels between 70 and 90 mg/dl (ADA, 2000). Glucose levels within this range will decrease the severity of neonatal hypoglycemia. IV fluids containing glucose are not given as a bolus to the woman who has gestational diabetes, although they may be necessary as maintenance fluids. Routine uterine activity and fetal heart rate assessments are done. Although gestational diabetes is not an indication for cesarean birth, it may be necessary in the presence of problems such as preeclampsia or macrosomia.

Postpartum Care. Most women with GDM will return to normal glucose levels after childbirth (Metzger & Coustan, 1998). However, GDM is likely to recur in future pregnancies, and, as previously stated, women with GDM are at significant risk of developing glucose intolerance later in life. Assessment for carbohydrate intolerance can be initiated 6 to 12 weeks postpartum or after breastfeeding has stopped and should be repeated at regular intervals throughout the woman's life (Metzger & Coustan, 1998). Obesity is a major risk factor for the later development of diabetes. Thus women with a history of GDM, particularly those who are overweight, should be encouraged to make lifestyle changes that include weight loss and exercise to reduce this risk (Hagay & Reece, 1999; Metzger & Coustan, 1998). Because offspring of women with GDM are at risk to develop obesity and diabetes in childhood or adolescence (Cunningham et al., 2001; Metzger & Coustan, 1998), regular health care for these children is essential.

HYPEREMESIS GRAVIDARUM

Nausea and vomiting complicate approximately 70% of all pregnancies and are usually confined to the first trimester (Gordon, 2002). Although these manifestations are distressing, they are typically benign, with no significant metabolic alterations or risks to the mother or fetus.

When vomiting during pregnancy becomes excessive enough to cause weight loss of at least 5% of prepregnancy weight and is accompanied by dehydration, electrolyte imbalance, ketosis, and acetonuria, the disorder is termed **hyperemesis gravidarum.** The estimated incidence varies from 0.5 to 10 per 1000 births (Snell et al., 1998). Hyperemesis gravidarum usually begins during the first 10 weeks of pregnancy. Women with hyperemesis tend to be younger than 20 years, obese, and nonsmokers. They also are more likely to have multifetal or molar pregnancies (Riely, 1999).

Several researchers have found that vomiting during pregnancy is associated with a decreased risk of miscarriage, but they could find no consistent association with perinatal mortality. Other studies reported an association between multiple hospital admissions for severe nausea and vomiting and decreased maternal weight gain and neonatal birth weight (Hill & Fleming, 1999; Snell et al., 1998).

Etiology

The etiology of hyperemesis gravidarum remains obscure. Several theories have been proposed as to the cause, although none of them adequately explains the disorder. Hyperemesis gravidarum may be related to high levels of estrogen or human chorionic gonadotropin (hCG) and may be associated with transient hyperthyroidism during pregnancy. It may be accompanied by liver dysfunction manifested by elevated transaminase and abnormal bilirubin level and prothrombin time. Other possible causes include vitamin B deficiencies and increased sensitivity to circulating sex steroid hormones (Hill & Fleming, 1999; Riely, 1999; Snell et al., 1998).

Psychologic factors also may play a part in the development of hyperemesis gravidarum, at least in some women. Ambivalence toward the pregnancy and difficult relationships with mothers or partners have been identified as causative factors. High stress levels are probably also associated with this condition (Hill & Fleming, 1999; Snell et al., 1998). Conflicting feelings regarding prospective motherhood, body changes, and lifestyle alterations may contribute to episodes of vomiting, particularly if these feelings are excessive or unresolved.

Clinical Manifestations

The woman with hyperemesis usually has significant weight loss and dehydration. She may have a decreased blood pressure, increased pulse rate, and poor skin turgor (Snell et al., 1998). She is almost always unable to keep down even clear liquids taken by mouth. Laboratory tests may reveal electrolyte imbalances.

Collaborative Care

Whenever a pregnant woman has a complaint of nausea and vomiting, the first priority is a thorough assessment to determine the severity of the problem. In most cases, the woman should be told to come immediately to the health care provider's office or to the emergency department, because the severity of the illness is often difficult to determine by telephone conversation.

The history includes information about the frequency, severity, and duration of episodes of nausea and vomiting. Other symptoms such as diarrhea, indigestion, and abdominal pain or distention also are identified. The woman is asked to report any precipitating factors relating to the onset of her symptoms. Any pharmacologic or nonpharmacologic treatment measures should be recorded. Prepregnancy weight and documented weight gain or loss during pregnancy are important to note.

The woman's weight and vital signs are measured, and a complete physical examination is performed, with attention to signs of fluid and electrolyte imbalance and nutritional status. The most important initial laboratory test to be obtained is a dipstick determination of ketonuria. Other laboratory tests that may be ordered are a urinalysis, a complete blood cell count, electrolytes, liver enzymes, and bilirubin levels. These tests help rule out the presence of underlying diseases such as gastroenteritis, pyelonephritis, pancreatitis, cholecystitis, hepatitis, and thyroid disease (Gordon, 2002; Steinlauf & Traube, 1999). Because of the recognized association between hyperemesis gravidarum and hyperthyroidism, thyroid function also may be assessed.

Psychosocial assessment includes asking the woman about anxiety, fears, and concerns related to her own health and the effects on pregnancy outcome. Family members should be assessed both for anxiety and in regard to their role in providing support for the woman.

Initial Care

Initially the woman who is unable to keep down clear liquids by mouth will require IV therapy for correction of fluid and electrolyte imbalances. She should be kept on nothing by mouth (NPO) status for 24 to 48 hours or until vomiting has been controlled (Cunningham et al., 2001; Gordon, 2002). In the past, women requiring IV therapy were admitted to the hospital. Today, however, they may be, and often are, successfully managed at home. Antiemetic medications may be used if nausea and vomiting are uncontrolled; commonly prescribed drugs in this category include promethazine, chlorpromazine, droperidol, diphenhydramine, and metoclopramide. Corticosteroids also have been used successfully to treat refractory hyperemesis gravidarum. In addition to medical management, some women can benefit from psychotherapy or stress reduction techniques (Gordon, 2002; Hill & Fleming, 1999; Snell et al., 1998). Once the vomiting has stopped, feedings are started in small amounts at frequent intervals, and the diet is slowly advanced as tolerated.

In severe cases of hyperemesis gravidarum, enteral nutrition via a feeding tube or parenteral nutrition may be necessary to correct maternal nutritional deprivation. Total parenteral nutrition (TPN) also has been used successfully (Hill & Fleming, 1999; Snell et al., 1998).

Initial care of the hyperemetic woman involves implementing the medical plan of care, whether in the hospital or home setting. Interventions may include initiating and monitoring IV therapy, administering drugs and nutritional supplements, and monitoring the woman's response to interventions. The nurse observes the woman for any signs of complications such as metabolic acidosis, jaundice, or hemorrhage and alerts the physician should these occur.

Accurate measurement of intake and output, including the amount of emesis, is an important aspect of care. Oral hygiene while the woman is receiving NPO, and after episodes of vomiting, helps allay associated discomforts. Assistance with positioning and providing a quiet, restful environment that is free from odors may increase the woman's comfort. When the woman begins responding to therapy, limited amounts of oral fluids and bland foods such as crackers or toast are begun. The diet is progressed slowly as tolerated by the woman until she is able to consume a nutritionally sound diet. Because sleep disturbances may accompany hyperemesis gravidarum, promoting adequate rest is important. The nurse can assist in coordinating treatment measures and periods of visitation to provide opportunity for rest periods (see Plan of Care).

Follow-Up Care

Most women are able to take nourishment by mouth after several days of treatment. Education at this time is very important to prevent rapid recurrence of nausea and vomiting. Women should be encouraged to eat small, frequent meals and low-fat protein foods, to avoid greasy and highly seasoned foods, and to increase their dietary intake of potassium and magnesium. Herbal teas such as chamomile or raspberry leaf may decrease nausea (Beal, 1998). Taking fluids between meals, rather than with them, sometimes helps decrease nausea. Many pregnant women find exposure to cooking odors nauseating. If other family members can take over cooking chores, even temporarily, the woman's nausea and vomiting may decrease. The woman is counseled to contact her health care provider immediately if the nausea and vomiting recurs, especially if accompanied by abdominal pain, dehydration, and/or significant weight loss (e.g., more than 2.3 kg [5 lbs] in 1 week) (Lowdermilk & Grohar, 1998).

A few women will continue to have intractable nausea and vomiting throughout pregnancy. Rarely it may be necessary to maintain a woman on enteral, parenteral, or TPN to provide adequate nutrition for the mother and fetus (Hill & Fleming, 1999; Snell et al., 1998). Many home health agencies are able to provide these services, and arrangements for service may be made depending on the woman's insurance coverage.

Regardless of the site of care, the nurse must remain calm, compassionate, and sympathetic, recognizing that the manifestations of hyperemesis can be physically and emotionally debilitating. Irritability, tearfulness, and mood changes are often consistent with this disorder. Fetal well-being is a primary concern of the woman. The nurse can provide an environment conducive to discussion of those concerns and assist the woman in identifying and mobilizing sources of

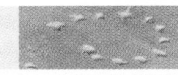

Plan of Care Hyperemesis Gravidarum

NURSING DIAGNOSIS Imbalanced nutrition: less than body requirements, related to nausea and persistent vomiting as evidenced by weight decrease as compared with prepregnant weight

Expected Outcomes *Client will exhibit no further weight losses, and weight will stabilize. Client will tolerate regular diet with adequate nutrients for pregnancy with no further nausea and vomiting.*

Nursing Interventions/*Rationales*

Ascertain client's prepregnant weight, and monitor client's current weight and intake and output *to provide a database for care planning.*

Resume oral diet as tolerated and prescribed by caregiver *to provide oral nutrition at optimal time.*

Provide small, frequent bland meals as client tolerates *to assess client's response to limited oral intake.*

Administer antiemetic medications as prescribed *to decrease or eliminate episodes of vomiting.*

Provide a quiet, restful environment *to decrease associated discomforts.*

Teach client the importance of a low-fat, high-protein diet with fluids between meals *to provide optimal nutrition for fetal growth and keep nausea to a minimum.*

Refer to dietitian to develop optimal diet plan individualized to client's current preferences, culture, and lifestyle *to encourage ongoing compliance.*

Discuss with client the importance of contacting health care provider if intractable nausea and vomiting recur *to provide prompt treatment and avoid complications.*

NURSING DIAGNOSIS Deficient fluid volume related to excessive vomiting as evidenced by fluid and electrolyte imbalance

Expected Outcome *Client's fluid and electrolyte balance will be restored.*

Nursing Interventions/*Rationales*

Assess and document skin turgor, condition of mucous membranes, vital signs, and urine specific gravity *to provide database for planning care.*

Obtain daily weight *to provide ongoing evaluation of care.*

Monitor laboratory values and report deviations from normal *to prevent complications.*

Maintain accurate intake and output record *to assess for evidence of fluid deficit.*

Initiate and maintain IV therapy carefully *to maintain fluid balance.*

Administer antiemetics as prescribed *to inhibit nausea and vomiting.*

Begin oral fluids slowly and carefully *to slowly increase tolerance and restore fluid balance.*

NURSING DIAGNOSIS Anxiety related to effects of hyperemesis on fetal well-being as evidenced by client statements of concern

Expected Outcome *Client will exhibit decreased incidence of anxiety.*

Nursing Interventions/*Rationales*

Use therapeutic communication to listen to client concerns *to maintain a relationship and feeling of trust.*

Provide information regarding any potential risks to the fetus *to alleviate anxiety.*

Assist client to identify personal strengths and previous coping mechanisms *to reinforce to client those strengths and coping mechanisms that may be of assistance during this illness.*

Help client identify sources of support and mobilize support person or group of her choice *to provide support as needed.*

Refer to social services as needed *for ongoing evaluation and assistance.*

support. The family should be included in the plan of care whenever possible. Encouraging their participation may help alleviate some of the emotional stress associated with this disorder. Psychologic counseling may be needed, as well as referral to a social worker. Education of the woman and her family about hyperemesis, its causes, potential complications, and a management plan is necessary at the onset because understanding enhances adherence to the treatment plan and influences maternal and fetal outcomes.

THYROID DISORDERS

Hyperthyroidism

Hyperthyroidism occurs in approximately 2 of every 1000 pregnancies (Seely & Burrow, 1999). In 90% to 95% of pregnant women, it is caused by Graves' disease. Other rare but possible causes are toxic nodular goiter and thyroiditis (Inzucchi & Burrow, 1999; Seely & Burrow, 1999). Clinical manifestations of hyperthyroidism are associated with an increased basal metabolism rate and increased sympathetic nervous system activity. Typical symptoms include fatigue, heat intolerance, warm skin, diaphoresis, emotional lability, tremulousness, and a wide pulse pressure. Many of these symptoms also occur with pregnancy, so the disorder can be difficult to diagnose. Signs that may help differentiate hyperthyroidism from normal pregnancy include unplanned weight loss, onycholysis (loose nails), and a pulse rate greater than 100 beats/min that does not decrease with the Valsalva maneuver (Diehl, 1998; Seely & Burrow, 1999). Laboratory findings include an elevated free thyroxine (T_4) level and a suppressed serum thyroid-stimulating hormone (TSH) level (Diehl, 1998; Seely & Burrow, 1999). Mild hyperthyroidism is not thought to impair fertility, although it is rare to find severe disease in early pregnancy. Hyperthyroidism should be treated during pregnancy; untreated or inadequately treated women give birth to infants with low birth weight and more minor fetal anomalies. Women with hyperthyroidism also are at increased risk to have severe preeclampsia (Diehl, 1998; Seely & Burrow, 1999). Hyperemesis gravidarum is often associated with elevated thyroid hormone levels (Mestman, 2002; Seely & Burrow, 1999).

The primary treatment of hyperthyroidism during pregnancy is drug therapy; the medication of choice is propylthiouracil (PTU). The usual starting dose is 100 to 150 mg every 8 hours. Clients generally show clinical improvement within 2 weeks of beginning therapy, but the medication requires 6 to 8 weeks to reach full effectiveness. During therapy, the woman's free T_4 levels are measured monthly and the results used to taper the drug to the smallest effective dosage to prevent unnecessary fetal hypothyroidism (Diehl, 1998; Mestman, 2002; Seely & Burrow, 1999). PTU is well tolerated by most clients. Rare side effects include pruritus, skin rash, fever, a metallic taste, nausea, bronchospasm, oral ulcerations, hepatitis, and a lupus-like syndrome (Seely & Burrow, 1999). The most severe side effect is agranulocytosis, which is more common in women older than 40 years and in those taking high doses of PTU (Seely & Burrow, 1999). Symptoms of agranulocytosis are fever and sore throat; these symptoms should be reported immediately to the health care provider, and the woman should stop taking the PTU. Transient, benign leukopenia may occur as a result of PTU therapy. PTU readily crosses the placenta and may induce fetal hypothyroidism and goiter (Mestman, 2002; Seely & Burrow, 1999).

Beta-adrenergic blockers such as propranolol may be used in severe hyperthyroidism. Long-term use is not recommended because of the potential for IUGR and altered response to anoxic stress, postnatal bradycardia, and hypoglycemia (Seely & Burrow, 1999).

Radioactive iodine must not be used in diagnosis or treatment of hyperthyroidism in pregnancy because it may compromise the fetal thyroid. If a mother taking hyperthyroid medication chooses to breastfeed, she should be aware that physiologically significant doses of the drug are passed to the infant through the breast milk. The infant's thyroid status should be monitored periodically so that hypothyroidism can be prevented (Seely & Burrow, 1999).

In severe cases, surgical treatment of hyperthyroidism, subtotal thyroidectomy, may be performed during the second or third trimester. Because of the increased risk of miscarriage and preterm labor associated with major surgery, this treatment is usually reserved for women with severe disease, those for whom drug therapy proves toxic, and those who are unable to adhere to the prescribed medical regimen. Postoperative hypothyroidism is common, occurring in at least 20% of women who were previously hyperthyroid.

NURSE ALERT

A serious but uncommon complication of undiagnosed or partially treated hyperthyroidism is thyroid storm, which may occur in response to stress such as infection, birth, or surgery. A woman with this emergency disorder may have fever, restlessness, tachycardia, vomiting, hypotension, or stupor. Congestive heart failure frequently occurs. Prompt treatment is essential; IV fluids and oxygen are administered along with high doses of PTU. Potassium iodide, antipyretics, glucocorticoids, and beta-adrenergic blockers also may be given; sedation may be necessary for extreme restlessness (Inzucchi & Burrow, 1999; Mestman, 2002).

Hypothyroidism

Hypothyroidism during pregnancy is a rare phenomenon because women with this disorder are often infertile. Hypothyroidism is usually caused by Hashimoto disease, thyroid gland ablation by radiation, previous surgery, or antithyroid medications. Reduced thyroid function resulting from hypothalamic or pituitary failure is rare, with only a few reported cases. Iodine deficiency in the United States also is rare (Diehl, 1998; Mestman, 2002).

Characteristic symptoms of hypothyroidism include weight gain; fatigue; cold intolerance; constipation; cool, dry skin; coarsened hair; and muscle weakness. Laboratory values in pregnancy include low or low-normal T_3 and T_4 levels and elevated levels of TSH (Diehl, 1998; Inzucchi & Burrow, 1999).

Pregnant women with untreated hypothyroidism are at risk for preeclampsia, placental abruption, and stillbirth. Infants born to mothers with hypothyroidism may be of low birth weight, but for the most part are healthy and without evidence of thyroid dysfunction (Diehl, 1998; Inzucchi & Burrow, 1999).

Thyroid hormone supplements are used to treat hypothyroidism. Levothyroxine (e.g., L-thyroxine [Synthroid]) is most often prescribed during pregnancy. The usual beginning dosage is 0.10 mg to 0.15 mg per day, in a single daily dose. The aim of drug therapy is to maintain the woman's TSH level within the normal range for pregnant women.

Dosage adjustments are made as necessary by measuring the woman's TSH levels periodically throughout pregnancy. Each dosage change should be followed by determining the TSH level 4 to 6 weeks later. Any woman with hypothyroidism who becomes pregnant should have her thyroid status checked as soon as pregnancy is confirmed. If her TSH level is normal, no dosage adjustment is necessary, although periodic determinations throughout pregnancy are recommended (Diehl, 1998; Inzucchi & Burrow, 1999).

NURSE ALERT

If taking iron supplementation, pregnant women should be told to take L-thyroxine 2 hours before or after iron tablets, because ferrous sulfate lowers the effectiveness of the medication (Diehl, 1998).

The fetus depends on maternal thyroid hormones until 12 weeks of gestation, when fetal production begins; thus maternal hypothyroidism does not cause fetal hypothyroidism. However, maternal treatment of hypothyroidism may result in increased fetal levels of thyroid hormones. Careful monitoring of the neonate's thyroid status is important to detect any abnormalities.

Collaborative Care

The pregnant woman with thyroid dysfunction often needs assistance from the nurse in coping with the discomforts and frustrations associated with symptoms of the disorder. For example, the woman with hyperthyroidism who has nervousness and hyperactivity concomitant with weakness and fatigue may benefit from suggestions to channel excess energies into quiet diversional activities such as reading or crafts. Discomfort associated with hypersensitivity to heat (hyperthyroidism) or cold intolerance (hypothyroidism) can be minimized by appropriate clothing and regulation of environmental temperatures, when possible, and by avoidance of temperature extremes.

Nutritional counseling with a registered dietitian may provide guidance in selecting a well-balanced diet. The woman with hyperthyroidism who has increased appetite and poor weight gain and the hypothyroid woman who has anorexia and lethargy need counseling to ensure adequate intake of nutritionally sound foods to meet both maternal and fetal needs.

Education of these women is essential to promote compliance with the plan of treatment. The woman is instructed regarding the disorder and its potential impact on herself and her fetus, the medication regimen and possible side effects, the need for continuing medical supervision, and the importance of compliance.

Psychologic and emotional implications of pregnancy complicated by thyroid dysfunction are similar to those of any high risk pregnancy. The woman is encouraged to verbalize feelings, concerns, and frustrations and is assisted in identifying support systems. The family is incorporated into the plan of care to foster mutuality and support among the members.

MATERNAL PHENYLKETONURIA

Phenylketonuria (PKU), a recognized cause of mental retardation, is an inborn error of metabolism caused by an autosomal recessive trait that creates a deficiency in the enzyme phenylalanine hydrolase. Absence of this enzyme impairs the body's ability to metabolize the amino acid phenylalanine, found in all protein foods. Consequently, there is toxic accumulation of phenylalanine in the blood, which interferes with brain development and function and also causes hypopigmented hair, eyes, and skin. PKU affects 1 in every 10,000 to 15,000 Caucasian infants (Cunningham et al., 2001).

PKU was the first inborn error of metabolism to be universally screened for in the United States. Beginning in 1961, all newborns were tested soon after birth for this disorder. Prompt diagnosis and therapy with a phenylalanine-restricted diet significantly decreased the incidence of mental retardation. Children with PKU were treated with the special diet up to age 6 years; after that time, further treatment was thought to be unnecessary (Luke, 1999). However, subtle but detrimental effects of elevated levels of phenylalanine on neurologic, behavioral, and intellectual function have been found in women who discontinued treatment in childhood; therefore dietary therapy for PKU has been recommended for continuation indefinitely (Cunningham et al., 2001).

Many women with PKU reach their childbearing years and start families. To have the best possible pregnancy outcomes, they must resume special dietary therapy before conception, although even then, a normal child cannot be guaranteed (Aminoff, 1999; Worthington-Roberts, 2000). Women with untreated PKU have an increased risk of miscarriage, and their children are more likely to be born with mental retardation, microcephaly, congenital heart disease, and low birth weight. These problems result from high maternal PKU levels, which cross the placenta and are teratogenic to the developing fetus (Aminoff, 1999; Luke, 1999).

The key to prevention of fetal anomalies caused by PKU is the identification of women in their reproductive years who have the disorder. Screening programs in the premarital period and even earlier, such as during school physical examinations, may help identify those individuals with PKU so that dietary therapy can be instituted before conception occurs. Before conception, these women and their families should be educated about the potential risks to the fetus if phenylalanine levels are not controlled.

Screening for undiagnosed maternal PKU at the first prenatal visit may be warranted, especially in individuals with a family history of the disorder, with low intelligence of uncertain etiology, or who have given birth to microcephalic infants. Ultrasound scans may be used to monitor fetal growth and identify anomalies. Although it may be too late to improve the current pregnancy outcome through diet therapy, the woman and her family will be aware of the problem and the necessary treatment should future pregnancies occur (Aminoff, 1999).

Infants born to women with PKU will either be homozygous or heterozygous for the trait. Homozygous infants definitely need phenylalanine-restricted diet therapy. Proper nutritional management of heterozygous infants is less clear. Women with PKU have been discouraged from breastfeeding because their milk contains a high concentration of phenylalanine (Aminoff, 1999). However, breastfeeding can be done safely if the amount of breast milk ingested is monitored so that phenylalanine levels do not get too high. Mothers who choose to breastfeed must still supplement the infant's diet with a special milk preparation that contains little or no phenylalanine. Monitoring amounts of phenylalanine can be tedious and frustrating. Health care providers can help parents in their decision making about how to feed their infant (Kirby, 1999).

KEY POINTS

- Lack of maternal glycemic control before conception and in the first trimester of pregnancy may be responsible for fetal congenital malformations.
- Maternal insulin requirements increase as the pregnancy progresses and may quadruple by term as a result of insulin resistance created by placental hormones, insulinase, and cortisol. At birth, levels decrease dramatically; breastfeeding will affect insulin needs.
- Poor glycemic control before and during pregnancy can lead to maternal complications such as miscarriage, infection, and dystocia caused by fetal macrosomia.
- Careful glucose monitoring, insulin administration when necessary, and dietary counseling are used to create a normal intrauterine environment for fetal growth and development in the pregnancy complicated by diabetes mellitus.
- Because gestational diabetes mellitus is asymptomatic in most cases, many women undergo routine screening during pregnancy.
- Hyperemesis gravidarum is frequently managed at home. The woman should receive IV fluids and electrolytes and remain on NPO status until nausea and vomiting have stopped. She can then slowly advance her diet as tolerated.
- Thyroid dysfunction during pregnancy requires close monitoring of thyroid hormone levels to regulate therapy and prevent fetal insult.
- High levels of PKU in the maternal bloodstream cross the placenta and are teratogenic to the developing fetus. Damage can be prevented or minimized by dietary restriction of phenylalanine before and during pregnancy.

CRITICAL THINKING EXERCISES

1. Janet, who has been a diabetic for more than 20 years, is admitted to your unit for blood sugar control at 26 weeks' gestation. About 4:30 PM, she calls the nurses' station and sounds hostile as she complains of having a headache and feeling "nervous."
   - **a.** What is the most likely cause of Janet's symptoms?
   - **b.** What assessments would you need to make to confirm your diagnosis?
   - **c.** What treatment measures would you institute? How could you determine if your treatment was effective?
2. Barbara goes to the Emergency Department by ambulance at 10 weeks' gestation with intractable nausea and vomiting.
   - **a.** What are possible causes for Barbara's nausea and vomiting?
   - **b.** What assessments will likely be ordered to diagnose the cause of Barbara's illness?
   - **c.** Assuming that Barbara is diagnosed with hyperemesis gravidarum, what orders would you expect to receive for her?
   - **d.** When Barbara's is again able to eat solid food, what advice would best help her avoid further vomiting?
3. Toni comes to the clinic for her yearly Pap smear. She has just been married, and she and her husband are anxious to start a family right away Toni tells you that she has PKU but has not followed a special diet since she was "just a little girl."
   - **a.** What dietary changes would you recommend before Toni attempts pregnancy?
   - **b.** Would your advice be different if Toni were already 6 weeks pregnant?

RESOURCES

American Diabetes Association
Diabetes Information Service Center
1660 Duke St.
Alexandria, VA 22314
800-342-2383
www.diabetes.org

COPE (Coping with the Overall Pregnancy/Parenting Experience)
37 Clarendon St.
Boston, MA 02116
617-357-5588

March of Dimes Birth Defects Foundation
1275 Mamaroneck Ave.
White Plains, NY 10605
914-428-7100
888-663-4637
www.modimes.org

Pregnancy and Infant Loss
1421 East Wayzata Blvd., Suite 40
Wayzata, MN 55391
614-473-9372

REFERENCES

American College of Obstetricians and Gynecologists. (1995). *Preconceptional care. ACOG Technical Bulletin Number 205,* Washington, DC: ACOG.

American College of Obstetricians and Gynecologists. (2001). *Gestational diabetes. ACOG Practice Bulletin Number 30.* Washington, DC: ACOG.

American Diabetes Association. (1998). *Medical management of type 1 diabetes* (3rd ed.). Alexandria, VA: The Association.

American Diabetes Association. (2000). *Medical management of pregnancy complicated by diabetes* (3rd ed.). Alexandria, VA: The Association.

American Diabetes Association. (2003). Position statement: Gestational diabetes mellitus. *Diabetes Care, 26*(suppl 1), S103-S105.

Aminoff, M. (1999). Neurologic disorders. In R. Creasy & R. Resnik (Eds.), *Maternal-fetal medicine* (4th ed.). Philadelphia: W.B. Saunders.

Beal, M. (1998). Women's use of complementary and alternative therapies in reproductive health care. *Journal of Nurse Midwifery, 43*(3), 224-234.

Becton Dickinson & Co. (1997). *Controlling low blood sugar reactions.* Franklin Lakes, NJ: Becton Dickinson & Co.

Cefalo, R., & Moos, M. (1995). *Preconceptional health care: A practical guide.* St. Louis: Mosby.

Cunningham, F. et al. (2001). *Williams obstetrics* (21st ed.). New York: McGraw-Hill.

Diehl, K. (1998). Thyroid dysfunction in pregnancy. *Journal of Perinatal and Neonatal Nursing, 11*(4), 1-12.

Expert Committee on the Diagnosis and Classification of Diabetes Mellitus. (2003). Report of the Expert Committee on the Diagnosis and Classification of Diabetes Mellitus. *Diabetes Care, 26*(suppl 1), S5-S20.

Gilbert, E., & Harmon, J. (2003). *Manual of high risk pregnancy and delivery* (3rd ed.). St. Louis: Mosby.

Gordon, M. (2002). Maternal physiology in pregnancy. In S. Gabbe, J. Niebyl, & J. Simpson (Eds.), *Obstetrics: Normal and problem pregnancies* (4th ed.). New York: Churchill Livingstone.

Hagay, A., & Reece, E. (1999). Diabetes mellitus in pregnancy. In E. Reece & J. Hobbins (Eds.), *Medicine of the fetus and mother* (2nd ed.). Philadelphia: Lippincott-Raven.

Hill, W., & Fleming, A. (1999). Gastrointestinal diseases complicating pregnancy. In E. Reece & J. Hobbins (Eds.), *Medicine of the fetus and mother* (2nd ed.). Philadelphia: Lippincott-Raven.

Inzucchi, S. (1999). Diabetes in pregnancy. In G. Burrow & T. Duffy (Eds.), *Medical complications during pregnancy* (5th ed.). Philadelphia: W.B. Saunders.

Inzucchi, S., & Burrow, G. (1999). Endocrine disorders in pregnancy. In E. Reece & J. Hobbins (Eds.), *Medicine of the fetus and mother* (2nd ed.). Philadelphia: Lippincott-Raven.

Jones, M., & Stone, L. (1998). Management of the woman with gestational diabetes mellitus. *Journal of Perinatal and Neonatal Nursing, 11(4)*, 13-24.

Kirby, R. (1999). Maternal phenylketonuria: A new cause for concern. *Journal of Obstetric, Gynecologic, and Neonatal Nursing, 28*(3), 227-234.

Korenbrot, C. et al. (2002). Preconception care: A systematic review. *Maternal and Child Health Journal, 6*(2), 75-88.

Landon, M.B., Catalano, P.M., & Gabbe, S.G. (2002). Diabetes mellitus. In S. Gabbe, J. Niebyl, & J. Simpson (Eds.), *Obstetrics: Normal and problem pregnancies* (4th ed.). New York: Churchill Livingstone.

Langer, O. (2000). Diabetes. In W. Cohen (Ed.), *Cherry and Merkatz's complications of pregnancy* (5th ed.). Philadelphia: Lippincott Williams & Wilkins.

Langer, O. et al. (2000). A comparison of glyburide and insulin in women with gestational diabetes mellitus. *New England Journal of Medicine, 343*, 1134-1138.

Lowdermilk, D., & Grohar, J. (1998). *High risk antepartal home care.* White Plains, NY: March of Dimes.

Luke, B. (1999). Maternal nutrition. In E. Reece & J. Hobbins (Eds.), *Medicine of the fetus and mother* (2nd ed.). Philadelphia: Lippincott-Raven.

Mestman, J. (2002). Endocrine diseases in pregnancy. In S. Gabbe, J. Niebyl, & J. Simpson (Eds.), *Obstetrics: Normal and problem pregnancies* (4th ed.). New York: Churchill Livingstone.

Metzger, B., & Coustan, D. (1998). Summary and recommendations of the fourth international workshop-conference on gestational diabetes mellitus. *Diabetes Care, 21*(suppl 2), B161-B167.

Moore, T. (1999). Diabetes in pregnancy. In R. Creasy & R. Resnik (Eds.), *Maternal-fetal medicine* (4th ed.). Philadelphia: W.B. Saunders.

Pagana, K., & Pagana, T. (2002). *Mosby's manual of diagnostic and laboratory tests* (2nd ed.). St. Louis: Mosby.

Riely, C. (1999). Liver diseases in pregnancy. In E. Reece & J. Hobbins (Eds.), *Medicine of the fetus and mother* (2nd ed.). Philadelphia: Lippincott-Raven.

Seely, L., & Burrow, G. (1999). Thyroid disease and pregnancy. In R. Creasy & R. Resnik (Eds.), *Maternal-fetal medicine* (4th ed.). Philadelphia: W.B. Saunders.

Snell, L. et al. (1998). Metabolic crisis: Hyperemesis gravidarum. *Journal of Perinatal and Neonatal Nursing, 12*(2), 26-37.

Steinlauf, A., & Traube, M. (1999). Gastrointestinal complications. In G. Burrow & T. Duffy (Eds.), *Medical complications during pregnancy* (5th ed.). Philadelphia: W.B. Saunders.

Worthington-Roberts, B. (2000). Nutrition. In W. Cohen (Ed.), *Cherry and Merkatz's complications of pregnancy* (5th ed.). Philadelphia: Lippincott Williams & Wilkins.

CHAPTER 33

Jane McAteer

Medical-Surgical Problems in Pregnancy

http://evolve.elsevier.com/Lowdermilk/MatWmnHlth/

LEARNING OBJECTIVES

- Describe the management of cardiovascular disorders in pregnant women.
- Identify nursing interventions for the pregnant woman with a cardiovascular disorder.
- Discuss anemia during pregnancy.
- Explain the care of pregnant women with pulmonary disorders.
- Examine the effect of a gastrointestinal disorder on gastrointestinal function during pregnancy.
- Identify the effects of neurologic disorders on pregnancy.
- Describe the care of women whose pregnancies are complicated by autoimmune disorders.
- Delineate the basic principles of care for a pregnant woman having surgery.

The effects of selected preexisting medical disorders on pregnancy and the nursing care that can lead to their effective management are presented in this chapter. These disorders, including cardiovascular, respiratory, gastrointestinal (GI), integumentary, and central nervous system (CNS) disorders, are sometimes first diagnosed during pregnancy. Abdominal surgery and the related nursing roles also are discussed.

CARDIOVASCULAR DISORDERS

During a normal pregnancy, the maternal cardiovascular system undergoes many changes that put a physiologic strain on the heart. The major cardiovascular changes that occur during a normal pregnancy and that affect the woman with cardiac disease are increased intravascular volume, decreased systemic vascular resistance, cardiac output changes occurring during labor and birth, and the intravascular volume changes that occur just after childbirth. The strain is present during pregnancy and continues for a few weeks after birth. The normal heart can compensate for the increased workload so that pregnancy, labor, and birth are generally well tolerated, but the diseased heart is hemodynamically challenged.

If the cardiovascular changes are not well tolerated, cardiac failure can develop during pregnancy, labor, or the postpartum period. In addition, if myocardial disease develops, valvular disease exists, or a congenital heart defect is present, **cardiac decompensation** (inability of the heart to maintain a sufficient cardiac output) is anticipated.

About 1% of pregnancies are complicated by heart disease (Cunningham et al., 2001), the leading cause of nonobstetric maternal mortality. Rheumatic fever is responsible for about 50% of cardiac complications; congenital diseases and mitral valve disease are the next most common causes. Other cardiac diseases are uncommon (Gilbert & Harmon, 2003). Cardiac disease ranks fourth overall as a cause of maternal death. A perinatal mortality of up to 50% is anticipated with persistent cardiac decompensation. See Box 33-1 for maternal cardiac disease risk groups.

The degree of disability experienced by the woman with cardiac disease is often more important in the treatment and prognosis of cardiac disease complicating pregnancy than is the diagnosis of cardiovascular disease. The New York Heart Association's (NYHA) (1964) functional classification of organic heart disease, a widely accepted standard, is as follows:

Class I: Asymptomatic at normal levels of activity
Class II: Symptomatic with increased activity
Class III: Symptomatic with ordinary activity
Class IV: Symptomatic at rest

No classification of heart disease can be considered rigid or absolute, but the NYHA classification offers a basic practical guide for treatment, assuming that frequent prenatal visits, good client cooperation, and appropriate obstetric care occur. Medical therapy is conducted by a team approach, including the cardiologist, obstetrician, and nurses. The functional classification may change for the pregnant woman because of the hemodynamic

BOX 33-1 Maternal Cardiac Disease Risk Groups

GROUP I (MORTALITY 1%)
- Corrected tetralogy of Fallot
- Pulmonic/tricuspid disease
- Mitral stenosis (classes I, II)
- Patent ductus arteriosus
- Ventricular septal defect
- Atrial septal defect
- Porcine valve

GROUP II (MORTALITY 5%-15%)
- Mitral stenosis with atrial fibrillation
- Artificial heart valves
- Mitral stenosis (classes III, IV)
- Uncorrected tetralogy of Fallot
- Aortic coarctation (uncomplicated)
- Aortic stenosis
- Marfan syndrome with normal aorta

GROUP III (MORTALITY 25%-50%)
- Aortic coarctation (complicated)
- Myocardial infarction (previous)
- Marfan syndrome with aortic involvement
- Pulmonary hypertension

From Gilbert, E., & Harmon, J. (2003). *Manual of high risk pregnancy and delivery* (3rd ed.). St. Louis: Mosby.

BOX 33-2 Contraindications to Pregnancy in a Woman with Heart Disease

- Pulmonary hypertension
- Shunt lesions associated with Eisenmenger syndrome
- Complex cyanotic congenital heart disease
- Aortic coarctation complicated by aortic dissection
- Poor ventricular function
- Marfan syndrome with marked aortic dilation

Adapted from Mendelson, M. (1997). Congenital cardiac disease and pregnancy. *Clinical Perinatology 24*(2), 467-482.

changes that occur in the cardiovascular system. A 30% to 50% increase in cardiac output occurs compared with nonpregnancy resting values, with most of the increase in the first trimester and the peak at 20 to 24 weeks of gestation (Cunningham et al., 2001). The functional classification of the disease is determined at 3 months and again at 7 or 8 months of gestation. Pregnant women may progress from class I or II to III or IV during the pregnancy. Women with cyanotic congenital heart disease do not fit into the NYHA classification because their exercise-induced symptoms have causes not related to heart failure. An Ability Index was developed for assessment of these clients (Gei & Hankins, 2001).

Contraindications to pregnancy in women with heart disease are listed in Box 33-2. The incidence of miscarriage is increased, and preterm labor and birth are more prevalent in the pregnant woman with cardiac problems. In addition, *intrauterine growth restriction (IUGR)* (impeded or delayed development of the fetus) is common, probably because of low oxygen pressure (Po_2) in the mother.

The incidence (4% to 16%) of congenital heart lesions is increased in children of mothers with congenital heart disease; thus preconception counseling is important (Mendelson, 1997).

A diagnosis of cardiac disease depends on the history, physical examination, radiographic findings, and, if indicated, ultrasonogram results. The differential diagnosis of heart disease also involves ruling out respiratory problems and other potential causes of chest pain.

Maternal mortality of more than 50% during pregnancy has been associated with pulmonary hypertension; it is vital that the woman with cardiac disease be assessed and the diagnosis established as soon as possible (Mendelson, 1997).

ASSOCIATED CARDIOVASCULAR DISORDERS

Nursing care of the woman with a cardiovascular disorder combines routine peripartum care with care specific for the cardiac diagnosis. Cardiac diseases vary in their impact on pregnancy because of acuteness or chronicity. The following discussion focuses first on congenital cardiac diseases, such as septal defects, patent ductus arteriosus, and cyanotic and acyanotic lesions. The second group of cardiac diseases are acquired diseases, specifically mitral stenosis, aortic stenosis, ischemic heart disease, and other cardiac diseases (pulmonary hypertension, Marfan syndrome, peripartum cardiomyopathy, and presence of artificial valves). A review of the care of the pregnant woman who has had a heart transplant concludes the discussion.

Congenital Cardiac Disease

Septal Defects

Atrial septal defect (ASD; abnormal opening between the atria), one of the causes of a left-to-right shunt, is the most common congenital defect seen during pregnancy. This defect may go undetected because the woman usually is asymptomatic. The pregnant woman with an ASD will most likely have an uncomplicated pregnancy. Some women may have right-sided heart failure or arrhythmias as the pregnancy progresses as a result of increased plasma volume.

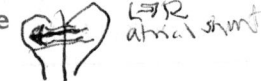

Ventricular septal defect (VSD; abnormal opening between the right and left ventricles), another cause of a left-to-right shunt, is usually diagnosed and corrected during infancy or childhood. As a result, a VSD is not very common in pregnancy. Women with a small uncomplicated VSD usually do not have pregnancy complications. For women with a large VSD, there is a higher risk for arrhythmias, heart failure, and pulmonary hypertension. Medical management includes rest and decrease of physical activity, as well as administration of anticoagulants.

Patent ductus arteriosus (PDA) is a cause of another left-to-right shunt that is usually diagnosed and corrected during infancy. Possible complications of a PDA include those of VSD as well as endocarditis and pulmonary emboli. Medical management is the same as for VSD.

Mortality rates for shunt defects are reported to be less than 1% (Gei & Hankins, 2001).

Acyanotic Lesions

Coarctation of the aorta (localized narrowing of the aorta near the insertion of the ductus) is an example of an acyanotic congenital heart lesion. Pregnancy is usually safe for the mother with uncomplicated coarctation (Warnes & Elkayam, 1998). Complications that can occur include hypertension, congestive heart failure, and aortic rupture. The mainstays of treatment for uncorrected coarctation of the aorta during pregnancy are rest and antihypertensive medications, preferably beta-adrenergic blocking agents. Vaginal birth is possible with epidural anesthesia and shortening of the second stage with vacuum extraction or use of forceps, if necessary. Beta-blockers should be continued throughout labor. Because of the risk of endocarditis, antibiotic prophylaxis is recommended at birth (see later discussion).

Cyanotic Lesions

Tetralogy of Fallot is the most common cyanotic heart disease present during pregnancy. Other cyanotic congenital heart diseases are rarely seen during pregnancy because women with these conditions rarely survive to adulthood. Components of tetralogy of Fallot include a VSD, pulmonary stenosis, overriding aorta, and right ventricular hypertrophy, leading to a right-to-left shunt. Women with corrected tetralogy of Fallot have less than 1% mortality; however, women with uncorrected tetralogy of Fallot have a 5% to 15% mortality rate (Gei & Hankins, 2001). Medical management for women with uncorrected tetralogy of Fallot includes anticoagulant therapy, high-concentration oxygen administration, and hemodynamic monitoring during labor and birth.

Acquired Cardiac Disease

Mitral Stenosis

Mitral valve stenosis (narrowing of the opening of the mitral valve caused by stiffening of valve leaflets, which obstructs blood flow from the atrium to the ventricles) is the characteristic lesion resulting from rheumatic heart disease (RHD) (Shabetai, 1999). Even though a history of rheumatic fever may be absent, it remains the most likely cause of mitral stenosis. As the mitral valve narrows, dyspnea worsens, occurring first on exertion and eventually at rest. A tight stenosis plus the increase in blood volume and thus cardiac output of normal pregnancy may cause ventricular failure and pulmonary edema; hemoptysis may occur. Maternal mortality rate in classes III and IV can be as high as 5%, and as high as 15% if atrial fibrillation occurs (Meller & Goldman, 2000).

Atrial fibrillation can precipitate a decrease in the cardiac output. Digoxin, a beta-adrenergic blocking agent, or a calcium channel–blocker agent may be needed to maintain a normal heart rate. A combination of these agents may be needed. In addition, anticoagulant therapy may be needed (Shabetai, 1999). About 25% of women with mitral valve stenosis may become symptomatic for the first time during pregnancy (Ramsey, Ramin, & Ramin, 2001). The care of the woman with mitral stenosis typically is managed by reducing her activity, restricting dietary sodium, and increasing bed rest. The pregnant woman with mitral stenosis should be monitored clinically for symptoms and with echocardiograms to monitor the atrial and ventricular size, as well as heart valve function. Prophylaxis for intrapartum endocarditis and pulmonary infections may be provided for women at high risk (Easterling & Otto, 2002) (Box 33-3).

Beta-blockers may be used to blunt heart rate response to exercise and anxiety. Effects of these drugs to the unstressed fetus are considered minimal, but in the stressed fetus, the response to fetal distress may be impaired (Hurst et al., 1998). Epidural analgesia for labor is preferred (Essop & Sareli, 1998). Even with close monitoring, the woman with moderate to severe mitral stenosis is at risk for pulmonary edema, right heart failure, and hypotension (Essop & Sareli, 1998). Intensive invasive

---

BOX 33-3 **Prophylaxis for Bacterial Endocarditis During Labor and Birth**

HIGH RISK CLIENTS

In active labor: ampicillin 2 g IV or IM plus gentamicin 1.5 mg/kg (not to exceed 120 mg)

6 hours later: ampicillin 1 g IV or IM or amoxacillin 1 g PO

Penicillin-Allergic Clients

In active labor: vancomycin 1 g IV over 1 to 2 hr plus gentamicin as above

MODERATE RISK CLIENTS

In active labor: amoxicillin 2 g PO or ampicillin 2 g IV or IM

Penicillin-Allergic Clients

In active labor: vancomycin 1 g IV over 1-2 hr

Sources: Dajani, A. et al. (1997). Prevention of bacterial endocarditis: Recommendation by the American Heart Association. *Journal of the American Medical Association, 277*, 1794-1801; Easterling, T., & Otto, C. (2002). Heart disease. In S. Gabbe, J. Niebyl, & J. Simpson (Eds.), *Obstetrics: Normal and problem pregnancies* (4th ed.). New York: Churchill-Livingstone.

pulmonary artery catheter monitoring should continue through labor, birth, and the postpartum period because fluid shifts can place the woman at risk for pulmonary edema (Kleinman, 1999).

For clients with NYHA class III or IV cardiac disease, mitral balloon valvuloplasty can be considered. This procedure should be considered only when symptoms cannot be controlled by standard means. Mitral balloon valvuloplasty is optimally performed after 20 weeks' gestation to decrease radiation risks to the fetus. Closed mitral valvotomy is an acceptable alternative if balloon valvuloplasty cannot be performed. Clients with pulmonary edema, hypotension, and right heart failure will require aggressive medical management with diuretics, beta-blockers, and digoxin. Mitral balloon valvuloplasty or closed mitral valvulotomy also may be considered. A fetal mortality of 10% to 30% is found for procedures requiring cardiopulmonary bypass (Essop & Sareli, 1998).

Aortic Stenosis

Aortic stenosis (narrowing of the opening of the aortic valve leading to an obstruction to left ventricular ejection) is rarely encountered as a complication of pregnancy. This defect is found more often in men than in women, and severe stenosis is uncommon in childbearing-age women (Comport & Seng, 1997). The reported maternal mortality rate is 17% (Essop & Sareli, 1998). Medical management is similar to that for mitral stenosis.

Ischemic Heart Disease

Myocardial infarction (MI; an acute ischemic event) is a rare event in childbearing-age women, estimated to occur in only 1 in 10,000 women during pregnancy (Roth & Elkayam, 1998). It is anticipated that the occurrence will increase, considering that an increase in the age of childbearing women and other risk factors such as stress, smoking, and cocaine use are increasing. Other risk factors for coronary artery disease that may affect childbearing women are familial hyperlipidemia, diabetes mellitus, family history of coronary artery disease, hypertension, multiple gestation, sickle cell anemia, and the use of oral contraceptives (Easterling & Otto, 2002; Kleinman, 1999). Finally, the cardiac changes that normally occur in a pregnant woman may provoke symptoms for the first time.

MI occurs most frequently in the last trimester and in women older than 32 years (Mendelson & Lang, 2000). Maternal mortality rates from MIs during pregnancy range from 19% to 35% (Poppas, 2000). Women who have MIs during pregnancy or the postpartum period should be assessed for thrombophilias (deficiency of proteins involved in coagulation inhibition), such as antiphospholipid antibody.

Medical management for pregnant women with MI is the same as for the nonpregnant woman and includes the administration of oxygen, aspirin, beta-blockers, nitrates, and heparin. Women who have had symptomatic cardiac disease during the pregnancy should continue cardiac medications and receive oxygen during labor. Because pain can lead to tachycardia and increased cardiac demands, pain control during labor is crucial. The side-lying position is preferred to avoid pressure on the vena cava. Vaginal birth is preferable, with avoidance of maternal pushing and a vacuum- or forceps-assisted birth. Postpartum diuretics usually are given (Easterling & Otto, 2002).

Other Cardiac Diseases

Pulmonary Hypertension. Women with **primary pulmonary hypertension (PPH)** have constriction of the arteriolar vessels in the lungs, leading to increase in the pulmonary artery pressure. As a result of this pathology, there is right ventricular hypertension, right ventricular hypertrophy and dilation, and finally, right ventricular failure with tricuspid regurgitation and systemic congestion.

Woman with PPH are usually young and have an increased incidence of Raynaud phenomenon. A connection may be found with recurrent pulmonary embolism, appetite suppressants, and cocaine use (Easterling & Otto, 2002; Meller & Goldman, 2000). The woman may have dyspnea, occasional chest pain, fatigue, edema, and ascites. Congestive heart failure may be evidenced by jugular vein distention, hepatomegaly, ascites, and edema.

Diagnostic tests performed are chest radiograph, electrocardiogram, echocardiogram, Doppler studies, and Swan-Ganz catheter. Mortality rates reported during pregnancy are as high as 50%, with half of these deaths occurring during the early postpartum period (Esterling & Otto, 2002). These women should be strongly discouraged from getting pregnant.

Medical management of pregnant women with PPH includes antepartal therapy with oral nifedipine or IV prostacyclin for pulmonary vasodilation; intrapartal intensive hemodynamic monitoring, use of antiembolic stockings, side-lying position, the administration of oxygen, and the use of epidural analgesia to promote hemodynamic stability. Anticoagulant therapy also is indicated to prevent pulmonary embolus. Clients with PPH are considered candidates for heart-lung transplants.

Marfan Syndrome. Marfan syndrome is an autosomal dominant genetic disorder characterized by generalized weakness of the connective tissue, resulting in joint deformities, ocular lens dislocation, and weakness of the aortic wall and root (Mendelson & Lang, 2000). About 90% of individuals with this syndrome have mitral valve prolapse (MVP), and 25% have aortic insufficiency, with an increased risk of aortic dissection and rupture during pregnancy (Mendelson & Lang, 2000). Excruciating chest pain is the most common symptom of aortic dissection. Aortic dissection most often occurs in the third trimester or postpartally (Elkayam et al., 1998). Marfan syndrome also may be responsible for cervical incompetence, placenta previa, and postpartum hemorrhage. Preconception genetic counseling is recommended to make women aware of the risks of pregnancy with this condition, with a 50% risk of inheritance of the syndrome (Mendelson & Lang, 2000). The woman should have baseline data gathered about the aortic root before pregnancy or at the first prenatal visit by noninvasive imaging with transesophageal echocardiography, computed tomography, or magnetic resonance imaging (MRI).

Management during pregnancy includes restricted activity and beta-blockers; surgery may be indicated in some women. Antibiotic prophylaxis is suggested for labor; regional analgesia is well tolerated. Mortality rates may be as high as 50% in women who have significant cardiac disease (Meller & Goldman, 2000).

Infective Endocarditis. **Infective endocarditis** (inflammation of the innermost lining–endocardium–of the heart caused by invasion of microorganisms) is an uncommon disorder during pregnancy (Mendelson & Lang, 2000). It may be seen in women taking IV street drugs. Bacterial endocarditis, leading to incompetence of heart valves and thus congestive heart failure and cerebral emboli, can result in death. Treatment is with antibiotics.

Eisenmenger Syndrome. **Eisenmenger syndrome** is a right-to-left or bidirectional shunting that can be at the atrial or ventricular level and is combined with elevated pulmonary vascular resistance (Easterling & Otto, 2002). The syndrome is associated with high mortality (30% to 50% in mothers and 50% in fetuses), and thus pregnancy is contraindicated (Kansaria & Salvi, 2000). Contraception is essential, and tubal ligation should be considered because oral contraceptives and intrauterine devices carry considerable risk (Mendelson & Lang, 2000). If pregnancy occurs, termination may be recommended if the woman has significant pulmonary hypertension (Easterling & Otto, 2002).

In women who continue pregnancy despite the risks, physical activity is strictly limited; prophylactic anticoagulation is considered (Mendelson & Lang, 2000). During labor and birth, Swan-Ganz monitoring is essential. Central hypovolemia should be avoided. Oxygen therapy is administered. Controversy exists about use of epidural analgesia. If it is used, serial determinations of arterial oxygen concentrations should be done.

Valve Replacement. Pregnant clients with mechanical or tissue prosthetic heart valves require specialized care for this high risk situation. Complications may affect both mother and fetus (Bonow et al., 1998). The primary medical management through the use of anticoagulants is controversial and complicated. A high risk for thromboembolism is present because of the hypercoagulability of pregnancy. In addition, the use of anticoagulants during pregnancy presents the possibility of maternal and fetal hemorrhage. Some oral anticoagulants pose a significant risk to the fetus, such as fetal abnormalities and fetal intracranial hemorrhage. Prosthetic heart valve thrombosis is a life-threatening emergency during pregnancy. This situation requires clot removal surgery, which has a high mortality rate. The use of recombinant tissue-type plasminogen activator (rtPA) has been described as a treatment for thrombosis in pregnancy (Mendelson & Lang, 2000). Women with porcine heterograft valves usually do not require anticoagulation during pregnancy. This type of valve is an ideal replacement for women of childbearing age. A disadvantage of this type of valve is premature valve failure, which may be exacerbated by pregnancy.

The current recommendation for pregnant women with mechanical prosthetic valves is subcutaneous heparin injected every 8 to 12 hours to achieve the goal of activated partial thromboplastin time (aPTT) of 1.5 to 2.0 times the control (Ramsey, Ramin, & Ramin, 2001). It also is recommended that women who are receiving coumadin therapy ideally change to heparin therapy before conception or as soon as possible after conception. The use of low-molecular-weight heparin has the advantage of a longer half-life than heparin, which may allow only daily injections in low risk situations. Low-molecular-weight heparin may prove to be advantageous for pregnant women with valve replacements when more studies confirm its effectiveness. Anticoagulation therapy should be discontinued at the time of active labor and reactivated within 6 hours of vaginal birth or 12 to 24 hours after cesarean birth. Because of the possibility of epidural hematoma, regional analgesia/anesthesia is not recommended.

Nursing care of the pregnant woman with a valve replacement is similar to care for any woman with a cardiac disorder. Emphasis should be placed on teaching the woman how to administer subcutaneous injections and how to monitor for adverse effects of anticoagulant therapy, primarily bleeding.

Peripartum Cardiomyopathy. The classical criteria for the diagnosis of **peripartum cardiomyopathy (PPCM)** include development of congestive heart failure in the last month of pregnancy or within the first 5 postpartum months, lack of another cause for heart failure, and absence of heart disease before the last month of pregnancy (Ramsey, Ramin, & Ramin, 2001). Some data suggest that this definition be expanded, because the diagnosis of PPCM has been made at other times during gestation (Lang et al., 1998). The etiology of the disease is unknown; theories suggest genetic predisposition, autoimmunity, and viral infections.

Associated risk factors include maternal age older than 35 years, multifetal gestation, preeclampsia, gestational hypertension, multiparity, and African-American race (Ramsey et al., 2001). Incidence is reported as 1 in 3000 to 1 in 4000 live births in the United States. Maternal mortality has been estimated in the range of 25% to 50% (Ramsey et al., 2001). Clinical findings are those of congestive heart failure (left ventricular failure). Clinical manifestations include dyspnea, fatigue, and edema, as well as radiologic findings of cardiomegaly (Rosene-Montella & Poppas, 2000) (Fig. 33-1). The prognosis is good if cardiomegaly does not persist for 6 months postpartum. There is no agreement on recommendations for future pregnancies; however, the mortality rate is greatly

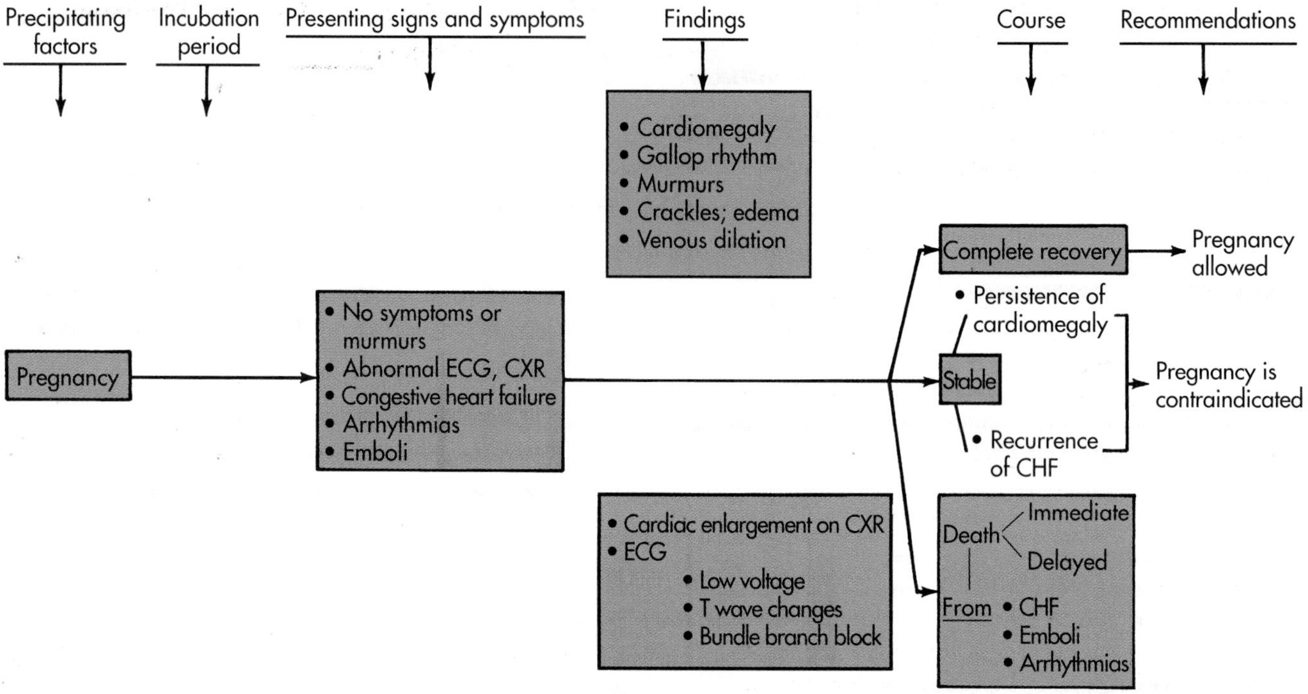
Precipitating factors
Incubation period
Presenting signs and symptoms
Findings
Course
Recommendations
• Cardiomegaly
• Gallop rhythm
• Murmurs
• Crackles; edema
• Venous dilation
Pregnancy
• No symptoms or murmurs
• Abnormal ECG, CXR
• Congestive heart failure
• Arrhythmias
• Emboli
Complete recovery
Pregnancy allowed
• Persistence of cardiomegaly
Stable
Pregnancy is contraindicated
• Recurrence of CHF
• Cardiac enlargement on CXR
• ECG
• Low voltage
• T wave changes
• Bundle branch block
Death
Immediate
Delayed
From
• CHF
• Emboli
• Arrhythmias

FIG. 33-1 Summary of course of peripartum cardiomyopathy. *CHF,* Congestive heart failure; *CXR,* chest x-ray; *ECG,* electrocardiogram.

increased for women whose hearts remain enlarged. PPCM tends to recur in subsequent pregnancies, even if cardiac function stabilizes. Women whose hearts remain enlarged 6 months postpartum will have PPCM in future pregnancies. Pregnancy is contraindicated for women with persistent cardiomegaly or cardiac dysfunction (Ramsey et al., 2001).

Medical management of cardiomyopathy during pregnancy includes a regimen used for congestive heart failure and the potential for thromboembolism: diuretics, sodium restriction, afterload-reducing agents, anticoagulants, and digoxin (Lang et al., 1998). Angiotensin-converting enzyme inhibitors can be used only in the postpartum period, because they are teratogenic agents. The nursing care of women with peripartum cardiomyopathy is essentially the same as for those with other types of cardiac problems.

Heart Transplantation

Increasing numbers of heart recipients are successfully completing pregnancies. Before conception, the woman should be assessed for quality of ventricular function and potential rejection of transplant. The woman should be considered to be stabilized on the immunosuppressant regimen. Conception should be postponed for at least 1 year after transplantation to avoid acute rejection episodes (Ramsey et al., 2001). Risks to the woman include hypertension, preeclampsia, preterm labor, renal insufficiency, small-for-gestational-age neonate, and infections. During labor, beta-blocking agents may be needed to prevent tachycardia due to vagal denervation from the transplant surgery. Vaginal birth is desired, but transplant recipients have an increased rate of cesarean births. Management of the intrapartal period requires the coordination of care among all health care providers involved in the care of the woman and her fetus.

After birth, the neonate may exhibit immunosuppressive effects during the first week of life. Breastfeeding is not advised for infants of mothers taking cyclosporine.

CARE MANAGEMENT

The presence of cardiac disease makes the decision to become pregnant more difficult (see Box 33-2). Planned pregnancy requires that the woman understand the peripartum risks. If the pregnancy is unplanned, the nurse should explore the woman's desire to continue the pregnancy after examining the risks in relation to the status of her cardiac condition. The nurse should review with the woman options for pregnancy termination if her cardiac status is tenuous and abortion is an acceptable alternative. The woman's significant other and family should be included in the discussion. Teaching sessions for the woman and her support people should be offered as indicated by their learning needs.

Care of these women at high risk requires a multidisciplinary approach. The multidisciplinary team includes a cardiologist who is familiar with expected cardiovascular changes in pregnancy; a perinatologist; an anesthesiologist (Mendelson, 1997); and nurses expert in labor and fetal and hemodynamic monitoring.

Assessment and Nursing Diagnoses

The pregnant woman with cardiac disease requires detailed assessment throughout the peripartum period to determine the potential for optimal maternal health and a viable fetus. If she chooses to continue the pregnancy, the high risk pregnant woman's condition may be assessed as often as weekly.

Interview

The nurse solicits information from the woman regarding her personal medical history and that of her family. Special notation is made of diseases of cardiovascular significance, including congenital heart disease, streptococcal infections, rheumatic fever, valvular disease, endocarditis, congestive heart failure, angina, or MI.

The nurse assesses for factors that would increase stress on the heart, such as anemia (see p. 918), infection, and edema. In reviewing for symptoms, the nurse should assess how the woman is adapting to the physiologic changes of pregnancy.

In assessing the pregnant woman with a cardiovascular disorder, special attention is given to the review of the cardiovascular and pulmonary systems. The nurse should determine whether the woman has had chest pain at rest or on exertion; edema of the face, hands, or feet; hypertension; heart murmurs; palpitations; paroxysmal nocturnal dyspnea; diaphoresis; pallor; or syncope. Pulmonary symptoms such as cough, hemoptysis, shortness of breath, and orthopnea also can be signs of cardiac disease. See Table 33-1 for normal and abnormal cardiovascular signs and symptoms during pregnancy.

TABLE 33-1 **Cardiovascular Signs and Symptoms During Pregnancy**

NORMAL	ABNORMAL
Signs	
Neck vein pulsation	Neck vein distention
Diffuse/displaced apical pulse	Cardiomegaly; heave
Split S_1, accentuated S_2	Loud P_2; wide split of S_2
Third heart sound	Summation gallop
Systolic murmur (1-2/6)	Loud systolic murmur (4-6/6)
Venous hum	Diastolic murmur
Sinus dysrhythmia	Sustained dysrhythmia
Peripheral edema	Clubbing/cyanosis
Symptoms	
Fatigue	Symptoms at rest
Chest pain	Exertional chest pain
Dyspnea	Exertional, severe dyspnea
Orthopnea	Orthopnea (progressive)
Hyperpnea	Paroxysmal nocturnal dyspnea
Palpitations	Tachycardia (>120 beats/min); dysrhythmia
Syncope (vasovagal)	Exertional syncope

Adapted from Mendelson, M. (1997). Congenital cardiac disease and pregnancy. *Clinical Perinatology 24*(2), 467-482.

The nurse documents all medication taken by the woman–including over-the-counter (OTC) medications such as supplemental iron–and is alert to their potential side effects and interactions. The woman also is assessed for undue emotional stress that might further compromise cardiac status. Examples of emotional stress are depression, anxiety or fear of morbidity or mortality for herself and the fetus, financial concerns related to extended hospitalization, anger because of impaired social interaction, and feelings of inadequacy regarding her inability to meet family and household demands. Women and their families may have a number of problems associated with the prescription of antepartum bed rest. Reported difficulties include anxiety over not being able to assume role functions, emotional stress for family and children, and financial difficulties (Maloni, Brezinski-Tomasi, & Johnson, 2001).

The woman's cultural background may affect the amount of support she is able to receive from significant others. Family size (number of children and extended family members in the home) as well as role expectations within the family may be dictated by cultural norms. For the woman with cardiac impairment, family expectations may be a cause of major stress if she is unable to bear the expected number of children or if it is unacceptable to receive help with domestic chores. The nurse should be aware of the cultural customs of the pregnant woman and her family.

Physical Examination

Routine assessments continue during the prenatal period, including monitoring the amount and pattern of edema, vital signs, oxygen saturation level, discomforts of pregnancy, and amount and pattern of weight gain. The woman is observed for signs of cardiac decompensation, that is, progressive generalized edema, crackles at the base of the lungs, or pulse irregularity (see Signs of Potential Complications box). Symptoms of cardiac decompensation may appear abruptly or gradually. Medical intervention must be instituted immediately to maintain optimal cardiac status. Dyspnea, palpitations, syncope, and edema occur commonly in pregnant women and can mask the symptoms of a developing or worsening cardiovascular disorder. A woman's sudden inability to perform activities that she previously was comfortable doing may indicate cardiovascular decompensation.

Laboratory and Diagnostic Tests

Routine urinalysis and blood work (complete blood cell count and blood chemistry) are done during the initial visit. The woman with cardiac impairment requires a

SIGNS OF **POTENTIAL COMPLICATIONS**

Cardiac Decompensation

PREGNANT WOMAN: SUBJECTIVE SYMPTOMS

- Increasing fatigue or difficulty breathing, or both, with usual activities
- Feeling of smothering
- Frequent cough
- Palpitations; feeling that her heart is racing
- Swelling of face, feet, legs, fingers (e.g., rings do not fit anymore)

NURSE: OBJECTIVE SIGNS

- Irregular weak, rapid pulse (≥100 beats/min)
- Progressive, generalized edema
- Crackles at base of lungs after two inspirations and exhalations
- Orthopnea; increasing dyspnea
- Rapid respirations (≥25 breaths/min)
- Moist, frequent cough
- Increasing fatigue
- Cyanosis of lips and nail beds

baseline 12-lead electrocardiogram (ECG) at the beginning of her pregnancy, if not before pregnancy, which permits vital diagnostic comparisons of subsequent ECGs. Echocardiograms and pulse oximetry studies may be performed as indicated. Chest films may be necessary during late pregnancy, provided the abdomen is carefully shielded. In addition, fetal ultrasound, fetal movement studies, or fetal nonstress tests may be used to determine fetal well-being.

The following lists nursing diagnoses that may be formulated. As always, individualization of diagnoses is vital.

- *Fear related to*
  - –increased peripartum risk
- *Risk for ineffective individual/family coping related to*
  - –woman's cardiac condition
  - –changes in role performance
- *Risk for altered tissue perfusion related to*
  - –hypotensive syndrome
- *Activity intolerance related to*
  - –cardiac condition
- *Deficient knowledge related to*
  - –cardiac condition
  - –pregnancy and how it affects cardiac condition
  - –medication, dosages and possible side effects
  - –requirements to alter self-care activities
- *Risk for self-care deficit (bathing, grooming, dressing) related to*
  - –fatigue or activity intolerance
  - –need for bed rest
- *Impaired home maintenance related to*
  - –woman's confinement to bed and/or limited activity level

Expected Outcomes of Care

The pregnant woman with cardiovascular problems faces curtailment of her activities. Bed rest during pregnancy affects all of the organ systems, but especially the cardiovascular and musculoskeletal. In addition, psychologic side effects can be debilitating, especially stress (Cunningham, 2001; Maloni et al., 2001). The community health nurse, social worker, and physical or occupational therapist are resource people whose services may be incorporated into the plan of care. Expected outcomes such as the following might be appropriate.

The pregnant woman (and family, if appropriate) will do the following:

- Verbalize understanding of the disorder, management, and probable outcome.
- Describe her role in management, including when and how to take medication, adjust diet, and prepare for and participate in treatment.
- Cope with emotional reactions to pregnancy and infant at risk.
- Adapt to the physiologic stressors of pregnancy and labor and birth.
- Identify and use support systems.
- Carry her fetus to viability or to term.
- Develop no complications in the postpartum period.

Plan of Care and Interventions

Antepartum Care

Therapy for the pregnant woman with heart disease is focused on minimizing stress on the heart, which is greatest between 28 and 32 weeks as the hemodynamic changes reach their maximum. Factors that increase the risk of cardiac decompensation are avoided. The workload of the cardiovascular system is reduced by appropriate treatment of any coexisting emotional stress, hypertension, anemia, hyperthyroidism, or obesity.

Signs and symptoms of cardiac decompensation are reviewed during the prenatal period. The woman with class I or II heart disease requires 8 to 10 hours of sleep every day and should take 30-minute naps after eating. Her activities are restricted, with housework, shopping, and exercise limited to the amount allowed for the functional classification of her heart disease. Information on how to cope with activity limitations is important in meeting the emotional needs of the woman. Referral to a support group may help the woman and her family to handle stress (Lowdermilk & Grohar, 1998).

The pregnant woman with class II cardiac disease should avoid heavy exertion and should stop any activity that causes even minor signs and symptoms of cardiac decompensation. She should also be admitted to the hospital near term (earlier if signs of cardiac overload or dysrhythmia develop) for evaluation and treatment.

Bed rest for much of each day is necessary for pregnant women with class III cardiac disease. About 30% of these women have cardiac decompensation during pregnancy.

With this possibility, a woman may require hospitalization for the remainder of the pregnancy. Because decompensation occurs even at rest in persons with class IV cardiac disease, a major initial effort must be made to improve the cardiac status of the pregnant woman in this category who chooses to continue her pregnancy (Box 33-4).

Infections are treated promptly because respiratory, urinary, or GI tract infections can complicate the condition by accelerating the heart rate and by direct spread of organisms (e.g., streptococci) to the heart structure. The woman should notify her physician at the first sign of infection or exposure to an infection. Vaccination against influenza and pneumococcus may be given. Prophylactic antibiotics against bacterial endocarditis during pregnancy are not recommended by the American Heart Association but may be needed by women with valvular disorders (Easterling & Otto, 2002).

Nutrition counseling is necessary, optimally with the woman's family present. The pregnant woman needs a well-balanced diet with iron and folic acid supplementation, high protein, and adequate calories to gain weight. Iron supplements tend to cause constipation. The pregnant woman should increase her intake of fluids and fiber. A stool softener may be prescribed. It is important that the woman with a cardiac disorder avoid straining during defecation, thus causing the Valsalva maneuver (forced expiration against a closed airway, which when released, causes blood to rush to the heart and overload the cardiac system). If sodium restriction is necessary, the amount should not be less that 2.5 g/day (Gilbert & Harmon, 2003). The woman's intake of potassium is monitored to prevent hypokalemia, especially if she is taking diuretics. A referral to a registered dietitian may be necessary.

Cardiac medications are prescribed as needed for the pregnant woman, with attention to fetal well-being. The physiologic changes that occur during pregnancy, labor, and the postpartum period can significantly alter how drugs are used and excreted by the body. Monitoring of the drug levels during the pregnancy is crucial to maintain effective therapy for the woman while minimizing risk to the fetus (Steinberg et al., 1998). Research on the effects of cardiovascular drugs on the fetus and pregnant woman has been limited. The nurse should review current pharmacologic literature, especially when administering any medication to a pregnant woman (Table 33-2).

Anticoagulant therapy may be needed during pregnancy in various situations, such as recurrent vein thrombosis, pulmonary embolus, rheumatic heart disease, prosthetic valves, or cyanotic congenital heart defects (Gei & Hankins, 2001).

If anticoagulant therapy is required during pregnancy, heparin may be used because this large-molecule drug does not cross the placenta. See the section on valve disorders for more discussion of anticoagulant therapy. The nurse should closely monitor the woman's blood tests, including clotting factors. The woman may need to learn to self-administer heparin. She also requires specific nutritional teaching to avoid foods high in vitamin K, such as raw, dark green, and leafy vegetables, which counteract the effects of the heparin. In addsition, she will require a folic acid supplement.

Tests for fetal maturity and well-being and placental sufficiency may be necessary. Other therapy is directly related to the functional classification of heart disease. The nurse may need to reinforce the need for close medical supervision.

Heart Surgery During Pregnancy. The ideal scenario is for a woman to have surgical correction of the cardiac lesion before pregnancy (Cohen & Castro, 1998); however, cardiac disease is diagnosed for the first time during pregnancy in some women. When medical therapy for a pregnant woman fails, cardiac surgery may be performed. Early in the second trimester is the best time for surgery. The woman, fetus, and uterine activity must be monitored carefully during surgery. Closed cardiac surgery, such as release of a stenotic mitral orifice, can be accomplished with little risk to mother or fetus. Open heart surgery requires

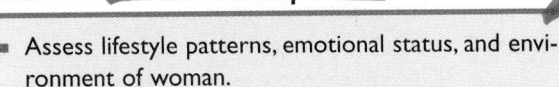

BOX 33-4 **The Pregnant Woman at Risk for Cardiac Decompensation**

- Assess lifestyle patterns, emotional status, and environment of woman.
- Arrange for consultations as needed (i.e., dietitian, home care, child care, social work).
- Determine woman's and her family's understanding of her heart disease and how the disease affects her pregnancy.
- Determine stressors in the woman's life. Assist woman in identifying effective coping strategies.
- Instruct woman to report signs of cardiac decompensation or congestive heart failure: generalized edema, distention of neck veins, dyspnea, pulmonary crackles, cough, palpitations, sudden weight gain.
- Instruct woman to be watchful for signs of thromboembolism, such as redness, tenderness, pain or swelling of the legs. Instruct woman to seek medical help immediately if such symptoms occur.
- Instruct woman to avoid constipation and thus straining with bowel movements (Valsalva maneuver) by taking in adequate fluids and fiber. A stool softener may be ordered.
- Explore with woman ways to obtain the needed rest throughout the day. Depending on the level of her cardiac disease, she may need to sleep 10 hr per night and rest 30 min after meals (class I or II) or rest for most of the day (class III or IV).
- Help woman make use of community resources, including support groups, as indicated.
- Emphasize the importance of keeping her prenatal visits.

From Gilbert, E., & Harmon, J. (2003). *Manual of high risk pregnancy and delivery* (3rd ed.). St. Louis: Mosby; Health Care Resources. (1997). *Handbook of high risk perinatal home care.* St. Louis: Mosby; Lowdermilk, D., & Grohar, J. (1998). *High risk antepartal home care.* White Plains, NY: March of Dimes.

TABLE 33-2 **Selected Drugs Used in Treatment of Cardiac Disorders in the Pregnant Woman**

CROSSES PLACENTA	CONSIDERATIONS	REFERENCES
Digoxin		
Yes	Fetal concentration of the drug is determined to avoid fetal toxicity (fetal toxicity existing with maternal overdose) Possible need to increase maternal dose because of increased blood volume while keeping in therapeutic range	Mendelson & Lang, 2000 Niebyl, 2002 Shabetai, 1999
Procainamide		
Yes	No known teratogenic effects Caution needed with use	Shotan et al., 1998
Verapamil		
Yes	Considered safe for use in pregnancy but can produce maternal hypotension with decreased uterine blood flow No controlled human studies on fetal effects	Elkayam & Dave, 1998 Shabetai, 1999
Propranolol		
Yes	Considered safe for use in pregnancy No known teratogenic effects Associated with fetal bradycardia, diminished uterine blood flow, IUGR, increased uterine irritability, and premature labor Associated with neonatal respiratory depression, hypoglycemia, hyperbilirubinemia	Roberts, 1999 Hurst et al., 1998
Heparin		
No	If anticoagulant therapy needed, heparin used Risk of maternal hemorrhage, preterm birth, stillbirth Prolonged IV use possibly inducing osteopenia in woman	McGehee, 1998 Shabetai, 1999
Warfarin		
Yes	Fetal anomalies and hemorrhage, congenital malformations, preterm birth, stillbirth Maternal hemorrhage Contraindicated in first trimester and at term	McGehee, 1998 Shabetai, 1999

extracorporeal circulation, and under these circumstances, hypoxia and fetal bradycardia may occur as a result of low blood-flow rates (Cohen & Castro, 1998). Periods of hypoxemia for the fetus can lead to various kinds of neurologic insults. Increase in flow rates on cardiopulmonary bypass may correct fetal bradycardia. Uterine contractions also increase in frequency before and during cardiopulmonary bypass and can be alleviated by medication.

Intrapartum Care

For all pregnant women, the intrapartum period is the one that evokes the most apprehension in clients and caregivers. The woman with impaired cardiac function has additional reasons to be anxious because labor and giving birth place an additional burden on her already compromised cardiovascular system.

Assessments include the routine assessments for all laboring women, as well as assessments for cardiac decompensation. In addition, arterial blood gases (ABGs) may be needed to assess for adequate oxygenation. A Swan-Ganz catheter may be inserted to monitor hemodynamic status accurately during labor and birth (see Chapter 34). ECG monitoring and continuous monitoring of blood pressure and pulse oximetry are usually instituted for the woman, and continuous fetal monitoring is used to monitor the fetus.

NURSE ALERT

A pulse rate of 100 beats/min or greater or respirations 25 breaths/min or greater are a concern. Respiratory status is checked frequently for developing dyspnea, coughing, or crackles at the base of the lungs. The color and temperature of the skin are noted. Pale, cool, clammy skin may indicate cardiac shock.

TABLE 33-2 **Selected Drugs Used in Treatment of Cardiac Disorders in the Pregnant Woman—cont'd**

CROSSES PLACENTA	CONSIDERATIONS	REFERENCES
Furosemide		
Yes	Fetal levels estimated to be equal to maternal levels No known teratogenic effects Limit use in first trimester Necessary to monitor for decreased plasma volume, which could lead to decreased placental perfusion	Cohen & Garity, 1998 Shabetai, 1999
Thiazides		
Yes	Neonatal jaundice, thrombocytopenia, hemolytic anemia, hypoglycemia, maternal electrolyte imbalances	Shabetai, 1999
Lidocaine		
Yes	Safe as long as toxic levels avoided Toxic dose—fetal CNS and cardiac toxicity Can cause maternal arrhythmia	Shabetai, 1999 Shotan et al., 1998 Mendelson & Lang, 2000
Quinidine		
Yes	No known teratogenic effects Neonatal thrombocytopenia reported	Shabetai, 1999 Shotan et al., 1998
Nifedipine		
Yes	Maternal orthostatic hypotension, headache, tachycardia Used with caution until potential fetal toxicity evaluated further May inhibit labor, may be synergistic with magnesium	Barron, 2000 Roberts, 1999 Shabetai, 1999
Diazoxide		
Yes	Fetal and maternal hyperglycemia possible Reserved for severe hypertension unresponsive to other medications Potent relaxant of uterine smooth muscle	Barron, 2000 Chari et al., 1998
Sodium Nitroprusside		
Yes	Use only in critical care unit for brief time with lowest possible therapeutic dose Low dose does not appear to cause toxic cyanide levels (fetal cyanide toxicity possibly occurring with higher doses)	Roberts, 1999 Siba, 2002

Nursing care during labor and birth focuses on the promotion of cardiac function. Anxiety is minimized by maintaining a calm atmosphere in the labor and birth rooms. The nurse provides anticipatory guidance by keeping the woman and her family informed of labor progress and events that will probably occur, as well as answering any questions they have. The woman's childbirth preparation method should be supported to the degree it is feasible for her cardiac condition. Nursing techniques that promote comfort, such as back massage, are used.

Cardiac function is supported by keeping the woman's head and shoulders elevated and body parts resting on pillows. The side-lying position usually facilitates hemodynamics during labor. Discomfort is relieved with medication and supportive care. Epidural regional analgesia provides better pain relief than narcotics and causes fewer alterations in hemodynamics (Cunningham et al., 2001). Hypotension must be avoided.

The woman may require other types of medication (e.g., anticoagulants, prophylactic antibiotics). If evidence of cardiac decompensation appears, the physician may order deslanoside (Cedilanid-D) for rapid digitalization, furosemide (Lasix) for rapid diuresis, and oxygen by intermittent positive pressure to decrease the development of pulmonary edema.

LEGAL TIP Cardiac and Metabolic Emergencies

The management of emergencies such as maternal cardiopulmonary distress or arrest or maternal metabolic crisis should be documented in policies, procedures, and protocols. Any independent nursing actions appropriate to the emergency should be clearly identified.

Beta-adrenergic agents (i.e., ritodrine and terbutaline) should not be used for tocolysis. These medications are associated with various cardiac side effects, including tachycardia and myocardial ischemia. A synthetic oxytocin (Syntocinon) can be used for induction of labor. This drug does not appear to cause significant coronary artery constriction in doses prescribed for labor induction or control of postpartum uterine atony. Cervical ripening agents containing prostaglandin are not contraindicated, but reports of use in pregnant women with cardiac disease are not available.

If there are no obstetric problems, vaginal birth is recommended and may be accomplished with the woman in the side-lying position to facilitate uterine perfusion. If the supine position is used, a pad is positioned under the hip to displace the uterus laterally and to minimize the danger of supine hypotension. The knees are flexed, and the feet are flat on the bed. To prevent compression of popliteal veins and an increase in blood volume in the chest and trunk as a result of the effects of gravity, stirrups are not used. Open-glottis pushing is recommended, and the Valsalva maneuver must be avoided during pushing in the second stage of labor because it reduces diastolic ventricular filling and obstructs left ventricular outflow. Mask oxygen is important. Episiotomy and vacuum extraction or outlet forceps may be used because these procedures decrease the length of the second stage of labor and decrease the workload of the heart in second stage labor. Cesarean birth is not routinely recommended for women who have cardiovascular disease because there is risk of dramatic fluid shifts, sustained hemodynamic changes, and increased blood loss.

Penicillin prophylaxis may be ordered for nonallergic pregnant women with class II or higher cardiac disease to protect against bacterial endocarditis in labor and during the early puerperium (see Box 33-3). Dilute IV oxytocin immediately after delivery of the placenta may be given to prevent postbirth hemorrhage. Ergot products should not be used because they increase blood pressure. Fluid balance should be maintained and blood loss replaced. If tubal sterilization is desired, surgery is delayed at least several days to ensure homeostasis.

Postpartum Care

Monitoring for cardiac decompensation in the postpartum period is essential. The first 24 to 48 postpartum hours are the most hemodynamically difficult for the woman. Hemorrhage or infection, or both, may worsen the cardiac condition. The woman with a cardiac disorder may continue to require a Swan-Ganz catheter and ABG monitoring.

NURSE ALERT

The immediate postbirth period is hazardous for a woman whose heart function is compromised. Cardiac output increases rapidly as extravascular fluid is remobilized into the vascular compartment. At the moment of birth, intraabdominal pressure is reduced drastically; pressure on veins is removed, the splanchnic vessels engorge, and blood flow to the heart is increased. When blood flow increases to the heart, a **reflex bradycardia** (slowing of the heart in response to the increased blood flow) may result.

Nursing diagnoses appropriate for the postpartum period include the following:

- *Anxiety related to*
  - –fear for infant's safety
- *Fear of dying related to*
  - –perceived physiologic inability to cope with stress of labor
- *Risk for impaired gas exchange related to*
  - –cardiac condition
- *Risk for excess fluid volume related to*
  - –extravascular fluid shifts
- *Situational low self-esteem related to*
  - –restriction placed on involvement in care of infant
  - –ineffective (compromised) family coping
- *Ineffective breastfeeding related to*
  - –fatigue from cardiac condition
- *Risk for altered mother/infant attachment related to*
  - –separation due to prematurity
  - –fatigue from cardiac condition

Care in the postpartum period is tailored to the woman's functional capacity. Postpartum assessment of the woman with cardiac disease includes vital signs, oxygen saturation levels, lung and heart auscultation, edema, amount and character of bleeding, uterine tone and fundal height, urinary output, pain (especially chest pain), the activity-rest pattern, dietary intake, mother-infant interactions, and emotional state. The head of the bed is elevated, and the woman is encouraged to lie on her side. Bed rest may be ordered, with or without bathroom privileges. Progressive ambulation may be permitted as tolerated. The nurse may help the woman meet her grooming and hygiene needs and other activities. Bowel movements without stress or strain for the woman are promoted with stool softeners, diet, and fluids.

The woman may need a family member to help in the care of the infant. Breastfeeding is not contraindicated, but not all women with heart disease (particularly those with life-threatening disease) will be able to do it (Lawrence, 1999). The woman who chooses to breastfeed will need the support of her family and the nursing staff to be successful. For example, the woman may need assistance in positioning herself and/or the infant for feeding. Further to conserve the woman's energy, the infant may be brought to the mother and taken from her after the feeding. Women who breastfeed may need less medication for their cardiac condition, especially diuretics. Because diuretics can cause neonatal diuresis that can lead to dehydration, lactating women must be monitored closely to determine if medication doses can be reduced and still be effective.

If the woman is unable to breastfeed and her energies do not allow her to bottle feed the infant, the baby can be kept at the bedside so she can look at and touch her baby to establish an emotional bond with her baby with a low expenditure of energy. The infant should be held at the mother's eye level and near her lips and brought to her fingers. At the same time, involving the mother passively in her infant's care helps the mother feel vitally important–as she is–to the infant's well-being (e.g., "You can offer something no one else can: provide your baby with your sounds, touch, and rhythms that are so comforting"). Perhaps the woman can be encouraged to make a tape recording of her talking, singing, or whispering, which can be played for the baby in the nursery to help the infant feel her presence and be in contact with her voice. This also enhances maternal-infant bonding.

Preparation for discharge is carefully planned with the woman and family. Provision of help for the woman in the home by relatives, friends, and others must be addressed. If necessary, the nurse refers the family to community resources (e.g., for homemaking services). Rest and sleep periods, activity, and diet must be planned. The couple may need information about reestablishing sexual relations and contraception or sterilization. Oral contraception, particularly combined estrogen-progestin pills, are usually avoided because of the risk for thrombophlebitis. Sterilization may be a risk for women with class III or IV heart disease. IUDs may put the woman at risk for infection, especially if she has a valve replacement. Injectable progestins are effective and safe (Easterling & Otto, 2002; Shabetai, 1999).

Monitoring for cardiac decompensation continues through the first few weeks after birth because of hormonal shifts that affect hemodynamics. Maternal cardiac output is usually stabilized by 2 weeks postpartum (Easterling & Otto, 2002).

Cardiopulmonary Resuscitation of the Pregnant Woman

Trauma, pulmonary embolism, anesthesia complications, drug overdose, hypovolemia, or septic shock may result in cardiopulmonary arrest. Preexisting disorders such as heart or pulmonary disease, hypertension, or autoimmune collagen vascular disease increase this risk (Luppi, 1999).

Various protocols exist for cardiopulmonary resuscitation (CPR) during pregnancy. The most widely used guide is the American Heart Association (AHA) ACLS Protocol (AHA, 1992). This protocol recommends 5 to 10 minutes of standard CPR with the uterus displaced laterally, fluid volume restoration, and defibrillation if indicated. If these measures are not successful within 15 minutes of the arrest, open chest heart massage is recommended if the fetus is viable. If there is still no change in maternal status after 15 minutes of open chest cardiac massage or there is fetal distress, immediate cesarean birth is recommended. Other protocols recommend cesarean birth within 5 minutes (Kloeck et al., 1997), whereas still others recommend cesarean birth based on the gestational age of the fetus (Luppi, 1999). No matter what protocol is used, nurses and other health care providers must be prepared if CPR is to be successful.

In the event of cardiac arrest, standard resuscitative efforts with a few modifications are implemented. To prevent supine hypotension, the pregnant woman is placed on a firm surface with the uterus displaced laterally either manually or with a wedge or rolled blanket or towel under one hip (Association of Women's Health, Obstetric, and Neonatal Nurses [AWHONN], 1998; Stapleton et al., 2001). If defibrillation is needed, the paddles need to be placed one rib interspace higher than usual because the heart is displaced slightly by the enlarged uterus. If possible, the fetus should be monitored during the cardiac arrest (Bajo, 1997) (see Emergency box).

Complications may be associated with CPR of a pregnant woman. These complications may include laceration,

EMERGENCY

Cardiopulmonary Resuscitation for the Pregnant Woman

AIRWAY

Determine unresponsiveness.

Activate emergency medical system and get the automated external defibrillator (AED) if available.

Position woman on flat, firm surface with uterus displaced laterally with a wedge (e.g., a rolled towel placed under her hip) or manually, or place her in a lateral position.

Open airway with head tilt–chin lift maneuver.

BREATHING

Determine breathlessness (look, listen, feel).

If the woman is not breathing, give two slow breaths.

CIRCULATION

Determine pulselessness by feeling carotid pulse.

If there is no pulse, begin chest compressions at rate of 100 per minute. Chest compressions may be performed slightly higher on the sternum if the uterus is enlarged enough to displace the diaphragm into a higher position.

After four cycles of 15 compressions and two breaths, check her pulse. If pulse is not present, continue CPR.

DEFIBRILLATION

Use an AED according to standard protocol to analyze heart rhythm and deliver shock if indicated.

RELIEF OF FOREIGN-BODY AIRWAY OBSTRUCTION

If the pregnant woman is unable to speak or cough, perform chest thrusts. Stand behind the woman and place your arms under her armpits to encircle her chest. Press backward with quick thrusts until the foreign body is expelled (Fig. 33-2). If the woman becomes unresponsive, follow the steps for victims who become unresponsive, but use chest thrusts instead of abdominal thrusts.

From Stapleton, E. et al. (2001). *Fundamentals of BLS for healthcare providers.* Dallas: American Heart Association.

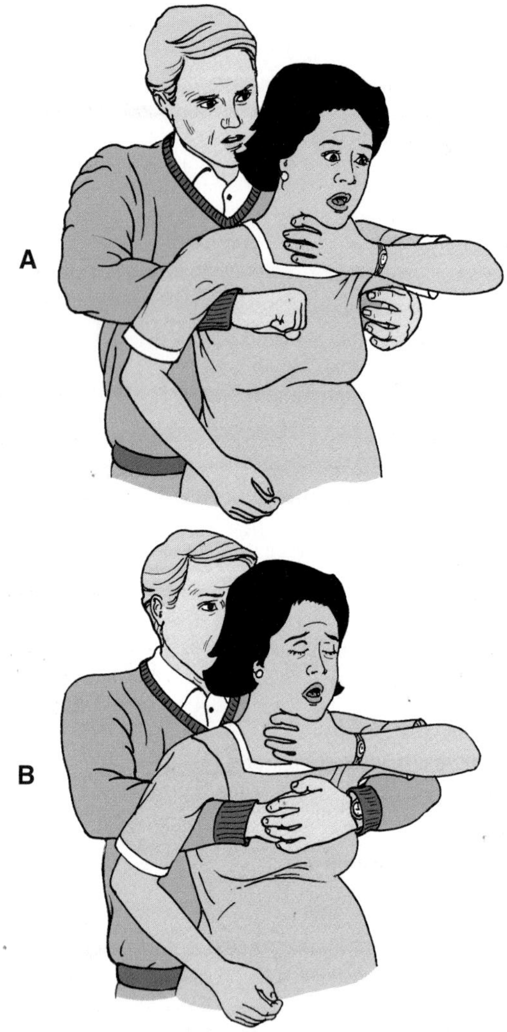
A
B

FIG. 33-2 Heimlich maneuver. Clearing airway obstruction in woman in late stage of pregnancy (can also be used in markedly obese victim). **A,** Standing behind victim, place your arms under woman's armpits and across chest. Place thumb side of your clenched fist against middle of sternum, and place other hand over fist. **B,** Perform backward chest thrusts until foreign body is expelled or woman becomes unconscious. If pregnant woman becomes unconscious because of foreign-body airway obstruction, place her on her back and kneel close to the victim's side. (Be sure uterus is displaced laterally by using, for example, a rolled blanket under her hip.) Open mouth with tongue-jaw lift, perform finger sweep, and attempt rescue breathing. If unable to ventilate, position hands as for chest compression. Deliver five chests thrusts firmly to remove obstruction. Repeat this sequence of Heimlich maneuver, finger sweep, and attempt to ventilate. Continue sequence until pregnant women's airway is clear of obstruction or help has arrived to relieve you (Stapleton et al., 2001). If woman is unconscious, give chest compressions as for woman without pulse.

of the liver, rupture of the uterus, hemothorax, or hemoperitoneum. Fetal complications also may occur. These include cardiac dysrhythmia or asystole related to maternal defibrillation and medications, CNS depression related to antidysrhythmic drugs and inadequate uteroplacental perfusion, and onset of preterm labor.

If there is successful resuscitation, the woman and her fetus must receive careful monitoring. The woman remains at increased risk for recurrent pulmonary arrest and dysrhythmias (ventricular tachycardia, supraventricular tachycardia, bradycardia). Therefore her cardiovascular, pulmonary, and neurologic status should be assessed continuously. Uterine activity and resting tone must be monitored. Fetal status and gestational age should be determined and used in decision making regarding the continuation of the pregnancy or the timing and route of birth.

Clearing an airway obstruction in a woman in the second or third trimester of pregnancy also requires a modification of the Heimlich maneuver (Fig. 33-2) (Stapleton, 2001).

Evaluation

The nurse uses the previously stated expected outcomes as criteria to evaluate the care of the woman with cardiac disease (see Plan of Care).

OTHER MEDICAL DISORDERS IN PREGNANCY

Anemia

Anemia is the most common medical disorder of pregnancy, affecting at least 20% of pregnant women. Women with anemia have a higher incidence of puerperal complications such as infection than do pregnant women with normal hematologic values.

Anemia results in reduction of the oxygen-carrying capacity of the blood, and the heart tries to compensate by increasing the cardiac output. This effort increases the workload of the heart and stresses ventricular function. Therefore anemia that occurs with any other complication (e.g., preeclampsia) may result in congestive heart failure.

An indirect index of the oxygen-carrying capacity is the packed red blood cell (RBC) volume, or hematocrit level. The normal hematocrit range in nonpregnant women is 38% to 45%. However, normal values for pregnant women with adequate iron stores may be as low as 34%. This has been explained by hydremia (dilution of blood), or the physiologic anemia of pregnancy.

At or near sea level, the pregnant woman is anemic when her hemoglobin level is less than 11 g/dl or the hematocrit is less than 33%. At high altitudes, much higher values indicate anemia; for example, at 1500 m (5000 ft) above sea level, a hemoglobin level less than 14 g/dl indicates anemia (Pagana & Pagana, 2001).

Plan of Care: The Pregnant Woman with Heart Disease

NURSING DIAGNOSIS Activity intolerance related to effects of pregnancy on the patient with rheumatic heart disease with mitral valve stenosis

Expected Outcome *Woman will verbalize a plan to change lifestyle throughout pregnancy in order to avoid risk of cardiac decompensation.*

Nursing Interventions/*Rationales*

Assist woman to identify factors that decrease activity tolerance and explore extent of limitations *to establish a baseline for evaluation.*

Help woman to develop an individualized program of activity and rest, taking into account the living and working environment as well as support of family and friends *to maintain sufficient cardiac output.*

Teach woman to monitor physiologic response to activity (i.e., pulse rate, respiratory rate) and reduce activity that causes fatigue or pain *to maintain sufficient cardiac output and prevent potential injury to fetus.*

Enlist family and friends to assist woman in pacing activities and to provide support in performing role functions and self-care activities that are too strenuous *to increase chances of compliance with activity restrictions.*

Suggest that woman maintain an activity log that records activities, time, duration, intensity, and physiologic response *to evaluate effectiveness of and adherence to activity program.*

Discuss various quiet diversional activities which could be done by the woman *to decrease the potential for boredom during rest periods.*

NURSING DIAGNOSIS Risk for ineffective therapeutic regimen management related to woman's first pregnancy and perceived sense of wellness

Expected Outcome *Woman will participate in an effective therapeutic regimen for pregnancy complicated by heart disease.*

Nursing Interventions/*Rationales*

Identify factors, such as insufficient knowledge about the effect of cardiac disease on pregnancy which could inhibit the woman from participating in a therapeutic regime *to promote early interventions, such as teaching about the importance of rest.*

Teach woman and family about factors such as lack of rest or not taking prescribed medications that could adversely affect the pregnancy *to provide information and promote empowerment over the situation.*

Encourage expression of feelings about the disease and its potential effect on the pregnancy *to promote a sense of trust.*

Identify resources in the community *to provide a shared sense of common experiences.*

Encourage woman to verbalize her plan for carrying out the regimen of care *to evaluate the effects of teaching.*

NURSING DIAGNOSIS Decreased cardiac output related to increased circulatory volume secondary to pregnancy and cardiac disease

Expected Outcome *The woman will exhibit signs of adequate cardiac output (i.e., normal pulse and blood pressure, normal heart and breath sounds, normal skin color, tone, and turgor, normal capillary refill, normal urine output, and no evidence of edema).*

Nursing Interventions/*Rationales*

Reinforce the importance of activity/rest cycles *to prevent cardiac complications.*

Plan with woman a frequent visit schedule to caregiver *to provide adequate surveillance of high risk pregnancy.*

Teach woman to lie in lateral position *to increase uteroplacental blood flow* and to elevate legs while sitting *to promote venous return.*

Monitor intake and output and check for edema *to assess for renal complications or venous return problems.*

Monitor FHR and fetal activity, perform NST as indicated *to assess fetal status and detect uteroplacental insufficiency.*

NURSING DIAGNOSIS Risk for altered tissue perfusion related to cardiac condition secondary to increased circulatory needs during pregnancy

Expected Outcomes *The woman will exhibit signs of hemodynamic stability (i.e., blood pressure, pulse, ABGs, and WBC counts are within normal limits). The fetus will exhibit signs of well-being (i.e., fetal activity and fetal heart rate [FHR] are within normal limits).*

Nursing Interventions/*Rationales*

Monitor heart rate and rhythm, blood pressure, skin color and temperature, WBCs, hemoglobin and hematocrit, and ABGs *to detect early signs of cardiac failure/hypoxia.*

Monitor fetal activity and FHR, and perform nonstress testing as indicated *to assess fetal status and detect uteroplacental insufficiency.*

Teach woman how to detect and report early signs of cardiac decompensation *to prevent maternal/fetal complications.*

When a woman has anemia during pregnancy, the loss of blood at birth, even if minimal, is not well tolerated. She is at an increased risk for requiring blood transfusions. Women with anemia have a higher incidence of puerperal complications, such as infection, than do pregnant women with normal hematologic values.

Nursing care of the anemic pregnant woman requires that the nurse be able to distinguish between the normal physiologic anemia of pregnancy and the disease states. About 90% of cases of anemia in pregnancy are of the iron-deficiency type. The remaining 10% embrace a considerable variety of acquired and hereditary anemias, including folic acid deficiency, sickle cell anemia, and thalassemia.

During prenatal visits, the nurse should take a diet history and provide dietary teaching as appropriate. Pregnancy may cause increased fatigue, stress, and financial difficulties for a woman with anemia as she copes with her activities of daily living. The nurse should assess the woman's needs and provide her with appropriate resources or referral.

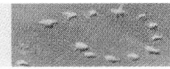

Iron Deficiency Anemia

Pathologic anemia of pregnancy is primarily caused by *iron deficiency* (Bormanis, 2000). Without iron therapy, even pregnant women who have excellent nutrition will end pregnancy with an iron deficit. Iron is actively transported across the placenta for fetal erythropoiesis. Diet alone cannot replace gestational iron losses. Inadequate nutrition without therapy will certainly mean iron deficiency anemia during late pregnancy and the puerperium. Successful iron therapy during pregnancy can be carried out in most cases with oral iron supplements (e.g., elemental iron of 60 to 80 mg/day). It is important to teach the woman the significance of the iron therapy (see Teaching for Self-Care box, Chapter 15, p. 379). In addition, the woman should be instructed in dietary ways to decrease the GI side effects of iron therapy. Some pregnant women cannot tolerate the prescribed oral iron because of nausea and vomiting. In such cases, the woman should receive parenteral iron such as an iron-dextran complex (Imferon).

Folic Acid Deficiency Anemia

Folic acid deficiency during conception and early pregnancy increases the incidence of neural tube defects, cleft lip, and cleft palate (Letsky, 2000). It is the second most common anemia of pregnancy. Even in well-nourished women, it is common to have a folate deficiency. Poor diet, cooking with large volumes of water, or home canning of food (especially vegetables) may lead to folate deficiency. Malabsorption may play a part in the development of anemia caused by a lack of folic acid. Folic acid deficiency anemia is common in multiple gestations. During pregnancy the recommended daily intake is 600 μg of folic acid per day; women who have a deficiency may need a supplement.

Sickle Cell Hemoglobinopathy

Sickle cell hemoglobinopathy is a disease caused by the presence of abnormal hemoglobin in the blood. *Sickle cell trait* (SA hemoglobin pattern), sickling of the RBCs but with a normal RBC life span, usually causes only mild clinical symptoms. *Sickle cell anemia* (sickle cell disease) is a recessive, hereditary, familial hemolytic anemia that affects those of African-American or Mediterranean ancestry. These individuals usually have abnormal hemoglobin types (SS or SC). People with sickle cell anemia have recurrent attacks (crises) of fever and pain in the abdomen or extremities. These attacks are attributed to vascular occlusion (from abnormal cells), tissue hypoxia, edema, and RBC destruction. Crises are associated with normochromic anemia, jaundice, reticulocytosis, a positive sickle cell test, and the demonstration of abnormal hemoglobin (usually SS or SC).

Almost 10% of African-Americans in North America have the sickle cell trait, but fewer than 1% have sickle cell anemia. The anemia is often complicated by iron and folic acid deficiency.

Women with sickle cell trait usually do well in pregnancy although they are at increased risk for urinary tract infections and may be deficient in iron (Kilpatrick & Laros, 1999). If the woman has sickle cell anemia, the anemia that occurs in normal pregnancies may aggravate the condition and bring on more crises. Fetal complications include being small for gestational age, IUGR, and skeletal changes. Pregnant women with sickle cell anemia are prone to pyelonephritis, leg ulcers, bone abnormalities, strokes, cardiopathy, congestive heart failure, and preeclampsia (O'Reilly-Green, 2000). Urinary tract infections (UTIs) and hematuria are common. An aplastic crisis may follow serious infection. Transfusions of the woman have been the usual treatment for symptomatic patients, however, partial exchange transfusions or prophylactic transfusions are common as well and significantly reduce the number of painful crises (Kilpatrick & Laros, 1999). Cesarean birth is warranted only for obstetric indications. Oral contraceptives are contraindicated.

Table 33-3 identifies some potential problems faced by the woman with sickle cell disease and some preventive and maintenance interventions.

Thalassemia

Thalassemia (Mediterranean or Cooley's anemia) is a relatively common anemia in which an insufficient amount of hemoglobin is produced to fill the RBCs. The condition eventually manifests itself in severe bone deformities caused by massive marrow tissue expansion. Thalassemia is a hereditary disorder that involves the abnormal synthesis of the alpha or beta chains of hemoglobin. Beta-thalassemia is the more common variety in the United States and often is diagnosed in persons of Italian, Greek, southern Chinese, Mediterranean, North African, African-American, Middle Eastern, southern Asian, or Indo-Pakistani descent. The unbalanced synthesis of hemoglobin leads to premature RBC death, resulting in severe anemia. Thalassemia major is the homozygous form of this disorder; thalassemia minor is the heterozygous form. Couples with the thalassemia trait should seek genetic counseling. Women with the thalassemia trait usually have an uncomplicated pregnancy.

Women with thalassemia major or minor have infertility problems, so few pregnancies will result. As many as 50% of these pregnancies have been complicated by stillbirth, IUGR, preeclampsia, and preterm birth. Medical management consists of ongoing monitoring and transfusion therapy (Hassell, 2000).

Women with thalassemia minor have a mild, persistent anemia, but the RBC level may be normal or even elevated. However, no systemic problems are caused by the anemia. Thalassemia minor must be distinguished from iron-deficiency anemia.

Pregnancy will neither worsen thalassemia minor nor be compromised by the disease. The anemia will not respond to iron therapy, and prolonged parenteral iron therapy can lead to harmful, excessive iron storage. People with thalassemia minor should have a normal life span despite a moderately reduced hemoglobin level.

TABLE 33-3 **Sickle Cell Anemia: Potential Problems, Prevention, and Maintenance**

POTENTIAL PROBLEM	PREVENTION AND MAINTENANCE
1. Inadequate oxygen to meet needs of labor and prevent sickling	1. a. Monitor Hb level and HCT to maintain Hb at ≥8 g and HCT at ≥20% b. Have typed and crossmatched blood available c. Assist with transfusions d. Administer oxygen continuously during labor e. Coach for relaxation and to lessen anxiety
2. Infection: UTI, pyelonephritis, pneumonia	2. a. Continue actions as under No. 1 b. Maintain adequate hydration c. Administer antibiotics as ordered d. Maintain strict asepsis e. Encourage frequent voiding to keep bladder empty
3. Sequestration crisis caused by need for and destruction of RBCs	3. Administer folic acid supplement (1 mg/day) to decrease erythropoietic demands and reduce probability of capillary stasis
4. Crisis caused by hypoxia, hypotension, acidosis, dehydration, exertion, sudden cooling, low-grade fever	4. a. Continue actions as under No. 1 b. Avoid supine hypotension c. Maintain adequate hydration d. Maintain comfortable room temperature: use warm blankets or cool cloths as needed e. Assist with analgesia and anesthesia
5. Pseudotoxemia (hypertension, proteinuria, no large weight gain); often accompanying bone pain crisis	5. a. If true PIH occurs, care is the same as for PIH b. Monitor blood pressure and urine
6. Thromboembolism (from increased blood viscosity)	6. a. Monitor for positive Homans' sign b. Initiate bed rest if Homans' sign is positive or if reddened, warm areas, or lump appears in the calf c. Maintain adequate hydration d. Administer heparin as ordered e. Apply warm compresses f. Apply antiembolism stockings
7. Congestive heart failure	7. a. Assess pulse, respiratory rate b. Place in semirecumbent position; lateral position for labor c. Auscultate for crackles in the lungs frequently d. Administer oxygen and medications (e.g., digitalis, antibiotics, diuretics, analgesics) e. Regional analgesia for pain relief in labor
8. Pulmonary infarction (hemoptysis, cough, temperature to 38.9° C, friction rub)	8. Assess for this possible complication to facilitate early diagnosis
9. Postpartum hemorrhage (resulting from heparin therapy)	9. Administer ordered oxytocic medication

Hb, Hemoglobin; *HCT,* hematocrit; *PIH,* pregnancy-induced hypertension; *RBCs,* red blood cells; *UTI,* urinary tract infection.

Pulmonary Disorders

As pregnancy advances and the uterus impinges on the thoracic cavity, any pregnant woman may have increased respiratory difficulty. This difficulty will be compounded by pulmonary disease. A pulmonary disorder in pregnancy requires assessment, planning, and interventions specific to the disease process, in addition to routine peripartum care. The nurse also must be alert to pulmonary complications precipitated by pregnancy.

Asthma

Bronchial asthma is an acute respiratory illness caused by allergens, marked change in ambient temperature, or emotional tension. In many cases the actual cause may be unknown. A family history of allergy is common in people with asthma. In response to stimuli, there is widespread but reversible narrowing of the hyperreactive airways, making it difficult to breathe. The clinical manifestations are expiratory wheezing, productive cough, thick sputum, and/or dyspnea.

From 1% to 4% of pregnant women have asthma (Schmidt & Hall, 2000), the most common respiratory crisis complicating pregnancy (Burton & Reyes, 2001). The effect of pregnancy on asthma is unpredictable. About one half will improve, one fourth will stay the same, and one fourth will worsen (Wendel, 2001). Physiologic alterations induced by pregnancy do not make the pregnant woman more prone to asthmatic attacks. Women often have few symptoms of asthma in the first trimester and in the last weeks of pregnancy. The severity of symptoms usually peaks between 29 and 36 weeks' gestation (Burton & Reyes, 2001).

Therapy for asthma has three objectives: (1) relief of the acute attack, (2) prevention or limitation of later attacks, and (3) adequate maternal and fetal oxygenation. These goals can be achieved in pregnancy by eliminating environmental triggers (e.g., dust mites, animal dander, pollen), drug therapy (e.g., bronchodilators and antiinflammatory agents), and client education. Respiratory infections should be treated, and mist or steam inhalation used to aid expectoration of mucus. Acute episodes may require albuterol, steroids, aminophylline, beta-adrenergic agents, and oxygen. Almost all asthma medications are considered safe in pregnancy (Burton & Reyes, 2001; Murdock, 2002) (Table 33-4).

Asthma attacks can occur in labor; thus medications for asthma are continued in labor and the postpartum period. Pulse oximetry should be instituted during labor. Epidurals are recommended for pain relief. Morphine and meperidine are histamine-releasing narcotics and should be avoided (Burton & Reyes, 2001).

During the postpartum period, women who have asthma are at increased risk for hemorrhage. If excessive bleeding occurs, oxytocin is the recommended drug. Asthma medications are usually safe for administration during the postpartum period and lactation. The woman usually returns to her prepregnancy asthma status within 3 months after giving birth.

Cystic Fibrosis

Cystic fibrosis is a common autosomal recessive genetic disorder in which the exocrine glands produce excessive viscous secretions, which causes problems with both respiratory and digestive functions. There is an increase in pulmonary capillary permeability, decrease of lung volume, and shunting, which results in arterial hypoxemia. Respiratory failure and early death (early twenties) may occur.

Since the gene for cystic fibrosis was identified in 1989, data can be collected for the purposes of genetic counseling for couples regarding carrier status (Pickard, 2000). All infants born to mothers with cystic fibrosis will be carriers of the gene; 2.5% of the infants born will have cystic fibrosis (Schmidt & Hall, 2000). Improvements in diagnosis and treatment have allowed an increasing number of women with cystic fibrosis to survive to adulthood. The median age of survival for clients with pancreatic insufficiency is 29 years (Pickard, 2000). Preconception counseling is essential for women with cystic fibrosis. Fewer than one in five women are able to become pregnant, as a result of very thick cervical mucus (Schmidt & Hall, 2000).

In women who do not have severe disease, pregnancy is usually tolerated well (Pickard, 2000). With data from clinical and radiologic findings, two classification scoring systems have been developed for assessing the risk of pregnancy in clients with cystic fibrosis. The Shwachmann-Kulcycki and Taussig scores range from 0 to 100. A score over 90 indicates an excellent outcome over the next few

TABLE 33-4 **Medications Used In Pregnancy in Clients with Asthma**

STAGE/CONDITION OF PREGNANCY	PREFERRED MEDICATION	MEDICATION(S) TO AVOID (RATIONALE)
Labor	Continue asthma medications	
Induction	Oxytocin	Prostaglandins (may cause bronchoconstriction or bronchospasm)
Pain relief	Fentanyl Epidural anesthesia	Morphine and meperidine (Demerol) (release histamine)
Preterm labor	Magnesium sulfate, nifedipine, β-agonist	β-Agonist if client is already taking one for her asthma (may cause respiratory distress) NSAIDs (may exacerbate asthma)
Postpartum hemorrhage	Oxytocin	Methylergonovine and 15-methyl prostaglandin $F_{2\alpha}$ (may worsen asthma)

NSAIDs, Nonsteroidal antiinflammatory drugs.
Data from Barbour, L. (2000). Asthma. In R. Lee et al. (Eds.), *Medical care of the pregnant patient.* Philadelphia: American College of Physicians; Wendel, P. (2001). Asthma in pregnancy. *Obstetrics and Gynecology Clinics of North America, 28*(3), 537-549.

years, whereas a score of less than 50 indicates likelihood of subsequent mortality. With scores of less than 80, pregnancy should be discouraged, and options discussed (Schmidt & Hall, 2000). Some clinicians use these scores, but others base their predictive findings on the pulmonary status, nutritional status, and pancreatic insufficiency (Pickard, 2000).

In those with severe disease, the pregnancy is often complicated by chronic hypoxia and frequent pulmonary infections. Women with cystic fibrosis show a decrease in their residual volume during pregnancy, as do normal pregnant women, and are unable to maintain vital capacity. Presumably the pulmonary vasculature cannot accommodate the increased cardiac output of pregnancy. The results are decreased oxygen to the myocardium, decreased cardiac output, and increased hypoxemia. A pregnant woman with less than 50% of expected vital capacity usually has a difficult pregnancy. Increased maternal and perinatal mortality is related to severe pulmonary infection. There is an increased incidence of preterm births, IUGR, and neonatal deaths in clients with cystic fibrosis. Predictors of adverse affects to the fetus and neonate are inadequate weight gain, dyspnea, and cyanosis.

In addition to the respiratory implications, women with cystic fibrosis may develop gestational diabetes and liver disease. Pancreatic insufficiency may put the woman at risk for malnutrition, because she cannot meet the increased nutritional requirements of pregnancy. Fat-soluble vitamins may not be used because of diminished absorption.

Weight and symptoms of malabsorption should be monitored at each prenatal visit, and pancreatic enzymes adjusted as necessary. Women with severe pancreatic insufficiency may require total parenteral nutrition. A glucose tolerance test should be done at 20 weeks' gestation. Routine respiratory management is continued throughout the pregnancy. Antibiotics such as cephalosporins, aminoglycosides, and antipseudomonal penicillins can be used safely in pregnancy (Pickard, 2000).

During labor, monitoring for fluid and electrolyte balance is required. The amount of sodium lost through sweat can be significant, and hypovolemia can occur. Conversely, if any degree of cor pulmonale is present, fluid overload is a concern. Oxygen is given by face mask during labor, and monitoring by pulse oximetry is recommended (de Swiet, 2000). Epidural or local analgesia is the preferred analgesic for birth.

Breastfeeding appears to be safe as long as the sodium content of the milk is not abnormal (Lawrence, 1999). Pumping and discarding the milk is done until the sodium content has been determined.

Adult Respiratory Distress Syndrome

Adult respiratory distress syndrome (ARDS), or shock lung, occurs when the lungs are unable to maintain levels of oxygen and carbon dioxide within normal limits. Severe hypoxemia, in spite of high levels of inspired oxygen, is accompanied by an increase in pulmonary capillary permeability, decrease in lung volume, and shunting of blood.

ARDS is not specific to pregnancy; it also can result from chest trauma, drug ingestion, or pneumonia. When ARDS is associated with pregnancy, inhalation of gastric contents during anesthesia, disseminated intravascular coagulation (DIC), preeclampsia, eclampsia, abruptio placentae, dead fetus syndrome, or amniotic fluid embolism may be the precipitating factors (de Swiet, 2000). An initial intervention is to find and correct the underlying cause, if possible. To provide the best fetal environment, early intubation and mechanical ventilation is recommended (Cunningham et al., 2001). With severe lung injury, positive end-expiratory pressure (PEEP) may be necessary. The administration of vasoactive agents, inotropic agents, and corticosteroids may be necessary. Maintaining fluid balance is a challenge and a key component of management. For the woman who is hypovolemic, administration of blood may help to increase cardiac output. For the woman who is hypervolemic, diuretics may be necessary to maintain adequate cardiac output.

The postpartum incidence of ARDS is affected not by the method of birth but by the amount of trauma occurring during pregnancy and birth. It also may occur after miscarriage or therapeutic abortion.

Laboratory reports are important in identifying the origin of acute pulmonary problems. Chest radiographs can indicate the presence of infiltrates in the lungs, and ABGs identify the status of acid-base balance. The priority assessments to note are vital signs, oxygen saturation, signs of thrombophlebitis, and hemorrhage. During the postpartum period, apprehension, distended neck veins, cyanosis, diaphoresis, or pallor may indicate hypoxemia. Mental confusion or disorientation also may be noted.

The pulse rate increases to compensate for respiratory insufficiency of any origin. The severity of the pulmonary problem increases as the pulse rate increases. An initial increase in blood pressure occurs as cardiac output increases in an attempt to supply the tissue with oxygen. When lung damage is severe, blood pressure decreases.

Respiratory changes are the most important indicators of ARDS. The rate, depth, respiratory pattern, symmetry of chest movement, and use of accessory muscles should be noted; therefore observation of respiratory characteristics after activity is important.

NURSE ALERT

If there is any indication of abnormality, respirations are counted for a full minute; an error in rate of plus or minus four respirations per minute may be highly significant.

On auscultation, crackles, rhonchi, wheezes, or a pleural friction rub should be reported, especially when they occur after an earlier assessment with normal findings. The pregnant woman should be positioned for breathing comfort. Oxygen and emergency equipment should be available. The woman should be reassured and coached in relaxation techniques to lessen her anxiety.

This syndrome has a high mortality rate. The prognosis is good if the woman is otherwise healthy and if ventilatory support can be maintained until the underlying disease can be treated (Cunningham et al., 2001).

Integumentary Disorders

The skin surface may exhibit many physiologic conditions during pregnancy. Dermatologic disorders induced by pregnancy include melasma (chloasma), vascular "spiders," palmar erythema, and striae gravidarum. Skin problems generally aggravated by pregnancy are acne vulgaris (in the first trimester), erythema multiforme, herpetiform dermatitis (fever blisters and genital herpes), granuloma inguinale (Donovan bodies), condylomata acuminata (genital warts), neurofibromatosis (von Recklinghausen disease), and pemphigus. Dermatologic disorders usually improved by pregnancy include acne vulgaris (in the third trimester), seborrheic dermatitis (dandruff), and psoriasis. An unpredictable course during pregnancy may be expected in atopic dermatitis, lupus erythematosus, and herpes simplex. Disease processes during and soon after pregnancy may be extremely difficult to diagnose and treat.

Pruritis is a common symptom in pregnancy-specific inflammatory skin diseases. The most common pregnancy-specific causes of pruritis are polymorphic eruption of pregnancy (also known as *pruritic urticarial papules and plaques of pregnancy [PUPPP]* (Fig. 33-3), prurigo gestationis, and cholestasis of pregnancy. Symptoms usually appear in the third trimester and usually subside in the postpartum period. The abdomen is usually affected, but lesions can spread to the arms, thighs, back, and buttocks. Topical steroid therapy usually provides relief, but some women may require systemic steroid therapy for severe symptoms (Stambuk & Colvin, 2002).

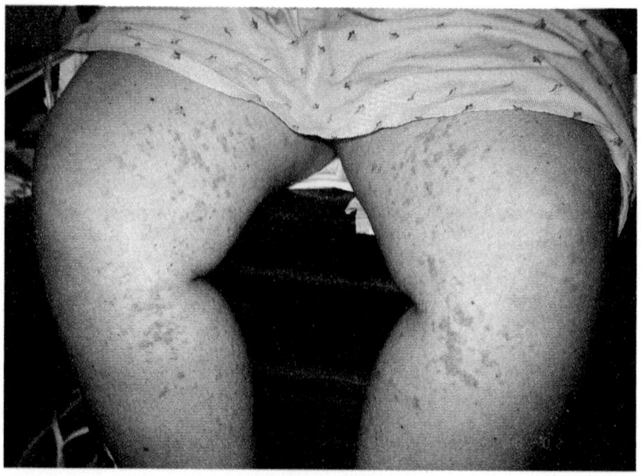

FIG. 33-3 Woman with pruritic urticarial papules and plaques of pregnancy. Lesions also are present on her arms, back, abdomen, and buttocks. (Courtesy Shannon Perry, San Jose, CA.)

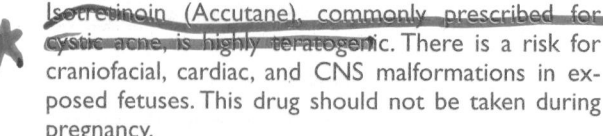

NURSE ALERT
Isotretinoin (Accutane), commonly prescribed for cystic acne, is highly teratogenic. There is a risk for craniofacial, cardiac, and CNS malformations in exposed fetuses. This drug should not be taken during pregnancy.

Pemphigoid gestationis and impetigo herpetiformis are rare complications that can cause fetal morbidity. Antepartal fetal assessments are recommended (Stambuk & Colvin, 2002).

Neurologic Disorders

The pregnant woman with a neurologic disorder must deal with potential teratogenic effects of prescribed medications, changes of mobility during pregnancy, and ability to care for the baby. The nurse should be aware of all drugs the client is taking and the associated potential for producing congenital anomalies. As the pregnancy progresses, the woman's center of gravity shifts and causes balance and gait changes. The nurse should advise the woman of these expected changes and suggest safety measures as appropriate. Family and community resources should be assessed to provide child care for the neurologically impaired woman.

Epilepsy

Epilepsy is a disorder of the brain causing recurrent seizures and is the most common neurologic disorder accompanying pregnancy (Barbour & Pickard, 2000). Epilepsy may result from developmental abnormalities or injury, as well as having no known cause. Convulsive seizures may be more frequent or severe during complications of pregnancy, such as edema, alkalosis, fluid-electrolyte imbalance, cerebral hypoxia, hypoglycemia, and hypocalcemia. They also may be related to hormonal changes, fatigue, or sleep deprivation.

The effect of epilepsy on pregnancy is unpredictable. Up to 80% of women have no change in seizure activity during pregnancy, whereas 20% have an increase, and up to 25% have a decrease in seizures (Gilmore, Pennell, & Stern, 1998).

The differential diagnosis between epilepsy and eclampsia may pose a problem. Epilepsy and eclampsia can coexist. However, a history of seizures and a normal plasma uric acid level, as well as the absence of hypertension, generalized edema, or proteinuria, point to epilepsy.

During pregnancy, the risk of vaginal bleeding is doubled, and there is a threefold risk of abruptio placentae. Abnormal presentations are more common in labor and birth, and there is an increased possibility that the fetus will experience seizures in utero (Aminoff, 1999).

Metabolic changes in pregnancy usually alter pharmacokinetics. In addition, nausea and vomiting may interfere with ingestion and absorption of medication. Failure to take medications is a common factor leading to worsening of seizure activity during pregnancy. This is largely owing to the message that drugs for epilepsy are harmful to the fetus (Gilmore et al., 1998). Teratogenicity of antiepileptic drugs (AEDs) has been described thoroughly, but the risk of occurrence of anomalies in the fetus has been exaggerated. Congenital anomalies that can occur with AEDs include cleft lip or palate, congenital heart disease, urogenital defects, and neural tube defects (Gilmore et al., 1998). AEDs should be monotherapeutic and should be used in the smallest therapeutic dose. Daily folic acid supplementation is important because of the depletion that occurs when taking AEDs (Cartlidge, 2000).

A 1% to 2% risk of seizure activity occurs during labor. If the woman cannot take oral AEDs, then phenytoin can be administered IV. Serum levels of AEDs should be checked within 48 hours and at 1 to 2 weeks after birth, because levels can change quickly, and toxicity can develop.

During the neonatal period, infants can have a hemorrhagic disorder associated with AED-induced vitamin K deficiency. Prophylaxis consists of administering vitamin K, 20 mg orally, daily during the last month of pregnancy and administering 1 mg IM to the newborn at birth (Gilmore et al., 1998). Neonates also should be monitored for drug withdrawal. With the exception of phenobarbital, clonazepam, and ethosuxamide, all other AEDs are compatible with breastfeeding (Barbour & Pickard, 2000).

Multiple Sclerosis

Multiple sclerosis (MS), a patchy demyelinization of the spinal cord and CNS, may be a viral disorder. MS has a greater prevalence in female subjects and is more common during the childbearing years, between ages 20 and 40 years (Cartlidge, 2000). Infertility, miscarriage, stillbirth, and fetal anomalies do not appear to be increased in women with MS (Eggum, 2001).

MS may occasionally complicate pregnancy, but exacerbations and remissions are unrelated to the pregnant state. Some women have flare-up in the third trimester and the postpartum period, whereas others have fewer symptoms. Bowel and bladder problems, increased difficulty in walking, and fatigue may be more pronounced in women with MS. Medications such as Avonex (interferon beta-1a), Betaseron (interferon beta-1b), and Copaxone (glatiramer acetate) that are given to reduce the frequency and intensity of attacks and slow the progression of disease should not be taken during pregnancy. Breastfeeding is contraindicated if these medications are resumed after the birth (National Women's Health Resource Center, 2001). Nursing care of the pregnant woman with MS is similar to the care of the normal pregnant woman.

Bell's Palsy

An association between **Bell's palsy** (idiopathic facial paralysis) and pregnancy was first cited by Bell in 1830. The incidence of Bell's palsy in pregnancy is about 57 per 100,000 per year. The clinical manifestations include the sudden development of a unilateral facial weakness, often discovered first thing in the morning. In addition, taste on the anterior two thirds of the tongue may be lost, depending on the location of the lesion. Pain may occur in and around the ear. The incidence usually peaks during the third trimester and the puerperium (Cartlidge, 2000). A causative relation does not seem to exist between the appearance of Bell's palsy and any complications of pregnancy.

No effects of maternal Bell's palsy have been observed in infants. Maternal outcome is generally good unless there is a complete block in nerve conduction. Steroids sometimes are prescribed for the condition, but they do not hasten recovery. In most affected women, 90% or more of facial function can be expected to return (Cunningham et al., 2001). Supportive care includes prevention of injury to the exposed cornea, facial muscle massage, careful chewing and manual removal of food from inside the affected cheek, and reassurance that return of total neurologic function is likely.

Autoimmune Disorders

Autoimmune disorders make up a large group of diseases that disrupt the function of the immune system of the body. In these types of disorders, the body develops antibodies that attack its normally present antigens, causing tissue damage. Autoimmune disorders have a predilection for women in their reproductive years; therefore associations with pregnancy are not uncommon (Bennett & Brown, 1999). Pregnancy may affect the disease process. Some disorders adversely affect the course of pregnancy or are detrimental to the fetus. Autoimmune disorders of concern in pregnancy include systemic lupus erythematosus (SLE) and myasthenia gravis (MG).

Systemic Lupus Erythematosus

One of the most common serious disorders of childbearing age, **systemic lupus erythematosus (SLE)** is a chronic, multisystem inflammatory disease characterized by autoimmune antibody production that affects the skin, joints, kidneys, lungs, CNS, liver, and other body organs (Classen, Paulson, & Zacharias, 1998). The exact cause is unknown, but viral infection and hormonal and genetic factors may be related.

Early symptoms such as fatigue, weight loss, skin rashes, and arthralgias may be overlooked. Pericarditis is often the presenting symptom. Eventually all organs become involved. The condition is characterized by a series of exacerbations and remissions.

If the diagnosis has been established and the woman desires a child, she is advised to wait until she has been in remission for at least 6 months before attempting to become pregnant (Gilbert & Harmon, 2003). An exacerbation of SLE during pregnancy or postpartum occurs in 50% of women.

SLE during pregnancy is associated with increased rates of miscarriage, fetal loss, IUGR, and prematurity (Rosene-Montella, 2000); risks for preeclampsia and HELLP syndrome also are increased (Bennett & Brown, 1999).

Medical therapy is kept to a minimum in women who are in remission or who have a mild form of SLE. Anti-inflammatory drugs such as prednisone and aspirin may be used. Immunosuppressive drugs are not recommended during pregnancy but may be used in some situations when there is more risk in not treating SLE. Nursing care focuses on early recognition of signs of SLE exacerbation and pregnancy complications, education and support of the woman and her family, and assessment of fetal well-being.

Vaginal birth is preferred, but cesarean birth is common because of maternal and fetal complications. During labor, efforts are aimed at reducing the risk of infection, which is the leading cause of death in women with SLE.

During the postpartum period, the mother should rest as much as possible to prevent an exacerbation of SLE. Breastfeeding is encouraged unless the mother is taking immunosuppressive agents. Women with SLE should limit their number of pregnancies because of increased adverse perinatal outcomes as well as the guarded maternal prognosis (Cunningham et al., 2001). Family planning is important. Oral contraceptives are used with caution because vascular disease commonly accompanies SLE. Intrauterine devices may increase the risk of infection. Barrier methods are the safest option (Bennett & Brown, 1999).

Myasthenia Gravis

Myasthenia gravis (MG), an autoimmune motor (muscle) end-plate disorder that involves acetylcholine use, affects the motor function at the myoneural junction. Muscle weakness, particularly of the eyes, face, tongue, neck, limbs, and respiratory muscles, results. In addition, women may experience ptosis, diplopia, and dysphagia. MG occurs at the rate of 1 in 20,000 pregnancies (Larson, 2000). The response of women with MG to pregnancy is unpredictable; remission, exacerbation, or remaining stable during pregnancy may occur (Cartlidge, 2000).

Treatment is the same as for a nonpregnant woman. Usual medications include immunosuppressive medications and acetylcholinesterase inhibitor. Monitoring blood glucose values is important because hyperglycemia may be the result of corticosteroid therapy. Thymectomy may result in remission of the disease but is best performed before or after pregnancy, if at all possible. For severe weakness, plasmapheresis or intravenous immunoglobulin therapy may be needed.

Women with MG usually tolerate labor well, but vacuum or forceps assistance for birth may be required because of muscle weakness. Oxytocin may be given, but magnesium sulfate is contraindicated because it inhibits the release of acetylcholine. Narcotic analgesia should be avoided because it may precipitate respiratory depression. Regional analgesia is preferred. After birth, women must be carefully supervised because relapses often occur during the puerperium (Cartlidge, 2000).

In approximately 10% to 20% of neonates, neonatal myasthenia develops, with symptoms of feeble cry, respiratory distress, and weak suck. These neonates may require ventilatory support. With proper management, complete recovery of the neonate should occur within 6 weeks.

Gastrointestinal Disorders

Compromise of GI function during pregnancy is a concern. Obvious physiologic alterations, such as the greatly enlarged uterus, and less apparent changes, such as hormonal differences and *hypochlorhydria* (deficiency of hydrochloric acid in the stomach's gastric juice), require understanding for proper diagnosis and treatment. Gallbladder disease is an example of a GI disorder that may occur during pregnancy.

Cholelithiasis and Cholecystitis

Women are twice as likely to have **cholelithiasis** (presence of gallstones in the gallbladder) as are men (Baker, 2000), and pregnancy seems to make the woman more vulnerable to gallstone formation. Decreased muscle tone allows gallbladder distention, thickening of the bile, and prolonged emptying time. Increased progesterone levels result in a slight hypercholesterolemia.

Cholecystitis (inflammation of the gallbladder) also is more common in pregnancy, probably because pressure of the enlarged uterus interferes with the normal circulation and drainage of the gallbladder. The incidence of acute cholecystitis is about 0.02% to 0.16%, most often in multiparous women who have a history of previous attacks (Berman & Friedman, 2000). Gallbladder disease is the second most common indication for nonobstetric surgical intervention in pregnancy (Angelini, 2002).

Women with acute cholecystitis usually have fatty food intolerance along with colicky abdominal pain radiating to the back or shoulder, nausea, and vomiting (see Teaching

TEACHING FOR SELF-CARE

Nutritional Counseling for the Pregnant Woman with Cholecystitis or Cholelithiasis

- Assess your diet for foods that cause discomfort and flatulence, and omit foods that trigger episodes.
- Reduce dietary fat intake to 40 to 50 g/day.
- Limit protein to 10% to 12% of total calories.
- Choose foods so that most of the calories come from carbohydrates.
- Prepare food without adding fats or oils as much as possible.
- Avoid fried foods.

for Self-Care box). Fever and an increased leukocyte count also may be present. Ultrasound is often used to detect the presence of stones or dilation of the common bile duct (Samuels, 2002). Obese multiparous women are usually without symptoms.

Generally, gallbladder surgery should be postponed until the puerperium. Usually the woman can be treated with medical therapy, consisting of antibiotics, analgesics, intravenous fluids, bowel rest, and nasogastric suctioning. Total parenteral nutrition (TPN) can be used in some cases as an alternative to surgery (Berman & Friedman, 2000). Morphine should not be used as an analgesic because it may cause ductal spasm. The woman's condition should improve significantly within 48 hours of beginning treatment. Surgery may be necessary if the woman has repeated attacks of biliary colic, acute cholecystitis, obstructive jaundice, peritonitis, or pancreatitis. Laparoscopic cholecystectomy performed in the second trimester poses minimal risk to both mother and fetus (Berman & Friedman, 2000). Other procedures performed may be endoscopic retrograde cholangiopancreatography (ERCP) or open cholecystectomy (Angelini, 2002).

Inflammatory Bowel Disease

Treatment of inflammatory bowel disease is the same for the pregnant woman as it is for the nonpregnant woman. Medicines include prednisone and sulfasalazine. Vitamin and folic acid supplementation is especially important because of problems with malabsorption. Effects of inflammatory bowel disease on pregnancy are usually minimal; however, if the woman is severely debilitated, miscarriage, preterm birth, or fetal death can occur.

Surgery During Pregnancy

The incidence of surgery requiring anesthesia during pregnancy ranges from 0.2% to 2.2% (Ludmir & Stubblefield, 2002). The need for abdominal surgery occurs as frequently among pregnant women as among nonpregnant women of comparable age. However, pregnancy may make the diagnosis more difficult. An enlarged uterus and displaced internal organs may make abdominal palpation more difficult, alter the position of an affected organ, and/or change the usual signs and symptoms associated with a particular disorder. The most common condition necessitating abdominal surgery during pregnancy is appendicitis.

Appendicitis

Appendicitis occurs approximately once in 2000 pregnancies. This condition occurs in approximately the same frequency during each trimester of pregnancy and the postpartum period (Ludmir & Stubblefield, 2002). The diagnosis of appendicitis is often delayed because the usual signs and symptoms mimic some normal changes of pregnancy such as nausea and vomiting and increased WBC count. As pregnancy progresses, the appendix is pushed upward and to the right from its usual anatomic location (see Fig. 14-14). Because of these changes, appendiceal rupture and peritonitis occur two to three times more often in pregnant women than in nonpregnant women.

The woman with appendicitis most commonly is first seen with right lower quadrant abdominal pain, nausea and vomiting, and loss of appetite. Approximately half of these affected women have muscle guarding. Moving the uterus tends to increase the pain. Temperature may be normal or mildly increased (to 38.3° C). Because of the physiologic increase in WBCs that occurs in pregnancy, elevated WBC counts are not clear indicators of appendicitis (Mourad et al., 2000).

The diagnosis of appendicitis requires a high level of suspicion because the typical signs and symptoms are similar to those found in many other conditions, including pyelonephritis, round ligament pain, placental abruption, torsion of an ovarian cyst, cholecystitis, and preterm labor (Ludmir & Stubblefield, 2002) (see Table 31-2).

Appendectomy before rupture usually does not require either antibiotic or tocolytic therapy. If surgery is delayed until after rupture, multiple antibiotics are ordered. Rupture is likely to result in preterm labor, perhaps necessitating the use of tocolytic agents.

Collaborative Care

Initial assessment of the pregnant woman requiring surgery focuses on her presenting signs and symptoms. A thorough history and physical examination are performed. Laboratory testing includes, at a minimum, a complete blood count with differential and a urinalysis. Additional laboratory and other diagnostic tests may well be necessary to reach a diagnosis. In addition, fetal heart rate (FHR) and activity, along with uterine activity, should be monitored, and constant vigilance for symptoms of impending obstetric complications maintained. The extent of presurgery assessment is determined by the immediacy of surgical intervention and the specific disorder that requires surgery.

Hospital Care. When surgery becomes necessary during pregnancy, the woman and her family are concerned about the effects of the procedure and medication on fetal well-being and the course of pregnancy. An important part of preoperative nursing care is encouraging the woman to express her fears, concerns, and questions.

Preoperative care for a pregnant woman differs from that for a nonpregnant woman in one significant aspect: the presence of at least one other person, the fetus. Continuous FHR and uterine contraction monitoring should be performed if the fetus is considered viable. Procedures such as preparation of the operative site and time of insertion of IV lines and urinary retention catheters vary with the physician and the facility. However, in every instance, there is a total restriction of solid foods and liquids or a clear specification of the type, amount, and time at which clear liquids may be taken before surgery. Some bowel preparation such as clear liquids and laxatives may be required before surgery (Wheeless, 2000). Food by mouth is restricted for several hours before a scheduled procedure. Even if she has had nothing by mouth–but more important, if surgery is unexpected–the woman is in danger of vomiting and aspirating, and special precautions are taken before anesthetic is administered (e.g., administering an antacid).

Intraoperatively, perinatal nurses may collaborate with the surgical staff to increase their knowledge about the special needs of pregnant women undergoing surgery. One intervention to improve fetal oxygenation is positioning the woman on the operating table with a lateral tilt to avoid maternal venacaval compression. Continuous fetal and uterine monitoring during the procedure is recommended because of the risk for preterm labor. Monitoring may be accomplished by using sterile aquasonic gel and a sterile sleeve for the transducer. During abdominal surgery, uterine contractions may be manually palpated.

In the immediate recovery period, general observations and care pertinent to postoperative recovery are initiated. Frequent assessments are carried out for several hours after surgery. Whether the woman is cared for in the surgical postanesthesia recovery area or in a labor and birth unit, continuous fetal and uterine monitoring will likely be initiated or resumed because of the increased risk of preterm labor. Tocolysis may be necessary if preterm labor occurs (see Chapter 36).

Home Care. Plans for the woman's return home and for convalescent care should be completed as early as possible before discharge. Depending on her insurance coverage, nursing care may be provided through a home health agency. If not, the woman and other support persons must be taught necessary skills and procedures, such as wound care. Ideally, the woman and other caregivers should have opportunities for supervised practice before discharge so that they can feel comfortable with their knowledge and ability before being totally responsible for providing care. Box 33-5 lists information that should be included in discharge teaching for the postoperative client. The woman also may need referrals to various community agencies for evaluation of the home situation, child care, home health care, and financial or other assistance.

BOX 33-5 Discharge Teaching for Home Care

- Care of incision site
- Diet and elimination related to GI function
- Signs and symptoms of developing complications; wound infection, thrombophlebitis, pneumonia
- Equipment needed and technique for assessing temperature
- Recommended schedule for resumption of activities of daily living
- Treatments and medications ordered
- List of resource persons and their telephone numbers
- Schedule of follow-up visits

If birth has not occurred:

- Assessment of fetal activity (kick counts)
- Signs of preterm labor

KEY POINTS

- The stress of the normal maternal adaptations to pregnancy on a heart whose function is already taxed may cause cardiac decompensation.
- In the case of a cardiac arrest in a pregnant woman, the standard advanced cardiac life support guidelines should be implemented with a few slight modifications: the uterus must be displaced laterally, and the defibrillation paddles should be placed one rib interspace higher.
- Maternal morbidity and mortality is a significant risk in a pregnancy complicated by mitral stenosis.
- The normal hemodynamic values are significantly altered as a result of pregnancy.
- Anemia, the most common medical disorder of pregnancy, affects at least 20% of pregnant women.
- Asthma is the most common respiratory crisis complicating pregnancy.
- Pruritis is a common symptom in pregnancy-specific inflammatory skin diseases.
- Epilepsy is the most common neurologic disorder of pregnancy and can be confused with eclampsia; however, a history of seizures and no signs of preeclampsia point to epilepsy.
- Cholecystitis and cholelithiasis are common gastrointestinal problems in pregnancy.
- Autoimmune disorders (e.g., SLE, MG) show a predilection for women in their reproductive years; therefore associations with pregnancy are not uncommon.
- In the pregnant woman, an enlarged uterus, displaced internal organs, and altered laboratory values may confound differential diagnosis when the need for immediate abdominal surgery occurs.
- Preoperative care for a pregnant woman differs from that for a nonpregnant woman in one significant aspect: the presence of at least one other person, the fetus.

CRITICAL THINKING EXERCISES

1. Anna, a 28-year-old woman pregnant with her first child, calls the advice nurse complaining of pain and redness in her lower calf. She has a history of cardiac disease.
   - **a.** What questions will you ask her?
   - **b.** What laboratory test will most likely be ordered to help determine the diagnosis?
   - **c.** Given a medical diagnosis of thrombophlebitis, what are your nursing diagnoses?
   - **d.** Formulate your plan of care, including client teaching for anticoagulant therapy.
2. Lisa, age 38 years and pregnant with her third child, has a history of peripartum cardiomyopathy, and is diagnosed as having class IV (NYHA) heart disease. She is in labor and discovered to be in cardiac arrest in the LDRP room.
   - **a.** What key assessments must be made now?
   - **b.** List the primary modifications that must be made in the CPR procedure.
   - **c.** Give examples of communications with family members that may assist with coping and decrease anxiety during this crisis.

RESOURCES

American Academy of Dermatology
www.aad.org

American Association of Critical Care Nurses
www.aacn.org

American Heart Association
Women's heart information: 888-MYHEART (888-694-3278)
800-242-8721
www.americanheart.org

Asthma and Allergy Foundation of America
www.aafa.org

Center for Sickle Cell Disease
2121 Georgia Ave., NW
Washington, DC 20059
202-636-7930

CPR Information
www.cpr-ecc.org

March of Dimes Birth Defects Foundation
1275 Mamaroneck Ave.
White Plains, NY 10605
914-428-7100
888-663-4637
www.modimes.org

National Association for Sickle Cell Disease
3345 Wilshire Blvd., Suite 1106
Los Angeles, CA 90010-1880
213-736-5455
800-421-8453

National Bed Rest Support Group
Sidelines
P.O. Box 1808
Laguna Beach, CA 92652
714-497-2265
www.sidelines.org

National Multiple Sclerosis Society
733 Third Ave
New York, NY 10017
800-344-4867
www.nmss.org

REFERENCES

American Heart Association (AHA). (1992). Subcommittee on Emergency Cardiac Care. Standards and guidelines for cardiopulmonary resuscitation and emergency cardiac care. *Journal of the American Medical Association, 268*, 2172, 2249.

Aminoff, M. (1999). Neurologic disorders. In R. Creasy & R. Resnik (Eds.), *Maternal-fetal medicine* (4th ed.). Philadelphia: W.B. Saunders.

Angelini, D. (2002). Gallbladder and pancreatic disease during pregnancy. *Journal of Perinatal and Neonatal Nursing, 15*(4), 1-12.

Association of Women's Health, Obstetric, and Neonatal Nurses (1998). *Standards and guidelines for professional nursing practice in the care of women and newborns* (5th ed). Washington, DC: The Association.

Bajo, T. (1997). Cardiopulmonary resuscitation of the pregnant patient. In M. Foley & T. Strong (Eds.), *Obstetric intensive care.* Philadelphia: W.B. Saunders.

Baker, A. (2000). Liver and biliary tract disease. In W. Barron & M. Lindheimer (Eds.), *Medical disorders during pregnancy* (3rd ed.). St. Louis: Mosby.

Barbour, L. (2000). Asthma. In R. Lee et al. (Eds.), *Medical care of the pregnant patient.* Philadelphia: American College of Physicians.

Barbour, L., & Pickard, J. (2000). Epilepsy. In R. Lee et al. (Eds.), *Medical care of the pregnant patient.* Philadelphia: American College of Physicians.

Barron, W. (2000). Hypertension. In W. Barron & M. Lindheimer (Eds.), *Medical disorders of pregnancy* (3rd ed.). St. Louis: Mosby.

Bennett, V., & Brown, L. (1999). *Myles textbook for midwives* (13th ed.). Edinburgh: Churchill Livingstone.

Berman, D., & Friedman, S. (2000). Diseases of the biliary tract and liver. In W. Cohen (Ed.), *Cherry and Merkatz's complications of pregnancy.* Philadelphia: Lippincott, Williams & Wilkins.

Bonow, R. et al. (1998). ACC/AHA guidelines for the management of clients with valvular heart disease: A report of the American College of Cardiology/American Heart Association Task Force on Practice Guidelines (Committee on Management of Patients with Valvular Heart Disease). *Journal of the American College of Cardiology, 32*, 1486-1588.

Bormanis, J. (2000). Anemia. In R. Lee et al. (Eds.), *Medical care of the pregnant patient.* Philadelphia: American College of Physicians.

Burton, J., & Reyes, J. (2001). Breathe in, breathe out, controlling asthma during pregnancy. *AWHONN Lifelines, 5*(1), 24-30.

Cartlidge, N. (2000). Neurologic disorders. In W. Barron & M. Lindheimer (Eds.), *Medical disorders during pregnancy* (3rd ed.). Philadelphia: Mosby.

Chari, R. et al. (1998). Hypertension during pregnancy: Diagnosis, pathophysiology, and management. In U. Elkayam & N. Gleicher (Eds.), *Cardiac problems in pregnancy.* New York: Wiley-Liss.

Classen, S., Paulson, P., & Zacharias, S. (1998). Systemic lupus erythematosus: Perinatal and neonatal implications. *Journal of Obstetric, Gynecologic, and Neonatal Nursing, 27*(5), 493-500.

Cohen, E., & Garity, M. (1998). Diuretics in pregnany. In U. Elkayam & N. Gleicher (Eds.), *Cardiac problems in pregnancy.* New York: Wiley-Liss

Cohen, R., & Castro, L. (1998). Cardiac surgery during pregnancy. In U. Elkayam & N. Gleicher (Eds.), *Cardiac problems in pregnancy.* New York: Wiley-Liss.

Comport, K.A., & Seng, J.K. (1997). Aortic stenosis in pregnancy. *Journal of Obstetric, Gynecologic, and Neonatal Nursing, 26*(1), 67-77.

Cunningham, F. et al (2001). *Williams obstetrics* (21st ed). New York: McGraw-Hill.

Dajani A. et al. (1997). Prevention of bacterial endocarditis: Recommendation by the American Heart Association. *Journal of the American Medical Association, 277*, 1794-1801.

de Swiet, M. (2000). Pulmonary disorders. In W. Barron & M. Lindheimer (Eds.), *Medical disorders in pregnancy* (3rd ed.). Philadelphia: Mosby.

Easterling, T., & Otto, C. (2002). Heart disease. In S. Gabbe, J. Niebyl, & J. Simpson (Eds.), *Obstetrics: Normal and problem pregnancies* (4th ed.). New York: Churchill-Livingstone.

Eggum, M. (2001). Breastfeeding with multiple sclerosis. *AWHONN Lifelines, 5*(1), 36-40.

Elkayam, U. et al. (1998). Marfan syndrome and pregnancy. In U. Elkayam & N. Gleicher (Eds.), *Cardiac problems in pregnancy.* New York: Wiley-Liss.

Elkayam, U., & Dave, R. (1998). Hypertrophic cardiomyopathy and pregnancy. In U. Elkayam & N. Gleicher (Eds.), *Cardiac problems in pregnancy.* New York: Wiley-Liss.

Essop, M., & Sareli, P. (1998). Rheumatic valvular disease and pregnancy. In U. Elkayam & N. Gleicher (Eds.), *Cardiac problems in pregnancy.* New York: Wiley-Liss.

Gei, A., & Hankins, G. (2001). Cardiac disease and pregnancy. *Obstetrics and Gynecology Clinics of North America, 28*(3), 465-512.

Gilbert, E., & Harmon, J. (2003). *Manual of high risk pregnancy and delivery* (3rd ed). St. Louis: Mosby.

Gilmore, J., Pennell, P., & Stern, B. (1998). Medication use during pregnancy for neurologic conditions. *Neurology Clinics of North America, 16*, 189-206.

Hassell, K. (2000). Hemoglobinopathies. In R. Lee et al. (Eds.), *Medical care of the pregnant patient.* Philadelphia: American College of Physicians.

Health Care Resources. (1997). *Handbook of high risk perinatal home care.* St. Louis: Mosby.

Hurst, A. et al. (1998). The use of beta-adrenergic blocking agents in pregnancy and lactation. In U. Elkayam & N. Gleicher (Eds.), *Cardiac problems in pregnancy.* New York: Wiley-Liss.

Kansaria, J., & Salvi, V. (2000). Eisenmenger syndrome in pregnancy. *Journal of Postgraduate Medicine, 46*(2),101-103.

Kilpatrick, S., & Laros, R. (1999). Maternal hemorrhagic disorders. In R. Creasy & R. Resnik (Eds.), *Maternal-fetal medicine* (4th ed.). Philadelphia: W.B. Saunders.

Kleinman, C. (1999). Cardiovascular disease. In J. Queenan (Ed.), *Management of high-risk pregnancy.* Malden, MA: Blackwell Science.

Kloeck, W. et al. (1997). Special resuscitation situations: An advisory statement from the International Liaison Committee on Resuscitation. *Circulation, 15*(8), 2196-2210.

Lang, R. et al. (1998). Peripartal cardiomyopathy. In U. Elkayam & N. Gleicher (Eds.), *Cardiac problems in pregnancy.* New York: Wiley-Liss.

Larson, L. (2000). Myasthenia gravis. In R. Lee et al. (Eds.), *Medical care of the pregnant patient.* Philadelphia: American College of Physicians.

Lawrence, R. (1999). *Breastfeeding: A guide for the medical profession* (5th ed.). St. Louis: Mosby.

Letsky, E. (2000). Hematologic disorders. In W. Barron & M. Lindheimer (Eds.), *Medical disorders during pregnancy* (3rd ed.). Philadelphia: Mosby.

Lowdermilk, D., & Grohar, J. (1998). *High risk antepartal home care.* White Plains, NY: March of Dimes.

Ludmir, J., & Stubblefield, P. (2002). Surgical procedures in pregnancy. In S. Gabbe, J. Niebyl, & J. Simpson (Eds.), *Obstetrics: Normal and problem pregnancies* (4th ed.). New York: Churchill Livingstone.

Luppi, C. (1999). Cardiopulmonary resuscitation in pregnancy. *AWHONN Lifelines, 3*(3), 41-45.

Maloni, J., Brezinski-Tomasi, J., & Johnson, L. (2001). Antepartum bed rest: effect upon the family. *Journal of Obstetric, Gynecologic, and Neonatal Nursing, 30*(2), 67-77.

McGehee, W. (1998) Anticoagulation in pregnancy. In U. Elkayam & N. Gleicher (Eds.), *Cardiac problems in pregnancy.* New York: Wiley-Liss.

Meller, J., & Goldman, M. (2000). Cardiovascular disease. In W. Cohen (Ed.), *Cherry and Merkatz's complications of pregnancy.* Philadelphia: Lippincott, Williams & Wilkins.

Mendelson, M. (1997). Congenital cardiac disease and pregnancy. *Clinical Perinatology, 24*(2), 467-482.

Mendelson, M., & Lang, R. (2000). Pregnancy and cardiovascular disease. In W. Barron & M. Lindheimer (Eds.), *Medical disorders during pregnancy* (3rd ed.). Philadelphia: Mosby.

Mourad, J et al. (2000). Appendicitis in pregnancy: New information that contradicts long-held beliefs. *American Journal of Obstetrics and Gynecology, 182*(5), 1027-1029.

Murdock, M. (2002). Asthma in pregnancy. *Journal of Perinatal and Neonatal Nursing, 15*(4), 27-36.

National Women's Health Resource Center. (2001). Multiple sclerosis and women's health. *National Women's Health Report, 23*(2), 1-7.

New York Heart Association (NYHA). (1964). *Diseases of the heart and blood vessels: Nomenclature and criteria for diagnosis* (6th ed.). Boston: Little, Brown.

Niebyl, J. (2002). Drugs in pregnancy and lactation. In S. Gabbe, J. Niebyl, & J. Simpson (Eds.), *Obstetrics: Normal and problems pregnancies* (4th ed.). New York: Churchill Livingstone.

O'Reilly-Green, C. (2000). Surgical considerations. In W. Cohen (Ed.), *Cherry and Merkatz's complications of pregnancy*. Philadelphia: Lippincott, Williams & Wilkins.

Pagana, K., & Pagana, T. (2003). *Mosby's diagnostic and laboratory test reference* (6th ed.). St. Louis: Mosby.

Pickard, J. (2000). Chronic lung disease. In R. Lee, et al. (Eds.), *Medical care of the pregnant patient*. Philadelphia: American College of Physicians.

Poppas, A. (2000). Congenital and acquired heart disease. In R. Lee et al. (Eds.), *Medical care of the pregnant patient*. Philadelphia: American College of Physicians.

Ramsey, P., Ramin, K., & Ramin, S. (2001). Cardiac disease in pregnancy. *American Journal of Perinatology, 18*(5), 245-262.

Roberts, J. (1999). Pregnancy-related hypertension. In R. Creasy & R. Resnik (Eds.), *Maternal-fetal medicine* (4th ed.). Philadelphia: W.B. Saunders.

Rosene-Montella, K. (2000). Systemic lupus erythematosus. In R. Lee et al. (Eds.), *Medical care of the pregnant patient*. Philadelphia: American College of Physicians.

Rosene-Montella, K, & Poppas, A. (2000). Peripartum cardiomyopathy. In R. Lee et al. (Eds.), *Medical care of the pregnant patient*. Philadelphia: American College of Physicians.

Roth, A., & Elkayam, U. (1998). Acute myocardial infarction and pregnancy. In U. Elkayam & N. Gleicher (Eds.), *Cardiac problems in pregnancy*. New York: Wiley-Liss.

Samuels, P. (2002). Hepatic disease. In S. Gabbe, J. Niebyl, & J. Simpson (Eds.), *Obstetrics: Normal and problems pregnancies* (4th ed.). New York: Churchill Livingstone.

Schmidt, G., & Hall, J. (2000). Pulmonary disease. In W. Barron & M. Lindheimer (Eds.), *Medical disorders during pregnancy* (3rd ed.). Philadelphia: Mosby.

Shabetai, R. (1999). Cardiac diseases. In R. Creasy & R. Resnik (Eds.), *Maternal-fetal medicine* (4th ed.). Philadelphia: W.B. Saunders.

Shotan, A. et al. (1998). Antiarrhythmic drugs during pregnancy. In U. Elkayam & N. Gleicher (Eds.), *Cardiac problems in pregnancy*. New York: Wiley-Liss.

Siba, B. (2002). Hypertension. In S. Gabbe, J. Niebyl, & J. Simpson (Eds.), *Obstetrics: Normal and problem pregnancies* (4th ed.). New York: Churchill Livingstone.

Stambuk, R., & Colvin, R. (2002). Dermatologic disorders. In S. Gabbe, J. Niebyl, & J. Simpson (Eds.), *Obstetrics: Normal and problems pregnancies* (4th ed.). New York: Churchill Livingstone.

Stapleton, E. et al. (2001). *Fundamentals of BLS for healthcare providers*. Dallas: American Heart Association.

Steinberg, I. et al. (1998). Pharmacokinetics of drugs in pregnancy and lactation. In U. Elkayam & N. Gleicher (Eds.), *Cardiac problems in pregnancy*. New York: Wiley-Liss.

Warnes, C., & Elkayam, U. (1998). Congenital heart disease in pregnancy. In U. Elkayam & N. Gleicher (Eds.), *Cardiac problems in pregnancy*. New York: Wiley-Liss.

Wendel, P. (2001). Asthma in pregnancy. *Obstetrics and Gynecology Clinics of North America, 28*(3), 537-549.

Wheeless, C. (2000). Surgical considerations. In W. Cohen (Ed.), *Cherry and Merkatz's complications of pregnancy*. Philadelphia: Lippincott, Williams & Wilkins.

CHAPTER 34

Karen F. Dorman and Mildred G. Harvey

Obstetric Critical Care

http://evolve.elsevier.com/Lowdermilk/MatWmnHlth/

LEARNING OBJECTIVES

- Discuss factors that have contributed to the development of the specialty of critical care obstetrics.
- Describe conditions that may place a pregnant woman in a critically ill state.
- Examine factors that affect the provision of obstetric critical care when a pregnant woman becomes critically ill.
- Describe significant cardiovascular, pulmonary, and hematologic alterations during pregnancy that affect critical care for the pregnant woman.
- Review cardiac anatomy and physiologic features, including location of chambers, valves, major vessels, and path of circulation.
- List the four determinants of cardiac output and relate the clinical significance of each.
- Describe the parameters measured and normal values for pulmonary artery monitoring.
- Describe the parameters measured and normal values for arterial pressure monitoring.
- Identify treatment strategies based on interpretation of hemodynamic profiles.
- Discuss implications of trauma on mother and fetus during pregnancy.
- Identify physiologic alterations of pregnancy that affect stabilization and treatment of the pregnant woman who has undergone trauma.
- Describe immediate assessment and stabilization measures for the pregnant victim of trauma.
- Compare components of the primary and secondary surveys for the pregnant woman who has undergone trauma.
- Discuss inclusion of the components of family-centered maternity care for the critically ill pregnant woman.
- Examine the impact of maternal death on families and nursing staff members who cared for the woman.

Obstetric and critical care units are equally challenged whenever presented with the multiple, complex needs of a critically ill pregnant woman and her fetus. Optimal outcome for mother and fetus depends on (1) swift recognition of severe complications and (2) delivery of critical care therapies adjusted for the physiologic alterations of pregnancy. Fetal effects of therapies also must be considered. Management of the critically ill pregnant woman includes measures to assess both maternal and fetal status continually, selection of therapeutic interventions appropriate for both mother and fetus, and careful management for the timing of birth.

The provision of critical care and hemodynamic monitoring for the seriously ill pregnant woman has developed slowly in many institutions. This seems to have been the result of two factors: (1) obstetric nurses and physicians, expert in the care of pregnant women, feel threatened by pressure transducers, alarms, hemodynamic monitoring, and ventilators; and (2) critical care nurses and physicians, expert in hemodynamic monitoring and mechanical ventilation, feel threatened by the pregnant uterus, labor, birth, the fetus, and fetal monitoring. The result is that few institutions have been able to provide optimal care whenever a sudden, acute, life-threatening complication has occurred in a pregnant woman.

A critical care unit, or intensive care unit, provides the setting where advanced care necessary to support life is immediately available. An expert medical, nursing, and technical staff uses sophisticated, state-of-the-art techniques and equipment for invasive hemodynamic monitoring and immediate life-saving interventions. The development of specialized critical care units has evolved in parallel with advances in invasive surgical and medical procedures and techniques.

Critical care obstetrics evolved as a subspecialty of perinatal medicine in response to the need for optimal care for the critically ill pregnant woman and her fetus. This subspecialty prepares the obstetric team, which has in-depth knowledge of pregnancy, to use critical care techniques in the management of the critically ill pregnant woman and her fetus. Obstetric intensive care units (OBICUs) have been developed in some centers so that expensive, specific equipment and individuals with special training and expertise in obstetric care and critical care are available to provide this care.

OBSTETRIC INTENSIVE CARE UNIT

Complications may develop during pregnancy that are so severe and life threatening that optimal maternal and fetal outcome, and many times survival, depend on the woman receiving critical care that meets her specific needs. Maternal adaptations that are normal for the pregnancy state alter physiologic status and make the pregnant woman hemodynamically different from the nonpregnant woman. Before the development of OBICUs, care for the critically ill pregnant woman was usually provided in an ICU for adults, where management modalities were based on hemodynamic values that are normal for the nonpregnant individual. Less than desirable outcomes in many cases led to studies that resulted in the development and establishment of OBICUs, which are set up to meet the specific needs of the critically ill pregnant woman.

Research in some of the first OBICUs reported on physical and hemodynamic differences during the pregnant state. Normal hemodynamic values for pregnancy were identified. Maternal and fetal outcomes improved when management of care was based on the enhanced hemodynamic state that accompanies normal pregnancy and care was provided in the specialized units (Mabie & Sibai, 1990).

PROVISION OF OBSTETRIC CRITICAL CARE

Anyone providing care for pregnant women may encounter the pregnant woman with a life-threatening complication and be challenged to recognize the need for immediate, critical care and to provide such care. This care may be delivered in a variety of ways. Problems can be decreased by development of a viable plan to provide care for the critically ill pregnant woman; adequate education of nursing, medical, and ancillary staff; provision of necessary equipment at the bedside; and liberal consultation between the obstetric and critical care units.

The most practical, efficient, economic method to provide care for the critically ill obstetric client who requires invasive hemodynamic monitoring, mechanical ventilation, or both depends primarily on the numbers of pregnant women cared for annually and the referral patterns in a specific facility. The ideal method to provide care for the pregnancy would be a specially trained team of obstetricians and obstetric nurses in an OBICU, augmented by anesthesiologists, pulmonologists, cardiologists, and intensivists as needed. The larger tertiary center is more likely to have this type of unit because the census of pregnant women cared for annually in the referral center would support development of the service. OBICUs are often small and may consist of one bed. Admissions may be limited only to the very sickest women and may not include all women eligible for a bed in the OBICU.

However, even in many large, tertiary centers, the number of truly critically ill pregnant women is not enough to warrant such an investment in equipment and training of medical staff. In these centers, collaborative practice between obstetrics and intensive care has been successful in providing the best care for these women (McCormack, 1998). If the woman remains pregnant, the optimal place for her is the labor and birth suite, with a critical care nurse in attendance. However, the ICU is the most usual site for this collaborative care. In this instance, obstetric practitioners serve a vital role in monitoring the woman as well as assessing the fetus. The institution must develop policies and procedures so that care is provided where it is most advantageous to the pregnant woman. Some institutions provide dual training for selected nurses (i.e., an ICU nurse receives advanced education in obstetrics or an obstetric nurse receives advanced education in intensive care nursing).

In still other institutions, an obstetric service may be established to provide care during the low risk pregnancy. The plan for the smaller unit or the low risk unit may be for the nursing and medical team to recognize the critical illness immediately, stabilize the woman, and initiate measures for transport to the tertiary center and/or the OBICU. *Standards and Guidelines for Professional Nursing Practice in the Care of Women and Newborns* (Association of Women's Health, Obstetric, and Neonatal Nurses [AWHONN], 1998) includes guidelines for the care of the pregnant woman requiring critical care.

LEGAL TIP Nursing Assignments

Continuous assignment of an obstetric and an intensive care nurse, or one nurse experienced in both specialties, is required in the care of the critically ill woman with a viable pregnancy.

LEGAL TIP Client Care Standards

Client care standards established for both obstetric care and intensive care must be met within the plan developed by an institution to provide complex, critical care for the critically ill pregnant woman. Standards of care from both specialties must be followed.

Obstetric clients requiring critical care are at risk for undesirable outcomes of the pregnancy because of the severity of complications, including decreased oxygen transport and multiple system organ failure and the possibility of long-term residual physical effects of the illness.

LEGAL TIP Legal Review

Because an optimal outcome is uncertain when the pregnant woman is critically ill, the medical records, with documentation of the medical and nursing care that mother, fetus, and neonate received, are more likely to be subjected to legal review than are medical records of other clients.

EQUIPMENT AND EXPERTISE

Appropriate care of the critically ill pregnant woman and her fetus depends on the availability of adequate, appropriate equipment and the presence of individuals educated in their use. The usual equipment for a labor, birth, and recovery suite is mandatory for an ICU or surgical suite where this woman may be admitted for care. Staff and equipment for neonatal resuscitation also must be available. The usual equipment for intensive care, including hemodynamic monitoring and mechanical ventilation, is equally necessary whenever the critically ill client is in the labor and birth unit.

Obstetric critical care may be delivered according to individual plans developed by individual institutions on the basis of a needs assessment. However, it is imperative that all institutions providing care for pregnant women have a plan and staff educated to care for the occasional woman who has a life-threatening complication during pregnancy. Pregnant women with a critical complication must receive the care needed; critical care must not be denied to pregnant women. Pregnancy is not a contraindication for invasive hemodynamic monitoring.

INDICATIONS FOR OBSTETRIC CRITICAL CARE

A severe complication of pregnancy may prompt the need for obstetric critical care with hemodynamic monitoring or mechanical ventilation. See Box 34-1 for a list of complications that indicate a need for critical care.

BOX 34-1 Complications of Pregnancy That Indicate the Need for Critical Care

1. Severe preeclampsia-eclampsia with complications
   a. Refractory pulmonary edema
   b. Refractory oliguria
   c. Hypertensive crisis
   d. Severe hemorrhage or disseminated intravascular coagulation (DIC)
   e. Renal failure
2. Hemorrhage or DIC that requires multiple transfusions
3. Cardiac problems
4. Chronic health problems
   a. Systemic lupus erythematosus
   b. Diabetic ketoacidosis
   c. Sickle cell disease
   d. Diabetes complicated by vascular changes
   e. Others
5. Trauma victim
   a. Motor vehicle crash
   b. Violence, battering

The number of pregnant women who need obstetric critical care has increased in recent years. This apparently is the result of women surviving childhood illnesses because of advances in pediatric care. These include the development of pediatric ICUs; improved surgical procedures for infants with congenital defects, such as cardiac lesions; and advanced knowledge in pediatric care for children with chronic health problems, including diabetes, cystic fibrosis, and pulmonary disorders. The wish to become a parent is not eliminated by a chronic health problem, and many women each year risk their lives to have a baby. Women have had successful pregnancies after kidney transplants (Sgro et al., 2002), after heart transplants (Branch et al., 1998), and after liver transplants (Miller, Mastrobattista, & Katz, 2000). More pregnant women with chronic health problems are predicted as graduates of neonatal ICUs reach adulthood.

Other pregnant women need critical care because of trauma resulting from automobile crashes or violence and battering. These causes account for most of the traumatic injuries during pregnancy.

The most common diagnosis for admission to an OBICU is severe preeclampsia with complications, including refractory pulmonary edema, refractory oliguria, hypertensive crisis, severe hemorrhage or disseminated intravascular coagulation (DIC), and renal failure. Massive hemorrhage or DIC is reported as the second most common reason for admission (Hazelgrove et al., 2001). Conditions that classify the parturient as critically ill and indicate the need for a pulmonary artery catheter include the following (American College of Obstetricians and Gynecologists [ACOG], 1992):

- Sepsis with refractory hypotension or oliguria
- Unexplained or refractory pulmonary edema, congestive heart failure, or oliguria
- Severe pregnancy-induced hypertension (PIH) with pulmonary edema or refractory oliguria
- Intraoperative or intrapartum cardiovascular decompensation
- Massive blood loss or volume replacement needs
- Adult respiratory distress syndrome
- Shock of undefined source
- Chronic disease, particularly when associated with labor or major surgery

The identification of women needing OBICU services merits careful consideration. It is important not to visualize just the "sickest client scenario"–that dramatic case, never to be forgotten. Instead, the typical picture of a critically ill pregnant woman is one with severe preeclampsia, whose condition has worsened and today has headache, high blood pressure (BP), oliguria, and low platelets. Or the woman may be sent in for referral from the level I center with a preexisting cardiac lesion exacerbated by pregnancy that has gradually deteriorated from class I to class III cardiac disease. Her presenting complaint may be "feeling extremely tired."

Approximately 0.9% to 1% of pregnant women giving birth in an institution require care in an OBICU. The percentage and numbers of pregnant women needing care in an OBICU are higher in an institution that receives referrals from a large area. As the number of high risk pregnant women served in an institution increases, the number of women likely to become critically ill also increases. More seriously ill pregnant women receive immediate critical care when an institution has an OBICU than when the pregnant woman must be transported to a medical-surgical ICU to receive care (Mabie & Sibai, 1990).

CARDIORESPIRATORY CHANGES OF PREGNANCY

The normal physiologic adaptations that accompany pregnancy and produce profound hemodynamic changes are the primary factors that make the pregnant woman a different type of critical care client and merit a separate critical care facility. Knowledge of the effects of the physiologic alterations during pregnancy is essential for optimal critical care management. Normal maternal alterations during pregnancy affect the major systems: the cardiovascular, pulmonary, renal, and hematologic systems (Harvey, 1999).

Cardiovascular Changes

The cardiovascular system changes dramatically during pregnancy. Pregnancy is a state of high flow, low resistance, so that pregnancy is hemodynamically similar to early sepsis. Hypervolemia is the result of the influence of estrogen and progesterone on aldosterone, which produces an increase in circulating blood volume. The increase in maternal blood volume begins with a 22% increase by 8 weeks of gestation. Total expansion increases progressively to a maximum of 45% by 32 to 34 weeks of gestation. This represents an increase of approximately 1570 ml for the singleton gestation. This includes a 40% to 50% increase in plasma volume and a 20% to 30% increase in red blood cell mass, a disproportional increase that results in a state of hemodilution. An increase in total body water of 6 to 8 L in the extravascular compartment, accompanied by an accumulation of 500 to 900 mEq of sodium, also occurs during pregnancy. Heart rate (HR) increases 20% (10 to 15 beats/min) with the major increase in the third trimester, and stroke volume increases to accommodate the increased circulating volume. See Table 34-1 for a summary of cardiovascular adaptations.

Colloid Osmotic Pressure

Colloid osmotic pressure (COP) is the gradient controlling whether fluid remains inside the capillary or moves into the interstitial space. The force to keep the fluid inside the vessel is the pulling pressure of the colloids, or proteins, present in the plasma. The most important plasma proteins are albumin, globulin, and fibrinogen. Pregnancy produces a decrease in COP values resulting from the hemodilution state that reduces the concentration of plasma proteins. Severe preeclampsia-eclampsia (PIH) usually produces renal damage, with a subsequent loss of proteins in the urine, further reducing the COP. The force exerted to push fluids through the membrane is the **capillary hydrostatic pressure** and is measured as the **pulmonary capillary wedge pressure (PCWP).** COP is measured with an oncometer. Colloid osmotic (oncotic) values in pregnancy are shown in Table 34-2. This measurement is not available

TABLE 34-1 **Cardiovascular Changes During Pregnancy**

PARAMETER	CHANGE
Blood volume	40%-50% increase
Plasma volume	40%-50% increase (1200-1300 ml)
Red blood cell mass	20%-30% increase (250-450 ml)
Heart	Displaced to the left and upward
Point of maximal impulse (PMI)	Fourth intercostal space and lateral
Rate	20% increase (10-15 beats/min)
Sounds	Exaggerated splitting first sound
	Systolic murmur usually present
	Third sound present
Stroke volume	32% increase by 20-24 wk
Cardiac output	Increases by 30%-50%
	22% increase by 28 wk
	43% increase by term
	Increases during labor
	≤3 cm, 17% increase
	4-7 cm, 23% increase
	≥8 cm, 34% increase

Source: Harvey, M. (1999). Physiologic changes during pregnancy. In L. Mandeville & N. Troiano (Eds.), *AWHONN's high risk and critical care intrapartum nursing* (2nd ed.). Philadelphia: J.B. Lippincott.

TABLE 34-2 **Colloid Osmotic (Oncotic) Pressure Values**

Nonpregnant	25.4 ± 2.3 mm Hg
Pregnant, antepartum	22.4 ± 0.54 mm Hg
Pregnant, postpartum	15.4 ± 2.1 mm Hg
Antepartum	17.9 ± 0.68 mm Hg
Postpartum	13.7 ± 0.46 mm Hg

in many institutions; however, knowledge of this key concept is helpful in understanding one of the basic differences between pregnant and nonpregnant women: that pulmonary edema tends to develop in pregnant women at a lower PCWP than in those who are not pregnant and have a normal COP.

The lower the COP and the higher the PCWP, the more likely pulmonary edema is to develop, as reflected by a lower COP-PCWP gradient. COP-PCWP gradient values are as follows: nonpregnant, 14.5 ± 2.5; pregnant, 10.5 ± 2.7.

Pulmonary edema is more likely to develop in pregnancy. For example, the normal PCWP is 6 to 10 mm Hg during pregnancy and 4 to 9 mm Hg in the nonpregnant state (Clark et al., 1989). With a PCWP of 8, calculations of the COP-PCWP gradient show:

Nonpregnant woman: COP of 25 − PCWP of 8 = 17 mm Hg
Pregnant woman with severe preeclampsia:
COP of 13 − PCWP of 8 = 5 mm Hg

Lower COP-PCWP gradients during pregnancy are usually caused by lower COP values occurring during pregnancy.

Respiratory Changes

Anatomic and physiologic alterations during pregnancy are necessary to supply adequate oxygenation to mother and fetus. A relative hyperventilation of pregnancy begins in the first trimester and increases 42% by term. Respiratory rate increases only slightly. Tidal volume and minute ventilations increase about 50% by term to meet increased oxygen consumption needs. The enlarging uterus pushes the diaphragm upward approximately 4 to 7 cm, reducing lung volume. Compensation is necessary to meet increased ventilatory demands, and the transverse diameter of the thorax increases 2 to 4 cm as the rib cage flares out. The functional residual capacity decreases 25% as more of the inhaled air is used, resulting in decreased reserve. These women become short of breath easily, as seen in walking or even light exercise. This can become critical if the oxygen demands of the pregnant women increase. The hyperventilation of pregnancy is associated with a resting arterial carbon dioxide tension less than 30 mm Hg. Maternal alkalosis is prevented by the compensatory decrease in serum bicarbonate of about 4 mEq/L, from 26 to 22 mEq. During gestation, respiratory acidosis and metabolic acidosis develop more rapidly than in the nonpregnant state.

Normal arterial blood gas values for pregnancy reflect a chronic state of compensated respiratory alkalosis, represented by a right shift in the oxyhemoglobin dissociation curve caused by the increased levels of 2,3-diphosphoglycerate from the high progesterone and estrogen levels present. Normal pregnancy values in comparison with those in the nonpregnant state are listed in Table 34-3.

Hematologic Changes

Pregnancy is a hypercoagulable state, as preparation is made for blood loss that accompanies childbirth. Table 34-4 gives a summary of alterations that enhance coagulation.

Bleeding and clotting times remain unchanged even when hypervolemia and hemodilution are present. The critically ill pregnant woman is at increased risk for thrombus formation whenever hemoconcentration develops, as occurs with preeclampsia-eclampsia or dehydration.

Systemic Vascular Resistance

Systemic vascular resistance (SVR) is a measure of the tension required for the ejection of blood into the circulation (afterload). To describe the physiologic relations between pressure and flow, measurements are made by the following formula as a ratio of pressure to flow:

$$SVR = [(MAP - CVP)/CO] \times 80$$

where MAP is mean arterial pressure (in millimeters of mercury), CVP is central venous pressure (in millimeters of mercury), and CO is cardiac output (in liters per minute).

Vasodilation of arterial vessels, a result of hormonal influences, and development of the uteroplacental circulation result in a decrease in SVR of 20% to 25% and a decrease in pulmonary vascular resistance of 40% during pregnancy. Systolic and diastolic blood pressures decrease during pregnancy, reaching the nadir at midtrimester, with a gradual return to prepregnancy values by term.

TABLE *34-3* **Arterial Blood Gas (ABG) Values**

ABGS	NONPREGNANT	PREGNANT
pH	7.35-7.45	7.40-7.45
Po_2 (mm Hg)	80-100	104-108
Pco_2 (mm Hg)	35-42	27-32
Bicarbonate (HCO_3) (mEq/L)	26	18-31

TABLE *34-4* **Gestational Changes That Enhance Coagulation**

Fibrinogen	Increased 30%-50% (from 300 to 480 mg/dl)
Coagulation factors VII-X	Increased
Fibrinolysis	Depressed

HEMODYNAMIC MONITORING

Anatomic and Physiologic Characteristics of Circulation

An in-depth knowledge of normal functioning and hemodynamics of the cardiovascular system is the basis for understanding hemodynamic monitoring; therefore a review of these functions is included. The purpose of the cardiopulmonary system is to deliver oxygenated blood to the tissues throughout the body and to remove waste products through the dynamics of normal circulation as follows (Fig. 34-1).

Deoxygenated blood flows from the capillaries into the veins and the right side of the heart through the superior vena cava, draining the upper part of the body, and from the inferior vena cava, draining the lower part of the body. Venous blood flows into the right atrium, a holding chamber for the right side of the heart. When the atrium is filled, the tricuspid valve opens, and blood flows through this valve into the right ventricle.

When the right ventricle is filled, its muscles (myocardium) contract, and blood is ejected through the pulmonic valve into the pulmonary artery. Blood is pushed through the pulmonary artery through its branches to the capillary beds (pulmonary beds) in both lungs. Gas exchange occurs in the capillary beds as carbon dioxide is released and oxygen enters the circulation across the alveolar membrane.

Oxygenated blood drains from the pulmonary beds into the pulmonary veins, two from each lung, into the left atrium, the holding chamber for the left side of the heart. When the left atrium is filled, the mitral valve opens, and blood flows through this valve into the left ventricle. After the left ventricle is filled, the muscles of the left ventricle contract, and the oxygenated blood is ejected through the aortic valve into the aorta and then pumped throughout the systemic arterial system so that oxygen is supplied to the organs and tissues of the body.

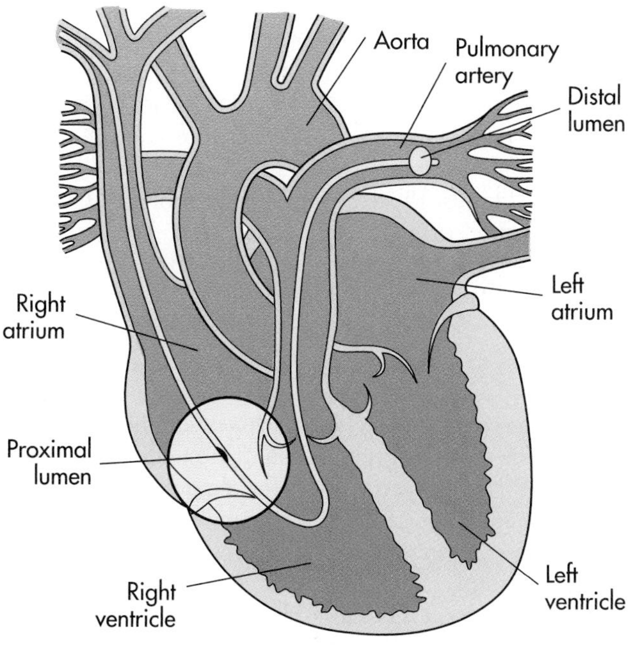
Aorta
Pulmonary artery
Distal lumen
Left atrium
Right atrium
Proximal lumen
Right ventricle
Left ventricle

FIG. 34-1 Diagram of heart with position of pulmonary artery catheter.

Synchronization by the electrical conduction system of the myocardium causes the right and left atrial and ventricular contractions to occur simultaneously. The period of the cardiac cycle when both ventricles are relaxed and filling is termed *diastole,* and the period of the cardiac cycle when both ventricles contract is termed *systole.*

Left ventricle contractions must generate enough force to pump blood throughout the systemic circulation. Force required for right ventricular work is less because the right ventricle has to exert only enough force for blood to flow through the pulmonary circulation. Therefore the left ventricle is referred to as the *hemodynamic ventricle,* and the left side of the heart is referred to as the *hemodynamic heart.* Hemodynamic monitoring with a pulmonary artery catheter (PAC) provides left heart values, and during a critical illness, values of left heart function are more significant than are values of right heart function.

Cardiac Output

Cardiac output (CO) is the volume of blood ejected from the left ventricle in 1 minute; it is measured in liters per minute. CO is the product of **stroke volume (SV),** the volume of blood ejected from the left ventricle during one cardiac cycle, and heart rate (HR) (CO = HR × SV). Because HR and SV increase during pregnancy, CO increases. The normal prepregnancy range of CO is 3 to 5 L/min. CO increases 40% to 50% during pregnancy, to produce a normal CO in the last trimester of 6 to 7 L/min at rest. Labor produces an additional 40% increase in CO because of catecholamine release in response to pain perception and the shunting of blood from the placental-fetal unit with uterine contractions, for a CO range during labor of 8 to 10 L/min. CO increases further after birth because of significant hemodynamic fluctuations that reflect the net effect of blood loss at birth and the autotransfusion with approximately 1000 ml of blood that occurs after the uterus is emptied. Soon after birth, the accumulated 6 to 8 L of extravascular fluid is mobilized into the intravascular compartment. The large increase in CO remains for 7 to 10 days after birth in the healthy woman but will continue longer if the usual diuresis fails to occur because of a complication.

Positional Changes

Maternal CO in the last trimester is position dependent. Clark et al. (1991) showed the effect of maternal position on CO output (Table 34-5).

The right or left lateral recumbent position provides optimal CO for the critically ill pregnant woman. Any time

TABLE 34-5 **Effect of Maternal Position on Cardiac Output**

Knee chest	6.9 (±2.1)
Right lateral	6.8 (±1.3)
Left lateral	6.6 (±1.4)
Sitting	6.2 (±2.0)
Supine	6.0 (±1.4)
Standing	5.4 (±2.0)

maternal CO is decreased, compensatory mechanisms are initiated. The first compensatory response is to shunt blood away from the peripheral circulation to the central circulation, to save the heart and brain. Peripheral circulation includes circulation to the skin, renal system, gastrointestinal system, lung beds, and reproductive system. Enhancing maternal CO enhances fetal perfusion.

NURSE ALERT

During the last trimester, CO decreases so significantly when the woman is supine that a hip wedge under one hip or manual displacement of the uterus to one side is necessary to prevent a sudden decrease in CO and a subsequent decrease in fetal perfusion.

Cardiac Output Determinants

The four determinants of CO are reflected in the calculation for cardiac output (CO = HR × SV) because SV is the result of preload, afterload, and contractility.

Preload is defined as the volume of blood in the ventricles at the end of diastole; preload is determined by intraventricular pressure and volume. Right preload is assessed by right atrial or CVP, and left preload is assessed by PCWP. The volume of blood in the ventricles stretches the myocardial muscle fibers and produces the intraventricular pressure. Measurements are made at end diastole, the time immediately preceding systole when the ventricles reach maximal stretch because of the extra amount of blood delivered into the ventricles when the tricuspid and mitral valves snap closed.

Right preload reflects the blood circulating through the right side of the heart, and left preload reflects the amount of blood circulating in the left side of the heart. The two sides of the heart are not equal when cardiac or pulmonary complications are present; therefore they are measured separately.

Preload must be adequate to maintain CO, and plotting of CO against preload gives a cardiac function curve (Fig. 34-2). As preload increases, CO increases up to the point of failure. The cardiac function curve shows that a heart in failure will require a higher preload than the healthy heart to produce the same CO. Bedside manipulations of preload are possible with continuous hemodynamic monitoring to determine effects on CO. A low preload can be increased by the administration of fluids,

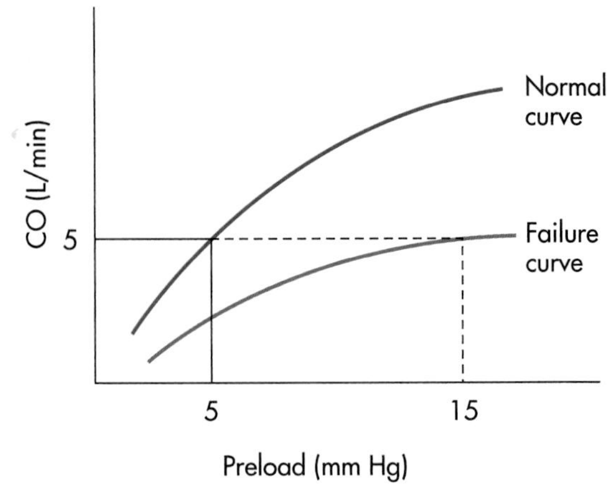
CO (L/min)
5
Normal curve
Failure curve
5
15
Preload (mm Hg)

FIG. 34-2 Relation of preload to cardiac output. Ventricular function (Starling) curve for heart showing both normal function and during failure.

including crystalloid, colloid, or blood, and by positioning with legs elevated. A high preload can be decreased by the administration of a vasodilator or diuretic or by phlebotomy and positioning in an upright position.

Afterload is defined as the ventricular wall tension during systole, or the resistance the blood meets as blood is ejected from the ventricles. Afterload is dependent on the end-diastolic radius of the ventricle, the aortic pressure, and the thickness of the ventricle wall. As afterload increases, CO decreases, and bedside manipulation of afterload is possible to achieve optimal cardiac output (Fig. 34-3). Right afterload is assessed by the **pulmonary vascular resistance (PVR),** and left afterload is assessed by the SVR. Arterial BP measurement does not give as accurate an indication of left ventricular work as the SVR but is used clinically as reflecting left afterload. The formula to calculate blood pressure (BP) is BP = CO × SVR. Therefore control of the woman's blood pressure is used to control left afterload.

Afterload must be adequate for circulation and CO; extremes of afterload may decrease CO. Increased left afterload occurs with hypertensive disease caused by the systemic arterial vasoconstriction. Increased right afterload occurs with pulmonary hypertension resulting from vasoconstriction in the pulmonary circulation.

Increased afterload can be corrected by the administration of vasodilator drugs. Hydralazine is commonly used as the first-line drug for hypertension. It is an arterial vasodilator that is usually effective, safe for mother and fetus, and has as an added bonus that the majority of obstetric personnel are comfortable in its use. However, many believe that the calcium channel blockers (such as nifedipine, orally) and the beta-blockers (such as labetalol) cause less hypotension (Dekker & Sibai, 2001). Sodium nitroprusside has the potential to produce such immediate changes in SVR that continuous intraarterial BP monitoring is required. Sodium

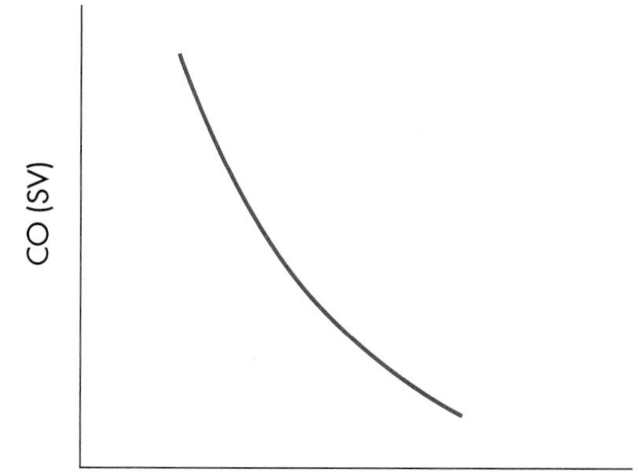
CO (SV)
Afterload
(SVR or PVR)

FIG. 34-3 Relation of afterload to cardiac output when preload is maintained constant. As afterload increases, cardiac output decreases.

nitroprusside produces cyanide as a metabolite; fetal cyanide toxicity must be a concern if this drug is administered during pregnancy. Of paramount importance is the correction of hypovolemia before administration of any antihypertensive to prevent acute hypotension (NIH, 2000).

NURSE ALERT

The continuous intravenous infusion of sodium nitroprusside is the vasodilator drug used most commonly in the adult intensive care setting, but it is saved for emergency use for pregnant women.

Severe vasodilation and loss of arterial resistance with a decreased afterload impedes venous return of blood to the right side of the heart and decreases CO. This situation is seen with septic shock. Decreased afterload can be corrected by fluid administration to fill the vascular space or by the administration of alpha-adrenergic drugs such as phenylephrine (Mandeville & Troiano, 1999).

Contractility (inotropic state of the heart) is defined as the force and velocity of ventricular contractions when preload and afterload are held constant. Contractility is governed by the Frank-Starling law, which states that the greater the length of the muscle fibers before contraction, the greater will be the contraction of the fibers, up to the point of failure. Fiber length is related to the maximal stretch of preload, because as more blood volume enters the ventricles, the more the fibers in the myocardium stretch to accommodate the increased volume.

Decreased contractility results in decreased CO. The first response to correct this problem is bedside manipulation to optimize both preload and afterload. If this fails to increase CO to the desired level, medications to increase myocardial contractility are indicated. Inotropic drugs such as dopamine hydrochloride or dobutamine are administered. Digitalis therapy also may be necessary.

Heart rate is the fourth determinant of cardiac output. The rate at which the ventricles fill and contract affects CO. Extremes of HR may decrease CO.

Sustained tachycardia can decrease CO as a result of myocardial ischemia or the decreased time for adequate filling of the ventricles during diastole and shortened systolic ejection times. The cause, such as fever, hypoxia, pain, hypovolemia, or hyperthyroidism, should be determined and treated. Drugs to correct tachycardia are seldom necessary for obstetric clients. However, propranolol, digoxin, or calcium-channel blockers such as verapamil are effective agents to decrease HR if needed.

Bradycardia can compromise CO when an inadequate number of ventricular contractions per minute occur to deliver the circulating volume needed to perfuse and oxygenate the body. If treatment is necessary for this problem, atropine or cardiac pacing is used.

Invasive Hemodynamic Monitoring

Invasive hemodynamic monitoring provides continuous measurements of preload, afterload, myocardial contractility, and HR in the critically ill pregnant woman so that therapeutic manipulations may be made quickly at the bedside in response to changes in client status. Monitoring may be done by use of a **pulmonary artery catheter (PAC)** (a balloon-tipped, multilumen catheter) or by CVP.

Although few adequate clinical studies at this time demonstrate the benefit of pulmonary artery catheterization for the critically ill client, most critical care bedside clinicians use the PAC to direct their therapy modalities; they believe that use of the PAC does improve outcomes in selected critically ill clients (Troiano, 1999). Conners and associates (1996) reported no benefit to right heart catheterization in the initial care of critically ill clients, and they even questioned whether the Food and Drug Administration should stop its use. The Society of Critical Care Medicine quickly held a consensus development conference and issued a consensus statement regarding the use of the PAC in critical care environments (Society of Critical Care Medicine, 1997). The consensus statement reiterated that, as with all other technology, the clinical usefulness of the PAC is dependent on correct interpretation of the data by clinicians. With respect to pregnancy, the ACOG guidelines (1992) for invasive hemodynamic monitoring were referenced. The statement also included a recommendation for additional research.

Use of a PAC allows the management of care to be based on immediate recognition of changes in hemodynamic values from the left ventricle. Immediate information is obtained, calculations are made, and management is adjusted quickly as needed. Results of therapeutic strategies can be calculated and evaluated (ACOG, 1992). The continuous hemodynamic measurements obtained will reinforce therapies in use or show that therapy should be changed. Use of a PAC or Swan-Ganz catheter in combination with an arterial pressure catheter and a pulse oximeter provides adequate data to assess cardiac, fluid, and pulmonary status of the client continuously. Indications for the use of invasive hemodynamic monitoring are the same in obstetrics as in any other area of medicine.

It is essential to evaluate risks and benefits of any procedure before use, especially because risks are associated with invasive techniques. The information obtained from hemodynamic monitoring is essential for management of critical, complex cases and is unavailable by other means; thus the benefits outweigh the risks in most cases. The overall complication rate in the obstetric population is low, approximately 1%. This low rate of complications is related to three factors: (1) the pregnant woman usually needs the device because of an acute event, (2) the duration of use is usually short, and (3) the majority of pregnant women requiring its use are young and healthy before the acute event.

It is essential that meticulous attention be paid to each step and detail of all procedures to decrease problems with the technique itself. The complications seen with invasive monitoring seem to be most closely correlated with the technical skill and experience of the clinician (Gonik, 1999).

Pulmonary Artery Catheter

A PAC, commonly called the Swan-Ganz catheter, provides continuous measurements of **pulmonary artery pressure (PAP)** and right atrial pressure (RAP) or CVP. Intermittent measurements of PCWP and CO also are possible. The standard flow-directed thermodilution PAC has three lumina and a thermistor connector (Fig. 34-4). The distal lumen or port is located in the pulmonary artery after insertion. It is connected to a transducer with a heparinized pressure line to measure a continuous PAP when the balloon is deflated and intermittent PCWP when the balloon is inflated. A continuous flush of 3 ml per hour of heparinized solution maintains patency of the lumen.

The proximal lumen or port exits approximately 30 cm from the tip of the catheter and is located in the right atrium after insertion. This port also is connected to a transducer with a heparinized line, and it can be used to measure continuous RAP, which is comparable to the CVP, or to administer fluid or drugs. Both the proximal and distal lumina of the catheter can be used to withdraw blood samples for laboratory studies.

The balloon lumen ends in a small latex balloon, located 0.5 inch from the tip of the PAC. Inflation of the balloon is used to assist in the insertion of the catheter and to obtain PCWP readings.

The thermodilution port is connected to a thermistor, a temperature sensor, located 5 cm proximal to the tip of the PAC. The thermistor continuously measures the temperature of the blood in the pulmonary artery.

Other types of PACs are available in addition to the standard PAC. Some have an extra right atrial port for intracardiac infusions. The small size of the ports makes them more effective for the administration of vasopressors or drugs such as antibiotics, rather than for the use of rapid administration of large volumes of blood or fluids. A fiberoptic PAC includes a sensor to measure the hemoglobin saturation of mixed venous blood, the $S\bar{v}O_2$, in the pulmonary artery continuously and is useful in cases of decreased oxygen transport, such as with preeclampsia-eclampsia. Another type for selected cases is modified PAC with a heated filament to provide continuous CO values (Medlin et al., 1998).

Venous Access

The internal or external jugular vein or the subclavian vein is most commonly used for venous access for invasive hemodynamic monitoring during pregnancy. Access with femoral or antecubital veins is not used so frequently for pregnant women because of the greater difficulty in positioning the catheter when this route is accessed. Furthermore, with use of a vein in the inguinal area, birth of the infant at a critical time can limit access to and manipulation of the catheter. With certain disorders, such as a coagulopathy, antecubital access may be preferred to decrease the possibility of intrathoracic bleeding (Gonik, 1999).

The flow-directed PAC is usually inserted at the bedside after preparations are complete. Meticulous attention to detail is critical when the equipment is prepared. Flushing the pressure tubing to eliminate any air, establishing a zero

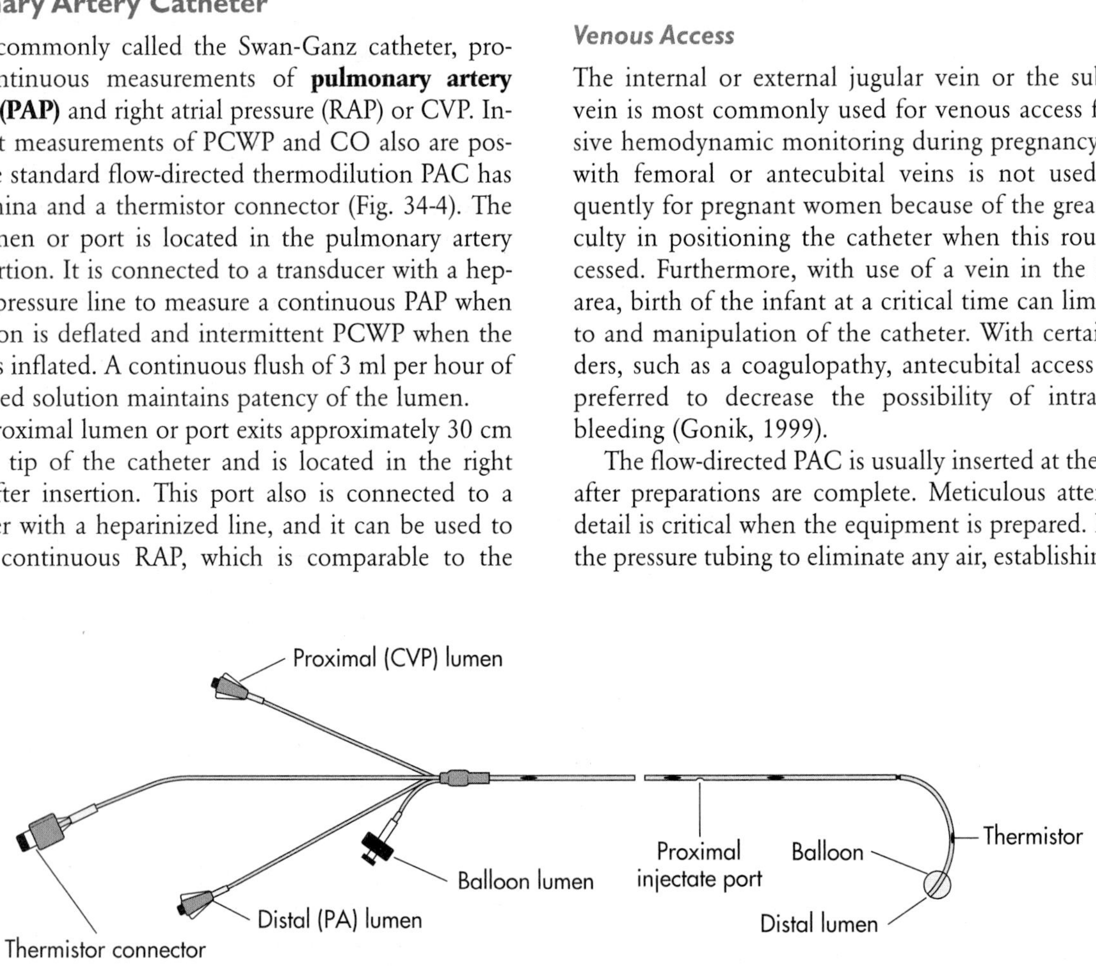
Proximal (CVP) lumen
Thermistor
Proximal injectate port
Balloon
Balloon lumen
Distal (PA) lumen
Distal lumen
Thermistor connector

FIG. 34-4 Standard triple-lumen flow-directed pulmonary artery catheter.

reference point, and both zeroing and calibrating the pressure transducer are done carefully before insertion. The Procedure box explains how to set up a pressure line and how to zero-reference and calibrate a pressure transducer. Box 34-2 describes nursing care during insertion and continuing care for a PAC.

Hemodynamic monitoring systems have three major components: (1) a pressure transducer that converts physiologic pressures into electrical energy, (2) an amplifier to magnify the volume of the signal being measured, and (3) a monitor screen to display in digital and graphic form the converted physiologic signal (Fig. 34-5).

Waveforms and Pressure Readings

The basis of interpretation of assessments obtained by hemodynamic monitoring is to understand the relation to cardiovascular status of the waveforms observed on the monitor screen and the pressure readings obtained.

Specific chambers in the heart have different pressures that are reflected by changing waveform patterns, and placement of the PAC is evaluated through the pressure and waveform changes that appear on the monitor screen to reflect the position of the catheter. Figure 34-6 displays pressure waveforms in different chambers of the heart.

PROCEDURE

How to Set Up, Calibrate, and Zero-Reference Pressure Lines

1. Connect pressure tubing to sterile disposable pressure transducer.
2. Check all connections for a tight fit to prevent leakage.
3. Heparinize flush solution of normal saline solution. Heparin is necessary for the pregnant client to prevent thrombus formation.
4. Connect the pressure tubing to the intravenous bag of heparinized solution.
5. Gently flush both pressure tubing and transducer to remove all air. Cap stopcocks with nonvented covers.
6. Connect transducer to hemodynamic monitor.
7. Place a pressure bag on the heparinized solution. Inflate to 300 mm Hg of pressure. (This allows a continuous rate of 3 ml/hr of heparinized solution to flow as a flush solution.) The heparinized solution and continuous flow of fluid prevent clot formation on the tip of the catheter.
8. Calibrate the pressure transducer by zeroing the line.
9. Zero-reference the transducer by positioning the woman supine with a hip wedge under the right hip, locating the phlebostatic axis at the fourth intercostal space at the midaxillary line, and marking on the chest wall.
10. Open stopcock to air. Push zero button on the monitor to identify zero. The transducer negates atmospheric pressure and establishes a baseline for subsequent readings. Close the stopcock to air.

Note: The phlebostatic axis is the physiologic reference point used when measuring pulmonary and arterial line pressures (see Fig. 34-7 for an illustration of this procedure).

Because the right atrium is a holding chamber with relatively small muscle mass, the waveform pattern for this chamber has a low amplitude. Right atrium pressures reflect intravascular volume and compliance of the right ventricle. Mean right atrium pressures in pregnancy are relatively low, 0 to 7 mm Hg.

When the catheter flows into the right ventricle, pressures change, and a distinct spiking waveform appears. The low-amplitude waveform of the right atrium converts to a high-amplitude waveform with distinct systolic and diastolic components in the right ventricle with a baseline pressure of 0 mm Hg. Right ventricular pressures are measured as systolic and diastolic. Normal right ventricle systolic pressure is 18 to 30 mm Hg, and the normal diastolic pressure is 0 to 7 mm Hg.

The catheter is then advanced into the pulmonary artery. This is reflected by a different spiking waveform with baseline pressures greater than 0 mm Hg. Pulmonary artery systolic pressures are equal to the systolic pressures in the right ventricle, but pulmonary artery diastolic pressures abruptly increase to the range of 6 to 10 mm Hg.

The catheter advances through the pulmonary artery as far as possible and becomes "wedged" in the vessel. This wedging is reflected by a distinct waveform of a dampened tracing with respiratory variation. This relatively low amplitude reflects the low pressures in the capillary beds of the lungs.

The PCWP is obtained when the balloon is inflated, with all pressures from the right side of the heart obstructed, so that the distal port now reads pressures from the left side of the heart across the lungs, because there are no valves in the pulmonary circulation. The PCWP measures left atrial filling pressures or left-sided preload. During right ventricular diastole, the pulmonic valve is closed, with the mitral valve open; the diastolic PAP is measured. In the absence of a problem, such as mitral valve disease or pulmonary edema, PAP diastolic readings reflect PCWP or left ventricular preload. The diastolic PAP is therefore used clinically to reflect left preload (Darovic, 2002). See the Procedure box for obtaining a PCWP reading.

The normal PCWP during pregnancy is 6 to 10 mm Hg. Pressures higher than 20 mm Hg are usually caused by abnormal left ventricular performance, such as left ventricular failure, mitral valve stenosis, or fluid volume overload. Lower-than-normal readings are seen usually with hypovolemia (see Fig. 34-6).

Box 34-3 describes nursing measures for managing selected problems that may arise with a PAC.

Arterial Pressure Catheter

Percutaneous arterial catheterization, in which a Teflon intravenous catheter, usually 20 gauge, is placed in an artery and connected to a hemodynamic monitor by a pressure line, provides continuous measurements of the systolic, diastolic, and mean arterial blood pressures. The **arterial**

BOX 34-2 **Pulmonary Artery Catheter Protocol**

SETUP

- Prepare two pressure lines for the distal and proximal ports as described in the Procedure box on how to set up, calibrate, and zero-reference pressure lines.
- Connect an intravenous line of normal saline solution, per infusion pump, to the introducer.
- Check PAC balloon for symmetric inflation, absence of air leak, and ease of spontaneous deflation.

CLIENT PREPARATION FOR INSERTION

- Assess woman's knowledge level and explain procedure to ensure her understanding, cooperation, and acceptance of the procedure.
- Confirm that informed consent form is signed and attached to chart.
- Provide support and encouragement throughout the procedure.
- Initiate electrocardiographic (ECG) monitoring. Obtain baseline ECG pattern.

NURSING MANAGEMENT DURING INSERTION

- Monitor ECG continuously as catheter passes through right ventricle to recognize any ventricular ectopy present.
- Use a slight Trendelenburg position with a hip wedge. This position engorges the neck veins and facilitates placement of the catheter. When the internal jugular approach is used, tilt head to the side away from the site of cannulation.
- Be available to provide assistance to the operator throughout the procedure.
- Adjust intravenous line connected to the introducer to maintain patency.
- Observe waveform patterns on the monitor screen and record pressures as the catheter advances through the chambers in the heart.
- Have lidocaine hydrochloride available for arrhythmias.
- Ensure that balloon is deflated. Deflate balloon passively.
- Anticipate orders for chest radiograph film to verify catheter placement.
- Apply dressing after physician secures introducer.
- Observe monitor screen for continuous tracing of pulmonary artery pressures.

NURSING ASSESSMENTS

- Verify that alarms are set at all times.
- Observe monitor screen closely for pressures and waveforms that denote placement of catheter. Be prepared to intervene when necessary (see Box 34-3).
- Record hemodynamic parameters according to client status and unit care protocols. Follow the procedure for obtaining a pulmonary capillary wedge pressure reading (see Procedure box).
- Inspect all connection sites every 2 hr and entire monitor system for presence of air or blood clots.
- Examine insertion site frequently for bleeding or signs of infection. Perform site care every shift or daily, as indicated by unit infection control policy.
- Change pressure and intravenous lines every 24 to 48 hr, as indicated by unit infection control policy.
- Monitor heparinized pressure flush for continuous correct pressure (300 mm Hg).
- Rezero and calibrate transducer every shift and as necessary.

NURSING MANAGEMENT FOR CATHETER REMOVAL

- Document vital signs and ECG pattern.
- Monitor for ECG arrhythmias during removal.
- After catheter removal, pressure to site must be applied for ≥5 min. Anticipate that physician may request application of pressure. Ensure that bleeding has stopped completely before pressure is removed.
- Apply pressure dressing to site, per unit protocol. Keep pressure dressing in place for 8 hr.

DOCUMENTATION

- Presence of signed informed consent form on chart.
- Date, time, site of insertion, type of introducer, and name of operator who performed procedure.
- Type of pulmonary catheter, number of attempts, confirmation of placement by x-ray studies, and any ventricular ectopy.
- Woman's tolerance of procedure.
- Zeroing and calibration of transducers and verification of alarm settings.
- Hemodynamic parameters obtained according to client status.
- Pertinent nursing assessments and medical and nursing care.
- Site assessments and care.
- Changes of pressure and intravenous lines.
- Date and time of removal of intact catheter, date and removal of introducer.
- Nursing care and assessments after catheter removal.

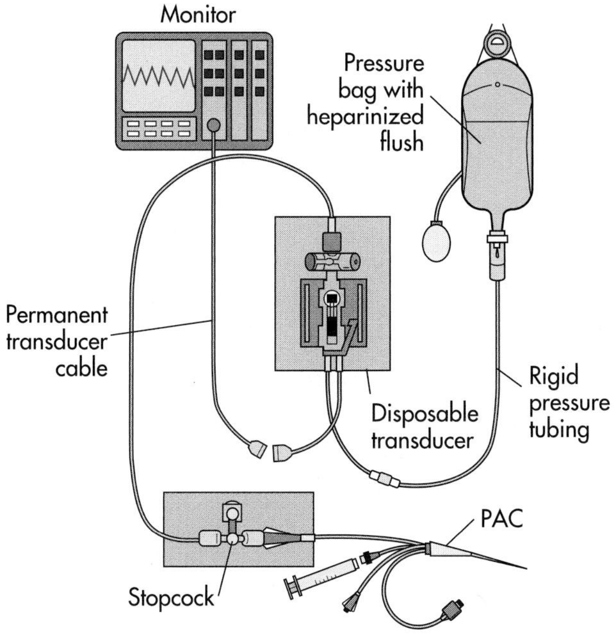
Monitor
Pressure bag with heparinized flush
Permanent transducer cable
Rigid pressure tubing
Disposable transducer
PAC
Stopcock

FIG. 34-5 Components of hemodynamic monitoring system: pressurized tubing, pressure transducer, and hemodynamic monitor.

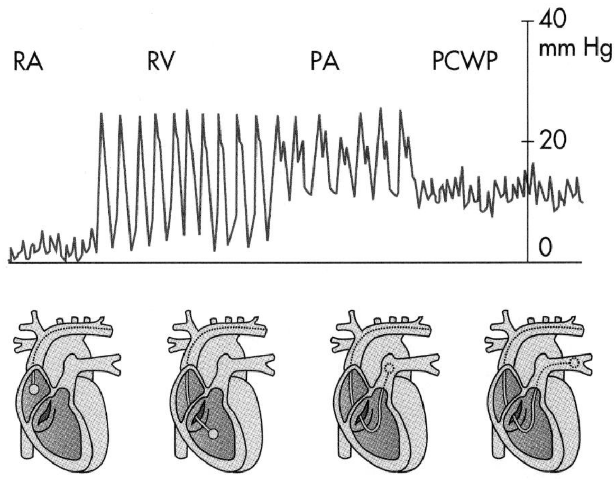
RA
RV
PA
PCWP
40
mm Hg
20
0

FIG. 34-6 Pressure waveforms in relation to catheter position from right atrium *(RA)*, to right ventricle *(RV)*, to pulmonary artery *(PA)*, to pulmonary capillary wedge pressure *(PCWP)*.

pressure catheter produces a waveform and also provides access for arterial blood gas sampling and analysis.

Indications for use of this type of hemodynamic monitoring include situations in which frequent and accurate BP measurements are needed, such as the administration of potent drugs (e.g., dopamine to treat septic shock or nitroprusside to treat severe hypertensive disease) or when frequent arterial blood gas determinations are needed. Characteristics of desirable arteries for an arterial line are (1) a vessel that has a diameter large enough for accurate measurement of pressure without occlusion of the artery by the catheter, (2) adequate collateral circulation, (3) ease of access to the site for care, and (4) a site not prone to infection. The most common vessels used in the pregnant woman are the radial, axillary, and pedal arteries, in that order.

In preparation for insertion of the arterial line into the radial artery, the procedure should be explained to the woman in simple terms, informed consent obtained, and Allen's test performed to validate collateral circulation into the hand by demonstrating a patent ulnar artery. Box 34-4 describes the steps to perform Allen's test.

The most common risk associated with an intraarterial line is infection. More serious, but less common, risks

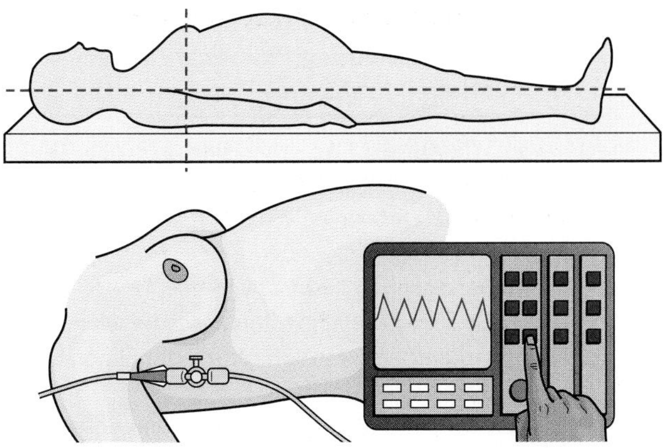

FIG. 34-7 Location of phlebostatic axis and zeroing.

PROCEDURE

Obtaining a Pulmonary Capillary Wedge Pressure Reading

1. Inflate balloon slowly while observing waveform on monitor screen. Stop inflation as soon as pulmonary artery waveform changes to pulmonary capillary wedge pressure waveform.
2. Note amount of air necessary to achieve wedge waveform. Do NOT inflate balloon further than necessary to obtain wedge waveform.
3. Keep balloon inflated only long enough to obtain pressure reading, about 5 sec. Complications associated with sustained wedging (>10 sec) are pulmonary infarction and pulmonary rupture.
4. Release syringe and allow balloon to deflate passively. Do NOT aspirate air from syringe. (Passive deflation of the balloon correlates with an intact balloon.)
5. Note return of pulmonary artery waveform after deflation of balloon.
6. Document assessments made.

BOX 34-3 Nursing Interventions Protocol: Trouble-Shooting Pulmonary Artery Catheter Problems

SPONTANEOUS WEDGING: PCWP WAVEFORM APPEARS ON MONITOR SCREEN

- Assess syringe. Determine if balloon is inflated or deflated.
- Have woman turn her head, cough deeply 2 to 3 times, and then take a few deep breaths while observing monitor screen for return of pulmonary artery waveform.
- If wedgeform continues, call physician immediately to the bedside to reposition catheter. (Catheter will need to be pulled back into larger-diameter vessel.)
- Monitor screen for return of pulmonary artery waveform.

MIGRATION OF CATHETER BACKWARD: RIGHT VENTRICULAR WAVEFORM ON SCREEN

- Call physician immediately to bedside to reposition catheter. (Balloon must be reinflated for catheter to flow back into the pulmonary artery.)
- Monitor ECG pattern for ventricle ectopy, especially premature ventricle contractions if catheter tip irritates wall of right ventricle.
- Have lidocaine hydrochloride available.

SUSPECTED BALLOON RUPTURE: ABSENCE OF RESISTANCE FELT WHEN INFLATING BALLOON OR INABILITY TO OBTAIN PCWP READING

- Confirm tight attachment of syringe. Do NOT inject air. Slowly withdraw plunger.
- If able to aspirate blood or fluid, balloon rupture is confirmed. Do NOT inject any air. Tape closed and label balloon inflation port, "balloon rupture."
- Rupture may be assumed if unable to aspirate blood or fluid because of absence of resistance in syringe. Do NOT inject any air. Tape closed and label balloon inflation port, "balloon rupture."
- Notify physician.
- Usually does not necessitate change of catheter, especially if diastolic PAP and PCWP readings have been similar. Diastolic PAP will be monitored to reflect left preload values.

include hemorrhage, thrombus formation, and embolization. The heparinized continuous flush solution of the pressure line helps prevent thrombus formation. Once the line is in place, a transparent occlusive dressing is applied. The transducer is then rezeroed, and an arm board is used to prevent movement of the wrist.

The hemodynamic monitor displays an arterial waveform and the systolic, diastolic, and MAPs for the health care team to interpret. Normal versus abnormal waveforms must be recognized at the bedside, and immediate intervention must be available as needed. The normal waveform should include the following (Fig. 34-8):

- Rapid upstroke to systole
- Clear dicrotic notch, which denotes closure of the aortic valve
- Definite end-diastolic wave

A blood pressure taken with a sphygmomanometer should be ascertained periodically to verify accuracy of the hemodynamic monitor.

Continuing assessments and documentation should include the following:

- Systolic and diastolic arterial pressures
- Cuff pressure readings
- Intraarterial strip recording
- Site care
- Dressing and line changes
- Transducer zeroing and calibration
- Description of the circulation in the extremity

BOX 34-4 Allen's Test Procedure

1. Determine the woman's dominant hand. Use opposite extremity.
2. Elevate woman's hand and occlude both radial and ulnar arteries.
3. Have woman clench and unclench fist to facilitate venous drainage.
4. Observe that palm is blanched.
5. Release pressure on the ulnar artery only. Radial artery remains occluded.
6. Observe and time the palm for capillary refill (normal time is $\leq$5 sec).
7. If it takes $>$5 sec, collateral circulation may be impaired.

Pressure Lines

All pressure lines use a specialized high-pressure tubing to transmit the physiologic signal to the transducer and monitor. The pressure tubing is rigid to prevent the dampening or absorption of pressure itself, so that the physiologic pressures are transmitted directly from the catheter tip to the transducer through the fluid that fills the length of the tubing. The line includes a continuous flushing mechanism to ensure patency (see Fig. 34-5).

Data Collection

Continuous measurements of the CVP and PAPs and intermittent PCWPs are obtained from the PAC. CO is also calculated intermittently by the use of a PAC with the thermodilution technique. ECG monitoring permits continuous evaluation of HR and rhythm. Newer ECG monitors

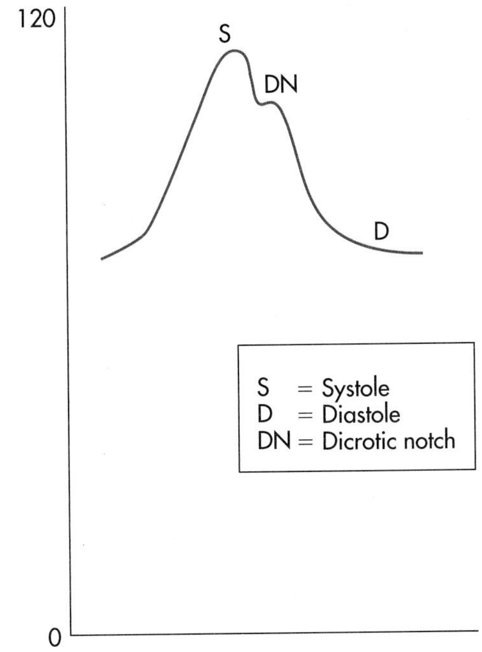
120
S
DN
D
0
S = Systole
D = Diastole
DN = Dicrotic notch

FIG. 34-8 Arterial waveform.

with sensitive leads connected to the chest wall also monitor respiratory rate. Systemic arterial BP can be evaluated by a manual or an automatic sphygmomanometer or by an arterial pressure line. Placement of an arterial pressure line also permits ready access for frequent arterial blood sampling and analysis, especially for arterial blood gases.

Mean pressure values are used to evaluate client status. They can be determined for the pulmonary arterial and systemic circulations by electronic dampening of the respective tracing or by use of the following calculation formula (Gonik, 1999):

$$\text{MAP} = \frac{\text{Systolic pressure} + 2\ (\text{Diastolic pressure})}{3}$$

The PCWP is reported as a mean value, determined by the average of its maximal and minimal deflections on the monitor screen or oscilloscope. Reading values from the oscilloscope is usually adequate for clinical management at the bedside; however, for complex cases, strip chart recordings are recommended. See the Procedure box for making and recording hemodynamic assessments.

When the thermodilution procedure to calculate CO in a pregnant woman is performed, the injectate should be chilled to obtain an accurate reading because of the high COs normal for pregnancy (Wallace & Winslow, 1993). The thermistor at the tip of the PAC measures the speed with which the blood temperature cools and returns to normal after the chilled fluid is injected. The time required for the temperature changes is computed, and a CO readout is given. The Procedure box describes the thermodilution procedure for measuring CO.

PROCEDURE

Making and Recording Hemodynamic Assessments

1. Position woman in supine position with a hip wedge.
2. Rezero all pressure transducers.
3. Print a strip recording of the PAC and arterial line blood pressures. Observe oscilloscope for mean values.
4. Record findings of the PAP, central venous pressure, and arterial BP.
5. Calibrate PCWP according to the Procedure box for obtaining a PCWP reading. Record the mean determination.
6. Calibrate cardiac output (CO) according to the Procedure box outlining the thermodilution procedure for measuring CO.
7. Document all findings and woman's tolerance of procedures.

PROCEDURE

Thermodilution Procedure for Measuring Cardiac Output

1. Enter the cardiac output (CO) coefficient into the computer.
2. Chill injectate in ice bath.
3. Use insulated syringe.
4. Flush coiled tubing with injectate solution to remove all air.
5. Connect syringe to three-way stopcock at the proximal port.
6. Draw injectate (5 or 10 ml per unit protocol) into insulated syringe.
7. Depress the CO control on the computer.
8. Inject the injectate as rapidly as possible with both hands. Observe oscilloscope for a smooth curve.
9. Repeat the procedure twice. Calculate results. If readings are within 15% of each other, average the three to determine CO. If not, omit the highest and lowest.

Oxygenation

Oxygen delivery to and use by the peripheral tissues must be adequate. Determination of oxygen transport is essential in the care of the critically ill pregnant woman. Oxygen delivery is directly proportional to CO; if CO decreases 50%, oxygen delivery decreases 50%. Conversely, increasing CO 50% doubles oxygen delivery. Oxygen delivery also can be improved by improving the hemoglobin value, which can be accomplished by the administration of red blood cells.

$Sa{O_2}$ Monitoring

Oxygen is transported to the tissues in two ways: dissolved in plasma and bound to hemoglobin. The oxygen dissolved in plasma (PaO_2) makes up only 1% to 2% of the total oxygen content, whereas the oxygen bound to hemoglobin

(SaO_2) makes up 98% to 99% of the total oxygen content. Results of arterial blood gas determination reflect the dissolved oxygen according to the PaO_2 value. The PaO_2 reflects the partial pressure that oxygen exerts when it is dissolved in blood; it is measured in millimeters of mercury. The normal PaO_2 for the pregnant state is 100 to 106 mm Hg, and it must be at least 60 mm Hg for fetal survival (Clark et al., 1991). The partial pressure of the oxygen tension is important because circulation transports the higher PaO_2 blood to organs with a lower PaO_2, and gas exchange occurs as gases move from the higher concentration to the lower concentration. The higher tension (PaO_2) pushes the oxygen molecule off the hemoglobin molecule through the cell membrane so that tissues receive a supply of oxygen.

The oxygen that cells can use are the oxygen molecules bound to hemoglobin (SaO_2). Each molecule of hemoglobin has four binding sites for oxygen; when all four sites are bound, an oxyhemoglobin molecule results. The saturation of hemoglobin with oxygen (SaO_2) is evaluated with the pulse oximeter (**SaO_2 monitoring**). The normal range for SaO_2 is 95% to 100%, and normal SaO_2 values for pregnancy are 97% to 100%. Critically ill pregnant women benefit from continuous SaO_2 monitoring.

SvO_2 Monitoring

The percentage of saturation of hemoglobin with oxygen in mixed venous and arterial blood is reflected as an SvO_2 value. **SvO_2 monitoring** involves insertion of a fiberoptic PAC that is connected to a bedside microprocessor to give a continuous SvO_2 value. Mixed venous blood saturation reflects the balance between oxygen delivery and oxygen use. It reflects tissue perfusion, the variation in oxygen requirements for different organs, and the affinity of hemoglobin to accept and then release oxygen (Cathelyn & Samples, 1998). The normal value of SvO_2 is 60% to 80%; values less than 60% are interpreted as abnormally low.

Fiberoptic PACs and bedside microprocessors provide the technology to plot the mixed venous blood oxygen saturation continuously. Plotting of mixed venous oxygen content is used as an early warning system because values may decrease before any other evidence of hemodynamic instability is seen (Cathelyn & Samples, 1998).

Use of pulse oximetry permits evaluation of the SaO_2, arterial blood saturation. Arterial blood usually has a saturation of 90% or greater. Because of the shape of the oxyhemoglobin dissociation curve, fluctuations at the high levels of oxygen tension, 90% and higher, are reflected by a small change in arterial oxygen saturation (SaO_2). However, the lower levels of oxygen tension in mixed venous blood (40% or less) produce a linear relation between saturation and tension, resulting in the SvO_2 becoming a sensitive alarm to detect physiologic instability.

Arterial blood analysis evaluates pulmonary oxygen exchange and ventilation but does not evaluate overall adequacy of oxygen delivery to the peripheral tissues. However, mixed venous blood analysis (SvO_2) reflects the end product of supply and demand and is used to evaluate overall adequacy of oxygen delivery to the peripheral tissues. This technique provides additional data and can be especially useful to support or change management strategies when used in conjunction with thermodilution CO calculations.

NURSE ALERT

Stable CO measurements in conjunction with an improvement in SvO_2 readings are associated with clinical improvement and are a good prognostic sign. The same improved SvO_2 readings in conjunction with a 100% increase in CO are a common first sign of the development of sepsis.

Continuous monitoring of SvO_2 is recommended for titration of vasoactive or inotropic drugs; during adjustments of positive end-expiratory pressure, evaluation of fluid administration, and routine care of critically ill pregnant women; and as an early warning system for changes in cardiopulmonary status (Cathelyn & Samples, 1998).

Central Venous Pressure Lines

Before the development of the flow-directed PAC in the early 1970s, CVP lines were used for the critically ill. Two primary problems with the use of CVP lines became apparent. First, CVP monitoring provides right-sided heart information only, the right preload. When a cardiac or pulmonary complication is present, right- and left-sided values are not equal. CVP monitoring gives no information about left ventricular function. Second, changes in CVP values occur much later with left ventricular dysfunction. This type of monitoring does not permit rapid calculation of effects of treatment modalities. Critically ill clients need a PAC monitoring that provides a continuous PAP and intermittent PCWP and CO calculations; therefore CVP monitoring is seldom used (Bolte et al., 2000).

Interpretation of Hemodynamic Data

Data obtained with hemodynamic monitoring techniques include values that reflect blood volume in the pulmonary and systemic circulations, which profoundly affect cardiac performance, in the following ways:

- Right atrial pressure or CVP indicates right end-diastolic pressure and reflects right preload.
- PAP: Pulmonary vascular resistance (PVR) is the calculation for right afterload. Clinically, mean PAP reflects right afterload.
- Diastolic PAP approximates PCWP and reflects left preload.
- PCWP indicates left end-diastolic pressure and reflects left preload.
- CO refers to the volume of blood ejected from the left ventricle in liters per minute.
- SVR is the calculation for left afterload; arterial BP reflects left afterload.

Hemodynamic profiles provide valuable data for evaluating status of the client and changing treatment strategies as needed. Normal hemodynamic values for calculation in the cases below are shown in Table 34-6. Table 34-7 compares normal nonpregnant hemodynamic values with normal values during pregnancy.

Oliguria is diagnosed if urine output is less than 25 to 30 ml for 2 consecutive hours. It may indicate severe renal dysfunction (Griffith, 1999). If oliguria is not corrected with fluid challenge, the woman is diagnosed as having oliguria refractory to conservative therapy.

Refractory oliguria caused by preeclampsia may be associated with three different hemodynamic subsets: hypovolemia, hypervolemia, and renal artery spasm. Treatment strategies for correction of oliguria are different for each hemodynamic subset. Noninvasive assessments do not differentiate the type of treatment that would be appropriate for the pregnant woman. Recognition of which hemodynamic subset has produced the refractory oliguria is obtained only by the use of a PAC. Failure to use PAC when refractory oliguria is present can result in inappropriate treatment.

Examples of three different pregnant women with preeclampsia complicated by refractory oliguria are included in Box 34-5 to demonstrate how useful hemodynamic monitoring is to determine the appropriate care for the individual woman with this complication. These three women, all with severe preeclampsia-eclampsia with similar noninvasive assessment findings, illustrate the need for use of a PAC when the pregnant woman with hypertensive disease and oliguria fails a fluid challenge test. Noninvasive parameters do not reflect volume status. Completely different treatment modalities to correct oliguria are indicated for each of these three women.

TABLE 34-6 **Normal Hemodynamic Values in Pregnancy**

Right atrial pressure (RAP) or central venous pressure (CVP)	0-7 mm Hg
Pulmonary artery pressure (PAP)	18-30 mm Hg (systolic) 6-10 mm Hg (diastolic)
Pulmonary capillary wedge pressure (PCWP)	6-10 mm Hg
Cardiac output (CO)	6-7 L/min
Systemic vascular resistance (SVR)	1210 ± 266
Pulmonary vascular resistance (PVR)	78 ± 22

TABLE 34-7 **Central Hemodynamic Normal Values**

PARAMETER	NONPREGNANT	PREGNANT
CO (L/min)	4.3 ± 0.9	6.2 ± 1.0
HR (beats/min)	71 ± 10.0	83 ± 10.0
SVR (dyne/cm/sec^{-5})	1530 ± 520	1210 ± 266
PVR (dyne/cm/sec^{-5})	119 ± 47.0	78 ± 22
PCWP (mm Hg)	6.3 ± 2.1	7.5 ± 1.8
CVP (mm Hg)	3.7 ± 2.6	3.6 ± 2.5
Left ventricular work index	41 ± 8	48 ± 6

Clark, S. et al. (1989). Central hemodynamic assessment of normal term pregnancy. *American Journal of Obstetrics and Gynecology, 161*(6), 1439-1442.

Pulmonary Edema

One of the most common uses of the PAC during pregnancy is the differentiation of cardiogenic (heart failure or hydrostatic) pulmonary edema from noncardiogenic (permeability or lung failure) pulmonary edema (Dorman, 1999). Optimal therapies for the two types of pulmonary edema are dramatically different; however, the correct diagnosis can be determined only by evaluation of the hemodynamic profile.

Cardiogenic or heart failure pulmonary edema develops as a result of left ventricular failure or acute fluid overload. The PCWP is elevated because of the increased volume of fluid in the pulmonary circulation. Therapy is focused on improvement of myocardial contractility with an inotropic drug, decreasing left afterload, if elevated, with an arterial vasodilator and reducing preload with a diuretic drug to a normal range. This type of pulmonary edema usually responds to therapy within a few hours, and a normal PCWP is restored.

Pulmonary edema also may result from damage to the pulmonary alveolar capillary membrane by numerous factors, the most common being sepsis. Disturbance of membrane permeability results in the leakage of both protein and fluid into the pulmonary interstitium and alveoli, in the presence of normal cardiac function and ventricular filling pressures (Dorman, 1999). The PCWP is normal. Alveolar membranes require days to heal, and adult respiratory distress disease may develop if the source of injury is not found and eradicated. The focus of therapy is to maintain the PCWP in the low-normal range to minimize transudation of protein and fluid into the lung and to eliminate the source of injury.

When radiography reveals pulmonary edema, evaluation of the hemodynamic profile is the only way to diagnose correctly the type of pulmonary edema present, as illustrated in the following two hemodynamic profiles (refer to Table 34-6 for the normal values):

Case I

CVP	4 mm Hg
PAP	44/21 mm Hg
PCWP	20 mm Hg
CO	6.1 L/min

BOX 34-5 Case Studies

CASE 1

Jessie is a 24-year-old woman, gravida 4, para 2, at 35 weeks of gestation, diagnosed with severe preeclampsia-eclampsia. She is scheduled for labor induction today because of the increasing severity of the disease.

Everything went well for the first 5 hr after admission. However, this hour, urine output is only 22 ml. The physician orders a fluid challenge of 1000 ml of lactated Ringer's solution (LR); 1 hr after this fluid infusion is completed, urine output is 24 ml.

This is a failed fluid challenge. A Swan-Ganz catheter (PAC) is inserted to determine volume status and to help determine why the kidneys are not excreting urine. The woman's hemodynamic profile was determined to be the following:

CVP	2 mm Hg
PAP	15/5 mm Hg
PCWP	4 mm Hg
CO	6.1 L/min

Evaluation

Evaluation of this profile shows a low PCWP of 4 mm Hg, which denotes decreased left preload and reflects hypovolemia. The low PAP reflects the decreased pulmonary circulating volume. CO is low for a laboring woman, probably as a result of the decreased preload. Her CO at 6.1 L/min is probably being maintained by her elevated HR; however, she is not in danger of dying with a CO of $\geq$ 6 L/min. This hemodynamic profile correlates with hypovolemia as the reason for oliguria. Urine is not being produced because the renal system is not adequately perfused. Additional fluids are needed rapidly. The oliguria is due to compensatory mechanisms that shunt the blood from the peripheral circulation to the central circulation in response to the extremely low preload. The 1000 ml of fluid given in the fluid challenge was not adequate to correct the hypovolemia. Additional fluid should be administered until left preload is adequate.

CASE 2

Shavone is an 18-year-old primigravid woman at 34 weeks of gestation with a diagnosis of severe preeclampsia-eclampsia. She is scheduled for induction of labor today because of increasing severity of disease.

Everything went well for the first 5 hr after admission. However, this hour urine output is only 23 ml. The physician orders a fluid challenge of 1000 ml of LR. One hour after this fluid is infused, urine output is 24 ml.

This is a failed fluid challenge. A Swan-Ganz catheter is inserted to determine volume status and to help determine the cause of the oliguria. Hemodynamic profile is determined to be the following:

CVP	2 mm Hg
PAP	22/9 mm Hg
PCWP	8 mm Hg
CO	7.8 L/min

Evaluation

Evaluation of this profile shows a normal PCWP of 8 mm Hg, a normal PAP, and a CO of 7.8 L/min. A normal hemodynamic profile in conjunction with refractory oliguria is associated with renal artery spasm that decreases perfusion and oxygenation to the kidneys and results in decreased urine output. Renal dose (low-dose) dopamine is used as the first-line management strategy to correct this type of oliguria. An arterial pressure line will be used during administration of the drug to monitor BP closely. Relaxation of the renal artery will improve renal system perfusion and correct the oliguria.

CASE 3

Bonnie is a 32-year-old woman, gravida 5, para 4, at 36 weeks of gestation with a diagnosis of severe preeclampsia-eclampsia. She is scheduled for labor induction today because of increasing severity of disease.

Everything went well for the first 5 hr after admission. However, this hour urine output is only 20 ml. The physician orders a fluid challenge of 1000 ml of LR. One hour after this fluid is completed, urine output is 22 ml.

This is a failed fluid challenge. A Swan-Ganz catheter is inserted to determine volume status and to help determine the cause of the oliguria. Hemodynamic profile is determined to be the following:

CVP	2 mm Hg
PAP	44/20 mm Hg
PCWP	18 mm Hg
CO	6.6 L/min

Evaluation

Evaluation of this profile shows a high PCWP of 18 mm Hg, which denotes an increased left preload. CO is adequate. This profile correlates with oliguria in the hypervolemic pregnant woman. Lack of urine excretion is probably due to renal damage from the ischemia accompanying the severe hypertensive disease. Intravenous fluids should be restricted to 50 ml/hr. The high wedge pressure correlates with pulmonary edema during pregnancy. With such severe preeclampsia, pulmonary edema is usually a combined cardiogenic and noncardiogenic type. Cardiogenic pulmonary edema is a result of the increased SVR, which increased the resistance that the left ventricle must overcome to eject blood. This can lead to congestive heart failure. The noncardiogenic pulmonary edema is a result of an extremely low COP, a result of renal disease and protein excretion. Reduction of left afterload with hydralazine is the initial management strategy to correct the pulmonary edema. CO is adequate, probably because of the increased HR and circulating volume. The high PAP reflects the increased pressures in the pulmonary circulation because of the excessive fluid that is present, produced by the increased left afterload. Immediate delivery will permit further renal studies to evaluate renal function. Dialysis may be indicated.

The high wedge pressure reflects a high left preload and correlates with cardiogenic pulmonary edema. Treatment would include an inotropic drug such as dobutamine, a vasodilator such as hydralazine if hypertension is present, and a diuretic such as furosemide (Lasix) because CO is adequate.

Case II

CVP	2 mm Hg
PAP	23/8 mm Hg
PCWP	7 mm Hg
CO	7.1 L/min

All readings are in the normal range, although pulmonary edema is present. This correlates with noncardiogenic pulmonary edema. A diuretic should not be administered. Preload is in the low-normal range. Reducing the preload with a diuretic drug could decrease CO and jeopardize the client's status. Instead, sepsis should be suspected, and treatment should focus on antibiotic therapy and elimination of foci of infection, continuing assessments, and support of vital systems while lung membranes heal.

TRAUMA DURING PREGNANCY

Trauma continues to be a common complication during pregnancy because of the continuation of usual activities by the majority of pregnant women in the United States.

Significance

Approximately 8% of pregnancies have been reported to be complicated by physical trauma (Van Hook, 2002). As pregnancy progresses, the risk of trauma seems to increase because more cases of trauma are reported in the third trimester than earlier in gestation. Most maternal injuries are a result of motor vehicle accidents. Falls, burns, gunshot wounds, and assault are other major sources (Daddario, 1999).

Acts of violence are a significant health problem in the United States. The risk of trauma caused by battering and abuse is increased during pregnancy, and rates of recurrence are high. The reported incidence of physical abuse during pregnancy ranges from 4% to 30% (Martin et al., 2001; Plichta & Falik, 2001). Up to 45% of women subject to domestic violence before pregnancy continue to be abused during the pregnancy. Abuse also may have its onset with the pregnant state (Biester et al., 1997). An even more frightening statistic is that women who are abused during pregnancy have a threefold risk of being murdered compared with their nonpregnant abused controls (McFarlane et al., 2002). The report goes on to say that African-American women have a threefold higher risk than Caucasion women in the same pregnancy group (McFarlane et al., 2002).

Trauma is the leading nonobstetric cause of maternal mortality and accounts for 20% of maternal deaths each year (ACOG, 1998). More than 70% of these fatal injuries result from motor vehicle accidents. Maternal death caused by trauma is usually the result of head injury or hemorrhagic shock. Fetal death usually occurs as a sequela to maternal death or as a result of placental abruption.

Fortunately, the majority of trauma injuries during pregnancy are minor and have no impact on pregnancy outcome. However, each case of trauma during pregnancy must be evaluated carefully because pregnancy can mask signs of severe injury. Research has not yet revealed an accurate "trauma score" to predict risk of adverse pregnancy outcome from the initial physical assessment (Biester et al., 1997). Therefore prolonged assessments are usually completed before discharge from the unit in seemingly "mild" cases of trauma.

Multisystem trauma during pregnancy is usually the result of a serious motor vehicle crash, especially if the woman is not wearing a seat belt with a shoulder harness and is ejected from the vehicle. Failure to wear restraining devices during pregnancy increases maternal and fetal risks (Pearlman et al., 2000; Reis, Sander, & Pearlman, 2000). ACOG (1998) recommends that pregnant women wear properly positioned restraints at all times when in a motor vehicle (see Fig. 16-17).

Trauma increases the incidence of miscarriage, preterm labor, abruptio placentae, and stillbirth (Furniss, 1997). The effect of trauma on pregnancy is influenced by the length of gestation, type and severity of the trauma, and degree of disruption of uterine and fetal physiologic features. Fetal death as a result of trauma is more common than the occurrence of both maternal and fetal death (Weiss, Songer, & Fabio, 2001). Less serious trauma is associated with numerous complications for pregnancy, including fetomaternal hemorrhage, abruptio placentae, intrauterine fetal death, and preterm labor and birth (Gilbert & Harmon, 2003). Careful evaluation of mother and fetus after all types of trauma is imperative (AAP & ACOG, 1997).

Special considerations for mother and fetus are necessary when trauma occurs during pregnancy because of the physiologic alterations that accompany pregnancy and because of the presence of the fetus. Fetal survival depends on maternal survival; therefore the pregnant woman must receive immediate stabilization and appropriate care for optimal fetal outcome.

Maternal Physiologic Characteristics

Optimal care for the pregnant woman after trauma is dependent on understanding the physiologic state of pregnancy and its effects on trauma. The pregnant woman's body will exhibit responses different from those of a nonpregnant person to the same traumatic insults. Because of the different responses to injury during pregnancy, management strategies must be adapted for appropriate resuscitation, fluid therapy, positioning, assessments, and most other interventions. Significant maternal adaptations and the relation to trauma are summarized in Table 34-8.

The uterus and bladder are confined to the bony pelvis during the first trimester of pregnancy and are at reduced

TABLE 34-8 **Maternal Adaptations During Pregnancy and Relation to Trauma**

SYSTEM	ALTERATION	CLINICAL RESPONSES
Respiratory	↑ Oxygen consumption	↑ Risk of acidosis
	↑ Tidal volume	
	↓ Functional residual capacity	
	Chronic compensated alkalosis	↑ Risk of respiratory mismanagement
	↓ $PaCO_2$	↓ Blood-buffering capacity
	↓ Serum bicarbonate	
Cardiovascular	↑ Circulating volume, 1600 ml	Can lose 1000 ml blood
	↑ CO	No signs of shock until blood loss >30% total blood volume
	↑ Heart rate	
	↓ SVR	↓ Placental perfusion in supine position
	↓ Arterial blood pressure	Point of maximal impulse, fourth intercostal space
	Heart displaced upward to left	
Renal	↑ Renal plasma flow	
	Dilation of ureters and urethra	↑ Risk of stasis, infection
	Bladder displaced forward	↑ Risk of bladder trauma
Gastrointestinal	↓ Gastric motility	↑ Risk of aspiration
	↑ Hydrochloric acid production	
	↓ Competency of gastroesophageal sphincter	Passive regurgitation of stomach acids if head lower than stomach
Reproductive	↑ Blood flow to organs	Source of ↑ blood loss
	Uterine enlargement	Vena caval compression in supine position
Musculoskeletal	Displacement of abdominal viscera	↑ Risk of injury, altered rebound response
	Pelvic venous congestion	Altered pain referral
	Cartilage softened	↑ Risk for pelvic fracture
		Center of gravity changed
	Fetal head in pelvis	↑ Risk of fetal injury
Hematologic	↑ Clotting factors	↑ Risk of thrombus formation
	↓ Fibrinolytic activity	

risk for injury in cases of abdominal trauma. After pregnancy progresses beyond the fourteenth week, the uterus becomes an abdominal organ, and the risk for injury increases in cases of abdominal trauma. During the second and third trimesters, the distended bladder becomes an abdominal organ and is at increased risk for injury and rupture. Bowel injuries occur less often during pregnancy because of the protection provided by the enlarged uterus.

The elevated levels of progesterone that accompany pregnancy relax smooth muscle and profoundly affect the gastrointestinal tract. Gastrointestinal motility decreases, with a resultant increased time required for gastric emptying, whereas the production of hydrochloric acid increases in the last trimester, and the gastroesophageal sphincter relaxes (Scott, 1999). Airway management of the unconscious pregnant woman is of critical importance.

NURSE ALERT

The unconscious pregnant woman is at increased risk for regurgitation of gastric contents and aspiration whenever her head is positioned lower than her stomach or if abdominal pressure is applied.

A pregnant woman has decreased tolerance for hypoxia and apnea because of her decreased functional residual capacity and increased renal loss of bicarbonate. Acidosis develops more quickly in the pregnant than in the nonpregnant state.

CO increases 44% to 50% over prepregnancy values and is positionally dependent in the third trimester. Because of compression of the inferior vena cava and descending aorta by the pregnant uterus, CO will decrease dramatically if the woman is placed in the supine position. The supine position must be avoided, even in women with cervical spine injuries. It is a primary priority that lateral uterine displacement be accomplished without any head movement. As soon as the neck is immobilized, the stretcher should be tilted laterally.

Circulating blood volume increases 50% during gestation, and pregnant women can tolerate a 1000-ml blood loss readily without demonstrating clinical signs. Hemodynamic instability that indicates the need for transfusion may not be apparent until blood loss nears 1500 to 2000 ml (Gonik, 1999). Clinical signs of hemorrhage do not appear until after a 30% loss of circulating volume occurs. Although HR increases with pregnancy, a maternal HR greater than 100 beats/min should be considered abnormal.

Fetal Physiologic Characteristics

Perfusion of the uterine arteries, which provide the primary blood supply to the uteroplacental unit, depends on adequate maternal arterial pressure because these vessels lack autoregulation. Therefore maternal hypotension decreases uterine and fetal perfusion. Maternal shock results in splanchnic and uterine artery vasoconstriction, which decreases blood flow and oxygen transport to the fetus. Electronic fetal monitoring (EFM) tracings can assist in the evaluation of maternal status after trauma. EFM tracings reflect fetal cardiac responses to hypoxia and hypoperfusion, including tachycardia or bradycardia, decreased or absent baseline variability, and late decelerations.

Careful monitoring of fetal status assists greatly in maternal assessment, because the fetal monitor tracing works as an "oximeter" of internal maternal well-being. Hypoperfusion may be present in the pregnant woman before the onset of clinical signs of shock. The EFM tracings show the first signs of maternal compromise, such as when maternal HR, BP, and color appear normal, yet the EFM printout shows signs of fetal hypoxia (Murray, 1997).

Mechanisms of Trauma

Blunt Abdominal Trauma

Blunt abdominal trauma is most commonly the result of motor vehicle crashes but also may be the result of battering or falls. Maternal and fetal mortality and morbidity rates are directly correlated with whether the mother remains inside the vehicle or is ejected. Maternal death is usually the result of a head injury or exsanguination from a major vessel rupture. Serious retroperitoneal hemorrhage after lower abdominal and pelvic trauma is reported more frequently during pregnancy. Serious maternal abdominal injuries are usually the result of splenic rupture or liver or renal injury.

When maternal survival of trauma occurs, fetal death is usually the result of abruptio placentae occurring within 48 hours of the accident (O'Keefe, 1997). Placental separation is thought to be a result of deformation of the elastic myometrium around the relatively inelastic placenta. Shearing of the placental edge from the underlying decidua basalis results and is worsened by the increased intrauterine pressure resulting from the impact. It is critical that all pregnant victims be carefully evaluated for signs and symptoms of abruptio placentae after even minor blunt abdominal trauma.

NURSE ALERT

Signs and symptoms of abruptio placentae include uterine tenderness or pain, uterine irritability, uterine contractions, vaginal bleeding, leaking of amniotic fluid, or a change in FHR characteristics.

Pelvic fracture may result from severe injury and may produce bladder trauma or retroperitoneal bleeding with the two-point displacement of pelvic bones that usually occurs. One point of displacement is commonly at the symphysis pubis, and the second point is posterior, because of the structure of the pelvis. Careful evaluation for clinical signs of internal hemorrhage is indicated.

Direct fetal injury as a complication of trauma during pregnancy most often involves the fetal skull and brain (Gilbert & Harmon, 2003). Most commonly this injury accompanies maternal pelvic fracture in late gestation, after the fetal head becomes engaged. When the force of the impact is great enough to fracture the maternal pelvis, the fetus will often sustain a skull fracture. Evaluation for fetal skull fracture or intracranial hemorrhage is indicated.

Uterine rupture as a result of trauma is rare, occurring in only 0.6% of all reported cases of trauma during pregnancy. Uterine rupture depends on numerous factors, including gestational age, the intensity of the impact, and the presence of a predisposing factor such as a distended uterus caused by polyhydramnios or multiple gestation or the presence of a uterine scar resulting from previous uterine surgery (Cunningham et al., 2001). When uterine rupture occurs, the force responsible is usually a direct, high-energy blow. Fetal death is common with traumatic uterine rupture. However, maternal death occurs less than 10% of the time, and when it occurs, it is usually the result of massive injuries sustained from an impact severe enough to rupture the uterus.

Penetrating Abdominal Trauma

Bullet wounds are the most frequent cause of penetrating abdominal injury, followed by stab wounds. Penetrating abdominal wounds have disparate prognoses for mother and fetus in almost 66% of cases; that is, the woman survives, but the fetus does not. The enlarged uterus may protect other maternal organs, but the fetus is more vulnerable (Cunningham et al., 2001).

Numerous factors determine the extent and severity of maternal and fetal injury from a bullet wound, including size and velocity of the bullet, anatomic region penetrated, angle of entry, path of the bullet, organs damaged, gestational age, and exit wound. Once the bullet enters the body, it may ricochet several times as it encounters organs or bone, or it may sever a large blood vessel. During the second half of pregnancy, the fetus usually sustains a direct injury from the bullet. Gunshot wounds require surgical exploration to determine the extent of injury and repair damage as needed (ACOG, 1998).

Stab wounds are limited by the length and width of the penetrating object and are usually confined to the pathway of the weapon. Maternal and fetal injury are less if the stab wound is located in the upper abdomen and from movement of the penetrating object from above the head downward toward the abdomen than from movement of the penetrating object from the ground upward toward the lower abdomen. Stab wounds usually require surgical exploration to clean out debris, determine extent of injury, and repair damage.

Thoracic Trauma

Thoracic trauma is reported to produce 25% of all trauma deaths. Pulmonary contusion results from nearly 75% of blunt thoracic trauma and is a potentially life-threatening condition (Keough & Pudelek, 2001). Pulmonary contusion can be difficult to recognize, especially if flail chest also is present or if there is no evidence of thoracic injury. Pulmonary contusion should be suspected in cases of thoracic injury, especially after blunt acceleration or deceleration trauma, such as that occurring when a rapidly moving vehicle crashes into an immovable object.

Penetrating wounds into the chest can result in pneumothorax or hemothorax. This type of injury is usually caused by a vehicular crash that results in impalement by the steering column or a loose article in the vehicle that became a projectile with the force of impact. Stab wounds into the chest also may occur as a result of violence.

Immediate Stabilization

Immediate priorities for stabilization of the pregnant woman after trauma should be identical to those of the nonpregnant trauma client. Pregnancy should not result in any restriction of the usual diagnostic, pharmacologic, or resuscitative procedures or maneuvers (ACOG, 1998). The initial response of many trauma team members when caring for the pregnant woman is to assess fetal status first because of the concern for a healthy neonate. The trauma team should follow a methodical evaluation of maternal status to ensure complete assessment and stabilization of the mother. Fetal survival depends on maternal survival, and stabilization of the mother improves fetal chance of survival.

NURSE ALERT

Priorities of care for the pregnant woman after trauma must be to resuscitate the woman and stabilize her condition first and then consider fetal needs.

Primary Survey

The systematic evaluation begins with a **primary survey** and the initial *ABCs* of resuscitation: establishment of and maintaining an *airway,* ensuring adequate *breathing,* and maintenance of an adequate *circulatory volume.*

Increased oxygen needs during gestation necessitate a rapid response. The presence of a cervical spine injury is always assumed.

NURSE ALERT

Hyperextension of the neck is avoided; instead jaw thrust is used to establish an airway for the trauma victim.

Once an airway is established, assessment should focus on adequacy of oxygenation. The chest wall is observed for movement. If breathing is absent, ventilations and endotracheal intubation are initiated. Supplemental oxygen should be administered with a tight-fitting, nonrebreathing face mask at 10 to 12 L per minute to maintain a maternal arterial oxygen tension (PaO_2) greater than 60 mm Hg and a hemoglobin saturation greater than 90% to maintain fetal status (Clark, 1991). The chest wall is assessed for penetrating chest wound or flail chest. Breathing with a flail chest will be rapid and labored; chest wall movements will be uncoordinated and asymmetric; crepitus from bony fragments may be palpated.

Rapid placement of two large-bore (14- to 16-gauge) intravenous lines is necessary in the majority of seriously injured clients. It is important to place the lines while veins are still distended. Cardiac arrest during the immediate stabilization period is usually the result of profound hypovolemia; massive fluid resuscitation is necessary when arrest is caused by hypovolemia. Infusion of crystalloids such as Ringer's solution or normal saline solution should be given as a 3:1 ratio; that is, 3 ml of crystalloid replacement to 1 ml of the estimated blood loss is given over the first 30 to 60 minutes of acute resuscitation (ACOG, 1998). Because of the 50% increase in blood volume during pregnancy, published formulas for nonpregnant adults used for estimating crystalloid and blood replacement to counter blood loss must be adjusted upward for pregnancy.

Replacement of red blood cells and other blood components is anticipated, and blood is drawn for type, crossmatch, complete blood cell count, and platelet count (Van Hook, 2002). Infusion of type-specific whole blood or packed red blood cells is usually necessary to improve fetal oxygenation status and to replace blood loss. During an extreme emergency, type O Rh-negative blood may be administered without matching.

Vasopressor drugs to restore maternal arterial BP should be avoided, if possible, until volume replacement is administered. Although vasopressor agents result in decreased perfusion to the uterus, they should be given, and not withheld, if needed for successful resuscitation of the mother (ACOG, 1998).

After 20 weeks of gestation, venous return to the heart is best accomplished by positioning the uterus to one side to eliminate the weight of the uterus compressing the inferior vena cava or the descending aorta. This facilitates efforts to establish the forward flow of blood through resuscitation and stabilization. If a lateral position is not possible because of resuscitative efforts or cervical spine immobilization, the uterus can be manually deflected to the left, or a wedge should be inserted underneath the right side of the backboard or stretcher.

Signs of bleeding may be more difficult to recognize in the pregnant woman because a 30% to 35% loss of maternal blood volume may produce only a minimal change in maternal MAP. Hypovolemia can be detrimental for the fetus because the vascular bed of the uterus is a low-resistance system that depends on adequate maternal arterial pressure to maintain uterine and fetal perfusion. Maternal hypovolemia can be fatal for the fetus.

Establishing a baseline neurologic status (level of consciousness, pupil size and reactivity) is essential. The Glasgow Coma Scale is commonly used at the scene of the accident to help determine the extent of the head injury. The scale is simple and easy to use (Box 34-6).

Secondary Survey

After immediate resuscitation and successful stabilization measures, a more detailed **secondary survey** of the mother and fetus should be accomplished. A complete physical assessment including all body systems is performed.

The maternal abdomen should be evaluated carefully, because a large percentage of serious injuries involve the uterus, intraperitoneal structures, and retroperitoneum. The pregnant woman's stomach is assumed to be full. A nasogastric tube can be used to empty the stomach to help prevent acid aspiration syndrome. An empty stomach facilitates respiratory efforts. The uterus should be evaluated for evidence of gross deformity, tenderness, irritability, or contractions (ACOG, 1998).

The greatest clinical concern after vehicular crashes is abruptio placentae, as up to 40% of these women will have an abruption (Van Hook, 2002). Assessments should focus on recognition of this complication, with careful evaluation of fetal monitor tracings, uterine tenderness, labor, or vaginal bleeding. Ultrasound examination may be performed to determine gestational age, viability of fetus, and placental location. However, ultrasound studies cannot exclude abruptio placentae.

Peritoneal lavage for the pregnant woman after blunt abdominal trauma has proved to be a safe procedure and can be helpful in the early diagnosis of intraperitoneal injury or hemorrhage. Under direct visualization, the peritoneum is incised, and a peritoneal dialysis catheter is positioned. If aspiration yields free-flowing blood, the test is considered positive, and a laparotomy should be performed. This procedure is not necessary before laparotomy if intraperitoneal bleeding is clinically apparent. Indications for peritoneal lavage include abdominal symptoms or signs suggestive of intraperitoneal bleeding, alteration in mental status, unexplained shock, and severe multiple injury (Cunningham et al., 2001).

If trauma is the result of a penetrating wound, the woman should be completely undressed and carefully examined for all entrance and exit wounds. A bullet may be located on x-ray films. Exploratory laparotomy is necessary after a gunshot wound to explore the abdominal cavity for organ damage and to repair any damage present, with careful examination of all organs, the entire bowel, and posterior vessels. If uterine injury is determined, a careful evaluation of the risks and benefits of cesarean birth is quickly accomplished. A cesarean birth is desirable if the fetus is alive and near term and may be necessary for the preterm fetus because of the high incidence of fetal injury in these cases. Tetanus prophylaxis guidelines are not changed by pregnancy. The fetus usually tolerates surgery and anesthesia if adequate uterine perfusion and oxygenation are maintained.

Electronic Fetal Monitoring

Use of electronic fetal monitoring (EFM) may be predictive of abruptio placentae in pregnant trauma victims beyond the twentieth week of gestation (ACOG, 1998). Continuous EFM may show early signs of abruptio placentae, including a change in baseline rate, loss of accelerations, or the presence of late decelerations. Fetal monitoring should be initiated soon after the woman is stable because abruptio placentae usually becomes apparent shortly after the injury. Fetal monitoring should be continued and further evaluation initiated if any of the aforementioned signs occur. The external device to monitor uterine activity, the tocodynamometer, is unable

BOX 34-6 **Glasgow Coma Scale**

Eyes	Open	Spontaneously	4
		To verbal command	3
		To pain	2
		No response	1
Best motor response	To verbal command	Obeys	6
	To painful stimulus	Localizes pain	5
		Flexion-withdrawal	4
		Flexion-abnormal (decorticate rigidity)	3
		Extension (decerebrate rigidity)	2
		No response	1
Best verbal response		Oriented and converses	5
		Disoriented and converses	4
		Inappropriate words	3
		Incomprehensible sounds	2
		No response	1
Total			3-15

to measure pressures, and the pattern made with this device shows the frequency and duration of contractions only. Palpation is required to evaluate the intensity of contractions and the uterine resting tone. It is important to palpate between contractions to verify that the uterus is well relaxed. If the uterus does not relax between contractions, abruptio placentae could be present.

Abruptio placentae occurring after trauma may be delayed up to 48 hours after the incident (O'Keefe, 1997). EFM periods of 2 to 6 hours after minor trauma are adequate if there are no uterine contractions, uterine tenderness, or bleeding (ACOG, 1998). However, fetal reassurance must be established after minor trauma before fetal monitoring is discontinued and the woman is discharged.

LEGAL TIP Care of Pregnant Woman Involved in Minor Trauma Situation

After minor trauma, the pregnant woman may be discharged after an adequate period of EFM that demonstrates fetal reassurance and absence of uterine contractions. However, clear instructions must be given for immediate return if vaginal bleeding, leaking of amniotic fluid, decreased fetal movement, or abdominal pain occurs (ACOG, 1998).

Fetal-Maternal Hemorrhage

The potential for fetal-maternal hemorrhage exists after trauma; hemorrhage can lead to fetal anemia, distress, or even death. If the pregnant trauma victim is Rh negative, fetal-maternal hemorrhage can result in sensitization and hemolytic disease of the neonate. The routine use of the Kleihauer-Betke assay in women with blunt abdominal trauma or multiple trauma helps identify cases with a hemorrhage of more than 30 ml (ACOG, 1998). Because most cases have less than 30 ml of hemorrhage, the routine administration of 300 μg (one ampule) of $Rh_0(D)$ immunoglobulin is appropriate because this practice would protect almost all pregnant trauma clients negative for $Rh_0(D)$ from isoimmunization (ACOG, 1998).

Ultrasound

Ultrasonography after trauma is not so sensitive as EFM for diagnosing abruptio placentae. Ultrasound may be useful to help establish gestational age, locate the placenta, evaluate cardiac activity (to determine whether the fetus is alive), and determine amniotic fluid volume (ACOG, 1998). Ultrasound may also be used to evaluate the presence of intraabdominal fluid that would suggest the presence of intraabdominal hemorrhage.

Radiation Exposure

If the pregnant woman has sustained serious injuries, any necessary radiographic examination should be performed, regardless of fetal exposure. If radiographic examination would be performed for the nonpregnant trauma victim, it also should be performed for the pregnant woman. Special efforts can minimize the dose to the lower abdomen. Shielding the uterus during irradiation procedures and eliminating duplicate films usually exposes the fetus to a radiation dose of less than 1 rad (ACOG, 1998).

In some victims with blunt abdominal trauma, abdominal-pelvic computed tomography is preferred to visualize extraperitoneal and retroperitoneal structures and the genitourinary tract. This procedure, in general, exposes the fetus to 5 to 10 rad and should not be withheld for the pregnant woman.

Blunt head trauma and loss of consciousness necessitate skull films and computed tomographic assessment with neurosurgical consultation. Magnetic resonance imaging also may be used to assess injuries (ACOG, 1998).

Perimortem Cesarean Delivery

In the presence of multisystem trauma, **perimortem cesarean delivery** may be indicated. Removal of the stressor of pregnancy early in the process of resuscitation may increase the chance for maternal survival. Fetal survival is unlikely if cesarean delivery is accomplished more than 20 minutes after maternal death. Therefore, to facilitate resuscitative efforts, consideration may be given to cesarean delivery for maternal benefit after 5 minutes of resuscitative efforts that produce no response in the mother (Gonik, 1999; Luppi, 1999).

Physical Assessment

Trauma may affect numerous systems in the maternal body and may affect more than the pregnancy. External signs of maternal trauma should suggest the possibility of internal trauma. Back and neck pain suggest spine injury, abrasions on the chest suggest chest injury, and limb pain and malposition suggest limb fractures. If head injury results in nonresponsiveness, suspect spinal, thoracic, and abdominal injuries. Hypovolemic shock can occur with internal hemorrhage, fracture of long bones, ruptured liver or spleen, hemothorax, or arterial dissection.

Once immediate stabilization is achieved, obstetric clients with severe trauma and massive blood loss that merits vigorous fluid resuscitation will usually benefit from the use of hemodynamic monitoring with a fiberoptic pulmonary catheter to determine cardiac and pulmonary function more precisely and to calculate volume and oxygen needs. The hemodynamic profile permits precise fluid resuscitation volumes. Oxygenation status calculations, including oxygen content, delivery, and consumption, will demonstrate which fluids are needed to enhance oxygen transport. Precise determinations can help prevent the potential sequelae of too little or too much fluid administration. With massive trauma, this care may be best provided in a regional trauma center with the obstetric team, working closely with the trauma team, providing the obstetric care while the trauma team provides the trauma care.

All female trauma victims of childbearing age should be considered pregnant until proven otherwise. Determination of the health history and a history of the events preceding the trauma are important components of care. If the pregnant woman was involved in a vehicular crash, it

BOX 34-7 Physical Examination of the Pregnant Trauma Victim

HEAD

Check scalp for signs of cuts, bruises, or edema. Examine skull for deformities, depressions, or lumps. Examine eyes and eyelids. Evaluate pupils for size, equality, and reaction to light. If contact lenses are present, remove them. Examine nose and ears, and observe for serous or bloody fluid. Open the mouth and look for blood, vomitus, loose teeth, and dentures.

Neurologic function should be evaluated frequently because the most frequent cause of death in women not using seat belts is head trauma (ACOG, 1998). If neurologic checks show a possible head trauma, a complete neurologic consultation and examination should be obtained quickly, including skull films and computed tomographic examination.

NECK

Palpate for tenderness over the cervical spine area. Immobilize with a cervical collar and backboard if complaints of tenderness are present or any injury is suspected. Tilt backboard to side as soon as the pregnant woman is placed on backboard.

CHEST

Observe for lacerations, contusions, wounds, or impaled objects. Observe chest wall movement for symmetry and equal expansion. Assess breath sounds and quality and rate of respirations. Observe for deviated trachea, sounds of sucking wounds, and flail chest. Palpate ribs, sternum, and clavicle.

ABDOMEN

Observe for lacerations, contusions, wounds, or impaled objects. Perform light and then deep palpation. Apply electronic fetal monitoring (EFM) devices, both the ultrasound Doppler device and tocodynamometer. Palpate for intensity of uterine contractions and determine uterine resting tone. Observe fetal heart rate tracing for signs of fetal reassurance or compromise.

LOWER BACK

Palpate for tenderness. Observe for contusions, deformities, or other signs of injury.

EXTREMITIES

Examine for deformities, edema, dislocation, bleeding, contusions, and fractures. Palpate for tenderness. Assess radial and pedal pulses. Request pregnant woman to move extremities; observe response.

VAGINA

Use digital examination for term gestation without vaginal bleeding; use sterile speculum examination for preterm gestation or if vaginal bleeding is present. Assess for signs of labor, injuries to tissues, or evidence of ruptured membranes.

URINARY TRACT

Observe for the presence of blood in the urine. Trauma to the lower urinary tract is usually accompanied by a fractured pelvis, requiring use of a Foley catheter. Rupture of the bladder may occur in late pregnancy without a pelvic fracture because the full bladder becomes an abdominal organ. Maintain accurate intake and output and observe color of urine.

should be determined whether she was the driver or a passenger and if she was ejected from the vehicle or used a restraining device and remained within the vehicle.

The physical examination should be performed in a systematic manner (Box 34-7).

FAMILY-CENTERED OBSTETRIC CRITICAL CARE

Obstetric critical care should include the components of family-centered maternity care because this critically ill woman also is experiencing pregnancy and birth.

Components of family-centered critical care include the following elements:

- Open visitation so that spouse, significant other, or family members are present and provide support during labor, birth, and the postpartum period.
- Facilitation of parent-infant contact and attachment. The neonate should be brought to the bedside frequently if the condition permits. When the infant's condition does not permit leaving the neonatal ICU, pictures of the infant should be placed within focus of the mother's eyes. Staff and family can talk about the infant and keep her updated on the infant's condition.
- Sibling visitation, reassuring the mother that the older child is included in the experience.
- Family visitation as the mother desires. This can be arranged around necessary care procedures. The critically ill mother needs this care, perhaps even more than the healthy mother does.

Obstetric nurses have become accustomed to family-centered maternity care. When the critically ill mother receives care in an OBICU, there seem to be fewer problems for inclusion of the components of family-centered care than when the mother has to be transported to the adult ICU, probably because the obstetric staff is accustomed to this care and the nursery is more readily available to the labor suite than to the ICU. However, obstetric and critical

care nurses can work together to include the components of family-centered care. Critical care nurses are supportive of these components.

Never assume that the mother is too ill to see and hold her infant. Encourage this and observe her body language to determine how much contact with the infant she desires. If perinatal loss occurs as a result of severe illness, provide grief support. Initiate all the components of grief support as usual for the institution. Burial plans can be delayed until the mother's condition improves so that her concerns are addressed (see Chapter 41).

Maternal Death

It is extremely rare for a woman to die in childbirth, but it does happen. The yearly occurrence of maternal deaths in the United States is 9.8 per 100,000 (Minino et al., 2000). The father and extended family who are faced with mourning not only the death of a wife and mother but also the death of the baby have a particularly difficult time. Conversely, the father may be faced with parenting a baby without a surviving mother. Death of a mother disrupts the family structure and leaves the father with the care of a baby when he is greatly distressed. Thus the father and extended family, especially other children and grandparents, need supportive grief counseling at the time of death and after discharge for them to heal after such a devastating loss.

The nursing care of families at this time is similar to that described in Chapter 41. Options need to be offered, memories made, and mementos obtained and held for the family until they are ready for them. These families are at risk for complicated bereavement and altered parenting of the surviving baby and other children in the family. Referral to social services to help the family mobilize support systems and for counseling can help combat potential problems before they develop. Such a referral may be beneficial not only at the time of the loss but also in the future.

The emotional toll that a maternal death can take on the nursing and medical staff also must be addressed. Guilt, anger, fear, sadness, and depression are all common responses to a maternal death. The staff may want to review the situation surrounding the events, the chart, and their responses in the forum of a mortality-morbidity review and a critical incident debriefing to help in coping with the feelings and emotions that result after a maternal death. Attending memorial or funeral services may benefit staff and family.

KEY POINTS

- The numbers of critically ill pregnant women are increasing, paralleling improvements in pediatric and neonatal care. Any nurse providing care for pregnant women may encounter the critically ill pregnant woman and must be able to initiate appropriate care.
- Nurses must recognize early signs of severe complications and expedite the institution's plan for the critically ill pregnant woman to receive necessary complex care.
- The institutional plan may consist of actual implementation of critical care procedures in a labor and birth unit, stabilization, and preparation for transport to a tertiary center or adult ICU, with obstetric consultation after transport.
- Normal physiologic alterations during pregnancy produce profound hemodynamic changes. The critical care team should base care on knowledge of normal hemodynamic values for the pregnant state.
- Pregnancy is not a contraindication for hemodynamic monitoring.
- Invasive hemodynamic monitoring is associated with potential complications. However, the benefits usually outweigh the risks when the woman is critically ill.
- Pulmonary artery catheterization provides continuous information about left ventricle function; this information is not available from any other method.
- Use of a PAC in combination with an arterial pressure catheter and pulse oximeter provides adequate data to assess continuously both cardiac and pulmonary status.
- The fiberoptic PAC provides a continuous SvO_2, which is a sensitive marker of physiologic instability because it reflects overall adequacy of oxygen delivery to the tissues.
- The active roles assumed by most pregnant women today place them at risk for vehicular crashes, falls, violence, and other injuries.
- Domestic violence and battering increase during pregnancy.
- Pregnancy does not limit or restrict resuscitative, diagnostic, or pharmacologic treatment after trauma.
- Fetal survival depends on maternal survival. After trauma the first priority is resuscitation and stabilization of the mother before consideration of fetal concerns.
- Optimal care for the pregnant victim of trauma depends on knowledge of the physiologic state of pregnancy.
- Minor trauma is associated with major complications for the pregnancy, including abruptio placentae, fetomaternal hemorrhage, preterm labor and birth, and fetal death.
- Trauma from accidents is the most common cause of death in women of childbearing age.
- Care of the critically ill pregnant woman should include the components of family-centered childbirth.
- Death of a woman in childbirth is rare; it disrupts family structure, and the family needs supportive grief counseling.

CRITICAL THINKING EXERCISES

1. Evaluate the plan in your institution for providing appropriate care for the critically ill pregnant woman. Compare your policies and procedures for hemodynamic monitoring with those outlined in this chapter.
   a. Will critically ill women receive care in your institution, or will they need to be transported to a tertiary care center?
   b. Are guidelines clear for immediate stabilization procedures?
   c. If care is to be provided in your institution, is the location an OBICU or an adult intensive care unit? If transport to the intensive care unit is necessary, are clear guidelines written for the obstetric nurse and fetal monitor to accompany the pregnant woman?
   d. Is the procedure for performing Allen's test before insertion of an arterial pressure line in the radial artery included in your policy and procedure manual?
   e. Are hemodynamic values for pregnancy readily available for all team members?
2. Louisa, an 18-year-old primigravida at 36 weeks of gestation, is brought to the emergency room by ambulance stretcher after a gunshot wound to the abdomen. Her BP is 90/50 mm Hg; HR, 156 beats/min; and respirations, 30 breaths/min. Mucous membranes are pale, and skin is clammy. Intravenous access is obtained with two large-bore catheters, and fluid resuscitation with 3 L of lactated Ringer's solution and 6 U of type O, Rh-negative packed red blood cells is rapidly administered. No fetal heart tones are present, and a hard, boardlike uterus is palpated. The diagnosis is abruptio placentae. She is taken to the OR for exploratory laparotomy and cesarean delivery under general anesthesia. A PAC is inserted, and the woman's hemodynamic profile reveals the following information:

CVP	2 mm Hg
PAP	13/4 mm Hg
PCWP	3 mm Hg
CO	4.8 L/min

   a. Is the CO adequate? Is the woman in danger of dying?
   b. Was the volume of fluid resuscitation adequate? Would it be safe to administer more volume rapidly?
   c. Is pulmonary edema developing from the massive fluid load?
   d. Should a beta-blocker be given to slow the HR?
3. Janna, a 32-year-old, gravida 2, para 0, is brought in by ambulance with complaints of a severe epigastric pain that she had when she awoke that morning. She is at 29 weeks' gestation. She has had no problems with her pregnancy but has not been compliant with her prenatal visits. Her BP is 170/112 mm Hg. An IV is started and blood drawn to rule out preeclampsia. Urine dipstick shows 4+ proteinuria, and magnesium sulfate is started for seizure prophylaxis. The laboratory results are indicative of severe preeclampsia with elevated liver enzymes. Induction of labor is started with oxytocin, and the NICU is notified to consult with the mother regarding care of the infant. As the NICU attending is talking with the woman, she becomes extremely agitated and complains of severe right upper quadrant pain. The FHR decreases, and she is taken to the OR for a STAT cesarean delivery for sustained fetal bradycardia. She is given general anesthesia and during the C/S, her BP decreases to 88/50, pulse 130. The baby is delivered. The physicians note a grossly enlarged liver during examination, but there is no overt bleeding. Janna's BP remains low, and she is given 3 L lactated Ringer's solution and 3 units packed red blood cells for the diagnosis of liver hematoma. She is stabilized and taken to the PACU where her urine output remains extremely low (less than 20 ml during the surgery). Her BP remains low, but she is complaining of shortness of breath. She has bilateral rales on auscultation. A PAC is inserted. The woman's hemodynamic profile reveals the following data:

CVP	2 mm Hg
PAP	16/8 mm Hg
PCWP	7 mm Hg
CO	4.4 L/min

   a. Is the CO adequate? Is the woman in danger of dying?
   b. Does this profile correlate with pulmonary edema? If yes, which type?
   c. According to a positive chest radiograph report of pulmonary edema, if furosemide (Lasix) had been given without benefit of a hemodynamic profile, what would be the potential effects?

RESOURCES

American College of Obstetricians and Gynecologists
409 12th St. SW
Washington, DC 20024
800-762-2264
www.acog.org

Association of Women's Health, Obstetric, and Neonatal Nurses
2000 L St. NW
Washington DC 20024
800-673-8499
www.awhonn.org

Centers for Disease Control and Prevention
1600 Clifton Rd. NE
Atlanta, GA 30333
404-329-1819
404-329-3286
www.cdc.gov

Family Violence Prevention Fund
383 Rhode Island St., Suite 304
San Francisco, CA 94103
415-252-8900
www.fvpf

REFERENCES

American Academy of Pediatrics & American College of Obstetricians and Gynecologists. (1997). *Guidelines for perinatal care* (4th ed.). Elk Grove Village, IL: AAP/ACOG.

American College of Obstetricians and Gynecologists. (1992). Invasive hemodynamic monitoring in obstetrics and gynecology. *ACOG Technical Bulletin No. 175.* Washington, DC: ACOG.

American College of Obstetricians and Gynecologists. (1998). Trauma during pregnancy. *ACOG Education Bulletin No. 251.* Washington, DC: ACOG.

Association of Women's Health, Obstetric, and Neonatal Nurses. (1998). *Standards and guidelines for professional nursing practice in the care of women and newborns* (5th ed.). Washington, DC: AWHONN.

Biester, E. et al. (1997). Trauma in pregnancy: Normal revised trauma score in relation to other markers of maternofetal status: A preliminary study. *American Journal of Obstetrics and Gynecology 176*, 1206-1212.

Bolte, A. et al. (2000). Lack of agreement between central venous pressure and pulmonary capillary wedge pressure in preeclampsia. *Hypertension in Pregnancy, 19*(3), 261-271.

Branch, K. et al. (1998). Risks of subsequent pregnancies on mother and newborn in female heart transplant recipients. *Journal of Heart and Lung Transplantation, 17*(7), 698-702.

Cathelyn, J., & Samples, D. (1998). SvO_2 monitoring tool for evaluating patient outcomes. *Dimensions in Critical Care Nursing, 17*(2), 58-63.

Clark, S. et al. (1989). Central hemodynamic assessment of normal term pregnancy. *American Journal of Obstetrics and Gynecology, 161*(6), 1439-1442.

Clark, S. et al. (1991). Position change and central hemodynamic profile during normal third-trimester pregnancy and postpartum. *American Journal of Obstetrics and Gynecology, 164*(3), 883-887.

Conners, A. et al. (1996). The effectiveness of right heart catheterization in the initial care of critically ill patients. *Journal of the American Medical Association, 18*, 889-897.

Cunningham, F. et al. (2001). *Williams obstetrics* (21st ed). New York: McGraw-Hill.

Daddario, J. (1999). Trauma in pregnancy. In L. Mandeville & N. Troiano (Eds.), *AWHONN's high risk and critical care intrapartum nursing* (2nd ed.). Philadelphia: J.B. Lippincott.

Darovik, G. (2002). *Hemodynamic monitoring: Invasive and noninvasive clinical application.* Philadelphia: W.B. Saunders.

Dekker, G., & Sibai, B. (2001). Primary, secondary, and tertiary prevention of pre-eclampsia. *Lancet, 357*, 209-215.

Dorman, K. (1999). Pulmonary disorders in pregnancy. In L. Mandeville & N. Troiano (Eds.), *AWHONN's high risk and critical care intrapartum nursing* (2nd ed.). Philadelphia: J.B. Lippincott.

Furniss, K. (1997). Battered women: How nurses can help. *AWHONN Lifelines, 1*(4), 12-18.

Gilbert E., & Harmon, J. (2003). *Manual of high risk pregnancy* (3rd ed.). St. Louis: Mosby.

Gonik, B. (1999). Intensive care monitoring of the critically ill pregnant patient. In R. Creasy & R. Resnik, (Eds.), *Maternal-fetal medicine* (4th ed.). Philadelphia: W.B. Saunders.

Griffith, S. (1999). Acute renal failure in pregnancy. In L. Mandeville & N. Troiano (Eds.), *AWHONN's high risk and critical care intrapartum nursing* (2nd ed.). Philadelphia: J.B. Lippincott.

Harvey, M. (1999). Physiologic changes during pregnancy. In L. Mandeville & N. Troiano (Eds.), *AWHONN's high risk and critical care intrapartum nursing* (2nd ed.). Philadelphia: J.B. Lippincott.

Hazelgrove, J. et al. (2001). Multicenter study of obstetric admissions to 14 intensive care units in southern England. *Critical Care Medicine, 29*(4), 770-775.

Keough, V., & Pudelek, B. (2001). Blunt chest trauma: Review of selected pulmonary injuries focusing on pulmonary contusion. *American Association of Critical Care Nursing Clinical Issues, 12*(2), 270-281.

Luppi, C. (1999). Cardiopulmonary resuscitation in pregnancy. In L. Mandeville & N. Troiano (Eds.), *AWHONN's high risk and critical care intrapartum nursing* (2nd ed.). Philadelphia: J.B. Lippincott.

Mabie, W., & Sibai, B. (1990). Treatment in an obstetric intensive care unit. *American Journal of Obstetrics and Gynecology, 162*(1), 1-4.

Mandeville, L., & Troiano, N. (Eds.). (1999). *AWHONN's high risk and critical care intrapartum nursing* (2nd ed.). Philadelphia: J.B. Lippincott.

Martin, S. et al. (2001). Physical abuse of women before, during, and after pregnancy. *Journal of the American Medical Association, 285*(12), 1581-1584.

McCormack, D. (1998). Care of the obstetric patient in the traditional intensive care unit. *Critical Care Nursing Quarterly, 21*(3), 1-22.

McFarlane, J. et al. (2002). Abuse during pregnancy and femicide: Urgent implications for women's health. *Obstetrics and Gynecology, 100*(1), 27-36.

Medlin, D. et al. (1998). Validation of continuous thermodilution cardiac output in critically ill patients with analysis of systematic errors. *Critical Care, 13*(4), 184-189.

Miller, J., Mastrobattista, J., & Katz, A. (2000). Obstetrical and neonatal outcome in pregnancies after liver transplantation. *American Journal of Perinatology, 17*(6), 299-302.

Minino, A. et al. (2002). Deaths: Final data for 2000. *National Vital Statistics Report, 50*(15), 1-119.

Murray, M. (1997). *Antepartal and intrapartal fetal monitoring* (2nd ed.). Albuquerque, NM: Learning Resources International.

National Institutes of Health & National Heart, Lung, Liver, Blood Institute. (2000). Classification of the hypertensive disorders of pregnancy. *Working report on hypertension in pregnancy*. Bethesda, MD: NIH.

O'Keefe, D. (1997). Trauma in pregnancy. In M. Foley & T. Strong (Eds.), *Obstetric intensive care: A practical approach*. St. Louis: Mosby.

Pearlman, M. et al. (2000). A comprehensive program to improve safety for pregnant women and fetuses in motor vehicle crashes: A preliminary report. *American Journal of Obstetrics and Gynecology, 182*(6), 1554-1564.

Plichta, S., & Falik, M. (2001). Prevalence of violence and its implications for women's health. *Womens' Health Issues, 11*(3), 244-258.

Reis, P., Sander, C., & Pearlman, M. (2000). Abruptio placentae after auto accidents: A case-control study. *Journal of Reproductive Medicine, 45*(1), 6-10.

Scott, L. (1999). Gastrointestinal disease in pregnancy. In R. Creasy & R. Resnik (Eds.), *Maternal-fetal medicine* (4th ed.). Philadelphia: W.B. Saunders.

Sgro, M. et al. (2002). Pregnancy outcome post renal transplantation. *Teratology, 65*(1), 5-9.

Society of Critical Care Medicine Consensus Development Conference. (1997). Pulmonary artery catheter consensus conference: Consensus statement. *New Horizons, 5*(3), 175-193.

Troiano, N. (1999). Invasive hemodynamic monitoring in obstetrics. In L. Mandeville & N. Troiano (Eds.), *AWHONN's high risk and critical care intrapartum nursing* (2nd ed.). Philadelphia: J.B. Lippincott.

Van Hook, J. (2002) Trauma in pregnancy. *Clinical Obstetrics and Gynecology, 45*(2), 414-424.

Wallace, D., & Winslow, E. (1993). Effects of iced and room temperature injectate on cardiac output measurements in critically ill patients with low and high cardiac outputs. *Heart and Lung, 32*(1), 2-12.

Weiss, H., Songer, T., & Fabio, A. (2001). Fetal deaths related to maternal injury. *Journal of the American Medical Association, 286*(15), 1863-1869.

CHAPTER 35

Anne Hopkins Fishel

Mental Health Disorders and Substance Abuse

http://evolve.elsevier.com/Lowdermilk/MatWmnHlth/

LEARNING OBJECTIVES

- Delineate emotional complications during pregnancy, including management of anxiety disorders and mood disorders.
- Examine substance abuse during pregnancy, including dual diagnosis, prevalence, risk factors, legal considerations, treatment programs, barriers to treatment, and care management
- Identify postpartum emotional complications, including incidence, risk factors, signs and symptoms, and management.
- Evaluate the role of the nurse in assessing and managing care of women with emotional complications during pregnancy and postpartum.

Management of mental health disorders takes place primarily in community settings. Women who have serious mental disorders have an opportunity for engaging in sexual activities that can result in pregnancy. Mental health disorders have implications for the pregnant woman, the fetus, the newborn, and the entire family. Between 10% and 15% of women have these disorders. The symptoms and treatment can complicate pregnancy, childbirth, and the postpartum period (Wintz, 1999).

MENTAL HEALTH DISORDERS DURING PREGNANCY

The pregnant woman may have a history of mood disorder, anxiety disorder, substance use disorder, schizophrenia, personality disorder, or developmental disorder. If she is not in treatment currently, assessment throughout pregnancy and the postpartum period is critical to the mother's and the baby's health. With a history of mental illness, referral to a mental health specialist for evaluation is recommended. Some psychiatric disorders, such as panic disorder, may improve or abate during pregnancy; in contrast, obsessive-compulsive disorder (OCD) appears to be more prevalent during pregnancy, with one study citing that more than 25% of women with OCD reported symptom onset during pregnancy (Stowe, Strader, & Nemeroff, 2001). Psychiatric disorders with a psychotic component, such as schizophrenia, generally worsen during pregnancy.

Mood Disorders

Women who are being treated for depression may become pregnant, either intentionally or accidentally. In approximately 6% of women, depression develops for the first time during their pregnancy. Depressive symptoms may be evident during the first trimester of pregnancy, as early as 10 to 14 weeks, in women who have no history of depression (Pederson, 1998). This finding dispels the myth that early pregnancy is a pleasant and happy event for all women.

Mood disorders are defined as disorders that have as their dominant feature a disturbance in the prevailing emotional state. To be diagnosed with major depression, at least five of the following must be present nearly every day: depressed mood, often with spontaneous crying; markedly diminished interest in all activities; insomnia or hypersomnia; weight changes (increases and decreases); psychomotor retardation or agitation; fatigue or loss of energy; feelings of worthlessness or inappropriate guilt; diminished ability to concentrate; and suicidal ideation with or without a suicidal plan (American Psychiatric Association [APA], 2000).

NURSE ALERT

Diagnostic assessment for depression in pregnant women is difficult because many of the symptoms of pregnancy mimic depression. Critical cues are the presence of psychologic symptoms, a suicide plan, and major disruptions in sleep pattern. Risk factors for developing depression in pregnancy include a prior history in self or family, a lack of social support, stressful life events, partner discord, and history of premenstrual syndrome (PMS).

Collaborative Care

Medical management of depression is usually a combination of antidepressants and cognitive-behavioral or interpersonal psychotherapy. Self-help strategies such as exercise, respite from caregiving, self-help groups, and making time for self can be helpful (Fishel, 1999). Nursing strategies include educating the woman about depression as an illness, about treatment success, and about antidepressant medications. For the woman who refuses medications during pregnancy, the nurse should discuss alternative treatments and respect her choice. The nurse also can be effective by maintaining a caring relationship, which includes being hopeful. The nurse can ask about a time when the woman was coping well and how she was able to combat the depression then.

If a woman becomes psychotic during pregnancy, usually because she has quit taking mood stabilizers or antipsychotics, or because she has a history of schizophrenia, this is a medical emergency. To treat a psychotic state, antipsychotic medication or electroconvulsive therapy is preferable to lithium or anticonvulsant medications (Kaplan & Sadock, 2000).

Antidepressant Medications. No consensus exists about safety in the use of antidepressant medications with pregnant women. To date, the U.S. Food and Drug Administration (FDA) has not approved any psychotropic medication for use during pregnancy. Because the majority of women are not aware of their pregnancy until at least 6 weeks of gestation, psychotropic medications may be discontinued after the period of greatest potential risk to the fetus has passed (Stowe et al., 2001). For women with severe depression who would be at risk of suicide without medication, clinical judgment usually dictates continued use of antidepressants. The commonly used antidepressant drugs are often divided into four groups: selective serotonin reuptake inhibitors (SSRIs), heterocyclics (including tricyclic antidepressants [TCAs]), monoamine oxidase inhibitors (MAOIs), and other antidepressant agents not in these classifications (Keltner & Folks, 2001) (Box 35-1).

None of these medications is rated as an FDA category A drug (controlled studies show no risk to the fetus). The only ones classified as category B (no evidence of risk in humans) are maprotiline (Ludiomil) and bupropion (Wellbutrin). Amitriptyline (Elavil), imipramine (Tofranil), and nortriptyline (Pamelor/Aventyl) are classified as D (positive evidence of risk to the fetus, but potential benefits may outweigh risk). The remaining antidepressant medications are rated as category C (risk cannot be ruled out, but potential benefits may justify potential risk).

Many scientists are reluctant to do research on the effects of psychotropic medications on fetuses. In a landmark study, Nulman (1997) reported that in utero exposure to fluoxetine or TCAs did not affect either neurodevelopment or behavior in preschool-age children. TCA dosage for women with depression during pregnancy may need to be increased over the course of pregnancy to maintain adequate therapeutic serum concentrations and response (Stowe et al., 2001). Kulin and others (1998) reported that fluvoxamine, paroxetine, and sertraline do not appear to increase the teratogenic risk when used in correct doses.

The SSRIs are prescribed more frequently today than other groups of antidepressant medications. They are relatively safe and carry fewer side effects than the TCAs. However, if an SSRI is taken with dextromethorphan, an agent found in cough syrup, the combination could trigger the serotonin syndrome (mental status changes, agitation, hyperreflexia, shivering, diarrhea, etc.) (Keltner & Folks, 2001). The most frequent side effects with the SSRIs are gastrointestinal (GI) disturbances (nausea, diarrhea), headache, and insomnia. In about one third of patients, the SSRIs reduce libido, arousal, or orgasmic function. SSRIs also can inhibit specific P-450 isoenzymes, resulting in marked elevations in drug concentrations and reduction in drug clearance.

The TCAs cause many central nervous system (CNS) and peripheral nervous system (PNS) side effects. Although some are simply annoying, others are significant or even dangerous (Keltner & Folks, 2001). In overdose, these

BOX 35-1 Antidepressant Medications

SELECTIVE SEROTONIN REUPTAKE INHIBITORS
Citalopram (Celexa)
Fluoxetine (Prozac)
Fluvoxamine (Luvox)
Paroxetine (Paxil)
Sertraline (Zoloft)

TRICYCLICS
Amitriptyline (Elavil)
Amoxapine (Asendin)
Clomipramine (Anafranil)
Desipramine (Norpramin)
Doxepin (Sinequan)
Imipramine (Tofranil)
Nortriptyline (Pamelor)
Protriptyline (Vivactil)

QUADRICYCLICS
Maprotiline (Ludiomil)
Mirtazepine (Remeron)

MONOAMINE OXIDASE INHIBITORS
Phenelzine (Nardil)
Tranylcypromine (Parnate)

OTHER AGENTS
Bupropion (Wellbutrin) IR & SR
Nefazodone (Serzone)
Trazodone (Desyrel)
Venlafaxine (Effexor)

medications can cause death. A common CNS effect is sedation, and this could easily interfere with mothers caring for their babies. A mother could doze off while holding the baby and drop him or her, or she could have trouble becoming fully awake during the night to care for the baby. Other side effects include weight gain, tremors, grand mal seizures, nightmares, agitation or mania, and extrapyramidal side effects. Anticholinergic side effects include dry mouth, blurred vision (usually temporary), difficulty voiding, constipation, sweating, and orgasm difficulty (Keltner & Folks, 2001).

The lack of research data on the use of MAOIs during pregnancy along with the dietary constraints and potential for hypertensive crisis generally discourage their use during pregnancy (Stowe et al., 2001).

Anxiety Disorders

Anxiety disorders are the most common mental disorder. They include phobias (irrational fears that lead a person to avoid common objects, events, or situations), panic disorder (repeated, unprovoked episodes of intense fear, which develop without warning and are not related to any specific event), generalized anxiety disorder (constant worry unrelated to any event), OCD, and posttraumatic stress disorder (APA, 2000).

OCD symptoms include recurrent, persistent, and intrusive thoughts that cause anxiety, which a person tries to control by performing repetitive behaviors or "compulsions" (APA, 2000). The pregnant woman may have persistent thoughts that something is wrong with the baby, or she may become very preoccupied with checking and rechecking to make sure the baby is all right. Although she recognizes that these rituals are excessive, she will still perform them because of the fear that harm will come to her or the baby if she does not. Treatment usually includes antidepressant medication such as fluvoxamine (Luvox), cognitive-behavioral therapy, and education about the illness and how to manage the symptoms (Fishel, 1998).

Posttraumatic stress disorder (PTSD) can occur as a result of rape (see Chapter 6). Symptoms include reexperiencing the traumatic event, persistent avoidance of stimuli, and numbing, as well as difficulty sleeping, irritability or angry outbursts, difficulty concentrating, hypervigilance, and exaggerated startle response (APA, 2000). Nurses can support the healing process of persons with PTSD by being alert to what the woman is experiencing during pregnancy and labor (Clark, 1997).

If the current pregnancy is a result of rape, the woman may be extremely ambivalent about the baby. If the rape occurred some time ago, the whole experience of pregnancy with prenatal examinations can trigger memories of the original trauma. She may avoid prenatal examinations because of the anxiety triggered by bodily touch and vaginal examinations. Some pregnant women with PTSD may feel more comfortable with a female nurse midwife or a female physician. Giving birth can trigger memories of being out of control, and she may lose contact with reality. The nurse can verbalize understanding of the anxiety and orient to current reality by saying, "You're having an examination to make sure the baby is okay" or "You're in labor preparing to give birth to your baby. I am your nurse. You're in the hospital. I will stay with you. You are safe here." Treatment usually includes psychotherapy and referral to support groups.

Collaborative Care

Benzodiazepines and antidepressants are the most commonly used drugs for the treatment of anxiety disorders, and benzodiazepines are the most widely prescribed psychotropic medications. Medicaid records revealed that at least 2% of pregnant women received one or more prescriptions for a benzodiazepine (Stowe et al., 2001). Some pregnant women who have been using benzodiazepines for "anxiety," "nervousness," or insomnia may not realize that these medications are teratogenic and that their use during pregnancy is not advised (Kaplan & Sadock, 2000). However, benzodiazepines should not be abruptly discontinued during pregnancy, and they should be tapered sufficiently before the birth to limit neonatal withdrawal syndrome (Stowe et al., 2001). Nurses should educate women about the dangers of benzodiazepines during pregnancy, assess for use during pregnancy, and help pregnant women find other ways to handle their anxiety and insomnia, or refer them to a psychiatrist who specializes in psychiatric disorders in pregnancy. Nursing strategies to reduce anxiety include empowerment through education; sensory interventions such as music therapy and aromatherapy; behavioral interventions such as breathing exercises, progressive muscle relaxation, guided imagery, and medication (Box 35-2); and cognitive strategies such as encouraging positive self-talk and questioning negative thinking (Fishel, 1998).

Medications to Avoid During Pregnancy. If the pregnant woman is receiving pharmacologic treatment, the nurse must make sure that the woman is being followed by a psychiatrist or an advanced practice psychiatric nurse. The basic rule is to avoid administering any medication to

BOX 35-2 Antianxiety Medications

- Alprazolam (Xanax)
- Chlordiazepoxide (Librium)
- Clonazepam (Klonopin)
- Clorazepate (Tranxene)
- Diazepam (Valium)
- Flurazepam (Dalmane)
- Lorazepam (Ativan)
- Midazolam (Versed)
- Temazepam (Restoril)
- Triazolam (Halcion)

a woman who is pregnant, particularly during the first trimester (Kaplan & Sadock, 2000). The administration of psychotherapeutic medications at or near birth may cause a baby to be overly sedated at birth and need a respirator, or to be physically dependent on the drug and to require detoxification and treatment of a withdrawal syndrome.

In addition to the benzodiazepines, all of the commonly used mood-stabilizing medications such as lithium carbonate, carbamazepine (Tegretol), gabapentin (Neurontin), and divalproex sodium (Depakote) appear to carry an increased risk of fetal malformations and a potentially deleterious effect on later cognitive development (Kaplan & Sadock, 2000; Stowe et al., 2001). Lithium administration during pregnancy is associated with an increase in cardiovascular malformations, particularly Ebstein anomaly (Stowe et al., 2001). Mood stabilizers are often taken over their lifetime by women with bipolar disorder. Women should receive prepregnancy counseling, and those with a single manic episode should have medication tapered gradually and an attempt at lithium-free pregnancy, or, if indicated, reinstitution of lithium after the first trimester. It is recommended that the clinician offer a fetal echocardiogram between weeks 16 and 18 of gestation for women who were treated with lithium during their first trimester of pregnancy (Stowe et al., 2001).

SUBSTANCE ABUSE DURING PREGNANCY

The damaging effects of alcohol and illicit drugs on pregnant women and their unborn babies are well documented (National Women's Health Resource Center, 1998). Alcohol and other drugs easily pass from a mother to her baby through the placenta. Smoking during pregnancy has serious health risks, including bleeding complications, miscarriage, stillbirth, prematurity, low birth weight, and sudden infant death syndrome (National Women's Health Resource Center, 1998). Prenatal exposure to nicotine may lead to dysregulation in neurodevelopment of the child and higher risk for psychiatric problems (Ernst, Moolchan, & Robinson, 2001). Congenital abnormalities have occurred in infants of mothers who have taken drugs (Stuart & Laraia, 2001). The safest pregnancy is one in which the mother is totally drug and alcohol free, with one exception: for pregnant women addicted to heroin, methadone maintenance is safer for the fetus than acute opiate detoxification (Stuart & Laraia, 2001).

Substance abuse refers to the continued use of substances despite related problems in physical, social, or interpersonal areas (APA, 2000). Recurrent abuse results in failure to fulfill major role obligations, and there may be substance-related legal problems. Any use of alcohol or illicit drugs during pregnancy is considered abuse (APA, 2000).

Dual diagnosis is the coexistence of substance abuse and psychiatric disorders within the same person. Approximately 4.7% of the population have a dual diagnosis (Naegle, 1997), but few data exist on the incidence of dual diagnoses in the pregnant, substance-abusing woman. Major depression and anxiety disorders are the psychiatric disorders that commonly occur with substance abuse.

Prevalence

Because many pregnant women are reluctant to reveal their use of substances or to reveal the extent of their use, data on prevalence are highly variable. One study of North Carolina prenatal clients reported that before pregnancy, 62% of the women had used one or more substances (cigarettes, alcohol, or illegal drugs); and during pregnancy, 31% had used one or more substances. This study is significant in that half of the women stopped using during their pregnancy (Finkelstein, 1999). The 1997 Household Survey revealed that 14% of pregnant women reported that they drank some alcohol, 1.3% engaged in binge drinking, 2.5% used some kind of illicit drug, 1.5% used marijuana, 0.2% used cocaine or crack, and 0.2% used heroin (Substance Abuse and Mental Health Services Administration, 1998). Although tobacco and alcohol were the substances of choice for pregnant women, public opinion seems to view illicit drugs as the bigger problem.

Risk Factors

Women have a clearer pattern of self-medication and are more likely than men to use a combination of alcohol and prescription drugs. Women begin to use after depression, to relax on dates, to feel more adequate, to lose weight, to decrease stress, or to help them sleep at night (National Women's Health Resource Center, 1998). Poor self-esteem is a major issue for most women with problems with drugs and alcohol. A history of psychiatric illness or a history of physical or sexual abuse greatly increases a woman's risk for developing substance-abuse problems (National Women's Health Resource Center, 1998). Both before and during pregnancy, victims of violence were significantly more likely to use multiple substances than were nonvictims. Continuation of substance use during pregnancy was significantly more likely among victims of violence than among nonvictims.

Barriers to Treatment

Fewer than 10% of pregnant women who are substance abusers receive treatment for their addictions. Women often do not seek help because of the fear of losing custody of the child or criminal prosecution (Corrarino et al., 2000). Pregnant women who abuse substances commonly have little understanding of the ways in which these substances affect them, their pregnancies, or their babies. Pregnant women who are substance abusers may not seek prenatal care until labor begins. Often, pregnant women who use psychoactive substances receive negative feedback from society, as well as from health care providers, who not only may condemn them for endangering the life of their fetus, but also may even withhold support as a result

(Selleck & Redding, 1998). Barriers within the drug treatment system may deter these women as well. Traditionally, substance-abuse treatment programs have not addressed issues that affect pregnant women, such as concurrent need for obstetric care and child care for other children; the long waiting lists and lack of health insurance present further barriers to treatment (Corrarino et al., 2000).

Legal Considerations

Because of the risks to the unborn children, pregnant women who abuse substances may now face criminal charges under expanded interpretations of child abuse and drug trafficking statutes. At least 24 states have attempted to prosecute a pregnant woman on a variety of charges for suspected harm to the fetus (Tillett & Osborne, 2001). Some policymakers have proposed that pregnant women who abuse substances should be jailed, placed under house arrest, or committed to psychiatric hospitals for the remainder of their pregnancies (Stuart & Laraia, 2001). In a survey of obstetricians, pediatricians, and family practice physicians in Michigan, 82% to 83% were in favor of compulsory treatment for illicit drug and alcohol use during pregnancy but opposed to criminal prosecution (Abel & Kruger, 2002). Nurses who screen for substance abuse in pregnancy and encourage prenatal care, counseling, and treatment will be of greater benefit to the mother and child than will prosecution (Foley, 2002).

LEGAL TIP Drug Testing During Pregnancy

There is no requirement the United States for a health care provider to test either the pregnant woman or the newborn for the presence of drugs. However, nurses need to know the practices of the states in which they are working. In some states, a woman whose urine drug screen test is positive at the time of labor and birth must be referred to child protective services. If the mother is not in a drug treatment program or is judged unable to provide care, the infant may be placed in foster care. In all states, the U. S. Supreme Court has ruled that it is unlawful to test for drug use without the pregnant woman's permission (Gottlieb, 2001).

Cigarette Smoking and Caffeine Consumption

Cigarettes and caffeine are two examples of legal substances that can be addicting or harmful to the pregnant woman and her fetus and the newborn. Effects of nicotine and caffeine on the fetus and newborn are discussed in Chapter 38.

Cigarette smoking is a major preventable cause of death and illness. Smoking is linked to cardiovascular heart disease, various types of cancers (especially lung and cervical), chronic lung disease, and negative pregnancy outcomes. Tobacco contains nicotine, which is an addictive substance that creates a physical and a psychologic dependence. Among adolescents and young adults, more women than men smoke (Grimes, 1998). Cigarette smoking impairs fertility in both women and men, may reduce the age for menopause, and increases the risk for osteoporosis after menopause. Passive or secondhand smoke contains similar hazards and presents additional problems for the smoker, as well as harm for the nonsmoker (Lee, 1998).

Smoking in pregnancy is known to cause a decrease in placental perfusion and is the cause of low birth weight (ACOG, 1997; Behrman & Shiono, 2002). The harmful effects of smoking are numerous because the oxygen-carrying capacity of hemoglobin is decreased when carbon monoxide passes through the placenta. Furthermore, nicotine causes vasoconstriction, and smokers generally have a nutrient-poor diet. Finally, smoking interferes with the body's ability to process essential vitamins and minerals, resulting in calcium loss from the bones, a decreased intestinal synthesis of vitamin B_{12}, and increased use of vitamin C. The woman who smokes during pregnancy is at risk for a variety of complications including ectopic pregnancy, miscarriage, premature rupture of membranes, preterm birth, placenta previa, abruptio placentae, and chorioamnionitis (ACOG, 1997; Lee, 1998).

Caffeine is found in society's most popular drinks: coffee, tea, and soft drinks. It is a stimulant that can affect mood and interrupt body functions by producing anxiety and sleep interruptions. Heart arrhythmias may be made worse by caffeine, and there can be interactions with certain medications such as lithium. Birth defects have not been related to caffeine consumption; however, high intake has been related to a slight decrease in birth weight and may also increase the risk of miscarriage (Cnattingius et al., 2000). The U.S. FDA recommends that pregnant women eliminate or limit their consumption of caffeine to less than 300 mg per day (3 cups of coffee or cola).

Alcohol

Prenatal alcohol exposure is the single greatest preventable cause of mental retardation (National Women's Health Resource Center, 1998). Fourteen percent to 20% of pregnant women report drinking alcohol sometime in pregnancy, with about 0.2% reporting heavy drinking (Morse & Hutchins, 2000). A 2010 national health objective is to have 94% of pregnant women abstain from alcohol use (USDHHS, 2000).

One of the greatest risks of alcohol use during pregnancy is fetal alcohol syndrome (FAS), as well as fetal alcohol effects (FAE). Low birth weight, mental retardation, behavioral problems, and learning and physical problems are some of the symptoms of FAS babies (see Chapter 38). Severe facial deformities of FAS occur at day 20 of conception–a time when women may not even suspect they are pregnant. Alcohol use during pregnancy can cause high blood pressure, miscarriage, premature birth, stillbirth, and anemia (National Women's Health Resource Center, 1998). In addition, women may experience nutritional deficiencies, pancreatitis, alcoholic hepatitis, deficient milk ejection, and cirrhosis (Cunningham et al., 2001).

Accurate data about alcohol abuse are difficult to obtain because alcohol is rapidly absorbed in the small intestine and metabolized in the liver, so it is difficult to test for its presence in blood. The underdiagnosing and underreporting of alcohol use in pregnancy is a major concern of health care providers (Hankin, McCaul, & Heussner, 2000).

Symptoms occurring during alcohol withdrawal can be managed with short-acting barbiturates or benzodiazepines; however, they are potentially teratogenic. Some clinicians recommend avoiding their use if at all possible. Disulfiram (Antabuse), a medication that acts as a deterrent to alcohol ingestion because it produces a dramatic, unpleasant reaction when small amounts of alcohol are consumed, is contraindicated during pregnancy because it is teratogenic (Woods, 1998). Two medications, naltrexone and acamprosate, have proven efficacious for decreasing alcohol intake; however, they have not been tested in pregnant women and therefore should be avoided (Keltner & Folks, 2001).

Marijuana

Marijuana is a substance derived from the cannabis plant. It is usually rolled into a cigarette and smoked, but it also may be mixed into food and eaten. Marijuana produces an altered state of awareness, relaxation, mild euphoria, and reduced inhibition (Stuart & Laraia, 2001). Prolonged use may lead to apathy, lack of energy, loss of desire to work or be productive, diminished concentration, poor personal hygiene, and preoccupation with marijuana–the amotivational syndrome (Stuart & Laraia, 2001). Marijuana readily crosses the placenta and causes increased carbon monoxide levels in the mother's blood, which reduces the oxygen supply to the fetus. Research findings regarding the effects of marijuana on pregnancy are inconsistent; however, it may cause fetal abnormalities (Stuart & Laraia, 2001).

Cocaine

Cocaine is a powerful CNS stimulant that blocks the reuptake of norepinephrine and dopamine at the nerve endings. Because more neurotransmitter is present at the synapse, the receptors are continuously activated. It is believed that this causes the euphoria. At the same time, presynaptic supplies of dopamine and norepinephrine are depleted. This causes the "crash" that happens when the effect of the drug wears off (Stuart & Laraia, 2001). The euphoria caused by cocaine is short acting, starting with a 10- to 20-second rush and followed by 15 to 20 minutes of less intense euphoria (Stuart & Laraia, 2001). A person who is high on cocaine feels euphoric, energetic, self-confident, and sociable. The relapse rate for clients who try to discontinue cocaine use is very high (Stuart & Laraia, 2001).

The smokable form of cocaine is produced by a process called freebasing. Crack is cocaine mixed with baking soda and heated until it reaches its purest form. It is sold in the form of "rocks," which are smoked in pipes. Crack is used by people from all cultures, and the low cost and availability make it the drug of choice among the economically disadvantaged. Because crack is highly addictive, it poses management problems for health care providers who care for pregnant addicts.

Predisposing factors and problems associated with cocaine use in pregnancy are polydrug use, poor nutrition, poverty, sexually transmitted infections, hepatitis B infection, dysfunctional family systems, employment difficulties, stress, anger, poor self-esteem, and previous or present physical, emotional, and sexual abuse (Woods, 1998). The clinical manifestations of cocaine use include tachycardia, pupillary dilation, and hypertension.

Medical complications of cocaine use in pregnancy range from mild to severe. Some of the less serious medical problems are lack of energy, insomnia, sinusitis, nosebleeds, sore throat, and decreased libido. More serious problems develop as the person's general health deteriorates. These include perforation of the nasal septum, increased cardiovascular stress, tachycardia, systemic hypertension, ventricular dysrhythmias, sudden coronary artery spasm, and myocardial infarction. Cocaine-associated complications also include liver damage, intestinal ischemia, pulmonary disease with acute pulmonary edema, seizures, hemorrhagic bronchitis, headache, and death. Needle-borne diseases such as hepatitis B and acquired immunodeficiency syndrome (AIDS) are common among cocaine users. Needle tracks, septic phlebitis, cellulitis, and superficial abscesses are seen in intravenous drug users. The tachycardia and subsequent increase in blood pressure is caused by the increasing levels of catecholamines produced by the cocaine. During pregnancy, uterine blood vessels are normally maximally dilated, but they vasoconstrict in the presence of catecholamines. The separation of the placenta (abruption) or the acute onset of preterm labor with long, hard contractions and precipitate birth seen in pregnant women after the intravenous administration of cocaine probably is secondary to acute spasm of uterine blood vessels. Maternal cocaine use also has been identified as a risk factor for abdominal pregnancy (Audain et al., 1999).

With consequences such as these, one wonders why pregnant women use cocaine. To begin to answer this question, a nurse researcher interviewed 60 women who reported using crack cocaine at least once a week during pregnancy (Kearney, 1997). A basic social psychologic process, "salvaging self," was identified. Threats that the pregnancy created led the women to delay acknowledging their pregnancies. As pregnancy progressed, women felt guilt, fear, and the need to take action. They used "facing the situation" and "evading harm" to salvage themselves and "maximize well-being" within their social worlds. They tried to reduce harm and manage stigma to decrease damage to the fetus and to their identities.

One of the newer and promising treatments for cocaine abuse in pregnancy is acupuncture. A component of traditional Chinese medicine, acupuncture is used to redirect energy flow (*chi*) within the body, reduce cravings, and enhance well-being. The pace and location of the flow of *chi* can be influenced by the insertion of needles at certain points along the meridians to facilitate harmony (Bennett, 1995). Evidence from controlled studies of the effectiveness of acupuncture alone or in combination with other therapies has been inconsistent (Avants et al., 2000; Margolin et al., 2002). Further investigation of this therapy is needed.

Opiates

The opiates include opium, heroin, meperidine, morphine, codeine, and methadone. Methadone is used to treat addiction to other opiates. It can be used either to aid withdrawal or to provide maintenance at a stable dose. Women taking methadone may work and live normally, although still addicted to narcotics. Heroin is one of the most commonly abused drugs of this class. It is usually taken by intravenous injection but can be smoked or "snorted." The signs and symptoms of heroin use are euphoria, relaxation, relief from pain, "nodding out" (apathy, detachment from reality, impaired judgment, and drowsiness), constricted pupils, nausea, constipation, slurred speech, and respiratory depression (APA, 2000).

The incidence of heroin use among pregnant women is unknown; however, those women with a dependency on heroin may use multiple drugs. Possible effects on pregnancy include preeclampsia, intrauterine growth restriction, miscarriage, premature rupture of membranes, infections, breech presentation, and preterm labor. Possible effects on the mother include poor nourishment with vitamin, iron, and folic acid deficiencies; medical complications from frequent use of dirty needles; sexually transmitted infections; and hypertension (Stuart & Laraia, 2001).

The recommended treatment is methadone maintenance combined with psychotherapy. This well-documented approach improves outcomes for both the woman and her fetus (Wang, 1999). The other approach is slow medical withdrawal with methadone, but the safety of this second approach is questionable (Hulse & O'Neill, 2001). In pregnancy, methadone is metabolized more rapidly, leading to withdrawal symptoms in less than 24 hours in many women. Withdrawal symptoms can include fetal hyperactivity and, if severe, preterm labor or fetal death. Women may resort to heroin to alleviate these uncomfortable symptoms. Doses of methadone that increase during the course of pregnancy and are delivered in split doses (morning and evening) are most effective in preventing withdrawal and subsequent heroin use (Kearney, 1997).

Methamphetamine

The active metabolite of methamphetamine is amphetamine, a CNS stimulant known as "speed" and "meth." Agents used as appetite suppressants or diet pills are closely related substances. The crystalline form of methamphetamine is known as "ice." When smoked, it produces a long, steady high and is more addictive than heroin. Ice enables a person to go without rest or food for 24 hours, only to "crash" for the next 24 hours.

Approximately 2% of the adult population has used methamphetamine at some time during their lives (APA, 2000). It is used by people from all levels of society, but its use is most common in the 18- to 30-year-old age group.

Clinical manifestations of methamphetamine use are euphoria, abrupt awakening, increased energy, talkativeness, agitation, tachycardia, tachypnea, hyperactivity, irritability, grandiosity, diaphoresis, weight loss, insomnia, hypertension, increased temperature, ectopic heartbeat, urinary retention, constipation, dry mouth, paranoid delusions, and violent behavior. Seizures, cardiac shock, and death may occur as a result of overdose (Stuart & Laraia, 2001). Most of the effects of amphetamines are similar to those of cocaine.

Although fewer maternal and neonatal complications have been attributed to this class of substances than to cocaine (APA, 2000), the rates of preterm births and of intrauterine growth restriction with smaller head circumference are higher in methamphetamine-exposed pregnant women than in pregnant women who abuse other substances.

Phencyclidine

Phencyclidine (PCP) is a synthetic drug known by various names (peace pill, elephant, angel dust, hog). Its use is more prevalent among ethnic minorities and in people between the ages of 18 and 40 years. Its effects are unpredictable and include hostility, aggressiveness, and other bizarre behavior (Stuart & Laraia, 2001). Signs and symptoms of PCP use include confusion, disorientation, euphoria, hallucinations, paranoia, grandiosity, agitation, a tendency toward violence, and antisocial behavior, but the severity of these symptoms depends on the dose. Clinical manifestations include red, dry skin; dilated pupils; nystagmus; ataxia; hypertension; rigidity; and seizures (Stuart & Laraia, 2001). Because some effects mimic the signs and symptoms of schizophrenia, a user may be admitted to a psychiatric unit.

After use, PCP persists in the brain and body fat for an extended period. In pregnant women, it crosses the placenta, and its concentration in fetal tissue tends to be higher than that in maternal tissue. However, an appreciation of the specific effects of PCP on pregnancy, the fetus, and the neonate has been limited by the fact that it tends to be used in various combinations with alcohol, cocaine, and marijuana. The major concerns regarding PCP use in pregnant women are its association with polydrug abuse and the neurobehavioral effects on the neonate (Woods, 1998). See Table 35-1 for psychologic and physiologic effects of selected illicit drugs.

TABLE 35-1 **Psychoactive Substance Effects**

DRUG	PSYCHOLOGIC SIGNS	PHYSIOLOGIC SIGNS
Alcohol		
Intoxication	Labile mood	Slurred speech
	Impaired attention	Flushed face
	Irritability	Unsteady gait
	Talkativeness	Nystagmus
Withdrawal	Anxiety	Nausea and vomiting
	Depressed mood	Malaise or weakness
	Maladaptive behavior	Hyperactivity
		Coarse tremor of hands, tongue, eyelids
		Orthostatic hypertension
Cocaine		
Intoxication	Psychomotor agitation	Tachycardia
	Elation	Pupillary dilation
	Grandiosity	Hypertension
	Hypervigilance	Perspiration, chills
	Maladaptive behaviors	Nausea; vomiting
Withdrawal	Depressed mood	Fatigue
	Disturbed sleep	Headache
	Increased dreaming	Convulsions
Heroin		
Intoxication	Euphoria	Pupillary constriction
	Psychomotor retardation	Drowsiness
	Apathy	Slurred speech
	Maladaptive behavior	
	Impaired attention	
Withdrawal	Insomnia	Lacrimation
		Rhinorrhea
		Pupillary dilation
		Sweating
		Diarrhea
		Yawning
		Mild hypertension
		Tachycardia
		Fever
Methamphetamine		
Intoxication	Hyperactivity	Tachycardia, palpitations
	Insomnia	Tachypnea
	Restlessness	Nausea, vomiting
	Irritability	Constipation
	Aggressiveness	Impotence
Withdrawal	Depression	Headache
	Increased sleeping	Nausea, vomiting
	Lethargy	Muscle pain
		Weakness
Phencyclidine (PCP)	Euphoria	Vertical or horizontal nystagmus
	Psychomotor agitation	Hypertension
	Increased anxiety	Increased heart rate
	Emotional lability	Numbness
	Grandiosity	Decreased response to pain
	Sensation of slowed time	Ataxia, dysarthria
	Synesthesias	
	Maladaptive behaviors	

CARE MANAGEMENT

Assessment and Nursing Diagnoses

The care of the substance-dependent pregnant woman is based on historical data, symptoms, physical findings, and laboratory results. All pregnant women should be asked screening questions for alcohol and drug abuse in the overall assessment at the first prenatal visit. Any judgmental attitude on the part of the health care provider will be evident to the client and will interfere with the development of trust and with an accurate report of consumption (Morse & Hutchins, 2000). Information about drug use should be obtained by first asking about the woman's intake of over-the-counter and prescribed medications. Next, her use of legal drugs, such as caffeine, nicotine, and alcohol, should be ascertained. Finally, the woman should be questioned about her use of illicit drugs, such as cocaine, heroin, and marijuana. The approximate frequency and amount should be documented for each drug used (Seidel et al., 2003).

A variety of screening tests are available to screen for alcohol abuse. The CAGE Questionnaire (Ewing, 1984) (Box 35-3) and the Brief Michigan Alcoholism Screening Test (MAST) (Pokorny, Miller, & Kaplan, 1972) are two well-known screens for alcohol use that are often administered by the nurse or included in the written previsit questionnaire. The CAGE is the most popular test used in primary care; however, both the CAGE and MAST focus on alcohol dependency and may not be sensitive to detect the levels of drinking that are considered harmful in pregnancy (USDHHS, 1997).

Urine screening for alcohol abuse is unreliable because alcohol is undetectable within a few hours after ingestion. Abnormal liver-function studies can provide diagnostic data about physical effects of alcohol abuse. Urine toxicology testing is often performed to screen for illicit drug use. Drugs may be found in urine days to weeks after ingestion, depending on how quickly they are metabolized and excreted from the body (Gilbert & Harmon, 2003).

In addition to screening for alcohol and drug abuse, the nurse should also screen for physical and sexual abuse and history of psychiatric illness, because these are risk factors in women who abuse substances. Substance-abusing women feel much stigma, shame, and guilt, which leads to denial of the abuse. If the nurse can help reduce those feelings, the woman will be more apt to confide in the nurse, and that is the first step in receiving help. Asking about how their spouses or partners feel about using substances can reveal whether there are family supports or barriers.

Initial and serial ultrasound studies may be performed to determine the gestational age, because amenorrhea, which is common among drug users, precludes dating on the basis of the history of the last menstrual period. Because of concerns about stillbirth and increased frequency of the birth of small-for-gestational-age infants, and the potential for hypoxia, nonstress testing may be performed, at least in the third trimester, in those pregnant women who are known substance abusers (Woods, 1998).

All states mandate that nurses report suspected child abuse or neglect, and these reports must be made in a timely manner and for each separate incident. Nurses who have filed a report with Children's Protective Services because of a mother's perinatal substance abuse have shared feelings of being torn between the mandated reporting law and trying to maintain some connectedness with the mother (Kovalesky & Flagler, 1997). Child custody loss can elicit feelings of grief, anger, or hopelessness in women and can promote or inhibit recovery from their addiction. Recurrent pregnancies in women who have lost custody of one or more children and who are not in recovery also are common. Information about the women's experiences and the various types of out-of-home placements for children can assist nurses in planning interventions that help mothers process their feelings about custody loss (Kovalesky & Flagler, 1997). Nursing diagnoses for the woman who is a substance abuser may include the following:

- *Risk for deficient fluid volume related to*
  - –effects of excessive use of psychoactive drugs
- *Risk for imbalanced nutrition: less than body requirements related to*
  - –effects of excessive use of psychoactive drugs
- *Risk for injury to self, fetus, or newborn related to*
  - –sensory effects of drug
- *Risk for infection related to*
  - –lifestyle
  - –dehydration and malnutrition
  - –method of administration of drug
- *Self-care deficit, bathing or hygiene, related to*
  - –effects of substance used
- *Denial related to*
  - –stigma
  - –shame
  - –guilt
- *Ineffective individual coping related to*
  - –lack of support system
  - –low self-esteem
  - –lack of anger management techniques

BOX 35-3 CAGE Questionnaire

C Have you ever felt you ought to CUT DOWN on your drinking?

A Have people ANNOYED you by criticizing your drinking?

G Have you ever felt bad or GUILTY about your drinking?

E Have you ever had a drink first thing in the morning to steady your nerves or get rid of a hangover? (EYE OPENER)

- *Risk for impaired parent-infant attachment related to*
  -guilt
  -continuance of substance use
- *Risk for violence related to*
  -maintenance of drug habit
  -effects of substance used
  -lifestyle
- *Hopelessness related to*
  -inability to stop using substances
- *Powerlessness related to*
  -lack of resources
  -relationship with abusive partners
- *Risk for suicide related to*
  -depression
  -impulsivity while taking substances

Expected Outcomes of Care

Planning the care for a pregnant woman who is a substance abuser must take into consideration the woman's lifestyle and habits. The ideal long-term outcome would be total abstinence, but the woman may be unable to face that level of commitment at that time. The thought of giving up the substance forever only provokes anxiety. A realistic goal may be to cut down on the use of substances. Short-term outcomes are necessary, and the woman must participate in the formulation of these expected outcomes. The outcomes must be stated as clear behavioral expectations. The expected outcomes may be written as a contract that is then signed by the woman and the nurse, and a copy is given to the woman. Short-term outcomes for the woman and her family may include the following:

- The woman will keep appointments for prenatal and postpartum care for herself and the well-baby care for the infant.
- Fetal effects will be minimized; the baby will be safe.
- The woman's physiologic symptoms will stabilize, and she will be able to care for herself and her infant.
- The woman will develop an attachment to her infant.
- The woman will become involved in a substance abuse treatment program.

Plan of Care and Interventions

An interdisciplinary model is essential when planning the care for women who abuse substances. Major issues that must be addressed in treatment for women that generally are not part of treatment for men are low self-esteem, stigmatization, high probability of sexual abuse and physical abuse, lack of social support, need for social services and child care, need for women's health services, and need for support and education in the mothering role (Kearney, 1997). Drug-free public housing or residential communities may offer an ideal route to stabilization in a safe environment. Treatment must demonstrate cultural sensitivity and responsiveness to recognize ethnicity and culture as an important part of her identity. Other needs of many women include relationship counseling, coping skills training, and vocational and legal assistance (Kearney, 1997).

Women for Sobriety may be a more helpful organization for women than Alcoholics Anonymous or Narcotics Anonymous, which are based on the 12-step program. The emphasis on powerlessness over addiction and avoidance of codependency found in 12-step programs may disempower and isolate women, particularly women of color (Saulnier, 1996). The confrontational techniques of the 12-step program, developed to break down denial in men, may be especially threatening to women, who often feel unworthy and full of shame and guilt.

Pregnancy presents a window of opportunity for motivating women to stop their abuse of substances (Selleck & Redding, 1998), but what specifically can the nurse do?

First, nurses must be knowledgeable about how to screen and identify women who abuse substances while pregnant. They also must maintain a nonjudgmental, nonpunitive attitude. Nurses can advocate for access to woman-centered drug treatment and harm reduction measures to minimize the damage caused by alcohol and drugs (Kearney, 1997) (see Research box). Collaboration with advanced practice psychiatric nurses will enable nurses to deal with their feelings and provide better care for this challenging group of women. Until the nurse can approach the patient with caring and concern, the therapeutic alliance, which is so important for any change to take place, will not occur. The nurse's role is aimed not only at promoting abstinence, but also at providing a caring, nurturing, and empowering environment in which women can rediscover their values and become authentic, independent decision makers (Kearney, 1997).

Second, the nurse should determine the individual's readiness for change. One model for doing this was developed by Prochaska and DiClemente (1992). The five stages of the model illustrate the readiness of women to change. Precontemplation is the earliest stage, in which individuals are unaware, unwilling, or discouraged about changing substance use behavior. They will be least responsive to interventions focused on change activities. First they need to take ownership of the problem. Contemplation involves an active consideration of the prospects of change. They engage in information seeking and begin to reevaluate themselves in light of their substance abuse behavior. Preparation indicates a readiness to change. They intend to change in the near future and have learned valuable lessons from past change attempts and failures. Action involves the overt modification of the problem behavior, and individuals must have the skills to carry out the changes. Maintenance is the final stage, and environmental supports are particularly important here, as well as supportive relationships with health care providers.

When working with pregnant adolescents with addictions, the nurse also must consider their developmental stage. A part of normal adolescence often includes

RESEARCH

Drug Abuse and Maternal-Fetal Attachment

Illicit drug use in pregnancy results in prematurity, low birth weight, or developmental delay, and it requires costly medical and community resources. Maternal-fetal attachment is a cumulative process throughout pregnancy. Many women who abuse drugs have had poor role models and may exhibit disturbed maternal attachment, which could lead to child abuse. Therefore early intervention when the maternal-fetal bond is stressed by drug use is likely to help with adaptation and transition to parenthood and maternal-infant bonding.

To explore maternal-fetal attachment in drug users, nurse researchers interviewed 40 pregnant women who had already felt fetal movement and who had been using illicit drugs during the pregnancy. Their responses were coded and categorized into three themes:

- Cognitive attachment themes included instilling characteristics in the baby based on his or her movement, acknowledging the fetus's individuality and feelings, and comparing the baby's perceived characteristics with partner and family.
- Affective attachment themes included reporting strong affection for the baby, tempered by ambivalence and guilt about the drugs and enjoying and/or being bothered by fetal movement. The women worried about retaining custody of the baby, and they wanted the baby to love them.
- Altruistic attachment themes included enduring normal discomforts of pregnancy, being motivated to improve health through diet and rest, and struggling to stay clean. Women alternated between uncertainty about their baby's health and hope that the baby would be healthy or that the baby's detoxification would be easy even if treatment was needed.

IMPLICATIONS FOR PRACTICE

The single most important intervention for addicted pregnant women is to get them into treatment so they can learn the skills and strategies to resist the emotional pain-drug cycle. Decreasing drug use is likely to improve their long-term health and their chances of being good parents. The nurse can provide them with praise and reinforcement on any positive lifestyle change, with a non-punitive and caring attitude. Prenatal education about fetal movement also may help pregnant drug abusers develop maternal-infant attachment.

Reference: Shieh, C., & Kravitz, M. (2002). Maternal-fetal attachment in pregnant women who use illicit drugs. *Journal of Obstetric, Gynecologic, and Neonatal Nursing, 31*(2), 156-164.

experimenting with drugs or alcohol, so how does the nurse know when alcohol or drug use is a problem? Certain patterns, such as drinking to escape reality or drinking to "get wasted," are more dangerous than others (Bragg, 1997). Drinking alone and being secretive about drugs and alcohol also are unhealthy patterns.

Third, the nurse uses supportive nursing interventions such as mutuality and avoidance of confrontation. In mutuality, the nurse conveys to women drug users that their perspective on their life situation is as valid as that of the nurse. Women should be encouraged to describe their views on the role of drug use in their lives, the degree of impairment they are experiencing, and the feasibility of change at this time (Kearney, 1997). Avoidance of confrontation is important because it can be damaging to the nurse-client relationship. The likely consequences of continued drug use can be presented in a warmly concerned, factual manner rather than as threats.

Fourth, the nurse uses principles of motivational interviewing (Miller & Rollnick, 1991) to effect change. These principles include the following:

- Displaying empathy
- Developing discrepancy between individuals' perceptions of where they are and where they want to be
- Avoiding argumentation
- Rolling with resistance
- Supporting the client's sense of self-efficacy

When problematic drug use is suspected, the nurse might ask in a noncritical way, "Are drugs or alcohol any part of this situation you have been describing?" By asking about the role of drugs in self-medication for stressors, the nurse can help the woman reflect on the degree of the problem and avenues for change. The woman can be helped to express the positive aspects of drug use that lead her to continue using and the harmful consequences that she has observed. She can be asked about times she tried to reduce or quit using her drug of choice. What interfered with her success? What times was she successful? What enabled her to succeed at those times? Praise can be given for being able to be successful at some time and optimism expressed that she can be successful again.

Treatment Programs for Alcohol- and Drug-Dependent Women

National concern regarding the problem of alcohol and drug use during pregnancy has brought to the forefront the lack of treatment programs specifically targeted to pregnant women. Traditional frameworks for substance abuse treatment include the psychodynamic model, cognitive-behavioral model, relapse-prevention model, 12-step self-help model, and medical model with medication treatment (Kearney, 1997). However, programs that provide comprehensive, coordinated, and "holistic" treatment are better able to draw pregnant women into care, as well as provide more effective treatment (Davis, 1997). Any discussion of treatment programs must start with the understanding that substance abuse in women is a complex problem surrounded by multiple individual, familial, and social issues that require many levels of intervention and treatment (Finkelstein, 1994). The powerlessness of the alcoholic condition and the powerlessness of the female condition act on each other, reinforcing the impotence and hopelessness of both, leaving the woman with few resources to regain a grip on her life.

Whereas the treatment approach of male substance abusers tends to be oriented toward the individual, substance-abusing women should be viewed within the context of their relationships to others. Women tend to find satisfaction, pleasure, and a sense of worth if they experience their life activities as arising from and leading back to a sense of connection with others (Finkelstein, 1994). Alcohol- and drug-abusing women experience multiple social and personal disconnections in their lives, and they may turn to alcohol or other drugs to relieve the pain and anxiety caused by these disconnections. Many alcoholic and drug-abusing women are involved in intimate relationships with other substance abusers. Their use is frequently dependent on the initiation, assistance, and encouragement of other people (Finkelstein, 1994). Women who use illicit drugs are likely to be introduced to and supplied with these drugs by men as part of an intimate or sexual relationship. Recognizing the complexities of treating substance-abusing pregnant women may explain why a recent study reported that pregnant women who received the most treatment in a residential/outpatient treatment program had higher birth weight infants than those treated in less intensive programs such as detox only (Daley et al., 2001).

An exciting pilot program (The Perinatal Outreach Project) involving public health nurses reported that outreach services provided to 10 pregnant substance-abusing women resulted in a 90% rate of entry into treatment (Corrarino et al., 2000). During a home visit, the public health nurse conducted a substance use assessment, and the nurse and the woman jointly agreed to a plan of care with an emphasis on the woman's readiness for change. Key elements of the project were the development of a trusting relationship, a nonjudgmental attitude of staff, and the development of a psychologically healthy and focused interpersonal approach. The other essential elements of the project were (Corrarino et al., 2000):

- Assignment of a primary public health nurse with a small caseload
- Flexible home visit plan
- Health education concerning pregnancy-related preventive health care
- Services of substance abuse counselor
- Follow-up at each contact of needs identified
- Referral to community and social services as needed
- Availability of medical social worker for social needs
- Referral to substance abuse treatment when the woman was ready
- Monthly meeting in an interdisciplinary team

Evaluation

Evaluation is difficult in pregnant women with substance abuse problems because the long-range effects cannot be projected. If the goals are realistic and short term, evaluation is easier. Short-term positive achievements are indicators of some success. Complete abstinence from drugs and assumption of mature adult behaviors within a short time are unrealistic. Long-term care is usually necessary (see Plan of Care).

POSTPARTUM PSYCHOLOGIC COMPLICATIONS

Mental health disorders in the postpartum period have implications for the mother, the newborn, and the entire family. Such conditions can interfere with attachment to the newborn and family integration, and some may threaten the safety and well-being of the mother, newborn, and other children. Because birth is usually thought to be a happy event, a new mother's emotional distress may puzzle and immobilize family and friends. When she most needs the caring attention of loved ones, they may either criticize or withdraw because of their anxiety.

Mood Disorders

Mood disorders are the predominant mental health disorder in the postpartum period (APA, 2000). Up to 70% of women experience a mild depression or "baby blues" after the birth of a child; however, functioning of the woman is usually not impaired. Other women can have more serious depressions that can eventually incapacitate them to the point of being unable to care for themselves or their babies. Postpartum depression exerts a moderate to large effect on the interaction of mothers and infants (Beck, 1995a), and disturbances in early mother-infant interactions are found to be predictive of poorer infant cognitive outcome (Murray, Fiori-Crowley, & Hooper, 1996). Nurses are strategically positioned to offer anticipatory guidance, to assess the mental health of new mothers, to offer therapeutic interventions, and to refer when necessary. Failure to do so may result in tragic consequences. In the rarest of cases, a disturbed mother may kill her infant, other family members, or herself.

The Diagnostic and Statistical Manual of Mental Disorders contains the official guidelines for the assessment and diagnosis of psychiatric illness (APA, 2000). However, specific criteria for postpartum depression (PPD) are not listed. Instead, postpartum onset can be specified for any mood disorder either without psychotic features (i.e., PPD) or with psychotic features (i.e., postpartum psychosis) if the onset occurs within 4 weeks of childbirth (APA, 2000).

Etiology and Risk Factors

The cause of PPD may be biologic, psychologic, situational, or multifactorial. Studies of levels of hormones including progesterone, estrogen, prolactin, thyroid, and

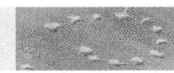

Plan of Care: Substance Abuse During Pregnancy

NURSING DIAGNOSIS Imbalanced nutrition: less than body requirements related to insufficient intake for prenatal metabolic needs as evidenced by insufficient weight gain for gestational age of fetus

Expected Outcome *Client will maintain steady weight gain appropriate for trimester of pregnancy.*

Nursing Interventions/*Rationales*

Compare current client weight to prepregnant weight *to assess if weight is appropriate for trimester of pregnancy.*

Assess client's current diet plan and caloric intake *to identify where modifications are necessary.*

Provide client with information regarding nutritional requirements during pregnancy *to assist client to provide modifications to diet and promote self-care.*

Weigh client frequently *to establish client compliance and effectiveness of plan.*

NURSING DIAGNOSIS Ineffective individual coping related to lack of support system as evidenced by client verbalization of concerns

Expected Outcome *Client will express satisfaction with identified effective coping methods.*

Nursing Interventions/*Rationales*

Remain nonjudgmental while listening to client express feelings and concerns *to promote trust.*

Assist client to identify positive coping methods and strengths *to promote involvement in self-care.*

Encourage client to take responsibility for activities leading to recovery *to promote self-care, self-esteem, and responsibility for self and fetus's well-being.*

Refer to appropriate health professionals and support groups *to promote involvement and responsibility in health and well-being of self and fetus.*

NURSING DIAGNOSIS Risk for delayed fetal growth and development related to maternal substance abuse

Expected Outcome *Fetus will exhibit appropriate growth and development during pregnancy.*

Nursing Interventions/*Rationales*

Provide information to woman regarding effects of substance abuse on fetus *to reinforce correlation.*

Monitor fundal height *to determine fetal growth pattern.*

Assess maternal nutrition and weight gain pattern *to verify potential for fetal growth.*

Monitor fetal assessment testing *to provide data concerning fetal well-being.*

NURSING DIAGNOSIS Situational low self-esteem related to loss of control during pregnancy

Expected Outcome *Woman will identify methods to increase self-esteem.*

Nursing Interventions/*Rationales*

Provide reinforcement for positive actions *to encourage woman to accept praise and continue positive actions throughout the pregnancy.*

Promote the expression of feelings through therapeutic communication *to facilitate ongoing support and trust.*

Discuss with the woman positive past coping mechanisms and experiences *to promote increase in current self-esteem.*

cortisol have been inconclusive (Abou-Saleh et al., 1998). Neurotransmitter deficiencies and psychosocial and marital adjustments in the postpartum period have been related to PPD (APA, 2000; Bergant et al., 1999; Huang & Mathers, 2001; Raskin, 1997). A personal history or a family history of mood disorder, mood and anxiety symptoms in the antepartal period, as well as postpartum blues increases the risk for PPD (APA, 2000). In a meta-analysis of 84 studies published in the 1990s, Beck (2001) found 13 risk factors for postpartum depression, four of which had not been identified previously as predictors. The effect sizes of the risk factors identified in an updated meta-analysis revealed that 10 predictors have a medium relation with postpartum depression, and three predictors have a small relation (Beck, 2002). A revised version of the Postpartum Depression Predictors Inventory has been published (Beck, 2002). Box 35-4 lists all 13 risk factors for PPD, with those having the greater effect size listed first.

In addition, recent research reported that fatigue is an important predictor of PPD (Bozoky & Corwin, 2002). As early as 7 postpartum days, fatigue is predictive of depression at postpartum day 28 (see Research box).

Postpartum Depression Without Psychotic Features

PPD is an intense and pervasive sadness with severe and labile mood swings and is more serious and persistent than postpartum blues. Intense fears, anger, anxiety, and despondency that persist past the baby's first few weeks are not a normal part of postpartum blues. Occurring in approximately 10% to 15% of new mothers, these symptoms rarely disappear without outside help. The majority of these mothers do not seek help from any source, and only about 20% consult a health professional. The occurrence of PPD among teenage mothers was more than 2.5 times that for older mothers (Herrick, 2002). African-American mothers were twice as likely as white mothers to experience PPD. Younger mothers (younger than 20 years) and those with less than a high school education were significantly less likely to seek help and had higher rates of PPD (Herrick, 2002). Mothers who had no one to talk to about their problems after giving birth had a high rate of PPD and low rate of help seeking.

The symptoms of postpartum major depression do not differ from the symptoms of nonpostpartum mood disorders, except that the mother's ruminations of guilt and in-

BOX 35-4 Risk Factors for Postpartum Depression

- Prenatal depression
- Low self-esteem
- Stress of child care
- Prenatal anxiety
- Life stress
- Lack of social support
- Marital relationship problems
- History of depression
- "Difficult" infant temperament
- Postpartum blues
- Single status
- Low socioeconomic status
- Unplanned/unwanted pregnancy

Source: Beck, C. (2002). Revision of the Postpartum Depression Predictors Inventory. *Journal of Obstetric, Gynecologic, and Neonatal Nursing, 31*(4), 394-402; Beck, C. (2001). Predictors of postpartum depression: An update. *Nursing Research, 50*(5), 275-282.

adequacy feed her worries about being an incompetent and inadequate parent. In PPD, there may be odd food cravings (often sweet desserts) and binges with abnormal appetite and weight gain. New mothers report an increased yearning for sleep, sleeping heavily, but awakening instantly with any infant noise, and an inability to go back to sleep after infant feedings.

A distinguishing feature of PPD is irritability. These episodes of irritability may flare up with little provocation, and they may sometimes escalate to violent outbursts or dissolve into uncontrollable sobbing. Many of these outbursts are directed against significant others ("He never helps me") or the baby ("She cries all the time, and I feel like hitting her"). Women with postpartum major depressive episodes often have severe anxiety, panic attacks, and spontaneous crying long after the usual duration of baby blues.

Many women feel especially guilty about having depressive feelings at a time when they believe they should be happy. They may be reluctant to discuss their symptoms or their negative feelings toward the child. A prominent feature of PPD is rejection of the infant, often caused by abnormal jealousy (APA, 2000). The mother may be obsessed by the notion that the offspring may take her place in her partner's affections. Attitudes toward the infant may include disinterest, annoyance with care demands, and blaming because of her lack of maternal feeling. When observed, she may appear awkward in her responses to the baby. Obsessive thoughts about harming the child are very frightening to her. Often she does not share these thoughts because of embarrassment, but when she does, other family members become very frightened.

Medical Management. The natural course is one of gradual improvement over the 6 months after birth. Supportive treatment alone is not efficacious for major postpartum depression. Pharmacologic intervention is needed in most instances. Treatment options include antidepressants, anxiolytic agents, and electroconvulsive therapy. Psychotherapy focuses on her fears and concerns regarding her new responsibilities and roles, as well as monitoring for suicidal or homicidal thoughts. For some women, hospitalization is necessary.

RESEARCH

Fatigue as a Predictor of Postpartum Depression

Women giving birth are expected to adapt without difficulty to changes in lifestyle and relationships, new dependent care demands, and multiple new roles. For many women, this is impossible. Instead, the demands of early infant care frequently result in symptoms of fatigue. The objective of the study was to examine whether and when fatigue in early postpartum is predictive of postpartum depression. A convenience sample of 38 healthy women was recruited from hospital maternity units within 24 hours after an uncomplicated birth. Outcome measures were the Modified Fatigue Symptom Checklist (MFSC) (administered at days 0, 7, 14, and 28 after childbirth) and the Center for Epidemiological Studies Depressive Symptomatology Scale (administered on day 28). After adjustments for multiple comparisons, significant correlations were found between fatigue and postpartum depression on days 7, 14, and 28. A limitation of this study is that the sample is relatively small and homogeneous, consisting mostly of Caucasian, married women. The depression screening tool also was not specific for PPD.

CLINICAL APPLICATION

PPD may hinder a new mother in developing her role. Nurses could use a simple fatigue screening tool such as the MFSC within the first 2 postpartum weeks to identify women who are at risk of later PPD and may greatly improve treatment outcome. Many women who are experiencing PPD do not realize it or do not discuss it with health care providers or family. By the time women return for their 6-week postpartum appointment, depression may be well established and may be overlooked. The earlier PPD is identified, the more effective is the treatment. The nurse could do a telephone screening at day 7 or 14, or the nurse in the pediatric office could do the screening at the 2-week newborn visit.

Source: Bozoky, I., & Corwin, E. (2002). Fatigue as a predictor of postpartum depression. *Journal of Obstetric, Gynecologic, and Neonatal Nursing, 31*(4), 436-443.

Postpartum Depression with Psychotic Features

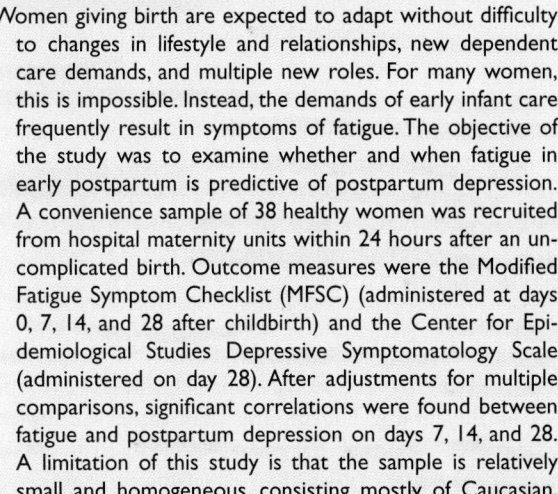

Postpartum psychosis is a syndrome most often characterized by depression (as described previously), delusions, and thoughts by the mother of harming either the infant or herself (Kaplan & Sadock, 2000). A postpartum mood disorder with psychotic features occurs in 1 to 2 per 1000 births and may occur more often in primiparas (Kaplan & Sadock,

2000). Once a woman has had one postpartum episode with psychotic features, there is a 30% to 50% likelihood of recurrence with each subsequent birth (APA, 2000).

Symptoms often begin within days after the birth, although the mean time to onset is 2 to 3 weeks and almost always within 8 weeks of birth (Kaplan & Sadock, 2000). Characteristically, the woman begins to complain of fatigue, insomnia, and restlessness and may have episodes of tearfulness and emotional lability. Complaints regarding the inability to move, stand, or work also are common. Later, suspiciousness, confusion, incoherence, irrational statements, and obsessive concerns about the baby's health and welfare may be present (Kaplan & Sadock, 2000). Delusions may be present in 50% of all women, and hallucinations, in about 25%. Auditory hallucinations that command the mother to kill the infant can also occur in severe cases. When delusions are present, they are often related to the infant. The mother may think the infant is possessed by the devil, has special powers, or is destined for a terrible fate (APA, 2000). Grossly disorganized behavior may be manifested as a disinterest in the infant or an inability to provide care. Some will insist that something is wrong with the baby or accuse nurses or family of hurting or poisoning their child. Nurses are advised to be alert for mothers who are agitated, overactive, confused, complaining, or suspicious.

A specific illness included in depression with psychotic features is bipolar disorder (formerly called manic depressive illness). This mood disorder is preceded or accompanied by manic episodes, characterized by elevated, expansive, or irritable moods. Clinical manifestations of a manic episode include at least three of the following symptoms that have been significantly present for at least 1 week: grandiosity, decreased need for sleep, pressured speech, flight of ideas, distractibility, psychomotor agitation, and excessive involvement in pleasurable activities without regard for negative consequences (APA, 2000). Because these women are hyperactive, they may not take the time to eat or sleep, which leads to inadequate nutrition, dehydration, and sleep deprivation. While in a manic state, mothers will need constant supervision when caring for their infant. Mostly they will be too preoccupied to provide child care.

Medical Management. A favorable outcome is associated with a good premorbid adjustment (before the onset of the disorder) and a supportive family network (Kaplan & Sadock, 2000). Because mood disorders are usually episodic, women may experience another episode of symptoms within a year or two of the birth. Postpartum psychosis is a psychiatric emergency, and the mother will probably need psychiatric hospitalization. Antipsychotics and mood stabilizers such as lithium are the treatments of choice. If the mother is breastfeeding, some sources recommend that no pharmacologic agents should be prescribed (Kaplan & Sadock, 2000), but other sources advise caution while prescribing some agents (Stowe et al., 2001). Antipsychotics and lithium should be avoided in breastfeeding mothers, but other mood stabilizers may be compatible with breastfeeding (see later discussion). It is usually advantageous for the mother to have contact with her baby if she so desires, but visits must be closely supervised. Psychotherapy is indicated after the period of acute psychosis is past.

CARE MANAGEMENT

Even though the prevalence of PPD is fairly well established, women are unlikely to seek help from a mental health care provider. Primary health care providers can usually recognize severe PPD or postpartum psychosis but may miss milder forms; even if it is recognized, the woman may be treated inappropriately or subtherapeutically (Gold, 2002; Straub et al., 1998).

Assessment and Nursing Diagnoses

To recognize symptoms of PPD as early as possible, the nurse should be an active listener and demonstrate a caring attitude (Beck, 1999b). Nurses cannot depend on women volunteering unsolicited information about their depression or asking for help. The nurse should observe for signs of depression and ask appropriate questions to determine moods, appetite, sleep, energy and fatigue levels, and ability to concentrate. Examples of ways to initiate conversation include the following: "Now that you have had your baby, how are things going for you? Have you had to change many things in your life since having the baby?" and "How much time do you spend crying?" If the nurse assesses that the new mother is depressed, she or he must ask if the mother has thought about hurting herself or the baby. The woman may be more willing to answer honestly if the nurse says, "Lots of women feel depressed after having a baby, and some feel so badly that they think about hurting themselves or the baby. Have you had these thoughts?"

Nurses can use screening tools in assessing whether the depressive symptoms have progressed from postpartum blues to PPD. Examples are the Edinburgh Postnatal Depression Scale (EPDS) (Cox, Holden, & Sagovsky, 1989) and the Postpartum Depression Predictors Inventory (PDPI) (Beck, 2002).

The EPDS is a self-report assessment designed specifically to identify women experiencing PPD. It has been used and validated in studies in numerous cultures (Eberhard-Gran et al., 2001) and has even been used to measure depression and anxiety in fathers (partners) (Matthey et al., 2001). The assessment tool asks the woman to respond to 10 statements about the common symptoms of depression. The woman is asked to choose the response that is closest to describing how she has felt for the past week.

Through focused research over at least a decade, Beck (1995a, 1995b, 1998a) continues to refine the Postpartum Depression Checklist (PDC) and the Postpartum Depression Screening Scale (PDSS) (Beck & Gable, 2000, 2001).

The latest revision (PDPI) is a checklist of 13 symptoms of PPD. The published tool is designed to be used by nurses and other health care providers to elicit information from the woman during an interview during pregnancy and continuing in the postpartum period to assess risk (Beck, 2002). Areas assessed include the predictors of depression as listed in Box 35-4.

If the initial interaction with the woman or analysis of her self-report reveals some question that she might be depressed, a formal screening is helpful in determining the urgency of the referral and the type of provider. Also important is the need to assess the woman's family, because they may be able to offer valuable information, as well as need to express how they have been affected by the woman's emotional disorder (Maley, 2002).

Planning is focused on meeting the individualized needs of the family to ensure safety, especially for the mother and infant and any other children, and to facilitate functional family coping. Nursing diagnoses may include the following:

- *Risk for violence toward self (mother) or children related to*
  -postpartum depression
- *Situational low self-esteem in the mother related to*
  -stresses associated with role changes
- *Ineffective family coping related to*
  -increased care needs of mother and infant
- *Risk for impaired parenting related to*
  -inability of depressed mother to attach to infant
- *Risk for injury to newborn related to*
  -mother's depression (inattention to infant's needs for hygiene, nutrition, safety) and psychotropic medications via breast milk

Expected Outcomes of Care

Specific measurable criteria can be developed based on the following general outcomes:

- The mother will no longer be depressed.
- The mother's and infant's physical well-being will be maintained.
- The family will cope effectively.
- Family members will demonstrate continued healthy growth and development.
- The infant will be fully integrated into the family.

Plan of Care and Interventions

On the Postpartum Unit

The postpartum nurse must observe the new mother carefully for any signs of tearfulness and conduct further assessments as necessary. Nurses must discuss PPD to prepare new parents for potential problems in the postpartum period (see Teaching for Self-Care box). The family must be able to recognize the symptoms and know where to go for help. Written materials that explain what the woman can do to prevent depression could be used as part of discharge planning.

TEACHING FOR SELF-CARE

Activities to Prevent Postpartum Depression

- Share knowledge about postpartum emotional problems with close family and friends.
- Take care of yourself: eat a balanced diet, exercise on a regular basis, and get enough sleep. Ask someone to take care of the baby so that you can get a full night's sleep.
- Share your feelings with someone close to you; don't isolate yourself at home with the TV.
- Don't overcommit yourself or feel like you need to be a superwoman.
- Don't place unrealistic expectations on yourself.
- Don't be ashamed of having emotional problems after your baby is born—it happens to approximately 15% of women.

Mothers are often discharged from the hospital before the blues or depression occurs. If the postpartum nurse is concerned about the mother, a mental health consult should be requested before the mother leaves the hospital. Routine instructions regarding PPD should be given to whoever comes to take the woman home; for example, "If you notice that your wife (or daughter) is upset or crying a lot, please call the postpartum care provider immediately—don't wait for the routine postpartum appointment."

NURSE ALERT

Because the newborn may be scheduled for a checkup before the mother's 6-week checkup, nurses in well-baby clinics or pediatrician offices should be alert for signs of PPD in new mothers and be knowledgeable about community referral resources.

In the Home and Community

Postpartum home visits can reduce the incidence of or complications from depression. A brief home visit or phone call at least once a week until the new mother returns for her postpartum visit may save the life of a mother and her infant; however, home visits may not be feasible or available. Supervision of the mother with emotional complications may become a prime concern. Because depression can greatly interfere with her mothering functions, family and friends may need to participate in the infant's care. This is a time for the extended family and friends to determine what they can do to help, and the nurse can work with them to ensure adequate supervision of and their understanding of the woman's mental illness.

When the woman has PPD, a partner often reacts with confusion, shock, denial, and anger and feels neglected and blamed. The nurse can talk with the woman about how her condition is hard for him too and that he is probably very worried about her. Men oftentimes withdraw or criticize when they are deeply worried about their significant others. The nurse can provide nonjudgmental opportunities for the partner to verbalize feelings and concerns, help the partner identify positive coping strategies, and be a source of encouragement for the partner to continue supporting the woman. Both the woman and her partner need an opportunity to express their needs, fears, thoughts, and feelings in a nonjudgmental environment.

Even if the mother is severely depressed, hospitalization can be avoided if adequate resources can be mobilized to ensure safety for both mother and infant. The nurse in home health care will need to make frequent phone calls or home visits to do assessment and counseling. Community resources that may be helpful are temporary child care or foster care, homemaker service, meals on wheels, parenting guidance centers, mother's-day-out programs, and telephone support groups (see Resource list at end of chapter).

Referral. Women with moderate to severe PPD should be referred to a mental health therapist, such as an advanced practice psychiatric nurse, for evaluation and therapy to avoid the effects that PPD can have on the woman and on her relationships with her partner, baby, and other children (Brown, 2001). Inpatient psychiatric hospitalization may be necessary. This decision is made when the safety needs of the mother or children are threatened.

Providing Safety. When depression is suspected, the nurse asks, "Have you thought about hurting yourself?" If delusional thinking about the baby is suspected, the nurse asks, "Have you thought about hurting your baby?" Four criteria measure the seriousness of a suicidal plan: method, availability, specificity, and lethality. Has the woman specified a method? Is the method of choice available? How specific is the plan? If the method is concrete and detailed, with access to it right at hand, the suicide risk increases. How lethal is the method? The most lethal method is shooting, with hanging a close second. The least lethal is slashing one's wrists. Medication overdose with TCAs does cause death. Avoid TCAs in suicidal women because of their danger in overdose.

NURSE ALERT

Suicidal thoughts or attempts are among the most serious symptoms of PPD and require immediate assessment and intervention (Appleby, Mortensen, & Faragher, 1998).

Psychiatric Hospitalization

Women with postpartum psychosis have a psychiatric emergency and must be referred immediately to a psychiatrist who is experienced in working with women with PPD, who can prescribe medication and other forms of therapy, and assess the need for hospitalization.

LEGAL TIP Commitment for Psychiatric Care

If a woman with PPD is experiencing active suicidal ideation or harmful delusions about the baby and is unwilling to seek treatment, legal intervention may be necessary to commit the woman to an inpatient setting for treatment.

Within the hospital setting, the reintroduction of the baby to the mother can occur at the mother's own pace. A schedule is set for increasing the number of hours the mother cares for the baby over several days, culminating in the infant staying overnight in the mother's room. This allows the mother to experience meeting the infant's needs and giving up sleep for the baby, a situation difficult for new mothers even under ideal conditions. The mother's readiness for discharge and caring for the baby is assessed. Her interactions with her baby also are carefully supervised and guided.

Nurses also should observe the mother for signs of bonding with the baby. Attachment behaviors are defined as eye-to-eye contact; physical contact that involves holding, touching, cuddling, and talking to the baby and calling the baby by name; and the initiation of appropriate care. A staff member is assigned to keep the baby in sight at all times. Indirect teaching, praise, and encouragement are designed to bolster the mother's self-esteem and self-confidence.

Psychotropic Medications

PPD is usually treated with antidepressant medications. If the woman with PPD is not breastfeeding, antidepressants can be prescribed without special precautions. In addition to the TCAs and SSRIs discussed previously, MAOIs, mood stabilizers, and antipsychotic medications may be prescribed for nonbreastfeeding women.

Hypertensive crisis is the main reason that MAOIs are not prescribed more frequently. The woman should be taught to watch for signs of hypertensive crisis—throbbing, occipital headache, stiff neck, chills, nausea, flushing, retroorbital pain, apprehension, pallor, sweating, chest pain, and palpitations (Keltner & Folks, 2001). This crisis is brought on by the client taking any of a large variety of over-the-counter medications or eating foods that contain tyramine, a sympathomimetic pressor amine, which normally is broken down by the enzyme monoamine oxidase. The nurse must do extensive teaching about avoidance of foods and medications that contain tyramine.

The woman taking mood stabilizers (Box 35-5) must be taught about the many side effects, and especially, for those taking lithium, the need to have serum lithium levels determined every 6 months. Women with severe psychiatric syndromes such as schizophrenia, bipolar disorder, or psychotic depression will probably require antipsychotic medications (Box 35-6). Most of these antipsychotic medications can cause sedation and orthostatic hypotension—both

BOX 35-5 Mood Stabilizers

Carbamazepine (Tegretol XR)
Clonazepam (Klonopin)
Divalproex (Depakote)
Lithium carbonate (Eskalith)

of which could interfere with the mother being able to care safely for her baby. They also can cause PNS effects such as constipation, dry mouth, blurred vision, tachycardia, urinary retention, weight gain, and agranulocytosis. CNS effects may include akathisia, dystonias, parkinsonism-like symptoms, tardive dyskinesia (irreversible), and neuroleptic malignant syndrome (potentially fatal). Medication education is especially important when caring for women who are taking antipyschotic medications. The nurse should use discretion in selecting the content to be shared because of the women's altered thought processes and the large number of side/toxic effects. The nurse may choose to do more extensive education with a close family member. The newer, atypical antipsychotic medications such as olanzapine, quetiapine, risperidone, and ziprasidone are usually safer and have fewer side effects than the older more traditional antipsychotics; however, their safety in pregnancy has not been established.

Psychotropic Medications and Lactation. A major clinical dilemma is the psychopharmacologic treatment of women with PPD who want to breastfeed their infants. In the past, women were told to discontinue lactation. Today, we know that 5% to 17% of all nursing mothers take a prescription medication (Stowe et al., 2001). The FDA has not approved any psychotropic medication for use during lactation. However, the American Academy of Pediatrics (AAP) has published reports on excretion of medications into human breast milk since 1983. The most current statement is an update of these reports, and the update for psychotropic drugs has been emphasized in this revision (AAP, 2001). Almost all of the psychotropic medications listed in this report are drugs for which the effects on the breastfeeding newborn are "unknown but still may be of concern." The reason for the concern is that although the medications appear to be in low concentrations in breast milk (commonly a milk-to-serum ratio of 0.5 to 1.0), many drugs have a long half-life, and levels may build up in plasma and tissue of nursing infants. Long-term effects on the newborn are unknown (AAP, 2001). Because all psychotropic medications pass through breast milk to the infant, the risks associated with the use of such medication must be weighed against the risks associated with maternal agitation and potentially self-destructive behavior (Wintz, 1999).

Breast milk–excretion studies have demonstrated that antidepressants are present in breast milk, with a milk-to-serum ratio that is typically greater than 1:1 (Stowe et al., 2001) and often in higher concentrations in the fatty hind milk (Newport, Wilcox, & Stowe, 2001). Most TCAs appear to be safe during breastfeeding, with the exception of doxepin, which is associated with respiratory depression (Wisner, Perel, & Findling, 1996). Minimal data are available concerning the SSRIs, so earlier reviews recommended using the secondary amine TCAs. In light of the increasing data on SSRIs, and the lack of adverse reports, these recommendations are likely to be revised (Stowe et al., 2001). MAOIs are usually avoided; no human data have been published on the newer antidepressants.

The elapsed time between maternal dosing and infant feeding has been shown to affect the amount of antidepressant medication to which the nursling is exposed. Amitriptyline, desipramine, and trazodone appear to reach a peak in breast milk at 4 to 6 hours after an oral dose; peak concentrations of sertraline occurred 7 to 10 hours after the maternal dose (Stowe et al., 2001). Adjusting both the schedule of dosing of the antidepressant and the infant's feeding schedule may considerably reduce the concentration of the drug to which the infant is exposed. In addition, discarding one daily feeding with the highest concentrations may be necessary (Stowe et al., 2001). Most of the drugs listed in Boxes 35-5 and 35-6 are classified as drugs whose effects on infants are unknown but may be of concern.

Antipsychotic medications are excreted into breast milk. None of these medications has been proven safe during lactation; the AAP does not rate any of the antipsychotic medications as compatible with breastfeeding because the Committee on Drugs found no reports in the literature (AAP, 2000).

Benzodiazepines at relatively low doses present no contraindications to nursing (Stowe et al., 2001). In contrast to other classes of psychotropic medications, benzodiazepines appear to have lower milk-to-maternal serum ratios.

Mood-stabilizing medications are present in breast milk. Lithium is usually not given to breastfeeding women because nursing infants can achieve serum lithium concentrations that are 40% to 50% of maternal levels (Stowe et al., 2001). Both carbamazepine and valproic acid appear in low concentrations in human milk, and both are considered compatible with breastfeeding (Stowe et al., 2001).

BOX 35-6 **Commonly Used Antipsychotic Medications**

PHENOTHIAZINES
- Chlorpromazine (Thorazine)
- Fluphenazine (Prolixin)
- Perphenazine (Trilafon)
- Thioridazine (Mellaril)
- Trifluoperazine (Stelazine)

OTHER
- Clozapine (Clozaril)
- Haloperidol (Haldol)
- Loxapine (Loxitane)
- Olanzapine (Zyprexa)
- Pimozide (Orap)
- Quetiapine (Seroquel)
- Risperidone (Risperdal)
- Thiothixene (Navane)
- Ziprasidone (Geodon)

The benefits of breastfeeding and the potential risks must be carefully considered before using lithium and other mood stabilizers.

In summary, all psychotropic medications studied to date are excreted in breast milk. The adverse effects of psychotropic agents on infants are limited to case reports. The nursing infant's daily dose of psychotropic agents is less than the maternal daily dose. Psychotropic medications are excreted into breast milk with a specific individual time course, allowing the minimization of infant exposure with continuation of breastfeeding. The long-term neurobehavioral effects of infant exposure to psychotropic medications through breastfeeding are unknown. When selecting psychotropic medications for breastfeeding women, choose those with greatest documentation of prior use, lower FDA risk category, few or no metabolites, and fewer side effects (Stowe et al., 2001).

Nursing Implications. When breastfeeding women have emotional complications and need psychotropic medications, referral to a mental health care provider who specializes in postpartum disorders is preferred. Depressed women will need the nurse to reinforce the need to take antidepressants as ordered. Because antidepressants do not exert any effect for about 2 weeks and usually do not reach full effect for 4 to 6 weeks, many women discontinue taking the medication on their own. Client and family teaching should reinforce the schedule for taking medications in conjunction with the infant's feeding schedule and to continue taking the medication until therapeutic effects occur.

Other Treatments for PPD

Other treatments for PPD include complementary/alternative therapies such as those listed in Box 35-7, electroconvulsive therapy (ECT), and psychotherapy. Alternative therapies may be used alone but often are used with other treatments for PPD. Safety and efficacy studies of these alternative therapies are needed to ensure that care and advice is based on evidence (Tiran & Mack, 2000).

NURSE ALERT

St. John's wort is often used to treat depression. It has not been proven safe for women who are breastfeeding.

ECT may be used for women with PPD who have not improved with antidepressant therapy. Psychotherapy in the form of group therapy or individual (interpersonal) therapy also has been used with positive results alone and in conjunction with antidepressant therapy (Beck, 1999a); however, more studies are needed to determine what types of professional support are most effective (Ray & Hodnett, 2001).

Evaluation

The nurse can be assured that care has been effective if the physical well-being of the mother and infant is maintained, the mother and family are able to cope effectively, and each family member continues to show a healthy adaptation to the presence of the new member of the family (see Plan of Care).

Postpartum Onset of Panic Disorder

Little is known about the risk for and course of panic disorder in the postpartum period. Hertzberg and Wahlbeck (1999) reviewed eight studies of pregnant and postpartum women with panic disorder and could not make any definite conclusion about effects of pregnancy or the postpartum period on panic disorder. In approximately 3% to 5% of women, panic disorder or OCD develops in the postpartum period. Panic attacks are discrete periods in which there is the sudden onset of intense apprehension, fearfulness, or terror (APA, 2000). During these attacks, symptoms such as shortness of breath, palpitations, chest pain, choking, smothering sensations, and fear of losing control are present. Women have reported having intrusive thoughts about terrible injury done to the infant, such as stabbing or burns, sometimes by themselves. Rarely do the women harm the baby. Nurses need only to listen to the mother to hear symptoms of panic disorder. Usually these women are so distraught that they will share with whomever will listen. Oftentimes the family has tried to tell them that what they are experiencing is normal, but they know differently. Potential nursing diagnoses for women experiencing postpartum panic disorder include the following:

- *Anxiety related to*
  –postpartum adaptations and expectations
- *Fear of harming others related to*
  –obsessions
- *Powerlessness related to*
  –feelings of losing control
- *Deficient knowledge related to*
  –postpartum mental health problems

BOX 35-7 Possible Alternative/Complementary Therapies for Postpartum Depression

Acupuncture
Acupressure
Aromatherapy
 Jasmine
 Ylang Ylang
 Rose
Herbal
 Lavender tea
Healing touch/Therapeutic touch
Massage
Relaxation techniques
Reflexology
Yoga

Source: Tiran, D., & Mack, S. (Eds.). (2000). *Complementary therapies for pregnancy and childbirth* (2nd ed.). Edinburgh: Bailliere Tindall.

Medical Management

Treatment is usually a combination of medications, education, psychotherapy, and cognitive behavioral interventions, along with an attempt to identify any medical or physiologic contributors. Antidepressants such as SSRIs may be prescribed (Brown, 2001), and sertraline (Zoloft) and paroxetine (Paxil) are approved in the United States for the treatment of panic disorder; fluvoxamine (Luvox) may be especially helpful with obsessions (Keltner & Folks, 2001).

Nursing Considerations

The following nursing interventions are suggested.

- Education is a crucial nursing intervention. New mothers should be provided with anticipatory guidance concerning the possibility of panic attacks during the postpartum period. Preparing for the attacks may help decrease their unexpected, terrifying nature (Beck, 1998b).
- Empowerment conveys to the woman that she can sort through her fears and expectations and take charge of her life. Women can be reassured that it is common to feel a sense of impending doom and fear of insanity during panic attacks. These fears are temporary and disappear once the panic attack is over (Beck, 1998b).
- Nurses can help women identify panic triggers that are particular to their own lives. Keeping a diary can help identify the triggers (Beck, 1998b).
- Family and social supports are helpful. The new mother is encouraged to put usual chores on hold and to ask for and accept help.
- Support groups allow these mothers to feel comfort in seeing others like themselves.
- Sensory interventions such as music therapy and aromatherapy are nonintrusive and inexpensive.
- Behavioral interventions such as breathing exercises and progressive muscle relaxation can be helpful (Fishel, 1998).
- Cognitive interventions such as positive self-talk training, reframing and redefining, and reassurance can alter the negative thinking (Fishel, 1998).

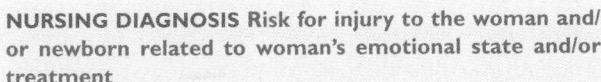

Plan of Care: Postpartum Depression

NURSING DIAGNOSIS Risk for injury to the woman and/or newborn related to woman's emotional state and/or treatment

Expected Outcomes *The mother and newborn will remain free of injury. The woman's family will verbalize understanding of the need for maternal and infant supervision and have a plan to provide that supervision.*

Nursing Interventions/*Rationales*

Assess the postpartum woman for risk factors for depression (before discharge) *to determine if she is at risk and in need of prompt interventions or referral.*

Provide information about signs of PPD to woman and family *to promote prompt recognition of problems.*

Observe maternal-infant interactions before discharge *to determine appropriateness.*

Maintain frequent contact with woman by telephone calls and home visits *to determine if further interventions are necessary, because most postpartum mothers are discharged early from the inpatient setting.*

Counsel woman and family to telephone health care provider if behaviors indicating depression, such as crying, increase *to provide prompt care and referral if necessary and avoid injury to newborn and mother.*

Provide opportunities for woman and family to verbalize feelings and concerns in a nonjudgmental setting *to promote a trusting relationship.*

Assess woman for any suicidal thoughts or plans *to provide for safety of woman and infant.*

Assist family to develop a plan for maternal and infant supervision *to provide for safety of woman and infant.*

Provide information about community resources for assistance *to ensure care if woman is unable to care for herself or infant.*

Reinforce teaching or refer breastfeeding mother to lactation consultant *to obtain information regarding effects of antidepressant and antipsychotic medications.*

NURSING DIAGNOSIS Disabled family coping related to postpartum maternal depression as evidenced by family members' denial of woman's illness

Expected Outcomes *Family will identify positive coping mechanisms and initiate a plan to cope with the woman's depression.*

Nursing Interventions/*Rationales*

Provide opportunity for family and significant others to verbalize feelings and concerns *to establish a trusting relationship.*

Give information to the family regarding postpartum depression *to clarify any misconceptions or misinformation.*

Assist family to identify positive coping mechanisms that have been effective during past crises *to promote active participation in care.*

Assist family to identify community sources of support *to provide additional resources as needed.*

Refer family to mental health counselor as needed *to provide further expertise from a mental health professional.*

NURSING DIAGNOSIS Risk for impaired parenting related to inability of mother to attach to infant

Expected Outcomes *Woman demonstrates appropriate attachment behaviors in infant interactions. Woman expresses satisfaction with infant.*

Nursing Interventions/*Rationales*

Observe maternal-infant interactions *to assess quality of interactions and to determine need for interventions.*

Encourage woman to express her anxiety, fears, or other feelings *to allow woman to ventilate her concerns and have them accepted.*

Encourage the woman to have as much contact with infant as possible *to minimize separation and to promote attachment.*

Demonstrate infant care and explain infant behaviors *to enhance mother's care abilities and understanding of infant's abilities.*

Make referrals as needed to community resources *to assist the woman in developing parenting skills or promoting confidence in infant care.*

KEY POINTS

- Because pregnant women may have a history of mental disorder or substance abuse, careful assessment is extremely important at the first and each subsequent prenatal and postnatal visit.
- Values clarification for health care workers may be necessary to assist them in providing nonjudgmental care for substance abusers.
- Alcohol abuse during pregnancy is the leading cause of mental retardation in the United States, and it is entirely preventable.
- Treatment programs must start with an understanding that substance abuse in women is a complex problem surrounded by multiple individual, familial, and social issues that require many levels of intervention and treatment.
- Mood disorders account for most mental health disorders in the postpartum period.
- Identification of women at greatest risk for substance abuse during pregnancy and depression in the postpartum period can be facilitated by use of various screening tools.
- Suicidal thoughts or attempts are among the most serious symptoms of PPD.
- Antidepressant medications are the usual treatment for PPD; however, specific precautions are needed for breastfeeding women.
- Treatment of postpartum onset of panic disorder requires a combination of medication, education, supportive measures, and psychotherapy.

CRITICAL THINKING EXERCISES

1. Review two websites listed in the Resources section of this chapter for PPD. Evaluate the sites for ease of use, accurate information, evidence of research, and links to other sources.
2. Identify resources in your community for pregnant women who are substance abusers. Develop criteria to evaluate these resources, and compare these resources according to the criteria.
3. You are assigned to a clinic to take maternal histories at the first prenatal visit. A 16-year-old gives the following history. She has missed one menstrual period, and her pregnancy test was positive. She smokes a half-pack of cigarettes a day and drinks beer every weekend. She has experimented with marijuana occasionally and tried cocaine twice in the past month. Her parents are divorced, and she currently lives with her mother, who is unaware of the pregnancy. She states that she plans to keep the baby and raise it by herself. She does not have a boyfriend at this time.
   a. Formulate nursing diagnoses.
   b. Assign priorities to the nursing diagnoses.
   c. Plan goals and expected outcomes of care.
   d. Plan interventions and give the rationale for each. Include referrals and community resources.

RESOURCES

American Psychological Association
202-336-5500
www.apa.org

Behavioral Health Care Information
www.behavenet.com

British Columbia Reproductive Mental Health Program
www.bcrmh.com/disorders/postpartum.htm

Depression After Delivery (DAD)
P.O. Box 1282
Morrisville, PA 19067
908-575-9121 or 800-944-4PPD
www.depressionafterdelivery.com

National Depressive & Manic Depressive Association
730 N. Franklin St., Suite 501
Chicago, IL 60610
800-826-3632
www.ndmda.org

National Women's Health Information Center
800-994-9662
www.4woman.gov

Office on Women's Health
202-690-7650
www.4woman.gov/own/about/index.htm

Postpartum Support International
927 North Kellogg Ave.
Santa Barbara, CA 93111
805-967-7636
www.chss.iup.edu/postpartum
www.postpartum.net

Women for Sobriety Support Group
www.womenforsobriety.org

REFERENCES

Abel, E., & Kruger, M. (2002). Physician attitudes concerning legal coercion of pregnant alcohol and drug abusers. *American Journal of Obstetrics and Gynecology, 186*(4), 768-772.

Abou-Saleh, M. et al. (1998). Hormonal aspects of postpartum depression. *Psychoneuroendocrinology, 23*(5), 465-475.

American Academy of Pediatrics Committee on Drugs. (2001). The transfer of drugs and other chemicals into human milk. *Pediatrics, 108*(3), 776-789.

American College of Obstetricians and Gynecologists. (1997). Smoking and women's health. *ACOG Technical Bulletin No. 240.* Washington, DC: ACOG.

American Psychiatric Association. (2000). *Diagnostic and statistical manual of mental disorders* (4th ed., rev.). Washington, DC: American Psychiatric Association Press.

Appleby, L., Mortensen, P., & Faragher, E. (1998). Suicide and other causes of mortality after post-partum psychiatric admissions. *British Journal of Psychiatry, 173,* 209-211.

Audain, L., et al. (1999). Cocaine and pregnancy: A deadly mix. *Epikrisis, 10*(1), 1-2.

Avants, B. et al. (2000). A randomized controlled trial of auricular acupuncture for cocaine dependence. *Archives of Internal Medicine, 160*(15), 2305-2312.

Beck, C. (1995a). Screening methods for postpartum depression. *Journal of Obstetric, Gynecologic, and Neonatal Nursing, 24*(4), 308-312.

Beck, C. (1995b). Perceptions of nurses' caring by mothers experiencing postpartum depression. *Journal of Obstetric, Gynecologic, and Neonatal Nursing, 24*(9), 819-825.

Beck, C. (1998a). A checklist to identify women at risk for developing postpartum depression. *Journal of Obstetric, Gynecologic, and Neonatal Nursing, 27,* 39-46.

Beck, C. (1998b). Postpartum onset of panic disorder. *Image: the Journal of Nursing Scholarship, 30*(2), 131-135.

Beck, C. (1999a). *Postpartum depression: Case studies, research, and nursing care.* Washington, DC: AWHONN.

Beck, C. (1999b). Postpartum depression: Stopping the thief that steals motherhood. *AWHONN Lifelines, 3*(4), 41-44.

Beck, C. (2001). Predictors of postpartum depression: An update. *Nursing Research, 50*(5), 275-282.

Beck, C. (2002). Revision of the Postpartum Depression Predictors Inventory. *Journal of Obstetric, Gynecologic, and Neonatal Nursing, 31*(4), 394-402.

Beck, C., & Gable, R. (2000). Postpartum Depression Screening Scale: Development and psychometric testing. *Nursing Research, 49*(5), 272-282.

Beck, C., & Gable, R. (2001). Further validation of the Postpartum Depression Screening Scale. *Nursing Research, 50*(3), 155-164.

Behrman, R., & Shiono, P. (2002). Neonatal risk factors. In A. Fanaroff & R. Martin. *Neonatal-perinatal medicine: Diseases of the fetus and infant* (7th ed.). St. Louis: Mosby.

Bennett, C. (1995). The tao, acupuncture, and crack cocaine. *Capsules and Comments in Psychiatric Nursing, 1*(4), 2-8.

Bergant, A. et al. (1999). Early postpartum depressive mood: Associations with obstetric and psychosocial factors. *Journal of Psychosomatic Research, 46*(4), 391-394.

Bozoky, I., & Corwin, E. (2001). Fatigue as a predictor of postpartum depression. *Journal of Obstetric, Gynecologic, and Neonatal Nursing, 31*(4), 436-443.

Bragg, E. (1997). Pregnant adolescents with addictions. *Journal of Obstetric, Gynecologic, and Neonatal Nursing, 26,* 577-584.

Brown, C. (2001). Depression and anxiety disorders. *Obstetrics and Gynecology Clinics of North America, 28*(2), 241-268.

Clark, C. (1997). PTSD: How to support healing. *American Journal of Nursing, 97*(8), 27-32.

Cnattingius, S. et al. (2000). Caffeine intake and the risk of first-trimester spontaneous abortion. *New England Journal of Medicine, 343*(25), 1839-1845.

Corrarino, J. et al. (2000). Linking substance-abusing pregnant women to drug treatment services: A pilot program. *Journal of Obstetric, Gynecologic, and Neonatal Nursing, 29*(4), 369-376.

Cox, J., Holden, J., & Sagovsky, R. (1989). Edinburgh Postnatal Depression Scale. *British Journal of Psychiatry, 150,* 782-786.

Cunningham, F. et al. (2001). *Williams obstetrics* (21st ed.). New York: McGraw-Hill.

Daley, M. et al. (2001). The impact of substance abuse treatment modality on birth weight and health care expenditures. *Journal of Psychoactive Drugs, 33*(1), 57-66.

Davis, S. (1997). Comprehensive interventions for affecting the parenting effectiveness of chemically dependent women. *Journal of Obstetric, Gynecologic, and Neonatal Nursing, 26*(5), 604-610.

Eberhard-Gran, M. et al. (2001). Review of validation studies of the Edinburgh Postnatal Depression Scale. *Acta Psychiatrica Scandinavica, 104*(4), 243-249.

Ernst, M., Moolchan, E., & Robinson, M. (2001). Behavioral and neural consequences of prenatal exposure to nicotine. *Journal of the American Academy of Child & Adolescent Psychiatry, 40*(6), 630-641.

Ewing, J. (1984). Detecting alcoholism: The CAGE questionnaire. *Journal of the American Medical Association, 22*(14), 1905-1907.

Finkelstein, N. (1994). Treatment issues for alcohol- and drug-dependent pregnant and parenting women. *Health and Social Work, 19*(1), 7-15.

Finkelstein, N. (1999). *Substance abuse and women.* Keynote address for the 8th Annual Statewide Conference of the NC Governor's Institute on Alcohol and Substance Abuse, Greensboro, NC.

Fishel, A. (1998). Nursing management of anxiety and panic. *Nursing Clinics of North America, 33*(1), 135-151.

Fishel, A. (1999). Evidence-based psychosocial therapies. In C. Shea (Ed.), *Advanced practice nursing in psychiatric and mental health care.* St. Louis: Mosby.

Foley, E. (2002). Drug screening and criminal prosecution of pregnant women. *Journal of Obstetric, Gynecologic, and Neonatal Nursing, 31*(2), 133-137.

Gilbert, E., & Harmon, J. (2003). *Manual of high risk pregnancy & delivery* (3rd ed.). St. Louis: Mosby.

Gold, L. (2002). Postpartum disorders in primary care: Diagnosis and treatment. *Primary Care, 29*(1), 27-41.

Gottlieb, S. (2001). Pregnant women cannot be tested for drugs without consent. *British Medical Journal, 322,* 753.

Grimes, D. (Ed.). (1998). Helping patients stop smoking: A new treatment option. *Contraceptive Report, 9*(3), 12.

Hankin, J., McCaul, M., & Heussner, J. (2000). Pregnant, alcohol-abusing women. *Alcoholism, Clinical and Experimental Research, 24*(8), 1276-1286.

Hankin, J., & Sokol, R. (1995). Identification and care of problems associated with alcohol ingestion in pregnancy. *Seminars in Perinatology, 19*(4), 286-292.

Herrick, H. (2002). *Postpartum depression: Who gets help?* Statistical Brief No. 24. Raleigh, NC: Department of Health and Human Services.

Hertzberg, T., & Wahlbeck, K. (1999). The impact of pregnancy and puerperium on panic disorder: A review. *Journal of Psychosomatic Obstetrics and Gynaecology, 20*(2), 590-564.

Huang, Y., & Mathers, N. (2001). Postnatal depression: Biological or cultural? A comparative study of postnatal women in the UK and Taiwan. *Journal of Advanced Nursing, 33*(3), 279-287.

Hulse, G., & O'Neill, G. (2001). Methadone and the pregnant user: A matter for careful clinical consideration. *Australian and New Zealand Journal of Obstetrics and Gynaecology, 41*(3), 329-332.

Kaplan, H., & Sadock, B. (2000). *Synopsis of psychiatry* (8th ed.). Baltimore: Williams & Wilkins.

Kearney, M. (1997). Drug treatment for women: Traditional modes and new directions. *Journal of Obstetric, Gynecologic, and Neonatal Nursing, 26*(4), 459-468.

Keltner, N., & Folks, D. (2001). *Psychotropic drugs.* St. Louis: Mosby.

Kovalesky, A., & Flagler, S. (1997). Child placement issues of women with addictions. *Journal of Obstetric, Gynecologic, and Neonatal Nursing, 26,* 585-592.

Kulin, N. et al. (1998). Pregnancy outcome following maternal use of the new selective serotonin reuptake inhibitors: A prospective controlled multicenter study. *Journal of the American Medical Association, 279*(8), 609-610.

Lee, M. (1998). Substance abuse in pregnancy: Marijuana and tobacco use in pregnancy. *Obstetrics and Gynecology Clinics of North America, 25*(19), 65-83.

Maley, B. (2002). Creating a postpartum depression support group. *AWHONN Lifelines, 6*(1), 62-65.

Margolin, A. et al. (2002). Acupuncture for the treatment of cocaine addiction: A randomized controlled trial. *Journal of the American Medical Association, 287*(1), 55-63.

Martin, S. et al. (1996). Violence and substance use among North Carolina pregnant women. *American Journal of Public Health, 86*(7), 991-998.

Matthey, S. et al. (2001). Validation of the Edinburgh Postnatal Depression Scale for men, and comparison of item endorsement with their partner. *Journal of Affective Disorders, 64*(2-3), 175-184.

Miller, W., & Rollnick, S. (1991). *Motivational interviewing: Preparing people to change addictive behaviour.* New York: Guilford Press.

Mills, J. (1999). Cocaine, smoking, and spontaneous abortion. *New England Journal of Medicine, 340*(5), 380-381.

Morse, B., & Hutchins, E. (2000). Reducing complications from alcohol use during pregnancy through screening. *Journal of the American Medical Women's Association, 55*(4), 225-227, 240.

Murray, L., Fiori-Crowley, A., & Hooper, R. (1996). The impact of postnatal depression and associated adversity on early mother-infant interactions and later infant outcome. *Child Development, 67*(5), 2512-2526.

Naegle, M. (1997). Understanding women with dual diagnoses. *Journal of Obstetric, Gynecologic, and Neonatal Nursing, 26,* 567-575.

National Women's Health Resource Center. (1998). Anxiety disorders and women' health. *National Women's Health Report, 20*(5), 1-6.

Newport, D., Wilcox, M., & Stowe, Z. (2001). Antidepressants during pregnancy and lactation: Defining exposure and treatment issues. *Seminars in Perinatology, 25*(3), 177-190.

Nulman, I. et al. (1997). Neurodevelopment of children exposed in utero to antidepressant drugs. *New England Journal of Medicine, 336*(4), 258-262.

Pederson, C. (1998). *Medical management of postpartum psychiatric disorders.* Psychiatric Nursing Institute presentation. Chapel Hill, NC.

Pokorny, A., Miller, B., & Kaplan, H. (1972). The Brief MAST: A shortened version of the Michigan Alcoholism Screening Test. *American Journal of Psychiatry, 129*(3), 342-345.

Prochaska, J., & DiClemente, C. (1992). Stages of change in the modification of problem behaviors. In M. Hersen, R. Eisler, & P. Miller (Eds.), *Progress in behavior modification,* Vol. 28. Sycamore, IL: Sycamore.

Raskin, V. (1997). *When words are not enough: The women's prescription for depression and anxiety.* New York: Broadway Books.

Ray, K., & Hodnett, E. (2001). Caregiver support for postpartum depression (Cochrane Review). In *The Cochrane Library, Issue 2.* Oxford: Update Software.

Saulnier, C. (1996). Images of the twelve-step model and sex and love addiction in an alcohol intervention group for black women. *Journal of Drug Issues, 26,* 95-123.

Seidel, H. et al. (2003). *Mosby's guide to physical examination* (5th ed.). St. Louis: Mosby.

Selleck, C., & Redding, B. (1998). Knowledge and attitudes of registered nurses toward perinatal substance abuse. *Journal of Obstetric, Gynecologic, and Neonatal Nursing, 27*(1), 70-77.

Stowe, J., Strader, J., & Nemeroff, C. (2001). Psychopharmacology during pregnancy and lactation. In A. Schartzberg & C. Nemeroff (Eds.), *Essentials of clinical psychopharmacology* (pp. 659-677). Washington, DC: American Psychiatric Publishing, Inc.

Straub, H. et al. (1998). Proactive nursing: The evolution of a task force to help women with postpartum depression. *MCN, American Journal of Maternal Child Nursing, 23*(5), 262-265.

Stuart, G., & Laraia, M. (2001). *Stuart and Sundeen's principles and practice of psychiatric nursing* (6th ed.). St. Louis: Mosby.

Substance Abuse and Mental Health Services Administration. (1998). *Preliminary results from the 1997 National Household Survey on Drug Abuse.* Rockville, MD: National Clearinghouse for Alcohol and Drug Information.

Tillett, J., & Osborne, K. (2001). Substance abuse by pregnant women: Legal and ethical concerns. *Journal of Perinatal and Neonatal Nursing, 14*(4), 1-11.

Tiran, D., & Mack, S. (Eds.). (2000). *Complementary therapies for pregnancy and childbirth* (2nd ed.). Edinburgh: Bailliere Tindall.

U.S. Department of Health and Human Services. (2000). *Healthy People 2010.* Washington, DC: Government Printing Office.

U.S. Department of Health and Human Services, Public Health Service. (1997). *Clinician's handbook of preventive services.* Washington, DC: U.S. Government Printing Office.

Wang, E. (1999). Methadone treatment during pregnancy. *Journal of Obstetric, Gynecologic, and Neonatal Nursing, 28*(6), 615-622.

Wintz, C. (1999). Difficult decisions: Women of childbearing age, mental illness, and psychopharmacologic therapy. *Journal of the American Psychiatric Nurses Association, 5*(1), 5-14.

Wisner, K., Perel, J., & Findling, R. (1996). Antidepressant treatment during breastfeeding. *Journal of the American Psychiatric Nurses Asociation, 153,* 1132-1137.

Woods, J. (1998). Substance abuse in pregnancy. *Obstetrics and Gynecology Clinics of North America, 25*(1), 169-191.

CHAPTER 36

Karen A. Piotrowski

Labor and Birth Complications

http://evolve.elsevier.com/Lowdermilk/MatWmnHlth/

LEARNING OBJECTIVES

- Differentiate between preterm birth and low birth weight.
- Identify the risk factors for preterm labor.
- Discuss current interventions to prevent preterm birth.
- Discuss the use of tocolytics and antenatal glucocorticoids in preterm labor and birth.
- Examine the effects of prescribed bed rest on pregnant women and their families.
- Define preterm premature rupture of membranes (PPROM).
- Describe the nursing care management for women with PPROM.
- Describe nursing management of a trial of labor, the induction and augmentation of labor, forceps- and vacuum-assisted birth, cesarean birth, and vaginal birth after a cesarean birth.
- Discuss the criteria for evaluating the nursing care of women with labor and birth complications.
- Describe the care of a woman with postterm pregnancy.
- Discuss obstetric emergencies and their appropriate management.

When complications arise during labor and birth, risk of perinatal morbidity and mortality increases. Some complications are anticipated, especially if the woman is identified as at high risk during the antepartum period; others are unexpected or unforeseen. The woman, her family, and the health care team can feel devastated when things go wrong. Nurses must recognize these feelings if they are to provide effective support. It is crucial for nurses to understand the normal birth process to prevent and detect deviations from normal labor and birth and to implement nursing measures when complications arise. Optimal care of the laboring woman, the fetus, and family with complications is possible only when the nurse and other members of the obstetric team use their knowledge and skills in a concerted effort to provide competent and compassionate care. This chapter focuses on the problems of preterm labor and birth, dystocia, postterm pregnancy, and obstetric emergencies.

PRETERM LABOR AND BIRTH

Preterm labor is defined as cervical changes and uterine contractions occurring between 20 and 37 weeks of pregnancy. Preterm birth is any birth that occurs before the completion of 37 weeks of pregnancy (ACOG/AAP, 1997). Preterm labor and birth are the most serious complications of pregnancy because they lead to about 90% of all neonatal deaths, with more than 75% of these deaths occurring in infants born at fewer than 32 weeks of gestation. Preterm birth is second only to congenital anomalies as a cause of infant mortality. In 2000, the preterm birth rate for all races in the United States was 11.6%. The **very preterm birth rate** (birth that occurs before the completion of 32 weeks of pregnancy) was 1.93% in 2000 (Martin et al., 2002).

Preterm Birth versus Low Birth Weight

Although they have distinctly different meanings, the terms *preterm birth* or *prematurity* and *low birth weight* are often used interchangeably. Preterm birth describes length of gestation (i.e., less than 37 weeks) regardless of the weight of the infant), whereas **low birth weight** describes only weight at the time of birth (i.e., 2500 g or less). Low birth weight is far easier to measure than preterm birth, and thus in many settings and publications, low birth weight has been used as a substitute term for preterm birth. Preterm birth, however, is a more dangerous health condition for an infant because a decreased length of time in the uterus correlates with immaturity of body systems. Low-birth-weight babies can be, but are not necessarily, preterm; low birth weight can be caused by conditions other than preterm birth, such as **intrauterine growth restriction (IUGR),** a condition of fetal growth not necessarily correlated with initiation of labor. Pregnant women who have various complications of pregnancy that interfere with uteroplacental perfusion, such as pregnancy-induced hypertension (PIH) or pregnant women who are poorly nourished, may give birth to a baby at term who is low birth weight because of IUGR.

The incidence of preterm birth in the United States varies according to race. The 2000 rate for African-American women was 17.3%, whereas the rate for Hispanic women was 11.2%, and the rate for non-Hispanic white women was 10.4%. The preterm birth rate for African-American women has been declining since a peak rate of 18.9% in 1991. The very preterm birth rate also has substantially decreased for these women to 4.04% in 2000. Anecdotal evidence suggests that sociodemographics may play a part in the race-based differences in preterm birth. Preterm birth rates are higher among socially disadvantaged populations, including minorities, women with low levels of education, and women who receive late or no prenatal care (Martin et al., 2002).

Predicting Preterm Labor and Birth

The known risk factors for preterm birth are shown in Box 36-1. The risk factors most commonly associated with preterm labor and birth are a history of preterm birth, race (i.e., African-American), and multiple gestation (Pschirrer & Monga, 2000). By using these risk factors, researchers have tried to determine which women might go into labor prematurely. Risk assessment schema were developed and used, and specialized interventions were developed for women considered at highest risk (Collaborative Group on Preterm Birth Prevention, 1993). None of these risk scoring systems has resulted in lowering the preterm birth rate in the United States, however, because at least 50% of all women who ultimately give birth prematurely have no identifiable risk factors. Programs aimed at decreasing preterm birth rates must include women labeled as "high risk for preterm birth" and women with no identifiable risk factors. Unless all women are included in prevention efforts that begin in the first trimester, a widespread reduction of preterm birth rates cannot be expected (Maloni, 2000; Pschirrer & Monga, 2000).

Biochemical Markers

The two most common biochemical markers used in an effort to predict who might experience preterm labor are fetal fibronectin and salivary estriol.

Fetal fibronectins are glycoproteins found in plasma and produced during fetal life. They appear in the cervical

BOX *36-1* **Risk Factors for Preterm Labor**

DEMOGRAPHIC RISKS
- Nonwhite race
- Age (<17, >35)
- Low socioeconomic status
- Unmarried
- Less than high school education

BIOPHYSICAL RISKS
- Previous preterm labor or birth
- Second-trimester abortion (more than two spontaneous or therapeutic); stillbirths
- Grand multiparity; short interval between pregnancies ≤1 year since last birth); family history of preterm labor and birth
- Progesterone deficiency
- Uterine anomalies or fibroids; uterine irritability
- Cervical incompetence, trauma, shortened length
- Exposure to DES or other toxic substances
- Medical diseases (e.g., diabetes, hypertension, anemia)
- Small stature (<1.19 cm in height; <45.5 kg or underweight for height)
- Current pregnancy risks:
  - Multifetal pregnancy
  - Hydramnios
  - Bleeding
  - Placental problems (e.g., placenta previa, abruptio placentae)
  - Infections (e.g., pyelonephritis, recurrent urinary tract infections, asymptomatic bacteriuria, bacterial vaginosis, chorioamnionitis)
  - Pregnancy-induced hypertension
  - Premature rupture of the membranes
  - Fetal anomalies
  - Inadequate plasma volume expansion; anemia

BEHAVIORAL-PSYCHOSOCIAL RISKS
- Poor nutrition; weight loss or low weight gain
- Smoking (>10 cigarettes a day)
- Substance abuse (e.g., alcohol; illicit drugs, especially cocaine)
- Inadequate prenatal care
- Commutes of more than 1½ hours each way
- Excessive physical activity (heavy physical work, prolonged standing, heavy lifting, young child care)
- Excessive lifestyle stressors

From Gilbert, E., & Harmon, J. (2003). *Manual of high risk pregnancy and delivery* (3rd ed.). St. Louis: Mosby; Iams, J. (2002). Preterm birth. In S. Gabbe, J. Niebyl, & G. Simpson (Eds.), *Obstetrics: Normal and problem pregnancies* (4th ed.). New York: Churchill Livingstone; Pschirrer, E., & Monga, M. (2000). Risk factors for preterm labor. *Clinics in Obstetrics and Gynecology, 43*(4), 727-734; Simpson, K. (1997). Preterm birth in the United States: Current issues and future perspectives. *Journal of Perinatal and Neonatal Nursing, 10*(4), 11-15; Varney, H. (1997). *Varney's textbook for midwives* (3rd ed.). Sudbury, MA: Jones & Bartlett.
DES, Diethylstilbestrol.

canal early in pregnancy, and then again in late pregnancy. Their appearance between 24 and 34 weeks of gestation could predict preterm labor (Moore, 1999). The negative predictive value of fetal fibronectins is high (up to 95%). The positive predictive value of the fetal fibronectin test is lower (25% to 40%) (Abrahams & Katz, 2002; Moore, 1999). This means that it may be possible to predict who will *not* go into preterm labor but not who will. The test is done during a vaginal examination.

Salivary estriol is a form of estrogen produced by the fetus that is present in plasma at 9 weeks of gestation. Levels of salivary estriol have been shown to increase before preterm birth. Specimens of salivary estriol are collected by the woman in the home; the testing is done every 2 weeks for about 10 weeks. This marker also has a high negative predictive value (98%) and a lower positive predictive value (7% to 25%) (Moore, 1999).

The cost of determining maternal levels of these biochemical markers is high. More research is needed before it will be known if these markers offer valuable assistance that is cost effective in the risk assessment for preterm labor.

Endocervical Length

Another possible predictor of imminent preterm labor is endocervical length. Some studies have suggested that a shortened cervix precedes preterm labor and can be determined by ultrasound measurement (Columbo & Iams, 2000; Niam et al., 2002). A shortened cervical length of less than 30 mm in a singleton pregnancy can predict some instances of preterm labor. When a woman has a short cervix combined with a positive fetal fibronectin result, her risk for spontaneous preterm birth is substantially higher than that for women positive for only one marker or none at all (Goldenberg et al., 2000).

Causes of Preterm Labor and Birth

The cause of preterm labor is unknown and is assumed to be multifactorial (Goldenberg & Rouse, 1998; Maloni, 2000) (Box 36-2). Infection is thought to be a major etiologic factor in some preterm labors, but trials of antibiotic therapy for all women at risk have not resulted in statistically significant reductions in preterm births (Creasy & Iams, 1999). When cervical, bacterial, or urinary tract infections are present, the risk of preterm birth is increased; thus early, continuous, and comprehensive prenatal care, which can detect and treat infection, is essential in dealing with this aspect of preterm birth prevention.

Not all preterm births can or even should be prevented. About 25% of all preterm births are iatrogenic, that is, babies are intentionally delivered prematurely because of pregnancy complications that put the life or health of the fetus or mother in danger, not because of preterm labor. Another 25% of all preterm births are preceded by spontaneous rupture of the membranes (preterm premature rupture of the membranes) followed by labor. These preterm births are not known to be preventable. About 50% of preterm births, therefore, are possibly amenable to prevention efforts and are considered idiopathic preterm births (Goldenberg & Rouse, 1998).

Sociodemographic factors such as poverty, low educational level, lack of social support, smoking, little or no prenatal care, domestic violence, and stress are thought to contribute to the 50% of preterm births that may be preventable (Curry, Perrin, & Wall, 1998; McFarlane & Gondolf, 1998; Moore & Freda, 1998). If prenatal care programs are to be effective in reducing the rate of preterm labor and birth, they must address these sociodemographic factors and develop strategies to attract all women to participate, including those at high risk for preterm labor (Maloni, 2000). Addressing the factors that contribute to preterm labor and birth can produce

BOX 36-2 **Multifactorial Etiology of Preterm Labor and Birth**

MATERNAL BEHAVIORS
- Smoking
- Substance use (alcohol or illegal drugs)
- Poor nutrition
- Work/fatigue
- Short interpregnancy interval
- Sexual activity

MATERNAL CHARACTERISTICS
- Young or older age
- Previous preterm birth
- Short stature
- Short cervix
- Uterine anomalies
- Diethylstilbestrol exposure
- Prematurely dilated cervix
- Low prepregnancy weight
- Race (e.g., African-American, Hispanic)
- Unmarried
- Low socioeconomic status
- Victim of domestic violence

OTHER FACTORS
- Inadequate support systems
- Stress
- Uterine irritability
- Multiple gestation
- Late or no prenatal care
- Preterm premature rupture of membranes (PROM)
- Anemia
- Infection
- Catecholamine release
- Decreased progesterone production
- Decidual cell disruption
- Prostaglandin synthesis
- Cytokine release

significant results. For example, Janke (1999) found that when women at risk for preterm birth participated in a daily program of relaxation to reduce stress and anxiety, they gave birth to larger newborns with significantly longer gestations.

CARE MANAGEMENT

Assessment and Nursing Diagnoses

Because all pregnant women must be considered at risk for preterm labor (as they are for any other pregnancy complication), nursing assessment begins at the time of entry to prenatal care. The onset of preterm labor is often insidious and can be easily mistaken for normal discomforts of pregnancy. It is essential that nurses teach pregnant women how to detect the early symptoms of preterm labor (Box 36-3) (Freston et al., 1997; Peck and Griffis, 1999; Witcher, 2002).

The nurse caring for women in a prenatal setting should use known successful modalities for teaching the pregnant woman about early recognition of preterm symptoms and then reassess the woman at each prenatal visit for the symptoms of preterm labor. Pregnant women also must be taught what to do if the symptoms of preterm labor occur. Some women wait hours or days before contacting a health care provider after preterm labor symptoms have begun. Women may ignore the symptoms because of ignorance regarding their significance or a belief that the symptoms are expected during pregnancy. The symptoms may be attributed to other factors such as the flu, incontinence of urine, or working too hard. Some women will become more vigilant waiting to see if the symptoms subside, go away, or become worse. They may take action by seeking advice about what to do from family or friends, resting more, increasing fluid intake, taking a bath, or rubbing the back or abdomen. Persistence of symptoms and increasing severity finally compel women to seek health care (Freston et al., 1997; Weiss, Saks, & Harris, 2002). Waiting too long to see a health care provider could result in inevitable preterm birth without the benefit of the administration of **antenatal glucocorticoids** (i.e., medication given to accelerate fetal lung maturity). In this event, the neonate is born at higher risk for respiratory distress syndrome and intraventricular hemorrhage.

The nurse must assess the psychosocial and emotional status of women in preterm labor and the impact that treatment (e.g., bed rest, hospitalization) can have on family dynamics. Factors influencing the impact of preterm labor treatment include stability of the support system, financial status, and availability of child support and assistance with household maintenance. Pregnant women who have risk factors for preterm birth are often offered special care with more frequent visits. Although there is no evidence in the literature that this enhanced care results in better outcomes, clinically it makes sense to evaluate at-risk women on a more frequent basis. Moore and colleagues (1998) found that telephone support to at-risk women by nurses can result in a 26% decrease in low-birth-weight births and a 27% decrease in preterm births in African-American women. This study demonstrates the power of nursing care, nursing support, and client education in the care of women at highest risk for preterm birth.

Nursing diagnoses relevant for women at risk for preterm birth include the following:

- *Risk for maternal excess fluid volume related to:*
  - administration of tocolytics to suppress preterm labor
- *Interrupted family processes related to:*
  - required limitation on maternal activity associated with preterm labor
- *Impaired mobility related to:*
  - prescribed bed rest
- *Anticipatory grieving related to:*
  - potential for birth of preterm infant
- *Risk for impaired parent-infant attachment related to:*
  - care requirements of preterm infant

BOX 36-3 Signs and Symptoms of Preterm Labor

UTERINE ACTIVITY
- Uterine contractions more frequent than every 10 minutes persisting for 1 hour or more
- Uterine contractions may be painful or painless

DISCOMFORT
- Lower abdominal cramping similar to gas pains; may be accompanied by diarrhea
- Dull, intermittent low back pain (below the waist)
- Painful, menstrual-like cramps
- Suprapubic pain or pressure
- Pelvic pressure or heaviness
- Urinary frequency

VAGINAL DISCHARGE
- Change in character and amount of usual discharge: thicker (mucoid) or thinner (watery), bloody, brown or colorless, increased amount, odor
- Rupture of amniotic membranes

Expected Outcomes of Care

The nurse develops a plan of care based on each woman's needs. Assessment of each pregnant woman's knowledge of the dangers of preterm birth, the symptoms of preterm labor, and what to do if symptoms should occur is the first step in working toward a positive outcome of pregnancy. Expected outcomes include that the woman will do the following:

- Learn the signs and symptoms of preterm labor and be able to assess herself and her need for intervention.

- Follow teaching suggestions and call her primary health care provider if symptoms occur.
- Not experience preterm symptoms, or if she does, she will take appropriate action.
- Maintain her pregnancy for at least 37 completed weeks.
- Give birth to a healthy, full-term infant.

Plan of Care and Interventions

Prevention

Prevention strategies that address risk factors associated with preterm labor and birth are less costly in human and financial terms than the high-tech and often lifelong care required by preterm infants and their families. Programs aimed at health promotion and disease prevention that encourage healthy lifestyles for the population in general and women of childbearing age in particular should be developed to prevent preterm labor and birth (Heaman, Sprague, & Stewart, 2001). One of the most important nursing interventions aimed at preventing preterm birth is the education of pregnant women about the early symptoms of preterm labor, so that if the symptoms occur, the woman can be referred promptly to her primary health care provider for more intensive care. Box 36-3 identifies the symptoms of preterm labor, and the Guidelines/Guías box identifies what the woman should do if the symptoms appear. Client education regarding any symptoms of uterine contractions or cramping between 20 and 37 weeks of gestation should be directed toward telling the woman that these symptoms are not normal discomforts of pregnancy, and that contractions or cramping that do not go away should prompt the woman to contact her primary health care provider. Because no one can discriminate between Braxton-Hicks contractions and the contractions of early preterm labor, Freda and Patterson (1995) suggest that the term "Braxton-Hicks contractions" be eliminated from teaching about pregnancy expectations (Fig. 36-1).

Early Recognition and Diagnosis

Early recognition of preterm labor is essential to implement interventions successfully, such as tocolytic therapy and administration of antenatal glucocorticoids. The

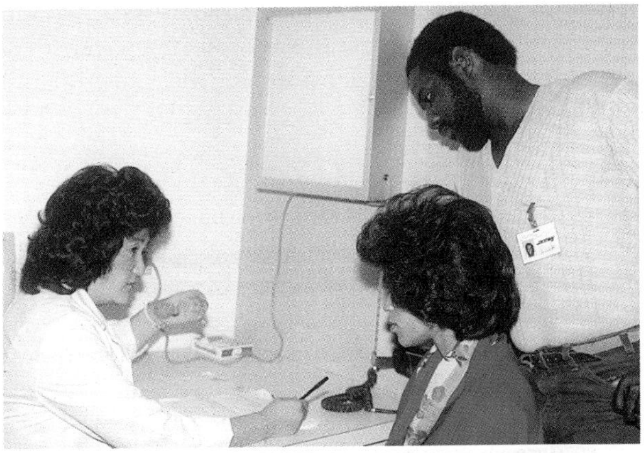

FIG. 36-1 Nurse teaching woman signs and symptoms of preterm labor. (Courtesy Marjorie Pyle, RNC, Lifecircle, Costa Mesa, CA.)

GUIDELINES/GUÍAS

What to Do if Symptoms of Preterm Labor Occur

Empty your bladder.
Vacíe su vejiga.

Drink 2 to 3 glasses of water or juice.
Bébase de dos o tres vasos de agua o jugo.

Lie down on your left side for 1 hour.
Acuéstese de lado izquierdo por una hora.

Palpate for contractions like this.
Palpe por contracciones así.

If symptoms continue, call your health care provider or go to the hospital.
Si le continuen los síntomas, llame a su proveedor de salud o vaya al hospital.

If symptoms abate, resume light activity but not what you were doing when the symptoms began.
Si se alivien los síntomas, resuma actividades leves pero no lo que hacía cuando le empezaron los síntomas.

If symptoms come back, call your health care provider or go to the hospital.
Si le regresen los síntomas, llame a su proveedor de salud o vaya al hospital.

If any of the following symptoms occur, call your health care provider immediately:
Si le continue cualquier de los síntomas siguientes, llame a su proveedor de salud inmediatamente:

Uterine contractions every 10 minutes or less for 1 hour or more
Contracciones uterinas cada diez minutos o menos por una hora o más

Vaginal bleeding
Sangrimiento vaginal

Odorous vaginal discharge
Desangre vaginal de muy mal olor

Fluid leaking from the vagina
Flujo que le gotea vaginal

diagnosis of preterm labor is based on three major diagnostic criteria:

- Gestational age between 20 and 37 weeks
- Uterine activity (e.g., contractions)
- Progressive cervical change (e.g., effacement of 80%, or cervical dilation of 2 cm or greater)

If the presence of fetal fibronectin is used as another diagnostic criterion, a sample of cervical mucus for testing should be obtained before an examination for cervical changes, because the lubricant used to examine the cervix can reduce the accuracy of the test for fetal fibronectin.

The pregnant woman at 30 weeks with an irritable uterus but no documented cervical change is not in preterm labor. Misdiagnosis of preterm labor can lead to inappropriate use of pharmacologic agents that can be dangerous to the health of the woman, the fetus, or both (Abrahams & Katz, 2002; ACOG/AAP, 1997).

Lifestyle Modifications

Nurses caring for women with symptoms of preterm labor should question the woman about whether she has symptoms when engaged in any of the following activities:

- Sexual activity
- Riding long distances in automobiles, trains, or buses
- Carrying heavy loads such as laundry, groceries, or a small child
- Standing more than 50% of the time
- Heavy housework
- Climbing stairs
- Hard physical work
- Being unable to stop and rest when tired

If symptoms occur when the woman is engaged in any of these activities, the woman should consider what she was doing when the symptoms began, and then consider stopping those activities until 37 weeks of pregnancy when preterm birth is no longer a risk. Counseling about lifestyle modification should be individualized; only women who have symptoms of preterm labor when they are engaged in certain activities need to alter their lifestyles. No specific rules describe which activities are safe for pregnant women and which are not. Each pregnant woman must understand which lifestyle factors might be contributing to her symptoms and be taught to modify only those factors. Sexual activity, for instance, is not contraindicated during pregnancy. If, however, symptoms of preterm labor occur after sexual activity, then that activity may need to be curtailed until 37 weeks of gestation.

Bed Rest

Bed rest is a commonly used intervention for the prevention of preterm birth. Although frequently prescribed, bed rest is not a benign intervention, and there is no evidence in the literature to support the efficacy of this intervention in reducing preterm birth rates. It is a form of care of unknown effectiveness (Enkin et al., 2000; Maloni, 1998). Maloni and colleagues (1993) described deleterious effects of bed rest on women: after 3 days there is decreased muscle tone, weight loss, calcium loss, and glucose intolerance. Weeks of bed rest lead to bone demineralization, constipation, fatigue, isolation, anxiety, and depression (Box 36-4). The father's sense of constant worry when bed rest is prescribed for his partner also has been documented. Bed rest is costly for society; the estimated economic costs are based on lost wages, household help and child care expenses, and hospital costs (Maloni, Brezinski-Tomasi, & Johnson, 2001; Youngblut, 2000). Prolongation of pregnancy does not necessarily occur despite the increased costs incurred. Women on bed rest need support and encouragement whether they are at home or are hospitalized. Nurses can create support groups of hospitalized women on bed rest. Internet resources including chat rooms for women on bed rest at home, as well as family and friends can be important sources of support for the women and reduce the sense of isolation they may feel. Interacting with other women experiencing preterm labor and bed rest has been found to be highly therapeutic (Adler & Zarchin, 2002; Maloni & Kutil, 2000). Durham (1998) found that women managed at home for preterm labor used certain strategies when de-

BOX 36-4 Adverse Effects of Bed Rest

MATERNAL EFFECTS (PHYSICAL)

- Weight loss; indigestion; loss of appetite
- Muscle wasting, weakness; aching muscles
- Bone demineralization and calcium loss
- Decreased plasma volume and cardiac output
- Increased clotting tendency; risk for thrombophlebitis
- Alteration in bowel function
- Sleep disturbance, fatigue
- Prolonged postpartum recovery

MATERNAL EFFECTS (PSYCHOSOCIAL)

- Loss of control associated with role reversals
- Dysphoria—anxiety, depression, hostility, and anger
- Guilt associated with difficulty complying with activity restriction and inability to meet role responsibilities
- Boredom, loneliness
- Emotional lability (mood swings); difficulty concentrating
- Increased stress

EFFECTS ON SUPPORT SYSTEM

- Stress associated with role reversals, increased responsibilities, and disruption of family routines
- Financial strain associated with loss of maternal income and cost of treatment
- Fear and anxiety regarding the well-being of the mother and fetus

mands from relationships, households, and careers competed with the prescription of bed rest. These strategies included cheating and testing the limits of their activity restriction. Exploring with these women the realities of their daily lives helps nurses work with them to set realistic guidelines for activity limitations that the women will follow, thereby avoiding feelings of cheating and its associated guilt.

Home Care

Women who are at high risk for preterm birth commonly are told that it would be best if they were at home on bed rest for weeks or months. The home care of the woman at risk for preterm birth is a challenge for the nurse, who must assist the woman and her family in dealing with the many difficulties faced by families in which one member is incapacitated. The scope of care given to women in their homes ranges from occasional visits to monitor the maternal and fetal condition, to daily telephone consultation and reading of uterine monitoring strips.

Regardless of the frequency of the visits, nursing care for the woman and family in the home demands organization and a sense of just how this family's life has been disrupted by the loss of activity of this essential family member. Families, who are often anxious regarding the health status of the mother and baby, may need help in learning how to organize time and space or to restructure family routines so that the pregnant woman can remain a part of family activity while still maintaining bed rest. It also is important for the nurse to work toward assisting all the family members to explore their feelings regarding the anxieties of preterm labor and help them to share their feelings with each other (Maloni et al., 2001). The Teaching for Self-Care boxes detail activities for women on bed rest and for their children.

The woman's environment can be modified for convenience by using tables and storage units around her bed to keep essential items within reach (e.g., telephone, television, radio, tape or CD player, computer with Internet access, snacks, books, magazines, and newspapers, items for hobbies) (Fig. 36-2). Ensuring that the bed or couch is near a window and the bathroom is also helpful. Covering the bed with an egg crate mattress can relieve discomfort. Women often find that a daily schedule of meals, activities, and hygiene and grooming (e.g., shower, dressing in street clothes, applying make-up) that they create reduces boredom and helps them maintain control and normalcy. Limiting naps, eating smaller but more frequent meals, and performing gentle range of motion exercises can help to reduce some of the detrimental effects of bed rest. It is essential that women and their families recognize that postpartum recovery will be slower as she works to regain strength and stamina (Maloni, 2002).

Home Uterine Activity Monitoring (HUAM)

Home care companies provide home uterine monitoring services for women diagnosed with preterm labor (Fig. 36-3); nurses are usually an integral part of the systems developed by the companies to educate the clients they serve. However, from the body of research over the past 15 years,

TEACHING FOR SELF-CARE

Suggested Activities for Women on Bed Rest

- Set a routine for daily activities (e.g., getting dressed, moving from the bedroom to a "day bed rest place," having social time, eating meals, self-monitoring fetal and uterine activity).
- Do passive exercises as allowed.
- Review childbirth education information or have a childbirth class at home, if this can be arranged.
- Plan menus and make up grocery shopping lists.
- Shop by phone.
- Read books about high risk pregnancy or other topics.
- Keep a journal of the pregnancy.
- Keep a calendar of your progress.
- Reorganize files, recipes, household budget.
- Update address book.
- Do mending, sewing.
- Listen to audiotapes, watch videos or television.
- Do crossword puzzles, jigsaw puzzles, etc.
- Do craft projects; make something for the baby.
- Put pictures in photo albums.
- Call a friend, family member, or support person each day or use e-mail.
- Treat yourself to a facial, manicure, neck massage, or other special treat when you need a lift.

From Gilbert, E., & Harmon, J. (2003). *Manual of high risk pregnancy and delivery* (3rd ed.). St. Louis: Mosby; Isennock, P. (1992). *Bed rest before baby: What's a mother to do?* Perry Hall, MD: Mustard Seed Publications; and Maloni, J. (1998). *Antepartum bedrest: Case studies, research, and nursing care.* Washington, DC: AWHONN.

TEACHING FOR SELF-CARE

Activities for Children of Women on Bed Rest

- Schedule brief play periods throughout the day.
- Keep a few favorite toys in a box or basket close to the bed or couch.
- Read to the child(ren).
- Put puzzles together.
- Watch videos, play video games (remote control for television is ideal).
- Play cards or board games.
- Color in coloring books.
- Cut out pictures from magazines and paste on cardboard.
- Play bed basketball with a soft (sponge) ball or rolled up sock and a trash can or empty laundry basket.

Adapted from Bolane, J., & Furlong, J. (1994). *Coping with bedrest in pregnancy.* Waco, TX: Childbirth Graphics; and Isennock, P. (1992). *Bed rest before baby: What's a mother to do?* Perry Hall, MD: Mustard Seed Publications.

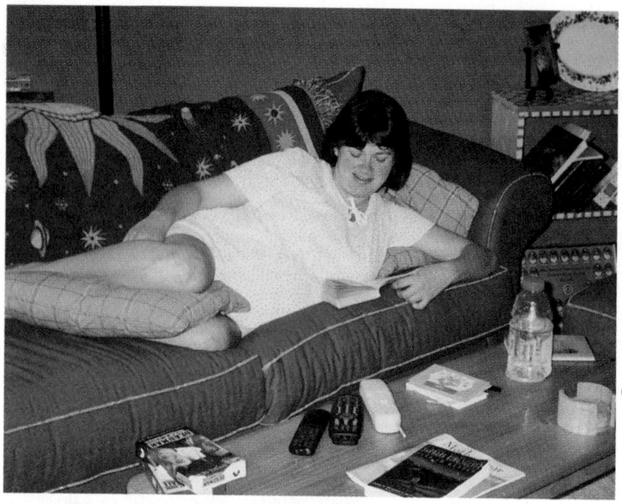

FIG. 36-2 Woman at home on restricted activity for preterm labor prevention. Note how she has arranged her daytime resting area so that needed items are close at hand. (Courtesy Amy Turner, Cary, NC.)

researchers have concluded that HUAM does not prevent preterm birth, and its prohibitive cost makes it an unacceptable intervention in the larger scheme of prenatal care (Dyson et al., 1998; Maloni, 2000). The use and effectiveness of HUAM remains controversial (Roberts & Morrison, 1998). It is a form of care unlikely to be beneficial in preventing preterm birth (Enkin et al., 2000). In addition, palpation of the uterus is more effective than a monitor for detecting uterine contractions when a woman is obese (e.g., excessive abdominal adipose tissue) or the gestational age is less than 26 weeks (Abrahams & Katz, 2000). Some research suggests that it is the nursing care offered by the home care nurses that helps the women the most (Moore et al., 1998).

Suppression of Uterine Activity

Tocolytics

Should preterm labor occur, women are usually admitted to the hospital for assessment; fetal monitoring; cervical/vaginal cultures; and assessment of cervical status, amniotic fluid leakage, and maternal temperature (an early sign of chorioamnionitis). The initiation of tocolytic therapy might be considered at this time. Once the pregnancy has progressed beyond 34 weeks' gestation, the benefits of prolonging the pregnancy do not justify the maternal risk of tocolytic therapy (Witcher, 2002). The use of **tocolytics** (medications that suppress uterine activity) in an attempt to prevent preterm birth has been the subject of research since the late 1970s. At first, it was thought that use of tocolytic therapy could prolong a threatened pregnancy indefinitely; research has demonstrated that a gain of 48 hours to several days is the best outcome that can be expected if the woman is less than 6 cm dilated. Once uterine contractions are suppressed, maintenance therapy may be implemented in an attempt to continue the suppression, or tocolytic treatment can be discontinued and resumed only if uterine contractions begin again. Research findings indicate that there is no significant difference in the mean gestational age when the two tocolytic treatment approaches are compared (Goldenberg & Rouse, 1998; Maloni, 2000; Witcher, 2002). It is now thought that the best reason to use tocolytics is that they afford the opportunity to begin administering antenatal glucocorticoids to accelerate fetal lung maturity and reduce the severity of sequelae in infants born preterm (Enkin et al., 2000; Goldenberg & Rouse, 1998). The use of tocolysis to suppress preterm labor has increased 50%, from 1.6% in 1990 to 2.3% in 2000 (Martin et al., 2002). The medications most commonly used for this purpose are ritodrine (Yutopar), terbutaline (Brethine), magnesium sulfate, indomethacin (Indocin), and nifedipine (Procardia). Ritodrine is the only medication approved by the Food and

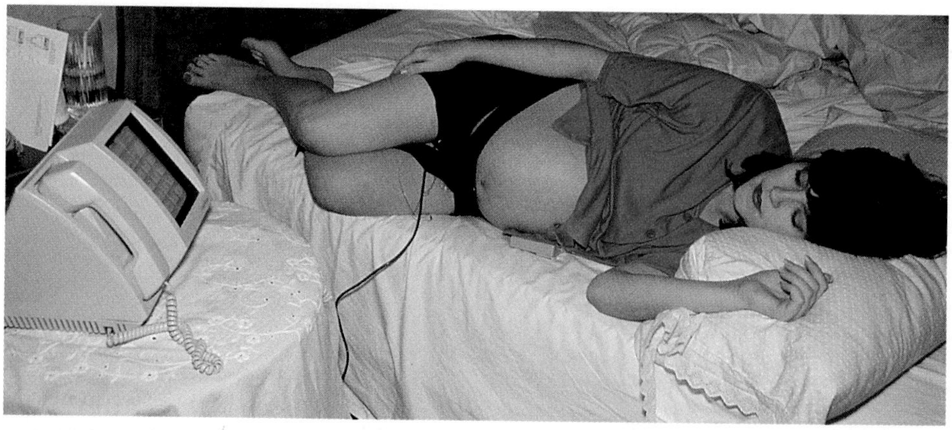

FIG. 36-3 Home uterine activity monitoring. Tocodynamometer is in place at center of abdomen below umbilicus. Recording unit and transmitter are on bedside table. (Courtesy Michael S. Clement, MD, Mesa, AZ.)

Drug Administration (FDA) specifically for the purpose of cessation of uterine contractions. The other drugs are used for this purpose on an "unlabeled" basis (i.e., drugs known to be effective for a specific purpose, although not specifically developed and tested for this purpose). Important contraindications exist to the use of all tocolytics (Box 36-5). Because these medications have the potential for serious adverse reactions for mother and fetus, close nursing supervision during treatment is critical (Lehne, 2001) (Box 36-6 and Table 36-1).

Magnesium sulfate is the most commonly used tocolytic agent, because maternal and fetal/neonatal adverse reactions are less common than with other tocolytic agents, especially the beta-adrenergic agonists. Although its exact mechanism of action on uterine muscle is unclear, magnesium sulfate does promote relaxation of smooth muscles (Iams, 2002; Witcher, 2002). At the onset of preterm labor, magnesium sulfate is administered via an intravenous infusion. Terbutaline, 0.25 mg, may be injected subcutaneously before the initiation of the magnesium sulfate infusion and then administered again by subcutaneous pump as the infusion is discontinued and the woman prepared for discharge to home care (see Table 36-1).

Ritodrine and terbutaline, beta-adrenergic agonist medications for tocolysis, work by relaxing uterine smooth muscle as a result of stimulation of $beta_2$ receptors on uterine smooth muscle. When used, ritodrine is usually administered intravenously as one of the first steps in suppressing preterm labor. Terbutaline is most commonly administered by a subcutaneous injection of 0.25 mg to suppress uterine hyperactivity or by a subcutaneous pump in the home setting. Effectiveness of pump therapy in prolonging gestation is controversial. Terbutaline also may be administered orally. Oral and pump therapy are similar in terms of effectiveness and adverse reactions (Guinn et al., 1998; Witcher, 2002). $Beta_2$-adrenergic agonists have many maternal and fetal cardiopulmonary and metabolic adverse reactions in part related to $beta_1$ stimulation and must always be used with extreme caution and careful, conscientious nursing care. Fewer neonatal adverse reactions occur if the administration of the beta-adrenergic agonist is discontinued at least 4 hours before birth (Witcher, 2002). Medication administration and nursing care are aimed at maintaining a therapeutic level of medication and avoiding the most serious side effects while maintaining optimal health of the fetus (see Table 36-1).

NURSE ALERT

Caution must be used when administering intravenous fluids to women in preterm labor because this practice can increase the risk for tocolytic-induced pulmonary edema, especially when a beta-adrenergic agonist or magnesium sulfate is used. It is recommended that the total oral and intravenous fluid intake in 24 hours should be restricted to 1500 to 2400 ml. Strict intake and output measurement, daily weight determination, and assessment of pulmonary function should be instituted (Gilbert & Harmon, 2003; Witcher, 2002).

Nifedipine, a calcium channel blocker, is another tocolytic agent that can suppress contractions. It works by inhibiting calcium from entering smooth muscle cells, thus reducing uterine contractions (Lehne, 2001). Mild maternal side effects and ease of administration have increased its use. When the tocolytic effects and maternal tolerance of nifedipine and beta-adrenergic agonists were compared, no significant differences in length of delay of

BOX 36-5 Contraindications to Tocolysis

MATERNAL

Severe pregnancy-induced hypertension or eclampsia
Active vaginal bleeding
Intrauterine infection (chorioamnionitis)
Cardiac disease
Medical or obstetric condition that contraindicates continuation of pregnancy
Dilation >6 cm

FETAL

Estimated gestational age >34 wk
Fetal death
Lethal fetal anomaly
Acute fetal distress
Chronic intrauterine growth restriction

BOX 36-6 Nursing Care for Women Receiving Tocolytic Therapy

- Explain the purpose and side effects of tocolytic therapy to woman and her family.
- Position woman on her side to enhance placental perfusion and reduce pressure on the cervix.
- Monitor maternal vital signs including lung sounds and respiratory effort, fetal heart rate (FHR) and pattern, and labor status according to hospital protocol and professional standards.
- Assess mother and fetus for signs of adverse reactions related to the tocolytic being administered.
- Determine maternal fluid balance by measuring daily weight and intake and output (I&O).
- Limit fluid intake to 1500-2500 ml/day, especially if a beta-adrenergic agonist or magnesium sulfate is being administered.
- Provide psychosocial support and opportunities for women and family to express feelings and concerns.
- Offer comfort measures as required.
- Encourage diversional activities and relaxation techniques.

TABLE 36-1 **Medication Guide: Tocolytic Therapy for Preterm Labor**

MEDICATION	DOSAGE AND ROUTE*	ADVERSE REACTIONS	MANAGEMENT CONSIDERATIONS
Ritodrine (Yutopar) $Beta_2$-adrenergic agonist Relaxes smooth muscles, inhibiting uterine activity and causing bronchodilation	Mix 150 mg in 500 ml isotonic intravenous solution Attach to controller pump and piggyback to primary infusion Begin infusion at 0.05 to 0.1 mg/min Increase rate by 0.05 mg q10 to 20 min until contractions stop, intolerable adverse reactions develop, or a maximum dose of 0.35 mg/min is reached Reduce rate gradually to lowest effective rate and maintain effective dose for 12 to 24 hr Oral dose: 10 to 20 mg, q3 to 4 hr (maximum oral dose is 120 mg/day) with meals to reduce GI distress	Maternal: Shortness of breath (SOB), coughing, tachypnea, pulmonary edema Tachycardia, palpitations, skipped beats Chest pain Hypotension Fluid retention and decreased urine production Tremors, dizziness, nervousness Muscle cramps and weakness Headache Hyperglycemia; hypokalemia; hypocalcemia; metabolic acidosis Nausea and vomiting Fetal/neonatal: mild tachycardia, hyperinsulinemia, hyperglycemia (fetal), hypoglycemia (neonatal), hyperbilirubinemia, hypotension, ileus	Women should be screened with ECG before therapy begins; maternal heart disease, severe hypertension including preeclampsia, hyperthyroidism, uncontrolled diabetes mellitus are contraindications Use cautiously if woman has type I diabetes, migraines Validate that woman is in PTL and is >20 wk and <35 wk gestation Assess woman and fetus to obtain baseline before beginning therapy and then before and after each increment; follow frequency of agency protocol Discontinue infusion and notify physician if the woman exhibits the following: Maternal heart rate >120 to 140 beats/min; dysrhythmias, chest pain BP <90/60 Signs of pulmonary edema (e.g., dyspnea, crackles, decreased SaO_2) Fetal heart rate >180 beats/min Ensure that propranolol (Inderal) is available to reverse adverse effects related to cardiovascular function
Terbutaline (Brethine)† $Beta_2$-adrenergic agonist Relaxes smooth muscles, inhibiting uterine activity and causing bronchodilation	Subcutaneous injection: 0.25 mg q20 to 30 min for 2 hr; then Maintenance dose: 0.25 mg q3-4 hr Subcutaneous pump: Maintenance dose 0.03-0.1 mg/hr Bolus: 0.25 mg q4-6 hr according to contraction pattern (peak uterine activity Maximum dose: 3 mg/24 hr Oral: 2.5 to 5 mg q4-6 hr	Similar to ritodrine but limited and less severe	Teach woman and family: Assessment measures: pulse, BP, respiratory effort, insertion site for infection, signs of PTL and adverse reactions of terbutaline Who to call if problems or concerns arise Site care and pump maintenance Activity restrictions Arrange for follow-up and home care

BP, Blood pressure; *DTRs,* deep tendon reflexes; *ECG,* electrocardiogram; *FHR,* fetal heart rate; *GI,* gastrointestinal; *PTL,* preterm labor; *NST,* nonstress test.
*NOTE: For variations in recommended administration protocols, always consult agency protocols, which should be evidence based.
†Caution: Not FDA approved for PTL (unlabeled use)

TABLE 36-1 **Medication Guide: Tocolytic Therapy for Preterm Labor—cont'd**

MEDICATION	DOSAGE AND ROUTE*	ADVERSE REACTIONS	MANAGEMENT CONSIDERATIONS
Magnesium sulfate† CNS depressant; relaxes smooth muscles including uterus	Mix 40 g in 1000 ml intravenous solution, piggyback to primary infusion, and administer using controller pump: Loading dose of 4 to 6 g over 15-30 min Maintenance dose: gradually increase from 2 g/hr to 4 g/hr as needed to suppress contractions; continue until contractions stop (or one contraction or less in 10 to 15 min) or intolerable adverse reactions develop	Maternal adverse reactions: Hot flushes, sweating, nausea and vomiting, drowsiness, and blurred vision, diplopia, headache, ileus, generalized muscle weakness, dizziness Hypocalcemia SOB, transient hypotension Some may subside when loading dose is completed Fetal/newborn (uncommon) Decreased breathing movement, reduced FHR variability, nonreactive NST Hypocalcemia, lethargy, hypotonia, respiratory depression Intolerable adverse reactions: Respiratory rate <12 Pulmonary edema Absent DTRs Chest pain Severe hypotension Altered level of consciousness Extreme muscle weakness Urine output <25-30 ml/hr or <100 ml/4 hr Serum magnesium level of ≥ 10 mEq/L (9 mg/dl)	Assess woman and fetus to obtain baseline before beginning therapy and then before and after each increment; follow frequency of agency protocol Monitor serum magnesium levels with higher doses; therapeutic range is between 4 to 7.5 mEq/L or 5 to 8 mg/dl Discontinue infusion and notify physician if intolerable adverse reactions occur Ensure that calcium gluconate (1 gm = 10 ml of 10% solution) is available for emergency administration to reverse magnesium sulfate toxicity
Nifedipine (Procardia; Adalat)† Calcium channel blocker; relaxes smooth muscles including the uterus by blocking calcium entry	Loading dose: 10-20 mg, po Maintenance dose: 20 mg, po, q6 hr for 24 hr; then 20 mg, po, q8 hr Do not use sublingual route	Maternal: Transient tachycardia, palpitations Hypotension Dizziness, headache, nervousness Peripheral edema Fatigue Nausea Facial flushing Fetal/newborn (rare): related to maternal hypotension, which would affect uteroplacental perfusion	Avoid use or use cautiously with magnesium sulfate because severe hypotension can result Assess woman and fetus according to agency protocol, being alert for adverse reactions

Continued

TABLE 36-1 **Medication Guide: Tocolytic Therapy for Preterm Labor—cont'd**

MEDICATION	DOSAGE AND ROUTE*	ADVERSE REACTIONS	MANAGEMENT CONSIDERATIONS
Indomethacin† Prostaglandin synthetase inhibitor; relaxes uterine smooth muscle	Loading dose: 50 mg (orally) or 50 to 100 mg rectally; repeat after 1 hr if no decrease in uterine activity is noted Maintenance dose: 25 to 50 mg, q4-6 hr for 24 to 48 hr (po or rectal)	Maternal: Nausea and vomiting, Dyspepsia, pyrosis Dizziness Oligohydramnios Reduced platelet aggregation increasing risk for hemorrhage Fetal: Constriction of ductus arteriosus progressing to premature closure Neonate: Bronchopulmonary dysplasia, respiratory distress syndrome Intracranial hemorrhage Necrotizing enterocolitis Hyperbilirubinemia	Used when other methods fail only if gestational age is <32 wk Administer for ≤48 hr Do not use for women with bleeding potential (coagulopathy), peptic ulcer disease, or oligohydramnios Assess woman and fetus according to agency policy, being alert for adverse reactions Determine amniotic fluid volume and function of ductus arteriosus before initiating therapy and within 48 hr of discontinuing therapy; assessment is critical if therapy continues for >48 hr Administer with food or use rectal route to decrease GI distress Monitor for signs of postpartum hemorrhage

BP, Blood pressure; *DTRs,* deep tendon reflexes; *ECG,* electrocardiogram; *FHR,* fetal heart rate; *GI,* gastrointestinal; *PTL,* preterm labor; *NST,* nonstress test.
*NOTE: For variations in recommended administration protocols, always consult agency protocols, which should be evidence based.
†Caution: Not FDA approved for PTL (unlabeled use).

birth were found, but significantly fewer maternal side effects occurred with nifedipine. Maternal side effects relate primarily to hypotension that occurs with administration. Concerns regarding adverse fetal effects have been reduced. Safety is achieved by following recommended dosages and maintaining maternal blood pressure, thereby preserving effective uteroplacental perfusion (Garcia-Velasco & Gonzalez-Gonzalez, 1998; Iams, 2002; Witcher, 2002) (see Table 36-1).

Indomethacin, a nonsteroidal antiinflammatory drug (NSAID), has been shown in some trials to suppress preterm labor by blocking the production of prostaglandins. Two prostaglandins are affected, prostacyclin and thromboxane. The decrease in prostacyclin suppresses uterine contractions, and the decrease in thromboxane suppresses platelet aggregation. However, both of these actions increase the risk for postpartum hemorrhage. The severity of fetal side effects associated with the use of indomethacin for tocolysis makes it less common than other classes of tocolytic drugs. Risk for premature closure of the ductus arteriosus increases if treatment goes beyond 48 hours or if the fetus is aged 32 or more weeks of gestation. Therefore, limiting the use of indomethacin to a short duration of treatment (e.g., 48 hours) or to women with less than 32 weeks of gestation is recommended (Iams, 2002; Lehne, 2001; Witcher, 2002). Macones and Robinson (1998) studied the risk of using indomethacin versus the benefit of delayed birth in 1000 women and found that it was more beneficial to the fetus to have received indomethacin and gained gestational age than was preterm birth at 32 weeks (see Table 36-1).

Promotion of Fetal Lung Maturity

Antenatal Glucocorticoids

Antenatal glucocorticoids given as intramuscular injections to the mother accelerate fetal lung maturity. It is viewed as a form of care likely to be beneficial (Enkin et al., 2000). This class of medications also seems to decrease rates of intraventricular hemorrhage in preterm infants (Goldenberg & Rouse, 1998). The National Institutes of Health consensus panel recommended that all women between 24 and 34 weeks of gestation should be given antenatal glucocorticoids when preterm birth is threatened, unless there is a medical indication for immediate delivery such as cord prolapse, chorioamnionitis, or abruptio placentae (National Institutes of Health, 2000). The regimen for administration of antenatal glucocorticoids is given in the Medication Guide.

MEDICATION GUIDE

Antenatal Glucocorticoid Therapy with Betamethasone, Dexamethasone

ACTION ▪ Stimulates fetal lung maturation by promoting release of enzymes that induce production or release of lung surfactant. NOTE: The FDA has not approved these medications for this use (i.e., this is an unlabeled use for obstetrics).

INDICATION ▪ To prevent or reduce the severity of respiratory distress syndrome in preterm infants between 24 and 34 weeks of gestation

DOSAGE AND ROUTE ▪ Betamethasone: 12 mg IM × 2 doses 24 hr apart
Dexamethasone: 6 mg IM × 4 doses 12 hr apart

ADVERSE REACTIONS ▪ Possible maternal infection, pulmonary edema (if given with beta-adrenergic medications), may worsen maternal condition (diabetes, hypertension)

NURSING CONSIDERATIONS ▪ Give deep IM in gluteal muscle. Teach signs of pulmonary edema. Assess blood glucose levels and lung sounds. Do not give if woman has infection. Use in women with PPROM not universally recommended.

NURSE ALERT

Nurses need to know that when any woman is admitted to the hospital and is 24 to 34 weeks pregnant, she should receive antenatal glucocorticoids unless she has chorioamnionitis. These drugs require a 24-hour period to become effective, so timely administration is essential.

Management of Inevitable Preterm Birth

Labor that has progressed to a cervical dilation of 4 cm is likely to lead to inevitable preterm birth. Preterm births in tertiary care centers lead to better neonatal and maternal outcomes. Women considered at risk for inevitable preterm birth should be transferred quickly to such a facility to ensure the best possible outcome. The first dose of antenatal glucocorticoids should be given before transfer.

Although maternal transport helps to ensure a better health outcome for the mother and the baby, it may have complications. Women may be transported to tertiary centers far from home, making visits by the family difficult, and increasing the anxiety levels of the woman and her family. Attention to the needs of the woman and her family before, during, and after the transport is essential to comprehensive nursing care for these families.

Evaluation

Evaluation of the nursing care provided for a woman at risk for preterm birth is based on achievement of the expected outcomes of care (see Plan of Care: Preterm Labor).

Preterm Premature Rupture of Membranes

Premature rupture of membranes (PROM) is the rupture of the amniotic sac and leakage of amniotic fluid beginning at least 1 hour before the onset of labor at any gestational age. **Preterm premature rupture of the membranes (PPROM)** (i.e., membranes rupture before 37 weeks of gestation) occurs in up to 25% of all cases of preterm labor. Infection often precedes PPROM, but the etiology of PPROM remains unknown. PPROM is diagnosed after the woman complains of either a sudden gush of fluid from the vagina, or a slow leak of fluid from the vagina.

Infection is the serious side effect of PPROM that makes it a major complication of pregnancy. **Chorioamnionitis** is an intraamniotic infection of the chorion and amnion that is potentially life-threatening for the fetus and the woman. Most cases of intrauterine infection respond well to antibiotics, yet sepsis can occur and can lead to maternal death. Fetal complications from chorioamnionitis include congenital pneumonia, sepsis, and meningitis (Garite, 1999). Even in the absence of infection, PPROM can precipitate cord prolapse or cause oligohydramnios, leading to cord compression, potentially life-threatening complications for the fetus.

Collaborative Care

Whenever PPROM is suspected, strict sterile technique should be used in any vaginal examination to avoid introduction of infection. A nitrazine or fern test is used to determine if the discharge is amniotic fluid or urine (see Chapter 21: Procedure box: Tests for Rupture of Membranes). A woman with this diagnosis can be cared for at home, with more frequent visits to her primary health care provider (see Teaching for Self-Care box). Expectant management will continue as long as there are no signs of infection or fetal distress. Nursing support of the woman and her family is critical at this time. She is often anxious about the health of her baby and may fear that she was responsible in some way for the membrane rupture. The nurse should encourage expression of feelings and concerns, provide information, and make referrals as needed (Weitz, 2001).

Frequent biophysical profiles are performed to determine fetal health status and estimate amniotic fluid volume. The woman with PPROM also should be taught how to count fetal movements daily, because a slowing of fetal movement has been shown to be a precursor to severe fetal compromise. Several methods are commonly used to count fetal movements; one method for fetal movement counting is described in the Teaching for Self-Care box (Freda et al., 1993). Antenatal glucocorticoids may be administered if chorioamnionitis is absent (ACOG, 1998a; Weitz, 2001).

Vigilance for signs of infection is a major part of the nursing care and client education after PPROM. The woman must be taught how to keep her genital area clean and that nothing should be introduced into her vagina. Signs of infection (e.g., fever, foul-smelling vaginal discharge, rapid pulse) should be reported to the primary health care provider immediately. Prophylactic antibiotic therapy may be ordered in an effort to improve perinatal outcome by preventing infection (ACOG, 1998b). However, use of prophylactic antibiotics for

Plan of Care Preterm Labor

NURSING DIAGNOSIS Deficient knowledge related to recognition of preterm labor

Expected Outcome *Woman and partner delineate the signs and symptoms of preterm labor.*

Nursing Interventions/*Rationales*

Assess what the woman and partner know about abnormal signs and symptoms during pregnancy *to identify areas of deficit.*

Discuss signs and symptoms that serve as warning signs of preterm labor *so that the woman or her partner has adequate information to identify problems early.*

Provide written supplemental materials that include a list of warning signs and instructions regarding what to do if any of the listed signs occur *so that the couple can reinforce and review learning and act swiftly and appropriately should a sign occur.*

Discuss and demonstrate how to assess and time the contractions *to provide needed skills to assess the signs of labor.*

NURSING DIAGNOSIS Risk for maternal/fetal injury related to recurrence of preterm labor

Expected Outcome *Woman demonstrates ability to assess self and fetus for signs of recurring labor; maternal-fetal well-being is maintained.*

Nursing Interventions/*Rationales*

Teach woman/partner how to monitor fetal and uterine contraction activity daily *to provide immediate evidence of a worsening condition.*

Have woman/partner report rupture of membranes, vaginal bleeding, cramping, pelvic pressure, or low backache to appropriate health care resource immediately *because such symptoms are signs of labor.*

If home uterine activity monitoring is to be used, teach woman/partner how to use the monitoring device and how to transmit the data to the health care provider via telephone *to enhance correct use of monitoring device and increase the accuracy of detection of early labor.*

Have woman monitor her weight, diet, fluid intake, and vital signs on a daily basis *to evaluate for potential problems.*

Limit activities to bed rest with bathroom privileges *to decrease the likelihood of onset of labor.*

Use a side-lying position *to enhance placental perfusion.*

Teach woman signs and symptoms of thrombophlebitis and encourage gentle exercise of lower extremities *because pregnancy and limited activity increase risk for clot formation.*

Abstain from sexual intercourse and nipple stimulation *because such activities may stimulate uterine contractions.*

Practice relaxation techniques *to decrease uterine tone and decrease anxiety and stress.*

Take tocolytic or other medications per physician's orders *to inhibit uterine contractions.*

Teach woman/partner about and have them report any medication side effects immediately *to prevent medication-induced complications.*

Have family arrange for alternative strategies in carrying out the woman's usual roles and functions *to decrease stress and limit temptations to increase activity.*

If small children are part of the household, encourage family to make alternative arrangements for child care *to enhance woman's adherence to bed rest protocol.*

NURSING DIAGNOSIS Anxiety related to preterm labor and potentially premature neonate

Expected Outcome *Feeling and symptoms of anxiety are reduced.*

Nursing Interventions/*Rationales*

Provide a calm, soothing atmosphere and teach family to provide emotional support *to facilitate coping.*

Encourage verbalization of fears *to decrease intensity of emotional response.*

Involve woman and family in the home management of her condition *to promote a greater sense of control.*

Help the woman identify and use appropriate coping strategies and support systems *to reduce fear/anxiety.*

Explore the use of desensitization strategies such as progressive muscle relaxation, visual imagery, or thought stopping *to reduce fear-related emotions and related physical symptoms.*

NURSING DIAGNOSIS Deficient diversional activity related to imposed bed rest

Expected Outcome *Verbalization of diminished feelings of boredom.*

Nursing Interventions/*Rationales*

Assist woman to creatively explore personally meaningful activities that can be pursued from the bed *to ensure activities that have meaning, purpose, and value to the individual.*

Maintain emphasis on personal choices of the woman *because doing so promotes control and minimizes imposition of routines by others.*

Evaluate what support and system resources are available in the environment *to assist in providing diversional activities.*

Explore ways for the woman to remain an active participant in home management and decision making *to promote control.*

Engage support of family and friends in carrying out chosen activities and making necessary environmental alterations *to ensure success.*

Encourage woman to use Internet to communicate with other women on bed rest *to obtain support and share feelings.*

Teach woman about stress management and relaxation techniques *to help manage tension of confinement.*

PROM before labor at term or preterm is a form of care of unknown effectiveness (Enkin et al., 2000).

DYSTOCIA

Dystocia is defined as long, difficult, or abnormal labor; it is caused by various conditions associated with the five factors affecting labor. It is estimated that dystocia occurs in approximately 8% to 11% of all births and is the primary cause for cesarean births (Gregory, 2000). Dystocia can be caused by any of the following:

- Dysfunctional labor, resulting in ineffective uterine contractions or maternal bearing-down efforts (the powers). It is the most common cause of dystocia (Cunningham et al., 2001).
- Alterations in the pelvic structure (the passage).

TEACHING FOR SELF-CARE

The Woman with PPROM

Take your temperature and assess pulse q4hr when awake
Report temperature of more than 38° C
Remain on modified bed rest
Insert nothing in the vagina
Do not engage in sexual activity
Assess for uterine contractions
Do fetal movement counts daily
Do not take tub baths
Watch for foul-smelling vaginal discharge
Wipe front to back after urinating or having a bowel movement
Take antibiotics if prescribed
See primary health care provider as scheduled

- Fetal causes, including abnormal presentation or position, anomalies, excessive size, and number of fetuses (the passenger).
- Maternal position during labor and birth.
- Psychologic responses of the mother to labor related to past experiences, preparation, culture and heritage, and support system.

These five factors are interdependent. In assessing the woman for an abnormal labor pattern, the nurse must consider the way in which these factors interact and influence labor progress. Dystocia is suspected when there is an alteration in the characteristics of uterine contractions, a lack of progress in the rate of cervical dilation, or a lack of progress in fetal descent and expulsion.

Research also documented a familial occurrence of dystocia. Laboring women whose mothers or sisters experienced dystocia during their labors had an increased risk for experiencing dystocia themselves, possibly related to a genetic factor affecting uterine activity (Berg-Lekas, Hogberg, & Winkvist, 1998).

Dysfunctional Labor

Dysfunctional labor is described as abnormal uterine contractions that prevent the normal progress of cervical dilation, effacement (primary powers), or descent (secondary powers). It is the fourth most common complication of labor and birth and occurs at an overall rate of 28.2 per 1000 live births. The highest rate (33.7) occurs among women 40 years of age and older, and the lowest rate (26.6) occurs among women 20 to 24 years of age (Martin et al., 2002).

Gilbert and Harmon (2003) cited several factors that seem to increase a woman's risk for uterine dystocia including the following:

- Body build (e.g., 30 pounds or more overweight, short stature)
- Uterine abnormalities (e.g., congenital malformations; overdistention, as with multiple gestation; or hydramnios)

TEACHING FOR SELF-CARE

Counting Fetal Movements (Kick Counts)

Choose a time of day when you can sit or lie quietly.
Choices for counting strategies:

- Starting at 9 AM, count the baby's movements until you have counted 10. If you have not counted 10 movements in 12 hours, notify your primary health care provider immediately.
- Count 4 movements, three times a day after meals. Most people count 4 movements in 1 hour. If you don't, then count for 1 more hour. If at the end of 2 hours, you still have not felt 4 movements, call your primary health care provider immediately.

- Malpresentations and positions of the fetus
- Cephalopelvic disproportion (CPD)
- Overstimulation with oxytocin
- Maternal fatigue, dehydration and electrolyte imbalance, and fear
- Inappropriate timing of analgesic or anesthetic administration

Dysfunction of uterine contractions can be further described as being hypertonic or hypotonic.

Hypertonic Uterine Dysfunction

The woman experiencing hypertonic uterine dysfunction, or primary dysfunctional labor, often is an anxious first-time mother who is having painful and frequent contractions that are ineffective in causing cervical dilation or effacement to progress. These contractions usually occur in the latent stage (cervical dilation of less than 4 cm) and are usually uncoordinated (Fig. 36-4). The force of the contractions may be in the midsection of the uterus rather than in the fundus, and the uterus is therefore unable to apply downward pressure to push the presenting part against the cervix. The uterus may not relax completely between contractions (Gilbert & Harmon, 2003; Varney, 1997).

Women with hypertonic uterine dysfunction may be exhausted and express concern about loss of control because of the intense pain they are experiencing and the lack of progress. **Therapeutic rest,** which is achieved with a warm bath or shower and the administration of analgesics such as morphine, meperidine (Demerol), or nalbuphine (Nubain) to inhibit uterine contractions, reduce pain, and encourage sleep, is usually prescribed for the management of hypertonic uterine dysfunction. After a 4- to 6-hour rest, these women are likely to awaken in active labor with a normal uterine contraction pattern (Gilbert & Harmon, 2003).

Hypotonic Uterine Dysfunction

The second and more common type of uterine dysfunction is hypotonic uterine dysfunction, or secondary uterine inertia. The woman initially makes normal progress into the

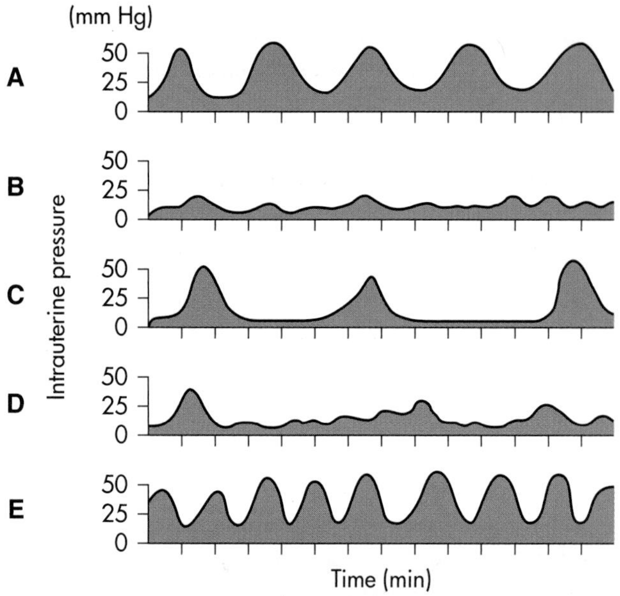

(mm Hg)
A
B
C
D
E
50
25
0
Intrauterine pressure
Time (min)

FIG. 36-4 Uterine contractility patterns in labor. **A,** Typical normal labor. **B,** Subnormal intensity, with frequency greater than needed for optimal performance. **C,** Normal contractions but too infrequent for efficient labor. **D,** Incoordinated activity. **E,** Hypercontractility.

active stage of labor; then the contractions become weak and inefficient or stop altogether (see Fig. 36-4). The uterus is easily indented, even at the peak of contractions. Intrauterine pressure (IUP) during the contraction (usually less than 25 mm Hg) is insufficient for progress of cervical effacement and dilation (Gilbert & Harmon, 2003). CPD and malpositions are common causes of this type of uterine dysfunction.

A woman with hypotonic uterine dysfunction may become exhausted and be at increased risk for infection. Management usually consists of performing an ultrasound or radiographic examination to rule out CPD and assessing the FHR and pattern, characteristics of amniotic fluid if membranes are ruptured, and maternal well-being. If findings are normal, then measures such as ambulation, hydrotherapy, enema, stripping or rupture of membranes, nipple stimulation, and oxytocin infusion can be used to augment the progress of labor (Varney, 1997).

Secondary Powers

Secondary powers, or bearing-down efforts, are compromised when large amounts of analgesia are given. Anesthesia may also block the bearing-down reflex and, as a result, alter the effectiveness of voluntary efforts (Mayberry et al., 1999). Exhaustion resulting from lack of sleep or long labor and fatigue resulting from inadequate hydration and food intake reduce the effectiveness of the woman's voluntary efforts. Maternal position can work against the forces of gravity and decrease the strength and efficiency of the contractions. Table 36-2 summarizes the characteristics of dysfunctional labor.

Alterations in Pelvic Structure

Pelvic Dystocia

Pelvic dystocia can occur whenever there are contractures of the pelvic diameters that reduce the capacity of the bony pelvis, including the inlet, midpelvis, outlet, or any combination of these planes.

Disproportion of the pelvis is the least common cause of dystocia (Cunningham et al., 2001). Pelvic contractures may be caused by congenital abnormalities, maternal malnutrition, neoplasms, or lower spinal disorders. An immature pelvic size predisposes some adolescent mothers to pelvic dystocia. Pelvic deformities also may be the result of automobile or other accidents or trauma.

An inlet contracture is diagnosed whenever the diagonal conjugate is less than 11.5 cm. The incidence of face and shoulder presentation is increased. Because these presentations interfere with engagement and fetal descent, the risk of prolapse of the umbilical cord is increased. Inlet contracture is associated with maternal rickets and a flat pelvis. Weak uterine contractions may be noted during the first stage of labor in affected women.

Midplane contracture, the most common cause of pelvic dystocia, is diagnosed whenever the sum of the interischial spinous and posterior sagittal diameters of the midpelvis is 13.5 cm or less. Fetal descent is arrested (transverse arrest of the fetal head) in such births because the head cannot rotate internally. These infants are usually born by cesarean, but vacuum-assisted birth has been used safely when the cervix is fully dilated. Midforceps-assisted birth usually is not done because of the increased perinatal morbidity associated with this intervention.

Outlet contracture exists when the interischial diameter is 8 cm or less. It rarely occurs in the absence of midplane contracture. Women with outlet contracture have a long, narrow pubic arch and an android pelvis, and this causes fetal descent to be arrested. Maternal complications include extensive perineal lacerations during vaginal birth because the fetal head is pushed posteriorly.

Soft-Tissue Dystocia

Soft-tissue dystocia results from obstruction of the birth passage by an anatomic abnormality other than that involving the bony pelvis. The obstruction may result from placenta previa (low-lying placenta) that partially or completely obstructs the internal os of the cervix. Other causes, such as leiomyomas (uterine fibroids) in the lower uterine segment, ovarian tumors, and a full bladder or rectum, may prevent the fetus from entering the pelvis. Occasionally cervical edema occurs during labor when the cervix is caught between the presenting part and the symphysis pubis or when the woman begins bearing-down efforts prematurely, thereby

TABLE 36-2 **Dysfunctional Labor: Primary and Secondary Powers**

HYPERTONIC UTERINE DYSFUNCTION	HYPOTONIC UTERINE DYSFUNCTION	INADEQUATE VOLUNTARY EXPULSIVE FORCES
Description		
Usually occurs before 4-cm dilation; cause unknown, may be related to fear and tension (primary powers)	Cause may be pelvic contracture and fetal malposition, overdistention of uterus (e.g., twins), or unknown (primary powers)	Involves abdominal and levator ani muscles Occurs in second stage of labor; cause may be related to nerve block anesthetic/analgesia, exhaustion
Change in Pattern of Progress		
Pain out of proportion to intensity of contraction Pain out of proportion to effectiveness of contraction in effacing and dilating the cervix Contractions increase in frequency Contractions uncoordinated Uterus is contracted between contractions, cannot be indented	Contractions decrease in frequency and intensity Uterus easily indentable even at peak of contraction Uterus relaxed between contractions (normal)	No voluntary urge to push or bear down or inadequate/ineffective pushing
Potential Maternal Effects		
Loss of control related to intensity of pain and lack of progress Exhaustion	Infection Exhaustion Psychologic trauma	Spontaneous vaginal birth prevented
Potential Fetal Effects		
Fetal asphyxia with meconium aspiration	Fetal infection Fetal and neonatal death	Fetal asphyxia
Care Management		
Initiate therapeutic rest measures • Administer analgesic (e.g., morphine, nalbuphine, meperidine) if membranes not ruptured or cephalopelvic disproportion not present • Relieve pain to permit mother to rest • Assist with measures to enhance rest and relaxation (e.g., hydrotherapy)	Rule out cephalopelvic disproportion Stimulate labor with oxytocin (augmentation) Perform amniotomy Assist with measures to enhance the progress of labor (e.g., position changes, ambulation, hydrotherapy)	Coach mother in bearing down with contractions; assist with relaxation between contractions Position mother in favorable position for pushing Reduce epidural infusion rate Apply low forceps or vacuum if assistance is needed Perform cesarean birth only if nonreassuring fetal status occurs

Brandl's Ring

inhibiting complete dilation. Sexually transmitted infections (e.g., human papillomavirus) can alter cervical tissue integrity and thus interfere with adequate effacement and dilation.

Bandl's ring, a pathologic retraction ring that forms between the upper and lower uterine segments (see Fig. 18-10), is associated with prolonged rupture of membranes, protracted labor, and increased risk for uterine rupture (Cunningham et al., 2001).

Fetal Causes

Dystocia of fetal origin may be caused by anomalies, excessive fetal size and malpresentation, malposition, or multifetal pregnancy. Complications associated with dystocia of fetal origin include neonatal asphyxia, fetal injuries or fractures, and maternal vaginal lacerations. Although spontaneous vaginal birth is possible in these instances, a low forceps-assisted, vacuum-assisted, or cesarean birth often is necessary.

Anomalies

Gross ascites, large tumors, and open neural tube defects (e.g., myelomeningocele, and hydrocephalus) are fetal anomalies that can cause dystocia. The anomalies affect the relation of the fetal anatomy to the maternal pelvic capacity, with the result that the fetus is unable to descend through the birth canal.

BOX 36-7 Back Labor—Occiput Posterior Position

MEASURES TO RELIEVE BACK PAIN AND FACILITATE ROTATION OF FETAL HEAD

Measures to Reduce Back Pain during a Contraction

- *Counterpressure:* apply fist or heel of hand to sacral area
- *Heat or cold applications:* apply to sacral area
- *Double hip squeeze:*
  Woman assumes a position with hip joints flexed such as knee-chest
  Partner, nurse, or doula places hands over gluteal muscles and presses with palms of hands up and inward toward the center of the pelvis
- *Knee press:*
  Woman assumes a sitting position with knees a few inches apart and feet flat on the floor or on a stool
  Partner, nurse, or doula cups a knee in each hand with heels of hands on top of tibia then presses the knees straight back toward the woman's hips while leaning forward toward the woman

Measures to Facilitate the Rotation of the Fetal Head (May Also Relieve Back Pain)

- *Lateral abdominal stroking:* stroke the abdomen in direction that the fetal head should rotate
- *Hands-and-knees position (all-fours):* can also be accomplished by kneeling while leaning forward over a birth ball, padded chair seat, bed, or over-the-bed table
- *Squatting*
- *Pelvic rocking*
- *Stair climbing*
- *Lateral position:* lie on side toward which the fetus should turn
- *Lunges:* widens pelvis on side toward which woman lunges
  Woman stands, facing forward, next to/alongside a chair so that she can lunge toward the side the fetal back is on or in the direction of the fetal occiput
  Places foot on seat of chair with toes pointed toward the back of the chair then lunges
  Alternative position for lunge: kneeling

Cephalopelvic Disproportion

Cephalopelvic disproportion (CPD), also called *fetopelvic disproportion* (FPD), is often related to excessive fetal size (i.e., 4000 g or more). It occurred at a rate of 17.2 per 1000 live births in 2000 (Martin et al., 2002).

When CPD is present, the fetus cannot fit through the maternal pelvis to be born vaginally. Excessive fetal size, or *macrosomia*, is associated with maternal diabetes mellitus, obesity, multiparity, or the large size of one or both parents. If the maternal pelvis is too small, abnormally shaped, or deformed, CPD may be of maternal origin. In this case, the fetus may be of average size or even smaller.

Malposition

The most common fetal malposition is persistent occipitoposterior position (i.e., right occipitoposterior [ROP] or left occipitoposterior [LOP]; see Chapter 18), occurring in about 25% of all labors. Labor, especially the second stage, is prolonged; the woman typically complains of severe back pain from the pressure of the fetal head (occiput) pressing against her sacrum. Box 36-7 identifies suggested measures to relieve back pain and facilitate rotation of the fetal occiput to an anterior position, which will facilitate birth (Gilbert & Harmon, 2003; Simkin & Ancheta, 2000).

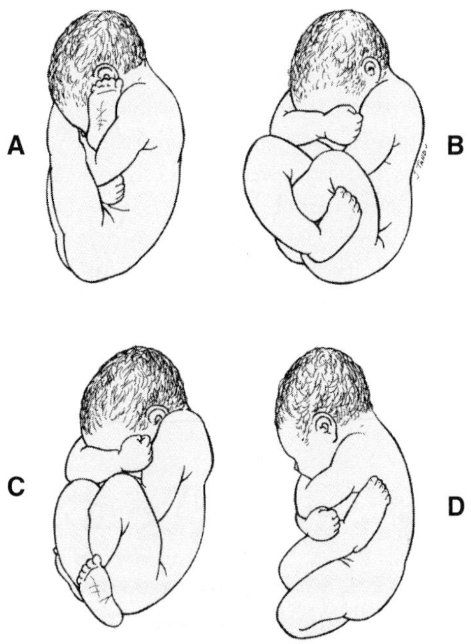
A
B
C
D

FIG. 36-5 Types of breech presentation. **A,** Frank breech: thighs are flexed on hips; knees are extended. **B,** Complete breech: thighs and knees are flexed. **C,** Incomplete breech: foot extends below the buttocks. **D,** Incomplete breech: knee extends below the buttocks.

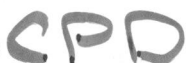

Malpresentation

Malpresentation is the third most commonly reported complication of labor and birth. In 2000, it occurred at a rate of 38.8 per 1000 live births, with the highest rate (i.e., 57.4) among women 40 to 54 years of age (Martin et al., 2002). Breech presentation is the most common form of malpresentation. The four main types of breech presentation are frank breech (thighs flexed, knees extended), complete breech (thighs and knees flexed), and two types of incomplete breech, one in which the knee extends below the buttocks and the other in which the foot extends below the buttocks (Fig. 36-5). Breech presentations are associated with multifetal gestation, preterm birth, fetal and maternal anomalies, hydramnios, and oligohydramnios. Diagnosis is made by abdominal palpation (e.g., Leopold maneuvers) and vaginal examination and usually is confirmed by ultrasound scan (Lanni & Seeds, 2002).

During labor, the descent of the fetus in a breech presentation may be slow because the breech is not so good a dilating wedge as is the fetal head; the labor itself usually is not prolonged. There is risk of prolapse of the cord if the membranes rupture in early labor. The presence of meconium in amniotic fluid is not necessarily a sign of fetal distress because it results from pressure on the fetal abdominal wall as it traverses the birth canal. Assessment of FHR and pattern should be used to determine whether the passage of meconium is an expected finding associated with breech presentation or is a nonreassuring sign associated with fetal hypoxia. The fetal heart tones of infants in a breech position are best heard at or above the umbilicus.

Vaginal birth is accomplished by mechanisms of labor that manipulate the buttocks and lower extremities as they emerge from the birth canal (Varney, 1997) (Fig. 36-6). Piper forceps sometimes are used to deliver the head (see Fig. 36-12). External cephalic version (ECV) may be tried to turn the fetus to a vertex presentation (see Fig. 36-9). Cesarean birth may be necessary (Lanni & Seeds, 2002).

Although opinions vary, a cesarean birth is commonly performed when the fetus is estimated to be larger than 3800 g or smaller than 1500 g, if this is a first pregnancy, if labor is ineffective, or if complications occur (Scott, 1999). Although cesarean birth reduces the risks to the fetus, the maternal risks are increased. ECV also poses risks and is not always successful. Women whose breech presentation occurs late in pregnancy need to be informed of the options for birth, as well as the risks associated with each option.

Face and brow presentations are uncommon and are associated with fetal anomalies, pelvic contractures, and CPD (Fig. 36-7). Vaginal birth is possible if the fetus flexes to a vertex presentation, although forceps often are used.

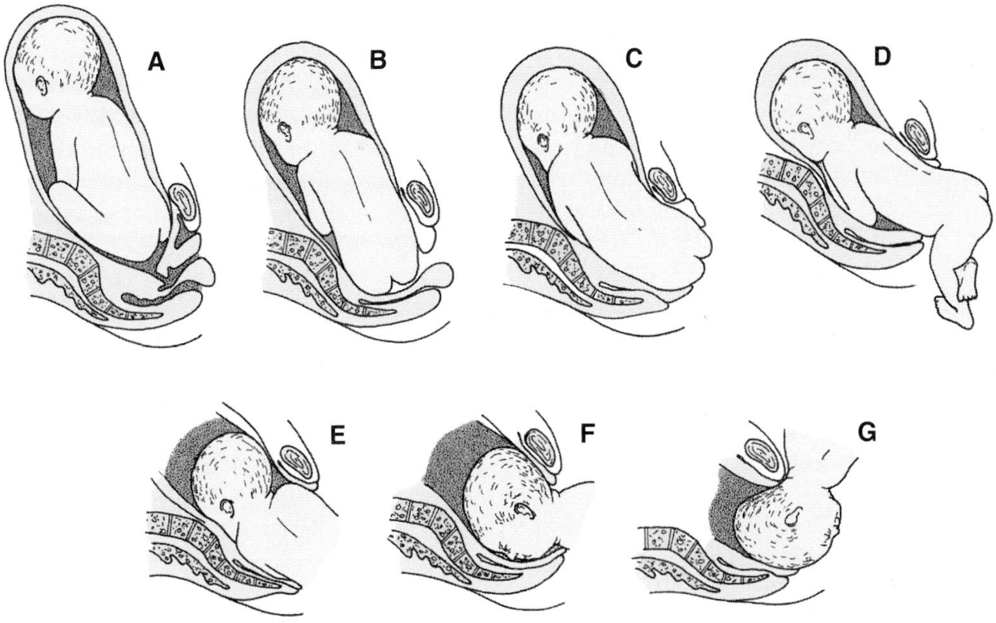
A
B
C
D
E
F
G

FIG. 36-6 Mechanism of labor in breech presentation. **A,** Breech before onset of labor. **B,** Engagement and internal rotation. **C,** Lateral flexion. **D,** External rotation or restitution. **E,** Internal rotation of shoulders and head. **F,** Face rotates to sacrum when occiput is anterior. **G,** Head is born by gradual flexion during elevation of fetal body.

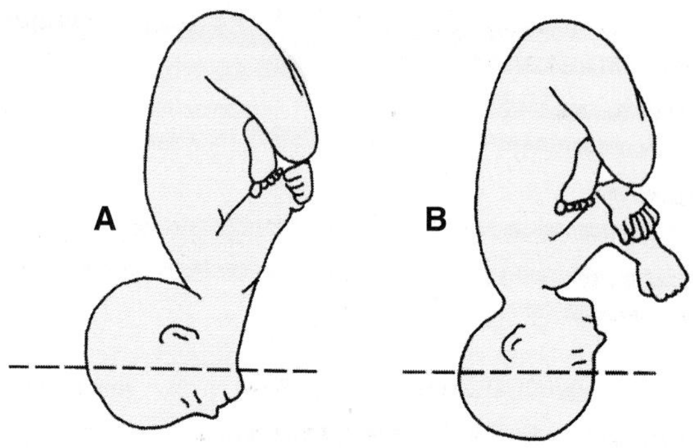
A
B

FIG. 36-7 Extension of normally flexed head. Face **(A)** and brow **(B)** presentations.

Cesarean birth is indicated if the presentation persists, if there is fetal distress, or if labor stops progressing.

Cesarean birth is usually necessary for a fetus in a shoulder presentation (i.e., the fetus is in a transverse lie), although ECV may be attempted after 38 weeks of gestation (Cunningham et al., 2001; Varney, 1997).

Multifetal Pregnancy

Multifetal pregnancy is the gestation of twins, triplets, quadruplets, or more infants. Since 1980, the twin birth rate has increased by 55%. The twin birth rate was 29.3 per 1000 live births in 2000. The higher-order multiple birth rate (i.e., triplet and more) was 180.4 per 100,000 live births in 2000, representing the second consecutive year of decline in what had been a rapid escalation since 1980 (Martin et al., 2002). It is likely that the rapid escalation was related to use of fertility-enhancing medications and procedures and the older age of childbearing women. When compared with younger women, women age 35 years and older are naturally more likely to have a multifetal pregnancy. Refinements in the treatments used to treat infertility may be responsible for the recent decline in higher-order multiple births.

Multiple births are associated with more complications (e.g., dysfunctional labor) than are single births. The higher incidence of fetal/newborn complications and higher risk of perinatal mortality primarily stem from the birth of low-birth-weight infants resulting from preterm birth and/or IUGR in part related to placental dysfunction and twin-to-twin transfusion. Fetuses may experience distress and asphyxia during the birth process as a result of cord prolapse and the onset of placental separation with the birth of the first fetus. As a result, the risk for long-term problems such as cerebral palsy is higher among multiple births.

In addition, fetal complications such as congenital anomalies and abnormal presentations can result in dystocia and an increased incidence of cesarean birth. For example, in only half of all twin pregnancies do both fetuses present in the vertex position, the most favorable for vaginal birth; in one third of the pregnancies, one twin may present in the vertex position and one in the breech (Cunningham et al., 2001; Ellings, Newman, & Bowers, 1998).

The health status of the mother may be compromised by an increased risk for hypertension, anemia, and hemorrhage associated with uterine atony, abruptio placentae, and multiple or adherent placentas. Duration of the phases and stages of labor may vary from the duration experienced with singleton births.

Teamwork and planning are essential components of the management of childbirth in multiple pregnancies, especially those of the higher-order multiples. The nurse plays a key role in coordinating the activities of many highly skilled health care professionals. Early detection and care of the maternal/fetal/newborn complications associated with multiple births are essential to achieve a positive outcome for mother and babies. Maternal positioning and active support are used to enhance labor progress and placental perfusion. Stimulation of labor with oxytocin, epidural anesthesia, forceps and vacuum assistance, and internal or ECV may be used to accomplish the vaginal birth of twins. Cesarean birth is most likely with higher-order multiple births. Each infant may have its own team of health care providers present at the birth. Emotional support that includes expression of feelings and full explanations of events as they occur and of the status of the mother and the fetuses/newborns is important to reduce the anxiety and stress the mother and her family experience (Ellings et al., 1998).

Position of the Woman

The functional relationship among the uterine contractions, the fetus, and the mother's pelvis are altered by the maternal position. In addition, the position can provide either a mechanical advantage or disadvantage to the mechanisms of labor by altering the effects of gravity and the body-part relations important to the progress of labor. For example, the hands-and-knees position facilitates rotation from a posterior occiput position more effectively than does the lateral position. Upright positions such as sitting and squatting facilitate fetal descent during pushing and shorten the second stage of labor (Mayberry et al., 2000; Simkin & Ancheta, 2000). Discouraging maternal movement or restricting labor to the recumbent or lithotomy position may compromise progress. The incidence of dystocia in women confined to these positions is increased, resulting in increased need for augmentation of labor or forceps-assisted, vacuum-assisted, or cesarean birth.

Psychologic Responses

Hormones and neurotransmitters released in response to stress (e.g., catecholamines) can cause dystocia. Sources of stress vary for each woman, but pain and the absence of a support person are two recognized factors. Confinement to bed and restriction of maternal movement can be a source of psychologic stress that compounds the physiologic stress caused by immobility in the unmedicated laboring woman. When anxiety is excessive, it can inhibit cervical dilation and result in prolonged labor and increased pain perception. Anxiety also causes increased levels of stress-related hormones (e.g., beta-endorphin, adrenocorticotropic hormone, cortisol, and epinephrine). These hormones act on the smooth muscles of the uterus; increased levels can cause dystocia by reducing uterine contractility.

Abnormal Labor Patterns

In 2000, prolonged labor patterns occurred at a rate of 7.8 per 1000 live births. The incidence of prolonged labor patterns was slightly higher (i.e., 8.6 per 1000) among women who were younger than 20 years (Martin et al., 2002).

Six abnormal labor patterns were identified and classified by Friedman (1989) according to the nature of the cervical dilation and fetal descent. The labor patterns seen in normal and abnormal labor are described in Table 36-3.

These patterns may result from a variety of causes, including ineffective uterine contractions, pelvic contractures, CPD, abnormal fetal presentations or position, early use of analgesics, nerve block analgesia/anesthesia, and anxiety and stress. Progress in either the first or second stage of labor can be protracted (prolonged) or arrested (stopped). Abnormal progress can be identified by plotting cervical dilation and fetal descent on a labor graph (partogram) at various intervals after the onset of labor and comparing the resulting curve with the expected labor curve for a nulliparous or multiparous labor. Figure 36-8, *A*, is a labor graph illustrating progress in a normal labor for a primigravida. Figure 36-8, *B*, illustrates major types of deviation from the normal progress of labor. If a woman exhibits an abnormal labor pattern, the primary health care provider should be notified.

Health care providers must be careful when diagnosing a labor pattern as prolonged and when intervening based on this diagnosis. Criteria defining the differences between false, latent, and active labor should be established. Using hospital admission areas to evaluate a woman's labor status is helpful in preventing the premature implementation of labor interventions such as administration of systemic opioid analgesics or induction of epidural analgesia/anesthesia. If a woman is found to be in false or latent (early) labor, she can be sent home or remain in the admissions area until labor becomes active. Women in active labor are admitted to the labor and birth unit (McNiven et al., 1998).

Maternal morbidity and death may occur as a result of uterine rupture, infection, severe dehydration, and postpartum hemorrhage. The fetus is at increased risk for hypoxia. A long and difficult labor can have an adverse psychologic effect on the mother, father, and family.

TABLE 36-3 Labor Patterns in Normal and Abnormal Labor

Normal Labor

1. Dilation: continues
   a. Latent phase: <4 cm and low slope
   b. Active phase: >5 cm or high slope
   c. Deceleration phase: ≥9 cm
2. Descent: active at ≥9 cm dilation

	ABNORMAL LABOR	
PATTERN	**NULLIPARAS**	**MULTIPARAS**
Prolonged latent phase	>20 hr	>14 hr
Protracted active phase dilation	<1.2 cm/hr	<1.5 cm/hr
Secondary arrest: no change	≥2 hr	≥2 hr
Protracted descent	<1 cm/hr	<2 cm/hr
Arrest of descent	≥1 hr	≥½ hr
Failure of descent	No change during deceleration phase and second stage	
Precipitous labor	>5 cm/hr	10 cm/hr

Precipitate Labor

Precipitate labor is defined as labor that lasts less than 3 hours from the onset of contractions to the time of birth. This abnormal labor pattern occurred at a rate of 19.6 per 1000 live births in 2000. Precipitate labor occurred at the highest rate (i.e., 23.5) among women aged 35 to 54 and at the lowest rate (i.e., 13.8) among women younger than 20 years (Martin et al., 2002).

Precipitate labor may result from hypertonic uterine contractions that are tetanic in intensity. Maternal and fetal complications can occur as a result. Maternal complications include uterine rupture, lacerations of the birth canal, amniotic fluid embolism, and postpartum hemorrhage. Fetal complications include hypoxia caused by decreased periods of uterine relaxation between contractions and intracranial hemorrhage related to rapid birth (Cunningham et al., 2001).

Women who have experienced precipitate labor often describe feelings of disbelief that their labor began so quickly, alarm that their labor progressed so rapidly, panic about the possibility they would not make it to the hospital on time to give birth, and finally, relief when they arrived at the hospital. In addition, women have expressed frustration when nurses would not believe them when they reported their readiness to push. Some women have difficulty remembering the details of their labor and birth and require others, including caregivers, to help them to fill in the gaps in their memory (Rippin-Sisler, 1996).

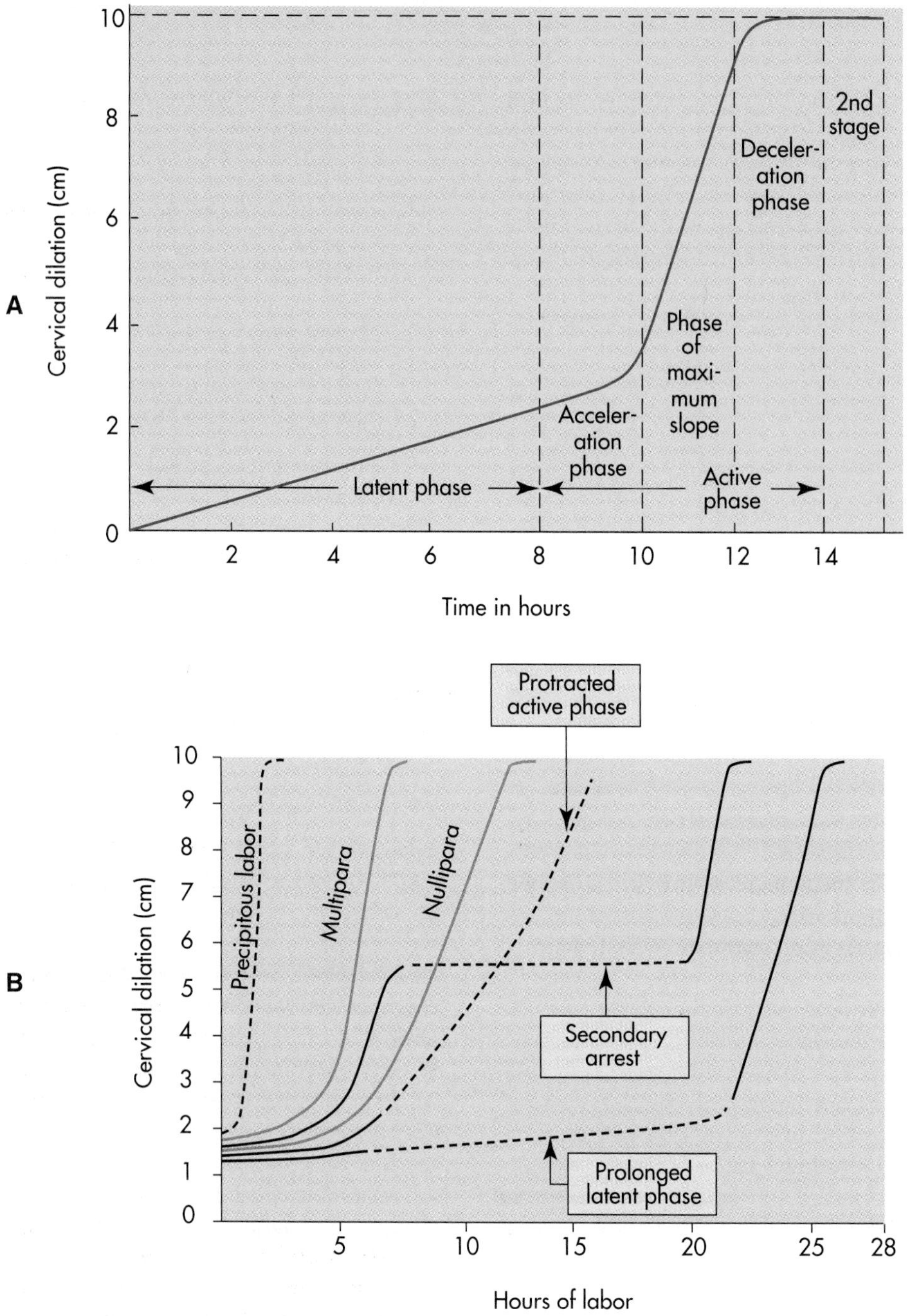

A
Cervical dilation (cm)
Time in hours
Latent phase
Acceleration phase
Phase of maximum slope
Deceleration phase
Active phase
2nd stage
B
Cervical dilation (cm)
Hours of labor
Protracted active phase
Precipitous labor
Multipara
Nullipara
Secondary arrest
Prolonged latent phase

FIG. 36-8 A, Depiction of a normal labor for a primigravida. **B,** Major types of deviation from normal progress of labor may be detected by noting dilation of cervix at various intervals after labor begins. If a woman exhibits an abnormal labor pattern, as depicted by *broken lines*, the primary health care provider should be notified.

CARE MANAGEMENT

The care management of the woman at risk for problems related to abnormal labor, birth, or both, involves all members of the health care team. Nursing care is facilitated through the use of the nursing process.

Assessment and Nursing Diagnoses

Risk assessment is a continuous process in the laboring woman. Review of the findings obtained during the initial interview conducted at the woman's admission to the labor unit and ongoing observations of her psychologic response to labor may reveal factors that can be a source of dysfunctional labor. These factors may include anxiety or fear, a complication of pregnancy, or previous labor complications. The initial physical assessment and ongoing assessments provide information about maternal well-being; status of labor in terms of the characteristics of uterine contractions and progress of cervical effacement and dilation; fetal well-being in terms of FHR and pattern, presentation, station, and position; and status of the amniotic membranes.

Laboratory data such as the scalp pH can be used to identify the degree of fetal distress. Ultrasound scanning can identify potential dysfunctional labor problems related to the fetus or maternal pelvis. All these assessments contribute to accurate identification of potential and actual nursing diagnoses related to dystocia and maternal-fetal compromise.

Nursing diagnoses that might be identified in women experiencing dystocia include the following:

- *Risk for maternal or fetal injury related to:*
  –interventions implemented for dystocia
- *Powerlessness related to:*
  –loss of control
- *Risk for infection related to:*
  –PPROM
- *Deficient knowledge related to:*
  –measures that can be used to enhance labor and facilitate birth
- *Ineffective individual coping related to:*
  –inadequate support system.
- *Risk for impaired parent-infant attachment related to:*
  –separation from infant associated with emergency cesarean birth

Expected Outcomes of Care

Expected outcomes for the woman with dystocia include the following. The woman will:

- Understand the causes and treatment of dysfunctional labor.
- Use measures recommended by the health care team to enhance the progress of labor and birth.
- Express relief of pain.
- Experience labor and birth with minimal or no complications, such as infection, injury, or hemorrhage.
- Exhibit diminished or a low level of anxiety.
- Give birth to a healthy infant who has experienced no fetal distress or birth injury.

Plan of Care and Interventions

Nurses assume many caregiving roles when labor is complicated. They also work collaboratively with other health care providers in providing care. Interventions that the nurse may implement or assist with include ECV, trial of labor, cervical ripening with prostaglandins, induction or augmentation with oxytocin, amniotomy, and operative procedures (e.g., forceps- or vacuum-assisted birth). The nursing role is identified with each of the procedures described.

LEGAL TIP Standard of Care—Labor and Birth Complications

- Document all assessment findings, interventions, and client responses on client record, and monitor strips according to unit protocols, procedures, and policies and professional standards.
- Assess whether the woman (and her family, if appropriate) is fully informed about procedures for which she is consenting.
- Provide full explanations regarding what is happening and what needs to be done to help her and her baby (see Guidelines/Guías: Labor and Birth Complications).
- Maintain safety in administering medications and treatments correctly.
- Have verbal orders signed as soon as possible.
- Provide care at the acceptable standard (e.g., according to hospital protocols and professional standards).
- If short staffing occurs in the unit and the nurse is assigned additional clients, the nurse should document that rejecting this additional assignment would have placed these clients in danger as a result of abandonment.
- Maternal and fetal monitoring continues until birth, according to the policies, procedures, and protocols of the birthing facility, even when a decision to carry out cesarean birth is made.

Version

Version is the turning of the fetus from one presentation to another and may be done either externally or internally by the physician.

External Cephalic Version. External cephalic version (ECV) is used to attempt to turn the fetus from a breech or shoulder presentation to a vertex presentation for birth. It may be attempted in a labor and birth setting after 37 weeks of gestation. ECV is accomplished by the exertion of gentle, constant pressure on the abdomen (Fig. 36-9). Before it is attempted, ultrasound scanning is done to determine the fetal position; locate the umbilical cord; rule out placenta previa; evaluate the adequacy of the maternal pelvis; and assess the amount of amniotic fluid, the fetal age, and the presence of any anomalies. A nonstress test (NST) is performed to confirm fetal well-being, or the FHR pattern is monitored for a period of time (i.e., 10 to 20 minutes). Informed consent is obtained. Contraindications to ECV include uterine anomalies, previous cesarean birth, CPD, placenta previa, multifetal gestation, and oligohydramnios (Cunningham et al., 2001; Lanni & Seeds, 2002). ECV performed at term to avoid breech birth is a beneficial form of care (Enkin et al., 2000).

Before the beginning of an attempted ECV, the nurse continuously monitors the FHR and pattern, especially for bradycardia and variable decelerations; checks the maternal vital signs; and assesses the woman's level of comfort because the procedure may cause discomfort. After the procedure is completed, the nurse continues to monitor maternal vital signs, uterine activity, and FHR and pattern, and assess for vaginal bleeding until the woman's condition is stable. Women who are Rh-negative should receive Rh immune globulin because the manipulation can cause fetomaternal bleeding (Cunningham et al., 2001; Lanni & Seeds, 2002).

Internal Version. With internal version, the fetus is turned by the physician who inserts a hand into the uterus and changes the presentation to cephalic (head) or podalic (foot). Internal version may be used in multifetal pregnancies to deliver the second fetus. The safety of this procedure has not been documented; maternal and fetal injury is possible. Cesarean birth is the usual method for managing malpresentation in multifetal pregnancies. The nurse's role is to monitor the status of the fetus and to provide support to the woman.

Trial of Labor

A **trial of labor (TOL)** is the observance of a woman and her fetus for a reasonable period (e.g., 4 to 6 hours) of spontaneous active labor to assess safety of vaginal birth for the mother and infant. It may be initiated if the mother's pelvis is of questionable size or shape, if the fetus is in an abnormal presentation, or if she wishes to have a vaginal birth after a previous cesarean birth. It is a form ❋ of care likely to be beneficial when implemented after a previous low-segment cesarean birth (Enkin et al., 2000). Fetal sonography, maternal pelvimetry, or both may be done before a TOL to rule out CPD. The cervix must be ripe (e.g., soft, dilatable). During a TOL, the woman is evaluated for the occurrence of active labor, including adequate contractions, engagement and descent of the presenting part, and effacement and dilation of the cervix.

The nurse assesses maternal vital signs and FHR and pattern and is alert for signs of potential complications. If complications develop, the nurse is responsible for initiating appropriate actions, including notifying the primary health care provider, and for evaluating and documenting the maternal and fetal responses to the interventions. Nurses must recognize that the woman and her partner are often anxious about her health and well-being and that of their baby. Supporting and encouraging the woman and her partner and providing information regarding progress can reduce stress and enhance the labor process and facilitate a successful outcome.

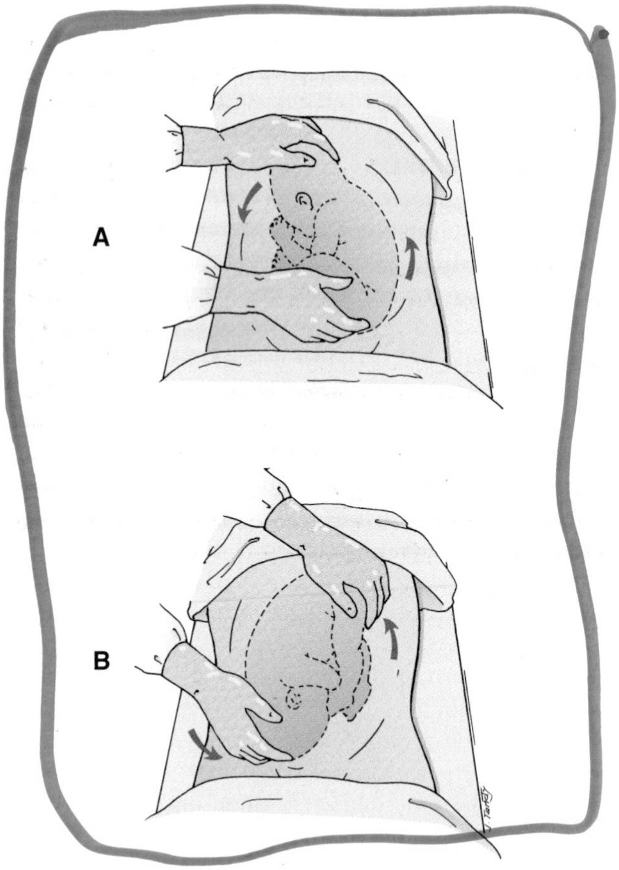
A
B

FIG. 36-9 External version of fetus from breech to vertex presentation. This must be achieved without force. **A,** Breech is pushed up out of pelvic inlet while head is pulled toward inlet. **B,** Head is pushed toward inlet while breech is pulled upward.

Induction of Labor

Induction of labor is the chemical or mechanical initiation of uterine contractions before their spontaneous onset for the purpose of bringing about the birth (see Guidelines/Guías: Labor and Birth Complications). In 2000, approximately 20% of women who gave birth had their labors induced, which is more than twice the labor induction rate of 9% in 1989 (Martin et al., 2002). Induction may be indicated for a variety of medical and obstetric reasons. These include PIH, diabetes mellitus, chorioamnionitis, and other medical problems, PROM, postdate gestation, suspected fetal jeopardy (e.g., IUGR), logistic factors such as history of previous rapid birth or distance of the woman's home from the hospital, and fetal death. Under such conditions, the risk to the mother or fetus is less than the risk of continuing the pregnancy (Mathews, 1998).

Both chemical and mechanical methods are used to induce labor. Intravenous oxytocin and amniotomy are the most common methods used in the United States. Prostaglandins are increasingly used for inducing labor. The most effective protocol (e.g., dose, frequency) to follow when using prostaglandins continues to be investigated (Simpson, 2002).

Less commonly used methods include stripping of membranes, nipple stimulation (manual or with a breast pump), and acupuncture. The ingestion of a laxative (e.g., castor oil), herbal preparations (e.g., green, chamomile, or raspberry tea; blue or black cohosh), or spicy food and administration of a soapsuds enema are other methods (Simpson, 2002; Summers, 1997). Many folk beliefs exist regarding methods to induce labor. These methods include activity (e.g., walking, exercise, strenuous work, intercourse), fasting, and increasing stress (e.g., frightening the woman). It is important for the nurse to know the practices a woman may believe in and follow, because some of these methods can be harmful (e.g., strenuous activity) (Schaffir, 2002).

Success rates for induction of labor are higher when the condition of the cervix is favorable, or inducible. A rating system such as the Bishop score (Table 36-4) can be used to evaluate inducibility. For example, a score of 9 or more on this 13-point scale indicates that the cervix is soft, anterior, 50% or more effaced, and dilated 2 cm or more; and that the presenting part is engaged. Induction of labor is likely to be more successful if the score is 9 or more for nulliparas and 5 or more for multiparas (Cunningham et al., 2001; Gilbert & Harmon, 2003; Simpson, 2002).

Cervical Ripening Methods

Chemical Agents. A prostaglandin E_2 gel (a cervical ripening agent) has been approved by the FDA since 1993. Preparations of prostaglandin E_1 and prostaglandin E_2 can be used before induction to "ripen" (soften and thin) the cervix (see Medication Guides). This treatment usually results in a higher success rate for the induction of labor, the need for lower dosages of oxytocin during the induction, and shorter induction times. The use of prostaglandins to increase cervical readiness for induction of labor is a beneficial form of care (Enkin et al., 2000). In some cases, women will go into labor after the administration of prostaglandin, thereby eliminating the need to administer oxytocin to induce labor (ACOG, 1999b; Gilbert & Harmon, 2003; Simpson, 2002; Summers, 1997; Wilson, 2000). Prostaglandin E_1, although less expensive and more effective than oxytocin or prostaglandin E_2 for inducing labor and birth, is associated with a higher risk for hyperstimulation of the uterus and nonreassuring changes in FHR and pattern (Goldberg, Greenberg, & Darney, 2001).

Mechanical Methods. Mechanical dilators ripen the cervix by stimulating the release of endogenous prostaglandins. Their use is a form of care with a trade-off between beneficial and adverse effects (Enkin et al., 2000). Balloon catheters (e.g., Foley catheter) can be inserted into the intracervical canal to ripen and dilate the cervix. Hydroscopic dilators (substances that absorb fluid from surrounding tissues and then enlarge) also can be used for cervical ripening. Laminaria tents (natural cervical dilators made from desiccated seaweed) and synthetic dilators containing magnesium sulfate (Lamicel) are inserted into the endocervix without rupturing the membranes. As they absorb fluid, they expand and cause cervical dilation. These dilators are left in place for 6 to 12 hours before being removed to assess cervical dilation. Fresh dilators are inserted if further cervical dilation is necessary. Synthetic dilators swell faster than natural dilators and become larger with less discomfort (ACOG, 1999b; Simpson, 2002). Amniotomy and membrane stripping also can be used to ripen the cervix (Norwitz, Robinson, & Repke, 2002).

Hydroscopic dilators compare favorably with prostaglandins in terms of their effectiveness in ripening the cervix but are associated with increased discomfort at insertion and during expansion and with a higher incidence of postpartum maternal and newborn infections. They are a reliable alternative when prostaglandins are contraindicated or are unavailable. Nursing responsibilities for women who have dilators inserted include documenting the number of dilators and sponges inserted during the procedure, as well as the number removed, and assessment for urinary retention, rupture of membranes, uterine tenderness/pain, contractions, vaginal bleeding, and fetal distress (Gilbert & Harmon, 2003; Norwitz et al., 2002; Simpson, 2002).

GUIDELINES/GUÍAS

Labor and Birth Complications

INDUCTION OF LABOR

Your labor is not progressing.
Su trabajo de parto no está progresando.

We need to stimulate the contractions.
Necesitamos provocar las contracciones.

I'm going to give you some medication to make your contractions stronger.
Le voy a dar una medicina para hacerle mas fuertes las contracciones.

I'm going to give you Pitocin through your IV.
Le voy a dar pitufina por medio del suero.

CESAREAN BIRTH

You need a cesarean.
Necesita una operación cesárea.

Do you understand why you need a cesarean?
¿Entiende usted por qué necesita una operación cesárea?

Please sign this consent form.
Por favor, firme esta forma de consentimiento.

TABLE 36-4 **Bishop Score**

	SCORE			
	0	1	2	3
Dilation (cm)	Closed	1-2	3-4	≥5
Effacement (%)	0-30	40-50	60-70	≥80
Station (cm)	−3	−2	−1, 0	+1, +2
Cervical consistency	Firm	Medium	Soft	
Cervix position	Posterior	Midposition	Anterior	

MEDICATION GUIDE

Cervical Ripening Using Prostaglandin E_1 (PGE_1): Misoprostol (Cytotec)

ACTION ▪ PGE_1 ripens the cervix, making it softer and causing it to begin to dilate and efface; stimulates uterine contractions.

INDICATIONS ▪ PGE_1 is used for preinduction cervical ripening (ripen cervix before oxytocin induction of labor when the Bishop score is ≤4) and to induce labor or abortion (abortifacient agent).

DOSAGE ▪ Insert 25 to 50 μg (¼ to ½ of a 100-μg tablet) intravaginally into the posterior fornix using the tips of index and middle fingers without the use of a lubricant. Repeat every 3 to 6 hr as needed to a maximum of 300 to 400 mg in a 24-hr period or until an effective contraction pattern is established (3 or more uterine contractions in 10 min), cervix ripens (Bishop score of ≥8), or significant adverse reactions occur. Administer: 50-100 μg, PO q4-6h (GI effects increased; there are insufficient data to support effectiveness, therefore oral administration is generally not recommended.)

ADVERSE REACTIONS ▪ Higher dosages are more likely to result in adverse reactions such as nausea and vomiting, diarrhea, fever, tachysystole (12 or more uterine contractions in 20 min without alteration of FHR pattern), hyperstimulation of the uterus (tachysystole with nonreassuring FHR patterns), or fetal passage of meconium. Risk for adverse reactions is reduced with lower dosages (i.e., 25 μg) and longer intervals between doses (i.e., q6h).

NURSING CONSIDERATIONS ▪ Explain procedure to woman and her family. Ensure that an informed consent has been obtained as per agency policy. Assess maternal-fetal unit, before each insertion and during treatment following agency protocol for frequency. Assess maternal vital signs and health status, FHR pattern, and status of pregnancy, including indications for cervical ripening or induction of labor, signs of labor or impending labor, and the Bishop score. Recognize that a nonreassuring FHR pattern; maternal fever, infection, vaginal bleeding, or hypersensitivity; and regular, progressive uterine contractions and history of cesarean birth or uterine scar; contraindicate the use of misoprostol. Use caution if the woman has a history of asthma, glaucoma, or renal, hepatic, or cardiovascular disorders. Have woman void before procedure. Assist woman to maintain a supine position with lateral tilt or a side-lying position for 30 to 40 min after insertion. Prepare to swab vagina to remove unabsorbed medication using a saline soaked gauze wrapped around fingers and to administer terbutaline 0.25 mg subcutaneously or intravenously if significant adverse reactions occur. Initiate oxytocin for induction of labor at least 4 hr after last dose of misoprostol was administered, following agency protocol, if ripening has occurred and labor has not begun. Document all assessment findings and administration procedures. Misoprostol (Cytotec) has not yet been approved by the FDA for cervical ripening or labor induction. It is a nonscored 100-μg tablet that must be cut in the pharmacy to ensure dosage accuracy.

MEDICATION GUIDE

Cervical Ripening Using Prostaglandin E_2 (PGE_2): Dinoprostone (Cervidil Insert; Prepidil Gel)

ACTION ▪ PGE_2 ripens the cervix, making it softer and causing it to begin to dilate and efface; stimulates uterine contractions.

INDICATIONS ▪ PGE_2 is used for preinduction cervical ripening (ripen cervix before oxytocin induction of labor when the Bishop score is ≤4), and to induce labor or abortion (abortifacient agent).

DOSAGE ▪ Place Cervidil insert (10 mg dinoprostone gradually released over 12 hr) intravaginally into the posterior fornix. Insert Prepidil gel (2.5-ml syringe containing 0.5 mg of dinoprostone) into cervical canal just below internal cervical os or into posterior fornix, a shield can be used to prevent insertion past internal os. Repeat gel insertion in 6 hr as needed to a maximum of 1.5 mg in a 24-hr period. Continue treatment until maximum dosage is administered or until an effective contraction pattern is established (3 or more uterine contractions in 10 min), cervix ripens (Bishop score of ≥8), or significant adverse reactions occur.

ADVERSE REACTIONS ▪ Potential adverse reactions include headache, nausea and vomiting, diarrhea, fever, hypotension, tachysystole (12 or more uterine contractions in 20 min without alteration of FHR pattern), hyperstimulation of the uterus (tachysystole with nonreassuring FHR patterns), or fetal passage of meconium. Adverse reactions are more common with intracervical administration.

NURSING CONSIDERATIONS ▪ Explain procedure to woman and her family. Ensure that an informed consent has been obtained as per agency policy. Assess maternal-fetal unit, before each insertion and during treatment following agency protocol for frequency. Assess maternal vital signs and health status, FHR pattern, and status of pregnancy, including indications for cervical ripening or induction of labor, signs of labor or impending labor, and the Bishop score. Recognize that a nonreassuring FHR pattern; maternal fever, infection, vaginal bleeding, or hypersensitivity; and regular, progressive uterine contractions and history of cesarean birth or uterine scar; contraindicate the use of dinoprostone. Use caution if the woman has a history of asthma; glaucoma; or renal, hepatic, or cardiovascular disorders. Bring gel to room temperature before administration. Do not force warming process by using a warm water bath or other source of external heat (e.g., microwave). Keep insert frozen until use (no rewarming needed). Have woman void before insertion. Assist woman to maintain a supine position with lateral tilt or a side-lying position for 30 to 60 min after insertion of gel or for 2 hr after placement of insert. Allow woman to ambulate after recommended period of bed rest and observation. Prepare to swab vagina to remove remaining gel using a saline-soaked gauze wrapped around fingers or pull string to remove insert and to administer terbutaline 0.25 mg subcutaneously or intravenously if significant adverse reactions occur. Initiate oxytocin for induction of labor within 6 to 12 hr after last instillation of gel or at least 30 to 60 min after removal of the insert. Follow agency protocol for induction if ripening has occurred and labor has not begun. Document all assessment findings and administration procedures. Dinoprostone is the only FDA-approved medication for cervical ripening or labor induction.

Amniotomy

Amniotomy (i.e., artificial rupture of membranes [AROM]) can be used to induce labor when the condition of the cervix is favorable (ripe) or to augment labor if progress begins to slow. Labor usually begins within 12 hours of the rupture; the duration of labor is decreased by up to 2 hours, especially if combined with oxytocin administration. However, if amniotomy does not stimulate labor, the resulting prolonged rupture may lead to infection and malposition of the fetus. Once an amniotomy is performed, the woman is committed to giving birth. For this reason, amniotomy often is used in combination with oxytocin induction. Evidence from controlled trials clearly demonstrates that amniotomy combined with oxytocin for induction is more effective than either amniotomy or oxytocin alone and is therefore a beneficial form of care (Enkin et al., 2000). Before the procedure, the woman should be told what to expect; she also should be assured that the actual rupture of the membranes is painless for her and the fetus, although she may experience some discomfort when the Amnihook or other sharp instrument is inserted through the vagina and cervix (see Procedure box).

The presenting part of the fetus should be engaged and well applied to the cervix to prevent cord prolapse. The woman should be free of active infection of the genital tract (e.g., herpes) and human immunodeficiency virus (HIV) infection (Norwitz et al., 2002; Summers, 1997). The membranes are ruptured with an Amnihook or other sharp instrument and the amniotic fluid allowed to drain slowly. The color, odor, and consistency of the fluid is assessed (i.e., for the presence or absence of meconium or blood). The time of rupture is recorded.

NURSE ALERT

The FHR is assessed before and immediately after the amniotomy to detect any changes (e.g., transient tachycardia is common, but bradycardia and variable decelerations are not) that may indicate cord compression or prolapse.

The woman's temperature should be checked at least every 2 hours to rule out possible infection. If her temperature is 38° C or higher, the primary health care provider should be notified. The nurse assesses for other signs and symptoms of infection, such as maternal chills, uterine tenderness on palpation, foul-smelling vaginal drainage, and fetal tachycardia (Simpson, 2002). Comfort measures, such as frequently changing the woman's underpads and perineal cleansing, are implemented.

Oxytocin

Oxytocin is a hormone normally produced by the posterior pituitary gland; it stimulates uterine contractions. It may be used either to induce labor or to augment a labor that is progressing slowly because of inadequate uterine contractions.

The indications for oxytocin induction or augmentation of labor may include, but are not limited to, the following:

- Suspected fetal jeopardy (e.g., IUGR)
- Inadequate uterine contractions; dystocia
- PROM
- Postterm pregnancy
- Chorioamnionitis
- Maternal medical problems (e.g., woman with severe Rh isoimmunization, inadequately controlled diabetes mellitus, chronic renal disease, or chronic pulmonary disease)
- PIH (e.g., eclampsia)
- Fetal death
- Multiparous women with a history of precipitate labor or who live far from the hospital

The management of stimulation of labor is the same regardless of the indication. Because of the potential dangers associated with the injection of oxytocin in the prenatal and intrapartal periods, the FDA has issued certain restrictions to its use.

Contraindications to oxytocin stimulation of labor include, but are not limited to, the following:

- CPD, prolapsed cord, transverse lie
- Nonreassuring FHR

PROCEDURE

Assisting with Amniotomy

PROCEDURE

Explain to the woman what will be done.

Assess woman for signs of infection, condition of cervix (e.g., ripeness, dilation), and station of the presenting part.

Assess FHR before procedure begins to obtain a baseline reading.

Place several underpads under the woman's buttocks to absorb the fluid.

Position the woman on a padded bed pan, fracture pan, or rolled up towel to elevate her hips.

Assist the health care provider who is performing the procedure by providing sterile gloves and lubricant for the vaginal examination.

Unwrap sterile package containing Amnihook or Allis clamp and pass instrument to the primary health care provider, who inserts it alongside the fingers and then hooks and tears the membranes.

Reassess the FHR and pattern.

Assess the color, consistency, and odor of the fluid.

Assess the woman's temperature every 2 hours or per protocol.

Evaluate the woman for signs and symptoms of infection.

DOCUMENTATION

Record the following:

- Indication for amniotomy
- Time of rupture
- Color, odor, consistency and clarity of the fluid
- FHR and pattern before and after the procedure
- Maternal status and how well procedure was tolerated

- Placenta previa or vasa previa
- Prior classic uterine incision or uterine surgery
- Active genital herpes infection
- Invasive cancer of the cervix

Certain maternal and fetal conditions, although not contraindications to the use of oxytocin to stimulate labor, do require special caution during its administration. These conditions include the following:

- Multifetal presentation
- Breech presentation
- Presenting part above the pelvic inlet
- Abnormal FHR pattern not requiring emergency birth
- Polyhydramnios
- Grand multiparity
- Maternal cardiac disease; hypertension

Oxytocin use can present hazards to the mother and fetus. These hazards are primarily dose related, with most problems caused by high doses that are given rapidly. Maternal hazards include water intoxication and tumultuous labor with tetanic contractions, which may cause premature separation of the placenta, rupture of the uterus, lacerations of the cervix, or postpartum hemorrhage. These complications can lead to infection, disseminated intravascular coagulation, or amniotic fluid embolism. Women may become anxious or fearful if the induction is not successful because they may then have concerns about the method of birth.

Uterine hyperstimulation reduces the blood flow through the placenta and results in FHR decelerations (bradycardia, diminished variability, late decelerations), fetal asphyxia, and neonatal hypoxia. If the estimated date of birth is inaccurate, physical injury, neonatal hyperbilirubinemia, and prematurity are other hazards.

The primary health care provider writes the order for the induction or augmentation of labor with oxytocin. The nurse implements the order by initiating the primary intravenous infusion and administering the oxytocin solution through a secondary line. The nurse's actions related to assessment and care of a woman whose labor is being induced are guided by hospital protocol and professional standards (Fig. 36-10; Box 36-8).

In the past, the aim of induction was to achieve a contraction pattern that simulates the active phase of labor as quickly as possible. However, research on uterine tolerance to oxytocin has now shown that lower physiologic doses (e.g., initial dose of 0.5 to 1 mU/min with increments of 1 to 2 mU/min) given over a longer time are as effective as previous protocols. A recommended dosage increment frequency is every 30 to 60 minutes because 30 to 40 minutes is required for a steady state of oxytocin to be reached and for the full effect of a dosage increment to be reflected in more intense, frequent, and longer contractions. Such an approach reduces the amount of oxytocin required to achieve a spontaneous vaginal birth and decreases the risk for uterine hyperstimulation, dysfunctional labor, fetal distress, and other adverse reactions such as water intoxication (ACOG, 1999b; Norwitz et al., 2002; Simpson, 2002; Summers, 1997).

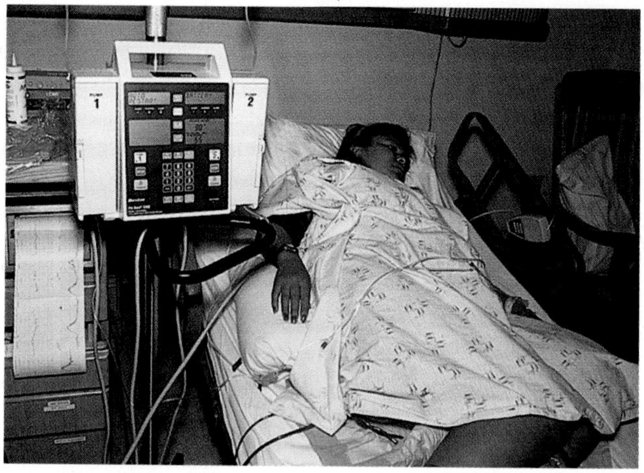

FIG. 36-10 Woman in side-lying position receiving oxytocin. (Courtesy Michael S. Clement, MD, Mesa, AZ)

Nursing Considerations. An evidence-based written protocol for the preparation and administration of oxytocin should be established by the obstetric department (physicians, nurses) in each institution. The procedure recommended for a woman who is eligible for induction of labor is discussed in Box 36-8.

NURSE ALERT

Oxytocin is discontinued immediately and the primary health care provider notified if uterine hyperstimulation, nonreassuring FHR and pattern, or both occur.

Other nursing interventions, such as administering oxygen by face mask, positioning the woman on her side, and infusing more intravenous fluids are implemented immediately (see Emergency box). Based on the status of the maternal-fetal unit, the primary health care provider may order that the infusion be restarted once the FHR and uterine activity return to acceptable levels. Depending on the length of time the infusion was discontinued, the induction may be restarted at half the rate that resulted in hyperstimulation (e.g., discontinued for 10 to 20 minutes) or at the same rate as the initial rate (e.g., discontinued for more than 30 to 40 minutes) (ACOG, 1999b; Simpson, 2002) (see Plan of Care: Dysfunctional Labor).

Augmentation of Labor

Augmentation of labor is the stimulation of uterine contractions after labor has started spontaneously but progress is unsatisfactory. Augmentation is usually implemented for the management of hypotonic uterine dysfunction, resulting in a slowing of the labor process (protracted active phase). Common augmentation methods

BOX 36-8 Protocol: Induction of Labor with Oxytocin

CLIENT/FAMILY TEACHING

Explain technique, rationale, and reactions to expect:

- Route and rate for administration of medication
- What "piggyback" is for
- Reasons for use:
  Induce labor, improve labor
- Reactions to expect concerning the nature of contractions: the intensity of contraction increases more rapidly, holds the peak longer, and ends more quickly; contractions will come regularly and more often
- Monitoring to anticipate:
  Maternal: blood pressure, pulse, uterine contractions, uterine tone
  Fetal: heart rate, activity/movements
- Success to expect: a favorable outcome will depend on inducibility of the cervix (e.g., Bishop score of 9)
- Keep woman and support person informed of progress

ADMINISTRATION

Position woman in side-lying or upright position

Assess status of maternal fetal unit

Prepare solution and administer with pump delivery system according to prescribed orders:

- Infusion pump and solution are set up (e.g., 10 U/1000 ml isotonic electrolyte solution)
- Piggyback solution is connected to IV line at proximal port (port nearest point of venous insertion)
- Solution with oxytocin is flagged with a medication label
- Begin induction at 0.5 to 2 mU/min
- Increase dose 1 to 2 mU/min at intervals of 30 to 60 min until a dose of up to 20 to 40 mU/min is reached

MAINTAIN DOSE IF

- Intensity of contractions results in intrauterine pressures of 40 to 90 mm Hg (shown by internal monitor)
- Duration of contractions is 60 to 90 sec
- Frequency of contractions is 2- to 3-min intervals
- Resting tone of 10 to 15 mm Hg
- Cervical dilation of 1 cm/hr in the active phase

MATERNAL/FETAL ASSESSMENTS

- Monitor blood pressure, pulse, and respirations every 30 to 60 min and with every increment in dose
- Monitor contraction pattern and uterine resting tone every 15 min and with every increment in dose
- Assess intake and output; limit IV intake to 1000 ml/8 hr; output should be 120 ml or more every 4 hr
- Perform vaginal examination as indicated
- Monitor for nausea, vomiting, headache, hypotension
- Assess fetal status using electronic fetal monitoring; evaluate tracing every 15 min and with every increment in dose
- Observe emotional responses of woman and her partner

REPORTABLE CONDITIONS

- Uterine hyperstimulation
- Nonreassuring FHR and pattern
- Suspected uterine rupture
- Inadequate uterine response at 20 mU/min

EMERGENCY MEASURES

Discontinue use of oxytocin per hospital protocol:

- Turn woman on her side
- Increase primary IV rate up to 200 ml/hr, unless woman has water intoxication, in which case, the rate is decreased to one that keeps the vein open
- Give woman oxygen by face mask at 8 to 10 L/min or per protocol or primary health care provider's order

DOCUMENTATION

- Medication: kind, amount, time of beginning, increasing dose, maintaining dose, and discontinuing medication
- Reactions of mother and fetus
  Pattern of labor
  Progress of labor
  FHR and pattern
  Maternal vital signs
  Nursing interventions and woman's response
- Notification of physician or nurse-midwife

From American College of Obstetricians and Gynecologists. (1999b). Induction of labor. *ACOG Practice Bulletin No. 10.* Washington, DC: ACOG; Pozaic, S. (1999). Induction and augmentation of labor. In L. Mandeville & N. Troiano (Eds.), *High-risk and critical care intrapartum nursing* (2nd ed.). Philadelphia: Lippincott; Simpson, K. (2002). *Cervical ripening and induction and augmentation of labor.* (2nd ed.). Washington, DC: AWHONN; and Summers, L. (1997). Methods of cervical ripening and labor induction. *Journal of Nurse Midwifery, 42*(2), 71-85.

include oxytocin infusion, amniotomy, and nipple stimulation. Noninvasive methods such as emptying the bladder, ambulation and position changes, relaxation measures, nourishment and hydration, and hydrotherapy should be attempted before invasive interventions are initiated. The administration procedure and nursing assessment and care measures for augmentation of labor with oxytocin are similar to those used for induction of labor with oxytocin; protocols for dosage and frequency of increments may vary (e.g., lower dosages may be needed to

EMERGENCY

Uterine Hyperstimulation with Oxytocin

SIGNS

Uterine contractions lasting >90 sec and occurring more frequently than every 2 min
Uterine resting tone >20 mm Hg
Nonreassuring FHR and pattern:
- Abnormal baseline (<110 or >160 beats/min)
- Absent variability
- Repeated late decelerations or prolonged decelerations

INTERVENTIONS

Maintain woman in side-lying position
Turn off oxytocin infusion; keep maintenance IV line open; increase rate
Start administering oxygen by face mask, per protocol or physician's order
Notify primary health care provider
Prepare to administer terbutaline (Brethine) 0.25 mg subcutaneously if ordered to decrease uterine activity
Continue monitoring FHR and pattern and uterine activity
Document responses to actions

achieve spontaneous vaginal birth (Gilbert & Harmon, 2003; Pozaic, 1999; Simpson, 2002).

Some physicians advocate active management of labor, that is, the augmentation of labor to establish efficient labor with the aggressive use of oxytocin so that the woman gives birth within 12 hours of admission to the labor unit. Advocates of active management believe that intervening early (as soon as a nulliparous labor is not progressing at least 1 cm/hr) with use of higher pharmacologic oxytocin doses administered at frequent increment intervals (e.g., a starting dose of 6 mU/min with increases of 6 mU/min every 15 minutes to a maximum dose of 40 mU/min) shortens labor and is associated with a lower incidence of cesarean birth (Norwitz et al., 2002; Simpson, 2002).

Additional components of the active management of labor include strict criteria to diagnose that the woman is in active labor with 100% effacement, amniotomy within 1 hour of admission of a woman in labor if spontaneous rupture of the membranes has not occurred, and continuous presence of a personal nurse who provides one-on-one care for the woman while she is in labor. When all components are fully implemented, active management of labor is associated with a lower incidence of cesarean birth. Active management of labor continues to be under study in the United States to determine effectiveness and impact on perinatal morbidity and mortality. Thus far results have been disappointing, especially in terms of reducing the rate of cesarean births. The disappointing results have been attributed, in part, to a greater than one-to-one nurse patient ratio and the high rate of epidural anesthesia. It is considered to be a form of care of unknown effectiveness (Enkin et al., 2000; Gilbert & Harmon, 2003; Simpson, 2000).

Forceps-Assisted Birth

A **forceps-assisted birth** is one in which an instrument with two curved blades is used to assist in the birth of the fetal head. The cephalic-like curve of the forceps commonly used is similar to the shape of the fetal head, with a pelvic curve to the blades conforming to the curve of the pelvic axis. The blades are joined by a pin, screw, or groove arrangement. These locks prevent the forceps from compressing the fetal skull. Maternal indications for forceps-assisted birth include the need to shorten the second stage of labor in the event of dystocia or to compensate for the woman's deficient expulsive efforts (e.g., if she is tired or has been given spinal or epidural anesthesia), or to reverse a dangerous condition (e.g., cardiac decompensation).

Fetal indications include birth of a fetus in distress or in certain abnormal presentations; arrest of rotation; or delivery of the head in a breech presentation. The use of forceps during childbirth has been decreasing. In 1999, forceps were used to assist 2.3% of births compared with 5.5% in 1989 (Ventura et al., 2001).

Certain conditions are required for a forceps-assisted birth to be successful. The woman's cervix must be fully dilated to avert lacerations and hemorrhage. The bladder should be empty. The presenting part must be engaged, and a vertex presentation is desired. Membranes must be ruptured so that the position of the fetal head can be determined and the forceps can firmly grasp the head during birth. In addition, CPD should not be present.

Different definitions of forceps applications are found. *Outlet forceps* are used if the fetal scalp is visible on the perineum without manually separating the labia (Fig. 36-11). Outlet forceps are used to shorten the second stage of labor. *Low forceps* refers to the application of forceps to the fetal head that is at least at the +2-cm station. *Midforceps* refers to the application of forceps to the fetal head that is engaged (no higher than station 0) but above the +2 station. In no instances should forceps be applied to an unengaged presenting part.

Nursing Considerations. When a forceps-assisted birth is deemed necessary, the nurse obtains the type of forceps requested by the primary health care provider (Fig. 36-12). The nurse may explain to the mother that the forceps blades fit like two tablespoons around an egg, with the blades coming over the baby's ears.

NURSE ALERT

Because compression of the cord between the fetal head and the forceps will cause a decrease in FHR, the FHR and pattern is assessed, reported, and recorded before and after application of the forceps.

If a decrease in FHR occurs, the primary health care provider removes and reapplies the forceps. Ordinarily traction is applied during contractions.

After birth, the mother is assessed for vaginal and cervical lacerations (e.g., bleeding that occurs even with a

Plan of Care: Dysfunctional Labor: Hypotonic Uterine Dysfunction with Protracted Active Phase

NURSING DIAGNOSIS Risk for injury to mother and/or fetus related to oxytocin augmentation secondary to dysfunctional labor

Expected Outcomes *Maternal-fetal well-being is maintained; labor progresses and birth occurs.*

Nursing Interventions/*Rationales*

Explain oxytocin protocol to woman and her labor partner *to allay apprehension and enhance participation.*

Encourage woman to void before beginning protocol *to prevent discomfort and remove a barrier to labor progress.*

Apply the electronic fetal monitor per hospital protocol and obtain a 15- to 20-min baseline strip *to ensure adequate assessment of FHR and contractions.*

Position woman in a side-lying position and administer the oxytocin per physician order using an IV infusion pump *to stimulate uterine activity and provide adequate control of the flow rate.*

Regulate the oxytocin per protocol (e.g., advancing the dose in increments of 1 to 2 mU/min every 30 to 60 min) *to allow adequate evaluation of the woman's response to stimulation and to prevent hyperstimulation and fetal hypoxia.*

Maintain oxytocin dose and rate when contractions occur every 2 to 3 min with a duration of 40 to 90 sec and intrauterine pressures of 60 to 90 mm Hg (if internal monitoring is used) *to produce effective uterine stimulation without risk of hyperstimulation.*

Monitor maternal vital signs every 30 to 60 min *to assess for oxytocin-induced hypertension.*

Monitor contractility pattern and FHR and pattern every 15 min *to assess uterine activity for possible hypertonicity or ineffective uterine response to oxytocin and to detect evidence of fetal distress.*

Monitor intake, output, and specific gravity (limit intake to 1000 ml/8 hr; output should be at least 120 ml/4 hr) *to assess for urinary retention and prevent water intoxication.*

Monitor cervical dilation, effacement, and station *to assess progress of labor.*

If hypertonicity or signs of fetal distress are detected, discontinue oxytocin immediately *to arrest the progress of hypertonicity;* turn woman on her side *to increase placental blood flow;* increase primary IV rate to 200 ml/hr (unless signs of water toxicity are present); administer oxygen per face mask *to enhance placental perfusion;* notify primary health care provider; and continuously monitor maternal vital signs and FHR *to provide ongoing assessment of maternal/fetal status.*

Maintain standard precautions and use scrupulous handwashing techniques when providing care *to prevent the spread of infection.*

NURSING DIAGNOSIS Acute pain related to increasing frequency, regularity, intensity, and prolonged peak of contractions

Expected Outcome *The woman exhibits signs of decreased discomfort.*

Nursing Interventions/*Rationales*

Prepare woman and labor partner for the change in the nature of the contractions once the oxytocin drip is initiated *to prepare them and allow for more effective coping.*

Review the use of specific techniques such as conscious relaxation, focused breathing, effleurage, massage, and application of sacral pressure *to increase relaxation, decrease intensity of pain of contractions, and promote use of controlled thought and direction of energy.*

Provide comfort measures such as frequent mouth care *to prevent dry mouth,* application of damp cloth to forehead and changing of damp gown or bed covers *to relieve discomfort of diaphoresis,* and positioning *to reduce stiffness.*

Encourage conscious relaxation between contractions *to prevent fatigue, which contributes to increased pain perceptions.*

Remind woman and labor partner that analgesics are available for use during labor *to provide knowledge to help them make decisions about pain control.*

NURSING DIAGNOSIS Anxiety related to prolonged labor, increased pain, and fatigue

Expected Outcomes *Woman's anxiety is reduced; woman actively participates in the labor process.*

Nursing Interventions/*Rationales*

Provide ongoing feedback to woman and partner *to allay anxiety and enhance participation.*

Present care options when possible *to increase feelings of control.*

Continue to provide comfort measures *to maintain a posture of support and caring and to aid woman in focusing on the labor process.*

Encourage woman and partner to continue to use those mechanisms that promote effective labor (e.g., breathing, activity, positioning) *to keep woman and partner actively involved in process.*

contracted uterus); urine retention, which may result from bladder or urethral injuries; and hematoma formation in the pelvic soft tissues, which may result from blood vessel damage. The infant should be assessed for bruising or abrasions at the site of the blade applications, facial palsy resulting from pressure of the blades on the facial nerve (cranial nerve VII), and subdural hematoma. Newborn and postpartum caregivers should be told that a forceps-assisted birth was performed.

Vacuum-Assisted Birth

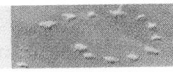

Vacuum-assisted birth, or vacuum extraction, is a birth method involving the attachment of a vacuum cup to the fetal head, using negative pressure to assist in the birth of the head. Indications for its use are similar to those for outlet forceps. Prerequisites for use include a vertex presentation, ruptured membranes, and absence of CPD (Cunningham et al., 2001). When an operative vaginal birth is required, vacuum assistance is preferred as a beneficial form of care when compared with forceps assistance (Enkin et al, 2002).

When the birth is to be vacuum assisted, the woman is prepared for a vaginal birth in the lithotomy position to allow sufficient traction. The cup is applied to the fetal head, and a caput develops inside the cup as the pressure is initiated (Fig. 36-13). Traction is applied to facilitate descent of the fetal head, and the woman is encouraged to push as suction is applied. As the head crowns, an episiotomy is performed if necessary. The vacuum cup is released and removed after birth of the head. If vacuum extraction is not successful, a forceps-assisted or cesarean birth is then performed.

Risks to the newborn include cephalhematoma, scalp lacerations, and subdural hematoma. Fetal complications can be reduced by strict adherence to the manufacturer's recommendations for method of application, degree of suction, and duration of application. Maternal complications are uncommon but can include perineal, vaginal, or cervical lacerations and soft-tissue hematomas.

Nursing Considerations. The nurse's role for the woman who has a vacuum- assisted birth is one of support person and educator. The nurse can prepare the woman for birth and encourage her to remain active in the birth process by pushing during contractions. The FHR should be assessed frequently during the procedure. After birth, the newborn should be observed for signs of trauma and infection at the application site and for cerebral irritation (e.g., poor sucking or listlessness). The newborn may be at risk for cephalhematoma and neonatal jaundice as bruising resolves. The parents may need to be reassured that the caput succedaneum will begin to disappear in a few hours. Neonatal caregivers should be told that the birth was vacuum assisted.

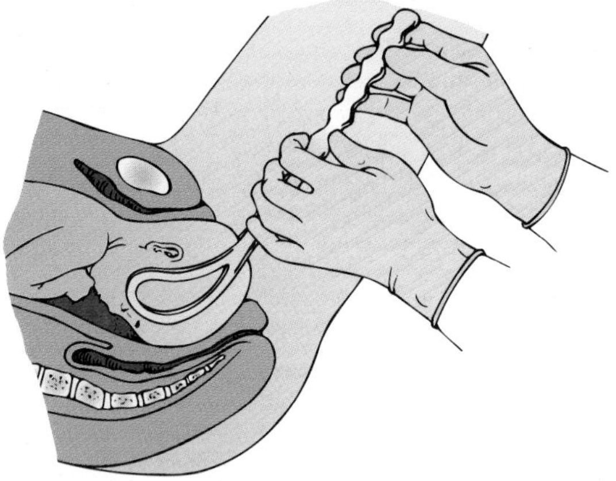

FIG. 36-11 Outlet forceps-assisted extraction of the head.

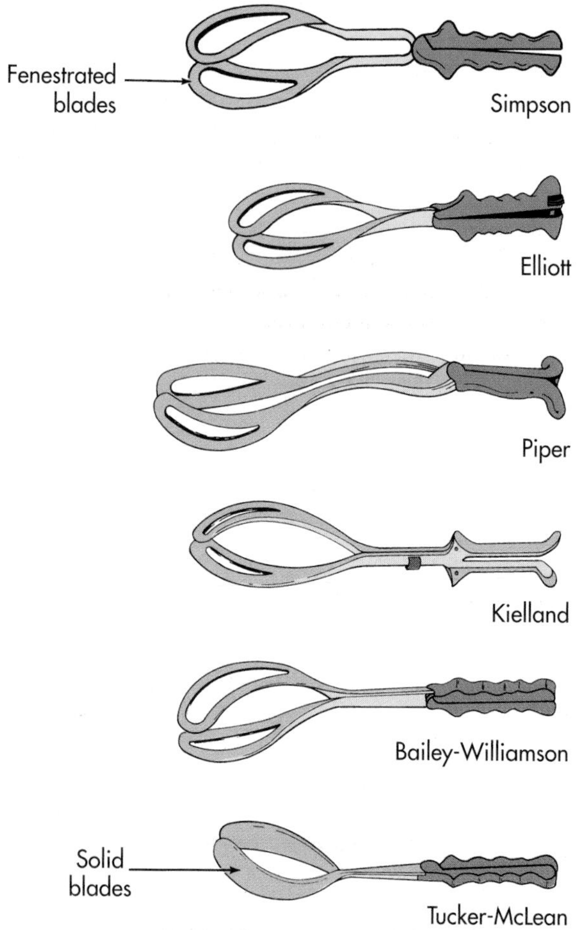
Fenestrated blades
Simpson
Elliott
Piper
Kielland
Bailey-Williamson
Solid blades
Tucker-McLean

FIG. 36-12 Types of forceps. Piper forceps are used to assist delivery of the head in a breech birth.

Cesarean Birth

Cesarean birth is the birth of a fetus through a transabdominal incision of the uterus. Whether cesarean birth is planned (scheduled) or unplanned (emergency), the loss of the experience of giving birth to a child in the traditional manner may have a negative effect on a woman's self-concept. An effort is therefore made to maintain the focus on the birth of a child rather than on the operative procedure.

The purpose of cesarean birth is to preserve the life or health of the mother and her fetus; it may be the best choice for birth when there is evidence of maternal or fetal complications. Since the advent of modern surgical methods and care, and the use of antibiotics, maternal and fetal morbidity and mortality have decreased. In addition, incisions are made into the lower uterine segment rather than into the muscular body of the uterus and thus promote more effective healing. However, despite these advances, cesarean birth still poses threats to the health of the mother and infant.

The incidence of cesarean births has increased from less than 5% in 1965 to 22.9% in 2000. Factors cited as sources of this increase include use of electronic fetal monitoring and epidural anesthesia; an increase in the number of first-time pregnancies, as well as pregnancies at an older age; and the high incidence of repeated cesarean births. A recent increase in cesarean birth is most likely associated with a decrease in the rate of vaginal births after cesarean birth (VBAC) (see later discussion). After increasing from 18.9% in 1989 to 28.3% in 1996, the rate of VBACs declined to 20.6% in 2000 (Martin et al., 2002).

In 2000, women age 35 years and older had a cesarean birth rate of more than 30%, approximately twice the rate for women younger than 20 years (Martin et al., 2002). Women who have private insurance, are of a higher socioeconomic status, or deliver in a private hospital are more likely to experience cesarean birth than are women who are poor, have no insurance, are receiving public assistance (e.g., Medicaid), or give birth in public hospitals (Scott, 1999).

Approaches for the management of labor and birth to reduce the rate of cesarean births, while increasing the rate of vaginal births after cesarean (VBAC) are presented in Box 36-9. These management approaches involve the combined efforts of health care professionals and pregnant women and their families (Flamm, Berwick, & Kabcenell, 1998; McNiven et al., 1998).

The type of nursing care given also may influence the rate of cesarean births. Radin, Harmon, and Hanson (1993) found that cesarean rates were lower for women whose nurses provided supportive care during labor. A labor management approach that uses one-to-one support and emphasizes ambulation, maternal position changes, relaxation measures, oral fluids and nutrition, hydrotherapy, and nonpharmacologic pain relief facilitates the progress of labor and reduces the incidence of dystocia (AWHONN, 2000; Hodnett, 2002; Miltner, 2000).

The labor management approach that most consistently reduced cesarean birth rates was one-to-one support of the laboring woman by another woman such as a nurse, nurse midwife, or doula (Cefalo & Bowes, 1998; Gabay & Wolfe, 1997).

Indications. Few absolute indications exist for cesarean birth. Today most are performed primarily for the benefit of the fetus. The most common indications for cesarean birth are related to labor and birth complications. The complications most closely associated with cesarean birth include CPD, malpresentations such as breech and shoulder, placental abnormalities (e.g., previa, abruptio), dysfunctional labor pattern, umbilical cord prolapse, fetal distress, and multiple gestation. Medical risk factors most closely associated with cesarean birth include hypertensive disorders, active genital herpes, positive HIV status, and diabetes (Martin et al., 2002).

Ethical Consideration: Forced Cesarean Birth. A woman's refusal to undergo cesarean birth when indicated for fetal reasons is often described as a maternal-fetal conflict. Health care providers are ethically obliged to protect the wellbeing of both the mother and the fetus; a decision for one affects the other. If a woman refuses a cesarean birth that is recommended because of fetal jeopardy, health care providers must make every effort to find out why she is refusing and provide information that may persuade her to change her mind. If the woman continues to refuse surgery, then health care providers must decide if it is ethical to get a court order for the surgery; however, every effort should be made to avoid this legal step.

Surgical Techniques. The two main types of cesarean operation are the classic and the lower-segment cesarean incisions. Classic cesarean birth is rarely performed today, although it may be used when rapid birth is necessary and in some cases of shoulder presentation and placenta previa. The incision is made vertically into the upper body of the uterus (Fig. 36-14, *A*). Because the procedure is associated with a higher incidence of blood loss, infection, and uterine rupture in subsequent pregnancies than is lower-segment cesarean birth, vaginal birth after a classic cesarean birth is contraindicated.

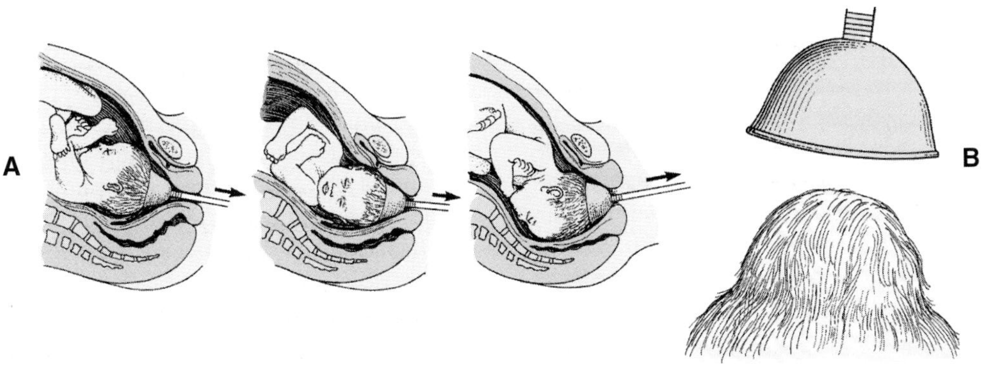
A
B

FIG. 36-13 Use of vacuum extraction to rotate fetal head and assist with descent. **A,** *Arrow* indicates direction of traction on the vacuum cup. **B,** Caput succedaneum formed by the vacuum cup.

BOX 36-9 Selected Measures to Reduce Cesarean Birth Rate and Increase Rate of VBAC

EDUCATE WOMEN REGARDING
- Advantages and safety of the home environment for early or latent labor
- Indicators for hospital admission
- Management techniques to use during labor to enhance progress
- Nonpharmacologic measures to reduce pain and discomfort and enhance relaxation
- Safety and effectiveness of TOL and VBAC

ESTABLISH ADMISSION CRITERIA FOR WOMEN IN LABOR THAT
- Distinguish clinical manifestations for false labor, latent/early labor, and active labor
- Conduct admission assessments in a separate admissions area
- Send women in false or early/latent labor home or keep them in the admissions area
- Admit women in active labor to the labor and birth unit

USE APPROPRIATE ASSESSMENT TECHNIQUES TO
- Determine status of the maternal-fetal unit
- Establish an individualized rationale for initiating labor interventions such as epidural anesthesia, induction/augmentation, amniotomy, cesarean birth

INITIATE A DOULA PROGRAM THAT
- Provides one-to-one support for women in labor

DEVELOP A PHILOSOPHY OF LABOR MANAGEMENT THAT
- Schedules admission during active labor
- Avoids automatic interventions such as routine induction for spontaneous rupture of membranes at term or postterm pregnancy and cesarean birth for breech presentation, twin gestation, genital herpes, or failure to progress
- Relies on assessment findings reflective of the status of the maternal-fetal unit rather than strict adherence to set ranges for the duration of the stages and phases of labor
- Employs intermittent rather than continuous electronic fetal monitoring of low risk pregnant women
- Focuses on measures that are known to enhance the progress of labor such as upright positions, frequent position changes, ambulation, oral nutrition and hydration, relaxation techniques, hydrotherapy
- Emphasizes nonpharmacologic measures to relieve pain
- Uses nonpharmacologic measures in a manner that reduces their labor-inhibiting effects
- Establishes criteria for elective cesarean birth and TOL
- Encourages women who have had a previous cesarean birth to participate in TOL to attempt a vaginal birth

TOL, Trial of labor; *VBAC*, vaginal birth after cesarean.

Lower-segment cesarean birth can be achieved through a vertical or transverse incision into the uterus (Fig. 36-14, *B* and *C*). The transverse incision is more popular, however, because it is easier to perform, is associated with less blood loss and fewer postoperative infections, and is less likely to rupture in subsequent pregnancies (Cunningham et al., 2001; Scott, 1999).

Complications and Risks. Cesarean births are not without complications for the mother and fetus. Maternal complications include aspiration, pulmonary embolism, wound infection, wound dehiscence, thrombophlebitis, hemorrhage, urinary tract infection, injuries to the bladder or bowel, and complications related to anesthesia. The fetus may be born prematurely if the gestational age has not been accurately determined; fetal injuries can occur during the surgery (Scott, 1999). Besides these risks, the woman is at economic risk because the cost of cesarean birth is higher than that of vaginal birth, and a longer recovery period may require additional expenditures.

Many women who have a cesarean birth speak of having feelings that interfere with their maintaining an adequate self-concept. These feelings include fear, disappointment, frustration at losing control, anger (the "why me" syndrome), and loss of self esteem related to a change in body image and perceived inability to give birth as they had expected and hoped. Often women experience a delay in their ability to interact with their newborns after birth. These women are less likely to breastfeed and may even have some difficulty expressing positive feelings about their newborns for some time after birth. They are often less satisfied with their childbirth experience and report more fatigue and poor physical functioning during the first few weeks after discharge. Success at mothering and in the recovery process can do much to restore the self-esteem of these women. Some women see the scar as mutilating, and worries concerning sexual attractiveness may surface. Some men are fearful of resuming intercourse because of the fear of hurting their partners. Parents may wonder if a cesarean birth was absolutely necessary, and such feelings may surface even years later. They should therefore be given opportunities to discuss the experience to try to understand and resolve concerns after the birth.

Anesthesia. Spinal, epidural, and general anesthetics are used for cesarean births. Epidural blocks are popular because women want to be awake for and aware of the

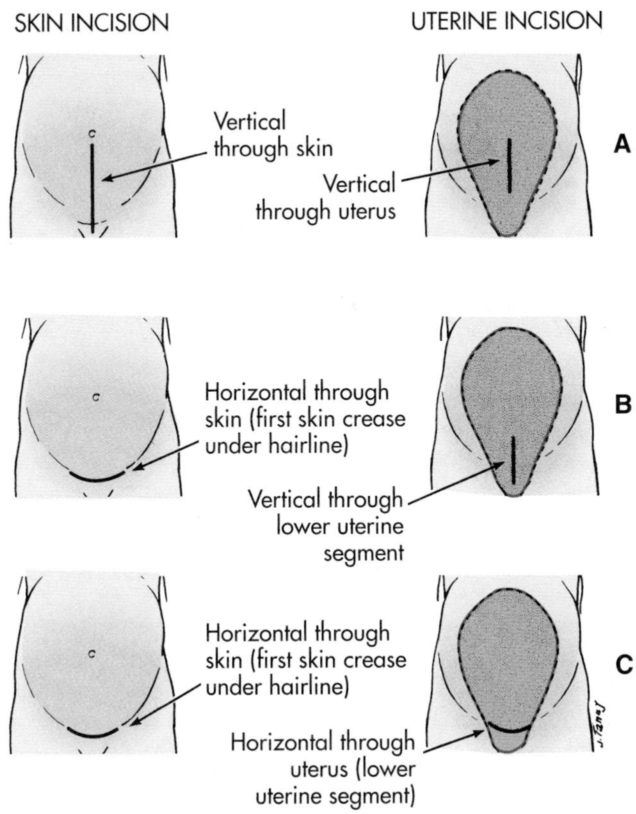
SKIN INCISION
UTERINE INCISION
Vertical through skin
Vertical through uterus
A
Horizontal through skin (first skin crease under hairline)
Vertical through lower uterine segment
B
Horizontal through skin (first skin crease under hairline)
Horizontal through uterus (lower uterine segment)
C

FIG. 36-14 Cesarean birth; skin and uterine incisions. **A,** Classic: vertical incisions of skin and uterus. **B,** Low cervical: horizontal incision of skin; vertical incision of uterus. **C,** Low cervical: horizontal incisions of skin and uterus.

birth experience. However, the choice of anesthetic depends on several factors. The mother's medical history or present condition, such as a spinal injury, hemorrhage, or coagulopathy, may rule out the use of regional anesthesia. Time is another factor, especially if there is an emergency and the life of the mother or infant is at stake. In such a case, general anesthesia will most likely be used unless the woman already has an epidural block in effect. The woman herself is a factor. Either she may not know all the options or may have fears about having "a needle in her back" or about being awake and feeling pain. She needs to be fully informed about the risks and benefits of the different types of anesthesia so that she can participate in the decision whenever there is a choice.

Scheduled Cesarean Birth. Cesarean birth is scheduled or planned if labor and vaginal birth is contraindicated (e.g., complete placenta previa, active genital herpes, positive HIV status), if birth is necessary but labor is not inducible (e.g., hypertensive states that cause a poor intrauterine environment that threatens the fetus), or if this has been decided on by the primary health care provider and the woman (e.g., a repeat cesarean birth).

Women who are scheduled to have a cesarean birth have time to prepare for it psychologically. However, the psychologic responses of these women may differ. Those having a repeat cesarean birth may have disturbing memories of the conditions preceding the initial surgical birth (primary cesarean birth) and of their experiences in the postoperative recovery period. They may be concerned about the added burdens of caring for an infant and perhaps other children while recovering from a surgical operation. Others may feel glad that they have been relieved of the uncertainty about the date and time of the birth and are free of the pain of labor.

Unplanned Cesarean Birth. The psychosocial outcomes of unplanned or emergency cesarean birth are usually more pronounced and negative when compared with the outcomes associated with a scheduled or planned cesarean birth (DiMatteo et al., 1996). Women and their families experience abrupt changes in their expectations for birth, postbirth care, and the care of the new baby at home. This may be an extremely traumatic experience for all.

The woman usually approaches the procedure tired and discouraged after an ineffective and difficult labor. Fear predominates as she worries about her own safety and well-being and that of her fetus. She may be dehydrated, with low glycogen reserves. Because preoperative procedures must be done quickly and competently, the time for explanation of the procedures and operation is often short. Because maternal and family anxiety levels are high at this time, much of what is said may be forgotten or misunderstood. The woman may experience feelings of anger or guilt in the postpartum period. Fatigue is often noticeable in these women, and they need much supportive care.

After surgery, therefore, time must be spent reviewing the events preceding the operation and the operation itself to ensure that the woman understands what has happened and that gaps in her recollections are filled. This approach will help create more realistic memories of the childbirth experience, thereby having a more positive influence on future pregnancies and labors (Ryding, Wijma, & Wijma, 1998).

Prenatal Preparation. Concerned professional and lay groups in the community have established councils for cesarean birth to meet the needs of these women and their families. Such groups advocate that a discussion of cesarean birth be included in all parenthood preparation classes. No woman can be guaranteed a vaginal birth, even if she is in good health and there is no indication of danger to the fetus before the onset of labor. For this reason, every woman needs to be aware of and prepared for this eventuality.

Childbirth educators stress the importance of emphasizing the similarities and differences between a cesarean and vaginal birth. In support of the philosophy of family-centered birth, many hospitals have instituted policies that permit fathers and other partners and family members to share in these births as they do in vaginal ones. Women who have undergone cesarean birth agree that the continued presence and support of their partners helped them respond positively to the entire experience. In addition to preparing women for the possibility of cesarean birth, childbirth educators should empower women to believe in their ability to give birth vaginally and to seek care measures during labor that will enhance the progress of their labors and reduce their risk for cesarean birth.

Preoperative Care. Family-centered care is the goal for the woman who is to undergo cesarean birth and for her family. The preparation of the woman for cesarean birth is the same as that done for other elective or emergency surgery. The primary health care provider discusses, with the woman and her family, the need for the cesarean birth and the prognosis for the mother and infant. The anesthesiologist assesses the woman's cardiopulmonary system and describes the options for anesthesia. Informed consent is obtained for the procedure.

Blood and urine tests are usually done a day or two before a planned cesarean birth or on admission to the labor unit. Laboratory tests, most commonly ordered to establish baseline data, include a complete blood cell count and chemistry, blood typing and crossmatching, and urinalysis. Maternal vital signs and blood pressure and FHR and pattern continue to be assessed per the hospital routine until the operation begins. Physical preoperative preparation usually includes inserting a retention catheter to keep the bladder empty and administering prescribed preoperative medications. Although uncommon, the primary health care provider may order an abdominal-mons shave or a clipping of pubic hair. In the event that general anesthesia will be used, an antacid, administered orally to neutralize gastric secretions in case of aspiration, is a beneficial form of care (Enkin et al., 2000). Intravenous fluids are started to maintain hydration and to provide an open line for the administration of blood or medications if needed.

Removal of dentures, nail polish, and jewelry may be optional, depending on hospital policies and type of anesthesia used. If the woman wears glasses and is going to be awake, the nurse should make sure her glasses accompany her to the operating room so she can see her infant. If the woman wears contact lenses, the nurse can find out whether they can be worn for the birth.

During the preoperative preparation, the support person is encouraged to remain with the woman as much as possible to provide continuing emotional support (if this action is culturally acceptable to the woman and support person). The nurse provides essential information about the preoperative procedures during this time. Although the nursing actions may be carried out quickly if a cesarean birth is unplanned, verbal communication, particularly

A B C

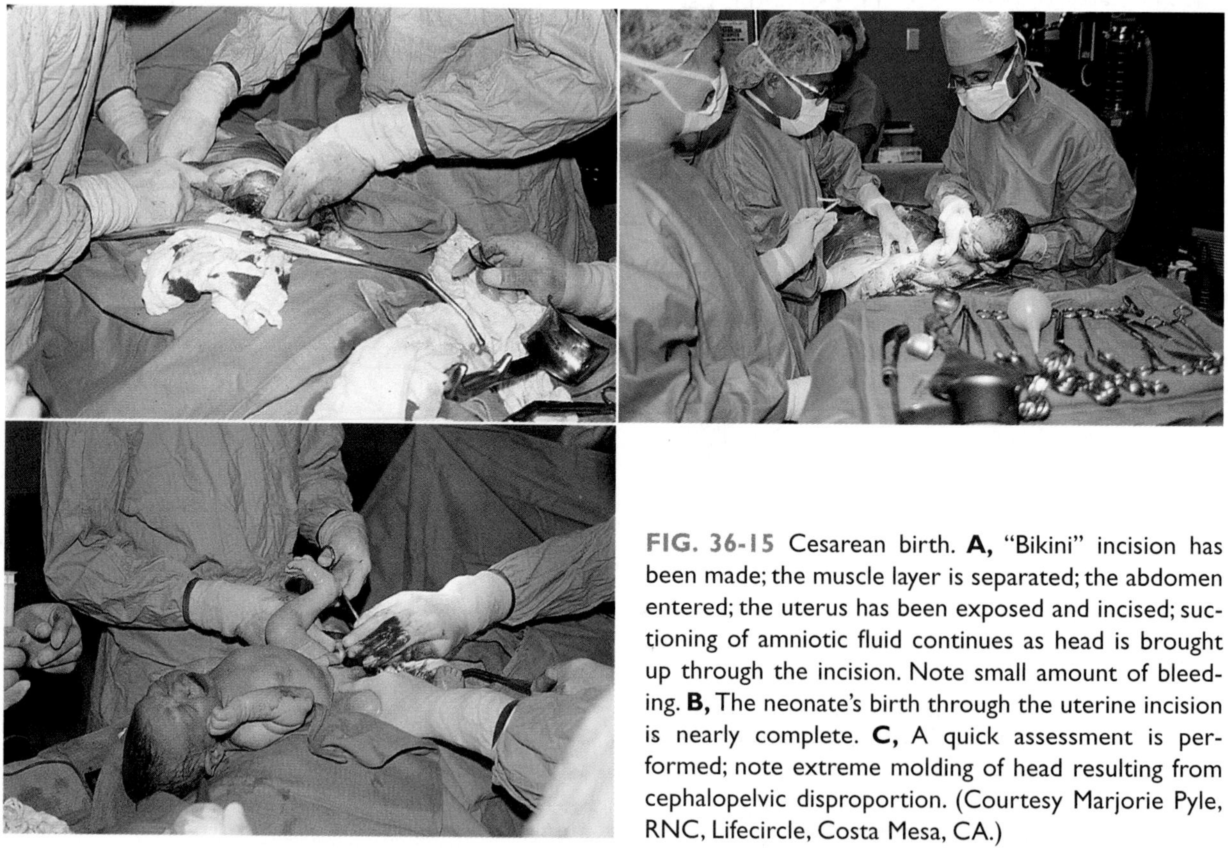

FIG. 36-15 Cesarean birth. **A,** "Bikini" incision has been made; the muscle layer is separated; the abdomen entered; the uterus has been exposed and incised; suctioning of amniotic fluid continues as head is brought up through the incision. Note small amount of bleeding. **B,** The neonate's birth through the uterine incision is nearly complete. **C,** A quick assessment is performed; note extreme molding of head resulting from cephalopelvic disproportion. (Courtesy Marjorie Pyle, RNC, Lifecircle, Costa Mesa, CA.)

explanations, is important. Silence can be frightening to the woman and her support person. The nurse's use of touch can communicate feelings of care and concern for the woman. The nurse can assess the woman's and her partner's perceptions about cesarean birth (e.g., the woman feels that she is a failure because she did not have a vaginal birth). As the woman expresses her feelings, the nurse may identify a potential for a disturbance in self-concept during the postpartum period that may need to be addressed. If there is time before the birth, the nurse can teach the woman about postoperative expectations and about pain relief, turning, coughing, and deep-breathing measures.

Intraoperative Care. Cesarean births occur in operating rooms in the surgical suite or in the labor and birth unit. Once the woman has been taken to the operating room, her care becomes the responsibility of the obstetric team, surgeon, anesthesiologist, pediatrician, and surgical nursing staff (Fig. 36-15). If possible, the partner, who is dressed appropriately for the operating room, accompanies the mother to the operating room and remains close to her so that continued support and comfort can be provided.

The nurse who is circulating may assist with positioning the woman on the birth (surgical) table. It is important to position her so that the uterus is displaced laterally to prevent compression of the inferior vena cava, which causes decreased placental perfusion. This is usually accomplished by placing a wedge under the hip. A Foley catheter is inserted into the bladder at this time if one is not already in place.

If the partner is not allowed or chooses not to be present, the nurse can stay in communication with him or her and give progress reports whenever possible. If the woman is awake during the birth, the nurse, anesthesiologist, or both can tell her what is happening and provide support. She may be anxious about the sensations she is experiencing, such as the coldness of solutions used to prepare the abdomen and pressure or pulling during the actual birth of the infant. She also may be apprehensive because of the bright lights or the presence of unfamiliar equipment and masked and gowned personnel in the room. Explanations by the nurse can help to decrease the woman's anxiety.

Care of the infant usually is delegated to a pediatrician or a nurse team skilled in neonatal resuscitation, because these infants are considered to be at risk until there is evidence of physiologic stability after the birth.

A crib with resuscitation equipment is readied before surgery. Those responsible for care are expert not only in resuscitative techniques but also in their ability to detect normal and abnormal infant responses. After birth, if the infant's condition permits and the mother is awake, the baby may be placed skin-to-skin on the mother or can be given to the woman's partner to hold (Fig. 36-16). The infant whose condition is compromised is transported after initial stabilization to the nursery for observation and the implementation of appropriate interventions. In some institutions, the partner may accompany the infant; if not, personnel keep the family informed of the infant's progress, and parent-infant contacts are initiated as soon as possible.

If the family cannot accompany the woman during surgery, the family is directed to the surgical or obstetric waiting room. The physician then reports on the condition of the mother and child to the family members after the

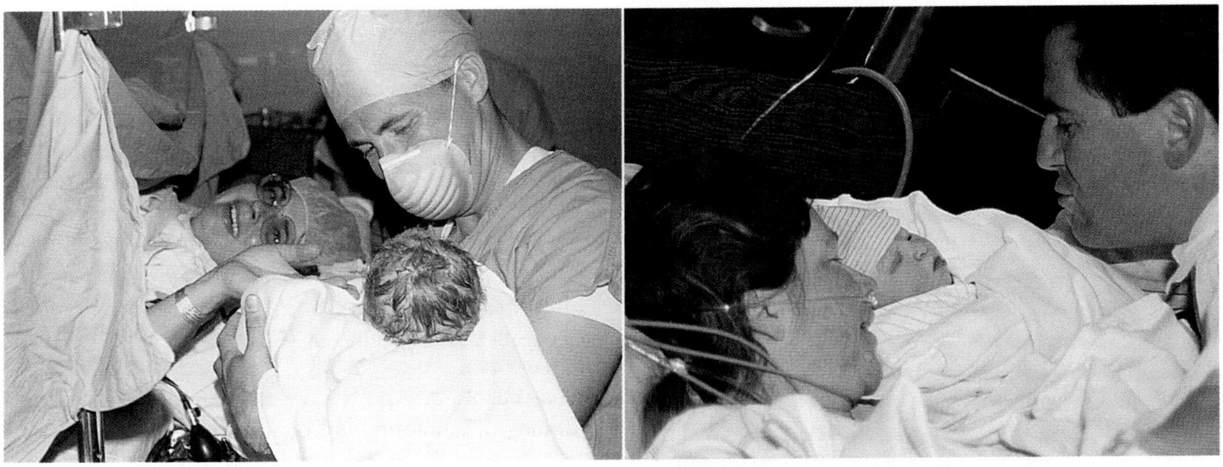
A
B

FIG. 36-16 **A,** Parents and their newborn. The physician manually removes the placenta, suctions the remaining amniotic fluid and blood from the uterine cavity, and closes the uterine incision, peritoneum, muscle layer, fatty tissue, and finally the skin, while the new family shares some private time. **B,** Parents become better acquainted with their newborn while mother rests after surgery. (Courtesy Marjorie Pyle, RNC, Lifecircle, Costa Mesa, CA.)

birth is completed. Family members may accompany the infant as she or he is transferred to the nursery, giving them an opportunity to see and admire the new baby.

NURSE ALERT

Some mothers/parents want the privilege of informing family and friends of the sex of the infant (if it was not known before birth). Before responding to requests for such information from people waiting outside the birthing area, the nurse should check with the mother (or ascertain the mother's wishes).

Immediate Postoperative Care. Once surgery is completed, the mother is transferred to a recovery room or back to her labor room. After a cesarean birth, women have both postoperative and postpartum needs that must be addressed. They are surgical clients as well as new mothers (Eakes & Brown, 1998). Nursing assessments in this immediate postbirth period follow agency protocol and include degree of recovery from the effects of anesthesia, postoperative and postbirth status, and degree of pain. A patent airway is maintained, and the woman is positioned to prevent possible aspiration. Vital signs are taken every 15 minutes for 1 to 2 hours, or until stable. The condition of the incisional dressing, the fundus, and the amount of lochia are assessed, as well as the intravenous intake and the urine output through the Foley catheter. The woman is helped to turn and do coughing, deep-breathing, and leg exercises. Medications to relieve pain may be administered.

If the baby is present, the mother and her partner are given some time alone with him or her to facilitate bonding and attachment. Breastfeeding can be initiated if the mother feels like trying. If the woman is in a recovery area or in her labor room, she usually is transferred to the postpartum unit after 1 to 2 hours, or once her condition is stable and the effects of anesthesia have worn off (i.e., she is alert, oriented, and able to feel and move extremities) (see Care Path).

Postoperative/Postpartum Care. The attitude of the nurse and other health team members can influence the woman's perception of herself after a cesarean birth. The caregivers should stress that the woman is a new mother first and a surgical client second. This attitude helps the woman perceive herself as having the same problems and needs as other new mothers, while requiring supportive postoperative care.

The women's physiologic concerns for the first few days may be dominated by pain at the incision site and pain resulting from intestinal gas, and hence the need for pain relief. If epidural anesthesia was used for the surgery, epidural opioids can be given in the immediate postoperative period to provide pain relief for approximately 24 hours. Otherwise, pain medications usually are given every 3 to 4 hours, or patient-controlled analgesia may be ordered instead. Other comfort measures such as position changes, splinting of the incision with pillows, and relaxation and breathing techniques (e.g., those learned in childbirth classes) may be implemented. Women are often the best judges of what their bodies need and can tolerate, including the postoperative ingestion of foods and fluids. If desired by the woman, the early introduction of solid food is safe. Women who eat early have been found to require less analgesia, and gastrointestinal problems do not occur (Burrows et al., 1995). Ambulation and rocking in a rocking chair may relieve gas pains, and avoiding the consumption of gas-forming foods and carbonated beverages may help minimize them (Thomas et al., 1990) (see Teaching for Self-Care: Postpartum Pain Relief After Cesarean Birth).

Nurses must be alert to a woman's physiologic needs, managing care to ensure adequate rest and pain relief. Mother-baby care (couplet care) for a cesarean birth mother must be modified according to her physiologic limitations as a surgical client (Eakes & Brown, 1998).

Daily care includes perineal care, breast care, and routine hygienic care, including showering after the dressing has been removed (if showering is acceptable according to the women's cultural beliefs and practices). The nurse assesses the woman's vital signs, incision, fundus, and lochia according to hospital policies, procedures, or protocols. Breath sounds, bowel sounds, circulatory status of lower extremities, and urinary and bowel elimination also are assessed. It is important to note maternal emotional status.

During the postpartum period, the nurse also can provide care that meets the psychologic and teaching needs of mothers who have had cesarean births. The nurse can explain postpartum procedures to help the woman participate in her recovery from surgery. The nurse can help the woman plan care and visits from family and friends that will allow adequate rest periods. Information on and assistance with infant care can facilitate adjustment to her role as a mother. The woman is supported as she breastfeeds her baby by receiving individualized assistance to comfortably hold and position the baby at her breast. The side-lying position and the use of pillows to support the newborn can enhance comfort and facilitate successful breastfeeding. The partner can be included in infant teaching sessions, and in explanations about the woman's recovery. The couple also should be encouraged to express their feelings about the birth experience. Some parents are angry, frustrated, or disappointed that a vaginal birth was not possible. Some women express feelings of low self-esteem or a negative self-image. Others express relief and gratitude that the baby is healthy and safely born. It may be helpful for them to have the nurse who was present during the birth visit and help fill in "gaps" about the experience. Other psychologic and lifestyle concerns that have been reported include depression, feeling limited in activities, and changes in family interactions (Ryding et al., 1998).

Discharge after cesarean birth is usually by the third postoperative day (Curtin & Kozak, 1998). The time is often determined by criteria established by the woman's insurance carrier or the federal government (e.g., diagnosis-related groups).

The Newborn's and Mother's Health Protection Act of 1996 provides for a length of stay of up to 96 hours for cesarean births. These criteria may not coincide with the woman's physical or psychosocial readiness for discharge. Some states have added home care provisions for mothers who meet appropriate criteria for discharge and choose to leave sooner than the allowed length of stay. This policy recognizes that home care is less costly than hospital care and in most cases is more beneficial for recovery (Carpenter, 1998).

Eakes and Brown (1998) studied the expressed postdischarge needs of women who experienced planned and unplanned cesarean births. Findings revealed that the three predominant needs expressed by both groups of women were for rest and sleep; relief of pain and discomfort; and assistance with household chores, infant care and feeding, and self-care. Women who experienced planned cesarean births also expressed a need for help with depression, socialization, and family closeness, especially with regard to the limited amount of time available to spend with their other children.

The nurse must provide discharge teaching to prepare women for self-care and newborn care in a limited time, while trying to ensure that the woman is comfortable and able to rest. The nurse must assess the woman's information needs and coordinate the health care team's efforts to meet them.

Discharge teaching and planning should include information about nutrition; measures to relieve pain and discomfort; exercise and specific activity restrictions; time management that includes periods of uninterrupted rest and sleep; hygiene, breast, and incision care; timing for resumption of sexual activity and contraception; signs of complications (see Teaching for Self-Care: Postpartum Pain Relief After Cesarean Birth and Teaching for Self-Care: Signs of Postoperative Complications After Discharge) and infant care. The nurse assesses the woman's need for continued support or counseling to facilitate her emotional recovery from the birth. The woman's family and friends should be educated regarding her needs during the recovery process, and their assistance should be coordinated before discharge. Referral to support groups or to community agencies may be indicated to promote the recovery process further. A postdischarge program of telephone follow-up and home visits can facilitate the woman's full recovery after cesarean birth.

Vaginal Birth After Cesarean

Indications for primary cesarean birth, such as dystocia, breech presentation, or fetal distress, often are nonrecurring. Therefore a woman who has had a cesarean birth may subsequently become pregnant and not have any contraindications to labor and vaginal birth in that pregnancy and may attempt a **vaginal birth after cesarean (VBAC).**

ACOG (1999a) encourages a TOL and VBAC attempt in women who have had one previous cesarean birth by low transverse incision. Vaginal birth is relatively safe, but there is risk for uterine rupture through a lower uterine segment scar. Increased reports of uterine rupture in the United States and Canada in the 1990s have raised concerns about the safety of VBAC. Recommendations for the use of VBAC are being reevaluated (ACOG, 1999a; Cunningham et al., 2001). A retrospective cohort analysis of more than 20,000 women who gave birth to a second child after a previous primary cesarean birth found that the incidence of uterine rupture was related to the method of the second labor and birth. The rate of uterine rupture was lowest when the women had a repeat cesarean birth without labor but highest when labor was induced with prostaglandins (Lydon-Rochelle et al., 2001). Labor and vaginal birth are not recommended if there are contraindications, such as a previous fundal classic cesarean scar, a scar from uterine surgery, or evidence of CPD.

According to Scott (1999), 60% to 88% of women can give birth vaginally after a TOL. Women are most often the primary decision makers with regard to choice of birth method. During the antepartal period, the woman should be given information about VBAC and encouraged to choose it as an alternative to repeat cesarean birth, as long as no contraindications exist. VBAC support groups and prenatal classes can help prepare the woman psychologically for labor and vaginal birth. Women need to believe not only that their efforts during a TOL will be successful but also that they are fully capable of doing what is necessary to give birth vaginally (self-efficacy). They must be given the opportunity to discuss their previous labor experience, including feelings of failure and loss of control, and to express concern they may have about how they will manage during their upcoming labor and birth (Dilks & Beal, 1997).

This labor should occur in a hospital facility that has the equipment and personnel available to begin the surgery within 30 minutes from the time a decision is made to perform cesarean birth. Ideally the woman is admitted to the labor and birth unit at the onset of spontaneous labor. In the latent phase of labor, the nurse encourages her to engage in normal activities such as ambulation. In the active phase of labor, FHR and pattern and uterine activity usually are monitored electronically, and intravenous access such as a saline lock may be established. The physician should be immediately available during active labor.

There is no evidence that administering oxytocin to induce or augment labor or the use of epidural anesthesia is contraindicated, although caution and close monitoring of the laboring woman are urged if these are used (Cunningham et al., 2001). However, use of prostaglandins, especially misoprostol (prostaglandin E_1), to ripen the cervix or induce labor is not recommended

Care Path Cesarean Birth Without Complications: Expected Length of Stay—48 to 72 Hours

	IMMEDIATE POSTOP CESAREAN	BY 4TH HOUR AFTER ADMISSION TO PP UNIT	5 TO 24 HOURS	25 TO 48 HOURS	BY DISCHARGE
ASSESSMENTS	Recovery room/ PACU admission assessment completed	PP admission assessment and care plan completed			
Vital Signs	q15min × 1 hr; q30min × 4 hr, WNL	q1h × 3, WNL	q4-8h, WNL	q8h, WNL	q8h, WNL
Postpartum Assessment	q15min × 1 hr, WNL	q1h × 3, WNL	q8h, WNL	q8-12h, WNL	q8-12h, WNL
Abdominal Incision	Dressing dry and intact	Dressing dry and intact	Dressing dry and intact	Dressing off or changed, incision intact	Incision intact; staples may be removed and Steri-Strips in place, incision WNL
Genitourinary	Retention catheter output >30 ml/hr	Retention catheter output >30 ml/hr	Retention catheter output >30 ml/hr	Catheter discontinued, output >100 ml/void or 240 ml/8 hr	Urine output >240 ml/8 hr
Gastrointestinal		Absent or hypoactive BS	Hypoactive to active BS	Active BS + flatus	Active BS + flatus; may or may not have BM
Musculoskeletal	Alert or easily aroused, can move legs	Alert and oriented, moving all extremities	Ambulating with help	Ambulating unassisted	Ambulating ad lib
Bonding	Evidence of parent-infant bonding; first breastfeeding if desired		Parent-infant bonding continues	Parent-infant bonding progressing	
Laboratory Tests			Intrapartal CBC results on chart/ computer; determine Rh status and need for anti-Rh globulin; check for rubella immunity	PP HCT WNL, all lab results on chart, give anti-Rh globulin if indicated	Give rubella vaccine if indicated
INTERVENTIONS					
IV	IV continues	IV continues	IV continues	IV may be discontinued	
Diet	NPO	Ice chips, sips of clear liquids	Clear liquids	Regular diet or as tolerated	Regular diet
Perineal		Pericare by nurse	Pericare with help	Self-pericare	
Activity	Bed rest	Bed rest	OOB × 3 with help, ADLs assisted, assisted to comfortable position to hold and feed baby	Holds baby comfortably, ambulates without assistance, ADLs unassisted	Activity ad lib

ADLs, Activities of daily living; *BM*, bowel movement; *BS*, bowel sounds; *CBC*, complete blood count; *HCT*, hematocrit; *IM*, intramuscular; *IV*, intravenous; *NPO*, nothing by mouth; *NSAIDs*, nonsteroidal antiinflammatory drugs; *OOB*, out of bed; *PACU*, postanesthesia care unit; *PCA*, patient-controlled analgesia; *PNV*, prenatal vitamins; *PP*, postpartum; *Rx*, prescription; *TCDB*, turn, cough, deep breathe; *WNL*, within normal limits.

Care Path Cesarean Birth Without Complications: Expected Length of Stay—48 to 72 Hours—cont'd

	IMMEDIATE POSTOP CESAREAN	BY 4TH HOUR AFTER ADMISSION TO PP UNIT	5 TO 24 HOURS	25 TO 48 HOURS	BY DISCHARGE
INTERVENTIONS—CONT'D					
Pulmonary Care	Patent airway; O_2 discontinued	TCDB q2h with splinting, incentive spirometry q1h if ordered, lungs clear	TCDB q2h while awake; lungs clear	TCDB as needed; lungs clear	
Medications	Oxytocin added to IV Pain control: analgesics, IV, or epidural narcotic	Oxytocin continued Pain control: analgesics—PCA, IM, PO, or epidural narcotic	Oxytocin may be discontinued Pain control: IM, PO, PCA narcotics or analgesics	Oxytocin discontinued Pain control: PO analgesics, NSAIDs; PCA discontinued; stool softener, PNV	Rx filled or given to take home
Teaching, Discharge Plan	Breastfeeding, positioning, leg exercises	Verbalize understanding/unit routines, how to achieve rest, TCDB, involution, pain control	*Self:* comfort measures and care; reinforce TCDB and positioning; introduce teaching videos, lactation promotion or suppression *Infant:* handwashing, infant safety, positioning for feeding and burping; if breastfeeding, then positioning baby, latching on, timing, removing from breast	*Self:* diet; activity/rest; bowel/bladder function *Infant:* bonding; parent concerns; feeding; infant bath, cord care; need for car seat; newborn characteristics; circumcision, if requested; answer questions	*Self:* home care, signs of complications (infections, bleeding), normal psychologic adjustments, normal ADLs; resumption of sexual activities; contraception; identification of support system at home; self-concept issues related to cesarean birth. Inform whom to call if problems; review need to keep follow-up appointment; provide information about community resources; provide copy of home care *Infant:* parents to demonstrate infant care; reinforce use of booklets for infant care, whom to call if problems; discuss immunization needs; review need to keep follow-up appointments

TEACHING FOR SELF-CARE

Postpartum Pain Relief After Cesarean Birth

INCISIONAL
- Splint incision with a pillow when moving or coughing.
- Use relaxation techniques such as music, breathing, and dim lights.

GAS
- Walk as often as you can.
- Do not eat or drink gas-forming foods, carbonated beverages, or whole milk.
- Do not use straws for drinking fluids.
- Take antiflatulence medication if prescribed.
- Lie on your left side to expel gas.
- Rock in a rocking chair.

TEACHING FOR SELF-CARE

Signs of Postoperative Complications After Discharge

Report the following signs to your health care provider:
- Temperature exceeding 38° C
- Painful urination
- Lochia heavier than a normal period
- Wound separation
- Redness or oozing at the incision site
- Severe abdominal pain

because they have been associated with an increased risk for uterine rupture.

Attention should be paid to the woman's psychologic, as well as physical, needs during the TOL. Anxiety increases the release of catecholamines and can inhibit the release of oxytocin, thus delaying the progress of labor and possibly leading to a repeat cesarean birth. To alleviate such anxiety, the nurse can encourage the woman to use breathing and relaxation techniques and to change positions to promote labor progress. The woman's partner can be encouraged to provide comfort measures and emotional support. Collaboration among the woman in labor, her partner, the nurse, and other health care providers often results in a successful VBAC. If a TOL does not proceed to vaginal birth, the woman will need support and encouragement to express her feelings about having another cesarean birth. It is very important that this outcome not be labeled a failed VBAC.

Evaluation

To evaluate the effectiveness of nursing care for a woman experiencing dystocia, the nurse reviews the expected outcomes of care that were met and assesses the woman's and the family's level of satisfaction with the care received.

POSTTERM PREGNANCY, LABOR, AND BIRTH

A **postterm** or **postdate pregnancy** is one that extends beyond the end of week 42 of gestation, or 294 days from the first day of the last menstrual period. The incidence of postterm pregnancy is estimated to be between 4% and 14%, with an average of 10% (Cunningham et al., 2001).

Many pregnancies are misdiagnosed as prolonged. This can occur because (1) the pregnancy is inaccurately dated because the woman has an irregular menstrual cycle pattern, (2) an accurate date of the last menstrual period is unknown, or (3) entry into prenatal care was delayed or did not occur.

Although the exact cause of postterm pregnancy is still unknown, a possible cause may be deficiency of placental estrogen and continued secretion of progesterone. Low levels of estrogen may result in a decrease in prostaglandin precursors and reduced formation of oxytocin receptors in the myometrium (Gilbert & Harmon, 2003). A woman who experiences one postterm pregnancy is 30% to 40% more likely to experience it again in subsequent pregnancies (Arulkumarian, 1997).

Clinical manifestations of postterm pregnancy include maternal weight loss (more than 1.4 kg/wk) and decreased uterine size (related to decreased amniotic fluid), meconium in the amniotic fluid, and advanced bone maturation of the fetal skeleton with an exceptionally hard fetal skull (Gilbert & Harmon, 2003).

Maternal and Fetal Risks

Maternal risks are often related to the birth of an excessively large infant. The woman is at increased risk for dysfunctional labor; birth canal trauma, including perineal lacerations and extension of episiotomy during vaginal birth; postpartum hemorrhage; and infection. Interventions such as induction of labor with prostaglandins or oxytocin, forceps- or vacuum-assisted birth, and cesarean birth are more likely to be necessary. The woman also may experience fatigue and psychologic reactions such as depression, frustration, and feelings of inadequacy as she passes her estimated date of birth (Arulkumarian, 1997; Gilbert & Harmon, 2003).

Fetal risks appear to be twofold. The first is the possibility of prolonged labor, shoulder dystocia, birth trauma, and asphyxia from macrosomia. Macrosomia occurs when the placenta continues to provide adequate nutrients to support fetal growth after 40 weeks of gestation. It is estimated to occur in approximately 25% of prolonged pregnancies (Divon, 2002). The second risk is the compromising effects on the fetus of an "aging" placenta. Spellacy (1999) notes that placental function gradually decreases after 37 weeks of gestation. Amniotic fluid volume (AFV) declines to approximately 800 ml by 40 weeks of gestation and to about 400 ml by 42 weeks of gestation. The resulting oligohydramnios can lead to fetal hypoxia related to cord compression. If placental

EVIDENCE-BASED PRACTICE

MANAGEMENT OF PROLONGED PREGNANCY

BACKGROUND

About 18% of pregnancies in the United States go beyond 41 weeks' and 7% go past 42 weeks' gestation. The risk of adverse maternal and perinatal outcomes is increased when pregnancy is prolonged. Maternal risks include pelvic injuries and risks related to induced labor and cesarean births. Perinatal risks may be related to uteroplacental insufficiency and include fetal hypoxia, meconium aspiration, and growth restriction. The continued growth of the fetus can lead to macrosomia and its related risks of labor abnormalities, including shoulder dystocia and brachial plexus injuries (ACOG, 1997a; ACOG, 2000).

OBJECTIVES

Controversy continues about the optimal time for delivery and the methods for managing postterm pregnancy. Available evidence about management of prolonged pregnancy was reviewed to assess the benefits, risks, and cost of different strategies.

SEARCH STRATEGY

Published literature on the management of postterm pregnancy was identified from the Cochrane Pregnancy and Childbirth Group trials register and through the review conducted by the Duke Evidence-based Practice Center for the Agency for Healthcare Research and Quality (Boulvain & Irion, 2001; Crowley, 2000; Myers, et al., 2002).

EVIDENCE

The searches yielded over 700 English language articles; however, fewer that 30 were randomized trials of interventions specifically for prolonged pregnancy. The principle findings include the following:

- There is no direct evidence that antepartal testing (e.g., ultrasound, biophysical profile) decreases perinatal mortality rates in prolonged pregnancy; however, morbidity rates may be reduced. There are no definitive conclusions about which test or combination of tests is best for predicting fetal compromise.
- Early pregnancy ultrasound examination and adjustment of estimated date of birth if needed may reduce the incidence of postterm pregnancy.
- Perinatal mortality rates appear to be reduced if women have labor induction after 41 weeks compared with women managed with antepartal testing. Cesarean birth rates do not appear to be different between women having elective induction and those managed expectantly.
- Sweeping or "stripping" of the membranes at 38 to 40 weeks' gestation was seen to promote spontaneous labor and reduce the number of women having induction at 41 or 42 weeks.
- Data about the different methods for induction consistently demonstrated tradeoffs between efficacy of the intervention and possible maternal and fetal effects; however, data about cost-effectiveness (medical and nonmedical) are lacking.
- There are almost no data regarding client values and preferences for management options or in epidemiologic differences in racial, ethnic, or sociologic subgroups.

CONCLUSIONS

These literature reviews do not provide a clear answer about prolonged pregnancy management. Induction at 41 or more weeks' gestation decreases perinatal mortality rates compared with antepartal testing, but there is not enough evidence to recommend any specific method. More clinical trials with adequate sample sizes are needed to detect clinically relevant outcomes.

Implications for nursing care include (1) educating women who are postterm to assess fetal activity on a daily basis, recognize signs of labor, and keep prenatal clinic appointments and (2) assisting these women to understand the management options so that they may make informed decisions.

Reference: American College of Obstetricians and Gynecologists. (1997a). ACOG practice patterns. Management of posterm pregnancy. No. 6, October 1997. *International Journal of Gynaecologists and Obstetricians, 60*(1), 86-91; American College of Obstetricians and Gynecologists. (2000). Fetal macrosomia. *ACOG Practice Bulletin No. 22.* Washington, DC: ACOG; Boulvain, M., & Irion, O. (2001). Stripping/sweeping the membranes for inducing labour or preventing postterm pregnancy (Cochrane Review). In *The Cochrane Library*, Issue 2. Oxford: Update Software; Crowley, P. (2000). Interventions for preventing or improving the outcome of delivery at or beyond term (Cochrane Review). In *The Cochrane Library*, Issue 2, Oxford: Update Software; Myers, E. et al. (2002). Management of prolonged pregnancy. *Evidence Report/technology Assessment No. 53* (AHRQ Publication No. 02-E018). Rockville, MD: Agency for Healthcare Research and Quality.

insufficiency is present, there is a high likelihood of fetal distress occurring during labor. Neonatal problems may include asphyxia, meconium aspiration syndrome, dysmaturity syndrome, hypoglycemia, polycythemia, and respiratory distress (Gilbert & Harmon, 2003). Whether an infant born after a postterm pregnancy has neurologic, behavioral, intellectual, or developmental problems must be further investigated.

Collaborative Care

The management of postterm pregnancy is still controversial (see Evidence-Based Practice box). The induction of labor at 41 to 42 weeks is suggested by some authorities as a means of reducing the rate of cesarean birth and stillbirth or neonatal death (Hannah et al., 1996).

Others follow a more individualized approach, allowing the pregnancy to proceed to 43 weeks of gestation as long as assessment of fetal well-being with a combination of tests is performed, and the results of the tests are normal. Tests are usually performed on a weekly or twice-weekly basis (Divon, 2002; Searing, 2001).

Antepartum assessments for postterm pregnancy may include daily fetal movement counts, nonstress tests (NSTs), AFV assessments, contraction stress tests (CSTs), biophysical profiles (BPPs), and Doppler flow measurements. The woman and her family should be fully informed regarding the tests, including why they are performed and the meaning of the results obtained in terms of the health of the mother and fetus.

The amniotic fluid index (AFI) should be greater than 8, with at least one pocket of amniotic fluid greater than 2 cm, and amniotic fluid should be present throughout the uterine cavity (Gilbert & Harmon, 2003; Schmidt, 1999). The BPP may be the best way of gauging fetal well-being because it combines nonstress testing with real-time ultrasound scanning to assess fetal movements, fetal breathing movements, and the AFV. Determining the AFV is critical in women with postterm pregnancies because a decreased AFV (i.e., oligohydramnios) has been associated with fetal stress as a result of umbilical cord compression.

Cervical checks usually are performed weekly after 40 weeks of gestation to determine whether the condition of the cervix is favorable for induction (5 or greater on the Bishop score for multiparas and 9 or more for nulliparas) (see Table 36-4). Vaginal secretions may be assessed for the amount of fetal fibronectin; a low concentration may predict increased risk for prolonged pregnancy, but results of studies have thus far been inconclusive (Divon, 2002; Gilbert & Harmon, 2003). Amniocentesis or amnioscopy may be performed to detect meconium in the amniotic fluid (Spellacy, 1999).

During the postterm period, the woman is encouraged to assess fetal activity daily, assess for signs of labor, and keep appointments with her primary health care provider (see Teaching for Self-Care: Postterm Pregnancy). The woman and her family should be encouraged to express their feelings (e.g., frustration, anger, impatience, fear) about the prolonged pregnancy and should be helped to realize that these feelings are normal. At times the emotional and physical strain of a postterm pregnancy may seem insurmountable. Referral to a support group or another supportive resource may be needed (Schmidt, 1999).

If the woman's cervix is ripe, labor is usually induced with oxytocin. If her cervix is not ripe, continued fetal surveillance or a cervical ripening agent (e.g., prostaglandin insert or gel) may be administered, followed by oxytocin induction (Gilbert & Harmon, 2003; Schmidt, 1999).

TEACHING FOR SELF-CARE

Postterm Pregnancy

- Perform daily fetal movement counts.
- Assess for signs of labor.
- Call your primary health care provider if your membranes rupture, or if you perceive a decrease in or no fetal movement.
- Keep appointments for fetal assessment tests or cervical checks.
- Come to the hospital soon after labor begins.

The fetus of a woman with a postterm pregnancy should be monitored electronically for a more accurate assessment of the FHR and pattern. Fetal scalp pH sampling or fetal oxygen saturation monitoring may be done to determine whether acidosis is occurring. Inadequate fluid volume leads to compression of the cord, which results in fetal hypoxia that is reflected in variable or prolonged deceleration patterns and passage of meconium. If oligohydramnios is present, an amnioinfusion may be performed to restore amniotic fluid volume to maintain a cushioning of the cord. The use of amnioinfusion to treat fetal distress associated with oligohydramnios in labor is a form of care likely to be beneficial.

However, it is likely to be ineffective or harmful to perform an amnioinfusion prophylactically (Enkin et al., 2000). Amnioinfusion may be used to prevent or minimize meconium aspiration syndrome (MAS) by diluting amniotic fluid thickened with meconium passed by a hypoxic fetus. Maternal-fetal risks related to amnioinfusion, although rare, can result from infection and overdistention of the uterine cavity with infused fluid (Gilbert & Harmon, 2003; Schmidt, 1997). Accurate assessment of the woman's labor pattern also is important because dysfunctional labor is common (Spellacy, 1999).

Emotional support is essential for the woman with a postterm pregnancy and her family. A vaginal birth is anticipated, but the couple should be prepared for a forceps-assisted, vacuum-assisted, or cesarean birth if complications arise. Expected outcomes of care include that the woman and her family use appropriate coping mechanisms to deal with the emotional aspects of her postterm pregnancy and that the woman and her newborn experience no injury during the birth.

OBSTETRIC EMERGENCIES

Shoulder Dystocia

Shoulder dystocia is an uncommon obstetric emergency that increases the risk for fetal/neonatal and maternal morbidity and mortality during the attempt to deliver the fetus vaginally. In this condition, the head is born, but the anterior shoulder cannot pass under the pubic arch. Fetopelvic disproportion related to excessive fetal size (greater than 4000 g) or maternal pelvic abnormalities may be a cause of shoulder dystocia, although shoulder dystocia can occur in the absence of any known risk factors. The nurse should be observant for signs that could indicate the presence of shoulder dystocia, including slowing of the progress of labor and formation of a caput succedaneum that increases in size. When the head emerges, it retracts against the perineum (turtle sign), and external rotation does not occur (Hall, 1997).

The fetus/newborn is more likely to experience birth injuries related to asphyxia, brachial plexus damage, and fracture, especially of the humerus or clavicle. The mother's primary risk stems from excessive blood loss as a result of uterine atony or rupture, lacerations, extension of the episiotomy, or endometritis. It is estimated that 0.6% to 1.4% of all vaginal births are complicated by shoulder dystocia (ACOG, 2000).

Collaborative Care

Many maneuvers such as suprapubic pressure and maternal position changes have been suggested and tried to free the anterior shoulder, although no one particular maneuver has been found to be most effective (ACOG, 1997b). Suprapubic pressure can be applied to the anterior shoulder by using the Mazzanti or Ruben technique (Fig. 36-17) in an attempt to push the shoulder under the symphysis pubis (ACOG, 1997b).

In the McRoberts maneuver (Fig. 36-18), the woman's legs are flexed apart, with her knees on her abdomen (ACOG, 1997b; Cunningham et al., 2001). This maneuver causes the sacrum to straighten, and the symphysis pubis rotates toward the mother's head; the angle of pelvic inclination is decreased, freeing the shoulder. Suprapubic pressure can be applied at this time. The McRoberts maneuver is the preferred method when a woman is receiving epidural anesthesia.

Having the woman move to a hands-and-knees position (the Gaskin maneuver), a squatting position, or lateral recumbent position also has been used to resolve cases of shoulder dystocia (Bruner et al., 1998; Hall, 1997).

Fundal pressure is usually not advised as a method of relieving shoulder dystocia (Nocon, 2000; Simpson & Knox, 2001).

When shoulder dystocia is diagnosed, the nurse helps the woman to assume the position(s) that may facilitate birth of the shoulders, assists the primary health care provider with these maneuvers and techniques during birth, and documents the maneuvers. The nurse also provides encouragement and support to reduce anxiety and fear.

Newborn assessment should include examination for fracture of the clavicle or humerus as well as brachial plexus injuries and asphyxia (Hall, 1997). Maternal assessment

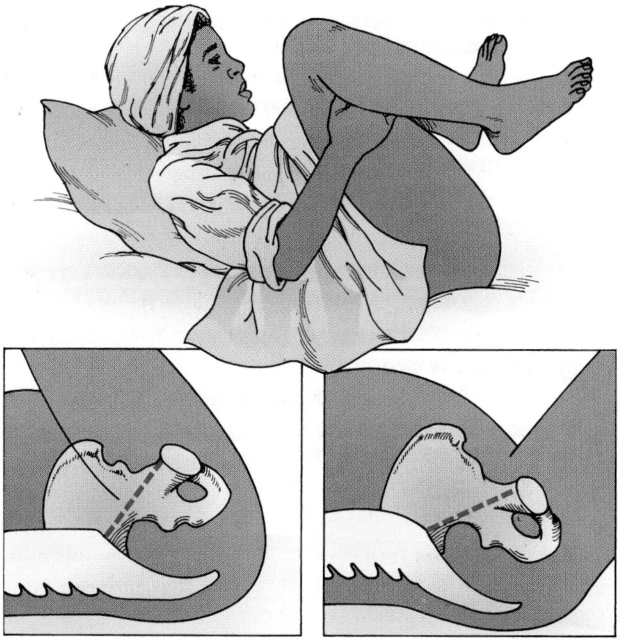

FIG. 36-18 McRoberts maneuver. (Modified from Gabbe, S., Niebyl, J., & Simpson, J. [2002]. *Obstetrics: Normal and problem pregnancies* [4th ed.]. New York: Churchill Livingstone, with permission.)

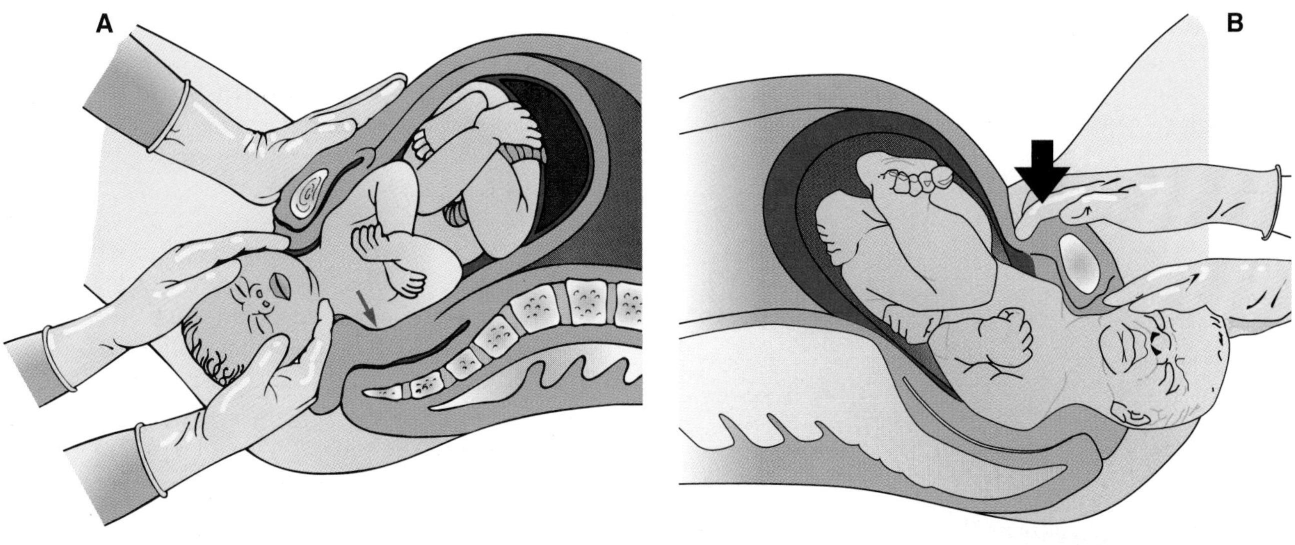
A
B

FIG. 36-17 Application of suprapubic pressure. **A,** Mazzanti technique: pressure is applied directly posteriorly and laterally above the symphysis pubis. **B,** Rubin technique: pressure is applied obliquely posteriorly against the anterior shoulder.

should focus on early detection of hemorrhage and trauma to the soft tissue of the birth canal.

Prolapsed Umbilical Cord

Prolapse of the umbilical cord occurs when the cord lies below the presenting part of the fetus. In 2000, prolapse of the umbilical cord occurred in 1.9% of 1000 live births (Martin et al., 2000). Umbilical cord prolapse may be occult (hidden, not visible) at any time during labor whether or not the membranes are ruptured (Fig. 36-19, *A* and *B*). It is most common to see frank (visible) prolapse directly after rupture of membranes, when gravity washes the cord in front of the presenting part (Fig. 36-19, *C* and *D*). Contributing factors include a long cord (longer than 100 cm), malpresentation (breech), transverse lie, or unengaged presenting part.

If the presenting part does not fit snugly into the lower uterine segment (e.g., as in hydramnios), when the membranes rupture, a sudden gush of amniotic fluid may cause the cord to be displaced downward. Similarly the cord may prolapse during amniotomy if the presenting part is high. A small fetus may not fit snugly into the lower uterine segment; as a result, cord prolapse is more likely to occur.

Collaborative Care

Prompt recognition of a prolapsed umbilical cord is important because fetal hypoxia resulting from prolonged cord compression (i.e., occlusion of blood flow to and from the fetus for more than 5 minutes) usually results in central nervous system damage or death of the fetus. Pressure on the cord may be relieved by the examiner putting a sterile gloved hand into the vagina and holding the presenting part off of the umbilical cord (Fig. 36-20, *A* and *B*). The woman is assisted into a position such as a modified Sims' (Fig. 36-20, *C*), Trendelenburg, or knee-chest (Fig. 36-20, *D*) position, in which gravity keeps the pressure of the presenting part off the cord. If the cervix is fully dilated, a forceps- or vacuum-assisted birth can be performed for the fetus in a cephalic presentation; otherwise, a cesarean birth is likely to be performed. Nonreassuring FHR patterns, inadequate uterine relaxation, and bleeding also can occur as a result of a prolapsed umbilical cord. Indications for immediate interventions are presented in the Emergency box. Ongoing assessment of the woman and her fetus is critical to determine the effectiveness of each action taken. The woman and her family are often aware of the seriousness of the situation; therefore the nurse must provide support by giving explanations for the interventions being implemented and their effect on the status of the fetus.

Rupture of the Uterus

Rupture of the uterus is a rare but very serious obstetric injury that occurs in 1 to 1500 to 2000 births. The most frequent causes of uterine rupture during pregnancy are separation of the scar of a previous classic cesarean birth, uterine trauma (e.g., accidents, surgery), and a congenital uterine anomaly. During labor and birth, uterine rupture may be caused by intense spontaneous uterine contractions, labor stimulation (e.g., oxytocin, prostaglandin), an overdistended uterus (e.g., multifetal gestation), malpresentation, external or internal version, or a difficult forceps-assisted birth. It occurs more commonly in multigravidas than in primigravidas (Varney, 1997).

A uterine rupture is classified as either complete or incomplete. A complete rupture extends through the entire uterine wall into the peritoneal cavity or broad ligament. An incomplete rupture extends into the peritoneum but not into the peritoneal cavity or broad ligament. Bleeding is

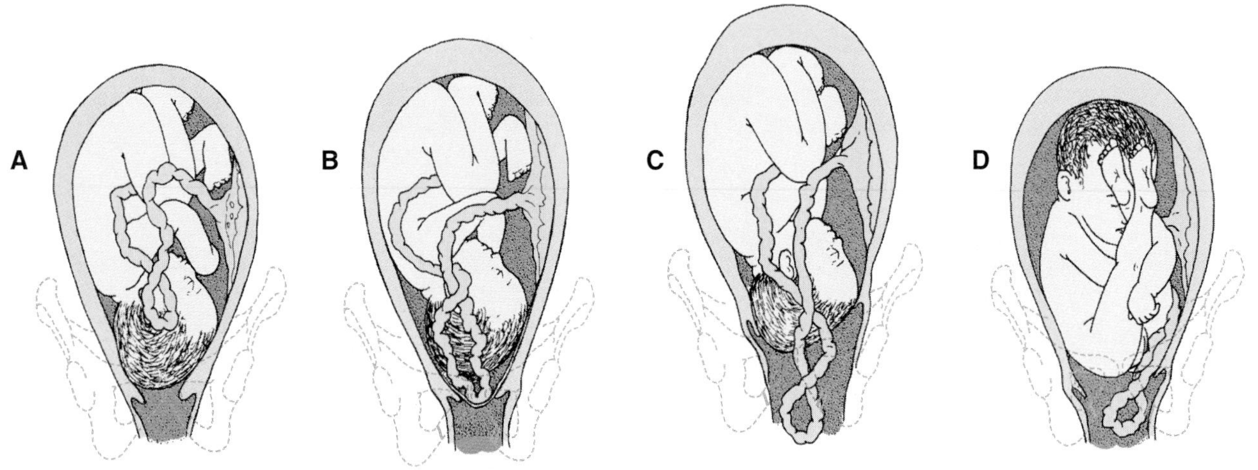
A
B
C
D

FIG. 36-19 Prolapse of umbilical cord. Note pressure of presenting part on umbilical cord, which endangers fetal circulation. **A,** Occult (hidden) prolapse of cord. **B,** Complete prolapse of cord. Note membranes are intact. **C,** Cord presenting in front of the fetal head may be seen in vagina. **D,** Frank breech presentation with prolapsed cord.

usually internal. An incomplete rupture also may be a partial separation at an old cesarean scar and may go unnoticed unless the woman undergoes a subsequent cesarean birth or other uterine surgery.

Signs and symptoms vary with the extent of the rupture and may be silent or dramatic. In an incomplete rupture, pain may not be present. The fetus may or may not have late decelerations, decreased variability, an increased or decreased heart rate, or other nonreassuring signs. The woman may experience vomiting, faintness, increased abdominal tenderness, hypotonic uterine contractions, and lack of progress. Eventually, bleeding and the effects of blood loss will be noted. Fetal heart tones may be lost. In a complete rupture, the woman may complain of sudden, sharp shooting abdominal pain and may state that "something gave way." If she is in labor, her contractions will cease, and pain is relieved. She may exhibit signs of hypovolemic shock caused by hemorrhage (i.e., hypotension, tachypnea, pallor, and cool, clammy skin). If the placenta separates, the FHR will be absent. Fetal parts may be palpable through the abdomen. The nurse should suspect pulmonary embolism if the woman complains of chest pain (Varney, 1997).

Collaborative Care

Prevention is the best treatment. Women who have had a previous classic cesarean birth are advised not to attempt vaginal birth in subsequent pregnancies. Women at risk

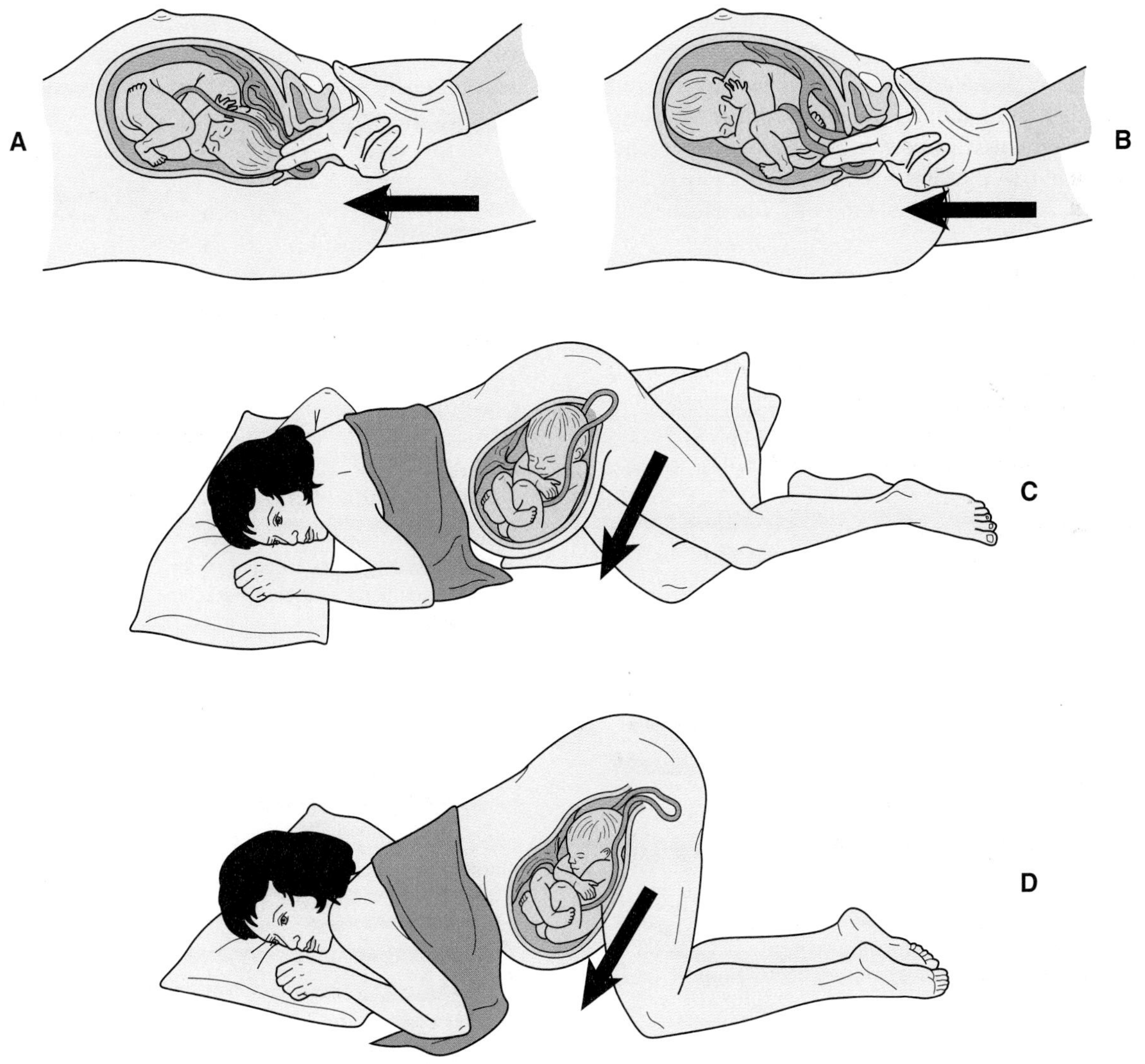
A
B
C
D

FIG. 36-20 *Arrows* indicate direction of pressure against presenting part to relieve compression of prolapsed umbilical cord. Pressure exerted by examiner's fingers in **A,** vertex presentation, and **B,** breech presentation. **C,** Gravity relieves pressure when woman is in modified Sims' position with hips elevated as high as possible with pillows. **D,** Knee-chest position.

for uterine rupture are assessed closely during labor. Women whose labor is induced with oxytocin or prostaglandin (especially if their previous birth was cesarean) are monitored for signs of uterine hyperstimulation, because this can precipitate uterine rupture. If hyperstimulation occurs, the oxytocin infusion is discontinued or decreased, and a tocolytic medication may be given to decrease the intensity of the uterine contractions. After giving birth, women are assessed for excessive bleeding, especially if the fundus is firm and signs of hemorrhagic shock are present.

If rupture occurs, the type of medical management depends on the severity. A small rupture may be managed with a laparotomy and birth of the infant, repair of the laceration, and blood transfusions, if needed. For a complete rupture, hysterectomy and blood replacement is the usual treatment.

The nurse's role may include starting intravenous fluids, transfusing blood products, administering oxygen, and assisting with the preparation for immediate surgery. Supporting the woman's family and providing information about the treatment is important during this emergency (Varney, 1997). The associated fetal mortality rate is high (50% to 75%), and the maternal mortality rate may be high if the woman is not treated immediately (Cunningham et al., 2001). Providing information about spiritual support services or suggesting that the family contact their own support system may be warranted.

Amniotic Fluid Embolism

Amniotic fluid embolism (AFE) occurs when amniotic fluid containing particles of debris (e.g., vernix, hair, skin cells, or meconium) enters the maternal circulation and obstructs pulmonary vessels, causing respiratory distress and circulatory collapse. This can occur because fluid can enter the maternal circulation any time there is an opening in the amniotic sac or maternal uterine veins, accompanied by enough intrauterine pressure to force the amniotic fluid into the veins (e.g., if the placenta separates or if there are rapid or strong contractions that

EMERGENCY
Prolapsed Cord

SIGNS

Fetal bradycardia with variable deceleration during uterine contraction.

Woman reports feeling the cord after membranes rupture.

Cord is seen or felt in or protruding from the vagina.

INTERVENTIONS

Call for assistance.

Notify primary health care provider immediately.

Glove the examining hand quickly and insert two fingers into the vagina to the cervix. With one finger on either side of the cord or both fingers to one side, exert upward pressure against the presenting part to relieve compression of the cord (Fig. 36-20, *A* and *B*). Place a rolled towel under the woman's right or left hip.

Place woman into the extreme Trendelenburg or a modified Sims' position (Fig. 36-20, *C*), or a knee-chest position (Fig. 36-20, *D*).

If cord is protruding from vagina, wrap loosely in a sterile towel saturated with warm sterile normal saline solution.

Administer oxygen to the woman by mask at 8 to 10 L/min until birth is accomplished.

Start IV fluids or increase existing drip rate.

Continue to monitor FHR by internal fetal scalp electrode, if possible.

Explain to woman and support person what is happening and the way it is being managed.

Prepare for immediate vaginal birth if cervix is fully dilated or cesarean birth if it is not.

EMERGENCY
Amniotic Fluid Embolism

SIGNS

Respiratory Distress

- Restlessness
- Dyspnea
- Cyanosis
- Pulmonary edema
- Respiratory arrest

Circulatory Collapse

- Hypotension
- Tachycardia
- Shock
- Cardiac arrest

Hemorrhage

- Coagulation failure: bleeding from incisions, venipuncture sites, trauma (lacerations); petechiae, ecchymoses, purpura
- Uterine atony

INTERVENTIONS

Oxygenate

- Administer oxygen by face mask (8-10 L/min) or resuscitation bag delivering 100% oxygen
- Prepare for intubation and mechanical ventilation
- Initiate or assist with cardiopulmonary resuscitation. Tilt pregnant woman 30 degrees to side to displace uterus

Maintain cardiac output and replace fluid losses

- Position woman on her side
- Administer IV fluids
- Administer blood: packed cells, fresh frozen plasma
- Insert indwelling catheter, and measure hourly urine output

Correct coagulation failure

Monitor fetal and maternal status

Prepare for emergency birth once woman's condition is stabilized

Provide emotional support to woman, her partner, and family

cause the uterus to lacerate or rupture). Although uncommon, this complication is estimated to be the cause of 10% of maternal deaths in the United States. The fetal mortality rate is estimated to be as high as 50% (Martin & Leaton, 2001).

Amniotic fluid is more damaging if it contains meconium and other particulate matter such as mucus, fat globules, lanugo, bacterial products, or debris from a dead fetus because emboli can then form more readily. Maternal death occurs most often when thick meconium is present in the amniotic fluid, because this clogs the pulmonary veins more completely than other debris. Even if death does not occur immediately, serious coagulation problems such as disseminated intravascular coagulopathy usually occur. The substances in the amniotic fluid also can affect pulmonary blood vessels, by causing venospasm or pulmonary hypertension, and cardiac function, by causing left ventricular failure.

Maternal factors (including multiparity, tumultuous labor, abruptio placentae, and oxytocin induction of labor) and fetal problems (including macrosomia, death, and meconium passage) have been associated with an increased risk for the development of AFE (Cunningham et al., 2001).

Collaborative Care

The immediate interventions for AFE are summarized in the Emergency box. Such medical management must be instituted immediately. Cardiopulmonary resuscitation is often necessary. The woman is usually placed on mechanical ventilation, and blood replacement is initiated; coagulation defects are treated. Although the incidence of possible complications is small, their immediate recognition and the prompt initiation of treatment is important.

The nurse's immediate responsibility is to assist with the resuscitation efforts. If the woman survives, she is usually moved to a critical care unit, where hemodynamic monitoring and blood replacement and coagulopathy treatment are implemented.

Support of the woman's partner and family is needed; they will be anxious and distressed. Brief explanations of what is happening are important during the emergency and can be reinforced after the immediate crisis is over. If the woman dies, emotional support and involvement of the perinatal loss support team or other resource for grief counseling is needed. Referral to grief and loss support groups would be appropriate (see Chapter 34). The nursing staff also may need help in coping with feelings and emotions that result from a maternal death.

KEY POINTS

- Preterm labor is cervical change and uterine contractions occurring between 20 weeks and 37 weeks of pregnancy; preterm birth is any birth that occurs before the completion of 37 weeks of pregnancy.
- The cause of preterm labor is unknown and is assumed to be multifactorial; therefore it is not possible to predict with certainty which women will experience preterm labor and birth.
- Because the onset of preterm labor is often insidious and can be mistaken for normal discomforts of pregnancy, nurses should teach all pregnant women how to detect the early symptoms of preterm labor and to call their primary health care provider when symptoms occur.
- Bed rest, a commonly prescribed intervention for preterm labor, has many deleterious side effects and has never been shown to decrease preterm birth rates.
- Research has demonstrated that a gain of 48 hours to several days is the best outcome that can be expected with the use of tocolytics; the best reason to use tocolytic therapy is to achieve sufficient time to administer glucocorticoids in an effort to accelerate fetal lung maturity and reduce the severity of respiratory complications in infants born preterm.
- Vigilance for signs of infection is a major part of the care for women with PPROM.
- Dystocia results from differences in the normal relations among any of the five factors affecting labor and is characterized by differences in the pattern of progress in labor.
- Dysfunctional labor occurs as a result of hypertonic uterine dysfunction, hypotonic uterine dysfunction, or inadequate voluntary expulsive forces.
- The functional relations among the uterine contractions, the fetus, and the mother's pelvis are altered by maternal positioning.
- Uterine contractility is increased by the effects of oxytocin and prostaglandin and is decreased by tocolytic agents.
- Cervical ripening using chemical or mechanical measures can increase the success of labor induction.
- Expectant parents benefit from learning about operative obstetrics (e.g., forceps-assisted, vacuum-assisted, or cesarean birth) during the prenatal period.
- The basic purpose of cesarean birth is to preserve the life or health of the mother and her fetus.
- Unless contraindicated, vaginal birth is possible after a previous cesarean birth.
- Labor management that emphasizes one-to-one support of the laboring woman by another woman (e.g., doula, nurse, nurse-midwife) can reduce the rate of cesarean birth and increase the rate of VBACs.
- A postterm pregnancy poses a risk to both the mother and the fetus.
- Obstetric emergencies (e.g., shoulder dystocia, prolapsed cord, rupture of the uterus, and amniotic fluid embolism) occur rarely but require immediate intervention to preserve the health or life of the mother and fetus/newborn.

CRITICAL THINKING EXERCISES

1. Imagine that you have just been appointed as the nurse manager of a labor and birth unit at a large University Medical Center. You are concerned regarding the high rate of cesarean births on your unit, especially those performed for failure to progress and unsuccessful VBAC attempts. Discuss the process you would use in an attempt to reduce the trend of increased cesarean births and unsuccessful VBAC attempts.
2. Shelly, a 36-year-old primigravida at 30 weeks of gestation, was admitted to your labor and birth unit with a diagnosis of preterm labor. She is accompanied by her husband; they are both distraught that their much anticipated baby may be born too soon. The woman tells you that she just thought she had a touch of the flu until her doctor told her that her cervix was changing, and she needed to be admitted right away. An order for a magnesium sulfate infusion and betamethasone IM have been ordered along with complete bed rest.
   - **a.** Explain to this couple the purpose for each component of the woman's treatment plan and how each will affect her and her baby.
   - **b.** Create an assessment protocol that you would follow when administering the magnesium sulfate infusion.
   - **c.** What care measures would you implement for this woman to ensure her comfort and emotional well-being during hospitalization? How would you help this father meet his emotional needs so that he can be a support for his wife?
   - **d.** This woman's statement that she did not know she was in labor, that she thought she just had the flu, prompts you to develop a teaching plan to alert pregnant women to the signs and symptoms of preterm labor and what to do should they occur. Prepare the content outline you would use when addressing the issue of preterm labor with a group of pregnant women and their partners at an expectant parents class.
   - **e.** Once her contractions subside, the magnesium sulfate infusion is discontinued, and Shelly begins treatment with nifedipine. Explain the rationale for using nifedipine as part of the treatment plan for her. What measures would you teach Shelly and her husband to ensure safe and effective treatment for her and her fetus?
   - **f.** Bed rest with bathroom privileges only will be continued at home. What suggestions would you give to Shelly, her husband, and their family to help reduce the stressors associated with prescribed antepartum bed rest?

RESOURCES

American College of Obstetricians and Gynecologists (ACOG)
409 12th St. SW
P.O. Box 96920
Washington, DC 20090-6920
800-762-2264
www.acog.org

Birthrites: Healing after Cesarean, Inc.
www.birthrites.org

C/SEC, Inc. (Cesarean/Support Education and Concern)
22 Forest Rd.
Framingham, MA 01701
508-877-8266

A Free Home for Moms on Bedrest
www.momsonbedrest.com

International Cesarean Awareness Network (ICAN)
1304 Kingsdale Ave.
Redondo Beach, CA 90278
310-542-6400
www.ican-online.org

Mothers of Supertwins (MOST)
MOST
P.O. Box 951
Brentwood, NY 11717
631-859-1110
www.mostonline.org

National Organization of Mothers of Twins Clubs, Inc. (NOMOTC)
P.O. Box 438
Thompsons Station, TN 37179-0438
615-595-0936
www.nomotc.org

National Perinatal Association
3500 East Fletcher Ave., Suite 205
Tampa, FL 33613-4712
813-971-1008
www.nationalperinatal.org

Pregnancy Bedrest: A Reading Room to Help You Survive and Thrive during Your Days of Waiting
Amy E. Tracy
445C E. Cheyenne Mtn. Blvd., #194
Colorado Springs, CO 80906
www.pregnancybedrest.com

Pregnancy Bedrest Web: Information on High-Risk Pregnancy for Women, Their Families, and Their Caregivers
Judy Maloni, PhD, RN, FAAN
Case Western Reserve University–Bolton School of Nursing
10900 Euclid Ave.
Cleveland, OH 44106
216-368-2912
fpb.cwru.edu/bedrest

RESOURCES—cont'd

Sidelines: High Risk Pregnancy Support Group
P.O. Box 1808
Laguna Beach, CA 92652
888-447-4754
www.sidelines.org

The Triplet Connection
P.O. Box 99571
Stockton, CA 95209
209-474-0885
www.tripletconnection.org

VBAC.com—A Woman-Centered Evidence Based Resource
Nicette Jukelevics
Center for Family
24050 Madison St., Suite 200
Torrance, CA 90505
310-375-3141
www.vbac.com

REFERENCES

Abrahams, C., & Katz, M. (2002). A perspective on the diagnosis of preterm labor. *Journal of Perinatal and Neonatal Nursing, 16*(1), 1-11.

Adler, C., & Zarchin, Y. (2002). The "Virtual Focus Group": Using the internet to reach pregnant women on home bed rest. *Journal of Obstetric, Gynecologic, and Neonatal Nursing, 31*(4), 418-427.

American College of Obstetricians and Gynecologists. (1997a). ACOG practice patterns. Management of posterm pregnancy. No. 6, October 1997. *International Journal of Gynaecologists and Obstetricians, 60*(1), 86-91.

American College of Obstetricians and Gynecologists (ACOG). (1997b). Shoulder dystocia. Preterm labor. *Practice Bulletin No. 7.* Washington, DC: ACOG.

American College of Obstetricians and Gynecologists (ACOG). (1998a). Antenatal corticosteroid therapy for fetal maturation. *ACOG Committee Opinion.* Washington, DC: ACOG.

American College of Obstetricians and Gynecologists (ACOG). (1998b). Premature rupture of membranes: Clinical management guidelines for obstetricians and gynecologists. *International Journal of Gynecology and Obstetrics, 63*(1), 75-84.

American College of Obstetricians and Gynecologists (ACOG). (1999a). Vaginal birth after a previous cesarean delivery. *Practice Bulletin No. 5.* Washington, DC: ACOG.

American College of Obstetricians and Gynecologists (ACOG). (1999b). Induction of labor. *Practice Bulletin No. 10.* Washington, DC: ACOG.

American College of Obstetricians and Gynecologists (ACOG). (2000). Fetal macrosomia. *Practice Bulletin No. 22.* Washington, DC: ACOG.

American College of Obstetricians and Gynecologists & American Academy of Pediatrics (ACOG/AAP). (1997). *Guidelines for perinatal care* (4th ed.). Washington, DC: ACOG.

Arulkumarian, S. (1997). Prolonged pregnancy. In D. James, et al. (Eds.), *High risk pregnancy management options.* London: WB Saunders.

Association of Women's Health, Obstetric, and Gynecologic Nurses. (2000). *Issue: Professional nursing support of laboring women.* Washington, DC: AWHONN

Berg-Lekas, M., Hogberg, U., & Winkvist, A. (1998). Familial occurrence of dystocia. *American Journal of Obstetrics and Gynecology, 179*(1), 117-121.

Bolane, J., & Furlong, J. (1994). *Coping with bedrest in pregnancy.* Waco, TX: Childbirth Graphics.

Boulvain, M., & Irion, O. (2001). Stripping/sweeping the membranes for inducing labour or preventing post-term pregnancy (Cochrane Review). In *The Cochrane Library*, Issue 2. Oxford: Update Software.

Bruner, J. et al. (1998). All-fours maneuver for reducing shoulder dystocia during labor. *Journal of Reproductive Medicine, 43*(5), 439-443.

Burrows, W. et al. (1995). Safety and efficacy of early postoperative solid food consumption after cesarean section. *Journal of Reproductive Medicine, 40*(6), 463-467.

Carpenter, J. (1998). Shortening the short stay. *AWHONN Lifelines, 2*(1), 28-34.

Cefalo, R., & Bowes, W. (1998). Managing labor: Never walk alone. *New England Journal of Medicine, 339*, 117-119.

Collaborative Group on Preterm Birth Prevention. (1993). Multicenter randomized controlled trial of a preterm birth prevention program. *American Journal of Obstetrics and Gynecology, 169*, 352-366.

Colombo D., & Iams, J. (2000). Cervical length and preterm labor. *Clinical Obstetrics and Gynecology, 43*(4), 735-745.

Creasy, R., & Iams, J. (1999). Preterm labor and birth. In R. Creasy & R. Resnik (Eds.). *Maternal- fetal medicine* (4th ed.). Philadelphia: W.B. Saunders.

Crowley, P. (2000). Interventions for preventing or improving the outcome of delivery at or beyond term (Cochrane Review). In *The Cochrane Library*, Issue 2, Oxford: Update Software.

Cunningham, F. et al. (2001). *Williams' obstetrics* (21st ed.). New York: McGraw-Hill.

Curry, M., Perrin, N., & Wall, E. (1998). Effects of abuse on maternal complications and birthweight in adult and adolescent women. *Obstetrics and Gynecology, 92*, 530-534.

Curtin, S., & Kozak, L. (1998). Decline in U.S. cesarean delivery rate appears to stall. *Birth, 25*(4), 259-262.

Dilks, F., & Beal, J. (1997). Role of self-efficacy in birth choice. *Journal of Perinatal and Neonatal Nursing, 11*(1), 1-9.

DiMatteo, M. et al. (1996). Cesarean childbirth and psychosocial outcomes: A meta-analysis. *Health Psychology, 15*(4), 303-314.

Divon, M. (2002). Prolonged pregnancy. In S. Gabbe, J. Niebyl, & J. Simpson (Eds.), *Obstetrics: Normal and problem pregnancies* (4th ed.). New York: Churchill Livingstone.

Durham, R. (1998). Strategies women engage in when managing preterm labor at home. *Journal of Perinatalogy, 18*(1), 61-64.

Dyson, D. et al. (1998). Monitoring women at risk for preterm labor. *New England Journal of Medicine, 338*, 15-19.

Eakes, M., & Brown, H. (1998). Home alone: Meeting the needs of mothers after cesarean birth. *AWHONN Lifelines, 2*(1), 36-40.

Ellings, J., Newman, R., & Bowers, N. (1998). Intrapartum care for women with multiple pregnancy. *Journal of Obstetric, Gynecologic, and Neonatal Nursing, 27*(4), 466-472.

Enkin et al. (2000). *A guide to effective care in pregnancy and childbirth* (3rd ed.). Oxford, NY: Oxford University Press.

Flamm, B., Berwick, D., & Kabcenell, A. (1998). Reducing cesarean section rates safely: Lessons from a "Breakthrough Series" Collaborative. *Birth, 25*(2), 117-124.

Freda, M., & Patterson, E. (1995). *Preterm birth: Prevention and nursing management: Nursing module.* New York: March of Dimes.

Freda, M. et al. (1993). Fetal movement counting: Which method? *MCN American Journal of Maternal Child Nursing, 18*, 314-321.

Freston, M. et al. (1997). Responses of pregnant women to potential preterm labor symptoms. *Journal of Obstetric, Gynecologic, and Neonatal Nursing, 26*, 35-41.

Friedman, E. (1989). Normal and dysfunctional labor. In W. Cohen et al. (Eds.), *Management of labor* (2nd ed.). Rockville, MD: Aspen.

Gabay, M., & Wolfe, S. (1997). The beneficial alternative. *Public Health Report, 112*, 386-394.

Gabbe, S., Niebyl, J., & Simpson, J. (2002). *Obstetrics: Normal and problem pregnancies* (4th ed.). New York: Churchill Livingstone.

Garcia-Velasco, J., & Gonzalez-Gonzalez, A. (1998). A prospective, randomized trial of nifedipine vs. ritodrine in threatened preterm labor. *International Journal of Gynecology and Obstetrics, 61*, 239-244.

Garite, T. (1999). Premature rupture of membranes. In R. Creasy & R. Resnik (Eds.), *Maternal-fetal medicine* (4th ed.). Philadelphia: W.B. Saunders.

Gilbert, E., & Harmon, J. (2003). *Manual of high risk pregnancy and delivery* (3rd ed.). St. Louis: Mosby.

Goldberg, A., Greenberg, M., & Darney, P. (2001). Drug therapy: Misoprostol and pregnancy. *New England Journal of Medicine, 344*(1), 38-47.

Goldenberg, R., & Rouse, D. (1998). Prevention of premature birth. *New England Journal of Medicine, 339*, 313-320.

Goldenberg, R. et al. (2000). The preterm prediction study: Sequential cervical length and fetal fibronectin testing for the prediction of spontaneous preterm birth. *American Journal of Obstetrics and Gynecology, 182*(3), 636-643.

Gregory, K. (2000). Monitoring risk adjustment and strategies to decrease cesarean rates. *Current Opinion in Obstetrics and Gynecology, 12*(6), 481-486.

Guinn, D. et al. (1998). Terbutaline pump maintenance therapy for prevention of preterm delivery: A double-blind trial. *American Journal of Obstetrics and Gynecology, 179*, 874-878.

Hall, S. (1997). The nurse's role in the identification of risks and treatment of shoulder dystocia. *Journal of Obstetric, Gynecologic, and Neonatal Nursing 26*(1), 25-32.

Hannah, M. et al. (1996). Postterm pregnancy: Putting the merits of a policy of induction of labor into perspective. *Birth, 23*(1), 13-19.

Heaman, M., Sprague, A., & Stewart, P. (2001). Reducing the preterm birth rate: a population health strategy. *Journal of Obstetric, Gynecologic, and Neonatal Nursing, 30*(1), 20-29.

Hodnett, E. (2002). Caregiver support for women during childbirth. (Cochrane Library). In *The Cochrane Library* Issue 1. Oxford: Update Software

Iams, J. (2002). Preterm birth. In S. Gabbe, J. Niebyl, & J. Simpson (Eds.), *Obstetrics: Normal and problem pregnancies* (4th ed.). New York: Churchill Livingstone.

Isennock, P. (1992). *Bed rest before baby: What's a mother to do?* Perry Hall, MD: Mustard Seed Publications.

Janke, J. (1999). The effect of relaxation therapy on preterm labor outcomes. *Journal of Obstetric, Gynecologic, and Neonatal Nursing, 28*(3), 255-263.

Lanni, S., & Seeds, J. (2002). Malpresentations. In S. Gabbe, J. Niebyl, & J. Simpson (Eds.), *Obstetrics: Normal and problem pregnancies* (4th ed.). New York: Churchill Livingstone.

Lehne, R. (2001). *Pharmacology for nursing care.* Philadelphia: W.B. Saunders.

Lydon-Rochelle, M. et al. (2001). Risk of uterine rupture during labor among women with a prior cesarean delivery. *New England Journal of Medicine, 345*(1), 3-8.

Macones, G., & Robinson, C. (1998). Is there justification for using indomethacin in preterm labor? An analysis of neonatal risks and benefits. *American Journal of Obstetrics and Gynecology, 178*, 873-874.

Maloni, J. (1998). *Antepartum bedrest: Case studies, research, and nursing care.* Washington, DC: AWHONN.

Maloni, J. (2000). *The prevention of preterm birth: Research-based practice, nursing interventions, and practice scenarios.* Washington, DC: Association of Women's Health, Obstetric, and Neonatal Nurses (AWHONN).

Maloni, J. (2002). Astronauts & pregnancy bed rest: What NASA is teaching us about inactivity. *AWHONN Lifelines, 6*(4), 318-323.

Maloni, J., Brezinski-Tomasi, J., & Johnson, L. (2001). Antepartum bedrest: Effect upon the family. *Journal of Obstetric, Gynecologic, and Neonatal Nursing, 30*(2), 165-173.

Maloni, J., & Kutil, R. (2000). Antepartum support group for women hospitalized on bedrest. *MCN American Journal of Maternal Child Nursing, 25*(4), 204-210.

Maloni, J. et al. (1993). Physical and psychosocial side effects of antepartum bed rest. *Nursing Research, 42*(4), 197-203.

Martin, J., et al. (2002). Births: Final data for 2000. *National Vital Statistics Report, 50*(5), 1-102.

Martin, R., & Leaton, M. (2001). Amniotic fluid embolism. *American Journal of Nursing, 101*(3), 43-44.

Mathews, T. (1998). Trends in stimulation and induction of labor, 1989-1995. *Statistical Bulletin, 78*(4), 20-26.

Mayberry, L. et al. (1999). Use of delayed pushing with epidural anesthesia: Findings from a randomized, controlled trial. *Journal of Perinatology, 19*(1), 26-30.

Mayberry, L. et al. (2000). Second stage labor management: Promotion of evidence-based practice and a collaborative approach to patient care. Washington, DC: AWHONN.

McFarlane, J., & Gondolf, E. (1998). Preventing abuse during pregnancy: A clinical protocol. (1998). *MCN American Journal of Maternal Child Nursing, 23*, 22-26.

McNiven, P. et al. (1998). An early labor assessment program: A randomized, controlled trial. *Birth, 25*(1), 5-10.

Miltner, R. (2000). Identifying labor support actions of intrapartum nurses. *Journal of Obstetric, Gynecologic, and Neonatal Nursing, 29*(5), 491-499.

Moore, M. (1999). Biochemical markers for preterm birth. *MCN American Journal of Maternal Child Nursing, 24*, 66-74.

Moore, M., & Freda, M. (1998). Reducing preterm and low birthweight births: Still a nursing challenge. *MCN American Journal of Maternal Child Nursing, 23*, 200-208.

Moore, M. et al. (1998). A randomized trial of nurse intervention to reduce preterm and low birthweight births. *Obstetrics and Gynecology, 91*, 656-661.

Myers, E. et al. (2002). Management of prolonged pregnancy. *Evidence Report/technology Assessment No. 53* (AHRQ Publication No. 02-E018). Rockville, MD: Agency for Healthcare Research and Quality.

National Institutes of Health. (2000). *Antenatal corticosteroids revisited. Consensus Development Conference Statement.* Maryland: NIH. Retrieved from http://consensus.nih.gov.

Niam, A. et al. (2002). Changes in cervical length and the risk of preterm labor. *American Journal of Obstetrics and Gynecology, 186*(5), 887-889.

Nocon, J. (2000). Shoulder dystocia and macrosomia. In L. Kean, P. Baker, & D. Edlestone (Eds.), *Best practice in labor ward management.* Philadelphia: W.B. Saunders.

Norwitz, E., Robinson, J., & Repke, J. (2002). Labor and delivery. In S. Gabbe, J. Niebyl, & J. Simpson (Eds.), *Obstetrics: Normal and problem pregnancies* (4th ed.). New York: Churchill Livingstone.

Peck, D., & Griffis, N. (1999). Preterm labor in the triage setting. *Journal of Nurse Midwifery, 44*(5), 449-457.

Pozaic, S. (1999). Induction and augmentation of labor. In L. Mandeville & N. Troiano (Eds.), *High-risk and critical care intrapartum nursing* (2nd ed.). Philadelphia: Lippincott.

Pschirrer, E., & Monga, M. (2000). Risk factors for preterm labor. *Clinics in Obstetrics and Gynecology, 43*(4), 727-734.

Radin, T., Harmon, J., & Hanson, D. (1993). Nurses' care during labor: Its effects on the cesarean birth rate of healthy nulliparous women. *Birth, 20*(1), 14-21.

Rippin-Sisler, C. (1996). The experience of precipitate labor. *Birth, 23*(4), 224-228.

Roberts, W., & Morrison, J. (1998). Has the use of home monitors, fetal fibronectin, and measurement of cervical length helped predict labor and/or prevent preterm delivery in twins? *Clinical Obstetrics and Gynecology, 41*, 94-102.

Ryding, E., Wijma, K., & Wijma, B. (1998). Experiences of emergency cesarean section: A phenomenological study of 53 women. *Birth, 25*(4), 246-251.

Schaffir, J. (2002). Survey of folk beliefs about induction of labor. *Birth, 29*(1), 47-51.

Schmidt, J. (1997). Fluid check: Making the case for intrapartum amnioinfusion. *AWHONN Lifelines, 1*(5), 46-51.

Schmidt, J. (1999). Prolonged pregnancy. In L. Mandeville & N. Troiano (Eds.), *High-risk and critical care intrapartum nursing* (2nd ed.). Philadelphia: Lippincott.

Scott, J. (1999). Cesarean delivery. In Scott, J. et al. (Eds.), *Danforth's obstetrics and gynecology* (8th ed.). Philadelphia: Lippincott, Williams & Wilkins.

Searing, K. (2001). Induction vs. post-date pregnancies: Exploring the controversy of who's really at risk. *AWHONN Lifelines, 5*(2), 44-48.

Simkin, P., & Ancheta, R. (2000). *The labor progress handbook.* Malden, MA: Blackwell Science.

Simpson, K. (1997). Preterm birth in the United States: Current issues and future perspectives. *Journal of Perinatal and Neonatal Nursing, 10*(4),11-15.

Simpson, K. (2002). *Cervical ripening and induction and augmentation of labor* (2nd ed.). Washington, DC: AWHONN.

Simpson, K., & Knox, G. (2001). Fundal pressure during second stage of labor. *MCM American Journal of Maternal Child Nursing, 26*(6), 64-70.

Spellacy, W. (1999). Postdate pregnancy. In J. Scott et al. (Eds.), *Danforth's obstetrics and gynecology* (8th ed.). Philadelphia: Lippincott, Williams & Wilkins.

Summers, L. (1997). Methods of cervical ripening and labor induction. *Journal of Nurse Midwifery, 42*(2), 71-85.

Thomas, L. et al. (1990). The effects of rocking, diet modifications, and antiflatulence medication on postcesarean section gas pain. *Journal of Perinatal and Neonatal Nursing, 4*(3), 12-24.

Varney, H. (1997). *Varney's textbook for midwives* (3rd ed.). Sudbury, MA: Jones & Bartlett.

Ventura, S. et al. (2001). Births: final data for 1999. *National Vital Statistics Report, 49*(1), 1-100.

Weiss, M., Saks, N., & Harris, S. (2002). Resolving the uncertainty of preterm symptoms: Women's experiences with the onset of preterm labor. *Journal of Obstetric, Gynecologic, and Neonatal Nursing, 31*(1), 66-76.

Weitz, B. (2001). Premature rupture of the fetal membranes: An update for advanced practice nurses. *MCN American Journal of Maternal Child Nursing, 26*(2), 86-92.

Wilson, C. (2000). The nurse's role in misoprostol induction: A proposed protocol. *Journal of Obstetric, Gynecologic, and Neonatal Nursing, 29*(6), 574-589.

Witcher, P. (2002). Treatment of preterm labor. *Journal of Perinatal and Neonatal Nursing, 16*(1), 25-46.

Wood, C. (1994). Postdate pregnancy update. *Journal of Nurse Midwifery, 39*(suppl 2), 110S-122S.

Youngblut, J., et al. (2000). Employment patterns and timing of birth in women with high-risk pregnancies. *Journal of Obstetric, Gynecologic, and Neonatal Nursing, 29*(2), 137-144.

CHAPTER 37

Deitra Leonard Lowdermilk

Postpartum Complications

http://evolve.elsevier.com/Lowdermilk/MatWmnHlth/

LEARNING OBJECTIVES

- Identify causes, signs and symptoms, and medical and nursing management of postpartum hemorrhage.
- Describe hemorrhagic shock as a complication of postpartum hemorrhage including management and hazards of therapy.
- Differentiate the causes of postpartum infection.
- Summarize assessment and care of women with postpartum infection.
- Describe thromboembolic disorders, including incidence, etiology, signs and symptoms, and management.
- Summarize the role of the nurse in the home setting in assessing potential problems and managing care of women with postpartum physiologic complications.

Collaborative efforts of the health care team are needed to provide safe and effective care to the woman and family experiencing postpartum physiologic complications including maternal death. This chapter focuses on hemorrhage and infection.

POSTPARTUM HEMORRHAGE

Definition and Incidence

Postpartum hemorrhage (PPH) continues to be a leading cause of maternal morbidity and mortality in the United States (Hoyert et al., 2001). It is a life-threatening event that can occur with little warning and is often unrecognized until the mother has profound symptoms. PPH has been traditionally defined as the loss of more than 500 ml of blood after vaginal birth and 1000 ml after cesarean birth. A 10% change in hematocrit between admission for labor and postpartum or the need for erythrocyte transfusion also has been used to define PPH (ACOG, 1998). However, defining PPH is not a clear-cut issue. The American College of Obstetricians and Gynecologists (ACOG) states that hemorrhage is difficult to define clinically. Diagnosis is often based on subjective observations, with blood loss often being underestimated by as much as 50% (ACOG, 1998).

Traditionally, PPH has been classified as early or late with respect to the birth. Early, acute, or primary PPH occurs within 24 hours of the birth. Late or secondary PPH occurs more than 24 hours but less than 6 weeks postpartum (ACOG, 1998). Today's health care environment encourages shortened stays after birth, thereby increasing the potential for acute episodes of PPH to occur outside the traditional hospital or birth center setting.

Etiology and Risk Factors

It is helpful to consider the problem of excessive bleeding with reference to the stages of labor. From birth of the infant until separation of the placenta, the character and quantity of blood passed may suggest excessive bleeding. For example, dark blood is probably of venous origin, perhaps from varices or superficial lacerations of the birth canal. Bright blood is arterial and may indicate deep lacerations of the cervix. Spurts of blood with clots may indicate partial placental separation. Failure of blood to clot or remain clotted indicates a pathologic condition or coagulopathy such as disseminated intravascular coagulation (DIC) (ACOG, 1998; Varner, 1998).

Excessive bleeding may occur during the period from the separation of the placenta to its expulsion or removal. Commonly, such excessive bleeding is the result of incomplete placental separation, undue manipulation of the fundus, or excessive traction on the cord. After the placenta has been expelled or removed, persistent or excessive blood loss usually is the result of atony of the uterus or prolapse of the uterus into the vagina. Late PPH may be the result of subinvolution of the uterus, endometritis, or retained placental fragments (ACOG, 1998). Predisposing factors for PPH are listed in Box 37-1.

Uterine Atony

Uterine atony is marked hypotonia of the uterus. Normally, placental separation and expulsion are facilitated by contraction of the uterus, which also prevents hemorrhage from the placental site. The corpus is in essence a basketweave of strong, interlacing smooth muscle bundles through which many large maternal blood vessels pass (see Fig. 5-3). If the uterus is flaccid after detachment of all or part of the placenta, brisk venous bleeding occurs, and normal coagulation of the open vasculature is impaired and continues until the uterine muscle is contracted.

Uterine atony is the leading cause of PPH, complicating approximately one in 20 births (Gonik, 1999). It is associated with high parity, hydramnios, a macrosomic fetus, and multifetal gestation. In such conditions, the uterus is "overstretched" and contracts poorly after the birth. Other causes of atony include traumatic birth, use of halogenated anesthesia (e.g., halothane) or magnesium sulfate, rapid or prolonged labor, chorioamnionitis, and use of oxytocin for labor induction or augmentation (ACOG, 1998; Varner, 1998).

Lacerations of the Genital Tract

Lacerations of the cervix, vagina, and perineum also are causes of PPH. Hemorrhage related to lacerations should be suspected if bleeding continues despite a firm, contracted uterine fundus. This bleeding can be a slow trickle, an oozing, or frank hemorrhage. Factors that influence the causes and incidence of obstetric lacerations of the lower genital tract include operative birth, precipitate birth, congenital abnormalities of the maternal soft parts, and contracted pelvis. Size, abnormal presentation, and position of the fetus; relative size of the presenting part and the birth canal; previous scarring from infection, injury, or operation; and vulvar, perineal, and vaginal varicosities also can cause lacerations.

Extreme vascularity in the labial and periclitoral areas often results in profuse bleeding if laceration occurs. Hematomas also may be present.

Lacerations of the perineum are the most common of all injuries in the lower portion of the genital tract. These are classified as first, second, third, and fourth degree (see Chapter 21). An episiotomy may extend to become either third- or fourth-degree laceration.

Prolonged pressure of the fetal head on the vaginal mucosa ultimately interferes with the circulation and may produce ischemic or pressure necrosis. The state of the tissues in combination with the type of birth may result in deep vaginal lacerations, with consequent predisposition to vaginal hematomas.

Pelvic **hematomas** may be vulvar, vaginal, or retroperitoneal in origin. Vulvar hematomas are the most common. Pain is the most common symptom, and most vulvar hematomas are visible. Vaginal hematomas occur more commonly in association with a forceps-assisted birth, an episiotomy, or primigravidity (Benedetti, 2002). During the postpartum period, if the woman reports a persistent perineal or rectal pain or a feeling of pressure in the vagina, a careful examination is made. However, a retroperitoneal hematoma may cause minimal pain, and the initial symptoms may be signs of shock (Benedetti, 2002).

Cervical lacerations usually occur at the lateral angles of the external os. Most are shallow, and bleeding is minimal. More extensive lacerations may extend into the vaginal vault or into the lower uterine segment.

BOX 37-1 Risk Factors and Causes of Postpartum Hemorrhage

Uterine atony
- Overdistended uterus
  - —Large fetus
  - —Multiple fetuses
  - —Hydramnios
  - —Distention with clots
- Anesthesia and analgesia
  - —Conduction anesthesia
- Previous history of uterine atony
- High parity
- Prolonged labor, oxytocin-induced labor
- Trauma during labor and birth
  - —Forceps-assisted birth
  - —Vacuum-assisted birth
  - —Cesarean birth

Lacerations of the birth canal
Retained placental fragments
Ruptured uterus
Inversion of the uterus
Placenta accreta
Coagulation disorders
Placental abruption
Placenta previa
Manual removal of a retained placenta
Magnesium sulfate administration during labor or postpartum period
Endometritis
Uterine subinvolution

Retained Placenta

Nonadherent Retained Placenta

Retained placenta may result from partial separation of a normal placenta, entrapment of the partially or completely separated placenta by an hourglass constriction ring of the uterus, mismanagement of the third stage of labor, or abnormal adherence of the entire placenta or a portion of the placenta to the uterine wall. Placental retention because of poor separation is common in very preterm births (20 to 24 weeks of gestation).

Management of nonadherent retained placenta is by manual separation and removal by the primary health care provider. Supplementary anesthesia is not usually needed for women who have had regional anesthesia for birth. For other women, administration of light nitrous oxide and oxygen inhalation anesthesia or intravenous thiopental facilitates uterine exploration and placental removal. After this removal, the woman is at continued risk for PPH and for infection.

Adherent Retained Placenta

Abnormal adherence of the placenta occurs for reasons unknown, but it is thought to result from zygotic implantation in an area of defective endometrium so that there is no zone of separation between the placenta and the decidua. Attempts to remove the placenta in the usual manner are unsuccessful, and laceration or perforation of the uterine wall may result, putting the woman at great risk for severe PPH and infection (Cunningham et al., 2001).

Unusual placental adherence may be partial or complete. The following degrees of attachment are recognized:

- *Placenta accreta*, slight penetration of myometrium by placental trophoblast
- *Placenta increta*, deep penetration of myometrium by placenta
- *Placenta percreta*, perforation of uterus by placenta

Bleeding with complete or total placenta accreta may not occur unless separation of the placenta is attempted. With more extensive involvement, bleeding will become profuse when delivery of the placenta is attempted. Treatment includes blood component replacement therapy, and hysterectomy may be indicated (Clark, 1999).

Inversion of the Uterus

Inversion of the uterus after birth is a potentially life-threatening complication. The incidence of uterine inversion is approximately 1 in 2000 to 2500 births (ACOG, 1998) and may recur with a subsequent birth. Uterine inversion may be partial or complete. Complete inversion of the uterus is obvious; a large, red, rounded mass (perhaps with the placenta attached) protrudes 20 to 30 cm outside the introitus. Incomplete inversion cannot be seen but must be felt; a smooth mass will be palpated through the dilated cervix. Contributing factors to uterine inversion include fundal implantation of the placenta, vigorous fundal pressure, excessive traction applied to the cord, uterine atony, leiomyomas, and abnormally adherent placental tissue (Bowes, 1999). Uterine inversion occurs most often in multiparous women and with placenta accreta or increta. The primary presenting signs of uterine inversion are hemorrhage, shock, and pain.

Prevention–always the easiest, cheapest, and most effective therapy–is especially appropriate for uterine inversion. The umbilical cord should not be pulled on strongly unless the placenta has definitely separated.

Subinvolution of the Uterus

Late postpartum bleeding may occur as a result of **subinvolution** of the uterus. Recognized causes of subinvolution include retained placental fragments and pelvic infection.

Signs and symptoms include prolonged lochial discharge, irregular or excessive bleeding, and sometimes hemorrhage. A pelvic examination usually reveals a uterus that is larger than normal and may be boggy.

CARE MANAGEMENT

Assessment and Nursing Diagnoses

PPH may be sudden and even exsanguinating. The nurse must therefore be alert to the symptoms of hemorrhage and hypovolemic shock and be prepared to act quickly to minimize blood loss (Fig. 37-1 and Box 37-2).

The woman's history should be reviewed for factors that cause predisposition to PPH (see Box 37-1). The fundus is assessed to determine whether it is firmly contracted at or near the level of the umbilicus. Bleeding should be assessed for color and amount. The perineum is inspected for signs of lacerations or hematomas to determine the possible source of bleeding.

Vital signs may not be reliable indicators of shock immediately postpartum because of the physiologic adaptations of this period. However, frequent vital sign measurements during the first 2 hours after birth may identify trends related to blood loss (e.g., tachycardia, tachypnea, decreasing blood pressure).

Assessment for bladder distention is important because a distended bladder can displace the uterus and prevent contraction. The skin is assessed for warmth and dryness; nail beds are checked for color and promptness of capillary refill. Laboratory studies include evaluation of hemoglobin and hematocrit levels.

Late PPH develops at least 24 hours after the birth or later in the postpartum period. The woman may be at home when the symptoms occur. Discharge teaching should emphasize the signs of normal involution, as well as potential complications. Nursing diagnoses for women experiencing PPH include the following:

- *Deficient fluid volume related to*
  - –excessive blood loss secondary to uterine atony, lacerations, or uterine inversion
- *Risk for imbalanced fluid volume related to*
  - –blood and fluid volume replacement therapy
- *Risk for infection related to*
  - –excessive blood loss or exposed placental attachment site
- *Risk for injury related to*
  - –attempted manual removal of retained placenta
  - –administration of blood products
  - –operative procedures
- *Fear/anxiety related to*
  - –threat to self
  - –deficient knowledge regarding procedures and operative management
- *Risk for impaired parenting related to*
  - –separation from infant secondary to treatment regimen
- *Ineffective peripheral tissue perfusion related to*
  - –excessive blood loss and shunting of blood to central circulation

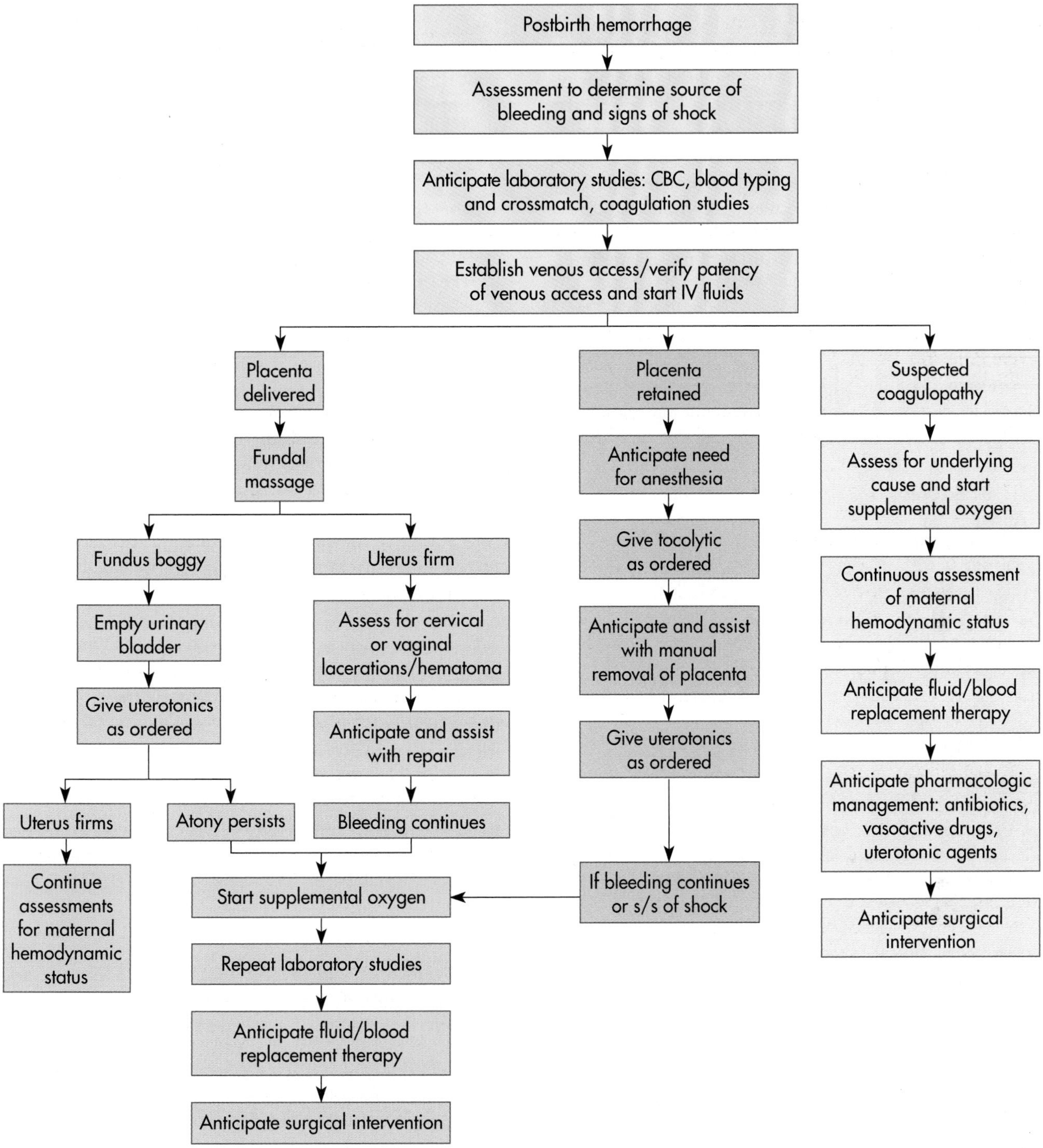
Postbirth hemorrhage
Assessment to determine source of bleeding and signs of shock
Anticipate laboratory studies: CBC, blood typing and crossmatch, coagulation studies
Establish venous access/verify patency of venous access and start IV fluids
Placenta delivered
Fundal massage
Fundus boggy
Empty urinary bladder
Give uterotonics as ordered
Uterus firms
Continue assessments for maternal hemodynamic status
Atony persists
Uterus firm
Assess for cervical or vaginal lacerations/hematoma
Anticipate and assist with repair
Bleeding continues
Start supplemental oxygen
Repeat laboratory studies
Anticipate fluid/blood replacement therapy
Anticipate surgical intervention
Placenta retained
Anticipate need for anesthesia
Give tocolytic as ordered
Anticipate and assist with manual removal of placenta
Give uterotonics as ordered
If bleeding continues or s/s of shock
Suspected coagulopathy
Assess for underlying cause and start supplemental oxygen
Continuous assessment of maternal hemodynamic status
Anticipate fluid/blood replacement therapy
Anticipate pharmacologic management: antibiotics, vasoactive drugs, uterotonic agents
Anticipate surgical intervention

FIG. 37-1 Nursing assessments for postpartum bleeding. *CBC*, Complete blood count; *IV*, intravenous; *s/s*, signs and symptoms; *uterotonics*, medications to contract the uterus.

Expected Outcomes of Care

Expected outcomes of care for the woman experiencing PPH may include that the woman will do the following:

- Maintain normal vital signs and laboratory values.
- Develop no complications related to excessive bleeding.
- Express understanding of her condition, its management, and discharge instructions.
- Identify and use available support systems.

Plan of Care and Interventions

Medical Management

Early recognition and acknowledgment of the diagnosis of PPH are critical to care management. The first step is to evaluate the contractility of the uterus. If the uterus is hypotonic, management is directed toward increasing contractility and minimizing blood loss.

The initial management of excessive postpartum bleeding is firm massage of the uterine fundus, expression of any clots in the uterus, eliminating any bladder distention, and continuous intravenous infusion of 10 to 40 units of oxytocin added to 1000 ml lactated Ringer's or normal saline solution. If the uterus fails to respond to oxytocin, a 0.2 mg dose of ergonovine (Ergotrate) or methylergonovine (Methergine) may be given intramuscularly to produce sustained uterine contractions. However, it is more common to administer a 0.25 mg dose of a derivative of prostaglandin $F_{2\alpha}$ (carboprost tromethamine) intramuscularly. It also can be given intramyometrially at cesarean birth or intraabdominally after vaginal birth (ACOG, 1998). See Table 37-1 for a comparison of drugs used to manage PPH. In addition to the medications used to contract the uterus, rapid administration of crystalloid solutions and or blood or blood products will be needed to restore the woman's intravascular volume (Mousa & Walkinshaw, 2001).

BOX 37-2 Noninvasive Assessments of Cardiac Output in Postpartum Clients Who Are Bleeding

Palpation of pulses (rate, quality, equality)
- Arterial
- Blood pressure

Auscultation
- Heart sounds/murmurs
- Breath sounds

Inspection
- Skin color, temperature, turgor
- Level of consciousness
- Capillary refill
- Urinary output
- Neck veins
- Pulse oximetry
- Mucous membranes

Presence or absence of anxiety, apprehension, restlessness, disorientation

NURSE ALERT

Use of ergonovine or methylergonovine is contraindicated in the presence of hypertension or cardiovascular disease. Prostaglandin $F_2\alpha$ should be used cautiously in women with cardiovascular disease or asthma (Bowes, 1999).

Hypotonic Uterus. Oxygen can be given to enhance oxygen delivery to the cells. A urinary catheter is usually inserted to monitor urine output as a measure of intravascular volume. Laboratory studies usually include a complete blood count with platelet count, fibrinogen, fibrin split products, prothrombin time, and partial thromboplastin time. Blood type and antibody screen are done if not previously performed (ACOG, 1998).

If bleeding persists, bimanual compression may be considered by the obstetrician or nurse midwife. This procedure involves inserting a fist into the vagina and pressing the knuckles against the anterior side of the uterus, and then placing the other hand on the abdomen and massaging the posterior uterus with it. If the uterus still does not become firm, manual exploration of the uterine cavity for retained placental fragments is implemented. If the preceding procedures are ineffective, surgical management may be the only alternative. Surgical management options include

TABLE 37-1 Drugs Used to Manage Postpartum Hemorrhage

	OXYTOCIN (PITOCIN)	METHYLERGONOVINE (METHERGINE)*	PROSTAGLANDIN $F_{2\alpha}$ (PROSTIN/15m; HEMABATE)
Action	Contraction of uterus; decreases bleeding	Contraction of uterus	Contraction of uterus
Side Effect	Infrequent; water intoxication; nausea and vomiting	Hypertension, nausea, vomiting, headache	Headache, nausea, vomiting, fever
Contraindications	None for PPH	Hypertension, cardiac disease	Asthma, hypersensitivity
Dosage; Route	10-40 U/L diluted in lactated Ringer's solution or normal saline at 125 to 200 mU/min IV or 10 to 20 U IM	0.2 mg IM q2-4hr up to five doses; 0.2 mg IV only for emergency	0.25 mg IM or intramyometrially q15-90 min up to eight doses
Nursing Considerations	Continue to monitor vaginal bleeding and uterine tone	Check blood pressure before giving and do not give if >140/90 mm Hg; continue monitoring vaginal bleeding and uterine tone	Continue to monitor vaginal bleeding and uterine tone

*Information about methylergonovine may also be used to describe ergonovine (Ergotrate).

vessel ligation (uteroovarian, uterine, hypogastric), selective arterial embolization, and hysterectomy (ACOG, 1998).

Bleeding with a Contracted Uterus. If the uterus is firmly contracted and bleeding continues, the source of bleeding still must be identified and treated. Assessment may include visual or manual inspection of the perineum, vagina, uterus, cervix, or rectum and laboratory studies (e.g., hemoglobin, hematocrit, coagulation studies, platelet count) (ACOG, 1998). Treatment depends on the source of the bleeding. Lacerations are usually sutured. Hematomas may be managed with observation, cold therapy, ligation of the bleeding vessel, or evacuation. Fluids and or blood replacement may be needed (Benedetti, 2002).

Uterine Inversion. Uterine inversion is an emergency situation requiring immediate recognition, replacement of the uterus within the pelvic cavity, and correction of associated clinical conditions. Tocolytics or halogenated anesthetics may be given to relax the uterus before attempting replacement (Hostetler & Bosworth, 2000). Medical management of this condition includes treating shock, repositioning the uterus, giving oxytocic agents after the uterus is repositioned, and initiating broad-spectrum antibiotics (Benedetti, 2002; Bowes, 1999).

Subinvolution. Treatment of subinvolution depends on the cause. Ergonovine, 0.2 mg every 4 hours for 2 or 3 days, and antibiotic therapy are the most common medications used (Cunningham et al., 2001). Dilation and curettage (D&C) may be needed to remove retained placental fragments or to debride the placental site.

Herbal Remedies

Herbal remedies have been used with some success to control PPH in some settings. Some herbs have homeostatic actions, whereas others work as oxytocic agents to contract the uterus (Beal, 1998; Schirmer, 1998). Box 37-3 lists herbs that have been used and their actions. However, published evidence of the safety and efficacy of herbal therapy is lacking. Evidence from well-controlled studies is needed before recommendation for practice should be made (Brucker, 2001).

Nursing Interventions

Immediate nursing care of the woman with PPH includes assessment of vital signs and uterine consistency and administration of oxytocin or other drugs to stimulate uterine contraction according to standing orders or protocols. The primary health care provider is notified if not present.

The woman and her family will be anxious about her condition. The nurse can intervene by calmly providing explanations about interventions being performed and the need to act quickly.

After the bleeding has been controlled, the care of the woman with lacerations of the perineum is similar to that for women with episiotomies (analgesia as needed for pain and hot or cold applications as necessary). The need for increased roughage in the diet and increased intake of fluids is emphasized. Stool softeners may be used to assist the woman in reestablishing bowel habits without straining and putting stress on the suture lines.

NURSE ALERT

To avoid injury to the suture line, a woman with third- or fourth-degree lacerations is not given rectal suppositories or enemas.

The care of the woman who has experienced an inversion of the uterus focuses on immediate stabilization of hemodynamic status. This requires close observation of her response to treatment to prevent shock or fluid overload. If the uterus has been repositioned manually, care must be taken to avoid aggressive fundal massage.

Discharge instructions for the woman who has had PPH are similar to those for any postpartum woman. In addition, she should be told that she will probably feel fatigue, even exhaustion, and will need to limit her physical activities to conserve her strength. She may need instructions in increasing her dietary iron and protein intake and iron supplementation to rebuild lost red cell (RBC) volume. She may need assistance with infant care and household activities until she has regained strength. Some women have problems with delayed or insufficient lactation and postpartum depression. Referrals for home care follow-up or to community resources may be needed (see Resources at the end of this chapter).

Evaluation

The nurse can be reasonably assured that care was effective to the extent that the expected outcomes were achieved (see Plan of Care).

BOX 37-3 Herbal Remedies for Postpartum Hemorrhage

HERB	ACTION
Witch hazel	Homeostatic
Lady's mantle	Homeostatic
Blue cohosh	Oxytocic
Cotton root bark	Oxytocic
Motherwort	Promotes uterine contraction; vasoconstrictive
Shepherd's purse	Promotes uterine contraction
Alfalfa leaf	Increases availability of vitamin K; increases hemoglobin
Nettle	Increases availability of vitamin K; increases hemoglobin
Red raspberry	Homeostatic; promotes uterine contraction

Source: Beal, M. (1998). Use of complementary and alternative therapies in reproductive medicine. *Journal of Nurse Midwifery 43*(3), 224-233; Schirmer, G. (1998). *Herbal medicine.* Bedford TX: MED2000 Inc.; Tiran, D., & Mack, S. (Eds.). (2000). *Complementary therapies for pregnancy and childbirth* (2nd ed.). Edinburgh: Bailliere Tindall.

Plan of Care: Postpartum Hemorrhage

NURSING DIAGNOSIS Deficient fluid volume related to postpartum hemorrhage

Expected Outcome *Patient will demonstrate fluid balance as evidenced by stable vital signs, prompt capillary refill time, and balanced intake and output.*

Nursing Interventions/*Rationales*

Monitor vital signs, oxygen saturation, urine specific gravity, and capillary refill *to provide baseline data.*

Measure and record amount and type of bleeding by weighing and counting saturated pads. If woman is at home, teach her to count pads and save any clots or tissue. If woman is admitted to hospital, save any clots and tissue for further examination *to estimate type and amount of blood loss for fluid replacement.*

Provide quiet environment *to promote rest and decrease metabolic demands.*

Give explanation of all procedures *to reduce anxiety.*

Begin IV access with 18-gauge or larger needle for infusion of isotonic solution as ordered *to provide fluid or blood replacement.*

Administer medications as ordered, such as oxytocin, methylergonovine, or prostaglandin $F_{2\alpha}$, *to increase contractility of the uterus.*

Insert indwelling urinary catheter *to provide most accurate assessment of renal function and hypovolemia.*

Prepare for surgical intervention as needed *to stop the source of bleeding.*

NURSING DIAGNOSIS Ineffective tissue perfusion related to hypovolemia

Expected Outcome *Woman will have stable vital signs, oxygen saturation, arterial blood gases, and adequate hematocrit and hemoglobin.*

Nursing Interventions/*Rationales*

Monitor vital signs, oxygen saturation, arterial blood gases, and hematocrit and hemoglobin *to assess for hypovolemic shock and decreased tissue perfusion.*

Assess for any changes in level of consciousness *to assess for evidence of hypoxia.*

Assess capillary refill, mucous membranes, skin temperature *to note indicators of vasoconstriction.*

Give supplementary oxygen as ordered *to provide additional oxygenation to tissues.*

Suction as needed, insert oral airway, *to maintain clear, open airway for oxygenation.*

Monitor arterial blood gases *to provide information about acidosis or hypoxia.*

Administer sodium bicarbonate if ordered *to reverse metabolic acidosis.*

NURSING DIAGNOSIS Anxiety related to sudden change in health status

Expected Outcome *Woman will verbalize the anxious feelings are diminished.*

Nursing Interventions/*Rationales*

Using therapeutic communication, evaluate woman's understanding of events *to provide clarification of any misconceptions.*

Provide calm, competent attitude and environment *to aid in decreasing anxiety.*

Explain all procedures *to decrease anxiety about the unknown.*

Allow woman to verbalize feelings *to permit clarification of information and promote trust.*

Continue to assess vital signs or other clinical indicators of hypovolemic shock *to evaluate if psychologic response of anxiety intensifies physiologic indicators.*

NURSING DIAGNOSIS Risk for infection related to blood loss and invasive procedures as a result of postpartum hemorrhage

Expected Outcomes *Woman will verbalize understanding of risk factors. Woman will demonstrate no signs of infection.*

Nursing Interventions/*Rationales*

Maintain Standard Precautions and use good handwashing technique when providing care *to prevent spread of infection.*

Teach woman to maintain good handwashing technique (particularly before handling her newborn) and to maintain scrupulous perineal care with frequent change and careful disposal of perineal pads *to avoid spread of microorganisms.*

Monitor vital signs *to detect signs of systemic infection.*

Monitor level of fatigue and lethargy, evidence of chills, loss of appetite, nausea and vomiting, and abdominal pain, *which are indicative of extent of infection and serve as indicators of status of infection.*

Monitor lochia for foul smell and profusion *as indicators of infection state.*

Assist with collection of intrauterine cultures or other specimens for laboratory analysis *to identify specific causative organism.*

Monitor laboratory values (i.e., WBC count, cultures) *for indicators of type and status of infection.*

Ensure adequate fluid and nutritional intake *to fight infection.*

Administer and monitor broad-spectrum antibiotics if ordered *to prevent infection.*

HEMORRHAGIC (HYPOVOLEMIC) SHOCK

Hemorrhage may result in **hemorrhagic (hypovolemic) shock.** Shock is an emergency situation in which the perfusion of body organs may become severely compromised and death may occur. Physiologic compensatory mechanisms are activated in response to hemorrhage. The adrenal glands release catecholamines, causing arterioles and venules in the skin, lungs, gastrointestinal tract, liver, and kidneys to constrict. The available blood flow is diverted to the brain and heart and away from other organs, including the uterus. If shock is prolonged, the continued reduction in cellular oxygenation results in an accumulation of lactic acid and acidosis (from anaerobic glucose metabolism). Acidosis (reduced serum pH) causes arteriolar vasodilation; venule vasoconstriction persists. A circular pattern is established; that is, decreased perfusion, increased tissue anoxia and acidosis, edema formation, and pooling of blood further decrease the perfusion. Cellular death occurs. See the Emergency box for assessments and interventions for hemorrhagic shock.

EMERGENCY

Hemorrhagic Shock

ASSESSMENTS	CHARACTERISTICS
Respirations	Rapid and shallow
Pulse	Rapid, weak, irregular
Blood pressure	Decreasing (late sign)
Skin	Cool, pale, clammy
Urinary output	Decreasing
Level of consciousness	Lethargy → coma
Mental status	Anxiety → coma
Central venous pressure	Decreased

INTERVENTION

Summon assistance and equipment.
Start IV infusion per standing orders.
Ensure patent airway; administer oxygen.
Continue to monitor status.

Medical Management

Vigorous treatment is necessary to prevent adverse sequelae. Medical management of hypovolemic shock involves restoring circulating blood volume and treating the cause of the hemorrhage (e.g., lacerations, uterine atony, or inversion). To restore circulating blood volume, a rapid intravenous infusion of crystalloid solution is given at a rate of 3 ml infused for every 1 ml of estimated blood loss (e.g., 3000 ml infused for 1000 ml of blood loss). Packed RBCs are usually infused if the woman is still actively bleeding and no improvement in her condition is noted after the initial crystalloid infusion. Infusion of fresh-frozen plasma may be needed if clotting factors and platelet counts are below normal values (Cunningham et al., 2001).

Nursing Interventions

Hemorrhagic shock can occur rapidly, but the classic signs of shock may not appear until the postpartum woman has lost 30% to 40% of blood volume. The nurse must continue to reassess the woman's condition, as evidenced by the degree of measurable and anticipated blood loss, and mobilize appropriate resources.

Most interventions are instituted to improve or monitor tissue perfusion. The nurse continues to monitor the woman's pulse and blood pressure. If invasive hemodynamic monitoring is ordered, the nurse may assist with the placement of the central venous pressure (CVP) or pulmonary artery (Swan-Ganz) catheter and monitor CVP, pulmonary artery pressure, or pulmonary artery wedge pressure as ordered (Troiano, 1999) (see Chapter 34).

Additional assessments to be made include evaluation of skin temperature, color, and turgor, as well as assessment of the woman's mucous membranes. Breath sounds should be auscultated before fluid volume replacement, if possible, to provide a baseline for future assessment. Inspection for oozing at the sites of incisions or injections and assessment of the presence of petechiae or ecchymosis in areas not associated with surgery or trauma are critical in the evaluation for DIC.

Oxygen is administered, preferably by nonrebreathing face mask, at 10 to 12 L/min to maintain oxygen saturation. Oxygen saturation should be monitored with a pulse oximeter, although measurements may not always be accurate in a woman with hypovolemia or decreased perfusion. Level of consciousness is assessed frequently and provides additional indications of blood volume and oxygen saturation. In early stages of decreased blood flow, the woman may report "seeing stars" or feeling dizzy or nauseated. She may become restless and orthopneic. As cerebral hypoxia increases, she may become confused and react slowly or not at all to stimuli. Some women complain of headaches. An improved sensorium is an indicator of improved perfusion.

Continuous electrocardiographic monitoring may be indicated for the woman who is hypotensive or tachycardic, continues to bleed profusely, or is in shock. A Foley catheter with a urometer is inserted to allow hourly assessment of urinary output. The most objective and least invasive assessment of adequate organ perfusion and oxygenation is urinary output of at least 30 ml/hr (Benedetti, 2002). Blood may be drawn and sent to the laboratory for studies that include hemoglobin and hematocrit levels, platelet count, and coagulation profile.

Fluid or Blood Replacement Therapy

Critical to successful management of the woman with a hemorrhagic complication is establishment of venous access, preferably with a large-bore IV catheter. The establishment of two IV lines facilitates fluid resuscitation. Vigorous fluid resuscitation includes the administration of crystalloids (lactated Ringer's, normal saline solutions), colloids (albumin), blood, and blood components (Benedetti, 2002). Fluid resuscitation must be carefully monitored because fluid overload may occur. Intravascular fluid overload occurs more frequently with colloid therapy. Transfusion reactions may follow administration of blood or blood components, including cryoprecipitates. Even in an emergency, each unit should be checked per hospital protocol. Complications of fluid or blood replacement therapy include hemolytic reactions, febrile reactions, allergic reactions, circulatory overload, and air embolism.

LEGAL TIP **Standard of Care for Bleeding Emergencies**

The standard of care for obstetric emergency situations such as PPH or hypovolemic shock is that provision should be made for the nurse to implement actions independently. Policies, procedures, standing orders or protocols, and clinical guidelines should be established by each health care facility in which births occur and should be agreed on by health care providers involved in the care of obstetric clients.

COAGULOPATHIES

When bleeding is continuous and there is no identifiable source, a coagulopathy may be the cause. The woman's coagulation status must be assessed quickly and continuously. The nurse may draw and send blood to the laboratory for studies. Abnormal results depend on the cause and may include increased prothrombin time, increased partial thromboplastin time, decreased platelets, decreased fibrinogen level, increased fibrin degradation products, and prolonged bleeding time. Causes of coagulopathies may be pregnancy complications such as idiopathic thrombocytopenic purpura or von Willebrand disease and disseminated intravascular coagulation.

Idiopathic Thrombocytopenic Purpura

Idiopathic or **immune thrombocytopenic purpura (ITP)** is an autoimmune disorder in which antiplatelet antibodies decrease the life span of the platelets. Thrombocytopenia, capillary fragility, and increased bleeding time are diagnostic findings. ITP may cause severe hemorrhage after cesarean birth or from cervical or vaginal lacerations. The incidence of postpartum uterine bleeding and vaginal hematomas also is increased. Neonatal thrombocytopenia, a result of the maternal disease process, occurs in about 50% of cases and is associated with high mortality (Kilpatrick & Laros, 1999).

Medical management focuses on control of platelet stability. If ITP was diagnosed during pregnancy, the woman likely was treated with corticosteroids or intravenous immunoglobulin. Platelet transfusions are usually given when there is significant bleeding. A splenectomy may be needed if the ITP does not respond to medical management.

von Willebrand Disease

von Willebrand disease, a type of hemophilia, is probably the most common of all hereditary bleeding disorders (Strozewski, 2000). Although von Willebrand disease is rare, it is among the most common congenital clotting defects in American women of childbearing age. It results from a factor VIII deficiency and platelet dysfunction that is transmitted as an incomplete autosomal dominant trait to both sexes. Symptoms include a familial bleeding tendency, previous bleeding episodes, prolonged bleeding time (the most important test), factor VIII deficiency (mild to moderate), and bleeding from mucous membranes. Although factor VIII increases during pregnancy, there is still a risk for postpartum hemorrhage as levels of von Willebrand factor begin to decrease (Roque, Funai, & Lockwood, 2000).

The woman may be at risk for bleeding for up to 4 weeks postpartum. Treatment of von Willebrand disease may include replacement of factor VIII, and administration of desmopressin or antifibrinolytics (Strozewski, 2000).

NURSE ALERT

Cryoprecipitate is no longer recommended by the Medical and Scientific Advisory Council of the National Hemophilia Association as a treatment for von Willebrand disease because it may contain donor viruses (Strozewski, 2000).

Disseminated Intravascular Coagulation

Disseminated intravascular coagulation (DIC) is a pathologic form of clotting that is diffuse and consumes large amounts of clotting factors, including platelets, fibrinogen, prothrombin, and factors V and VII. Widespread external bleeding, internal bleeding, or both can result. DIC also causes vascular occlusion of small vessels resulting from small clots forming in the microcirculation. In the obstetric population, DIC may occur as a result of abruptio placentae, amniotic fluid embolism, dead fetus syndrome (fetus has died but is retained in utero for at least 6 weeks), severe preeclampsia, septicemia, cardiopulmonary arrest, and hemorrhage.

The diagnosis of DIC is made according to clinical findings and laboratory markers. Physical examination reveals unusual bleeding; spontaneous bleeding from the woman's gums or nose may be noted. Petechiae may appear around a blood pressure cuff placed on the woman's arm. Excessive bleeding may occur from the site of a slight trauma (e.g., venipuncture sites, intramuscular or subcutaneous injection sites, nicks from shaving of perineum or abdomen, and injury from insertion of a urinary catheter). Symptoms also may include tachycardia and diaphoresis. Laboratory tests reveal decreased levels of platelets, fibrinogen, proaccelerin, antihemophiliac factor, and prothrombin (the factors consumed during coagulation). Fibrinolysis is increased at first but is later severely depressed. Degradation of fibrin leads to the accumulation of fibrin split products in the blood; these have anticoagulant properties and prolong the prothrombin time. Bleeding time is normal, coagulation time shows no clot, clot-retraction time shows no clot, and partial thromboplastin time is increased. DIC must be distinguished from other clotting disorders before therapy is initiated.

Primary medical management in all cases of DIC involves correction of the underlying cause (e.g., removal of the dead fetus, treatment of existing infection or of preeclampsia or eclampsia, or removal of a placental abruption). Volume replacement, blood component therapy, optimization of oxygenation and perfusion status, and continued reassessment of laboratory parameters are the usual forms of treatment. Plasma levels usually return to normal within 24 hours after birth. Platelet counts usually return to normal within 7 days (Kilpatrick & Laros, 1999).

Nursing interventions include assessment for signs of bleeding and signs of complications from the administration of blood and blood products, administering fluid or blood replacement as ordered, and protecting from injury. Because renal failure is one consequence of DIC, urinary output is monitored, usually by insertion of an indwelling urinary catheter. Urinary output must be maintained at more than 30 ml/hr.

The woman and her family will be anxious or concerned about her condition and prognosis. The nurse offers explanations about care and provides emotional support to the woman and her family through this critical time.

THROMBOEMBOLIC DISEASE

A thrombosis results from the formation of a blood clot or clots inside a blood vessel and is caused by inflammation **(thrombophlebitis)** or partial obstruction of the vessel. Three thromboembolic conditions are of concern in the postpartum period:

- *Superficial venous thrombosis*: Involvement of the superficial saphenous venous system
- *Deep venous thrombosis*: Involvement varies but can extend from the foot to the iliofemoral region
- *Pulmonary embolism*: Complication of deep venous thrombosis occurring when part of a blood clot dislodges and is carried to the pulmonary artery where it occludes the vessel and obstructs blood flow to the lungs

Incidence and Etiology

The incidence of thromboembolic disease in the postpartum period varies from about 0.5 to 3 per 1000 women (Laros, 1999). The incidence has declined in the last 20 years because early ambulation after childbirth has become the standard practice. The major causes of thromboembolic disease are venous stasis and hypercoagulation, both of which are present in pregnancy and continue into the postpartum period. Other risk factors include cesarean birth, history of venous thrombosis or varicosities, obesity, maternal age older than 35 years, multiparity, and smoking (Falter, 1997; Weiss & Bernstein, 2000).

Clinical Manifestations

Superficial venous thrombosis is the most frequent form of postpartum thrombophlebitis. It is characterized by pain and tenderness in the lower extremity. Physical examination may reveal warmth, redness, and an enlarged, hardened vein over the site of the thrombosis. Deep vein thrombosis is more common in pregnancy and is characterized by unilateral leg pain, calf tenderness, and swelling (Fig. 37-2). Physical examination may reveal redness and warmth, but women also may have a large amount of clot and have few symptoms (Stenchever et al., 2001). A positive Homans' sign may be present, but further evaluation is needed because the calf pain may be attributed to other causes such as a strained muscle resulting from the birthing position. Pulmonary embolism is characterized by dyspnea and tachypnea. Other signs and symptoms frequently seen include apprehension, cough, tachycardia, hemoptysis, elevated temperature, and pleuritic chest pain (Laros, 1999).

Physical examination is not a sensitive diagnostic indicator for thrombosis. Venography is the most accurate method for diagnosing deep venous thrombosis; however, it is an invasive procedure that exposes the woman and fetus to ionizing radiation and is associated with serious complications. Noninvasive diagnostic methods are more commonly used; these include real-time and color Doppler ultrasound. Cardiac auscultation may reveal murmurs with pulmonary embolism. Electrocardiograms are usually normal. Arterial P_{O_2} may be lower than normal. A ventilation/perfusion scan, Doppler ultrasound, and pulmonary arteriogram may be used for diagnosis (Laros, 1999).

Medical Management

Superficial venous thrombosis is treated with analgesia (nonsteroidal antiinflammatory agents), rest with elevation of the affected leg, and elastic stockings (Falter, 1997). Local application of heat also may be used. Deep venous thrombosis is initially treated with anticoagulant (usually continuous intravenous heparin) therapy, bed rest with the affected leg elevated, and analgesia. After the symptoms have decreased, the woman may be fitted with elastic stockings to use when she is allowed to ambulate. Intravenous heparin therapy continues for 5 to 7 days. Oral anticoagulant therapy (warfarin) is started during this time and will be continued for about 3 months. Contin-

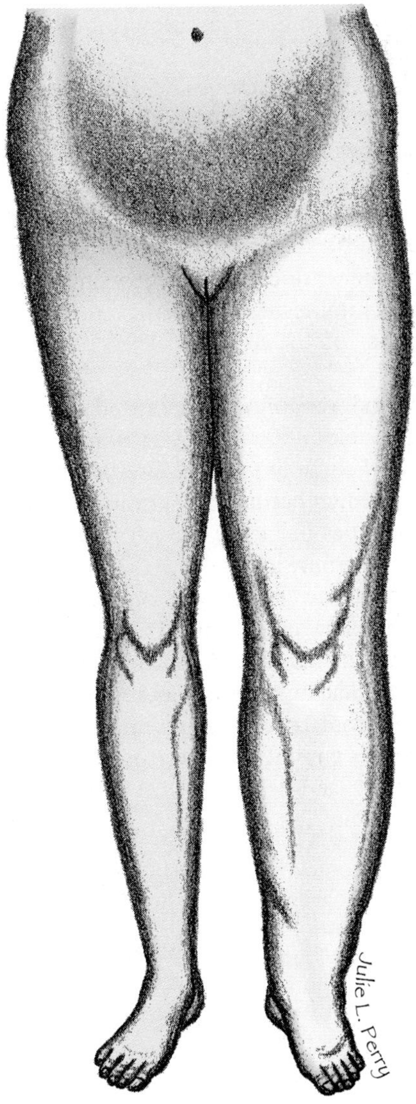
Julie L. Perry

FIG. 37-2 Deep vein thrombophlebitis.

uous intravenous heparin therapy is used for pulmonary embolism until symptoms have resolved. Intermittent subcutaneous heparin or oral anticoagulant therapy is usually continued for 6 months.

Nursing Interventions

In the hospital setting, nursing care of the woman with a thrombosis consists of continued assessments: inspection and palpation of the affected area; palpation of peripheral pulses; checking Homans' sign; measurement and comparison of leg circumferences; inspection for signs of bleeding; monitoring for signs of pulmonary embolism including chest pain, coughing, dyspnea, and tachypnea; and respiratory status for presence of crackles. Laboratory reports are monitored for prothrombin or partial thromboplastin times. The woman and her family are assessed for their level of understanding about the diagnosis and their ability to cope during the unexpected extended period of recovery.

Interventions include explanations and education about the diagnosis and the treatment. The woman will need assistance with personal care as long as she is on bed rest; the family should be encouraged to participate in the care if that is what she and they wish. While the woman is on bed rest, she should be encouraged to change positions frequently but not to place the knees in a sharply flexed position that could cause pooling of blood in the lower extremities. She also should be cautioned not to rub the affected area, as this action could cause the clot to dislodge. Once the woman is allowed to ambulate, she is taught how to prevent venous congestion by putting on the elastic stockings before getting out of bed.

Heparin and warfarin are administered as ordered, and the physician is notified if clotting times are outside the therapeutic level. If the woman is breastfeeding, she is assured that neither heparin nor warfarin is excreted in significant quantities in breast milk. If the infant has been discharged, the family is encouraged to bring the infant for feedings as permitted by hospital policy; the mother also can express milk to be sent home.

Pain can be managed with a variety of measures. Position changes, elevating the leg, and application of moist warm heat may decrease discomfort. Administration of analgesics and antiinflammatory medications may be needed.

NURSE ALERT

Medications containing aspirin are not given to women receiving anticoagulant therapy because aspirin inhibits synthesis of clotting factors and can lead to prolonged clotting time and increased risk of bleeding.

The woman is usually discharged home with oral anticoagulants and will need explanations about the treatment schedule and possible side effects. If subcutaneous injections are to be given, the woman and family are taught how to administer the medication and about site rotation. The woman and her family also should be given information about safe care practices to prevent bleeding and injury while she is receiving anticoagulant therapy, such as using a soft toothbrush and using an electric razor. She also will need information about follow-up with her health care provider to monitor clotting times and to make sure the correct dose of anticoagulant therapy is maintained (Lowdermilk & Grohar, 1998). The woman also should use a reliable method of contraception if taking warfarin, because this medication is considered teratogenic (Toglia & Nolan, 1997).

POSTPARTUM INFECTIONS

Postpartum or **puerperal infection** is any clinical infection of the genital canal that occurs within 28 days after miscarriage, induced abortion, or childbirth. The definition used in the United States continues to be the presence of a fever of 38° C or more on 2 successive days of the first 10 postpartum days (not counting the first 24 hours after birth) (Cunningham et al., 2001). Puerperal infection is probably the major cause of maternal morbidity and mortality throughout the world; however, it occurs after about 6% of births in the United States (5 to 10 times higher after cesarean births than after

BOX 37-4 Predisposing Factors for Postpartum Infection

PRECONCEPTION OR ANTEPARTAL FACTORS

- History of previous venous thrombosis, urinary tract infection, mastitis, pneumonia
- Diabetes mellitus
- Alcoholism
- Drug abuse
- Immunosuppression
- Anemia
- Malnutrition

INTRAPARTAL FACTORS

- Cesarean birth
- Prolonged rupture of membranes
- Chorioamnionitis
- Prolonged labor
- Bladder catheterization
- Internal fetal/uterine pressure monitoring
- Multiple vaginal examinations after rupture of membranes
- Epidural anesthesia
- Retained placental fragments
- Postpartum hemorrhage
- Episiotomy or lacerations
- Hematomas

vaginal births) (Gibbs & Sweet, 1999). Common postpartum infections include endometritis, wound infections, mastitis, urinary tract infections (UTIs), and respiratory tract infections.

The most common infecting organisms are the numerous streptococcal and anaerobic organisms. *Staphylococcus aureus*, gonococci, coliform bacteria, and clostridia are less common but serious pathogenic organisms that also cause puerperal infection. Postpartum infections are more common in women who have concurrent medical or immunosuppressive conditions or who had a cesarean or other operative birth. Intrapartal factors such as prolonged rupture of membranes, prolonged labor, and internal maternal or fetal monitoring also increase the risk of infection (Varner, 1998). Factors that predispose the woman to postpartum infection are listed in Box 37-4.

Endometritis

Endometritis is the most common cause of postpartum infection. It usually begins as a localized infection at the placental site (Fig. 37-3) but can spread to involve the entire endometrium. Incidence is higher after cesarean birth. Assessment for signs of endometritis may reveal a fever (usually greater than 38° C); increased pulse; chills; anorexia; nausea; fatigue and lethargy; pelvic pain; uterine tenderness; or foul-smelling, profuse lochia (Duff, 2002).

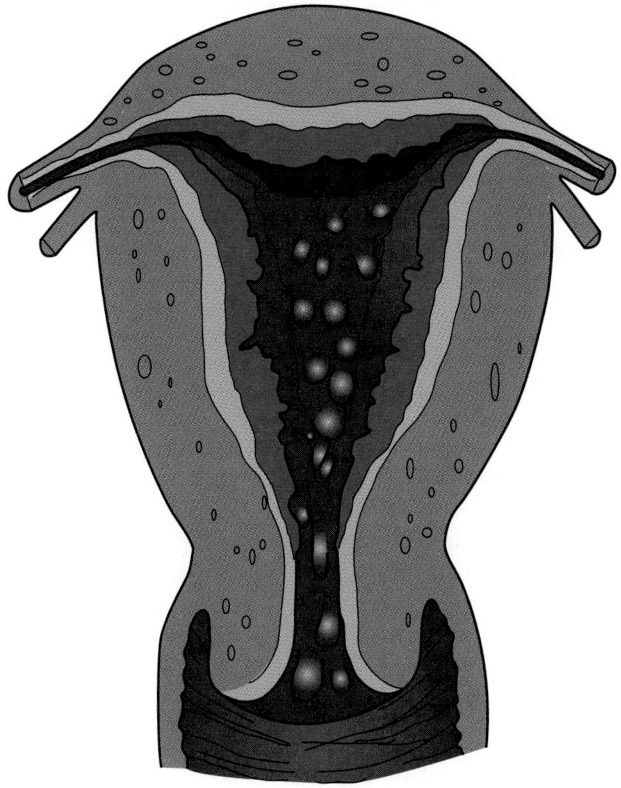

FIG. 37-3 Postpartum infection: endometriosis.

Leukocytosis and a markedly increased RBC sedimentation rate are typical laboratory findings of postpartum infections. Anemia also may be present. Blood cultures or intracervical or intrauterine bacterial cultures (aerobic and anaerobic) should reveal the offending pathogens within 36 to 48 hours.

Wound Infections

Wound infections also are common postpartum infections but often develop after the woman is at home. Sites of infection include the cesarean incision and the episiotomy or repaired laceration site. Predisposing factors are similar to those for endometritis (see Box 37-4). Signs of wound infection include erythema, edema, warmth, tenderness, seropurulent drainage, and wound separation. Fever and pain also may be present.

Urinary Tract Infections

Urinary tract infections (UTIs) occur in 2% to 4% of postpartum women. Risk factors include urinary catheterization, frequent pelvic examinations, epidural anesthesia, genital tract injury, history of UTI, and cesarean birth. Signs and symptoms include dysuria, frequency and urgency, low-grade fever, urinary retention, hematuria, and pyuria. Costovertebral angle (CVA) tenderness or flank pain may indicate upper UTI. Urinalysis results may reveal *Escherichia coli*, although other gram-negative aerobic bacilli also may cause UTIs.

Mastitis

Mastitis affects about 1% of women soon after childbirth, most of whom are first-time mothers who are breastfeeding. Mastitis almost always is unilateral and develops well after the flow of milk has been established (Fig. 37-4). The

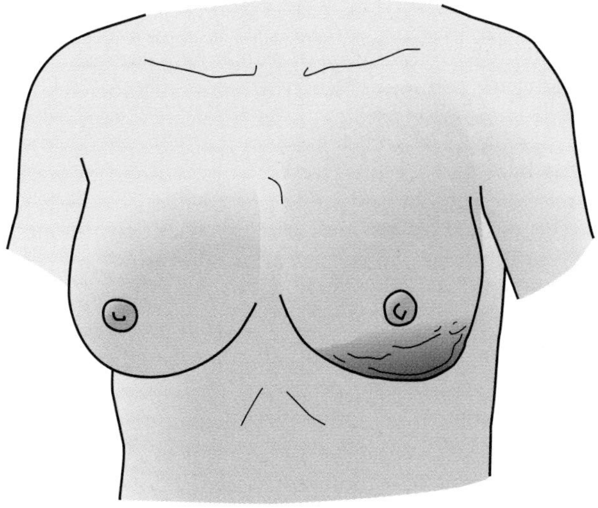

FIG. 37-4 Mastitis.

infecting organism generally is the hemolytic *S. aureus*. An infected nipple fissure usually is the initial lesion, but the ductal system is involved next. Inflammatory edema and engorgement of the breast soon obstruct the flow of milk in a lobe; regional, then generalized, mastitis follows. If treatment is not prompt, mastitis may progress to a breast abscess.

Symptoms rarely appear before the end of the first postpartum week and are more common in the second to fourth weeks. Chills, fever, malaise, and local breast tenderness are noted first. Localized breast tenderness, pain, swelling, redness, and axillary adenopathy also may occur. Antibiotics are prescribed. Lactation can be maintained by emptying the breasts every 2 to 4 hours by breastfeeding, manual expression, or breast pump.

CARE MANAGEMENT

Prenatal and intrapartal factors that can predispose a woman to postpartum infection are listed in Box 37-4. Signs and symptoms associated with postpartum infection were discussed with each infection. Laboratory tests usually performed include a complete blood count, venous blood cultures, and uterine tissue cultures. Nursing diagnoses for women experiencing postpartum infection include the following:

- *Deficient knowledge related to*
  - –etiology, management, course of infection
  - –transmission and prevention of infection
- *Impaired tissue integrity related to*
  - –effects of infection process
- *Acute pain related to*
  - –mastitis
  - –puerperal infection
  - –UTI
- *Interrupted family processes related to*
  - –unexpected complication to expected postpartum recovery
  - –possible separation from newborn
  - –interruption in process of realigning relationships after the addition of the new family member
- *Risk for impaired parenting related to*
  - –fear of spread of infection to newborn.

The most effective and least expensive treatment of postpartum infection is prevention. Preventive measures include good prenatal nutrition to control anemia and intrapartal hemorrhage. Good maternal perineal hygiene with thorough handwashing is emphasized. Strict adherence by all health care personnel to aseptic techniques during childbirth and the postpartum period is very important.

Management of endometritis consists of intravenous broad-spectrum antibiotic therapy (cephalosporins, penicillins, or clindamycin and gentamicin) and supportive care, including hydration, rest, and pain relief (French & Smaill, 2002). Antibiotic therapy is usually discontinued 24 hours after the woman is asymptomatic (Gibbs & Sweet, 1999). Assessments of lochia, vital signs, and changes in the woman's condition continue during treatment. Comfort measures depend on the symptoms and may include cool compresses, warm blankets, perineal care, and sitz baths. Teaching should include side effects of therapy, prevention of spread of infection, signs and symptoms of worsening condition, and adherence to the treatment plan and the need for follow-up care. Women may need to be encouraged or assisted to maintain mother-infant interactions and breastfeeding (if allowed during treatment).

Postpartum women are usually discharged to home by 48 hours after birth. This is often before signs of infection are evident. Nurses in birth centers and hospital settings must be able to identify women at risk for postpartum infection and to provide anticipatory teaching and counseling before discharge. After discharge, telephone follow-up, hot lines, support groups, lactation counselors, home visits by nurses, and teaching materials (videos, written materials) are all interventions that can be implemented to decrease the risk of postpartum infections. Home care nurses must be able to recognize signs and symptoms of postpartum infection so that the woman can contact her primary health care provider. These nurses also must be able to provide the appropriate nursing care for women who need follow-up home care.

Treatment of wound infections may combine antibiotic therapy with wound debridement. Wounds may be opened and drained. Nursing care includes frequent wound and vital sign assessments and wound care. Comfort measures include sitz baths, warm compresses, and perineal care. Teaching includes good hygiene techniques (i.e., changing perineal pads front to back, handwashing before and after perineal care), self-care measures, and signs of worsening conditions to report to the health care provider. The woman is usually discharged to home for self-care or home nursing care after treatment is initiated in the inpatient setting.

Medical management for UTIs consists of antibiotic therapy, analgesia, and hydration. Postpartum women are usually treated on an outpatient basis; therefore teaching should include instructions on how to monitor temperature, bladder function, and appearance of urine. The woman also should be taught about signs of potential complications and the importance of taking all antibiotics as prescribed. Other suggestions for prevention of UTIs include proper perineal care, wiping from front to back after urinating or having a bowel movement, and increasing fluid intake.

Because mastitis rarely occurs before the postpartum woman is discharged, teaching should include warning signs of mastitis and counseling about prevention of cracked nipples. Management includes intensive antibiotic therapy (e.g., cephalosporins and vancomycin, which are particularly useful in staphylococcal infections), support of breasts, local heat (or cold), adequate hydration, and analgesics.

Almost all instances of acute mastitis can be avoided by proper breastfeeding technique to prevent cracked nipples. Missed feedings, waiting too long between feedings, and abrupt weaning may lead to clogged nipples and mastitis. Cleanliness practiced by all who have contact with the newborn and new mother also reduces the incidence of mastitis. See Chapter 27 for further information.

KEY POINTS

- Postpartum hemorrhage is the most common and most serious type of excessive obstetric blood loss.
- Hemorrhagic (hypovolemic) shock is an emergency situation in which the perfusion of body organs may become severely compromised, leading to significant morbidity or mortality rates for the mothers.
- The potential hazards of the therapeutic interventions may further compromise the woman with a hemorrhagic disorder.
- Clotting disorders are associated with many obstetric complications.
- The first symptom of postpartum infection is usually fever greater than 38° C on 2 consecutive days in the first 10 postpartum days (after the first 24 hours).
- Prevention is the most effective and inexpensive treatment of postpartum infection.

CRITICAL THINKING EXERCISES

1. Develop a concept care map (see example in Study Guide that accompanies this text) for a breastfeeding woman who has a wound infection after a cesarean birth. This is the woman's first pregnancy. She carried to term. The cesarean was performed for failure to progress. It has been 2 days since the surgery. Include the problems you think might be present, the assessments needed, outcome criteria, and interventions. Be sure to show links between the problems.
2. Review the literature for studies about assessing for thromboembolism using Homans' sign. In a clinical conference, debate the efficacy of performing this assessment for all postpartum clients.

RESOURCES

AHCPR website
www.hcfa.gov/medicaid/siq/siqipg/htm

National Center for Complementary and Alternative Medicine (NCCAM)
P.O. Box 8218
Silver Spring, MD 20907-8218
888-644-6226
www.nccam.nih.gov

Postpartum Support International
927 North Kellog Ave.
Santa Barbara, CA 93111
805-967-7636
www.chss.iup.edu/postpartum

REFERENCES

American College of Obstetricians and Gynecologists (ACOG). (1998). Postpartum hemorrhage. *AGOG Educational Bulletin Number 243.* Washington, DC: ACOG.

Beal, M. (1998). Use of complementary and alternative therapies in reproductive medicine. *Journal of Nurse Midwifery, 43*(3), 224-233.

Benedetti, T. (2002). Obstetric hemorrhage. In S. Gabbe, J. Niebyl, & J. Simpson (Eds.), *Obstetrics: Normal and problem pregnancies* (4th ed.). New York: Churchill Livingstone.

Bowes, W. (1999). Clinical aspects of normal and abnormal labor. In R. Creasy & R. Resnick (Eds.), *Maternal-fetal medicine* (4th ed.). Philadelphia: W.B. Saunders.

Brucker, M. (2001). Management of the third stage of labor: An evidence-based approach. *Journal of Midwifery and Women's Health, 46*(6), 381-392.

Clark, S. (1999). Placenta previa and abruptio placentae. In R. Creasy & R. Resnick (Eds.), *Maternal-fetal medicine* (4th ed.). Philadelphia: W.B. Saunders.

Cunningham, F. et al. (2001). *Williams obstetrics* (21st ed.). New York: McGraw-Hill.
Duff, P. (2002). Maternal and perinatal infection. In S. Gabbe, J. Niebyl, & J. Simpson (Eds.), *Obstetrics: Normal and problem pregnancies* (4th ed.). New York: Churchill Livingstone.
Falter, H. (1997). Deep vein thrombosis in pregnancy and the puerperium: A comprehensive review. *Journal of Vascular Nursing, 15*(2), 58-62.
French, L., & Smaill, F. (2002). Antibiotic regimens for endometritis after delivery (Cochrane Review). In: *The Cochrane Library*, Issue 2. Oxford: Update Software.
Gibbs, R., & Sweet, R. (1999). Maternal and fetal infectious disorders. In R. Creasy & R. Resnick (Eds.), *Maternal-fetal medicine* (4th ed.). Philadelphia: W.B. Saunders.
Gonik, B. (1999). Intensive care monitoring of the critically ill pregnant patient. In R. Creasy & R. Resnick (Eds.), *Maternal-fetal medicine* (4th ed.). Philadelphia: W.B. Saunders.
Hostetler, D., & Bosworth, M. (2000). Uterine inversion: A life-threatening obstetric emergency. *Journal of American Board of Family Practice, 13*(2), 120-123.
Hoyert, D. et al. (2001). Deaths: Final data for 1999. *National Vital Statistics Report, 49*(8), 1-113.
Kilpatrick, S., & Laros, R. (1999). Maternal hematologic disorders. In R. Creasy & R. Resnick (Eds.), *Maternal-fetal medicine* (4th ed.). Philadelphia: W.B. Saunders.
Laros, R. (1999). Thromboembolic disease. In R. Creasy & R. Resnick (Eds.), *Maternal-fetal medicine* (4th ed.). Philadelphia: W.B. Saunders.
Lowdermilk, D., & Grohar, J. (1998). *High-risk antepartal home care.* White Plains, NY: March of Dimes.
Mousa, H., & Walkinshaw, S. (2001). Major postpartum haemorrhage. *Current Opinions in Obstetrics and Gynecology, 13*(6), 595-603.
Roque, H., Funai, R., & Lockwood, C. (2000). von Willebrand disease and pregnancy. *Journal of Maternal and Fetal Medicine, 9*(5), 257-266.
Schirmer, G. (1998). *Herbal medicine.* Bedford, TX: MED2000 Inc.
Stenchever, M. et al. (2001). *Comprehensive gynecology* (4th ed.). St. Louis: Mosby.
Strozewski, S. (2000). Von Willebrand's disease: What you need to know about this inherited bleeding disorder. *American Journal of Nursing, 100* (2), 24AA-24DD.
Tiran, D., & Mack, S. (Eds.). (2000). *Complementary therapies for pregnancy and childbirth* (2nd ed.). Edinburgh: Bailliere Tindall.
Toglia, M., & Nolan, T. (1997). Venous thromboembolism during pregnancy: A review of diagnosis and management. *Obstetrics and Gynecology Survey, 52*(1), 60-72.
Troiano, N. (1999). Invasive hemodynamic monitoring in obstetrics. In L. Mandeville & N. Troiano (Eds.). *AWHONN's high risk and critical care intrapartum nursing* (2nd ed.). Philadelphia: Lippincott.
Varner, M. (1998). Medical conditions of the puerperium. *Clinical Perinatology, 25*(2), 403-416.
Weiss, N., & Bernstein, P. (2000). Risk factor scoring for predicting venous thromboembolism in obstetric patients. *American Journal of Obstetrics and Gynecology, 182*(5), 1073-1075.

CHAPTER 38

Debbie Fraser Askin

Acquired Problems of the Newborn

http://evolve.elsevier.com/Lowdermilk/MatWmnHlth/

LEARNING OBJECTIVES

- Summarize the care of the newborn with soft tissue, skeletal, and nervous system injuries.
- Describe assessment of infants for birth trauma and for sequelae of a diabetic pregnancy.
- Develop nursing care plans for complications typically seen in infants of mothers with diabetes.
- Describe in detail the assessment of a newborn with a suspected infection.
- Formulate nursing diagnoses for the infant and family for common bacterial and viral infections.
- Interpret the evidence available to guide the care of the infant at risk for group B streptococcus (GBS) sepsis.
- Review implementation and evaluation of care of infants with infections; include their families.
- Distinguish between the effects of maternal use of alcohol, heroin, methadone, marijuana, cocaine, and smoking on the fetus and newborn.
- Describe the assessment and care of a newborn experiencing drug withdrawal; include the infant's family.

This chapter deals with acquired problems of the newborn. *Acquired problems* refer to those conditions resulting from environmental factors rather than genetic circumstances. The focus is on birth trauma, the infant of a mother with diabetes, neonatal infections, and effects of maternal substance abuse.

BIRTH TRAUMA

Birth trauma (injury) is physical injury sustained by a neonate during labor and birth. The significance of birth injuries is assessed most accurately by review of recent mortality data. These data show a modest decline in fatal birth injuries. In 1981 birth injuries ranked sixth among major causes of infant mortality in the United States, resulting in 23.8 deaths per 100,000 live births. In 2000 birth injuries ranked seventh and caused 20.3 deaths per 100,000 live births (Hoyert et al., 2001). This improvement is attributed to refinements in obstetric techniques, increased use of cesarean birth for births that would be difficult vaginally, and decreased use of vacuum extraction and version and extraction. Despite this decrease, birth injuries still are an important source of neonatal morbidity. Therefore the clinician should consider the broad range of birth injuries in the differential diagnosis of neonatal clinical disorders (Mangurten, 2002).

In theory, most birth injuries may be avoidable, especially if careful assessment of risk factors and appropriate planning of birth occur. The use of ultrasonography allows antepartum diagnosis of macrosomia, hydrocephalus, and unusual presentations. Elective cesarean birth can be chosen for some pregnancies to prevent significant birth injury (Paige & Carney, 2002). A small percentage of significant birth injuries are unavoidable despite skilled and competent obstetric care, as in especially difficult or prolonged labor or when the infant is in an abnormal presentation (Mangurten, 2002). Some injuries cannot be anticipated until the specific circumstances are encountered during childbirth. Emergency cesarean birth may provide a last-minute salvage, but in these circumstances, the injury may be truly unavoidable. The same injury might be caused in several ways. For example, a cephalhematoma could result from an obstetric technique such as forceps birth or vacuum extraction or from pressure of the fetal skull against the maternal pelvis.

Many injuries are minor and resolve readily in the neonatal period without treatment. Other traumas require some degree of intervention. A few are serious enough to be fatal. The nurse's contribution to the welfare of the newborn begins with early observation and accurate recording. The prompt reporting of signs that

TABLE 38-1 **Types of Birth Injuries**

SITE OF INJURY	TYPE OF INJURY
Scalp	Caput succedaneum
	Subgaleal hemorrhage
	Cephalhematoma
Skull	Linear fracture
	Depressed fracture
	Occipital osteodiastasis
Intracranial	Epidural hematoma
	Subdural hematoma (laceration of falx, tentorium, or superficial veins)
	Subarachnoid hemorrhage
	Cerebral contusion
	Cerebellar contusion
	Intracerebellar hematoma
Spinal cord (cervical)	Vertebral artery injury
	Intraspinal hemorrhage
	Spinal cord transection or injury
Plexus	Erb palsy
	Klumpke paralysis
	Total (mixed) brachial plexus injury
	Horner syndrome
	Diaphragmatic paralysis
	Lumbosacral plexus injury
Cranial and peripheral nerve	Radial nerve palsy
	Medial nerve palsy
	Sciatic nerve palsy
	Laryngeal nerve palsy
	Diaphragmatic paralysis
	Facial nerve palsy

Source: Moe, P., & Paige, L. (2002). Neurologic disorders. In G. Merenstein & S. Gardner (Eds.), *Handbook of neonatal intensive care* (5th ed.). St. Louis: Mosby.

indicate deviations from normal permits early initiation of appropriate therapy. Table 38-1 provides an overview of neurologic birth injuries and the sites in which they occur.

CARE MANAGEMENT

Assessment and Nursing Diagnoses

Several factors predispose an infant to birth injuries (Mangurten, 2002; Paige & Carney, 2002). Maternal factors include uterine dysfunction that leads to prolonged or precipitate labor, preterm or postterm labor, and cephalopelvic disproportion. Injury may result from dystocia caused by fetal macrosomia, multifetal gestation, abnormal or difficult presentation (not caused by maternal uterine or pelvic conditions), and congenital anomalies. Intrapartum events that can result in scalp injury include the use of intrapartum monitoring of fetal heart rate (FHR) and collection of fetal scalp blood for acid-base assessment. Obstetric birth techniques can cause injury. Forceps birth, vacuum extraction, version and extraction, and cesarean birth are potential contributory factors. Often more than one factor is present, and multiple predisposing factors may be related to a single maternal condition.

The Apgar score may alert the caregiver to birth injuries and help in identifying infants in need of immediate resuscitation. Flaccid muscle tone, regardless of cause, increases the risk of joint dislocations and separation during the birth process. Flaccid tone in extremities may be traced to nerve plexus injuries or long-bone fractures. A weak or hoarse cry is characteristic of laryngeal nerve palsy as a result of excessive traction on the neck during birth. Pronounced bruising of the skin may preclude accurate assessment for color.

A complete physical assessment of the newborn is performed soon after birth. Because evidence of birth injury may not be apparent at the initial examination, assessment continues during each contact with the neonate. The nursing diagnoses depend on the particular injury incurred; thus the following list represents examples only.

Infant

- *Impaired physical mobility related to*
  –brachial plexus injury
- *Impaired gas exchange related to*
  –diaphragmatic paralysis (partial or complete)
- *Acute pain related to*
  –injury
- *Injury related to*
  –bruising, cephalhematoma, hyperbilirubinemia

Parents and family

- *Anxiety related to deficient knowledge regarding*
  –injury and its cause
  –management and therapy
  –prognosis
- *Anticipatory grieving related to*
  –possible sequelae of the birth injury

Expected Outcomes of Care

Meeting the unique needs of the birth-injured newborn requires constant vigilance. Expected outcomes are established and priorities assigned. Nursing actions are selected in terms of the particular disorder and individual needs of the infant and family. The overall outcomes for care of infants with birth trauma include the following:

- The newborn will have minimal or no sequelae of trauma.
- The infant will receive prompt and appropriate treatment.
- The parents will initiate and maintain a positive parent-child relationship.
- The parents' and family's educational needs regarding the injury and its management will be met.

Plan of Care and Interventions

Soft-Tissue Injuries

Caput succedaneum is a localized edematous swelling of the scalp that is not confined within the suture lines of the skull. The swelling persists for a few days after birth and then disappears without treatment. It is most often seen after vertex vaginal births and has no pathologic significance (see Fig. 25-5, *A*).

Cephalhematoma is a collection of blood from ruptured blood vessels between the periosteum and the surface of the skull. Because blood collects beneath the periosteum, it does not cross the cranial suture lines (see Fig. 25-5, *B*). The swelling may appear unilaterally or bilaterally, usually is minimal or absent at birth, increases over the first 3 days of life, and disappears gradually in 2 to 3 weeks. Occasionally hyperbilirubinemia may result from breakdown of the accumulated blood.

Subconjunctival (scleral) and **retinal hemorrhages** result from rupture of capillaries caused by increased intracranial pressure (ICP) during birth. They clear within 5 days after birth and usually present no problems; however, parents need reassurance about their presence.

Erythema, ecchymoses, petechiae, abrasions, lacerations, and edema of buttocks and extremities may be present. Localized discoloration may appear over presenting or dependent parts. Ecchymoses and edema may appear anywhere on the body and especially on the presenting body part from the application of forceps. They also may result from manipulation of the infant's body during birth.

Bruises over the face may be the result of face presentation (Fig. 38-1). In a breech presentation, bruising and swelling may be seen over the buttocks or genitalia (Fig. 38-2). The skin over the entire head may be ecchymotic and covered with petechiae caused by a tight nuchal cord. Petechiae, or pinpoint hemorrhagic areas, acquired during birth may extend over the upper portion of the trunk and face. These lesions are benign if they disappear within 2 days of birth and no new lesions appear. Ecchymoses and petechiae may be signs of a more serious disorder, such as thrombocytopenic purpura. If the hemorrhagic areas do not disappear spontaneously in 2 days, the physician is notified. To differentiate hemorrhagic areas from skin rashes and discolorations such as mongolian spots, the nurse blanches the skin with two fingers. Because extravasated blood remains within the tissues, petechiae and ecchymoses do not blanch.

Forceps injury occurs at the site of application of the instrument. Forceps injury typically has a linear configuration across both sides of the face, outlining the placement of the forceps. The affected areas are kept clean to minimize the risk of secondary infection. These injuries usually resolve spontaneously within several days with no specific therapy.

Accidental lacerations may be inflicted with a scalpel during cesarean birth or with scissors during an episiotomy. These cuts may occur on any part of the body but most often are found on the scalp, buttocks, and thighs. Usually they are superficial, needing only to be kept clean. Butterfly adhesive strips will hold together the edges of more serious lacerations. Rarely are sutures needed.

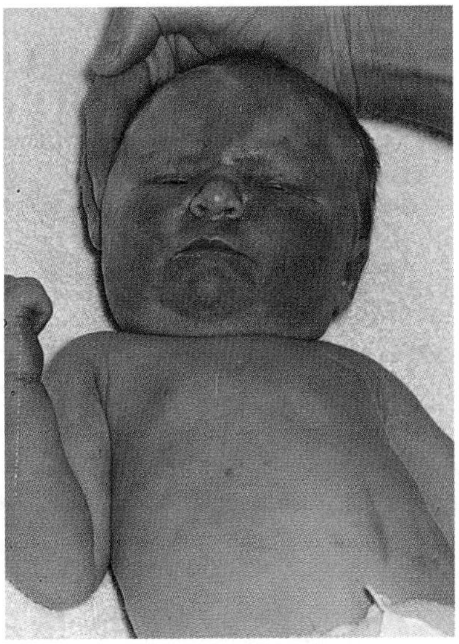

FIG. 38-1 Marked bruising on the entire face of an infant born vaginally after face presentation. Less severe ecchymoses were present on the extremities. Phototherapy was required for treatment of jaundice resulting from the breakdown of accumulated blood. (From O'Doherty, N. [1986]. *Neonatology: Micro atlas of the newborn.* Nutley, NJ: Hoffmann-La Roche.)

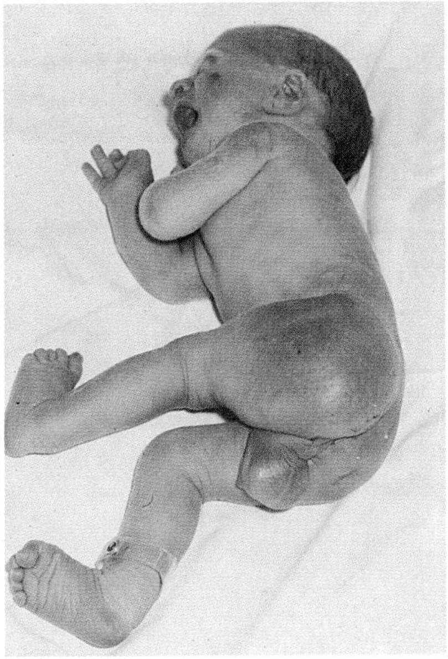

FIG. 38-2 Swelling of the genitals and bruising of the buttocks after a breech delivery. (From O'Doherty, N. [1986]. *Neonatology: Micro atlas of the newborn.* Nutley, NJ: Hoffmann-La Roche.)

Skeletal Injuries

The newborn's immature, flexible skull can withstand a great degree of deformation (molding) before fracture results. Considerable force is required to fracture the newborn's skull. Two types of skull fractures typically are identified in the newborn: linear fractures and depressed fractures. The location of the fracture and involvement of underlying structures determine its significance.

If an artery lying in a groove on the undersurface of the skull is torn as a result of the fracture, increased ICP will ensue. Unless a blood vessel is involved, linear fractures (which account for 70% of all fractures for this age group) heal without special treatment. The soft skull may become indented without laceration of either the skin or the dural membrane. These depressed fractures, or "ping-pong ball" indentations, may occur during difficult births from pressure of the head on the bony pelvis (Fig. 38-3). They also can occur as a result of injudicious application of forceps. Spontaneous or nonsurgical elevation of the indentation by using a hand breast pump or vacuum extractor has been reported (Mangurten, 2002).

The clavicle is the bone most often fractured during birth. Generally the break is in the middle third of the bone (Fig. 38-4). Dystocia, particularly shoulder impaction, is a risk factor in clavicular fracture (Hsu et al., 2002). Others believe that maternal age and birthweight greater than 4000 g are more significant risk factors (Beall & Ross, 2001). Limitation of motion of the arm, crepitus over the bone, and the absence of the Moro reflex on the affected side are diagnostic. Except for use of gentle rather than vigorous handling, no accepted treatment for fractured clavicle exists, and the prognosis is good. A sign posted on the bassinet will alert care providers to the need for careful handling. The figure-of-eight bandage appropriate for the older child should not be used for the newborn.

The humerus and femur may be fractured during a difficult birth. Fractures in newborns generally heal rapidly. Immobilization is accomplished with slings, splints, swaddling, and other devices.

The parents need support in handling these infants because they often are fearful of hurting them. Parents are encouraged to practice handling, changing, and feeding the affected neonate under the guidance of nursery personnel. This increases their confidence and knowledge and facilitates attachment. A plan for follow-up therapy is developed with the parents so that the times and arrangements for therapy are acceptable to them.

Peripheral Nervous System Injuries

Erb-Duchenne paralysis (**brachial paralysis** of the upper portion of the arm) is the most common type of paralysis associated with a difficult birth, occurring at rates of 0.5 to 2.0 per 1000 live births (Paige & Carney, 2002) (Fig. 38-5). Injury to the upper plexus results from stretching or pulling the head away from the shoulder during the difficult birth. Typical symptoms are a flaccid arm with the elbow extended and the hand rotated inward, absence of the Moro reflex on the affected side, sensory loss over the lateral aspect of the arm, and an intact grasp reflex.

Treatment is by intermittent immobilization, proper positioning, and range-of-motion (ROM) exercises. Gentle manipulation and ROM exercises are delayed until about the tenth day to prevent additional injury to the brachial plexus.

Immobilization may be accomplished with a brace or splint or by pinning the infant's sleeve to his or her shirt.

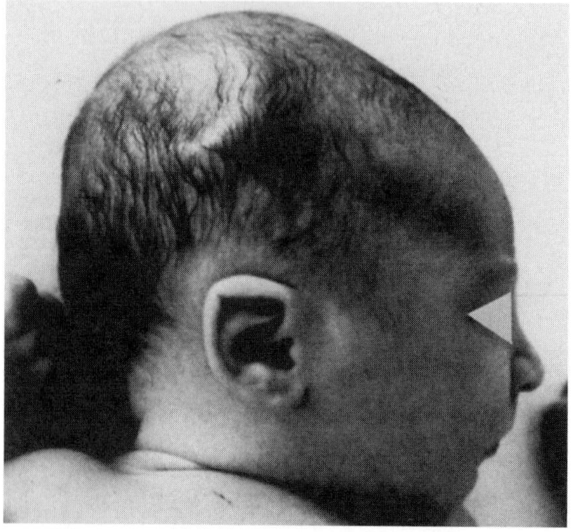

FIG. 38-3 Depressed skull fracture in a full-term boy born after rapid (1-hour) labor. The infant was delivered by occiput-anterior presentation after rotation from occiput-posterior position. (From Mangurton, H. [2002]. Birth injuries. In A. Fanaroff & R. Martin (Eds.), *Neonatal-perinatal medicine: Diseases of the fetus and infant* [7th ed.]. St. Louis: Mosby.)

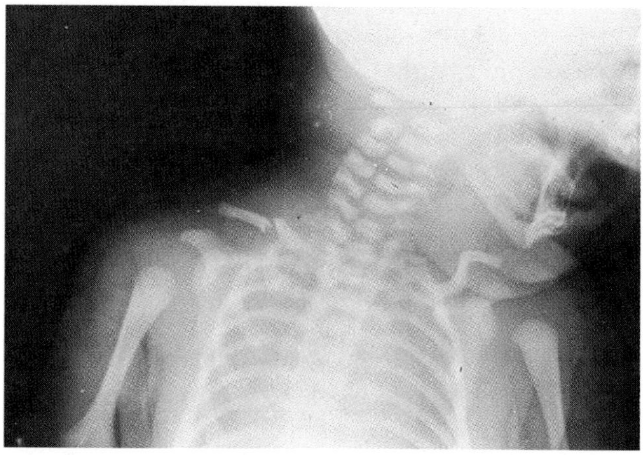

FIG. 38-4 Fractured clavicle after shoulder dystocia. (From O'Doherty, N. [1986]. *Neonatology: Micro atlas of the newborn.* Nutley, NJ: Hoffmann-La Roche.)

The infant should be positioned for 2 or 3 hours at a time as follows:

- Abduct the arm 90 degrees.
- Externally rotate the shoulder.
- Flex the elbow 90 degrees.
- Supinate the wrist with the palm directed slightly toward the face (Fig. 38-6).

Damage to the lower plexus, *Klumpke palsy*, is less common. With lower arm paralysis, the wrist and hand are flaccid, the grasp reflex is absent, deep tendon reflexes are present, and dependent edema and cyanosis may be apparent (in the affected hand). Treatment consists of placing the hand in a neutral position, padding the fist, and gently exercising the wrist and fingers.

Parents are taught to position and immobilize the arm or wrist or both. They can gently massage and manipulate the muscles to prevent contractures while the arm is healing. If edema or hemorrhage is responsible for the paralysis, the prognosis is good, and recovery may be expected in a few weeks. If laceration of the nerves has occurred and healing does not result in return of function within a few months (4 to 6 months or 2 years at the most), surgery may be indicated; however, return of function is variable. Full recovery is expected in 88% to 92% of infants (Paige & Carney, 2002).

Facial paralysis (palsy) (Fig. 38-7) generally is caused by pressure on the facial nerve during birth. The face on the affected side is flattened and unresponsive to the grimace that accompanies crying or stimulation, and the eye will remain open. Moreover, the forehead will not wrinkle. Often the condition is transitory, resolving within hours or days of birth. Permanent paralysis is rare.

Treatment involves assistance with feeding, prevention of damage to the cornea of the open eye, and supportive care of the parents. Usually the infant's face appears distorted, especially when crying. Feeding may be prolonged, with the

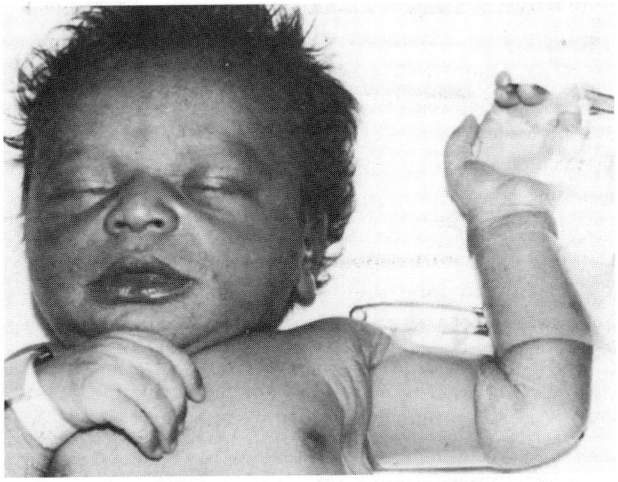

FIG. 38-6 Recommended corrective positioning for treatment of Erb-Duchenne paralysis. Notice abduction and external rotation at shoulder, flexion at elbow, supination of forearm, and slight dorsiflexion at wrist. (From Behrmann, R. [1973]. *Neonatology: Diseases of the fetus and infant.* St. Louis: Mosby.)

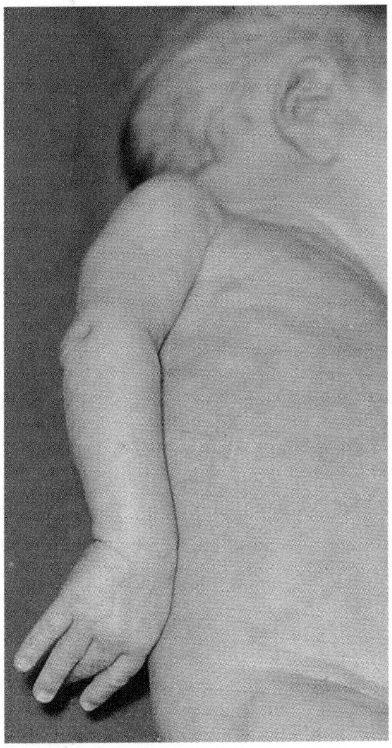

FIG. 38-5 Erb-Duchenne paralysis in newborn infant. The Moro reflex was absent in right upper extremity. Recovery was complete. (From O'Doherty, N. [1986]. *Neonatology: Micro atlas of the newborn.* Nutley, NJ: Hoffmann-La Roche.)

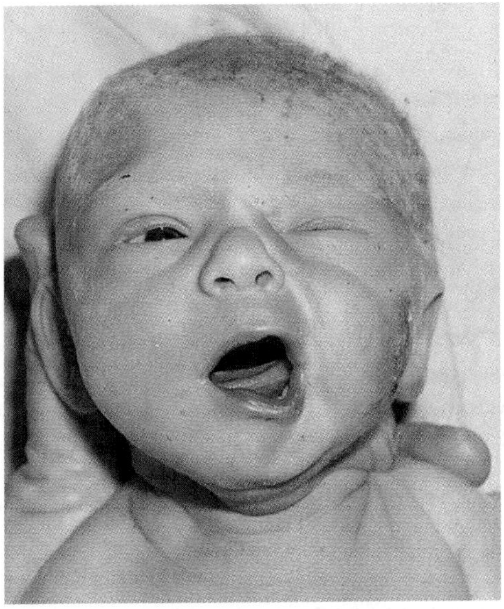

FIG. 38-7 Facial paralysis 15 minutes after forceps birth. Absence of movement on affected side is especially noticeable when infant cries. (From O'Doherty, N. [1986]. *Neonatology: Micro atlas of the newborn.* Nutley, NJ: Hoffmann-La Roche.)

milk flowing out the newborn's mouth around the nipple on the affected side. The mother will need understanding and sympathetic encouragement while learning how to feed and care for the infant, as well as how to hold and cuddle the baby.

Phrenic nerve injury almost always occurs as a component of brachial plexus injury rather than as an isolated problem. Injury to the phrenic nerve may be unilateral or bilateral and results in diaphragmatic paralysis. Cyanosis and irregular thoracic respirations, with no abdominal movement on inspiration, are characteristic of paralysis of the diaphragm. Babies with diaphragmatic paralysis usually require mechanical ventilatory support, at least for the first few days after birth. Other treatments include diaphragmatic pacing or surgical correction.

Central Nervous System Injuries

All types of **intracranial hemorrhage (ICH)** occur in newborns. ICH as a result of birth trauma is more likely to occur in the term, large infant. The frequency and degree of severity of ICH are different in the newborn than in older children or adults. In the newborn, more than one type of hemorrhage can and frequently does occur (Hockenberry et al., 2003).

Subdural hemorrhages (hematomas), life-threatening collections of blood in the subdural space, most often are produced by the stretching and tearing of the large veins in the tentorium of the cerebellum, the dural membrane that separates the cerebrum from the cerebellum. When this type of bleeding occurs, the typical history includes a nulliparous mother, with the total labor and birth occurring in less than 2 or 3 hours; a difficult birth involving high forceps or midforceps application; or a large-for-gestational-age (LGA) infant. Subdural hematoma occurs infrequently today because of improvements in obstetric care. However, it is especially serious because of its inaccessibility to aspiration by subdural tap (Hockenberry et al., 2003).

Subarachnoid hemorrhage, the most common type of ICH, occurs in term infants as a result of trauma and in preterm infants as a result of hypoxia. Small hemorrhages are the most common. Bleeding is of venous origin, and underlying contusion also may occur (Hockenberry et al., 2003).

The clinical presentation of hemorrhage in the term infant can vary considerably. In many infants, signs are absent, and hemorrhaging is diagnosed only because of abnormal findings on lumbar puncture (e.g., red blood cells in the cerebrospinal fluid [CSF]). The initial clinical manifestations of neonatal subarachnoid hemorrhage may be the early onset of alternating depression and irritability, with refractory seizures. Occasionally the infant appears normal initially and then has seizures on the second or third day of life, followed by no apparent sequelae.

In general, nursing care of an infant with ICH is supportive and includes monitoring of ventilatory and intravenous therapy, observation and management of seizures, and prevention of increased ICP. Minimal handling to promote rest and reduce stress should guide nursing care (Hockenberry et al., 2003).

Spinal cord injuries are usually the result of breech births, especially those difficult ones in which version and extraction were used. Brow and face presentations, dystocia, preterm birth, maternal nulliparity, and precipitate birth also have been identified as predisposing factors in these types of injuries. Stretching of the spinal cord, usually by forceful longitudinal traction on the trunk while the head is still firmly engaged in the pelvis, is the most common mechanism of injury. This injury is rarely seen today because cesarean birth is often used for breech presentation (Mangurten, 2002).

Clinical manifestations depend on the severity and location of the injury. High cervical cord injuries are more likely to cause stillbirths or rapid death of the neonate. Lower lesions cause an acute spinal cord syndrome. Common signs of spinal shock include flaccid extremities, diaphragmatic breathing, paralyzed abdominal movements, atonic anal sphincter, and distended bladder. Therapy is supportive and usually unsatisfactory. Infants who survive present a therapeutic challenge that requires combined treatment from many health care providers, including the pediatrician, neurologist, neurosurgeon, urologist, orthopedist, nurse, physical therapist, and occupational therapist. Parents need to understand fully the implications of severe injury to the spinal cord and the overwhelming implications it presents for the family.

Evaluation

The nurse can be assured that care has been effective if the outcomes for care have been achieved. That is, the injury receives prompt and appropriate therapy, the newborn has no or minimal sequelae of trauma, and the parents understand how to care for the infant.

INFANTS OF DIABETIC MOTHERS

No single physiologic or biochemical event can explain the diverse clinical manifestations seen in the **infants of diabetic mothers (IDMs)** or **infants of gestational diabetic mothers (IGDMs).** A better understanding of maternal and fetal metabolism, resulting in stricter control of maternal diabetes and improved obstetric and neonatal intensive care, has led to a decrease in the perinatal mortality rate in diabetic pregnancy. However, maternal diabetes continues to play a significant role in neonatal morbidity and mortality. Of infants born to mothers with gestational diabetes, 35% will weigh more than 4000 g, and 11% will be of low birth weight (McMahon, Ananth, & Liston, 1998). IDMs account for approximately 5% of NICU admissions annually (McKenna, 2000).

All infants born to mothers with diabetes are at some risk for complications. The degree of risk is affected by the severity and duration of maternal disease. Problems seen in IDMs include congenital anomalies, macrosomia, birth trauma and perinatal asphyxia, respiratory distress syndrome (RDS), hypoglycemia, hypocalcemia and hypomagnesemia, cardiomyopathy, and hyperbilirubinemia and polycythemia.

Pathophysiology

The mechanisms responsible for the problems seen in IDMs are not fully understood. In early pregnancy, fluctuations in blood glucose levels and episodes of ketoacidosis are believed to cause congenital anomalies. Later in pregnancy, when the mother's pancreas cannot release sufficient insulin to meet increased demands, maternal hyperglycemia results. Increased amounts of glucose cross the placenta and stimulate the fetal pancreas to release insulin. The combination of the increased supply of maternal glucose and other nutrients and increased fetal insulin results in excessive fetal growth called macrosomia (see later discussion).

Hyperinsulinemia accounts for many of the problems of the fetus or infant. In addition to fluctuating glucose levels, maternal vascular involvement or superimposed maternal infection adversely affects the fetus. Normally, maternal blood has a more alkaline pH than does the carbon dioxide–rich fetal blood. This phenomenon encourages the exchange of oxygen and carbon dioxide across the placental membrane. When the maternal blood is more acidotic than the fetal blood, such as during ketoacidosis, little carbon dioxide or oxygen exchange occurs at the level of the placenta. The mortality rate for unborn babies resulting from an episode of maternal ketoacidosis may be as high as 50% or more (Kalhan & Parimi, 2002).

Some neonatal conditions–macrosomia, hypoglycemia, polyhydramnios, preterm birth, and perhaps fetal lung immaturity–may be eliminated or the incidence decreased by maintaining control over maternal glucose levels within narrow limits (Reece et al., 1998).

Congenital Anomalies

Congenital anomalies occur in about 7% to 10% of IDMs. Their incidence is 2 to 3 times that for infants born to mothers without diabetes. The incidence is greatest among small-for-gestational-age (SGA) newborns. Intrauterine growth restriction (IUGR) leading to SGA infants is seen in IDMs with severe vascular disease. The most frequently occurring anomalies involve the cardiac, musculoskeletal, and central nervous systems. In most defects associated with diabetic pregnancies, the structural abnormality occurs before the eighth week after conception. This reinforces the importance of control of blood glucose both before conception and in the early stages of pregnancy.

The incidence of congenital heart lesions in these infants is 3 to 5 times higher than that in the general population (Montoya & Washington, 2002). Coarctation of the aorta, transposition of the great vessels, and atrial or ventricular septal defects are the most common lesions encountered in the IDM. Maternal diabetic control is correlated with the incidence of lesions; that is, the better the control, the fewer the lesions.

CNS anomalies include anencephaly, encephalocele, meningomyelocele, and hydrocephalus. The musculoskeletal system may be affected by *caudal regression syndrome* (*sacral agenesis*, with weakness or deformities of the lower extremities; malformation and fixation of the hip joints; and shortening or deformity of the femurs). Other defects noted in this population include gastrointestinal atresia and urinary tract malformations.

Neonatal small left colon syndrome, also called lazy colon syndrome, occurs in up to 50% of IDMs and IGDMs (McCollum & Thigpen, 1998). This syndrome is suspected when failure to pass meconium, abdominal distention, and bile-stained vomitus are noted. Contrast enemas show a greatly diminished caliber of the left colon from the splenic flexure to the anus. The syndrome is transient, with normal bowel function developing early in infancy.

Macrosomia

Despite improvements in the control of maternal blood sugar levels, the incidence of **macrosomia** is 50% in women with gestational diabetes and 40% in women with type 1 diabetes (Landon, Catalano, & Gabbe, 2002). At birth, the typical LGA infant has a round, cherubic ("tomato" or cushingoid) face, a chubby body, and a plethoric or flushed complexion (Fig. 38-8). The infant has enlarged internal organs (hepatosplenomegaly, splanchnomegaly, cardiomegaly)

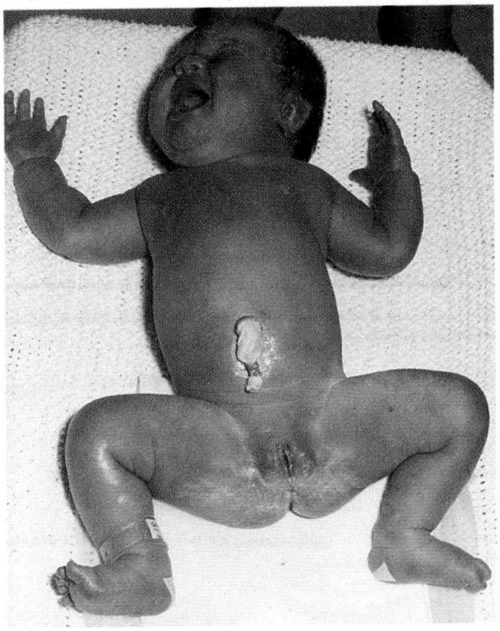

FIG. 38-8 Macrosomia. (From O'Doherty, N. [1986]. *Neonatology: Micro atlas of the newborn.* Nutley, NJ: Hoffmann-La Roche.)

and increased body fat, especially around the shoulders. The placenta and umbilical cord are larger than average. The brain is the only organ that is not enlarged. IDMs may be LGA but physiologically immature.

Insulin has been implicated as the primary growth hormone for intrauterine development. Maternal diabetes results in elevated maternal levels of amino acids and free fatty acids along with hyperglycemia. As the nutrients cross the placenta, the fetal pancreas responds by producing insulin to match the fuel supply. The resulting accelerated protein synthesis, together with a deposition of excessive glycogen and fat stores, is responsible for the typical macrosomic infant. This is the infant most at risk for the neonatal complications of hypoglycemia, hypocalcemia, hyperviscosity, and hyperbilirubinemia. The excessive amounts of metabolic fuels presented to the fetus from the mother and the consequent fetal hyperinsulinism are now understood to represent the basic pathologic mechanism in the diabetic pregnancy (Lindsay, 2002).

The excessive shoulder size in these infants often leads to dystocia, particularly because the head may be smaller in proportion to the shoulders than in a nonmacrosomic infant. Macrosomic infants, born vaginally or by cesarean birth after a trial of labor, may incur birth trauma.

Birth Trauma and Perinatal Hypoxia

Birth injury (resulting from macrosomia or method of birth) and perinatal hypoxia occur in 20% of IGDMs and 35% of IDMs. Examples of birth trauma include cephalhematoma; paralysis of the facial nerve (cranial nerve VII) (see Fig. 38-7); fracture of the clavicle or humerus; brachial plexus paralysis, usually Erb-Duchenne (right upper arm) palsy (see Fig. 38-5); and phrenic nerve paralysis, invariably associated with diaphragmatic paralysis.

Respiratory Distress Syndrome

IDMs and IGDMs are 4 to 6 times more likely than normal infants to develop RDS. With improved maternal glucose control, this risk has been substantially reduced.

In the fetus exposed to high levels of maternal glucose, synthesis of surfactant may be delayed because of the high fetal serum level of insulin (Jones, 2001). Fetal lung maturity, as evidenced by a lecithin/sphingomyelin (L/S) ratio of 2:1, is not reassuring if the mother has diabetes mellitus or gestation-induced diabetes mellitus. For the infants of such mothers, an L/S ratio of 3:1 or more or the presence of **phosphatidylglycerol** (a component of surfactant) in the amniotic fluid is more indicative of adequate lung maturity.

Hypoglycemia

Hypoglycemia (blood glucose levels less than 40 mg/dl in term infants) affects many IDMs, with a reported incidence of 25% to 40%. LGA and preterm infants have the highest risk (Cordero et al., 1998; Hagay & Reece, 1999). After constant exposure to high circulating levels of glucose, hyperplasia of the fetal pancreas occurs, resulting in hyperinsulinemia. Disruption of the fetal glucose supply occurs with the clamping of the umbilical cord, and the neonate's blood glucose level decreases rapidly in the presence of fetal hyperinsulinism. Hypoglycemia is most common in the macrosomic infant, but blood glucose levels should be monitored in all infants of known or suspected mothers with diabetes.

Asymptomatic or symptomatic hypoglycemia most frequently manifests within the first 1 to 3 hours after birth. Signs of hypoglycemia include jitteriness, apnea, tachypnea, and cyanosis. Significant hypoglycemia may result in seizures. Hypoglycemia is worsened by the presence of hypothermia or respiratory distress.

Hypocalcemia and Hypomagnesemia

Hypocalcemia and hypomagnesemia have been reported to occur in as many as 50% of IDMs (Kalhan & Parimi, 2002). A number of these cases are related to hypoxia or prematurity; however, the overall incidence of hypocalcemia is higher than in nondiabetic pregnancies. Hypomagnesemia is believed to develop because of maternal renal losses that occur in diabetes. Hypocalcemia is associated with preterm birth, birth trauma, and perinatal asphyxia. Signs of hypocalcemia are similar to those of hypoglycemia, but they occur between 24 and 36 hours of age. Hypocalcemia should be considered if therapy for hypoglycemia is ineffective.

Cardiomyopathy

All IDMs need careful observation for **cardiomyopathy** (disease affecting the structure and function of the heart) because an increased heart size is often found in these infants. Two types of cardiomyopathy can occur. Clinicians must be alert to identify the type of lesion correctly so that appropriate therapy is instituted. Both types of lesions are associated with respiratory symptoms and congestive heart failure.

Hypertrophic cardiomyopathy (HCM) is characterized by a hypercontractile and thickened myocardium. The ventricular walls are thickened, as is the septum, which in severe cases results in outflow tract obstructions. The mitral valve is poorly functioning. In *nonhypertrophic cardiomyopathy* (non-HCM), the myocardium is poorly contractile and overstretched. The ventricles are increased in size, and no outflow obstruction is found. Most infants are asymptomatic, but severe outflow obstruction may cause left ventricular heart failure. HCM may be treated with a beta-adrenergic blocker (such as propranolol) to decrease contractility and heart rate. A cardiotonic agent is used to treat non-HCM (such as digoxin, to increase contractility and decrease heart rate). The abnormality usually resolves in 3 to 12 months.

Hyperbilirubinemia and Polycythemia

IDMs are at increased risk of developing hyperbilirubinemia. Many IDMs also are polycythemic. Polycythemia increases blood viscosity, thereby impairing circulation. In addition, this increased number of red blood cells to be hemolyzed increases the potential bilirubin load that the neonate must clear. The excessive red blood cells are produced in extramedullary foci (liver and spleen) in addition to the usual sites in bone marrow; therefore both liver function and bilirubin clearance may be adversely affected. Bruising associated with birth of a macrosomic infant will contribute further to high bilirubin levels.

Nursing Care

Nursing care depends on the neonate's particular problems. General care of the compromised infant is addressed in Chapter 40. If the maternal blood glucose level was well controlled throughout the pregnancy, the infant may require only monitoring. Because euglycemia (normal blood glucose levels) is not always possible, the nurse must promptly recognize and treat any consequences of maternal diabetes that arise. The most common problems of IDMs that require intervention include birth trauma and perinatal asphyxia; RDS; difficult metabolic transition, including hypoglycemia and hypocalcemia; and congenital anomalies (see previous sections and Plan of Care).

NEONATAL INFECTIONS

Sepsis

Sepsis (presence of microorganisms or their toxins in blood or other tissues) continues to be one of the most significant causes of neonatal morbidity and mortality. The newborn infant is susceptible to infection. Maternal immunoglobulin (IgM) does not cross the placenta. IgA and IgM require time to reach optimal levels after birth. Phagocytosis is less efficient. Serum complement levels are inadequate; serum complement (C1 through C6) is involved in immunologic reactions, some of which kill or lyse bacteria and enhance phagocytosis. Dysmaturity seen with IUGR

Plan of Care — Infant of Mother with Gestational Diabetes

NURSING DIAGNOSIS Risk for injury related to hypoglycemia, hypocalcemia, polycythemia, or hyperbilirubinemia secondary to maternal gestational diabetes

Expected Outcome *Infant will exhibit blood glucose, serum calcium, hematocrit, and serum bilirubin levels that are within normal limits.*

Nursing Interventions/*Rationales*

Monitor blood glucose levels (<40 mg/dl indicative of hypoglycemia); and serum calcium levels (<7 mg/dl indicative of hypocalcemia); and serum bilirubin levels (>15 mg/dl indicative of hyperbilirubinemia) *to assess and detect early onset to prevent complications.*

Observe for signs of hypoglycemia (jitteriness, twitching, lethargy, apathy, convulsions, cyanosis, sweating, eye rolling, refusal to eat); hypocalcemia (jitters, apnea, high-pitched cry, abdominal distention); polycythemia (plethora); and hyperbilirubinemia (jaundice) *to assess and detect signs of onset to prevent complications.*

Early feeding of infant, glucose supplements as prescribed *to prevent or treat early hypoglycemia;* increased milk feedings/calcium supplements per physician order *to prevent or treat early hypocalcemia;* early and frequent feedings *to reduce hematocrit and enhance excretion of bilirubin in stool.*

Reduce adverse environmental factors (e.g., stimuli such as jarring or shaking, cold stress, and respiratory distress) *that can predispose infant to hypoglycemia or precipitate a seizure.*

NURSING DIAGNOSIS Risk for impaired gas exchange related to lung immaturity or cardiomyopathy secondary to maternal gestational diabetes

Expected Outcomes *Infant will exhibit signs of adequate oxygen supply (respiratory rate, rhythm, and amplitude, and blood gas levels within normal limits).*

Nursing Interventions/*Rationales*

Monitor infant vital signs, blood gas levels per order, patency of airway *to evaluate pulmonary and circulatory status.*

Avoid activities that may reduce body temperature and lead to cold stress, *which can induce respiratory distress.*

Suction as needed *to keep airway patent and prevent aspiration.*

Position infant on side *to facilitate mucus drainage.*

Have resuscitation equipment and oxygen available *for quick treatment of respiratory distress.*

NURSING DIAGNOSIS Risk for ineffective thermoregulation related to physiologic immaturity; potential for infection related to immature immunologic defenses/environmental exposure

See the Nursing Plan of Care for the normal newborn in Chapter 26.

NURSING DIAGNOSIS Anxiety (risk for powerlessness, situational low self-esteem, ineffective coping) related to neonate's condition, management, and prognosis

Expected Outcome *Parents demonstrate understanding of prognosis and therapy for infant.*

Nursing Interventions/*Rationales*

Explain potential effects of maternal diabetic condition on newborn *to relieve fear of unknown and support ability to cope.*

Encourage open communication (e.g., inform parents of ongoing condition, procedures, and treatment; answer questions; correct misperceptions; actively listen to parental concerns) *to provide support and help provide sense of control.*

Encourage parents to interact with infant and to become involved in care routines *to foster emotional connection.*

and preterm and postdate birth further compromises the neonate's immune system.

Table 38-2 outlines risk factors for neonatal sepsis. Special precautions for preventing infection, as well as prompt recognition when it occurs, are necessary for optimal newborn care. Neonatal infections may be acquired in utero, during birth, during resuscitation, and nosocomially.

Prenatal acquisition of infection occurs by organisms placentally transferred directly into the fetal circulatory system and from infected amniotic fluid, such as with herpes simplex virus (HSV), cytomegalovirus (CMV), and rubella. Microorganisms also may ascend from the vagina and pass through the cervix. The membranes become infected and may rupture. Infection of the fetal skin and respiratory or gastrointestinal tract may result.

During birth, contact with an infected birth canal can result in generalized or local infection. The upper airway and gastrointestinal tract are the principal pathways for generalized infections. The conjunctiva and oral cavity are the usual sites of local infection.

Postnatal infection may be acquired during resuscitation or through the introduction of foreign objects such as indwelling catheters or endotracheal tubes. Nursery-acquired infections may be transferred to the infant by the hands of the parents or health care personnel or spread from contaminated equipment. The umbilicus is a receptive site for cutaneous infection leading to sepsis (Edwards, 2002).

TABLE 38-2 **Risk Factors for Neonatal Sepsis**

SOURCE	RISK FACTORS
Maternal	Low socioeconomic status
	Poor prenatal care
	Poor nutrition
	Substance abuse
Intrapartum	Premature rupture of fetal membranes
	Maternal fever
	Chorioamnionitis
	Prolonged labor
	Premature labor
	Maternal urinary tract infection
Neonatal	Twin gestation
	Male
	Birth asphyxia
	Meconium aspiration
	Congenital anomalies of skin or mucous membranes
	Galactosemia
	Absence of spleen
	Low birth weight or prematurity
	Malnourishment
	Prolonged hospitalization

From Askin, D. (1995). Bacterial and fungal sepsis in the neonate. *Journal of Obstetric, Gynecologic, and Neonatal Nursing, 24*(7), 635-643.

Neonatal bacterial infection is classified into two patterns according to the time of presentation. Early-onset or congenital sepsis usually manifests within 24 to 72 hours after birth, progresses more rapidly than later-onset infection, and has a mortality rate between 5% and 50% (Klein, 2001). Early-onset infection is usually caused by microorganisms from the normal flora of the maternal vaginal tract, including group B streptococci, *Haemophilus influenzae, Listeria monocytogenes, Escherichia coli,* and *Streptococcus pneumoniae* (Merenstein, Adams, & Weisman, 2002). It is associated with a history of obstetric complications, such as preterm labor, premature rupture of membranes, maternal fever during labor, and chorioamnionitis (Klein, 2001).

Acquired infection is most frequently seen after 1 to 2 weeks of age and is slower in progression. Bacteria responsible for late-onset sepsis are varied, may be acquired from the birth canal or from the external environment, and include *Staphylococcus aureus, S. epidermidis, Pseudomonas* organisms, and group B streptococci. The mortality rate for late-onset infection varies between 2% and 6% (Klein, 2001).

Viral infections may cause miscarriage, stillbirth, intrauterine infection, congenital malformations, and acute disease. These pathogens also may cause chronic infection, with subtle manifestations that may be recognized only after a prolonged period. It is important to recognize the manifestations of infections in the neonatal period to treat the acute infection and to prevent nosocomial infections in other infants, and to anticipate effects on the infant's subsequent growth and development.

Fungal infections are of greatest concern in the immunocompromised or premature infant. Occasionally, fungal infections such as thrush are found in otherwise healthy term infants.

Septicemia refers to a generalized infection in the bloodstream. Pneumonia, the most common form of neonatal infection, is one of the leading causes of perinatal death and is caused by many of the same organisms that cause sepsis (Edwards, 2002). Bacterial meningitis affects 1 in 2500 liveborn infants. Gastroenteritis is sporadic, depending on epidemic outbreaks. Local infections such as conjunctivitis and omphalitis occur frequently, but incidence rates are unavailable. Infection continues to be a significant factor in fetal and neonatal morbidity and mortality.

CARE MANAGEMENT

Assessment and Nursing Diagnoses

The prenatal record is reviewed for risk factors associated with infection and signs and symptoms suggestive of it. Maternal vaginal or perineal infection may be transmitted directly to the infant during passage through the birth canal. Psychosocial history and history of sexually transmitted infections (STIs) may indicate possible human immunodeficiency virus (HIV), hepatitis B virus (HBV), or CMV infection.

Perinatal events also are reviewed. Premature rupture of membranes (PROM) may be caused by maternal or intrauterine infection. Ascending infection may occur after prolonged PROM, prolonged labor, or intrauterine fetal monitoring. A maternal history of fever during labor or the presence of foul-smelling amniotic fluid also may indicate the presence of infection. Antibiotic therapy initiated during labor should be noted. Resuscitation that requires intubation and deep suctioning may result in infection. The neonate's gestational age, maturity, birth weight, and gender all affect the incidence of infection. Sepsis occurs about twice as often and results in a higher mortality rate in male than in female infants. The neonate is assessed for respiratory distress, skin abscesses, rashes, and other indications of infection.

During the postnatal period, the time of onset of suggestive signs is noted. Onset within the first 48 hours of life is more often associated with prenatal or perinatal predisposing factors. Onset after 2 or 3 days more frequently reflects disease acquired at or subsequent to birth.

The earliest clinical signs of neonatal sepsis are characterized by a lack of specificity. The nonspecific signs include lethargy, poor feeding, poor weight gain, and irritability. The nurse or parent may simply note that the infant is just not doing as well as before. Differential diagnosis may be difficult because signs of sepsis are similar to signs of noninfectious neonatal problems such as anemia or hypoglycemia. Additional clinical and laboratory information and appropriate cultures supplement the findings described. Table 38-3 outlines signs of sepsis.

Laboratory studies are performed. Specimens for cultures include blood, nasopharyngeal or oropharyngeal specimens, CSF, stool, and urine. Increased direct (conjugated) bilirubin levels may be found, especially if the infecting microorganism is gram negative. Complete blood cell count with differential is performed to determine the presence of anemia, increased white blood cell count, or decreased white blood cell count (an ominous sign). C-reactive protein may or may not be elevated.

Vigilant assessment continues during and after treatment. The newborn continues to be assessed for sequelae to septicemia. Before the advent of antibiotics, 90% of newborns with sepsis died. Antibiotic therapy decreased mortality rates to between 13% and 45%, depending on the causative organism.

Sequelae to septicemia include meningitis, disseminated intravascular coagulation (DIC), and septic shock.

Septic shock results from the toxins released into the bloodstream. The most common sign is a decrease in blood pressure, a vital sign often not assessed in the care of the neonate. The infant will often appear gray or mottled and may be noted to have cool extremities. Other signs are rapid, irregular respirations and pulse (similar to septicemia in general).

Any number of nursing diagnoses are possible, depending on the infant's gestational age and birth weight, the organ systems involved, and the nature of the infection. Examples of nursing diagnoses related to neonatal infections include the following:

Newborn

- *Infection related to*
  - –maternal vaginal (or other) infection
  - –need for resuscitation or ventilation therapy
  - –need for indwelling umbilical catheters, total parenteral nutrition (TPN), parenteral fluids
  - –intrauterine electronic fetal monitoring
  - –dysmaturity, IUGR, gestational age
- *Ineffective thermoregulation related to*
  - –infection
- *Impaired tissue integrity related to*
  - –need for multiple supportive measures (e.g., biometric monitoring, TPN, inhalation therapy)
- *Acute pain related to*
  - –need for multiple supportive measures

Parents and family

- *Anxiety, fear, or anticipatory grieving related to*
  - –uncertainty about infant's prognosis
  - –poor prognosis
- *Risk for impaired parenting related to*
  - –separation of parent and newborn
  - –feelings of inadequacy in caring for infant
- *Powerlessness or spiritual distress related to*
  - –perinatal events or newborn's condition
- *Anxiety related to knowledge deficit regarding*
  - –newborn's condition, its course, and its management

Expected Outcomes of Care

Planning begins with the development of standards for preventive measures in nurseries and protocols for diagnosis and treatment of infections. Individual assessment findings are used to plan care for each infant. Parents and family are encouraged to participate in planning. Expected outcomes include the following:

- The newborn will remain free of sepsis.
- The newborn's early signs of sepsis will be recognized, and appropriate therapy will be instituted.
- If therapy is necessary, the newborn will have no harmful sequelae.
- Parents will begin bonding with and attachment to newborn.
- Parents will maintain self-esteem.
- Staff members will establish caring relationship with parents to foster their trust and to encourage continuing, active, positive interactions of family with members of the health care system.

Plan of Care and Interventions

Preventive Measures

Virtually all controlled clinical trials have demonstrated that effective handwashing is responsible for the prevention of nosocomial infection in nursery units. Nursing is

TABLE 38-3 **Signs of Sepsis***

SYSTEM	SIGNS
Respiratory	Apnea, bradycardia
	Tachypnea
	Grunting, nasal flaring
	Retractions
	Decreased oxygen saturation
	Acidosis
Cardiovascular	Decreased cardiac output
	Tachycardia
	Hypotension
	Decreased perfusion
Central nervous	Temperature instability
	Lethargy
	Hypotonia
	Irritability, seizures
Gastrointestinal	Feeding intolerance
	Abdominal distention
	Vomiting, diarrhea
Integumentary	Jaundice
	Pallor
	Petechiae

From Askin, D. (1995). Bacterial and fungal sepsis in the neonate. *Journal of Obstetric, Gynecologic, and Neonatal Nursing, 24*(7), 635-643.
*Laboratory findings include neutropenia, increased bands, hypoglycemia or hyperglycemia, metabolic acidosis, and thrombocytopenia.

directly or indirectly responsible for minimizing or eliminating environmental sources of infectious agents in the nursery. Measures to be taken include Standard Precautions, careful and thorough cleaning, frequent replacement of used equipment (e.g., changing intravenous tubing per hospital protocol, cleaning resuscitation and ventilation equipment), and disposal of excrement and linens in an appropriate manner. Overcrowding must be avoided in nurseries.

Instillation of antibiotic ointment in newborns' eyes 1 to 2 hours after birth is done to prevent infection, such as from gonorrhea and chlamydiosis. The skin, its secretions, and its normal flora are natural defenses that protect against invading pathogens. Warm water may be used to remove blood and meconium from the neonate's face, head, and body. A mild nonmedicated soap (in single-use container or in a small bar reserved for a single newborn) can be used with careful water rinsing. The vernix caseosa is left in place. The cord can be left to air dry. The stump and base of the cord should be assessed for edema, redness, and purulent drainage.

Curative Measures

Breastfeeding or feeding the newborn breast milk from the mother is encouraged. Protective mechanisms exist in breast milk. Colostrum contains immunoglobulin A (IgA), which offers protection against infection in the gastrointestinal tract. Human milk contains iron-binding protein that exerts a bacteriostatic effect on *E. coli.* Human milk also contains macrophages and lymphocytes. The vulnerability of infants to common mucosal pathogens such as respiratory syncytial virus (RSV) may be reduced by passive transfer of maternal immunity in the colostrum and breast milk.

Administering medications, taking precautions when performing treatments, and following isolation procedures also are interventions to be considered when a newborn has an infection.

Monitoring the intravenous infusion rate and administering antibiotics are the nurse's responsibility. It is important to administer the prescribed dose of antibiotic within 1 hour after it is prepared to avoid loss of drug stability. If the intravenous fluid the infant is receiving contains electrolytes, vitamins, or other medications, the nurse should check with the hospital pharmacy before adding antibiotics. The antibiotic (or other medication) may be deactivated or may form a precipitate when combined with other substances. In that case, a piggyback solution of the prescribed fluid is attached with a three-way stopcock at the infusion site.

Care must be taken in suctioning secretions from any newborn's oropharynx or trachea. These secretions may be infected.

Isolation procedures are implemented according to hospital policy as indicated. Isolation protocols are changing rapidly, and the nurse is urged to participate in continuing education and in-service programs to remain up to date.

Rehabilitative Measures

Rehabilitative measures vary with the individual needs of the neonate. Some neonates will need to be weaned from ventilatory support systems. Those who have sequelae such as mental retardation and epilepsy will require a knowledgeable family and supportive community resources. Some children will require corrective care for problems with dentition, vision, and hearing.

Evaluation

The nurse can be reasonably assured that care was effective if the outcomes for care are achieved: the newborn remains free of sepsis or the newborn's early signs of sepsis are recognized and appropriately treated (see Care Path).

TORCH Infections

The occurrence of certain maternal infections during early pregnancy is known to be associated with various congenital malformations and disorders. The most common and best understood infections are traditionally represented by the acronym **TORCH,** for *t*oxoplasmosis, *o*ther (gonorrhea, syphilis, varicella, HBV, and HIV), *r*ubella, *c*ytomegalovirus, and *h*erpes simplex virus (Box 38-1). Additional organisms known to cause congenital infection include enteroviruses and parvovirus, leading some clinicians to

Care Path Suspected Neonatal Sepsis

ASSESSMENTS	1. Potential maternal risk factors and unstable vital signs, especially temperature instability. 2. Sepsis screen in first hour (complete blood count with differential, platelets, and C-reactive protein [CRP] level) if significant maternal risk factors (prolonged rupture of membranes, maternal temperature) are found or if infant demonstrates physiologic signs of sepsis.
TREATMENT	1. Start IV administration of antibiotics by peripheral IV. 2. Provide other treatments as needed for additional physiologic problems (ventilator for respiratory distress, incubator for temperature instability).
POSSIBLE CONSULTATIONS	1. Neonatologists and advanced practice nurses for care of unstable infants. 2. Medical specialists for care of infants with additional problems (congenital deformities). 3. Lactation consultant, interpreter, social worker, and chaplain as needed or requested.
ADDITIONAL ASSESSMENTS	1. Weight and measurements. 2. Blood culture, chest radiograph study, urinalysis, and lumbar puncture, if infant is symptomatic or CRP level is positive. 3. Repeat determination of CRP level in the morning for 2 days. If negative and infant not symptomatic, stop antibiotic treatment. 4. Continuous cardiac and oxygen saturation monitor assessment if infant's condition is unstable.
DIRECT INFANT CARE	1. Vital signs every 1 to 2 hours for the first 4 hours, and then every 4 hours. 2. Advance oral feedings as tolerated (infant takes nothing by mouth only if condition is physiologically unstable). 3. Bath and cord care done per unit protocols.
TEACHING AND DISCHARGE PLANNING	1. Initiate on admission. Provide parents with written and oral information on suspected sepsis. 2. Reinforce information and determine parents' understanding of information before discharge. Include information on well-baby care and community follow-up with the family's primary health care provider.

Courtesy Lucile Salter Packard Children's Hospital at Stanford, California.

suggest the need for a new more comprehensive acronym (Klein & Remington, 2001). HSV may result in a severe, often fatal systemic illness in neonates. Survivors of herpetic infection may have residual neurologic defects and chorioretinitis. The other congenital infections also may result in encephalopathy with various anomalies, including microcephaly, chorioretinitis, intracranial calcifications, microphthalmos, and cataracts. To a certain extent, the varied clinical manifestations of these infections overlap, but a specific diagnosis can be made by the clustering of clinical findings, as well as specific antibody studies.

BOX 38-1 TORCH Infections Affecting Newborns

T Toxoplasmosis
O Other: gonorrhea, syphilis, varicella, hepatitis B virus (HBV), human immunodeficiency virus (HIV)
R Rubella
C Cytomegalovirus (CMV) infections or cytomegalic inclusion disease (CMID)
H Herpes simplex virus (HSV) infection

Toxoplasmosis

Toxoplasmosis is a multisystem disease caused by the protozoan *Toxoplasma gondii* parasite, commonly found in cats, dogs, pigs, sheep, and cattle, with cats being the definitive host. About 30% of women who contract toxoplasmosis during gestation transmit the disease to their offspring (Lynfield & Guerina, 1997). Fetal infection occurs in 0.07% to 0.11% of all pregnancies (Beazley & Egerman, 1998). The diagnosis of toxoplasmosis in the neonate is supported by elevated levels of cord blood serum IgM.

Most (80% to 90%) neonates infected with *T. gondii* in utero may be asymptomatic at birth, but in approximately 50%, progressive chorioretinitis develops, and in 40%, CNS involvement such as hydrocephalus develops in the weeks and months after birth (Martin, 2001; Remington et al., 2001). In some cases, chorioretinitis may develop during school age or adolescent stages. Others are born with severe manifestations at birth. Clinical features ascribed to *T. gondii* infection include four key findings first described by Sabin (1942): hydrocephalus or microcephaly; chorioretinitis; seizures or other neurologic manifestations; and cerebral calcifications. Transmission of toxoplasmosis from an infected mother to her fetus can be significantly reduced by maternal treatment with spiramycin (Lynfield & Guerina, 1997).

Severe toxoplasmosis is associated with preterm birth, growth restriction, microcephaly or hydrocephaly, microphthalmos, chorioretinitis, CNS calcification, thrombocytopenia, jaundice, and fever. Petechiae or a maculopapular rash also may be evident. The affected infant may be treated with pyrimethamine, as well as oral sulfadiazine; folic acid supplement will be required to prevent anemia.

Gonorrhea

With the prophylactic use of silver nitrate or antibiotics, the incidence of gonococcal conjunctivitis is less than 0.5% (Cowles & Gonik, 2002). After rupture of membranes, ascending infection can result in orogastric contamination of the fetus. The organism also may invade mucosal surfaces such as the conjunctiva (ophthalmia neonatorum), rectal mucosa, and pharynx. Contamination may occur as the infant passes through the birth canal, or it may occur postnatally from an infected adult. Neonatal gonococcal arthritis, septicemia, meningitis, vaginitis, and scalp abscesses also can develop.

Eye prophylaxis (e.g., with 0.5% erythromycin ointment) is administered at or shortly after birth to prevent ophthalmia neonatorum. The infant with a mild infection often recovers completely with appropriate treatment, such as neonatal ceftriaxone. Rarely infants die of overwhelming infection in the early neonatal period.

Syphilis

Congenital and neonatal syphilis have reemerged in recent years as significant health problems. It is estimated that for every 100 women diagnosed with primary or secondary disease, two to five infants will contract congenital syphilis. If syphilis during pregnancy is untreated, 40% to 50% of neonates born to these women will have symptomatic congenital syphilis. Treatment failure can occur, particularly when treatment is given in the third trimester; therefore infants born to women treated within 4 weeks of birth should be investigated for congenital syphilis. The following factors have been identified as placing the neonate at high risk for exposure to syphilis: inadequate prenatal care, single or teenage mother, substance abuse in mother or partner, multiple sexual partners or partner with known STI, history of STI, poverty, homelessness, and HIV infection (Cloherty, 1998).

The mode of transmission in adults is sexual. The infant is usually infected in utero by transplacental infection, but infection of the amniotic fluid also may occur (Ingall & Sanchez, 2001). The risk to the fetus and neonate varies according to the stage of maternal infection, but it is generally recognized that untreated maternal disease poses a significant risk of stillbirth (12%) and live births with congenital infection (29%) (Sheffield et al., 1999). Prompt maternal treatment will eliminate most fetal infections; however, delayed treatment or a failure to obtain treatment may result in fetal effects that range from minor anomalies to preterm birth or fetal death. Damage to the fetus depends on when in gestation the infection occurred and the time that has elapsed before treatment. Silent infection may be present at birth but may not be expressed for up to 2 years of age (AAP, 2000).

Early congenital syphilis may result in prematurity, hydrops fetalis, and failure to thrive. Hepatosplenomegaly is common, as is lymphadenopathy. Hematologic findings include anemia, leucopenia, and thrombocytopenia. Characteristic bony lesions occur in the long bones, cranium, and spine and include osteochondritis, osteomyelitis, and periostitis (Ingall & Sanchez, 2001). Other findings include snuffles, mucocutaneous lesions, edema, and a copper-colored maculopapular dermal rash first noticeable on the palms of the hands, soles of the feet, and in the diaper area (AAP, 2000). *Condylomata* (elevated wartlike lesions) may be seen around the anus. Other involvement results in exfoliation (separation, flaking) of nails and loss of hair. Iritis and choroiditis are characteristic of infection of the eyes. Nephrotic syndrome secondary to renal infection; hepatitis with jaundice, lymphadenopathy, and inflammation of the pancreas, testes, and colon; and a pseudoparalysis of the extremities may be noted. Laboratory tests may show a pleocytosis (usually lymphocytosis) and elevated CSF protein levels.

In some infants, signs of congenital syphilis do not appear until late in the neonatal period. In these newborns, early signs such as poor feeding, slight hyperthermia, and snuffles may be nonspecific. *Snuffles* refers to the copious clear mucous discharge from the nose.

Medical Management. If the mother was adequately treated before giving birth and serologic testing of the infant does not show syphilis, generally the infant is not treated with antibiotics. The infant is checked for antibody titer (received from the mother through the placenta) every 2 weeks for 3 months, at which time, the test result should be negative. Some physicians recommend antibiotic therapy for asymptomatic or inconclusive cases.

Treatment should be carried out in the following situations: when the diagnosis of congenital syphilis is confirmed or suspected, when maternal treatment status is unknown, when the mother is treated within 4 weeks of giving birth or does not respond to treatment, when medications other than penicillin are used to treat the mother, and when inadequate neonatal follow-up is anticipated (Hollier & Cox, 1998).

For antibiotic treatment to be effective, an "adequate" blood level must be maintained for an "adequate" period. The suggested medication protocol in the presence of symptomatic systemic disease differs from author to author and from physician to physician. Penicillin is the usual treatment (Hollier & Cox 1998). After 12 hours of antibiotic therapy, the child's condition is not considered contagious. It generally is accepted that erythromycin is the substitute antibiotic of choice for infants sensitive to penicillin.

Prognosis. In general, treatment of syphilis is more effective if it is begun early rather than late in the course of the disease. However, a recurrence rate of 5% can be expected. Even adequate treatment of congenital syphilis after birth does not always prevent late (5 to 15 years after initial infection) complications. Potential complications include neurosyphilis, deafness, Hutchinson teeth (notched incisors), saber shins, joint involvement, saddle nose (depressed bridge), gummas (soft, gummy tumors) over the skin and other organs, interstitial keratitis (inflammation of the cornea), rhagades (circumoral radiating scars around the lips), frontal bossing, and mulberry molars (AAP, 2000).

Varicella-Zoster

The varicella-zoster virus responsible for chickenpox and shingles is a member of the herpes family. Approximately 90% of women in the childbearing years are immune; therefore the risk of infection in pregnancy is low, 0.7 to 3 per 1000 deliveries (Birthistle & Carrington, 1998; Chapman, 1998).

Varicella transmission to the fetus may occur across the placenta when the disease is contracted in the first half of pregnancy, but this is relatively infrequent. When transmission to the fetus does occur in the early part of pregnancy, the effects on the fetus include limb atrophy, neurologic abnormalities, eye abnormalities, and IUGR.

When maternal infection occurs in the last 3 weeks of pregnancy, 25% of infants born to these mothers will develop clinical varicella (Nathwani et al., 1998). The severity of the infant's illness will increase greatly if maternal infection occurred within 5 days before or 2 days after birth. The mortality rate in severe illness is 30% (Chapman, 1998).

Seroimmune pregnant women exposed to active chickenpox can be given varicella-zoster immune globulin (VZIG), which does not reduce the incidence of infection but should decrease the effects of the virus on the fetus. The immunoglobulin must be given within 72 hours of exposure to be effective.

Infants born to mothers in whom chickenpox develops between 5 days before birth and 48 hours after should be given VZIG at birth because of the risk of severe disease. Acyclovir can be used to treat infants with generalized involvement and pneumonia (Chapman, 1998; Nathwani et al., 1998).

Term infants exposed to chickenpox after birth will have a mild or no infection if they are born to immune mothers. In those born to nonimmune mothers, chickenpox may develop, but the course is not usually severe. Experts are divided as to whether this group of infants should receive VZIG. Infants younger than 28 weeks are at risk regardless of their mother's status and probably benefit from VZIG if exposed to chickenpox.

Hepatitis B Virus

HBV infection during pregnancy is not associated with an increase in malformations, stillbirths, or IUGR; however, approximately 35% will be born before term (Baley & Toltzis, 2002). The transmission rate of HBV to the newborn is as high as 85% when the mother is seropositive for both hepatitis B surface antigen (HBsAg) and hepatitis B e antigen (HBeAg) (Baley & Toltzis, 2002). Transmission occurs transplacentally, serum to serum, and by contact with contaminated urine, feces, saliva, semen, or vaginal secretions during birth. Infants are most frequently infected during birth or in the first few days of life. The rate of transmission is highest when the mother contracts the virus immediately before birth. These mothers will be positive for HBsAg. Transmission may occur through breast milk, but antigens also develop in formula-fed infants at the same or higher rate. Diagnosis is made by viral culture of amniotic fluid, as well as the presence of HBsAg and IgM in the cord or baby's serum.

Neonatal and fetal effects are serious. Preterm birth exposes the neonate to the problems of prematurity. Infants may be symptom free at birth or show evidence of acute hepatitis with changes in liver function. The mortality rate for full-blown hepatitis is 75%. Infants who become carriers are at high risk for chronic hepatitis, cirrhosis of the liver, or liver cancer even years later.

Infants whose mothers have antibodies for HBsAg or in whom hepatitis developed during pregnancy or the postpartum period should be treated with hepatitis B immunoglobulin (HBIG), 0.5 ml intramuscularly, as soon as possible after birth–within the first 12 hours of life. The hepatitis B vaccine also should be given at the same time but in a different site (AAP, 2002; Baley & Toltzis, 2002). The second dose of vaccine is given at 1 month, and the third dose, at 6 months. The vaccine should protect the child for up to 9 years. After the infant has been cleansed thoroughly and has received the vaccine, breastfeeding may be initiated. Vaccination for infants not exposed to HBV is recommended before discharge but may be given by 2 months of age; breastfeeding for these infants may begin before the vaccine is given (Baley & Toltzis, 2002).

Human Immunodeficiency Virus and Acquired Immunodeficiency Syndrome

Maternal infection with the retrovirus HIV is discussed in Chapter 8. The focus of this discussion is the neonate at risk for infection with HIV. It is estimated that globally, more than 1 million children born to HIV-infected women will acquire the virus (Mofenson, 1997). The majority of cases of pediatric AIDS result from maternal-fetal transmission. Since 1994, when research demonstrated that prenatal treatment of HIV-positive women reduced the vertical transmission of the HIV virus to the fetus, there has been an almost 70% decrease in the risk of transmission, from 25% to 8% (Minkoff, 1998). The risk of perinatal transmission can be further reduced to about 2% when maternal zidovudine prophylaxis is combined with elective cesarean birth (International Perinatal HIV Group, 1999). Universal counseling and screening of pregnant women is recommended in the United States and Canada (American College of Obstetricians and Gynecologists, 1997; Workowsky & Levine, 2002).

Transmission of HIV from the mother to the infant may occur transplacentally at various gestational ages. Transmission close to or at the time of birth is thought to account for 50% to 80% of cases (Baley & Toltzis, 2002; Franck & Johnson, 1998; Mofenson, 1997). Postnatal transmission through breastfeeding also may occur, with an additional risk of 16% to 21% attributed to breast-milk contact (John et al., 2001; Nduati et al., 2000). The risk of breast-milk transmission appears to be greatest early in the postpartum period (Nduati et al., 2000).

Prevention. A number of factors increase the risk of HIV transmission from mother to fetus. A high viral load correlates strongly with increased transmission, as does a low maternal CD4 T-lymphocyte count, indicative of severe disease. Asymptomatic women can transmit infection but are less likely than symptomatic women to do so. Chorioamnionitis, rupture of membranes more than 4 hours before birth, and preterm birth also have been shown to increase the risk of HIV transmission to the fetus (Franck & Johnson, 1998; Minkoff, 1998; Mofenson, 1997).

Strategies to prevent HIV acquisition in the fetus and newborn should address these risk factors. Antenatal and postnatal treatment with antiretroviral agents such as zidovudine has been shown to reduce the infant's risk of acquiring HIV. Combination therapy with several anti-HIV medications is of additional benefit in reducing transmission rates and preventing the development of drug resistance. Vaginal birth within 4 hours of rupture of membranes and cesarean birth have been shown to reduce contact with maternal virus (Working Group, 2001). HIV-positive women should be counseled to avoid breastfeeding.

Diagnosis. Diagnosis of HIV infection in the neonate is complicated by the presence of maternal IgG antibodies, which cross the placenta after 32 weeks of gestation. Three methods to detect HIV virus or its components are available for use in neonates. Viral cultures detect the presence of HIV in the neonate's blood. This sensitive but expensive test requires 4 to 6 weeks for a result. Detection of core protein antigen p24 is less expensive but also less sensitive in neonates. Polymerase chain reaction (PCR) detects HIV DNA or RNA in peripheral blood. This test has reduced sensitivity in the first 6 months of age, and a negative result does not necessarily rule out infection.

The accuracy of all HIV tests varies according to the infant's age and is dependent on the viral load in the blood. The Centers for Disease Control and Prevention (CDC) recommends that at least two PCR assays or viral cultures be done before a definitive diagnosis is made (Franck & Johnson, 1998; McGowan, Crane, & Wiznia, 1999). Testing should be done in the first 48 hours of life, at age 1 to 2 months, and at age 3 to 6 months (Working Group, 2001).

Typically the HIV-infected neonate is asymptomatic at birth. In the past, these infants tend to be of lower birth weight than those born to noninfected mothers. No difference is found in the incidence of preterm birth or IUGR between the offspring of zidovudine-treated mothers and those born to HIV-negative women (European Collaborative Study, 1998; Lambert et al, 2000). Some will have physical stigma from concurrent exposure to substance abuse using injectable drugs or other STIs.

About 5% of infants infected with HIV at birth deteriorate rapidly over the first 10 to 18 months of life (Cole, 1998). In these babies, **opportunistic infections** (caused by an organism that usually does not cause illness) and rapid progression of immunodeficiency develop, which progresses to death in the first 1 to 2 years of life (Franck & Johnson, 1998). Another 30% of infants have nonspecific findings such as failure to thrive, parotitis, oral candidiasis, developmental delay, and recurrent or persistent upper respiratory infections. Common secondary infections include *Pneumocystis carinii* pneumonia, candidiasis, CMV infection, cryptosporidiosis, HSV or herpes zoster, and disseminated varicella.

Of newborns who are seropositive for HIV at birth, 70% remain free of symptoms at 18 to 24 months of age (Cole, 1998). The median age of survival of HIV-infected children in Europe and the United States is 8 to 13 years (Kuhn et al., 1998). The age at onset of symptoms predicts the length of survival.

Care Management. Although it is rare for an infant to be born with symptoms of HIV infection, all infants born to seropositive mothers should be presumed to be HIV positive. Management begins by implementing Standard Precautions. Measures should be undertaken to protect the infant from further exposure to maternal blood and body fluids. The infant's skin should be cleansed with soap and water and alcohol before invasive procedures such as vitamin K administration or heel punctures. Umbilical cord stumps are cleaned meticulously every day until healing is complete. Isolation is not required, and the infant can usually be cared for in the normal nursery. The use of gloves is not required for routine care activities such as dressing or feeding the infant.

Regimens for the prevention of HIV transmission include treatment of the neonate for 6 weeks after birth with zidovudine until the infant's HIV status is determined (Working Group, 2001). If a diagnosis of HIV infection in the infant is made, the family should be counseled about conventional and investigational treatment options. The Pediatric AIDS Clinical Trials group sponsors research studies that allow infants to receive the latest investigational treatments and follow-up care. The efficacy of treating asymptomatic infants with antiretroviral drugs has not yet been demonstrated in clinical trials; however, early initiation of treatment is thought to be advantageous (Working Group, 2001). Aggressive therapy with a combination of antiretroviral drugs is currently being investigated. Monotherapy is no longer recommended for the treatment of known HIV infection, regardless of the age of the client.

Counseling regarding the care of the mothers themselves, the family's care of the infant, and future pregnancies challenges the caregiver. Some parents opt to place the infected infants in foster homes despite the low risk for transmission among members of the same household. Social services are required in these cases. If the parent chooses to keep the infant, home health care may be arranged. For more information and updated information, parents are offered the following resource: the National AIDS hotline, 800-342-AIDS.

The family must be counseled about vaccinations. Children with symptomatic or asymptomatic HIV infection should receive all routine vaccines except varicella vaccine and oral polio vaccine because of their immunocompromised status (AAP, 2000). (Note: Only inactivated polio vaccine has been given in the United States since 1999.)

Rubella Infection

Since the rubella vaccination program was begun in 1969, cases of **congenital rubella infection** have been reduced dramatically; however, it is still seen occasionally in the newborn. Vaccination failures, lack of compliance, and the migration of nonimmunized persons result in periodic outbreaks of rubella, also known as German measles.

The risk of a congenitally infected infant varies with the gestational age of the fetus when maternal infection occurs. Abnormalities are most severe if the mother contracts the virus during the first trimester.

More than two thirds of infected infants show no apparent symptoms at birth, but sequelae may develop years later. Hearing loss, the most common result, appears to be progressive after birth. Congenital rubella syndrome comprises cataracts or glaucoma, hearing loss, and cardiac defects (pulmonary artery stenosis, patent ductus arteriosus, or coarctation of the aorta) (Baley & Toltzis, 2002). Multiple other abnormalities also are present, including IUGR, microphthalmia, hypotonia, hepatosplenomegaly, thrombocytopenic purpura (Fig. 38-9), dermatoglyphic abnormalities, bony radiolucencies, and brain wave abnormalities. Severe infection may result in fetal death. Delayed effects of infection manifest as thyroid dysfunction, diabetes mellitus, growth hormone deficiency, myocarditis, glaucoma, and microcephaly (Baley & Toltzis, 2002).

The rubella virus has been cultured in infants for up to 18 months after their birth. These infants are a serious source of infection to susceptible individuals, particularly women in the childbearing years. Extended pediatric isolation is mandatory until the noncontagious stage of rubella has been reached. The infant should be isolated until pharyngeal mucus and urine are free of virus.

Cytomegalovirus Infection

CMV infection during pregnancy may result in miscarriage, stillbirth, or congenital or neonatal cytomegalic inclusion disease (CMID). It is the most common cause of congenital viral infections in humans, occurring in 1% of newborns (Baley & Toltzis, 2002). Most (90%) affected infants are asymptomatic at birth; however, hearing loss and learning disabilities have been reported in previously asymptomatic infants (Baley & Toltzis, 2002).

The neonate with classic, full-blown CMID displays IUGR and has microcephaly. The neonate also has a rash, jaundice, and hepatosplenomegaly (Fig. 38-10). Anemia, thrombocytopenia, and hyperbilirubinemia are to be expected. Intracranial, periventricular calcification often is

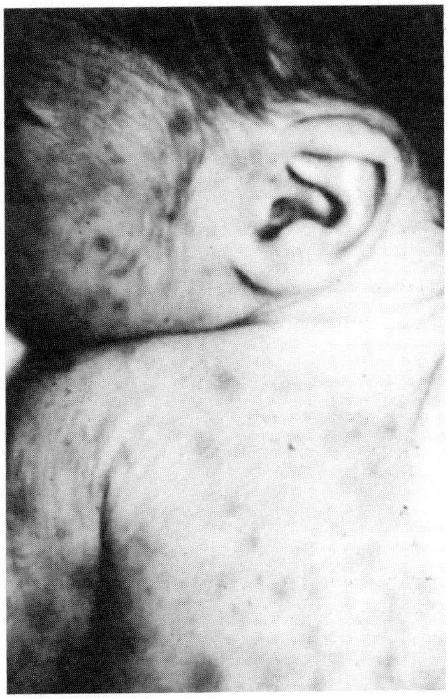

FIG. 38-9 Newborn with congenital rubella syndrome, showing multiple purpuric lesions over face and trunk. (Courtesy Donald C. Anderson, Baylor College of Medicine, Houston, TX.)

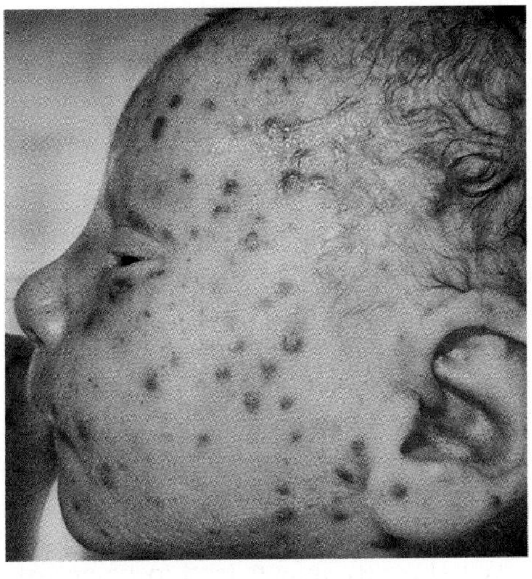

FIG. 38-10 Neonatal cytomegalovirus infection. Typical rash seen in a severely affected infant. (Courtesy David A. Clarke, Philadelphia, PA.)

noted on x-ray films. Inclusion bodies ("owl's eye" figures) in cells sedimented from freshly voided urine or in liver biopsy specimens are typical.

Elevated levels of cord blood IgM are suggestive of disease. The virus may be isolated from urine or saliva of the newborn. Differential diagnosis includes other causes of jaundice, syphilis (positive Venereal Disease Research Laboratories [VDRL] findings), toxoplasmosis (positive Sabin-Feldman dye test result), hemolytic disease of the newborn (positive Coombs test reaction), or coxsackievirus infection (positive culture).

Despite the extensive, endemic nature of the disease in women and men and its potential for havoc in perinatal life, critically affected newborns are born only occasionally. Milder forms of the disease often may result when the fetus is affected late in pregnancy. CMV can be transmitted through breast milk while the mother has acute CMV infection. CMV infections acquired after birth are often asymptomatic and have no sequelae. Exceptions to this occur in preterm infants in whom postnatal acquisition of CMV can result in pneumonia, hepatitis, thrombocytopenia, and long-term neurologic sequelae.

Antenatally infected infants who are asymptomatic at birth are at risk for late sequelae. Hearing loss may not be apparent until after the first year of life. Chorioretinitis, microcephaly, mental retardation, and neuromuscular deficits may occur by 2 years of age. Some children are at risk for a defect in tooth enamel, resulting in severe caries.

Herpes Simplex Virus

HSV infections among newborns are being diagnosed more frequently. The incidence of neonatal herpes simplex infection is estimated to occur in 1 in every 1500 to 2000 live births (Baley & Toltzis, 2002).

The neonate may acquire the virus by any of four modes of transmission:

- Transplacental infection
- Ascending infection by way of the birth canal
- Direct contamination during passage through an infected birth canal
- Direct transmission from infected personnel or family

Transplacental transmission of HSV infection to the neonate may occur during maternal viremia; however, an ascending transcervical infection first involves the intact fetal membranes, causing chorioamnionitis. Transcervical infection can be accelerated by fetal monitoring scalp electrodes. The electrodes break the fetal skin barrier and increase the risk of infection.

Congenital infection is rare and characterized by in utero destruction of normally formed organs. Affected infants are growth restricted. They have severe psychomotor delays, with intracranial calcifications, microcephaly, hypertonicity, and seizures. They have eye involvement, including microphthalmos, cataracts, chorioretinitis, blindness, and retinal dysplasia. Some infants have patent ductus arteriosus, limb anomalies, and recurrent skin vesicles, with a short life expectancy.

Most infants are infected directly during passage through the birth canal. The risk of infection during vaginal birth in the presence of genital herpes has not been clearly delineated. It may be as high as 40% to 60%, with active primary infection at term. Primary maternal infections after 32 weeks of gestation have a higher risk for the fetus and newborn than do recurrent infections (Baley & Toltzis, 2002). The transmission rate of chronic vaginal herpes from the pregnant woman to her newborn is low, 2% or less (Arvin & Whitley, 2001). Passive intrauterine immunity to herpes may be responsible. In more than 75% of cases of neonatal HSV infection, the mother has no history or symptoms of infection at the time of birth (AAP, 2000), but serologic testing reveals evidence of the herpes virus (Ashley & Wald, 1999).

Postnatal acquisition of the virus and spread within a nursery have been documented by DNA analysis. Both mother and father, as well as maternal breast lesions, have been implicated in neonatal infections. There also is concern regarding symptomatic and asymptomatic shedding among hospital personnel. Nursery personnel with cold sores should practice strict handwashing and wear a mask, but no evidence indicates that they should be removed from the nursery unless they have a herpetic whitlow (primary HSV infection of the terminal segment of a finger) (Baley & Toltzis, 2002).

Clinically, neonatal HSV infections are classified as disseminated infection; encephalitis; or localized infection of the skin, eye, or mouth. Disseminated infections may involve virtually every organ system, but the liver, adrenal glands, and lungs are primarily involved. Affected infants exhibit initial symptoms usually in the first week of life but sometimes in the second week, with signs of bacterial sepsis or shock. Clinical manifestations include skin vesicles in about 50% of infants. Death results from progression of CNS involvement, respiratory distress and pneumonitis, shock, DIC, and bleeding.

Encephalitis may occur. Blood-borne seeding of the brain results in multiple lesions of cortical hemorrhagic necrosis. It also can occur alone or in association with oral, eye, or skin lesions. Brain involvement usually manifests in the second to fourth week of life. Only 60% of the infants have skin lesions, and the CSF of fewer than 50% will reveal the virus. The presenting manifestations include lethargy, poor feeding, irritability, and local or generalized seizures. Almost half of the infants die of neurologic deterioration as late as 6 months after onset, and virtually all survivors have severe sequelae, including microcephaly and blindness (Baley & Toltzis, 2002).

Localized HSV infections most often occur with skin findings or rarely with isolated oral cavity lesions (Fig. 38-11). CNS or disseminated disease develops in 70% of the infants with skin vesicles. Ocular involvement, which can occur alone, may be secondary to either HSV-1 or HSV-2.

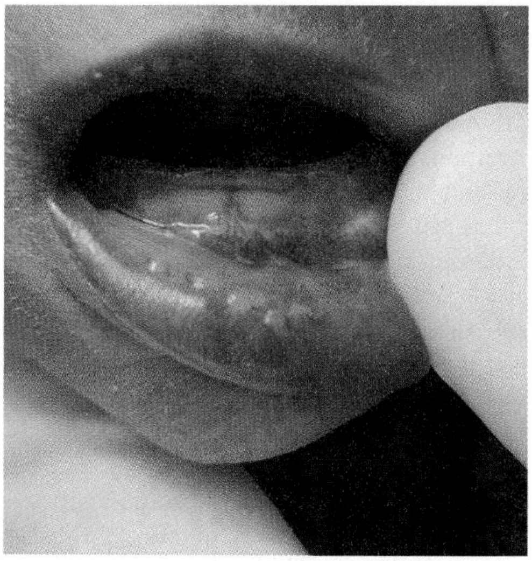

FIG. 38-11 Neonatal herpes simplex virus oral lesions. (Courtesy David A. Clarke, Philadelphia, PA.)

Ocular disease may not be discovered for months. Microphthalmos, cataracts, optic atrophy, and corneal scarring may result from chorioretinitis, keratitis, and retinal hemorrhage (Baley & Totlzis, 2002).

Care Management. Gloves should be worn when caregivers are in contact with these infants. The neonate's eyes, oral cavity, and skin are inspected carefully for the presence of any lesions. Cultures are obtained from the mouth, the eyes, and any possible lesions. Circumcision, if performed, is delayed until the infant is ready to be discharged. The infant may be discharged with the mother if the infant's cultures are negative for the virus. As long as no suspicious lesions are on the mother's breasts, breastfeeding is allowed. For the infant at risk, prophylactic topical eye ointment (vidarabine) is administered for 5 days for prevention of keratoconjunctivitis. No current recommendations exist for prophylactic systemic therapy; each case should be considered individually. Blood, urine, and CSF specimens should be cultured when indicated clinically. If herpetic lesions first occur after 6 weeks of life, the risk of dissemination and severe illness is very low (Baley & Toltzis, 2002).

Therapy includes general supportive measures, as well as treatment with vidarabine or acyclovir. Acyclovir is the most frequently used drug. It is considered safe because only viral replication is inhibited, although long-term sequelae are not yet known. Acyclovir is easier to administer; however, a randomized controlled trial has shown no difference between vidarabine and acyclovir for treatment of HSV. The current recommended dose of acyclovir is 10 mg/kg/day intravenously every 8 hours for at least 14 days. Continuing therapy may be required in case of recurrence. Ophthalmic ointment should be administered simultaneously (Baley & Toltzis, 2002).

Bacterial Infections

Group B Streptococcus

The most common cause of neonatal sepsis and meningitis in the United States is GBS. From 15% to 28% of pregnant women are colonized at the time of birth. Colonization rates are higher in sexually active women, those younger than 21 years, those with an intrauterine contraceptive device, those of African-American descent, and in women of lower parity (Cowles & Gonik, 2002).

The incidence of early-onset GBS infection is 1.3 to 3 per 1000 live births (Cowles & Gonik, 2002). Early-onset GBS infection in the neonate occurs in the first 7 days of life but most commonly manifests in the first 24 hours after birth. Risk factors for the development of early-onset GBS include low birth weight, preterm birth, rupture of membranes of more than 18 hours, maternal fever, previous GBS infant, maternal GBS bacteriuria, and multiple gestation. Usually resulting from vertical transmission from the birth canal, early-onset disease results in a respiratory illness that mimics the symptoms of severe respiratory distress. The infant may rapidly develop septic shock, which has a significant mortality rate. In recent years, prophylactic antibiotics given to mothers with risk factors during labor significantly reduced the incidence and severity of early-onset GBS infection in the newborn (Cowles & Gonik, 2002).

Late-onset GBS infections occur between 1 week and 3 months of age, with an average age at onset of 24 days. Eighty-five percent of infants with late-onset GBS have meningitis and have a mortality rate of none to 23%. Fifty percent of the survivors develop neurologic damage. No recent data are available to determine if changes in care have altered these figures (Edwards & Baker, 2001).

Escherichia coli

Escherichia coli is the second most common cause of neonatal sepsis and meningitis in the United States. The stated incidence of *E. coli* sepsis is 1 to 2 cases per 1000 births; however, this rate may be declining. *Escherichia coli* is found in the gastrointestinal tract soon after birth and makes up the bulk of human fecal flora. In addition to meningitis, *E. coli* also can cause infections in other body systems, including the urinary tract. Increasing use of ampicillin in labor as prophylaxis against GBS disease may result in more virulent *E. coli* disease resulting from ampicillin-resistant organisms (Joseph, Pyati, & Jacobs, 1998).

Tuberculosis

The incidence of tuberculosis (TB), caused by *Mycobacterium tuberculosis,* is once again increasing in Canada and the United States. It is found primarily in those of lower socioeconomic status, those with HIV infection, and in immigrants from countries where TB is endemic. Outbreaks in first-nations communities also are common. Of particular concern is the emergence of antibiotic-resistant strains found in some people with HIV.

Congenitally acquired TB, although rare, can cause otitis media, pneumonia, hepatosplenomegaly, enlarged lymph glands, or disseminated disease. After birth, exposed infants contract TB through droplets expelled by infected individuals, which results in pneumonia and necrosis of lung tissue. Signs of TB in the neonate relate to the site and size of the lesion. Occasionally present at birth, signs and symptoms are more likely to present by the second or third week of life. These signs include hepatosplenomegaly, respiratory distress, fever, lymphadenopathy, ear discharge, irritability or lethargy, and abdominal distention (Starke & Smith, 2001).

Untreated neonatal TB is almost always fatal. When maternal treatment is initiated early in pregnancy, however, neonatal morbidity and mortality rates are similar to those in pregnancies unaffected by TB (Edwards, 2002).

Listeriosis

Listeria monocytogenes is a bacterium capable of producing significant intrapartum illness. Prenatal infection causes chorioamnionitis or endometritis and should be suspected in cases of meconium-stained amniotic fluid in infants younger than 37 weeks of gestation. It also has been implicated as a cause of miscarriage and stillbirth (Guerina, 1998; Nolla-Salas et al., 1998). With disseminated fetal infection, microabscesses have been reported in the liver, lungs, and adrenal glands of stillborn infants. Live-born infants demonstrate granulomas on the skin and posterior pharyngeal wall. Listeriosis also can manifest as meningitis in a late-onset infection (Pong & Bradley, 1999).

Chlamydia Infection

Chlamydia trachomatis is an intracellular bacterium that causes neonatal conjunctivitis (20% to 50% of exposed infants) and pneumonia (10% to 20% of exposed infants) (Schachter & Grossman, 2001). The conjunctivitis (congestion and edema), with minimal discharge, develops 5 days to 2 weeks after birth. Inclusion conjunctivitis is usually self-limiting, but if untreated, chronic follicular conjunctivitis, with conjunctival scarring and corneal microgranulations (Schachter & Grossman, 2001), has been reported.

Chlamydial pneumonia has a gradual onset, between 2 and 12 weeks of age, beginning with rhinorrhea and progressing to tachypnea and coughing. It is speculated that pneumonia may occur as a result of movement of the organism from the conjunctiva into the lower respiratory tract; however, conjunctivitis is not a prerequisite to pneumonia (Schachter & Grossman, 2001).

Silver nitrate is not effective against *C. trachomatis,* but erythromycin or tetracycline ointment may prevent ophthalmic infection (Edwards, 2002). Eye prophylaxis is not sufficient to prevent the development of chlamydial pneumonia; therefore infants at risk also should be treated with systemic antibiotics such as oral erythromycin syrup.

Fungal Infections

Candidiasis

Candida infections, formerly known as moniliasis, may occur in the newborn. *Candida albicans,* the organism usually responsible, may cause disease in any organ system. It is a yeastlike fungus (producing yeast cells and spores) that can be acquired from a maternal vaginal infection during birth; by person-to-person transmission; or from contaminated hands, bottles, nipples, or other articles. It usually is a benign disorder in the neonate, often confined to the oral and diaper regions (Hockenberry et al., 2003).

Candidal diaper dermatitis appears on the perianal area, inguinal folds, and lower portion of the abdomen. The affected area is intensely erythematous, with a sharply demarcated, scalloped edge, frequently with numerous satellite lesions that extend beyond the larger lesion. The source of the infection is through the gastrointestinal tract. Treatment is with applications of an antifungal ointment, such as nystatin (Mycostatin) or miconazole 2% (Monistat), with each diaper change. The infant also may be given an oral antifungal preparation to eliminate any gastrointestinal source of infection (Hockenberry et al., 2003).

Oral candidiasis (**thrush,** or mycotic stomatitis) is characterized by the appearance of white plaques on the oral mucosa, gums, and tongue. The white patches are easily differentiated from milk curds; the patches cannot be removed and tend to bleed when touched. In most cases, the infant does not seem to be in discomfort from the infection. A few infants seem to have some difficulty swallowing.

Infants who are sick, debilitated, or receiving antibiotic therapy are more susceptible to thrush. Those with conditions such as cleft lip or palate, neoplasms, and hyperparathyroidism seem to be more vulnerable to mycotic infection.

The objectives of management are to eradicate the causative organism, to control exposure to *C. albicans,* and to improve the infant's resistance. Interventions include maintenance of scrupulous cleanliness to prevent reinfection (nursing personnel, parents, others). Good handwashing technique is always essential. Clean surfaces should be provided for neonates. Proper cleanliness of the equipment and environment is ensured. If the infant is breastfeeding, the mother also is treated with topical nystatin.

Medications are administered as ordered. Nystatin is instilled into the newborn's mouth with a medicine dropper after the infant is given sterile water to wash out any residual milk. Nystatin also may be swabbed over mucosa, gums, or tongue. Less frequently, an aqueous solution of gentian violet (1% to 2%) is applied with a swab to oral mucosa, gums, and tongue. The nurse should guard against staining the skin, clothes, and equipment and should warn parents about the purple staining of the baby's mouth.

SUBSTANCE ABUSE

Certain maternal behaviors result in perinatal risk. Maternal habits hazardous to the fetus and neonate include drug addiction, smoking, and alcohol abuse. Occasional withdrawal reactions have been reported in neonates of mothers who use to excess such drugs as barbiturates, alcohol, or amphetamines. Serious reactions are seen in neonates whose mothers abuse psychoactive drugs or are treated with methadone. Almost 50% of pregnancies of women addicted to opioids result in low-birth-weight (LBW) infants who are not necessarily preterm. Alcohol is a teratogen; maternal ethanol abuse during gestation can lead to a readily identifiable fetal alcohol syndrome (FAS). Maternal substance abuse is discussed in Chapter 35.

The adverse effects of exposure of the fetus to drugs are varied. They include transient behavioral changes such as fetal breathing movements or irreversible effects such as fetal death, IUGR, structural malformations, or mental retardation. Critical determinants of the effect of the drug on the fetus include the specific drug, the dosage, the route of administration, the genotype of the mother or fetus, and the timing of the drug exposure. Fig. 38-12 shows critical periods in human embryogenesis and the teratogenic effects of drugs. Table 38-4 summarizes the effects of commonly abused substances on the fetus and neonate.

Alcohol

Documentation of the **fetal alcohol syndrome (FAS)** has been reported in the literature since the early part of the eighteenth century. The incidence of FAS in the United States is about 2 per 1000 population (Rosen & Bateman, 2002).

FAS is based on minimal criteria of signs in each of three categories: prenatal and postnatal growth restriction; CNS malfunctions, including mental retardation; and craniofacial features such as microcephaly, small eyes or short palpebral fissures, thin upper lip, flat midface, and an indistinct philtrum. Neurologic problems in FAS children include some degree of IQ deficit, attention-deficit disorder, diminished fine motor skills, and poor speech. These children have been shown to lack inhibition, have no stranger anxiety, and lack appropriate judgment skills. Infants exposed prenatally to alcohol who are affected but do not meet the criteria for FAS may be said to have **fetal alcohol effects (FAEs).** These effects run the gamut from learning disabilities and behavioral problems to speech or language problems and hyperactivity. Often these problems are not detected until the child goes to school and learning problems become evident. FAEs can be seen with other disorders, such as fetal hydantoin syndrome; therefore a careful history is needed.

Predictable abnormal patterns of fetal and neonatal morphogenesis are attributed to severe, chronic alcoholism in women who continue to drink heavily during pregnancy. The pattern of growth deficiency begun in prenatal

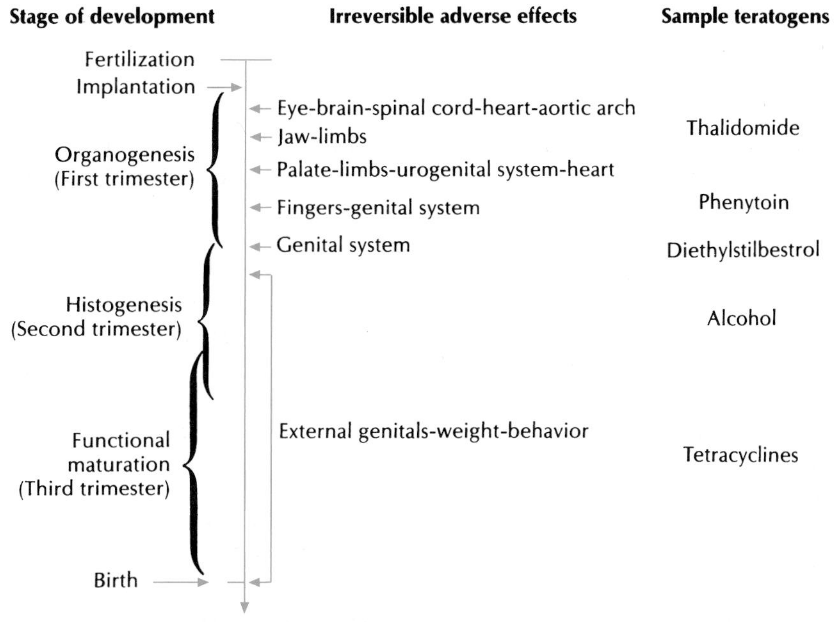

Stage of development
Irreversible adverse effects
Sample teratogens
Fertilization
Implantation
Organogenesis
(First trimester)
Eye-brain-spinal cord-heart-aortic arch
Jaw-limbs
Palate-limbs-urogenital system-heart
Fingers-genital system
Genital system
Thalidomide
Phenytoin
Diethylstilbestrol
Histogenesis
(Second trimester)
Alcohol
Functional
maturation
(Third trimester)
External genitals-weight-behavior
Tetracyclines
Birth

FIG. 38-12 Critical periods in human embryogenesis. (From Aranda, J. et al. [2002]. In A. Fanaroff & R. Martin (Eds.), *Neonatal-perinatal medicine: Diseases of the fetus and infant* [7th ed.]. St. Louis: Mosby.)

TABLE 38-4 **Summary of Neonatal Effects of Commonly Abused Substances**

SUBSTANCE	NEONATAL EFFECTS
Alcohol	*Fetal alcohol syndrome* (FAS): craniofacial anomalies, including short eyelid opening, flat midface, flat upper lip groove, thin upper lip; microcephaly; hyperactivity; developmental delays; attention deficits *Fetal alcohol effects:* milder forms of FAS, cardiac anomalies, failure to thrive
Cocaine	Prematurity, small for gestational age, microcephaly, poor feeding, irregular sleep pattern, diarrhea, visual attention problems, hyperactivity, difficult to console, hypersensitivity to noise and external stimuli, irritability, developmental delays, congenital anomalies such as prune belly syndrome (distended, flabby, wrinkled abdomen caused by lack of abdominal muscles)
Heroin	Low birth weight, small for gestational age, neonatal abstinence syndrome (see Table 38-6)
Amphetamines	Small for gestational age, prematurity, poor weight gain, lethargy
Tobacco	Prematurity, low birth weight, increased risk for sudden infant death syndrome, increased risk for bronchitis, pneumonia, developmental delays
Marijuana	Possible neonatal tremors, possible low birth weight

life persists after birth, especially in the linear growth rate, rate of weight gain, and growth of head circumferences.

Ocular structural anomalies are common findings (Fig. 38-13). Limb anomalies and a variety of cardiocirculatory anomalies, especially ventricular septal defects, pose problems for the child. Table 38-5 outlines physical findings in FAS. Mental retardation (IQ of 79 or less at age 7 years), hyperactivity, and fine motor dysfunction (poor hand-to-mouth coordination, weak grasp) add to the handicapping problems that maternal alcoholism can impose. Genital abnormalities are seen in daughters of alcohol-addicted mothers. Two thirds of newborns with FAS are girls; the cause of this altered fetal sex ratio is unknown. Severe and chronic alcoholism (ethanol toxicity), not maternal malnutrition, is responsible for the severity and consistency of postnatal performance problems (Rosen & Bateman, 2002). High alcohol levels are lethal to the developing embryo. Lower levels cause brain and other malformations. Long-term prognosis (no studies are available) is discouraging even in an optimal psychosocial environment, when one considers the combination of growth failure and mental retardation.

Alcohol effects, however, depend not only on the amount of alcohol consumed but also on the interaction of quantity, frequency, type of alcohol, and other drug abuse. Other drugs, such as cigarettes, caffeine, and marijuana, may potentiate the fetal effects of alcohol consumption during gestation.

The infant of a mother who abuses alcohol is faced with many clinical problems. Identification of the problems leads to the medical diagnosis of FAS. The infant may have respiratory distress related to preterm birth, neurologic damage, and a "floppy" epiglottis and small trachea. Tracheoepiglottal anomalies may cause cardiopulmonary arrest. Other disorders include recurrent otitis media and hearing loss. Craniofacial features may be important in diagnosing craniofacial and oral anomalies, dental development abnormalities, and long-term body growth patterns. Feeding difficulties are related to preterm birth, poor sucking ability, and possible cleft palate. The infant may exhibit brain dysfunction, microcephaly, and grand mal seizures.

Long-term effects into childhood may include impaired visuomotor perception and performance, lowered IQ scores, and delayed receptive and expressive language, as well as reduced capacity to process and store factual data. It is now recognized as one of the leading causes of mental retardation in the United States. Although the distinctive facial features of the infant tend to become less evident, the mental capacities never become normal.

Nursing care involves many of the same strategies used for the care of preterm infants (see Chapter 40). Special efforts are made to involve the parents in their child's care and to encourage opportunities for parent-child attachment.

Placing infants in a warm, caring environment with understanding caregivers who can deal with the infant's hyperirritability can lead to improved emotional development and social functioning (D'Apolito, 1998; Wagner et al., 1998). These caregivers provide extensive cuddling and human contact and can deal with the eating problems that typically lead to a diagnosis of failure to thrive. However, these infants may not go home to such an environment. Often the family is dysfunctional.

Heroin

Heroin crosses the placenta and frequently results in IUGR. Heroin may have a direct growth-inhibiting effect on the fetus, but the exact mechanisms of growth inhibition are not clear. There is an increased rate of stillbirths but not of congenital anomalies.

Many of the medical complications attributed to heroin result from prematurity. Other risks include physi-

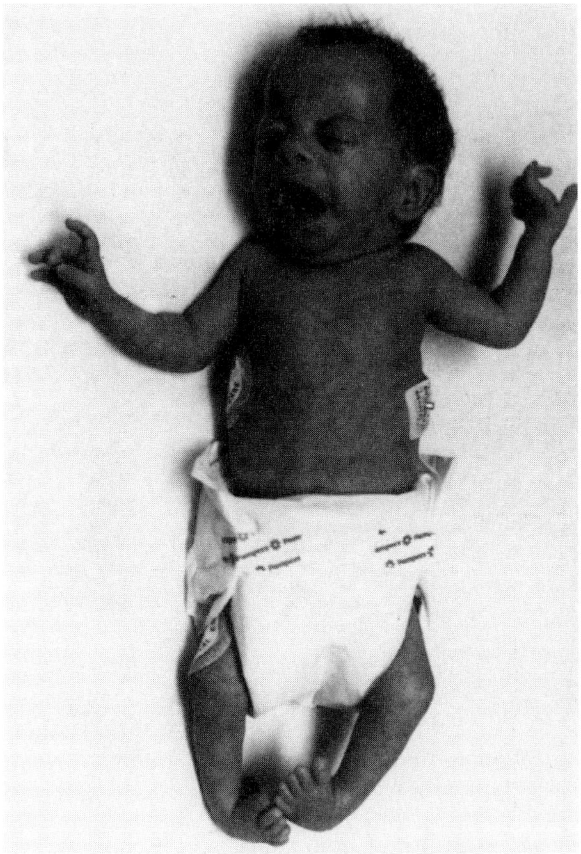

FIG. 38-13 Infant with fetal alcohol syndrome. (From Hockenberry, M. et al. [2003]. *Wong's nursing care of infants and children* [7th ed.]. St. Louis: Mosby.)

TABLE 38-5 **Features of Fetal Alcohol Syndrome**

AFFECTED PART	CHARACTERISTICS
Eyes	Epicanthal folds, strabismus, ptosis, hypoplastic retinal vessels
Mouth	Poor suck, cleft lip, cleft palate, small teeth
Ears	Deafness
Skeleton	Radioulnar synostosis, fusion of cervical vertebrae, restricted bone growth
Heart	Atrial and ventricular septal defects, tetralogy of Fallot, patent ductus arteriosus
Kidney	Renal hypoplasia, hydronephrosis, urogenital sinus
Liver	Extrahepatic biliary atresia, hepatic fibrosis
Immune system	Increased infections: otitis media, upper respiratory infections, immune deficiencies
Tumors	Nonspecific neoplasms
Skin	Abnormal palmar creases, irregular hair, whorls

From Weiner, L., & Morse, B. (1991). FAS: Clinical perspectives and prevention. In I. Chasnoff (Ed.), *Drugs, alcohol, pregnancy and parenting*. Boston: Kluwer.

cal dependence in the fetus and the risk of exposure to infections, including hepatitis B and C virus and HIV. Drug withdrawal in the mother is accompanied by fetal withdrawal, which can lead to fetal death (Kaltenbach, Berghella, & Finnegan, 1998; Wagner et al., 1998).

Maternal detoxification in the first trimester carries an increased risk of miscarriage. Detoxification is not recommended after the thirty-second week because of possible withdrawal-induced fetal distress (Kaltenbach et al., 1998).

Heroin withdrawal occurs in 50% to 80% of infants born to addicted mothers, usually within the first 48 to 72 hours of life (Wagner et al., 1998). The signs depend on the length of maternal addiction, the amount of drug taken, and the time of injection before birth. The infant whose mother is taking methadone may not demonstrate signs of withdrawal until a week or so after birth. The symptoms of infants whose mothers used heroin or methadone are similar in nature. Initially the infant may be depressed. The withdrawal syndrome may manifest as a combination of any of the following signs. The infant may be jittery and hyperactive. Usually the infant's cry is shrill and persistent. The infant may yawn or sneeze frequently. The tendon reflexes are increased, but the Moro reflex is decreased. The neonate may exhibit poor feeding and sucking, tachypnea, vomiting, diarrhea, hypothermia or hyperthermia, and sweating. In addition, an abnormal sleep cycle, with absence of quiet sleep and disturbance of active sleep, has been described in these infants (Rosen & Bateman, 2002).

If withdrawal is not treated, vomiting, diarrhea, dehydration, apnea, and convulsions may develop. Death may follow. Therapy is individualized. Dehydration and electrolyte imbalance are prevented or treated. Usually one of the following drugs is ordered: phenobarbital, methadone, morphine syrup, or diazepam, singly or in combination.

The use of naloxone (Narcan) is contraindicated in infants born to narcotic addicts because it may cause severe signs and symptoms of narcotic abstinence syndrome and seizures.

The long-term effect on these infants is now being studied. The risk of sudden infant death syndrome (SIDS) is 5 to 10 times higher for infants with significant withdrawal problems than for infants in the general population.

Methadone

Methadone, a synthetic opiate, has been the therapy of choice for heroin addiction since 1965. Methadone crosses the placenta. An increasing number of infants have been born to methadone-maintained mothers, who seem to have better prenatal care and a somewhat better lifestyle than those taking heroin (Rosen & Bateman, 2002).

Methadone withdrawal resembles heroin withdrawal but tends to be more severe and prolonged. In addition, the incidence of seizures is higher. Seizures usually occur between days 7 and 10. The infants exhibit a disturbed sleep pattern similar to that seen in heroin withdrawal. The infants have a higher birth weight than that in heroin withdrawal, usually appropriate for gestational age. No increased incidence of congenital anomalies is seen.

Late-onset withdrawal occurs at 2 to 4 weeks and may continue for weeks or months. A higher incidence of SIDS also has been reported in these infants (Rosen & Bateman, 2002). This factor is important for perinatal nurses who coordinate follow-up care for the infant and education for the mother or other caregiver. Community health nurses must know about the potential for withdrawal symptoms to occur.

Therapy for methadone withdrawal is similar to that for heroin withdrawal. The few available follow-up studies of these infants reveal a high incidence of hyperactivity, learning and behavior disorders, and poor social adjustment (Rosen & Bateman, 2002).

BOX 38-2 Neonatal Effects of Maternal Cocaine Use

PHYSICAL

- Preterm birth
- Decreased length
- Decreased head circumference
- Intrauterine growth restriction
- Ileal atresia
- Prune belly syndrome
- Cryptorchidism
- Hypospadias
- Hydronephrosis
- Seizures
- Fever
- Congenital heart disease
- Skull defects
- Hypertension
- Cerebral infarction
- Vomiting
- Diarrhea
- Sudden infant death syndrome
- Tachypnea

BEHAVIORAL

- Irritability
- Tremors
- Poor feeding
- Abnormal sleep patterns
- Increased startles
- Disorganized behavior
- Lability
- Poor visual processing
- Difficult to console

Marijuana

Marijuana crosses the placenta. Its use during pregnancy may result in a shortened gestation and a higher incidence of IUGR. Some investigators have found a higher incidence of meconium staining (Rosen & Bateman, 2002). Some association has been reported between the use of marijuana and a decrease in infant birth weight and length and the occurrence of congenital anomalies; however, the findings have been inconsistent. No differences were detected on infant follow-up at 6, 12, and 24 months in general measures of physical growth and development. At 4 years of age, children had poorer scores on memory and verbal tests compared with a control group. Compounding the issue of the effects of marijuana is multidrug use, especially among adolescents, thus combining the harmful effects of marijuana, tobacco, alcohol, and cocaine. Long-term follow-up studies on exposed infants are needed.

Cocaine

Cocaine crosses the placenta and is found in breast milk. Considerable controversy exists regarding the effects of cocaine on the fetus and neonate. Fetal brain, kidney, and urogenital system malformations have been associated with maternal cocaine ingestion (Bellini, Massocco, & Serra, 2000; Nzerue, Hewan-Lowe, & Riley, 2000). Other reported effects include infarctions to developing organs, resulting in defects such as congenital heart disease, skull defects, ileal atresia, and limb reduction. Infants born to cocaine-abusing mothers show a high rate of perinatal morbidity, IUGR, preterm birth, and placental or cerebral infarction (Rosen & Bateman, 2002).

Cocaine-dependent neonates do not experience a process of withdrawal seen in narcotic-exposed infants but rather have neurotoxic effects of the drug (Askin & Diehl-Jones, 2001). Signs of exposure have some of the same characteristics as those of heroin withdrawal but can be highly varied. There may be an increased risk for SIDS. The effects of prenatal exposure to cocaine on neonatal behavior have been studied extensively. Findings indicate that cocaine-exposed infants have limited ability to habituate to stimuli. As these children enter school, they demonstrate a reduced capacity for verbal reasoning and difficulties maintaining attention (Rosen & Bateman, 2002). Box 38-2 summarizes neonatal effects of maternal cocaine use.

Miscellaneous Substances

The fetal and neonatal effects of maternal use of methamphetamines in pregnancy are not well known. The effects appear to be dose related. LBW, preterm birth, and perinatal mortality may be consequences of higher doses used throughout pregnancy. A higher incidence of cleft lip and palate and cardiac defects has been reported in infants exposed to amphetamines in utero (Plessinger, 1998). After birth, infants may have bradycardia or tachycardia that resolves as the drug is cleared from the infant's system. Lethargy may continue for several months, along with frequent infections and poor weight gain. Emotional disturbances and delays in gross and fine motor coordination may be seen during early childhood.

Phenobarbital crosses the placenta readily and is subsequently found in high levels in the fetal liver and brain. Because of its slow metabolic rate, when withdrawal does occur, onset is generally at 2 to 14 days after birth, and duration is about 2 to 4 months. Irritability, crying, hiccoughs, and sleepiness mark the initial response. During the second stage, the infant is extremely hungry, regurgitates and gags frequently, and demonstrates episodic irritability, sweating, and a disturbed sleep pattern.

Treatment consists of swaddling, frequent feedings, and protection from noxious external stimuli. If no improvement occurs, the neonate should be given phenobarbital and then slowly withdrawn from this drug after control of symptoms (Rosen & Bateman, 2002).

Caffeine has not been implicated as a teratogen in humans. Fernandes et al. (1998) reported that caffeine consumption of more than 150 mg per day was associated with IUGR and LBW. Santos et al. (1998) reported no adverse effects in the fetus with consumption of less than 300 mg of caffeine per day.

Tobacco

Cigarette smoking in pregnancy has been found to be associated with birth-weight deficits in the full-term neonate (Aranda et al., 2002). Maternal cigarette smoking is implicated in 21% to 39% of LBW infants. Passive exposure to secondhand smoke by a pregnant woman also may result in the birth of an LBW infant.

The rate of miscarriage and preterm birth is increased in the smoking population. When other variables have been controlled for, no clear association has been found between maternal smoking and congenital anomalies (Aranda et al., 2002). Nicotine and cotinine, the two pharmacologically active substances in tobacco, are found in higher concentrations in infants whose mothers smoke. These substances can be secreted in breast milk for up to 2 hours after the mother has smoked. Cigarette smoke contains more than 2000 compounds, including carbon monoxide, dioxin, cyanide, and cadmium. Long-term studies show residual effects beyond the neonatal period (Aranda et al., 2002). Deficits in growth, in intellectual and emotional development, and in behavior have been documented. These include poor auditory responsiveness, increased fine motor tremors, hypertonicity, and decreased verbal comprehension.

Pregnant women need to be aware of the harmful effects of smoking on their unborn baby's health. These include IUGR, miscarriage, PROM, placenta previa, and SIDS (Lee, 1998). Increasing concern surrounds secondhand smoke and its potential effects on infants and siblings. Mothers and all others should refrain from smoking near the infant. It is not clear whether the association between smoking and SIDS reflects in utero exposure or passive exposure postnatally, or both.

CARE MANAGEMENT

Assessment of the newborn requires a review of the mother's prenatal record. A medical and social history of drug abuse and detoxification is noted. The infant may have IUGR or be preterm with LBW.

The woman who is addicted to narcotics may have infections that compound the risk to the infant, including hepatitis, septicemia, and STIs, including AIDS (Wagner et al., 1998).

The nurse often is the first to observe the signs of drug dependence in the infant. The nurse's observations help the physician differentiate between drug dependence and other conditions, such as tracheoesophageal fistula, CNS disorder, sepsis, hypoglycemia, and electrolyte imbalance.

The infant is assessed by means of the guidelines discussed in Chapter 26. The infant's gestational age and maturity are noted. In utero exposure to some drugs results in observable malformations or dysmorphism (abnormality of shape). Neonatal behavior may arouse suspicion. **Neonatal abstinence syndrome** is the term given to the group of signs and symptoms associated with drug withdrawal in the neonate (Table 38-6). Figure 38-14 provides an example of a scoring system for assessing withdrawal symptoms. Because many women are multidrug users, the newborn initially may exhibit a confusing complex of signs.

Urine or meconium screening may be used to identify substances abused by the mother. Initially costly and of limited availability, tests of meconium collected on day 1 or 2 of life have been shown to be both sensitive and reliable in detecting the metabolites of several street drugs, including cocaine (Buchi, 1998; Kwong & Shearer, 1998).

TABLE *38-6* **Signs of Neonatal Abstinence Syndrome**

SYSTEM	SIGNS
Gastrointestinal	Poor feeding, vomiting, regurgitation, diarrhea, excessive sucking
Central nervous	Irritability, tremors, shrill cry, incessant crying, hyperactivity, little sleep, excoriations on knees and face, convulsions
Metabolic, vasomotor, respiratory	Nasal congestion; tachypnea; sweating; frequent yawning; increased respiratory rate, >60 breaths/min; fever, >37.2° C

NEONATAL ABSTINENCE SCORING SYSTEM

SYSTEM	SIGNS AND SYMPTOMS	SCORE	AM	PM	COMMENTS
CENTRAL NERVOUS SYSTEM DISTURBANCES	Excessive High Pitched (Or other) Cry Continuous High Pitched (Or other) Cry	2 3			Daily Weight:
	Sleeps <1 Hour After Feeding Sleeps <2 Hours After Feeding Sleeps <3 Hours After Feeding	3 2 1			
	Hyperactive Moro Reflex Markedly Hyperactive Moro Reflex	2 3			
	Mild Tremors Disturbed Moderate-Severe Tremors Disturbed	1 2			
	Mild Tremors Undisturbed Moderate-Severe Tremors Undisturbed	3 4			
	Increased Muscle Tone	2			
	Excoriation (Specific Area)	1			
	Myoclonic Jerks	3			
	Generalized Convulsions	5			
METABOLIC/VASOMOTOR/RESPIRATORY DISTURBANCES	Sweating	1			
	Fever <101 (99-100.8 F./37.2-38.2C.) Fever >101 (38.4C. and Higher)	1 2			
	Frequent Yawning (>3-4 Times/Interval)	1			
	Mottling	1			
	Nasal Stuffiness	1			
	Sneezing (>3-4 Times/Interval)	1			
	Nasal Flaring	2			
	Respiratory Rate >60/min Respiratory Rate >60/min with Retractions	1 2			
GASTROINTESTINAL DISTURBANCES	Excessive Sucking	1			
	Poor Feeding	2			
	Regurgitation Projectile Vomiting	2 3			
	Loose Stools Watery Stools	2 3			
	TOTAL SCORE				
	INITIALS OF SCORER				

FIG. 38-14 Neonatal Abstinence Scoring (NAS) system, developed by L. Finnegan. (From Nelson, N. [1990]. *Current therapy in neonatal-perinatal medicine* [2nd ed.]. St. Louis: Mosby.)

Plan of Care: Infant Undergoing Drug Withdrawal

NURSING DIAGNOSIS Risk for injury related to hyperactivity, seizures secondary to passive narcotic addiction resulting from maternal substance abuse during pregnancy

Expected Outcome *Infant exhibits no signs of seizure activity.*

Nursing Interventions/*Rationales*

Administer phenobarbital, diazepam per physician order *to decrease central nervous system (CNS) irritability and control seizure activity.*

Decrease environmental stimuli *that may trigger irritability and hyperactive behaviors.*

Plan care activities carefully *to allow minimal stimulation.*

Wrap infant snugly and hold infant tightly *to reduce self-stimulation behaviors and protect skin from abrasions.*

If infant is cocaine addicted, position to avoid eye contact, swaddle infant, use vertical rocking techniques, and use a pacifier *to counter poor organizational response to stimuli and depressed interactive behaviors.*

Monitor activity level, note the relation between activity level and external stimulation, and stop external stimulation *if it causes activity increase.*

NURSING DIAGNOSIS Altered nutrition, less than body requirements related to CNS irritability, poor suck reflex, vomiting, and diarrhea

Expected Outcome *Infant exhibits ingestion and retention of adequate nutrients and appropriate weight gain.*

Nursing Interventions/*Rationales*

Feed in frequent small amounts, elevate head during and after feeding, and burp well *to diminish vomiting and aspiration.*

Experiment with various nipples *to find one most effective in compensating for poor suck reflex.*

Monitor weight daily, and maintain strict intake and output *to evaluate success of feeding.*

If intake is insufficient, feed by oral gavage per physician order *to ensure ingestion of needed nutrients.*

Have suction available as required *to reduce chances of aspiration.*

NURSING DIAGNOSIS Risk for fluid volume deficit related to diarrhea and vomiting

Expected Outcome *Infant exhibits evidence of fluid homeostasis.*

Nursing Interventions/*Rationales*

Administer oral and parenteral fluids per physician order and regulate *to maintain fluid balance.*

Monitor hydration status (skin turgor, weight, mucous membranes, fontanels, urine specific gravity, electrolytes) and intake and output *to evaluate for evidence of dehydration.*

NURSING DIAGNOSIS Ineffective maternal coping, anxiety, powerlessness related to drug use, infant distress during withdrawal, and single-parent status

Expected Outcomes *Woman will accept newborn's condition and participate in care activities, showing evidence of maternal-infant bonding process.*

Nursing Interventions/*Rationales*

Explain effects of maternal drug use on newborn and the withdrawal process *to provide understanding and reality concerning effects of drug use.*

Encourage open communication (e.g., inform mother of ongoing condition, procedures, and treatment; answer questions; correct misperceptions; actively listen to her concerns) *to provide a sense of respect, provide support, and encourage a sense of control.*

Encourage mother to interact with infant and to become involved in care routines *to foster emotional connection.*

Explain how to do care procedures, how to avoid excess stimulation, and how to hold and rock infant *to enhance mother's care abilities and her sense of confidence and control.*

If the mother is addicted to cocaine, explain infant's inability to interact, gaze aversion, arching back, and lack of response to cuddling *to enhance understanding of infant behaviors.*

Make appropriate referrals to social agencies for treatment of maternal drug addiction, infant development programs, and other needed support services *to ensure adequate resources for care of self and infant.*

LEGAL TIP Neonatal Drug Screening

Testing of neonatal urine or meconium for the presence of drug metabolites is a sensitive and reliable means of identifying neonates at risk for withdrawal symptoms. Controversy arises over whether universal drug screening should be instituted and whether informed consent is needed for screening neonates. Ethical issues include the cost versus benefit of universal testing and the rights of parents versus the medical need to diagnose withdrawal.

Nursing diagnoses, which depend on the assessment findings, are tailored to the individual needs of the neonate and the family.

Nursing Care

Planning for care of the infant born to a substance-abusing mother presents a challenge to the health care team. Parents are included in the planning for the newborn's care and also are encouraged to plan for their own care. A multidisciplinary approach includes home health or community resource personnel (e.g., regulatory agencies such as child protective services).

Education and social support to prevent the abuse of drugs provide the ideal approach. However, given the scope of the drug abuse problem, total prevention is unrealistic.

Nursing care of the drug-dependent neonate involves supportive therapy for fluid and electrolyte balance, nutrition, infection control, and respiratory care. Swaddling, holding, reducing stimuli, and feeding as necessary may be helpful in easing withdrawal (see Plan of Care). Specific suggestions for providing care to infants experiencing withdrawal are listed in the Teaching for Self-Care box.

Pharmacologic treatment is usually based on the severity of withdrawal symptoms, as determined by an assessment tool (see Fig. 38-14). When indicated, medications are

TEACHING FOR SELF-CARE

Care of Infant Experiencing Withdrawal

- Place the infant in a side-lying position with the spine and legs flexed.
- Position the infant's hands in midline with the arms at the side.
- Carry the infant in a flexed position.
- When interacting with the infant, introduce one stimulus at a time when the infant is in a quiet, alert state.
- Watch for time out or distress signals (gaze aversion, yawning, sneezing, hiccoughs, arching, mottled color).
- When the infant is distressed, swaddle in a flexed position and rock in a slow, rhythmic fashion.
- Put the infant in a sitting position with chin tucked down for feeding.

given as ordered. Neonatal morphine solution (0.4 mg/ml), phenobarbital, and less commonly, paregoric may be used to control symptoms. Treatment may be needed for 2 weeks or more.

Drug dependence in the neonate is physiologic, not psychologic. Thus a predisposition to dependence later in life is not believed to be a factor. However, the psychosocial environment in which the infant is raised may create a tendency to addiction.

The mother requires considerable support. Her need for and her abuse of drugs result in a decreased capacity to cope. The infant's withdrawal signs and decreased consolability stress her coping abilities even further. Home health care, treatment for addiction, and education are important considerations. Sensitive exploration of the woman's options for the care of her infant and herself and for future fertility management may help her see that she has choices. This approach helps communicate respect for the new mother as a person who can make responsible decisions.

The issue of breastfeeding in this population is a difficult one. Although breast milk remains the optimal source of nutrition for these infants, care must be taken to avoid exposing the infant to additional drugs through the breast milk. The American Academy of Pediatrics has compiled a list of drugs contraindicated in breastfeeding (Table 38-7).

TABLE 38-7 **Drugs of Abuse Contraindicated During Breastfeeding***

DRUG	REPORTED EFFECT OR REASONS FOR CONCERN
Amphetamine†	Irritability, poor sleeping pattern
Cocaine	Cocaine intoxication
Heroin	Tremors, restlessness, vomiting, poor feeding
Marijuana	Only one report in literature; no effect mentioned; at risk for inhaling smoke
Nicotine (smoking)	Shock, vomiting, diarrhea, rapid heart rate, restlessness, decreased milk production
Phencyclidine	Potent hallucinogen

Modified from American Academy of Pediatrics. (2001). The transfer of drugs and other chemicals into human milk. *Pediatrics, 108*(3), 776-789; also in Lawrence, R. (1999). *Breastfeeding: A guide for the medical profession* (5th ed.). St. Louis: Mosby.

*AAP Committee on Drugs strongly believes that breastfeeding mothers should not ingest any substances listed here. Not only are they hazardous to the nursing infant, but they also are detrimental to the physical and emotional health of the mother. This list is obviously not complete; no drug of abuse should be ingested by breastfeeding mothers even though adverse reports are not in the literature.

†Drug is concentrated in human milk.

KEY POINTS

- A small percentage of significant birth injuries may occur despite skilled and competent obstetric care.
- The same birth injury may be caused in several ways.
- The nurse's primary contribution to the welfare of the neonate begins with early observation, accurate recording, and prompt reporting of abnormal signs.
- Metabolic abnormalities of diabetes mellitus in pregnancy adversely affect embryonic and fetal development.
- Prepregnancy planning and good diabetic control, coupled with strict diabetic control during pregnancy, may prevent the embryonic, fetal, and neonatal conditions associated with pregnancies complicated by diabetes mellitus.
- Regardless of the infant's disorder or condition, the care provider must remember that the infant belongs to a family that also has many needs.
- Infection in the neonate may be acquired in utero, during birth, during resuscitation, and from within the nursery.
- The most common maternal infections during early pregnancy that are associated with various congenital malformations are caused by viruses.
- HIV transmission from mother to infant occurs transplacentally at various gestational ages, perinatally by maternal blood and secretions, and by breast milk.
- The nurse often is the first to observe signs of newborn drug withdrawal.
- Providing high-quality perinatal care to a varied population with multiple conditions is complicated by the special needs of high risk drug-dependent clients.
- Signs and symptoms of infant withdrawal vary in time of onset depending on the type and dose of drug involved.
- Rehabilitative measures must be included in the plan for care for the infant and parents to offer the infant an opportunity for optimal development after discharge.

CRITICAL THINKING EXERCISES

1. In providing care for Monica during her labor and birth, her sister tells you that Monica used cocaine during this pregnancy. Describe the potential implications for Monica's newborn. Monica denies that she has used drugs. What methods of drug screening can be used to identify cocaine metabolites in her newborn? Outline the ethical implications of testing the baby for cocaine.

2. Timothy and Barbara are preparing to take home their 2-week-old infant who was diagnosed with herpes encephalitis. Develop a home care plan for this infant. Identify community resources that can be used for this infant.

RESOURCES

AIDS Network Hotline
800-342-2437

American Academy of Pediatrics
141 Northwest Point Blvd.
Elk Grove, IL 60007-1098
847-228-5005
www.aap.org

Centers for Disease Control and Prevention
1600 Clifton Rd. NE
Atlanta, GA 30333
404-329-1819
404-329-3286
www.cdc.gov

National AIDS Information Clearinghouse
P.O. Box 6003
Rockville, MD 20849-6003
800-458-5231 (English and Spanish)

National Clearinghouse for Alcohol and Drug Abuse Information
P.O. Box 426
Dept. DQ
Kensington, MD 20795
800-729-6686
www.health.org

REFERENCES

American Academy of Pediatrics. (2000). *Red book: Report of the Committee on Infectious Diseases.* Elk Grove, IL: AAP.

American Academy of Pediatrics. (2001). The transfer of drugs and other chemicals into human milk. *Pediatrics, 108*(3), 776-789.

American Academy of Pediatrics Committee on Infectious Diseases. (2002). Recommended childhood immunization schedule, United States, 2002. *Pediatrics, 109,* 162-164.

American College of Obstetricians and Gynecologists. (1997). Human immunodeficiency virus infection in pregnancy. *International Journal of Gynecology and Obstetrics, 57,* 73-80.

Aranda, J. et al. (2002). Developmental pharmacology. In A. Fanaroff & R. Martin (Eds.), *Neonatal-perinatal medicine: Diseases of the fetus and infant.* St. Louis: Mosby.

Arvin, A., & Whitley, R. (2001). Herpes simplex virus infections. In J. Remmington & J. Klein (Eds.), *Infectious diseases of the fetus and newborn infant.* Philadelphia: W.B. Saunders.

Ashley, R., & Wald, A. (1999). Genital herpes: Review of the epidemic and potential use of type-specific serology. *Clinical Microbiology Review, 12,* 1-8.

Askin, D. (1995). Bacterial and fungal sepsis in the neonate. *Journal of Obstetric, Gynecologic, and Neonatal Nursing, 24*(7), 635-643.

Askin, D., & Diehl-Jones, B. (2001). Cocaine: Effects of in utero exposure on the fetus and neonate. *Journal of Perinatal and Neonatal Nursing, 14*(4), 83-102.

Baley, J., & Toltzis, P. (2002). Viral infections. In A. Fanaroff & R. Martin (Eds.), *Neonatal-perinatal medicine: Diseases of the fetus and infant* (7th ed.). St. Louis: Mosby.

Beall, M., & Ross, M. (2001). Clavicle fracture in labor: Risk factors and associated morbidities. *Journal of Perinatology, 21*(8), 513-515.

Beazley, D., & Egerman, R. (1998). Toxoplasmosis. *Seminars in Perinatology, 22*(4), 332-338.

Behrmann, R. (1973). *Neonatology: Diseases of the fetus and infant.* St. Louis: Mosby

Bellini, C., Massocco, D., & Serra, G. (2000). Prenatal cocaine exposure and the expanding spectrum of brain malformations. *Archives of Internal Medicine, 160*(15), 2393.

Birthistle, K., & Carrington, D. (1998). Fetal varicella syndrome–a reappraisal of the literature. *Journal of Infection, 36*(51), 25-29.

Buchi, K. (1998). The drug exposed infant in the well baby nursery. *Clinics in Perinatology, 25*(2), 335-348.

Chapman, S. (1998). Varicella in pregnancy. *Seminars in Perinatology, 22*(4), 339-346.

Cloherty, J. (1998). Syphilis. In J. Cloherty & A. Stark (Eds.), *Manual of neonatal care* (4th ed.). Boston: Little, Brown.

Cole, F. (1998). Fetal/Newborn human immunodeficiency virus infection. In H. Taeusch & R. Ballard (Eds.), *Avery's diseases of the newborn.* Philadelphia: W.B. Saunders.

Cordero, L. et al. (1998). Management of infants of diabetic mothers. *Archives of Pediatric and Adolescent Medicine, 152*(3), 249-254.

Cowles, T., & Gonik, B. (2002). Perinatal infections. In A. Fanaroff & R. Martin (Eds.), *Neonatal-perinatal medicine: Diseases of the fetus and infant* (7th ed.). St. Louis: Mosby.

D'Apolito, K. (1998). Substance abuse: Infant and childhood outcomes. *Journal of Pediatric Nursing, 13*(5), 307-316.

Edwards, M. (2002). Postnatal bacterial infections. In A. Fanaroff & R. Martin (Eds.), *Neonatal-perinatal medicine: Diseases of the fetus and infant* (7th ed.). St. Louis: Mosby.

Edwards, M., & Baker, C. (2001). Group B streptococcal infections. In J. Remmington & J. Klein (Eds.), *Infectious diseases of the fetus and newborn infant.* Philadelphia: W.B. Saunders.

European Collaborative Study. (1998). Is zidovudine therapy in pregnant HIV-infected women associated with gestational age and birthweight? *AIDS, 13,* 119-124.

Fernandes, O. et al. (1998). Moderate to heavy caffeine consumption during pregnancy and relationship to spontaneous abortion and abnormal fetal growth: A meta-analysis. *Reproduction Toxicology, 12*(4), 435-444.

Finnegan, L. (1991). Drug addiction and pregnancy: The newborn. In I. Chasnoff (Ed.), *Drugs, alcohol, pregnancy and parenting.* Boston: Kluwer.

Franck, L., & Johnson, L. (1998). Recognition and management of neonates at risk for perinatally acquired infection with human immunodeficiency virus. *Critical Care Nurse, 18*(4), 74-85.

Guerina, N. (1998). Bacterial and fungal infections. In J. Cloherty & A. Stark (Eds.), *Manual of neonatal care* (4th ed.). Boston: Little, Brown.

Hagay, Z., & Reece, E. (1999). Diabetes mellitus in pregnancy. In E. Reece & J. Hobbins (Eds.), *Medicine of the fetus and mother* (2nd ed.). Philadelphia: Lippincott-Raven

Hockenberry, M. et al. (2003). *Wong's nursing care of infants and children* (7th ed.). St. Louis: Mosby.

Hollier, L., & Cox, S. (1998). Syphilis. *Seminars in Perinatology, 22*(4), 323-331.

Hoyert, D., Freedman, M., Strobino, D., & Guyer, B. (2001). Annual summary of vital statistics: 2000. *Pediatrics, 108*(6), 1241-1255.

Hsu, T. et al. (2002). Neonatal clavicular fracture: Clinical analysis of incidence, predisposing factors, diagnosis and outcome. *American Journal of Perinatology, 19*(1), 17-21.

Ingall, D., & Sanchez, P. (2001). Syphilis. In J. Remington & J. Klein (Eds.), *Infectious diseases of the fetus and newborn infant.* Philadelphia: W.B. Saunders.

International Perinatal HIV Group. (1999). The mode of delivery and the risk of vertical transmission of human immunodeficiency virus type 1: A meta-analysis of 15 prospective cohort studies. *New England Journal of Medicine, 340,* 977-987.

John, G. et al. (2001). Timing of breast milk HIV-1 transmission: A meta-analysis. *East Africa Medicine, 78*(2), 75-79.

Jones, C. (2001). Gestational diabetes and its impact on the neonate. *Neonatal Network, 20*(6), 17-23.

Joseph, T., Pyati, S., & Jacobs, N. (1998). Neonatal early-onset *Escherichia coli* disease. *Archives of Pediatrics and Adolescent Medicine, 152*(1), 35-40.

Kalhan, S., & Parimi, P. (2002). Disorders of carbohydrate metabolism. In A. Fanaroff & R. Martin (Eds.), *Neonatal-perinatal medicine: Diseases of the fetus and infant* (7th ed.). St. Louis: Mosby.

Kaltenbach, K., Berghella, V., & Finnegan, L. (1998). Opioid dependence during pregnancy. Effects and management. *Obstetrics and Gynecology Clinics of North America, 25*(1), 139-151.

Klein, J. (2001). Bacterial sepsis and meningitis. In J. Remington & J. Klein (Eds.), *Infectious diseases of the fetus and newborn infant.* Philadelphia: W.B. Saunders.

Klein, J., & Remington, J. (2001). Current concepts of infections of the fetus and newborn infant. In J. Remington & J. Klein (Eds.), *Infectious diseases of the fetus and newborn infant.* Philadelphia: W.B. Saunders.

Kuhn, L. et al. (1998). Long-term survival of children with human immunodeficiency virus infection in New York City: Estimates from population-based surveillance data. *American Journal of Epidemiology, 47*(9), 846-854.

Kwong, T., & Shearer, D. (1998). Detection of drug use during pregnancy. *Obstetrics and Gynecology Clinics of North America, 25*(1), 43-64.

Lambert, J. et al. (2000). Risk factors for preterm birth, low birth weight, and intrauterine growth retardation in infants born to HIV-infected pregnant women receiving zidovudine: Pediatric AIDS Clinical Trials Group 185 Team. *AIDS, 14*(10), 1389-1399.

Landon, M., Catalano, & Gabbe, S. (2002). In S. Gabbe, J. Niebyl, & J. Simpson (Eds.), *Obstetrics: Normal and problem pregnancies* (4th ed.). New York: Churchill Livingstone.

Lawrence, R. (1999). *Breastfeeding: A guide for the medical profession* (5th ed.). St. Louis: Mosby.

Lee, M. (1998). Marijuana and tobacco use in pregnancy. *Obstetrics and Gynecology Clinics of North America, 25*(1), 65-83.

Lindsay, C. (2002). Pregnancy complicated by diabetes mellitus. In A. Fanaroff & R. Martin (Eds.), *Neonatal-perinatal medicine: Diseases of the fetus and infant* (7th ed.). St. Louis: Mosby.

Lynfield, R., & Guerina, N. (1997). Toxoplasmosis. *Pediatric Review, 18*(3), 75-83.

Mangurten, H. (2002). Birth injuries. In A. Fanaroff & R. Martin (Eds.), *Neonatal-perinatal medicine: Diseases of the fetus and infant* (7th ed.). St. Louis: Mosby.

Martin, S. 2001. Congenital toxoplasmosis. *Neonatal Network, 20*(4), 23-30.

McCollum, L., & Thigpen, J. (1998). Assessment and management of gastrointestinal dysfunction. In C. Kenner, J. Lott, & A. Flandermeyer (Eds.), *Comprehensive neonatal nursing.* Philadelphia: W.B. Saunders.

McGowan, J., Crane, M., & Wiznia, A. (1999). Combination antiretroviral therapy in human immunodeficiency virus-infected pregnant women. *Obstetrics and Gynecology, 94,* 641-646.

McKenna, L. (2000). Pancreatic disorders in the newborn. *Neonatal Network, 19*(4),13-20.

McMahon, M., Ananth, C., & Liston, R. (1998). Gestational diabetes mellitus: Risk factors, obstetric complications, and infant outcomes. *Journal of Reproductive Medicine, 43*(4), 372-378.

Merenstein, G., Adams, K., & Weisman, L. (2002). Infection in the neonate. In G. Merenstein & S. Gardner (Eds.), *Handbook of neonatal intensive care* (5th ed.). St. Louis: Mosby.

Minkoff, H. (1998). Human immunodeficiency virus infection in pregnancy. *Seminars in Perinatology, 22*(4), 293-308.

Mofenson, L. (1997). Mother-child HIV-1 transmission: Timing and determinants. *Obstetrics and Gynecology Clinics of North America, 24*(4), 759-784.

Montoya, K., & Washington, R. (2002). Cardiovascular disease and surgical interventions. In G. Merenstein & S. Gardner (Eds.), *Handbook of neonatal intensive care* (5th ed.). St. Louis: Mosby.

Nathwani, D. et al. (1998). Varicella infections in pregnancy and the newborn. *Journal of Infection, 36*(S1), 59-71.

Nduati, R. et al. (2000) Effects of breastfeeding and formula feeding on transmission of HIV-1: A randomized clinical trial. *Journal of the American Medical Association, 283*(9), 1167-1174.

Nelson, N. (1990). *Current therapy in neonatal-perinatal medicine* (2nd ed.). St. Louis: Mosby.

Nolla-Salas, J. et al. (1998). Perinatal listeriosis: A population based multicenter study in Barcelona, Spain. *American Journal of Perinatology, 15*(8), 461-467.

Nzerue, C., Hewan-Lowe, K., & Riley, L. (2000). Cocaine and the kidney: A synthesis of pathophysiologic and clinical perspectives. *Americal Journal of Kidney Disease, 35*(5), 783-795.

O'Doherty, N. (1986). *Neonatology: Micro atlas of the newborn.* Nutley, NJ: Hoffmann-La Roche.

Paige, P., & Carney, P. (2002). Neurologic disorders. In G. Merenstein & S. Gardner (Eds.), *Handbook of neonatal intensive care* (5th ed.). St. Louis: Mosby.

Plessinger, M. (1998). Prenatal exposure to amphetamines. *Obstetrics and Gynecology Clinics of North America, 25*(1), 119-138.

Pong, A., & Bradley, J. (1999). Bacterial meningitis and the newborn infant. *Infectious Disease Clinics of North America, 13*(3), 771-733.

Reece, E. et al. (1998). Pregnancy outcomes among women with and without diabetic microvascular disease (White's classes B to FR) versus nondiabetic controls. *American Journal of Perinatology, 15*(9), 549-555.

Remington, J. et al. (2001). Toxoplasmosis. In J. Remington & J. Klein (Eds.), *Infectious diseases of the fetus and newborn infant.* Philadelphia: W.B. Saunders.

Rosen, T., & Bateman, D. (2002). Infants of addicted mothers. In A. Fanaroff & R. Martin (Eds.), *Neonatal-perinatal medicine: Diseases of the fetus and infant* (7th ed.). St. Louis: Mosby.

Sabin, A. (1942). Toxoplasmosis: Recently recognized disease of human beings. V. Clinical manifestations of toxoplasmosis in man. *Advances in Pediatrics, 1,* 1-56.

Santos, I. et al. (1998). Caffeine intake and low birth weight: A population-based case-control study. *American Journal of Epidemiology, 147*(7), 620-627.

Schachter, J., & Grossman, M. (2001). Chlamydia. In J. Remington & J. Klein (Eds.), *Infectious diseases of the fetus and newborn.* Philadelphia: W.B. Saunders.

Sheffield, J. et al. (1999). Congenital syphilis: The influence of maternal stage of syphilis on vertical transmission. *American Journal of Obstetrics and Gynecology, 180,* S85.

Starke, J., & Smith, M. (2001). Tuberculosis. In J. Remington & J. Klein (Eds.), *Infectious diseases of the fetus and newborn infant.* Philadelphia: W.B. Saunders.

Wagner, C. et al. (1998). The impact of prenatal drug exposure on the neonate. *Obstetrics and Gynecology Clinics of North America, 25*(1), 169-194.

Weiner, L., & Morse, B. (1991). FAS: Clinical perspectives and prevention. In I. Chasnoff (Ed.), *Drugs, alcohol, pregnancy and parenting.* Boston: Kluwer.

Working Group on Antiviral Therapy. (2001). *Guidelines for the use of antiretroviral agents in pediatric HIV infection,* Dec. 14, 2001 [Online]. Available URL: www.hivatis.org/guidelines/Pediatric Dec 12_01/peddec.pdf.

Workowsky, K., & Levine, W. Sexually transmitted diseases treatment guidelines–2002. *MMWR, 51*(RR06), 1-8.

CHAPTER 39

Gayle Tart Davis

Hemolytic Disorders and Congenital Anomalies

http://evolve.elsevier.com/Lowdermilk/MatWmnHlth/

LEARNING OBJECTIVES

- Discuss assessment of the newborn for hyperbilirubinemia.
- Develop a nursing plan of care for the prevention, identification, and management of hyperbilirubinemia in a newborn.
- Compare Rh and ABO incompatibility.
- Explain nursing management to prevent the pathologic consequences of hyperbilirubinemia.
- Review prenatal diagnosis of neonatal disorders.
- Present assessment strategies during the postnatal period to aid in diagnosis of congenital disorders.
- Describe each congenital disorder presented in this chapter and identify the priority of nursing care for each.
- Describe preoperative and postoperative nursing care of the newborn.
- Develop a nursing plan of care for parents of a newborn with a defect or disorder.

The physiologic alterations that occur in infants during the newborn period differ and have varying effects. The nurse must be alert to the presence of any deviations from normal, ranging from an obvious congenital anomaly, such as myelomeningocele, to a less obvious deviation such as a congenital heart defect that may not be symptomatic at birth. The nurse must possess the assessment skills necessary to detect any deviation from normal, as well as the knowledge base necessary to participate in the skilled care needed for affected infants. The nurse also must be cognizant of the special needs of the family with a child who is born with or acquires an abnormal condition.

The complications that affect newborns can stem from three basic problems: problems relating to gestational age or intrauterine growth that does not follow normal patterns, such as a preterm birth; acquired problems resulting from maternal or newborn physiologic factors, such as ABO incompatibility or respiratory distress syndrome; and physical problems, such as congenital anomalies or birth defects.

HYPERBILIRUBINEMIA

In **hyperbilirubinemia,** the bilirubin level in the blood is increased. It is characterized by a yellow discoloration of the skin, mucous membranes, sclera, and various organs. This yellow discoloration is referred to as **jaundice,** or *icterus.* Jaundice is caused primarily by the accumulation in the skin of unconjugated bilirubin, a breakdown product of hemoglobin formed after its release from hemolyzed RBCs. Physiologic jaundice, discussed in Chapters 25 and 26, is the most common abnormal finding in newborns and is usually benign. The challenge in the care of neonates with hyperbilirubinemia is to distinguish physiologic jaundice from a serious clinical pathologic condition.

Physiologic Jaundice

Physiologic jaundice occurs in about half of all healthy term newborns and in 80% of preterm infants (Halamek & Stevenson, 2002). It typically arises more than 24 hours after birth. In both Caucasian and African-American infants, it is manifested by a progressive increase in the unconjugated bilirubin level in cord blood of from 2 mg/dl to a mean peak of 5 to 6 mg/dl between 60 and 72 hours of age. In Asian and Native American infants, the level may increase to 10 to 14 mg/dl between 72 and 120 hours of age. Resolution in Caucasian and African-American newborns is evidenced by a rapid decline in the unconjugated bilirubin level to 2 mg/dl by 5 days after birth; in Asian and Native American infants, this takes 7 to 10 days.

Physiologic jaundice is more common and severe in preterm infants, in whom the serum bilirubin level typically reaches a mean peak of 10 to 12 mg/dl by the fifth day of life. It takes longer for the maximal concentration to be reached in preterm than in full-term infants because the livers of preterm infants are immature, and hence liver function is not fully developed.

Pathologic Jaundice

Pathologic jaundice, or hyperbilirubinemia, is the level of serum bilirubin that, if left untreated, can result in kernicterus. These findings support a diagnosis of pathologic jaundice and, if encountered in an infant, warrant further investigation (Halamek & Stevenson, 2002):

- Serum bilirubin concentrations of greater than 4 mg/dl in cord blood
- Clinical jaundice evident within 24 hours of birth
- Total serum bilirubin levels increasing by more than 5 mg/dl in 24 hours or increasing at a rate of 0.5 mg/dl or more over a 4- to 8-hour period
- A serum bilirubin level in a term newborn that exceeds 15 mg/dl at any time or clinical jaundice lasting more than 10 days
- A serum bilirubin level in a preterm newborn that exceeds 10 mg/dl at any time
- Any case of visible jaundice that persists for more than 10 days of life in a term infant or 21 days in a preterm infant, unless the infant is receiving breast milk

Many potential causes of pathologic hyperbilirubinemia are found in neonates (Box 39-1). The most common are hemolytic disorders of the newborn.

BOX 39-1 Potential Causes of Pathologic Hyperbilirubinemia in Neonates

MATERNAL FACTORS

Rh and ABO incompatibility
Maternal infections
Maternal diabetes
Oxytocin administration during labor
Maternal ingestion of sulfonamides, diazepam, or salicylates near time of birth

FETAL/NEWBORN FACTORS

Prematurity
Hepatic cell damage by infection or drugs
Neonatal hyperthyroidism
Polycythemia
Intestinal obstruction such as meconium ileus
Pyloric stenosis
Biliary atresia
Sequestered blood (e.g., from cephalhematomas, ecchymosis, or hemangiomas)
Maternal blood swallowed by neonate

Hemolytic Disease of the Newborn

Hemolytic diseases of the newborn occur most often if the blood groups of the mother and baby are different; the most common of these are ABO and Rh factor incompatibilities.

The four major blood groups in the ABO system are A, B, AB, and O. People with type A blood have A antigen; those with type B have B antigen; those with type AB have both A and B antigens; and those with type O have no antigen. In turn, people with type A blood have plasma antibodies to type B blood; those with type B blood have antibodies to type A blood; those with type AB blood have no antibodies; and those with type O blood have antibodies to type A and B blood. If a person is administered or exposed to an incompatible blood type, he or she will form antibodies against the antigen in that blood, with an agglutination, or clumping, occurring as the antibodies in the plasma mix with the antigens of the different blood group.

The Rh factor, a genetically determined factor present on RBCs, can be a major source of incompatibility. Of the several forms of the Rh antigen, the D antigen is the most significant because it causes the most antibody production in a person who is Rh negative. Rh positivity is a dominant trait, so one must inherit the recessive gene from both parents to be Rh negative. A person who has the Rh factor is considered Rh positive; a person without it is considered Rh negative. For example, a mother who has A-negative blood has the A antigen, plasma antibodies to the B antigen, and no Rh factor on her RBCs.

Hemolytic disorders occur because maternal antibodies are present naturally or form in response to an antigen from the fetal blood crossing the placenta and entering the maternal circulation. The maternal antibodies of the immunoglobulin G (IgG) class in turn cross the placenta, causing hemolysis of the fetal RBCs, resulting in hyperbilirubinemia and jaundice.

Rh Incompatibility

Rh incompatibility, or **isoimmunization,** occurs when an Rh-negative mother has an Rh-positive fetus who inherits the dominant Rh-positive gene from the father. If the mother is Rh negative and the father is Rh positive and homozygous for the Rh factor, all the offspring will be Rh positive. If the father is heterozygous for the factor, there is a 50% chance that each infant born of the union will be Rh positive and a 50% chance that each will be born Rh negative (see Fig. 3-3). An Rh-negative fetus is in no danger because it has the same Rh factor as the mother. An Rh-negative fetus with an Rh-positive mother also is in no danger. Only the Rh-positive offspring of an Rh-negative mother is at risk. From 10% to 15% of all Caucasian couples and about 5% of African-American couples have Rh incompatibility. It is rare in Asian couples.

The incidence of Rh sensitization and resulting hemolytic disease of the newborn has decreased dramatically since the development of $Rh_0(D)$ immune globulin in 1968. New treatment modalities, including early detection and fetal blood transfusions, have improved the outcome of affected fetuses. However, despite continuing research and advances in management modalities, a 1% isoimmunization rate is found among women who are Rh negative, and it continues to be a major factor in fetal and neonatal morbidity and mortality (Neal, 2001).

The pathogenesis of Rh incompatibility is as follows. Hematopoiesis in the fetus, or the formation of blood cells, begins as early as the eighth week of gestation and, in up to 40% of pregnancies, these cells pass through the placenta into the maternal circulation. If the fetus is Rh positive and the mother Rh negative, the mother forms antibodies against the fetal blood cells–first IgM antibodies that are too large to pass through the placenta, and then later, IgG antibodies that can cross the placenta. The process of antibody formation is called *maternal sensitization.* Sensitization may occur during pregnancy, birth, miscarriage, abortion, or amniocentesis. Usually women become sensitized in their first pregnancy with an Rh-positive fetus but do not produce enough antibodies to cause lysis of fetal blood cells. During subsequent pregnancies, antibodies form in response to repeated contact with the antigen from the fetal blood, resulting in lysis or destruction of fetal RBCs.

Severe Rh incompatibility results in marked fetal hemolytic anemia, because the fetal erythrocytes are destroyed by maternal Rh-positive antibodies. Although the placenta usually clears the bilirubin generated by the RBC breakdown, in extreme cases, fetal bilirubin levels increase. This results in fetal jaundice, also known as *icterus gravis.*

The fetus compensates for the anemia by producing large numbers of immature erythrocytes to replace those hemolyzed; thus the name for this condition is **erythroblastosis fetalis.** In the most severe form of this disease, **hydrops fetalis,** the fetus has marked anemia, together with cardiac decompensation, cardiomegaly, and hepatosplenomegaly. Hypoxia results from the severe anemia. In addition, because of the decreased intravascular oncotic pressure involved, fluid leaks out of the intravascular space, resulting in generalized edema, as well as effusions into the peritoneal (ascites), pericardial, and pleural (hydrothorax) spaces. The placenta is often edematous, which, along with the edematous fetus, can cause the uterus to rupture.

Intrauterine or early neonatal death may occur as a result of hydrops fetalis, although intrauterine exchange transfusions and early birth of the fetus may avert this. **Intrauterine transfusion** involves the infusion of Rh-negative, type O blood into the umbilical vein. Such transfusions are administered as needed until birth, prolonging the intrauterine period available to the developing fetus. Studies of the use of intrauterine transfusions have demonstrated a high survival rate and low risk of disabilities in the surviving infant (Neal, 2001).

ABO Incompatibility

ABO incompatibility is more common than Rh incompatibility but causes less severe problems in the affected infant. It occurs if the fetal blood type is A, B, or AB, and the maternal type is O. It occurs rarely in infants with type B blood born to mothers with type A blood. The incompatibility arises because naturally occurring anti-A and anti-B antibodies are transferred across the placenta to the fetus. Unlike the situation that pertains to Rh incompatibility, firstborn infants may be affected, because mothers with type O blood already have anti-A and anti-B antibodies in their blood. Such a newborn may show a weakly positive result to a direct Coombs test. The cord bilirubin level usually is less than 4 mg/dl, and any resulting hyperbilirubinemia usually can be treated with phototherapy. Exchange transfusions are required only occasionally. Although ABO incompatibility is a common cause of hyperbilirubinemia, it rarely precipitates significant anemia resulting from the hemolysis of RBCs.

Kernicterus

The goal of the care given the infant with hyperbilirubinemia is the prevention of kernicterus. **Kernicterus,** or bilirubin encephalopathy, has also been defined by a new term, bilirubin-induced neurologic dysfunction (BIND) by some pediatricians (Poland, 2002). It is caused by the deposition of bilirubin in the brain, especially within the basal ganglia, cerebellum, and hippocampus. This deposition can occur because unconjugated bilirubin is highly lipid soluble, making it capable of crossing the blood-brain barrier if it is not bound to protein. If the concentration of unconjugated bilirubin reaches toxic levels, it results in the yellowish staining of the brain tissue and the necrosis of neurons.

Kernicterus, which can develop in newborns who show no apparent signs of clinical jaundice, is generally considered to be directly related to the total serum bilirubin level, although these levels alone do not predict the risk of brain injury. In a term infant, a serum bilirubin level of 25 mg/dl is considered the upper limit, beyond which the risk for kernicterus increases, although the condition may occur at much lower levels in premature infants or infants with other complications. In some high risk, low-birth-weight infants, a mean peak level of unconjugated bilirubin of even 10 to 12 mg/dl may be associated with the development of kernicterus (Halamek & Stevenson, 2002). Some of the perinatal events that increase the likelihood of kernicterus developing, even at these lower bilirubin levels, include hypoxia, asphyxia, acidosis, hypothermia, hypoglycemia, sepsis, treatment with certain medications, and hypoalbuminemia. These conditions interfere with the conjugation of bilirubin or compete for albumin-binding sites. The resulting unconjugated bilirubin can pass through the blood-brain barrier and enter the brain, resulting in kernicterus.

Kernicterus has been associated with acute and long-term symptoms of neurologic damage; it is never present at birth. The clinical manifestations typically appear between 2 and 6 days after birth and go through several phases as the disease progresses, generally beginning after the bilirubin level has peaked. During the first phase, the newborn is hypotonic and lethargic and shows a poor suck and depressed or absent Moro reflex. These more subtle signs are followed by the appearance of a high-pitched cry, opisthotonos (severe muscle spasm that causes the back to arch acutely), spasticity, hyperreflexia, and often by fever and seizures. All of this occurs over a period of about 24 hours. About half of the affected infants survive, although they often have permanent kernicteric sequelae including extrapyramidal movement disorders (especially dystonia and athetosis), gaze abnormalities (especially an upward gaze), auditory disturbances (especially sensorineural hearing loss), intellectual deficits (rarely in the mentally retarded range), and the posticteric sequelae of enamel dysplasia of the deciduous teeth. Movement abnormalities and auditory disturbances are almost always present. The minimal requirement for a diagnosis of kernicteric sequelae is an abnormality in two or more of the five categories listed, with the impairment in at least one area being severe enough to necessitate ongoing specialized therapy and assistance with skills of living (Johnson, Bhutani, & Brown, 2002).

Choreoathetoid cerebral palsy is the athetosis type of extrapyramidal movement disorder. This chronic condition is characterized by both choreiform (jerky, ticlike twitching) and athetoid (slow, writhing) movements. Fortunately, because it is now possible to identify the problem early and institute timely treatment with phototherapy and exchange transfusions, the classic bilirubin encephalopathy just described is not so prevalent as it once was. However, in the recent past, the incidence of kernicterus in the United States has increased, after a long period when it appeared to be waning. Researchers note that there is a need for (1) increased awareness of the problems inherent in the management of neonatal jaundice, especially as associated with early hospital discharge and medical care cost constraints; (2) strategies to improve prenatal and postnatal jaundice management; (3) education of physicians, nurses, and parents; and (4) a universal screening predischarge examination with targeted, individualized postnatal follow-up (Johnson et al., 2002).

NURSE ALERT

Several cases of kernicterus were reported in infants of mothers who were discharged early after birth. The discharge teaching for and follow-up of infants who are discharged early is therefore imperative.

In May 2001 the Joint Commission on Accreditation of Healthcare Organizations (JCAHO) issued a sentinel alert warning health care providers about the dangerous and potentially fatal consequences of kernicterus. JCAHO indicated that a combination of the following factors may place a neonate at risk for hyperbilirubinemia: jaundice appearing in the first 24 hours after birth, preterm infants (born 3 to 5 weeks early), inadequate nutrition and hydration resulting from insufficient breastfeeding, bruising and cephalhematomas, unrecognized hemolysis (e.g., ABO incompatibility), glucose-6-phosphate dehydrogenase (G6PD) deficiency, and genetic or ethnic risk factors (e.g., siblings with jaundice; East-Asian or Mediterranean descent). To protect newborns from developing kernicterus, it is recommended that hospitals evaluate all cases of jaundice appearing before age 24 hours, provide medical follow-up for newborns within 24 to 48 hours after hospital discharge, develop policies and procedures to measure serum or transcutaneous bilirubin level before discharge to determine need for follow-up, educate parents about jaundice, and provide adequate equipment for treatment (JCAHO, 2001).

CARE MANAGEMENT

Assessment and Nursing Diagnoses

It is important to determine the blood type and Rh factor of the pregnant woman prenatally. A thorough history must then be obtained in the Rh-negative pregnant woman to assess for the existence of events that could have caused her to develop antibodies to the Rh factor. Such events include (1) previous pregnancy with an Rh-positive fetus; (2) transfusion with Rh-positive blood, which causes immediate sensitization; (3) miscarriage or abortion after 8 or more weeks of gestation; (4) amniocentesis performed for any reason; (5) premature separation of the placenta; and (6) trauma.

Because hematopoiesis begins in the fetus during the eighth gestational week, a woman who has had a miscarriage or induced abortion after this time or has previously given birth to a child may have been inoculated with fetal blood at the time of placental separation. During amniocentesis, the needle may cause localized damage to the single layer of cells that separates the maternal and fetal circulation in the placenta, thereby allowing fetal RBCs to enter the maternal circulation.

If any of these events has occurred, the woman's record is checked to determine whether she has received **Rh_0(D) immune globulin,** such as RhoGam, which is a commercial preparation of passive antibodies against the Rh factor. This injection of anti-Rh antibodies destroys any fetal RBCs in the maternal circulation by causing the cells to be phagocytosed before the woman's immune system is activated to produce antibodies.

At the first prenatal visit of an Rh-negative woman with a fetus who may be Rh positive, an indirect **Coombs test** should be done to determine whether she has antibodies to the Rh antigen. In this test, the maternal blood serum is mixed with Rh-positive erythrocytes (RBCs). If the Rh-positive RBCs agglutinate or clump, this indicates that maternal antibodies are present. The dilution of the specimen of blood at which clumping occurs determines the titer, or level, of maternal antibodies, which indicates the degree of maternal sensitization. A level of 1:8 rarely results in fetal jeopardy. If the titer reaches 1:16, amniocentesis is performed to determine optical density (ΔOD) of amniotic fluid to estimate fetal hemolytic process (see Chapter 29). Increasing bilirubin levels may indicate the need for an intrauterine transfusion.

The indirect Coombs test is repeated at 28 weeks, and if the result remains negative, indicating that sensitization has not occurred, the woman is given an intramuscular injection of Rh_0(D) immune globulin. If the test result is positive, showing that sensitization has occurred, it is then repeated every 4 to 6 weeks to monitor the maternal antibody titer as just described. Examples of nursing diagnoses pertinent to newborns at risk because of hyperbilirubinemia include the following:

- *Risk for injury to neurons and cells in the kidney, pancreas, and intestine related to*
  -hyperbilirubinemia
- *Impaired gas exchange related to*
  -hemolytic anemia
- *Risk for deficient fluid volume related to*
  -phototherapy
- *Risk for parental anxiety related to*
  -hyperbilirubinemia, its management, and potential sequelae
- *Risk for impaired skin integrity related to*
  -increased stooling while undergoing phototherapy
- *Risk for ineffective thermoregulation (increased or decreased) related to*
  -phototherapy

Expected Outcomes of Care

Hospital protocols for the care of infants with hyperbilirubinemia are developed as a collaborative effort of the health care team. These protocols are then used in individualizing care for the infant and parents. Expected outcomes for care are stated in client-centered terms, as in the following:

- The infant's prenatal and perinatal risk factors will be identified, and intervention will be implemented when appropriate.
- The infant will not develop hyperbilirubinemia or its sequela, kernicterus.
- The infant will have minimal or no sequelae from hyperbilirubinemia and its treatment.
- The infant's serum bilirubin levels will return to normal.
- The infant's parents will demonstrate an understanding of the infant's condition, the therapies, and the possible sequelae of the condition.

Plan of Care and Interventions

Prevention of hyperbilirubinemia is the primary prenatal focus of care. The implementation of interventions focused on the care of the woman whose fetus is considered at risk for hyperbilirubinemia is essential to prevent problems in the newborn. Prenatal control of diabetes mellitus, prevention of maternal infection, avoidance of drugs such as diazepam and salicylates near the time of birth, and prevention of preterm birth reduce the risk.

BOX 39-2 Indications for Amount of Rh_0(D) Immune Globulin to Be Administered

50 μg
- After chorionic villus sampling, ectopic pregnancy, miscarriage, or abortion before 13 weeks of gestation

300 μg
- After any of the following events:
  Miscarriage or elective abortion after 13 weeks of gestation
  Percutaneous umbilical sampling
  - Amniocentesis
  - Abruptio placentae or placenta previa
  - Trauma
- At 28 weeks of gestation
- Within 72 hours of the preterm or term birth of an Rh-positive infant

More than 300 μg
- After a large transplacental hemorrhage
- After a mismatched blood transfusion

Early identification of the Rh-negative woman must occur, and care must be taken to prevent sensitization. The Rh-negative woman should be asked about any blood transfusion or any of the other factors already cited that would predispose her to sensitization. Rh_0(D) immune globulin is administered to Rh-negative women whose Coombs tests are negative (Halamek & Stevenson, 2002) (Box 39-2).

The fetus and maternal antibody titers are monitored prenatally. If amniocentesis reveals that the ΔOD is high and the fetus is in jeopardy, intrauterine transfusion may be done every 1 to 2 weeks between 26 and 32 weeks. If the endangered fetus is at more than 32 weeks of gestation, a preterm birth may be indicated, usually by cesarean.

Postpartum interventions focus on preventing sensitization in the mother, if it has not occurred already, and treating any complications in the neonate resulting from the hemolysis of RBCs (see Plan of Care). The unsensitized Rh-negative mother whose baby is Rh positive should receive 300 μg of Rh_0(D) immune globulin within 72 hours of birth. This should prevent her from producing antibodies to the fetal blood cells that entered her bloodstream during the birth.

At birth, the neonate's cord blood is sent to the laboratory to determine the infant's blood type and Rh status. A direct Coombs test is performed on this cord blood to determine whether there are maternal antibodies in the fetal blood. If antibodies are present, the titer, indicating the degree of maternal sensitization, is measured. If the titer is 1:64, an exchange transfusion is indicated. In addition, the prevention of or prompt therapy for perinatal asphyxia, acidosis, cold stress, sepsis, and hypoglycemia will decrease the newborn's risk for severe hemolytic disease and his or her susceptibility to kernicterus. Early, frequent feedings also are initiated to stimulate the gastrocolic reflex and thus facilitate the removal of bilirubin through stooling.

If pathologic jaundice is present, the cause is determined, and therapeutic management is begun. This includes monitoring and reducing the elevated bilirubin level. The bilirubin level also can be measured noninvasively by using transcutaneous bilirubinometry. This screening test for neonatal jaundice uses as its basis the relation between the yellow color of the skin and the total serum bilirubin level.

Various techniques are used to administer phototherapy to reduce the serum bilirubin levels, particularly if the jaundice is physiologic rather than pathologic, the jaundice occurs past the 24-hour period after birth, and the bilirubin levels are generally less than 15 mg/dl (see Chapter 26 and Fig. 26-17).

Exchange transfusions are needed less frequently today because of the decrease in the incidence of hemolytic disease in newborns resulting from isoimmunization. However, it is still the treatment of choice for some infants, with recommendations for treatment based on the total serum bilirubin and the age of the infant. For example, it is recommended that a healthy term newborn between 25 and 48 hours old receive an exchange transfusion after intensive phototherapy has failed to produce a decrease in total serum bilirubin of 1 to 2 mg/dl within 4 to 6 hours, with the total serum bilirubin continuing to decrease and remaining below 20 mg/dl (Frank, Cooper, & Merenstein, 2002). Other indications for transfusion include a positive direct Coombs test performed on cord blood; a hemoglobin concentration of less than 12 g/dl, indicating hemolytic disease in the newborn; hydrops fetalis; or signs of cardiac failure. In addition, because premature infants are thought to be more susceptible to bilirubin toxicity than are term infants, treatment strategies have been aimed at keeping serum bilirubin levels lower in these infants. Other factors must always be considered as well, particularly the clinical condition of the infant, because it is a procedure with many potential complications and a mortality risk of about 0.5% (Frank et al., 2002).

Exchange transfusion is accomplished by alternately removing a small amount of the infant's blood and replacing it with an equal amount of donor blood. Exchange transfusion replaces the RBCs that would otherwise be hemolyzed by circulating maternal antibodies, removes the antibodies responsible for hemolysis, and corrects the anemia caused by hemolysis of the infant's sensitized RBCs. It also reduces the serum bilirubin level in infants who have severe hyperbilirubinemia from any cause. If the infant has Rh incompatibility, type O Rh-negative blood is used for transfusion, so the maternal antibodies still present in the infant do not hemolyze the transfused blood. Depending on the infant's size, maturity, and condition, amounts of 5 to 20 ml of the infant's blood are removed at one time and replaced with donor blood. The total amount of blood exchanged approximates 170 ml/kg of body weight, or 75% to 85% of the infant's total blood volume. The amount exchanged is limited to 500 ml. During the procedure, the health care team members observe the infection control precautions for invasive procedures.

The infant is monitored closely during and after the procedure, including the heart rate and rhythm, respirations, blood pressure, temperature, pedal pulses, and the presence of edema. Hypervolemia or hypovolemia, as well as air emboli, may be a complication of the procedure. Symptoms of hypocalcemia, such as jitteriness, irritability, convulsions, tachycardia, and electrocardiogram changes, may be triggered by preservatives in the donor blood that reduce the infant's serum calcium level. This may necessitate an infusion of calcium gluconate to correct the deficit. The nurse also monitors the infusion site for hemorrhage and is constantly alert for any other complications that may occur, such as embolization or thrombosis, volume overload and cardiac arrest, other electrolyte abnormalities, and overheparinization and bleeding (Frank et al., 2002).

The treatment of hyperbilirubinemia by using a drug to decrease bilirubin production is the focus of ongoing clinical trials. Heme oxygenase (HO) is the first enzyme in the heme catabolic sequence that results in bilirubin. Inhibition of HO activity therefore prevents the production of bilirubin. A metalloporphyrin, such as tin mesoporphyrin (SnMP), is an HO inhibitor. When bilirubin production is suppressed by the administration of SnMP, heme is excreted directly into bile. Infants receiving a single dose of SnMP have lower peak bilirubin levels and a decreased need for phototherapy. In clinical studies, side effects have been minimal, and dosages used in the studies appear to be safe for administration to newborns for the management of hyperbilirubinemia. Metalloporphyrins are not approved by the FDA for use in humans, and work remains to be done with regard to safety, efficacy, and clinical dosing (Dixit & Gartner, 1999).

Phenobarbital is effective in reducing serum bilirubin levels in newborns. It is not commonly used, however, primarily because it requires up to 6 days of treatment for maximal effect (Dixit & Gartner, 1999).

A device that measures carbon monoxide production, which is an index of bilirubin production, is being evaluated. This noninvasive device measures carbon monoxide by sampling expired air with a small nasal catheter. Hemolysis can be identified before anemia and hyperbilirubinemia develop (Augustine, 1999).

Planning for rehabilitative measures is necessary if kernicterus occurs. The family will need the services of many community resources to care for the affected child. An interdisciplinary approach that includes social services must be taken (Box 39-3).

Plan of Care: Infant with Hyperbilirubinemia

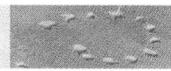

NURSING DIAGNOSIS Risk for injury related to hemolytic disease and treatment effects

Expected Outcomes *Bilirubin levels decrease with treatment; no evidence exists of harmful effects from phototherapy (e.g., no eye irritation, dehydration, temperature instability, or skin breakdown); and no complications occur from exchange transfusions.*

Nursing Interventions/*Rationales*

Initiate early feedings *to enhance excretion of bilirubin in stools.*

Observe skin and mucous membranes for signs of jaundice, *indicative of increasing bilirubin levels;* monitor serum bilirubin levels *to determine rate of increase and treatment response.*

Note time of jaundice onset *to help distinguish physiologic from other causes of jaundice.*

Observe for signs of hypoxia, hypothermia, hypoglycemia, and metabolic acidosis, *which occur as a result of hyperbilirubinemia and increase the risk of brain damage.*

Initiate phototherapy per physician order *to decrease bilirubin levels.*

During phototherapy, shield infant's eyes *to prevent damage to corneas and retinas;* keep infant nude and change positions frequently *for maximal body surface exposure;* cleanse skin frequently *to prevent irritation;* maintain adequate fluid intake *to prevent dehydration;* monitor body temperature *to prevent hyperthermia.*

Before exchange transfusion, keep infant on nothing-by-mouth (NPO) status (2 to 4 hours) *to prevent aspiration;* check donor blood for compatibility *to prevent transfusion reaction;* have resuscitation equipment (oxygen, Ambu bag, endotracheal tubes, laryngoscope) at bedside *in preparation for emergency action.*

Assist physician with exchange transfusion procedure; track amounts of blood withdrawn and transfused *to maintain balanced blood volume;* maintain body temperature *to avoid hypothermia and cold stress;* monitor vital signs and observe for rash *for indicators of transfusion reaction.*

After transfusion, continue to monitor vital signs *for transfusion reaction or other complications;* check umbilical cord *for bleeding or signs of infection.*

NURSING DIAGNOSIS Interrupted breastfeeding related to discharge of mother and continued hospitalization of infant

Expected Outcome *Mother expresses desire to continue breastfeeding as much as possible and expresses and stores milk when she cannot come to the hospital to nurse the infant.*

Nursing Interventions/*Rationales*

Encourage the mother to come to hospital to nurse infant as often as feasible for her *to maintain milk supply and encourage bonding.*

Provide private and comfortable space for nursing that is available 24 hours per day *to support the mother in breastfeeding.*

Instruct the mother in methods to express and store breast milk *to ensure a safe and adequate milk supply.*

Provide written educational materials and audiovisual aids *to demonstrate proper techniques for expressing and storing milk and to allow the mother to learn at her own pace.*

Recommend use of a breast pump and pump according to recommended guidelines (e.g., pump a minimum of five times a day; pump a minimum of 100 minutes a day; pump long enough to soften breasts) *to provide maximum stimulation for milk production.*

Reassure the mother that infant's nutritional needs will be met through expressed milk or other methods *to allay anxiety.*

Review the daily routine of the mother to advise her on ways *to incorporate pumping into her daily schedule.*

Provide information about breastfeeding support groups *to help the mother obtain emotional support from other breastfeeding mothers.*

NURSING DIAGNOSIS Parental role conflict related to separation from hospitalized infant and interruptions of family life due to travel to hospital to see infant.

Expected Outcomes *Parents will share responsibilities for child care and home maintenance; parents will visit infant in hospital as often as feasible.*

Nursing Interventions/*Rationales*

Suggest to parents that they mutually establish a routine for child care for siblings and home maintenance *to enhance communication and provide necessary home activities.*

Encourage parents to seek assistance and support from friends, relatives, and community groups such as their church, *to meet their needs and ensure that a minimal level of appropriate functioning is maintained.*

Encourage parents travel to hospital as often as is desirable and feasible *to promote breastfeeding and bonding with infant.*

NURSING DIAGNOSIS Risk for knowledge deficit related to administration of home phototherapy

Expected Outcome *Family demonstrates ability to provide home therapy.*

Nursing Interventions/*Rationales*

Explore family's willingness to try home phototherapy *to evaluate feasibility of home therapy option.*

Explore family's understanding of jaundice and proposed therapy *to establish baseline for teaching.*

Teach family with demonstration–return demonstration, allowing for several practice sessions, and supplement with written materials with pictorial representations *to ensure safe and optimal results.*

Include the following in your instructions: placement of lamp or fiberoptic unit; proper eye care and patching; proper skin care; proper positioning under lamp; provision of increased fluid intake; monitoring of time under lamp; monitoring of vital signs, skin, eyes, feeding patterns, stooling and voiding patterns; observation for complications *to ensure that the family understands and implements safe and effective use of phototherapy.*

Stress importance of obtaining the prescribed bilirubin tests on schedule *as a way of tracking success of therapy.*

Give parents a contact if they have any questions while carrying out therapy *to offer ongoing support and increase parent comfort.*

BOX 39-3 **Monitoring for Jaundice After Early Discharge**

If the infant is discharged from the hospital before 48 hours of age, the parents should receive teaching regarding adequate hydration and assessment of the infant for the appearance of jaundice. Appropriate testing and follow-up of the infant should be available. A program of home phototherapy, where available, allows infants to receive treatment of uncomplicated hyperbilirubinemia after discharge from the hospital. For these infants, nurses provide monitoring of treatment and of serum bilirubin levels as outlined by hospital or agency policy.

Evaluation

On a short-term basis, the nurse can consider nursing care to be effective to the degree that the previously described outcomes for care are achieved.

CONGENITAL ANOMALIES

The desired and expected outcome of every wanted pregnancy is a normal, functioning infant with a good intellectual potential. Fulfillment of this hope depends on numerous hereditary and environmental factors. Probably all human characteristics have a genetic component, including those that produce symptoms or physical abnormalities that impair the fitness of the person. Some disorders or diseases occur through the influence of a single gene or the combined action of many genes inherited from the parents; others result from the action of the intrauterine environment. Many defects appear to occur as the result of multifactorial inheritance, the interaction of multiple genes with environmental factors that affect the embryonic development of the affected system. Examples of these include neural tube defects, congenital heart defects, developmental dysplasia of the hip, and cleft lip or palate. Researchers are adding information about factors that might cause congenital anomalies (Chuangsuwanich et al., 1998; Hoek, Brown, & Susser, 1998; Yerkes et al., 1998).

A **congenital** disorder is present at birth and can be caused by genetic or environmental factors, or both. Some congenital disorders such as inborn errors of metabolism and mental retardation are not malformations.

Congenital anomalies are evident in 3% of all live births (Brent, 2001), but this number increases to about 6% by age 5 years, when more anomalies are diagnosed. Major congenital defects are the leading cause of death in infants younger than 1 year in the United States and account for 20% of neonatal deaths. Although there has been a decrease in the incidence of other causes of neonatal mortality, the death rate associated with most congenital anomalies has essentially remained stable for the last 70 years.

The most common major congenital anomalies that cause serious problems in the neonate are congenital heart disease, neural tube defects, cleft lip or palate, clubfoot, and developmental dysplasia of the hip. These are thought to result from the interaction of multiple genetic and environmental factors. Minor anomalies are less apparent but are important to identify because they may be a part of a characteristic pattern of malformations. That is, they may point to the presence of a more serious major anomaly and aid in its diagnosis. For example, about 15% of newborns have a minor anomaly; of these, only 1.4% also have a major anomaly. In contrast, only 0.5% of newborns have three or more minor anomalies, but the probability of these infants also having a major anomaly is 90% (Hudgins & Cassidy, 2002). Minor malformations are more common in areas of the body that have variable features, such as the face and distal extremities. Some of the most common malformations include the lack of a helical fold of the pinna, complete or incomplete simian creases, and a capillary hemangioma other than on the face or posterior aspect of the neck.

The seriousness of congenital anomalies in terms of their effect on society is reflected in the more than six million hospital days and $200 billion a year required for the care and treatment of these neonates. Ways of preventing and detecting these anomalies are being improved continuously, as are techniques for the care of the fetus with certain anomalies. Promoting the availability of these services to populations at risk challenges community health care systems. An interdisciplinary team approach is vital for providing holistic care: the surgical treatment, rehabilitation, and education of the child, as well as psychosocial and financial assistance for the parents. Parental disappointment and disillusion add to the complexity of the nursing care needed for these infants.

Cardiovascular System Anomalies

During fetal development, cell division and differentiation of the organs and tissues of a particular body system sometimes occur rapidly. During these various sensitive, or critical, periods, particular body systems are more susceptible to environmental influences than they are later in gestation. For example, the critical period for the cardiovascular system is from week 3 of embryonic development to week 8, when many women may not be aware that they are pregnant.

Congenital heart defects (CHDs) are anatomic abnormalities in the heart that are present at birth, although they may not be diagnosed immediately. Some type of cardiologic problem occurs in 8 to 10 of every 1000 live births (Lewin, 2000) or 32,000 to 35,000 children born per year (Smith, 2001). Ventricular septal defects, constituting more than 20% of all CHDs, are the most common type of acyanotic lesion, and 10% of all CHDs are atrial septal defects (McDaniel, 2001). Tetralogy of Fallot, constituting 10% of all CHDs, is the most common type resulting in cyanosis. After prematurity, CHDs are the next major cause of death in the first year of life.

The etiology of CHDs is unknown in more than 90% of the cases. This is important for parents to know, because they often feel guilty that they have done something to cause the defect. Maternal factors that are associated with a higher incidence of CHD include the following:

- Viral infections such as rubella
- Ingestion of folic acid antagonists or anticonvulsants such as phenytoin, progesterone, estrogen, lithium, or warfarin (Coumadin)
- Use of the acne medication isotretinoin (Accutane)
- Alcoholism
- Poor nutrition
- Radiation exposure
- Complications of pregnancy such as antepartal bleeding
- Metabolic disorders such as diabetes mellitus and phenylketonuria
- Maternal age ≥40 years

There also is an increased likelihood of cardiac disease in low-birth-weight infants, especially those small for gestational age, as well as in premature infants and those with congenital infections. In addition, CHDs may be associated with other extracardiac defects such as renal agenesis, tracheoesophageal fistula, and diaphragmatic hernias.

Genetic factors are implicated in the pathogenesis of CHD. As a general rule, these defects are thought to be multifactorial in origin, involving both genetic and environmental influences; however, a familial occurrence of virtually all forms of CHD has been noted. If a family has one affected child, the risk for having a second child with CHD has been thought to be 1% to 3%; the risk for the acquisition of some defects is greater than this. For example, the risk for left-sided lesions such as hypoplastic left heart syndrome and coarctation of the aorta is higher (Hockenberry et al., 2003). If the father is affected, the risk of having a child with CHD is 1% to 3%; it is 2% to 10% if the mother is affected. This inherited risk will become more important as children with CHD live longer and reproduce; therefore continuing epidemiologic studies are needed in this area.

Additionally, it now appears that a much greater percentage than believed to be true in the past can be attributed to single gene mutations. This recognition is based on animal models, studies of human familial patterns of inheritance, and the finding of cardiovascular defects as a part of syndromes exhibiting mendelian patterns of inheritance. An example of this is the identification of chromosome 22q11 deletions in infants with DiGeorge syndrome. This syndrome affects an estimated 1 in 4000 live births, making this one of the most frequent genetic disorders with congenital heart defects. The gene or genes located in the chromosomal region involved with DiGeorge syndrome appear to play a major role in the development of cardiovascular defects, particularly truncus arteriosus, absent pulmonary valve syndrome, tetralogy of Fallot, pulmonary atresia, and other abnormalities involving the aortic arch (Lewin, 2000).

Chromosomal abnormalities also may be associated with CHDs. For example, 45% of children with trisomy 21, or Down syndrome, have a cardiac defect. All children who have trisomy 18, the second most common chromosomal abnormality, have cardiac anomalies. About 95% of trisomy 18 fetuses miscarry, and the survivors usually die within the first year of life. Approximately 80% of infants born with trisomy 13 have cardiac defects. In general, cardiovascular surgical intervention has not been offered to infants with trisomies 13 and 18 because of their overall poor prognosis.

Although traditionally CHD has been classified as either cyanotic or acyanotic, a classification that categorizes cardiac defects physiologically is now considered more descriptive. The first of the four categories in this classification includes defects that result in increased pulmonary blood flow, often with congestive heart failure. Examples of the CHDs in this category are atrial and ventricular septal defects and patent ductus arteriosus. The second category includes defects that involve decreased pulmonary blood flow and typically result in cyanosis. The most common example of this type of defect is tetralogy

TABLE *39-1* **Physiologic Classification of Cardiac Defects**

CATEGORIES	EXAMPLES
Defects that result in increased pulmonary blood flow, often with congestive heart failure	Atrial and ventricular septal defects Patent ductus arteriosus
Defects that involve decreased pulmonary blood flow and typically result in cyanosis	Tetralogy of Fallot Tricuspid atresia
Defects that cause obstruction to blood flow out of the heart	Pulmonary stenosis; causes cyanosis Coarctation of the aorta; congestive heart failure, no cyanosis Subaortic stenosis; congestive heart failure, no cyanosis
Complex cardiac anomalies that involve a flow of mixed saturated and desaturated blood in the heart or great vessels	Transposition of the great vessels Total anomalous venous return

of Fallot; tricuspid atresia is a less common defect in this category. The third category includes those defects that cause obstruction to blood flow out of the heart. Pulmonary stenosis is an example of an obstruction to the flow of blood out of the right side of the heart that causes cyanosis. Coarctation of the aorta and subaortic stenosis are examples of obstructions to the flow of blood out of the left side of the heart that can result in congestive heart failure but not cyanosis. The fourth category comprises those complex cardiac anomalies that involve a flow of mixed saturated and desaturated blood in the heart or great vessels. These include such defects as transposition of the great vessels and total anomalous venous return (Table 39-1; Fig. 39-1).

Severe CHDs often are evident immediately after birth, especially defects that cause cyanosis such as transposition of the great vessels. Infants with these anomalies are transferred directly to special care nurseries or pediatric units. Even though the structural or functional anomalies are always present at birth, some affected newborns may be asymptomatic. Some CHDs, such as a small coarctation of the aorta, become apparent only as the infant or child is exposed to stresses such as growth demands or infection.

If symptoms are present at birth, they may be obvious with the first cry, which may be weak and muffled or loud and breathless. Affected newborns may be cyanotic and unrelieved by oxygen treatment, with the cyanosis increasing whenever the child is in the supine position or cries. The bluish gray, dusky color of cyanotic infants may be mild, moderate, or severe. Other infants may be acyanotic and pale, with or without mottling on exertion, which includes crying, feeding, or stooling.

The affected newborn's activity level varies from restlessness to lethargy, and possibly unresponsiveness, except to

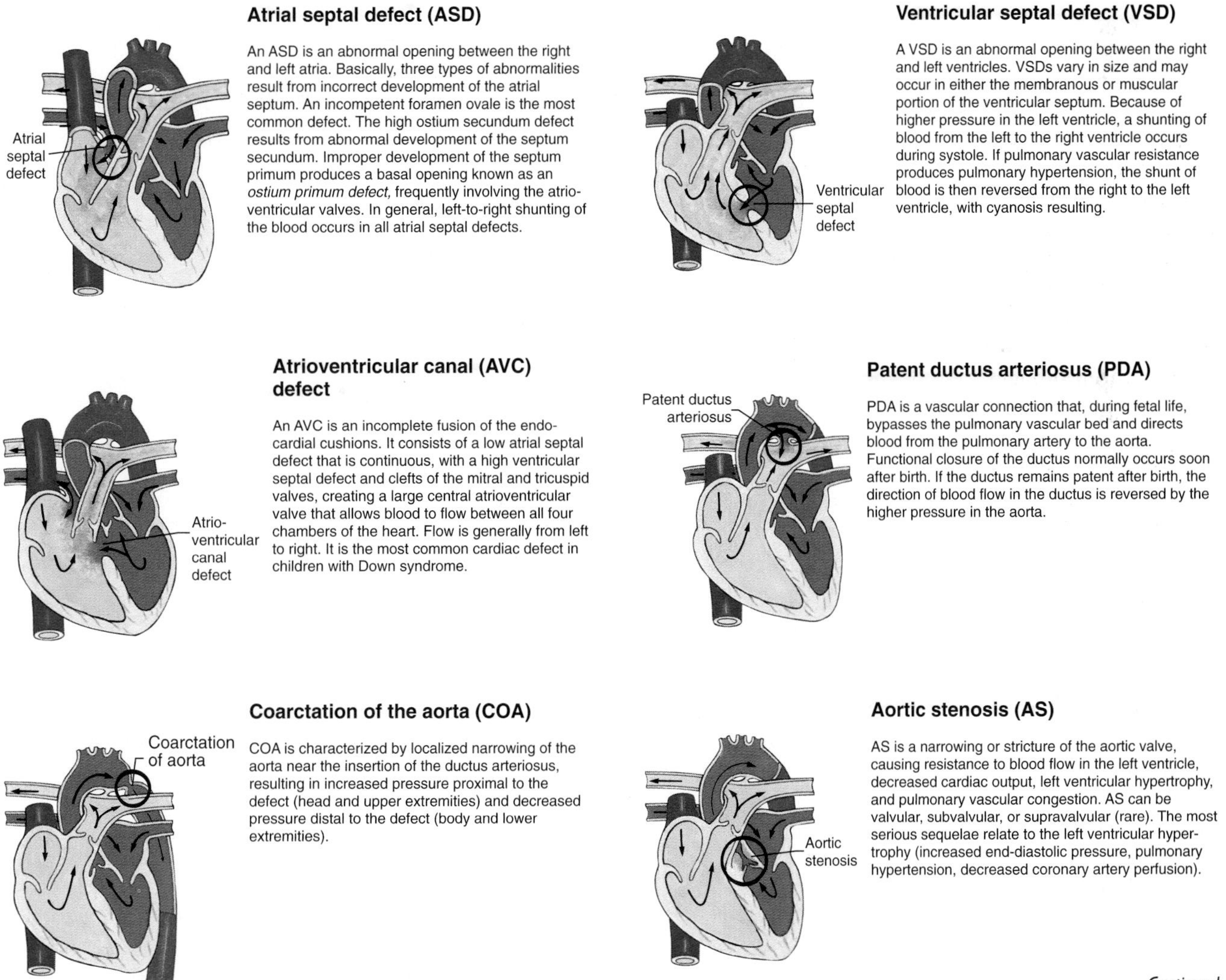
Atrial septal defect (ASD)
An ASD is an abnormal opening between the right and left atria. Basically, three types of abnormalities result from incorrect development of the atrial septum. An incompetent foramen ovale is the most common defect. The high ostium secundum defect results from abnormal development of the septum secundum. Improper development of the septum primum produces a basal opening known as an *ostium primum defect,* frequently involving the atrioventricular valves. In general, left-to-right shunting of the blood occurs in all atrial septal defects.
Atrial septal defect
Ventricular septal defect (VSD)
A VSD is an abnormal opening between the right and left ventricles. VSDs vary in size and may occur in either the membranous or muscular portion of the ventricular septum. Because of higher pressure in the left ventricle, a shunting of blood from the left to the right ventricle occurs during systole. If pulmonary vascular resistance produces pulmonary hypertension, the shunt of blood is then reversed from the right to the left ventricle, with cyanosis resulting.
Ventricular septal defect
Atrioventricular canal (AVC) defect
An AVC is an incomplete fusion of the endocardial cushions. It consists of a low atrial septal defect that is continuous, with a high ventricular septal defect and clefts of the mitral and tricuspid valves, creating a large central atrioventricular valve that allows blood to flow between all four chambers of the heart. Flow is generally from left to right. It is the most common cardiac defect in children with Down syndrome.
Atrioventricular canal defect
Patent ductus arteriosus (PDA)
PDA is a vascular connection that, during fetal life, bypasses the pulmonary vascular bed and directs blood from the pulmonary artery to the aorta. Functional closure of the ductus normally occurs soon after birth. If the ductus remains patent after birth, the direction of blood flow in the ductus is reversed by the higher pressure in the aorta.
Patent ductus arteriosus
Coarctation of the aorta (COA)
COA is characterized by localized narrowing of the aorta near the insertion of the ductus arteriosus, resulting in increased pressure proximal to the defect (head and upper extremities) and decreased pressure distal to the defect (body and lower extremities).
Coarctation of aorta
Aortic stenosis (AS)
AS is a narrowing or stricture of the aortic valve, causing resistance to blood flow in the left ventricle, decreased cardiac output, left ventricular hypertrophy, and pulmonary vascular congestion. AS can be valvular, subvalvular, or supravalvular (rare). The most serious sequelae relate to the left ventricular hypertrophy (increased end-diastolic pressure, pulmonary hypertension, decreased coronary artery perfusion).
Aortic stenosis

Continued

FIG. 39-1 Congenital heart abnormalities. (Modified from Hockenberry, M. et al. [2003]. *Wong's nursing care of infants and children* [7th ed.]. St. Louis: Mosby.)

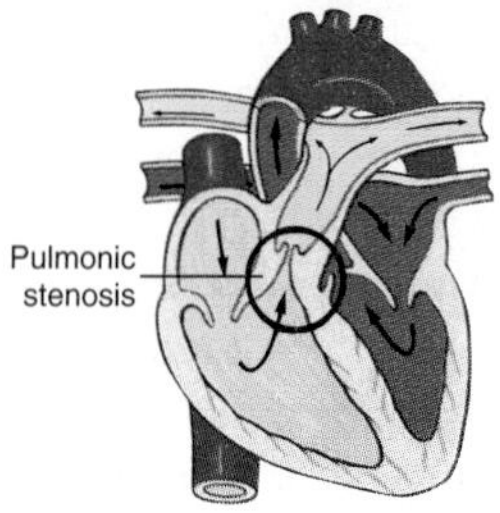

Pulmonic
stenosis

Pulmonic stenosis (PS)

PS is a narrowing at the entrance to the pulmonary artery. Resistance to blood flow causes right ventricular hypertrophy and decreased pulmonary blood flow. Pulmonary atresia is the extreme form of PS; no blood flows to the lungs.

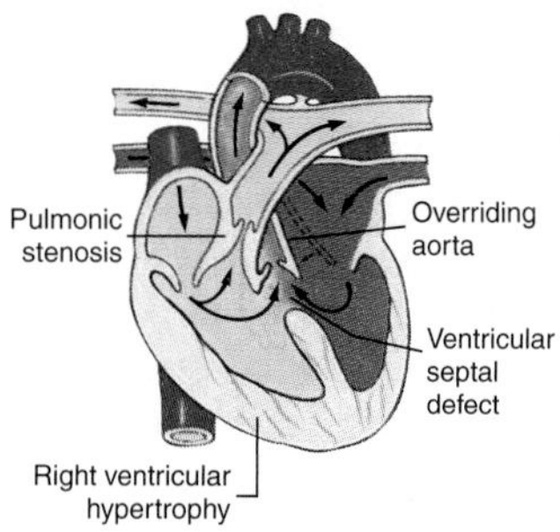

Pulmonic
stenosis
Overriding
aorta
Ventricular
septal
defect
Right ventricular
hypertrophy

Tetralogy of Fallot (TOF)

TOF is characterized by the combination of four defects: (1) pulmonary stenosis, (2) ventricular septal defect, (3) overriding aorta, and (4) hypertrophy of the right ventricle. It is the most common defect, causing cyanosis in children surviving beyond 2 years of age. The severity of symptoms depends on the degree of pulmonary stenosis, the size of the ventricular septal defect, and the degree to which the aorta overrides the septal defect.

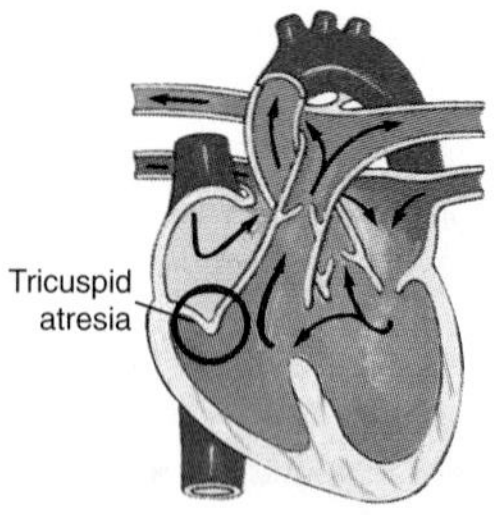

Tricuspid
atresia

Tricuspid atresia

Tricuspid valvular atresia is characterized by a small right ventricle, a large left ventricle, and usually a diminished pulmonary circulation. Blood from the right atrium passes through an atrial septal defect into the left atrium, mixes with oxygenated blood returning from the lungs, flows into the left ventricle, and is propelled into the systemic circulation. The lungs may receive blood through one of three routes: (1) a small ventricular septal defect, (2) a patent ductus arteriosus, or (3) bronchial vessels.

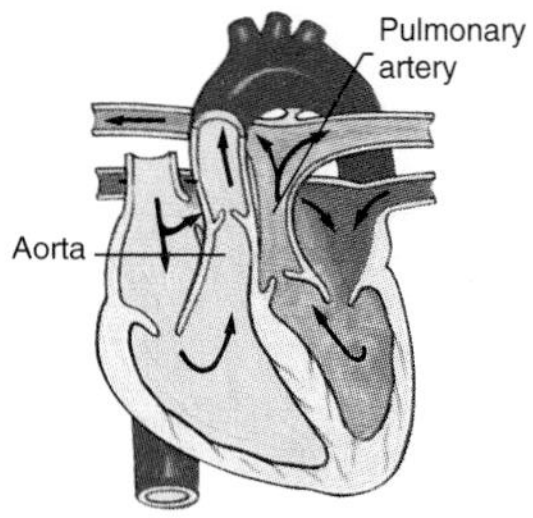

Pulmonary
artery
Aorta

Transposition of the great vessels (TGV)

TGV is an embryologic defect caused by a straight division of the bulbar trunk without normal spiraling. As a result, the aorta originates from the right ventricle and the pulmonary artery from the left ventricle. An abnormal communication between the two circulations must be present to sustain life.

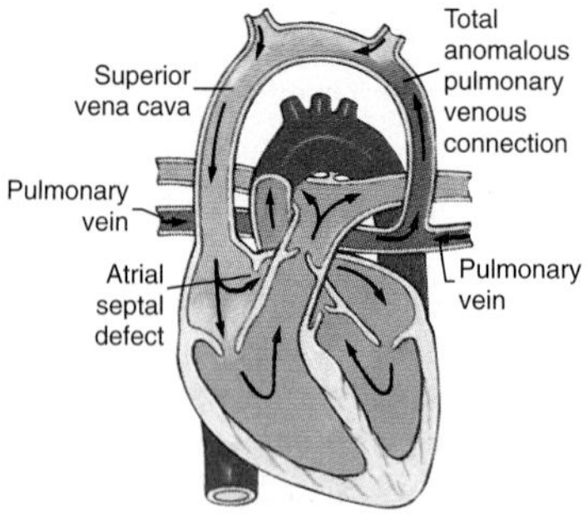

Superior
vena cava
Total
anomalous
pulmonary
venous
connection
Pulmonary
vein
Atrial
septal
defect
Pulmonary
vein

Total anomalous pulmonary venous connection (TAPVC)

TAPVC is a rare defect characterized by a failure of the pulmonary veins to join the left atrium. Instead, the pulmonary veins are abnormally connected to the systemic venous circuit via the right atrium or various veins draining toward the right atrium (e.g., superior vena cava). The abnormal attachment results in mixed blood being returned to the right atrium and shunted from the right to the left through an atrial septal defect.

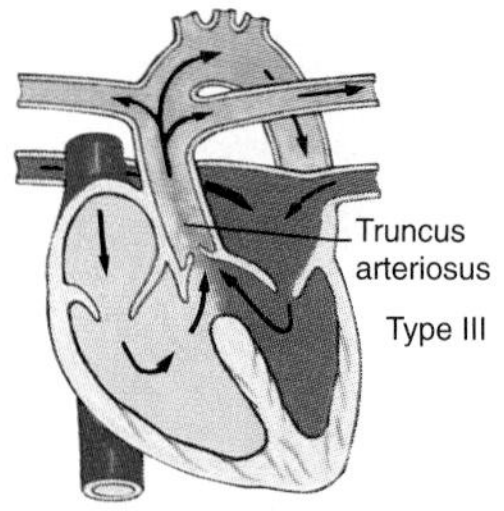

Truncus
arteriosus
Type III

Truncus arteriosus (TA)

TA is a retention of the embryologic bulbar trunk. It results from the failure of normal septation and division of this trunk into an aorta and pulmonary artery. This single arterial trunk overrides the ventricles and receives blood from them through a ventricular septal defect. The entire pulmonary and systemic circulation is supplied from this common arterial trunk.

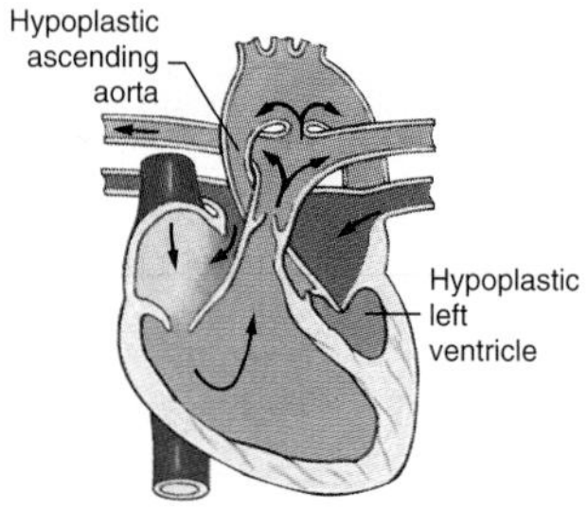

Hypoplastic
ascending
aorta
Hypoplastic
left
ventricle

Hypoplastic left heart syndrome (HLHS)

HLHS is characterized by underdevelopment of the left side of the heart, resulting in a hypoplastic left ventricle and aortic atresia. Most blood from the left atrium flows across the patent foramen ovale to the right atrium, to the right ventricle, and out the pulmonary artery. The descending aorta receives blood from the patent ductus arteriosus supplying systemic blood flow.

FIG. 39-1, cont'd

pain. Persistent bradycardia (resting heart rate of less than 80 beats/min) or tachycardia (rate exceeding 160 beats/min) may be noted (Askin, 2002). The cardiac rhythm may be abnormal, and murmurs may be heard. Signs of congestive heart failure, diminished cardiac output, and decreased tissue perfusion may be evident (Suddaby, 2001).

Because the cardiac and respiratory systems function together, cardiac disease may be manifested by respiratory signs and symptoms. The respiratory rate should be determined when the newborn is in a resting state. Abnormal findings may include tachypnea, which is a rate of 60 to 120 breaths/min; retractions with nasal flaring; grunting occurring with or without exertion; and dyspnea, which may worsen when the infant is supine or exerting itself.

A major role of the nurse is to assess infants for abnormal findings, which, if observed, must be reported immediately. Newborns exhibiting these symptoms require prompt diagnosis and appropriate therapy in a neonatal or pediatric intensive care unit. Interventions planned if a nursing diagnosis of decreased cardiac output is made include administering oxygen as ordered, as well as cardiotonic and other medications such as diuretics that rid the body of accumulated fluid, decreasing the workload of the heart by maintaining a thermoneutral environment, feeding with the gavage method if necessary, and preventing crying if this precipitates cyanosis. Various diagnostic tests such as echocardiography and cardiac catheterization are performed to obtain specific information about the defect and the need for surgical intervention. Significant improvements in diagnosis, medical management, and surgical treatment of CHD have caused the death rate to decrease by approximately 23% between 1987 and 1997. Surgical mortality is currently about 5%. The result is that more of these children are growing up (Smith, 2001).

Central Nervous System Anomalies

Most congenital anomalies of the central nervous system (CNS) result from defects in the closure of the neural tube during fetal development. These include spina bifida, occurring in 1 per 1000 to 2000 births; encephalocele involving the brain, which is one tenth as common as neural tube closure defects involving the spine; and anencephaly, which occurs in 1 per 8000 births (Haslam, 2000). Although the cause of **neural tube defects** is unknown, they are thought to stem from the interaction of many genes that are in turn influenced by factors in the fetal environment. Environmental influences such as treatment with valproic acid (an anticonvulsant), treatment with methotrexate (a chemotherapeutic medication), and alcohol consumption have been implicated. Excessive maternal body heat exposure during the early first trimester, such as from a significant febrile illness or extensive hot-tub exposure, also may increase the risk of a neural tube defect (Elias & Hobbs, 1998). Studies have shown that a maternal folic acid deficit has a direct bearing on failure of the neural tube to close; therefore in 1993, the American Academy of Pediatrics issued recommendations that folic acid be taken by women of childbearing age (Morrow & Kelsey, 1998). Despite an abundance of information about folic acid, many women of childbearing age are unaware of the importance of folic acid intake or chose to ignore it (see Research box). Neural tube defects also continue to occur because of unplanned pregnancies and planned pregnancies, of which 30% are thought to be folic acid resistant (Rintoul et al., 2002).

Although a neural tube defect is usually an isolated defect, it can occur with some chromosomal abnormalities and syndromes and also with other defects such as cleft palate, ventricular septal defect, tracheoesophageal fistula, diaphragmatic hernia, imperforate anus, and renal anomalies. Some neural tube defects can be diagnosed prenatally with fetal ultrasonography and the finding of elevated levels of alpha-fetoprotein in the amniotic fluid and maternal serum.

RESEARCH

Preconception Counseling: Young Women and Folic Acid

Research since the 1980s has demonstrated that inadequate maternal folic acid intake can lead to neural tube defects (NTDs). During fetal development, the neural tube normally closes from the middle to both ends by the 25th through the 27th day after fertilization. NTD is a failure to close normally. Results range from mild spinal curvature to spina bifida to anencephaly (absence of part of the brain, which is always fatal). In the United States approximately 4000 pregnancies are affected each year, resulting in about 2500 infants born with NTD. The U.S. Public Health Service and the March of Dimes have recommended that all women in the childbearing years take 0.4 mg of folic acid every day, starting at least 3 months prior to conception. Young women ages 18-24 frequently diet for weight control and consequently lack adequate nutrients. Most (80%) pregnancies in this age group are unintended, making it likely that their folic acid intake was inadequate and thereby increasing their risk for NTD.

To measure the knowledge and intake of folic acid by young women, a nurse researcher surveyed 42 nursing majors ages 19 to 24. Approximately one in five thought that folic acid would prevent Down syndrome, 10% thought it would prevent cerebral palsy, and 62% correctly identified that it would help prevent spina bifida. Slightly more than half of the students knew that folic acid was one of the vitamin B complexes. All the participants had inadequate folic acid in their diets, and only one in three took multivitamin supplements.

IMPLICATIONS FOR PRACTICE

Nurses have many resources to use in helping to increase public awareness of folic acid, such as the March of Dimes and the Folic Acid campaign. Information about nutrition and folic acid and NTDs needs to be available in settings where young women get health care, such as college student health clinics, public health clinics, physician offices, and in the workplace. Adequate family planning counseling is also essential.

Reference: Hilton, J. (2002). Folic acid intake of young women. *Journal of Obstetric, Gynecologic, and Neonatal Nursing, 31*(2), 172-177.

Encephalocele and Anencephaly

Encephalocele and anencephaly are abnormalities resulting from failure of the anterior end of the neural tube to close. An **encephalocele** is a herniation of the brain and meninges through a skull defect. Treatment consists of surgical repair and shunting to relieve hydrocephalus, unless a major brain malformation is present. Most of these infants will have some degree of cognitive deficit. **Anencephaly** is the absence of both cerebral hemispheres and of the overlying skull. This condition is incompatible with life; many of the infants are stillborn or die within a few days of birth. Comfort measures are provided until the infant eventually dies of respiratory failure.

Spina Bifida

Spina bifida, the most common defect of the CNS, results from failure of the neural tube to close at some point. The two categories of spina bifida are spina bifida occulta and spina bifida cystica. Spina bifida occulta is a malformation in which the posterior portion of the laminas fails to close, but the spinal cord or meninges do not herniate or protrude through the defect (Fig. 39-2). It is usually asymptomatic and may be not diagnosed unless there are associated problems. Spina bifida cystica includes meningocele and myelomeningocele. A meningocele is an external sac that contains meninges and cerebrospinal fluid (CSF) and that protrudes through a defect in the vertebral column. A **myelomeningocele** is similar, except that it also contains nerves, resulting in motor and sensory deficits below the lesion. Myelomeningocele occurs in approximately 0.4 to 1 per 1000 live births in the United States each year, with this number varying by region of the country (Ball & Bindler, 1999).

A myelomeningocele, which is visible at birth and most often in the lumbosacral area, is usually covered with a very fragile, thin membrane (see Fig. 39-2). The sac can tear easily, allowing CSF to leak out, as well as providing an entry for infectious agents into the CNS. Myelomeningocele usually is associated with an Arnold-Chiari malformation, which results from the improper development and downward displacement of part of the brain into the cervical spinal canal. This in turn results in the development of hydrocephalus, which affects about 90% of children with myelomeningocele, although it may not be present at birth. The long-term prognosis in an affected infant can be determined to a large extent at birth, with the degree of neurologic dysfunction related to the level of the lesion, which determines the nerves involved (Bowman et al., 2001). Although decisions regarding closure of the sac and treatment traditionally have been a matter of controversy, many physicians now recommend that treatment be instituted regardless of the level of the lesion, unless there is a severe CNS anomaly, advanced hydrocephalus at birth, severe anoxic brain damage, active CNS infection, or a congenital malformation or syndromes incompatible with long-term survival. Prenatal diagnosis of myelomeningocele by maternal serum alpha-fetoprotein, ultrasonography, and amniocentesis has made possible a scheduled cesarean birth, allowing more careful delivery of the infant's back to try to prevent rupture of the meningeal sac.

A major preoperative nursing intervention for a neonate with a myelomeningocele is protection of the protruding sac from injury to prevent its rupture and resultant risk of CNS infection. Such infants should be positioned in a side-lying or prone position to prevent pressure on the sac until surgical repair is done. If the infant is allowed to be held, the nurse or parent must be careful to prevent injury to the sac. The sac should be covered with a sterile, moist, nonadherent dressing, and sterile techniques used in its care. The skin around the defect must be cleansed and dried carefully to prevent breakdown, which would establish a portal of entry for infectious agents. Because a lack of normal innervation may prevent the bladder from emptying completely, the Credé method is used at regular intervals to express urine from the bladder.

Other nursing care involves an assessment of the infant's neurologic function that includes the status of the following: apparent paralysis of lower extremities; the flaccidity and spasticity of muscles below the defect; and sphincter control, as evidenced by the number and char-

A

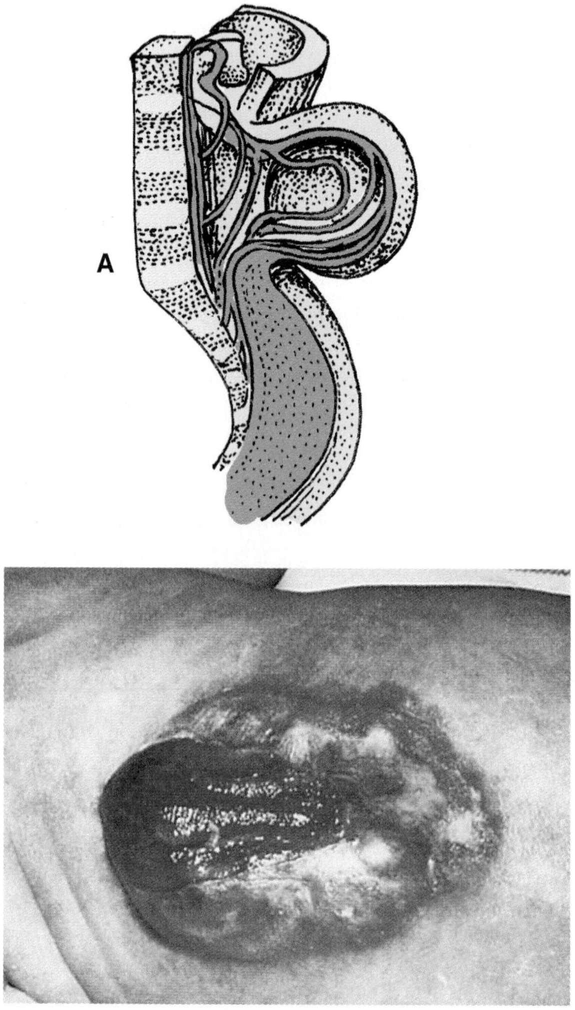

B

FIG. 39-2 **A,** Myelomeningocele. Note absence of vertebral arches. **B,** Myelomeningocele (spina bifida). (From Zitelli, B., & Davis, H. [1997]. *Atlas of pediatric physical diagnosis.* [3rd ed.]. St. Louis: Mosby.)

acter of voidings and stools, as well as the leakage of urine and stool. The infant's head circumference is measured, and other neurologic assessments are performed to determine the presence and degree of hydrocephalus.

A major nursing intervention is providing support and needed information to parents as they begin to learn to cope with an infant who has immediate needs for intensive care and probably will have long-term needs as well. Surgical repair is often done in the neonatal period, preferably within the first 24 hours. Early closure can prevent CNS infection and trauma to the exposed nerves. It also can prevent stretching of other nerve roots, which can occur as the sac continues to enlarge after birth. Surgical shunt procedures to prevent increasing hydrocephalus may be needed. Other problems, such as infection, are treated as they occur. Additionally, these infants are at increased risk for developing latex sensitivity, so latex precautions should be enforced.

Maternal-fetal surgery to repair a fetal myelomeningocele is a significant new development in maternal-fetal intervention. The rationale for this intervention is based on direct and indirect evidence that some of the neural damage resulting from the myelomeningocele is acquired in the later part of gestation, caused by amniotic fluid exposure or trauma to the exposed neural elements. It is believed that closure of the defect will prevent this damage, resulting in less hydrocephalus, lower extremity impairment, and bowel and bladder incontinence (Flake, 2001). Although this seems to be a good treatment option, a number of issues are debated, the most important being that because of the nature and complexity of myelomeningocele, it is difficult to prove benefits that offset the significant maternal risk involved. Second, there is a significant likelihood that maternal-fetal surgery will increase the mortality rate and the probability of premature birth with its accompanying problems. The term birth of an infant with myelomeningocele is a viable alternative to fetal repair. Numerous other significant issues have been addressed in the consideration of maternal-fetal surgery for this and other nonlethal anomalies. The National Institutes of Health (NIH) is sponsoring a randomized, multi-institution trial to investigate the open fetal repair of myelomeningocele compared with standard postnatal treatment (Flake, 2001).

Hydrocephalus

Hydrocephalus is a condition in which the ventricles of the brain are enlarged as a result of an imbalance between the production and absorption of the CSF. It is almost always caused by interference with the circulation and absorption of CSF. Congenital hydrocephalus usually arises as a result of a malformation in the brain or an intrauterine infection. It occurs in approximately 3 to 4 per 1000 live births (Jackson & Harvey, 2000). Approximately one third of all cases of congenital hydrocephalus result from stenosis of the aqueduct of Sylvius in the brain. Hydrocephalus commonly occurs in conjunction with a myelomeningocele, which blocks the flow of CSF.

An infant with congenital hydrocephalus will initially have a bulging anterior fontanel and a head circumference that increases at an abnormal rate, resulting from the increase in CSF pressure (Fig. 39-3). Enlargement of the forehead with depressed eyes that are rotated downward, causing a "setting sun" sign, occurs as the condition worsens. If the surgical shunting of excess CSF from the brain is not done soon after birth, the resulting increasing intracranial pressure will lead to irreversible neurologic damage, as evidenced by palpably widening sutures and fontanels, lethargy, poor feeding, vomiting, irritability, opisthotonos, and a high-pitched, shrill cry.

Nursing actions appropriate to the needs of a newborn with hydrocephalus include careful documentation of the ongoing observations. The occipitofrontal circumference of the head is measured daily at its largest point, and neurologic assessments are done frequently. If the infant's head is large, the placement of sheepskin or a flotation mattress under the infant and frequent position changes are necessary to prevent skin breakdown resulting from the pressure.

The infant's heavy head should be supported carefully during holding or turning, and positioning in the crib should be done in such a way that a patent airway is maintained. The method, amount, and frequency of feeding are determined by the infant's tolerance and energy level. The nurse should be alert to the possibility of projectile vomiting, which is a frequent occurrence in the presence of increased intracranial pressure, and maintain aspiration precautions. Nonnutritive sucking, touching, and cuddling needs should be met.

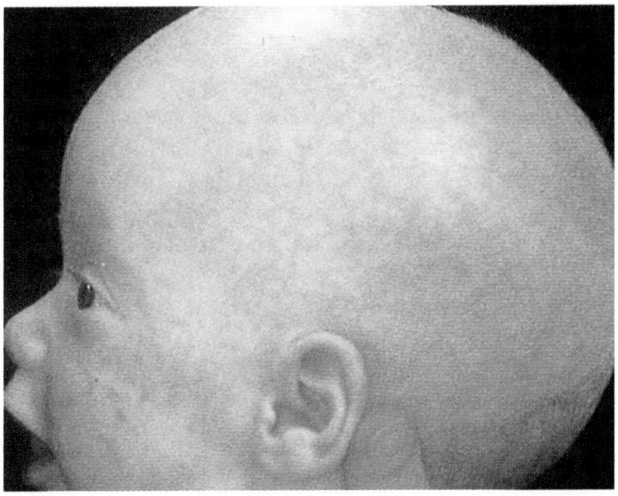

FIG. 39-3 Infantile hydrocephalus. The characteristic appearance is an enlarged head, thinning of the scalp, distended scalp veins, and a full fontanel. (From Booth, I., & Wozniak, E. [1984]. *Pediatrics*. Baltimore: Williams & Wilkins.)

Diagnosis is made by computed tomography and magnetic resonance imaging; antenatal diagnosis can be made by fetal ultrasonography. The surgical correction of hydrocephalus involves the placement of a shunt that goes from the ventricles of the brain usually to the peritoneum to allow the drainage of excess CSF. Damaged or destroyed brain tissue cannot be restored; the long-term prognosis in affected infants depends on the presence and extent of such tissue damage, along with the cause of the hydrocephalus; the presence of concurrent neurologic problems; and the long-term success of the shunt procedure.

Microcephaly

Microcephaly refers to a small brain in a generally normally formed head. It can be an autosomal recessive disorder or the result of a chromosomal abnormality; exposure of the woman to x-rays; alcohol ingestion; or rubella, cytomegalovirus, or other maternal infections. Microcephalic infants require supportive nursing care and medical observation to determine the extent of the psychomotor retardation that almost always accompanies this abnormality. There is no treatment. Parents need support to learn to care for a child with such cognitive impairment.

Respiratory System Anomalies

Screening for congenital anomalies of the respiratory system is necessary even in infants who are apparently normal at birth. Respiratory distress at birth or shortly thereafter may be the result of lung immaturity or anomalous development. Congenital laryngeal web and bilateral choanal atresia are readily apparent at birth. Respiratory distress caused by diaphragmatic hernia and tracheoesophageal fistula may appear immediately or be delayed, depending on the severity of the defect.

Choanal Atresia and Laryngeal Web

Choanal atresia (Fig. 39-4) is the most common congenital anomaly of the nose; it is a bony or membranous septum located between the nose and the pharynx. Inability to pass a suction catheter through the nose into the pharynx usually leads to its detection. Nearly half of the infants with choanal atresia have other anomalies. Infants with either a laryngeal web or choanal atresia require emergency surgery. A laryngeal web, which is uncommon, results from the incomplete separation of the two sides of the larynx and is most often between the vocal cords.

Congenital Diaphragmatic Hernia

Congenital diaphragmatic hernia (CDH) results from a defect in the formation of the diaphragm, allowing the abdominal organs to be displaced into the thoracic cavity. It occurs in approximately 1 in 2500 live births (Lockridge, Caldwell, & Jason, 2002); however, if stillbirths resulting from this defect are included, the incidence increases to 1 in 2000. Herniation of the abdominal viscera into the thoracic cavity may cause severe respiratory distress and represent a neonatal emergency (Fig. 39-5). The defect and herniation may be minimal and easily repaired, or the defect may be so extensive that the viscera present in the thoracic cavity during embryonic life have prevented the normal development of pulmonary and sometimes cardiac tissue. The defect is usually on the left because that is the side of the diaphragm that fuses last.

Most congenital diaphragmatic hernias are discovered prenatally on ultrasound studies and may be repaired by fetal surgery in some research institutions. At birth, most affected infants have severe respiratory distress, and respiratory assessment reveals worsening distress as the bowels fill with air. Typically the breath sounds are diminished, and bowel sounds are heard in the chest. Heart sounds may be heard on the right side of the chest because the heart has been displaced there by the abdominal contents. Physical examination reveals a flat or scaphoid abdomen and a prominent ipsilateral chest. Diagnosis can be made on the basis of the radiographic study finding of loops of intestine in the thoracic cavity and the absence of intestine in the abdominal cavity.

Surgical repair is performed as soon as is feasible. There appears to be no difference in mortality rate if the surgical repair is done before or after 24 hours of age (Moyer et al., 2001). Preoperative nursing interventions include participating in the stabilization of the infant's condition until surgical repair can be done. The infant should be positioned with the head and chest elevated and the af-

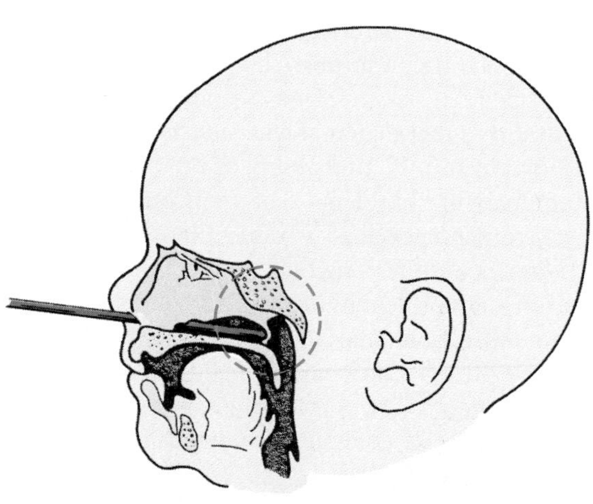

FIG. 39-4 Choanal atresia. Posterior nares are obstructed by membrane or bone either bilaterally or unilaterally. Infant becomes cyanotic at rest. With crying, newborn's color improves. Nasal discharge is present. Snorting respirations often are observed with increased respiratory effort. Newborn may be unable to breathe and eat at the same time. Diagnosis is made by noting inability to pass small feeding tube through one or both nares. (Used with permission of Ross Products Division, Abbott Laboratories, Inc., Columbus, OH 43216. From Clinical Education Aid #6, Copyright 1963, Ross Products Division, Abbott Laboratories, Inc.)

fected side downward to allow the normal lung to expand. Gastric contents are aspirated and suction applied to decompress the gastrointestinal tract and prevent further cardiothoracic compromise. Oxygen therapy, mechanical ventilation, and the correction of acidosis are necessary in infants with large defects. As a result of the lung hypoplasia that affected infants sometimes have, pulmonary hypertension occurs. Extracorporeal membrane oxygenation (ECMO) or high-frequency oscillatory ventilation may be used in infants with severe circulatory and respiratory complications (see Chapter 40). The prognosis for these infants depends largely on the degree of lung hypoplasia and the success of surgical diaphragmatic closure, but the prognosis in severe cases is poor. The Extracorporeal Life Support Organization (ELSO) registry, which is the largest registry of infants with congenital diaphragmatic hernia, reports on the outcome of infants treated with ECMO. A 59% survival rate was found in the 2627 infants who were registered by mid-1997. Of those survivors, a significant number had chronic lung disease with long-term oxygen dependency, feeding difficulties, and gastroesophageal reflux (Finer et al., 1998). Other preoperative management modalities include use of surfactant; steroids such as dexamethasone; and inhaled nitric oxide (NO), which acts as a selective pulmonary dilator and is FDA approved for use in newborns older than 34 weeks of gestation (Juretschke, 2001). Another new therapy is the use of partial liquid ventilation with oxygenated perfluorocarbon (Perflubron) to attain better gas exchange (Boloker et al., 2002).

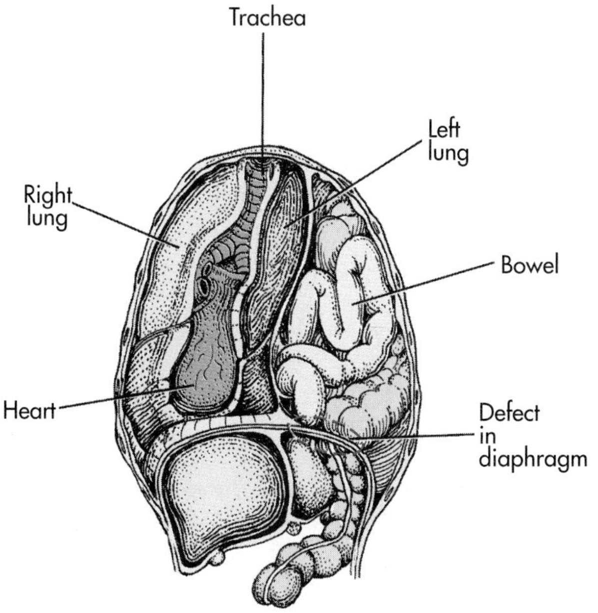
Trachea
Left lung
Right lung
Bowel
Heart
Defect in diaphragm

FIG. 39-5 Diaphragmatic hernia. (Used with permission of Ross Products Division, Abbott Laboratories, Inc., Columbus, OH 43216. From Clinical Education Aid #6, Copyright 1963, Ross Products Division, Abbott Laboratories, Inc.)

Some success was reported with fetal repair, but the mortality rate associated with it is higher than that associated with current conventional management, including ECMO. A current NIH-sponsored randomized study investigates prenatal treatment compared with standard postnatal treatment (Flake, 2001).

Gastrointestinal System Anomalies

Anomalies in the gastrointestinal system can occur anywhere along the gastrointestinal tract, from the mouth to the anus. Some anomalies, such as cleft lip, omphalocele, and gastroschisis, are apparent at birth. Others, including cleft palate, esophageal atresia, pyloric stenosis, intestinal obstructions, and imperforate anus, become apparent as the infant is further assessed or becomes symptomatic. These anomalies arise as a result of the interrupted development of that particular organ at a crucial point during organogenesis.

Cleft Lip and Palate

Cleft lip or palate is a commonly occurring congenital midline fissure, or opening, in the lip or palate resulting from failure of the primary palate to fuse (Fig. 39-6). One or both deformities may occur, and nasal deformity may also be present. Multiple genetic and, to a lesser extent, environmental factors, such as maternal infection, radiation exposure, alcohol ingestion, and treatment with medications such as corticosteroids, some tranquilizers, and anticonvulsants, appear to be involved in their development.

Cleft lip with or without cleft palate occurs in approximately 1 in 800 live births (Bender, 2000; Mitchell & Wood, 2000). It is more common in Native American and Asians and less common in African-Americans. Cleft lip is more common in male infants. Smoking during pregnancy increases the risk of cleft lip and palate by 50%; the risk is in direct proportion to the number of cigarettes smoked (Chung et al., 2000). The defect can range from a simple notch in the lip to complete separation of the lip that extends to the floor of the nose. The treatment for a cleft lip is surgical repair, which usually is done between ages 6 and 12 weeks, if the infant is healthy and free of infection. Advances in surgical techniques have made it possible for some infants, particularly those with unilateral cleft lip, to have a near-normal appearance. The results of the repair depend on the severity of the defect, with more severe bilateral cleft lip requiring surgical repair done in stages.

Anomalies of the palate often occur in association with cleft lip. Cleft palate alone occurs in approximately 1 in 2000 live births (Bender, 2000; Mitchell & Wood, 2000). It is more common in female infants and occurs more frequently as a constituent of certain syndromes. This defect can range from a cleft in the uvula to a complete cleft of the hard and soft palates that may be unilateral, bilateral, or midline. Feeding is difficult because the cleft lip renders the newborn unable to maintain a seal around a nipple, and the cleft palate renders the infant unable to form a vacuum to maintain suction when feeding. In addition, the inability to suck and swallow normally allows milk to pool in the nasopharynx, which increases the likelihood of aspiration. Furthermore, as the infant attempts to suck, milk often comes out through the cleft and out of the nares. Although the degree of difficulty depends on the size of the cleft, feeding problems are greater in infants with a cleft palate than in those with a cleft lip. Regardless of the extent and type of defect, feeding may become a very frustrating experience for parents. Breastfeeding can be successful in some infants, particularly if the infant has a cleft lip alone. Infants with cleft palate can be put to the breast, but because they are unable to obtain sufficient suction will be ineffective in obtaining adequate nutrition without supplements or specialized techniques (Glass & Wolf, 1999). Special nipples, bottles, and appliances are available to aid in feeding (Fig. 39-6, *E*; Fig. 39-7). In general, parents of infants with these defects need education and support as they learn to feed their baby, to prevent what should be a normal part of infant care from becoming a very frustrating experience.

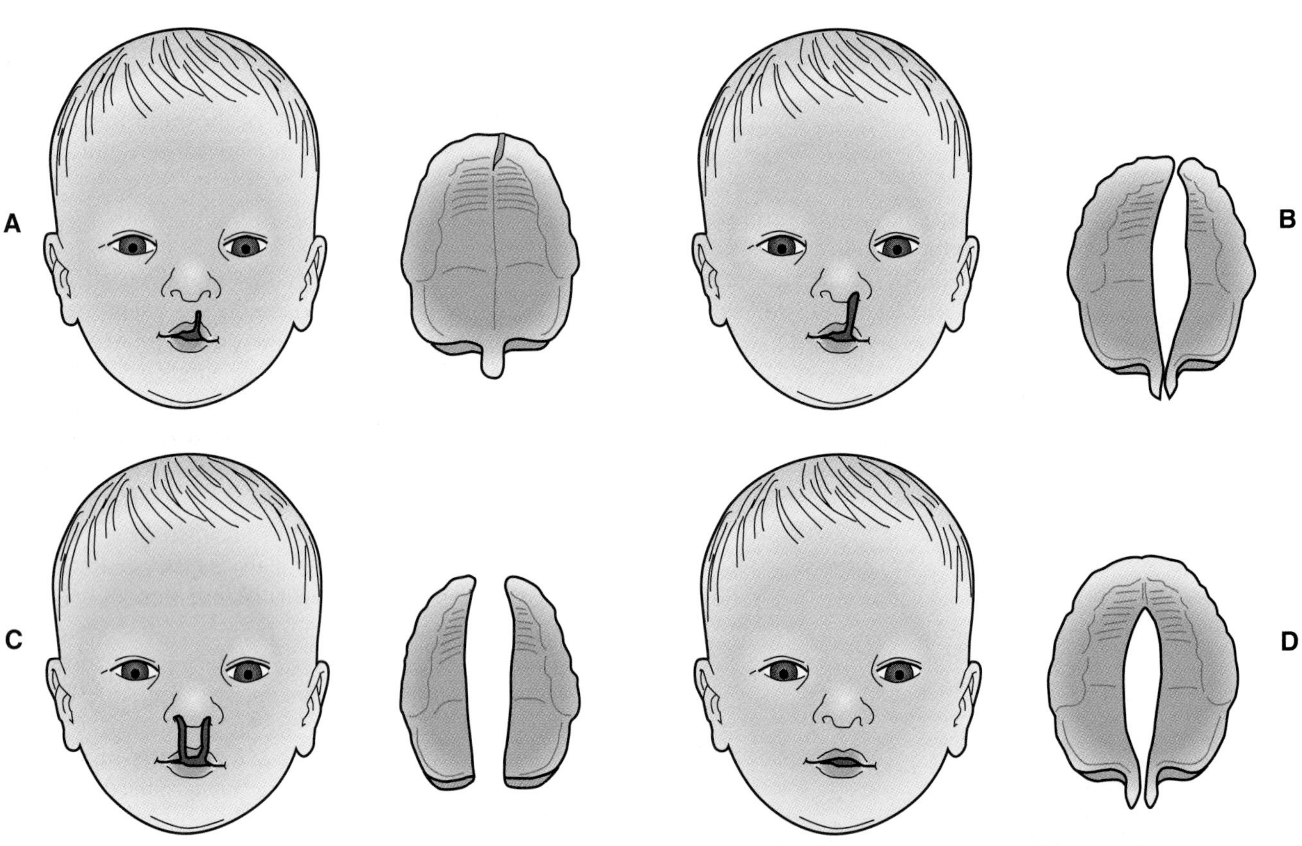
A
B
C
D

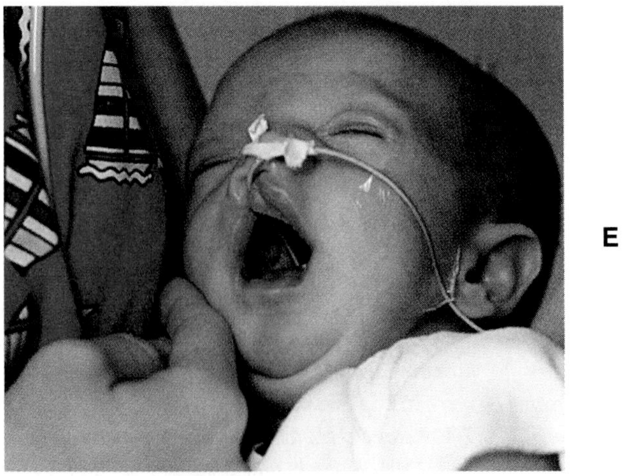
E

FIG. 39-6 Variations in clefts of lip and palate at birth. **A,** Notch in vermilion border. **B,** Unilateral cleft lip and cleft palate. **C,** Bilateral cleft lip and cleft palate. **D,** Cleft palate. **E,** Infant with complete unilateral cleft lip. Note the feeding tube. (**A-D,** From Hockenberry, M. et al. [2003]. *Wong's nursing care of infants and children* [7th ed.]. St. Louis: Mosby. **E,** From Dickason, E., Silverman, B., & Kaplan J. [1998]. *Maternal-infant nursing care* [3rd ed.]. St. Louis: Mosby.)

The type of surgical repair done to close the cleft palate is based on the degree of the cleft and, as with a cleft lip, if severe, may necessitate repair done in stages. Repair is begun at 6 to 18 months, after some development of the affected area has occurred. Early repair helps avert some of the speech problems that may occur in people with palate defects. Long-term care is often necessary for children with a cleft palate and involves the combined efforts of a health care team comprising acute care and community nurses; social workers; ear, nose, and throat and plastic surgeons; speech therapists; and orthodontists.

Parents of infants with a cleft lip or palate need much support, particularly in the case of a cleft lip, because this is both a cosmetic and functional defect. Recognizing that this may interfere with normal parent-infant bonding in the neonatal period, the nurse must assess for this and intervene appropriately.

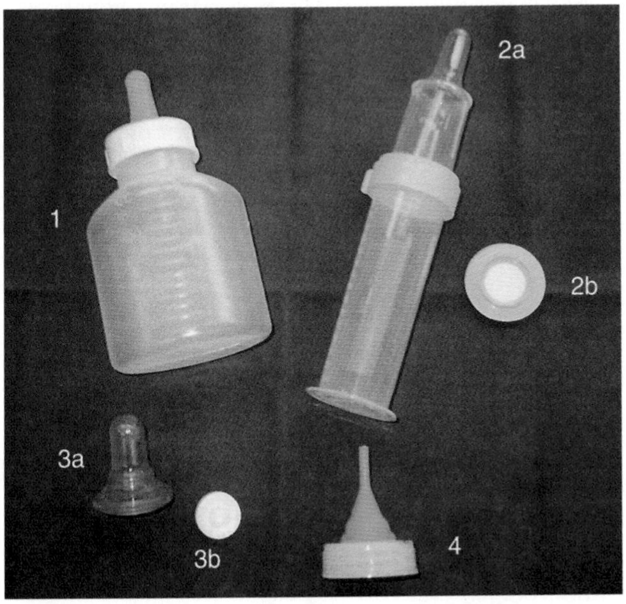
1
2a
2b
3a
3b
4

FIG. 39-7 *1*, Mead Johnson bottle and nipple for cleft palate. Cleft palate nipple system (*2a*) with valve (*2b*) to regulate flow. Haberman feeder (*3a*) with disc (*3b*) to control flow of milk. *4*, Ross cleft palate assembly. Nipple can be trimmed to accommodate palate size. (Courtesy Shannon Perry, San Jose, CA.)

Esophageal Atresia and Tracheoesophageal Fistula

Esophageal atresia (EA) and tracheoesophageal fistula (TEF), the most life-threatening anomalies of the esophagus, often occur together, although they can occur singly. **Esophageal atresia** is a congenital anomaly in which the esophagus ends in a blind pouch or narrows into a thin cord, thus failing to form a continuous passageway to the stomach. TEF is an abnormal connection between the esophagus and trachea.

Hydramnios is a common maternal finding, particularly if the fetus has an EA without a TEF. Variations of the anomalies are possible, depending on the presence or absence of a TEF, the site of the fistula, and the location and degree of the esophageal obstruction. The most common variant is the combination of a proximal EA, in which the esophagus ends in a blind pouch, with a distal TEF, in which the lower esophagus exits the stomach and is connected to the trachea by a fistula, rather than forming a continuous tube to the upper esophagus (Fig. 39-8). This defect occurs in approximately 1 in 4000 live births (Adzick &

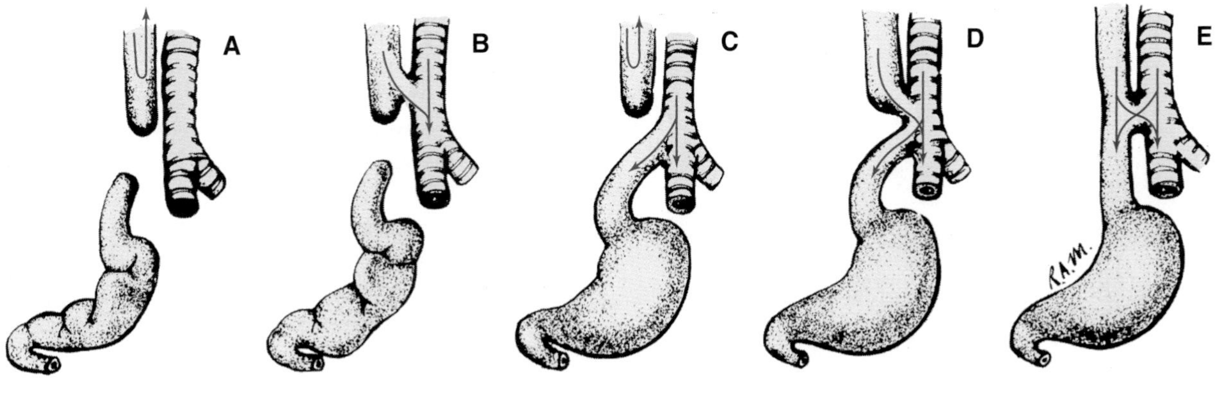
A
B
C
D
E

FIG. 39-8 Congenital atresia of esophagus and tracheoesophageal fistula. **A,** Upper and lower segments of esophagus end in blind sac, occurring in 5% to 8% of such infants. **B,** Upper segment of esophagus ends in atresia and connects to trachea by fistulous tract, occurring rarely. **C,** Upper segment of esophagus ends in blind pouch; lower segment connects with trachea by small fistulous tract, occurring in 80% to 95% of such infants. **D,** Both segments of esophagus connect by fistulous tracts to trachea, occurring in less than 1% of such infants. Infant may aspirate with first feeding. **E,** Esophagus is continuous but connects by fistulous tract to trachea; known as *H-type*. (From Hockenberry, M. et al. [2003]. *Wong's nursing care of infants and children* [7th ed.]. St. Louis: Mosby.)

Nance, 2000). More than half of the infants have associated anomalies, which are usually cardiac or gastrointestinal.

Infants with the life-threatening anomaly EA with TEF show significant respiratory difficulty immediately after birth. EA with or without TEF results in excessive oral secretions, drooling, and feeding intolerance. When fed, the infant may swallow, but then cough and gag and return the fluid through the nose and mouth. Respiratory distress can result from aspiration or from the acute gastric distention produced by the TEF. Choking, coughing, and cyanosis occur after even a small amount of fluid is taken by mouth.

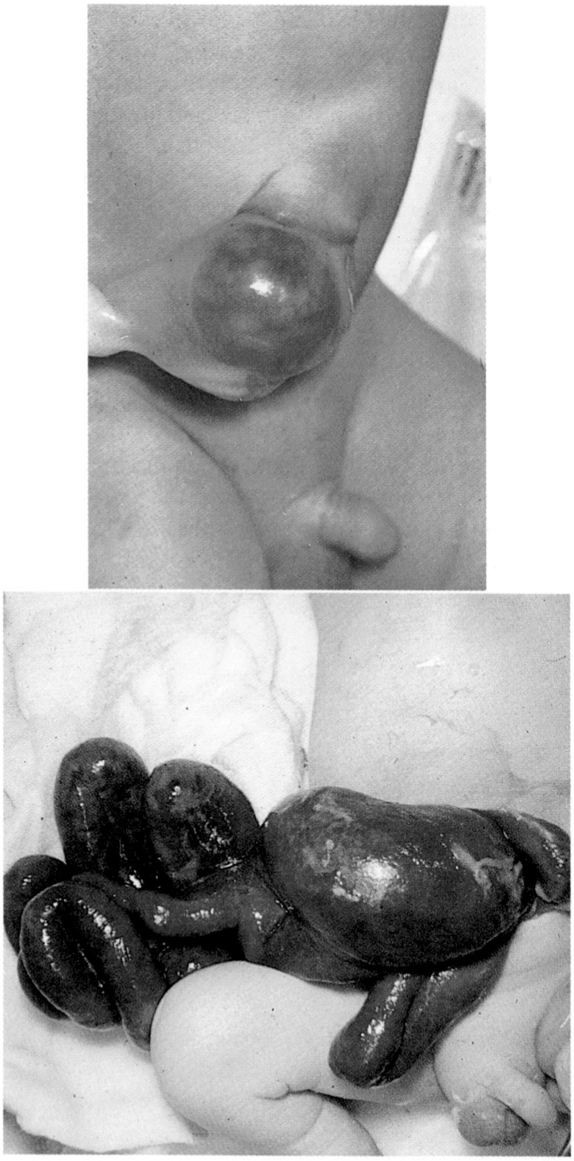

A

B

FIG. 39-9 **A,** Omphalocele. **B,** Gastroschisis of bowel and stomach. (**A,** From O'Doherty, N. [1986]. *Neonatology: Micro atlas of the newborn.* Nutley, NJ: Hoffmann-La Roche. **B,** Courtesy Wyeth-Ayerst Laboratories, Philadelphia, PA.)

Nursing interventions are supportive until surgery is performed.

NURSE ALERT

Any infant with excessive oral secretions and respiratory distress should not be fed orally until a physician is consulted.

The infant with EA and TEF is placed in a semi-Fowler position, which facilitates respiratory efforts and diminishes the reflux of gastric contents into the trachea. A double-lumen catheter is placed in the proximal esophageal pouch and attached to continuous suction to remove secretions and decrease the possibility of aspiration. The infant requires close observation and intervention to maintain a patent airway. Other supportive measures include maintaining fluid and electrolyte balance intravenously, and thermoregulation. Surgical correction, done in one stage if possible, consists of ligating the fistula and anastomosing the two segments of the esophagus. Prematurity increases the risk of poor outcome. In addition, major congenital cardiac and chromosomal anomalies have been found to be predictors of a poor outcome (Chondhury et al., 1999). The mortality rate for these infants is reported as high as 50%. The survival rate for infants in a good risk category exceeds 95% (Adzick & Nance, 2000).

Omphalocele and Gastroschisis

Although uncommon, omphalocele and gastroschisis are two of the more frequently occurring congenital defects of the abdominal wall. The incidence of omphalocele is approximately 1 in 5000 live births, and the incidence of gastroschisis is about 1 to 3 in 10,000 live births (Hockenberry et al., 2003). An **omphalocele** is a covered defect of the umbilical ring into which varying amounts of the abdominal organs may herniate (Fig. 39-9, *A*). Although it is covered with a peritoneal sac, the sac may rupture during or after birth. More than half of the infants born with an omphalocele are premature and have other serious syndromes or anomalies involving the gastrointestinal, cardiac, genitourinary, musculoskeletal, and nervous systems.

Gastroschisis is the herniation of the bowel through a defect in the abdominal wall to the right of the umbilical cord (Fig. 39-9, *B*), and no protective sac covers the intestines. These infants rarely have associated anomalies. Nearly all are of low birth weight and more than half are premature (Howell, 1998).

The preoperative nursing care for infants with either defect is similar. Exposure of the viscera causes problems with thermoregulation and fluid and electrolyte balance. A common method to prevent evaporative heat loss from the exposed bowel preoperatively is to place the infant immediately after birth into a sterile bag covering the lower two thirds of the body (Howell, 1998). Antibiotics, fluid and electrolyte replacement, gastric decompression, and thermoregulation are needed for physiologic support. If complete closure is impossible because of the small size of the defect and the large amount of viscera to be replaced, a polymeric silicone (Silastic; Dow Corning, Midland, MI) silo pouch is created and sewn to the fascia of the abdominal defect. This protects the contents as they are gradually placed back into the abdominal cavity. The defect is closed surgically after the reduction of the contents that have been exposed is completed, which usually takes 7 to 10 days. Preoperative gastric decompression is necessary to prevent aspiration pneumonia and to allow as much bowel as possible to be placed into the abdomen during surgery. Surgery is usually performed soon after birth. With improved surgical treatment, nutritional support, and medical management, the prognosis has improved for infants born with an abdominal wall defect. It is estimated that more than 71% of infants born with an omphalocele survive, as do more than 90% of those born with gastroschisis (Hockenberry et al., 2003). It is thought that minimizing septic complications would contribute significantly to reducing the mortality (Driver et al., 2000).

Parental support is essential, because the infant has an obvious disfiguring anomaly that can be shocking and repulsive in appearance. Depending on the size of the defect, the infant may also be critically ill before surgery. The nurse must be aware of the effect this may have on parental bonding and intervene appropriately as the parents cope with this crisis.

Gastrointestinal Obstruction

Congenital intestinal obstruction can occur anywhere in the gastrointestinal tract and occurs in the form of atresia, which is a complete obliteration of the passage; partial obstruction, in which the symptoms may vary in severity and sometimes not be detected in the neonatal period; or malrotation of the intestine, which leads to twisting of the intestine (volvulus) and obstruction. EA, discussed previously, is a type of gastrointestinal obstruction. Duodenal atresia, midgut malrotation and volvulus, jejunoileal atresia, necrotizing enterocolitis, and meconium ileus are the most common causes of neonatal intestinal obstruction (Kimura, 2000). Meconium ileus is an obstruction caused by impacted meconium and is the earliest symptom of cystic fibrosis, a life-threatening chronic illness. Infants with this type of obstruction should be tested for cystic fibrosis, because 95% of infants with meconium ileus have cystic fibrosis. Meconium ileus occurs in 7% to 25% of patients with cystic fibrosis (Bensard et al., 2002).

The infant shows the following cardinal signs and symptoms: bilious vomiting, abdominal distention, and failure to pass normal amounts of meconium in the first 24 hours. High intestinal obstruction is characterized by vomiting, even if the infant is not being fed orally. A low obstruction is characterized primarily by distention, with vomiting occurring later. Abdominal distention can elevate the diaphragm, which causes respiratory difficulties. Careful evaluation must be done to make a correct diagnosis.

Nursing care is aimed at supporting the infant until surgical intervention can be carried out to eliminate the obstruction. Oral feedings are discontinued, a nasogastric tube is placed for suction, and intravenous therapy is initiated to provide needed fluid and electrolytes. In infants with an intestinal obstruction, surgery consists of resecting the obstructed area of bowel and anastomosing the nonaffected bowel. In recent years, the survival rate for these infants has increased to 85% to 90% as a result of better treatments, better neonatal intensive care, and a better understanding of the total problem.

Imperforate Anus

Imperforate anus describes a wide range of congenital disorders involving the anus and rectum (Fig. 39-10). More common in male infants, it occurs in approximately 1 in 5000 live births (Bensard et al., 2002). It results from the failure of anorectal development in weeks 7 and 8 of gestational life. Such infants have no anal opening, and frequently a fistula from the rectum to the perineum or genitourinary system also is found (Fig. 39-11). The defect can be further classified according to its location as a "high" or "low" type, which determines the treatments necessary, as

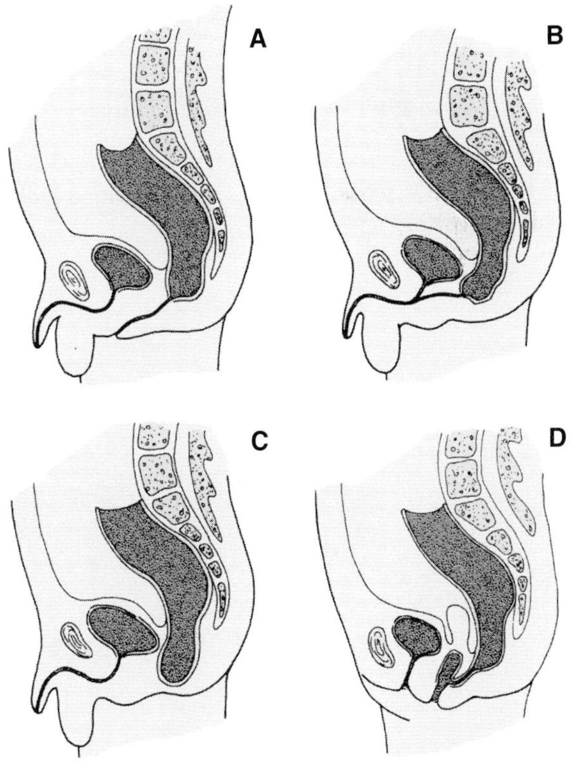
A
B
C
D

FIG. 39-10 Types of imperforate anus. Anal sphincter muscle may be present and intact. **A,** High lesion opening onto perineum through narrow fistulous tract. **B,** High lesion ending in fistulous tract to urinary tract. **C,** Low lesion in bowel passes through puborectal muscle. **D,** High lesion ending in fistulous tract to vagina.

well as the prognosis. Infants with high defects, which occur primarily in male infants, require a colostomy in the neonatal period, with corrective surgery done in stages over time. Low anomalies may involve stenotic areas, or a thin translucent membrane may cover the anal opening. Treatment for such a membrane is excision followed by daily dilation, which parents are taught to do. Other low lesions are surgically corrected by anoplasty. The preoperative nursing care is similar to that described for other gastrointestinal obstructions. Imperforate anus is often associated with other anomalies, with nearly half having additional genitourinary anomalies, which may complicate long-term care.

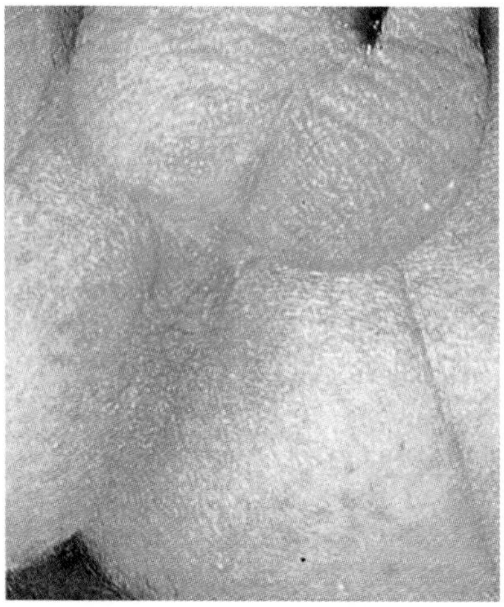

FIG. 39-11 Imperforate anus. (From Chessell, G. et al. [1984]. *Diagnostic picture tests in clinical medicine* [vol. 2]. St. Louis: Mosby.)

Musculoskeletal System Anomalies

The two most common musculoskeletal system anomalies seen in neonates are developmental dysplasia of the hip and congenital clubfoot. Both of these conditions must be detected and treated early for successful correction.

Developmental Dysplasia of the Hip

Developmental dysplasia of the hip (DDH) consists of disorders that result from the abnormal development of one or all of the components of the hip joint, resulting in instability of the hip. This causes one or both of the femoral heads to be displaced from the hip socket, or acetabulum. The dislocated femoral head does not exert pressure on the acetabulum, causing delayed development of the femoral head and failure of the acetabulum to form normally. The etiology is considered to be multifactorial, with genetic factors involved, and female infants are more often affected than are male infants. Risk factors for the defect include breech presentation, a family history, the birth order (firstborn), and prenatal maternal oligohydramnios with fetal compression and deformation. The effect of maternal hormones during pregnancy may foster hip joint capsule laxity, especially in the female infant. Some newborn screening surveys suggest evidence of instability in as many as 1 in 100 newborns and 1 to 1.5 cases of dislocation per 1000 newborns (Goldberg, 2001). Nearly one fourth of infants presenting in the breech position have DDH.

The examiner tests for an unstable or actually dislocated femoral head by abducting the hips and feeling for a click when the femoral head passes back into the acetabulum (see Fig. 25-12). Other diagnostic clues include an asymmetric number of skinfolds, one knee higher than the other when the hips and knees are flexed to

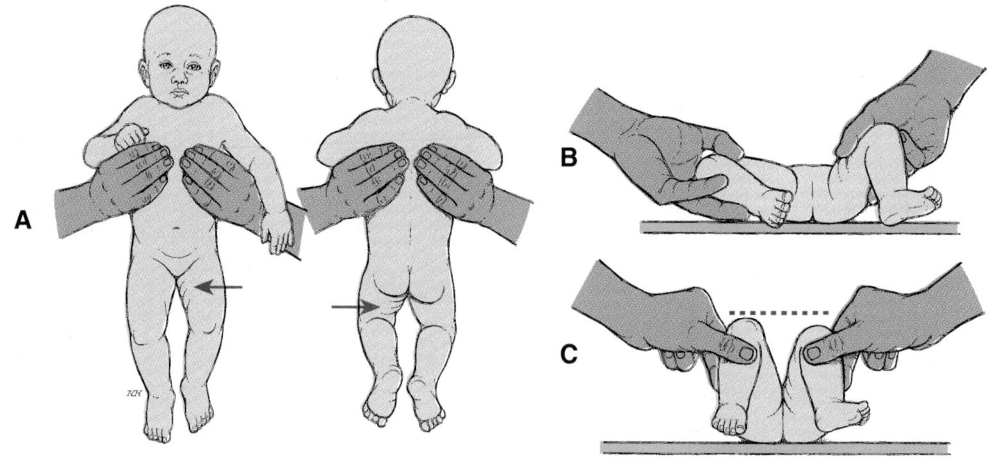
A
B
C

FIG. 39-12 Developmental dysplasia of hip. **A,** Asymmetry of gluteal and thigh folds. **B,** Limited hip abduction as seen in flexion. **C,** Apparent shortening of femur as indicated by the level of the knees in flexion. Femoral head is displaced. (From Hockenberry, M. et al. [2003]. *Wong's nursing care of infants and children* [7th ed.]. St. Louis: Mosby.)

90 degrees (Allis or Galeazzi sign), and limited hip abduction (Fig. 39-12).

Early detection, often by the nurse during a routine newborn assessment, allows early treatment, which is more effective than later treatment and can prevent complications. Treatment involves the use of a Pavlik harness, a dynamic device that keeps the hips and knees flexed, the hips abducted, and the femoral head in the acetabulum (Fig. 39-13). Worn continuously for 3 to 6 months, it promotes the development of muscle and cartilage, resulting in a stable hip. If the infant is treated between ages 1 and 8 months, the harness is effective 80% to 90% of the time (Hockenberry et al., 2003). If not effective, traction, casting, and even surgery may be necessary to stabilize the hip.

In addition to the major intervention of assessing and helping identify the disorder, another key nursing intervention is teaching the parents about the care of the infant, who will remain in the harness continuously during the treatment. Because this occurs during a time of maximal growth, it will be necessary for them to adjust the infant's care to accommodate the infant's changing needs. Continuing thorough follow-up care is necessary, as is psychosocial support for the family.

Clubfoot

Clubfoot is a congenital deformity in which portions of the foot and ankle are twisted out of a normal position. These can be of varying degrees of severity and assume a variety of combinations of abnormal positions. The most common, seen in approximately 95% of infants with clubfoot, is *talipes equinovarus*. In this abnormality, the foot appears C shaped, pointing downward and inward; the ankle is inverted; and the Achilles tendon is shortened. The foot appears small, wide, and stiff, and the lower leg appears small because of hypoplasia of the calf muscles. Unless treated, further stiffening occurs, and bony changes will result.

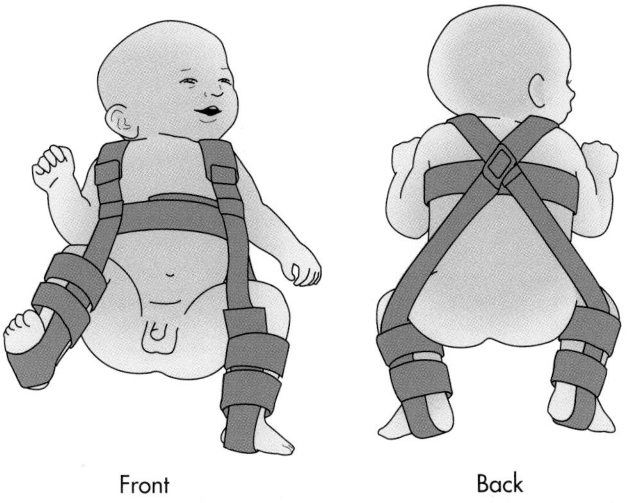
Front
Back

FIG. 39-13 Treatment for developmental dysplasia of the hip by application of the Pavlik harness. (From Ball, J. [1998]. *Mosby's pediatric patient teaching guides*. St. Louis: Mosby.)

Clubfoot is one of the most common congenital anomalies, occurring in approximately 1.5 per 1000 live births, with two times more male than female infants affected (Trilling & Potts, 2002). The condition is bilateral in about half of affected infants. The exact cause is unknown, but possibilities include a genetic predisposition, in utero compression, and abnormal embryonic development. Treatment begins soon after birth. This consists of manipulation and frequent serial casting, which is necessary because of the rapid growth of the infant. If this is ineffective, surgical correction is necessary. Although a controversial issue, the optimal age for surgery is generally acknowledged to be between 4 and 12 months. Treatment, which may continue into adolescence, often results in good function of the foot, although the feet may differ in size. The deformity may recur, and repeated surgery may be necessary.

Because these infants are often placed in a cast before discharge, the nurse must teach parents necessary care, including how to protect the cast and assess the toes for neurovascular compromise. This is particularly important because of the potential for the infant to outgrow the cast. As is true with the birth of any child with an anomaly, the nurse should be supportive of the parents as they learn the ways in which to meet the infant's normal needs, as well as those brought about by the infant's physical problem.

Polydactyly

Extra digits on the hands or feet occur occasionally. In some instances, polydactyly is hereditary. If there is little or no bone involvement, the extra digit is tied with silk suture soon after birth. The finger or toe falls off within a few days, leaving a small scar. When there is bone involvement, surgical repair is indicated.

Genitourinary System Anomalies

Anomalies involving the genitourinary system can be distressing to parents because they may be readily apparent and, in the case of some conditions, because of the concern about sexuality and reproductive functioning. These anomalies range from obvious anomalies of the external genitalia, such as hypospadias, to those involving internal organs that may not be detected but may cause damage to the urinary tract. An example of the latter is an obstruction in the urinary tract that can cause hydronephrosis, which is the abnormal collection of urine in the renal pelvis, which can eventually destroy the kidney.

Hypospadias and Epispadias

Hypospadias constitutes a range of penile anomalies associated with an abnormally located urinary meatus. The meatus can open below the glans penis or anywhere along the ventral surface of the penis, the scrotum, or the perineum. One of the most common congenital anomalies, it is thought to affect approximately 1 in 250 male births, although the exact incidence is unknown (Bergstein, 2000). It is classified according to the location of the meatus and the presence or absence of chordee, which is a ventral curvature of the penis. The cause is unknown, although it is thought to be of multifactorial inheritance. One large retrospective study found hypospadias to be significantly more prevalent in infants who had uniformly poor intrauterine growth (lower than the 10th percentile) in weight, length, and head circumference (Hussain et al., 2002).

Mild cases of hypospadias are often repaired for cosmetic reasons and involve a single surgical procedure. In more severe cases, several operations are required to reconstruct the urethral opening and correct the chordee, thereby straightening the penis. The goals are to improve the appearance of the genitalia, to enable the child to urinate in a standing position, and to provide a sexually adequate organ. It is vital that these infants not be circumcised, because the foreskin may be needed during surgical repair. Repair is done early, often during or soon after the first year of life, so that the child's body image is not impaired.

Epispadias, a rare anomaly affecting approximately 1 in 117,000 male infants and 1 in 480,000 female infants, results from failure of urethral canalization. Affected male infants have a widened pubic symphysis and a broad spadelike penis with the urethra opening on the dorsal surface. Female infants have a wide urethra and a bifid clitoris. Severity ranges from a mild to a severe anomaly that is associated with exstrophy of the bladder. Surgical correction is necessary, and affected male infants should not be circumcised.

Exstrophy of the Bladder

The most common bladder anomaly is exstrophy (Fig. 39-14), which often occurs in conjunction with epispadias. It is rare, occurring in approximately 1 in 35,000 to 40,000 live births (Bergstein, 2000). It results from the abnormal development of the bladder, abdominal wall, and pubic symphysis that causes the bladder, urethra, and ureteral orifices to all be exposed. The bladder is visible in the suprapubic area as a red mass with numerous folds, with urine draining from it onto the infant's skin. The bladder is covered with a sterile, nonadherent dressing to protect its delicate surface until closure can be performed. It is recommended that reconstructive surgery be started in the neonatal period, preferably with the bladder being closed during the first or second day of life. Parents will need much support as they deal with caring for an infant who has such an obvious defect. Repair is completed before school age, if possible, although some children never attain normal voiding patterns and later may be considered for surgery for urinary diversion.

Sexual Ambiguity

Sexual ambiguity in the newborn (Fig. 39-15) often is discovered by the nurse during a physical assessment. Erroneous or abnormal sexual differentiation may be a genetic aberration, such as congenital adrenal hypoplasia, which can be life threatening because of the deficiency of all adrenal cortical hormones involved. Other possible causes of sexual ambiguity include chromosomal abnormalities, defective sex hormone synthesis in male infants, and the placental transfer of masculinizing agents to female fetuses. Gender assignment should be based on data gathered from the following sources: maternal and family history, including the ingestion of steroids during pregnancy, and relatives with ambiguous genitalia or who died during

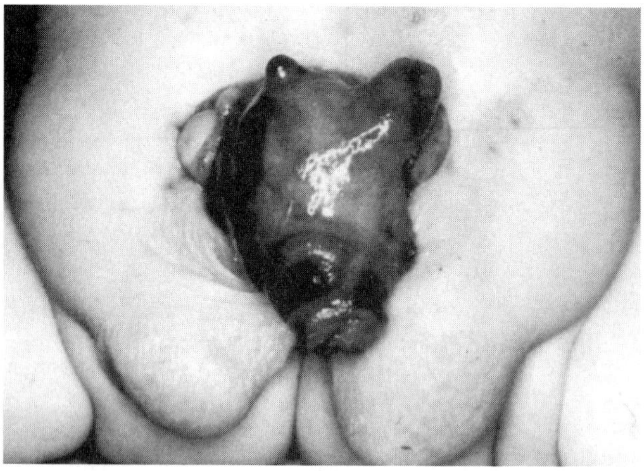

FIG. 39-14 Exstrophy of bladder. (Courtesy Edward S. Tank, M.D., Division of Urology, Oregon Health Science University, Portland, OR.)

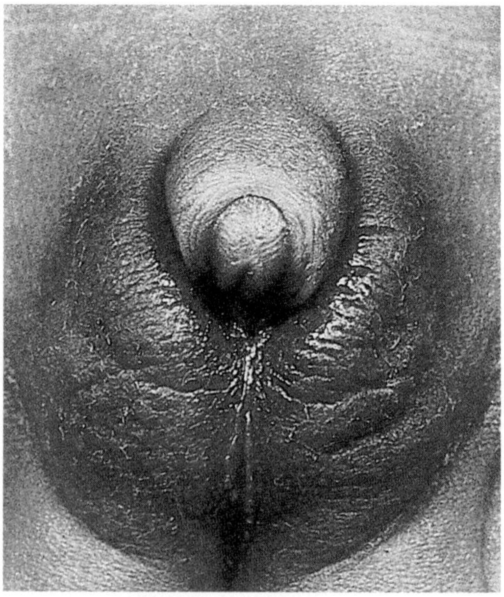

FIG. 39-15 Ambiguous external genitals (i.e., structure can be enlarged clitoral hood and clitoris or malformed penis). (Courtesy Edward S. Tank, M.D., Division of Urology, Oregon Health Science University, Portland, OR.)

the neonatal period; physical examination; chromosomal analysis (results are available in 2 to 3 days); endoscopy, ultrasonography, and radiographic contrast studies; biochemical tests, such as analysis of urinary steroid excretion, which helps detect several of the adrenal cortical syndromes; and, in some instances, laparotomy or gonad biopsy.

Therapeutic intervention, including any surgery, should be started as soon as possible. Any child born with ambiguous genitalia should not receive a sex assignment until the appropriate sex of rearing may be properly assessed and assigned. An appropriate sex assignment should be based on the following: potential for mature sexual function, potential fertility, and the long-term psychologic and intellectual impact on the child and family (Finegold, 1997). Parents need much support as they learn to deal with this very challenging situation.

Teratoma

A **teratoma** is an embryonal tumor that may be solid, cystic, or mixed. It is composed of at least two and usually three types of embryonal tissue: ectoderm, mesoderm, and endoderm. This rare tumor in the neonate may occur in the skull, cervical area, mediastinum, abdomen, or sacral area, with more than half located in the sacrococcygeal area. A cervical teratoma may compress the esophagus in utero and produce polyhydramnios. After birth, compression of the upper airway from the mass may create a surgical emergency (Nakayama, 1997). The treatment of choice is complete surgical resection. Approximately 80% of all teratomas are benign, and no additional therapy is needed after complete resection done in the neonatal period. If the tumor is not surgically resected before the infant is 1 to 2 months old, the likelihood of the teratoma becoming malignant increases rapidly.

CARE MANAGEMENT

Prenatal Diagnosis

Refined testing procedures are available to monitor fetal development. Prenatal diagnostic techniques such as amniocentesis, ultrasonography, alpha-fetoprotein measurements, chorionic villus sampling, percutaneous umbilical cord blood sampling, fetal nuchal translucency (FNT) screening (Beamer, 2001), and gene probes contribute information to the database (see Chapter 29). Although they are a valuable adjunct to prenatal care, these tests cannot identify all congenital disorders. Furthermore, ethical issues surround such testing (Flake, 2001), and the nurse must be prepared to support the family's decision regarding these tests. If a disorder is detected and the family decides to proceed with the pregnancy, the advantage is that appropriate care can be made available for the infant immediately at birth.

In addition to testing, the history and medical information in the prenatal record is reviewed for factors associated with congenital disorders. These factors include various medical, surgical, and social conditions and their treatments (see Chapter 33); maternal infection (see Chapter 8); maternal endocrine and metabolic disorders (see Chapter 32); and infection and drug dependence in the newborn (see Chapter 38).

Perinatal Diagnosis

Many congenital anomalies require intervention soon after birth. By careful observations in the birth room or nursery, the nurse can identify most of these conditions. An excessive amount of amniotic fluid, **hydramnios,** is commonly associated with congenital anomalies in the newborn, and such infants should be examined closely at the earliest possible time.

Oligohydramnios, an insufficient amount of amniotic fluid, is associated primarily with anomalies of the urinary tract that prevent normal micturition in utero. It is most often associated with renal agenesis or dysplasia and obstructive lesions in the lower urinary tract. Anomalies of the ears sometimes occur with renal abnormalities. Bilateral renal agenesis, resulting in oligohydramnios, commonly manifests as Potter syndrome, which is characterized by atypical facial appearance consisting of a flat nose, recessed chin, epicanthal folds, and low-set abnormal ears; limb abnormalities; pulmonary hypoplasia; and fetal growth restriction. These conditions may be diagnosed prenatally.

Postnatal Diagnosis

Apgar scoring and a brief assessment are completed for all neonates after birth. Any deviations from normal are reported to the physician or midwife immediately. A thorough assessment of all body systems follows, with identification both of visible anomalies and of those that might not be visible. Some infants have multiple congenital anomalies. A recognized pattern of malformations is referred to as a *syndrome.* The most common, affecting about 1 in every 900 births (Beamer, 2001), is Down syndrome (Fig. 39-16), with diagnosis confirmed early in the neonatal period.

Genetic Diagnosis

Diagnostic procedures for the detection of genetic disorders are performed after birth at any time from the postnatal period through adulthood. Many tests exist for various disorders; only the most frequently used tests are discussed here.

Biochemical Tests. The most widespread use of postnatal testing for genetic disease is the routine screening of newborns for inborn errors of metabolism such as phenylketonuria (PKU), which is mandatory in most states in the United States. **Inborn errors of metabolism** is the term applied to a large group of disorders caused by a metabolic defect that results from the absence of or change in a protein, usually an enzyme, and mediated by

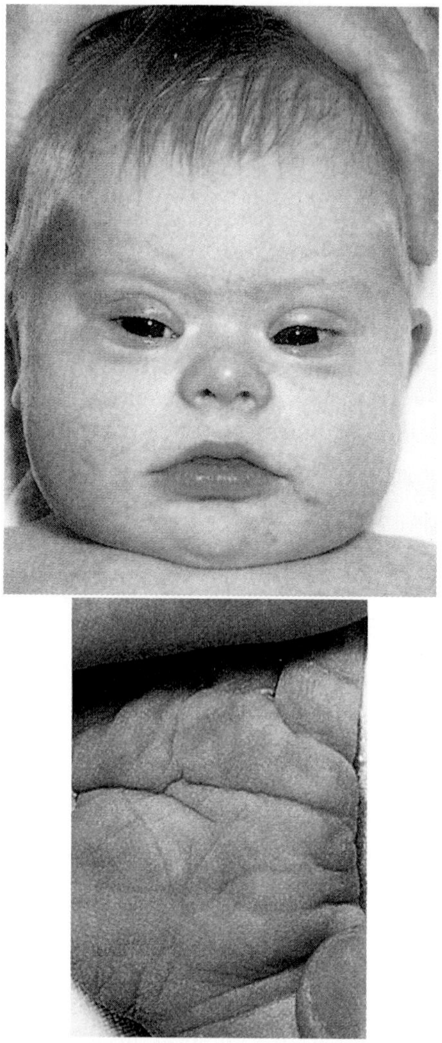

A

B

FIG. 39-16 **A,** Clinical features of Down syndrome. **B,** Simian crease. (From Zitelli, B., & Davis, H. [1997]. *Atlas of pediatric physical diagnosis* [3rd ed.]. St. Louis: Mosby.)

the action of a certain gene. These defects can involve any substrate produced from protein, carbohydrate, or fat metabolism. Inborn errors of metabolism are recessive disorders, so a person must receive a defective gene from each parent. The parents usually are unaffected because their normal dominant gene directs the synthesis of sufficient protein to meet their metabolic needs under normal circumstances. With the advent of new biochemical techniques, it is now possible to detect the abnormal gene responsible for causing an increasing number of these disorders.

Phenylketonuria results from a deficiency of the enzyme phenylalanine dehydrogenase (see Chapter 3). The test for PKU is not reliable, however, until the newborn has ingested an ample amount of the amino acid phenylalanine, a constituent of both human and cow milk.

NURSE ALERT

The nurse must document the initial ingestion of milk and perform the test at least 24 hours after that time.

The current trend toward early infant discharge from the hospital has the potential to cause neonates with a disorder such as PKU not to be screened so frequently as in the past. In response to this, the American Academy of Pediatrics (1996) made the following recommendations:

- Obtain a subsequent sample before age 2 weeks if the initial specimen is collected before the newborn is 24 hours old.
- Designate a primary care provider for all newborns before discharge for adequate newborn screening follow-up.
- Collect the initial specimen as close as possible to discharge or no later than 7 days after birth.

If the infant is found to have PKU, a diet low in phenylalanine is begun soon after birth. Breastfeeding or partial breastfeeding may be possible for some infants if the phenylalanine levels are monitored carefully and remain within acceptable limits (Kirby, 1999). Although severe mental retardation is seen less in affected children living in countries where there is neonatal screening for PKU, many affected children have some intellectual impairment.

Galactosemia, caused by a deficiency of the enzyme galactose 1-phosphate uridyltransferase, results in the inability to convert galactose to glucose. Galactosemia can be detected by measuring the blood levels of galactose in the urine of newborns suspected of having the disease who have ingested formula containing galactose. Early symptoms are vomiting, weight loss, and CNS symptoms, including poor feeding, drowsiness, and seizures. If the disorder goes untreated, the galactose levels will continue to increase, and the affected infant will show failure to thrive, mental retardation, cataracts, jaundice, hepatomegaly, and cirrhosis of the liver, with death possibly occurring in the first month of life. Therapy consists of eliminating galactose from the diet.

Congenital hypothyroidism results from a deficiency of thyroid hormones and affects approximately 1 of every 4000 newborns (Poblenz et al., 2001). All states in the United States routinely screen for hypothyroidism. This can be done by measuring thyroxine (T_4) in a drop of blood obtained from a heel stick at 2 to 5 days of age. At this time the normally expected increase in T_4 would be lacking in newborns with hypothyroidism. It is more often included as part of the newborn screen done in the first 24 to 48 hours or before discharge. Early screening may have false-positive results, but this is better than failure to detect infants with hypothyroidism. Treatment is thyroid hormone replacement. If the baby is untreated, symptoms usually appear after 6 weeks and include bradycardia; hypothermia; hypotension; hyporeflexia; abdominal distention; umbilical hernia; coarse, dry hair; thick, dry skin that feels cold; anemia; widely patent cranial sutures; and retarded bone age beginning at birth. The most disabling problem, however, is delayed development of the nervous system, leading to severe mental retardation (Hockenberry et al., 2003).

Cytologic Studies. Abnormalities can occur in either the autosomes or the sex chromosomes (Matthews, 1999). Chromosomal disorders often can be diagnosed on the basis of the clinical manifestations alone; however, an infant may have a clinical appearance that is only suggestive of a problem. Cytologic studies must be done to confirm or rule out a suspected diagnosis.

Disorders in the number or structure of chromosomes can be diagnosed by a *karyotype* (see Fig. 3-1), which is a photographic enlargement of the chromosomes arranged by their numbered pairs.

Abnormalities of the sex chromosomes make up about half of all the chromosomal abnormalities occurring in the newborn. The most common test for sex chromosome abnormalities is the buccal smear, using cells scraped from the mucosa inside the mouth. When prepared and stained, these show the number of inactive X chromosomes, also known as an *X-chromatin mass* or a *Barr body.* Each cell, whether male or female, has one genetically active X chromosome. Therefore a normal female has one active X chromosome and one Barr body, which is on the inactive X chromosome. A normal male has no Barr bodies, because he has only one genetically active X chromosome.

Dermatoglyphics. *Dermatoglyphics* is the study of the patterns formed by the ridges in the skin on the digits, palms, and soles. Development of these ridges begins during week 13 of gestation and is complete by week 19. Thus many genetic and chromosomal disorders also will affect the ridges. The addition or deletion of genetic material produces alterations in the loops, swirls, and arches of the finger and toe prints, in the palm lines, and in the flexion creases on the palms of the hands and soles of the feet. Characteristic dermatoglyphic patterns have been noted for almost all the chromosomal abnormalities, such as Down syndrome.

An infant with Down syndrome may have a single, palmar crease (see simian crease in Fig. 39-16, *B*), a single flexion crease of the fifth digit, and an open-field pattern on the ball of the foot (Matthews & Robin, 2002). The characteristic dermatoglyphic feature in a child with Turner syndrome is the large size of the dermal patterns on the fingers and toes. Certain fingerprint patterns also may be found in those people who have cardiac valvular problems later in life. Asymmetry of palmar ridges has been reported in congenital anomalies such as cleft lip and palate and congenital vertebral anomaly (Goldberg et al., 1997).

The nursing diagnoses formulated for an infant born with a congenital anomaly depend on the anomaly the infant has. For example, the diagnoses in an infant born with a CHD causing cyanosis will relate to inadequate oxygenation of body tissues, such as "activity intolerance related to imbalance between oxygen supply and demand." General nursing diagnoses pertaining to the care of neonates with congenital abnormalities include the following:

Newborn

- *Risk for injury or death related to*
  –presence of a congenital disorder
- *Risk for infection related to*
  –anomaly or its treatment
- *Risk for impaired gas exchange, imbalanced nutrition: less than body requirements, or impaired physical mobility related to*
  –congenital anomaly
- *Risk for delayed growth and development related to*
  –inborn error of metabolism

Parents and family

- *Dysfunctional grieving or spiritual distress related to*
  –birth of a child with a defect
- *Risk for ineffective individual or family coping related to*
  –birth of a child with a defect
- *Deficient knowledge related to*
  –cause of disorder, its management, alternative courses of action, community resources, prognosis, and the care needed by the child after discharge
- *Anxiety related to*
  –uncertainty regarding prognosis or ability to care for child
- *Risk for impaired parenting related to*
  –birth of a child with a disorder or defect

Collaborative Care

Newborn

A collaborative health team approach that includes specialists (e.g., orthodontists, physical therapists, geneticists) and community service representatives is needed in the care of infants with some disorders. Surgical intervention in the neonatal period may be necessary for the infant requiring either immediate correction or a palliative procedure to relieve the symptoms of the anomaly until definitive correction can be done. However, the complications induced by the stress of surgery may upset the delicate metabolic balance in a neonate already attempting to adapt to its extrauterine environment. This is compounded by the fact that only a limited amount of nutrient reserves is normally present in the neonate, and these reserves are already being drawn on by the energy-expending processes involved in rapid growth. Any surgical procedures performed during this time of growth place additional demands on these reserves. Although neonatal surgical mortality has decreased steadily over the last 50 years, a higher morbidity and mortality rate is found in neonates than in older children or adults undergoing similar procedures (Rowe & Rowe, 2000). However, despite these problems unique to neonates, advances in surgical techniques, anesthesia, and the nursing care given in intensive care nurseries have together been responsible for lessening the risk of surgery in neonates.

The health care team must be highly skilled to meet the needs of these infants. These needs are similar to those of the compromised infant. In addition to stabilization of the infant's condition, other preoperative interventions, such as orogastric tube placement for abdominal decompression, the management of open lesions, and the maintenance of fluid and electrolyte balance, are implemented to manage specific anomalies.

Postoperatively the infant is returned to the intensive care nursery, where close monitoring is maintained. The infant's respiratory efforts are supported; this often requires suctioning and usually mechanical ventilation. Constant surveillance is necessary to detect any respiratory complications resulting from the anesthesia. A pulse oximeter is attached to measure the oxygen saturation in hemoglobin, which closely correlates with arterial oxygen saturation. Oxygen is provided as needed. An indwelling gastric catheter attached to intermittent suction is placed to remove gastric secretions, thereby preventing aspiration and the abdomen from becoming distended. The infant's fluid, electrolyte, and acid-base status are monitored and adjusted as needed. Urinary output is monitored and should equal 1 to 2 ml/kg/hr. Other nursing interventions are focused on caring for the surgical site, maintaining thermoregulation, and promoting comfort.

Parents and Family

While the infant is receiving optimal care, the parents, too, have needs that must be met as they deal with the crisis of having an infant with an abnormal condition. Their reactions are carefully assessed and are likely to be those typical of a grief response. Facilitating their understanding of the information given them about their infant's condition is a vital nursing intervention. A newly diagnosed disorder often implies the need for the implementation of a therapeutic regimen. For example, the disorder may be an inborn error of metabolism, such as PKU, which requires consistent and rigid adherence to a diet. The family of such an infant may need help with securing the required formula and receiving counseling from the clinical dietitian. The importance of maintaining the diet, keeping an adequate supply of special preparations, and avoiding the use of unauthorized substitutions must be impressed on the family.

Referral to appropriate agencies is another essential component of the follow-up management, and the nurse should make the parents aware of all possible sources of aid, including pertinent literature, parent groups, and national organizations (see Resources at the end of the chapter). Many organizations and foundations, such as the Cystic Fibrosis Foundation and the Muscular Dystrophy Association, provide services and equipment for affected children. Numerous parent groups exist for the family to share experiences and derive mutual support in coping with problems similar to those of other group members. Nurses should be familiar with the services available in their community that provide assistance and education to families with these special problems.

A major nursing function is providing emotional support to the family during all aspects of the care of the child born with a defect or disorder. The feelings stemming from the real or imagined threat posed by a congenital anomaly are as varied as the people being counseled (Baumann & Braddick, 1999). Responses may include apathy, denial, anger, hostility, fear, embarrassment, grief, and loss of self-esteem (see Chapter 41).

Parents benefit from seeing before-and-after pictures of other babies born with the same defect. Coupled with other verbal and nonverbal supportive care, this visual reassurance may be effective in allaying their concerns.

Families need much information, guidance, and support as they make decisions regarding the care of their infants. Once they have been given the facts and possible consequences and all the assistance they need in problem solving, the final decision regarding a course of action must be their own. It is then incumbent on health care providers to support the decision of the family.

KEY POINTS

- Hyperbilirubinemia is caused by a variety of factors, including maternal-fetal Rh and ABO incompatibility.
- Erythroblastosis fetalis leads to anemia, edema, and the cytotoxic effects of unconjugated bilirubin.
- The injection of $Rh_0(D)$ immune globulin in Rh-negative and Coombs test–negative women bestows passive immunity and also minimizes the possibility of isoimmunization.
- Neonatal exchange transfusion with type O, Rh-negative RBCs serves to treat anemia and acidosis and to remove bilirubin, maternal antibodies, and fetal RBCs that are beginning to hemolyze.
- Major congenital defects are the leading cause of death in infants younger than 1 year in the United States and account for 20% of neonatal deaths.
- The most common major congenital anomalies that cause serious problems in the neonate are congenital heart disease, neural tube defects, cleft lip or palate, clubfoot, and developmental dysplasia of the hip.
- Minor anomalies may be part of a characteristic pattern of malformations.
- Hydramnios and oligohydramnios are associated with the occurrence of many congenital anomalies.

KEY POINTS—cont'd

- Current technology permits the prenatal diagnosis of many congenital anomalies and disorders.
- The most widespread use of postnatal testing for genetic disease is the routine screening of newborns for inborn errors of metabolism.
- The curative and rehabilitative problems of an infant with a congenital disorder are often complex and require a multidisciplinary approach to care.
- The supportive care given to the parents of infants with an abnormal condition must begin at birth or at the time of diagnosis and continue for years.

CRITICAL THINKING EXERCISES

1. Baby Eugene, a newborn who had an uneventful birth and has a normal appearance, shows symptoms of a gastrointestinal obstruction.
   - **a.** What are classic symptoms of a gastrointestional obstruction in a newborn?
   - **b.** Based on your knowledge, what type of obstruction do you think this infant might have?
   - **c.** Identify nursing diagnoses based on your analysis of this situation.
   - **d.** Develop a plan of care, including interventions and rationale.
2. It was determined that Eugene has a meconium ileus, and he had surgery.
   - **a.** What are your priority nursing diagnoses at this time?
   - **b.** Develop a plan of care, including interventions and rationale.
   - **c.** Identify additional needs and resources for Eugene's parents.
3. Baby Jennifer has a myelomeningocele, which had been detected prenatally. A few hours after birth, a nursing student is preparing to care for Jennifer's mother. How would she address these potential questions:
   - **a.** "I took folic acid during my pregnancy—why did this happen?"
   - **b.** "When will she have it closed?"
   - **c.** "Tell me again what a myelomeningocele is."
   - **d.** "Can I breastfeed her?"
   - **e.** "When will I know if she'll be able to walk?"

RESOURCES

American Cleft Palate Association
1218 Grandview Ave.
Pittsburgh, PA 15211
412-681-1376
800-242-5338 (800-24-CLEFT)
www.cleftline.org

American Society of Plastic Surgeons
Plastic Surgery Educational Foundation
Plastic Surgery Information Service: FAQs
www.plasticsurgery.org/faq/cleft.htm

Cystic Fibrosis Foundation
6931 Arlington Rd.
Bethesda, MD 20814
800-344-4832 (800-FIGHTCF)
www.cff.org

HEST (Helga's European Specialty Toys)
www.downsyndromedolls.com
(Down syndrome dolls used to teach children about disabilities and for children with Down syndrome)

March of Dimes Birth Defects Foundation
National Foundation/March of Dimes
1275 Mamaroneck Ave.
White Plains, NY 10605
914-663-4637 (800-MODIMES)
www.modimes.org

National Down Syndrome Congress
1800 Dempster St.
Park Ridge, IL 60069-1146
708-823-7550
800-232-6372
www.ndsccenter.org

National Down Syndrome Society Hotline
666 Broadway
New York, NY 10012
800-221-4602
www.ndss.org

Spina Bifida Association of America
4590 McArthur Blvd. NW, Suite 250
Washington, DC 20007-4226
800-621-3141
www.sbaa.org

REFERENCES

Adzick, N., & Nance, M. (2000). Pediatric surgery. *New England Journal of Medicine, 342*, 1651-1657.

American Academy of Pediatrics Committee on Genetics. (1996). Newborn screening facts. *Pediatrics, 98*, 473-481.

Askin, D. (2002). Complications in the transition from fetal to neonatal life. *Journal of Obstetric, Gynecologic, and Neonatal Nursing, 31*, 328-339.

Augustine, M. (1999). Hyperbilirubinemia in the healthy term newborn. *Nursing Practice, 24*, 24-41.

Ball, J. (1998). *Mosby's pediatric patient teaching guides.* St. Louis: Mosby.

Ball, J., & Bindler, R. (1999). *Pediatric nursing: Caring for children* (2nd ed.). Stamford, CT: Appleton & Lange.

Baumann, S., & Braddick, M. (1999). Out of their element: Fathers of children who are "not the same." *Journal of Pediatric Nursing, 14*, 369-373.

Beamer, L. (2001). Fetal nuchal translucency: A prenatal screening tool. *Journal of Obstetric, Gynecologic, and Neonatal Nursing, 31*, 376-385.

Bender, P. (2000). Genetics of cleft lip and palate. *Journal of Pediatric Nursing, 15*(4), 242-249.

Bensard, D. et al. (2002). Neonatal surgery. In G. Merenstein & S. Gardner (Eds.), *Handbook of neonatal intensive care* (5th ed.). St. Louis: Mosby.

Bergstein, J. (2000). Anomalies of the bladder. In R. Behrman, R. Kliegman, & H. Jenson (Eds.), *Nelson textbook of pediatrics* (16th ed.). Philadelphia: W.B. Saunders.

Boloker, J. et al. (2002). Congenital diaphragmatic hernia in 120 infants treated consecutively with permissive hypercapnia/spontaneous respiration/elective repair. *Journal of Pediatric Surgery, 137*, 357-366.

Booth, I., & Wozniak, E. (1984). *Pediatrics.* Baltimore: Williams & Wilkins.

Bowman, R. et al. (2001). Spina bifida outcome: A 25-year prospective. *Pediatric Neurosurgery, 34*, 114-120.

Brent, R. (2001). Addressing environmentally caused human birth defects. *Pediatrics in Review, 22*, 132-138.

Chessell, G. et al. (1984). *Diagnostic picture tests in clinical medicine* (vol. 2). St. Louis: Mosby.

Chondhury, S. et al. (1999). Survival of patients with esophageal atresia: Influence of birth weight, cardiac anomaly, and late respiratory complications. *Journal of Pediatric Surgery, 34*, 70-74.

Chuangsuwanich, A. et al. (1998). Epidemiology of cleft lip and palate in Thailand. *Annals of Plastic Surgery, 41*, 7-10.

Chung, K. et al. (2000). Maternal cigarette smoking during pregnancy and the risk of having a child with a cleft lip/palate. *Plastic Reconstructive Surgery, 105*, 485-491.

Dickason, E., Silverman, B., & Kaplan, J. (1998). *Maternal-infant nursing care* (3rd ed.). St. Louis: Mosby.

Dixit, R., & Gartner, L. (1999). The jaundiced newborn: Minimizing the risks. *Contemporary Pediatrics, 16*, 166-183.

Driver, C. et al. (2000). The contemporary outcome of gastroschisis. *Journal of Pediatric Surgery, 35*, 1719-1723.

Elias, E., & Hobbs, N. (1998). Spina bifida: Sorting out the complexities of care. *Contemporary Pediatrics 15*, 156-171.

Finegold, D. (1997). Endocrinology. In B. Zitelli & H. Davis (Eds.), *Atlas of pediatric physical diagnosis* (3rd ed.). St. Louis: Mosby.

Finer, N. et al. (1998). Congenital diaphragmatic hernia: Developing a protocolized approach. *Journal of Pediatric Surgery, 33*, 1331-1337.

Flake, A. (2001). Prenatal intervention: Ethical considerations for life-threatening and non life-threatening anomalies. *Seminars in Pediatric Surgery, 10*, 212-221.

Frank, C., Cooper, S., & Merenstein, G. (2002). Jaundice. In G. Merenstein & S. Gardner (Eds.), *Handbook of neonatal intensive care* (5th ed.). St. Louis: Mosby.

Glass, R., & Wolf, L. (1999). Feeding management of infants with cleft lip and palate and micrognathia. *Infants and Young Children, 12*, 70-81.

Goldberg, C. et al. (1997). Fluctuating asymmetry and vertebral malformation: A study of dermatoglyphics in congenital spine deformities. *Spine, 22*, 775-779.

Goldberg, M. (2001). Early detection of developmental hip dysplasia: Synopsis of the AAP clinical practice guideline. *Pediatrics in Review, 22*, 131-134.

Halamek, L., & Stevenson, D. (2002). Neonatal jaundice and liver disease. In A. Fanaroff & R. Martin (Eds.), *Neonatal-perinatal medicine: Diseases of the fetus and infant* (7th ed.). St. Louis: Mosby.

Haslam, R. (2000). Congenital anomalies of the central nervous system: Folic acid intake of young women. *Journal of Obstetric, Gynecologic, and Neonatal Nursing, 31*, 172-177.

Hockenberry, M. et al. (2003). *Wong's nursing care of infants and children* (7th ed.). St. Louis: Mosby.

Hoek, H., Brown, A., & Susser, E. (1998). The Dutch famine and schizophrenia spectrum disorders. *Social Psychiatry and Psychiatric Epidemiology, 33*, 373-379.

Howell, K. (1998). Understanding gastroschisis: An abdominal wall defect. *Neonatal Network, 17*, 17-25.

Hudgins, L., & Cassidy, S. (2002). Congenital anomalies. In A. Fanaroff & R. Martin (Eds.), *Neonatal-perinatal medicine: Diseases of the fetus and infant* (7th ed.). St. Louis: Mosby.

Hussain, N. et al. (2002). Hypospadius and early gestation growth restriction in infants. *Pediatrics, 109*, 473-478.

Jackson, P., & Harvey, J. (2000). Hydrocephalus. In P. Jackson & J. Vessey (Eds.), *Primary care of the child with a chronic condition* (3rd ed.). St. Louis: Mosby.

Johnson, L., Bhutani, V., & Brown, A. (2002). System-based approach to management of neonatal jaundice and prevention of kernicterus. *Journal of Pediatrics, 140*, 396-403.

Joint Committee of Accreditation of Healthcare Organizations. (April 2001). Kernicterus threatens healthy newborns. *Sentinel Event Alert, 18*, 1.

Juretschke, L. (2001). Congenital diaphragmatic hernia: Update and review. *Journal of Obstetric, Gynecologic, and Neonatal Nursing, 30*, 259-268.

Kimura, K. (2000). Bilious vomiting in the newborn: Rapid diagnosis of intestinal obstruction. *American Family Physician, 61*, 2791-2798.

Kirby, R. (1999). Maternal phenylketonuria: A new cause for concern. *Journal of Obstetric, Gynecologic, and Neonatal Nursing, 28*, 227-234.

Lewin, M. (2000). The genetic basis of congenital heart disease. *Pediatric Annals, 29*, 469-480.

Lockridge, T., Caldwell, A., & Jason, P. (2002). Neonatal surgical emergencies: Stabilization and management. *Journal of Obstetric, Gynecologic, and Neonatal Nursing, 31*, 328-339.

Matthews, A. (1999). Chromosomal abnormalities: Trisomy 18, trisomy 13, deletions and microdeletions. *Journal of Perinatal and Neonatal Nursing, 13*, 59-75.

Matthews, A., & Robin, N. (2002). Genetic disorders, malformations, and inborn errors of metabolism. In G. Merenstein & S. Gardner (Eds.), *Handbook of neonatal intensive care* (4th ed.). St. Louis: Mosby.

McDaniel, N. (2001). Ventricular and atrial septal defects. *Pediatrics in Review, 22*, 265-270.

Mitchell, J., & Wood, R. (2000). Management of cleft lip and palate in primary care. *Journal of Pediatric Health Care, 14*(1), 13-19.

Morrow, J., & Kelsey, K. (1998). Folic acid for prevention of neural tube defects: Pediatric anticipatory guidance. *Journal of Pediatric Health Care 12*, 55-59.

Moyer, V. et al. (2001). Late versus early surgical correction for congenital diaphragmatic hernia in newborn infants. *The Cochrane Library*, Issue 1, Oxford: Update Software.

Nakayama, D. (1997). Surgery. In B. Zitelli & H. Davis (Eds.), *Atlas of pediatric physical diagnosis* (3rd ed.). St. Louis: Mosby.

Neal, J. (2001). Isoimmunization and current management modalities. *Journal of Obstetric, Gynecologic, and Neonatal Nursing, 30*, 589-603.

Nora, J., & Fraser, F. (1989). *Medical genetics: Principles and practice* (3rd ed.). Philadelphia: Lea & Febiger.

O'Doherty, N. (1986). *Neonatology: Micro atlas of the newborn.* Nutley, NJ: Hoffmann-La Roche.

Poblenz, J. et al. (2001). Congenital hypothyroidism in a child with unsuspected familial dysalbuminemic hyperthyroxinemia caused by a mutation (R218H) in the human albumin gene. *Journal of Pediatrics, 139*, 887-891.

Poland, R. (2002). Preventing kernicterus: Almost there. *Journal of Pediatrics, 140*, 385-386.

Rintoul, N. et al. (2002). A new look at myelomeningoceles: Functional level, vertebral level, shunting, and the implications for fetal interventions. *Pediatrics, 109*, 409-413.

Rowe, M., & Rowe, S. (2000). The last fifty years of neonatal surgical management. *American Journal of Surgery, 180*, 345-352.

Smith, P. (2001). Primary care in children with congenital heart disease. *Journal of Pediatric Nursing, 16*, 308-319.

Suddaby, E. (2001). Contemporary thinking for congenital heart disease. *Pediatric Nursing, 27*, 233-240.

Trilling, J., & Potts, N. (2002). Musculoskeletal alterations. In N. Potts & B. Mandleco (Eds.), *Pediatric nursing: Caring for children and their families*. Clifton Park, NY: Delmar.

Yerkes, E. et al. (1998). Role of angiotensin in the congenital anomalies of the kidney and urinary tract in the mouse and the human. *Kidney International Supplement, 67*, S75-S77.

Zitelli, B., & Davis, H. (1997). *Atlas of pediatric physical diagnosis* (3rd ed.). St. Louis: Mosby.

CHAPTER 40

Carole Kenner

Nursing Care of the High Risk Newborn

http://evolve.elsevier.com/Lowdermilk/MatWmnHlth/

LEARNING OBJECTIVES

- Analyze the differences in the characteristics of preterm, term, postterm, and postmature neonates.
- Discuss respiratory distress syndrome and the approach to treatment.
- Compare methods of oxygen therapy.
- Analyze the appropriate nursing interventions for nutritional care of the preterm infant.
- Discuss the pathophysiology of retinopathy of prematurity and bronchopulmonary dysplasia (BPD) and the risk factors that predispose preterm infants to these problems.
- Discuss pain assessment and management in the preterm infant.
- Describe the signs and symptoms of perinatal asphyxia.
- Analyze the pathophysiology of meconium aspiration syndrome and its clinical signs.
- Plan developmentally appropriate care.
- Discuss the needs of parents of high risk infants.
- Evaluate a neonatal transport plan.
- Explain appropriate responses and interventions the nurse can use in caring for families experiencing anticipatory grief or loss and grief in the neonatal period.

Modern technology and expert nursing care have made important contributions to improving the health and overall survival of high risk infants. However, infants who are born considerably before term and survive are particularly susceptible to the development of sequelae related to their preterm birth. These conditions, which also can occur in term and near-term infants, but not so frequently, include necrotizing enterocolitis, BPD, intraventricular and periventricular hemorrhage, and retinopathy of prematurity. The focus of this chapter is on care of the preterm infant. Care of other high risk infants with gestational age–related problems also is discussed.

PRETERM INFANTS

Preterm infants are at risk because their organ systems are immature and they lack adequate reserves of bodily nutrients. The potential problems and care needs of the preterm infant weighing 2000 g differ from those of the term, postterm, or postmature infant of equal weight. If these infants have physiologic disorders and anomalies as well, these affect the infant's response to treatment. In general, the closer infants are to term from the standpoint of both gestational age and birth weight, the easier their adjustment to the external environment. The cost of the care required by low birth weight (LBW) infants is estimated to be in the billions of dollars each year and is increasing as technology use increases.

Varying opinions exist about the practical and ethical dimensions of resuscitation of **extremely low birth weight** infants (those infants whose birth weight is 1000 g or less). Some of the ethical issues associated with resuscitation of these infants are in the Ethical Considerations box.

CARE MANAGEMENT

Assessment and Nursing Diagnoses

For the high risk infant, an accurate assessment of gestational age (see Chapter 26) is critical in helping the nurse identify the potential problems the newborn is likely to have. The response of the preterm or postterm infant to extrauterine life is different from that of the term infant. By understanding the physiologic basis of these differences, the nurse can assess these infants, determine the response of the preterm or postterm infant, and discern which potential problems are most likely to occur.

Respiratory Function. The preterm infant is likely to have difficulty making the pulmonary transition from intrauterine to extrauterine life. Numerous problems may affect the respiratory systems of preterm infants and may include the following:

- Decreased number of functional alveoli
- Deficient surfactant levels

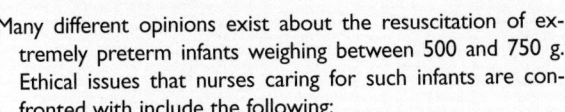

ETHICAL CONSIDERATIONS

Resuscitation of Extremely Premature Infants

Many different opinions exist about the resuscitation of extremely preterm infants weighing between 500 and 750 g. Ethical issues that nurses caring for such infants are confronted with include the following:

- Whether to resuscitate?
- Who should decide?
- Is the cost of resuscitation justified?
- Do the benefits of technology outweigh the burdens in relation to the quality of life?

All people involved (health care providers and parents) should participate in the discussions in which these controversial issues are resolved.

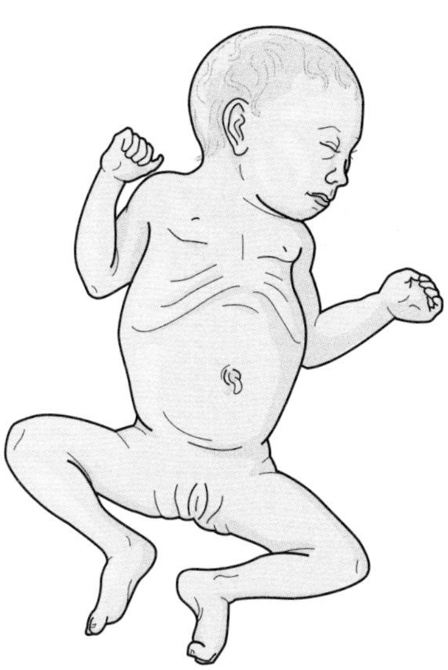

FIG. 40-1 Retractions: Substernal, subcostal, and intercostal retractions are evident. (Courtesy Ross Laboratories, Columbus, OH.)

- Smaller lumen in the respiratory system
- Greater collapsibility or obstruction of respiratory passages
- Insufficient calcification of the bony thorax
- Weak or absent gag reflex
- Immature and friable capillaries in the lungs
- Greater distance between functional alveoli and the capillary bed

In combination, these deficits severely hinder the infant's respiratory efforts and can produce respiratory distress or apnea.

Respiratory difficulty often follows a progressive pattern. Infants normally breathe between 30 to 60 breaths/min, relying significantly on their abdominal muscles to accomplish this (Cavalieri & Sansouci, 2003). However, the respiratory rate may increase without a change in rhythm. Early signs of respiratory distress include flaring of the nares and an expiratory grunt. Depending on the cause, retractions may begin as subcostal, suprasternal, or clavicular retractions (Fig. 40-1). If the infant shows increasing respiratory effort, for example, seesaw breathing patterns, retraction, flaring of the nares, expiratory grunts, and apneic spells (Fig. 40-2), this indicates deepening distress. A compromised infant's color progresses from pink to circumoral cyanosis and then to generalized cyanosis. Acrocyanosis deepens. (Acrocyanosis is a normal finding in the neonate, but central cyanosis indicates the existence of an underlying problem.)

Periodic breathing is a respiratory pattern commonly seen in premature infants. Such infants exhibit 5- to 10-second respiratory pauses followed by 10 to 15 seconds of compensatory rapid respirations. Such periodic breathing should not be confused with apnea, which is a 15- to 20-second cessation of respiration. The nurse must be prepared to provide oxygen and ventilation as necessary.

Cardiovascular Function. Evaluation of heart rate and rhythm, skin color, blood pressure, perfusion, pulses, oxygen saturation, and acid-base status provides information on the cardiovascular status. The nurse must be prepared to intervene if symptoms of hypovolemia, shock, or both, are found. These symptoms include hypotension, slow capillary refill (longer than 3 seconds), and continued respiratory distress despite the provision of oxygen and ventilation.

An accurate and timely blood pressure reading can assist in making an early diagnosis of cardiorespiratory disease and in monitoring the effects of fluid therapy. Blood pressure readings can be obtained by the Doppler method or by an electronic monitor.

Maintaining Body Temperature. Preterm infants are susceptible to temperature instability as a result of numerous factors. Preterm infants are at high risk for heat loss because of their large body surface area in relation to weight. Other factors that place preterm infants at risk for temperature instability include the following:

- Minimal insulating subcutaneous fat
- Limited stores of brown fat (an internal source for the generation of heat present in normal term infants)
- Friable (easily damaged) capillaries
- Decreased or absent reflex control of skin capillaries (shiver response)
- Inadequate muscle mass activity (rendering the preterm infant unable to produce its own heat)
- Poor muscle tone resulting in more body surface area being exposed to the cooling effects of the environment
- An immature temperature regulation center in the brain

The goal of thermoregulation is to create a **neutral thermal environment (NTE),** which is the environmental temperature at which oxygen consumption is minimal but adequate to maintain the body temperature (Kenner, 2003). Armed with the knowledge of the four mechanisms

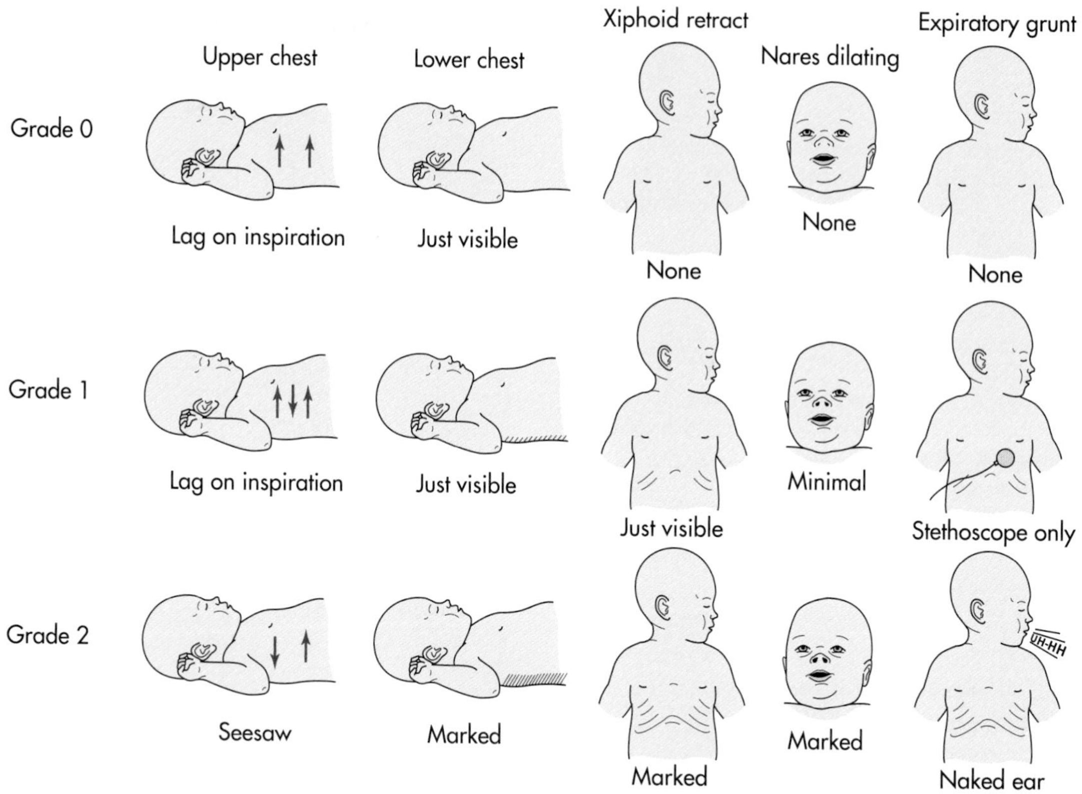
Upper chest
Lower chest
Xiphoid retract
Nares dilating
Expiratory grunt
Grade 0
Lag on inspiration
Just visible
None
None
None
Grade 1
Lag on inspiration
Just visible
Just visible
Minimal
Stethoscope only
Grade 2
Seesaw
Marked
Marked
Marked
Naked ear

FIG. 40-2 Observation of retractions. Silverman-Anderson index of respiratory distress is determined by grading each of five arbitrary criteria: *grade 0*, no respiratory difficulty; *grade 1*, moderate difficulty; *grade 2*, maximum difficulty. The retraction score is a sum of these values; a total score of 0 indicates no dyspnea, whereas a total score of 10 indicates maximal respiratory distress. (Modified from Silverman, W., & Anderson, D. [1956]. A controlled clinical trial of effects of water mist on obstructive respiratory signs, death rate and necropsy findings among premature infants. *Pediatrics, 17*, 1.)

of heat transfer (convection, conduction, radiation, and evaporation), the nurse can then create an environment for the preterm infant that prevents temperature instability (see Chapter 25). The infant will be kept in a radiant warmer or isolette with control settings at a temperature to maintain the NTE. Because the premature infant has few reserves (extra energy calories, minimal or no fat stores), cold sensitivity is a problem. This infant can easily lose heat and experience stress from the cold. Physiologically the infant tries to conserve heat, burns more calories, and the metabolic system goes into overdrive, further stressing the already compromised neonate. The nurse's role is to prevent or minimize cold stress by recognizing the risk factors and using intervention strategies to prevent and treat such stress. Signs of cold stress are listed in Box 40-1.

Central Nervous System Function. The preterm infant's central nervous system (CNS) is susceptible to injury as a result of the following problems:

- Birth trauma that includes damage to immature structures
- Bleeding from fragile capillaries
- An impaired coagulation process, including prolonged prothrombin time
- Recurrent anoxic episodes
- Predisposition to hypoglycemia

Research evidence indicates that the developing nervous system has the ability to reorganize neural connection after injury, meaning that some injuries that would be permanent in adults are not so in infants. Certain neurologic signs appear to be predictive of later neurologic abnormalities. These signs include hypotonia, a decreased level of activity, weak cry for more than 24 hours, and an inability to coordinate suck and swallow (Vanucci & Yager, 2002). Ongoing assessment and documentation of these neurologic signs is needed for the purpose of discharge teaching and making follow-up recommendations, as well as for their predictive value.

Maintaining Adequate Nutrition. The goal of neonatal nutrition is to promote normal growth and development. However, the maintenance of adequate nutrition in the preterm infant is complicated by problems with intake and metabolism. The preterm infant has the following dis-

BOX 40-1 Signs of Cold Stress

Skin temperature	Decreases before other signs
Respiratory rate	Initially increases, then apneic spells occur
Heart rate	Initially increases, then bradycardia occurs
Skin color	Mottled with acrocyanosis increasing to cyanosis
Physical activity	Increased in term infants without respiratory distress Decreased in term infants with respiratory distress Decreased in premature infants
Thermoregulatory control	Unstable in premature infants

advantages with regard to intake: weak or absent suck, swallow, and gag reflexes; a small stomach capacity; and weak abdominal muscles. The preterm infant's metabolic functions are compromised by a limited store of nutrients, a decreased ability to digest proteins or absorb nutrients, and immature enzyme systems.

The nurse must continuously assess the infant's ability to take in and digest nutrients. Some preterm infants require gavage or intravenous (IV) feedings instead of oral feedings. An area of research that holds promise for premature infants is use of minimal enteral nutrition (MEN) that may only be 1 ml/hr (Tyson & Kennedy, 2002). These feedings stimulate the gastrointestinal system with minute amounts of formula or breast milk, usually given via gavage, so that when enteral feedings can really begin, the gastrointestinal system is primed for nutrient absorption.

Maintaining Renal Function. The preterm infant's immature renal system is unable to (1) adequately excrete metabolites and drugs; (2) concentrate urine; or (3) maintain acid-base, fluid, or electrolyte balance. Therefore intake and output, as well as specific gravity, must be assessed. Laboratory tests must be done to assess acid-base and electrolyte balance. Medication levels also are monitored in preterm infants because certain medications can overwhelm the immature system's ability to excrete them.

Maintaining Hematologic Status. The preterm infant also is particularly predisposed to hematologic problems because of the following problems:

- Increased capillary friability
- Increased tendency to bleed (prolonged prothrombin time and partial thromboplastin time)
- Slowed production of red blood cells resulting from rapid decrease in erythropoiesis after birth
- Loss of blood due to frequent blood sampling for laboratory tests

BOX 40-2 Signs and Symptoms of Infection

Temperature instability
- Hypothermia
- Hyperthermia

Central nervous system changes
- Lethargy
- Irritability

Changes in color
- Cyanosis, pallor
- Jaundice

Cardiovascular instability
- Poor perfusion
- Hypotension
- Bradycardia/tachycardia

Respiratory distress
- Tachypnea
- Apnea
- Retractions, nasal flaring, grunting

Gastrointestinal problems
- Feeding intolerance
- Vomiting
- Diarrhea
- Glucose instability

Metabolic acidosis

- Decreased red blood cell survival related to the relatively larger size of the red blood cell and its increased permeability to sodium and potassium

The nurse assesses such infants for any evidence of bleeding from puncture sites and the gastrointestinal (GI) tract. Infants also are examined for signs of anemia (decreased hemoglobin and hematocrit levels, pale skin, increased apnea, lethargy, tachycardia, and poor weight gain) (Luchtman-Jones, Schwartz, & Wilson, 2002).

Resisting Infection. Preterm infants are at increased risk for infection because they have a shortage of stored maternal immunoglobulins, an impaired ability to make antibodies, and a compromised integumentary system (thin skin and fragile capillaries). Preterm infants exhibit various nonspecific signs and symptoms of infection (Box 40-2). Early identification and treatment of sepsis are essential (see Chapter 38). As with all aspects of care, strict handwashing is the single most important measure to prevent iatrogenic infections.

Growth and Development Potential

Although it is impossible to predict with complete accuracy the growth and development potential of each preterm infant, some findings support an anticipated favorable outcome in the absence of ongoing medical sequelae that can affect growth, such as BPD, necrotizing enterocolitis, and CNS problems. The lower the birth weight, the greater the likelihood of negative sequelae.

The growth and development milestones (e.g., motor milestones, vocalization, growth) are corrected for gestational age until the child is approximately $2\frac{1}{2}$ years old (Avery, Fletcher, & MacDonald, 1999).

The age of a preterm newborn is corrected by adding the gestational age and the postnatal age. For example, an infant born at 32 weeks of gestation 4 weeks ago would now be considered 36 weeks of age. The infant's **corrected age** at 6 months after the birth date is then 4 months, and the infant's responses are accordingly evaluated against the norm expected for a 4-month-old infant.

Certain measurable factors predict normal growth and development. The preterm infant experiences catch-up body growth during the first 2 to 3 years of life. The maximal growth occurs between 36 and 40 weeks of postconceptional age (Kliegman & Das, 2002). The head is the first to experience catch-up growth, followed by a gain in weight and height. At the infant's discharge from the hospital, which usually occurs between 37 and 40 weeks of postconceptional age, the infant should exhibit the following characteristics:

- An ability to raise the head when prone and to hold the head parallel with the body when tested for the head-lag response
- An ability to cry with vigor when hungry
- An appropriate amount and pattern of weight gain according to a growth grid
- Neurologic responses appropriate for corrected age

At 39 to 40 weeks of corrected age, the infant should be able to focus on the examiner's or parent's face and to follow with his or her eyes.

Of very low-birth-weight (VLBW) survivors, approximately 15% to 25% will have neurologic and/or cognitive disabilities in varying degrees of severity (Avery et al., 1999). Research is focused on examining other factors including environmental ones that may affect adverse cognitive and neurodevelopmental outcomes for VLBW and extremely low-birth-weight (ELBW) babies by the time they reach school age (Taylor, Klein, & Hack, 2000).

Parental Adaptation to Preterm Infant

The experience of parents whose infant is born prematurely or is otherwise high risk is different from the experience of parents whose infant is born at term and is normal (Holditch-Davis & Miles, 2000). This may cause parental attachment and the adaptation to the parental role to differ as well.

Parental Tasks. Parents of preterm infants must accomplish numerous psychologic tasks before effective relationships and parenting patterns can evolve. These tasks include the following:

- Experiencing **anticipatory grief** over the potential loss of an infant. The parent grieves in preparation for the infant's possible death, although the parent clings to the hope that the child will survive. This process begins during labor and lasts until the infant dies or shows evidence of surviving. Anticipatory grief occurs when families have knowledge of an impending loss, such as when a baby is admitted to a neonatal intensive care unit (NICU) with problems or when a diagnosis of an anencephalic fetus is made with ultrasonography. The baby is still alive, but the prognosis is poor. Being able to anticipate the loss gives families an opportunity to plan, feel more in control of their situation, and say good-bye in a special way. However, some individuals or family members may distance or detach themselves from the experience or from their loved ones as a way of protecting themselves from the pain of loss and grief. How a parent responds to this situation is dependent on the religious, spiritual, and cultural beliefs. These must be considered when planning care. The nurse's role is to advocate for the family so that other health professionals realize that the family is grieving. Being fully present for these families and practicing active listening is important.
- The mother's acceptance of her failure to give birth to a healthy, full-term infant. Grief and depression typify this phase, which persists until the infant is out of danger and is expected to survive.
- Resuming the process of relating to the infant. As the baby's condition begins to improve and the baby gains weight, feeds by nipple, and is weaned from the isolette or radiant warmer, the parent can begin the process of developing an attachment to the infant that was interrupted by the infant's critical condition at birth.
- Learning about the ways in which this baby differs in terms of his or her special needs and growth patterns, care-giving needs, and growth and development expectations.
- Adjusting the home environment to accommodate the needs of the new infant. Parents are encouraged to limit the number of visitors to minimize exposure of the infant to pathogens. The environmental temperature may need to be altered to optimize conditions for the infant. Grandparents and siblings also react to the birth of the preterm infant. Parents must deal with the grief of grandparents and the bewilderment and anger of the infant's siblings at the seemingly disproportionate amount of parental time spent on the newborn.

Parental Responses. Parents progress in interactions with their infants from maintaining an *en face* position, stroking, and touching their infant to assuming some child care activities, such as feeding, bathing, and changing the infant (Fig. 40-3). Parents go through numerous phases of adjustment as they learn to parent their infant. Nurses assist the transition to parenthood through their teaching and support of parental efforts.

Parenting Disorders. The incidence of physical and emotional abuse has been found to be greater in infants who, because of preterm birth or illness, are separated from their parents for a time after birth. Physical abuse includes varying degrees of poor nutrition, poor hygiene, and battering. Emotional abuse ranges from subtle disinterest to outright dislike of the infant to abandonment. **Shaken baby syndrome** is another possibility with premature infants.

This problem occurs when the child is shaken so violently that brain damage and retinal hemorrhages occur.

NURSE ALERT

Parents may show preferential treatment toward the brothers and sisters of the infant, discipline the infant harshly for normal behaviors, have extremely high expectations of the infant, or show other types of overt or covert negative parental responses.

Factors surrounding the birth may predispose parents to treat their infant this way because subconsciously they have rejected the infant. These factors might include parental pain and anxiety, a heavy financial burden because of the cost of the infant's care, unresolved anticipatory grief, a threat to self-esteem, or the fact that the infant was the product of an unwanted pregnancy. The goal of health professionals is to identify abuse and neglect early so that further problems can be prevented and, in turn, the incidence of such abuse can be reduced.

Potential nursing diagnoses for high risk infants and their parents include the following:

- *Impaired gas exchange related to*
  - –decreased number of functional alveoli
  - –deficiency of surfactant
- *Ineffective breathing pattern related to*
  - –inadequate chest expansion, secondary to infant position
- *Ineffective thermoregulation related to*
  - –immature thermoregulation center
- *Risk for infection related to*
  - –invasive procedures
  - –decreased immune response
- *Anxiety (parental) related to*
  - –lack of knowledge regarding infant condition
  - –lack of knowledge regarding infant development
- *Risk for impaired parent/infant attachment*
  - –lack of knowledge regarding infant cues

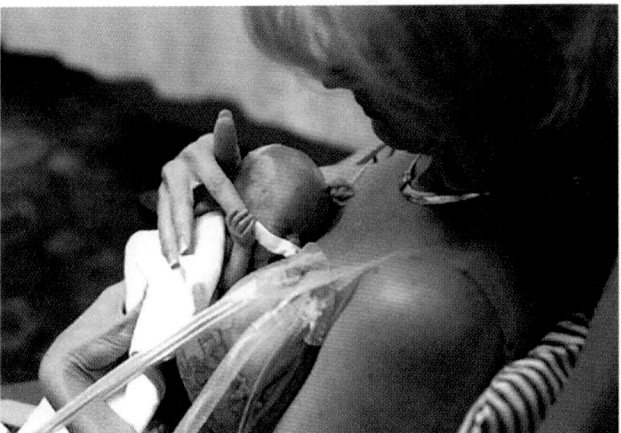

FIG. 40-3 Mother interacts with her premature infant. (Courtesy Children's Medical Ventures, Norwell, MA.)

Expected Outcomes of Care

The plan of nursing care for the preterm infant is directed by the physiologic needs of the infant's immature systems and often involves emergency treatments and procedures. Nursing care is a critical element in determining the infant's chances for survival, as well as normal development. In addition to meeting the infant's physical needs, nursing care is planned in conjunction with parents to promote parent-infant attachment and interaction. Expected outcomes are presented in client-centered terms and include that the infant will do the following:

- Maintain physiologic functioning.
- Maintain adequate nutrition.
- Experience no or minimal hematologic problems.
- Remain free of infection.
- Develop no retinal problems.
- Have no trauma to the immature musculoskeletal system.
- Experience attachment to parents.

Expected outcomes for the parents include that they will do the following:

- Perceive the infant as potentially normal (if this is medically substantiated).
- Provide care competently and comfortably.
- Experience pride and satisfaction in the care of their infant.
- Organize their time and energies to meet the love, attention, and care needs of the other members of the family, as well as their own needs.

Plan of Care and Interventions

The best environment for fetal growth and development is the uterus of a healthy, well-nourished woman. The goal of care for the preterm infant is to provide an extrauterine environment that approximates the healthy intrauterine environment to promote normal growth and development. Physicians, nurses, nurse practitioners, infant developmental specialists, and respiratory therapists work together as a team to provide the intensive care needed.

The admission of a preterm newborn to the intensive care nursery usually represents an emergency situation. Immediately after admission, a rapid initial evaluation is done to determine the infant's need for lifesaving treatment. Resuscitation is started in the birthing unit, and the newborn's need for warmth and oxygen is provided for during transfer to the nursery.

Nursing care is focused on the continuous assessment and analysis of the infant's physiologic status. Nurses fulfill many roles in providing the intensive and extended care that these infants require. In addition, they are the support persons and teachers during the first phase of the parents' adjustment to the birth of their preterm infant.

The nurse uses many technologic support systems to monitor the body responses and maintain the body functions of the infant. Technical skill must be combined with a gentle touch and concern about the traumatic effects of harsh lighting and the volume of machinery noise. The NICU environment may be a major contributing factor to learning and behavioral problems in preterm infants (Symington & Pinelli, 2001).

Physical Care

The environmental support measures for the preterm infant typically consist of the following equipment and procedures:

- An isolette or radiant warmer placed over the infant to control body temperature (NTE)
- Oxygen administration, depending on the infant's cardiopulmonary and circulatory status
- Electronic monitors as needed for the observation of respiratory and cardiac functions
- Assistive devices for positioning the infant in neutral flexion and with boundaries
- Clustering of care and minimization of stimulation according to infant cues

Various metabolic support measures that may be instituted consist of the following:

- Parenteral fluids to help support nutrition and maintain normal arterial blood gas (ABG) levels and acid-base balance
- IV access to facilitate the administration of antibiotic therapy if sepsis is a concern
- Blood work to monitor ABG levels, pH, blood glucose levels, electrolytes, and the status of blood cultures

Maintaining Body Temperature

The high risk infant is susceptible to heat loss and its complications. In addition, LBW infants may be unable to increase their metabolic rate because of impaired gas exchange, caloric intake restrictions, or poor thermoregulation. Transepidermal water loss is greater because of skin immaturity in very premature infants (those at less than 28 weeks of gestation) and can contribute to temperature instability.

High risk infants are cared for in the thermoneutral environment created by use of an external heat source. A probe to an external heat source supplied by a radiant warmer or a servocontrolled incubator is attached to the infant. The infant acts as a thermostat to regulate the amount of heat supplied by the external source. This idealized environment maintains an infant's normal body temperature between 36.5° C and 37.2° C. Maintaining a thermoneutral condition in the youngest, most immature infants decreases the need for them to generate additional heat. As a result, excessive oxygen consumption is prevented in such compromised infants (Blake & Murray, 2002).

Oxygen Therapy

Clinical criteria for identifying the need for oxygen administration include increased respiratory effort, respiratory distress with apnea, tachycardia, bradycardia, and central cyanosis with or without hypotonia. In addition, the need for oxygen should be substantiated by biochemical data (arterial oxygen pressure [$Pa{O_2}$] of less than 60 mm Hg or an oxygen saturation of less than 92%). High risk infants often require saturations of more than 95% to maintain respiratory stability because their hemoglobin levels are frequently low. As the $Pa{O_2}$ decreases, less oxygen is released from the hemoglobin, which increases the risk for cellular hypoxia.

Oxygen administered to an infant is warmed and humidified to prevent cold stress and drying of the respiratory mucosa. During the administration of oxygen, the concentration, volume, temperature, and humidity of the gas are carefully controlled. Delivery of oxygen for more than a few minutes requires the use of special equipment (hood, nasal cannula, positive-pressure mask, or endotracheal tube) because the concentration of free-flow oxygen cannot be monitored accurately. Free-flow oxygen into an incubator should not be used because the concentration fluctuates dramatically each time the doors or portholes are opened. The indiscriminant use of oxygen may be hazardous. Possible complications of oxygen therapy include retinopathy of prematurity and BPD.

NURSE ALERT

Administration of a therapeutic level of oxygen for a severely depressed infant could cause significant physiologic harm if given to an infant with mild respiratory disease.

Infants who need oxygen should have their respiratory status assessed accurately every 1 to 2 hours; this includes a continuous pulse oximetry reading and at least one ABG measurement (Cifuentes, Segars, & Carlo, 2003). The interventions implemented are then determined on the basis of the findings yielded by the clinical assessment, including telemetry (pulse oximetry or $tcP{O_2}$ monitoring) and laboratory tests (Cifuentes et al., 2003). The interventions ordered are those that can directly manage the underlying disease process and range from hood oxygen administration to ventilator therapy.

Hood Therapy. A hood can be used to administer oxygen to infants who do not require mechanical pressure support. The hood is a clear plastic cover that is sized to fit over the head and neck of the infant (Fig. 40-4). Inside the hood the infant receives the correct amount of oxygen. The nurse checks the oxygen level every 1 to 2 hours because the concentration must be adjusted in response to the infant's condition.

Nasal Cannula. Infants requiring low-flow amounts of oxygen can benefit from the use of a nasal cannula (Fig. 40-5). These are of particular value for older infants who are recuperating but still require supplemental oxygen. They are the preferred method for home oxygen administration. They permit the infant to receive an adequate, continuous flow of oxygen while allowing optimal vision, positioning, and parental holding. Infants also can breastfeed while receiving oxygen by this method. However, the nasal prongs must be inspected frequently to make sure they are not partially obstructed by milk or

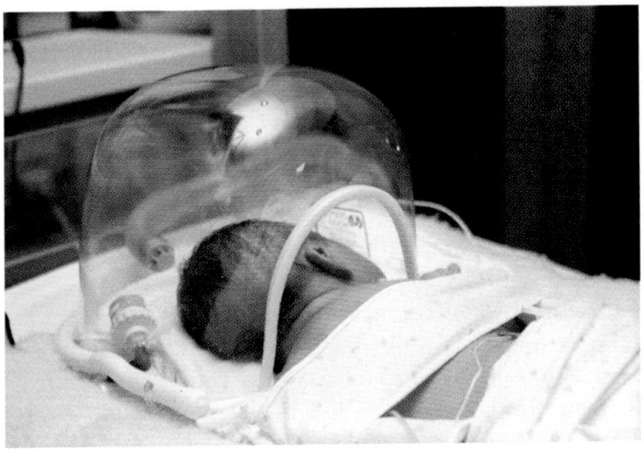

FIG. 40-4 Infant receiving oxygen therapy. (Courtesy Leslie Altimier, MSN, RN, TriHealth, Cincinnati, OH.)

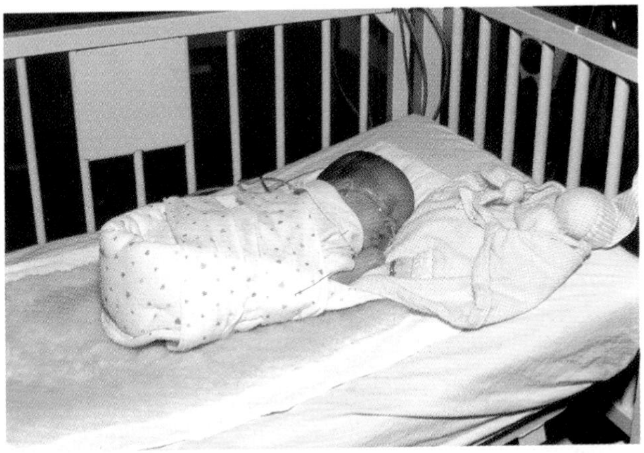

FIG. 40-5 Positioning of infant while receiving neonatal care. (Courtesy Leslie Altimier, MSN, RN, TriHealth, Cincinnati, OH.)

secretions. Nasal cannulas allow easier feedings and psychosocial interactions.

Continuous Positive Airway Pressure Therapy. Infants who are unable to maintain an adequate PaO_2 despite the administration of oxygen by hood or nasal cannula may require the delivery of oxygen by using **continuous positive airway pressure (CPAP).** CPAP infuses oxygen or air under a preset pressure by means of nasal prongs, a face mask, or an endotracheal tube. An orogastric tube should be used for decompression of the stomach during use of nasal prongs. CPAP increases the functional residual capacity, improves the diffusion time of pulmonary gases, including oxygen, and can decrease pulmonary shunting. If implemented early enough, CPAP may preclude the need for mechanical ventilation (Cifuentes et al., 2003). CPAP can cause vascular shunting in the pulmonary beds, which can lead to persistent pulmonary hypertension and severe respiratory distress.

Mechanical Ventilation. **Mechanical ventilation** must be implemented if other methods of therapy cannot correct abnormalities in oxygenation. Its use is indicated whenever blood gas values reveal the existence of severe hypoxemia or severe hypercapnia. The condition of the infant with apnea with bradycardia, ineffective respiratory effort, shock, asphyxia, infection, meconium aspiration syndrome, respiratory distress syndrome, or congenital defects that affect ventilation also may deteriorate and require intubation to reverse the process (Cifuentes et al., 2003). Dexamethasone may be administered to prevent chronic lung disease (Garland et al., 1999).

The ventilator settings are determined by the infant's particular needs. The ventilator is set to provide a predetermined amount of oxygen to the infant during spontaneous respirations and also to provide mechanical ventilation in the absence of spontaneous respirations.

Surfactant Administration. Surfactant can be administered as an adjunct to oxygen and ventilation therapy. Before 34 weeks of gestation, most infants do not produce enough surfactant to survive extrauterine life (American Academy of Pediatrics, 1999). As a result, lung compliance is decreased, and not enough gas exchange occurs as the lungs become atelectatic and require greater pressures to expand. With administration of artificial surfactant, respiratory compliance is improved until the infant can generate enough surfactant on his or her own. Exogenous surfactant is either artificial or natural and is given in several doses through an endotracheal tube. As with any drug therapy, the infant must be monitored for the occurrence of potential side effects such as a patent ductus arteriosus (PDA) and pulmonary hemorrhage. Use of this drug has been associated with a significantly reduced length of time on ventilators and oxygen therapy, and an increased survival rate in premature infants (see Medication Guide).

Extracorporeal Membrane Oxygenation Therapy. Infants with severe pulmonary dysfunction who are older than 34 weeks of gestation may be candidates for **extracorporeal membrane oxygenation (ECMO)** therapy. ECMO makes use of cardiopulmonary bypass to oxygenate the infant's blood outside the body through a membrane oxygenator. The membrane oxygenator serves as an artificial lung while the infant's lungs heal. Because of the massive systemic anticoagulation therapy required in the pump tubing and the increased risk for hemorrhage, the criteria for its use are very strict, and the use of this therapy is therefore limited (Schwartz, 2003). The risk for intraventricular hemorrhages in premature infants is particularly high, and for this reason, ECMO therapy cannot be used in them. ECMO has been successful in the treatment of various acute and chronic lung diseases, including meconium aspiration syndrome and persistent pulmonary hypertension of the newborn (Cifuentes et al., 2003).

High-Frequency Ventilation. Other modes of ventilator therapies include high-frequency oscillator ventilation, jet ventilation, flow interruption ventilation, and liquid

MEDICATION GUIDE

Surfactant Replacement: Bovine Lung Extract: Beractant (Survanta) Artificial Surfactant: Colfosceril (Exosurf)

ACTION ▪ These medications provide exogenous surfactant to correct deficiency in lung immaturity.

INDICATIONS ▪ Surfactants are used in the prevention and treatment of respiratory distress syndrome in premature infants. For *prevention,* drug is administered within 15 minutes of birth to infants with clinical manifestations of surfactant deficiency or with a birth weight less than 1250 g. For *treatment,* drug is administered to infants with confirmed diagnosis of respiratory distress syndrome, preferably within 8 hours of birth.

DOSAGE ▪ Dosage depends on drug used. Administer via endotracheal tube

ADVERSE REACTIONS ▪ Adverse reactions include respiratory distress immediately after administration and bradycardia and oxygen desaturation.

NURSING CONSIDERATIONS ▪ Observe infant's condition for changes. Diuresis may occur with improvement. Ventilator settings may need changing as the infant's ability to oxygenate increases.

ventilation (Cools & Offringa, 1999; Plavka et al., 1999; Schwartz, 2003). These methods of high-frequency ventilation work by providing smaller volumes of oxygen at a significantly more rapid rate (more than 300 breaths/min) than do traditional mechanical ventilators. As a result, the intrathoracic pressure is decreased, and along with this, the risk of barotrauma. In liquid ventilation, the surface tension is reduced while oxygenation is improved through the recreation of a fetal lung environment. Instead of air pressure, an experimental oxygenated lipid solution is pumped continuously through the lungs.

Nitric Oxide Therapy. Inhaled nitric oxide (NO), delivered as a gas, causes potent and sustained pulmonary vasodilation in the pulmonary circulation (Schwartz, 2003). NO binds with hemoglobin in red blood cells and is inactivated after metabolism. In the few studies conducted with human infants, positive results were seen: oxygen saturation improved, and no toxic effects from methemoglobin or increased levels of nitrogen oxide were documented. Several multicenter studies are currently being conducted (Finer & Barrington, 2001; Schwartz, 2003). NO shows much promise in reducing adverse respiratory sequelae of being born prematurely. Its use has reduced the need for invasive technologies such as ECMO.

Weaning from Respiratory Assistance

Respiratory assistance is weaned slowly as the infant's status improves. The infant is ready to be weaned from respiratory assistance once the ABG and oxygen saturation levels are maintained within normal limits. A spontaneous, adequate respiratory effort must be present, and the infant must show improved muscle tone during increased activity. Weaning is done in a stepwise and gradual manner. This may consist of the infant being extubated, placed on CPAP, and then weaned to oxygen by means of a hood or nasal cannula. Throughout the weaning process, the infant's oxygen levels are monitored by pulse oximetry, $tcPo_2$ monitoring, and blood gas levels.

The goal of weaning is the withdrawal of all oxygen support. However, some infants do not achieve this before discharge from the hospital and may require home oxygen therapy for several months. Throughout the weaning period, the infant is assessed for signs and symptoms indicating poor tolerance of the process. These include an increased pulse, respiratory distress, or cyanosis, or a combination of these. If these occur, the amount of oxygen being delivered is increased, and weaning proceeds more slowly while further assessments are done. Underlying causes of intolerance of weaning may be BPD, a PDA, or CNS damage.

Nutritional Care

It is not always possible to provide enteral (by the GI route) nourishment to a high risk infant. Such infants are often too ill or weak to breastfeed or bottle feed because of respiratory distress or sepsis. Early enteral feeding of the asphyxiated neonate with a low Apgar score also is avoided to prevent bowel necrosis. In such cases, nutrition is provided parenterally. Those infants who require parenteral nutrition may have one or more of the following problems:

- Lack of a coordinated suck-and-swallow reflex
- Inability to suck because of a congenital anomaly
- Respiratory distress requiring aggressive ventilator support
- Asphyxiation with a potential for necrotizing enterocolitis

Type of Nourishment. The types of formulas used, the mode and volume of feeding, and the feeding schedule of the infant are determined on the basis of the findings yielded by assessment of the following variables:

- Initially, the birth weight, and then the current weight of the preterm infant
- Pattern of weight gain or loss (infants weighing less than 1500 g require more energy for growth and thermoregulation and may gain weight poorly with either breastfeedings or bottle feedings)
- Presence or absence of suck-and-swallow reflex in all infants at less than 35 weeks of gestation
- Behavioral readiness to take oral feedings
- Physical condition, including presence or absence of bowel sounds, abdominal distention, or bloody stools, as well as presence and degree of respiratory distress or apneic episodes
- Residual from previous feeding, if being gavage fed

- Malformations (especially GI defects such as gastroschisis, omphalocele or esophageal atresia), including the need for a gastrostomy feeding tube
- Renal function, including urinary output and laboratory values (nitrogen balance, electrolyte balance, glucose level); premature infants are especially susceptible to altered renal function

Weight and Fluid Loss or Gain. For many reasons, the caloric, nutrient, and fluid requirements of high risk infants are greater than those of the term, normal newborn. One reason is that premature or dysmature (malnourished) newborns often have limited stores of nutrients and fluids. In addition, symptomatic or asymptomatic hypoglycemia, electrolyte imbalances, or other metabolic disturbances can develop in an infant whose nutritional intake is poor. Such hypoglycemia may cause serious damage to carbohydrate-dependent brain cells.

The infant's weight is measured and recorded daily, and the rate of weight loss or gain is calculated. Further depletion of weight and metabolic stores can occur as a result of one or a combination of the following factors:

- Birth asphyxia
- Increased respirations or respiratory effort
- PDA
- Hypothermic environment
- Insensible fluid loss caused by evaporation (with radiant heat or phototherapy)
- Vomiting, diarrhea, and dysfunctional absorption from the GI tract
- Growth demands (a premature infant's growth rate approximates that of fetal growth during the last trimester and is at least 2 times faster than a term infant's growth rate after birth)
- Inability of the renal system to concentrate urine and maintain an adequate rate of urea excretion, as well as infant's inadequate response to antidiuretic hormone

The high risk newborn is predisposed to have weight and fluid losses because of the greater amount of fluid needed to meet the demands of the increased cellular metabolic processes (resulting from stress, repair, or growth). The body weight of premature infants weighing less than 1500 g consists of 83% to 89% water, compared with the term infant's water content of 71% (Denne et al., 2002). Most of this water is in the extracellular fluid compartment. Even with the early institution of fluid and nutrition intake, the premature infant's weight and fluid losses seem exaggerated. Inadequate fluid intake, resulting from either delayed administration or insufficient volume, can further cause weight and fluid losses in the premature infant.

BOX 40-3 Calculation of a Weight Loss or Gain

EXAMPLE 1

Day 4 1750 g
Day 5 1730 g
20 g loss

$$\frac{20}{1750} = \frac{X\%}{100\%}$$

$$1750X = 2000$$

$$1750\overline{)2000.0} = 1.1$$

$$X = 1.1\% \text{ weight loss}$$

EXAMPLE 2

Day 4 1750 g
Day 5 1790 g
40 g gain

$$\frac{40}{1750} = \frac{X\%}{100\%}$$

$$1750X = 4000$$

$$1750\overline{)4000.00} = 2.3$$

$$X = 2.3\% \text{ weight gain}$$

Insensible water loss (IWL) is an evaporative loss that occurs largely through the skin. Approximately 30% of this IWL comes from the respiratory tract. The total IWL in a normal infant ranges anywhere from 30 to 60 ml/kg/24 hr. The effects of radiant warmers, incubators, phototherapy, and other factors can augment the IWL. Humidifying the respiratory gases administered can prevent some of this loss.

During the first week of extrauterine life, the premature infant can lose up to 15% of his or her birth weight. In contrast, a weight loss of up to only 10% is acceptable in a term appropriate-for-gestational age (AGA) infant. After the initial week, a premature infant's loss or gain during each 24-hour period should not exceed 2% of the previous day's weight. (To calculate a weight loss or gain, see Box 40-3.) Increased stooling or voiding, increased evaporative losses, inadequate volume or incorrect fluid administration, and problems with malabsorption may cause weight loss. Implementation of interventions and frequent reassessment of the infant and its environment are necessary to correct the problems. Such interventions include adjusting the incubator temperature; "swamping" or providing high levels of humidity under a cover over the radiant warmer; monitoring and adjusting the volume and type of fluids being administered; assessing the urinary output, including the specific gravity; and assessing the blood glucose levels. The glucose determinations are used to assess urine osmolarity and hence renal function. High glucose levels (greater than 125 mg/dl) can stimulate an excessive osmotic diuresis (Hockenberry et al., 2003). Weight gain may be due to overfeeding or fluid retention. The nurse reports and records the findings and continues to assess the infant's fluid status, urinary output, and blood glucose levels. The interventions implemented are determined by the infant's specific disorder and nutritional needs.

Elimination Patterns. The infant's elimination patterns also are assessed. This includes the frequency of urination, as well as the amount, color, pH, and specific gravity of the urine. The assessment of the infant's bowel movements includes the frequency of stooling and the character of the stool, as well as whether there is constipation, diarrhea, or loss of fats (steatorrhea). All of these

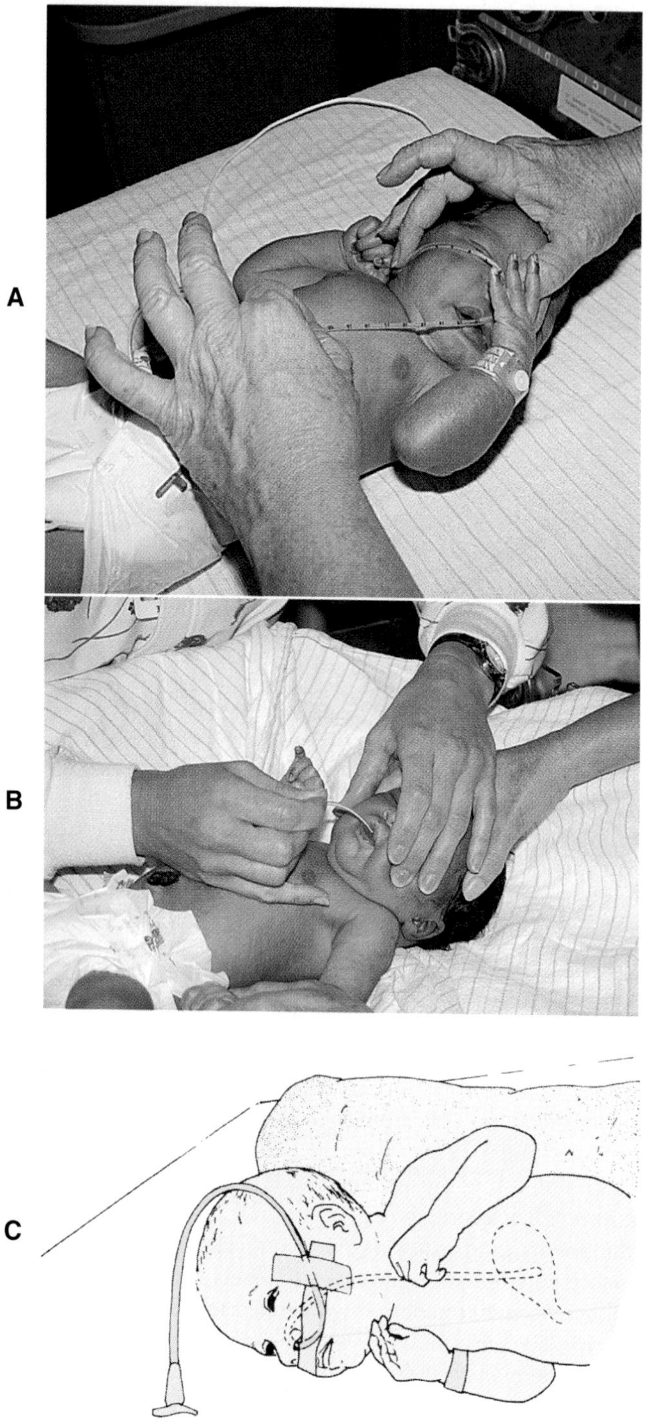
A
B
C

FIG. 40-6 Gavage feeding. **A,** Measurement of gavage feeding tube from tip of nose to earlobe and to midpoint between end of xyphoid process and umbilicus. Tape may be used to mark correct length on tube. **B,** Insertion of gavage tube by using orogastric route. **C,** Indwelling gavage tube, nasogastric route. After feeding by orogastric or nasogastric tube, infant is propped on right side for 1 hour to facilitate emptying of stomach into small intestine. Note rolled towel for support. (**A** and **B,** courtesy Marjorie Pyle, RNC, Lifecircle, Costa Mesa, CA.)

findings are documented. The nurse may request guaiac tests to assess for blood in the stool, tests to detect stool-reducing substances, and a pH determination to assess for malabsorption. Infants with unexplained abdominal distention are assessed carefully to rule out the presence of hypomotility or obstructions of the GI tract.

Oral Feeding. Nourishment by the oral route is preferred for the infant who has adequate strength and GI function. The best milk for an infant is that of its mother. Breast milk may be fed by breast or bottle. Formula may be fed by bottle or a supplementer (see Fig. 27-2). Throughout the feeding, the nurse assesses the newborn's tolerance of the procedure. When the infant breastfeeds, the nurse assists the mother by providing support and help, as necessary.

The needs of the high risk infant must be considered when determining the type and frequency of the feedings. Many high risk infants cannot suck well enough to breastfeed or bottle feed until they have recovered from their initial illness or matured physically (older than 32 weeks of gestation). Mothers of high risk infants are encouraged to continue pumping breast milk, especially if theirs is a very premature infant who may not breastfeed for many weeks. Because of the significant breastfeeding attrition rates among these mothers, they need support and encouragement every few days to continue pumping while their infant is not yet able to nurse. If no breast milk is available (from the mother or a milk bank), commercial formula is used. The calories, protein, and mineral content of commercial formulas vary (see Chapter 27). The type of nipple selected ("preemie," regular, orthodontic) depends on the infant's ability to suck from the specific type of nipple. The nurse also considers the energy the infant needs to expend in the process.

Overfeeding of the preterm infant should be avoided because this can lead to abdominal distention, with apnea, vomiting, and possibly aspiration of the feeding. The nurse monitors the infant's abdominal girth when distention is obvious.

Gavage Feeding. Gavage feeding is a method of providing nourishment to the infant who is compromised by respiratory distress, the infant who is too immature to have a coordinated suck-and-swallow reflex, or the infant who is easily fatigued by sucking. In gavage feeding, breast milk or formula is given to the infant through a nasogastric or orogastric tube (Fig. 40-6). This spares the infant the work of sucking.

Gavage feeding can be done either with an intermittently placed tube providing a bolus feeding or continuously through an indwelling catheter. Infants who cannot tolerate large-bolus feedings (those on ventilators for more than a week) are given continuous feedings. **Minimal enteral nutrition (MEN)** may be used to stimulate or prime the GI tract to achieve better absorption of nutrients when bolus or regular intermittent gavage feedings can be given (Tyson & Kennedy, 2002). Breast milk or formula can be supplied intermittently by using a syringe with gravity-controlled flow or can be given continuously by using an infusion pump. The type of fluid instilled is recorded with every syringe change. The volume of the continuous feedings is recorded hourly, and the residual gastric aspirate is measured every 4 hours. Residuals of less than a fourth of a feeding can be refed to the infant to prevent the loss of gastric electrolytes. Feeding is usually stopped if the residual is greater than a quarter of the feeding and is not resumed until the infant can be assessed for a possible feeding intolerance.

The orogastric route for gavage feedings is preferred because most infants are preferential nose breathers. Also when indwelling nasogastric tubes are used, there is a tendency towards nares necrosis; however, some infants do not tolerate oral tube placement. A small nasogastric feeding tube can be placed in older infants who would otherwise gag or vomit or in ones who are learning to suck. To insert the tube and give the feeding, the nurse should follow the sequence given in the Procedure boxes.

Gastrostomy Feedings. Infants with certain congenital malformations require gastrostomy feedings. This involves the surgical placement of a tube through the skin of the abdomen into the stomach. The tube is then taped in an upright position to prevent trauma to the incision site. After the site heals, the nurse initiates small bolus feedings per the physician's orders. Feedings by gravity are done slowly over 20- to 30-minute periods. Special care must be taken to prevent rapid bolusing of the fluid because this may lead to abdominal distention, GI reflux into the esophagus, or respiratory compromise. Meticulous skin care at the tube insertion site is necessary to prevent skin breakdown or infections. In addition, intake and output are monitored scrupulously because these infants are prone to diarrhea until regular feedings are established.

Parenteral Fluids. Feeding supplemental parenteral fluids is indicated for infants who are unable to obtain sufficient fluids or calories by enteral feeding (Fig. 40-7). Some of these infants are dependent on **total parenteral nutrition (TPN)** for extensive periods. The nurse assesses and documents the following in infants receiving parenteral fluids or TPN:

- Type and infusion rate of the solution
- Functional status of the infusion equipment, including the tubing and infusion pump
- Infusion site for possible complications (phlebitis, infiltration, dislodgment)
- Caloric intake
- Infant's responses to therapy

The physician or nurse practitioner orders TPN per the hospital protocol. These orders must specify the electrolytes and nutrients desired, as well as the volume and rate of infusion. The amounts of calories, protein, and fat are determined on the basis of the individual infant's energy needs (Wyckoff et al., 2003).

While caring for the infant receiving parenteral fluids or TPN, the nurse secures and protects the insertion site

PROCEDURE
Gavage Feeding

- To begin the feeding, connect the barrel of a syringe to the gavage tube. While crimping the feeding tube, pour the specified amount of breast milk or formula into the syringe.
- Release the crimp in the tube and allow the feeding to flow down by gravity (Fig. 40-7). The infant usually tolerates the feeding better if the rate approximates that of an oral feeding (about 1 ml/min).
- The parent or nurse can swaddle or hold the infant to help the infant associate the feeding with positive interactions. Some parents like to do kangaroo care while gavage feeding their infant. The parents are encouraged to talk to their infant during the feedings.
- Once the prescribed volume has been delivered, the nurse crimps or pinches the tube and removes the syringe.
- The gavage tube is capped (or the nurse continues to pinch it) while removing it in one steady motion. Capping the tube (or pinching it off) prevents breast milk or formula from leaking from the tube and being aspirated during removal of the tube.
- After the feeding, position the infant on the right side to prevent aspiration.
- Document the procedure: the size of the feeding tube, the amount and quality of the residual from the previous feeding, the type and quantity of fluid instilled (sterile water, breast milk, or formula), and the infant's response to the procedure.

PROCEDURE
Inserting a Gavage Feeding Tube

1. Measure the length of the gavage tube from the tip of the nose to the lobe of the ear to the midpoint between the xiphoid process and the umbilicus (Fig. 40-6, *A*). Mark the tube with a piece of tape.
2. Lubricate the tip of the tube with sterile water and insert gently through the nose or mouth (Fig. 40-6, *B*) until the predetermined mark is reached. Placement of the tube in the trachea will cause the infant to gag, cough, or become cyanotic.
3. Check correct placement of the tube by
   a. Pulling back on the plunger to aspirate stomach contents. Lack of fluid is not necessarily evidence of improper placement. Respiratory secretions may be mistaken for stomach contents; however, the pH of the stomach contents is much lower (more acidic) than the pH of respiratory secretions.
   b. Injecting a small amount of air (1 to 3 ml) into the tube while listening for gurgling or by using a stethoscope placed over the stomach. Ensure that the tube is inserted to the mark; it is possible to hear air entering the stomach even if the tube is positioned above the gastroesophageal (cardiac) sphincter.
4. Tape the tube in place and also tape it to the cheek to prevent accidental dislodgment and incorrect positioning (Fig. 40-6, *C*).
   a. Assess the infant's skin integrity before taping the tube.
   b. Edematous or very premature infants should have a pectin barrier placed under the tape to prevent abrasions (Lund & Durand, 2003).
5. Tube placement must be assessed before each feeding.

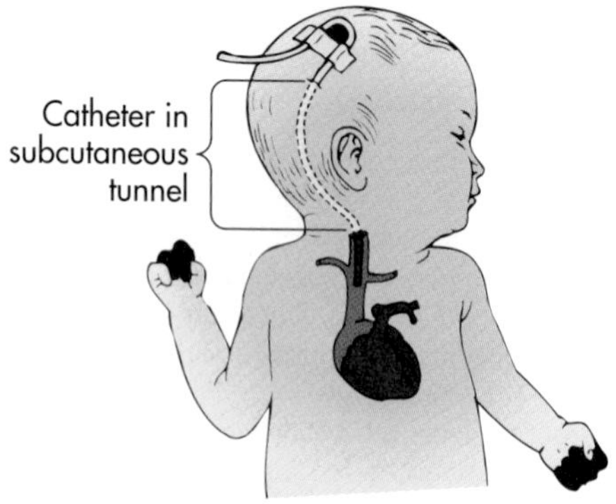
Catheter in
subcutaneous
tunnel

FIG. 40-7 Total parenteral nutrition (TPN). Close-up showing infusion site and internal placement of catheter into descending vena cava.

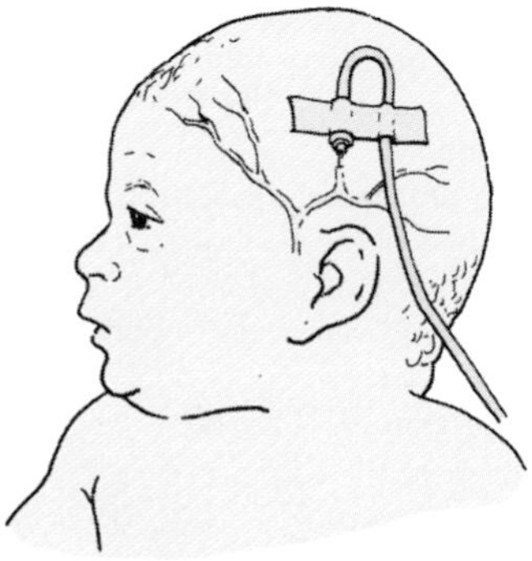

FIG. 40-8 Venipuncture of scalp vein.

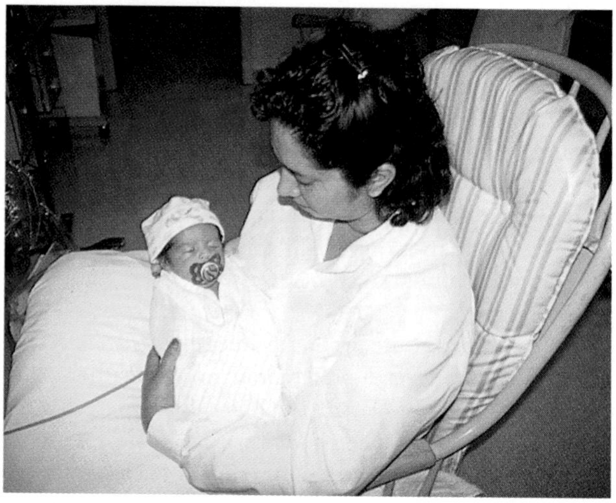

FIG. 40-9 Nonnutritive sucking by infant. (Courtesy Marjorie Pyle, RNC, Lifecircle, Costa Mesa, CA.)

(Fig. 40-8). In addition to observing the principles of asepsis, the nurse must observe the principles of neonatal skin care (Lund & Kuller, 2003). The nurse also should inspect the infusion site for signs of infiltration and reposition the infant frequently to maintain body alignment and protect the site. Parents of infants need to be given explanations about TPN and the way in which the IV equipment and solutions affect their infant.

Advancing Infant Feedings. Feedings are advanced as assessment data and the infant's ability to tolerate the feedings warrant it. Documentation of a premature infant's sucking patterns also can be used to determine its readiness to nipple feed. Feedings are advanced from passive (parenteral and gavage) to active (nipple and breastfeeding). At each step, the nurse must carefully assess the infant's response to prevent overstressing the infant.

The infant receiving nutrition parenterally is gradually weaned off of this type of nutrition. To do this, the nourishment given by continuous or intermittent gavage feedings is increased while the parenteral fluids are decreased. Even the smallest infant is sometimes now given MEN to stimulate the GI system to mature and to enhance caloric intake (Wyckoff et al., 2003).

Feedings are advanced slowly and cautiously because, if feedings are advanced too rapidly, the infant may vomit (with an attendant risk of aspiration), with diarrhea, abdominal distention, and apneic episodes. Rapid advancement of feedings also may cause fluid retention with cardiac compromise or a pronounced diuresis with hyponatremia.

If the infant needs additional calories, a commercial human milk fortifier can be added to the gavaged breast milk, or the number of calories per 30 ml of commercial formula can be increased. Soy and elemental formulas are used only for infants with very special dietary needs, such as allergies to cow's milk or chronic malabsorption. Calories in breast milk can be lost if the cream separates and adheres to the tubing during continuous infusion. This problem is decreased if microbore tubing is used for both continuous and intermittent gavage feedings.

The infant receiving gavage feedings progresses to bottle feeding or breast milk feedings. To do this, the gavage feedings are decreased as the infant's ability to suckle breast milk or formula improves. Often during this transition, the infant is fed by both nipple and gavage feeding to ensure the intake of both the prescribed volume of food and nutrients. However, when there is an indwelling tube, during nipple feedings, some infants experience an increased respiratory effort, so nurses must watch for this. The parents need support during this transition because many families measure their parenting competence by how well they can feed their infant.

As the time of discharge nears, the appropriate method of feeding, as well as the assessments pertaining to the method (e.g., tolerance of feedings, status of gavage tube placement), are reviewed with the parents. The parents should be encouraged to interact with the infant by talking and making eye contact with the infant during the

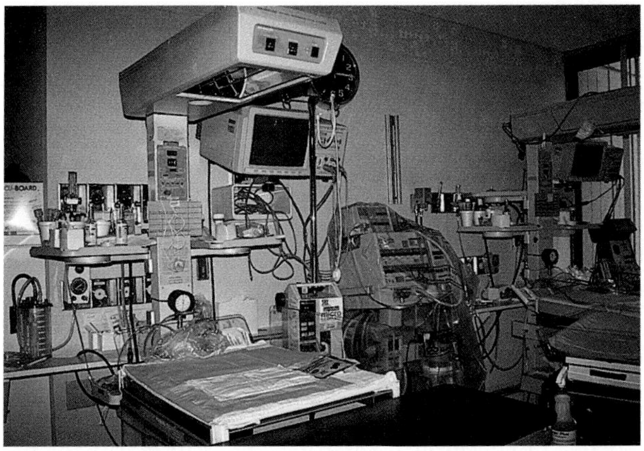

FIG. 40-10 Significant environmental stimulation. Note bed, wall oxygen attachments, monitor, ventilator, incubator, and pumps, all of which have alarm systems. (Courtesy Marjorie Pyle, RNC, Lifecircle, Costa Mesa, CA.)

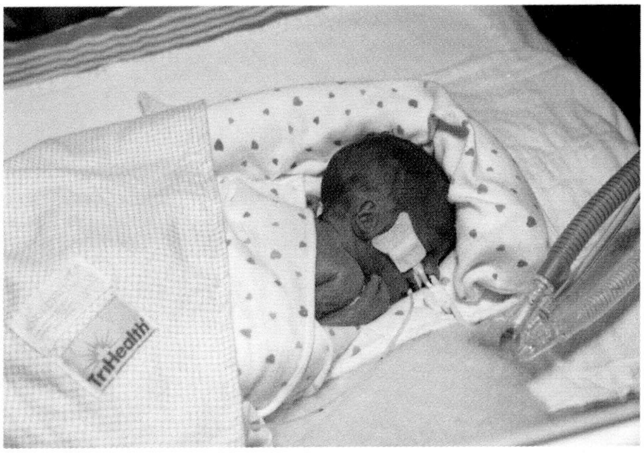

FIG. 40-11 Ventilator-dependent infant. (Courtesy Leslie Altimier, MSN, RN, TriHealth, Cincinnati, OH.)

feeding. This interaction is encouraged to stimulate the psychosocial development of the infant and to facilitate bonding and attachment.

Nonnutritive Sucking. If the gavage or the parenteral route nourishes the infant, **nonnutritive sucking** is encouraged (Fig. 40-9) for several reasons. Allowing the infant to suck on a pacifier during gavage or between oral feedings may improve oxygenation. In addition, such nonnutritive sucking may lead to a decreased energy expenditure with less restlessness, positive weight gain, and promote faster attachment to the nipple when oral feedings are initiated (Wyckoff et al., 2003).

Mothers of premature infants should be encouraged to let their premature infants start sucking at the breast during kangaroo care (skin-to-skin) because some infant's suck-and-swallow reflexes may be coordinated as early as 32 weeks of gestation.

Infants with intrauterine growth restriction (IUGR) may have an age-appropriate sucking reflex but require thermoregulatory support, making it difficult to breastfeed. These infants also may benefit from nonnutritive sucking at the breast for short periods.

Environmental Concerns

Infants in NICUs also are exposed to high levels of auditory input from the various machine alarms, and this can have adverse effects (Fig. 40-10). In addition, continuous noise levels of 45 to 85 decibels (db) are common in NICUs. An incubator alone produces a constant noise level of 60 to 80 db (Haubrich, 2003), and each new piece of life-support equipment used adds another 20 db to the background noise. The infant's hearing may be damaged if it is exposed to a constant decibel level of 90 db or frequent decibel swings higher than 110 db. Cochlear damage has been recognized as a side effect of the NICU environment. Thus both conductive and sensorineural hearing losses have been identified in NICU graduates; these losses lead to long-term speech and language deficits (Haubrich, 2003).

Respiratory equipment (Fig. 40-11) or a phototherapy mask, making it difficult for the infant to interact with caregivers and family members, may alter the infant's vision. The infant also may be unable to establish diurnal and nocturnal rhythms because of the continuous exposure to overhead lighting. In addition, sedation or pain medications affect the way in which the infant perceives the environment.

An additional concern in the care of infants is that some drugs used for infant therapy can potentiate environmental hazards. Diuretics (especially furosemide [Lasix]), antibiotics (gentamicin), and antimalarial agents can potentiate noise-induced hearing loss (Haubrich, 2003).

Research is ongoing to determine effects of light and noise on the premature infant. Long-term problems are the focus of much research (Symington & Pinelli, 2001; Walsh-Sukys, et al., 2001). Cycling of light and covering of isolettes to reduce direct light hitting the retina are two areas of research. The retina of the immature infant has little protection from the nearly translucent eyelid, thus allowing light to almost continuously penetrate the retina unless it is artificially protected with dimming of the lights or isolette covers. Light and sound are known adverse stimuli that add to an already stressed premature infant. The result is stress cues, increased metabolic rates, increased oxygen and caloric use, and depression of the immune system. The nurse must monitor the macro and microenvironment (unit and immediate environments) for sources of overstimulation. Providing a developmentally supportive environment can lead to decreased complications and lengths of stay. There are national recommendations for sound and light levels in the NICU (see Resources at end of chapter).

NURSE ALERT

Routine hearing screening should be performed in all infants before discharge, with universal screening completed by no later than the third month of life.

Nurses can modify the environment to provide a developmentally supportive milieu. In that way, the infant's neurobehavioral and physiologic needs can be met better, the infant's developing organization can be supported, and growth and development fostered (Symington & Pinelli, 2002).

EVIDENCE-BASED PRACTICE

Developmental Care and Its Effect on Preventing Morbidity in Preterm Infants

This review focused on developmental care and its effect on morbidity of preterm infants. The rationale for the review was that environmental stimuli are known factors in adding to morbidity of this population. Developmental care tends to reduce adverse stimuli and should theoretically decrease morbidity and mortality in preterm infants.

Objectives: To determine if developmental care reduced neurodevelopmental delay, poor weight gain, length of stay, use of mechanical ventilation, physiologic instability, and other clinically relevant adverse outcomes known to be associated with preterm birth and an NICU hospitalization.

Methods: Studies from 1990 to July 2000 were reviewed. The review was limited to randomized controlled trials for infants <37 weeks' gestation and that involved use of developmental care and were published in English. A meta-analysis was done on each intervention identified. Outcome measures and/or instruments had to be comparable in the studies on each variable.

Findings: Thirty-one studies were included accounting for four major developmental care interventions with 19 subgroups and varied clinical outcomes. The outcomes were positive for short-term growth, decreased need for mechanical ventilation, decrease in length of stay when compared with average length of stay for similar gestational age infants, cost savings, and neurodevelopmental outcomes at 24 months corrected age.

Limitations: For each of the developmental interventions, only two to three studies fit the criteria, which resulted in very small sample sizes. In none of the studies were the health professionals doing the assessments blinded to the intervention, which created the potential for bias in the results. No consideration of personnel or intervention costs were included in the calculation of cost savings.

Conclusions: Although evidence appears to support practice using developmental interventions, more research is needed with larger samples and with more stringent controls including blinding of the examiner of infant outcomes and costs of personnel and interventions included in the cost factor. This area of neonatal care looks very promising. Some low-level evidence supports its incorporation into care, as the neurobehavioral outcomes were better than expected compared with average comparable gestational age infants. More research is needed before one can definitively say that these interventions are appropriate and positive for all preterm infants.

Reference: Symington, A., & Pinelli, J. (2002). Developmental care for promoting development and preventing morbidity in preterm infants. (Cochrane Review). *The Cochrane Library,* 2. Oxford: Update Software, Ltd.

Developmental Care

The goal of developmental care is to support each infant's efforts to become as well-organized, competent, and stable as possible. Developmental care includes all care procedures and the physical and social aspects of care in the NICU (Als, 1998). The caregiver uses the infant's own behavior and physiologic functioning as the basis for planning care and providing interventions (see Evidence-Based Practice box). Through caregiver observation, the infant's strengths, thresholds for disorganization, and areas in which the infant is vulnerable can be identified (Als, 1998). The family is included in developmental care as the primary coregulators (Als, 1998). Working together, the family and other caregivers provide opportunities to enhance the strengths of the family and the infant and to reduce the stress that is associated with the birth and care of high risk infants. In some settings, a "cuddler" (specially trained adult volunteer who holds, reads, talks to, and consoles infant when the parents are unable to visit) (Steuber, Carroll, McCoy, & Nurney, 2002) participates in the care.

Reducing light and noise levels by instituting "quiet hours" during each 8-hour shift and positioning are just two of the ways in which nurses can support infants in their development (Gray et al., 1998). Sleep interruptions are minimized, and positioning and bundling the infant help promote self-regulation and prevent disorganization (Symington & Pinelli, 2002).

Positioning. The motor development of preterm infants permits less flexion than that in their term counterparts. Caregivers can provide a variety of positions for infants; side-lying and prone are preferred to supine. Body containment with use of blanket rolls, swaddling, holding the infant's arms in a crossed position, and secure holding provide boundaries and promote self-regulation during feeding, procedures, and other stressful interventions (Hendricks-Munoz et al., 2002). The prone position encourages flexion of the extremities; a sling or hip roll assists in maintenance of flexion. Use of a sheepskin prevents abrasion of the knees. However, there is some concern that fibers from sheepskin can be breathed in if the infant's face is positioned near the sheepskin itself, so it should be used with caution. Holding the limbs close to the body when the infant is moved decreases stimulation that produces jerky, uncoordinated movements (Hockenberry et al., 2003). Proper body alignment is necessary to prevent developmental problems that may affect the ability to walk as the child matures.

Reducing Inappropriate Stimuli. Staff can reduce unnecessary noise by closing doors or portholes on incubators quietly, placing only necessary objects gently on top of incubators, keeping radios at low volume, speaking quietly, and handling equipment noiselessly. Earmuffs also may reduce auditory input (Hockenberry et al., 2003).

Infants can be protected from light by dimming the lights during the night, placing a blanket over the incubator (Fig. 40-12), or covering the infant's eyes with a mask. Sleep-wake cycles can be induced with such measures. Infants need periods when they are completely undisturbed (Hockenberry et al., 2003).

Infant Communication. Infants communicate their needs and ability to tolerate sensory stimulation through physiologic responses. The nurses and parents of high risk infants must therefore be alert to such cues. Although term infants may thrive on stimulation, this same stimulation in high risk infants can instead provoke physical symptoms of stress and anxiety (Symington & Pinelli, 2002).

Problems with noxious stimuli and barriers to normal contact may cause anxiety and tension. Clues to overstimulation include averting the gaze, hiccuping, gagging, or regurgitating food. Term infants exhibit a startle reflex, and premature infants move all of their limbs in an uncoordinated fashion in response to noxious stimuli. An irregular respiratory rate or an increased heart rate may develop in severely distressed infants, and they may then be unable to regain a calm state.

A relaxed infant state is indicated by stabilization of vital signs, closed eyes, and a relaxed posture. Nonintubated infants may make soothing verbal sounds when they are relaxed. Infants requiring artificial ventilation cannot cry audibly and often show their distress through posturing; they then relax once their needs are met. As high risk infants heal and mature, they increasingly respond to stimuli in a self-regulated manner rather than with a dissociated response. Infants who do not show increased self-regulation should be evaluated for a neurologic problem.

Infant Stimulation. A neonatal individualized developmental care and assessment program (NIDCAP) routinely integrates aspects of neurodevelopmental theory with caregivers' observations, environmental interventions, and parental support (Hendricks-Munoz et al., 2002). Routine reassessment is built into the program's design. Developmental stimuli may consist of such simple measures as placing a waterbed mattress on the top of the infant's mattress or kangaroo (skin-to-skin) holding. The simplest calming technique is to contain the infant's extremities close to the body with both hands. The care of the infant is organized to allow extended periods of undisturbed rest and sleep. Pain medications or sedatives should be administered consistently, per the unit's protocol.

Infants acquire a sense of trust as they learn the feel, sound, and smell of their parents. High risk infants also must learn to trust their caregivers to obtain comfort. However, caregivers in the nursery also may inflict pain as part of the care they must give. For this reason, it is important for both the parents and the caregivers of such infants to use comforting interventions such as removing painful stimuli, stopping hunger, and changing wet or soiled clothing to foster trust. They can offer nonnutritive sucking opportunities or use oral sucrose for pain relief and topical creams before procedures to avoid the sensation of pain. All of these techniques are part of developmental, supportive care.

When the infant is ready for stimulation, the nurse has many options. All infants can tolerate being held, even if only for short periods. Additional ways for the nurse or parents to stimulate infants include cuddling, rocking, singing, use of music therapy, and talking to the infant (Fig. 40-13). These activities are beneficial, increase weight gain, and decrease time to discharge (Standley, 1998, 2002). Stroking the infant's skin during medical therapy can provide tactile stimulation. The caregiver responds to the infant's cues by offering reassurance, providing nonnutritive sucking, stroking the infant's back, and talking to the infant.

Mobiles and decals that can be changed frequently also may be placed within the infant's visual range to stimulate the infant visually. Wind-up musical toys provide rhythmic distractions as long as they are not too loud. If the infant is

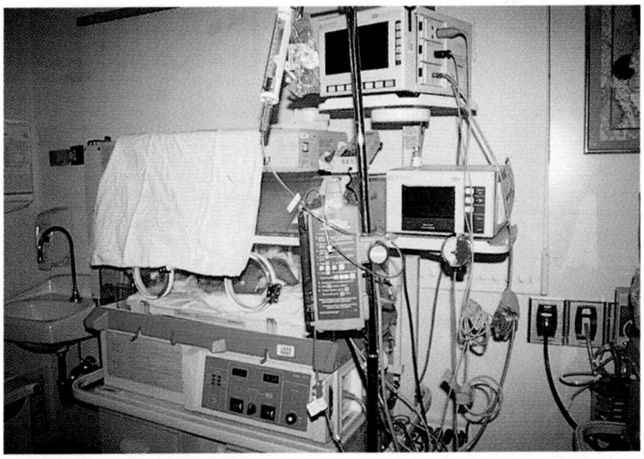

FIG. 40-12 Infant in double-walled incubator with a blanket for a light shield. (Courtesy Marjorie Pyle, RNC, Lifecircle, Costa Mesa, CA.)

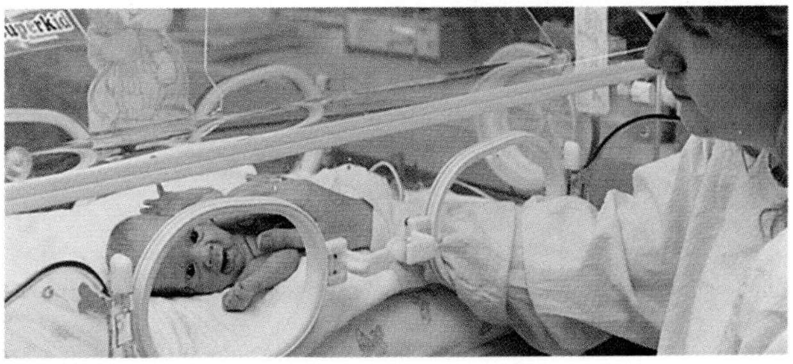

FIG. 40-13 A tiny preterm infant in the NICU. (Courtesy Children's Medical Ventures, Norwell, MA.)

receiving phototherapy, the protective eye patches are removed periodically (e.g., during feeding) so that the infant can see the caregiver's face for short, comforting sessions.

Kangaroo Care. Kangaroo care (skin-to-skin holding) helps infants to interact directly with their parents (Gale & VandenBerg, 1998). In this technique, the infant, dressed only in a diaper, is placed directly on the parent's bare chest and then covered with the parent's clothing or a warmed blanket (Fig. 40-14). In this way, the parent's body temperature also functions as an external heat source that enhances the infant's temperature regulation. Even ventilator-dependent infants weighing less than 1000 g have been found to benefit from this measure, although they usually tolerate it for only 30 minutes or less at a time (see Research box).

Kangaroo holding was originally developed in Bogota, Colombia, where radiant warmers and incubators were in severely short supply. Although such care has its roots in severe economic hardships, it stems from a deep respect for natural processes. Infants and parents who participate in such kangaroo care have been observed to have dramatically better outcomes. The mothers report increased breast milk output and fewer feelings of helplessness related to their experiences in the NICU (Anderson, Dombrowski, & Swinth, 2001). The infants have been found to maintain their temperatures and oxygenation levels better and to experience fewer episodes of crying, apnea, and periodic respirations. They also have been observed to be alert and quiet longer and to have slightly higher heart rates. Kangaroo care also meets developmental needs by fostering neurobehavioral development.

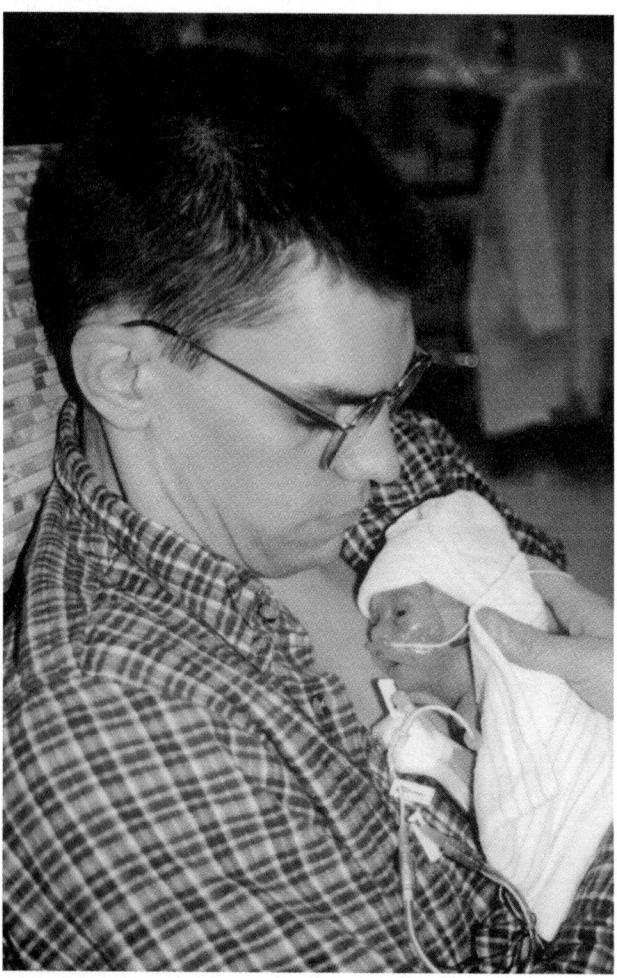

FIG. 40-14 Father providing kangaroo care. (Courtesy Judy Meyr, St. Louis, MO.)

Parental Support

The nurse as the support person and teacher is responsible for shaping the environment and making the care-giving responsive to the needs of the parents and infant. Nurses are instrumental in helping parents learn who their infant is and to recognize behavioral cues in his or her development (VandenBerg, 1999).

RESEARCH

Kangaroo Care in the NICU

Kangaroo care (KC) is an intervention in which a diaper-clad preterm infant is held skin-to-skin next to the parent's chest. It has been useful for infants even below 1000 grams. Infant benefits include improvement in thermoregulation, oxygenation, breathing pattern stability, weight gain, and increased quiet sleep. Breastfeeding is enhanced with KC, with increased maternal milk production and longer feeding time. Parents report increased closeness to their infant and increased feelings of competence. Symptoms of depression are reportedly lower when mothers practice KC.

Parents have generally initiated KC, according to a survey of neonatal intensive care units (NICUs) reported by a group of 12 nurse researchers. The investigators sent surveys to nurse managers of all 1006 NICUs in the United States and received responses from 537 (59%). Over 82% of the respondents reported practicing KC in their unit. Nurses on these units were more positive about its value and worth than nurses on non-KC NICUs. Barriers to practicing KC included infant safety concerns (such as concern for lines and tubes), lack of guidelines, lack of enough time to implement, lack of physician support, and staff reluctance. KC was practiced with infants with a variety of ongoing treatments, with the exception of vasopressors and oscillators. Some nurses did not have an accurate understanding of KC.

IMPLICATIONS FOR PRACTICE

Even though parents tend to initiate use of KC, NICU nurses can advocate for implementing this intervention. Published reports show that KC may lighten the nurses' workload by stabilizing the infant and involving the parents in care. Nurses wanting to incorporate KC could benefit from visiting units that practice KC and learning hands-on skills such as techniques for infant transfer to parent. Protocols for KC practice also are available through the WHO KC Network.

Reference: Engler, A. et al. (2002). Kangaroo care: National survey of practice, knowledge, barriers, and perceptions. *MCN The American Journal of Maternal Child Nursing, 27*(3), 146-153.

If a high risk birth has been anticipated, the family can be given a tour of the NICU or shown a video to prepare them for the sights and activities of the unit. After the birth, the parents can be given a booklet, be shown a video, or have someone describe what they will see when they go to the unit to see their infant. As soon as possible, the parents should see and touch their infant so that they can begin to acknowledge the reality of the birth and the infant's true appearance and condition. They will need encouragement as they begin to accomplish the psychologic tasks imposed by the high risk birth. For the following reasons, a nurse or physician should be present during the parents' first visit to see the infant:

- To help them "see" the infant rather than focus on the equipment. The importance and purpose of the apparatus that surrounds their infant also should be explained to them.
- To explain the characteristics normal for an infant of their baby's gestational age; in this way parents do not compare their child with a term, healthy infant.
- To encourage the parents to express their feelings about the pregnancy, labor, and birth and the experience of having a high risk infant.
- To assess the parents' perceptions of the infant to determine the appropriate time for them to become actively involved in care (see Guidelines/Guías box).

As soon as possible after the birth, the parents are given the opportunity to meet the infant in the *en face* position, to touch the infant, and to see his or her favorable characteristics. Mothers often state that their greatest source of stress is the appearance of their baby (Miles et al., 2002). As soon as possible, depending primarily on her physical condition, the mother is encouraged to visit the nursery as desired and help with the infant's care. When the family cannot be present physically, staff members devise appropriate methods to keep them in almost constant touch with the newborn, such as with daily phone calls, notes written as if by the infant, or photographs of the infant.

Some hospitals have support groups for the parents of infants in NICUs. These groups help parents experiencing anxiety and grief by encouraging them to share their feelings. Hospitals also often arrange to have an experienced NICU parent make contact with a new group member to provide additional support. The volunteer parents provide support by making hospital visits, phone calls, and home visits.

Many NICUs use volunteers in varying capacities. After they have gone through the orientation program, volunteers can perform tasks such as holding the infants, stocking bedside cabinets, assembling parent packets, and, in some nurseries, feeding the infants.

Some high risk infants can be discharged earlier than the expected time (Gamblian, Hess, & Kenner, 1998). The criteria showing an infant's readiness for early discharge are that the infant's physiologic condition is stable, the infant is receiving adequate nutrition, and the infant's body temperature is stable. The parents, or other caregivers, also need to exhibit a physical, emotional, and educational readiness to assume responsibility for the care of the infant. Ideally, the home environment is adequate for meeting the needs of the infant. The parents also need to show that they know the way to take the infant's temperature, know the signs and symptoms to report, and understand the dietary needs of the infant.

Parent Education

Cardiopulmonary Resuscitation. Sudden infant death syndrome (SIDS) is 8 to 10 times more likely to develop in preterm infants than in term infants. Furthermore, it has been found that infants discharged from an NICU are about twice as likely to die unexpectedly during the first year of life as are infants in the general population. Instruction in cardiopulmonary resuscitation (CPR) is essential for parents of all infants but especially for those of infants at risk for life-threatening events (see Chapter 28). Infants considered at risk include those who are premature, have apnea or bradycardia spells, or have a tendency to choke. Before taking their infant home, parents must be able to administer CPR. All parents should be encouraged to obtain instruction in CPR at their local Red Cross or other community agency if it is not provided by the NICU.

Evaluation

The nurse uses the previously stated expected outcomes of care to evaluate the effectiveness of the physical and psychosocial aspects of care (see Plan of Care).

GUIDELINES/GUÍAS

Intensive Care Nursery—Parent Teaching on First Visit

He/she is small but strong.
Él/ella es pequeño/pequeña pero fuerte.

This is a special bed that keeps the baby warm with radiant heat.
Esta es una cama especial que mantiene al bebé caliente con calor radiante.

The baby is breathing by himself on room air.
El bebé está respirando solo en el aire ambiente.

The baby has an IV so we can give him fluids.
El bebé tiene un cateter intrevenoso para administrarle líquidos.

The baby has an umbilical catheter so that we may administer fluids and nutrients and so we may draw blood for laboratory testing.
El bebé tiene un cateter umbilical que nos permite administrar líquidos y nutrimentos al bebé y nos permite obtener muestras de sangre para hacer pruebas.

This nasogastric tube allows us to feed the baby.
Este tubo nasogastrica nos permite alimentar a su bebé.

This endotracheal tube delivers air directly to the lungs.
Este tubo endotraqueal entrega aire directamente a los pulmones.

Plan of Care High Risk Premature Newborn

NURSING DIAGNOSIS **Ineffective breathing pattern related to pulmonary and neuromuscular immaturity, decreased energy, fatigue**

Expected Outcomes *Infant exhibits adequate oxygenation (i.e., ABGs and acid-base within normal limits [WNL], oxygen saturations 92% or greater, respiratory rate and pattern WNL, breath sounds clear, absence of grunting, nasal flaring, minimal retractions, skin color WNL).*

Nursing Interventions/*Rationales*

Position neonate prone or supine, avoiding neck hyperextension *to promote optimum air exchange.* Use a side-lying position after feeding or in cases of excessive mucous production *to avoid aspiration.* Avoid Trendelenburg's position *because it can cause increased intracranial pressure and reduce lung capacity.*

Suction nasopharynx, trachea, and endotracheal tube as indicated *to remove mucus.* Avoid oversuctioning *because it can cause bronchospasm, bradycardia, hypoxia, and predispose neonate to intraventricular hemorrhage.*

Administer percussion, vibration, and postural drainage as prescribed *to facilitate drainage of secretions.*

Administer oxygen and monitor neonatal response *to maintain oxygen saturation.*

Maintain a neutral thermal environment *to conserve oxygen use.*

Monitor arterial blood gases, acid-base balance, oxygen saturation, respiratory rate and pattern, breath sounds, and airway patency; observe for grunting, nasal flaring, retractions, and cyanosis *to detect signs of respiratory distress.*

NURSING DIAGNOSIS **Ineffective thermoregulation related to immature temperature regulation and minimal subcutaneous fat stores**

Expected Outcome *Infant exhibits maintenance of stable body temperature within normal range for postconceptional age (36.5° C to 37.2° C).*

Nursing Interventions/*Rationales*

Place neonate in a prewarmed radiant warmer *to maintain stable temperature.*

Place temperature probe on neonatal abdomen *to control heat levels in radiant warmer.*

Take axillary temperature periodically *to monitor temperature and cross-check functioning of warmer unit.*

Avoid infant exposure to cool air and drafts, cold scales, cold stethoscopes, cold examination tables, and prolonged bathing *that predispose the infant to heat loss.*

Monitor probe frequently *as detachment can cause overheating or warmer-induced hyperthermia.*

Transfer infant to a servocontrolled open warmer bed or incubator *when temperature has stabilized.*

NURSING DIAGNOSIS **Risk for infection related to immature immune system**

Expected Outcome *Infant exhibits no evidence of nosocomial infection.*

Nursing Interventions/*Rationales*

Institute scrupulous handwashing techniques before and after handling neonate, ensure all supplies and/or equipment are clean before use, and ensure strict aseptic technique with invasive procedures *to minimize exposure to infective organisms.*

Prevent contact with persons who have communicable infections and instruct parents in infection control procedures *to minimize infection risk.*

Administer prescribed antibiotics *to provide coverage for infection during sepsis workup.*

Continuously monitor vital signs for stability *as instability, hypothermia, or prolonged temperature elevations serve as indicators for infection.*

NURSING DIAGNOSIS **Risk for imbalanced nutrition: less than body requirements related to inability to ingest nutrients secondary to immaturity**

Expected Outcomes *Infant receives adequate amount of nutrients with sufficient caloric intake to maintain positive nitrogen balance; demonstrates steady weight gain.*

Nursing Interventions/*Rationales*

Administer parenteral fluid/total parenteral nutrition (TPN) as prescribed *to provide adequate nutrition and fluid intake.*

Monitor for signs of intolerance to TPN, *which can interfere with effective replenishment of nutrients.*

Periodically assess readiness to orally feed (i.e., strong suck, swallow, and gag reflexes) *to provide appropriate transition from TPN to oral feeding as soon as neonate is ready.*

Advance volume and concentration of formula when orally feeding per unit protocol *to avoid overfeeding and feeding intolerance.*

If mother desires to breastfeed when neonate is stable, demonstrate how to express milk *to establish and maintain lactation until infant can breastfeed.*

NURSING DIAGNOSIS **Risk for deficient/excess fluid volume related to immature physiology**

Expected Outcome *Infant exhibits evidence of fluid homeostasis.*

Nursing Interventions/*Rationales*

Administer parenteral fluids as prescribed and regulate carefully *to maintain fluid balance.* Avoid hypertonic fluids such as undiluted medications, and concentrated glucose because *they can cause excess solute load on immature kidneys.*

Implement strategies (e.g., use of plastic covers and increase of ambient humidity) *that minimize insensible water loss.*

Monitor hydration status (i.e., skin turgor, blood pressure, edema, weight, mucous membranes, fontanels, urine specific gravity, electrolytes) and intake and output *to evaluate for evidence of dehydration or overhydration.*

NURSING DIAGNOSIS **Risk for impaired skin integrity related to immature skin structure, immobility, or invasive procedures**

Expected Outcome *Infant's skin remains intact with no evidence of irritation or injury.*

Nursing Interventions/*Rationales*

Cleanse skin as needed with plain warm water and apply moisturizing agents to skin *to prevent dryness and reduce friction across skin surface.*

When performing procedures: minimize use of tape and apply a skin barrier between tape and skin; use transparent elastic film for securing central and peripheral lines; use limb electrodes for monitoring or attach with hydrogel and rotate electrodes frequently; remove adhesives with soap and water rather than alcohol or acetone-based adhesive removers *to minimize skin damage.*

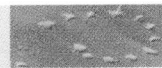

Plan of Care High Risk Premature Newborn—cont'd

Monitor use of thermal devices such as warmers or heating pads carefully *to prevent burns.*

Monitor skin closely for evidence of redness, rash, irritation, bruising, breakdown, ischemia, and infiltration *to detect and treat potential complications early.*

NURSING DIAGNOSIS Risk for injury related to increased intracranial pressure and intraventricular hemorrhage secondary to immature central nervous system

Expected Outcome *Infant will exhibit normal intracranial pressure (ICP) with no evidence of intraventricular hemorrhage.*

Nursing Interventions/*Rationales*

Institute minimum stimulation protocol (i.e., minimal handling, clustering care techniques, avoidance of sudden head movements to one side, undisturbed sleep periods, light variations to simulate day and night, limiting personnel and equipment noise in environment) *to decrease stress responses, which can increase ICP.*

Institute ordered pharmacologic and nonpharmacologic pain control methods *to manage pain and reduce physical stress.*

Avoid hypertonic solutions and medications *as they increase cerebral blood flow.*

Elevate head of bed 15 to 20 degrees *to decrease ICP.*

Monitor vital signs *for evidence of ICP.*

Recognize signs of overstimulation (i.e., flaccidity, yawning, irritability, crying, staring, active averting) *so stimulation can be stopped to allow rest.*

NURSING DIAGNOSIS Impaired parenting related to separation and interruption of parent/infant attachment secondary to premature birth

Expected Outcomes *Parents establish contact with neonate; demonstrate competent parenting skills and willingness to care for neonate.*

Nursing Interventions/*Rationales*

Before parents' first visit to the NICU, prepare them by explaining what the neonate will look like, what the equipment will look like and its function *to diminish fear and decrease sense of shock.*

Keep parents informed about infant's condition (improvements and setbacks) and important aspects of infant's care; encourage and answer parental questions; actively listen to parent concerns *to establish trust, open communication, and caring atmosphere to aid in coping.*

Encourage parents to visit the NICU often; to name infant (if that is culturally appropriate); to touch, hold, or caress infant as physical condition permits; to be actively involved in infant's care; to bring personal items (i.e., clothing, stuffed animals, or pictures of family) *to allow for formation of emotional bond.*

Reinforce parent involvement and praise care endeavors *to increase self-confidence in their contribution.*

Encourage parents to bring other siblings to visit; explain to siblings what they are seeing; encourage siblings to draw pictures or write letters for infant and place in or near infant's crib *to promote family involvement, help ease sibling fears, and let them contribute to infant's care.*

Refer parents to social services as needed *to ensure comprehensive care.*

NURSING DIAGNOSIS Anticipatory grieving related to perceived loss of premature infant

Expected Outcome *Parents express feelings about the potential loss and seek support from staff, family, clergy, and other support systems.*

Nursing Interventions/*Rationales*

Encourage parents to express feelings about perceived loss of infant *to reinforce reality and help alleviate guilt.*

Encourage parents to use family, friends, clergy, and other support persons *to enhance coping ability.*

Plan time on each shift to sit and listen to parents *to demonstrate concern, empathy, and support.*

Inform parents about support groups in the facility and the community *to encourage parents to use available resources.*

COMPLICATIONS IN HIGH RISK INFANTS

Respiratory Distress Syndrome

Respiratory distress syndrome (RDS) refers to a lung disorder usually affecting premature infants. Maternal and fetal conditions associated with a decreased incidence and severity of RDS include female infant, African-American race, maternal pregnancy-induced hypertension, maternal drug abuse, maternal steroid therapy (betamethasone), chronic retroplacental abruption, prolonged rupture of membranes, and IUGR. The incidence and severity of RDS increase with a decrease in the gestational age. Perinatal asphyxia, hypovolemia, male infant, white race, maternal diabetes (types 1 and 2), second-born twin, familial predisposition, maternal hypotension, cesarean birth without labor, hydrops fetalis, and third-trimester bleeding are all factors that place an infant at increased risk for RDS. The incidence of RDS in infants weighing less than 1500 g is between 40% and 60% (Cifuentes et al., 2003; Schwartz, 2003).

RDS is caused by a lack of pulmonary surfactant, which leads to progressive atelectasis, loss of functional residual capacity, and a ventilation-perfusion imbalance with an uneven distribution of ventilation. This surfactant deficiency may be caused by insufficient surfactant production, abnormal composition and function, disruption of surfactant production, or a combination of these factors. The weak respiratory muscles and an overly compliant chest wall common to premature infants further compromise the sequence of events that occurs. Lung capacity is further compromised by the presence of proteinaceous material and epithelial debris in the airways. The resulting decreased oxygenation, cyanosis, and metabolic or respiratory acidosis can

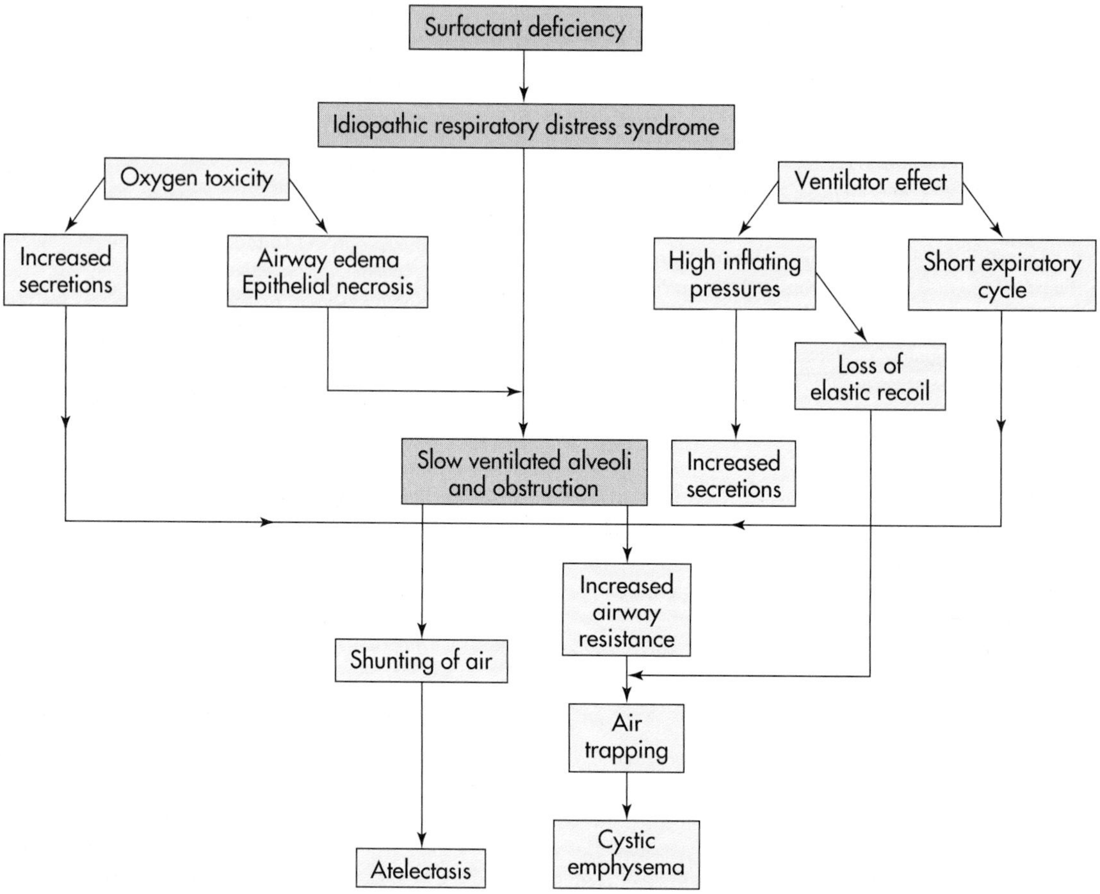

Surfactant deficiency
Idiopathic respiratory distress syndrome
Oxygen toxicity
Ventilator effect
Increased secretions
Airway edema
Epithelial necrosis
High inflating pressures
Short expiratory cycle
Loss of elastic recoil
Slow ventilated alveoli and obstruction
Increased secretions
Increased airway resistance
Shunting of air
Air trapping
Atelectasis
Cystic emphysema

FIG. 40-15 Pathogenesis of respiratory distress syndrome (RDS). (From Hagedorn, M., Gardner, S., & Abman, S. (2002). Respiratory diseases. In G. Merenstein & S. Gardner. [Eds.], *Handbook of neonatal intensive care* [5th ed.]. St. Louis: Mosby.)

BOX 40-4 Clinical Signs of Respiratory Distress Syndrome

- Tachypnea
- Grunting
- Flaring
- Retractions
- Cyanosis
- Increased work of breathing
- Hypercapnia
- Respiratory or mixed acidosis
- Hypotension and shock

cause the pulmonary vascular resistance (PVR) to be increased. This increased PVR can lead to right-to-left shunting and a reopening of the ductus arteriosus and foramen ovale (Hagedorn, Gardner, & Abman, 2002) (Fig. 40-15).

Clinical symptoms of RDS are listed in Box 40-4. These respiratory symptoms usually appear immediately after birth or within 6 hours of birth. Physical examination reveals crackles, poor air exchange, pallor, the use of accessory muscles (retractions), and occasionally apnea. Radiographic findings include a uniform reticulogranular appearance and air bronchograms (Rodriguez, Martin, & Fanaroff, 2002). The infant's clinical course typically is variable, with usually an increased oxygen requirement and increased respiratory effort as atelectasis, a loss of functional residual capacity, and ventilation-perfusion imbalance worsen.

However, RDS is a self-limiting disease, with the respiratory symptoms abating after 72 hours. This disappearance of respiratory symptoms coincides with the production of surfactant in the type 2 cells of the alveoli.

The treatment for RDS is supportive. Adequate ventilation and oxygenation must be established and maintained in an attempt to prevent ventilation-perfusion mismatch and atelectasis. Exogenous surfactant may be administered at birth or shortly after birth, and this has the effect of altering the typical course of RDS. Positive-pressure ventilation, bubble CPAP, and oxygen therapy

TABLE 40-1 **Normal Arterial Blood Gas Values for Neonates**

VALUE	RANGE
pH	7.32-7.49
Arterial oxygen pressure (PaO_2)	60-70 mm Hg
Carbon dioxide pressure ($PaCO_2$)	26-41 mm Hg
Bicarbonate (HCO_3)	16-24 mEq/L
Oxygen saturation	40%-90%

From Pagana, K., & Pagana, T. (2003). *Mosby's diagnostic and laboratory test reference* (6th ed.). St. Louis: Mosby.

may be needed during the respiratory illness. However, the prevention of complications associated with mechanical ventilation also is critical. These complications include pulmonary interstitial emphysema, pneumothorax, pneumomediastinum, and pneumopericardium. The mortality and morbidity rates associated with RDS are attributed to the immature organ systems of the infant and the complications associated with the treatment of the disease (Rodriguez et al., 2002).

Acid-base balance is evaluated by monitoring the ABG values (Table 40-1). Frequent blood sampling requires arterial access accomplished either by umbilical artery catheterization or by a peripheral arterial line. Pulse oximetry and transcutaneous carbon dioxide and oxygen monitors document trends in ventilation and oxygenation. Capillary blood gas values indicate the pH and PCO_2 status in infants who are in more stable condition.

The maintenance of an NTE continues to be of critical importance in infants with RDS because infants with hypoxemia are unable to increase their metabolic rate when cold stressed (Rodriguez et al., 2002).

The clinical and radiographic presentation (radiodense lung fields and air bronchograms) of neonatal pneumonia may be similar to that of RDS. Fluid in the minor tissue also may be noted in infants with neonatal pneumonia. Therefore sepsis evaluation, including blood culture and complete blood count (CBC) with differential, is done in infants with RDS to rule out neonatal pneumonia. Occasionally a lumbar puncture is done as part of the evaluation. Broad-spectrum antibiotics are begun while the results of cultures are awaited.

Fluid and nutrition must be maintained in the critically ill infant with RDS. Parenteral nutrition can be implemented to provide protein and fats to promote a positive nitrogen balance. Daily monitoring of the electrolyte values, urinary output, specific gravity, and weight help evaluate the infant's hydration status.

Frequent blood sampling may make blood transfusions necessary. The critically ill infant usually needs to have a venous hematocrit level of more than 40% to maintain adequate oxygen-carrying capacity.

NURSE ALERT

Directed-donor blood may be requested. This donor blood usually is obtained from a family member or close friend of the family who has the same blood type as the infant or a compatible blood type. It may be necessary to notify the infant's family of the potential need for blood transfusion on admission to allow for the processing of directed-donor blood.

Reassuring the family that stringent testing of all blood products is done may alleviate some of their anxiety about the transmission of blood-borne pathogens such as human immunodeficiency virus (HIV) and hepatitis B. Because some religions prohibit the use of blood transfusions, it is critical to obtain a complete history from the family, including their religious preference. Alternative strategies for maintaining the hematocrit may be used in these instances.

Complications Associated with Oxygen Therapy

Retinopathy of Prematurity

Retinopathy of prematurity (ROP) is a complex multicause disorder that affects the developing retinal vessels of premature infants. The normal retinal vessels begin to form in utero at approximately 16 weeks in response to an unknown stimulus. These vessels continue to develop until they reach maturity at approximately 42 to 43 weeks after conception. Once the retina is completely vascularized, the retinal vessels are not susceptible to ROP. The mechanism of injury in ROP is unclear. Oxygen tensions that are too high for the level of retinal maturity initially result in vasoconstriction. After oxygen therapy is discontinued, neovascularization occurs in the retina and vitreous, with capillary hemorrhages, fibrotic resolution, and possible retinal detachment. Cicatricial (scar) tissue formation and consequent visual impairment may be mild or severe. The entire disease process in severe cases may take as long as 5 months to evolve. Examination by an ophthalmologist before discharge and a schedule for repeated examinations thereafter are recommended for the parents' guidance.

The key to the management of ROP is prevention and early detection of premature birth. Circumferential cryopexy, laser photocoagulation, vitamin E therapy, and decreasing the intensity of ambient light are used in the prevention and treatment of ROP, with varying results (Phelps, 2002). More research is being done to examine the impact of the NICU environment on the development of ROP in relation to light that shines directly through the very thin eyelid of very immature infants. Ambient lighting in the NICU is known to have an effect on the developing eye; whereas it may not directly cause ROP, it does contribute to other visual problems for the premature infant (Fielder & Moseley, 2000).

Bronchopulmonary Dysplasia

Bronchopulmonary dysplasia (BPD) is a chronic pulmonary iatrogenic condition caused by barotrauma from pressure ventilation and oxygen toxicity. The etiology of BPD is multifactorial and includes pulmonary immaturity, surfactant deficiency, lung injury and stretch, barotrauma, inflammation caused by oxygen exposure, fluid overload, ligation of a PDA, and a familial predisposition. With the advent of prenatal use of maternal steroids when premature birth is expected coupled with use of exogenous surfactant in the neonate, most BPD or chronic lung disease (CLD) has been eliminated.

Clinical symptoms of BPD include tachypnea, retractions, nasal flaring, increased work of breathing, exercise intolerance (to handling and feeding), and tachycardia. Auscultation of the lung fields in affected infants typically reveals crackles, decreased air movement, and occasionally expiratory wheezing. The treatment for BPD includes oxygen therapy, nutrition, fluid restriction, and medications (diuretics, corticosteroids, bronchodilators). However, the key to the management of BPD is prevention by preventing prematurity and RDS and by using surfactant and other less toxic therapies. Use of high-frequency ventilation and nitric oxide have contributed to the decline of this condition.

The prognosis for infants with BPD depends on the degree of pulmonary dysfunction. Most deaths occur within the first year of life as a result of cardiorespiratory failure, sepsis, or respiratory infection; in some infants, the deaths are sudden and unexplained (Cifuentes et al., 2003; Schwartz, 2003).

Patent Ductus Arteriosus

The ductus arteriosus is a normal muscular contractile structure in the fetus connecting the left pulmonary artery and the dorsal aorta. The duct constricts after birth as oxygenation, the levels of circulating prostaglandins, and the muscle mass increase. Other factors that promote ductal closure include catecholamines, low pH, bradykinin, and acetylcholine. When the fetal ductus arteriosus fails to close after birth, **patent ductus arteriosus (PDA)** occurs. During the first few days of life when a premature or sick infant is under stress, this ductus arteriosus can reopen, leading to mottling and cyanosis. It may last only a few minutes until the stress is past, or it may remain open if the infant is quite unstable. The incidence of PDA in premature infants weighing less than 1500 g is 40% to 60%, with an increased percentage of cases occurring in premature infants weighing less than 1000 g (Gomella, Cunningham, & Eyal, 1999).

The clinical presentation in an infant with a PDA includes systolic murmur, active precordium, bounding peripheral pulses, tachycardia, tachypnea, crackles, and hepatomegaly. The systolic murmur is heard best at the second or third intercostal space at the upper left sternal border. An increased left ventricular stroke volume causes an active precordium. In addition, a widened pulse pressure may result in an increase in peripheral pulses.

Radiographic studies in infants with PDA typically show cardiac enlargement and pulmonary edema. ABG findings reveal hypercapnia and metabolic acidosis. Echocardiography can demonstrate a PDA and can quantitate the amount of blood shunting across the PDA (Montoya & Washington, 2002).

The PDA can be managed medically or surgically. Medical management consists of ventilatory support, fluid restriction, and the administration of diuretics and indomethacin. Indomethacin is a prostaglandin synthetase inhibitor that blocks the effect of the arachidonic acid products on the ductus and causes the PDA to constrict (Montoya & Washington, 2002). Some evidence indicates that use of indomethacin may contribute to the incidence of ROP, but further research must be done. Ventilatory support is adjusted based on the ABG values. Fluid restriction is implemented to decrease cardiovascular volume overload in association with the diuretic therapy. Surgical ligation is done when a PDA is clinically significant and medical management has failed (Montoya & Washington, 2002).

The nursing care of the infant with PDA focuses on supportive care. The infant needs an NTE, adequate oxygenation, meticulous fluid balance, and parental support.

Periventricular-Intraventricular Hemorrhage

Periventricular-intraventricular hemorrhage (PV-IVH) is one of the most common types of brain injury that occurs in neonates and is among the most severe from the standpoint of both short- and long-term outcomes. The true incidence of PV-IVH is unknown, but approximately 50% of infants who die in the first few days of life have hemorrhage (Paige & Carney, 2002). Use of prenatal corticosteroids can reduce the incidence to about 25% (Reed & Blumer, 2002). The general estimate is 20% to 30% in infants younger than 32 weeks of gestation or less than 1500 g (Paige & Carney, 2002).

The pathogenesis of PV-IVH includes intravascular factors (fluctuating or increasing cerebral blood flow, increases in cerebral venous pressures, and coagulopathy), vascular factors, extravascular factors, and nursery care. PV-IVH events typically occur within the first hours or days of life. The exact location of this hemorrhage varies with gestational age. In the very immature infant (younger than 28 weeks), it usually occurs in or adjacent to the germinal matrix.

PV-IVH is classified according to a grading system of I to IV, with grade I being the least severe, and grade IV, the most severe (Blackburn, 2003) (Table 40-2).

The long-term neurodevelopmental outcome is determined by the severity of the PV-IVH. Infants with grade I or II usually have good outcomes; infants with grade

TABLE 40-2 **Grading of Severity of Germinal Matrix—Intraventricular Hemorrhage by Ultrasound Scan**

GRADE	SEVERITY	DESCRIPTION
I	Small	Isolated germinal matrix hemorrhage
II	Small	Intraventricular hemorrhage with normal ventricular size
III	Moderate	Intraventricular hemorrhage with acute ventricular dilation
IV	Severe	Intraventricular hemorrhage with parenchymal hemorrhage

From Papile, L. (2002). Intracranial hemorrhage. In A. Fanaroff & R. Martin, *Neonatal-perinatal medicine: Diseases of the fetus and infant* (7th ed.). St. Louis: Mosby.

III and IV often have long-term morbidity (Blackburn, 2003). This hemorrhage often is associated with a lesion in the area of the periventricular white matter. The result is a necrosis that alters cerebral brain flow in the affected area. This condition is referred to as periventricular leukomalacia (PVL).

Nursing care focuses on recognition of factors that increase the risk of PV-IVH and PVL, interventions to decrease the risk of bleeding, and supportive care to infants who have bleeding episodes. The infant is positioned with the head in midline and the head of the bed elevated slightly to prevent or minimize fluctuations in intracranial blood pressure. NTE is maintained, as well as oxygenation. Rapid infusions of fluids should be avoided. Blood pressure is monitored closely for fluctuations. The infant is monitored for signs of pneumothorax because it often precedes PV-IVH.

Necrotizing Enterocolitis

Necrotizing enterocolitis (NEC) is an acute inflammatory disease of the GI mucosa, commonly complicated by perforation. This often fatal disease occurs in about 2% to 5% of newborns in NICUs. Although the cause is unknown, the factors listed in Box 40-5 are known to contribute to its development. Breastfeeding seems to lower the incidence of NEC, as does use of minimal enteral nutrition.

Reversal of perinatal asphyxia within 30 minutes may prevent GI tract insult and thus prevent the pathophysiologic events that trigger NEC. After 30 minutes, the distribution of cardiac output tends to be directed more toward the heart and brain and away from the abdominal organs. Therefore prompt birth of the intrauterine-asphyxiated fetus or ventilation of the asphyxiated newborn may be beneficial to the GI tract, as well as to other organs.

The onset of NEC in the term infant usually occurs between 4 and 10 days after birth. In the preterm infant, the onset may be delayed for up to 30 days. The signs of developing NEC are nonspecific, which is characteristic of many neonatal diseases. Some generalized signs include decreased activity, hypotonia, pallor, recurrent apnea and bradycardia, decreased oxygen saturation values, respiratory distress, metabolic acidosis, oliguria, hypotension, decreased perfusion, temperature instability, and cyanosis. GI symptoms include abdominal distention, increasing or bile-stained residual gastric aspirates, vomiting (bile or blood), grossly bloody stools, abdominal tenderness, and erythema of the abdominal wall.

A diagnosis of NEC is confirmed by a radiographic examination that reveals bowel loop distention, pneumatosis intestinalis, pneumoperitoneum, portal air, or a combination of these findings. The abnormal radiographic findings are caused by the bacterial colonization of the GI tract associated with NEC, resulting in ileus. Pneumatosis intestinalis, pneumoperitoneum, and portal air are caused by gas produced by the bacteria that invade the wall of the intestines and escape into the peritoneum and portal system when perforation occurs. The laboratory evaluation in such infants consists of a CBC with differential, coagulation studies, ABG analysis, measurement of serum electrolyte levels, and blood culture. The white blood cell count on the CBC may be either increased or decreased. The platelet count and coagulation study findings may be abnormal, showing thrombocytopenia and disseminated intravascular coagulation (DIC). Electrolyte levels may be abnormal, with leaking capillary beds and fluid shifts with the infection.

BOX 40-5 **Proposed Risk Factors for Necrotizing Enterocolitis**

- Asphyxia
- Respiratory distress syndrome
- Umbilical artery catheter
- Exchange transfusion
- Early enteral feedings/hyperosmolar feedings
- Patent ductus arteriosus
- Congenital heart disease
- Polycythemia
- Anemia
- Shock
- Gastrointestinal infection

Treatment in such infants is supportive. Oral or tube feedings are discontinued to rest the GI tract. An orogastric tube is placed and attached to low wall suction to provide gastric decompression. Parenteral therapy (often TPN) is begun. Because NEC is an infectious disease, control of the infection is imperative, with an emphasis on careful handwashing before and after infant contact. Antibiotic therapy may be instituted, and surgical resection is performed if perforation or clinical deterioration occurs. Therapy is usually prolonged, and recovery may be delayed by the formation of adhesions, the development of the complications associated with bowel resection, the occurrence of short-bowel syndrome (especially if the ileocecal valve is removed), or the development of intolerance to oral feedings. Some of these infants are candidates for intestinal transplants if they truly have short-bowel syndrome.

A decrease in the incidence of NEC correlates with the use of nonnutritive sucking during gavage feedings (Pickler & Terrell, 1994). The authors hypothesized that nonnutritive sucking has this effect because it makes the GI tract less susceptible to the factors that precipitate NEC by promoting gastric motility and thus increasing the release of gastric enzymes. The improvement in the infant's behavioral organization brought about by nonnutritive sucking also appears to play a role in this. Other researchers have not supported this finding, and more research is needed before a definitive linkage can be made between nonnutritive sucking and a decreased incidence of NEC (Pinelli & Symington, 2000).

Infant Pain Responses

The physiology of pain and pain assessment in the newborn were discussed in Chapter 26. This discussion focuses on pain assessment and management in the preterm infant.

Pain Assessment

Assessment of pain in the neonate is difficult because evaluation must be based on physiologic changes and behavioral observations. Pain is now considered as the fifth vital sign, and its assessment is a requirement of the Joint Commission on Accreditation of Healthcare Organizations (JCAHO). A scale that examines multiple dimensions is more accurate (Stevens & Koren, 1998). Although behaviors such as vocalizations, facial expressions, body movements, and general state are common to all infants, they vary with different situations. Crying associated with pain is more intense and sustained. Facial expression is the most consistent and specific characteristic; scales are available for systematic evaluation of facial features, such as eye squeeze, brow bulge, and open mouth and taut tongue (Walden & Franck, 2003). Most infants respond with increased body movements, but the infant may be experiencing pain even when lying quietly with eyes closed. The preterm infant's response to pain may be behaviorally blunted or absent. An infant who receives a muscle-paralyzing agent such as vecuronium also will be incapable of mounting a behavioral or visible pain response (Box 40-6), yet the infant still feels the pain.

NURSE ALERT

When in doubt about the presence of pain in infants, base your decision for the need for intervention on the following rule: Whatever is painful to an adult or child is painful to an infant unless proved otherwise. Anticipate pain; do not wait for pain symptoms to appear before intervening.

Several tools have been developed for the assessment of pain in the neonate. One pain assessment tool used by nurses in the NICU is called the *CRIES* (Table 40-3). Nurses who work with premature and term infants developed this tool. CRIES is an acronym for the physiologic and behavioral indicators of pain. The indicators include crying, requiring increased oxygen, increased vital signs, expression, and sleeplessness. Each indicator is scored from 0 to 2–similar to the Apgar score for neonates. The total possible pain score, which represents the worst pain, is 10. A pain score that is greater than 4 should be considered significant. This tool has been tested for reliability and validity for postoperative pain in infants between the ages of 32 weeks of gestation and 20 weeks postterm (Bildner & Krechel, 1996; Krechel & Bildner, 1995). Other instruments that are used are the Pain Assessment Tool (PAT) (Hodgkinson et al., 1994), Scale for Use in Newborns (SUN) (Blauer & Gerstmann, 1998), Behavioral Pain Score (BPS) (Pokela, 1994); Distress Scale for Ventilated Newborn Infants (DSVNI) (Sparshott, 1995), Neonatal Infant Pain Scale (NIPS) (Lawrence et al., 1993), and the Premature Infant Pain Profile (PIPP) (Stevens et al., 1996). The PIPP is one of the most widely used scales for premature infants as it considers behavioral, physiologic, and contextual indicators (Stevens et al., 1999; Walden & Franck, 2003).

Memory of Pain

Premature infants are subjected to a variety of repeated noxious stimuli, including multiple heel sticks, venipuncture, endotracheal intubation and suctioning, arterial sticks, chest tube placement, and lumbar puncture. The effects of pain caused by such procedures are not fully known, but researchers have begun to investigate potential consequences. From preliminary reports, it appears that a rewiring of the pain responses occurs in premature infants who have been subjected to multiple painful treatments early in their lives. The nervous system networks of the premature infant appear more dense and have more branches than those in the average infant, leading to the conclusion that the pain threshold and sensitivity in once premature infants is heightened for life (Anand & Scalzo, 2000).

Nurses' anecdotal reports suggest that infants show memory by exhibiting defensive behaviors when painful

BOX 40-6 Manifestations of Acute Pain in the Neonate

PHYSIOLOGIC RESPONSES

Vital Signs: Observe for Variations
Increased heart rate
Increased blood pressure
Rapid, shallow respirations

Oxygenation
Decreased transcutaneous O_2 saturation ($tcPO_2$)
Decreased arterial O_2 saturation (SaO_2)

Skin: Observe Color and Character
Pallor or flushing
Diaphoresis
Palmar sweating

Other Observations
Increased muscle tone
Dilated pupils
Decreased vagal nerve tone
Increased intracranial pressure
Laboratory evidence of metabolic or endocrine changes
- Hyperglycemia
- Lowered pH
- Elevated corticosteroids

BEHAVIORAL RESPONSES

Vocalizations: Observe Quality, Timing, and Duration
Crying
Whimpering
Groaning

Facial Expression: Observe Characteristics, Timing, and Orientation of Eyes and Mouth (see Fig. 40-16)
Grimaces
Brow furrowed
Chin quivering
Eyes tightly closed
Mouth open and squarish

Body Movements and Posture: Observe Type, Quality, and Amount of Movement or Lack of Movement; Relationship to Other Factors
Limb withdrawal
Thrashing
Rigidity
Flaccidity
Fist clenching

Change in State: Observe Sleep, Appetite, Activity Level
Changes in sleep/wake cycles
Changes in feeding behavior
Changes in activity level
Fussiness, irritability
Listlessness

From Hockenberry M. et al. (2003). *Wong's nursing care of infants and children* (7th ed.). St. Louis: Mosby.

procedures are repeated. Nurses often describe infants who stiffen and withdraw when touched because human touch has repeatedly been associated with pain. Such infants often become hypervigilant and gaze intently at the hands rather than at the eyes of people who approach them.

These reports not only indicate that infants remember painful events but also show that continual exposure to pain affects development, especially in response to human contact.

Consequences of Untreated Pain in Infants

Despite current research on the neonate's experience of pain, infant pain remains inadequately managed. The mismanagement of infant pain is partially due to misconceptions regarding the effects of pain on the neonate, as well as a lack of knowledge of immediate and long-term consequences of untreated pain. Infants respond to noxious stimuli through physiologic indicators (increased heart rate and blood pressure, variability in heart rate and intracranial pressure, and decreases in arterial oxygen saturations and skin blood flow) and behavioral indicators (muscle rigidity, facial expression, crying, withdrawal, and sleeplessness) (Anand, Grunau, & Oberlander, 1997; Bildner & Krechel, 1996). The physiologic and behavioral indicators, as well as a variety of neurophysiologic responses to noxious stimulation, are responsible for short- and long-term consequences of pain.

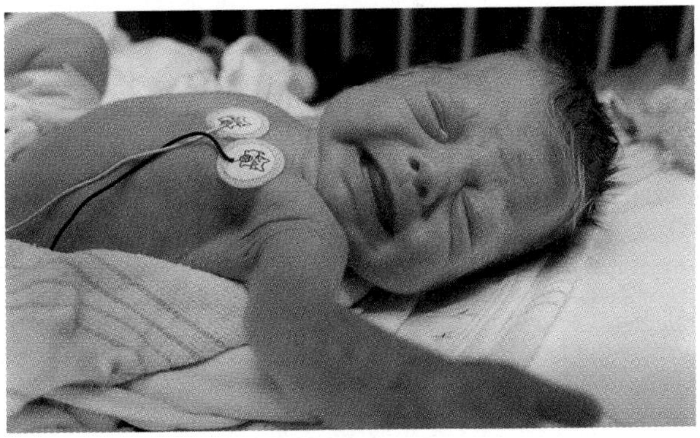

FIG. 40-16 The face of pain after heelstick. Note eye squeeze, brow bulge, nasolabial furrow, and wide-spread mouth. (Courtesy Paul Vincent Kuntz, Houston, TX.)

TABLE 40-3 **CRIES Neonatal Postoperative Pain Scale**

	0	1	2
Crying	No	High pitched	Inconsolable
Requires O_2 for sat >95%	No	<30%	>30%
Increased vital signs	Heart rate and blood pressure equal or less than preoperative state	Heart rate and blood pressure <20% of preoperative state	Heart rate and blood pressure >20% of preoperative state
Expression	None	Grimace	Grimace/grunt
Sleepless	No	Wakes at frequent intervals	Constantly awake

CODING TIPS FOR USING CRIES

Crying	The characteristic cry of pain is *high pitched* If no cry or cry that is not high pitched, score 0 If cry high pitched but infant is easily consoled, score 1 If cry is high pitched and infant is inconsolable, score 2
Requires O_2 for saturation >95%	Look for *changes* in oxygenation. Infants experiencing pain manifest decreases in oxygenation as measured by tCO_2 or oxygen saturation. (Consider other causes of changes in oxygenation, such as atelectasis, pneumothorax, oversedation.) If no oxygen is required, score 0 If <30% O_2 is required, score 1 If >30% O_2 is required, score 2
Increased vital signs	Note: measure blood pressure last because this may wake child, causing difficulty with other assessments. Use baseline preoperative parameters from a non-stressed period. Multiply baseline HR × 0.2, then add this to baseline HR to determine the HR that is 20% over baseline. Do likewise for BP. Use mean BP If HR and BP are both unchanged or less than baseline, score 0 If HR or BP is increased but increase is <20% of baseline, score 1 If either one is increased >20% over baseline, score 2
Expression	The facial expression most often associated with pain is a grimace This may be characterized by brow lowering, eyes squeezed shut, deepening of the nasolabial furrow, open lips and mouth If no grimace is present, score 0 If grimace alone is present, score 1 If grimace and noncry vocalization grunt is present, score 2
Sleepless	This parameter is scored based on the infant's state during the hour preceding this recorded score If the child has been continuously asleep, score 0 If he/she has awakened at frequent intervals, score 1 If he/she has been awake constantly, score 2

BP, Blood pressure; *HR,* heart rate.
Neonatal pain assessment tool developed at the University of Missouri-Columbia.
From Krechel, S., & Bildner, J. (1995). CRIES: A new neonatal postoperative pain measurement score: Initial testing of validity and reliability, *Pediatric Anaesthesia 5,* 53-61.

Pain Management

The International Evidence-Based Group for Neonatal Pain developed a Consensus Statement for the Prevention and Management of Pain in the Newborn (Anand, 2001). This statement states that pain must be anticipated and prevented to avoid long-term consequences. Nonpharmacologic measures to alleviate pain include repositioning, swaddling, containment, cuddling, rocking, music, reducing environmental stimulation, tactile comfort measures, nonnutritive sucking, and use of oral sucrose (Walden & Franck, 2003). However, nonpharmacologic measures may not be sufficient to decrease physiologic distress, even if behavioral responses such as crying are lessened (Walden & Franck, 2003). In premature infants, additional stimulation such as stroking or environmental light or noise may *increase* physiologic distress (Walden & Franck, 2003). The impact of the NICU environment must be considered along with other forms of stimuli that may produce stress and pain.

Morphine is the most widely used opioid analgesic for pharmacologic management of neonatal pain, with fentanyl as an effective alternative. Continuous or bolus epidural or IV infusion of opioids provides effective and safe pain control (Walden & Franck, 2003). Other methods of relieving pain are epidural/intrathecal infusion, local and regional nerve blocks, and topical anesthetics (Walden & Franck, 2003).

Parents are universally concerned that their infants are feeling pain during procedures. Nurses need to address these concerns and encourage the parents to speak with the health care professionals involved. Parents have the right to withhold consent for invasive procedures and are entitled to honest answers from those responsible for the infant's care. When appropriate, they also can help provide comfort measures for the infant. Kangaroo care is one method of parental intervention that comforts and calms the infant. Parents want to know that nurses recognize pain in their infants and that the infants will be comfortable when they, the parents, are not present. They want to know that the nurse will advocate for comfort care for their baby. Although pain is considered a fifth vital sign, it cannot be assessed only at the time of vital signs. It must receive an ongoing evaluation of the pain level and the effectiveness of comfort measures used. This assessment is not lengthy but can be as simple as walking to the bedside and really looking at the infant's color, posture, movements, and breathing. Pain is a real phenomenon that is preventable in many instances. Pain management is a standard of care, and it is considered unethical not to prevent and effectively treat pain. Another growing area of neonatal nursing is end-of-life and palliative care. Most of this care centers on pain management. Palliative care is really comfort care that supports the needs of the premature, sick neonate.

Postmature Infants

A pregnancy that is prolonged beyond 42 weeks is a postterm pregnancy, and the infant who is born is called *postmature.* Postmaturity can be associated with placental insufficiency, resulting in a fetus that has a wasted appearance (dysmaturity) at birth because of loss of subcutaneous fat and muscle mass. Meconium staining of the fingernails may be noted, and the hair and nails may be long. The skin may peel off. Not all postmature infants will show signs of dysmaturity; some will continue to grow in utero and be large at birth.

The perinatal mortality rate is significantly higher in the postmature fetus and neonate. One reason for this is that during labor and birth, the increased oxygen demands of the postmature fetus may not be met. Insufficient gas exchange in the postmature placenta also increases the likelihood of intrauterine hypoxia, which may result in the passage of meconium in utero, thereby increasing the risk for meconium aspiration syndrome (MAS). Of all the deaths that occur in postmature newborns, half occur during labor and birth, about one third occur before the onset of labor, and one sixth occur during the postpartum period.

Meconium Aspiration Syndrome (MAS)

Meconium staining of the amniotic fluid can be indicative of nonreassuring fetal status, especially in a vertex presentation. It appears in 8% to 20% of all births. Many infants with meconium staining exhibit no signs of depression at birth; however, the presence of meconium in the amniotic fluid necessitates careful supervision of labor and close monitoring of fetal well-being. Use of amniofusion has decreased some of the incidence of MAS (Yoder et al., 2002). This procedure thins any meconium particles that may be present in the amniotic fluid, thus decreasing the chance of thick meconium being aspirated at the time of birth. Because these infants are surfactant deficient, one method of prevention of MAS is to use surfactant lavages in the delivery room. The findings indicate that outcomes for these infants are better than those of their counterparts who received no surfactant lavages (i.e., they were weaned from mechanical ventilation quicker, had less full-blown MAS, and had better oxygenation patterns) (Wiswell et al., 2002). This was a randomized multicenter trial, so more research is needed. In any case, the presence of a team skilled at neonatal resuscitation is required at the birth of any infant with meconium-stained amniotic fluid. The mouth and nares of the infant should be suctioned on the perineum before the infant's first breath. The use of endotracheal suctioning of meconium below the cords in a vigorous infant is controversial. This treatment used to be standard of care, but little evidence supports the need to do this in a *vigorous infant* (American Academy of Pediatrics, 2002). Research is ongoing on this topic.

If the infant is very depressed and the meconium is not removed from the airway at birth, it can migrate down to the terminal airways, causing mechanical obstruction leading to MAS. It also is possible that the fetus aspirated meconium in utero. Such meconium aspiration can cause a chemical pneumonitis. These infants may develop persistent pulmonary hypertension of the newborn (PPHN), further complicating their management.

Persistent Pulmonary Hypertension of the Newborn

The term *persistent pulmonary hypertension of the newborn (PPHN)* is applied to the combined findings of pulmonary hypertension, right-to-left shunting, and a structurally normal heart. PPHN may be either a single entity or the main component of MAS, congenital diaphragmatic hernia, RDS, hyperviscosity syndrome, or neonatal pneumonia or sepsis. PPHN also is called *persistent fetal circulation* (PFC) because the syndrome includes a reversion to fetal pathways for blood flow.

A brief review of the characteristics of fetal blood flow can help in the visualization of the problems with PPHN (see Fig. 13-9). In utero, oxygen-rich blood leaves the placenta via the umbilical vein, goes through the ductus venosus, and enters the inferior vena cava. From there it empties into the right atrium and is mostly shunted across the foramen ovale to the left atrium, effectively bypassing the lungs. This blood enters the left ventricle, leaves via the aorta, and preferentially perfuses the carotid and coronary arteries. Thus the heart and brain receive the most oxygenated blood. Blood drains from the brain into the superior vena cava, reenters the right atrium, proceeds to the right ventricle, and exits via the main pulmonary artery. The lungs are a high-pressure circuit, needing only enough perfusion for growth and nutrition. The ductus arteriosus (connecting the main pulmonary artery and the aorta) is the path of least resistance for the blood leaving the right side of the fetal heart, shunting most of the cardiac output away from the lungs and toward the systemic system. This *right-to-left shunting* is the key to fetal circulation.

After birth, both the foramen ovale and the ductus arteriosus close in response to various biochemical processes, pressure changes within the heart, and dilation of the pulmonary vessels. This dilation allows virtually all of the cardiac output to enter the lungs, become oxygenated, and provide oxygen-rich blood to the tissues for normal metabolism. Any process that interferes with this transition from fetal to neonatal circulation may precipitate PPHN. PPHN characteristically proceeds into a downward spiral of exacerbating hypoxia and pulmonary vasoconstriction. Prompt recognition and aggressive intervention are required to reverse this process.

The infant with PPHN is typically born at term or after term and has tachycardia and cyanosis. Management depends on the underlying cause of the persistent pulmonary hypertension. The use of ECMO has improved the chances of survival in these infants (see earlier discussion); however, it is considered a very invasive procedure. Use of nitric oxide (NO) as a pharmacologic intervention has increased in the last few years with great success. NO acts as a vasodilator to decrease the pulmonary hypertension while increasing oxygenation (Zehka & Patel, 2002). This therapy is proving to work well either alone or with high-frequency ventilation. Another pharmacologic treatment is use of exogenous surfactant, as some of these infants appear to be surfactant deficient. Use of environmental strategies such as decreasing adverse stimuli (excessive light and noise) to decrease stress is another area of ongoing research. This intervention is used in conjunction with other therapies.

Another mode of treatment for PPHN and other respiratory disorders of the newborn is high-frequency ventilation, a group of assisted ventilation methods that deliver small volumes of gas at high frequencies and limit the development of high airway pressure, thus reducing barotrauma. High-frequency ventilation decreases carbon dioxide while increasing oxygenation. It can be effectively used in conjunction with NO (Zehka & Patel, 2002). It is important to understand that PPHN is considered a cardiovascular and a respiratory problem. The lungs of these infants are healthy, but the hypertension of the cardiovascular system leads to their oxygenation problems.

CARE MANAGEMENT

To ensure the safe birth of the fetus, it becomes important to determine whether the pregnancy is actually prolonged and also whether there is any evidence of fetal jeopardy as a result.

Most postmature infants are oversized but otherwise normal, with advanced development and bone age. A postmature infant will have some, but not necessarily all, of the following physical characteristics:

- Generally a normal skull, but the reduced dimensions of the rest of the body make the skull look inordinately large
- Dry, cracked (desquamating), parchment-like skin at birth
- Hard nails extending beyond the fingertips
- Profuse scalp hair
- Depleted subcutaneous fat layers, leaving the skin loose and giving the infant an "old person" appearance
- Long and thin body
- Absent vernix
- Often meconium staining (golden yellow to green) of skin, nails, and cord, indicative of a hypoxic episode in utero or a perinatal infection such as listeriosis (this is practically the only time a preterm infant has meconium staining)
- May have an alert, wide-eyed appearance symptomatic of chronic intrauterine hypoxia

Possible nursing diagnoses for the postmature infant include the following:

- *Impaired gas exchange related to*
  - –decreased number of functional alveoli
  - –deficiency of surfactant
  - –cardiovascular hypertension in the pulmonary tree
- *Ineffective breathing pattern related to*
  - –inadequate chest expansion, secondary to infant position
  - –environmental stimuli
  - –pain
  - –pulmonary hypertension

- *Ineffective thermoregulation related to*
  - –immature thermoregulation center
  - –exposure to cold air or increased factors promoting thermal loss
  - –lack of subcutaneous tissue and fat stores
- *Risk for infection related to*
  - –invasive procedures
  - –decreased immune response
  - –immature skin or very thin, friable skin
- *Anxiety (parental) related to*
  - –lack of knowledge regarding infant condition
  - –lack of knowledge regarding infant cues
  - –fear of death of infant
  - –feeling powerless in the situation/inability to protect infant from harm
- *Anticipatory grieving (parental) related to*
  - –fear of infant's death
  - –lack of knowledge about what to expect
  - –lack of clear communication on part of health care team

Immediate outcomes of care are that the postmature newborn will do the following:

- Initiate and maintain respirations.
- Experience no CNS trauma or infection.
- Have any birth trauma identified and treated promptly without sequelae.

The long-term expected outcome is that the infant will not experience adverse effects of postmaturity.

The immediate care rendered to postmature infants is similar to that given to preterm infants. Potential complications experienced by postmature infants include polycythemia, hypothermia, hypoglycemia, and meconium aspiration. See other sections for the management and care of these complications.

The nurse can be assured that care was effective when the short-term outcomes for care have been achieved. Long-term follow-up will be needed to evaluate whether any adverse effects are a result of postmaturity.

OTHER PROBLEMS RELATED TO GESTATION

Small for Gestational Age and Intrauterine Growth Restriction

Infants who are small for gestational age (SGA; e.g., weight is below the 10th percentile expected at term) and infants who have IUGR (rate of growth does not meet expected growth pattern) are considered high risk, with the perinatal mortality rate 5 to 20 times greater than that for the normal term infant (Kliegman & Das, 2002). In some cases, a genetic linkage is possible, as maternal genes have been implicated when infants who are SGA run in families. The maternal genes must regulate the fetal growth potential through uteroplacental circulation effects (Kliegman & Das, 2002). Women with chronic illness or suboptimal nutrition also are at risk for producing an SGA infant, as the nutrients to the fetus are diminished. So the underlying cause of the SGA can affect the condition of the infant; however, common problems are predictable.

Common problems that affect SGA IUGR infants are perinatal asphyxia, meconium aspiration, hypoglycemia, polycythemia, and heat loss.

Perinatal Asphyxia

Commonly, IUGR infants have been exposed to chronic hypoxia for varying periods before labor and birth. Labor is a stressor to the normal fetus, but it is an even greater stressor for the growth-restricted fetus. The chronically hypoxic infant is severely compromised even by a normal labor and has difficulty compensating after birth. The alert, wide-eyed appearance of such newborns is attributed to the prolonged fetal hypoxia. Appropriate management and resuscitation are essential for these depressed infants.

The birth of SGA babies with perinatal asphyxia may be associated with a maternal history of heavy cigarette smoking; preeclampsia; low socioeconomic status; multifetal gestation; gestational infections such as rubella, cytomegalovirus, and toxoplasmosis; advanced diabetes mellitus; and cardiac problems. The nursing staff must be alert to and prepared for possible perinatal asphyxia during the birth of an infant in a woman with such a history. Sequelae to perinatal asphyxia include MAS and hypoglycemia.

Hypoglycemia

All stressed infants are at risk for the development of hypoglycemia. Such stress may include perinatal asphyxia and IUGR. The definition of **hypoglycemia** differs for the term and the preterm infant. Hypoglycemia occurring within the first 3 days of life in the term infant is defined as a blood glucose level of less than 40 mg/dl; that occurring in the preterm infant within the same time frame is defined as a blood glucose level of less than 25 mg/dl. Symptoms of hypoglycemia include poor feeding, hypothermia, and diaphoresis. CNS symptoms can include tremors and jitteriness, weak cry, lethargy, floppy posture, convulsions, or coma. Diagnosis is confirmed by blood glucose determinations performed by the laboratory when suspected or by unit visual methods with reagent strips such as Chemstrip-BG or Dextrostix (Kliegman & Das, 2002).

Polycythemia

Polycythemia or hyperviscosity of the blood is another common problem of the SGA infant. The plasma volume may be on average 52 ml/kg (normal, 43 ml/kg) (Kliegman & Das, 2002). This condition is a result of fetal hypoxia and intrauterine stress that forces the body to produce more red blood cells in an attempt to provide oxygen to the developing fetus. This condition can compromise blood circulation and oxygenation, and lead to further hypoglycemia and hypoxia in extrauterine life. A partial exchange transfusion to reduce the viscosity of the blood may be necessary.

Heat Loss

For numerous reasons, SGA infants are particularly susceptible to temperature instability, and close attention must be paid to them to maintain thermoneutrality. They have less muscle mass, less brown fat, less heat-preserving subcutaneous fat, and little ability to control skin capillaries. Nursing considerations in these infants focus on the maintenance of thermoneutrality to promote recovery from perinatal asphyxia, because cold stress jeopardizes such recovery (Kliegman & Das, 2002).

CARE MANAGEMENT

Several physical findings are characteristic of the SGA neonate:

- Generally a normal skull, but the reduced dimensions of the rest of the body make the skull look inordinately large
- Reduced subcutaneous fat stores
- Loose and dry skin
- Diminished muscle mass, especially over buttocks and cheeks
- Sunken abdomen (scaphoid) as opposed to the well-rounded abdomen seen in normal infants
- Thin, yellowish, dry, and dull umbilical cord (normal cord is gray, glistening, round, and moist)
- Sparse scalp hair
- Wide skull sutures (inadequate bone growth)

The nursing care given to the SGA infant is determined by the nature of the clinical problems and is the same as that given to the preterm infant with the same problems. Maintaining a clear airway and preventing cold stress support gas exchange. Hypoglycemia is treated with oral feedings (e.g., breast milk, formula, dextrose solution) per the hospital protocol. Parenteral infusions may be necessary. If polycythemia is present, assessment of the cardiovascular circulation is important, and assistance with a partial exchange transfusion may be necessary. To assist with thermoregulation, an external heat source is used until the infant's temperature is stabilized (radiant warmer or isolette). The nursing support given to parents is similar to that given to parents of preterm infants.

Large for Gestational Age

The large-for-gestational age (LGA), or oversized, infant traditionally has been regarded as one weighing 4000 g or more at birth. An infant is considered LGA despite gestation when the weight is above the 90th percentile on growth charts or two standard deviations above the mean weight for gestational age. Certain fetal disorders also can result in LGA infants. These include transposition of the great vessels and Beckwith-Wiedemann syndrome.

Birth trauma, especially in infants with a breech or shoulder presentation, is a serious hazard for the oversized neonate. Asphyxia or CNS injury, or both, may occur. All pregnancies of more than 42 weeks of gestation must be carefully evaluated. All large fetuses are monitored during a trial of labor, and preparation is made for cesarean birth if a nonreassuring fetal status or poor progress of labor occurs. LGA newborns may be preterm, term, or postterm; they may be the infants of mothers who are diabetic (or prediabetic); and they may be postmature. Each of these problems has special concerns. Regardless of any coexisting potential problems, the oversized infant is at risk just by virtue of its size.

CARE MANAGEMENT

The nurse assesses the LGA infant for gestational age, hypoglycemia, and trauma resulting from vaginal or cesarean birth. The blood glucose levels of LGA infants are monitored, and any hypoglycemia is corrected. Any specific birth injuries are identified and treated appropriately. Care depends on the LGA infant's condition.

DISCHARGE PLANNING

Discharge planning for the high risk infant begins at the time of admission. Throughout the infant's hospitalization, the discharge planning coordinator gathers information from all of the health care team members. This information is used to determine the infant's and family's readiness for discharge. Nurses are very influential members of the planning team because as the direct caregivers throughout the infant's hospitalization, they have a first-hand knowledge of the infant and the family.

As the home care needs of the infant's parents are assessed, steps are taken to eliminate any knowledge deficits. Information is provided about infant care, especially as it pertains to the particular infant's home needs (e.g., the administration of oxygen, gastrostomy feedings). Parent education includes having them give return demonstrations of their infant care skills to show whether they are becoming increasingly independent in the provision of this care. Parents also should obtain an age-appropriate car seat before the discharge of their infant. Instruction in infant CPR should be offered to all parents before discharge. With the emphasis on the American Academy of Pediatrics (AAP) Back-to-Sleep program to reduce the incidence of SIDS, it may be necessary to place the infant in this position before discharge to challenge the infant's ability to tolerate the position. Because the parents saw their infant in a prone or side-lying position while sick; they need to understand the importance of use of the new positioning on the back once the infant is stable and at home.

As the home care of medically fragile clients is expanded to the pediatric population, early teaching and planning become a necessity. With the advent of managed care and cost-effective care strategies, more facilities using vertical integration of services thus provide home care as part of their inpatient continuum of care. These institutions are investigating such home care options as one way to provide long-term care for the compromised infant. If the infant requires palliative care or is considered to be dying, hospice and palliative care are available in some areas of the country. Some problems still exist with insurance coverage for these services in some states, but many discharge coordinators are able to obtain payment when the services are coupled with home care (American Academy of Pediatrics, 2000; Association of Pediatric Oncology Nurses, National Association of Neonatal Nurses, & Society of Pediatric Nurses, 2002).

Referrals for appropriate resources should be made whether the infant just needs follow-up or is going home to die. Social service involvement is especially important for young or psychosocially high risk parents (e.g., substance abusers or those with a mental illness). Social services also can provide parents with information about financial assistance (Aid to Families with Dependent Children, Medicaid, Crippled Children's Program, Social Security Disability). As our understanding of genetics increases, appropriate counseling, referral, and follow-up will become more important.

Infants with developmental disabilities, or those infants who may be at risk for further problems (premature infants), are referred to appropriate community programs. Federal Public Law 102-119 mandates that community resources be available to those children and families with special educational and medical needs (Robinson & Driscoll, 2003). Such services range from family counseling to physical therapy. Some hospitals also offer infant stimulation and development programs for the parents of at-risk infants. This law recognizes nursing as one of the 10 qualified disciplines that can provide these services.

Referrals are made for home health assistance, as appropriate (some medical plans cover these services). These health care providers can perform actual nursing functions, as well as provide some relief from the emotional burden of caring for an infant with medical problems. Special attention should be given to parents' feelings of uncertainty, anxiety, and overwhelming frustration. Parents often have these emotions during the planning for an infant's home care, especially if the infant has had a severe or prolonged illness (Holditch-Davis & Miles, 2000; Miles et al., 2002).

TRANSPORT TO A REGIONAL CENTER

If a hospital is not equipped to care for a high risk mother and fetus or a high risk infant, transfer to a specialized perinatal or tertiary care center is arranged. Maternal transport ideally occurs with the fetus in utero because this has two distinct advantages: (1) The associated neonatal morbidity and mortality are decreased; and (2) infant-parent attachment is supported, thereby avoiding separation of the parents and infant.

For a variety of reasons, however, it is not always possible to transport the mother before the birth. These reasons include imminent birth and unanticipated problems; therefore, physicians and nurses in level 1 and 2 facilities must have the skills and equipment necessary for making an accurate diagnosis and implementing emergency interventions to stabilize the infant's condition until transport can occur (Box 40-7) (Pettett, Sewell, & Merenstein, 2002). The goal of these interventions is to maintain the infant's condition within the normal physiologic range. Specific attention is given to the following areas:

- Vital signs
- Oxygen and ventilation
- Thermoregulation
- Acid-base balance
- Fluid and electrolyte levels
- Glucose level
- Developmental interventions

The transport team may consist of physicians, nurse practitioners, nurses, and respiratory therapists. Commonly the team consists of a nurse trained in neonatal intensive care and a respiratory therapist. The team must have expertise in resuscitation, stabilization, and provision of critical care during the transport (Fig. 40-17). In a neonatal transport, the team should provide information for the parents about the tertiary center (Box 40-8). Transport teams can integrate an individual developmental plan of care into their caregiving efforts, thereby initiating multidisciplinary interventions early in the infant's life.

The birth of any high risk infant can cause profound parental stress. Such parents can grieve the loss of the ideal infant. They are fearful of the possible eventual outcomes for the infant. They also must deal with the technologic world surrounding their infant, and amid all the equipment, it is sometimes difficult for them to perceive the infant and respond to its needs. Parents of high risk infants who have been transported to regional centers therefore need special support. As one way to deal with this problem, many intensive care units provide the family with a handbook or pictures of the tertiary care unit to help them understand what is going on around them.

TRANSPORT FROM A REGIONAL CENTER

Infants may need to be transferred back to the referring facility. Often premature infants who require thermoregulation and gavage feedings can be cared for in community hospitals closer to the parents' home. This back transfer allows parents to visit their infant more easily and to work

BOX 40-7 **Neonatal Resuscitation Supplies and Equipment**

SUCTION EQUIPMENT
Bulb syringe
Mechanical suction and tubing
Suction catheters, 5F or 6F, 8F, 10F, or 12F
8F feeding tube and 20-ml syringe
Meconium aspirator

BAG-AND-MASK EQUIPMENT
Neonatal resuscitation bag with a pressure-release valve or pressure manometer (the bag must be capable of delivering 90% to 100% oxygen)
Face masks, newborn and premature sizes (cushioned-rim masks preferred)
Oxygen source with flowmeter (flow rate up to 10 L/min) and tubing

INTUBATION EQUIPMENT
Laryngoscope with straight blades, No. 0 (preterm) and No. 1 (term)
Extra bulbs and batteries for laryngoscope
Endotracheal tubes, 2.5-, 3.0-, 3.5-, 4.0-mm internal diameter (ID)
Stylet (optional)
Scissors
Tape or securing device for endotracheal tube
Alcohol sponges
CO_2 detector (optional)
Laryngeal mask airway (optional)

MEDICATIONS
Epinephrine, 1:10,000 (0.1 mg/ml): 3-ml or 10-ml ampoules
Isotonic crystalloid (normal saline or Ringer's lactate) for volume expansion: 100 or 250 ml
Sodium bicarbonate, 4.2% (5 mEq/10 ml): 10-ml ampoules
Naloxone hydrochloride, 0.4 mg/ml: 1-ml ampoules; or 1.0 mg/ml: 2-ml ampoules
Dextrose, 10%: 250 ml
Normal saline for flushes
Feeding tube, 5F (optional)
Umbilical vessel catheterization supplies
Sterile gloves
Scalpel or scissors
Povidone-iodine solution
Umbilical tape
Umbilical catheters, 3.5F, 5F
Three-way stopcock
Syringes: 1, 3, 5, 10, 20, 50 ml
Needles: 25, 21, 18 gauge, or puncture device for needle-less system

MISCELLANEOUS
Gloves and appropriate personal protection
Radiant warmer or other heat source
Firm, padded resuscitation surface
Clock (timer optional)
Warmed linens
Stethoscope (neonatal head preferred)
Tape, ½ or ¾ inch
Cardiac monitor and electrodes or pulse oximeter and probe (optional for delivery room)
Oropharyngeal airways (0, 00, and 000 sizes or 30-, 40-, and 50-mm lengths)

Used with permission of the American Academy of Pediatrics. (2000). *Textbook of neonatal resuscitation* (4th ed.). Elk Grove Village, IL: American Academy of Pediatrics.

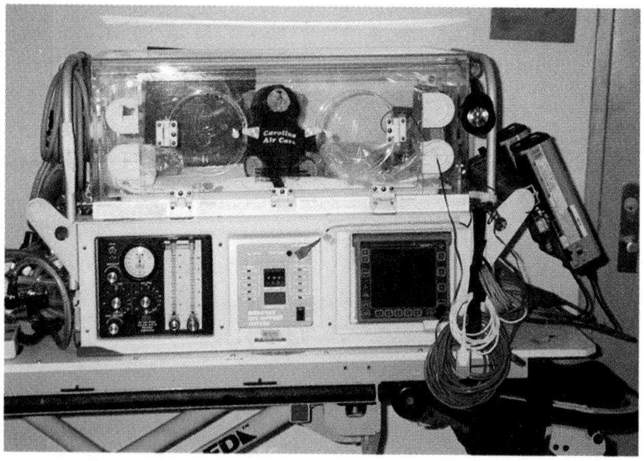
Carolina
Air Care

FIG. 40-17 Total life support system for transport of high risk newborns. (Courtesy UNC Hospitals, Carolina Air Care, Chapel Hill, NC.)

BOX 40-8 **Information for Parents About the Tertiary Center**

Exact location of the unit—address, map
Visiting hours and hospital rules
Telephone numbers
Names of individuals likely to be involved with the baby's care
Information of the special care unit—what it is, what it does
Location of parking facilities, nearby lodging, and rules regarding young children (siblings)
Any particular rules or regulations regarding the special care unit

From Pettett, G., Sewell, S., & Merenstein, G. (2002). Regionalization and transport in perinatal care. In G. Merenstein & S. Gardner (Eds.), *Handbook of neonatal intensive care* (5th ed.). St. Louis: Mosby.

with their personal health care provider on the long-range expected outcomes for the infant. Specialized incubators make these trips possible (see Fig. 40-17). However, parents may express mixed feelings about such return transports and may be reluctant to adapt to a different facility and group of caregivers. To minimize some of these concerns, it is important to give the parents very clear information about return transports during the initial discharge planning.

Although at the time of discharge, parents may not recognize the need for information on the various resources available to help them in the care of their infant, they can be given such lists of agencies and telephone numbers for later use. Providing them with a client-specific directory covering special programs, social support, community, and funding resources can help them make the transition to the home care of their infants. As the nurse continually reinforces the idea that the infant will go home, this will prompt the parents to plan for the days ahead and therefore be ready to take their infant home when the time comes.

ANTICIPATORY GRIEF

Families experience anticipatory grief when they are told of the impending death of their infant. Anticipatory grief prepares and protects parents who are facing a loss. Parents who have an infant with a debilitating disease (with or without a congenital deformity), but one that may not necessarily threaten the life of the child, also may experience anticipatory grief. An alteration in relationships, a change in lifestyle, and a very real threat to their hopes and dreams for the future may affect the day-to-day interaction of the family with their infant and the staff. Nurses can help facilitate the family's grieving process. If the nurse observes that a family member's day-to-day interactions with the infant change, the nurse should assess the situation and request psychosocial support or intervention by a chaplain or social worker, if necessary.

Loss of an Infant

Parents who know their infant is going to die have a very difficult time. Before the infant's death, the parents need to direct their attention, energy, and caregiving activities toward the dying infant (Fig. 40-18). However, some parents find it difficult to visit their infant even for short periods once a terminal diagnosis has been made. Grandparents also grieve but often are unsure how to comfort their own child (the infant's parent) during the period of impending death. Health care professionals can help by involving the family in the infant's care, providing privacy, answering questions, and preparing them for the inevitability of the death (see Chapter 41). Today there is a growing emphasis on hospice and palliative care for infants and their families (End-of-Life Nursing Education Consortium, 2002).

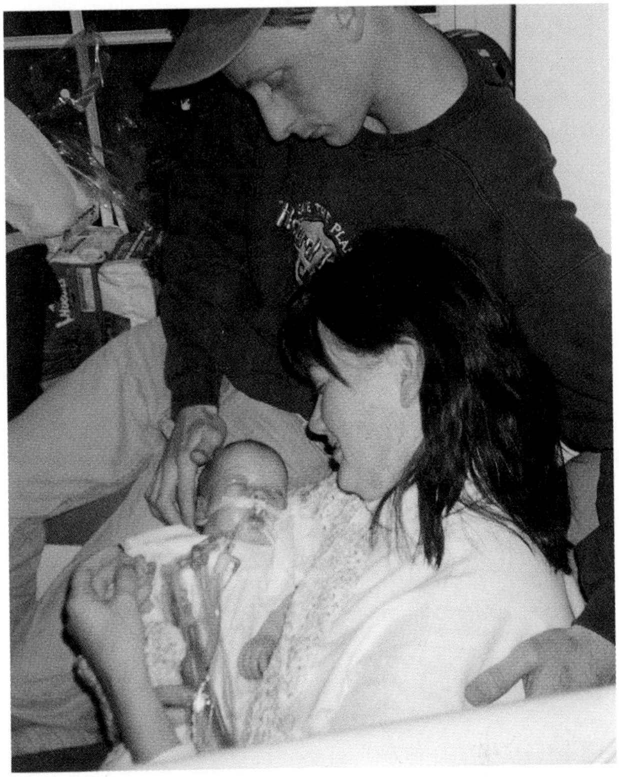

FIG. 40-18 Parents comfort their dying infant. (Courtesy family of Laura Turner, Cary, NC.)

The nursing staff also experiences grief. Many primary staff nurses find themselves grieving as if the infant were their own because they often have been the health professional that has worked closely with the infant and family for weeks, or even months. Managers and other staff members must acknowledge this grief. Talking about the infant or attending the funeral may help the affected staff members resolve their feelings about the infant's death (End-of-Life Nursing Education Consortium, 2002).

KEY POINTS

- Preterm infants are at risk for problems stemming from the immaturity of their organ systems.
- Nurses who work with preterm and other high risk infants observe them for respiratory distress and other early symptoms of physiologic disorders.
- The adaptation of parents to preterm or high risk infants differs from that of parents to normal term infants.
- Nurses can facilitate the development of a positive parent-child relationship.
- Nurses' skills in interpreting data, making decisions, and initiating therapy in newborn intensive care units are crucial to ensuring infants' survival.
- Pain management requires vigilant ongoing assessment, anticipation of painful events, and early interventions to prevent and diminish such a response.
- Nurses' need to assess the macroenvironments and microenvironments of the infant and family to create a developmentally positive atmosphere.
- Developmental care is a philosophy that embraces family-centered care and awareness of the impact of environmental stimuli on the physical and psychologic well-being of the infant and family
- Parents need special instruction (e.g., CPR, oxygen therapy, suctioning, developmental care) before they take home a high risk infant.
- SGA infants are considered at risk because of fetal growth restriction.
- The high incidence of nonreassuring fetal status among postmature infants is related to the progressive placental insufficiency that can occur in a postterm pregnancy.
- Specially trained nurses may transport high risk infants to and from special care units.
- Parents need assistance with coping with anticipatory grief or loss and grief.

CRITICAL THINKING EXERCISES

1. Madeline is born at 23 weeks' gestation; after 2 months in the NICU, the infant is ready to be discharged on oxygen. The family lives 25 miles from the medical center, but there is a local community hospital nearby. What discharge teaching should be done with this family? What community assessment should be done before the discharge? What community resources will this infant and family need? What is your role as the nurse in this discharge?
2. Identify an infant with IUGR. Is the growth restriction symmetric or asymmetric? Review the prenatal and postnatal history. Identify reasons that an infant is growth restricted. Identify problems that might occur with this infant. If this problem appears to have a genetic linkage what referrals should be made for this infant and family?
3. Danielle is a 3-day-old infant born at 32 weeks' gestation and has mild sepsis. Each time anyone walks by her bed, the oxygen saturation is noted to decrease. What is likely to be the cause of these changes? What environmental changes might you institute to safeguard Danielle from stress? What would you teach the parents about developmental care?

RESOURCES

Journal of Perinatal and Neonatal Nursing
Lippincott Williams & Wilkins
Philadelphia, PA

National Association of Neonatal Nurses
4700 W. Lake Ave.
Glenview, IL 60025-145
800-451-3795
888-477-6266 (fax)
www.nann.org
E-mail: info@nann.org

Neonatal Network
1410 Neotomas Ave., Suite 107
Santa Rosa, CA 95405
707-569-1415
www.neonatalnetwork.com

Parents of Prematures
13613 NE 26th Place
Bellevue, WA 98005
206-283-7466

Recommended Standards for NICU Design
www.nd.edu/~kkolberg/frmain.htm

See also Resources list in Chapters 38 and 39

REFERENCES

Als, H. (1998). Developmental care in the newborn intensive care unit. *Current Opinion in Pediatrics, 10*(2), 138-142.

American Academy of Pediatrics. (2002). *ECC Evidence-Based Guidelines: Worksheet for proposed guideline recommendations.* Retrieved from www.aap.org/profed/nrp/docs/meconium.doc, June 16, 2002.

American Academy of Pediatrics Committee on Bioethics and Committee on Hospital Care. (2000). Palliative care for children. *Pediatrics, 106*(2) 351-357.

American Academy of Pediatrics Committee on Fetus and Newborn. (1999). Surfactant replacement therapy for respiratory distress syndrome. *Pediatrics, 103*(3), 684-685.

American Heart Association/American Academy of Pediatrics. (2000). *Textbook of neonatal resuscitation* (4th ed.). Dallas: American Heart Association.

Anand, K. (2001). Consensus statement for the prevention and management of pain in the newborn: International Evidence-Based Group for Neonatal Pain. *Archives of Pediatric and Adolescent Medicine, 155*(2), 173-180.

Anand, K., Grunau, R., & Oberlander, T. (1997). Developmental character and long-term consequences of pain in infants and children. *Child and Adolescent Psychiatric Clinics of North America, 6*(4), 703-724.

Anand, K., & Scalzo, F. (2000). Can adverse neonatal experiences alter brain development and subsequent behavior? *Biology of the Neonate, 77*(2), 69-82.

Anderson, G., Dombrowski, M., & Swinth, J. (2001). Kangaroo care: Not just for stable preemies anymore. *Reflections on Nursing Leadership*, Second Quarter, 32-34, 45.

Association of Pediatric Oncology Nurses (APON), National Association of Neonatal Nurses (NANN), & Society of Pediatric Nurses (SPN). (2002). *Precepts of palliative care for children/adolescents and their families.* Chicago, IL: Last Acts.

Avery, G., Fletcher, M., & MacDonald, M. (1999). *Neonatology: Pathophysiology and management of the newborn* (5th ed.). Philadelphia: Lippincott.

Bildner, J., & Krechel, S. (1996). Increasing staff nurse awareness of postoperative pain management in the NICU. *Neonatal Network, 15*(1), 11-16.

Blackburn, S. (2003). Assessment and management of the neurologic system. In C. Kenner & J. Lott (Eds.), *Comprehensive neonatal nursing care: A physiologic perspective* (3rd ed.). St. Louis: Mosby.

Blake, W., & Murray, J. (2002). Heat balance. In G. Merenstein & S. Gardner. (Eds.), *Handbook of neonatal intensive care* (5th ed.). St. Louis: Mosby.

Blauer, T., & Gerstmann, D. (1998). A simultaneous comparison of three neonatal pain scales during common NICU procedures. *Clinical Journal of Pain, 14*(1), 39-47.

Cavalieri, T., & Sansouci, D. (2003). Newborn and infant assessment. In C. Kenner & J. Lott (Eds.), *Comprehensive neonatal nursing care: A physiologic perspective.* St. Louis: Mosby.

Cifuentes, J., Segars, A., & Carlo, W. (2003). Assessment and management of neonatal respiratory system disorders. In C. Kenner, & J. Lott (Eds.), *Comprehensive neonatal nursing care: A physiologic perspective.* St. Louis: Mosby.

Cools, F., & Offringa, M. (1999). Meta-analysis of elective high frequency ventilation in preterm infants with respiratory distress syndrome. *Archives of Disease in Childhood: Fetal and Neonatal Edition, 80*(1), F15-20.

Denne, S. et al. (2002). Nutrition and metabolism in the high-risk neonate. In A. Fanaroff & R. Martin (Eds.). *Neonatal-perinatal medicine: Diseases of the fetus and infant* (7th ed.). St. Louis: Mosby.

Dickason, E., Silverman, B., & Kaplan, J. (1998). *Maternal-infant nursing care* (3rd ed.). St. Louis: Mosby.

End-of-Life Nursing Education Consortium (ELNEC) (Pediatric). (2002). *End-of-Life Nursing Education Corsortium Training (Pediatric).* Washington, DC: American Association of Colleges of Nursing and City of Hope.

Fielder, A., & Moseley, M. (2000). Environmental light and the preterm infant. *Seminars in Perinatology, 24*(4), 291-298.

Finer, N., & Barrington, K. (2002). Nitric oxide for respiratory failure in infants born at or near term. *Cochrane Database of Systematic Reviews,* Issue 4.

Gale, G., & VandenBerg, K. (1998). Kangaroo care. *Neonatal Network, 17*(5), 69-71.

Gamblian, V., Hess, D., & Kenner, C. (1998). Early discharge from the NICU. *Journal of Pediatric Nursing, 13*(5), 296-301.

Garland, J. et al. (1999). A three-day course of dexamethasone therapy to prevent chronic lung disease in ventilated neonates: A randomized trial. *Pediatrics, 104* (1 pt 1), 91-99.

Gomella, T., Cunningham, M., & Eyal, F. (1999). *Neonatology: Management, procedure, on-call problems, diseases and drugs* (4th ed.). Norfolk, CT: Appleton & Lange.

Gray, K. et al. (1998). Developmentally supportive care in a neonatal intensive care unit: A research utilization project. *Neonatal Network, 17*(2), 33-38.

Hagedorn, M., Gardner, S., & Abman, S. (2002). Respiratory diseases. In G. Merenstein & S. Gardner (Eds.), *Handbook of neonatal intensive care* (5th ed.). St. Louis: Mosby.

Haubrich, K. (2003). Assessment and management of auditory dysfunction. In C. Kenner & J. Lott (Eds.), *Comprehensive neonatal nursing: A physiologic perspective* (3rd ed.). St. Louis: Mosby.

Hendricks-Munoz, K. et al. (2002). Developmental care: The impact of Wee Care developmental care training on short-term infant outcome and hospital costs. *Newborn and Infant Nursing Reviews, 2*(1), 39-45.

Hockenberry, M. et al. (2003). *Wong's nursing care of infants and children* (7th ed.). St. Louis: Mosby.

Hodgkinson, K. et al (1994). Measuring pain in neonates: Evaluating an instrument and developing a common language. *Australian Journal of Advances in Nursing, 12*(1), 17-22.

Holditch-Davis, D., & Miles, M. (2000). Mothers' stories about their experiences in the neonatal intensive care unit. *Neonatal Network, 19*(3), 13-21.

Kenner, C. (2003). Resuscitation and stablization of the newborn. In C. Kenner & J. Lott (Eds.), *Comprehensive neonatal nursing care: A physiologic perspective* (3rd ed.). St. Louis: Mosby.

Kliegman, R., & Das, U. (2002). Intrauterine growth retardation. In A. Fanaroff & R. Martin (Eds.), *Neonatal-perinatal medicine: Diseases of the fetus and infant* (7th ed.). St. Louis: Mosby.

Krechel, S., & Bildner, J. (1995). CRIES: A new neonatal post-operative pain measurement score: Initial testing of validity and reliability. *Pediatric Anaesthesia, 5*, 53-61.

Lawrence, J. et al. (1993). The development of a tool to assess neonatal pain. *Neonatal Network, 12*(6), 59-66.

Luchtman-Jones, L., Schwartz, & Wilson, D. (2002). The blood and hematopoietic system: Part one, Hematologic problems in the fetus and neonate. In A. Fanaroff & R. Martin (Eds.), *Neonatal-perinatal medicine: Diseases of the fetus and infant* (7th ed.). St. Louis: Mosby.

Lund, C., & Durand, D. (2002). Skin and skin care. In G. Merenstein & S. Gardner (Eds.), *Handbook of neonatal intensive care* (5th ed.). St. Louis: Mosby.

Lund, C., & Kuller, J. (2003). Assessment and management of the integumentary system. In C. Kenner & J. Lott (Eds.), *Comprehensive neonatal nursing care: A physiologic perspective* (3rd ed.). St. Louis: Mosby.

Merenstein, G., & Gardner, S. (Eds.). (2002). *Handbook of neonatal intensive care* (5th ed.). St. Louis: Mosby.

Miles, M. et al. (2002). Perceptions of stress, worry, and support in black and white mothers of hospitalized, medically fragile infants. *Journal of Pediatric Nursing, 17*(2), 82-88.

Montoya, K., & Washington, R. (2002). Cardiovascular diseases and surgical interventions. In G. Merenstein & S. Gardner (Eds.), *Handbook of neonatal intensive care* (5th ed.). St. Louis: Mosby.

Pagana, K., & Pagana, T. (2003). *Mosby's diagnostic and laboratory test reference* (6th ed.). St. Louis: Mosby.

Paige, P., & Carney, P. (2002). Neurologic disorders. In G. Merenstein & S. Gardner (Eds.), *Handbook of neonatal intensive care* (5th ed.). St. Louis: Mosby.

Papile, L. (2002). Intracranial hemorrhage. In A. Fanaroff & R. Martin (Eds.), *Neonatal-perinatal medicine: Diseases of the fetus and infant* (7th ed.). St. Louis: Mosby.

Pettett, G., Sewell, S., & Merenstein, G. (2002). Regionalization and transport in perinatal care. In G. Merenstein & S. Gardner (Eds.), *Handbook of neonatal intensive care* (5th ed.). St. Louis: Mosby.

Phelps, D. (2002). The eye: Part three, Retinopathy of prematurity. In A. Fanaroff & R. Martin (Eds.), *Neonatal-perinatal medicine: Diseases of the fetus and infant* (7th ed.). St. Louis: Mosby.

Pickler, R., & Terrell, B. (1994). Nonnutritive sucking and necrotizing enterocolitis. *Neonatal Network, 13*(8), 15-18.

Pinelli, J., & Symington, A. (2000). How rewarding can a pacifier be? A systematic review of nonnutritive sucking in preterm infants. *Neonatal Network, 19*(8), 41-48.

Plavka, R. et al. (1999). A prospective randomized comparison of conventional mechanical ventilation and very early high frequency oscillatory ventilation in extremely premature newborns with respiratory distress syndrome. *Intensive Care Medicine, 25*(1), 68-75.

Pokela, M. (1994). Pain relief can reduce hypoxemia in distressed neonates during routine treatment procedures. *Pediatrics, 93*(3), 379-383.

Reed, M., & Blumer, J. (2002). Pharmacologic treatment of the fetus. In A. Fanaroff & R. Martin (Eds.), *Neonatal-perinatal medicine: Diseases of the fetus and infant* (7th ed.). St. Louis: Mosby.

Robinson, T., & Driscoll, K. (2003). Legal and ethical issues of neonatal care. In C. Kenner & J. Lott (Eds.), *Comprehensive neonatal nursing care: A physiologic perspective* (3rd ed.). St. Louis: Mosby.

Rodriguez, R., Martin, R., & Fanaroff, A. (2002). Respiratory distress syndrome and its management. In A. Fanaroff & R. Martin (Eds.), *Neonatal-perinatal medicine: Diseases of the fetus and infant* (7th ed.). St. Louis: Mosby.

Schwartz, J. (2003). New technologies applied to the management of the respiratory system. In C. Kenner & J. Lott (Eds.), *Comprehensive neonatal nursing care: A physiologic perspective* (3rd ed.). St. Louis: Mosby.

Silverman, W., & Anderson, D. (1956). A controlled clinical trial of effects of water mist on obstructive respiratory signs, death rate, and necropsy findings among premature infants. *Pediatrics, 17*(1), 1-10.

Sparshott, M. (1995). Assessing the behaviour of the newborn infant. *Paediatric Nursing*, 7(7), 14-16, 36.

Standley, J. (1998). The effect of music and multimodal stimulation on responses of premature infants in neonatal intensive care. *Pediatric Nursing, 24*(6), 532-538.

Standley, J. (2002). A meta-analysis of the efficacy of music therapy for premature infants. *Journal of Pediatric Nursing, 17*(20), 107-114.

Steuber, K. et al. (2002). Cuddler volunteers: A very special part of the NICU team. *Central Lines, 18*(4), 4-6.

Stevens, B., & Koren, G. (1998). Evidence-based pain management for infants. *Current Opinions in Pediatrics, 10*(2), 203-207.

Stevens, B. et al. (1996). Premature infant pain profile: Development and initial validation. *Clinical Journal of Pain, 12*, 13-22.

Stevens, B. et al. (1999). The efficacy of developmentally sensitive interventions and sucrose for relieving procedural pain in very low birth weight neonates. *Nursing Research, 48*, 35-43.

Symington, A., & Pinelli, J. (2002). Developmental care for promoting development and preventing morbidity in preterm infants. (Cochrane Review). *The Cochrane Library*, 2. Oxford: Update Software, Ltd.

Taylor, H., Klein, N., & Hack, M. (2000). School-age consequences of birth weight less than 740 g: A review and update. *Developmental Neuropsychology, 17*(3), 289-321.

Tyson, J., & Kennedy, K. (2002). Minimal enteral nutrition for promoting feeding tolerance and preventing morbidity in parenterally fed infants. [Systematic Review]. Cochrane Neonatal Group. *Cochrane Database of Systematic Review*, Issue 4.

VandenBerg, K. (1999). What to tell parents about the developmental needs of their baby at discharge. *Neonatal Network, 18*(1), 57-59.

Vanucci, R., & Yager, J. (2002). The central nervous system: Part one, Newborn neurologic assessment. In A. Fanaroff & R. Martin (Eds.), *Neonatal-perinatal medicine: Diseases of the fetus and infant* (7th ed.). St. Louis: Mosby.

Walden, M., & Franck, L. (2003). Identification, management, and prevention of newborn/infant pain. In C. Kenner & J. Lott (Eds.), *Comprehensive neonatal nursing care: A physiologic perspective* (3rd ed.). St. Louis: Mosby.

Walsh-Sukys, M. et al. (2001). Reducing light and sound in the neonatal intensive care unit: An evaluation of patient safety, staff satisfaction and costs. *Journal of Perinatology, 21*(4), 230-235.

Wiswell, T. et al. (2002). A multicenter randomized, controlled trial comparing Surfaxin (Lucinactant) lavage with standard care for treatment of meconium aspiration syndrome. *Pediatrics, 109*(6), 1081-1087.

Wyckoff, M. et al. (2003). Nutrition: Physiologic basis of metabolism and management of enteral and parenteral nutrition. In C. Kenner & J. Lott (Eds.), *Comprehensive neonatal nursing: A physiologic perspective* (3rd ed.). St. Louis: Mosby.

Yoder, B. et al. (2002). Changing obstetric practices associated with decreasing incidence of meconium aspiration syndrome (1). *Obstetrics and Gynecology, 99*(5), 731-739.

Zehka, K., & Patel, C. (2002). Cardiovascular problems of the neonate. In A. Fanaroff & R. Martin (Eds.), *Neonatal-perinatal medicine: Diseases of the fetus and infant* (7th ed.). St. Louis: Mosby.

CHAPTER 41

Margaret Shandor Miles and Kelly A. Pelosi

Grieving the Loss of a Newborn

http://evolve.elsevier.com/Lowdermilk/MatWmnHlth/

LEARNING OBJECTIVES

- Describe emotional, behavioral, cognitive, and physical responses commonly experienced during the grieving process associated with perinatal loss.
- Understand the personal and societal issues that may complicate responses to perinatal loss.
- Formulate appropriate nursing diagnoses for parents experiencing perinatal loss.
- Identify specific nursing interventions to meet the special needs of parents and their families related to perinatal loss and grief.
- Differentiate among helpful and nonhelpful responses in caring for parents experiencing loss and grief.

Becoming a parent is an important developmental milestone that is anticipated by most men and women in our society. Becoming a parent gives one social status, expands one's capacity for caring and loving for another, and adds immense responsibility to one's life. However, loss can be associated with pregnancy and birth. During pregnancy, parents plan for the birth, imagine what the birth will be like, and develop an image of the appearance of the baby. The reality of childbirth may not be what the parents have dreamed of or hoped for. In particular, the experience of premature labor and preterm birth or cesarean birth all involve a loss of the expected pregnancy and birth plans. Parents also may grieve over the sex or appearance of their child. For some parents, loss is associated with the birth of an infant who has a birth defect or chronic illness.

Although having children can be a strong desire and goal for women and men, not everyone is successful in achieving parenthood. For some couples, infertility may thwart their plans and desires for parenthood and cause intense feelings of grief. When couples undergo infertility treatments, feelings of loss may intensify, especially when treatments fail and/or a pregnancy ends in a miscarriage (Lukse & Vacc, 1999). Women, in particular, experience high distress during this time (Mori et al., 1997).

Many women and their partners, whether infertile or not, experience miscarriage in the early months of pregnancy. Miscarriage affects the personal identity of the woman and causes guilt, depression, and anxiety (Frost & Condon, 1996). Others may have an ectopic pregnancy or experience a fetal death. Women and their partners also may suddenly be confronted with stillbirth, the birth of an infant who is not alive. All of these experiences may be called **perinatal loss.** Others may experience intense grief after infant death (Kavanaugh, 1997). These others include women who give birth prematurely to an infant who survives only a few hours or who dies after days, weeks, or months in an intensive care unit. In addition, a woman may give birth to an infant with severe congenital anomalies or other serious health problems; these infants also may die after a few hours, days, weeks, or months in an intensive care unit.

The statistics on perinatal loss and death of an infant are grim. Approximately 19.7 of each 1000 pregnancies are ectopic pregnancies, taking place outside the uterus, usually in a uterine tube (Pisarska & Carson, 1999). Ectopic pregnancies accounted for 9% of maternal deaths in 1992 (Pisarska & Carson, 1999). A **miscarriage**–a pregnancy that ends before 20 weeks of gestation–is reported to account for 15% to 20% of all pregnancies (Zinaman et al., 1996). In addition, each year approximately 5 of every 1000 births end in stillbirth or fetal deaths (those occurring after 20 weeks of gestation). Newborn death, death of a baby born showing signs of life such as respiratory effort, heart rate, pulsating cord at birth, and/or muscle irritability, regardless of gestational age, accounts for almost 28,000 deaths per year in the United States (Hoyert et al., 2001). Of those, 19,000 infants die in the early postpartum period of prematurity, birth defects, and other acute illnesses (Hoyert et al., 2001). African-American women experience pregnancy and infant losses at rates twice those of Caucasian women and women of other ethnic minority groups (Van, 2001).

Thus parents can experience grief before or during the childbearing experience. **Grief** involves the painful emotions and related behavioral and physical responses to a major loss. Grief can be particularly difficult with perinatal losses for a number of reasons: the societal belief that there are no barriers to getting pregnant, and the expectation that once a woman is pregnant, the result will be a healthy live infant. As a result, our society tends to minimize perinatal loss and to lack understanding of the associated pain. Women and men who undergo perinatal losses struggle with these issues themselves, and because of these societal attitudes, they may not receive the support they need. In addition, many perinatal losses are hidden or private, in that others may not know about the infertility or the early pregnancy that ended in miscarriage. Perinatal losses may be intensified for couples who delay pregnancy until the woman's career and the family's financial status is at the right point to take on the responsibilities of a child. Feelings of helplessness and loss of control can be very difficult when the couple experiences infertility or miscarriage. In many instances of perinatal loss, the lack of an identified cause for the loss can complicate grief. This is particularly difficult for women, who often feel personally responsible for infertility, miscarriage, and infant death. Some couples endure repeated losses, which can be devastating. Further, society allows much too little time for mothers grieving a perinatal loss and even less for men. All of these issues can reduce the support to bereaved parents. Parents in a Canadian study reported that social support from families and friends fell short of expectations, and they interpreted this inattention as an indication that the death of their baby was not an important life event (Malacrida, 2000). Some also reported a lack of understanding and support from health care professionals.

Nurses have a powerful influence on how parents experience and cope with perinatal loss (Corbet-Owen & Kruger, 2001). Nurses encounter these parents in a variety of settings, including the antepartum, labor and birth, neonatal, postpartum, and gynecologic units of hospitals, and obstetric, gynecologic, and infertility outpatient clinics and offices. In these settings, nurses have opportunities to provide sensitive and caring interventions to parents. Parents have reported that their nurses were an important resource in helping them cope with their grief. Nurses in many inpatient settings have developed protocols that provide clear direction to all staff in how to help parents through this difficult process. In some units, experienced nurses or social workers who are particularly comfortable in helping bereaved parents are designated as perinatal grief consultants. They are available to help parents but also to help prepare the staff for their role with parents. In addition, many institutions now have follow-up programs involving telephone calls, home visits, and support groups that are effective in helping parents after discharge. It is important, then, that dealing with perinatal loss be included in nursing curricula and in-service training for staff nurses.

The focus of this chapter is to prepare the beginning nurse to provide sensitive, supportive, and therapeutic interventions to parents experiencing perinatal loss in a variety of settings. An overview of the grief process is presented as a guide for assessing and understanding the responses of bereaved women, men, and their families. Guidelines for intervention are given, and specific intervention approaches are discussed.

GRIEF RESPONSES

Grief or **bereavement** has been described as a cluster of painful responses experienced by individuals coping with the death of someone with whom they had a close relationship, generally a relative or close friend (Lindemann, 1944; Osterweis, Solomon, & Green, 1984; Parkes, 1972; Parkes & Weiss, 1983). Many authors believe there are overlapping phases in the grief process, but most do not believe that grief is experienced in "stages." There is an early period of acute distress and shock followed by a period of intense grief that includes emotional, cognitive, behavioral, and physical responses. The phase of reorganization is reached when the individuals return to their usual level of functioning in society, although the pain associated with the death remains. The duration of grief varies with the individual, but there is general agreement that grief is a long-term process that can extend for months and years. With a very close relationship such as with one's baby, some aspects of grief never truly end. Another way of conceptualizing the grief process is through the achievement of certain tasks of mourning. Worden (1991) identified four tasks: (1) Accepting the loss, (2) working through the pain, (3) adjusting to the environment, and (4) moving on. He proposed that these four "tasks of mourning" must be completed to resolve grief.

Miles (1984) and Miles and Demi (1986, 1997) proposed a conceptual model of parental grief, based on the work of Lindemann (1944), Parkes (1972, 1983), and Worden (1991). In addition, the model proposes that the grief responses of a parent are closely linked to the self-image as a mother or father. Parental grief responses occur in three overlapping phases of grief–acute distress, intense grief, and reorganization (Box 41-1).

Acute Distress

The loss of a pregnancy or death of an infant is an acute and distressing experience for mothers and fathers who planned for and expected a normal healthy infant as the outcome. The loss encompasses a loss of their identity as a mother or father and the loss of their many dreams related to parenthood. The immediate reaction to news of a perinatal loss or infant death encompasses a period of **acute distress.** Parents generally are in a state of shock and numbness. They may feel a sense of unreality and confusion, as though they were in a bad dream or in a fog or trancelike state. Disbelief and denial can occur. However,

BOX 41-1 Conceptual Model of Parental Grief

PHASE OF ACUTE DISTRESS
Shock
Numbness
Intense crying
Depression

PHASE OF INTENSE GRIEF
Loneliness, emptiness, and yearning
Guilt
Anger, resentment, bitterness, irritability
Fear and anxiety (especially about getting pregnant again)
Disorganization
Difficulties with cognitive processing
Sadness and depression
Physical symptoms

REORGANIZATION
Search for meaning
Reduction of distress
Reentering normal life activities with more enthusiasm
Can make future plans, including decision about another pregnancy

Adapted from Miles, M. (1980). *The grief of parents...when a child dies.* Oak Brook, IL: Compassionate Friends, Inc.; Miles, M. (1984). Helping adults mourn the death of a child. In H. Wass & C. Corr (Eds.), *Childhood and death.* New York: Hemisphere.

parents also feel very sad and depressed. Intense outbursts of emotion and crying are common. However, lack of affect, euphoria, and calmness may occur and may reflect numbness, denial, or a personal way of coping with stress.

Much of the literature and research on grief after perinatal loss and infant death has focused on the mother. Likewise, much of the attention during the time of a loss is on the mother; the father is expected to be her main support but is often not acknowledged as grieving, too. The response of fathers may be more variable than that of mothers and depends on the level of identification with the pregnancy. With early miscarriage or ectopic pregnancy, some fathers may not have a strong investment in the wished-for child. However, many fathers do grieve deeply for a miscarriage (Puddifoot & Johnson, 1997; Schaap et al., 1997). Fathers are profoundly affected by a stillbirth or death of an infant. Fathers also are distressed by the grief of the mother and often feel helpless as to how to help her with the intense pain. Some fathers appear stoic and unemotional to maintain the societal expectation that they be "strong" for the mother and other family members. It is important to realize that fathers may be experiencing deep pain beneath their calm and quiet appearance and need help in acknowledging these feelings. Because fathers do not easily share feelings or ask for help, special efforts are needed to help them realize that they too have a right to support from others in their pain.

During this time of acute distress, parents face the first task of grief, accepting the reality of the loss. The pregnancy has ended or the baby has died, and their life has changed. Although parents are often required to make many decisions, such as having an autopsy, naming the infant, and funeral arrangements, normal functioning is impeded, and decisions are difficult to make. These decisions are especially painful and difficult for young couples who have limited or no previous experience with death. Grandparents are often called on to help make difficult decisions regarding funeral arrangements and/or disposition of the body because they have more life experience with taking care of these painful, yet required arrangements. However, some well-meaning grandparents and other family members may try to take over with all the decisions that must be made. It is critical that the nurse remember that a very important role is always to be a client advocate and that the parents themselves should approve the final decisions.

Intense Grief

The phase of **intense grief** encompasses many difficult emotions, including loneliness, emptiness, yearning; guilt, anger, and fear; disorganization and depression; and physical symptoms. During this time, parents are working on two additional tasks of mourning: working through the pain and adjusting to life without the wished-for child. Being able to adjust to the environment after the loss means learning how to accommodate the changes that the loss has brought.

In the early months after the loss, parents often experience feelings of loneliness, emptiness, and yearning. The mother may report that her arms ache to hold or nurse her baby and that she wakes to the sound of a baby crying. When her milk comes in, it is particularly poignant when there is no baby to take to breast. Both mothers and fathers may be preoccupied with thoughts about the wished-for child. Some women cope with these feelings by avoiding memories and by not talking about the baby, whereas others want to reminisce and discuss their loss over and over. Deciding what to do about the nursery and baby clothes is particularly difficult during this period. Some women want the room taken down before they go home, whereas others want the room left intact until they have had time to grieve their loss. It is not unusual for a grandparent or other family member to want to rush home to take down the nursery with the thought that they would be sparing additional painful grief. In fact, their actions might only complicate the grief if parents were not involved in the decision. The bereaved parents, in their own time frame, must go through these types of experiences so that healing can take place.

During this phase of intense grief, guilt may emerge from the deep feelings of helplessness in not somehow preventing the pregnancy loss or the death of the infant.

Mothers are particularly vulnerable to feel guilt because of their sense of responsibility for the well-being of the fetus and baby. With many perinatal losses, there is no clear cause of the event, leaving the woman to speculate about what she might have done or not done to cause the loss. Guilt also may be intense if a mother thinks she is being punished for some unrelated event such as having had a prior induced abortion. Such self-blame is torture for mothers, and they need repeated emotional reassurance that they were not at fault. Guilt can occur when one is enjoying life again and experiencing happiness despite the loss of the infant.

Another common response during this phase of grief is anger, resentment, bitterness, or irritability. Anger is particularly poignant if the loss is perceived as senseless, and there is a need to blame others. Anger may be focused on the health care team who failed to save the pregnancy or infant. For some parents, anger is vented toward a God who allowed the loss to occur. This can lead to a spiritual crisis. Anger also occurs toward family, friends, and peers when they do not provide the support bereaved parents need and want. Some parents focus their resentment on parents who do not appreciate their children or who neglect and abuse them. A sense of bitterness or generalized irritability, rather than frank anger, may be another response.

Fear and anxiety can occur during the grief process as a profound worry that something else bad might happen to another. Fear and anxiety are particularly poignant when the couple thinks about another pregnancy. Whereas some parents, especially mothers, are almost obsessed with the desire to become pregnant again, others struggle with whether they can cope with another potential loss.

Deep sadness and depression occur when the parent is faced with the full awareness of the reality of the loss. This often occurs several months after a perinatal loss and can continue for some time. Sadness and depression are often accompanied by **disorganization** and problems with cognitive processing. This leads to behavioral changes such as difficulty in getting things done, an inability to concentrate, restlessness, confused thought processes, difficulty in solving problems, and poor decision making. Disorganization and depression often cause difficulties in keeping up with work and family expectations. Additionally, parents returning to work face issues such as handling well-meaning but painful comments or the silence of co-workers.

Physical symptoms of grief include fatigue, headaches, dizziness, or backaches. Parents are at risk for developing health problems, such as colds or hypertension. The grieving process makes it difficult for bereaved parents to sleep. Their appetites may be depressed or voracious. Lack of sleep and inadequate nutrition and fluids can complicate other grief responses.

Grief responses are very personal, ongoing, and difficult to cope with. Some parents may suppress or deny their feelings because of societal indifference toward pregnancy loss and infant death. Suppression of feelings may, on the surface, be more socially acceptable. However, denying the pain of grief may lead to eventual physical and emotional distress or illness. Many parents, especially mothers, want to tell their story over and over. This helps them actualize the loss and face their feelings. Sometimes parents begin to think they are the only individuals who have ever had such a rough time and that they may be going crazy. Although bereaved parents have many ups and downs for many months and even years after a child's death, few parents actually become mentally ill or commit suicide. Knowing that these feelings are normal and that others have felt the same is helpful. The grief process during this phase is often difficult for fathers. Some may continue to have difficulty sharing their feelings. A rift can occur if one parent, usually the mother, wants to talk about the loss and pain, and the other parent, often but not always the father, withdraws. Other signs of problems include reliance on alcohol and drugs, extramarital affairs, prolonged hours at work, and overinvolvement in diversional and other activities outside the home as an escape.

Reorganization

From the time of the pregnancy loss or infant death, parents attempt to understand "why?" This leads to a long and intense **search for meaning.** At first the "why" is focused on the cause of death. Finding few good answers, parents focus next on "why me, why mine?" These questions lead some parents into an existential search about the meaning of life and death. "What does my loss mean to my life?" "What is life all about?" "What do I do with the rest of my life?" This search continues into the phase of reorganization and may lead to profound changes in the parents' views about the fragility of life.

Time helps to ease slowly the painful feelings of grief. Over time, the pain becomes less frequent. **Reorganization** occurs when the parent is better able to function at home and work, experiences a return of self-esteem and confidence, can cope with new challenges, and has placed the loss in perspective. Reorganization begins to peak sometime after the first year as parents begin to achieve the task of moving on with their lives. Enjoying the simple pleasures of life without feeling guilty, nurturing self and others, developing new interests, and reestablishing relationships are all signs of moving on. For some women and families, another pregnancy and the birth of a subsequent child is an important step in moving on with their lives; however, the term "recovery" is used because the grief related to perinatal loss can continue in varying degrees for life. Parents have shared that they will never forget the baby who has died, and they are not the same persons as before the loss. The term **"bittersweet grief,"** coined by Kowalski (1984), refers to the grief response that occurs with reminders of the loss. This typically happens at special anniversary dates related to the loss. Grief feelings also can be triggered after a subsequent live birth (Box 41-2).

BOX 41-2 Bittersweet Grief

To Jessica Mayo—on her eleventh birthday
Sunday, November 18, 1990
"The child who is born on the Sabbath day,
is bonny and blithe and good and gay."
Sundays are special days.
. . . a day of rest, a day to play.
A day to reflect on days past.
. . . a day to thank God for all that we bless.
I bless your memory.
I wish you were here.
On your eleventh birthday I still want to share.
. . . Your dreams of the future.
. . . Our memories past.
My baby's first cry.
My daughter's first laugh.
I was told you were an angel in heaven above.
Eleven years later, I'm an expert . . .
At long-distance love.
On your third birthday I wrote my first poem
to you.
Eight years later, it's still true
". . . no birthday cake,
no presents unwrapped . . .
no pictures of you in your party hat.
But the candles are lit,
Never to go out
For they burn forever in my heart.
Love, Mom"
Kathie Rataj Mayo
1990

Resuming the sexual relationship is an extremely important aspect of recovery but can be very complicated. Many parents are comforted with the belief that their babies were conceived in love, lived in love, and died in love. The result of their love and intimacy created this child, and parents may believe that they may never experience joy and closeness again. Once the doctor has given permission for resumption of sexual activities, parents may find it emotionally very difficult. Some couples may have an increased need for sexual activity in an attempt for closeness and healing, whereas others have a decreased desire for sexual intimacy. It is important that clients be aware of some possible deep need from inside themselves to stop the emotional pain. Difficulties arise when the needs of the couple differ.

Sexuality also brings with it decisions about a future pregnancy. Some are eager to have another child, although one child cannot replace the one who died, and the grief will continue despite being pregnant. Other parents have a deep fear of experiencing the pain of loss again, which can make the resumption of sexual activity difficult. These ambivalent feelings are normal, and couples will find themselves moving back and forth between the emotions of exhilaration and fear. The subsequent pregnancy after a loss is often filled with guarded emotions and great anxiety (Cote-Arsenault & Mahlangu, 1999). The excitement that many others experience with a pregnancy is very different for previously bereaved parents. Fathers also reported anxiety about the outcome of the next pregnancy and increased their vigilance (Armstrong, 2001). Couples often mark the progress of the pregnancy in terms of fetal development, waiting anxiously until the number of weeks of the previous loss are passed (Cote-Arsenault & Mahlangu, 1999). In some cases, the fear of repeated loss, especially after a stillbirth, is so great that induction of labor is considered if lung maturity studies can confirm that the baby is mature.

FAMILY ASPECTS OF GRIEF: GRANDPARENTS AND SIBLINGS

It is extremely important for the nurse taking care of these clients to keep in mind that they have an entire family to minister to, including especially grandparents and siblings. Grandparents have hopes and dreams for a grandchild; these have been shattered. The grief of grandparents is often complicated by the fact that they are experiencing intense emotional pain by witnessing and feeling the immense grief of their own child. It is extremely difficult to watch their son or daughter experience unimaginable emotional trauma with very few ways to comfort and end their pain. As a result, the grief response may be complicated or delayed for grandparents. On occasions, some grandparents experience immense "survival guilt" because they feel the death is out of order. They are angry that they are alive and their grandchild is not.

The siblings of the expected infant also experience a profound loss. Most children have been prepared for having another child in the family once the pregnancy is confirmed. These children come in all ages and stages of development, and this must be considered in understanding how they view the event and their loss experience. A young child will respond more to the response of their parents, picking up on the fact that they are behaving differently and are extremely sad. This can cause clinging, altered eating and sleeping patterns, or acting out behaviors, yet it is a time when parents have limited patience for responding to and meeting the needs of the child. Older children have a more complete understanding of the loss. School-aged children may be frightened by the entire event, whereas teens may understand fully but feel awkward in responding. Older siblings need to be included in grieving rituals to the extent the parents and the child feel comfortable. They may need to see the baby to actualize the loss. Nurses need to have a basic understanding about how children view death and grieve to reach out to siblings in an appropriate and sensitive manner. Nurses also need to help parents understand and be sensitive to the needs of their other children despite their own deep pain.

CARE MANAGEMENT

Nursing care of mothers and fathers experiencing a perinatal loss begins the first time the parents are faced with the potential loss of their pregnancy or death of their infant. Supportive interventions are important both at the time of the loss and after the parents have returned home.

Assessment and Nursing Diagnoses

An important step in the nursing process involves assessment. Several key areas to address include the following:

- *The nature of the parental attachment with the pregnancy or infant, the meaning of the pregnancy and infant to the parent, and the related losses they are experiencing.* Each pregnancy and birth has a special meaning to parents. Whether a woman has experienced a miscarriage or ectopic pregnancy, stillbirth, or death of an infant, it is important to gain some understanding of parents' perceptions of their unique loss. The meaning of the loss is determined by familial and cultural systems of the parents. In one study, feelings about perinatal loss ranged from feeling devastated to feeling relieved (Corbet-Owen & Kruger, 2001). Listening to parents tell their story and being sensitive to the language used to describe their experience can help one gain an understanding of the meaning of the loss. Open-ended questions are helpful: "Tell me about your labor and birth with Mia." Or "When did you know you were miscarrying?" Mothers who have had a previous pregnancy loss may feel less attached, which can increase their feelings of guilt when a loss occurs.
- *The circumstances surrounding the loss, including the level of preparation for the loss and the parents' level of understanding about the cause of the loss or death, and any related unresolved issues are important.* While listening to the parents' stories, it is important to uncover any special experiences that may make their losses even more poignant. A history of infertility, repeated pregnancy losses, a previous stillbirth, or infant death can make this loss even more painful. In addition, other life circumstances such as illness of another family member, loss of a job, or other family stresses can increase the distress of parents. It also is helpful to know whether the mother and father perceived the loss to be totally unexpected or whether they had some forewarning or preparation.
- *The immediate response of the mother and father to the loss, whether their responses are complementary or problematic, and how their responses match with their past experiences, personalities, and behavioral and cultural backgrounds.* An understanding of the usual responses to grief described earlier can be helpful in attempting to understand the unique grief responses of the mother and father and other family members. As nurses work with families, they may uncover information about how the individual or family responded to a previous loss, or a personality or behavioral trait that may interact in their responses to this grief. In particular, it is important to know about any history of infertility, previous pregnancy losses, or infant deaths and evaluate how that might affect parental responses (Armstrong & Hutti, 1998; Lukse & Vacc, 1999). It also is important to be sensitive to different expectations during grief for men and women from different cultural groups (see section on cultural and spiritual needs of parents later in this chapter).
- *The social support network of the parent (e.g., extended family, friends, co-workers, church) and the extent to which it has been activated.* Support during a perinatal loss is important to most couples. However, it is important to assess the amount of support and the type of support from others that a couple wants. Some prefer to handle the tragedy alone for a time. Others want assistance in calling other family members, friends, and clergy to be with them and to help them with decisions.

Nursing diagnoses may include physiologic and psychosocial problems experienced by the individual mother or father, or problems occurring within the couple or family because of the loss and subsequent grief. Examples of nursing diagnoses include the following:

- *Anxiety related to*
  - –lack of experience regarding how to manage the loss
  - –worry about the partner
  - –intense concern over not achieving a pregnancy
  - –becoming pregnant again with risk of another loss
- *Ineffective family or individual coping related to*
  - –inability to make decisions as a family
  - –difficulties in communication within the family
  - –conflicting coping patterns between mother and father
- *Powerlessness related to*
  - –high risk pregnancy and birth
  - –unexpected cesarean birth
  - –inability to prevent the infant's death
- *Interrupted family processes related to*
  - –maternal depression leading to changes in role function
  - –inadequate communication of feelings between the grieving mother and father
  - –lack of expected support from family
  - –behavioral and emotional reactions of siblings
  - –grief within the family system including grandparents and other relatives
- *Ineffective sexuality patterns between the mother and father related to*
  - –guilt and fear associated with sexuality
  - –loss of pleasure in sexual intercourse
  - –differences in desires of each partner
  - –fear of getting pregnant again

- *Fatigue and disturbed sleep pattern related to*
  - –inability to fall asleep because of grief
  - –waking in the night and thinking about the loss
  - –loss of sleep
- *Dysfunctional grieving related to*
  - –prolonged denial or avoidance of the loss
  - –intense guilt related to the loss
  - –continued anger about the loss
  - –serious depressive symptoms and despair
  - –loss of self-esteem
  - –intense grieving patterns that continue for more than a year
  - –social isolation due to grief
- *Situational low self-esteem related to*
  - –prolonged feelings of poor self-worth because of the loss
  - –feeling unworthy of having a child
- *Spiritual distress related to*
  - –anger with God
  - –confusion about why prayers were not answered
- *Disturbed thought processes related to*
  - –difficulty making decisions
  - –inability to get organized
  - –poor work performance
  - –confused thinking

Expected Outcomes of Care

Expected outcomes are set and priorities assigned in client-centered terms according to the mutual goals chosen by the client and the nurse. Nursing actions are then selected to meet the expected outcomes, which may include that the woman/family will do the following:

- Actualize the loss.
- Share experiences and verbalize feelings of grief as much as is culturally and personally appropriate.
- Understand the normal grief responses they and others in the family may experience at the time of and after the loss.
- Demonstrate increasing independence in participating in and making decisions that meet their needs and reflect their religious and cultural beliefs.
- Identify family, spiritual, health care, and community resources for support.
- Discuss problems or issues involving relationships with each other and family.
- Verbalize satisfaction with the care and support provided by their health care professionals.

Plan of Care and Interventions

Interventions and support for parents from the nursing and medical staff after a perinatal loss or infant death are extremely important in their healing. Although parents often cannot recall details of their experiences at the time of death, they may recall vividly minor events that were perceived as particularly painful or particularly helpful. However, care must be individualized to each parent and family. In a large longitudinal study of parents after a perinatal death, Rand and associates (1998) found that parents appreciated the opportunity to make choices about their needs. The authors suggested that providers should not bias parents or make presumptions that would limit their choices or force them to make choices they do not want. Furthermore, the cultural and spiritual beliefs and practices of individual parents and families must be considered. The interventions discussed later are general ideas about what may be helpful to parents.

Help the Mother, Father, and Other Family Members Actualize the Loss

When a loss or death occurs, the nurse should be sure that parents have been honestly told about the situation by their physician or others on the health care team. It is important for their nurse to be with them during this time. With infant death, caregivers must use the words "dead" and "died," rather than "lost" or "gone," to assist the bereaved in accepting this reality. Parents need opportunities to tell their story about the events, experiences, and feelings surrounding the loss. This can help them come to terms with the reality of their loss. Listening to their pain and allowing time for them to absorb the information are important.

One way of actualizing the loss is to tell the parents the sex of the baby and give them the option of naming the fetus or to help them to name an infant who has died. Choosing a name helps make the baby a member of their family so that the baby can be remembered in a special way. Once the baby is named, the nurse should use the name when referring to the baby. Although naming can be helpful, it is important not to create the sense that the parents have to name the "baby," especially in the case of a miscarriage when the sex is not known.

NURSE ALERT

A caution about naming is important. Cultural taboos and rules in some religious faiths prohibit the naming of an infant who has died. It is very important to be sensitive to this possibility and not impose naming on such parents.

It may be helpful for mothers and fathers to see the fetus or baby. Many professionals, based on vast clinical experiences with parents, believe that seeing the fetus/baby helps parents face the reality of the loss, reduces painful fantasies, and offers an opportunity for closure. This has recently been questioned as the result of a longitudinal study of a small group of mothers in England (Hughes et al., 2002). These authors suggest that the wishes of the parents should be respected. Parents should never be made to feel they "should" see or hold their baby when this is something that they do not really want. Encouraging reluctant parents to hold or see their dead child by telling them that not seeing the child could make mourning more difficult is inappropriate. Obviously, this subject must be approached very carefully. A question such as, "Some parents have found it helpful to see their baby. Would you like time to consider this?" Because the need or willingness to see also may vary between the mother and father, it is extremely important to determine what each parent really wants. This should not be a joint decision made by one person or a decision made for the parents by grandparents or others. It is a good policy for the nurse to first tell them about this option and then give them time to think about it. Later the nurse can return and ask each parent individually what they decided.

In preparation for the visit with the baby, parents appreciate explanations about what to expect. Descriptions of how their baby looks is important. For example, babies may have red, peeling skin like a bad sunburn, dark discoloration similar to bruises, molding of the head that makes the head look soft and swollen, or birth defects. The nurse should make the baby look as normal as possible, and remember that parents see their baby with different eyes from health care professionals. Bathing the baby, applying lotion to the baby's skin, combing hair, placing identification bracelets on the arm and leg, dressing the baby in a diaper and special outfit, sprinkling powder in the baby's blanket, and wrapping the baby in a pretty blanket conveys to the parents that their baby has been cared for in a special way (Fig. 41-1). The use of powder and lotion stimulates the parent's senses and provides pleasant memories of their baby.

It is more complicated if the fetus died several days or weeks before birth or if decapitation or dismemberment occurred. Consultation with a local funeral director can help the nurse prepare the baby to be seen by his or her parents. If the baby has been in the morgue, he or she can be placed underneath a warmer for 20 to 30 minutes and wrapped in a warm blanket before being brought to the parents. Cold cream rubbed over stiffened joints can help in positioning the baby.

When bringing the baby to the parents, it is important to treat the baby as one would a live baby. Holding the baby close, touching a hand or cheek, using the baby's name, and talking with the parents about the special features of their child conveys that it is all right for them to do likewise. If a baby has a congenital anomaly, the nurse can desensitize the family by pointing out aspects of the baby that are normal. Nurses can help parents explore the baby's body as they desire. Parents often seek to identify family resemblance. A good question might be: "Who in your family does Michael resemble?"

Some families may like to have the opportunity to bathe and dress their baby. Although the skin may be fragile, parents can still apply lotion with cotton balls, sprinkle powder, tie ribbons, fasten the diaper, and place amulets, medallions, rosaries, or special toys or mementos in their baby's hands or alongside their baby. They may want to perform other parenting activities, such as combing hair, dressing the baby in a special outfit, wrapping the baby in a blanket, or placing the baby in a crib.

Parents need to be offered time alone with their baby if they wish. They also need to know when the nurse will return and how to call if they should need anything. If at all possible, the family should be placed in a private room, and when possible, the room should have a rocking chair for the parents to sit in when holding their baby. This offers the mother and father special time together with their baby and with other family members (Fig. 41-2). Marking the door to the room with a special card can be helpful in reminding the staff that this family has experienced a loss (Fig. 41-3).

It is difficult to predict how long and how often parents will need to spend time with their baby. These moments are the only ones they will have to parent their child while their child's physical presence is still with them. Some parents need only a few minutes; others need hours. It is extremely painful for some parents to say good-bye to their baby. They will tell the nurse when they are ready verbally and nonverbally. The nurse should watch for cues that the parents have had enough time with their baby, such as when parents are no longer holding their child close to them or have placed the baby back in the crib. Asking parents whether they have had enough time may make parents feel that the nurse thinks they have had enough time, which may not be the case. When a baby is taken too soon from parents, it leaves them feeling as though the baby was "ripped from their arms too soon." Heiman, Yankowitz, and Wilkins (1997) found that 85% of parents in their study would have appreciated additional opportunities to see their baby, and 44% felt they did not have adequate time with the baby. Thus sensitivity to parental needs in actualizing the loss and coping with the reality of the

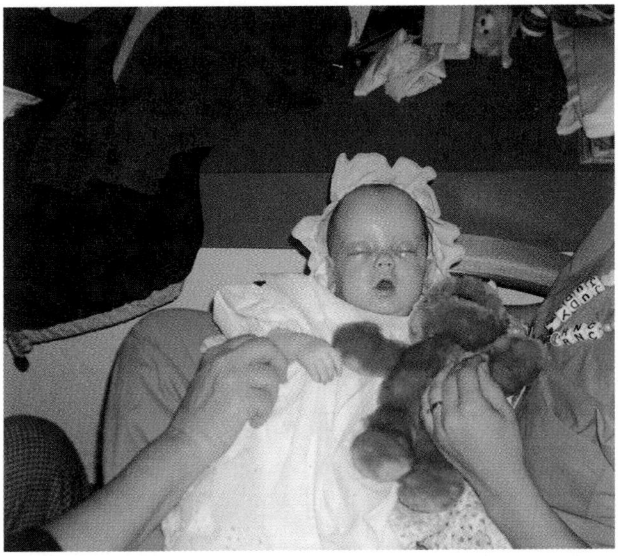

FIG. 41-1 Laura. (Courtesy Amy and Ken Turner, Cary, NC.)

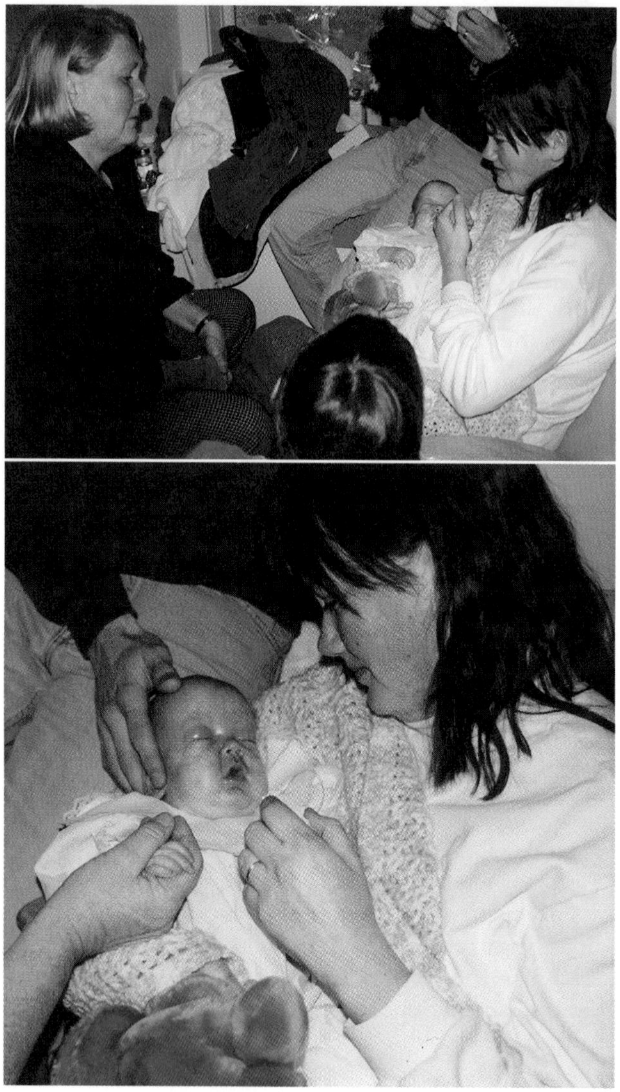

FIG. 41-2 Laura's family members say a special good-bye. (Courtesy Amy and Ken Turner, Cary, NC.)

death is essential for their healing. Grandparents should be offered the same opportunities to hold, rock, swaddle, and love their grandchildren so that their grief is started in a healthy way.

Help the Parents with Decision Making

At the time of a perinatal loss, and especially if the loss was of an infant, parents have many decisions to make when they are experiencing great distress. Mothers, fathers, and extended families look to the medical and nursing staff for guidance in knowing what decisions they must and can make, and in understanding the options related to those decisions. Thus it is a primary responsibility of the nurse to help them and to advocate for them because decisions made during the time of their loss will provide their memories for a lifetime.

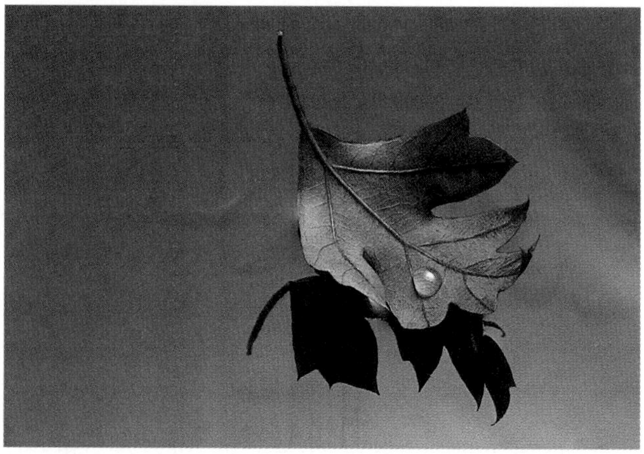

FIG. 41-3 Door card for room of mother who has had a perinatal loss. (Used with permission of Bereavement Services. Copyright Lutheran Hospital—La Crosse, Inc., A Gundersen Lutheran Affiliate, La Crosse, WI.)

One decision might be related to conducting an autopsy. An autopsy can be very important in answering the question "why" if there is a chance that the cause of death can be determined. This information can be helpful in processing grief and perhaps preventing another loss. However, the cost of an autopsy must be considered. Autopsies are not covered by insurance and are expensive. However, if the autopsy is done under the jurisdiction of the medical examiner's office, there is no charge. Some parents may feel that their baby has been through enough and prefer not to have further information about the cause of death. Some religions prohibit autopsy or limit the choice to times when it may help prevent another loss. Options for the type of autopsy, such as excluding the head, are available to parents. Parents may need time to make this decision. There is no need to rush them, unless there was evidence of contagious disease or maternal infection at the time of death.

Organ donation can be an aid to grieving and an opportunity for the family to see something positive associated with their experience. The federal "Gift of Life Act" and HCFA-3005-F, enacted in 1998, shifted the responsibility for determining organ donation potential from the hospital staff to the state's organ procurement organization (OPO). States and hospitals have clear procedures for how and when to call OPO. Generally, if a death certificate is issued, a call must be made to OPO. Once contacted, they will decide whether to talk to the family, and either an OPO representative or a designated requester will contact them. This allows requests to be made by trained personnel in a consistent and compassionate manner. The most common donation is of cornea; donation of cornea from a baby can occur if the baby was born alive at 36 weeks of gestation or later.

Another important decision relates to spiritual rituals that may be helpful and important to parents. Support from the clergy is an option that should be offered to all parents. Parents may wish to have their own pastor, priest, rabbi, or spiritual leader contacted, or they may wish to see the hospital's chaplain. They may choose to do neither. Members from the clergy may offer the parents the opportunity for baptism when appropriate. Other rituals that may be important include a blessing, a naming ceremony, anointing, ritual of the sick, memorial service, or prayer.

One of the major decisions parents must make has to do with disposition of the body. Parents should be given information about the choices for the final disposition of their baby, regardless of gestational age. The nurses must be aware, however, of cultural and spiritual beliefs that may dictate the choices of parents. A baby younger than 20 weeks of gestation is considered a product of conception, whereas embryos, uterine tubes removed with an ectopic pregnancy, and tissue from a pregnancy obtained during a dilation and curettage are all considered tissue. Many hospitals will make arrangements for the cremation of these infants. The nurse should know the hospital's policies and procedures and answer the parents' questions honestly. In most states, if a baby is at least 20 weeks and 1 day of gestational age or is born alive, it is the parents' responsibility to make the final arrangements for their baby, although some hospitals will offer free cremation. In this case, the family would not get the ashes.

LEGAL TIP

Laws in all states govern what constitutes a live birth. In most states a live birth is considered to be any products of conception expelled from a woman that show any signs of life. Signs of life are considered to be any muscle irritability, respiratory effort, or heart rate, regardless of gestational age. All nurses should be knowledgeable about their state laws regarding what constitutes a live birth and what forms must be completed and filed in the case of fetal death, stillbirth, or newborn death.

Final disposition of all identifiable babies, regardless of gestational age, includes burial or cremation. Depending on the cemetery's policies, babies in caskets or the ashes from cremated babies can be buried in a special place designated for babies, at the foot of a deceased relative, in a separate plot, or in a mausoleum. Ashes also may be scattered in a designated area; many states have regulations regarding where ashes can be scattered. A local funeral director or a state's Vital Statistics Bureau should have information about the state's rules, codes, and regulations regarding live births, burial requirements, transportation of the deceased by parents, and cremation.

In making final arrangements for their baby, parents may want a special service. They may choose to have a service in the hospital chapel, visitation at a funeral home or their own home, a funeral service, or a graveside service. Parents can make any of these services as special, personal, and memorable as they like. They can choose special music, poetry, or prose written by themselves or others.

If the family has decided on a funeral and burial, they still have decisions about what funeral home to call and where to bury the baby. Many couples may be living in an area distant from their family homes, and they may want to bury their child in their hometown or family cemetery. If the family desires cremation, they may want to have the option of obtaining the ashes. It is important to determine whether this will be done by the facility conducting the cremation.

Parents' hopes, dreams, self-esteem, and role expectations have been shattered with a perinatal loss; thus they may have many needs. Unmet needs can form the basis of "if only" that may plague a mother or family for a lifetime and can be the foundation for the development of complicated bereavement. However, it is difficult for parents to know exactly what they can expect or what they need; thus the nurse as an advocate should lead by offering various options that might meet specific needs. When a mother or family is able to verbalize needs, it is extremely important for the nurse to respond positively and do everything to see that the request is met (see Research box).

Families become unaware of time frames and do not care about the change of shifts or any needs the hospital system might have in "moving things along." When families are pushed or rushed into making decisions, in most cases, they make a decision in response to the health care system's needs, not their own. The timing for actions such as naming the baby, seeing and holding the baby, disposition of the body, and funeral arrangements should never be rushed. In some cases, the mother may be discharged home before these decisions are made. Then the family can think about them in the comfort of their home and contact the hospital in the following days to give their answers.

Help the Bereaved to Acknowledge and Express Their Feelings

One of the most important goals of the nurse is to validate the experience and feelings of the parents by encouraging them to tell their stories and listening with care (Corbet-Owen & Kruger, 2001). At the very least, the nurse should acknowledge the loss with a simple but sincere comment such as "I'm sorry about the baby." Helping the parents to talk about their loss and the meaning it has for their lives and to share their emotional pain is the next step. "Tell me about what happened." Because nurses tend to be very focused on the physical and emotional needs of the mother, it is especially important to ask the father directly about his views of what happened and his feelings of loss.

The nurse should listen patiently during the story of loss or grief, but listening is hard work and can be painful for the helper. The feelings and emotions of expressed grief can overwhelm health care professionals. Being with someone who is terribly sad and crying or sobbing can be extremely difficult. The initial impulse to reduce one's sense of helplessness is to say or do something that you think will reduce

RESEARCH

Neonatal Death and Mother's Interactions with Health Care Professionals

The death of a newborn is for most parents the most traumatic event of their lives. Into the stress of birth comes uncertainty, fear, and then overwhelming grief. Health care professionals must tend to both the dead baby's needs and the parents' needs. The nurse may draw on research, experience, and intuition to guide him or her. For example, some neonatal loss studies state that encouraging the parents to touch or hold their baby is greatly appreciated later, but mothers in other studies found the experience too painful. Most parents in these studies wanted time and individualized, sensitive care from the professional.

Swedish nurse researchers asked 16 mothers who had lost a newborn about their perceptions of experiences with health professionals. Themes of both powerlessness and empowerment arose. The mothers felt empowered when the health personnel attended to them without being asked, when information was accurate and gradual, and when they were able to make treatment decisions, even though they were overwhelmed. Mothers were especially grateful to nurses who complimented their mothering, showed sympathy with touch, and accommodated family wishes. All but one were glad that they were persuaded to hold their infant and treasured their mementos.

Powerlessness occurred when health care professionals rigidly enforced the rules, withheld information, and questioned the mothers' decisions. Mothers would become uncommunicative and not ask for the guidance or time to become involved in the babies' care. Mothers were left wanting the approval of the staff yet not wanting the staff to make their decisions. Despite this, mothers were generally forgiving of the staff.

IMPLICATIONS FOR PRACTICE

Parents who lose a newborn may not be able to identify or articulate their needs. They may be comforted if they know that the professionals are "seeing it through the parent's eyes." Involving the parents in decisions and encouraging meaningful good-byes can be profoundly comforting to the grieving parents.

Reference: Lundqvist, A., Nilstrun, T., & Dykes, A. (2002). Both empowered and powerless: Mother's experiences of professional care when their newborn dies. *Birth, 29*(3), 192-199.

their pain. Although such a response may seem supportive at the time, it can stifle the further expression of emotion. Bereaved parents have identified many unhelpful responses made to them by well-meaning health care professionals, family, and friends. The nurse should resist the temptation to give advice or to use clichés in offering support to the bereaved (Box 41-3). Nurses need to be comfortable with their own feelings of grief and loss to support and care for bereaved persons effectively. The nurse should have a presence of self, the willingness to be alongside, quietly supporting the bereaved in whatever expressions of feelings or emotions are appropriate for them. This presence leaves

BOX 41-3 What to Say and What Not to Say to Bereaved Parents

WHAT TO SAY

"I'm sad for you."
"How are you doing with all of this?"
"This must be hard for you."
"What can I do for you?"
"I'm sorry."
"I'm here, and I want to listen."

WHAT NOT TO SAY

"God had a purpose for her."
"Be thankful you have another child."
"The living must go on."
"I know how you feel."
"It's God's will."
"You have to keep on going for her sake."
"You're young; you can have others."
"We'll see you back here next year, and you'll be happier."
"Now you have an angel in heaven."
"This happened for the best."
"Better for this to happen now, before you knew the baby."
"There was something wrong with the baby anyway."

parents feeling that they were cared for. Leaning forward, nodding the head, and saying "Uh-huh" or "Tell me more" is often encouragement enough for the bereaved person to tell his or her story. Sitting through the silence can be therapeutic; silence gives the bereaved person an opportunity to collect thoughts and to process what he or she is sharing. Furthermore, careful assessment is important before using touch as a therapeutic technique. For some, touch is a meaningful expression of concern, but for others it is an invasion of privacy.

Bereaved parents have many questions surrounding the event of their loss that can leave them feeling guilty. This is particularly true for mothers. Such questions include "What did I do?" "What caused this to happen?" "What do you think I should have, could have done?" Part of the grief process for bereaved parents is figuring out what happened, their role in the loss, why it happened to them, and why it happened to their baby. The nurse should recognize that the answers to these questions must be answered by the bereaved themselves; it is part of their healing. For example, a bereaved mother might ask, "Do you think that this was caused by painting the baby's room?" An appropriate response might be, "I understand you need to find an answer for why your baby died, but we really don't know why she died. What are some of the other things you have been thinking about?" Trying to give bereaved parents answers when there are no clear answers or trying to squelch their guilt feelings by telling them they should not feel guilty does not help them process their grief. In reality, many times there are no definite answers to the question of why this terrible thing has happened to them. However, factual information, such as data about the frequency of miscarriages in pregnant women or the fact that there usually is no clear cause of a stillbirth, can be helpful.

Feelings of anger, guilt, and sadness can occur immediately but often become more problematic in the early days and months after a loss. When a bereaved person expresses feelings of anger, it can be helpful to identify the feeling by simply saying, "You sound angry," or "You look angry." The nurse's willingness to sit down and listen to these feelings of anger can help the bereaved move past those surface feelings into the underlying feelings of powerlessness and helplessness in not being able to control the many aspects of the situation.

Normalize the Grief Process and Facilitate Positive Coping

While helping parents share their feelings of pain, it is critical to help them understand their grief responses and feel they are not alone in these painful responses. Most parents are not prepared for the raw feelings that they experience or the fact that these painful, complex feelings and related behavioral reactions continue for many weeks or months. Thus reassuring them of the normality of their responses and preparing them for the length of their grief is important. The nurse can help the parent be prepared for the emptiness, loneliness, and yearning; for the feelings of helplessness that can lead to anger, guilt, and fear; and for the cognitive processing problems, disorganization, difficulty making decisions; and sadness and depression that are part of the grief process. Books and pamphlets about grief, if short and sensitive, can be given to parents to take home. Many parents have reported feelings of fear that they were going crazy because of the many emotions and behavioral responses that leave them feeling totally out of control in the months after the loss. It is essential for the nurse to reassure and educate bereaved parents about the grief process, including the physical, social, and emotional responses of individuals and families. Offering health teaching on the bereavement process alone is not enough, however. In the initial days after a loss, other strategies might include follow-up phone calls, referrals to a perinatal grief support group, or providing a list of publications or web sites intended for helping parents who have experienced a perinatal loss. As with any referral, however, the nurse should first read the materials or check out the websites (see Resources at the end of the chapter).

To reduce relationship problems that can occur in couples who are grieving, it is particularly important to help them understand that they may respond and grieve in very different ways (Wallerstedt & Higgins, 1996). Discongruent grieving can lead to serious marital problems and be a risk factor for complicated bereavement (Schaap et al., 1997). Remind the couple of the importance of being understanding and patient with each other. Fathers may need to be encouraged to share their grief with their wives because of the desire to protect the woman from his pain or the need to appear strong.

Nurses can reinforce positive coping efforts and attempt to prevent negative coping. They can remind the parents of the importance of being patient and being good to themselves during the grief process. Additional suggestions are to encourage attempts to resume normal activities; reinforce and encourage positive ways to hold onto memories of the pregnancy or baby, while letting go; and help the parent to organize a plan for daily activities, if needed. In particular, nurses should discourage overdependence on drugs and alcohol.

Meet the Physical Needs of the Postpartum Bereaved Mother

Coping with loss and grief after childbirth can be an overwhelming experience for the woman and her family. One particularly difficult aspect of the loss is the sound of crying babies and the happiness of other families on the unit who have given birth to healthy infants. The mother should be given the opportunity to decide if she wants to remain on the maternity unit or be moved to another hospital unit. She also should be helped to understand the pluses and minuses of each choice. Postpartum care as well as grief support may not be as good on another hospital unit where the staff are not experienced in postpartum and bereavement care. The physical needs of a bereaved mother are the same as those of any woman who has given birth. The cruel reality for many bereaved mothers is that their milk may come in with no baby to nurse, their afterpains remind them of their emptiness, and gas pains feel as though a baby is still moving inside. The nurse should assure that the mother receives appropriate medications to reduce these physical symptoms. Adequate rest, diet, and fluids must be offered to replenish her physical strength. Mothers need postpartum care instructions on discharge. They also need ideas about how to cope with problems with sleep such as decreasing food or fluids that contain caffeine, limiting alcohol and nicotine consumption, exercising regularly, using strategies for rest, taking a warm bath or drinking warm milk before bedtime, relaxation exercises, restful music, or a massage. Furthermore, the couple needs to be encouraged and supported in maintaining their relationship and keeping open channels of communication. They also need to be prepared for some of the issues related to resuming sexuality after perinatal loss.

Assist the Bereaved in Communicating with, Supporting, and Getting Support from Family

Providing sensitive care to bereaved parents means including their families in the grief process. Grandparents and siblings are particularly important when a perinatal loss has occurred. However, it is up to the parents to decide to what extent they want family involved in their grief process. If it is the parents' desire, children, grandparents, extended family members, and friends should be allowed to be involved in the rituals surrounding the death, such as seeing and holding the baby. Such visits afford others the opportunity to become acquainted with the baby, to understand the parents' loss, to offer their support, and to say good-bye (see Fig. 41-2). This experience helps parents explain to their surviving children who their brother or sister was and what death means, offers the children answers to their questions in a concrete manner, and helps the children in expressing their grief. Involving extended family and friends enables the parents to mobilize their social support system of people who will support the family not only at the time of loss but also in the future.

Parents also need information about how grief affects a family. They may need help in understanding and coping with the potential differing responses of various family members. Frustrations may arise because of the insensitive or inadequate responses of other family members. Parents may need help in determining ways to let family members know how they feel and what they need.

Create Memories for Parents to Take Home

Parents may want tangible mementos of their baby to allow them to actualize the loss. Some may want to bring in a previously purchased baby book. Special memory books, cards, and information on grief and mourning are available for purchase by parents or hospitals or clinics through national perinatal bereavement organizations (Fig. 41-4).

The nurse can provide information about the baby's weight, length, and head circumference to the family. Footprints and handprints can be taken and placed with the other information on a special card or in a memory or baby book. Sometimes it is difficult to obtain good handprints or footprints. Application of alcohol or acetone on the palms or soles can help the ink adhere to make the prints clearer, especially for small babies. When making prints, have a hard surface underneath the paper to be printed. The baby's heel or palm is placed down first, the foot or hand is rolled forward, keeping the toes or fingers extended. It may be helpful to have a partner to assist in this procedure. If the print does not turn out, tracing around the baby's hands and feet can be done, although this distorts the actual size. A form of plaster of paris can also be used to make an imprint of the baby's hand or foot.

Parents often appreciate articles that were in contact with or used in caring for the baby. This might include the tape measure used to measure the baby, baby lotions, combs, clothing, hats, blankets, crib cards, and identification bands. The identification band helps the parents remember the size of the baby and personalizes the mementos. The nurse should ask parents if they wish to have these articles before giving them to the parents. A lock of hair may be another important keepsake. Parents must be asked for permission before cutting a lock of hair, which can be removed from the nape of the neck where it is not noticeable.

For some, pictures are the most important memento. Photographs should be taken whenever there is an identifiable baby and when it is culturally acceptable to the family. It does not matter how tiny the baby is, what the baby looks like, or how long the baby has been dead. Pictures should be taken by an instant-print camera as well as a 35-mm camera. Pictures should include close-ups of the baby's face, hands, and feet. Pictures should be taken of the baby clothed and wrapped in a blanket as well as unclothed. If there are any congenital anomalies, close-ups of the anomalies also should be taken. Flowers, blocks, stuffed animals, or toys can be placed in the background to make the picture more special. Parents may want their pictures taken holding the baby. Keeping a camera nearby and taking pictures when parents are spending special time with their baby can provide special memories. Some parents may have their own camera or video camera and would like the nurse to record them as they bathe, dress, hold, or diaper their baby.

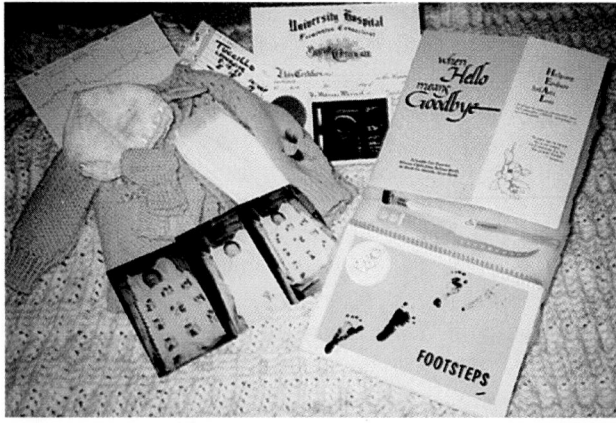
when Hello means Goodbye
FOOTSTEPS

FIG. 41-4 A memory kit assembled at the University of Connecticut Health Center, Farmington, CT. It includes pictures of the infant, clothing, death certificate, footprints, ID bands, fetal monitor printout, and ultrasound picture. (From Dickason, E., Silverman, B., & Kaplan, J. [1998]. *Maternal-infant nursing care* [3rd ed.]. St. Louis: Mosby.

Communicate Using a Caring Framework

Mothers, fathers, and extended families look to the nursing staff for support and understanding during the time of loss. Nurses have an important role in providing sensitive care to parents at the time of a perinatal loss. One model for conceptualizing intervention is that developed by Swanson-Kauffman based on her research with women experiencing perinatal loss (Swanson-Kauffman, 1986, 1988). The framework identifies five components in a caring concept:

1. Knowing
2. Being with
3. Doing for
4. Enabling
5. Maintaining belief

Knowing implies that the nurse has taken the time to understand the perception of the loss and its meaning to the woman and her family. *Being with* involves how the nurse conveys acceptance of the various feelings and perceptions of each family member. *Doing for* refers to the activities performed by the nurse that provide physical care, comfort, and safety for the woman and her family. This may include offering pain medication or sitz baths, maintaining the patency of the intravenous line, performing postpartum checks, and giving back rubs. *Enabling* occurs when the nurse offers the woman and her family options for care. Offers of information, anticipatory guidance, choices for decision making, and support during hospitalization and after discharge help the family feel more in control of a situation in which they feel very much out of control. Enabling raises their self-esteem and allows them to feel more comfortable in asking for options according to their needs for memories and closure, rather than to the nurse's perception of their needs. *Maintaining belief* involves encouraging the woman and her family to believe in their own ability to pick up the pieces and begin to heal. The nurse spends time with the family, learns their inner strengths and coping abilities, and points out these inner resources to the family by saying, "I know this is a difficult time for you, but I have seen some of your inner strength and know that you will be able to make it through all of this."

Be Concerned About Cultural and Spiritual Needs of Parents

Parents who experience perinatal loss can be from widely diverse cultural and ethnic groups. In addition, parents belong to many different religious groups. Many of the responses that were described and the interventions suggested in this chapter are based on Euro-American views of perinatal grief and loss (Hebert, 1998). Although it is thought that there are no particular differences in the individual, intrapersonal experiences of grief based on culture, ethnicity, or religion, many differences are found in mourning rituals, traditions, and behavioral expressions of grief that are often ignored or misunderstood (Cowles, 1996; Hebert, 1998). Thus the practices suggested earlier may not be appropriate for parents from other cultural, ethnic, and religious groups, and the nurse must consider the potential unique responses and needs of parents from different groups. This involves understanding the cultural orientation and beliefs of the individual parent, the partner, the extended family, and the larger community to which they belong.

Cultural and religious differences can affect the way parents respond to a perinatal loss. This includes their way of communicating with health care professionals, as well as their emotional and behavioral responses and family interaction patterns. Some groups, such as Orthodox Jews, may not support the notion of grieving for perinatal loss because the fetus or stillborn infant is not considered a person. African-American women were found to use self-healing strategies that reflect inner processes, resources, and remedies (Van, 2001). Mothers from some cultural groups may have intense somatic symptoms. In some cultures such as Muslims, decisions are communal (Hebert, 1998). Expressions of grief may range from quiet and stoic to dramatic and hysterical for different Native American groups. Native Americans from many tribes would not respond well to an "interviewing" or "questioning" approach (Lawson, 1990). Mexican mothers may be very demonstrative in their grief, while also struggling with the view that hardship is "God's will" (Lawson, 1990).

With perinatal loss, culture and religious beliefs can affect issues such as seeing the child, naming the child, and taking pictures. Some cultural and religious groups do not believe in naming an infant who dies before 30 days of age. Picture taking can conflict with beliefs of some cultures, such as some Native Americans, Eskimos, Amish, Hindu, and Muslim. Families from these cultures should be sensitively offered this opportunity but not pushed into having a picture taken.

Many different taboos and expectations are related to death for different religious groups. Autopsies are not allowed by some religions except under unusual circumstances. Cremation is forbidden by the Jewish religion, Baha'is, and the Greek Orthodox Church (Harakas, 1999). It is discouraged or allowed only under unusual circumstances in the Church of Jesus Christ of Latter-Day Saints. Embalming is not allowed for Jews, Baha'is, and Muslims.

Culture and religious beliefs also influence the customs surrounding death. Many religious groups have rituals, such as prayers, ritualistic washing and shrouding, or anointing with oil, that are performed at the time of death. Baptism is extremely important for Roman Catholics and some Protestant groups. Baptism can be performed by a lay person, such as a nurse, in an emergency situation when a priest cannot be there in a timely fashion (Box 41-4).

Many Protestant groups believe that baptism is conducted at the age of reason, and parents from these religions

BOX 41-4 Infant Baptism

In an emergency, baptism may be performed by anyone by pouring water over the forehead (or products of conception) and saying "I baptize you in the name of the Father and of the Son and of the Holy Spirit." The person performing the baptism needs only to have the intention of baptizing and does not necessarily have to believe in infant baptism for the baptism to be valid. If the infant has no signs of life, the person performing the baptism can add "If you are alive, I baptize you..." In the Greek Orthodox tradition, baptism is only for the living; thus a miscarried or stillborn infant would not be baptized. If the infant is born alive and in serious danger of death, the infant can be lifted up while saying "The servant of God is baptized in the name of the Father and the Son and the Holy Spirit" (Harakas, 1999).

would not want their baby baptized. When bereaved parents need a referral for grief counseling, cultural considerations are paramount. Native Americans, for example, are best referred to native healers and counselors rather than to Western biomedical therapists (Lawson, 1990).

Provide Sensitive Care at and After Discharge

When leaving the hospital, mothers are often taken out in a wheelchair. This can be a devastating experience for the mother who has experienced a pregnancy loss. Leaving the hospital without a baby in her arms is a very empty and painful experience. It is especially difficult if others are seen leaving with babies; thus the discharge of mothers and fathers who have experienced a perinatal loss should be done with great sensitivity to their feelings. They should not be discharged at a time when other mothers with live babies are leaving. Giving the mother a special flower to carry in her arms can be a thoughtful gesture.

The grief of the mother and her family does not end with discharge; rather it really begins once they return home, attend the funeral, and start to live their lives without their baby. Follow-up phone calls after a loss may be helpful to some parents. However, it must be determined when parents do not want a follow-up call, which often is the case after early loss. Follow-up calls let the parents know they are still thought of and cared about. The calls are made at predictably difficult times such as the first week at home, 1 month to 6 weeks later, 4 to 6 months after the loss, and at the anniversary of the death. Families who experienced a miscarriage, ectopic pregnancy, or death of a premature baby may appreciate a phone call on the estimated date of birth. The calls provide an opportunity for parents to ask questions, share their feelings, seek advice, and receive information to help them in processing their grief.

A grief conference can be planned when parents return for an appointment with their doctor, nurses, and other health care providers. At the conference, the loss or death of the infant is discussed in detail, parents are given information about the baby's autopsy report and genetic studies, and they have opportunities to ask the questions that have arisen since their baby's death. Parents appreciate the opportunity to review the events of hospitalization, go over the baby's and/or mother's chart with their primary health care provider, and talk with those who cared for them and their baby during hospitalization. This is an important time to help parents understand the cause of the loss, or to accept the fact that the cause will forever be unknown. This gives health care professionals the opportunity to assess how the family is coping with their loss and provide additional information and education on grief.

Some parents are very interested in finding a perinatal or parent grief support group. They appreciate the opportunity to talk with others who have been through similar experiences. A grief support group also can be helpful in sharing feelings and gaining an understanding of the normality of the grief process. Over time, it may be the only place where bereaved parents can talk about the wished-for child and their grief. However, not all parents find such groups helpful. When referring to a group, it is important to know something about the group and how it operates. For example, if a group has a religious base for their interventions, a nonreligious parent would not likely find the group to be helpful. If parents experiencing a perinatal loss are referred to a parental grief group, they might feel overwhelmed with the grief of parents whose older children have died of cancer, suicide, or homicide. In addition, their grief might be minimized by participants; thus the needs of the parents must be matched with the focus of the group.

Provide Postmortem Care

Preparation of the baby's body and transport to the morgue depends on the procedures and protocols developed by individual hospitals. The Joint Committee on Accreditation of Healthcare Organizations requires that we offer appropriate care to the body after death. A sensitive and respectful approach for taking the fetus or infant to the morgue is the use of a "burial cradle." These miniature coffins have a quilted lining and replace wrapping the baby in a Chux pad. These can be obtained from Bay Memorials (321 South 15th Street, Escanaba, MI 49829, 906-786-2609). Postmortem care can be an emotional and sometimes difficult task for the nurse. However, nurses may find that providing postmortem care helps them find closure in their own grief related to a perinatal loss. This is particularly true for neonatal intensive care nurses who have cared for an infant for several hours, days, or weeks. The use of a "burial cradle" makes the process more dignified and is helpful to the staff in coping with the death.

Evaluation

The evaluation of nursing care is made more difficult by the shock and numbness of the bereavement process and the varied grief responses of the parents and other family members during hospitalization. The achievement of expected outcomes is assured when the positive integration of the perinatal loss is expressed by the family (see Plan of Care).

One approach to evaluation is the use of checklists. Many hospitals have checklists used in providing care, mobilizing members of the multidisciplinary health care team, communicating options the family has chosen, and keeping track of all the details in meeting the needs of bereaved parents (Figs. 41-5 and 41-6). Such checklists may be a permanent part of the chart. Documentation in the nursing notes of primary concerns, grief responses, health teaching, health care advice, and any referrals of the mother or other family members is essential to ensure continuity and consistency of care.

Plan of Care: Fetal Death: 20 Weeks of Gestation

NURSING DIAGNOSIS Dysfunctional grieving related to fetal death, as evidenced by intense expressions of grief for prolonged period of time

Expected Outcome *Parents will identify appropriate ways to deal with grief.*

Nursing Interventions/*Rationales*

Prepare family for viewing fetus by cleaning body and wrapping in clean blanket *to initiate and support the grieving process in a supportive setting.*

Allow family quiet time to hold and view fetus. Take pictures for family to keep *to provide reality to death and support the grieving process.*

Provide a certificate for the family with vital statistics, along with identification bands, lock of hair, and footprints *to provide reality of situation and support the grieving process.*

Provide spiritual support as needed to assist with religious services, such as baptism and memorial services *to provide spiritual support and assist with religious practices.*

Refer to appropriate community support groups to facilitate grieving with group input and *to share experiences.*

NURSING DIAGNOSIS Situational low self-esteem related to fetal death as evidenced by mother's/family's intense feelings of guilt

Expected Outcomes *Mother/family will exhibit positive self-comments and adapt to death of fetus in a timely manner.*

Nursing Interventions/*Rationales*

Provide private time for expressions of feelings through therapeutic communication and active listening *to validate feelings.*

Identify mother's/family's perception and feelings about fetal death *to correct any misconceptions and alleviate guilt.*

Assist mother/family to identify positive coping mechanisms and support systems *to promote feelings of self-worth.*

Refer to appropriate health professionals for further evaluation and counseling, such as social service *to provide ongoing assistance as needed.*

NURSING DIAGNOSIS Spiritual distress related to perinatal loss

Expected Outcome *Parents will verbalize a decrease in spiritual distress.*

Nursing Interventions/*Rationales*

Assess parent's spiritual preference *to reinforce parent's own beliefs.*

Assist with spiritual rituals for parents and infant *to promote comfort for parents.*

Provide opportunity for parents to express feelings about perinatal loss *to facilitate the grief process.*

Assist parents in contacting the facility's chaplain or personal spiritual advisor *to provide spiritual support.*

NURSING DIAGNOSIS Risk for maternal injury related to perinatal loss

Expected Outcome *Woman will not experience any injury during labor or birth.*

Nursing Interventions/*Rationales*

Monitor maternal vital signs and contraction pattern *to provide baseline data.*

Monitor woman for any excessive bleeding *to prompt immediate interventions.*

Provide pain medication as needed *to prevent alteration in maternal vital signs and promote comfort.*

Confirm presence of emergency equipment and medications *to provide immediate maternal assistance and prevent maternal injury.*

SPECIAL LOSSES

Prenatal Diagnoses with Negative Outcome

Early prenatal diagnostic tests such as ultrasonography, chorionic villi sampling, and amniocentesis can determine the well-being of the embryo or fetus. Reasons for prenatal testing include history of chromosomal abnormality in the family; three or more miscarriages; maternal age over 35 years; lack of fetal growth, movement, or heartbeat; and diabetes mellitus or other chronic illnesses. If the health care provider is certain that the baby has a serious genetic defect that would lead to death in utero or after birth (congenital anomalies incompatible with life or genetic disorders with severe mental retardation), the choice of interruption of a pregnancy may be offered. Abortion is controversial, and this may prevent parents from sharing this decision with other family members or friends. This limits their support systems after their loss (Lorenzen & Holzgreve, 1995).

The decision to terminate a pregnancy paves the way for feelings such as guilt, despair, sadness, depression, and anger. The nurse's role is to be a good listener. It is important to assess how these families feel about the experience and to offer options for their memories as appropriate. Healing can take place when words can be given to feelings and needs can be met.

The parent who decides to continue the pregnancy also requires emotional support. The time of labor and birth can be particularly difficult. The nurse should remember that parents may be grieving not only the loss of the perfect child but the loss of expectations for their child's future.

Loss of One in a Multiple Birth

The death of a twin or baby in a multifetal gestation during pregnancy, labor, birth, or after birth requires parents to parent and grieve at the same time. Such a death imposes a confusing and ambivalent induction into parenthood (Swanson-Kauffman, 1988). Parents feel that they cannot do anything right. They cannot parent their surviving child with all the joy and enthusiasm of new parents because their surviving child reminds them of what they have lost. They cannot give over completely and grieve in

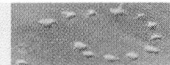

RTS Bereavement Services

CHECKLIST FOR ASSISTING PARENT(S) EXPERIENCING MISCARRIAGE/ECTOPIC PREGNANCY

SAMPLE

RTS Counselor ______	Date ______
Mother's name ______	Age ______ Due date ______
Date of beginning of miscarriage ______	Date of surgery ______
# of Miscarriages ______ # of Children ______	Religion ______
Address ______	Occupation ______
Phone number ( ) ______	Marital status ______
Father's name ______	Age ______ Occupation ______
Address ______	Phone number ( ) ______
Baby's name ______	Sex ______
Support people available ______	Children's names: ______
Problem areas ______	Physician ______
OK to send written material to home address ☐ Yes ☐ No	

Date	Time	See Miscarriage Protocol RTS Manual	Comments	Initials
		Notify/Assign RTS counselor ☐ Yes ☐ No		
		Pastoral Care ☐ Yes ☐ No		
		Offered: ☐ Blessing ☐ Memorial Service ☐ Naming Ceremony ☐ Burial		
		Asked: "Would you like someone with you now?" ☐ Yes ☐ No		
		D&C/Surgical procedure discussed ☐ Yes ☐ No		
		Saw baby or tissue ☐ Mother ☐ Father		
		Touched and/or held baby ☐ Mother ☐ Father		
		If RH negative, RhoGAM given within 72 hrs ☐ Yes ☐ No		
		Patient's room flagged with door card ☐ Yes ☐ No		
		Photos taken: ☐ 35 mm ☐ Polaroid ☐ Given to parents ☐ On file		
		Footprints & handprints/weight & length: ☐ Given to parents ☐ On file		
		Grief process discussed ☐ Yes ☐ No		
		Incongruent grief discussed ☐ Yes ☐ No		
		Grief packet given ☐ Yes ☐ No		
		Info Brochure given to parents re: RTS PSG ☐ Yes ☐ No		
		Name/business card given ☐ Yes ☐ No		
		Regular OB/Midwife notified ______ ☐ Memo ☐ Verbally		
		Childbirth Educator notified ______ ☐ Yes ☐ No		
		Telephone number verified ☐ Yes ☐ No Optimal call time ______		
		Preg & Inf Loss Card sent to RTS Secretary ☐ Yes ☐ No		
		Given option to transfer from Maternity Unit ☐ Yes ☐ No		
		Genetic Studies ordered ☐ Yes ☐ No		
		Sex determination desired (tissue in NS only) ☐ Yes ☐ No		
		Would like another parent to call: ☐ Yes ☐ No ☐ Ask later		
		Parent contact: ______ Follow-up calls: eg. ☐ 1 wk, ☐ 3 wk, ☐ 4 mo, ☐ due date/anniv. date		

Forms for burial or cremation of:

a) Products of conception - 2 copies of "Request for Return of Products of Conception to Patients" (1 copy-chart, 1 copy-lab). Obtain forms from histology.

b) Identifiable baby less than 20 wk or less than 350 gm - 2 copies of "Request for Return of Products of Conception to Patients" (1-chart, 1-lab). "Notice of Removal" #DOH 5043 - Responsible party for burial signs this form (either parent or a funeral director). Pink copy goes to responsible party. "Final Disposition of a Human Corpse" #DOH 5045 is required for any age identifiable baby that goes across state lines.

Note: Some cemeteries may require a "Final Disposition of a Human Corpse" report for their own recordkeeping.

FIG. 41-5 Sample checklist for assisting parents experiencing miscarriage/ectopic pregnancy. (Used with permission of Bereavement Services. Copyright Lutheran Hospital—La Crosse, Inc., A Gundersen Lutheran Affiliate, La Crosse, WI.)

SAMPLE

RTS Bereavement Services
CHECKLIST FOR ASSISTING PARENT(S) EXPERIENCING STILLBIRTH OR NEWBORN DEATH

Mother's discharge date: ______	Age ______ Gr ___ Para ___ L.C. ___ Due date ______
Mother's name: ______	Previous loss: ______
Address: ______	Date/Time delivered: ______
Phone number: ( ) ______	Date/Time death: ______
Father's name: ______	Baby's name: ______ Sex: ______
Address: ______	Children's name(s): ______ Age: ______
Phone number: ( ) ______	______ Age: ______
Optimal call time: ______	______ Age: ______
RTS Counselor: ______	Support people
Unit: ______ Ext ______	Attending MD &/or Pediatrician ______
Regular OB MD/Midwife: ______	Notify Peds Nurse Practitioner ______
Religion: ______	

Date	Time		Comments	Initials
		Notify/Assign RTS counselor ☐ Yes ☐ No		
		Pastoral Care notified ☐ Yes ☐ No		
		Funeral Home notified: ☐ Yes ☐ No Family Burial: ☐ Yes ☐ No		
		Saw baby when born and/or after delivery: ☐ Mother ☐ Father		
		Touched and/or held baby: ☐ Mother ☐ Father ☐ Siblings ☐ Grandparents ☐ Friends		
		Offered private time with their baby: ☐ Yes ☐ No		
		Baptism offered: (use seashell as vessel, give to parents) ☐ Yes ☐ No		
		Remembrance of Blessing offered: ☐ Yes ☐ No (can offer for any perinatal loss) ☐ Given to parents		
		Given option to transfer off Maternity Unit: ☐ Yes ☐ No		
		Patient's room flagged with door card ☐ Yes ☐ No		
		Autopsy: ☐ Yes ☐ No Genetic studies: ☐ Yes ☐ No Genetic Associate notified: ☐ Yes ☐ No		
		Regular Physician/Midwife notified of death: ☐ Yes ☐ No Memo sent to Physician/Midwife: ☐ Yes ☐ No		
		Section of Fetal monitor strip: ☐ Given to parents ☐ On file		
		ID Bands/Crib cards/Tape measure: ☐ Given to parents ☐ On file		
		Footprints/Handprints/Weight/Length recorded on "In Memory Of" sheet: ☐ Given to parents ☐ On file		
		Lock of hair offered: (ask permission) ☐ Yes ☐ No ☐ Given to parents ☐ On file		
		Mementos (clothing, hat , blanket, pacifier, crib cards, basin, baby ring, bear, thermometer, silk flower) ☐ Given to parents ☐ On file		
		Complimentary birth keepsake ☐ Given to parents ☐ On file		
		RTS Photos taken: (clothed, unclothed, w. props, family photo) 1) Polaroid - 3 or more ☐ Given to parents ☐ On file 2) 35 mm (6-12 pictures) ☐ Given to parents ☐ On file 3) Medical photos: ☐ Yes ☐ No		

Continued

FIG. 41-6 Sample checklist for assisting parents experiencing stillbirth or newborn death. (Used with permission of Bereavement Services. Copyright Lutheran Hospital—La Crosse, Inc., A Gundersen Lutheran Affiliate, La Crosse, WI.)

Date	Time		Comments	Initials
		Informed about postponing funeral until mother is able to attend: ☐ Yes ☐ No		
		Services/Funeral arrangements, options discussed: ☐ Self-transport ☐ Gravesite service ☐ Visitation ☐ Hospital chapel ☐ Cremation ☐ Funeral home ☐ Burial at foot or head of relative's grave ☐ Specific area for babies in cemetery ☐ Plan own service		
		Funeral arrangements made by: ☐ Mother ☐ Father Discussed: ☐ Seeing baby at funeral home ☐ Taking pictures there ☐ Providing outfit/toy for baby ☐ Dressing baby at funeral home		
		Grief information packet given to: ☐ Mother ☐ Father		
		Discussed grief process/incongruent grief with: ☐ Mother ☐ Father		
		Discussed grief conference: ☐ Yes ☐ No		
		RTS Parents Support Group brochure given to: ☐ Mother ☐ Father		
		RTS business card given to: ☐ Mother ☐ Father		
		Pregnancy & Infant Loss Card sent to RTS secretary: ☐ Yes ☐ No		
		Follow-up calls: 1 week: . . . . 3 weeks:. . . . . Due date: . . . . 6-10 months: . . . . Anniversary date:		
		Grief conference planned with parents: Date ________ Time _________ Place ____________________ Letter of confirmation sent: ☐ Yes ☐ No		
		Parent Support Group, first meeting attended: Date: ______________ Follow-up meetings attended: Dates ____		
		Would like another parent to call: ☐ Yes ☐ No ☐ Ask later Parent contact: _____________________________________		

Forms Needed: Report of fetal death (Photocopy and save for mother.)
Autopsy if ordered
Record of death
Genetics protocol (folder) if ordered
Notice of removal of a human corpse from an institution
Final disposition form
If funeral home involved - Final disposition will be completed by them.
Original certificate of death (for NB death only)

Note: Family Burial - Check with your funeral home.

** You may wish to list your hospital and state forms that are necessary, as required by your state laws and your institution.

FIG. 41-6, cont'd For legend see page 1167.

the manner they need to because their surviving child demands their attention. These parents are at risk for altered parenting and complicated bereavement.

It is important to help the parents acknowledge the birth of all their babies. Parents should be treated as bereaved families, and all the options previously discussed should be offered. Pictures should be taken of the babies and parents should be offered the opportunity to hold their babies in their arms and have time to say good-bye to the baby who has died.

Bereaved parents should be warned that well-meaning family members or friends may say, "Well, at least you have the other baby," implying that there should be no grief because they are lucky to have one at all. Parents need to be able to anticipate insensitivity to their loss and be empowered to say to those people, "That is not how I feel." By simply setting a boundary on what their feelings are, they are able to acknowledge the baby who died and then have an opportunity to share more about their feelings if they so choose.

Bereaved parents of multiples have special problems in coping with life without their anticipated "extra special" family, telling their surviving child about his or her twin, dealing with the possibility of that child's feelings of survivor guilt, and deciding on how to celebrate birthdays, death days, or special holidays.

Adolescent Grief

Adolescent pregnancy accounts for many births in the United States. Each year, many adolescents experience perinatal loss, particularly as elective abortion or miscarriage. Although adolescent participants have been included in the samples of research done in all areas of perinatal bereavement, their particular responses to perinatal loss have not been specifically identified. Adolescents grieve the loss of their babies through miscarriage, stillbirth, or newborn death and need the emotional support from the nurses who care for them. However, nurses and other health care professionals, as well as family members, often believe that the adolescent's loss of her baby was for the best, so that the adolescent can move on with her life. Adolescent girls, then, may not receive the support they need from staff and family. In addition, adolescent girls usually do not have the support from the father of the baby as compared with older women who have a perinatal loss; thus there is a great need to provide sensitive care to all adolescents who experience any type of perinatal loss.

The first step for the nurse in caring for a bereaved adolescent is to acknowledge the significance of giving birth, no matter what age the mother might be. Second, the nurse should make additional efforts to develop a trusting relationship in working with the adolescent. Third, the nurse should offer options for saying good-bye, anticipatory guidance, support, and information to meet the adolescent at the point of her need. It may take longer for adolescents to process their grief because of their level of cognitive and emotional maturation. Being patient, saving mementos, and giving the adolescent information on how to contact the nurse are interventions that can help the adolescent accept the reality of the loss and process her grief.

COMPLICATED BEREAVEMENT

Although most parents cope adequately with the pain of their grief and return to some level of normal functioning, some parents have extremely intense grief reactions that last for a very long time; this response is **complicated bereavement.** Other parents have grief from one loss that is exaggerated or intensified by other past losses. A long pre-loss pregnancy (i.e., the fetus/infant died in late gestation), a more neurotic personality, more preexisting psychiatric symptoms, and not having other living children are important risk factors for stronger grief reactions (Janssen et al., 1997).

Evidence of complicated grief includes continued obsession with yearning and loneliness, intense and continued guilt or anger, relentless depression or anxiety that interferes with role functioning, abuse of drugs (including prescription medications) or alcohol, severe relationship difficulties, continued feelings of inadequacy and low self-esteem, and suicidal thoughts or threats (Hunfeld, Wladimiroff, & Passchier, 1997). Hunfeld and co-workers (1997) also found that feelings of inadequacy, in particular, were strongly and positively related to distress after 4 years.

Parents showing signs of complicated grief should be referred for counseling. It is the responsibility of a qualified mental health professional to determine whether the parents are experiencing a normal, albeit intense grief response or whether they are also having a serious mental health problem such as depression. However, it is important to refer to a therapist or counselor who is experienced in grief counseling and knows how to help the bereaved, because some therapists and counselors do not have an understanding of the special needs related to grief.

Therapy is a big step. The highest number of cancellations and "no shows" in a therapist's practice are intakes, or first visits; therefore, anything the nurse can do for a family or individual to help with that major hurdle would be helpful. However, it also is important to remember that people may have symptoms but may not, for whatever reason, be ready to deal directly with these symptoms or may not have the energy to make the call. Enlisting a family member to encourage parents to seek such assistance may be helpful.

KEY POINTS

- Parental and infant attachment can begin before pregnancy with many hopes and dreams for the future.
- The gestational age of the baby influences neither the severity of the grief response nor the bereavement process.
- When a baby dies, all members of a family are affected, but no two family members grieve in the same way.
- When birth represents death, the role of the nurse is critical in caring for the woman and her family, regardless of the age of the woman or stage of gestation.
- An understanding of the grief process is fundamental in the implementation of the nursing process.
- Assessment of each family member's perception and experience of the loss is important.
- Therapeutic communication and counseling techniques can help families identify their feelings, feel comfortable in expressing their grief, and understand their bereavement process.
- Follow-up after discharge can be an important component in providing care to families who have experienced a loss.
- Nurses need to be aware of their own feelings of grief and loss to provide a nonjudgmental environment of care and support for bereaved families.

CRITICAL THINKING EXERCISES

1. Identify community resources and support groups for parents who have experienced the following:
   a. Infertility
   b. Birth of a less than perfect child
   c. Death of a baby through miscarriage, stillbirth, or newborn death.

   What services do each of these resources/groups provide?
2. Interview a mother or father (or a couple) who has experienced a perinatal loss.
   a. Ask them to tell you their story and then listen intently for their story lines
   b. Ask them who or what helped them the most
   c. Ask who or what made their experience more difficult
   d. Ask what they would want nursing students caring for such parents to know so they may help parents
3. Role play a situation in which a family has experienced a newborn death and the nurse is bringing their baby to them.
   a. Discuss how it felt to be the nurse.
   b. Discuss how it felt to be the parents.

RESOURCES

American Association of Pastoral Counselors (AAPC)
www.aapc.org

The Compassionate Friends
A self-help organization for bereaved parents and siblings
www.compassionatefriends.org

Griefnet
A collection of resources of value to those who are experiencing loss and grief
www.griefnet.org

Growth House, Inc.
Grief related to pregnancy, including miscarriage, stillbirth, termination of pregnancy, and neonatal death
www.growthhouse.org

Hannah's Prayer
Christian support for fertility challenges
www.hannah.org

Houston's Aid in Neonatal Death (HAND): Supporting grieving parents in the greater Houston area with the rest of the world via the Internet
www.hern.org/~hand

Hygeia
An online journal for pregnancy and neonatal loss: Dr. Michael Berman
www.connix.com/~hygeia/

Miscarriage Support and Information Resources
Comprehensive resource list
www.pinelandpress.com/support/miscarriage.html

OBGYN.net
List of resources for loss and bereavement
www.obgyn.net/woman/loss/loss.htm

Pen-Parents, Inc.
An international nonprofit support network for bereaved parents
www.penparents.org

A Place to Remember
Uplifting resources for those who have been touched by a crisis in pregnancy or the birth of a baby
www.aplacetoremember.com

SHARE
Pregnancy and Infant Loss Support, Inc.
www.nationalshareoffice.com

SIDS NETWORK
Sudden infant death syndrome (SIDS) information website
www.sids-network.org

REFERENCES

Armstrong, D. (2001). Exploring fathers' experiences of pregnancy after a prior perinatal loss. *MCN American Journal of Maternal Child Nursing, 26,* 147-153.

Armstrong, D., & Hutti, M. (1998). Pregnancy after perinatal loss: The relationship between anxiety and prenatal attachment. *Journal of Obstetric, Gynecologic, and Neonatal Nursing, 27,* 183-189.

Corbet-Owen, C., & Kruger, L. (2001). The health system and emotional care: Validating the many meanings of spontaneous pregnancy loss. *Family Systems of Health, 19,* 411-417.

Cote-Arsenault, D., & Mahlangu, N. (1999). Impact of perinatal loss on the subsequent pregnancy and self: Women's experiences. *Journal of Obstetric, Gynecologic, and Neonatal Nursing, 28,* 274-282.

Cowles, K. (1996). Cultural perspectives of grief: An expanded concept analysis. *Journal of Advanced Nursing, 23*, 287-294.
Dickason, E., Silverman, B., & Kaplan, J. (1998). *Maternal-infant nursing care* (3rd ed.). St. Louis: Mosby.
Frost, M., & Condon, J. (1996). The psychological sequelae of miscarriage: A critical review of the literature. *Australian and New Zealand Journal of Psychiatry, 30*(1), 54-62.
Harakas, S. (1999). E-mail to M. Miles.
Hebert, M. (1998). Perinatal bereavement in its cultural context. *Death Studies, 22*, 61-78.
Heiman, J., Yankowitz, J., & Wilkins, J. (1997). Grief support programs: Patients' use of services following the loss of a desired pregnancy and degree of implementation in academic centers. *American Journal of Perinatology, 14*, 587-591.
Hoyert, D. et al. (2001). Annual summary of vital statistics: 2000. *Pediatrics, 108*(6), 1241-1255.
Hughes, P. et al. (2002). Assessment of guidelines for good practice in psychosocial care of mothers after stillbirth: A cohort study. *Lancet, 360*, 1-11.
Hunfeld, J., Wladimiroff, J., & Passchier, J. (1997). Prediction and course of grief four years after perinatal loss due to congenital anomalies: A follow-up study. *British Journal of Medicine and Psychology, 70*, 85-91.
Janssen, H. et al. (1997). A prospective study of risk factors predicting grief intensity following pregnancy loss. *Archives of General Psychiatry, 54*, 56-61.
Kavanaugh, K. (1997). Parents' experience surrounding the death of a newborn whose birth is at the margin of viability. *Journal of Obstetric, Gynecologic, and Neonatal Nursing, 26*, 43-51.
Kowalski, K. (1984). *Perinatal death: An ethnomethodological study of factors influencing parental bereavement.* Doctoral dissertation, University of Colorado.
Lawson, L. (1990). Culturally sensitive support for grieving parents. *MCN American Journal of Maternal Child Nursing, 15*, 76-79.
Lindemann, E. (1944). Symptomatology and management of acute grief. *American Journal of Psychiatry, 101*, 141-148.
Lorenzen, J., & Holzgreve, W. (1995). Helping parents to grieve after second trimester termination of pregnancy for fetopathic reasons. *Fetal Diagnosis and Therapy, 10*(3), 147-156.
Lukse, M., & Vacc, N. (1999). Grief, depression, and coping in women undergoing infertility treatment. *Obstetrics and Gynecology, 93*, 245-251.
Malacrida, C. (1999). Complicating mourning: The social economy of perinatal death. *Qualitative Health Research, 9*, 504-519, 1999.
Miles, M. (1980). *The grief of parents. . .when a child dies.* Oak Brook, IL: Compassionate Friends, Inc.
Miles, M. (1984). Helping adults mourn the death of a child. In H. Wass & C. Corr (Eds.), *Childhood and death.* New York: Hemisphere Publishing.
Miles, M., & Demi, A. (1986). Guilt in bereaved parents. In T. Rando (Ed.), *Parental loss of a child: Clinical and research considerations.* Champaign, IL: Research Press.
Miles, M., & Demi, A. (1997). Historical and contemporary theories of grief. In I. Corless, B. Germino, & M. Pittman-Lindeman (Eds.), *Dying, death and bereavement.* Boston, MA: Jones & Bartlett.
Mori, E. et al. (1997). Anxiety of infertile women undergoing IVF-ET: Relation to the grief process. *Gynecology and Obstetrics Investigation, 44*, 157-162.
Osterweis, M., Solomon, F., & Green, M. (Eds.). (1984). *Bereavement: Reactions, consequences, and care.* Washington, DC: National Academy Press.
Parkes, C. (1972). *Bereavement: Studies of grief in adult life.* New York: International Universities Press.
Parkes, C., & Weiss, R. (1983). *Recovery from bereavement.* New York: Basic Books.
Pisarska, M., & Carson, S. (1999). Incidence and risk factors for ectopic pregnancy. *Clinical Obstetrics and Gynecology, 42*(1), 2-8.
Puddifoot, J., & Johnson, M. (1997). The legitimacy of grieving: The partner's experience at miscarriage. *Social Science and Medicine, 45*, 837-845.
Rand, C. et al. (1998). Parental behavior after perinatal death: Twelve years of observations. *Journal of Psychosomatic Obstetrics and Gynaecology, 19*, 44-48.
Schaap, A. et al. (1997). Long-term impact of perinatal bereavement: Comparison of grief reactions after intrauterine versus neonatal death. *European Journal of Obstetrics, Gynecology, and Reproductive Biology, 74*, 161-167.
Swanson-Kauffman, K. (1986). Caring in the instance of unexpected early pregnancy loss. *Topics in Clinical Nursing, 8*, 37-46.
Swanson-Kauffman, K. (1988). There should have been two: Nursing care of parents experiencing perinatal death of a twin. *Journal of Perinatal and Neonatal Nursing, 2*, 78-85.
Van, P. (2001). Breaking the silence of African American women: Healing after pregnancy loss. *Health Care for Women International, 22*, 229-243.
Wallerstedt, C., & Higgins, P. (1996). Facilitating perinatal grieving between the mother and the father. *Journal of Obstetric, Gynecologic, and Neonatal Nursing, 25*, 389-394.
Worden, W. (1991). *Grief counseling and grief therapy: A handbook for the mental health practitioner.* New York: Springer.
Zinaman, M. et al. (1996). Estimates of human fertility and pregnancy loss. *Fertility and Sterility, 65*(3), 503-509.

APPENDIX A

Standard Laboratory Values: Pregnant and Nonpregnant Women

http://evolve.elsevier.com/Lowdermilk/MatWmnHlth/

	NONPREGNANT	PREGNANT
Hematologic Values		
Complete Blood Count (CBC)		
Hemoglobin, g/dl	12 to 16*	>11*
Hematocrit, PCV, %	37 to 47	>33*
Red blood cell (RBC) volume, per ml	1600	1500 to 1900
Plasma volume, per ml	2400	3700
RBC count, million/mm^3	4.2 to 5.4	5 to 6.25
White blood cells, total per mm^3	5000 to 10,000	5000 to 15,000
Polymorphonuclear cells, %	55 to 70	60 to 85
Lymphocytes, %	20 to 40	15 to 40
Erythrocytes sedimentation rate, mm/hr	20/hr	Elevated second and third trimesters
MCHC, g/dl packed RBCs (mean corpuscular hemoglobin concentration)	32 to 36	No change
MCH (mean corpuscular hemoglobin) per picogram (less than a nanogram)	27 to 31	No change
MCV/μm^3 (mean corpuscular volume) per cubic micrometer	80 to 95	No change
Blood Coagulation and Fibrinolytic Activity†		
Factors VII, VIII, IX, X		Increase in pregnancy, return to normal in early puerperium; factor VIII increases during and immediately after birth
Factors XI, XIII		Decrease in pregnancy
Prothrombin time (PT)	11 to 12.5 sec	Slight decrease in pregnancy
Partial thromboplastin time (PTT)	60 to 70 sec	Slight decrease in pregnancy and again decrease during second and third stage of labor (indicates clotting at placental site)
Bleeding time	1 to 9 min (Ivy)	No appreciable change
Coagulation time	6 to 10 min (Lee/White)	No appreciable change
Platelets	150,000 to 400,000/mm^3	No significant change until 3 to 5 days after birth and then a rapid increase (may predispose woman to thrombosis) and gradual return to normal
Fibrinolytic activity		Decreases in pregnancy and then abrupt return to normal (protection against thromboembolism)
Fibrinogen	200 to 400 mg/dl	Increased levels late in pregnancy

Continued

	NONPREGNANT	PREGNANT
Hematologic Values—cont'd		
Mineral/Vitamin Concentrations		
Vitamin B_{12}, folic acid, ascorbic acid	Normal	Moderate decrease
Serum proteins		
Total, g/dl	6.4 to 8.3	5.5 to 7.5
Albumin, g/dl	3.5 to 5.0	Slight increase
Globulin, total, g/dl	2.3 to 3.4	3 to 4
Blood glucose		
Fasting, mg/dl	70 to 105	Decreases
2-hour postprandial, mg/dl	<140	Under 140 after a 100 g carbohydrate meal is considered normal
Hepatic Values		
Bilirubin total	Not more than 1 mg/dl	Unchanged
Serum cholesterol	120 to 200 mg/dl	Increases from 16 to 32 weeks of pregnancy; remains at this level until after birth
Serum alkaline phosphatase	42 to 128 U/L	Increases from week 12 of pregnancy to 6 weeks after birth
Serum globulin albumin	2.3 to 3.4 g/dl	Slight increase
Renal Values		
Bladder capacity	1300 ml	1500 ml
Renal plasma flow (RPF), ml/min	490 to 700	Increases by 25%
Glomerular filtration rate (GFR), ml/min	88 to 128	Increases by 50%
Nonprotein nitrogen (NPN), mg/dl	25 to 40	Decreases
Blood urea nitrogen (BUN), mg/dl	10 to 20	Decreases
Serum creatinine, mg/dl	0.5 to 1.1	Decreases
Serum uric acid, mg/dl	2.0 to 6.6	Decreases
Urine glucose	Negative	Present in 20% of pregnant women
Intravenous pyelogram (IVP)	Normal	Slight-to-moderate hydroureter and hydronephrosis; right kidney larger than left kidney

From Pagana, K., & Pagana, T. (1997). *Mosby's diagnostic and laboratory test reference* (3rd ed.). St Louis: Mosby.
*At sea level. Permanent residents of higher levels (e.g., Denver) require higher levels of hemoglobin.
†Pregnancy represents a hypercoagulable state.

APPENDIX B

Standard Laboratory Values in the Neonatal Period

http://evolve.elsevier.com/Lowdermilk/MatWmnHlth/

	NEONATAL
1. Hematologic Values	
Clotting factors	
Activated clotting time (ACT)	2 min
Bleeding time (Ivy)	2 to 7 min
Clot retraction	Complete 1 to 4 hr
Fibrinogen	125 to 300 mg/dl*

	TERM	PRETERM
Hemoglobin (g/dl)	14.5 to 22.5	15 to 17
Hematocrit (%)	44 to 72	45 to 55
Reticulocytes (%)	0.4 to 6	Up to 10
Fetal hemoglobin (% of total)	40 to 70	80 to 90
Red blood cells (RBCs)/mm^3	4.0^6 to 6.0^6	
Platelet count/mm^3	84,000 to 478,000	120,000 to 180,000
White blood cells (WBCs)/mm^3	9000 to 30,000	10,000 to 20,000
Neutrophils (%)	54 to 62	47
Eosinophils and basophils (%)	1 to 3	
Lymphocytes (%)	25 to 33	33
Monocytes (%)	3 to 7	4
Immature WBC (%)	10	16

*dl refers to deciliter (1 dl = 100 ml); this conforms to the SI system (standardized international measurements).

			NEONATAL
2. Biochemical Values			
Bilirubin, direct			0 to 1 mg/dl
Bilirubin, total	Cord:		<2 mg/dl
	Peripheral blood:	0 to 1 day	6 mg/dl
		1 to 2 days	8 mg/dl
		3 to 5 days	12 mg/dl
Blood gases		Arterial:	pH 7.31 to 7.45
			P_{CO_2} 33 to 48 mm Hg
			P_{O_2} 50 to 70 mm Hg
		Venous:	pH 7.28 to 7.42
			P_{CO_2} 38 to 52 mm Hg
			P_{O_2} 20 to 49 mm Hg
α_1-Fetoprotein			0
Fibrinogen			150 to 300 mg/dl
Serum glucose			40 to 60 mg/dl

Continued

	NEONATAL
3. Urinalysis	
Color	Clear, straw
Specific gravity	1.001 to 1.018
pH	5 to 7
Protein	Negative
Glucose	Negative
Ketones	Negative
RBCs	Rare
WBCs	0 to 4
Casts	Rare
17-Ketosteroids	Under 1
17-Hydroxycorticosteroids	Same
Urinary calcium	5 mg/kg of body weight
Urinary sodium	20% of adult values
Urinary vanillylmandelic acid (VMA)	$<$1.0 mg/24 hr

Volume: 20 to 40 ml excreted daily in the first few days; by week 1, 24-hr urine volume close to 200 ml
Protein: may be present in first 2 to 4 days
Osmolarity (mOsm/L): 100 to 600

4. Urine Screening Tests for Inborn Errors of Metabolism

Benedict's test: for reducing substances in the urine—glucose, galactose, fructose, lactose; phenylketonuria (PKU), alkaptonuria, tyrosyluria, and tyrosinosis may give a positive Benedict's test result.

Ferric chloride test: an immediate green color for PKU, histidinemia, and tyrosinuria; a gray to green color for presence of phenothiazines, isoniazid; red to purple color for presence of salicylates or ketone bodies.

Dinitrophenylhydrazine test: for PKU, maple syrup urine disease, Lowe's syndrome.

Cetyltrimethylammonium bromide test: for mucopolysaccharides: immediate positive reaction in gargoylism (Hurler syndrome); delayed, moderately positive reaction for Marfan, Morquio-Ullrich, and Murdoch syndromes.

Metachromatic stain (or urine sediment): granules (free or as inclusion bodies in cells) are seen in metachromatic leukodystrophy; may also be seen rarely in Tay-Sachs and other lipid diseases of central nervous system.

Amino acid chromatography: aminoaciduria may be normal in newborns; chromatography may be helpful to detect hypophosphatasia and argininosuccinicaciduria.

Diaper test, Phenistix test, and Dinitrophenylhydrazine (DNPH) test: simple, inexpensive tests for PKU; used for screening; most useful when infant is at least 6 weeks of age.

5. Blood Serum Phenylalanine Tests

Guthrie inhibition assay methods: drops of blood placed on filter paper; laboratory uses bacterial growth inhibition test; phenylalanine level above 8 mg/dl blood: diagnostic of PKU. Effective in newborn period; used also to monitor PKU diet; blood easily obtained by heel or finger puncture; inexpensive; used for wide-scale screening.

APPENDIX C

Relationship of Drugs to Breast Milk and Effect on Infant

http://evolve.elsevier.com/Lowdermilk/MatWmnHlth/

The drugs listed in this appendix have been categorized by their major use. The ratings given are those published by the American Academy of Pediatrics (AAP) Committee on Drugs. These ratings label drugs that transfer into human milk. Drugs without a rating were not included in the AAP list. The ratings are described as follows:

1. Drugs that are contraindicated during breastfeeding
2. Drugs of abuse that are contraindicated during breastfeeding
3. Radioactive compounds that require temporary cessation of breastfeeding
4. Drugs with unknown effects on breastfeeding but may be of concern
5. Drugs that have been associated with significant effects on some breastfeeding infants and should be given to breastfeeding mothers with caution
6. Maternal medication usually compatible with breastfeeding
7. Food and environmental agents: effect on breastfeeding

DRUG	EXCRETED IN MILK	% ADULT DOSE IN MILK	AAP RATING	COMMENTS
Analgesics and Antiinflammatory Drugs (Nonnarcotic)				
Acetaminophen (Datril, Tylenol)	Yes	0.04 to 1.85	6	Detoxified in liver. Avoid in immediate postbirth period; otherwise no problems with therapeutic dose.
Aspirin (Bayer, Anacin, Bufferin, Excedrin, etc.)	Yes	10.55 ± 10.45	6	Long history of experience shows complications rare. Can cause interference with platelet aggregation and diminished factor XII (Hageman factor) at birth. When mother requires high, continuing level of medication for arthritis, aspirin is drug of choice. Observe infant for bruisability. Platelet aggregation can be evaluated. Salicylism seen only in maternal overdosing. Mother should increase vitamin C and vitamin K intake.
Ibuprofen (Advil, Nuprin, Motrin, etc.)	Yes	<0.8	6	No apparent effects in therapeutic doses.
Indomethacin (Indocin)	Yes	0.11 to 0.98	6	Convulsions in breastfed neonate (case report). Used to close patent ductus arteriosus. Insufficient data as to ef[illegible] on other vessels. May be ne[illegible]

DRUG	EXCRETED IN MILK	% ADULT DOSE IN MILK	AAP RATING	COMMENTS
Analgesics and Antiinflammatory Drugs (Nonnarcotic)—cont'd				
Mefenamic acid (Ponstel)	Yes	0.036 to 0.8	6	No apparent effect on infant at therapeutic doses; infant able to excrete via urine.
Naproxen (Naproxyn, Anaprox, Naprosyn, Aleve)	Yes	1.1		Less toxic in adults than some other organic derivatives.
Propoxyphene (Darvon)	Yes	Trace amounts	6	Only symptoms detectable would be failure to feed and drowsiness. On daily, around-the-clock dosage, infant could consume 1 mg/day.
Antiinfectives (May change intestinal flora of infant and sensitize for later allergic reaction)				
Acyclovir (Zovirax)	Yes	5.6 ± 4.4	6	Minimal absorption through maternal skin.
Ampicillin (Polycillin, Amcill, Omnipen, Penbritin)	Yes	0.05 to 0.04		Sensitivity resulting from repeated exposure; diarrhea or secondary candidiasis.
Carbenicillin (Pyopen, Geopen)	Yes	0.001		Levels not significant. Drug is given to neonate. Not well absorbed from gastrointestinal (GI) tract.
Cefazolin (Ancef, Kefzol)	Yes	0.075	6	Probably not significant. Detected in milk if given intravenously (IV).
Cephalexin (Keflex)	Yes	0.86 ± 0.35		Completely gone by 8 hours; absorption less in first few months.
Cephalothin (Keflin)	Yes	0.4		Negligible.
Chloramphenicol (Chloromycetin)	Yes	1.6	4	Gray syndrome. Infant does not excrete drug well, and small amounts may accumulate. Contraindicated. May be tolerated in older infant with mature glycuronide system.
Colistin (Colymycin)	Yes	0.07		Not absorbed orally.
Demeclocycline (Declomycin)	Yes	Trace		Not significant in therapeutic doses. Can be given to infants. Drug remains in milk 3 days after dose.
Erythromycin (Ilosone, E-Mycin, Erythrocin)	Yes	0.1 to 2.1	6	Higher concentrations have been reported in milk than in plasma. Should not be given under 1 month of age because of risk of jaundice. Dose in milk higher when given IV to mother.
Gentamicin	Yes			Not absorbed from GI tract, may change gut flora. Drug is given to newborns directly.
Isoniazid (Nydrazid)	Yes	2.3		Infant at risk for toxicity, but need for breast milk may outweigh risk.
Kanamycin (Kantrex)	Yes	0.95	6	Infant absorbs little from GI tract. Infants can be given drug.
Metronidazole (Flagyl)	Yes	0.13 to 36	4	Caution should be exercised because of its high milk concentrations. Contraindicated when infant under 6 months; may cause neurologic disorders and blood dyscrasia. AAP says to discard milk for 12 hours if mother takes 2-g dose.

DRUG	EXCRETED IN MILK	% ADULT DOSE IN MILK	AAP RATING	COMMENTS
Antiinfectives—cont'd				
Nitrofurantoin (Furadantin, Macrodantin)	Yes	0.6	6	No significant effect in therapeutic doses except in infant with G6PD deficiency.
Novobiocin (Albamycin, Cathomycin)	Yes	0.15		Infant can be given drug directly.
Nystatin (Mycostatin)	No	Not absorbed orally		Can be given to infant directly.
Oxacillin (Prostaphlin)	No	Trace		
Penicillin G, benzathine (Bicillin)	Yes	0.8		Clinical need should supersede possible allergic responses.
Penicillin G, potassium	Yes	0.8		Infant can be given penicillin directly. Parents should be told to inform physician that infant has been exposed to penicillin because of potential sensitivity.
Streptomycin	Yes	0.5	6	Not to be given more than 2 weeks. Ototoxic and nephrotoxic with long use. Is given to infants directly.
Sulfisoxazole (Gantrisin)	Yes	0.45	6	To be avoided during first month after birth; may cause kernicterus.
Tetracycline HCl (Achromycin, Panmycin, Sumycin)	Yes	0.3 to 4.8	6	Not enough to treat an infection in an infant. May cause discoloration of the teeth in the infant; the antibiotic, however, may be largely bound to the milk calcium. Do not give longer than 10 days or repeatedly.
Anticoagulants				
Coumarin derivatives Dicumarol (bishydroxycoumarin), warfarin (Panwarfin)	Yes	6.5	6	Monitor prothrombin time. Give vitamin K to infant. Discontinue if surgery or trauma occurs. Drug of choice if mother to continue breastfeeding. May cause bleeding.
Heparin	No			Heparin ineffective orally.
Anticonvulsants and Sedatives (Barbiturates may pass into milk but do not sedate infant)				
Magnesium sulfate	Yes	0.5	6	May produce sedation in infant.
Pentobarbital (Nembutal)	Yes	Traces		Depends on liver for detoxification so may accumulate in first week of life until infant is able to detoxify. No problem for older infant in usual doses.
Phenytoin (Dilantin)	Yes	1.4 to 7.2	6	No problem if mother's dose is in therapeutic range.
Phenobarbital (Luminal)	Yes	1.5		Sleepiness and decreased sucking possible. On usual analeptic doses, infants alert and feed well. On hypnotic doses, infants depressed and difficult to rouse.
Sodium bromide (Bromo-Seltzer and over-the-counter sleeping aids)	Yes	6, 7		Drowsy, decreased crying, rash, decreased feeding. No longer available in the United States.

Continued

DRUG	EXCRETED IN MILK	% ADULT DOSE IN MILK	AAP RATING	COMMENTS
Antihistamines (May suppress lactation; administer after breastfeeding; all pass into breast milk)				
Brompheniramine (Dimetane)	Yes	Unknown		Drugs used in neonates. May cause sedation or decreased feeding, or may produce stimulation and tachycardia. Should avoid long-acting preparations, which may accumulate in infant.
Diphenhydramine (Benadryl)	Yes	Unknown		When combined with decongestants, may cause decrease in milk.
Promethazine (Phenergan)	Yes	Unknown	6	Passage into breast is expected; increases serum prolactin levels.
Autonomic Drugs				
Atrophine sulfate*	Yes	Traces	6	Hyperthermia, atropine toxicity, infants especially sensitive; also inhibits lactation. Infant dose 0.01 mg/kg.
Ergotamine	Yes	Unknown	1	May inhibit lactation.
Neostigmine	No	No known harm to infant		
Propantheline bromide (Pro-Banthine)	No	Uncontrolled data indicate no measurable levels		Drug rapidly metabolized in maternal system to inactive metabolite. Mother should avoid long-acting preparations, however.
Cardiovascular Drugs				
Diazoxide (Hyperstat)	Possible			Arteriolar dilators and antihypertensive, given only IV, not active orally.
Digoxin	Yes	0.07 to 14	6	Not detected in infant's plasma.
Hydralazine (Apresoline)	Yes	0.8	6	Jaundice, thrombocytopenia, electrolyte disturbances possible.
Methyldopa (Aldomet)	Yes	0.02 to 0.09		Galactorrhea. No specific data except as affects mother's milk production.
Propranolol (Inderal)	Yes	Traces		Risk of effect almost nonexistent.
Quinidine	Yes	4.1	6	Arrhythmia may occur.
Cathartics				
Cascara	Yes	Low	6	Causes colic and diarrhea in infant.
Milk of magnesia	No	None	6	No effect.
Mineral oil	No	None	6	No effect.
Phenolphthalein	Unknown	Unknown	6	Reported to cause symptoms in some.
Rhubarb	Unknown	None	6	None in syrup form. Fresh rhubarb may give symptoms of colic and diarrhea.
Saline cathartics	No	None	6	No effect.
Senna	No	None	6	None
Stool softeners and bulk-forming laxatives	No	None	6	No effect.
Suppositories (for constipation)	No	None	6	Not absorbed.
Diuretics				
Furosemide (sulfamoylanthranilic acid) (Lasix)	Possible	Not found in all samples		Drug is given to children under medical management.
Spironolactone (Aldactone)	Yes	Canrenone, a metabolite, appears	6	Acts as antagonist of aldosterone; causes sodium excretion and potassium retention. The metabolite apparently has some activity.

*An ingredient in many prescription and nonprescription drugs.

DRUG	EXCRETED IN MILK	% ADULT DOSE IN MILK	AAP RATING	COMMENTS
Diuretics—cont'd				
Thiazides (Diuril, Enduron, Esidrix, HydroDiuril, Oretic, Thiuretic tablets)	Yes	0.25 to 0.43	6	Risk of dehydration and electrolyte imbalance, especially sodium loss, which would require monitoring. Watch weight and wet diapers and take an occasional specific gravity reading of urine and serum sodium to indicate status of infant. Risk, however, is extremely low. May suppress lactation because of dehydration in mother.
Hormones and Contraceptives				
Contraceptives (oral) Ethinyl estradiol, mestranol, 19-nortestosterone, norethindrone (Norlutin)	Yes	0.16 ± 0.14	6	May diminish milk supply. May decrease vitamins, protein, and fat in milk. Most significant concern is long-range influence of hormone on young infant, which is not certain. Reports of feminization of infant.
Corticotropin	Yes	1.1	6	May decrease quantity and quality of milk.
Cortisone	Yes	Significant amounts		May affect infant in therapeutic doses.
Epinephrine (Adrenalin)	Yes			Destroyed in GI tract of infant.
Estrogen	Yes	0.1	6	Risks as with oral contraceptives. May alter quality and quantity of milk.
Insulin	No			Destroyed in intestinal tract.
Medroxyprogesterone acetate (Provera)	Yes	0.86 to 5	6	6-month injection may affect milk supply; 3-month injection should not decrease supply.
Prednisone	Yes	0.06 to 3.6	6	Minimum amount not likely to cause effect on infant in short course.
Tolbutamide (Orinase)	Yes	18	6	Watch for jaundice.
Narcotics				
Cocaine	Yes	Significant levels in milk	1, 2	No metabolites or drug found in milk after 36 hours or in infant's urine after 60 hours.
Codeine	Yes	5 ± 2	6	No effect in therapeutic level and transient use. Can accumulate. Individual variation. Watch for neonatal depression. Asians metabolize drug less than Caucasians do.
Heroin	Yes		2	Level in milk enough to cause addiction in infant.
Marijuana (*Cannabis sativa* L.)	Yes		2	Shown in laboratory animals to produce structural changes in nursling's brain cells; impairs DNA and RNA formation. Infant at risk of inhaling smoke during feeding or when held by person who is smoking.
Meperidine (Demerol)	Yes	Trace		Trace amounts may accumulate if drug taken around the clock when infant is neonate. Watch for drowsiness and poor feeding.

Continued

DRUG	EXCRETED IN MILK	% ADULT DOSE IN MILK	AAP RATING	COMMENTS
Narcotics—cont'd				
Methadone	Yes	2.2	6	When dosage not excessive, infant can be breastfed if monitored for evidence of depression and failure to thrive. Suggest mother take daily dose after evening feeding and supplement formula at next feeding.
Morphine	Yes	0.8 to 1.2	6	Single doses have minimum effect. Potential for accumulation. May be addicting to neonate. Amounts in breast milk too variable to consider breastfeeding as means of treating withdrawal symptoms.
Percodan (oxycodone [derived from opiate thebaine], aspirin, phenacetin, caffeine)	Yes	Unknown		Consider for its component parts. In neonatal period, sleepiness and failure to feed, which increase maternal engorgement and neonatal weight loss, have been observed, probably caused by oxycodone.
Psychotropic and Mood-Changing Drugs				
Alcohol (Ethanol)	Yes	1 to 19.5	6	Milk may smell like alcohol. Ethanol in doses of 1 to 2 g/kg to mother causes depression of milk-ejection reflex (dose dependent). No acetaldehyde found because infant cannot metabolize ethanol.
Amphetamine	Yes	6.1 ± 0.1	2	Has caused stimulation in infants with jitteriness, irritability, sleeplessness. Long-acting preparations cumulative.
Benzodiazepines* Chlordiazepoxide (Librium)	Yes			Not sufficient to affect infant first week when glucuronyl system needed for detoxification. May accumulate. May cause jaundice. Older infant, no apparent problem.
Diazepam (Valium)	Yes	2 to 4.7	4	Detoxified in glucuronyl system. In first weeks of life may contribute to jaundice. Metabolite active. Effect on infant: hypoventilation, drowsiness, lethargy, weight loss. Single doses over 10 mg contraindicated during breastfeeding. Accumulation in infant possible.
Haloperidol (Haldol)	Yes	0.15 to 2	4	An antipsychotic: animal studies in nurslings show behavior abnormalities.
Lithium carbonate (Eskalith, Lithane, Lithonate)	Yes	1.8		Measurable lithium in infant's serum. Infant kidney can clear lithium; however, lithium inhibits adenosine 3′,5′-cyclic monophosphate, significant for brain growth. Also affects amine metabolism. Report of cyanosis and poor muscle tone and ECG changes in nursing infant.
Meprobamate (Miltown, Equanil)	Yes	2 to 4 times maternal plasma level		If therapy continued, infant should be followed closely.

*Alcohol enhances the effects of these drugs.

DRUG	EXCRETED IN MILK	% ADULT DOSE IN MILK	AAP RATING	COMMENTS
Psychotropic and Mood-Changing Drugs—cont'd				
Phencyclidine (PCP)	Yes		1	Animal studies show PCP in milk even after drug has been discontinued for 40 days.
Phenothiazines				
Chlorpromazine (Thorazine)	Yes	0.07 to 0.2		Drowsiness and lethargy in infants.
Thioridazine (Mellaril)	Yes	No information		Thioridazine is less potent in general than other phenothiazines. Probably safe.
Trifluoperazine (Stelazine)	Yes	Minimum		
Tricyclic antidepressants				Apparently no accumulation. No infants who have been observed showed symptoms.
Amitriptyline (Elavil)	Yes	0.8 ± 0.2	4	Watch for depression or failure to feed; increases maternal prolactin secretion.
Desipramine (Norpramin, Pertofrane)		1	4	
Imipramine (Tofranil)	Yes	0.1	4	
Stimulants				
Caffeine	Yes	0.66 to 10	6	Accumulates when intake moderate and continual. Causes jitteriness, wakefulness, and irritability. Caffeine present in many hot and cold drinks. Consider if infant very wakeful.
Theobromine	Yes	20	7	No adverse symptoms observed in the infants. Chocolate the most common cause of exposure.
Theophylline	Yes	<1 to 15	6	Irritability, fretfulness.
Thyroid and Antithyroid Medications				
Thiouracil	Yes	0.3 to 2.6	6	Get baseline levels of T_3, T_4, and TSH before and 6 weeks after mother starts medication.
Thyroid and thyroxine	Yes	0.3 to 2.6	6	Does not produce adverse symptoms on long-range follow-up study. Noted to improve milk supply of hypothyroid mothers. No contraindication.
Miscellaneous				
DPT	Yes	Minimum		Does not interfere with immunization schedule.
Methotrexate	Yes	0.93	1	Antimetabolite. Infant would receive 0.26 g/dl, which researchers consider nontoxic for infant.
Nicotine	Yes		2	Decreases milk production. Smoking may interfere with let-down reflex if smoking started before onset of a feeding. Smoke exposure may be a concern.
Poliovirus vaccine	No			Live vaccine taken orally. Not necessary to withhold breastfeeding 30 minutes before and after dose. Provide booster after infant no longer breastfeeding.

Continued

DRUG	EXCRETED IN MILK	% ADULT DOSE IN MILK	AAP RATING	COMMENTS
Miscellaneous—cont'd				
Rh antibodies	Yes			Destroyed in GI tract; not effective orally.
Rubella virus vaccine	Yes	Minimum		Will not confer passive immunity. Mother should not be given vaccine when at risk for pregnancy.
Tuberculin test	No			Tuberculin-sensitive mothers can adaptively immunize their infants through breast milk, and that immunity may last several years.
Chest x-rays	No			No effect.

Compiled from Lawrence, R. (1999). *Breastfeeding: A guide for the medical profession* (5th ed.). St. Louis: Mosby; The Committee on Drugs, American Academy of Pediatrics. (1994). The transfer of drugs and other chemicals into human breast milk. *Pediatrics* 93(1), 137-150.

APPENDIX D

Resources

http://evolve.elsevier.com/Lowdermilk/MatWmnHlth/

This appendix includes community and national resources, national clearinghouses, journals, and nursing organizations of interest to maternity and women's health nurses.

COMMUNITY AND NATIONAL RESOURCES

Academy for Guided Imagery
P.O. Box 2070
Mill Valley, CA 94942
(800) 726-2070
http://www.healthy.net/agi/

AIDS Network Hotline
(800) 342-2437 (AIDS)

AIDS Resource List
http://www.hivnet.org/aidsres.html

American Academy of Husband-Coached Childbirth
P.O. Box 5224
Sherman Oaks, CA 91413
(800) 422-4784

American Academy of Pediatrics
141 Northwest Point Blvd.
Elk Grove, IL 60007-1098
(847) 228-5005
http://www.aap.org

American Association of Acupuncturists and Oriental Medicine
4104 Lake Boone Trail, Suite 201
Raleigh, NC 27607-6518
(919) 787-5181

American Cancer Society
1599 Clifton Rd., NE
Atlanta, GA 30329
(800) ACS-2345
http://www.cancer.org

American Cleft Palate Association
1218 Grandview Ave.
Pittsburgh, PA 15211
(412) 681-1376
(800) 24-CLEFT

American College of Obstetricians and Gynecologists
409 12th St., SW
Washington, DC 20024
(800) 762-2264
http://www.acog.com

American Diabetes Association
Diabetes Information Service Center
1660 Duke St.
Alexandria, VA 22314
(800) 342-2383
http://www.diabetes.org

American Fertility Foundation
2131 Magnolia Ave., Suite 201
Birmingham, AL 35256
(205) 251-9764

American Heart Association
Women's heart information: 1-888-MYHEART
(1-888-694-3278)
(800) 242-8721
http://www.americanheart.org

American Red Cross
430 17th St., NW
Washington, DC 20006
(202) 737-8300
http://www.redcross.org

American Society for Reproductive Medicine
1209 Montgomery Hwy.
Birmingham, AL 35316
(205) 978-5000
http://www.asrm.com

Anorexia Nervosa and Related Eating Disorders Inc.
http://www.amred.com

Association for Childbirth at Home, International
P.O. Box 39498
Los Angeles, CA 90039
(213) 667-0839

Association of Maternal and Child Health Programs
1220 19th St., NW, Suite 801
Washington, DC 20036
(202) 775-0436
http://www.amchp.org

Baby Center
(Source for expectant parents)
http://www.babycenter.com

Bereavement Services/RTS
Lutheran Hospital–La Crosse
1910 South Ave.
La Crosse, WI 54601
(608) 791-4747
(800) 362-9567

Cancernet
http://www.cancernet.nei.nih.gov

CDC National Prevention Information Network
http://www.cdcnpin.org

Center for Sickle Cell Disease
2121 Georgia Ave., NW
Washington, DC 20059
(202) 636-7930

Centers for Disease Control and Prevention
1600 Clifton Rd., NE
Atlanta, GA 30333
(404) 329-1819
(404) 329-3286
http://www.cdc.gov

Childbirth Graphics
P.O. Box 21207
Waco, TX 76702
(800) 229-3366

Compassionate Friends
(Following death of an infant)
P.O. Box 1347
Oak Brook, IL 60521
(312) 990-0010

COPE (Coping with the Overall Pregnancy/Parenting Experience)
37 Clarendon St.
Boston, MA 02116
(617) 357-5588

C/SEC, Inc. (Cesarean/Support Education and Concern)
22 Forest Rd.
Framingham, MA 01701
(508) 877-8266

Doulas of North America (DONA)
1100 23rd Ave. East
Seattle, WA 98112
(206) 324-5440
http://www.dona.com

Endometriosis Association
8585 North 76th Place
Milwaukee, WI 53223
(414) 355-2200
(800) 992-3636
http://www.ivf.com/endohtml.html

Environmental Protection Agency (EPA)
Public Information Center
Room PM 211-B
401 M St., SW
Washington, DC 20460
(202) 382-7550
http://www.epa.gov

Gynecologic Cancer Foundation
http://www.sgo.org/gcf

Harvard Eating Disorders Center
356 Boylston St.
Boston, MA 02166
(888) 236-1188
http://www.hedc.org

Healing Touch International, Inc.
12477 W. Cedar Drive, Suite 202
Lakewood, CO 80228
(303) 989-7982
http://www.healingtouch.net

Health Web: Evidence Based Health Care
http://www.uic.edu/depts/lib/health/hw/ebhc

Healthy Mothers, Healthy Babies Coalition
409 12th St., SW
Washington, DC 20024
(202) 863-2458

Human Genome Project and ELSI (Ethical, Legal, and Social Implications in Genetics)
http://www.nhgri.nih.gov

Hysterectomy Educational Resource and Services (HERS)
422 Byrn Mawr Ave.
Bala Cynwyd, PA 19004
(215) 667-7757
http://www.ccon.com/hers

Institute for Women's Policy Research
1400 20th St., NW, Suite 104
Washington, DC 20036
(202) 785-5100
http://www.iwpr.org

International Association of Infant Massage
http://www.infantmassage.com

International Childbirth Education Association (ICEA)
P.O. Box 20048
Minneapolis, MN 55420
(612) 854-8660
http://www.icea.org

International Lactation Consultant Association
201 Brown Ave.
Evanston, IL 60202-3601
(708) 260-8874

Lact-Aid
(Provides information and services to promote breastfeeding)
P.O. Box 1066
Athens, TN 37303
(614) 744-9090

La Leche League
1400 N. Meacham Rd.
Schaumburg, IL 60173
(800) 525-3243 (24-hour line)
http://www.lalecheleague.org

Lamaze International
1200 19th St., NW, Suite 300
Washington, DC 20036-2422
(800) 368-4404
(202) 857-1128
http://www.lamaze-childbirth.com

March of Dimes Birth Defects Foundation
National Foundation/March of Dimes
1275 Mamaroneck Ave.
White Plains, NY 10605
(914) 428-7100
(888) 663-4637 (MODIMES)
http://www.modimes.org

Maternity Center Association, Inc.
281 Park Ave. South, 5th Floor
New York, NY 10010
(212) 777-5000

Mining Company Guide to Pregnancy and Birth
http://pregnancy/miningco.com

National Abortion Federation Consumer Hotline
1156 15th St., NW, Suite 700
Washington, DC 20005
(800) 772-9100

National Alliance of Breast Cancer Organizations
9 East 37th St., 10th Floor
New York, NY 10016
(800) 719-0154
http://www.nabco.org

National Association for Sickle Cell Disease
3345 Wilshire Blvd., Suite 1106
Los Angeles, CA 90010-1880
(213) 736-5455
(800) 421-8453

National Association of Childbearing Centers
3123 Gottschall Rd.
Perkiomenville, PA 18074
(215) 234-8068

National Association of Parents and Professionals for Safe Alternatives in Childbirth (NAPSAC)
P.O. Box 267
Marble Hill, MO 63764
(314) 238-2010

National Breast Cancer Coalition
P.O. Box 66373
Washington, DC 20035
(202) 296-7477
(800) 935-0434

National Cancer Institute Cancer Information Service
(800) 4-CANCER
http://www.nci.nih.gov

National Center for Complementary and Alternative Medicine (NCCAM)
P.O. Box 8218
Silver Spring, MD 20907-8218
(888) 644-6226
http://altmed.od.nih.gov/nccam/

National Cervical Cancer Coalition
http://www.nccc-online.org

National Coalition Against Sexual Assault
912 North 2nd St.
Harrisburg, PA 17102
(717) 232-6771

National Coalition of Feminist and Lesbian Cancer Projects
P.O. Box 90437
Washington, DC 20090
(202) 332-5536

National Coalition of Hispanic Health and Human Services Organizations (COSSMHO)
1030 15th St., NW, Suite 1053
Washington, DC 20005
(202) 387-5000
http://www.cossmho.org

National Council of Women's Organizations
Women's Health
1126 16th St., NW, Suite 411
Washington, DC 20036
(202) 331-7343
http://womensorganizations.org/healthtopic_toc.cfm

National Domestic Violence and Abuse Hotline
(800) 799-SAFE

National Down Syndrome Congress
1800 Dempster St.
Park Ridge, IL 60068-1146
(708) 823-7550
(800) 232-6372

National Down Syndrome Society Hotline
666 Broadway
New York, NY 10012
(800) 221-4602

National Foundation for Jewish Genetic Diseases, Inc.
250 Park Ave., Suite 1000
New York, NY 10177
(212) 371-1030

National Institute of Child Health and Human Development (NICHD)
National Institutes of Health
9000 Rockville Pike
Bldg. 31, Room 2A32
Bethesda, MD 20892
(301) 496-4000
http://www.nih.gov

National Institutes of Health Information Page
http://www.nih.gov/health

National Organization of Mothers of Twins Clubs, Inc.
P.O. Box 23188
Albuquerque, NM 87192
(505) 275-0955

National Organization on Adolescent Pregnancy, Parenting, and Prevention
2401 Pennsylvania Ave., Suite 350
Washington, DC 20037
(202) 293-8370
http://www.noappp.org

National Organization for Women (NOW) Legal Defense and Education Fund
99 Hudson St.
New York, NY 10013-2871
(212) 925-6635

National Osteoporosis Foundation
1150 17th St., NW, Suite 500
Washington, DC 20036
(800) 223-9994
http://www.nof.org

National Ovarian Cancer Coalition
2335 East Atlantic Blvd., #401
Pompano Beach, FL 33062
(888) 682-7426
http://ww.ovarian.org

National Perinatal Association
101½ South Union St.
Alexandria, VA 22314-3323
(703) 549-5523

National Resource Center for Domestic Violence
(800) 537-2238

National Right to Life Committee
419 7th St., NW, Suite 500
Washington, DC 20004
(202) 626-8800

National Sexually Transmitted Diseases Hotline
(800) 227-8922

National Sudden Infant Death Syndrome Foundation
10500 Little Patuxent Parkway, Suite 420
Columbia, MD 21044
(301) 964-8000
(800) 221-7437

National Women's Health Resource Center
120 Albany St., Suite 820
New Brunswick, NJ 08901
(877) 986-9472
http://www.healthywomen.org

New York Times on the Web Women's Health
http://www.nytimes.com/specials/women/whome/index.html

Office of Minority Health Resource Center
P.O. Box 37337
Washington, DC 20013-7337
(301) 587-1938

Parent Care, Inc.
(Neonatal intensive care unit family support)
101½ South Union St.
Alexandria, VA 22314-3323
(703) 836-4678

Parenthood After Thirty
451 Vermont
Berkeley, CA 94707
(415) 524-6635

Parents of Prematures
13613 NE 26th Place
Bellevue, WA 98005
(206) 883-6040

Parents Without Partners
8807 Colesville Rd.
Silver Spring, MD 20910
(301) 588-9354
(800) 637-7974

Planned Parenthood Federation of America, Inc.
810 Seventh Ave.
New York, NY 10019
(800) 230-PLAN
http://www.plannedparenthood.org

Pregnancy and Infant Loss
1421 East Wayzata Blvd., Suite 40
Wayzata, MN 55391
(614) 473-9372

Premenstrual Syndrome Action
P.O. Box 16292
Irving, CA 92713
(714) 854-4407

Reach to Recovery
(*see* American Cancer Society)
(breast cancer)

Read Natural Childbirth Foundation
P.O. Box 956
San Rafael, CA 94915
(415) 456-8462

Resolve, Inc.
(Impaired fertility)
1310 Broadway, Dept. GM
Summerville, MA 02144-1713
(617) 623-0744
(888) 299-1585
http://www.resolve.org

Sex Information and Education Council of the United States
(Provides publications [e.g., "Sexual relations in pregnancy and postpartum"] and teaching aids)
130 W. 42nd St., Suite 350
New York, NY 10036
http://www.siecus.org

Society for Women's Health Research
1828 L St., NW, Suite 625
Washington, DC 20036
(202) 223-8224
http://www.womens-health.org

Soy Protein Council
(202) 467-6610
http://spcouncil.com

Special Supplemental Nutrition Program for Women, Infants, and Children (WIC)
Food and Consumer Service
3101 Park Center Dr., Room 819
Alexandria, VA 22302
(703) 305-2286
http://www.usda.gov/fns/wic.html

Spina Bifida Association of America
4590 McArthur Blvd., NW, Suite 250
Washington, DC 20007-4226
(800) 621-3141

Susan G. Koman Breast Cancer Foundation
(800) 462-9273

The Touch Research Institute
http://www.miami.edu/touch-research/home.html

NATIONAL CLEARINGHOUSES

Breastfeeding Resources
http://www.parentsplace.com/expert/lactation/

Food and Drug Administration (FDA)
Office of Consumer Affairs
Public Inquiries
5600 Fishers Lane (HFE-88)
Rockville, MD 20857
(301) 443-3170
http://www.fda.gov

Infertility Resources
http://www.ihr.com/infertility/index.html

International Council on Infertility Information Dissemination
(703) 379-9178
http://www.inciid.org

National AIDS Information Clearinghouse
P.O. Box 6003
Rockville, MD 20849-6003
(800) 458-5231 (English and Spanish)

National Clearinghouse for Alcohol and Drug Abuse Information
P.O. Box 426
Dept DQ
Kensington, MD 20795
(800) 729-6686
http://www.health.org

National Clearinghouse for Family Planning Information
P.O. Box 10716
Rockville, MD 20850
(703) 558-4990

National Clearinghouse for Human Genetic Disease
(Provides information about inherited diseases)
National Center for Education in Maternal and Child Health
38th and R Sts., NW
Washington, DC 20057

Sudden Infant Death Syndrome Clearinghouse
8201 Greensboro Dr., Suite 600
McLean, VA 22102
(723) 821-8955

NURSING JOURNALS

Alternative Therapies in Health and Medicine
101 Columbia
Aliso Viejo, CA 92656
(800) 899-1712
http://www.alternative-therapies.com

AWHONN's Lifelines
2000 L St., NW, Suite 740
Washington, DC 20036
(202) 261-2400
http://www.awhonn.org

Birth: Issues in Prenatal Care and Education
(Formerly Birth and Family Journal)
Blackwell Scientific Publications, Inc.
3 Cambridge Center, Suite 208
Cambridge, MA 02142
(617) 876-7000

Bookmarks
(Complimentary annotated catalog of book reviews)
ICEA Supplies Center
P.O. Box 20048
Minneapolis, MN 55420

Canadian Nurse
The Canadian Nurses Association
50 The Driveway
Ottawa, Canada K2P1E2

The Female Patient
Division Excerpta Medica
301 Gibraltar Dr.
P.O. Box 528
Morris Plains, NJ 07950

Journal of Nurse-Midwifery
Elsevier Science, Inc.
655 Avenue of the Americas
New York, NY 10010
(212) 989-5800

Journal of Obstetric, Gynecologic, and Neonatal Nursing (JOGNN)
J.B. Lippincott Co.
12107 Insurance Way
Hagerstown, MD 21740

Journal of Perinatal and Neonatal Nursing
Aspen Publishers, Inc.
7201 McKinney Circle
Frederick, MD 21701
(800) 234-1660

Maternal/Newborn Advocate
The National Foundation/March of Dimes
P.O. Box 2000
White Plains, NY 10602

MCN The American Journal of Maternal Child Nursing
555 W. 57th St.
New York, NY 10019

Mother-Baby Journal/Neonatal Network
1410 Neotomas Ave., Suite 107
Santa Rosa, CA 95405
(707) 569-1415
www.neonatalnetwork.com

Nurse Practitioner: A Journal of Primary Nursing Care
3845 42nd Ave., NE
Seattle, WA 98105

Nursing Research
555 W. 57th St.
New York, NY 10019

Women's Health Issues
The Jacob's Institute for Women's Health
409 12th St., SW
Washington, DC 20024
(888) 4ES-INFO

NURSING ORGANIZATIONS

American College of Nurse Midwives
818 Connecticut Ave., NW, Suite 900
Washington, DC 20006
(202) 728-9860
http://www.midwife.org

American Holistic Nurses' Association
P.O. Box 2130
Flagstaff, AZ 86003
http://www.ahna.org

American Nurses Association
600 Maryland Ave., SW
Suite 100 W
Washington, DC 20024
(800) 274-4262
http://www.ana.org

The Association of Women's Health, Obstetric, and Neonatal Nurses (AWHONN)
2000 L St., NW, Suite 740
Washington, DC 20036
(800) 673-8499 (United States)
(800) 245-0231 (Canada)
http://www.awhonn.org

Canadian Nurses Association
50 The Driveway
Ottawa, Ontario K2P 1E2
(613) 237-2133
http://www.cna-nurses.ca

Midwives Alliance of North America
United States and Canada
c/o Concord Midwifery Service
30 South Main St.
Concord, NH 03301
(603) 225-9586

National Association of Neonatal Nurses (NAAN)
701 Lee St., Suite 450
Des Plaines, IL 60016
(800) 451-3795
http://www.nann.org

National League for Nursing (NLN)
61 Broadway
New York, NY 10006
(800) 669-9656
http://www.nln.org

National Perinatal Association
3500 E. Fletcher Ave., Suite 205
Tampa, FL 33613
(813) 971-1008

HUMAN MILK BANKING ASSOCIATION OF NORTH AMERICA (HMBANA) MEMBER BANKS

HMBANA Executive Office
P.O. Box 370464
West Hartford, CT 06137-0464
(860) 232-8809

Community Human Milk Bank
Georgetown University Hospital
Washington, DC 20007
(202) 784-2177

Lactation Support Service
British Columbia Children's Hospital
Vancouver, British Columbia, Canada V6H 3V4
(604) 875-2345, ext. 7607

Mothers' Milk Bank
Medical Center of Delaware
Wilmington, DE 19579
(302) 733-2340

Mothers' Milk Bank
Central Baptist Hospital
Lexington, KY 40503
(606) 275-6502

Mothers' Milk Bank
Presbyterian/St. Luke's Medical Center
Denver, CO 80218
(303) 869-1888

Mothers' Milk Bank
Valley Medical Center
San Jose, CA 95128
(408) 998-4550

Regional Milk Bank
The Medical Center of Central Massachusetts
Worcester, MA 01605
(508) 793-6005

Triangle Mothers' Milk Bank
Wake Medical Center
Raleigh, NC 27610
(919) 250-8599

Glossary

http://evolve.elsevier.com/Lowdermilk/MatWmnHlth/

abdominal Belonging or relating to the abdomen and its functions and disorders.

a. birth Birth of a child through a surgical incision made into the abdominal wall and uterus; cesarean birth.

a. gestation Implantation of a fertilized ovum outside the uterus but inside the peritoneal cavity.

ABO incompatibility Hemolytic disease that occurs when the mother's blood type is O and the newborn's is A, B, or AB.

abortion Termination of pregnancy before the fetus is viable and capable of extrauterine existence, usually less than 20 weeks of gestation (or when the fetus weighs less than 500 g); miscarriage.

complete a. Abortion in which fetus and all related tissue have been expelled from the uterus.

elective a. Termination of pregnancy chosen by the woman that is not required for her physical safety.

habitual (recurrent) a. Loss of three or more successive pregnancies for no known cause.

incomplete a. Loss of pregnancy in which some but not all the products of conception have been expelled from the uterus.

induced a. Intentionally produced loss of pregnancy by woman or others.

inevitable a. Threatened loss of pregnancy that cannot be prevented or stopped and is imminent.

missed a. Loss of pregnancy in which the products of conception remain in the uterus after the fetus dies.

septic a. Loss of pregnancy in which there is an infection of the products of conception and the uterine endometrial lining, usually resulting from attempted termination of early pregnancy.

spontaneous a. Loss of pregnancy that occurs naturally without interference or known cause; preferred term is *miscarriage.*

therapeutic a. Pregnancy that has been intentionally terminated for medical reasons.

threatened a. Possible loss of a pregnancy; early symptoms are present (e.g., the cervix begins to dilate).

abruptio placentae Partial or complete premature separation of a normally implanted placenta.

abstinence Refraining from sexual intercourse periodically or permanently.

access to care Opportunity to receive health care services.

accreta, placenta See *placenta accreta.*

acid mantle Covering of skin formed by uppermost horny layer of epidermis, sweat, superficial fat, metabolic products, and external substances.

acidosis Increase in hydrogen ion concentration resulting in a lowering of blood pH below 7.35.

acini cells Milk-producing cells in the breast.

acme Highest point (e.g., of a contraction).

acoustic stimulation test Antepartum test to elicit fetal heart rate response to sound; performed by applying sound source (laryngeal stimulator) to maternal abdomen over the fetal head.

acquaintance Process used by parents to get to know or become familiar with their new infant; an important step in attachment.

acrocyanosis Peripheral cyanosis; blue color of hands and feet in most infants at birth that may persist for 7 to 10 days.

acromion Projection of the spine of the scapula (forming the point of the shoulder); used to explain the presentation of the fetus.

active phase Phase in first stage of labor from 4 to 7 cm dilation.

acupressure Massage technique applied to specific points along certain energy pathways of the body called meridians. A form of treatment based in the theories of traditional Chinese medicine.

acupuncture A form of treatment using slender needles to stimulate points along energy pathways to correct, enhance, and rebalance the flow of body energy.

adequate intakes (AIs) Recommended nutrient intakes estimated to meet the needs of almost all healthy people in the population. They are provided for nutrients or age-group categories where the available information is not sufficient to warrant establishing recommended dietary allowances.

adnexa Adjacent or accessory parts of a structure.

uterine a. Ovaries and uterine (fallopian) tubes.

adolescence That period of an individual's transformation from a child to an adult.

adult respiratory distress syndrome (ARDS) Set of symptoms including decreased compliance of lung tissue, pulmonary edema, and acute hypoxemia. The condition is similar to respiratory distress syndrome of the newborn.

afibrinogenemia Absence or decrease of fibrinogen in the blood such that the blood will not coagulate. In obstetrics, this condition occurs from complications of abruptio placentae or retention of a dead fetus.

afterbirth Lay term for the placenta and membranes expelled after the birth of the child.

afterbirth pains (afterpains) Painful uterine cramps that occur intermittently for approximately 2 or 3 days after birth and that result from contractile efforts of the uterus to return to its normal involuted condition.

afterload Ventricular wall tension during systole, or the resistance the blood meets as blood is ejected from the ventricles.

AGA Appropriate (growth) for gestational age.

agenesis Failure of an organ to develop.

agonist-antagonist compounds An *agonist* is an agent that activates something; an *antagonist* is an agent that blocks something.

albuminuria Presence of readily detectable amounts of albumin in the urine.

alkalosis Abnormal condition of body fluids characterized by a tendency toward an increased pH, such as from an excess of alkaline bicarbonate or a deficiency of acid.

allopathic, standard, or Western medicine Interchangeable terms used to describe the current U.S. health care system. With foundations in germ theory and reductionism, standard medical practice often focuses on one body system or disease complex. Treatments are often pharmaceutical or surgical and produce effects that are different from those of the disease complex.

alpha-fetoprotein (AFP) Fetal antigen; elevated levels in amniotic fluid are associated with neural tube defects.

alternative and complementary therapies Nontraditional approaches to health care and healing, often philosophically different from Western medicine. Often involve interventions that are said to induce healing from within the client or improve the internal environment so that the body, mind, or spirit can heal. Often referred to as "natural healing." Might be used in place of or in conjunction with standard health care practices. Also defined as therapeutic modalities not commonly taught by U.S. medical schools or available in U.S. hospitals. *Alternative therapy* often refers to those modalities used in place of conventional (or other) health care. *Complementary therapy* refers to those modalities used in conjunction with conventional (or other) health care. Many therapies can be either alternative or complementary.

amenorrhea Absence or suppression of menstruation.

amniocentesis Procedure in which a needle is inserted through the abdominal and uterine walls into the amniotic fluid; some fluid is withdrawn; used for assessment of fetal health and maturity.

amnioinfusion Infusion of normal saline warmed to body temperature through an intrauterine catheter into the uterine cavity in an attempt to increase the fluid around the umbilical cord and prevent compression during uterine contractions.

amnion Inner membrane of two fetal membranes that form the sac and contain the fetus and the fluid that surrounds it in utero.

amnionitis Inflammation of the amnion, occurring most frequently after early rupture of membranes.

amniotic Pertaining or relating to the amnion.

a. fluid Fluid surrounding fetus derived primarily from maternal serum and fetal urine.

a. fluid embolism Embolism resulting from amniotic fluid entering the maternal bloodstream during labor and birth after rupture of membranes; this is often fatal to the woman if it is a pulmonary embolism.

a. fluid index (AFI) Estimation of amount of amniotic fluid by means of ultrasound to determine excess or decrease.

a. sac Membrane "bag" that contains the fetus and fluid before birth.

amniotomy Artificial rupture of the fetal membranes (AROM), using a plastic Amnihook or surgical clamp.

analgesia Absence of pain without loss of consciousness.

analgesic Any medication or agent that relieves pain.

anaphylaxis Immediate hypersensitivity reaction characterized by local reactions such as urticaria or by systemic reactions; may be fatal.

android pelvis Male type of pelvis; heart-shaped inlet.

anencephaly Congenital deformity characterized by the absence of cerebrum, cerebellum, and flat bones of skull.

anesthesia Partial or complete absence of sensation with or without loss of consciousness.

aneuploidy Having an abnormal number of chromosomes.

announcement phase The first developmental task experienced by expectant fathers as identified by May. During this phase the expectant father accepts the biologic fact of pregnancy.

anomaly Organ or structure that is malformed or in some way abnormal with reference to form, structure, or position.

anovulatory Failure of the ovaries to produce, mature, or release eggs.

anoxia Absence of oxygen.

antenatal Occurring before or formed before birth (newborn).

a. glucocorticoids Medications given 24 hours before a preterm birth between 24 and 34 weeks of gestation to accelerate fetal lung maturation.

antepartal Before labor (maternal).

anthropoid pelvis Pelvis in which the anteroposterior diameter is equal to or greater than the transverse diameter; oval inlet.

antibody Specific protein substance made by the body that exerts restrictive or destructive action on specific antigens, such as bacteria, toxins, or Rh factor.

anticipatory grief Grief that predates the loss of a beloved object.

antigen Protein foreign to the body that causes the body to develop antibodies (e.g., bacteria, dust, Rh factor).

Apgar score Numeric expression of the condition of a newborn obtained by rapid assessment at 1 and 5 minutes of age; developed by Dr. Virginia Apgar.

apnea Cessation of respirations for more than 15 seconds associated with generalized cyanosis.

Apt test Differentiation of maternal and fetal blood when there is vaginal bleeding. It is performed as follows: Add 0.5 ml of blood to 4.5 ml of distilled water. Shake. Add 1 ml of 0.25 N sodium hydroxide. Fetal and cord blood remain pink for 1 or 2 minutes. Maternal blood becomes brown in 30 seconds.

areola Pigmented ring of tissue surrounding the nipple.

secondary a. During the fifth month of pregnancy, a second faint ring of pigmentation seen around the original areola.

arterial pressure catheter A Teflon intravenous catheter, usually 20 gauge, that is placed in an artery and connected to a hemodynamic monitor by means of a pressure line to provide continuous measurements of the systolic, diastolic, and mean arterial blood pressures.

arteriolar vasospasm Diameter of arteriolar vessels diminishes, impeding blood flow to all organs and raising blood pressure.

Asherman's syndrome Intrauterine adhesions after inflammation and infection; one cause of impaired fertility.

asphyxia Decreased oxygen with or without excess of carbon dioxide in the body.

perinatal a. Condition occurring in utero with the following biochemical changes: hypoxemia (lowering of PO_2), hypercapnia (increase in PCO_2), and respiratory and metabolic acidosis (reduction of blood pH).

aspiration pneumonia Inflammatory condition of the lungs and bronchi caused by the inhalation of vomitus containing acid gastric contents.

assisted reproductive therapies (ARTs) Treatments for infertility, including in vitro fertilization procedures, embryo adoption, embryo hosting, and therapeutic insemination.

asynclitism Oblique presentation of the fetal head at the superior strait of the pelvis; the pelvic planes and those of the fetal head are not parallel.

ataractics Drugs capable of promoting tranquility; a tranquilizer.

atelectasis Pulmonary pathosis involving alveolar collapse.

atony Absence of muscle tone.

atresia Absence of a normally present passageway.

biliary a. Absence of the bile duct.

choanal a. Complete obstruction of the posterior nares, which open into the nasopharynx, with membranous or bony tissue.

esophageal a. Congenital anomaly in which the esophagus ends in a blind pouch or narrows into a thin cord, thus failing to form a continuous passageway to the stomach.

attachment A specific and enduring affective tie to another person.

attitude Body posture or position.

fetal a. Relation of fetal parts to each other in the uterus (e.g., all parts flexed, all parts flexed except neck is extended).

augmentation of labor Stimulation of ineffective uterine contractions after labor has started spontaneously but is not progressing satisfactorily.

autoimmune disorders Body produces antibodies against itself, causing tissue damage.

autoimmunization Development of antibodies against constituents of one's own tissues (e.g., a man may develop antibodies against his own sperm).

autolysis "Self-digestive" process by which the uterus returns to a nonpregnant state after childbirth. The decrease in estrogen and progesterone levels after childbirth results in this destruction of excess hypertrophied uterine tissue.

autosomal inheritance Characteristics transmitted by genes on the autosomes, not the sex chromosomes.

autosomes Any of the paired chromosomes other than the sex (X and Y) chromosomes.

azoospermia Absence of sperm in the semen.

bacteremic shock Shock that occurs in septicemia when endotoxins are released from certain bacteria into the bloodstream.

bag of waters Lay term for the sac containing amniotic fluid and fetus.

ballottement (1) Movability of a floating object, such as a fetus. (2) Diagnostic technique using palpation: a floating object, when tapped or pushed, moves away and then returns to touch the examiner's hand.

Bandl's ring Abnormally thickened ridge of uterine musculature between the upper and lower segments that occurs after a mechanically obstructed labor, with the lower segment thinning abnormally.

barotrauma Tissue damage caused by pressure, often applied to the lungs.

Bartholin's glands Two small glands situated on either side of the vaginal orifice that secrete small amounts of mucus during coitus and that are homologous to the bulbourethral glands in the male.
basal body temperature Lowest body temperature of a healthy person taken immediately after awakening and before getting out of bed.
basalis, decidua See *decidua basalis.*
bearing-down effort "Secondary powers"; energy exerted by the woman during contractions to push out the baby.
behavioral assessment Assessment of activity, feeding and sleeping patterns, and responsiveness.
behavioral repertoire A set of behaviors (actions and reactions) that both parent and infant use to facilitate interactions.
Bell's palsy See *palsy, Bell's.*
bereavement The feelings of loss, pain, desolation, and sadness that occur after the death of a loved one.
best practice A program or service that has been recognized for excellence.
bicornuate uterus Anomalous uterus that may be either a double or single organ with two horns.
biliary atresia See *atresia, biliary.*
bilirubin Yellow or orange pigment that is a breakdown product of hemoglobin. It is carried by the blood to the liver, where it is chemically changed and excreted into the bile or is conjugated and excreted by the kidneys.
Billings method See *ovulation method.*
bimanual Performed with both hands.
  b. palpation Examination of a woman's pelvic organs done by placement of one hand on the abdomen and one or two fingers of the other hand into the vagina.
biofeedback Technique that teaches the client to consciously control certain body functions usually thought of as unconscious (e.g., breathing, heart rate). Often involves electronic instrumentation that provides immediate visual and auditory feedback to assist the learning process.
biophysical profile (BPP) Noninvasive assessment of the fetus and its environment using ultrasonography and uterine fetal monitoring; includes fetal breathing movements, gross body movements, fetal tone, reactive fetal heart rate, and qualitative amniotic fluid volume.
biopsy Removal of a small piece of tissue for microscopic examination and diagnosis.
biorhythmicity Cyclic changes that occur with established regularity, such as sleeping and eating patterns.
biparietal diameter Largest transverse diameter of the fetal head; extends from one parietal bone to the other.
bipolar disorders Depression with previous or current manic episodes.
birth plan A tool by which parents can explore their childbirth options and choose those that are most important to them.
birth rate Number of live births per 1000 population per year. See also *fertility.*
Bishop score Rating system to evaluate inducibility of the cervix; a higher score increases the rate of successful induction of labor.
bittersweet grief The resurgence of feelings and emotions that occur on remembering a loved one after the bereavement process has lessened.
blastocyst Stage in the development of a mammalian embryo, occurring after the morula stage, that consists of an outer layer, or trophoblast, and a hollow sphere of cells enclosing a cavity.
blended family Family form that includes stepparents and stepchildren.
bloody show Vaginal discharge that originates in the cervix and consists of blood and mucus; increases as cervix dilates during labor.
body boundaries Boundaries that serve to separate the self from the nonself and provide a feeling of safety.
body image Person's subjective concept of his or her physical appearance.
bonding A process by which parents, over time, form an emotional relationship with their infant.
Bradley method Husband-coached childbirth using labor breathing techniques.
Braxton Hicks sign Mild, intermittent, painless uterine contractions that occur during pregnancy. These contractions occur more frequently as pregnancy advances but do not represent true labor.
Brazelton assessment Method for assessing the interactional behavior of a newborn.
breakthrough bleeding Escape of blood occurring between menstrual periods; may be noted by women using chemical contraception (birth control pills).
breast self-examination (BSE) Self-examination of the breasts.
breast shells Rigid plastic cups that are worn inside a bra to put pressure on the areola to help a nipple protrude or to protect sore nipples from the pressure of clothing.
breech presentation Presentation in which buttocks or feet are nearest the cervical opening and are born first; occurs in approximately 3% of all births.
  complete b.p. Simultaneous presentation of buttocks, legs, and feet.
  footling (incomplete) b.p. Presentation of one or both feet.
  frank b.p. Presentation of buttocks, with hips flexed so that thighs are against abdomen.
bregma Point of junction of the coronal and sagittal sutures of the skull; the area of the anterior fontanel of the fetus.
brim Edge of the superior strait of the true pelvis; the inlet.
bronchopulmonary dysplasia (BPD) Pulmonary condition affecting preterm infants who have experienced respiratory failure and have been oxygen dependent for more than 28 days.
brown fat Source of heat unique to neonates that is capable of greater thermogenic activity than ordinary fat.

Deposits are found around the adrenals, kidneys, and neck, between the scapulas, and behind the sternum for several weeks after birth.

bruit, uterine See *uterine bruit.*

calendar method See *rhythm method.*

Candida vaginitis Vaginal, fungal infection; formerly called *moniliasis.*

candidiasis Infection of the skin or mucous membrane by a yeastlike fungus, *Candida albicans*; see *thrush.*

capacitation Enzymatic process resulting in removal of plasma protein over acrosome of sperm; prerequisite for sperm to fertilize an ovum.

capillary hydrostatic pressure Pressure in the arterial capillary system to promote the movement of fluid across the semipermeable membrane of the capillary wall from the vessel into the interstitial space. Measured as the pulmonary capillary wedge pressure (PCWP).

capsularis, decidua See *decidua capsularis.*

caput Occiput of fetal head appearing at the vaginal introitus preceding birth of the head.

c. succedaneum Swelling of the tissue over the presenting part of the fetal head caused by pressure during labor.

carcinoma Malignant, often metastatic epithelial neoplasm; cancer.

cardiac decompensation A condition of heart failure in which the heart is unable to maintain a sufficient cardiac output.

cardiac output (CO) Volume of blood ejected from the left ventricle in 1 minute, measured in liters per minute. Cardiac output is the product of stroke volume and heart rate ($CO = HR \times SV$).

cardinal movements of labor The mechanism of labor in a vertex presentation; includes engagement, descent, flexion, internal rotation, extension, external rotation (restitution), and expulsion.

carpal tunnel syndrome Pressure on the median nerve at the point at which it goes through the carpal tunnel of the wrist. It causes soreness, tenderness, and weakness of the muscles of the thumb.

carrier Individual who carries a gene that does not exhibit itself in physical or chemical characteristics but that can be transmitted to children (e.g., a female carrying the trait for hemophilia, which is expressed in male offspring).

caul Hood of fetal membranes covering fetal head during birth.

cephalhematoma NOTE: This is spelled *cephalohematoma* in some sources. Extravasation of blood from ruptured vessels between a skull bone and its external covering, the periosteum. Swelling is limited by the margins of the cranial bone affected (usually parietals).

cephalic Pertaining to the head.

c. presentation Presentation of the fetal head.

cephalocaudal development Principle of maturation that development progresses from the head to tail (rump).

cephalopelvic disproportion (CPD) Condition in which the infant's head is of such a shape, size, or position that it cannot pass through the mother's pelvis; can also be caused by maternal pelvic problems.

cerclage Use of nonabsorbable suture to keep a premature dilating cervix closed; released when pregnancy is at term to allow labor to begin.

cervical cap Individually fitted contraceptive barrier for the cervix.

cervical cauterization Destruction (usually by heat or electric current) of the superficial tissue of the cervix.

cervical conization Excision of a cone-shaped section of tissue from the endocervix.

cervical funneling Effacement of the internal cervical os.

cervical intraepithelial neoplasm (CIN) Uncontrolled and progressive abnormal growth of cervical epithelial cells.

cervical mucus method See *ovulation method.*

cervical os "Mouth" or opening to the cervix.

cervical ripening Process of effecting physical softening and distensibility of the cervix in preparation for labor and birth

cervicitis Cervical infection.

cervix Lowest and narrow end of the uterus; the "neck." The cervix is situated between the external os and the body, or corpus, of the uterus, and its lower end extends into the vagina.

cesarean birth Birth of a fetus by an incision through the abdominal wall and uterus.

cesarean hysterectomy Removal of the uterus immediately after the cesarean birth of an infant.

Chadwick's sign Violet color of vaginal mucous membrane that is visible from about the fourth week of pregnancy; caused by increased vascularity.

chloasma Increased pigmentation over bridge of nose and cheeks of pregnant women and some women taking oral contraceptives; also known as *mask of pregnancy.*

choanal atresia See *atresia, choanal.*

cholecystitis Acute or chronic inflammation of the gallbladder.

cholelithiasis Presence of gallstones in the gallbladder.

choreoathetoid cerebral palsy Condition characterized by both choreiform (jerky, ticlike, twitching) and athetoid (slow, writhing) movements.

chorioamnionitis Inflammatory reaction in fetal membranes to bacteria or viruses in the amniotic fluid, which then become infiltrated with polymorphonuclear leukocytes.

chorion Fetal membrane closest to the intrauterine wall that gives rise to the placenta and continues as the outer membrane surrounding the amnion.

chorionic villus (villi) Tiny vascular protrusions on the chorionic surface that project into the maternal blood sinuses of the uterus and that help form the placenta and secrete human chorionic gonadotropin.

chorionic villus sampling (CVS) Removal of fetal tissue from placenta for genetic diagnostic studies.

chromosome Element within the cell nucleus carrying genes and composed of DNA and proteins.

circumcision

female c. Religious or cultural removal of a portion of the clitoris and labia; practiced in some Third World countries but illegal in the United States. Mutilating procedure that can cause problems in childbirth.

male c. Excision of the prepuce (foreskin) of the penis, exposing the glans; may be done for religious or cultural reasons.

claiming process Process by which the parents identify their new baby in terms of likeness to other family members, differences, and uniqueness.

cleft lip Incomplete closure of the lip. Lay term used is harelip.

cleft palate Incomplete closure of the palate or roof of mouth; a congenital fissure.

climacteric The period of a woman's life when she is passing from a reproductive to a nonreproductive state, with regression of ovarian function. The cycle of endocrine, physical, and psychosocial changes that occurs during the termination of the reproductive years. Also called climacterium.

clinical benchmark Process used to compare one's own performance against the performance of the best in an area of service.

clitoris Female organ analogous to male penis; a small, ovid body of erectile tissue situated at the anterior junction of the vulva.

clonus (ankle) Spasmodic alternation of muscular contraction and relaxation; counted in beats.

clubfoot Congenital deformity in which portions of the foot and ankle are twisted out of a normal position.

coitus Penile-vaginal intercourse.

c. interruptus Intercourse during which penis is withdrawn from vagina before ejaculation.

cold stress Excessive loss of heat that results in increased respirations and nonshivering thermogenesis to maintain core body temperature.

colloid osmotic pressure (COP) Pressure in the arterial capillary system to prevent the movement of fluid across the semipermeable membrane of the capillary wall from the vessel into the interstitial space. The COP measures the "pulling" pressure of proteins in the plasma to retain fluid inside the vessel.

colostrum The fluid in the breast from pregnancy into the early postpartal period. It is rich in antibodies, which provide protection from many diseases; high in protein, which binds bilirubin; and laxative acting, which speeds the elimination of meconium and helps loosen mucus.

colporrhaphy Procedure of suturing the vagina for the purpose of narrowing the vagina, as in anterior or posterior vaginal repair surgery.

colposcopy Examination of vagina and cervix with a colposcope to identify neoplastic or other changes.

complement Naturally occurring blood component that is a factor in the destruction of bacteria.

complete abortion See *abortion, complete.*

complete breech presentation See *breech presentation, complete.*

complicated bereavement The persistent feelings of anger, guilt, loss, pain, and sadness over time that lead to feelings of hopelessness, helplessness, and diminishing self-worth. Signs and symptoms of clinical depression, which is different from the normal depression of bereavement.

conception Union of the sperm and ovum resulting in fertilization; formation of the one-celled zygote.

conceptional age In fetal development the number of completed weeks since the moment of conception. Because the moment of conception is almost impossible to determine, conceptional age is estimated at 2 weeks less than gestational age.

conceptus Embryo or fetus, fetal membranes, amniotic fluid, and the fetal portion of the placenta.

condom Mechanical barrier worn on the penis for contraception or to protect against STIs; a "rubber."

condyloma acuminatum (plural condylomata acuminata) Wartlike growth on the skin usually seen near the anus or external genitals caused by human papillomavirus (HPV); genital warts. (Must be differentiated from condyloma latum seen in secondary syphilis.)

congenital Present or existing before birth as a result of either hereditary or prenatal environmental factors.

congenital rubella syndrome Complex of problems, including hearing defects, cardiovascular abnormalities, and cataracts, caused by maternal rubella in the first trimester of pregnancy.

conjoined twins See *twins, conjoined.*

conjugate

diagonal c. Radiographic measurement of distance from inferior border of symphysis pubis to sacral promontory; may be obtained by vaginal examination; 12.5 to 13 cm.

true c. (conjugata vera) Radiographic measurement of distance from upper margin of symphysis pubis to sacral promontory; 1.5 to 2 cm less than diagonal conjugate.

conjunctivitis Inflammation of the mucous membrane that lines the eyelids and is reflected onto the eyeball.

conscious relaxation Technique used to release the mind and body from tension through conscious effort and practice.

contraception Prevention of impregnation or conception.

contractility Force and velocity of ventricular contractions when preload and afterload are held constant.

contraction ring See *Bandl's ring.*

contractions

duration Period from the beginning of the contraction to the end.

frequency How often the contractions occur–the period from the beginning of one contraction to the beginning of the next.

intensity Strength of the contraction at its peak.

interval Period between uterine contractions, timed from the end of one contraction to the beginning of the next.

resting tone The tension in the uterine muscle between contractions.

contraction stress test (CST) Test to stimulate uterine contractions for the purpose of assessing fetal response; a healthy fetus does not react to contractions, whereas a compromised fetus demonstrates late decelerations in the fetal heart rate that are indicative of uteroplacental insufficiency.

Coombs' test Indirect: determination of Rh-positive antibodies in maternal blood; direct: determination of maternal Rh-positive antibodies in fetal cord blood. A positive test result indicates the presence of antibodies or titer.

coping mechanism Any effort directed at stress management. It can be task oriented and involve direct problem-solving efforts to cope with the threat itself or be intrapsychic or ego-defense oriented with the goal of regulating one's emotional distress.

copulation Coitus; sexual intercourse.

corpus luteum Yellow body. After rupture of the graafian follicle at ovulation, the follicle develops into a yellow structure that secretes progesterone and some estrogen in the second half of the menstrual cycle, atrophying about 3 days before sloughing of the endometrium in menstrual flow. If impregnation occurs, it continues to produce the hormones until the placenta can take over this function.

cotyledon One of the 15 to 28 visible segments of the placenta on the maternal surface, each made up of fetal vessels, chorionic villi, and an intervillous space.

counterpressure Pressure to sacral area of back during uterine contractions.

couplet care One nurse, educated in both mother and infant care, functions as the primary nurse for both mother and infant (also known as mother-baby care or single-room maternity care).

Couvade syndrome The phenomenon of expectant fathers' experiencing pregnancy-like symptoms.

Couvelaire uterus See *uterus, Couvelaire.*

CPAP Continuous positive airway pressure.

cradle cap Common seborrheic dermatitis of infants consisting of thick, yellow, greasy scales on the scalp.

craniotabes Localized softening of cranial bones.

creatinine Substance found in blood and muscle; measurement of levels in maternal urine correlates with amount of fetal muscle mass and therefore fetal size.

crib death Unexpected and sudden death of an apparently normal and healthy infant that occurs during sleep and with no physical or autopsic evidence of disease. Also referred to as *sudden infant death syndrome (SIDS).*

cri-du-chat syndrome Rare congenital disorder recognized at birth by a kitten-like cry, which may prevail for weeks and then disappear. Other characteristics include low birth weight, microcephaly, "moon face," wide-set eyes, strabismus, and low-set misshapen ears. Infants are hypotonic; heart defects and mental and physical retardation are common. Also called *cat-cry syndrome.*

critical path The exact timing of all key incidents that must occur to achieve the standard outcomes within the diagnosis related group (DRG)–specific length of stay.

crowning Stage of birth when the top of the fetal head can be seen at the vaginal orifice as the widest part of the head distends the vulva.

cryosurgery Local freezing and removal of tissue without injury to adjacent tissue and with minimum blood loss, done with special equipment.

cryptorchidism Failure of one or both of the testicles to descend into the scrotum. Also called undescended testis.

cul-de-sac of Douglas Pouch formed by a fold of the peritoneum dipping down between the anterior wall of the rectum and the posterior wall of the uterus; also called *Douglas's cul-de-sac, pouch of Douglas,* and *rectouterine pouch.*

culdocentesis Puncture of cul-de-sac of Douglas through the vagina for aspiration of fluid.

Cullen's sign Faint, irregularly formed, hemorrhagic patches on the skin around the umbilicus. The discolored skin is blue-black and becomes greenish brown or yellow. Cullen's sign may appear 1 to 2 days after the onset of anorexia and the severe, poorly localized abdominal pains characteristic of acute pancreatitis. Cullen's sign is also present in massive upper gastrointestinal hemorrhage and ruptured ectopic pregnancy.

cultural context Setting in which one considers the individual's and the family's beliefs and practices (culture).

curettage (curet or curette) Scraping of the endometrium lining of the uterus with a curet to remove the contents of the uterus (as is done after an incomplete miscarriage or induced abortion) or to obtain specimens for diagnostic purposes.

cycle of violence Pattern of three phases: period of increasing tension, the abusive episode, and a period of contrition and kindness.

cystocele Bladder hernia: injury to the vesicovaginal fascia during labor and birth may allow herniation of the bladder into the vagina.

cytology Study of cells, including their formation, origin, structure, function, biochemical activities, and pathology.

daily fetal movement counts (DFMCs) Maternal assessment of fetal activity; the number of fetal movements within a specific time are counted.

death Cessation of life.
fetal d. Intrauterine death; death of a fetus weighing 500 g or more of 20 weeks of gestation or more.
infant d. Death during the first year of life.
maternal d. Death of a woman as a result of a pregnancy or birth-related problem.
neonatal d. Death of a newborn within the first 28 days after birth.
perinatal d. Death of a fetus of 20 weeks of gestation or older or death of a neonate 28 days old or younger.

decidua Mucous membrane, lining of uterus, or endometrium of pregnancy that is shed after giving birth.
d. basalis Maternal aspect of the placenta made up of uterine blood vessels, endometrial stroma, and glands. It is shed in lochial discharge after delivery.
d. capsularis That part of the decidual membranes surrounding the chorionic sac.
d. vera Nonplacental decidual lining of the uterus.

decrement Decrease or stage of decline, as of a contraction.

deep tendon reflexes (DTRs) Reflex caused by stimulation of tendons, such as elbow, wrist, knee, triceps, and ankle jerk reflexes.

delivery (birth) Expulsion of the child with placenta and membranes by the mother or their extraction by the obstetric practitioner.
abdominal d. See *abdominal birth.*

ΔOD_{450} (delta OD_{450}) Delta optical density (or absorbance) at 450 nm, obtained by spectral analysis of amniotic fluid. This prenatal test is used to measure the degree of hemolytic activity in the fetus and to evaluate fetal status in women sensitized to the Rh factor.

demand feeding Feeding a newborn every third hour or when the baby cries to be fed, whichever comes first.

deoxyribonucleic acid (DNA) Intracellular complex protein that carries genetic information, consisting of two purines (adenine and guanine) and two pyrimidines (thymine and cytosine).

depression An intense and pervasive sadness with severe and labile mood swings.

depressive reactions Depression related to the postpartum period including postpartum blues, postpartum nonpsychotic depression, and postpartum psychosis.

DES Diethylstilbestrol; female fetus is predisposed to reproductive tract malformations and (later) dysplasia if her mother ingested this medication during pregnancy.

desquamation Shedding of epithelial cells of the skin and mucous membranes.

developmental crisis Severe, usually transient, stress that occurs when a person is unable to complete the tasks of a psychosocial stage of development and is therefore unable to move on to the next stage.

developmental task Physical or cognitive skill that a person must accomplish during a particular age period to continue developing, such as walking, which precedes the development of the sense of autonomy in the toddler period.

developmental theory Theoretic approach for viewing the family. The developmental perspective sees family members pass through phases of growth from dependence through active independence to interdependence.

diabetes mellitus Systemic disorder of carbohydrate, protein, and fat metabolism; caused by deficient insulin production or ineffective use of insulin at the cellular level.

diaphragmatic hernia Congenital malformation of diaphragm that allows displacement of the abdominal organs into the thoracic cavity.

diastasis recti abdominis Separation of the two rectus muscles along the median line of the abdominal wall. This is often seen in women with repeated childbirths or with a multiple gestation (e.g., triplets). In the newborn it is usually attributable to incomplete development.

Dick-Read method An approach to childbirth based on the premise that fear of pain produces muscular tension, producing pain and greater fear. The method includes teaching physiologic processes of labor, exercise to improve muscle tone, and techniques to assist in relaxation and prevent the fear-tension-pain mechanism.

dietary reference intakes (DRIs) New nutritional recommendations being prepared for the United States, consisting of the recommended dietary allowances, adequate intakes, and tolerable upper intake levels, the upper limit of intake associated with low risk in almost all members of a population.

dilation and curettage (D&C) Vaginal procedure in which the cervical canal is stretched enough to admit passage of an instrument called a *curet* (or *curette*). The endometrium of the uterus is scraped with the curet to empty the uterine contents or to obtain tissue for examination.

dilation of cervix Stretching of the external os from an opening a few millimeters in size to an opening large enough to allow the passage of the infant.

diploid number Having two sets of chromosomes; found normally in somatic (body) cells; 23 sets or 46 chromosomes.

discordance Discrepancy in size (or other indicator) between twins.

disorganization A dimension of bereavement characterized by depression, anorexia, difficulty in concentration, and a generalized feeling of not feeling good about oneself physically and emotionally.

disparate twins See *twins, disparate.*

disseminated intravascular coagulation (DIC) Pathologic form of coagulation in which clotting factors are consumed to such an extent that generalized bleeding can occur; associated with abruptio placentae, eclampsia, intrauterine fetal demise, amniotic fluid embolism, and hemorrhage.

dizygotic Related to or proceeding from two zygotes (fertilized ova).

dizygotic twins See *twins, dizygotic.*

Döderlein's bacillus Gram-positive bacterium occurring in normal vaginal secretions.

dominant trait Gene that is expressed whenever it is present in the heterozygous gene state (e.g., brown eyes are dominant over blue).

Doppler blood flow analysis Device for measuring blood flow noninvasively in the fetus and placenta to detect intrauterine growth restriction.

Douglas's cul-de-sac See *cul-de-sac of Douglas.*

doula Experienced assistant hired to give the woman support during labor and birth.

Down syndrome Abnormality involving the occurrence of a third chromosome, rather than the normal pair (trisomy 21), that characteristically results in a typical picture of mental retardation and altered physical appearance. This condition was formerly called mongolism.

drug dependence (addiction) Physical or psychologic dependence or both on a substance.

dry labor Lay term referring to labor in which amniotic fluid has already escaped. A "dry birth" does not exist.

Dubowitz assessment Estimation of gestational age of a newborn based on criteria developed for that purpose.

ductus arteriosus In fetal circulation an anatomic shunt between the pulmonary artery and arch of the aorta. It is obliterated after birth by a rising PO_2 and a change in intravascular pressures in the presence of normal pulmonary function. It normally becomes a ligament after birth but in some instances remains patent.

ductus venosus In fetal circulation, a blood vessel carrying oxygenated blood between the umbilical vein and the inferior vena cava, bypassing the liver. It is obliterated and becomes a ligament after birth.

Duncan's mechanism Delivery of placenta with the maternal surface presenting, rather than the shiny fetal surface.

dys- Prefix meaning abnormal, difficult, painful, faulty.

dysfunctional labor Abnormal uterine contractions that prevent normal progress of cervical dilation and effacement.

dysfunctional uterine bleeding (DUB) Abnormal bleeding from the uterus for reasons that are not readily established.

dysmaturity See *intrauterine growth restriction (IUGR).*

dysmenorrhea

- **primary d.** Painful menstruation beginning 2 to 6 months after menarche, related to ovulation.
- **secondary d.** Painful menstruation related to organic disease such as endometriosis, pelvic inflammatory disease, or uterine neoplasm.

dyspareunia Painful sexual intercourse, for either sex.

dysplasia Any abnormal development of tissues or organs.

dystocia Prolonged, painful, or otherwise difficult birth because of mechanical factors produced by the passenger (the fetus) or the passage (the pelvis and soft tissues of the birth canal of the mother), inadequate powers (uterine and other muscular activity), or maternal position.

ecchymosis Bruise; bleeding into tissue caused by direct trauma, serious infection, or bleeding diathesis.

eclampsia Severe complication of pregnancy of unknown cause and occurring more often in the primigravida; characterized by tonic and clonic convulsions, coma, high blood pressure, albuminuria, and oliguria occurring during pregnancy or shortly after birth.

ectoderm Outer layer of embryonic tissue giving rise to skin, nails, and hair.

ectopic Out of normal place.

- **e. pregnancy** Implantation of the fertilized ovum outside of its normal place in the uterine cavity. Locations include the abdomen, uterine tubes, and ovaries.

edema Generalized accumulation of interstitial fluid.

- **dependent e.** Edema of lower or most dependent parts of body where hydrostatic pressure is greater.
- **pitting e.** Edema that leaves a small depression or pit when pressure is applied to a swollen area.

effacement Thinning and shortening or obliteration of the cervix that occurs during late pregnancy or labor or both.

effleurage Gentle stroking used in massage.

Eisenmenger syndrome Pulmonary hypertension characterized by elevated pulmonary vascular resistance and right-to-left (or bidirectional) shunting in either atria or ventricles.

ejaculation Sudden expulsion of semen from the male urethra.

elective abortion See *abortion, elective.*

electronic fetal monitoring (EFM) Electronic surveillance of fetal heart rate by external and internal methods.

embolus Any undissolved matter (solid, liquid, or gaseous) that is carried by the blood to another part of the body and obstructs a blood vessel.

embryo Conceptus from the second or third week of development until about the eighth week after conception, when mineralization (ossification) of the skeleton begins. This period is characterized by cellular differentiation and predominantly hyperplastic growth.

emotional lability Rapid mood changes from irritability to anger or sadness to joy and cheerfulness; often seen in the first trimester of pregnancy.

endocarditis Inflammation of the inner layer of the heart muscle (endocardium).

endocervical Pertaining to the interior of the canal of the cervix of the uterus.

endocrine glands Ductless glands that secrete hormones into the blood or lymph.

endometriosis Tissue closely resembling endometrial tissue but located outside the uterus in the pelvic cavity. Symptoms may include pelvic pain or pressure, dysmenorrhea, dyspareunia, abnormal bleeding from the uterus or rectum, and sterility.

endometritis Postpartum uterine infection, often beginning at the site of the placental implantation.
endometrium Inner lining of the uterus that undergoes changes caused by hormones during the menstrual cycle and pregnancy; decidua.
endorphins Endogenous opioids secreted by the pituitary gland that act on the central and peripheral nervous systems to reduce pain.
energy healing A variety of techniques and disciplines that are said to augment, modulate, stimulate, or remedy certain deficiencies or blocks in the human energy system.
en face Face-to-face position in which the parent's and infant's faces are approximately 20 cm apart and on the same plane.
engagement In obstetrics, the entrance of the fetal presenting part into the superior pelvic strait and the beginning of the descent through the pelvic canal.
engorgement Distention or vascular congestion. In obstetrics, the process of swelling of the breast tissue brought about by an increase in blood and lymph supply to the breast, which precedes true lactation. It lasts about 48 hours and usually reaches a peak between the third and fifth postbirth days.
engrossment A parent's absorption, preoccupation, and interest in his or her infant; term typically used to describe the father's intense involvement with his newborn.
enterocele Herniation of the peritoneum of the posterior cul-de-sac between the uterosacral ligaments into the rectovaginal septum.
entoderm Inner layer of embryonic tissue giving rise to internal organs such as the intestine.
entrainment Phenomenon observed in the microanalysis of sound films in which the speaker moves several parts of the body and the listener responds to the sounds by moving in ways that are coordinated with the rhythm of the sounds. Infants have been observed to move in time to the rhythms of adult speech but not to random noises or disconnected words or vowels. Entrainment is believed to be an essential factor in the process of maternal-infant bonding.
epicanthus Fold of skin covering the inner canthus and caruncle that extends from the root of the nose to the median end of the eyebrow; characteristically found in certain races but may occur as a congenital anomaly.
epidural block Type of regional anesthesia produced by injection of a local anesthetic into the epidural (peridural) space.
epidural blood patch A patch formed by a few millimeters of the mother's blood occluding a tear or hole in the dura mater around the spinal cord.
episiotomy Surgical incision of the perineum at the end of the second stage of labor to facilitate birth and to avoid laceration of the perineum.
epispadias Defect in which the urethral canal terminates on the dorsum of the penis or above the clitoris (rare).
Epstein's pearls Small, white blebs found along the gum margins and at the junction of the soft and hard palates. They are a normal manifestation and are typically seen in the newborn. Similar to Bohn's nodules.
epulis Tumorlike benign lesion of the gingiva seen in pregnant women.
equilibrium State of balance or rest resulting from the equal action of opposing forces, as with calcium and phosphorus in the body. In psychiatry, a state of mental or emotional balance.
Erb-Duchenne paralysis Paralysis caused by physical injury to the upper brachial plexus, occurring most often in childbirth from forcible traction during birth. The signs of Erb's paralysis include loss of sensation in the arm and paralysis and atrophy of the deltoid, the biceps, and the branchialis muscles. Also called *Erb's palsy.*
ergot Drug obtained from *Claviceps purpurea*, a fungus, which stimulates the smooth muscles of blood vessels and the uterus, causing vasoconstriction and uterine contractions.
erythema toxicum Innocuous pink papular neonatal rash of unknown cause, with superimposed vesicles appearing within 24 to 48 hours after birth and resolving spontaneously within a few days.
erythroblastosis fetalis Hemolytic disease of the newborn usually caused by isoimmunization resulting from Rh incompatibility or ABO incompatibility.
esophageal atresia See *atresia, esophageal.*
estimated date of birth (EDB) Approximate date of birth. Usually determined by calculation using Nägele's rule; "due date."
estradiol An estrogen.
estriol Major metabolite of estrogen that increases during the second half of pregnancy with an intact fetoplacental unit (normal placenta, normal fetal liver and adrenals) and normal maternal renal function.
estrogen Female sex hormone produced by the ovaries and placenta.
estrogen replacement therapy (ERT) Exogenous estrogen given to women during and after menopause to prevent hot flashes, mood changes, osteoporosis, and genitourinary symptoms.
ethics Systematic inquiry into the principles of right and wrong conduct, of virtue and vice, and of good and evil as they relate to conduct.
eutocia Normal or natural labor or birth.
evidence-based practice Practice based on analysis of research findings.
exchange transfusion Replacement of 75% to 85% of circulating blood by withdrawal of the recipient's blood and injection of a donor's blood in equal amounts, the purposes of which are to prevent an accumulation of bilirubin in the blood above a dangerous level, to prevent the accumulation of other by-products of hemolysis in hemolytic disease, and to correct anemia and acidosis.
expressive style Expectant father's strong emotional response to partner's pregnancy.

expulsive Having the tendency to drive out or expel.
e. contractions Labor contractions that are characteristic of the second stage of labor.
extended family Family form that includes the nuclear family and other blood-related persons.
external cephalic version (ECV) Turning the fetus to a vertex position by exertion of pressure on the fetus externally through the maternal abdomen.
extracorporeal membrane oxygenation (ECMO) Oxygenation of blood external to body using cardiopulmonary bypass and a membrane oxygenator. Used primarily for newborns with refractory respiratory failure or meconium aspiration syndrome.
extrauterine Occurring outside the uterus.
e. pregnancy Pregnancy in which the fertilized ovum implants itself outside the uterus.
extrusion reflex Infant automatically extends tongue when it is stimulated.
facies Pertaining to the appearance or expression of the face; certain congenital syndromes typically cause a specific facial appearance.
FAD Fetal activity determination; also called *fetal activity test (FAT).*
failure to thrive Condition in which neonate's or infant's growth and development patterns are below the norms for age.
fallopian tubes Two canals or oviducts extending laterally from each side of the uterus through which the ovum travels, after ovulation, to the uterus; also called uterine tubes.
false labor Uterine contractions that do not result in cervical dilation, are irregular, are felt more in front, often do not last more than 20 seconds, and do not become longer or stronger.
false pelvis Part of the pelvis superior to a plane passing through the linea terminalis (brim or outlet).
family dynamics Process by which family members assume varying social roles.
family functions Activities carried out within families for the well-being of family members, including biologic, economic, educational, psychologic, and sociocultural aspects.
family stress theory Theory that explains how families react and adapt to stressors that they experience.
family systems theory Theory that conceptualizes the family as a unit and focuses on observing interactions among family members.
family violence Interpersonal violence, including child, elder, sibling, and spouse.
fantasy child The imagined dream child; the "ideal" unborn child.
fantasy mom A composite of the ideal mother ("supermom") whom a woman envisions in her mind's eye but who may have enviable but totally unrealistic accomplishments to her credit.
feeding readiness cues Infant responses that indicate optimal times to begin a feeding. The baby may make mouthing motions, suck a fist, or awaken and cry.
Ferguson reflex Reflex contractions of the uterus after stimulation of the cervix.
ferning (arborization) test The appearance of a fernlike pattern found on slides of certain fluids.
ovulation f.t. Test in which cervical mucus, placed on a slide, dries in a branching pattern in the presence of high estrogen levels at the time of ovulation.
fertile period Period before and after ovulation during which the human ovum can be fertilized; usually 3 days before and 4 days after ovulation.
fertility Quality of being able to reproduce; also number of births per 1000 women ages 15 through 44 years. See also *birth rate.*
fertilization Union of an ovum and a sperm.
fetal Pertaining or relating to the fetus.
f. alcohol effect (FAE) Lesser set of the same symptoms that make up fetal alcohol syndrome.
f. alcohol syndrome (FAS) Congenital abnormality or anomaly resulting from excessive maternal alcohol intake during pregnancy. It is characterized by typical craniofacial and limb defects, cardiovascular defects, intrauterine growth restriction, and developmental delay.
f. asphyxia See *asphyxia, fetal.*
f. attitude See *attitude, fetal.*
f. compromise Evidence such as a nonreassuring fetal heart rate pattern that indicates the fetus may be in jeopardy.
f. death See *death, fetal.*
f. lie Relation of the fetal spine to the maternal spine; that is, in vertical lie, maternal and fetal spines are parallel and the fetal head or breech presents; in transverse lie, fetal spine is perpendicular to the maternal spine and the fetal shoulder presents.
f. membrane See *membrane.*
f. presentation The part of the fetus that enters the pelvic inlet first.
f. heart rate (FHR) Beats per minute of the fetal heart. Normal range is 110 to 160 beats per minute.
acceleration Increase in fetal heart rate, usually seen as a reassuring sign.
baseline Average fetal heart rate between uterine contractions.
bradycardia Baseline fetal heart rate below 110 beats per minute.
deceleration Slowing of fetal heart rate attributed to a parasympathetic response and described in relation to uterine contractions.
early d. Onset corresponding to onset of uterine contraction, related to fetal head compression.
late d. Onset after peak of contraction, continuing into interval after contraction; caused by uteroplacental insufficiency.
prolonged d. Slowing of fetal heart rate lasting longer than 2 minutes.
variable d. Onset at any time unrelated to contraction; caused by cord compression.

tachycardia Baseline fetal heart rate above 160 beats per minue.

f. scalp spiral electrode Internal signal source for electronically monitoring the fetal heart rate.

f. tobacco syndrome Diagnostic term applicable to infants who fit the following criteria: mother who smoked more than 5 cigarettes a day during pregnancy and had no prenatal evidence of hypertension; infant has symmetric growth restriction, weighs less than 2500 g, and has no other cause of intrauterine growth restriction.

fetotoxic Poisonous or destructive to the fetus.

fetus Child in utero from approximately the eighth week after conception until birth.

fibroid Fibrous, encapsulated connective tissue tumor, especially of the uterus.

fimbria Structure resembling a fringe, particularly the fringelike end of the uterine tube.

first stage Stage of labor from the onset of regular uterine contractions to full dilation of the cervix.

fissure Groove or open crack in tissue.

fistula Abnormal tubelike passage that forms between two normal cavities, possibly congenital or caused by trauma, abscesses, or inflammatory processes.

flaccid Having relaxed, limp, or absent muscle tone.

flaring of nostrils Widening of nostrils (alae nasi) during inspiration in the presence of air hunger; sign of respiratory distress.

flexion Opposite of extension. In obstetrics, resistance to the descent of the baby down the birth canal causes the head to flex, or bend, so that the chin approaches the chest. Thus the smallest diameter (suboccipitobregmatic) of the vertex presents.

focusing phase Third developmental task experienced by expectant fathers as identified by May. This phase is characterized by the father's active involvement in both the pregnancy and his relationship with his infant.

follicle Small secretory cavity or sac.

graafian f. Mature, fully developed ovarian cyst containing the ripe ovum. The follicle secretes estrogens, and after ovulation the corpus luteum develops within the ruptured graafian follicle and secretes estrogen and progesterone.

follicle-stimulating hormone (FSH) Hormone produced by the anterior pituitary during the first half of the menstrual cycle. Stimulates development of the graafian follicle.

fomites Nonliving material on which disease-producing organisms may be conveyed (e.g., bed linen).

fontanel Broad area, or soft spot, consisting of a strong band of connective tissue contiguous with cranial bones and located at the junctions of the bones.

anterior f. Diamond-shaped area between the frontal and two parietal bones just above the baby's forehead at the junction of the coronal and sagittal sutures.

mastoid f. Posterolateral fontanel, usually not palpable.

posterior f. Small, triangular area between the occipital and parietal bones at the junction of the lambdoidal and sagittal sutures.

sagittal f. Soft area located in the sagittal suture, halfway between the anterior and posterior fontanels; may be palpated in normal newborns and in some neonates with Down syndrome.

sphenoid f. Anterolateral fontanel usually not palpable.

footling (incomplete) breech presentation See *breech presentation, footling.*

foramen ovale Septal opening between the atria of the fetal heart. The opening normally closes shortly after birth, but if it remains patent, surgical repair usually is necessary.

forceps Curved-bladed instruments used to protect head of fetus during birth and to apply traction to assist birth.

forceps-assisted birth Birth in which forceps are used to assist in delivery of the fetal head.

foreskin Prepuce, or loose fold of skin covering the glans penis.

fornix Any structure with an arched or vaultlike shape.

f. of the vagina Anterior and posterior spaces, formed by the protrusion of the cervix into the vagina, into which the upper vagina is divided.

fourth stage of labor Initial period of recovery from childbirth. It is usually considered to last for the first 1 to 2 hours after the expulsion of the placenta.

fourth trimester Another term for the puerperium; the 3-month interval after the birth of the newborn that includes return of the reproductive organs to their nonpregnant state and psychologic adaptation to parenthood.

frank breech presentation See *breech presentation, frank.*

fraternal twins Nonidentical twins that come from two separate fertilized ova.

free-standing birth center A center that provides prenatal care, labor and birth, and postbirth care outside of a hospital setting.

frenulum Thin ridge of tissue in midline of undersurface of tongue extending from its base to varying distances from the tip of the tongue.

friability Easily broken. May refer to a fragile condition of the cervix, especially during pregnancy, that causes the cervix to bleed easily when touched.

Friedman's curve Labor curve; pattern of descent of presenting part and of dilation of cervix; partogram.

FSH See *follicle-stimulating hormone.*

fundus Dome-shaped upper portion of the uterus between the points of insertion of the uterine tubes.

funic souffle See *souffle, funic.*

funis Cordlike structure, especially the umbilical cord.

galactorrhea Lactation not associated with childbirth or breastfeeding; a symptom of a pituitary gland tumor.

galactosemia Inherited, autosomal recessive disorder of galactose metabolism, characterized by a deficiency of the enzyme galactose-1-phosphate uridyltransferase.

gamete Mature male or female germ cell; the mature sperm or ovum.

gastroschisis Abdominal wall defect at base of umbilical stalk.

gastrostomy Surgical creation of an artificial opening into the stomach through the abdominal wall, performed to feed a client when oral feeding is not possible.

gate control theory Proposed in 1965 by Melzack and Wall, this theory explains the neurophysical mechanism underlying the perception of pain: the capacity of nerve pathways to transmit pain is reduced or completely blocked by using distraction techniques.

gavage Feeding by means of a tube passed through the nose or mouth to the stomach.

gender identity Sense or awareness of knowing to which sex one belongs. The process begins in infancy, continues throughout childhood, and is reinforced during adolescence.

gene Factor on a chromosome responsible for hereditary characteristics of offspring.

genetic Dependent on the genes. A genetic disorder may or may not be apparent at birth.

genetic counseling Process of determining the occurrence or risk of occurrence of a genetic disorder within a family and of providing appropriate information and advice about the courses of action that are available, whether care of a child already affected, prenatal diagnosis, termination of a pregnancy, sterilization, or artificial insemination is involved.

genitalia Organs of reproduction.

genome Complete copy of genetic material in an organism.

genotype Hereditary combinations in an individual determining physical and chemical characteristics. Some genotypes are not expressed until later in life (e.g., Huntington's chorea); some hide recessive genes, which can be expressed in offspring; and others are expressed only under the proper environmental conditions (e.g., diabetes mellitus appearing under the stress of obesity or pregnancy).

gestation Period of intrauterine fetal development from conception through birth; the period of pregnancy.

gestational age In fetal development, the number of completed weeks counting from the first day of the last normal menstrual cycle.

gestational diabetes Glucose intolerance first recognized during pregnancy.

gestational trophoblastic neoplasia (GTN) Persistent trophoblastic tissue that is presumed to be malignant.

GIFT Gamete intrafallopian transfer of ova and washed sperm into uterine tubes.

gingivitis Inflammation of the gums characterized by redness, swelling, and tendency to bleed.

glans penis Smooth, round head of the penis, analogous to the female glans clitoris.

glomerulonephritis Noninfectious disease of the glomerulus of the kidney, characterized by proteinuria, hematuria, decreased urine production, and edema.

glucose tolerance test A test of the body's ability to use carbohydrates; used as a screening measure for gestational diabetes.

glycosuria Presence of glucose (a sugar) in the urine.

glycosylated hemoglobin (Ghb) Glycohemoglobin, a minor hemoglobin with glucose attached. Ghb A1c concentration represents the average blood glucose level over the previous several weeks and is a measurement for glycemic control in diabetic therapy.

gonad Gamete-producing, or sex, gland; the ovary or testis.

gonadotropic hormone Hormone that stimulates the gonads.

gonadotropin-releasing hormone (GnRH) Hormone released from hypothalamus that stimulates pituitary gland to produce FSH and LH.

Goodell's sign Softening of the cervix, a probable sign of pregnancy, occurring during the second month.

graafian follicle (vesicle) See *follicle, graafian.*

gravida Pregnant woman.

gravidity Number of times a woman has been pregnant.

grief responses The physical, emotional, social, and cognitive responses to the death of a loved one.

grieving process A complex of somatic and psychologic symptoms associated with some extreme sorrow or loss, specifically the death of a loved one.

growth spurts Times of increased neonatal growth that usually occur at approximately 6 to 10 days, 6 weeks, 3 months, and 4 to 5 months. The increased caloric needs necessitate more frequent feedings to increase the amount of milk needed.

grunt, expiratory Sign of respiratory distress (hyaline membrane disease [respiratory distress syndrome, or RDS] or advanced pneumonia) indicative of the body's attempt to hold air in the alveoli for better gaseous exchange.

guided imagery The use of imagination and thought processes in a purposeful way to change certain physiologic and emotional conditions.

gynecoid pelvis Pelvis in which the inlet is round instead of oval or blunt; typical female pelvis.

gynecology Study of the diseases of the female, especially of the genital, urinary, and rectal organs.

habitual (recurrent) abortion See *abortion, habitual.*

habituation An acquired tolerance from repeated exposure to a particular stimulus. Also called *negative adaptation*; a decline and eventual elimination of a conditioned response by repetition of the conditioned stimulus.

haploid number Having half the normal number of chromosomes found in somatic (body) cells; 23 chromosomes.

harlequin sign Rare color change of no pathologic significance occurring between the longitudinal halves of the neonate's body. When infant is placed on one side, the dependent half is noticeably pinker than the superior half.

healing The integrating and balancing of the body, mind, and spirit. May or may not affect physical healing from illness. Often perceived as improved sense of well-being, acceptance, and inner peace and harmony.

healing touch A combination of energetic healing techniques used by nurses and other health care professionals.

health promotion Motivation to increase well-being and actualize health potential.

Hegar's sign Softening of the lower uterine segment that is classified as a probable sign of pregnancy and that may be present during the second and third months of pregnancy and is palpated during bimanual examination.

HELLP syndrome Condition characterized by hemolysis, elevated liver enzymes, and low platelet count; a form of severe preeclampsia.

hematocrit Volume of red blood cells per deciliter (dl) of circulating blood; packed cell volume (PCV).

hematoma Collection of blood in a tissue; a bruise or blood tumor.

hematopoiesis Production of blood cells.

hemoconcentration Increase in the number of red blood cells in proportion to the volume, resulting from either a decrease in plasma volume or increased erythropoiesis.

hemodilution An increase in fluid content of blood, resulting in diminution of the proportion of formed elements.

hemoglobin Component of red blood cells consisting of globin, a protein, and hematin, an organic iron compound.

- **h. electrophoresis** Test to diagnose sickle cell disease in newborns. Cord blood is used.

hemolytic disease of the newborn Breakdown of fetal red blood cells by maternal antibodies, usually from an Rh-negative mother.

hemorrhagic disease of newborn Bleeding disorder during first few days of life based on a deficiency of vitamin K.

hemorrhagic shock Clinical condition in which the peripheral blood flow is inadequate to return sufficient blood to the heart for normal function, particularly oxygen transport to the organs or tissue.

hereditary Pertaining to a trait or characteristic transmitted from parent to offspring by way of the genes; used synonymously with the term *genetic.*

hermaphrodite Person having genital and sexual characteristics of both sexes.

heterozygous Having two dissimilar genes at the same site, or locus, on paired chromosomes (e.g., at the site for eye color, one chromosome carrying the gene for brown, the other for blue).

high risk Increased possibility of suffering harm, damage, loss, or death. See also *risk factor.*

hirsutism Condition characterized by the excessive growth of hair.

holism Philosophy that states that the whole is greater than the sum of its parts. In healing, refers to consideration and treatment of the whole client as a unified being. May include alternative and complementary modalities, but it is more a philosophical base than a modality in and of itself.

holistic medicine Health care treatment with techniques not commonly taught in U.S. medical schools or widely available in U.S. hospitals. May include a variety of disciplines involving diet, exercise, vitamin and nutritional supplements, bodywork, or alternative pharmacologic agents. Philosophy of medicine that encompasses holism.

holistic nursing Nursing practice that stems from the philosophy of holism, one that views the client as an integrated whole, and influenced by a variety of internal and external factors, including the biopsychosocial and spiritual dimensions of the person.

Homans' sign Early sign of phlebothrombosis of the deep veins of the calf in which there are complaints of pain when the leg is in extension and the foot is dorsiflexed.

home birth Planned birth of the child at home, usually done under the supervision of a midwife.

homologous Similar in structure or origin but not necessarily in function.

homologous insemination Insemination in which the semen specimen is provided by the husband. The procedure is used primarily in cases of impotence or when the husband is incapable of sexual intercourse because of some physical disability.

homosexual family Family in which parents form a homosexual union. Children may be the offspring of a previous heterosexual union, adopted, or conceived by one or both members of a homosexual couple through artificial insemination.

homozygous Having two similar genes at the same locus, or site, on paired chromosomes.

hormone Chemical substance produced in an organ or gland that is conveyed through the blood to another organ or part of the body, stimulating it to increased functional activity or secretion. See also specific hormones.

hormone replacement therapy (HRT) Progestin and estrogen given for menopausal symptoms. See *estrogen replacement therapy.*

hot flash (flush) Transient sensation of warmth experienced by some women during or after menopause, resulting from autonomic vasomotor disturbances that accompany changes in the neurohormonal activity of the ovaries, hypothalamus, and pituitary gland.

human chorionic gonadotropin (hCG) Hormone that is produced by chorionic villi; the biologic marker in pregnancy tests.

hyaline membrane disease (HMD) See *respiratory distress syndrome (RDS).*

hydatidiform mole (molar pregnancy) Gestational trophoblastic neoplasm usually resulting from fertilization of egg that has no nucleus or an inactivated nucleus.

hydramnios (polyhydramnios) Amniotic fluid in excess of 1.5 liters; often indicative of fetal anomaly and frequently seen in poorly controlled, insulin-dependent, diabetic pregnant women even if there is no coexisting fetal anomaly.

hydrocele Collection of fluid in a saclike cavity, especially in the sac that surrounds the testis, causing the scrotum to swell.

hydrocephalus Accumulation of fluid in the subdural or subarachnoid spaces.

hydrops fetalis Most severe expression of fetal hemolytic disorder, a possible sequela to maternal Rh isoimmunization; infants exhibit gross edema (anasarca), cardiac decompensation, and profound pallor from anemia, and seldom survive.

hymen Membranous fold that normally partially covers the entrance to the vagina.

hymenal tag Normally occurring redundant hymenal tissue protruding from the floor of the vagina of a newborn female that disappears spontaneously within a few weeks after birth.

hyperbilirubinemia Elevation of unconjugated serum bilirubin concentrations.

hyperemesis gravidarum Abnormal condition of pregnancy characterized by protracted vomiting, weight loss, and fluid and electrolyte imbalance.

hyperesthesia Unusual sensibility to sensory stimuli, such as pain or touch.

hyperglycemia Excess glucose in the blood.

hyperplasia Increase in number of cells; formation of new tissue.

hyperreflexia Increased action of the reflexes.

hyperthyroidism Excessive functional activity of the thyroid gland.

hypertonic uterine dysfunction Uncoordinated, painful, frequent uterine contractions that do not cause dilation and effacement; primary dysfunctional labor.

hypertrophic cardiomyopathy Enlargement and loss of elasticity of the heart muscle, that is, the septum and the left ventricle, causing impaired filling during diastole resulting in decreased cardiac output.

hypertrophy Enlargement, or increase in size, of existing cells.

hyperventilation Rapid, shallow (or prolonged, deep) respirations resulting in respiratory alkalosis: a decrease in H^+ concentration and PCO_2 and an increase in the blood pH and the ratio of $NaHCO_3$ to H_2CO_3. Symptoms may include faintness, palpitations, and carpopedal (hands and feet) muscular spasms.

hypocalcemia Deficiency in calcium often seen in preterm infants, in infants of diabetic mothers, or after long stressful labor in full-term infants.

hypofibrinogenemia Deficient level of a blood-clotting factor, fibrinogen, in the blood; in obstetrics, it occurs after complications of abruptio placentae or retention of a dead fetus.

hypogastric arteries Branches of the right and left iliac arteries carrying deoxygenated blood from the fetus through the umbilical cord, where they are known as umbilical arteries, to the placenta.

hypoglycemia Less than normal amount of glucose in the blood, usually caused by administration of too much insulin, excessive secretion of insulin by the islet cells of the pancreas, or dietary deficiency.

hypospadias Anomalous positioning of urinary meatus on undersurface of penis or close to or just inside the vagina.

hypothalamus Portion of the diencephalon of the brain forming the floor and part of the lateral wall of the third ventricle. It activates, controls, and integrates the peripheral autonomic nervous system, endocrine processes, and many somatic functions, such as body temperature, sleep, and appetite.

hypothermia Temperature that falls below normal range, that is, below 35° C, usually caused by exposure to cold.

hypothyroidism Deficiency of thyroid gland activity with underproduction of thyroxine.

hypotonic uterine dysfunction Weak, ineffective uterine contractions usually occurring in the active phase of labor; often related to cephalopelvic disproportion (CPD) or malposition of the fetus.

hypoxemia Reduction in arterial PO_2 resulting in metabolic acidosis by forcing anaerobic glycolysis, pulmonary vasoconstriction, and direct cellular damage.

hypoxia Insufficient availability of oxygen to meet the metabolic needs of body tissue.

hysterectomy Surgical removal of the uterus.

- **TAH-BSO** Total abdominal hysterectomy and bilateral salpingo-oophorectomy; removal of uterus, both tubes, and both ovaries.
- **TVH** Total vaginal hysterectomy.

hysterosalpingography Recording by x-rays of the uterus and uterine tubes after they are injected with radiopaque material.

hysterotomy Surgical incision into the uterus.

iatrogenic Caused by a health care provider's words, actions, or treatment.

icterus neonatorum Jaundice in the newborn.

idiopathic peripartum cardiomyopathy A primary disease of the heart muscle with no apparent cause, occurring during the peripartum period.

IDM Infant of a diabetic mother.

immunity

- **acquired i.** Protection against microorganisms that develops in response to actual infection or transfer of antibody from an immune donor.
- **active i.** Protection against specific microorganisms that develops in response to actual infection or vaccination.

natural i. Nonspecific protection against microorganisms. Natural immunity is the first line of defense and includes skin and phagocytic cells.

passive i. Protection against specific microorganisms that develops in response to the transfer of antibody or lymphocytes from an immune donor.

immunocompetent Ability of the immune system to respond appropriately to foreign antigens and to develop antigen-specific antibodies.

immunoglobin

IgA Primary immunoglobulin in colostrum.

IgG Transplacentally acquired immunoglobulin that confers passive immunity to the fetus against the infections to which the mother is immune.

IgM Immunoglobulin neonate can manufacture soon after birth. Fetus produces it in the presence of amnionitis.

immunology The study of the components essential to the recognition and disposal of foreign (nonself or antigenic) material and maintenance of body defenses.

impaired fertility Inability to conceive or to carry fetus to live birth at a time a couple chooses to do so.

implantation Embedding of the fertilized ovum in the uterine mucosa; nidation.

impotence Term designating a man's inability, partial or complete, to perform sexual intercourse or to achieve orgasm; erectile dysfunction.

inborn error of metabolism Hereditary deficiency of a specific enzyme needed for normal metabolism of specific chemicals (e.g., deficiency of phenylalanine hydroxylase results in phenylketonuria [PKU]; a deficiency of hexosaminidase results in Tay-Sachs disease).

incompetent cervix Cervix that is unable to remain closed until a pregnancy reaches term because of a mechanical defect in the cervix resulting in dilation and effacement usually during the second or early third trimester of pregnancy. *Premature dilation of the cervix* is the preferred term.

incomplete abortion See *abortion, incomplete.*

increment Increase, or buildup, as of a contraction.

induced abortion See *abortion, induced.*

induction Stimulation of uterine contractions before the spontaneous onset of labor.

inertia Sluggishness or inactivity; in obstetrics, refers to the absence or weakness of uterine contractions during labor.

inevitable abortion See *abortion, inevitable.*

infant Child who is under 1 year of age.

infective endocarditis Inflammation of the inner layer of the heart muscle (endocardium), caused by a bacterial infection.

infertility Decreased capacity to conceive.

informed consent Choice based on full comprehension of relevant information.

inhalation analgesia Reduction of pain by administration of anesthetic gas. Occasionally given during the second stage of labor. Consciousness is retained to allow the woman to follow instructions and to avoid the adverse effects of general anesthesia.

inlet Passage leading into a cavity.

pelvic i. Upper brim of the pelvic cavity.

insemination Introduction of semen into the vagina or uterus for impregnation.

therapeutic donor i. Introduction of donor semen by instrument injection into the vagina or uterus for impregnation.

instrumental style Characteristic style displayed by expectant fathers that emphasizes tasks to be accomplished.

insulin Hormone produced by the beta cells of the pancreatic islets of Langerhans; promotes glucose transport into the cells; aids in protein and lipid synthesis.

integrative health care Encompasses complementary and alternative therapies in combination with conventional Western modalities of treatment.

internal os Inside mouth or opening.

intertuberous diameter Distance between ischial tuberosities. Measured to determine dimension of pelvic outlet.

intervillous space Irregular space in the maternal portion of the placenta, filled with maternal blood and serving as the site of maternal-fetal gas, nutrient, and waste exchange.

intoxication Development of a reversible substance-specific syndrome caused by the recent ingestion of or exposure to a substance. The symptoms of intoxication are attributable to the direct physiologic effects of the substance on the central nervous system.

intrapartum During labor and birth.

intrathecal Within the subarachnoid space.

intrauterine device (IUD) Small plastic or metal form placed in the uterus to prevent implantation of a fertilized ovum.

intrauterine growth restriction (IUGR) Fetal undergrowth of any cause, such as deficient nutrient supply or intrauterine infection, or associated with congenital malformation; birth weight below population 10th percentile corrected for gestational age.

intrauterine pressure catheter (IUPC) Catheter inserted into uterine cavity to assess uterine activity and pressure by electronic means.

intrauterine resuscitation Interventions initiated when nonreassuring fetal heart rate patterns are noted and are directed at improving intrauterine blood flow.

introitus Entrance into a canal or cavity such as the vagina.

intussusception Prolapse of one segment of bowel into the lumen of the adjacent segment.

in utero Within or inside the uterus.

in vitro fertilization Fertilization in a culture dish or test tube.

inversion Turning end for end, upside down, or inside out.

i. of uterus Condition in which the uterus is turned inside out so that the fundus intrudes into the cervix or vagina, caused by a too vigorous removal of the placenta before it is detached by the natural process of labor.

involution (1) Rolling or turning inward. (2) Reduction in size of the uterus after birth and its return to its nonpregnant condition.

isoimmune hemolytic disease Breakdown (hemolysis) of fetal/neonatal Rh-positive red blood cells because of Rh antibodies formed by an Rh-negative mother who had been previously exposed to Rh-positive red blood cells.

isoimmunization Development of antibodies in a species of animal with antigens from the same species (e.g., development of anti-Rh antibodies in an Rh-negative person).

ITP Idiopathic thrombocytopenic purpura.

IVF-ET In vitro fertilization and embryo transfer

jaundice Yellow discoloration of the body tissues caused by the deposit of bile pigments (unconjugated bilirubin); icterus.

breast milk j. Term used by some clinicians to describe late-onset (after day 5) jaundice in the breastfed infant. A cause for this phenomenon has not been conclusively identified. See *physiologic j.*

pathologic j. Jaundice usually first noticeable within 24 hours after birth; caused by some abnormal condition such as an Rh or ABO incompatibility and resulting in bilirubin toxicity (e.g., kernicterus).

physiologic j. Yellow tinge to skin and mucous membranes in response to increased serum levels of unconjugated bilirubin; not usually apparent until after 24 hours; also called *neonatal jaundice, physiologic hyperbilirubinemia.*

kangaroo care Skin-to-skin infant care, especially for preterm infants, which provides warmth to infant. Infant is placed naked or diapered against mother's or father's bare chest and is covered with parent's shirt or a warm blanket.

karyotype Schematic arrangement of the chromosomes within a cell to demonstrate their numbers and morphology.

Kegel exercises Pelvic muscle exercises to strengthen the pubococcygeal muscles.

kernicterus Bilirubin encephalopathy involving the deposit of unconjugated bilirubin in brain cells, resulting in death or impaired intellectual, perceptive, or motor function and adaptive behavior.

ketoacidosis The accumulation of ketone bodies in the blood as a consequence of hyperglycemia; leads to metabolic acidosis.

Kleihauer-Betke test Laboratory test that detects the presence of fetal blood cells in the maternal circulation.

labia majora Two folds of skin containing fat and covered with hair that lie on either side of the vaginal opening and form each side of the vulva. (Singular, *labium majus.*)

labia minora Two thin folds of delicate, hairless skin inside the labia majora. (Singular, *labium minus.*)

labor Series of processes by which the fetus is expelled from the uterus; parturition; childbirth.

active phase Phase in first stage of labor from 4 to 7 cm in dilation.

first stage Stage of labor from the onset of regular uterine contractions to full dilation of the cervix.

latent phase Phase in first stage of labor from none to 3 cm in dilation.

second stage Stage of labor from full dilation of the cervix to the birth of the baby.

third stage Stage of labor from the birth of the baby to the expulsion of the placenta.

transition phase Phase in first stage of labor from 8 to 10 cm in dilation.

labor, delivery, recovery (LDR) A single room where all steps of the birth process occur. Avoids having to move the woman to different rooms for each phase of the birth process. The woman is moved to a postpartum room after recovery.

labor, delivery, recovery, postpartum (LDRP) A single room where all steps of the birth process and hospitalization occur. The woman stays in the same room throughout her hospitalization.

laceration Irregular tear of wound tissue; in obstetrics, it usually refers to a tear in the perineum, vagina, or cervix caused by childbirth.

lactase Enzyme necessary for the digestion of lactose.

lactation Function of secreting milk or period during which milk is secreted.

l. consultant A health care professional who has specialized training in breastfeeding.

l. suppression Stopping the production of breast milk through the use of medication (rare) or nonpharmacologic interventions.

lactogen Medication or other substance that enhances the production and secretion of milk.

lactogenesis stage I Initial synthesis of milk components (colostrum) that begins during pregnancy.

lactogenesis stage II Beginning of milk production 2 to 5 days postpartum.

lactose intolerance Inherited absence of the enzyme lactose.

lactosuria Presence of lactose in the urine during late pregnancy and during lactation. Must be differentiated from glycosuria.

Lamaze (psychoprophylaxis) method Method of preparation for childbirth developed in the 1950s by a French obstetrician, Fernand Lamaze, that gained popularity in the United States in the 1960s. It requires practice at home and coaching during labor and birth. The goals are to minimize fear and the perception of pain and to promote positive family relationships by using both mental and physical preparation.

lambdoid suture Suture line extending across the posterior third of the skull, separating the occipital bone from the two parietal bones, and forming the base of the triangular posterior fontanel.

Laminaria tent Cone of dried seaweed that swells as it absorbs moisture. Used to dilate the cervix nontraumatically in preparation for an induced abortion or in preparation for induction of labor.

lanugo Downy, fine hair characteristic of the fetus between 20 weeks of gestation and birth that is most noticeable over the shoulder, forehead, and cheeks but is found on nearly all parts of the body except the palms of the hands, soles of the feet, and the scalp.

laparoscopy Examination of the interior of the abdomen by insertion of a small telescope through the anterior abdominal wall.

large for gestational age (LGA) Exhibiting excessive growth for gestational age.

last menstrual period (LMP) Date of the first day of the last menstrual bleeding.

latch-on Attachment of the infant to the breast for feeding.

latent phase Phase in first stage of labor from none to 3 cm in dilation.

lecithin A phospholipid that decreases surface tension; surfactant.

lecithin/sphingomyelin ratio Ratio of lecithin to sphingomyelin in the amniotic fluid. It is used to assess maturity of the fetal lung.

leiomyoma Benign smooth muscle tumor.

Leopold's maneuvers Four maneuvers for diagnosing the fetal position by external palpation of the mother's abdomen.

letdown or letdown reflex See *milk ejection reflex.*

letting-go phase Interdependent phase after birth in which the mother and family move forward as a system with interacting members.

leukorrhea White or yellowish mucous discharge from the cervical canal or the vagina that may be normal physiologically or caused by pathologic states of the vagina and endocervix (e.g., *Trichomonas vaginalis* infections).

LH See *luteinizing hormone (LH).*

libido Sexual drive.

lie Relationship existing between the long axis of the fetus and the long axis of the mother. In a longitudinal lie, the fetus is lying lengthwise or vertically, whereas in a transverse lie, the fetus is lying crosswise or horizontally in the uterus.

lightening Sensation of decreased abdominal distention produced by uterine descent into the pelvic cavity as the fetal presenting part settles into the pelvis. It usually occurs 2 weeks before the onset of labor in nulliparas.

linea nigra Line of darker pigmentation seen in some women during the latter part of pregnancy that appears on the middle of the abdomen and extends from the symphysis pubis toward the umbilicus.

linea terminalis Line dividing the upper (false) pelvis from the lower (true) pelvis.

lithotomy position Position in which the woman lies on her back with her knees flexed and with abducted thighs drawn up toward her chest.

live birth Birth in which the neonate, regardless of gestational age, manifests any heartbeat, breathes, or displays voluntary movement.

living ligature Configuration of smooth muscle fibers of the uterus that gives them the capacity to ligate blood vessels and control blood loss after abortion, miscarriage, and childbirth.

local infiltration anesthesia Process by which a substance such as a local anesthetic drug is deposited within the tissue to anesthetize a limited region.

lochia Vaginal discharge during the puerperium consisting of blood, tissue, and mucus.

l. alba Thin, yellowish to white, vaginal discharge that follows lochia serosa on about the tenth day after birth and that may last from 2 to 6 weeks postpartum.

l. rubra Red, distinctly blood-tinged vaginal flow that follows birth and lasts 2 to 4 days.

l. serosa Serous, pinkish brown, watery vaginal discharge that follows lochia rubra until about the tenth day after birth.

low birth weight (LBW) An infant birth weight of less than 2500 g.

low spinal (saddle) block anesthesia Type of regional anesthesia produced by injection of a local anesthetic solution into the cerebrospinal fluid intrathecal (subarachnoid) space in the spinal canal.

L/S ratio See *lecithin/sphingomyelin ratio.*

lunar month Four weeks (28 days).

luteinizing hormone (LH) Hormone produced by the anterior pituitary that stimulates ovulation and the development of the corpus luteum.

luteotropin (LTH) Lactogenic hormone; prolactin; an adenohypophyseal hormone.

lysozyme Enzyme with antiseptic qualities that destroys foreign organisms and that is found in blood cells of the granulocytic and monocytic series and is also normally present in saliva, sweat, tears, and breast milk.

maceration (1) Process of softening a solid by soaking it in a fluid. (2) Softening and breaking down of fetal skin from prolonged exposure to amniotic fluid as seen in a postterm infant. Also seen in a dead fetus.

macroglossia Hypertrophy of tongue or tongue large for oral cavity; seen in some preterm neonates and in neonates with Down syndrome.

macrophage Any phagocytic cell of the reticuloendothelial system, including Kupffer cells in the liver, splenocytes in the spleen, and histocytes in the loose connective tissue.

macrosomia Large body size as seen in neonates of diabetic or prediabetic mothers.

magnetic resonance imaging (MRI) Noninvasive nuclear procedure for imaging tissues with high fat and water content; in obstetrics, uses include evaluation of fetal structures, placenta, and amniotic fluid volume.

malpractice Professional negligence that is the proximate cause of injury or harm to a client, resulting from a lack of professional knowledge, experience, or skill that can be expected in others in the profession or from a failure to exercise reasonable care or judgment in the application of professional knowledge, experience, or skill.

mammary gland Compound gland of the female breast that is made up of lobes and lobules that secrete milk for nourishment of the young. Rudimentary mammary glands exist in the male.

mammography X-ray examination technique used to screen for and evaluate breast lesions.

managed care System of guiding care to promote efficiency and cost-effectiveness.

Marfan syndrome An inherited disorder that is an autosomal dominant trait resulting in an abnormal condition characterized by elongation of the bones, causing significant musculoskeletal disturbances. Also usually associated with cardiovascular and eye abnormalities.

mask of pregnancy See *chloasma.*

mastectomy Excision, or removal, of the mammary gland.

- **modified radical m.** Removal of breast tissue, skin, and axillary nodes.

mastitis Infection in a breast, usually confined to a milk duct, characterized by influenza-like symptoms and redness and tenderness in the affected breast.

maternal adaptation Process that a woman goes through in adjusting to her version of the maternal role; includes three phases: taking in, taking hold, and letting go.

maternal mortality Death of a woman related to childbearing.

maturation (1) Process of attaining maximum development. (2) In biology, a process of cell division during which the number of chromosomes in the germ cells (sperm or ova) is reduced to one half the number (haploid) characteristic of the species.

maturational crisis Crisis that arises during normal growth and development, such as puberty.

McDonald's sign Easy flexion of the fundus on the cervix.

mean arterial pressure (MAP) Average of systolic and diastolic blood pressures. An MAP of greater than 90 mm Hg in the second trimester is associated with an increase in the incidence of pregnancy-induced hypertension in the third trimester.

meatus Opening from an internal structure to the outside (e.g., urethral meatus).

mechanical ventilation Technique used to provide predetermined amount of oxygen; requires intubation.

meconium First stools of infant: viscid, sticky; dark greenish brown, almost black; sterile; odorless.

- **m. aspiration syndrome (MAS)** Function of fetal hypoxia: with hypoxia, the anal sphincter relaxes and meconium is released; reflex gasping movements draw meconium and other particulate matter in the amniotic fluid into the infant's bronchial tree, obstructing the airflow after birth.
- **m. ileus** Lower intestinal obstruction by thick, puttylike, inspissated (dried) meconium that may be the result of deficiency of trypsin production in the newborn with cystic fibrosis.
- **m.-stained fluid** In response to hypoxia, fetal intestinal activity increases and anal sphincter relaxes, resulting in the passage of meconium, which imparts a greenish coloration.

meditation Any activity that focuses the attention in the present moment and quiets and relaxes the mind and body in the process.

meiosis Process by which germ cells divide and decrease their chromosomal number by one half.

membrane(s) Thin, pliable layer of tissue that lines a cavity or tube, separates structures, or covers an organ or structure; in obstetrics, the amnion and chorion surrounding the fetus.

- **artificial rupture of m. (AROM)** Rupture of membranes using a plastic Amnihook or surgical clamp.
- **premature rupture of m. (PROM)** Rupture of amniotic sac and leakage of amniotic fluid beginning at least 1 hour before onset of labor at any gestational age.
- **preterm premature rupture of m. (PPROM)** PROM that occurs before 37 weeks of gestation.
- **spontaneous rupture of m. (SROM)** Rupture of membranes by natural means.

menarche Onset, or beginning, of menstrual function.

meningomyelocele Saclike protrusion of the spinal cord through a congenital defect in the vertebral column.

menopausal hormone therapy (MHT) Hormonal therapy for menopausal symptoms, usually estrogen and progestin.

menopause From the Greek word *mēn* (month) and Greek word *pausis* (cessation), the actual permanent cessation of menstrual cycles; so diagnosed after 1 year without menses.

menorrhagia Abnormally profuse or excessive menstrual flow.

menses (menstruation) (Latin plural of *mensis* "month.") Periodic vaginal discharge of bloody fluid from the nonpregnant uterus that occurs from the age of puberty to menopause.

mentum Chin, a fetal reference point in designating position (e.g., "left mentoanterior" [LMA], meaning that the fetal chin is presenting in the left anterior quadrant of the maternal pelvis).

mesoderm Embryonic middle layer of germ cells giving rise to all types of muscles, connective tissue, bone marrow, blood, lymphoid tissue, and urogenital system.

metastasis Process by which tumor cells spread from site of origin to distant parts of the body.

metrorrhagia Abnormal bleeding from the uterus, particularly when it occurs at any time other than the menstrual period.

microcephaly Congenital anomaly characterized by abnormal smallness of the head in relation to the rest of the body and by underdevelopment of the brain, resulting in some degree of mental retardation.

midwife One who practices the art of helping and aiding a woman to give birth.

certified nurse m. Registered nurse with advanced education in midwifery.

lay m. Midwife who learned skills through practice; has no formal education in midwifery

milia Unopened sebaceous glands appearing as tiny, white, pinpoint papules on forehead, nose, cheeks, and chin of a neonate that disappear spontaneously in a few days or weeks.

milk ejection reflex (MER) Release of milk caused by the contraction of the myoepithelial cells within the milk glands in response to oxytocin; also called *letdown.*

milk-leg Thrombophlebitis of femoral vein resulting in edema of leg and pain; may occur after difficult vaginal birth.

milk transfer Infant's removal of milk from the breast, which is dependent on correct latch-on and the efficiency of the baby's suck, as well as the mother's milk ejection reflex.

miscarriage Spontaneous abortion; lay term usually referring to the loss of the fetus.

missed abortion See *abortion, missed.*

mitleiden "Suffering along," or the psychosomatic symptoms of fathers-to-be.

mitosis Process of somatic cell division in which a single cell divides, but both of the new cells have the same number of chromosomes as the first.

mitral valve prolapse (MVP) A disorder in which one or both of the cusp(s) of the mitral valve protrude backward into the left atrium during ventricular systole, resulting in incomplete closure of the valve. A midsystolic click or a late systolic murmur may be heard.

mitral valve stenosis Narrowing of the opening of the mitral valve caused by stiffening of valve leaflets, obstructing the blood flow from the atrium to the ventricle.

mittelschmerz Abdominal pain in the region of an ovary during ovulation that usually occurs midway through the menstrual cycle. Present in many women, mittelschmerz is useful for identifying ovulation, thus pinpointing the fertile period of the cycle.

molding Overlapping of cranial bones or shaping of the fetal head to accommodate and conform to the bony and soft parts of the mother's birth canal during labor.

mongolian spot Bluish gray or dark nonelevated pigmented area usually found over the lower back and buttocks present at birth in some infants, primarily nonwhite. The spot usually fades by school age.

mongolism See *Down syndrome.*

moniliasis See *candidiasis.*

monosomy Chromosomal aberration characterized by the absence of one chromosome from the normal diploid complement.

monozygotic Originating or coming from a single fertilized ovum, such as identical twins.

monozygotic twins See *twins, monozygotic.*

mons veneris Pad of fatty tissue and coarse skin that overlies the symphysis pubis in the woman and that, after puberty, is covered with hair.

Montgomery's glands (tubercles) Small, nodular prominences (sebaceous glands) on the areolas around the nipples of the breasts that enlarge during pregnancy and lactation.

mood disorders Disorders that have a disturbance in the prevailing emotional state as the dominant feature. Cause is unknown.

moratorium phase The second developmental task experienced by expectant fathers as identified by May. During this phase the expectant father adjusts to the reality of pregnancy.

morbidity (1) Condition of being diseased. (2) Number of cases of disease or of sick persons in relationship to a specific population; incidence.

morning sickness Nausea and vomiting that affect some women during the first few months of their pregnancy; may occur at any time of day.

Moro's reflex Normal, generalized reflex in a young infant elicited by a sudden loud noise or by striking the table next to the child, resulting in flexion of the legs, an embracing posture of the arms, and usually a brief cry. Also called startle reflex.

mortality (1) Quality or state of being subject to death. (2) Number of deaths in relation to a specific population; incidence.

fetal m. Number of fetal deaths per 1000 births (or per live births). See also *death, fetal.*

infant m. Number of deaths per 1000 children 1 year of age or younger.

maternal m. Number of maternal deaths per 100,000 births.

neonatal m. Number of neonatal deaths per 1000 births (or per live births). See also *neonatal mortality.*

perinatal m. Combined fetal and neonatal mortality. See also *death, perinatal.*

morula Developmental stage of the fertilized ovum in which there is a solid mass of cells resembling a mulberry.

mosaicism Condition in which some somatic cells are normal, whereas others show chromosomal aberrations.

mourning The process of finding the answers to the questions surrounding the loss, coping with grief responses, and determining how to live again.

multifetal pregnancy Pregnancy in which there is more than one fetus in the uterus at the same time; multiple pregnancy.

multigravida Woman who has been pregnant two or more times.
multipara Woman who has carried two or more pregnancies to viability, whether they ended in live infants or stillbirths.
mutation Change in a gene or chromosome in gametes that may be transmitted to offspring.
mutuality Component of parent-infant attachment; infant behaviors and characteristics call forth corresponding parent behaviors and characteristics.
myelomeningocele External sac containing meninges, spinal fluid, and nerves that protrudes through defect in vertebral column.
Nägele's (or Naegele's) rule Method for calculating the estimated date of birth (EDB) or "due date."
narcotic antagonist A compound such as naloxone (Narcan) that promptly reverses the effects of narcotics such as meperidine (Demerol).
natal Relating or pertaining to birth.
navel Depression in the center of the abdomen, where the umbilical cord was attached to the fetus; umbilicus.
necrotizing enterocolitis (NEC) Acute inflammatory bowel disorder that occurs primarily in preterm or low-birth-weight neonates. It is characterized by ischemic necrosis (death) of the gastrointestinal mucosa, which may lead to perforation and peritonitis; formula-fed infants are at higher risk for this disease.
negligence Commission of an act that a prudent person would not have done or the omission of a duty that a prudent person would have fulfilled, resulting in injury or harm to another person. In particular, in a malpractice suit a professional person is negligent if harm to a client results from such an act or such a failure to act, but it must be proved that other prudent persons of the same profession would ordinarily have acted differently under the same circumstances.
neonatal abstinence syndrome Signs and symptoms associated with drug withdrawal in the neonate.
neonatal mortality Statistical rate of infant death during the first 28 days after live birth, expressed as the number of such deaths per 1000 live births in a specific geographic area or institution in a given period of time.
neonatal narcosis Central nervous system depression in the newborn caused by a narcotic; may be exhibited by respiratory depression, hypertonia, lethargy, and delay in temperature regulation.
neonatology Branch of medicine that studies care of the neonate.
neoplasia Growth of new tissue; tumor that serves no physiologic function; may be benign or malignant.
neural tube Tube formed from fusion of the neural folds from which develop the brain and spinal cord.
  n. t. defect Improper development of tube resulting in malformation of brain or spinal cord; see alpha-fetoprotein.
neutral thermal environment (NTE) Environment that enables the neonate to maintain a body temperature of at least 36.5° C with minimum use of oxygen and energy.
nevus Natural blemish or mark; a congenital circumscribed deposit of pigmentation in the skin; mole.
  n. flammeus Port-wine stain; reddish, usually flat, discoloration of the face or neck. Because of its large size and color, it is considered a serious deformity.
  n. vasculosus (strawberry hemangioma) Elevated lesion of immature capillaries and endothelial cells that regresses over a period of years.
nidation Implantation of the fertilized ovum in the endometrium, or lining, of the uterus.
nipple confusion Difficulty experienced by some infants in mastering breastfeeding after having been given a pacifier or bottle. This problem appears to be more related to tactile sensation than flow of liquid.
nipple cup A device used to make inverted nipples erectile.
nonmaleficence The principle in bioethics directing us to act so as to avoid causing harm.
nonnutritive sucking Use of a pacifier by infants.
nonreassuring fetal heart rate pattern Fetal heart rate pattern that indicates the fetus is not well oxygenated and requires intervention.
nonshivering thermogenesis Infant's method of producing heat from brown fat by increasing metabolic rate.
nonstress test (NST) Evaluation of fetal response (fetal heart rate) to natural contractile uterine activity or to an increase in fetal activity.
normoglycemia Blood glucose level within normal limits; glycemic control.
nosocomial Pertaining to a hospital.
nuchal cord Encircling of fetal neck by one or more loops of umbilical cord.
nuclear family Family form consisting of parents and their dependent children.
nulligravida Woman who has never been pregnant.
nullipara Woman who has not yet carried a pregnancy to viability.
nurse-practitioner Registered nurse who has additional education to practice nursing in an expanded role.
observer style Characteristic style described by May that is displayed by expectant fathers who show a detached approach to involvement in their partner's pregnancy.
occipitobregmatic Pertaining to the occiput (the back part of the skull) and the bregma (junction of the coronal and sagittal sutures) or anterior fontanel.
occiput Back part of the head or skull.
oligohydramnios Abnormally small amount or absence of amniotic fluid; often indicative of fetal urinary tract defect.
oliguria Urine output below 25 to 30 ml by the kidneys for 2 consecutive hours (in adults).

omphalitis Inflammation of the umbilical stump characterized by redness, edema, and purulent exudate in severe infections.

omphalocele Congenital defect resulting from failure of closure of the abdominal wall or muscles and leading to hernia of abdominal contents through the navel.

oocyte Primordial or incompletely developed ovum.

oogenesis Formation and development of the ovum.

operculum Plug of mucus that fills the cervical canal during pregnancy.

ophthalmia neonatorum Infection in the neonate's eyes usually resulting from gonorrheal or other infection contracted when the fetus passes through the birth canal (vagina).

opisthotonos Tetanic spasm resulting in an arched, hyperextended position of the body.

oral glucose tolerance test Test for blood glucose after oral ingestion of a concentrated sugar solution.

orchitis Inflammation of one or both of the testes, characterized by swelling and pain, often caused by mumps, syphilis, or tuberculosis.

orifice Normal mouth, entrance, or opening, to any aperture.

os Mouth, or opening.

- **external o. (o. externum)** External opening of the cervical canal.
- **internal o. (o. internum)** Internal opening of the cervical canal.
- **o. uteri** Mouth, or opening, of the uterus.

ossification Mineralization of fetal bones.

osteoporosis Deossification of bone tissue resulting in structural weakness; decreased bone mass increasing risk of fractures, especially after menopause.

outlet Opening by which something can leave.

- **pelvic o.** Lower aperture, or opening, of the true pelvis.

ovary One of two glands in the female situated on either side of the pelvic cavity that produces the female reproductive cell, the ovum, and two known hormones, estrogen and progesterone.

ovulation Periodic ripening and discharge of the ovum from the ovary, usually 14 days before the onset of menstrual flow.

- **o. method** Control of fertility using evaluation of cervical mucus throughout the menstrual cycle; ovulation occurs just after the appearance of the peak mucus sign; Billings method.

ovum Female germ, or reproductive cell, produced by the ovary; egg.

oxygen toxicity Oxygen overdosage that results in pathologic tissue changes (e.g., retinopathy of prematurity, bronchopulmonary dysplasia).

oxytocics Drugs that stimulate uterine contractions, thus accelerating childbirth and preventing postbirth hemorrhage. They may be used to increase the letdown reflex during lactation.

oxytocin Hormone produced by the posterior pituitary that stimulates uterine contractions and the release of milk in the mammary gland (letdown reflex).

- **o. challenge test (OCT)** Evaluation of fetal response (fetal heart rate) to contractile activity of the uterus stimulated by exogenous oxytocin (Pitocin).

$Paco_2$ Partial pressure of carbon dioxide in arterial blood.

palmar erythema Rash on the surface of the palms sometimes seen in pregnancy.

palsy Permanent or temporary loss of sensation or ability to move and control movement; paralysis.

- **Bell's p.** Peripheral facial paralysis of the facial nerve (cranial nerve VII), causing the muscles of the unaffected side of the face to pull the face into a distorted position.
- **Erb's p.** See *Erb-Duchenne paralysis.*

Pao_2 Partial pressure of oxygen in arterial blood.

Papanicolaou (Pap) smear Microscopic examination using scrapings from the cervix, endocervix, or other mucous membranes that will reveal, with a high degree of accuracy, the presence of premalignant or malignant cells.

para Usually expressed as a number that refers to parity. See *parity.*

paracervical block Type of regional anesthesia produced by injection of a local anesthetic into the lower uterine segment just beneath the mucosa adjacent to the outer rim of the cervix (3 and 9 o'clock positions).

parental adjustment Process that a person goes through in adapting to the parental role; includes three stages: expectations, reality, and transition to mastery.

parity Number of past pregnancies that have reached viability, regardless of whether the infant or infants were alive or stillborn. See *para.*

parturient Woman giving birth.

parturition Process or act of giving birth.

patent Open.

pathogen Substance or organism capable of producing disease.

pathologic jaundice See *jaundice, pathologic.*

peau d'orange Orange peel–like skin secondary to cancerous lesions and seen over edematous breasts.

pedigree Shorthand method of depicting family lines of individuals that is usually used for tracing manifestations of a physical or chemical disorder.

pelvic Pertaining or relating to the pelvis.

- **p. exenteration** Surgical removal of all reproductive organs and adjacent tissues
- **p. inflammatory disease (PID)** Infection of internal reproductive structures and adjacent tissues usually secondary to sexually transmitted infections.
- **p. inlet** See *inlet, pelvic.*
- **p. outlet** See *outlet, pelvic.*
- **p. relaxation** Refers to the lengthening and weakening of the fascial supports of pelvic structures.

p. tilt (rock) Exercise used to help relieve low back discomfort during menstruation and pregnancy.

pelvimetry Measurement of dimensions and proportions of the pelvis to determine its capacity and ability to allow the passage of the fetus through the birth canal.

pelvis Bony structure formed by the sacrum, coccyx, innominate bones, and symphysis pubis and the ligaments that unite them.
  android p. See *android pelvis.*
  anthropoid p. See *anthropoid pelvis.*
  gynecoid p. See *gynecoid pelvis.*
  platypelloid p. See *platypelloid pelvis.*
  true p. Pelvis below the linea terminalis.

penis Male organ used for urination and copulation.

percutaneous umbilical blood sampling (PUBS) Procedure during which the fetal umbilical vessel is accessed for blood sampling or for transfusions.

perimenopause Period of transition of changing ovarian activity before menopause and through first few years of amenorrhea.

perinatal Of or pertaining to the time and process of giving birth or being born.

perinatal period Period extending from the twentieth or twenty-eighth week of gestation through the end of the twenty-eighth day after birth.

perinatologist Physician who specializes in fetal and neonatal care.

perineum Area between the vagina and rectum in the female and between the scrotum and rectum in the male.

periodic breathing Sporadic episodes of cessation of respirations for periods of 10 seconds or less not associated with cyanosis typically noted in preterm infants.

periods of reactivity (newborn infant) First period (within 30 minutes after birth): brief cyanosis, flushing with crying; crackles, nasal flaring, grunting, retractions; heart sounds loud, forceful, irregular; alert; mucus; no bowel sounds; followed by period of sleep. Second period (4 to 8 hours after birth): swift color changes; irregular respiratory and heart rates; mucus with gagging; meconium passage; temperature stabilizing.

peripartum heart failure Inability of the heart to maintain an adequate cardiac output. Heart failure occurring during pregnancy.

periventricular Intraventricular hemorrhage, a common type of brain injury in preterm infants; prognosis depends on severity of hemorrhage.

pessary Device placed inside the vagina to function as a supportive structure for the uterus.

petechiae Pinpoint hemorrhagic areas caused by numerous disease states involving infection and thrombocytopenia and occasionally found over the face and trunk of the newborn because of increased intravascular pressure in the capillaries during birth.

pH Hydrogen ion concentration.

phenotype Expression of certain physical or chemical characteristics in an individual resulting from interaction between genotype and environmental factors.

phenylketonuria (PKU) Recessive hereditary disease that results in a defect in the metabolism of the amino acid phenylalanine caused by the lack of an enzyme, phenylalanine hydroxylase, that is necessary for the conversion of the amino acid phenylalanine into tyrosine. If PKU is not treated, brain damage may occur, causing severe mental retardation.

phimosis Tightness of the prepuce, or foreskin, of the penis.

phlebitis Inflammation of a vein with symptoms of pain and tenderness along the course of the vein, inflammatory swelling and acute edema below the obstruction, and discoloration of the skin because of injury or bruise to the vein, possibly occurring in acute or chronic infections or after procedures or childbirth.

phlebothrombosis Formation of a clot or thrombus in the vein; inflammation of the vein with secondary clotting.

phocomelia Developmental anomaly characterized by the absence of the upper portion of one or more limbs so that the feet or hands or both are attached to the trunk of the body by short, irregularly shaped stumps, resembling the fins of a seal.

phosphatidylglycerol A phospholipid, a component of pulmonary surfactant; its presence in amniotic fluid is considered a sign of fetal lung maturity when the pregnancy is complicated by maternal diabetes.

phototherapy Utilization of lights to reduce serum bilirubin levels by oxidation of bilirubin into water-soluble compounds that are then processed in the liver and excreted into bile and urine.

physiologic jaundice See *jaundice, physiologic.*

phytoestrogens Plant compounds that have a weak estrogenic effect in the human body; used in the management of menopause as an alternative or complement to conventional hormone replacement therapy.

pica Unusual craving during pregnancy (e.g., of laundry starch, dirt, red clay).

pinch test Determines if nipples are everted or inverted by placing thumb and forefinger on areola and pressing inward. The nipple will stand erect or invert.

placenta Latin, flat cake; afterbirth, specialized vascular disk-shaped organ for maternal-fetal gas and nutrient exchange. Normally it implants in the thick muscular wall of the upper uterine segment.
  abruptio p. See *abruptio placentae.*
  battledore p. Umbilical cord insertion into the margin of the placenta.
  circumvallate p. Placenta having a raised white ring at its edge.
  p. accreta Invasion of the uterine muscle by the placenta, thus making separation from the muscle difficult if not impossible.

p. increta Deep penetration in myometrium by placenta.
p. percreta Perforation of uterus by placenta.
p. previa Placenta that is abnormally implanted in the thin, lower uterine segment and that is typed according to proximity to cervical os: total–completely occludes os; partial–does not occlude os completely; and marginal–placenta encroaches on margin of internal cervical os.
p. succenturiata Accessory placenta.
placental Pertaining or relating to the placenta.
p. infarct Localized, ischemic, hard area on the fetal or maternal side of the placenta.
p. souffle See *souffle, placental.*
platypelloid pelvis Broad pelvis with a shortened anteroposterior diameter and a flattened, oval, transverse shape.
plethora Deep, beefy-red coloration of a newborn caused by an increased number of blood cells (polycythemia) per volume of blood.
plugged ducts Milk ducts blocked by small curds of dried milk.
podalic Concerning or pertaining to the feet.
p. version Shifting of the position of the fetus so as to bring the feet to the outlet during labor.
polycythemia Increased number of erythrocytes per volume of blood, which may be caused by large placental transfusion, fetus transfusion, or maternal-fetal transfusion, or it may be attributable to hypovolemia resulting from movement of fluid out of vascular into interstitial compartment.
polydactyly Excessive number of digits (fingers or toes).
polyhydramnios See *hydramnios.*
polyp Small tumorlike growth that projects from a mucous membrane surface.
polyuria Excessive secretion and discharge of urine by the kidneys.
position Relationship of an arbitrarily chosen fetal reference point, such as the occiput, sacrum, chin, or scapula on the presenting part of the fetus to its location in the front, back, or sides of the maternal pelvis.
positive signs of pregnancy Definite indication of pregnancy (e.g., hearing the fetal heartbeat, visualization and palpation of fetal movement by the examiner, sonographic examination).
posterior Pertaining to the back.
p. fontanel See *fontanel, posterior.*
postmature infant Infant born at or after the beginning of week 43 of gestation or later and exhibiting signs of dysmaturity.
postnatal Happening or occurring after birth (newborn).
postpartum Happening or occurring after birth (mother).
p. blues A letdown feeling, accompanied by irritability and anxiety, which usually begins 2 to 3 days after giving birth and disappears within a week or two. Sometimes called the "baby blues."
p. depression Depression occurring within 6 months of childbirth, lasting longer than postpartum blues and characterized by a variety of symptoms that interfere with activities of daily living and care of the baby.
p. hemorrhage Excessive bleeding after childbirth; traditionally defined as a loss of 500 ml or more after a vaginal birth
p. psychosis Symptoms begin as postpartum blues or depression but are characterized by a break with reality. Delusions, hallucinations, confusion, delirium, and panic can occur.
postterm pregnancy Pregnancy prolonged past 42 weeks of gestation (also called *postdate pregnancy*).
posttraumatic stress disorder An anxiety disorder characterized by an acute emotional response to a traumatic event or situation such as sexual abuse.
precipitous labor Rapid or sudden labor of less than 3 hours beginning from onset of cervical changes to completed birth of neonate.
preconception care Care designed for health maintenance before pregnancy.
preeclampsia Disease encountered after 20 weeks of gestation or early in the puerperium; a vasospastic disease process characterized by increasing hypertension, proteinuria, and hemoconcentration.
pregestational diabetes Diabetes mellitus type 1 or type 2 that exists before pregnancy.
pregnancy Period between conception through complete birth of the products of conception. The usual duration of pregnancy in the human is 280 days, 9 calendar months, or 10 lunar months.
abdominal p. See *abdominal gestation.*
ectopic p. See *ectopic pregnancy.*
extrauterine p. See *extrauterine pregnancy.*
pregnancy-induced hypertension (PIH) Hypertensive disorders of pregnancy including preeclampsia, eclampsia, and transient hypertension.
preload The stretch of myocardial fiber at end-diastole. The ventricular end-diastole pressure and volume reflect this parameter.
premature dilation of the cervix See *incompetent cervix.*
premature infant Infant born before completing week 37 of gestation, irrespective of birth weight; preterm infant.
premature rupture of membranes (PROM) See *membrane(s).*
premenstrual syndrome Syndrome of nervous tension, irritability, weight gain, edema, headache, mastalgia, dysphoria, and lack of coordination occurring during the last few days of the menstrual cycle preceding the onset of menstruation.
premonitory Serving as an early symptom or warning.
prenatal Occurring or happening before birth.
prepartum Before birth; before giving birth.

prepuce Fold of skin, or foreskin, covering the glans penis of the male.
p. of the clitoris Fold of the labia minora that covers the glans clitoris.
presentation That part of the fetus that first enters the pelvis and lies over the inlet: may be head, face, breech, or shoulder.
breech p. See *breech presentation.*
cephalic p. See *cephalic presentation.*
presenting part That part of the fetus that lies closest to the internal os of the cervix.
pressure edema Edema of the lower extremities caused by pressure of the heavy pregnant uterus against the large veins; edema of fetal scalp after cephalic presentation (caput succedaneum).
presumptive signs of pregnancy Manifestations that are suggestive of pregnancy but are not absolutely positive. These include the cessation of menses, Chadwick's sign, morning sickness, and quickening.
preterm birth Birth occurring before 37 weeks of gestation.
preterm premature rupture of membranes (PPROM) See *membrane(s).*
prevention Desire to avoid illness, detect it early, or maintain optimal functioning when illness is present.
previa, placenta See *placenta previa.*
primary survey The immediate response after trauma: the ABCs of resuscitation: establishment and maintenance of an airway, ensuring adequate breathing, and maintenance of an adequate circulatory volume.
primigravida Woman who is pregnant for the first time.
primipara Woman who has carried a pregnancy to viability whether the child is dead or alive at the time of birth.
primordial Existing first or existing in the simplest or most primitive form.
probable signs of pregnancy Manifestations or evidence that indicates that there is a definite likelihood of pregnancy. Among the probable signs are enlargement of abdomen, Goodell's sign, Hegar's sign, Braxton Hicks sign, and positive hormonal tests for pregnancy.
prodromal Serving as an early symptom or warning of the approach of a disease or condition (e.g., prodromal labor).
progesterone Hormone produced by the corpus luteum and placenta whose function is to prepare the endometrium of the uterus for implantation of the fertilized ovum, develop the mammary glands, and maintain the pregnancy.
prolactin A pituitary hormone that triggers milk production.
prolapsed cord Protrusion of the umbilical cord in advance of the presenting part.
proliferative phase of menstrual cycle Preovulatory, follicular, or estrogen phase of the menstrual cycle.
promontory of the sacrum Superior projecting portion of the sacrum at the junction of the sacrum and L5.
prophylactic (1) Pertaining to prevention or warding off of disease or certain conditions. (2) Condom, or "rubber."
proscription Forbidden; taboo.
prostaglandin (PG) Substance present in many body tissues; has a role in many reproductive tract functions; used to induce abortions, cervical ripening for labor induction.
proteinuria Presence of protein in urine.
pruritus Itching.
pseudocyesis Condition in which the woman has all the usual signs of pregnancy, such as enlargement of the abdomen, cessation of menses, weight gain, and morning sickness, but is not pregnant; phantom or false pregnancy.
pseudopregnancy See *pseudocyesis.*
psychoprophylaxis Mental and physical education of the parents in preparation for childbirth, with the goal of minimizing fear and pain and promoting positive family relationships.
ptyalism Excessive salivation.
puberty Period in life in which the reproductive organs mature and one becomes functionally capable of reproduction.
pubic Pertaining to the pubis.
pubis Pubic bone forming the front of the pelvis.
pudendal block Injection of a local anesthetizing drug at the pudendal nerve root to produce numbness of the genital and perianal region.
puerperal infection Infection of the pelvic organs during the postbirth period; childbed fever.
puerperium Period after the third stage of labor and lasting until involution of the uterus takes place, usually about 3 to 6 weeks.
pulmonary artery catheter (PAC) A flow-directed, balloon-tipped multilumen catheter made of polyvinyl chloride that is inserted into the pulmonary artery to provide continuous measurements of pulmonary artery pressure when the balloon is deflated and pulmonary capillary wedge pressures when the balloon is inflated. Sometimes called a Swan-Ganz catheter.
pulmonary artery pressure (PAP) Systolic and diastolic pressures of blood in the pulmonary artery; reflects right afterload.
pulmonary capillary wedge pressure (PCWP) Pressure when the balloon of the pulmonary artery catheter (PAC) is inflated to obstruct right-sided pressures and to reflect left-sided pressures. Value is obtained during diastole, with the mitral valve open; it reflects left preload.
pulmonary vascular resistance A measure for the tension required for the ejection of blood from the right ventricle into the circulation (afterload).
pulse oximetry Noninvasive method of monitoring oxygen levels by detecting the amount of light absorbed by oxygen-carrying hemoglobin.

pyrosis A burning sensation in the epigastric and sternal region from stomach acid (heartburn).

quickening Maternal perception of fetal movement; usually occurs between weeks 16 and 20 of gestation.

radioimmunoassay Pregnancy test that tests for the beta subunit of human chorionic gonadotropin using radioactively labeled markers.

rape-trauma syndrome Characteristic symptoms seen in victims of rape and consisting of several phases; similar to posttraumatic stress syndrome.

recessive trait Genetically determined characteristic that is expressed only when present in the homozygotic state.

reciprocity Type of body movement or behavior that provides the observer with cues, such as the behavioral cues infants provide to parents and parents' responses to cues.

recommended dietary allowances (RDAs) Recommended nutrient intakes estimated to meet the needs of almost all (97% to 98%) of the healthy people in the population.

reconstituted family See *blended family*.

rectocele Herniation or protrusion of the rectum into the posterior vaginal wall.

referred pain Discomfort originating in a local area such as cervix, vagina, or perineal tissues but felt in the back, flanks, or thighs.

reflection Looking within for solutions and answers to certain dilemmas, using intuition and inner wisdom as guides for attainment of healing.

reflex Automatic response built into the nervous system that does not need the intervention of conscious thought (e.g., in the newborn, rooting, gagging, grasp).

reflex bradycardia Slowing of the heart in response to a particular stimulus.

refractory oliguria Oliguria not corrected with fluid challenge.

regional anesthesia Anesthesia of an area of the body by injection of a local anesthetic to block a group of sensory nerve fibers.

regurgitate Vomiting or spitting up of solids or fluids.

relaxation The absence or alleviation of mental, physical, and emotional tension through purposeful activities that quiet the mind and body.

residual urine Urine that remains in the bladder after urination.

respiratory distress syndrome (RDS) Condition resulting from decreased pulmonary gas exchange, leading to retention of carbon dioxide (increase in arterial P_{CO_2}). Most common neonatal causes are prematurity, perinatal asphyxia, and maternal diabetes mellitus; hyaline membrane disease (HMD).

restitution In obstetrics, the turning of the fetal head to the left or right after it has completely emerged from the introitus as it assumes a normal alignment with the infant's shoulders.

resuscitation Restoration of consciousness or life in one who is apparently dead or whose respirations or cardiac function or both have ceased.

retained placenta Retention of all or part of the placenta in the uterus after birth.

retinopathy of prematurity (ROP) Associated with hyperoxemia, resulting in eye injury and blindness in premature infants.

retraction (1) Drawing in or sucking in of soft tissues of chest, indicative of an obstruction at any level of the respiratory tract from the oropharynx to the alveoli. (2) Retraction of uterine muscle fiber. After contracting, the muscle fiber does not return to its original length but remains slightly shortened, a unique attribute of uterine muscle that aids in preventing postdelivery hemorrhage and results in involution.

retroflexion Bending backward.

r. of uterus Condition in which the body of the uterus is bent backward at an angle with the cervix, the position of which usually remains unchanged.

retrolental fibroplasia (RLF) See *retinopathy of prematurity*.

retroversion Turning or a state of being turned back.

r. of uterus Displacement of the uterus; the body of the uterus is tipped backward with the cervix pointing forward toward the symphysis pubis.

Rh factor Inherited antigen present on erythrocytes. The individual with the factor is known as positive for the factor.

Rh immune globulin (RhIG) Solution of gamma globulin that contains Rh antibodies. Intramuscular administration of Rh immune globulin (trade name RhoGAM) prevents sensitization in Rh-negative women who have been exposed to Rh-positive red blood cells.

rheumatic heart disease Permanent damage of the heart muscle and valves secondary to an autoimmune reaction in the heart tissue precipitated by rheumatic fever.

rhythm method Contraceptive method in which a woman abstains from sexual intercourse during the ovulatory phase of her menstrual cycle; calendar method.

ribonucleic acid (RNA) Element responsible for transferring genetic information within a cell; a template, or pattern.

ring of fire Burning sensation as vagina stretches and fetal head crowns.

risk factors Factors that cause a person or a group of people to be particularly vulnerable to an unwanted, unpleasant, or unhealthful event.

risk taking Intentional behaviors with uncertain outcomes.

rite of passage Significant life event indicating movement from one maturational level to another.

Ritgen maneuver Procedure used to control the birth of the head.

rooming-in unit Maternity unit designed so that the newborn's crib is at the mother's bedside or in a nursery adjacent to the mother's room.

rooting reflex Normal response of the newborn to move toward whatever touches the area around the mouth and to attempt to suck. This reflex usually disappears by 3 to 4 months of age.
rotation In obstetrics, the turning of the fetal head as it follows the curves of the birth canal downward.
rubella vaccine Live attenuated rubella virus given to clients who have not had rubella or who are serologically negative. Exposure to the rubella virus through vaccination causes the client to form antibodies, producing active immunity.
Rubin's test Transuterine insufflation of the uterine tubes with carbon dioxide to test their patency; infrequently used.
rugae Folds in the vaginal mucosa and scrotum.
sac, amniotic See *amniotic sac.*
sacroiliac Of or pertaining to the sacrum and ilium.
sacrum Triangular bone composed of five united vertebrae and situated between L5 and the coccyx; forms the posterior boundary of the true pelvis.
safe passage Normal uneventful birth process for mother and child.
safe period The days in the menstrual cycle that are not designated as fertile days, that is, before and after ovulation.
safer sex Use of protection whenever body fluids (semen, blood, vaginal secretions) are exchanged.
sagittal suture Band of connective tissue separating the parietal bones, extending from the anterior to the posterior fontanel.
salpingo-oophorectomy Removal of a uterine tube and an ovary.
Schultze's mechanism Delivery of the placenta with the fetal surfaces (shiny in appearance) presenting.
scrotum Pouch of skin containing the testes and parts of the spermatic cords.
second stage Stage of labor from full dilation of the cervix to the birth of the baby.
secondary areola See *areola, secondary.*
secondary survey A complete physical assessment of all body systems after immediate resuscitation and stabilization after trauma to mother and fetus.
secretory phase of menstrual cycle Postovulatory, luteal, progestational, premenstrual phase of menstrual cycle; 14 days in length.
secundines Fetal membranes and placenta expelled after childbirth; afterbirth.
self-care Client provides care for self as part of plan of care.
semen Thick, white, viscid secretion discharged from the urethra of the male at orgasm; the transporting medium of the sperm.
semen analysis Examination of semen specimen to determine liquefaction, volume, pH, sperm density, and normal morphology.
sensitization Development of antibodies to a specific antigen.
sensory behavior Responses of the five senses; indicate a readiness for social interaction.
sepsis Bacterial infections of the bloodstream.
septic abortion See *abortion, septic.*
sex chromosome Chromosome associated with determination of gender: the X (female) and Y (male) chromosomes. The normal female has two X chromosomes, and the normal male has one X and one Y chromosome.
sexual decision making Selection of choices concerned with intimate and sexual behavior.
sexual history Past and present health conditions, lifestyle behaviors, knowledge, and attitudes related to sex and sexuality.
sexual response cycle The phases of physical changes that occur in response to sexual stimulation and sexual tension release.
sexuality The part of life that has to do with being male or female.
sexually transmitted infections (STIs) Infections transmitted as a result of sexual activity with an infected individual; also called sexually transmitted diseases (STDs).
shake test "Foam" test for lung maturity of fetus; more rapid than determination of lecithin/sphingomyelin ratio.
Sheehan syndrome Postpartum necrosis of the pituitary gland resulting from hypovolemic shock and disseminated intravascular coagulation.
sibling rivalry Negative behaviors exhibited by siblings in response to the addition of a new baby in the family.
sickle cell hemoglobinopathy Abnormal crescent-shaped red blood corpuscles in the blood.
Sims' position Position in which the client lies on the left side with the right knee and thigh drawn upward toward the chest.
single-parent family Family form characterized by one parent (male or female) in the household. This may result from loss of spouse by death, divorce, separation, desertion, or birth of a child to a single woman.
single-room maternity care (SRMC) Variation of care sites where one nurse provides care to a mother and infant, that is, mother-baby units, LDRPs.
singleton A single fetus.
situational crisis Crisis that arises suddenly in response to an external event or a conflict concerning a specific circumstance. The symptoms are transient, and the episode is usually brief.
sitz bath Application of moist heat to the perineum by sitting in a tub or basin filled with warm water.
sleep-wake cycles Variations in states of newborn consciousness.
small for gestational age (SGA) Inadequate growth for gestational age.
smegma Whitish secretion around labia minora and under foreskin of penis.
somatic pain Perineal discomfort resulting from stretching of perineal tissues.

sonogram See *ultrasonography.*

souffle Soft, blowing sound or murmur heard by auscultation.

funic s. Soft, muffled, blowing sound produced by blood rushing through the umbilical vessels and synchronous with the fetal heart sounds.

placental s. Soft, blowing murmur caused by the blood current in the placenta and synchronous with the maternal pulse.

uterine s. Soft, blowing sound made by the blood in the arteries of the pregnant uterus and synchronous with the maternal pulse.

sperm Male sex cell. Also called *spermatozoon, spermatozoa.*

spermatogenesis Process by which mature spermatozoa are formed, during which the diploid chromosome number (46) is reduced by half (haploid, 23).

spermicide Chemical substance that kills sperm by reducing their surface tension, causing the cell wall to break down by a bactericidal effect or by creating a highly acidic environment. Also called *spermatocide.*

spina bifida occulta Congenital malformation of the spine in which the posterior portion of laminas of the vertebrae fails to close but there is no herniation or protrusion of the spinal cord or meninges through the defect. The newborn may have a dimple in the skin or growth of hair over the malformed vertebrae.

spinnbarkeit Formation of a stretchable thread of cervical mucus under estrogen influence at time of ovulation.

spirituality The individual's connection to one's own values, purpose, and meaning of life. May encompass organized religion or belief in higher power or authority. Recognition of wisdom, imagination, spirit, intuition. A perception of the unity of nature and the interconnectedness of all beings. Inner strength.

splanchnic engorgement Excessive filling or pooling of blood within the visceral vasculature that occurs after the removal of pressure from the abdomen, such as birth of an infant, removal of an excess of urine from bladder, removal of large tumor.

spontaneous abortion See *abortion, spontaneous.*

spontaneous rupture of membranes (SROM) Rupture of membranes by natural means.

squamocolumnar junction Site in the endocervical canal where columnar epithelium and squamous epithelium meet; also called *transformation zone.*

squamous intraepithelial lesion (SIL) Term used to describe neoplastic changes of the cervix.

square window Angle of wrist between hypothenar prominence and forearm; one criterion for estimating gestational age of neonate.

standard body weight An appropriate weight for height; a body mass index (BMI) within the normal range.

state-related behavior Behavioral responses dependent on current state of infant.

station Relationship of the presenting fetal part to an imaginary line drawn between the ischial spines of the pelvis.

sterility (1) State of being free from living microorganisms. (2) Complete inability to reproduce offspring.

sterilization Process or act that renders a person unable to produce children.

stillbirth The birth of a baby after 20 weeks of gestation and 1 day or weighing 350 g (depending on the state code) that does not show any signs of life.

stress urinary incontinence (SUI) Loss of urine occurring with increased abdominal pressure (e.g., with coughing or sneezing).

striae gravidarum ("stretch marks") Shining reddish lines caused by stretching of the skin, often found on the abdomen, thighs, and breasts during pregnancy. These streaks turn to a fine pinkish white or silver tone in time in fair-skinned women and brownish in darker-skinned women.

stroke volume Volume of blood ejected from the left ventricle during one cardiac cycle.

subinvolution Failure of a part (e.g., the uterus) to reduce to its normal size and condition after enlargement from functional activity (e.g., pregnancy).

suboccipitobregmatic diameter Smallest diameter of the fetal head–follows a line drawn from the middle of the anterior fontanel to the undersurface of the occipital bone.

supine hypotension Shock; fall in blood pressure caused by impaired venous return when gravid uterus presses on ascending vena cava, when woman is lying flat on her back; vena cava syndrome.

supply meets demand Physiologic basis for determining milk production. The volume of milk produced equals the amount of milk removed from the breast.

support systems Network from which people receive help in times of crisis.

surfactant Phosphoprotein necessary for normal respiratory function that prevents the alveolar collapse (atelectasis). See also lecithin and L/S ratio.

suture (1) Junction of the adjoining bones of the skull. (2) Procedure uniting parts by their being sewn together.

Svo_2 monitoring Percentage of saturation of hemoglobin with oxygen in mixed venous and arterial blood monitored with a fiberoptic pulmonary artery catheter that is connected to a bedside microprocessor. The Svo_2 reflects the balance between oxygen delivery and oxygen use.

symphysis pubis Fibrocartilaginous union of the bodies of the pubic bones in the midline.

synchrony Fit between an infant's cues and the parent's response.

syndactyly Malformation of digits, often seen as a fusion of two or more toes to form one structure.

systemic analgesia Analgesics administered either intramuscularly or intravenously that cross the blood-brain barrier and provide central analgesic effects.

systemic lupus erythematosus (SLE) A chronic inflammatory connective tissue disease affecting many systems, that is, the integumentary, renal, and nervous systems.

systemic vascular resistance (SVR) A measure of the tension required for the ejection of blood from the left ventricle into the circulation (afterload) and is derived by calculation as follows: SVR = [(MAP − CVP)/CO] × 80.

taboo Proscribed (forbidden) by society as improper and unacceptable; a proscription.

tachypnea Excessively rapid respiratory rate (e.g., in neonates, respiratory rate of 60 breaths/min or more).

taking-hold phase Period after birth characterized by a woman becoming more independent and more interested in learning infant care skills; learning to be a competent mother is an important task.

taking-in phase Period after birth characterized by the woman's dependency; maternal needs are dominant, and talking about the birth is an important task.

talipes equinovarus Deformity in which the foot is extended and the person walks on the toes.

telangiectasia Permanent dilation of groups of superficial capillaries and venules.

telangiectatic nevi ("stork bites") Clusters of small, red, localized areas of capillary dilation frequently seen in neonates at the nape of the neck or lower occiput, upper eyelids, and nasal bridge that can be blanched with pressure of a finger.

teratogenic agent Any drug, virus, or irradiation, the exposure to which can cause malformation of the fetus.

teratogens Nongenetic factors that cause malformations and disorders in utero.

teratoma Tumor composed of different kinds of tissue, none of which normally occurs together or at the site of the tumor.

term infant Live infant born between weeks 38 and 42 of completed gestation.

term pregnancy Gestation that continues until at least 38 weeks.

testis One of the glands contained in the male scrotum that produces the male reproductive cell, or sperm, and the male hormone, testosterone; testicle.

tetany, uterine Extremely prolonged uterine contractions.

thalassemia An anemia affecting Mediterranean and Southeast Asian populations in which there is an insufficient amount of globin produced to fill the red blood cells.

therapeutic abortion See *abortion, therapeutic.*

therapeutic donor insemination See *insemination, therapeutic donor.*

therapeutic rest Administration of analgesics to decrease pain and induce rest for management of hypertonic uterine dysfunction.

therapeutic touch A modern interpretation of the laying-on-of-hands for healing, as interpreted by Dolores Krieger, PhD, RN, and Dora Kunz, a noted healer. Originally taught within nursing programs.

thermal shift Drop and subsequent rise in basal body temperature around the time of ovulation.

thermistor probe Automatic sensor used to monitor skin temperature of infant under radiant warmer.

thermogenesis Creation or production of heat, especially in the body.

thermoregulation Control of temperature.

third stage Stage of labor from the birth of the baby to the expulsion of the placenta.

threatened abortion See *abortion, threatened.*

thrombocytopenia Abnormal hematologic condition in which the number of platelets is reduced, usually by destruction of erythroid tissue in bone marrow because of certain neoplastic diseases or an immune response to a drug.

thrombocytopenic purpura Hematologic disorder characterized by prolonged bleeding time, decreased number of platelets, increased cell fragility, and purpura, which result in hemorrhages into the skin, mucous membranes, organs, and other tissue.

thromboembolism Obstruction of a blood vessel by a clot that has become detached from its site of formation.

thrombophlebitis Inflammation of a vein with secondary clot formation.

thrombus Blood clot obstructing a blood vessel that remains at the place it was formed.

thrush Fungal infection of the mouth or throat that is characterized by the formation of white patches on a red, moist, inflamed mucous membrane and is caused by *Candida albicans.*

toco- (toko-) Combining form that means childbirth or labor.

tocolysis See *tocolytic therapy.*

tocolytic therapy Medications used to relax the uterus, to suppress preterm labor, or for version.

tocotransducer Electronic device for measuring uterine contractions.

TORCH infections Infections caused by organisms that damage the embryo or fetus; acronym for *t*oxoplasmosis, *o*ther (e.g., syphilis), *r*ubella, *c*ytomegalovirus, and *h*erpes simplex.

toxemia Term previously used for hypertensive states of pregnancy.

toxicology screen Laboratory analysis of blood or urine to test for alcohol or drug content. Urine drug screening is the most common because it is noninvasive.

toxic shock syndrome A severe acute disease usually caused by *Staphylococcus aureus*; associated with high-absorbency tampon use during menstruation.

tracheoesophageal fistula Congenital malformation in which there is an abnormal tubelike passage between the trachea and esophagus.

traditional Chinese medicine Ancient methods of healing that combine herbs, energy healing, and movement as a pathway to health. Seeks to heal on deeper levels, rather than just treat symptoms.

transformation zone See *squamocolumnar junction.*

transition–labor See *transition phase.*

transition period–newborn Period from birth to 4 to 6 hours later; infant passes through period of reactivity, sleep, and second period of reactivity.

transition phase Phase in first stage of labor from a cervical dilation of 8 to 10 cm.

transition to parenthood Period of time from the preconception parenthood decision through the first months after birth of the baby during which parents define their parental roles and adjust to parenthood.

translocation Condition in which a chromosome breaks and all or part of that chromosome is transferred to a different part of the same chromosome or to another chromosome.

trial of labor (TOL) Period of observation to determine if a laboring woman is likely to be successful in progressing to a vaginal birth.

Trichomonas vaginitis Inflammation of the vagina caused by *Trichomonas vaginalis*, a parasitic protozoon, and characterized by persistent burning and itching of the vulvar tissue and a profuse, frothy, white discharge.

trimester One of 3 periods of about 3 months each into which pregnancy is divided.

trisomy Condition whereby any given chromosome exists in triplicate instead of the normal duplicate pattern.

trophoblast Outer layer of cells of the developing blastodermic vesicle that develops the trophoderm or feeding layer, which will establish the nutrient relationships with the uterine endometrium.

trophoblastic disease A condition in which trophoblastic cells covering the chorionic villi proliferate and undergo cystic changes, which may be malignant.

tubal ligation Abdominal procedure in which the uterine tubes are tied off and a section is removed to interrupt tubal continuity and thus sterilize the woman.

tubercles of Montgomery Small papillae on surface of nipples and areolae that secrete a fatty substance that lubricates the nipples.

twins Two neonates from the same impregnation developed within the same uterus at the same time.

- **conjoined t.** Twins who are physically united; Siamese twins.
- **disparate t.** Twins who are different (e.g., in weight) and distinct from one another.
- **dizygotic t.** Twins developed from two separate ova fertilized by two separate sperm at the same time; fraternal twins.
- **monozygotic t.** Twins developed from a single fertilized ovum; identical twins.

ultrasonography Use of high-frequency sound waves for a variety of obstetric diagnoses and for fetal surveillance.

ultrasound transducer External signal source for monitoring fetal heart rate electronically.

umbilical cord (funis) Structure connecting the placenta and fetus and containing two arteries and one vein encased in a tissue called Wharton's jelly. The cord is ligated at birth and severed; the stump falls off in 4 to 10 days.

umbilicus Navel, or depressed point in the middle of the abdomen that marks the attachment of the umbilical cord during fetal life.

urethra Small tubular structure that drains urine from the bladder.

urinary frequency Need to void often or at close intervals.

urinary meatus Opening, or mouth, of the urethra.

uterine Referring or pertaining to the uterus.

- **u. adnexa** See *adnexa, uterine.*
- **u. atony** Relaxation of uterus; leads to postpartum hemorrhage.
- **u. bruit** Abnormal sound or murmur heard while auscultating the uterus.
- **u. ischemia** Decreased blood supply to the uterus.
- **u. prolapse** Falling, sinking, or sliding of the uterus from its normal location in the body.
- **u. souffle** See *souffle, uterine.*

uteroplacental insufficiency (UPI) Decline in placental function–exchange of gases, nutrients, and wastes–leading to fetal hypoxia and acidosis; evidenced by late fetal heart rate decelerations in response to uterine contractions.

uterus Hollow muscular organ in the female designed for the implantation, containment, and nourishment of the fetus during its development and expulsion of fetus during labor and birth; also organ of menstruation.

- **Couvelaire u.** Interstitial myometrial hemorrhage after premature separation (abruption) of placenta. A purplish-bluish discoloration of the uterus and board-like rigidity of the uterus are noted.
- **inversion of u.** See *inversion of uterus.*
- **retroflexion of u.** See *retroflexion of uterus.*
- **retroversion of u.** See *retroversion of uterus.*

vaccination Intentional injection of antigenic material given to stimulate antibody production in the recipient.

vacuum-assisted birth Birth involving attachment of vacuum cup to fetal head and using negative pressure to assist in birth of the fetus.

vacuum curettage Uterine aspiration method of early abortion.

vagina Normally collapsed musculomembranous tube that forms the passageway between the uterus and the entrance to the vagina.

vaginal birth after cesarean (VBAC) Giving birth vaginally after having had a previous cesarean birth.

vaginismus Intense, painful spasm of the muscles surrounding the vagina.

Valsalva maneuver Any forced expiratory effort against a closed airway such as holding one's breath and tightening the abdominal muscles (e.g., pushing during the second stage of labor).

variability Normal irregularity of fetal cardiac rhythm; short term–beat-to-beat changes; long term–rhythmic changes (waves) from the baseline value.

varicocele Enlargement of veins of the spermatic cord.

varicosity (varicose veins) Swollen, distended, and twisted veins that may develop in almost any part of the body but are most commonly seen in the legs, caused by pregnancy, obesity, congenital defective venous valves, and occupations requiring much standing.

vasectomy Ligation or removal of a segment of the vas deferens, usually done bilaterally to produce sterility in the male.

VDRL test Abbreviation for Venereal Disease Research Laboratories test, a serologic flocculation test for syphilis.

vernix caseosa Protective gray-white fatty substance of cheesy consistency covering the fetal skin.

version Act of turning the fetus in the uterus to change the presenting part and facilitate birth.

external cephalic v. See *external cephalic version.*

podalic v. Shifting of the fetus's position so as to bring the feet to the outlet during birth.

vertex Crown or top of the head.

v. presentation Presentation in which the fetal head is nearest the cervical opening and is born first.

very low birth weight (VLBW) Refers to infant weighing 1500 g or less at birth.

viable, viability Capable, capability of living, as in a fetus that has reached a stage of development, usually 22 menstrual weeks (20 weeks of gestation), which will permit it to live outside the uterus.

visceral pain Discomfort from cervical changes and uterine ischemia located over the lower portion of the abdomen and radiating to the lumbar area of the back and down the thighs.

vulva External genitalia of the female that consist of the labia majora, labia minora, clitoris, urinary meatus, and vaginal introitus.

vulvar self-examination (VSE) Systematic examination of the vulva by the woman.

vulvectomy Surgical removal of all or parts of the vulva.

warm line A help line, or consultation service, for families to access; most often for support of newborn care and postpartum care after hospital discharge.

weaning Process of changing from breastfeeding or bottle feeding to drinking from a cup.

Wharton's jelly White, gelatinous material surrounding the umbilical vessels within the cord.

witch's milk Secretion of a whitish fluid for about a week after birth from enlarged mammary tissue in the neonate, presumably resulting from maternal hormonal influences.

withdrawal (1) Physiologic or cognitive changes that occur after removal of the substance in the substance-dependent person; (2) removing penis from vagina before ejaculation (coitus interruptus).

womb See *uterus.*

X chromosome Sex chromosome in humans existing in duplicate in the normal female and singly in the normal male.

X linkage Genes located on the X chromosome.

Y chromosome Sex chromosome in the human male necessary for the development of the male gonads.

ZIFT Zygote intrafallopian transfer.

zona pellucida Inner, thick membranous envelope of the ovum.

zygote Cell formed by the union of two reproductive cells or gametes; the fertilized ovum resulting from the union of a sperm and an ovum.

INDEX

Page numbers with "t" denote tables; those with "f" denote figures; and those with "b" denote boxes

C

E

G

H

M

O

Q

R

T

W

RESEARCH

PROCEDURE

EMERGENCY

SIGNS OF POTENTIAL COMPLICATIONS

GUIDELINES/GUÍAS

Care Path

MEDICATION GUIDE

CULTURAL CONSIDERATIONS